Contents

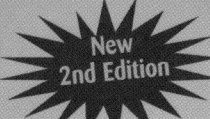
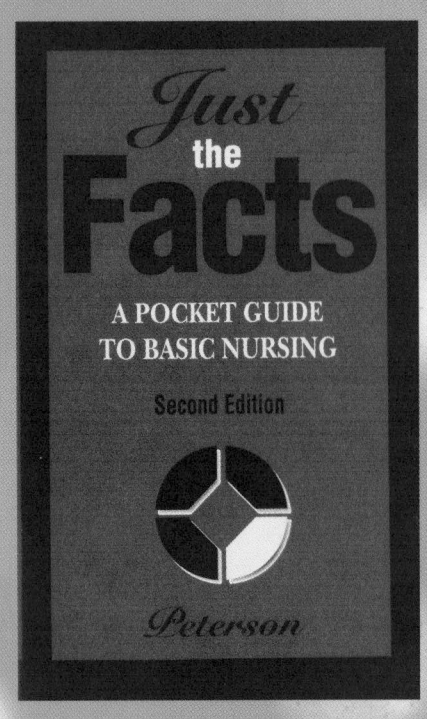
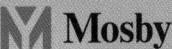
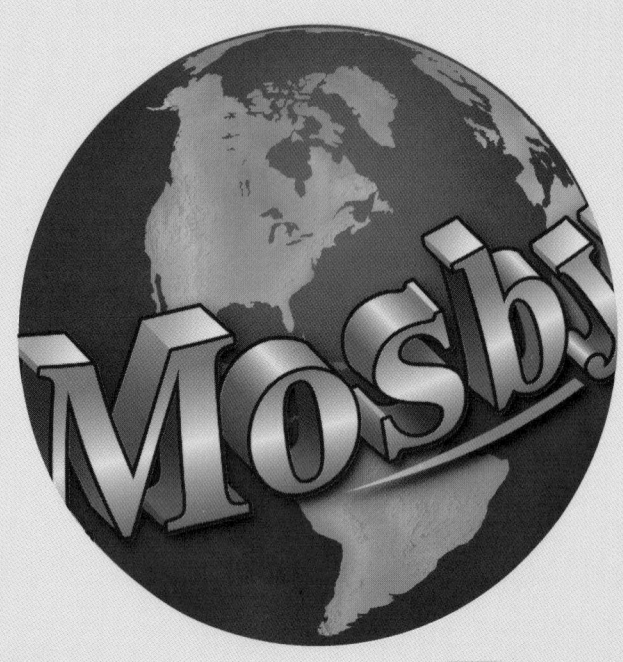

Basic Nursing

ing Approach

Basic
Nursing

A Critical Thinking Approach

Fourth Edition

with 700 illustrations

Patricia A. Potter, RN, MSN
(formerly) Director of Nursing Practice
Barnes-Jewish Hospital
Doctoral Student
Saint Louis University School of Nursing
St. Louis, Missouri

Anne Griffin Perry, RN, MSN, EdD
Professor and Coordinator, Adult Health Specialty
Saint Louis University School of Nursing
Saint Louis University Health Sciences Center
St. Louis, Missouri

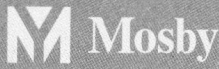 Mosby

St Louis Baltimore Boston Carlsbad Chicago Minneapolis New York Philadelphia Portland
London Milan Sydney Tokyo Toronto

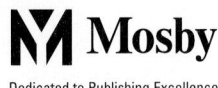

Mosby

Dedicated to Publishing Excellence

A Times Mirror Company

Vice President and Publisher: Sally Schrefer
Senior Editor: Susan Epstein
Developmental Editor: Billi Carcheri
Project Manager: John Rogers
Production Editor: Cheryl Abbott
Book Designer: Yael Kats
Manufacturing Manager: Linda Ierardi

Printed in the United States of America
Composition by Graphic World, Inc.
Printing/binding by Von Hoffmann Press

Mosby, Inc.
11830 Westline Industrial Drive
St. Louis, Missouri 63146

Library of Congress Cataloging in Publication Data
Basic nursing : a critical thinking approach / [edited by] Patricia A.
   Potter, Anne Griffin Perry. — 4th ed.
      p.   cm.
   Includes bibliographical references and index.
   ISBN 0-323-00099-1
   1. Nursing. I. Potter, Patricia Ann. II. Perry, Anne Griffin.
   [DNLM: 1. Nursing. 2. Nursing Care. 3. Nursing Process. WY 100
B3117 1999]
RT41.B288 1999
610.73—dc21
DNLM/DLC
for Library of Congress   98–23777
                                   CIP

98 99 00 01 02 / 9 8 7 6 5 4 3 2 1

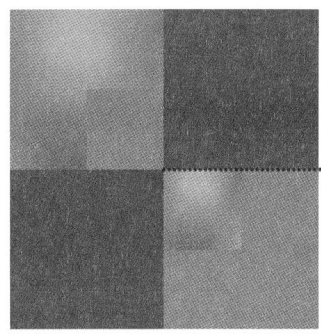

Contributors

Elizabeth A. Ayello, RN, BSN, MS, PhD, CS, CETN
Clinical Assistant Professor of Nursing
New York University School of Education;
Nursing Clinical Associate
Enterostomal Therapy Service
New York University Medical Center
New York, New York

Peggy Breckinridge, MSN, FNP
Associate Professor of Nursing
College of Health Sciences
Roanoke, Virginia

Judith C. Brostron, RN, BA, JD
Attorney, Health Care Law
Lashly and Baer
St. Louis, Missouri

Victoria M. Brown, RN, BSN, MSN, PhD
Associate Professor of Nursing
School of Health Sciences
Milledgeville, Georgia

Gale Carli, RN, BSN, MSN, MSHEd
Instructor of Nursing
Ohlone College
Fremont, California

Rick Daniels, RN, BSN, MSN, PhD
Professor of Nursing
Oregon Health Sciences University at Southern
Ashland, Oregon

Carolyn Ruppel d'Avis, RN, BSN, MSN
Director, Baccalaureate Program
Adjunct Assistant Professor
The Catholic University of America
School of Nursing
Washington, DC

Margaret Ecker, RN, MS, PNP
Clinical Nurse Specialist, Pediatrics
University of California at Los Angeles Children's
　Hospital
Los Angeles, California

Linda Fasciani, RN, BSN, MSN
Assistant Professor of Nursing
County College of Morris
Randolph, New Jersey

Susan Jane Fetzer, RN, BSN, MSN, MBA, PhD, CCRN
Assistant Professor of Nursing
University of New Hampshire
Durham, New Hampshire

Cynthia S. Goodwin, RN, BSN, MSN
Instructor, School of Nursing at Health Professions
University of Southern Indiana
Evansville, Indiana

Lois C. Hamel, BS, MS
Assistant Professor of Nursing
Westbrook College–University of New England
Portland, Maine

Judith Kilpatrick, MSN, RNC
Lecturer
Widener University
Chester, Pennsylvania

Carl A. Kirton, RN-C, BSN, MA, ACRN, ANP
Clinical Assistant Professor;
Adult Nurse Practitioner
New York University
New York, New York

Kristine L'Ecuyer, BSN, MSN
Adjunct Assistant Professor of Nursing
Saint Louis University School of Nursing
St. Louis, Missouri

Ruth Ludwick, RN, BSN, MSN, PhD, RN-C
Associate Professor
Kent State University, School of Nursing
Kent, Ohio

Mary Kay Knight Macheca, RN, BSN, MSN(R), CS, CDE
Certified Adult Nurse Practitioner
The Health Care Group of St. Louis/Unity Medical
    Group
St. Louis, Missouri

Mary Dee Miller, RN, BSN, MS, CIC
Regional Director, Epidemiology Services
Mercy Regional Health System
Cincinnati, Ohio

Elaine K. Neel, RN, BSN, MSN
Nursing Instructor
Methodist Medical Center of Illinois
Peoria, Illinois

Geralyn A. Ochs, RN, ADN, BSN, MSN
Assistant Professor of Nursing
Saint Louis University School of Nursing
St. Louis, Missouri

Marsha Evans Orr, RN, MS, CS, CNSN
Division Clinical Manager
Apria Healthcare
Phoenix, Arizona

Janice J. Rumfelt, BSN, MSN, RNC, EdD
Assistant Professor of Nursing
Southern Illinois University at Edwardsville
Edwardsville, Illinois

Sharon Souter, RN, BSN, MSN
Nursing Program Director
New Mexico State University at Carlsbad
Carlsbad, New Mexico

Elizabeth Speakman, RN, MEd
Assistant Professor of Nursing
Community College of Philadelphia
Philadelphia, Pennsylvania

Rachel E. Spector, BS, MS, PhD, CTN, FAAN
Associate Professor
Boston College, School of Nursing
Chestnut Hill, Massachusetts

Susan Speraw, RN, PhD, CNP
Associate Professor of Pediatrics
University of Tennessee College of Medicine–
    Chattanooga Unit
Chattanooga, Tennessee

Pamela Becker Weilitz, RN, MSN(R), CS, ANP
Adult Nurse Practitioner
University Care, Washington University
    School of Medicine
St. Louis, Missouri

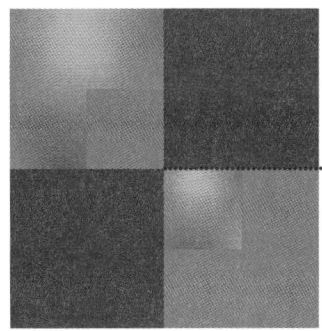

Reviewers

Marianne Adam, RN, MSN
Instructor
St. Luke's School of Nursing
Bethlehem, Pennsylvania

Filippa Bahl, MSN
Associate Professor
Broward Community College
Pembroke Pines, Florida

Margaret W. Bellak, RN, BSN, MN
Associate Professor
Indiana University of Pennsylvania
Indiana, Pennsylvania

Mary Lou Bennett, BA, MA, PhD
Pastoral Care Director
Saint Louis University Hospital
St. Louis, Missouri

Linda Berry, RN, BSN, MSN
Associate Professor
Front Range Community College, Larimer Campus
Fort Collins, Colorado

Teri Boese, BSN, MSN
Learning Resource Services Coordinator
University of Iowa
Iowa City, Iowa

Raylawni G. Branch, BSN, MSN, CNOR
Freshman Instructor of Nursing
Pearl River Community College
Poplarville, Mississippi

Peggy Breckinridge, MSN, FNP
Associate Professor of Nursing
College of Health Sciences
Roanoke, Virginia

Sister Mary Rosita Brennan, RN, MSN, MA, CSSF, DNSc
Chair, Department of Associate Nursing
Felician College
Lodi, New Jersey

Elaine E. Brown, BSN, MSN
Director/Coordinator
Big Bend Community College
Moses Lake, Washington

Margie Brown, MS, RNC, ANP
Professor of Nursing
Long Beach City College, School of Health and
    Science
Long Beach, California

Jerri Bryant, RN, MPH
Director, Quality Assessment/Improvement
Emerald Health
Cleveland, Ohio

Susan Burchiel, MSN, RNC
Instructor of Nursing
Cuesta College, Nursing Division
San Luis Obispo, California

Catherine B. Burke, RN, MS
Nursing Instructor
Kankakee Community College
Kankakee, Illinois

Susan Burkett, RN, MSN, CPNP, CPN
Administrator
T.C. Thompson Children's Hospital at Erlanger
    Medical Center
Chattanooga, Tennessee

Jeanie Burt, RN, BSN, MA
Assistant Professor of Nursing
Harding University School of Nursing
Searcy, Arkansas

Darlene Nebel Cantu, MSN, RNC
Assistant Director, Baptist Health System School of
    Professional Nursing
Adjunct Faculty, San Antonio College
San Antonio, Texas

Gale Carli, RN, BSN, MSN, MSHEd
Instructor of Nursing
Ohlone College
Fremont, California

Sandra Luz Martinez de Castillo, RN, MA, PHN
Instructor of Nursing
Contra Costa College
San Pablo, California

Judith Chovanec-Toy, RN, BSN, MS
Assistant Professor of Nursing
Kauai Community College
Lihue, Hawaii

Denise Demers, MS
Assistant Professor of Nursing
St. Joseph's College
Standish, Maine

Janet Duffy Dionne, RN, BSN, MS, ANP
Clinical Nurse Specialist/Certified Biofeedback
    Therapist
MedCare Program at the Denver Urology Clinic
Denver, Colorado

Patricia A. Eagan, RN, BSN, MSN
Doctoral Student
University of Arkansas at Little Rock
Little Rock, Arkansas

Carol E. Feingold, RN, MS
Senior Lecturer
University of Arizona, College of Nursing
Tucson, Arizona

Leah Frederick, RN, MS, CIC
Infection Control Consultant
Infection Control Consultants
Phoenix, Arizona

Mary Ann Fritz, BSN, MS, EdD
Chair, Nursing Education
South Florida Community College
Avon Park, Florida

Jean Foret Giddens, RN, MSN, CS
Instructor
University of Texas at El Paso, College of Nursing and
    Health Sciences
El Paso, Texas

Denise Goldy, MSN, ARNP, CFNP
Assistant Professor of Nursing
Morehead State University
Morehead, Kentucky

Gayle Gransberry, BSN, MSN, CRN
Assistant Professor
Montana State University–Northern Nursing
    Department
Harve, Montana

Denise A. Hahn, MSN, MEd, ARNP
Professor, Nursing Education
Miami-Dade Community College
Miami, Florida

Heidi Hahn, MHS, PT
Physical Therapist
Barnes-Jewish Hospital
St. Louis, Missouri

Lois C. Hamel, BS, MS
Assistant Professor of Nursing
Westbrook College–University of New England
Portland, Maine

Kathleen Harvey, BSN, MS, CRRN
Instructor of Nursing
Kansas City Kansas Community College
Kansas City, Kansas

Mary Reuther Herring, BSN, MSN, COHN-S
Senior Occupational Health Nurse, Motorola, Inc.;
Nursing Faculty, University of Phoenix
Phoenix, Arizona

Janice J. Hoffman, BSN, MSN, CCRN
Assistant Professor
Anne Arundel Community College
Arnold, Maryland

Lou Ella Humphrey, BS, MSN, EdD, RNCS
Professor of Nursing
Texarkana College
Texarkana, Arkansas

Patricia Jacobson, BSN, MSN
Nursing Instructor
Bullard Havens RVTS, State of Connecticut
Bridgeport, Connecticut

Sharon Johnson, RN, PhD, FNP, CS
Associate Professor of Nursing
San Francisco State University
San Francisco, California

Allison B. Jones, RN, MSN
Assistant Professor
Troy State University
Montgomery, Alabama

Christine R. Kuntz, AAS
Registered Respiratory Therapist
Memorial Medical Center
Springfield, Illinois

Maryanne Lachat, RNC, PhD
Associate Professor of Nursing
Georgetown University
Washington, DC

Virginia Lester, RN, BSN, MSN
Adult Med-Surg Clinical Nurse Specialist
Assistant Professor of Nursing, Angelo State
    University
San Angelo, Texas

Chaplain Arthur M. Lucas, BA, MDiv
Board Certified Chaplain, Certified Supervisor
Director, Spiritual Care Services
Barnes-Jewish Hospital at Washington University
    Medical Center
St. Louis, Missouri

Maureen McHatton, RN, MBA
Assistant Administrator, Acute Care Services
Chief Nurse Executive, St. Mary Medical Center
Long Beach, California

Maria Menendez, RN, RD
High-Tech Cardiac Home Care Nurse
Columbia Olsten Kimberly Homecare
Miami Beach, Florida

Rita Mertig, BSN, MS, RNC
Nursing Educator
John Tyler Community College
Chester, Virginia

Ramona Midamba, RN, MS, CNM
Director of Nursing Programs
Valley Grande College of Health and Technology
Weslaco, Texas

Mary E. Newell, RN, MSN
Program Director
Highline Community College
Des Moines, Washington

Susan K. Odom, RN, MS, CCRN
Assistant Professor of Nursing
Lewis and Clark State College
Lewiston, Idaho

Donna Y. Ortega, RN, BSN, MSN
Professor of Nursing
Community College of Denver
Denver, Colorado

Sharon Pero, MSN, RNCS, CIC
Administrator, Brockton Hospital School of Nursing
Nurse Consultant, U.S. Laboratory
Brockton, Massachusetts

Beth Hogan Quigley, RN, MSN, CRNP
Clinical Lecturer and Consultant
University of Pennsylvania School of Nursing
Philadelphia, Pennsylvania

Marsha L. Ray, BSN, MSN, AA
Instructor of Nursing
Shasta Community College
Redding, California

Vince Salyers, RN, MSN
Assistant Professor and Learning Resources
    Coordinator
Dominican College
San Rafael, California

Ruth Schumacher, MSN, RNC
Instructor of Nursing
University of Illinois at Chicago
Chicago, Illinois

Kathleen G. Stilling, BSN, MS, RNC
Instructor
Johnston School of Practical Nursing, Union
    Memorial Hospital
Baltimore, Maryland

Sylvia Tatman, RN, MSN, CS
Associate Professor of Nursing
Palomar College
San Marcos, California

Rowena Tessman, RN-CS, DCur
Assistant Professor
University of Maine at Fort Kent
Fort Kent, Maine

Susanne M. Tracy, RN, MSN, MA
Associate Professor of Nursing
Rivier–St. Joseph School of Nursing
Nashua, New Hampshire

Kathleen Upham, BSN, MSN, ONC
Assistant Professor of Nursing
Coastal Georgia Community College
Brunswick, Georgia

Rosemary H. Wittstadt, RN, BSN, MS, EdD
Assistant Professor of Nursing
Towson University
Towson, Maryland

Thomas Worms, MSN, CCRN
Assistant Professor of Nursing
Truman College
Chicago, Illinois

To Anne, for her mentorship, intellectual excellence, and commitment to our profession. I thank her for her support during my educational adventure.

Patricia A. Potter

To professional nurses, nurse educators, and nurse researchers, who embrace the standards of excellence in clinical scholarship while meeting the contemporary challenges of health care.

Anne Griffin Perry

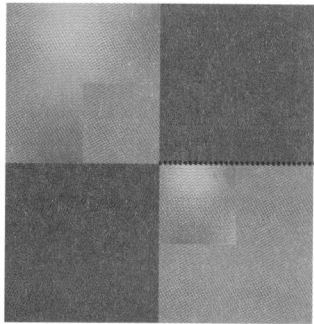

Preface to the Student

Basic Nursing was developed to provide you with all of the fundamental nursing concepts and skills in a visually appealing, easy-to-use format. We know how busy you are and how precious your time is. As you begin your nursing education, it is very important that you have a resource that includes all the information you need to prepare for lectures, classroom activities, clinical rotations, and exams. We've designed this text to meet all of those needs.

This book has been designed to help you succeed in this course, and prepare you for more advanced study. In addition to the readable writing style and abundance of full-color photographs and drawings, we've incorporated numerous features to help you study and learn. We've made it easy for you to pull out important content. Check out the following special learning aids:

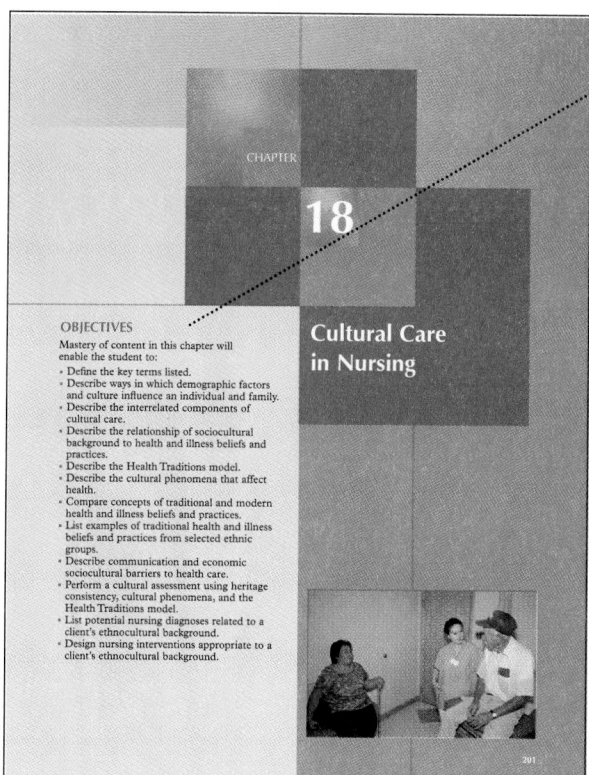

Learning **Objectives** begin each chapter to help you focus on the key information that follows.

Chapters end with **Key Concepts** and **Critical Thinking Activities** that will help you review and apply the essential content from the chapter.

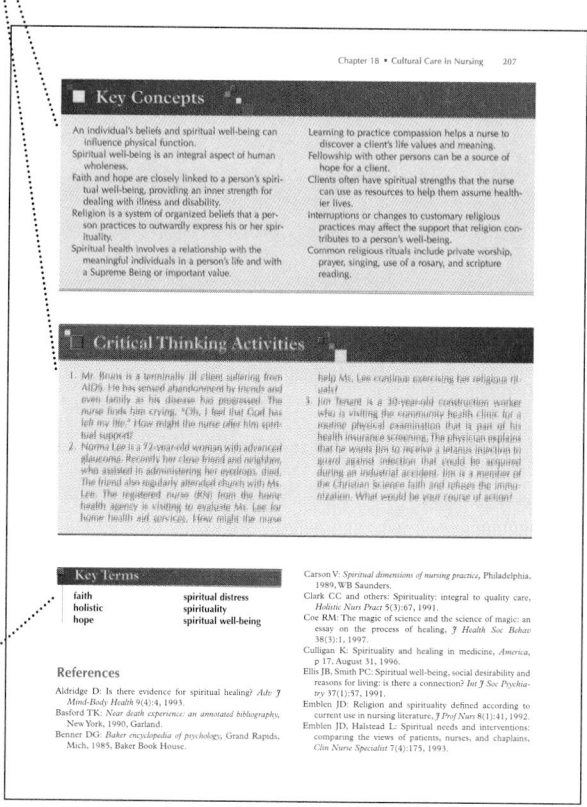

Key Terms are listed, boldfaced within the chapter, and defined in the Glossary to ensure that you understand important vocabulary.

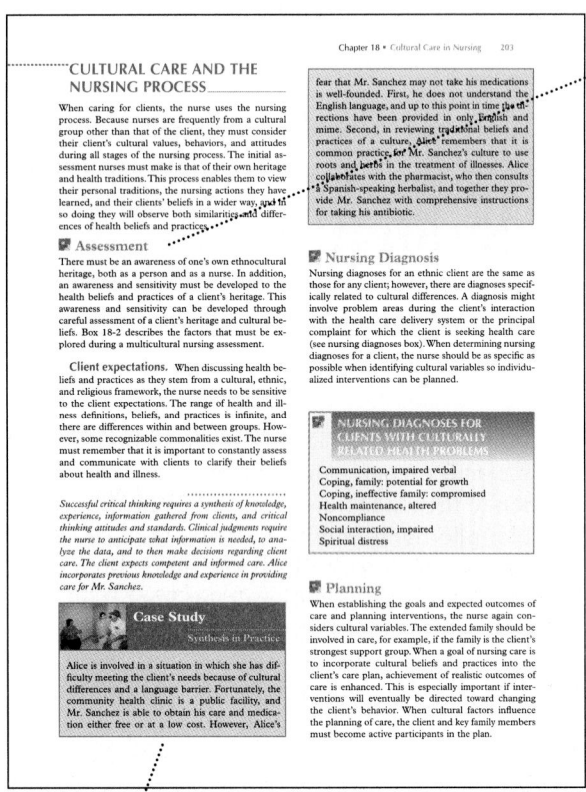

Nursing Process provides a consistent framework that is easy to follow. Headings, boxes, and care plans are all color-keyed for easy recognition.

The Critical Thinking model shows you how to use this thought process along with the nursing process to provide competent, thorough care for your clients. We've made it easy to understand and show you just how to use it.

Ongoing **Case Studies** in all of the clinical chapters introduce you to real-life clients, families, and nurses and follow them through the chapter. These engaging scenarios bring the critical thinking approach to life.

Nursing **Skills** are presented in a clear, two-column format that includes steps and rationale so you learn *why* as well as how. Clear, close-up photos help you learn to perform important techniques.

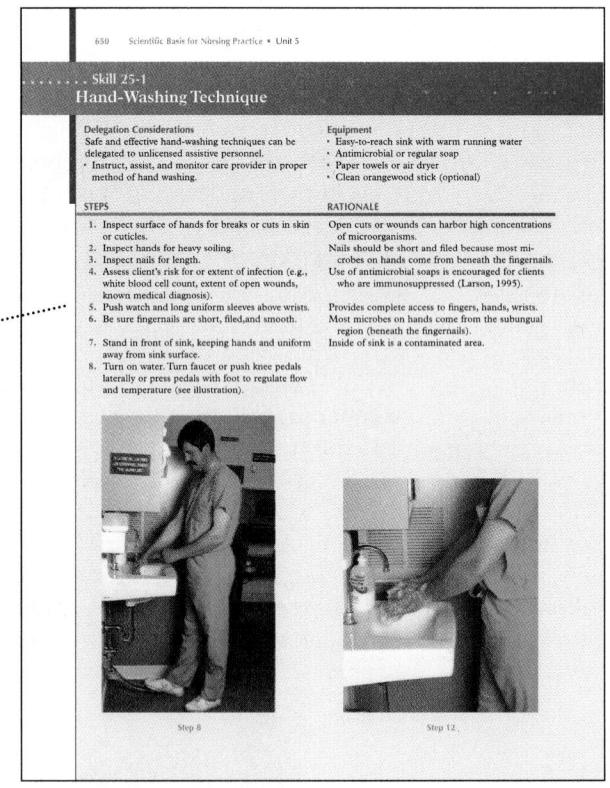

The free CD-ROM included with this text contains the innovative program, **Butterfield's Fluids and Electrolytes,** to help you understand and apply this often difficult content. Also on this CD are elements from the text, including Client Teaching boxes, Case Study boxes, Procedural Guidelines boxes, Skills Performance Checklists, Normal Reference Laboratory Values, Common Abbreviations, NANDA Nursing Diagnoses, and the CDC Isolation Guidelines. It's easy to use and a fun way to learn.

We hope you find this book helpful as you begin your nursing education and wish you much success. Be sure to visit our website at www.mosby.com!

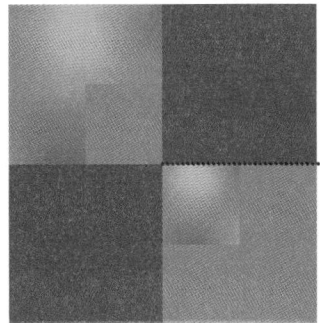

Preface to the Instructor

"Traditional nursing" is a thing of the past. Today's nurse must be prepared to adapt to continual changes in the very nature of health care. Roles and responsibilities are expanding—in addition to caring for clients, nurses function more and more as managers and team leaders. They continue to play a vital role in the delivery of multidisciplinary health care. The practice arena is changing—moving more and more to the community setting. The focus of care is changing—more emphasis is being placed on health promotion and restorative care. Even the clients are changing—more cultural diversity exists and more are older adults. Clients are far more involved in and informed about health care. But the basics of nursing must remain the foundation of practice. Nurses must be knowledgeable and professional. They must be both technically proficient and personally caring. And they must be able to synthesize all they know and all they are when providing care for their clients.

It is this building of the new on the old that serves as the foundation for the 4th edition of *Basic Nursing.* We continue to cover all of the fundamental nursing concepts, skills, and techniques that students must master before moving on to more advanced areas of study. We address the changes in practice that affect how those skills and techniques are used. Critical thinking lies at the heart of this revision. Although the term may be new, nurses have always been critical thinkers. This text takes the mystery out of the process and helps students develop the ability to think critically within the framework of the nursing process.

FEATURES

We have designed this text to welcome the new student to nursing, communicate our own love for the profession, and promote learning and understanding. We want to ensure that students are ready to continue with advanced courses and will ultimately be prepared for all of the challenges of practice. Key features of this text include the following:

- Students will appreciate the **clear, engaging writing style.** Even complex technical and theoretical concepts are presented in language that is easy to understand.
- The book's **visual appeal** has been carefully planned. The clear, readable type and bold headings make the content easy to read and follow. Each special element is consistently color-keyed with attractive icons so students can readily identify important information. Hundreds of large, clear, full-color photographs and drawings reinforce and clarify key concepts and techniques.
- The **five-step nursing process** serves as the organizing framework for all clinical chapters. The narrative discussions are supported by special boxes that highlight NANDA diagnoses and case study nursing care plans.
- The **critical thinking model** provides a practical, clinical decision-making guide that is applied to the nursing process in a way that is easy even for the beginning student to understand.
- **Ongoing case studies** in each clinical chapter introduce "real-world" clients, families, and nurses. The chapter follows the case study through the nursing process, helping students see how to apply the process, along with critical thinking, to the care of clients. Cases take place in both acute and community settings and include clients and nurses from a variety of cultural backgrounds.
- Nursing care focuses on **expected outcomes** and **client satisfaction** to prepare the students for the realities of today's practice.
- Implementation narrative consistently addresses **health promotion, acute care,** and **restorative care** to reflect the current focus on community-based nursing and health promotion.
- **Skills** are presented in a clear, two-column format with steps and rationale. *New* to this edition, skills include guidelines to assist nurses when **delegating to unlicensed assistive personnel** and **critical decision points** that alert students to steps that require special assessment or a particular technique. Skills also include recording and reporting guidelines and home care considerations.
- *New* **procedural guidelines** provide streamlined step-by-step instructions for performing basic skills.

- Each chapter incorporates a **cultural perspective** to highlight the importance of cultural sensitivity in client care.
- **Care of the older adult client** and **client teaching** are stressed in the narrative and in special boxes.
- **Collaborative care** is addressed in the narrative and in care paths/maps to reflect the multidisciplinary approach to health care today.
- **Learning aids** to help students identify, review, and apply important content in each chapter include Objectives, Key Terms, Key Concepts, and Critical Thinking Activities.
- Key terms are boldfaced in each chapter and defined in the **Glossary** at the end of the book.

TEACHING AND LEARNING PACKAGE

In recognition of the incredible challenges faced by both students and educators, we have developed an unsurpassed array of teaching/learning materials.

For faculty, we provide the following:

- **Instructor's Resource Manual with Test Bank** that includes a Topical Outline, answers to the Critical Thinking Activities in the text, Educational Strategies, Independent Learning, Student Resources, a Cross Curriculum Guide, Multimedia Resources, and a bank of questions in NCLEX format.
- **Computerized Test Bank** for Windows or Mac that includes the questions from the Instructor's Resource Manual.

- **Mosby's Electronic Image Collection** conveys key content from the text to enhance classroom lectures.
- **Mosby's Nursing Skills Video Series** provides visual reinforcement to enhance learning. Contact your Mosby sales representative for ordering information.
- Mosby/FITNE **APPLYING CRITICAL THINKING TO NURSING SKILLS Interactive Videodisc Series** helps students learn to incorporate critical thinking in the performance of basic skills. For information or to order, please contact FITNE, Inc., at 800-337-4107.

For the student, we offer two NEW and exciting learning aids with this edition:

- **Study Guide** to Accompany BASIC NURSING provides a myriad of activities and exercises that include Study Charts, additional case studies with critical thinking questions, Independent Learning activities, a Self-Test with multiple choice questions, matching, and completion, and Study Group Questions.
- A free CD-ROM is included with each text. This CD includes **Butterfield's FLUIDS and ELECTROLYTES,** an innovative, easy-to-use program to help students learn and apply the basic principles of fluid and electrolyte balance. Also included on this CD are elements from the text: Client Teaching boxes, Case Study boxes, Procedural Guidelines boxes, Skills Performance Checklists, Normal Reference Laboratory Values, Common Abbreviations, NANDA Nursing Diagnoses, and the CDC Isolation Guidelines.

ACKNOWLEDGMENTS

This edition of *Basic Nursing* is the result of an innovative collaborative effort among the authors, nursing editorial, design, production editing, and marketing, each of whom contributed their talents and time to creating what we think is a unique text. The advanced planning and design has ensured our readers a quality textbook.

- We wish to acknowledge Suzi Epstein, Senior Editor, for spearheading the effort to develop a text that offers a new approach to the presentation of *Basic Nursing*. Her enthusiasm and support, along with her creativity, attention to detail, and thoughtful editing, kept us focused and on track, resulting in a comprehensive, well-designed textbook.
- To Billi Carcheri, Developmental Editor, who undertook this project after its inception. Her patience, commitment to excellence, gracious manner, and a good sense of humor was a catalyst in making this project a very enjoyable one. We appreciate her support and professionalism.
- Yael Kats, our book designer, contributed a clear, crisp, and visually distinctive design for *Basic Nursing*. Involved from the beginning, her work helped us to avoid numerous pitfalls and achieve a finished product that is visually appealing.
- Thanks also goes to the production team of Project Manager John Rogers and Production Editor Cheryl Abbott, who collaborated on the project from the beginning to ensure a well-coordinated and accurate production process.
- The sales and marketing team of Mary Hamby, Senior District Sales Manager, and Janet Blanner, Nursing Marketing Manager, offered insight into design elements that would enhance the quality of the text.
- To our contributors, excellent clinicians and educators, who share invaluable experiences and knowledge in the chapters they have created. Their attention to detail within their areas of specialization helped us achieve a state-of-the-art textbook. We are fortunate to be associated with excellent nurse authors who are able to convey standards of nursing excellence through the printed word.
- To Mike Clement, MD and Rick Brady for their photographic excellence.
- We wish to acknowledge many nursing professionals who influence us everyday in our careers. They enable us to envision what excellence in nursing practice truly means. In addition, our reviewers lend us their expertise, candor, and astute comments to assist in developing a text with high standards that reflects professional nursing practice today.

We continue to enjoy and respect our collaborative work as co-authors. However, more important is our rewarding friendship. This friendship encourages each of us to seek new professional challenges and to extend our boundaries. A friendship built on caring, consideration, respect, and compassion is unbeatable, and for that we are truly blessed.

Patricia A. Potter
Anne Griffin Perry

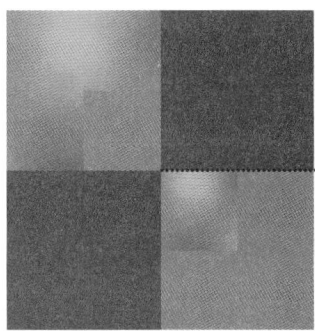

Contents

13 Communication, 200

Cynthia S. Goodwin, RN, BSN, MSN

14 Documentation and Reporting, 223

Rick Daniels, RN, BSN, MSN, PhD

15 Client Education, 244

Mary Kay Knight Macheca, RN, BSN, MSN(R), CS, CDE

The Client and the Health Care Environment

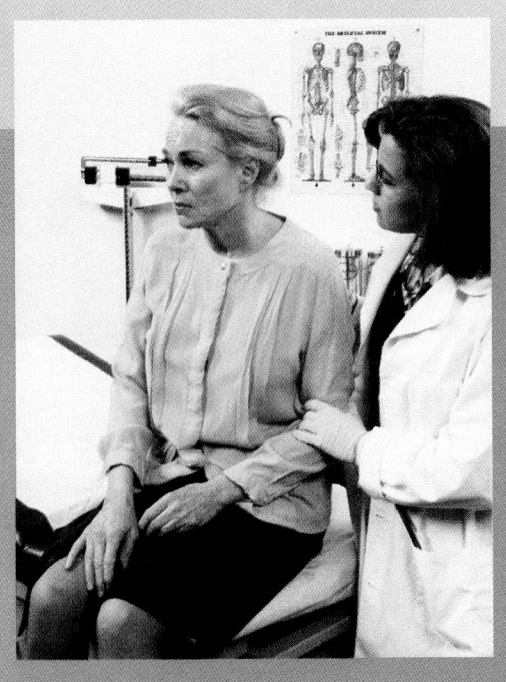

UNIT

1

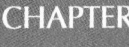

1

Health and Wellness

OBJECTIVES

Mastery of content in this chapter will enable the student to:

- Define the key terms listed.
- List the three Healthy People 2000 public health goals for Americans.
- Discuss the definition of health and related concepts.
- Discuss the health-illness continuum, health belief, health promotion, basic human needs, and holistic health models of health and illness to understand the relationship between clients' attitudes toward health and health practices.
- Describe health promotion and illness prevention activities.
- Discuss the three levels of preventive care and four types of risk factors.
- Describe the variables influencing health beliefs and practices.
- Describe the variables influencing illness behavior.
- Discuss the stages of illness behavior.
- Describe the impact of illness on the client and family.
- Discuss the nurse's role in health and illness.

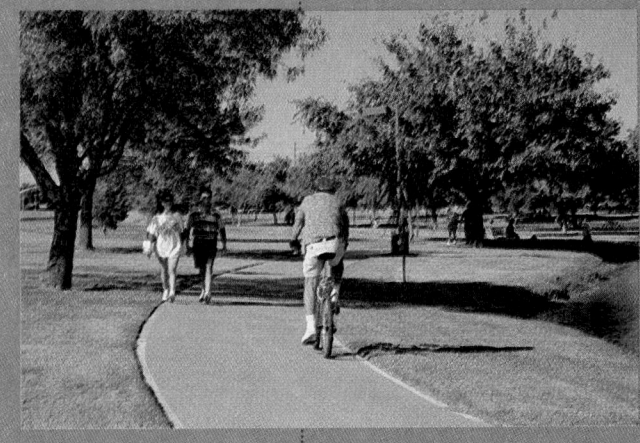

In the past most individuals and societies viewed good health or **wellness** as the opposite or absence of disease. This simple attitude ignores states of health between disease and good health. In the approaching twenty-first century, health will be viewed from a broader perspective. The broader aspect of health may include such elements as a feeling of empowerment, loving relationship, zest for living, strong social support network, sense of meaning in life, or certain level of independence (Haber, 1994).

Nurses identify actual and potential risk factors that predispose a person or a group to illness. Nursing actions utilizing wellness activities and involving health promotion and illness prevention strategies assist the client to achieve and maintain an optimal level of health.

People also have different attitudes about illness and react in different ways to illness. Medical sociologists call the reaction to illness **illness behavior.** The nurse who understands how clients react to illness can minimize the effects of illness and assist the client and family to maintain or return to the highest level of functioning. The nurse assesses the whole person in all dimensions and observes all interactions with family and community (Edelman and Mandle, 1994).

HEALTHY PEOPLE 2000

In 1979 an influential document, *Healthy People: The Surgeon General's Report on Health Promotion and Disease Prevention,* was published; it introduced national goals for improving the health of Americans by 1990 (USDHHS, 1990, 1996). This report outlined priority objectives for preventive services, health protection, and health promotion to address improvements in health status, risk reduction, public and professional awareness of prevention, health services and protective measures, and surveillance and evaluation. The report served as a framework for the 1990s as the United States began to focus more on health promotion and disease prevention instead of illness care. The strategy announced by the Secretary of Health and Human Services requires a cooperative effort by government, voluntary and professional organizations, businesses, and individuals. Widely cited by popular media, in professional journals, and at health conferences, it has inspired health promotion programs throughout the country.

In 1990, *Healthy People 2000: National Health Promotion and Disease Prevention Objectives* was published as a follow-up effort to reduce preventable deaths, disabilities, and diseases for Americans by the year 2000. The *Healthy People 2000* initiative focused on three broad public health goals for Americans: (1) to increase the span of healthy life, (2) to reduce health disparities, and (3) to achieve access to preventive services. Specific objectives to achieve these goals are organized into 22 pri-

ority areas (Box 1-1). In 1995 a midcourse review was published to report progress toward the targets in more than two thirds of the objectives (USDHHS, 1996).

DEFINITION OF HEALTH

Defining good health is difficult, because each person has a personal concept of health. Individual views of health can vary among different age groups, gender, race, and culture (Pender, 1996). Pender (1996) explains that "all people free of disease are not equally healthy." **Health** is a state of being that people define in relation to their own values, personality, and lifestyle.

No current definition of health is acceptable to all health care workers. The World Health Organization (WHO) defines health as a "state of complete physical, mental and social well-being, not merely the absence of disease or infirmity" (WHO, 1947). The following characteristics of this definition promote a more holistic concept of health (Edelman and Mandle, 1994):

1. A concern for the individual as a total system
2. A view of health that identifies internal and external environments
3. An acknowledgment of the importance of an individual's role in life

To help clients identify and reach health goals, the nurse must discover and use information about their concepts of health to set individual goals. Pender (1996) suggests that for many people it is "conditions of life" rather than "pathologic states" that define health.

Health and illness must be defined in terms of the individual. Health can include conditions previously considered to be illness. For example, a person with epilepsy who has learned to control seizures with medication and who functions at home and at work may no longer consider himself ill. Nurses' attitudes toward health and illness should consider the total person, as well as the environment in which the person lives, to individualize nursing care and enhance meaningfulness in the client's future health status.

MODELS OF HEALTH AND ILLNESS

A model is a theoretical way of understanding a concept or idea. Models represent different ways of approaching complex issues. Because health and illness are complex concepts, models are used to understand the relationships between these concepts and the client's attitudes toward health and health practices.

Health beliefs are a person's ideas, convictions, and attitudes about health and illness. They may be based on factual information or misinformation, common sense or myths, or reality or false expectations. Because health beliefs usually influence health behavior, they can

Box 1-1
Healthy People 2000: Priority Areas

1. Physical activity
   More people exercising regularly
   Fewer people never exercising
2. Nutrition
   Fewer people overweight
   Lower fat diets
3. Tobacco
   Fewer people smoking cigarettes
   Fewer youths beginning to smoke
4. Alcohol and other drugs
   Fewer alcohol-related automobile deaths
   Less alcohol use among youth age 12 to
   17 years
   Less marijuana use among youth age 12 to
   17 years
5. Family planning
   Fewer teen pregnancies
   Fewer unintended pregnancies
6. Mental health and mental disorders
   Fewer suicides
   Fewer people reporting stress-related
   problems
7. Violent and abusive behavior
   Fewer homicides
   Fewer assault injuries
8. Educational and community-based programs
   More schools with comprehensive health
   education
   More workplaces with health promotion
   programs
9. Unintentional injuries
   Fewer unintentional injury deaths
   More people using automobile restraints
10. Occupational safety and health
    Fewer work-related deaths
    Fewer work-related injuries
11. Environmental health
    No children with blood lead 25 μg/dl
    More people with clear air in their
    communities
    More people in radon-tested houses

12. Food and drug safety
    Fewer salmonella outbreaks
13. Oral health
    Fewer children with dental caries
    Fewer older people without teeth
14. Maternal and infant health
    Fewer newborns with low weight
    More mothers with first trimester care
15. Heart disease and stroke
    Fewer coronary heart disease deaths
    Fewer stroke deaths
    Better control of high blood pressure
    Lower cholesterol levels
16. Cancer
    Decrease cancer deaths
    Increase screening for breast cancer
       (age > 50)
    Increase screening for cervical cancer
       (age > 18)
    Increase fecal occult blood testing (age > 50)
17. Diabetes and chronic disabling conditions
    Fewer people disabled by chronic conditions
    Fewer diabetes-related deaths
18. HIV infection
    Slower increase in HIV infection
19. Sexually transmitted diseases
    Fewer gonorrhea infections
    Fewer syphilis infections
20. Immunization and infectious disease
    No measles cases
    Fewer pneumonia and influenza deaths
    Higher immunization levels (ages 19 to
    35 months)
21. Clinical preventive services
    No financial barrier to recommended preven-
    tive services
22. Surveillance and data systems
    Common and comparable health status indi-
    cators in use

Modified from U.S. Department of Health and Human Services, PHS: *Healthy people 2000: midcourse review and 1995 revisions*, Sudbury, Mass, 1996, Jones & Bartlett; www.jbpub.com. Reprinted with permission.

positively or negatively affect a client's level of health. **Positive health behaviors** are activities related to maintaining, attaining, or regaining good health and preventing illness. Common positive health behaviors include immunizations, proper sleep patterns, adequate exercise, and nutrition. **Negative health behaviors** in-

clude activities that are actually or potentially harmful to health, such as smoking, drug or alcohol abuse, poor diet, and refusal to take necessary medications.

Nurses have developed the following health models to understand clients' attitudes and values about health and illness so that effective health care can be provided.

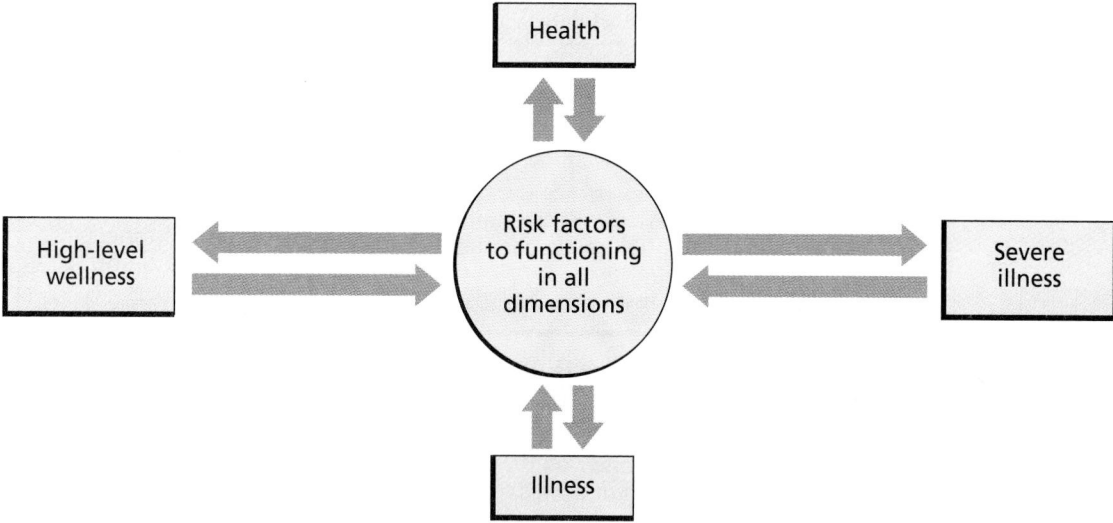

Figure 1-1. The health-illness continuum, ranging from high-level wellness to severe illness, provides a method of identifying a client's level of health. Level of health is a reflection of the client's level of functioning in all dimensions.

These nursing models allow nurses to understand and predict clients' health behavior, including how they use health services and adhere to recommended therapy.

Health-Illness Continuum Model

According to a **health-illness continuum model,** health is a dynamic state that fluctuates as a person adapts to changes in the internal and external environments to maintain a state of physical, emotional, intellectual, social, developmental, and spiritual well-being. Illness is a process in which the functioning of a person is diminished or impaired in one or more dimensions when compared with the person's previous condition. Because health and illness are relative qualities, existing in varying degrees, it may be more useful to consider health and illness in terms of a point on a scale or continuum rather than as an absolute state (Figure 1-1).

High-level wellness and severe illness are at opposite ends of the continuum. According to Neuman (1990), "health on a continuum is the degree of client wellness that exists at any point in time, ranging from an optimal wellness condition, with available energy at its maximum, to death, which represents total energy depletion."

Central to the health-illness continuum model are risk factors, which are important in identifying level of health. Risk factors include genetic and physiological variables such as age, lifestyle, and environment. As a person progresses through the developmental stages, certain risk factors are more common than others. An adolescent, for example, is more likely than an adult to experience stressors related to body image and self-concept, and an older adult is more likely than a child to develop cardiac illness.

The way clients view their levels of health depends on their attitudes toward health, values, beliefs, and per-

ceptions of their physical, emotional, intellectual, social, developmental, and spiritual well-being. Stubblefield (1995) notes that "nurses are intuitively aware of the positive effects of an optimistic outlook on their clients' response to illness."

The drawback of the health-illness continuum is that it is not always easy to describe a client's level of health in terms of one point between two extremes. For example, is a man with a broken leg who has adapted to limited mobility more or less healthy than a physically healthy man experiencing severe depression after the death of his spouse? The health-illness continuum is most effective when used to compare a client's present level of health with his or her own previous level of health. Subsequently it is useful as the nurse helps the client set goals to attain a future level of health.

Health Belief Model

Rosenstoch's (1974) and Becker and Maiman's (1975) **health belief model** (Figure 1-2) addresses the relationship between a person's belief and behaviors. It provides a way of understanding and predicting how clients will behave in relation to their health and how they will comply with health care therapies.

The first component of this model involves the individual's perception of susceptibility to an illness. For example, a client needs to recognize the familial link for coronary artery disease. After this link is recognized, particularly when one parent and two siblings have died in the fourth decade from myocardial infarction, the client may perceive the personal risk of heart disease.

The second component is the individual's perception of the seriousness of the illness. This perception is influenced and modified by demographic and sociopsychological variables, perceived threats of the illness, and

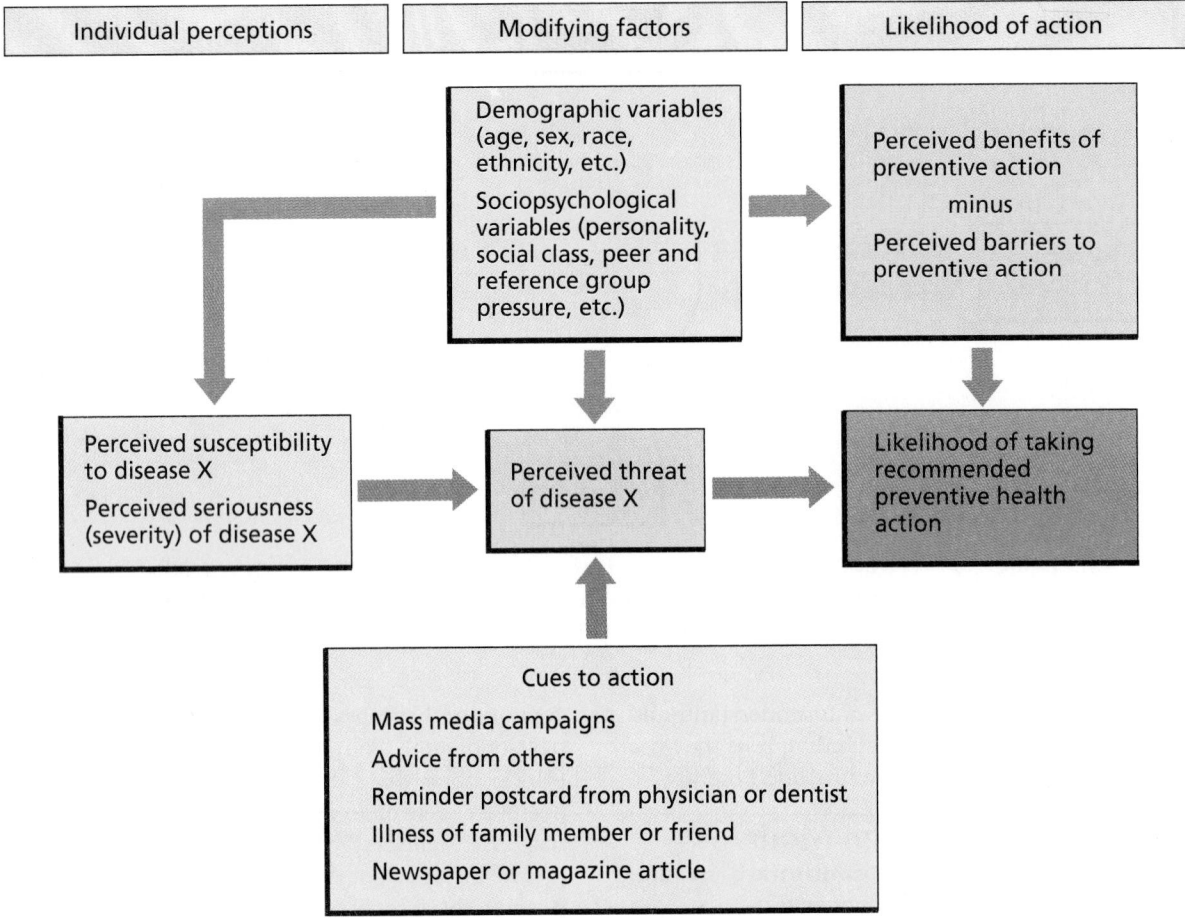

Figure 1-2.   Health belief model. (Data from Becker MH, Maiman LA: Sociobehavioral determinants of compliance with health and medical care recommendations, *Med Care* 13[1]:12, 1975.)

cues to action (e.g., mass media campaigns and advice from family, friends, and medical professionals).

The third component—the likelihood that a person will take preventive action—results from the person's perception of the benefits of and barriers to taking action. Preventive action may include lifestyle changes, increased adherence to medical therapies, or a search for medical advice or treatment.

The health belief model helps nurses to understand factors influencing clients' perceptions, beliefs, and behavior to plan care that will most effectively assist clients in maintaining or restoring health and preventing illness.

Health Promotion Model

The **health promotion model** proposed by Pender (1982, 1993, 1996) (Figure 1-3) defines health as a positive, dynamic state, not merely the absence of disease. The health promotion model emphasizes well-being, personal fulfillment, and self-actualization rather than reacting to the threat of illness (Duffy, 1993). The health promotion model was designed to be a "complementary counterpart to models of health protection"

(Pender, 1993, 1996). Health promotion is directed at increasing a client's level of well-being (Pender, 1993, 1996). The health promotion model describes the multidimensional nature of persons as they interact within their environment to pursue health (Pender, 1996). The model focuses on the three functions of client's cognitive-perceptual factors (individual perceptions), modifying factors (demographic and social), and participation in health promoting behaviors (likelihood of action). The model also organizes cues into a pattern to explain the likelihood of a client's developing health promotion behaviors (Pender, 1993, 1996). The focus of this model is to explain the reasons that individuals engage in health activities. It is not designed for use with families or communities. Revisions to the health promotion model were made in 1996 to increase its potential use for prediction and intervention of health promotion.

Basic Human Needs Model

Basic human needs are elements necessary for human survival and health (e.g., food, water, safety, love). Although each person has other unique needs, the ba-

INDIVIDUAL
CHARACTERISTICS
AND EXPERIENCES

BEHAVIOR-SPECIFIC
COGNITIONS
AND AFFECT

BEHAVIORAL
OUTCOME

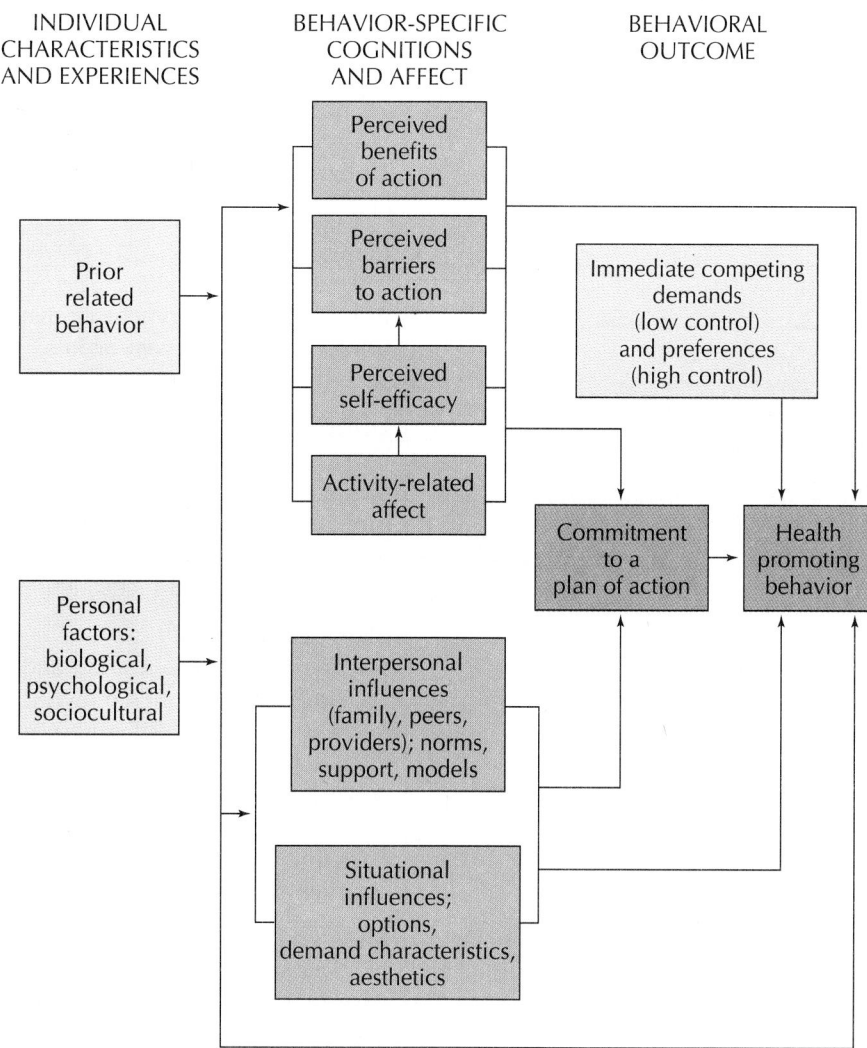

Figure 1-3. Health promotion model. (Redrawn from Pender NJ: *Health promotion and nursing practice,* ed 3, Stamford, Conn, 1996, Appleton & Lange.)

sic human needs are shared by all people, and the extent to which basic needs are met is a major factor in determining a person's level of health.

Maslow's hierarchy of human needs is a model nurses can use to understand the interrelationships of basic human needs (Figure 1-4). According to this model, certain human needs are more basic than others; that is, some needs must be met before other needs (e.g., fulfilling the physiological needs before the needs of love and belonging). The major goal is to restore the client as much as possible to a self-actualized state.

This model can provide a basis for nursing clients of all ages in all health settings. However, when the model is applied, the focus of care is on the client's needs rather than strict adherence to the hierarchy. In all cases, an emergent physiological need takes precedence over a higher-level need. In some situations it is unrealistic to expect a client's basic needs to occur in the fixed

hierarchical order. To provide the most effective care, the nurse needs to understand the relationships of different needs and the factors that determine the priorities for the client.

Holistic Health Models

The **holistic health model** of nursing attempts to create conditions that promote optimal health. The client's current belief system is the beginning framework from which the nurse helps the client find healthy ways to meet individual needs (Rawlins and others, 1993). In this model, nurses utilizing the nursing process consider clients the ultimate experts regarding their own health and respect clients' subjective experience as relevant in maintaining health or assisting in healing. Clients in the holistic model are coparticipants in health promotion, working closely with the nurse to determine necessary and appropriate interventions (Rawlins and others,

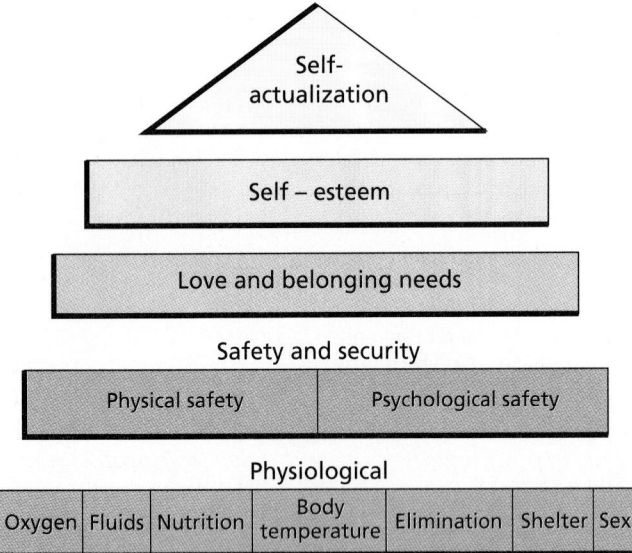

Figure 1-4. Maslow's hierarchy of needs.

Box 1-2
Holistic Nursing Interventions

Music Therapy

Utilizes music of client's taste to reduce anxiety, decrease pain, provide distraction, or induce sleep.

Reminiscence

The process of recalling past events or experiences to provide entertainment or distraction or to assist in coping with an event or loss.

Relaxation Therapy

Utilizes nursing taught skills such as breathing exercises, visualization, guided imagery, meditation, or prayer to decrease anxiety, tension, or pain or to promote a sense of well-being. Relaxation therapy works by decreasing the arousal of the sympathetic nervous system and focusing attention inward.

Therapeutic Touch

Involves deep concentration and modulation of energy fields on a client's body. Assessment of energy fields is based on differences in temperature, tingling, and size, while treatment "unruffles" the energy field. The purpose of therapeutic touch is to decrease pain; increase circulating hemoglobin; and decrease headaches, anxiety, and stress. Advance training in therapeutic touch is required.

Massage Therapy

Involves a variety of massage techniques that increase oxygen to muscle groups to induce relaxation, decrease stress, and relieve muscle tension. Certification is required in many states to be a massage therapist.

Data from Mornhinweg GC, Voignier RR: Holistic nursing interventions, *Orthop Nurs* 14(4):20, 1995; and Petersen B: The mind-body connection, *Can Nurs* 92(1):29, 1996.

1993). Edelman and Mandle (1994) add that health and vitality can be achieved only through the client's own action. The power to bring about healing comes from the client, not the health professional.

Nurses use holistic nursing interventions (Box 1-2) because they are economical, noninvasive, nonpharmacological alternatives to traditional medical care. Holistic interventions can be used to augment standard treatments, to replace interventions that are ineffective or debilitating, and to promote or maintain health (Mornhinweg and Voignier, 1995). These holistic strategies are integral in the expanding role of nursing.

Most holistic therapies are easily learned and can be applied to almost any nursing setting and to all stages of health and illness. For example, reminiscence may be used in the geriatric population to help relieve anxiety for a client dealing with memory loss or for a cancer patient dealing with the difficult side effects of chemotherapy. Music therapy may be used in the operating room to create a soothing environment. Relaxation therapy may be useful in any setting to distract a client during a painful procedure, such as a dressing change. Breathing exercises are commonly taught to help clients deal with the shortness of breath that accompanies some chronic respiratory diseases.

Nurses can help clients recognize the many options available and assist them in making choices to enhance health. Holistic nurses' most powerful healing and teaching come from who they are and how they relate to others. Holistic nurses who pursue their own personal growth and strive toward optimal health for themselves are better able to facilitate healing and optimal health in others.

Emerging Models of Health

The wellness-illness model. Jensen and Allen (1993) propose a **wellness-illness model** that describes the relationship between health, disease, wellness, and illness as distinct parts of a process involving the changing person in the changing world. In this model, health is viewed as an objective process characterized by stability, balance, and integrity of functioning. Disease, also an objective process, is viewed as a dysfunction or alteration in functioning. Disease is measured by laboratory tests and direct observation. In contrast, wellness is the subjective experience of health (Benner and Wrubel, 1989). Thus illness is the human experience of disease and may be perceived as loss, challenge, threat, punishment, or gain (Lipowski, 1969, 1983).

In this model, wellness-illness is affected by intrapersonal, interpersonal, health-disease–related, and extrapersonal factors. Intrapersonal factors include personality, past experiences, and emotional state. Interpersonal factors include social supports and relationships. Health-disease–related factors include health promotion orientation, functional status, visibility of disease-health, and severity and prognosis of disease. Extrapersonal factors are sociocultural and economic (Jensen and Allen, 1993).

Simplified, wellness-illness is viewed as the human experiences of actual or perceived function-dysfunction states that are influenced by the way the individual perceives or views the experience of health-disease.

The HEALTH-Healing/Disordering model.
McCabe (1995) constructed a model of healing based on current literature on the phenomenon of healing and the lived experiences of nurses who use holistic and complementary therapies in their practice of nursing. The proposed model may have significance for any health care practitioner as a means to understand the health care provider's role in the process of healing. In the model (Figure 1-5), health is a dynamic process conceptualized as a functional state. Illness is deviation from a normal state, in which disordering processes occur.

The **HEALTH-Healing/Disordering model** is a conceptual map. It is not to be interpreted as a fixed sequence of events, but rather as an energy field wherein health processes are seen as dynamic potentials. Out of these potentials events may arise sequentially or spontaneously. The HEALTH-Healing/Disordering model denotes a concept of health *which incorporates both healing and disordering processes as aspects of health* (McCabe, 1995).

In the model, the middle circle represents a normal state of health where minor fluctuations occur on a daily basis and can be perceived as temporary fatigue, constipation, indigestion, or a headache. A normal state of health is challenged (shifting) by any disordering influence that renders an individual susceptible to illness. Symptoms of an illness are known as signaling and act to summon the healing response. The healing response corrects everyday fluctuations in physical and nonphysical health status; its strength is dependent on the total health of the individual. This model views healing as purposeful with a goal to recreate integrated function in an impaired system. The choices made by the individual during the illness phase or disordering phase will affect the individual's adaptation and ability to return to a previous or improved state of health. As health returns, a reordering process occurs. An adapting-compromising pattern exists when care is not taken to treat an illness, and an adapting-evolving pattern exists when an individual chooses to act on the signals of an illness to return to a healthy state.

By actively supporting and enhancing the healing process, nurses can improve client outcomes. Nurses assist clients in choosing health promoting behaviors. Nurses also educate clients to recognize the symptoms of an illness and how to respond to a disordering process.

⋯VARIABLES INFLUENCING HEALTH BELIEFS AND PRACTICES

There are many variables that can influence clients' health beliefs and practices. Internal and external variables can influence how a person thinks and acts. As previously stated, health beliefs usually influence health behavior or health practices and likewise can positively or negatively affect a client's level of health. Therefore, understanding the effects of these variables allows the nurse to plan and deliver individualized care.

Internal Variables
Internal variables include a person's developmental stage, intellectual background, perception of functioning, and emotional and spiritual factors.

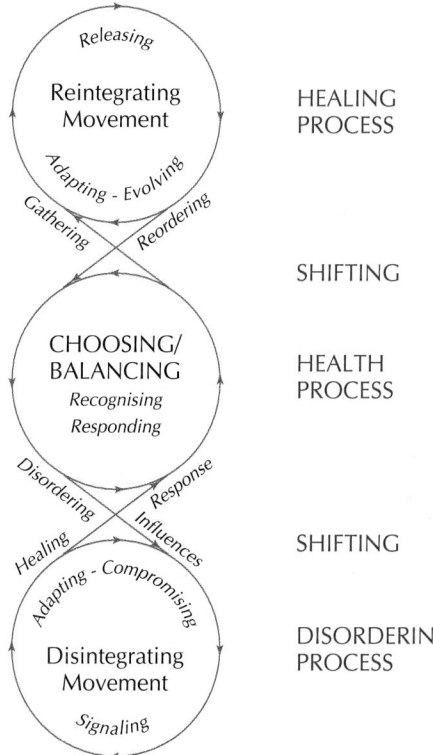

Figure 1-5. The HEALTH-Healing/Disordering model. (Redrawn from McCabe P: Exploring the phenomenon of healing: healing as a health capacity, *Aust J Holistic Nurs* 2[1]:13, 1995.)

Developmental stage. A person's thought and behavior patterns change throughout life. The nurse must consider the client's level of growth and development when using his or her health beliefs and practices as a basis for planning care. The concept of illness of a child, adolescent, or adult is dependent on the person's developmental stage. Fear and anxiety are common among ill children, especially if thoughts about illness, hospitalization, or procedures are based on lack of information or lack of clarity of information. Good communication by providing age-appropriate explanations aimed at increasing a client's understanding and knowledge of illness or procedures provides the foundation for effective treatment (Moss-Morris and Paterson, 1995). Emotional development may also influence personal beliefs about health-related matters. For example, the nurse uses different techniques of teaching about contraception to an adolescent than would be used for an adult. Knowledge of the stages of growth and development helps the nurse predict the client's response to the present illness or the threat of future illness. The planning of nursing care is then adapted to these expectations, as well as to the client's abilities to participate in self-care.

Intellectual background. A person's beliefs about health are shaped in part by knowledge (or misinformation) about body functions and illnesses, educational background, and past experiences. These variables influence how a client thinks about health. In addition, cognitive abilities shape the *way* a person thinks, including the ability to understand factors involved in illness and to apply knowledge of health and illness to personal health practices. Cognitive abilities also relate to a person's developmental stage. A nurse considers intellectual background so that these variables can be incorporated into nursing care (Edelman and Mandle, 1994).

Perception of functioning. The way people perceive their physical functioning affects health beliefs and practices. When nurses assess a client's level of health, they gather subjective data about the way the client perceives physical functioning, such as level of fatigue, shortness of breath, or pain. They also obtain objective data about actual functioning, such as blood pressure, height measurements, and lung sound assessment. This information allows nurses to more successfully plan and implement individualized care.

Emotional factors. The client's degree of calm or stress can influence health beliefs and practices. The manner in which a person handles stress throughout each phase of life will influence the way the person reacts to illness. A person who generally is very calm may have little emotional response during illness, whereas an individual unable to cope emotionally with the threat of

illness may either overreact to illness and assume it is life threatening or may deny the presence of symptoms and not take therapeutic action (see Chapter 22).

Spiritual factors. Spirituality is reflected in how a person lives his or her life, including the values and beliefs exercised, the relationships established with family and friends, and the ability to find hope and meaning in life. Spirituality serves as an integrating theme in peoples' lives (see Chapter 17). Religious practices are one way people exercise spirituality. There are some religions that restrict the use of certain forms of medical treatment. Nurses must understand clients' spiritual dimensions to involve them effectively in nursing care. Ross (1995) suggests that hospitalization can precipitate spiritual distress; therefore a client's spiritual needs should be addressed, because the spiritual dimension is important for the attainment of an overall sense of health, well-being, and quality of life.

External Variables

External variables influencing a person's health beliefs and practices include family practices, socioeconomic factors, and cultural background.

Family practices. The way that clients' families use health care services generally affects their health practices. Their perceptions of the seriousness of diseases and their history of preventive care behaviors (or lack of them) can influence how clients will think about health.

Socioeconomic factors. Social and psychosocial factors can increase the risk for illness and influence the way that a person defines and reacts to illness. Psychosocial variables include the stability of the person's marital or intimate relationship, lifestyle habits, and occupational environment. A person generally seeks approval and support from social networks (neighbors, peers, and co-workers), and this desire for approval and support affects health beliefs and practices. Najman (1993) suggests that the five social categories that comprise the majority of those in poverty are single parents and their children, the aged, the unemployed, racial and ethnic minorities, and the disabled. Additionally, data point to a consistent pattern of higher mortality rates for the economically most disadvantaged.

Social variables partly determine how the health care system provides medical care. Because the health system is organized in certain ways, it determines how clients can obtain care, the treatment method, the economic cost to the client, and potential reimbursement to the health care agency or client.

Like social variables, economic variables may affect a client's level of health by increasing the risk for disease and influencing how or at what point the client enters the health care system.

A person's compliance with the treatment that is designed to maintain or improve health is also affected by economic status. A person who has high utility bills, a large family, and a low income tends to give a higher priority to food and shelter than to costly drugs or treatment or expensive foods for special diets.

Cultural background. Cultural background influences beliefs, values, and customs. It influences the approach to the health care system, personal health practices, and the nurse-client relationship. If nurses are not aware of their own and other cultural patterns of behavior and language, they may not be able to recognize and understand a client's behavior and beliefs and may have difficulty interacting with the client. As with family and socioeconomic variables, cultural variables must be incorporated into a client's care plan (see Chapter 18).

HEALTH PROMOTION, WELLNESS, AND ILLNESS PREVENTION

Health care has become increasingly focused on health promotion, wellness, and illness prevention. The rapid rise of health care costs has motivated people to seek ways of decreasing the incidence and minimizing the results of illness or disability.

Health promotion activities can be passive or active. With **passive strategies of health promotion,** individuals gain from the activities of others without acting themselves. The fluoridation of municipal drinking water and the fortification of homogenized milk with vitamin D are examples of passive health promotion strategies. With **active strategies of health promotion,** individuals are motivated to adopt specific health programs. Weight-reduction and smoking-cessation programs require clients to be actively involved in measures to improve their present and future levels of wellness while decreasing the risk of disease.

Nurses emphasize health promotion, wellness-enhancing strategies, and illness prevention activities as important forms of health care because they assist clients in maintaining and improving health. Health promotion activities such as routine exercise and good nutrition help clients maintain or enhance their present levels of health. Wellness education teaches people how to care for themselves in a healthy way and includes topics such as physical awareness, stress management, and self-responsibility. **Illness prevention** activities such as immunization programs protect clients from actual or potential threats to health. The concepts of health promotion, wellness, and illness prevention are closely related and in practice overlap to some extent. All are focused on the future; the difference between them involves motivations and goals. Health promotion

activities motivate people to act positively to reach more stable levels of health. Wellness strategies are designed to help persons achieve new understanding and control of their lives. Illness prevention activities motivate people to avoid declines in health or functional levels.

The goal of a total health program is to improve a client's level of well-being in all dimensions, not just physical health. Total health programs are based on the belief that many factors can affect level of health. Health can be influenced by individual practices such as poor eating habits and little or no exercise. It can also be affected by physical stressors, a poor living environment, exposure to air pollutants, and an unsafe environment. Psychological stressors and heredity factors can also influence level of health. Total health programs are directed at changing lifestyle by developing habits that can improve level of health. The following categories are identified as important determinants of health status (Edelman and Mandle, 1994):

1. Tobacco use
2. Nutrition
3. Alcohol use
4. Habituating drug use
5. Driving
6. Exercise
7. Sexuality and contraceptive or barrier use
8. Family relationships
9. Risk-factor modification
10. Coping and adaptation

Other programs are aimed at specific health care problems. For example, support groups exist to help people with acquired immunodeficiency syndrome (AIDS). Exercise programs encourage participants to exercise regularly to reduce their risk of cardiac disease. Stress-reduction programs teach participants to cope with stressors and reduce their risks for multiple illnesses, such as infections, gastrointestinal disease, and cardiac disease.

Some health promotion, wellness education, and illness prevention programs are operated by health care agencies; others are independently operated. Many corporations have developed on-site health promotion activities for employees. Likewise, colleges and community centers offer health promotion and illness prevention programs. Nurses may be actively involved in these programs or may be consultants or give referrals. The goal of these activities is to improve the client's level of health through preventive health services, environmental protection, and health education.

The cornerstone of a wellness lifestyle is self-responsibility for health (Walker, 1992). Nurses assist clients in accepting responsibility for their own health by teaching them about health and health-enhancing behavior and avoidance of high-risk behavior while adopting desirable behavior patterns (Walker, 1992). Health promotion, wellness education, and illness prevention activities are important to the consumer and the health care provider. Nurses in all areas of practice often have opportunities to assist clients in adopting activities to promote health and decrease risks of illness.

Levels of Preventive Care

Nursing care oriented to health promotion, wellness, and illness prevention can be understood in terms of health activities on the primary, secondary, and tertiary levels (Table 1-1).

Primary prevention. Primary prevention is true prevention; it precedes disease or dysfunction and is applied to clients considered physically and emotionally healthy. It is not therapeutic, does not use therapeutic treatments, and does not involve symptom identification (Edelman and Mandle, 1994). Primary prevention includes health education programs, immunization, and physical and nutritional fitness activities. It can be provided to an individual or to a general population, or it can focus on individuals at risk for developing specific diseases. Wellness activities (Edelman and Mandle, 1994) are synonymous with the activities identified for primary prevention by Leavell and Clark (1965) in Table 1-1.

Secondary prevention. Secondary prevention focuses on individuals who are experiencing health problems or illnesses and who are at risk for developing complications or worsening conditions. Activities are directed at diagnosis and prompt intervention, thereby reducing severity and enabling the client to return to a normal level of health as early as possible (Pender, 1993; Edelman and Mandle 1994). A large portion of secondary level nursing care is delivered in homes, hospitals, or skilled nursing facilities. It includes screening techniques and treating early stages of disease to limit disability by averting or delaying the consequences of advanced disease.

Tertiary prevention. Tertiary prevention occurs when a defect or disability is permanent and irreversible. It involves minimizing the effects of long-term disease or disability by interventions directed at preventing complications and deterioration (Edelman and Mandle, 1994). Activities are directed at rehabilitation rather than diagnosis and treatment (Pender, 1993). Care at this level aims to help clients achieve as high a level of functioning as possible, despite the limitations caused by illness or impairment. This level of care is called *preventive care* because it involves preventing further disability or reduced functioning.

TABLE 1-1
The Three Levels of Prevention

Primary Prevention		Secondary Prevention		Tertiary Prevention
Health Promotion	**Specific Protection**	**Early Diagnosis and Prompt Treatment**	**Disability Limitations**	**Restoration and Rehabilitation**
Health education	Use of specific immunizations	Case-finding measures: individual and mass	Adequate treatment to arrest disease process and prevent further complications	Provision of hospital and community facilities for retraining and education to maximize use of remaining capacities
Good standard of nutrition adjusted to developmental phases of life	Attention to personal hygiene	Screening surveys	Provision of facilities to limit disability and prevent death	Education of the public and industries to use rehabilitated persons to the fullest possible extent
Attention to personality development	Use of environmental sanitation	Selective examinations		
Provision of adequate housing and recreation and agreeable working conditions	Protection against occupational hazards	Cure and prevention of disease process to prevent spread of communicable disease, prevent complications, and shorten period of disability		Selective placement
Marriage counseling and sex education	Protection from accidents			Work therapy in hospitals
Genetic screening	Use of specific nutrients			Use of sheltered colony
Periodic selective examinations	Protection from carcinogens			
	Avoidance of allergens			

Modified from Leavell HR, Clark AE: *Preventive medicine for doctors in the community*, ed 3, New York, 1965, McGraw-Hill.

RISK FACTORS

A **risk factor** is any situation, habit, environmental condition, physiological condition, or other variable that increases the vulnerability of an individual or group to an illness or accident. The presence of risk factors does not mean that a disease will develop, but risk factors increase the chances that the individual will experience a particular disease. Nurses and other health care professionals are concerned with risk factors, sometimes called *health hazards,* for several reasons. Risk factors play a major role in how a nurse identifies a client's health status. They can also influence health beliefs and practices if a person is aware of their presence. Risk factors can be placed in the following interrelated categories: genetic and physiological factors, age, physical environment, and lifestyle.

Genetic and Physiological Factors

Physiological risk factors involve the physical functioning of the body. Certain physical conditions, such as being pregnant or overweight, place increased stress on physiological systems (e.g., the circulatory system), increasing susceptibility to illness in these areas. Heredity, or genetic predisposition to specific illness, is a major physical risk factor. For example, a person with a family history of diabetes mellitus is at risk for developing the disease later in life. Other documented genetic risk factors include family histories of cancer, heart disease, or kidney disease.

Age

Age increases susceptibility to certain illnesses (e.g., the risk of heart disease increases with age for both sexes). The risks of birth defects and complications of pregnancy increase in women bearing children after age 35. Many kinds of cancer pose a greater risk for persons over age 45 than for younger persons. Age risk factors are often closely associated with other risk factors such as family history and personal habits. Nurses need to educate their clients about the importance of regularly scheduled checkups for their age group (Figure 1-6).

Environment

The physical environment in which a person works or lives can increase the likelihood that certain illnesses will occur. For example, some kinds of cancer and other diseases are more likely to develop when industrial workers are exposed to certain chemicals or when people live near toxic waste disposal sites. Screening for

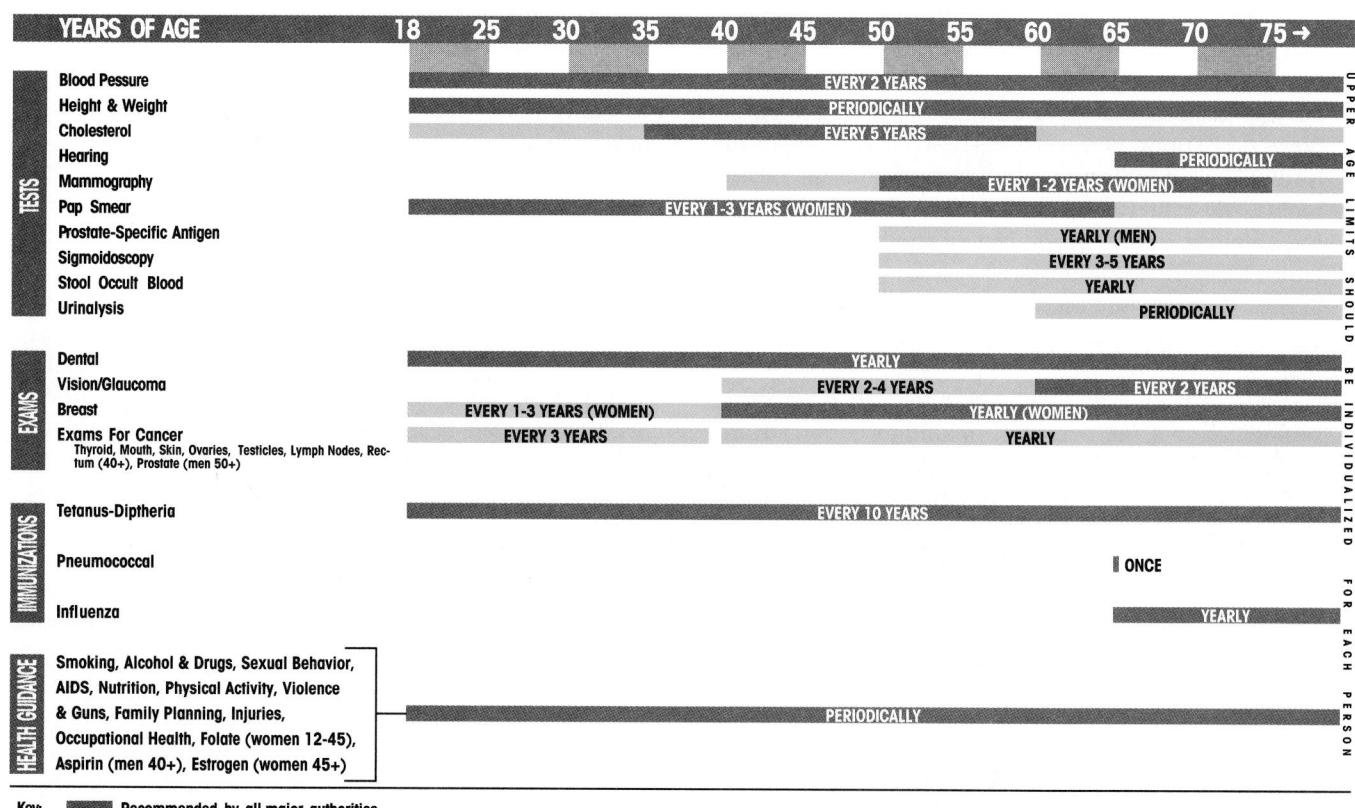

Figure 1-6. Adult preventive care timetable: recommendation of major authorities. (Redrawn from American Nurses Association: *Clinician's handbook of preventive services: put prevention into practice,* Washington, DC, 1994, The Association; modified from *Healthy People 2000.*)

these environmentally based risk factors is directed at the short-term effects of the exposure and the potential for long-term effects (Edelman and Mandle, 1994).

Blackburn (1994) reports that researchers have demonstrated how low income acts as a key health hazard by increasing exposure to health hazards such as poor housing, pollution (air, water, noise), lack of safe play areas, and poor social support networks. For example, in the home, the environment may include conditions that pose risks to an individual or family such as unclean, poorly heated or cooled, or overcrowded dwellings. These conditions can increase the likelihood that infections and other diseases will be contracted and spread.

Lifestyle

Many activities, habits, and practices involve risk factors; the stresses of life crises and frequent lifestyle changes are also risk factors. Lifestyle practices and behaviors can have positive or negative effects on health. Practices with potential negative effects are risk factors; these include overeating or poor nutrition, insufficient rest and sleep, and poor personal hygiene. Other habits that put a person at risk for illness include tobacco use, alcohol or drug abuse, and activities involving a threat of injury such as skydiving or mountain climbing. Some habits are risk factors for specific diseases. For example, excessive sunbathing increases the risk of skin cancer, and being overweight increases the risk of cardiovascular disease. These lifestyle risk factors have gained increased attention because it is known that many of the leading causes of death in the United States are related to lifestyle patterns or habits. This also represents a huge impact on the economics of the health care system. Therefore it is important to understand the impact of lifestyle behaviors on health status. Nurses can educate their clients and the public on wellness promoting lifestyle behaviors.

Stress can be a lifestyle risk factor if it is severe or prolonged or if the person is unable to cope with life events adequately. Stress can threaten mental health (emotional stress), as well as physical well-being (physiological stress). Both may influence the development of an illness, the ability to adapt to potential changes associated with an illness, and the ability to survive a life-threatening illness. Stress may also interfere with health promotion activities and the ability to implement needed lifestyle modifications. Emotional stressors may result from life events such as divorce, pregnancy, death of a spouse or family member, and financial instabilities. Job-related stressors, for example, may overtax a person's cognitive skills and decision-making ability, leading to "mental overload" or "burnout" (see Chapter 22). Stress can also threaten physical well-being and has been associated with illnesses such as heart disease, cancer, and gastrointestinal disorders (Pender, 1996).

Life stressors should be reviewed as a part of a comprehensive risk factor analysis.

The goal of risk factor identification is to merely assist clients to visualize those areas in their lives that can be modified or even eliminated to promote wellness and prevent illness. More comprehensive health risk appraisals, utilizing a variety of available health risk appraisal forms, can be done to estimate a person's specific health threats based on the presence of various risk factors (Edelman and Mandle, 1994). It is important to understand that implementation of a health risk appraisal must be linked with educational programs and other community resources to result in necessary lifestyle changes and risk reduction (Pender, 1996).

···RISK FACTOR MODIFICATION AND CHANGING HEALTH BEHAVIORS

Identifying risk factors is the first step in health promotion, wellness education, and illness prevention activities. Health hazards should be discussed with the client following a comprehensive nursing assessment; then the client can decide if he or she wants to maintain or improve his or her health status by taking risk reduction actions (Edelman and Mandle, 1994). Risk factor modification can be considered a wellness strategy in that it teaches clients to care for themselves in a healthier way. Modification of risk factors often involves a health behavior change.

Despite the knowledge that certain lifestyle behaviors (risk behaviors) may lead to illness or other problems, some individuals continue to engage in them (McKie and others, 1993). Changing health behavior is difficult, especially those behaviors that are ingrained in lifestyle patterns. Changing more than one behavior at a time is even more difficult, for example, losing weight and quitting smoking (McKie and others, 1993); however, "improved health, for many people, depends on their ability to change behaviors" (Conn, 1994). Many chronic health problems of older adults are often manageable or preventable through behavioral change (Haber and Lacy, 1993). This has important implications for nurses, who spend the greatest amount of time in direct contact with clients. Risk factor modification, health promotion or illness prevention activities, or any program that attempts to change unhealthy lifestyle behaviors can be considered a wellness strategy. Wellness strategies need to be emphasized because they have the ability to decrease the potential high costs of unmanaged health problems.

Attempts to change may be aimed at the cessation of a health damaging behavior (tobacco use, alcohol misuse) or at the adoption of a healthy behavior (healthy diet) (Pender, 1996). It has been assumed that change in behavior (especially risky behavior) is achieved through information about the potentially adverse effects of engaging in such activity (McKie and others, 1993). However, information alone most likely will not lead to behavior change. Supplementation of an information giving health promotion program with sociobehavioral modalities can result in greater benefits to participants (Haber and Lacy, 1993). These sociobehavioral modalities can include support groups, behavioral contracting, and advanced practice nurse and physician guidance. A behavioral contract is a written set of guidelines for changing health behaviors that is mutually agreed on by the health professional and the client. The contract stipulates a specific plan of action the client agrees to follow to meet a desired goal (Box 1-3).

An understanding of the process of changing behaviors can help nurses support difficult health behavior change in their clients. It is believed that change involves movement through a series of stages (Figure 1-7). Five stages of change ranging from no intention to change (precontemplation) to maintaining a changed behavior (maintenance stage) have been identified (Prochaska and DiClemente, 1992). Nursing implications for each stage are discussed in Table 1-2, p. 16. As individuals attempt change in behavior, relapse and recycling through the stages occur frequently. When relapse occurs, the person will return to the contemplation or precontemplation stage before attempting change again. Relapse can be viewed as a learning process, and what is learned from relapse can be applied to the next attempt to change. It is important to understand what occurs at the various stages of the change process to time the wellness strategies adequately and to provide appropriate care at each stage (Pender, 1996).

Most behavior change programs are designed for those people who are ready to take action on their health behavior problems. Only a minority of people are actually in this action stage (Prochaska, 1991). Further work needs to be done to design interventions and wellness strategies for people in all stages of health behavior change. The goal of any health promotion program is to assist individuals to change their health-related behaviors for the better, whether it is to reduce risks or improve level of wellness (Redland and Stuifbergen, 1993). Changes will be maintained over time only if the health behavior changes are integrated into an individual's overall lifestyle. Maintenance of healthy lifestyles can prevent hospitalizations and potentially lower the cost of health care. Nurses can assist clients with their adaptation to a changed and healthier lifestyle.

···ILLNESS

Illness is a state in which a person's physical, emotional, intellectual, social, developmental, or spiritual functioning is diminished or impaired compared with previous experience. Cancer is a disease process, but one client with leukemia who is responding to treatment may continue to function as usual, whereas another client with breast cancer who is preparing for surgery may be affected in dimensions other than the physical.

Illness, therefore, is not synonymous with disease; although nurses must be familiar with different kinds of diseases and their treatments, they are concerned more with illness, which may include not only disease but also the effects on functioning and well-being in all dimensions.

Box 1-3
Steps of Behavioral Contracting

1. *Set a goal:* Describe the behavior change that is desired.
2. *List the benefits:* What will be gained from achievement of the goal?
3. *Know the barriers:* What things might interfere with achievement of the goal?
4. *Plan of action:* Detail the steps required to achieve the goal. Acknowledge barriers, time, and required resources.
5. *Evaluation:* Regularly evaluate progress. Make revisions to plan of action if needed.

Data from Haber D, Lacy MG: Evaluation of a sociobehavioral intervention for changing health behaviors of older adults, *Behav Health Aging* 3(2):73, 1993.

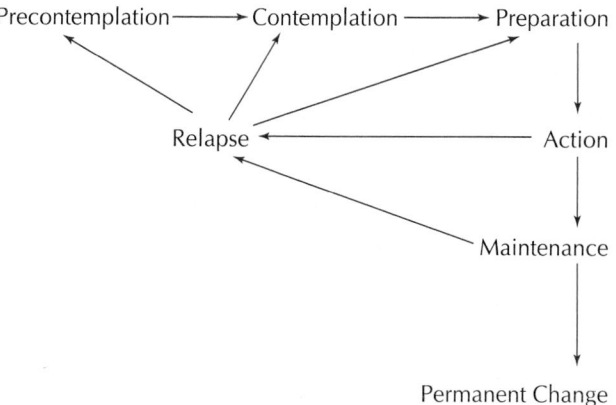

Figure 1-7. Stages of health behavior change. (Redrawn from Conn VS: A stage-based approach to helping people change health behaviors, *Clin Nurs Spec* 8[4]:187, 1994; and Prochaska JO and others: In search of how people change: applications and addictive behaviors, *Am Psychol* 47[9]: 1102, 1992.)

TABLE 1-2		
Stages of Health Behavior Change		
	Definition	Nursing Implications
Precontemplation	Not intending to make changes within the next 6 months.	Client will not be interested in information about the behavior, and may be defensive when confronted with the information.
Contemplation	Considering a change within the next 6 months.	Ambivalence may be present, but clients will more likely accept information as they are developing more belief in the value of change.
Preparation	Make small changes in preparation for a change in the next month.	Client believes advantages outweigh disadvantages of behavior change. May need assistance in planning for the change.
Action	Actively engaged in strategies to change behavior. This stage may last up to 6 months.	Be aware of previous habits that may prevent action on new behaviors. Identify barriers and facilitators of change.
Maintenance Stage	Sustained change over time. This stage begins 6 months after action has started and continues indefinitely.	Changes need to be integrated into the client's lifestyle.

Modified from Prochaska JO, DiClemente CC: Stages of change in the modification of problem behaviors, *Prog Behav Modif* 28:184, 1992; and Conn VS: A staged-based approach to helping people change health behaviors, *Clin Nurs Spec* 8(4):187, 1994.

Acute and Chronic Illness

Acute and chronic illness are two general classifications of illness used in this chapter. An **acute illness** is usually short term and severe. The symptoms appear abruptly, are intense, and often subside after a relatively short period. An acute illness may affect functioning in any dimension. A **chronic illness** persists, usually longer than 6 months, and can also affect functioning in any dimension. The client may fluctuate between maximal functioning and serious health relapses that may be life threatening. A person with a chronic illness is similar to a person with a disability, in that both have limitations (of varying degrees) in function resulting from either a pathological process or an injury. Mechanic (1995) notes that "a chronic disabling disease interferes with ongoing life adaptations by making the performance of routine tasks more challenging." Additionally, the social surroundings and physical environment in which the individual lives can affect the abilities, motivation, and psychological maintenance of the disabled person.

Chronic illnesses and disabilities remain a leading health problem in North America for older adults and children. Nurses can greatly influence the care of these clients by utilizing a holistic approach to promote healing in the physical, emotional, mental, and spiritual dimensions of the person (Lindsey, 1995). A major role for nursing is to provide client education aimed at helping clients manage their illness or disability to reduce the occurrence of symptoms and improve the tolerance of symptoms, as well as to enhance wellness and improve quality of life for clients living with chronic illnesses or disabilities.

⋯ILLNESS BEHAVIOR

People who are ill generally act in a way medical sociologists call *illness behavior*. It involves how people monitor their bodies, define and interpret their symptoms, take remedial actions, and use the health care system (Mechanic, 1982). Personal history, social situations, social norms, and the opportunities and constraints of community institutions can all affect illness behavior (Mechanic, 1995). Although there is a large variability in the way people react to an illness, illness behavior displayed in sickness can be used to manage life adversities (Mechanic, 1995). In other words, if people perceive themselves to be ill, illness behaviors can be coping mechanisms. For example, illness behavior can result in clients being released from roles, social expectations, or responsibilities. For a homemaker, for example, the "flu" may be viewed as an added stressor, or it may be a temporary release from child care and household responsibilities.

Variables Influencing Illness Behavior

Just as health behavior is affected by internal and external variables, so is illness behavior. The influences of these variables, as well as the stage of illness behavior the client is in, may affect the likelihood of seeking health care, compliance with therapy, and therefore health outcomes. Based on an understanding of these variables and behaviors, nurses can plan individualized care to assist clients in coping with their illness at various stages. The goal of nursing is to promote optimal functioning in all dimensions throughout an illness.

Internal variables. Internal variables influencing the way clients behave when they are ill are their perceptions of symptoms and the nature of the illness. If clients believe that the symptoms of their illnesses disrupt their normal routine, they are more likely to seek health care assistance than if they do not perceive the symptoms to be disruptive. If clients believe that the symptoms are serious or perhaps life threatening, they are also more likely to seek assistance. Persons awakened by crushing chest pains in the middle of the night generally view this symptom as potentially serious and life threatening and will probably be motivated to seek assistance. However, such a perception can also have the opposite effect. Individuals may fear serious illness, react by denying it, and not seek medical assistance.

The nature of the illness, either acute or chronic, can also affect a client's illness behavior. Clients with acute illnesses are likely to seek health care and comply readily with therapy. On the other hand, a client with a chronic illness, in which the symptoms may not be cured but only partially relieved, may not be motivated to comply with the therapy plan. Chronically ill clients may become less actively involved in their care, may experience greater frustration, and may comply less readily with care. Because nurses generally spend more time than other health care professionals with chronically ill clients, they are in the unique position of being able to assist these clients in overcoming problems related to illness behavior.

External variables. External variables influencing a client's illness behavior include the visibility of symptoms, social group, cultural background, economic variables, accessibility of the health care system, and social support. The visibility of the symptoms of an illness can affect body image and illness behavior. A client with a visible symptom may be more likely to seek assistance than a client without such a visible symptom.

Clients' social groups may assist them in recognizing the threat of illness or support the denial of potential illness. Families, friends, and co-workers all may influence clients' illness behavior. Clients often react positively to social support while practicing positive health behaviors. Cultural and ethnic background teaches a person how to be healthy, how to recognize illness, and how to be ill. The effects of disease and its interpretation vary according to cultural circumstances.

Economic variables influence the way a client reacts to illness. Because of economic constraints, a client may delay treatment and in many cases may continue to carry out daily activities. Clients' access to the health care system is closely related to economic factors. The health care system is a socioeconomic system that clients must enter, interact within, and exit. For many clients, entry into the system is complex or confusing, and some clients may seek nonemergency medical care in an emergency room because they do not know how otherwise to obtain health services. The physical proximity of clients to a health care agency often influences how soon they enter the system after deciding to seek care.

IMPACT OF ILLNESS ON CLIENT AND FAMILY

Illness is never an isolated life event. The client and family must deal with changes resulting from illness and treatment. Each client responds uniquely to illness, and therefore nursing interventions must be individualized. The client and family commonly experience behavioral and emotional changes, as well as changes in roles, body image, self-concept, and family dynamics.

Behavioral and Emotional Changes

People react differently to illness or the threat of illness. Individual behavioral and emotional reactions depend on the nature of the illness, the client's attitude toward it, the reaction of others to it, and the variables of illness behavior.

Short-term, non–life-threatening illnesses evoke few behavioral changes in the functioning of the client or family. A husband and father who has a cold, for example, may lack the energy and patience to spend time in family activities and may be irritable and prefer not to interact with his family. This is a behavioral change, but the change is subtle and does not last long. Some may even consider such a change a normal response to illness.

Severe illness, particularly one that is life threatening, can lead to more extensive emotional and behavioral changes, such as anxiety, shock, denial, anger, and withdrawal. These are common responses to the stress of illness. The nurse can develop interventions to assist the client and the family in coping with and adapting to this stress, because the stressor itself cannot usually be changed.

Impact on Family Roles

People have many roles in life, such as wage earner, decision maker, professional, and parent. When an illness occurs, the roles of client and family may change (see Chapter 19). Such a change may be subtle and short term or drastic and long term. An individual and family generally adjust more easily to subtle, short-term changes. In most cases they know that the role change is only temporary and will not require prolonged adjustment phases. Long-term changes, however, require an adjustment process similar to the grief process (see Chapter 21). The client and family often require specific counseling and guidance to assist them in coping with the role changes.

Impact on Body Image

Body image is the subjective concept of physical appearance (see Chapter 16). Some illnesses result in changes in physical appearance, and clients and families react differently to these changes. These reactions of clients and families to changes in body image depend on the following:

1. The type of changes (e.g., the loss of a limb, a special sense, or an organ)
2. Their adaptive capacity
3. The rate at which changes take place
4. Support services available

When a change in body image occurs, such as results from a leg amputation, the client generally adjusts in the following phases: shock, withdrawal, acknowledgment, acceptance, and rehabilitation. Initially the client may be shocked by the change or impending change and may depersonalize it and talk about it as though it were happening to someone else. As the client and family recognize the reality of the change, they become anxious and may withdraw, refusing to discuss it. Withdrawal is an adaptive coping mechanism that can assist the client in making the adjustment. As the client and family acknowledge the change, they move through a period of grieving. At the end of the acknowledgment phase, they accept the loss. During rehabilitation, the client is ready to learn how to adapt to the change in body image through use of a prosthesis or changing lifestyles and goals.

Impact on Self-Concept

Self-concept is a mental self-image of strengths and weaknesses in all aspects of personality. Self-concept depends in part on body image and roles but also includes other aspects of psychology and spirituality (see Chapters 16 and 17). The impact of illness on the self-concepts of clients and family members may be more complex and less readily observed than role changes.

Self-concept is important in relationships with other family members. A client whose self-concept changes because of illness may no longer meet family expectations, leading to tension or conflict. As a result, family members may change their interactions with the client. In the course of providing care, a nurse is able to observe changes in the client's self-concept (or in the self-concepts of family members) and develop a care plan to help the client adjust to the changes resulting from the illness.

Impact on Family Dynamics

Because of the effects of illness on the client and family, family dynamics often change. Family dynamics is the process by which the family functions, makes decisions, gives support to individual members, and copes with everyday changes and challenges. If a parent in a family becomes ill, family activities and decision making often come to a halt as the other family members wait for the illness to pass, or they delay action because they are reluctant to assume the ill person's roles or responsibilities. Because of the effects of illness, family dynamics often change. Role reversal is common, as parents and children try to adapt to major changes resulting from a family member's illness. If a parent of an adult becomes ill and cannot carry out usual activities, the adult child often assumes many of the parent's responsibilities and in essence becomes a parent to the parent. Such a reversal of the usual situation can lead to stress, conflicting responsibilities for the adult child, or direct conflict over decision making. The nurse must view the whole family as a client under stress, planning care to help the family regain the maximal level of functioning and well-being (see Chapter 19).

Key Terms

active strategies of health promotion
acute illness
basic human needs
chronic illness
health
health belief model
health beliefs
health promotion model
HEALTH-Healing/Disordering model
health-illness continuum model
holistic health model

illness
illness behavior
illness prevention
negative health behaviors
passive strategies of health promotion
positive health behaviors
primary prevention
risk factor
secondary prevention
tertiary prevention
wellness
wellness-illness model

■ Key Concepts

Health and wellness are not merely the absence of disease and illness.

A person's state of health, wellness, or illness depends on individual values, personality, and lifestyle.

According to the health-illness continuum model, health and illness are in a dynamic, relative relationship.

The health-belief model considers factors influencing health beliefs.

The health promotion model increases individual well-being and self-actualization.

Holistic health models of nursing promote optimal health by incorporating active participation of the client in improving the health state.

Holistic nursing interventions can be used by nurses to augment standard medical therapy.

Health beliefs and practices are influenced by internal and external variables and should be considered when planning care.

Health promotion activities help maintain or enhance health.

Wellness education teaches clients how to care for themselves.

Illness prevention activities protect against health threats and thus maintain an optimal level of health.

Nursing incorporates health promotion, wellness, and illness prevention activities rather than simply treating illness.

The three levels of preventive care are primary, secondary, and tertiary.

Risk factors threaten health, influence health practices, and are important considerations in illness prevention activities.

Risk factors involve genetic or physiological variables, age, environment, and lifestyle.

Improvement in health may involve a change in health behaviors.

Illness behavior, like health practices, is influenced by many variables and must be considered by the nurse when planning care.

Illness can have many effects on the client and family, including changes in behavior and emotions, family roles and dynamics, body image, and self-concept.

■ Critical Thinking Activities

1. How would you describe your current state of health: excellent, good, fair, or poor? What definition of health did you use to make this judgment? List the current health promotion, wellness, and illness prevention activities in which you regularly engage. Are there any areas that need to be improved or changed? What will influence your ability to adopt any needed changes?

2. Assess the lifestyle patterns of someone you know. Identify risk factors that increase the person's vulnerability to illness or susceptibility to disease. Are there risk factors present that could be modified?

3. Using the same individual chosen for the previous activity, how could you approach the subject of risk factor modification? What influences exist that will assist the individual in making a change? What barriers exist that may prevent maintenance of a change in health behavior? What is the major nursing implication in the maintenance stage of health behavior change? What resources are available to you and to this individual that may assist in the change process?

References

American Nurses Association: *Clinician's handbook of preventive services: put prevention into practice,* Washington, DC, 1994, The Association.

Becker MH, Maiman LA: Sociobehavioral determinants of compliance with health and medical care recommendations, *Med Care* 33(1):1021, 1975.

Benner P, Wrubel J: *The primacy of caring: stress and coping in health and illness,* Con Mills, Ont, 1989, Addison-Wesley.

Blackburn C: Low income, inequality and health promotion, *Nurs Times* 90(39):42, 1994.

Conn VS: A staged-based approach to helping people change health behaviors, *Clin Nurs Spec* 8(4):187, 1994.

Duffy ME: Determinants of health-promoting lifestyles in older persons, *Image* 25(1):23, 1993.

Dunn H: What high level wellness means, *Health Values* 1:9, 1977.

Dunn HL: High-level wellness for man and society, *Am J Public Health* 49:789, 1959.

Edelman CL, Mandle CL: *Health promotion throughout the life span,* ed 3, St. Louis, 1994, Mosby.

Haber D: *Health promotion and aging,* New York, 1994, Springer.

Haber D, Lacy MG: Evaluation of a socio-behavioral intervention for changing health behaviors of older adults, *Behav Health Aging* 3(2):73, 1993.

Jensen L, Allen M: Wellness: the dialectic of illness, *Image* 25(3):220, 1993.

Leavell HR, Clark AE: *Preventive medicine for doctors in the community,* ed 3, New York, 1965, McGraw-Hill.

Lindsey E: The gift of healing chronic illness/disability, *J Holistic Nurs* 13(4):287, 1995.

Lipowski ZJ: Psychological aspects of disease, *Ann Intern Med* 71:1197, 1969.

Lipowski ZJ: Psychosocial reactions to physical illness, *Can Med Assoc J* 128:1069, 1983.

McCabe P: Exploring the phenomenon of healing: healing as a health capacity, *Aust J Holistic Nurs* 2(1):13, 1995.

McKie L and others: Defining and assessing risky behaviours, *J Adv Nurs* 18:1911, 1993.

Mechanic D: The epidemiology of illness behavior and its relationship to physical and psychological distress. In Mechanic D: *Symptoms, illness behavior, and help seeking,* New York, 1982, Prodist.

Mechanic D: Sociological dimensions of illness behavior, *Soc Sci Med* 41(9):1207, 1995.

Mornhinweg GC, Voignier RR: Holistic nursing interventions, *Orthop Nurs* 14(4):20, 1995.

Moss-Morris R, Paterson J: Understanding children's concepts of health and illness: implications for developmental therapists, *Phys Occup Ther Pediatr* 14(3/4):95, 1995.

Najman JM: Health and poverty: past, present and prospects for the future, *Soc Sci Med* 36(2):157, 1993.

Neuman B: Health as a continuum based on the Neuman Systems Model, *Nurs Sci Q* 3:129, 1990.

Pender NJ: Health promotion and illness prevention. In Werley HH, Fitzpatrick JJ, editors: *Annual review of nursing research,* New York, 1993, Springer.

Pender NJ: *Health promotion and nursing practice,* Norwalk, Conn, 1982, Appleton-Century-Crofts.

Pender NJ: *Health promotion and nursing practice,* ed 3, Stamford, Conn, 1996, Appleton & Lange.

Peterson B: The mind-body connection, *Can Nurs* 92(1):29, 1996.

Prochaska JO: Assessing how people change, *Cancer* 67(3):805, 1991.

Prochaska JO, DiClemente CC: Stages of change in the modification of problem behaviors, *Prog Behav Modif* 28:184, 1992.

Prochaska JO and others: In search of how people change: applications and addictive behaviors, *Am Psychol* 47(9):1102, 1992.

Rawlins R and others: *Mental health-psychiatric nursing: a holistic life cycle approach,* St. Louis, 1993, Mosby.

Redland AR, Stuifbergen AK: Strategies for maintenance of health-promoting behaviors, *Nurs Clin North Am* 28(2):427, 1993.

Rosenstoch I: Historical origin of the health belief model, *Health Educ Monogr* 2:334, 1974.

Ross (nee Waugh) L: The spiritual dimension: its importance to patients' health, well-being and quality of life and its implications for nursing practice, *Soc Sci Med* 32(5):457, 1995.

Stubblefield C: Optimism: a determinant of health behavior, *Nurs Forum* 39(1):19, 1995.

U.S. Department of Health and Human Services, PHS: *Healthy people 2000: midcourse review and 1995 revisions,* Sudbury, Mass, 1996, Jones & Bartlett.

U.S. Department of Health and Human Services, PHS: *Healthy people 2000: national health promotion and disease prevention objectives,* Washington, DC, 1990, U.S. Government Printing Office.

Walker SN: Wellness for elders, *Holistic Nurs Pract* 7(1):38, 1992.

World Health Organization Interim Commission: *Chronicle of WHO,* Geneva, 1947, The Organization.

CHAPTER

2

The Health Care Delivery System

OBJECTIVES

Mastery of content in this chapter will
enable the student to:

- Define the key terms listed.
- Describe the six levels of health care.
- Explain the relationship between levels of care
  and levels of prevention.
- Discuss the types of settings where various
  levels of health care are provided.
- Discuss the role of nurses in different health
  care delivery settings.
- Explain the advantages and disadvantages of
  managed health care.
- Describe the meaning of a seamless system of
  health care.
- Describe the quality measures used to evaluate
  health care delivery performance.
- Compare the various methods for financing
  health care.
- Discuss the implications that changes in the
  health care system have on nursing.
- Discuss nursing's role within delivery of care
  and work redesign methodologies.

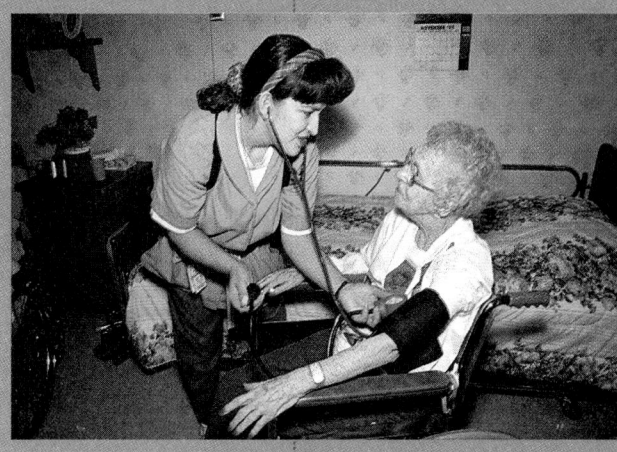

Gloria is a 56-year-old married woman who was diagnosed with diabetes over 15 years ago. She lives in Healthland, USA. Gloria has a nurse case manager, Eric, who visits her monthly at home or more often if she begins to develop any problems. Gloria and her husband attended classes many years ago on diabetes self-management. They have become very reliable in managing Gloria's diet and exercise, administering her daily insulin injections, and measuring her blood glucose daily. If any new forms of insulin are introduced to the market, the hospital's pharmacist knows to give Gloria a call to discuss information about the new drug. When the nearby community clinic has a lecture on new trends in diabetes, Gloria always receives a flyer and an invitation to attend. Her physician scans Gloria's blood glucose values routinely on his office computer, which links to Gloria's home computer. One year ago she was admitted to the hospital for complications. Eric was there to inform the nursing staff about her case. Her personal physician managed her medical care during hospitalization. When asked about her satisfaction with her health care, Gloria says she is very pleased and believes she can access any service quickly, when she needs it.

Gloria's story unfortunately is fictitious. It describes what is called a **seamless care delivery** model. In such a model, fragmentation of health care services has been eliminated, and clients receive a continuum of health care services when they need it, with minimal inconvenience and with a limited number of health professionals involved. It is a model that the most progressive health care systems are trying to achieve. In reality, however, many health care systems within the United States are highly fragmented. Clients often meet barriers in trying to access health care and are frequently forced to see a variety of different health care providers. The health care system within the United States is facing the need for unprecedented change to improve care delivery. McCloskey and Grace (1994) note that the challenge to nursing in the face of current health care change is to bring continuity to a chaotic and fragmented system.

The U.S. health care system is being challenged to reduce costs while maintaining quality of care. Pressures to reduce costs come from declining reimbursement by **third-party payers** and health care institutions being managed more as businesses rather than service organizations. Many clients who would have been hospitalized for a condition 10 years ago now receive care in outpatient facilities. Hospitalized clients are sicker, and their treatment involves a higher level of technological care. Clients are discharged from hospitals sooner, often leaving families with the burden of providing care in the home setting that used to be provided in the hospital. Fragmentation of services coupled with changes in funding sources creates demands for better coordination of services if individuals and their families are to receive adequate health care (McCloskey and Grace, 1994).

The practice of nursing is changing to keep up with changes within our health care systems. It is important to understand the issues facing health care professionals today and how these issues influence the manner in which health care services are organized and delivered. The nurse's role is different depending on the setting where health care services are provided. However, a common theme found in any setting is the nurse's goal of helping clients maintain or achieve an optimal level of health with the client as an active participant. The nurse must be at the center of any innovation occurring within health care to remain an advocate of quality care to all.

FINANCING HEALTH CARE SERVICES

The climate in health care has changed because of changes in the way in which health care services are paid. Health care spending in the United States has been growing for many years. Before 1985, health insurers basically paid whatever a client was charged for medical care. There was little incentive for hospitals to control costs. By 1994 nearly 14% of the gross domestic product was spent on health care (Solovy, 1994). In contrast, health care made up only 8.6% of Canada's gross national product in 1990 (Harrington, 1990). Despite the differences in spending between the two countries, studies have failed to show clear differences in outcomes. Spending more money does not necessarily mean a higher quality of care.

Experts estimate that by the year 2000, health care spending in the United States will increase to 16% to 18% of the gross domestic product (Solovy, 1994). Because business, industry, and the government are paying the majority of health care bills, they are demanding greater controls over use of resources and evidence that quality health care is being received by clients (Sovie, 1990). Health care institutions are scrambling to find better ways to provide health care at a lower cost. At the same time, they are being evaluated very closely by regulatory agencies such as the Joint Commission on Accreditation of Healthcare Organizations (JCAHO), professional review organizations (PROs), and state health departments. The reviews focus on the outcomes of health care and whether clients leave health care institutions in an improved state of health with the capacity to manage their continued health care needs.

How does this affect nursing? In many ways. The demands for cost control are affecting nurses at the bedside: more control over supply utilization, greater emphasis on coordinating clients' timely discharge from health care agencies, and fewer numbers of staff to manage client care. Because nursing care is directly affected by health care financing, it is important for nurses to understand the types of finance mechanisms that exist. This is not always easy because in any given health care market, a variety of finance mechanisms can exist.

Private Insurance Plans

Traditionally, health care systems operated on a fee-for-service basis, receiving payment for each episode of care. Even though this trend has changed dramatically, there are still "private-pay" insurance options that support fee-for-service activities. The policies are expensive. Such an insurance policy can be obtained by an individual or through a group plan offered by employers. This type of plan is a retrospective fee-for-service option. Payment is computed after services are provided on the basis of the number of services used. Health insurance programs pay for some, most, or all of the health care expenses. Such payments are called third-party reimbursements because the costs of health care services are met, not by the health care agency or the client, but by the third party, the insurer. Ultimately, of course, consumers bear the costs through insurance premiums. The problem with private insurance plans is that there are no incentives for reducing health care costs. More companies are changing their fee-for-service payment structures to methods similar to those used by Medicare.

Medicare

Medicare is a nationwide health insurance program authorized under Title 18 of the Social Security Act, which provides benefits to persons 65 years of age or older. Medicare Part A is the hospital insurance program; Part B is the supplementary medical insurance program, covering physician and certain outpatient services (Box 2-1). The Omnibus Budget Reconciliation Act of 1990 covers services of nurse practitioners and clinical nurse specialists performed in collaboration with a physician in the rural setting (Streff, 1994). Persons entitled to **Medicare** coverage include adults who are 65 years of age or older, persons of any age with permanent kidney failure, and select individuals with disabling illnesses. The program is administered by the Health Care Financing Administration (HCFA) and is funded in part through Social Security (FICA) taxes, paid by all employed individuals. Most recipients of Medicare do not pay monthly premiums directly for Medicare because of deductions of premiums from monthly Social Security checks.

Medicare does not pay for the full cost of certain services. For example, a diagnostic test such as a mammogram will only be reimbursed for a flat amount of $50. If a radiological center charges more than the flat rate, the client must pay the remainder. Hospitals and physicians voluntarily choose to participate in Medicare, although many states make it mandatory for licensure. When a physician agrees to participate in Medicare, a percentage of the fee (e.g., 10%) is paid directly by the

---

Box 2-1
Examples of Health Care Services Covered and Not Covered by Medicare

Examples of Covered Services
Acute hospital care
Selected skilled nursing care
Home health care within defined limits
Diagnostic laboratory testing
Diagnostic radiological testing
Physical therapy
Speech pathology services
Ambulance (when health is at risk)
Kidney dialysis or transplant
Medications given in the hospital or skilled nursing facility
Selected outpatient medications
Physician care for medical and surgical services, treatments, tests, and procedures
Outpatient and emergency care for illness or accidents
Prosthetic devices
Durable medical equipment (e.g., oxygen, wheelchairs, home dialysis)
Medical supplies (e.g., syringes, dressings)
Hospice benefits
Respite care under specific conditions
Mental health services (only 180 days paid for a lifetime)
Selected immunizations

Examples of Services Not Covered
Long-term care
Preventive health services (e.g., immunizations, physical examinations)
Hearing examinations and hearing aids
Dental care (nonserious)
Eye examinations and eyeglasses

---

client. Participants in the program are encouraged to purchase supplemental insurance plans through private insurers. Coverage by Medicare can be confusing to a client. The Social Security Administration offers pamphlets explaining all benefits.

Medicare pays for hospital care through **prospective payment.** The health care agency receives a predetermined or fixed rate per discharge, depending on the **diagnosis-related group (DRG)** in which the client is classified. DRGs make up a classification system of 23 major diagnostic categories (e.g., diseases of the respiratory system, diseases of the circulatory system). Most of the categories contain a medical and surgical division. Each division is then further broken down into DRGs, totaling 494. The specific DRG assigned depends primarily on a client's principal medical diagnosis. However, secondary diagnoses, operating room procedures, age, discharge status, complications, and comorbidities (preexisting conditions) are also considered. A hospital receives one payment for each Medicare discharge based on the DRG classification, regardless of actual cost for caring for a client. The formula for determining a DRG payment is weighted, depending on the intensity and changes in resource consumption. For example, certain DRGs receive higher weights if they involve extensive diagnostic procedures or more complex therapies. Each DRG is assigned an average length of stay.

Because Medicare reimburses a hospital a fixed amount, regardless of actual costs, the hospital is at risk for operating at a loss. The hospital is given the incentive to find other methods of providing quality care to recover costs and make a profit. The hospital is also motivated not to keep the client hospitalized longer than necessary because the reimbursement is the same regardless of the client's actual length of stay.

In theory, prospective payments should help contain costs and even be an incentive for improved quality. Hospitals know the projected length of stay for each DRG and the anticipated payment. Opportunities to reduce system delays and inefficiencies, find better diagnostic measures, coordinate care more efficiently, and reduce unnecessary procedures should improve quality care. On the other hand, there is public concern that prospective payments might reduce the quality of care in certain cases. Regulatory mechanisms within the Medicare system protect clients from premature discharge and reduced standards of care.

◼ Clinical Scenario

Mr. Truman was admitted to the hospital on November 1 after experiencing chest pain and shortness of breath. He had undergone cardiac surgery almost 10 years before but was beginning to have recurrent chest pain, even at rest. He was scheduled for a cardiac catheterization, but it was delayed until November 3. The physician also referred Mr. Truman for diet counseling for a low-cholesterol diet. The cardiac catheterization proceeded without complications, and surgery was unnecessary. Mr. Truman remained hospitalized overnight to ensure that no problems developed. He was discharged on November 4.

Principal diagnosis: Heart ischemia

Secondary diagnosis: Disturbances of heart, functional, long-term effect of cardiac surgery

DRG assigned: DRG 125: circulatory disorders except acute myocardial infarction with cardiac catheterization without complex diagnosis

Assigned or allowed length of stay: 2.2 days

Actual length of stay: 3.1 days

Payment calculation (based on 2.2 days): Payment per discharge × DRG weight = $3400 × 0.7015 = $2385

Acutal hospital costs for Mr. Truman: $2960

Loss for hospital: $575

Medicaid

Medicaid is a federally assisted and state-administered program providing medical assistance to members of families with dependents who are older adults, blind, disabled, or under the age of consent (minors). Each state designs and administers its own program. Nationally, the average income eligibility requirement for Medicaid is less than that of the federal poverty level (nationally defined income level below which a family is considered "poor").

Medicaid has financed a large portion of maternal and child care for the poor. Since 1963 the Medicaid program has helped improve child health and reduce infant mortality rates through prenatal care. Nurse-midwifery services to Medicaid subscribers have been reimbursable since 1982. Twenty-eight states reimbursed nurses in advanced practice roles under Medicaid and 31 states reimbursed certified nurse anesthetists as of 1994 (Streff, 1994).

An increased number of impoverished people who fail to qualify for Medicaid struggle to access health care. With the growing number of poor, the funds for Medicaid are dwindling. Many hospitals and other agencies are taking measures to minimize treatment of Medicaid clients because they are not reimbursed for their costs. Obvious reforms to the Medicaid system are needed. Many enter **health maintenance organization (HMO)** plans for better managed medical care.

Managed Care

A **managed care** program is one that is designed to control the cost of health care services delivered to members while still maintaining quality of care. A wide variety of health care financing and delivery structures make up managed care programs. A managed care program is a model of health care delivery in which all of the health care needs of a client are funneled through one party—the case manager or gatekeeper (Vruwink and Mitchell, 1997). The program limits an enrollee's ability to choose any **provider** and to self-refer through the health care system. Specific guidelines exist for levels of health care service, length of hospitalization, and medical specialist access. The case manager or often a primary care provider is the gatekeeper in the system and must approve any referrals to specialty care. For example, if a client develops an acute muscle sprain and perhaps wishes to see an orthopedic physician, it will be necessary to first see the primary care physician (such as a medical internist) or be screened by a case manager (often a nurse) before an orthopedist can be seen. The aim in managed care is to reduce unnecessary use of health care resources (e.g., specialized medical care, unnecessary diagnostic tests) and to manage the client so that hospitalization is not required. If the client has a problem requiring treatment, **precertification** authorization is conducted to determine whether the treatment is covered by the managed care plan and what is the most appropriate setting for the treatment to be delivered. There are select procedures and diagnoses that must be treated on an outpatient basis only. Table 2-1 outlines types of managed care programs.

Capitation. **Capitation** is a payment mechanism in which a provider (e.g., health care network, HMO) receives a fixed amount per enrollee (Appleby, 1996). The aim of capitation is to build a payment plan for select diagnoses or surgical procedures that includes the best standards of care, including essential diagnostic and treatment procedures at the lowest cost. For example, if heart surgery is to be capitated, the health care plan will develop practice protocols for common medical services (e.g., pharmaceuticals, diagnostic tests, surgical treatment). The protocols will ensure thoroughness and a measure of consistency in the way physicians covered by the capitated plan deliver care.

The plan will also decide what tests and procedures will and will not be included in the primary care physician's portion of the capitated rate. The role of specialists and hospitals will also be defined so that each provider receives a "piece of the pie." It does a hospital no good to bill for additional services in an attempt to increase revenue. Payment is capped. No additional monies are available if the client's care requires more than what is typically included in the capitated rate. The risk of capitation is clients' receiving less care than might be optimal, particularly if standards of care change. However, the aim is to establish payment on strong clinical standards. If physicians involved in a capitated plan do not have input in developing the guidelines for payment, serious problems can arise. Tests or procedures deemed necessary by physicians might not be included in guidelines if financial advisors recommend clinical standards. In that case, clients clearly might not receive necessary services.

TABLE 2-1

Types of Managed Care Programs

Type	Definition	Characteristics
Preferred provider organization (PPO)	One that limits an enrollee's choice to a list of "preferred" hospitals, physicians, and providers. An enrollee pays more out of pocket for using a provider not on the list.	Contractual agreement exists between a set of providers and one or more purchasers (self-insured employers or insurance plans). Comprehensive health services at a discount to companies under contract.
Exclusive provider organization (EPO)	One that limits an enrollee's choice to providers belonging to one organization. May or may not be able to use outside providers at additional expense.	Focus on health maintenance. Limited contractual agreement. Less access to select specialists.
Health maintenance organization (HMO)	Provides comprehensive, preventive, and treatment services to a specific group of voluntarily enrolled persons. Structures include a variety of models: Staff model—physicians are salaried employees of the HMO. Group model—HMO contracts with single group practice. Network model—HMO contracts with multiple group practices and/or integrated organizations. **Independent practice association (IPA)**— HMO contracts with physicians who usually are not members of groups and whose practices include fee for service and capitated clients.	Focus on health maintenance, primary care. All care provided by a primary care physician.
Medicare HMO	Program same as HMO but designed to cover health care costs of senior citizens.	

Fixed payment. Most reimbursement through managed care programs occurs through a fixed payment system. The program provides comprehensive preventive and treatment services to a specific group of voluntarily enrolled persons under a fixed, prepaid plan. Members of an HMO, for example, pay periodic payments in advance for expected costs of benefits for a population group. The HMO's promise to deliver specifically defined services within a fixed, prepaid system offers providers an incentive to contain costs and unnecessary use of services. Providers receive a fixed payment based on an individual client's medical condition or surgical procedure. The formulas are similar to those seen in Medicare DRG payments. Typically an acute care payment is based on the anticipated number of days required for treatment of a specific condition or surgical procedure. Home health reimbursement is often based on the number of required visits.

Direct contracting. Employers are looking for ways to reduce health care costs. This is particularly true for large self-insured organizations, which may spend millions of dollars paying a portion of their employees' medical insurance. Many companies are looking at direct contracting with providers, such as hospitals and health care systems. The employer contracts at a package price for all needed care and services and agrees to work cooperatively on improving efficiency and outcomes (Meyer, 1996). Contracting may be established with selected high-quality health care systems anywhere in the country. The key is managing high-cost cases like organ transplantation or respiratory failure. Employees have more choices in selecting a contracting physician because the company usually contracts with a wide variety of physicians and hospitals who have established evidence of excellent clinical care. The direct contract approach bypasses the middleman in HMOs (the gatekeepers) to improve efficiency and lower administrative costs.

Long-Term Insurance

About 75% of older adults in the United States are covered by some type of private health insurance. This is necessary to cover the percentage of costs not covered by Medicare. However, most plans cover the same expenditures as Medicare, and as a result, there are large gaps in coverage for chronic health problems and long-term care. It appears that annual health care expenditures for older adults are about $3000, or two and one-half times the national average (Ebersole and Hess, 1994). Most persons who are 50 years or older will also need some form of long-term care for themselves or their parents. The expense for long-term care is high; for example, families pay an average of $25,000 to $60,000 annually for nursing home care (Ebersole and Hess, 1994). The unavailability of long-term care insurance is a national concern.

Private insurance companies have begun to offer long-term care policies. The policy will provide an insured person a set amount of dollars for an unlimited time or for as little as 2 years (Ebersole and Hess, 1994). At one time the U.S. legislature was considering a plan to offer long-term care benefits through a national health care plan, although this initiative has been stalled. A concern regarding long-term care insurance is the number of exclusions. Many insurance companies will not offer plans to clients with certain disabilities. A good long-term care insurance policy has a minimum waiting period for eligibility; maximum benefit for one stay of at least 4 years; payment for skilled nursing, intermediate care, or custodial care; and home care benefits (Ebersole and Hess, 1994).

Catastrophic Health Insurance

More people are surviving illness and living longer. The high costs associated with major and chronic illness are not covered by most insurance programs. In July 1988 the Medicare Catastrophic Coverage Act was passed to provide protection against the overwhelming out-of-pocket costs of major lengthy illnesses. Medicare recipients must pay flat premiums for the coverage. In addition, Medicare recipients who file income tax returns pay an additional fee based on taxable income.

The catastrophic coverage includes benefits for clients hospitalized over 60 days. There is also a limit on the amount that clients will be required to pay for physician fees. Expanded coverage for medications has also been added.

Canadian Government Health Insurance

The Canadian government has an integrated health care system with national health insurance. All citizens of Canada are covered by the mandatory program financed with tax dollars. Benefits are comprehensive, including short- and long-term care, and involve use of private-sector providers of services. The tax-supported program remains one of the most highly valued and popular initiatives of the Canadian government (Kerr, 1997). The government negotiates directly with providers to establish reasonable health care rates. Canada has substantially lower health care costs than the United States. For example, expenses for physicians' services make up approximately 16% of health expenditures, a figure that is higher (20%) in the United States (Kerr, 1997). The Canadian health care plan is more cost-effective in that it has fewer expenditures on insurance, prepayment, and administration costs, and the costs to hospitals and physicians are also lower.

Access to specialized medical care has been strictly limited in Canada, and as a result half of all Canadian physicians are general practitioners or primary care physicians (Terris, 1991). During that same year, only 10% of physicians practicing in the United States were primary care physicians (Terris, 1991). Since that time, the number of primary care physicians in the United States has grown to approximately 40% (Hospitals and Health Networks, 1997). Unlike in the United States, clients in Canada may experience long waiting periods for elective procedures. The emphasis within the system has been on disease prevention. To ensure the survival of the Canadian system, measures are needed to ensure that universal availability and access to needed services are balanced by the provision of reasonably comprehensive services in a publicly funded, nonprofit, affordable system (Kerr, 1997). Like the United States, Canada is seeing the need to place more emphasis on health promotion through a community-based model.

LEVELS OF HEALTH CARE

It is important to understand the variety of settings and services available for health care delivery. The health care system provides six levels of care (Figure 2-1). Levels of care describe the scope of services and settings where health care is offered to clients in all stages of health and illness. For example, the secondary level of care is the traditional **acute care** setting where clients who present signs and symptoms of disease are diagnosed and treated. **Restorative care** includes those settings and services where clients who are recovering from illness or disability receive rehabilitation and supportive care. Levels of care are not the same as levels of prevention (see Chapter 1). Levels of prevention instead describe the focus of health-related activities: avoiding disease (health promotion and disease prevention), curing disease (secondary prevention), and diminishing complications (tertiary prevention). At any level of care, nurses and other health care providers might offer a variety of levels of prevention. The nurse working in an acute care setting, for example, might monitor the recovery of a postoperative open heart surgery client while also providing health promotion information to the family concerning diet and exercise.

It is important to understand how levels of care are organized and delivered. Each level creates different requirements and opportunities for the role of the nurse (Table 2-2). In addition, changes unique to each level of care have developed as a result of health care reform. For example, there is greater emphasis being placed on the importance of wellness and primary and preventive care. More resources are being dedicated to these levels of care, particularly health promotion. Pender (1996) calls for health empowerment in all settings so that people of all ages and cultures can benefit from quality health-promotive care. Nursing has the chance to provide leadership to communities and health care systems that are aligning resources to better serve their populations. Critical to the success of improving health care

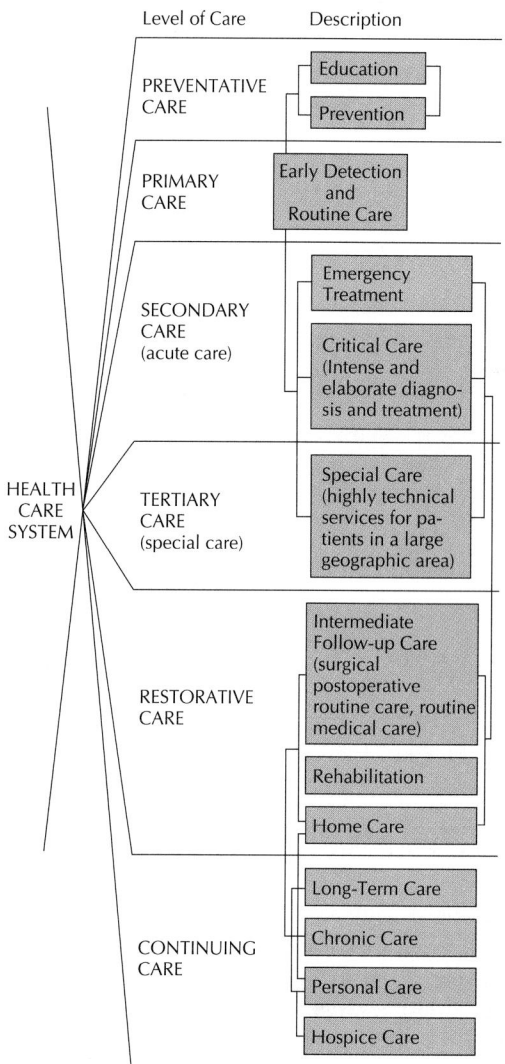

Figure 2-1. ■ Spectrum of health services delivery. (Modified from Cambridge Research Institute: *Trends affecting the U.S. health care system,* 262, Health Planning Information Series, Human Resources Administration, Public Health Service, Department of Health, Education, and Welfare, Washington, DC, 1976, revised and updated 1992, U.S. Government Printing Office.)

delivery will be the ability to find strategies that better address client needs at all levels of care.

A broad variety of health care services (Box 2-2) are available to clients and families, depending on the nature and extent of a health problem and the level of care required. The types of services offered also depend on the site in which clients seek health care.

Preventive and Primary Health Care Services

In the settings where preventive and **primary care** are delivered, health promotion is a major theme. Health promotion services are a key to quality health care. Successful programs help clients to acquire healthier

TABLE 2-2

Nursing Opportunities in the Health Care System

Level of Care	Nursing Opportunity
Preventive and primary health care	Clinic educator School health nurse Occupational health nurse Nurse practitioner Nurse-midwife Nurse entrepreneur: child care, older adult care, breast-feeding counseling
Secondary and tertiary care	Staff nurse: critical care, medicine, surgery, and specialty nursing units, operating room, emergency department Infection control specialist Case manager Risk management Clinical nurse specialist Nurse entrepreneur: patient classification systems, quality management, staff development, computer information management, documentation systems, temporary staffing agency
Restorative Care	Home health nurse Hospice nursing Staff nurse: long-term care, extended care Clinical nurse specialist Nurse entrepreneur: home health agency, chronic pain management

lifestyles and achieve a decent standard of living. The focus of health promotion is to keep people healthy through personal hygiene, good nutrition, clean living environments, regular exercise, rest, and the adoption of positive health attitudes. Health promotion programs can lower the overall costs of health care by reducing the incidence of disease, minimizing complications, and thus reducing the need to use more expensive health care resources. Preventive care is more disease oriented and focused on reducing and controlling risk factors for disease through activities such as immunization and occupational health programs. Community health promotion and illness prevention require education and involvement of the public. The nurse works in a variety of settings with programs designed to help clients reduce the risk of illness, maintain maximal function, and promote habits related to good health.

School health services.
Often we think of school health services as the school nurse sitting in an office and offering first aid and symptom management to children who become ill during class sessions. In fact, effective school health services are comprehensive programs that integrate health promotion principles throughout a school's educational program. School health services are designed to protect and promote the health of all students and school personnel. School health nurses are specialized in school nursing practice. The American Nurses Association (ANA) (1983) pub-

lished *Standards of School Nursing Practice,* which addresses issues such as program management, interdisciplinary collaboration, and community health systems. The school nurse helps to develop programs that foster children's growth, self-actualization, positive life skills for successful coping, and acquisition of knowledge and skills for self-care and that reinforce positive health attitudes (Pender, 1996). Specific nursing interventions in the school setting include health education, parent programming and counseling, communicable disease control, physical assessment, screening, crisis intervention, environmental safety, nutrition planning, and emergency care. The school nurse's role is rewarding when one is able to contribute to the overall process of education within a school.

Occupational health services.
Recently, occupational health in the work setting has gained importance as employers seek to reduce the costs of health insurance benefits for injured or ill workers. Occupational health is a national concern, affecting individuals, families, and communities. A comprehensive occupational health program geared toward health promotion and accident or illness prevention can increase worker productivity, decrease absenteeism, reduce use of expensive medical care, and lower disability claims (Pender, 1996). The aim in occupational health is to increase the health-enhancing potential of social and physical environments. When such programs are effective, busi-

Box 2-2
Examples of Health Care Services

Health Promotion
Prenatal care
Well-baby care
Nutrition counseling
Exercise classes
Family planning

Illness Prevention
Blood pressure and cancer screening
Immunizations
Poison control information
Community legislation (seat belts, air bags, safety helmets)
Mental health counseling and crisis prevention

Acute and Tertiary Care
Radiological procedures
Serum testing
Surgical outpatient and inpatient services
Laser therapies
Emergencies care

Restorative Care
Cardiovascular and pulmonary rehabilitation
Sports medicine
Spinal cord injury programs
Home health care

Continuing Care
Domiciliary homes
Psychiatric day care

nesses have little difficulty in recruiting and retaining employees.

Occupational health nurses conduct environmental surveillance (hazardous equipment, types of injuries occurring in the workplace, potential stressors) and direct nursing care (physical assessment, screening, emergencies and first aid), health education, communicable disease control, counseling, administration, and research (Clemen-Stone and others, 1995). Frequently recurring issues that nurses face in the workplace are drug testing, right-to-know issues, concerns related to acquired immunodeficiency syndrome (AIDS), and exposure to environmental hazards. One of the nurse's roles is not only to work to improve conditions in the workplace but also to help ensure that workers who have been injured are recovered and able to return to the workplace safely. Some businesses try to reintroduce employees into the workforce as soon as possible following illness or injury, even if they assume a different job temporarily. The workplace is a point of social contact and of personal growth and expression (Clemen-

Stone and others, 1995). The nurse can help to optimize the work experience by creating programs that involve workers in health promotion and in creating a safe work environment.

Physicians' offices. Physicians' offices have traditionally provided primary care for a large segment of the population. Physicians in office practices tend to focus on the diagnosis and treatment of specific illnesses rather than on health promotion. However, this trend is slowly changing. More health care plans require enrollees to have regular physical examinations or "checkups" with their primary care physician. During these visits physicians screen for possible health problems, identify clients' health promotion practices, and make recommendations to minimize or control risk factors. Many physicians are hiring advanced practice nurses to complement their office staff (see Chapter 10). Advanced practice nurses assume responsibility for groups of clients within the joint physician-nurse practice. The advanced practice nurse can conduct physical examinations and diagnose and treat conditions under the guidelines of established collaborative practice protocols. When clients develop problems outside the scope of the nurse's practice, the physician is called in to consult or intervene. Advanced practice nurses provide follow-up care to their clients. The nurse looks beyond diagnosis and treatment to the holistic needs of the client. The advanced practitioner's time spent with a client addresses education, counseling, and community referrals to promote wellness.

Managed care now dictates that primary care physicians provide expanded services in their offices. This includes a wider range of diagnostic and therapeutic services. Some offices have complete laboratory facilities for analyzing specimens and equipment for obtaining electrocardiograms (ECGs) and x-ray films. Diagnostic procedures such as sigmoidoscopy and ultrasound may be performed. Simple surgical procedures such as biopsies and removal of skin lesions are offered.

Registered nurses (RNs) are employed in physicians' offices to assume a more traditional role of office activity coordinator. This may include registering clients, taking vital signs, preparing the client for examination or laboratory studies, and providing health educational information. The role of the RN within an office setting should not be undervalued. The nurse provides an important bridge to the physician in becoming closely familiar with clients, identifying trends in the types of problems clients present, and recognizing opportunities to increase health promotion activities.

Clinics. Clinics, which are often called **ambulatory health services,** assess and treat ambulatory clients on an outpatient basis. A clinic may be affiliated with a hospital, medical school, group practice, HMO, church, or community organization (Clemen-Stone and others, 1995). The nature of the clinic affiliation often determines the type of services the clinic provides. For example, hospital clinics offer diagnostic and treatment services. A clinic in a church or community organization may offer primary care such as immunizations or screening services (e.g., high blood pressure, tuberculosis testing, glaucoma, mammography). There are also clinics that serve only specific client populations (e.g., well-baby care, mental health, allergies). Frequently, hospital emergency departments serve as ambulatory clinics for neighborhoods or towns with no formal outpatient clinic facility or primary care physicians. The type of care offered through clinics may be episodic, in which only the acute needs of clients are managed, or comprehensive, providing all levels of preventive services, primary care, and rehabilitation.

Community health nurses play an important role in planning and providing clinic health care services. A comprehensive assessment of community needs is critical to ensure that clinic programs address the health status, lifestyle patterns, and cultural diversity of the clients. Nurses can provide valuable input regarding the appropriate setting for a clinic, selection of professional staff, establishing appropriate services, securing volunteers, and developing marketing strategies (Clemen-Stone and others, 1995). Often a neighborhood clinic becomes a focal point for a community. The successful clinic recognizes the work and lifestyle patterns of its clients and establishes a strong network of relationships with churches, schools, and businesses. Those networks become important for clients' continued care following hospitalization.

Nursing centers. Nurse-managed clinics or nursing centers (Figure 2-2) have developed over the past 20 years to provide high-quality nursing services with a focus on health promotion and health education, disease prevention, chronic disease management, and support for self-care and care givers (Aydelotte and Gregory, 1992; Riesch, 1992). The clinics are organizations where nurses control practice and client care. Riesch (1992) identified three criteria for nursing centers: direct access by client to the nurse, a nursing model of care, and holistic reimbursed services. Nurses in advanced practice roles such as nurse practitioners and clinical nurse specialists typically manage the nursing center. However, registered nurses in traditional roles also are actively involved in the centers. Many of the centers operate in association with academic centers to combine teaching and research in a nurse-controlled environment (Phillips and Steel, 1994). The clinics maintain a collaborative and consultative relationship with physicians. This is necessary in most states to guarantee reimbursement for nursing services. The services offered in a nurse-managed clinic are varied (Box 2-3). It is how the services are delivered that makes a nurse-managed clinic unique. The nurse in an advanced practice role combines nursing and medical knowledge within a perspective of client-centered care (Phillips and Steel, 1994). The advanced practice nurse stresses education and self-care. Clients with chronic illness are taught to partner with family members or friends to do the work of managing their illness. A nurse-managed clinic designs services to help people assume more responsibility for their health and to acquire necessary coping skills. Scott and Moneyham (1995) learned that the design of the services and actions of the nurses in a nursing center supported clients' need for respect, which helped to build the confidence needed for self-care. Over the long term, advanced practice nurses are very effective in improving client outcomes by enabling clients to maintain maximal function within their home and community.

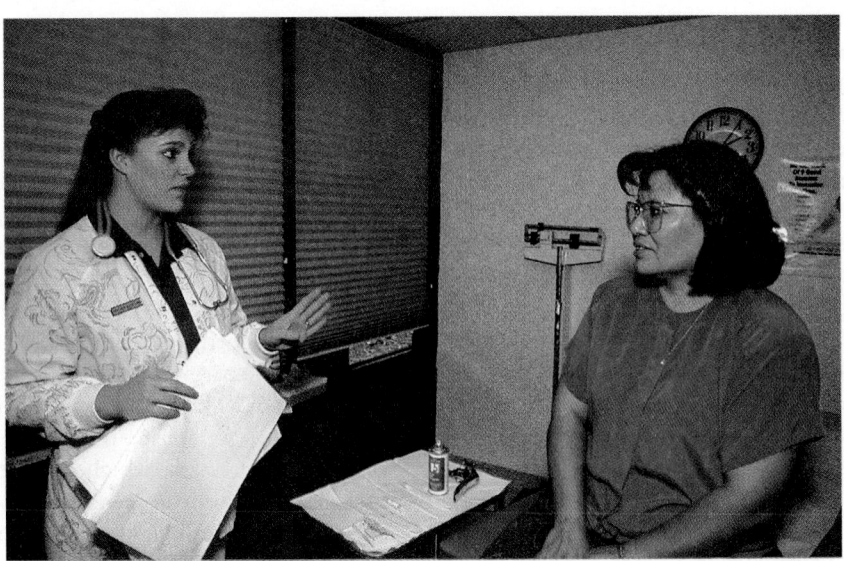

Figure 2-2. Nursing center.

> **Box 2-3**
> **Nurse-Managed Clinic Services**
>
> Physical and developmental assessment
> Health risk appraisal
> Wellness counseling
> Health education
> Psychosocial counseling
> Care and prevention of common diseases
> Acute and chronic care management
> Home care services
> Imaging, visualization, and therapeutic touch

Block and parish nursing. Two nontraditional settings where preventive and primary care can be found are in block nursing and parish nursing. Both fill in gaps of the formal health care system, usually involving older clients or those unable to leave the home (Clemen-Stone and others, 1995). Block nursing happens where the nurse lives, and services are available based on need rather than on the availability of reimbursement (Jamieson, 1990). Nurses who live within a neighborhood, through networks of friends, church groups, Girl Scouts, or Boy Scouts, collaborate to offer services to people in the community. These services might include running errands to the grocery store or pharmacy, transporting clients to a physician's office, providing respite care to family members, and being homemaker aides. Parish nursing is the same as block nursing, except churches and synagogues offer the site and support system for the program's activities.

Volunteer agencies. **Volunteer agencies** are not-for-profit health care agencies established nationally or within a community to meet a specific need. Examples are the American Lung Association and the American Cancer Society and, in Canada, the Canadian Lung Association and the Canadian Heart Foundation. Most volunteer agencies do not provide treatment but have programs designed to provide education for the prevention and detection of specific illnesses. In addition, some volunteer agencies provide financial support for training of physicians and nurses, as well as for biomedical research directed at the prevention, detection, or treatment of certain diseases.

Volunteer agencies depend on professional and lay volunteers. Financial support generally comes from fund-raising activities, federal grants, and donations from individuals. Many health professionals donate time and resources to agencies within their specialty.

The community. The environment of the community in which one lives has a significant impact on a person's health. The health problems that commonly affect members of a lower socioeconomic level can often be traced to poor community services, such as water treatment, waste disposal, air quality, and transportation services. Pender (1996) notes that community-wide collaboration in health care delivery is a key to developing a system of health promotion services that is user-friendly, well integrated, and responsive to the needs of citizens. Nurses in occupational and school health roles, as well as nurses in business, education, and public policy, can influence the conditions of their community at large.

Making a community healthy requires the work of many people. Individual citizens, community organizations, the journalistic media, schools, churches, and businesses must all collaborate to meet the needs of the whole community. Community-based intervention enhances opportunities for information exchange and social support. Costs of health promotion programming are reduced because large groups rather than small ones are the recipients of services. A community-based health promotion program offers comprehensive instead of fragmented approaches to health promotion and illness prevention (Weiss, 1984).

Green (1996) has described a three-pronged approach used by several community health departments across the country. The first approach involves completion of an expanded health assessment. This is an elaborate "history and physical" of the community and its residents. It includes such information as how often people exercise, whether children are exposed to lead, who wears seat belts, where is the source of water, and whether there is an adequate sewage treatment system. Such a comprehensive database gives hospitals, health departments, community service groups, and government leaders the information they need to select community health priorities. The second approach requires involvement of the community in program planning. Sometimes this requires a rethinking as to what role institutions play in a community. Often institutions must change if the needs identified in the assessment are to be met. Innovative and ambitious programs may evolve from the planning effort. For example, Green (1996) reports that a New Jersey hospital chose to respond to community concerns over high stress levels and implemented a mobile van manned by hospital staff and volunteers. The van goes to town events, schools, and shopping centers to offer resources to the community's residents about stress management. The final approach requires monitoring and measuring program effectiveness. It is very important for a community to know the outcomes of health programs to determine if resources are being effectively utilized.

At an interventional level, communities might institute a variety of programs aimed at health promotion and illness prevention. Environmental programs can reduce the threat of illness or disability. For example, public health departments may regularly spray insecticides to control the breeding of mosquitoes to reduce the risk of encephalitis. Community-wide immunization programs are designed to improve the status of childrens' health. Public education programs on issues such as drug abuse, AIDS awareness, and drinking while driving can at least make the public aware of health risks. Local legislation can support illness and injury prevention programs. Laws requiring the use of seat belts, approved infant or toddler restraint seats, and motorcycle helmets are a few examples. The community can make a difference in the lives of its people. Health promotion and illness prevention should be at the core of any community's philosophy.

Secondary and Tertiary Care

The diagnosis and treatment of illness are traditionally the most commonly used services of the health care delivery system. With the arrival of managed care, these services can be delivered in primary care settings. For example, more physicians are performing simple surgeries in office surgical suites. However, once a client develops a more complicated problem and the primary care provider is not able to care for a particular condition, a medical specialist is often needed. This often requires hospitalization of the client. Typically secondary and tertiary care (also called acute care) are quite costly, particularly if clients wait to have health care after symptoms have developed.

Hospital emergency departments, urgent care centers, critical care units, and inpatient medical-surgical units are the sites where secondary and tertiary levels of care are provided. In these settings, nurses are challenged to work more closely with all members of the health care team. Planning and coordination of care are necessary to deliver services in a competent and timely manner. Nurses must constantly evaluate whether care is effective and how it can be improved. In addition, nurses are recognizing that in a busy, stress-filled location such as an inpatient nursing unit, client satisfaction is a priority. Clients expect to be treated courteously and respectfully and to be involved in daily care decisions. Acute care nurses must be responsive to learning client needs and expectations early to form effective partnerships that ultimately enhance the level of nursing care given.

Hospitals. Hospitals traditionally have been the major agency of the health care system. Typically, a client would come to a hospital for diagnosis and treatment and stay there until almost fully recovered. This has changed with the arrival of prospective payment and DRGs. A client with a given medical diagnosis or who undergoes surgery is expected to be cared for and discharged within a projected time period. The amount paid for medical care is based on that projected time period, regardless of how long the client remains in the hospital. For example, a client who has coronary bypass surgery without complications is expected to be discharged home within 5 to 7 days (if not sooner) in most hospitals. If the client is not fully recovered, alternative care sites are found as soon as possible (see discussions of restorative and continuing care).

Even the hospital environment has changed. As institutions adjust to reimbursement limitations, traditional service designs are a thing of the past. Hospitals now offer better public access to outpatient treatment services, and many have redesigned nursing units. Now more services are available on nursing units, thus minimizing the need to transfer and transport clients across multiple diagnostic and treatment areas. Customer service is the philosophy of most acute care organizations.

At present, clients who are hospitalized are acutely ill and need comprehensive and specialized tertiary health care. The services provided by hospitals vary considerably. Small rural hospitals may only offer limited emergency and diagnostic services, as well as general inpatient services. In comparison, large urban medical centers offer comprehensive, state-of-the-art diagnostic services, trauma and emergency care, surgical intervention, intensive care units, inpatient services, and rehabilitation facilities. Larger hospitals also offer professional staff from a variety of specialties such as social service, respiratory therapy, physical and occupational therapy, and speech therapy. The focus in hospitals is to provide the highest quality of care possible so that clients can be discharged early but safely to the home or a facility that can adequately manage remaining health care needs.

Hospitals are classified as public or private and as for-profit or not-for-profit. Public hospitals are not-for-profit institutions that exist throughout Canada and the United States. A public hospital is financed and operated by a government agency at the local, state, provincial, or national level. Many clients in public hospitals either cannot afford to pay for care or are underinsured. Many public hospitals have charity budgets to offset such medical costs. The hospitals provide services at a not-for-profit rate. Private hospitals may be for-profit or not-for-profit and are operated by groups such as churches, corporations or businesses, or charitable organizations. Many are merging together to form large hospital system networks (e.g., Kaiser Permanente, Allina Health system, Henry Ford Health system). The majority of clients who enter private hospitals have some type of personal health insurance or health care plan. The profit status of a hospital influences how revenue can be used for services and taxation purposes. Many large corporations such as Humana and Columbia Hospital Corporation of America (HCA) operate groups of for-profit hospitals across the United States.

Two other types of hospitals include military and Veterans Administration (VA) hospitals. Military hospitals are located throughout the United States and in countries around the world to provide medical care for members of the armed forces and their families. VA hospitals provide health care to veterans with service-related and non–service-related illnesses or disabilities.

A nurse who works within a hospital has the opportunity to work in a variety of roles and different departments (see Chapter 10). The care of hospitalized clients requires the nurse to have the knowledge and skills for using critical thinking and applying the nursing process (see Unit 2) to deliver appropriate nursing therapies, provide client education, facilitate family support, and coordinate health care services and discharge planning. As their depth of nursing knowledge increases, many nurses specialize in an area of practice. This allows them to become experts in the care of select client populations. Many hospitals have, for example, specialized units for the care of clients with oncological, orthopedic, pulmonary, or cardiac problems. Other opportunities for nurses within a hospital setting may include the role of client educator, nurse manager, clinical nurse specialist, and infection control coordinator.

Intensive care. An intensive care unit (ICU) or critical care unit is a hospital unit in which clients receive close monitoring and intensive medical care. The units are equipped with the most advanced technologies such as computerized cardiac monitors, intravenous infusion devices, mechanical ventilators, and blood perfusion devices. Although many of these devices can be found on regular nursing units, the clients hospitalized within ICUs are being monitored and maintained on multiple devices. Nursing and medical staff within an ICU are educated on critical care principles and techniques. An ICU is the most expensive delivery site for medical care because of the staffing pattern required to deliver care and the related volume of treatments and procedures the clients must undergo.

Subacute care. Subacute care units are designated sites that provide medical specialty care for clients who need a greater intensity of care than generally provided in a skilled nursing facility but who no longer require acute care (Stahl, 1994). Generally clients who have suffered an acute illness, injury, or worsening of a disease and require continued hospitalization are candidates for subacute care. The clients require a transitional phase of stabilization and often still have intensive medical, social, and familial needs. Clients receive goal-oriented treatment given immediately after or instead of acute hospitalization to treat one or more specific active, complex medical conditions or to administer technically complex treatments (Stahl, 1994). Many of the clients who require subacute care are **outliers** (clients with extended lengths of stay, well beyond allowed inpatient DRG days). Thus a hospital can transfer a client to a subacute unit and reduce its financial burden, because the stay on the unit meets different reimbursement guidelines. In addition, physicians worry less over releasing clients to an outside setting when a hospital-based subacute unit is available. Subacute units are located in hospitals and in skilled nursing and rehabilitation facilities. The typical clients seen on subacute units include those being rehabilitated after cerebrovascular accidents, trauma, and respiratory failure.

Psychiatric facilities. Clients who suffer emotional and behavioral problems such as depression, violent behavior, and eating disorders often require special counseling and treatment in psychiatric facilities. Located in hospitals, independent outpatient clinics, or private mental health hospitals, psychiatric facilities offer inpatient and outpatient services, depending on the seriousness of the problem. Clients may enter these facilities voluntarily or involuntarily. Hospitalization involves relatively short stays with the purpose of stabilizing clients and then transferring them to outpatient treatment centers. A comprehensive multidisciplinary treatment plan involving clients and families is established for clients with psychiatric illness. Medicine, nursing, social work, and activity therapy collaborate to develop a plan of care that will enable clients to return to functional states within the community. At discharge from inpatient facilities, clients are usually referred for follow-up care at clinics or with counselors.

Crisis intervention centers. Crisis intervention centers provide emergency psychiatric care and counseling to clients experiencing extreme stress or conflict, often involving suicide attempts or drug or alcohol abuse. These centers, which are usually self-contained units within a hospital or community health care center, provide services 24 hours a day. The services may be delivered directly on the premises, or counseling may be provided over the telephone. The primary objectives of crisis intervention centers are to help the person cope with the immediate problem and to offer guidance and support for long-term therapy.

Rural hospitals. Access to health care in rural areas has been a serious problem. Most rural hospitals have had a severe shortage of primary care providers. Many have been forced to close because of economic failure. In 1989 the Omnibus Budget Reconciliation Act (OBRA) directed the Department of Health and Human Services to create a new health care entity, rural primary care hospitals (RPCHs). An RPCH provides 24-hour emergency care, with no more than six inpatient beds for providing temporary care for 72 hours or less to clients needing stabilization before transfer to a larger hospital. Physicians, nurse practitioners, or physician assistants staff the RPCH (Sharp, 1991). The RPCH can provide inpatient care to acutely ill or injured persons before they are transferred to better-equipped facilities. Basic radiological and laboratory services are also available.

With health care reform, more big-city health care systems are branching out and establishing affiliations or mergers with rural hospitals. The rural hospitals provide a referral base to the larger tertiary care medical centers. Recently federal laws have granted higher cost-based rates of payment from Medicare and Medicaid to certified rural health clinics (Montague, 1994). This improves the hospitals' financial standing. The number of these clinics has grown significantly in the last few years. Better partnerships and reimbursement should ensure survival of rural health care and improve access for millions of citizens.

Nurses who work in rural hospitals or clinics often function independently in the absence of a physician. Competence in physical assessment, clinical decision making, and emergency care are essential. Nurse practitioners use medical protocols or work under collaborative agreements with staff physicians.

Restorative Care

Clients recovering from acute illnesses or who have chronic illnesses or disabilities usually require a continuing level of care. This is necessary until they return to their previous level of function or reach a new level of function limited by their illness or disability. The goal of restorative care is to assist an individual to regain maximal functional status, thereby enhancing the individual's quality of life. The intent is to promote client independence and self-care. With the emphasis on early discharge from hospitals, there are few clients who do not require some level of restorative care. For example, surgical clients will require ongoing wound care, activity and exercise management, and sometimes diet interventions until they have recovered to a point where they can independently resume normal activities of daily living.

The intensity of care has increased in restorative care settings, since clients leave hospitals earlier. It is not uncommon to have clients in the home setting still receiving intravenous fluids (see Chapter 31), enteral nutrition (see Chapter 34), and pain control therapy (see Chapter 33). The restorative health care team is an interdisciplinary group of health professionals that includes the client and family or significant others. In restorative settings, nurses recognize early that success is dependent on effective partnering with clients and their families. Clients and families require a clear understanding of goals for physical recovery, the rationale for any physical limitations, and the purpose and potential risks associated with therapies. The more clients and families are involved in restorative care, the more likely that they will be motivated to follow treatment plans and that clients will be able to achieve optimal functioning.

The restorative care team functions as a unit to assist clients in achieving a level of function that will enable them to return to their community. As a whole, the team engages in clinical decision making involving assessment, diagnosis, planning, implementation, and evaluation (American Congress of Rehabilitation Medicine, 1992). All health care professionals on the team participate and contribute from the specific focus of their respective disciplines (McCourt, 1993). For example, if the team is concerned with a functional problem related to mobility, the physical therapist focuses on the physical adjustments to enhance mobility while the nurse focuses on planning activities to increase activity tolerance during mobility.

The home setting. Home health care is the provision of medically related professional and paraprofessional services and equipment to clients and families in their homes for health maintenance, education, illness prevention, diagnosis and treatment of disease, palliation, and rehabilitation. Nursing is the one service most often used as a result of client needs; however, home health care might also include medical services; physical, occupational, speech, and respiratory therapy; and nutritional therapy. Home health equipment, or durable medical equipment (DME), is any medically related product adapted for home use.

Home health care agencies provide almost every type of health care service in the client's home. Health promotion and education are traditionally the primary objective of home care, yet at present, most clients receive professional services on the basis of some medically related need (Figure 2-3). The focus is on client and family independence. Recovery and stabilization of illness must be addressed in the home, where problems related to lifestyle, safety, environment, family dynamics, and health care practices can be identified.

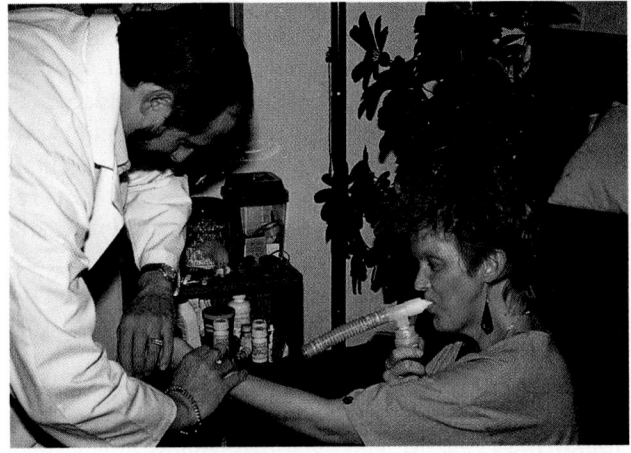

Figure 2-3.   Home health nurse providing aerosol therapy. (From Elkin MK and others: *Nursing interventions and clinical skills,* St. Louis, 1996, Mosby.)

Home health care agencies provide skilled and intermittent professional services and home health aide services. These services usually are delivered once or twice a day, up to 7 days a week. Some of the services offered by home health care agencies are summarized in Box 2-4. Approved home health care agencies usually receive reimbursement for services from the government (such as Medicare and Medicaid in the United States), private insurance, and private pay. The government has strict, elaborate regulations for governing reimbursement for home health care services. An agency cannot simply charge for a service and expect to receive full reimbursement. Most professional services are reimbursed at the costs for providing the service by government programs. Commercial payers, such as Blue Cross, often negotiate contract rates or provide reimbursement for billed charges.

Home health nurses provide individualized care and have one-on-one contact with clients and families. They are independent and have their own caseloads. The home health nurse helps clients adapt to any permanent or temporary physical limitations so that a more normal daily home routine can be assumed.

Rehabilitation. **Rehabilitation** is the restoration of a person to the fullest physical, mental, social, vocational, and economic usefulness possible (Clemen-Stone and others, 1995). Clients require rehabilitation after a physical or mental illness, injury, or chemical addiction. Rehabilitation was once available primarily for clients with illnesses or injury to the nervous or musculoskeletal system, but the health care delivery system has expanded its scope of such services. At present, specialized rehabilitation services, such as cardiovascular and pulmonary rehabilitation programs, help clients and families adjust to necessary changes in lifestyle and learn to function with the limitations of their disease. **Drug rehabilitation centers** help the client become free from drug dependence and return to the community.

Rehabilitation services include physical, occupational, and speech therapy. Ideally rehabilitation begins the moment a client enters a health care setting for treatment. For example, some orthopedic programs now have clients undergo physical therapy exercises before major joint repair to enhance their recovery postoperatively. Initially rehabilitation may focus on the prevention of complications related to the illness or injury. As the condition stabilizes, rehabilitation is directed at maximizing the client's functioning and level of independence.

Rehabilitation occurs in many health care settings, including specific rehabilitation institutions, outpatient settings, and the home. Frequently clients needing long-term rehabilitation (e.g., stroke and spinal injury clients) have severe disabilities affecting their ability to carry out the activities of daily living. When rehabilitation services are provided in outpatient settings, clients receive treatment at specified times during the week but remain at home the rest of the time. Specific rehabilitation strategies are applied to the home environment so that maximal levels of function and independence can be achieved. Nurses and other members of the health care team visit homes and help clients and families learn to adapt to illness or injury.

Box 2-4
Home Health Care Services

Wound Care
Sterile dressing changes, debridement and irrigations, packing, and instructing clients and families in wound care techniques.

Respiratory Care
Oxygen therapy, mechanical ventilation, suctioning, and care of tracheotomies.

Vital Signs
Monitoring blood pressure and cardiopulmonary status. Instructing clients and families in vital sign measurement.

Elimination
Ostomy care, appliance application, skin care, and irrigation. Insertion of indwelling and intermittent urinary catheters, irrigations, and instructing families in catheter management. Home dialysis.

Nutrition
Administration of tube feedings and enteral feedings. Assessment of nutrition and hydration status. Instructing clients and families in tube feedings.

Rehabilitation
Ambulation and gait training, use of assistive devices, range of motion exercises, and instructing clients and families on transfer techniques.

Medications
Monitoring compliance, administering injections, and instructing clients and families on drug information, medication preparation, and steps to take in the event of side effects.

Intravenous Therapy
Administration of blood products, analgesic and chemotherapeutic agents, and long-term hydration. Instructing clients and families on use of intravenous devices, steps to take in the event of disconnection or accidental fluid infusion, and side effects.

Laboratory Studies
Blood glucose monitoring (including client and family instruction) and drawing blood for specific diagnostic purposes.

Extended care facilities. An **extended care facility** provides intermediate medical, nursing, or custodial care for clients recovering from acute illness or clients with chronic illnesses or disabilities. Extended care facilities include intermediate care and skilled nursing facilities. Some include long-term care and nursing homes, and some retirement community institutions (see discussion of continuing care). At one point, extended care facilities primarily cared for older adults. However, as hospitals manage clients toward early discharge, there is a greater need for intermediate care settings for clients of all ages. For example, a young client who has experienced a stroke or traumatic accident may be transferred to an extended care facility for rehabilitative or supportive care until discharge to the home becomes a safe option. The growth of extended care facilities will increase as the number of older adults grows. With a "graying" population on the rise, more extended care facilities are needed.

An intermediate care or **skilled nursing facility** offers skilled care from a licensed nursing staff. This may include administration of intravenous fluids, wound care, long-term ventilator management, and physical rehabilitation. Extensive supportive care is provided until clients can move back into the community or into residential care. Extended care facilities provide around-the-clock nursing coverage. Nurses employed in such a setting have expertise similar to that of nurses working in acute care inpatient settings. In addition, the nurse should have a background in gerontological nursing principles.

Continuing Care

Clients across the life span who have long-term health care needs are the chronically ill and disabled. Continuing care describes a collection of health, personal, and social services provided over a prolonged period to persons who are disabled, who never were functionally independent, or who suffer a terminal disease. The need for continuing health care services is growing in the United States and Canada. People are living longer, and many of those with continuing health care needs have no immediate family members to care for them. A decline in the number of children families choose to have, the aging of care providers, and the increasing rates of divorce and remarriage complicate this problem. Continuing care may be provided within institutional settings (nursing homes, group homes, and retirement communities), communities (adult day care and senior centers), or within the home (home health, home-delivered meals, and hospice) (Lueckenotte, 1996).

Long-term care. A long-term care facility or nursing home provides 24-hour intermediate and custodial care such as bathing, dressing, feeding, and exercise therapy for clients of any age with chronic or debilitating illnesses. The majority of clients in long-term care facilities are older adults. Long-term care has been under attack for years because of claims regarding inadequate care and abuse. Many of the claims have been justified. However, much of the negative public opinion about nursing homes is based on misconceptions about the level of care provided. Box 2-5 compares nursing functions in long-term and acute care institutions. The philosophy of care in a long-term care facility is that a person's life continues with meaning and value. Clients are provided recreational, social, and physical therapy to help them remain as functional as possible. The nurse plays a key role in assisting the client to attain or retain positive meaning and value in life.

Respite care. The need to care for family members within the home can create great physical and emotional burdens for adult care givers. The care giver is usually an adult who not only has the responsibility for providing care to a loved one (e.g., spouse, parent, sibling) but often must maintain a full-time job and manage the routines of daily living as well. **Respite care** is a service that provides short-term relief or time off for persons providing home care to an ill, disabled, or frail older adult (Lueckenotte, 1996). Adult day care is one form of respite care. However, respite care can also be provided within the home by health professionals and trained volunteers. The care giver is able to leave the home for errands or just some social time while a responsible person stays in the home to care for the loved one.

Adult day care centers. **Adult day care centers** provide a variety of health and social services to specific client populations who live alone or with family in the community. Services offered during the day allow family members to maintain their lifestyles and employment and still provide home care for their relatives (Lueckenotte, 1996). Day care centers may be associated with a hospital or nursing home or exist as independent centers. Frequently the clients of such centers do not require hospitalization but need continuous health care services while their families or support persons work. These clients include older adults needing daily physical rehabilitation, individuals with emotional illnesses needing daily counseling, and individuals with chemical dependence problems who are involved in rehabilitation programs. The centers usually operate 5 days per week during typical business hours and usually charge on a per diem basis. Adult day care centers reduce the cost of health care and allow clients to retain more independence by living at home.

Services offered in day care settings include transportation to and from the facility, assistance with personal care, nursing and therapeutic services (e.g., counseling, rehabilitation), meals, and recreational activities (Lueckenotte, 1996). Nurses working in day care centers provide continuity between care delivered in the home and in the center. For instance, nurses can ensure

Box 2-5
Nursing Functions in Caring for Older Adults in Institutions

Long-Term Care

Provide a milieu for living rather than illness and dying.

Teach clients and families.

Counsel clients and family.

Learn about and use community resources, advise family and client of same.

Establish short-term and long-term goals; evaluate progress toward both periodically.

Secure and maintain health, recreation, and social history.

Plan and coordinate care.

Teach ancillary personnel.

Communicate clients' needs in written and verbal form.

Give treatments, medications, and rehabilitative exercises.

Observe and evaluate client response to treatment, medications, and care plan.

Teach health care maintenance to staff and clients.

Keep physician aware of changes in clients' condition.

Institute life-saving measures in the absence of a physician.

Perform physical assessment of clients.

Ensure adequate medical, dental, and podiatric care for clients.

Maintain hydration, nutrition, aeration, and comfort.

Acute Care

Support client in achieving highest level of autonomy possible in situation.

Provide appropriate information to client and family about treatment plan, medications, and diagnosis in collaboration with physician.

Collaborate with multiprofessionals, client, and family to develop a comprehensive care plan.

Supervise ancillary personnel.

Recognize implications of syndromes for client care (e.g., renal failure, coronary disease, emphysema).

Protect clients from injury or iatrogenic disease.

Perform physical and psychosocial assessments and integrate in nursing care plan.

Initiate action as outlined in nursing protocols regarding various conditions.

Provide emergency treatment as needed (e.g., cardiopulmonary resuscitation, amelioration of shock, hemorrhage, convulsions, poisoning).

Alert physician to changes in client status and abnormal findings of tests.

Maintain hydration, nutrition, aeration, and comfort.

From Ebersole P, Hess P: *Toward healthy aging: human needs and nursing response*, ed 4, St. Louis, 1994, Mosby.

---

that the client continues to take prescribed medication and administer specific treatments. Knowledge of community needs and resources is essential in providing adequate support of clients, who often spend only a few hours a week in the day care setting (Ebersole and Hess, 1994).

Residential community. Another type of continuing care facility is a residential or retirement community. Clients live in separate apartments or condominiums that compose a residential center. The clients remain relatively independent within a partially protective setting. Usually people keep all personal possessions in their residences. Services available within retirement communities include 24-hour nursing care, emergency medical care, housekeeping, laundry, transportation, social activities, and food service. The residential community bridges the gap between independent living and placement in a nursing home.

Hospice. A **hospice** is a system of family-centered care designed to allow clients to live and remain at home with comfort, independence, and dignity while alleviating the strains caused by terminal illness. The focus of hospice care is palliative care, not curative treatments (see Chapter 21). A hospice can benefit a client in the terminal phases of any disease, such as cardiomyopathy, multiple sclerosis, AIDS, and cancer.

A client entering a hospice has reached the terminal phase of illness (generally the final 6 weeks), and the client, family, and physician have agreed that no further treatment could reverse the disease process. An attempt is made to provide care that ensures death with dignity in the client's home. Occasionally a client must be admitted to a hospice unit within a hospital. The client and family must accept the fact that the hospice will not use emergency measures such as cardiopulmonary resuscitation to prolong life. Instead, the hospice, utilizing a multidisciplinary approach, provides pain control and comfort measures.

Hospice nurses work in institutional and community settings. They are committed to the philosophy and objectives of the facilities for which they work. They provide care and support for the client and family during the terminal phase and at the time of death and continue to offer bereavement counseling and follow-up to the family after the client's death. Many hospice programs provide respite care, which is important in maintaining the health of the primary care giver and family.

ISSUES IN HEALTH CARE DELIVERY

The climate in health care today is influencing health care professionals and consumers. Health care professionals, such as nurses, are worried about being able to provide quality care while being asked to control costs through tight restrictions in resource use. There are health care organizations that have often responded to the challenge by cutting nursing staff, reducing support services (e.g., transporters, dietitians), and limiting resources for staff education and development. However, there are also organizations that have looked to the future in developing innovative approaches for reorganizing care delivery and making client expectations of health care a priority.

Consumers of health care want to access appropriate, cost-effective, quality health care. Society generally believes that all people have a right to health care. Access to care refers to the consumer's ability to easily use a broad range of health care providers at a variety of community health care sites (AONE, 1994). Furthermore, access should not be limited to those individuals who are healthy or who can afford insurance. It is important for clients to be able to acquire needed health services easily, in cost-effective settings. Consumers also want health care institutions to be accountable for quality and to be able to show the influence interaction with health care systems has on clients' overall lives and their functional health status.

Nursing plays a major role in the health care delivery system. Nursing services are necessary for virtually every client seeking care at any level. Because nursing is such an important part of the health care delivery system, the nurse needs to understand the issues affecting health care delivery. Every nurse practicing today needs to appreciate that health care is a business. The success of any health care business depends on nursing's participation in being accountable for high-quality care and collaborating to help create the systems and strategies to ensure that clients receive cost-effective and efficient care.

Competency of Health Care Providers

As the health care system changes, so must the competencies of its professionals. A consumer of health care should expect that the standards of nursing care and practice in any health care setting are appropriate, safe, and efficacious. There are two principal mechanisms designed to ensure competent professional nursing

practice. An established nursing education program must set professional standards for its students and meet educational outcomes based on national accreditation guidelines. Graduates of these programs should be able to assume entry-level positions within health care settings and perform competently within their defined responsibilities. Health care organizations, such as hospitals or home care agencies, ensure quality by establishing policies, procedures, and protocols that meet national accrediting standards. Competency is further promoted with organizations' providing appropriate, ongoing in-service education. An additional assurance that high-quality standards are met by professionals is in certification of individuals in general and specialty practices.

The Pew Health Professions Commission (Shugars and others, 1991) investigated the trends in health care and the preparation of professionals and identified six critical competencies needed for health professions by the year 2005:

- Provide care for the community's health
- Practice primary care and prevention
- Promote healthy lifestyles
- Involve clients and families in health care decision making
- Assess and use technology appropriately
- Accommodate expanded accountability

Changes are occurring in professional education curriculums. Students are receiving more clinical opportunities in "nontraditional" settings such as clinics, neighborhood health centers, and day care facilities. Students are learning to understand the variables influencing a person's willingness and ability to remain healthy rather than just the factors that cause illness and disease. Nurses will play a key role in primary care and health promotion. Thus graduates of professional nursing programs must acquire the knowledge and skills needed to build strong relationships with clients and family members so that they may actively participate in the plan of care.

Work Redesign

The changes that are occurring, particularly in secondary and tertiary care settings, are requiring a rethinking as to how the work of client care is performed. Organizations are looking for ways to reduce costs, gain efficiencies, reduce the duplication of tasks, and reduce the overall size of the workforce. **Work redesign** is a concept that refers to changing the actual structure and ultimately the responsibilities of the jobs people perform (Tonges, 1992). Specifically, health care institutions are looking at how care is delivered to clients. Are there ways to make work more efficient, help care providers become more productive, and improve clients' satisfaction with the level of care delivered?

Most hospitals can point to inefficiencies in services

as a source of increasing costs. The work of client care involves a variety of care providers, each duplicating the work of others. In work redesign, an analysis is made of the work process being performed (e.g., the admission of clients). Each task or activity (e.g., nursing history, delivering supplies, gathering specimens) associated with the process is reviewed to determine if it is necessary or appropriate. Then the analysis asks who is performing the task and whether that person should be doing it (Tonges, 1992).

In many work redesign efforts it becomes obvious that indirect or nonnursing care activities (e.g., gathering supplies, delivering meals, cleaning client units) take up a good amount of the nurses' time. Work redesign on a client care unit involves identifying care activities that can be safely and appropriately assigned to nonlicensed staff. Many hospitals have developed positions such as the patient service representative. This staff member provides no direct client care but assumes a role that combines the elements of housekeeping, dietary, supply clerk, and unit maintenance aspects of a nurse's aide role (Tonges, 1992). Services formerly centralized in hospital departments are often redistributed to client units. Well-planned work redesign can improve efficiency and both staff and client satisfaction.

Delegation in Care Delivery

Professional nurses are finding themselves in situations where more support is needed to do the daily, repetitive tasks of care. The RN is needed to coordinate care delivery for groups of clients, make the assessments and professional judgments needed to deliver and change therapies as needed, deliver complex therapies, and provide client counseling and education. A professional nurse simply cannot do all of the work necessary to care for groups of clients.

Professional nurses are being asked to redesign care delivery to allow them adequate time for the activities that require their advanced knowledge and skills. The best use of the RN's time requires efficient use of ancillary personnel, including licensed practical nurses (LPNs), **unlicensed assistive personnel** such as nurse assistants, and nursing unit clerks. The best approach is redesigning delivery of care to involve all levels of staff in the redesign process. RNs and LPNs, for example, identify the types of activities and tasks that require their knowledge and experience. Licensure issues, as well as state nurse practice acts, are reviewed and clarified. Then the RNs and LPNs identify the types of tasks they believe can be safely delegated to multiskilled unlicensed assistive personnel. This process helps all staff understand their unique role so as to minimize duplication of effort and ensure better teamwork.

Delegation has been defined by the American Nurses Association (1995) as transferring responsibility for the performance of an activity or task while retaining accountability for the outcome. When delegating responsibilities to a competent individual, the RN still remains accountable for the overall nursing care of the client (Parkman, 1996). Thus the nurse must exercise good judgment at all times in deciding what tasks to delegate and in what situations. The National Council of State Boards of Nursing have provided some guidelines for delegation of tasks in accordance with RNs' legal scopes of practice (Box 2-6). It is important to recognize that in regard to **delegation** to unlicensed assistive personnel, tasks are delegated, not clients. Leah Curtin (1994) wrote that unlicensed personnel should not be at the bedside but at the nurse's side. The RN is the one in most settings who makes judgments during client care as to when delegation is appropriate. The LPN directs care in many long-term care facilities. Once a redesign team identifies the roles of licensed professionals and those of unlicensed assistive personnel in care delivery, training on delegation, interpersonal communication, decision making, and conflict resolution is important for the entire team. As the leader of the health care team, the RN must know how to give clear instructions, effectively prioritize client needs and therapies, and be able to give staff members timely and meaningful feedback. Unlicensed personnel should receive necessary skill training with an opportunity for supervised demonstration. A well-planned redesign of care delivery improves collaboration and teamwork between all staff members and improves client and staff satisfaction (Gould and others, 1996).

■ Box 2-6
The Five Rights of Delegation

Right Task
One that is delegable for a specific client, such as tasks that are repetitive, require little supervision, and are relatively noninvasive.

Right Circumstances
Appropriate client setting, available resources, and other relevant factors considered.

Right Person
Right person is delegating the right tasks to the right person to be performed on the right person.

Right Direction/Communication
Clear, concise description of the task, including its objective, limits, and expectations.

Right Supervision
Appropriate monitoring, evaluation, intervention as needed, and feedback.

Modified and reprinted with permission from National Council of State Boards of Nursing, Inc: *Delegation: concepts and decision-making process*, Chicago, 1995, The Council.

Quality Measures of Performance

Quality health care has often been difficult to define. Unless health care providers can define quality, the purchasers of health care (e.g., employers, insurers, HMOs) will buy services based on price alone. The health care system that can deliver a given service (e.g., delivery of a baby and mother-infant care) for the cheapest price will become the primary provider of that service. Health care providers are trying to define and measure quality in terms of outcomes. An outcome is a measure of what actually does or does not happen as a result of a process of care; it is the end result (desirable or undesirable) of care delivered (Donabedian, 1966; Bernstein and Hilborne, 1993). Examples of outcomes are the readmission rates for sickle cell clients, functional health status of clients after discharge (e.g., ability and time frame for returning to work), and the rate of infection after surgery. One of the most common outcome measures is client satisfaction. The JCAHO (1997) requires health care organizations to determine how well an organization meets client needs and expectations. Organizations are using outcomes such as client satisfaction as a basis to redesign how care is managed and delivered in hopes of improving quality in the long term.

Client satisfaction. Almost every major health care organization measures certain aspects of client satisfaction. The Picker/Commonwealth Program for Patient-Centered Care was established in 1987 to explore clients' needs and concerns, as defined by clients, and to promote models of care that make the experience of illness and hospitalization more humane (Gerteis and others, 1993). Seven dimensions of patient-centered care were defined (Box 2-7). The seven dimensions cover much of what is the scope of nursing practice. This should be no surprise because nurses are involved in almost every aspect of a client's care in a hospital. A close look shows that most of the dimensions that can be reflected in client satisfaction can be applied to almost any health care setting.

The Picker/Commonwealth Program has developed a tool that measures client satisfaction along the seven dimensions. The survey looks globally at client perceptions of care in an attempt to understand how all hospital departments influence client satisfaction. The survey is conducted through telephone interviews after the client is discharged from the health care setting. Many other companies have developed similar client satisfaction surveys that are distributed in the mail to clients. Staff involved in client care receive the satisfaction scores as feedback regarding their success in meeting client expectations. It is the responsibility of staff to identify the unique issues that influence client satisfaction for their area. For example, nurses working on an oncology unit will have different client satisfaction issues around physical comfort than nurses caring for new mothers. Client satisfaction findings become the basis for many quality improvement studies (see Chapter 9).

It is important for nurses to recognize the need to identify client expectations. The seven dimensions of care can be a useful guide. By learning early what a client expects in regard to information, comfort, and availability of family and friends, the nurse can better plan client care. When should the nurse ask about a client's expectations? It should become a routine question when the client first enters a health care setting and episodically as care continues. Client expectations are an important measure of the evaluation of nursing care.

Care Delivery Innovations

Professional nurses must never forget the importance of being involved in the decisions that direct client care. As the health care system changes, the delivery of client care is a critical issue. Nurses have been key players in the development of several important new approaches to care delivery.

Care management and critical pathways. In the past, care givers from all disciplines such as nursing, medicine, and social work managed a client's care within a hospital by contributing their own plans of care. There has always been an objective to coordinate the work of all care givers so that a single plan was followed with favorable outcomes. This was not always easy to do, depending on the nursing delivery of care model or the collaboration of all care givers. For example, team nursing was so focused on the tasks of nursing care that little effort was given to ensure continuity of discharge planning and participation by all care givers. Frequently, members of the team were unaware of each discipline's plan.

A new approach that has been met with success is **care management:** structuring accountability for client outcomes at the care delivery level within a unit or area of care (Zander, 1994). With care management, typically one care giver coordinates care from admission through discharge within an acute care setting. A single, multidisciplinary plan is implemented so that all care givers work with one plan to achieve the same client outcomes. A popular tool used in care management is a **critical pathway.** A critical pathway is a multidisciplinary treatment plan that sequences clinical interventions over a projected length of stay or a projected time frame (e.g., home health visits) for specific case types (Figure 2-4), such as normal vaginal delivery, total hip replacement, or congestive heart failure. A pathway is developed by members of all disciplines that normally care for the particular client type. The interdisciplinary team reviews best practice patterns in determining the type of interventions and desired outcomes that should compose a critical pathway. One model for a pathway is the **CareMap.** Initially developed at the New England

---

Box 2-7

The Dimensions of Patient-Centered Care

1. Respect for clients' values, preferences, and expressed needs

   Clients expect to be treated with dignity and respect.

   Clients want to be informed and involved in decisions about their care.

   Clients' perception of needs should not be completely different from those identified by a care provider.

2. Coordination and integration of care

   Clients' feelings of powerlessness can be reduced by a competent and caring staff.

   Clients look for someone to be in charge of care and to communicate clearly with other health team members.

   Clients look to have services and procedures well coordinated.

   Clients need to know at all times whom to call for help.

3. Information, communication, and education

   Clients expect to receive accurate and timely information about their clinical status, progress, or prognosis.

   Clients and families need to be informed of major changes in therapies or status.

   Tests and procedures must be explained clearly in language clients understand.

   Clients and family members want to know how to manage care on their own to the extent they desire or are able.

4. Physical comfort

   Physical care that comforts clients is one of the most elemental services care givers can provide.

   Nurses should respond in a timely and effective way to any request for pain medication, explain the extent of pain clients can expect, and offer alternatives for pain management.

   Clients expect privacy and to have their cultural values respected.

   The health care setting environment should be clean and comfortable.

5. Emotional support and relief of fear and anxiety

   Clients look to care providers to share their fears and concerns.

   Clients need to understand the impact illness will have on their ability to care for themselves and their family.

   Clients worry about their ability to pay for their medical care. Are there staff who can help with those worries?

6. Involvement of family and friends

   Care providers must recognize and respect the family and friends on whom clients rely for support.

   Clients have the right to determine if family members are to be involved in decisions about their care.

   Clients expect those family or friends who will provide physical support and care after discharge to be properly informed.

7. Transition and continuity

   Clients want information about medications to take, dietary or treatment plans to follow, and danger signals to look for after hospitalization or treatment.

   Clients expect to have their continuing health care needs met after discharge with well-coordinated services.

   Clients and family members expect access to any necessary health care resources after discharge.

Data from Gerteis M and others: *Through the patient's eyes*, San Francisco, 1993, Jossey-Bass.

Medical Center in Boston, a CareMap describes the clinical work of each professional discipline and department as it relates to clients' and families' measurable outcomes of care (Zander, 1992). A CareMap is unique in that it does incorporate day-to-day expected outcomes, as well as those outcomes anticipated at discharge or at the end of a treatment phase.

Each day the CareMap outlines clinical assessments, treatments and procedures, dietary interventions, activity and exercise therapies, patient education, and other discharge planning activities necessary to ensure a smooth, uneventful course of recovery. The CareMap tells care givers what care needs to be given and when so that a client is discharged on time and in as healthy a condition as possible. Outcomes incorporated into a CareMap give nurses, physicians, and other care providers important signs for determining if care is appropriate and if the client is responding as desired. Of course there will always be clients who do not follow the CareMap's course of recovery. If a client does not proceed as predicted and if interventions or outcomes do not occur as planned, the team analyzes these

BARNES

CARE PATH
100 CHEMOTHERAPY

SERVICE		PHYSICIAN	
PRIMARY NURSE		PRIMARY NURSE	
DC DATE	ADM DATE	DATE OF SURGERY	

A-8

(1)

PROBLEM NUMBER	*IF APPLICABLE	PATIENT PROBLEMS / NURSING DIAGNOSES
#1	LACK OF KNOWLEDGE	
#2	ALTERATION IN NUTRITION R/T DECREASED INTAKE, NAUSEA, VOMITING, ANOREXIA, INCREASED CALORIC REQUIREMENT	
#3	POTENTIAL FOR INFECTION R/T MYELOSUPPRESSION, IMMUNO-SUPPRESSION	
#4	POTENTIAL ALTERATION IN MUCOUS MEMBRANES R/T STOMATITIS, ESOPHAGITIS, VAGINITIS	
#5	ALTERATION IN URINARY ELIMINATION R/T NEPHROTOXIC EFFECTS OF CHEMOTHERAPY, POTENTIAL FOR HEMORRHAGIC CYSTITIS	
#6	POTENTIAL FOR INJURY R/T THROMBOCYTOPENIA, SEDATION	

PROBLEM NUMBER		PRE-ADMIT	DAY 1	DAY 2
#2 #3 #4 #5 #6 #7 #8	ASSESSMENT / MONITORING	Evaluate IV access Evaluate response to previous treatment **Patient tolerated previous treatment without complications** Patient has adequate IV access (peripheral or VAD)	Nutritional status Nausea, vomiting Weight Bowel Function I & O Pain / comfort Skin / mucous membrane integrity Fall prevention Understanding of therapy / knowledge deficits Emotional response / coping mechanisms IV / vascular access site condition / type Results of CBC, SMA6 Vital signs **Pt will have stable vital signs** **Pt will have adequate urinary output without evidence of hematuria**	Nausea, vomiting Effectiveness of antiemetics Bowel Function I & O Pain / comfort Skin / mucous membrane integrity Patient response to treatment Emotional response / coping mechanisms IV / vascular access site condition Vital signs **Pt will have stable vital signs** **Pt will have adequate urinary output without evidence of hematuria**
#2 #7	CONSULTS	*Surgery for access placement	*SW - Emotional support, community resources, financial resources *Dietary - If patient has lost 5% of TBW within one month BHH / *BHIV - IF portion of tx to be done at home. If nursing required at home. *CNS *Pastoral Care *Psychological Resource Nurse (Gyn / Onc only)	*SW-consult completed *Dietary consult completed *CNS consult completed
	PROC. TEST	CBC *SMA 6 *Cr Cl	**CBC / SMA6 results adequate for chemotherapy administration**	*SMA 6 *Mg
#4 #5 #8	TREATMENT		Initiate and monitor IV fluid Administer antiemetic therapy Initiate Chemotherapy Regimen Initiate oral hygiene	Monitor IV fluid Administer antiemetic Rx Continue Chemotherapy Regimen Continue oral hygiene Determine accuracy of IV rate - determine if rate needs to be increased with MD approval to facilitate DC

Figure 2-4.   Chemotherapy care path. (Courtesy Barnes-Jewish Hospital, St. Louis, Mo.)

③

				DAY 1	DAY 2
	ACTIVITY			Up with assistance	Up with assistance
				Institute fall prevention protocol	Continue fall prevention protocol
	MEDS / IV			Initiate IV access within 2 hours of admission	
				IV site / VAD without redness, swelling, tenderness and with adequate blood return	**IV site / VAD without redness, swelling, tenderness and with adequate blood return**
#2	NUTRITION			Diet as tolerated	Diet as tolerated
				Pt will have 2 or less episodes of nausea / vomiting.	**Pt will have 2 or less episodes of nausea / vomiting.**
				Pt will have 2 or less episodes of diarrhea	**Pt will have 2 or less episodes of diarrhea**

#1 #7	PATIENT / FAMILY EDUCATION			**Develop and Initiate Teaching Plan**
				1. Reason for and implication of chemotherapy
				2. Method of administration
				3. Anticipated length of therapy
				4. Names of drugs
				5. Review of each drug
				6. Side effects / management
				   A. Nausea / Vomiting
				   B. Anorexia
				   C. Diarrhea
				   D. Constipation
				   E. Alopecia
				   F. Stomatitis
				   G. Skin Changes
				   H. Fatigue
				   I. Myelosuppression
				   J. Sexuality implications
				  *K. Renal Toxicity
				  *L. Hemorrhagic Cystitis
				  *M. Cardiotoxicity
				  *N. Neurotoxicity
				  *O. Ototoxity
				7. Resources:
				   Cancer Information Center (CIC)
				   American Cancer Society
				   Support Groups (refer to CIC)
				*Care of VAD
				Informed consent signed (If chemotherapy is investigational)
				 Give drug information and symptom management sheets to pt
				Pt will have written information outlining chemotherapy drug names, method of administration, common side effects and their management.
				Pt will have information regarding support groups, community resources and Cancer Information Center
					Reassess Comprehension
					Reinforce teaching.
					Teach signs and symptoms to report to MD after discharge
					1. Severe nausea, vomiting, diarrhea, constipation
					2. Temperature greater than 38.5C
					3. Sore which will not heal
					4. Spontaneous bleeding / bruising
					5. Cough which does not resolve
					6. Frequent, painful urination or blood in urine
					7. Rash of any kind
					8. Sudden weight gain or loss
					9. Pain of unusual intensity or distribution.
					
					Medications to **AVOID** without MD order.
					Aspirin
					Antibiotics
					Anticonvulsants
					Anticoagulants
					Barbiturates
					Antihypertensives
					Cough Medications
					Darvon
					Hypoglycemics
					Diuretics
					Hormones
					Tranquilizers
					Nasal Spray
					Vitamins

	DISCHARGE PLANNING	Evaluate for appropriateness of home infusional therapy		**Pt / Family verbalizes understanding of Care Path. Plan of care mutually set with pt / family.**	
#1 #7	PSYCHOSOCIAL / EMOTIONAL NEEDS			Provide opportunity to discuss implications / issues relating to disease / treatment **Patient / family exhibits positive coping skills related to disease / treatment**	Provide opportunity to discuss implications / issues relating to disease / treatment **Patient / family exhibits positive coping skills related to disease / treatment**
	SIGNATURES				

100

3100-22 REV. 9/92

Figure 2-4, cont'd   Chemotherapy care path.

variances (see Chapter 9) to decide how to revise the CareMap. When a CareMap is used 24 hours a day by each professional caring for a client, care management toward outcomes is tightly structured (Zander, 1992). In many hospitals a primary nurse coordinates a client's progress through a CareMap. The nurse is responsible for communicating with other care givers so that a client's progress is uninterrupted.

Case management.
Case management is a delivery of care approach that coordinates and links health care services to clients and their families. Various models have been used in the past to arrange and connect health and social services for clients who have ongoing health problems. Case management is defined by Zander (1994) as the coordination of client care across care areas, between agencies, and (where possible) extending into wellness. What is unique about case management is that clinicians, either as individuals or as part of collaborative groups, are overseeing the management of case type–based care (e.g., clients with specific diagnoses) and are usually held accountable to some standard of cost management and quality.

Case management involves managing a client's care across a continuum and is one approach that comes close to providing seamless integration of services. For example, in one model a client with a chronic disease such as congestive heart failure may be assigned a nurse as a case manager in a medicine outpatient clinic. Whenever the client is hospitalized, the same case manager coordinates care so that all providers understand the client's unique needs. When the client is discharged, the case manager will determine if home care or other services are necessary to sustain and support the clients' health status. The case manager may visit the client in the home to ensure that health promotion behaviors are being maintained. All institutions have different models based on their services and needs of clients.

All clients need their health care managed, but not all require case management. Typically formal case management is needed for approximately 20% of clients who enter acute health care settings (Zander, 1994). Clients requiring case management are high risk, usually are experiencing complicated medical problems, and have limited resources for ongoing health care.

In many institutions, case managers are often clinical nurse specialists or primary nurses who have demonstrated an expert level of nursing practice. The case manager, once assigned a client, becomes accountable for short- and long-range clinical outcomes, as well as overall financial outcomes. In other words, the case manager partners with the physician and other care providers to ensure diagnostic and treatment approaches are appropriate and delivered promptly. Duplication of services and use of unnecessary resources are effectively managed by a case manager. In addition, the case manager establishes a plan of care with the client, coordinates any consults, updates the client and family on progress in care, and facilitates discharge to an appropriate health care facility or the home. In many cases the case manager is accountable for placing clients on a CareMap and utilizing the clinical guidelines for effective management of client care. A nurse who assumes the role of a case manager must have skills and knowledge in negotiating, obtaining and coordinating services and resources, intervening at key points for clients, and analyzing the trends in care that create negative clinical outcomes. Case managers are an extremely important part of managed care.

Patient-focused care.
The process of caring for clients is a complex one. Many different types of professionals and nonprofessionals are involved. Too often in the past, attention has focused primarily on the tasks, functions, and structures involved in caring for clients. However, this has created numerous inefficiencies in care delivery. The focus instead should be on client need.

The concept of **patient-focused care** was first implemented in 1989 (Clouten and Weber, 1994). It involves bringing all care providers and services to the client. Cross-trained care givers from multidisciplinary backgrounds form self-governed teams, responsible for the "whole" work process that delivers care to clients (Clouten and Weber, 1994). The assumption is that if the tasks that are normally provided by ancillary personnel (e.g., phlebotomy, ECG testing, physical therapy, respiratory therapy) are moved closer to clients, the number of staff involved and number of steps to get the work done will be reduced. Thus hospitals will realize cost savings, and clients will perceive better overall care and service. A typical patient-focused care unit has its own admitting, pharmacy, laboratory, and radiology areas. Variations of patient-focused care models exist within different hospitals.

In a patient-focused care model, the nurse is still a key player in coordinating client care. Nurses are more likely performing professional nursing activities, such as education and clinical assessment, than ancillary functions, such as bed making or specimen collection. Cross-trained care providers can deliver multiple services and reduce the number of personnel a client must see. This can significantly add to client satisfaction and staff satisfaction.

To develop a patient-focused care model, all staff members must be able to participate in the redesign of their work. In addition, staff must be ready and willing to change. The process involves cross training of staff, giving staff more decision-making power on their unit, grouping similar client populations together, and designing streamlined documentation systems. Nursing's challenge is to take the care production process apart and to recombine its elements into a new, more adaptable delivery system that achieves favorable outcomes (Tonges, 1992).

Discharge Planning Across the Continuum

In secondary and tertiary care settings, as well as restorative care settings, nursing plays an important role in coordinating client care across a continuum of services. As nurses prepare clients for the transition to different services in different settings, **discharge planning** becomes a priority. Discharge planning is a centralized, coordinated, multidisciplinary process that ensures that the client has a plan for continuing care after leaving a health care agency. The process helps in the transition of the client from one environment to another, for example, from hospital to rehabilitation facility, from rehabilitation facility to home.

There are certain clients more in need of discharge planning because of the risks they present. However, any client who is being discharged from a health care facility with remaining functional alterations or who must follow certain restrictions or therapies for recovery needs discharge planning. All care givers who care for a client with a specific health problem must participate in discharge planning. The process is truly multidisciplinary. For example, the diabetic client visiting an education center requires the collaboration of a nurse educator, dietitian, and physician to ensure that the client returns home with the right information to manage the condition. A client who has experienced a stroke will not be discharged from a hospital until plans have been established with physical and occupational therapists to begin a program of rehabilitation.

Effective discharge planning often requires referrals to various health care disciplines. The nurse is often the first to recognize the client's needs. In many agencies a physician's order is needed for a referral, especially when specific therapies are planned (e.g., physical therapy). It is best to have clients participate in referral processes so that they are involved early in any necessary decision making. Some tips on making the referral process successful include the following:

- Make a referral as soon as possible. Always think and anticipate the client's needs.
- Inform the care provider receiving the referral of as much information about the client as possible. This avoids duplication of effort and exclusion of important information.
- Involve the client and family in the referral process, including selecting the necessary referral. Explain the service to be provided, the reason for the referral, and what to expect from the referral's services.
- Determine what the referral discipline recommends for the client's care, and incorporate this into the treatment plan as soon as possible.

Another important aspect of discharge planning is client and family education (see Chapter 15). All members of the health care team participate in client educa-tion. The JCAHO (1997) has the following standards for the education of hospitalized clients.

Clients and, when appropriate, family are provided with the specific knowledge and skills required to meet the client's ongoing health care needs. Such instruction includes, but is not limited to:

- Safe and effective use of medications
- Instruction on potential food-drug interactions, nutrition intervention, and modified diets
- Rehabilitation techniques to support adaptation to and/or functional independence in the environment
- Access to available community resources as needed
- When and how to obtain further treatment
- The client's and family's responsibilities in the client's care

Wherever a client might be within the health care system, the nurse plays an important role in minimizing any difficulties the client might have in moving from one service to another. Consider your own feelings if you were to be in a clinic or medical center and not know what the care providers have planned for you. Powerlessness, anxiety, and even anger are common emotions when one does not know what to expect and feels a loss of control in life events. Good discharge planning involves the client from the beginning, uses the strengths of the client in planning, provides resources to meet the client's limitations, and is focused on improving the client's long-term outcomes.

The Future of Health Care

This chapter began with a story about Gloria. In a perfect world, Gloria was able to access whatever health care resources she needed with minimal effort. The health care system was well adapted to meet Gloria's needs, regardless of her situation. The system was not only illness oriented but also wellness oriented. Resources were easily accessible and available to keep Gloria as healthy as possible.

Health care in the United States and Canada has not yet created Gloria's world. However, many health care organizations are striving to find ways to redesign their services, reduce unnecessary costs, and improve access to the services clients need. The American Nurses Association (1991) published Nursing's Agenda for Health Care Reform (Box 2-8). The document offers useful strategies designed to provide better quality of health care services to the population. The American Nurses Association was futuristic and challenged nurses to become active participants in developing a better health care system.

The components of the agenda still apply as nursing strives to participate in the leadership needed to influence the future of health care. The traditional medical model for health care is no longer responsive to the holistic needs of clients. Successful achievement of nursing's agenda will shift the focus of health care from illness and cure to wellness and care (American Nurses Association, 1991).

Box 2-8
Nursing's Agenda for Health Care Reform

The basic components of nursing's "core of care" include:

A restructured health care system that:

Enhances consumer access to services by delivering primary health care in community settings

Fosters consumer responsibility for personal health, self-care, and informed decision making in selecting health care services

Facilitates the use of the most cost-effective providers and therapeutic options

A federally defined standard package of essential health care services available to all citizens and residents of the United States, provided and financed through an integration of public and private plans and sources

A phase-in of essential services, so that the health care delivery system can be fiscally responsible in the:

Coverage of pregnant women and children, which is critical

Design of services that specifically assist vulnerable populations who have had limited access to the health care delivery system (A "Healthstart Plan" is proposed to improve the health status of these individuals.)

Planned change to anticipate health care service needs that correlate with changing national demographics

Steps to reduce health care costs, including:

Required use of managed care in a public health plan and encouraged in private plans

Incentives for consumers and providers to use managed care arrangements

Controlled growth of the health care delivery system through planning and prudent resource allocation

Incentives for consumers and providers to be more cost efficient in exercising health care options

Development of health care policies based on effectiveness and outcomes research

Ensurance of direct access to a full range of qualified providers

Elimination of unnecessary bureaucratic controls and administrative procedures

Case management required for clients with continuing health care needs

Provisions for long-term care, including:

Public and private funding for services of short duration to prevent personal impoverishment

Public funding for extended care

Emphasis on the consumers' responsibility to financially plan for long-term care needs

Insurance reforms to ensure improved access to coverage

Access to services ensured by no payment at the point of service and elimination of balance billing in public and private plans

Establishment of public or private-sector review—operating under federal guidelines and including payers, providers, and consumers—to determine resource allocation, cost reduction approaches, allowable insurance premiums, and fair and consistent reimbursement levels (This review would progress in a climate sensitive to ethical issues.)

Modified from American Nurses Association: *Nursing's agenda for health care reform*, Kansas City, Mo, 1991, The Association.

Key Terms

acute care
adult day care centers
ambulatory health services
capitation
care management
CareMap
case management
crisis intervention centers
critical pathway
delegation

diagnosis-related group (DRG)
discharge planning
drug rehabilitation centers
extended care facility
health maintenance organization (HMO)
home health care
hospice
Independent Practice Association (IPA)

managed care
Medicaid
Medicare
outliers
patient-focused care
precertification
preferred provider organizations (PPO)
primary care
prospective payment
provider
rehabilitation

respite care
restorative care
seamless care delivery
skilled nursing facility
subacute care
unlicensed assistive personnel
third-party payers
variances
volunteer agencies
work redesign

Changes in health care are being driven by increased costs and decreasing reimbursement, forcing health care institutions to deliver care more efficiently without sacrificing quality.

Levels of health care describe the scope of services and settings where health care is offered to clients in all stages of health and illness.

Health promotion occurs in home, work, and community settings.

Occupational health nursing includes reducing exposure to environmental hazards, health education, and helping workers return to work safely.

Community-wide collaboration in health care delivery is needed to develop appropriate health promotion services.

Hospitalized clients are more acutely ill than in the past, requiring better coordination of services before discharge.

Rehabilitation allows an individual to return to a level of normal or near-normal function after a physical or mental illness, injury, or chemical dependency.

Nurse-managed clinics offer primary care delivered by advanced practice nurses with a focus on helping clients assume more responsibility for their health.

Home health care agencies provide almost every type of health care service with an emphasis on client and family independence.

Capitation forces providers to assume the risk to keep clients healthy.

The Medicare prospective reimbursement system is based on payment calculated on the basis of DRG assignment.

Access to specialized medical care has been more limited in Canada than in the United States.

The redesign of care delivery can involve identifying aspects of traditional nursing care that can be safely and appropriately assigned to unlicensed staff.

The registered nurse makes decisions about delegation in regard to the tasks that can be appropriately delegated in the right situation, with the right direction and support.

Health care organizations are being evaluated on the basis of outcomes such as prevention of complications, clients' functional outcomes, and client satisfaction.

Managed care plans establish specific guidelines for covered medical benefits available to enrollees, length of hospitalization for which the plan will pay, and access to medical specialists.

Consumers of health care should be guaranteed competent health care professionals.

A CareMap is an example of a multidisciplinary plan of care for each day of a client's expected length of stay or episode of treatment.

1. Mr. Wilson is a 62-year-old client who will have major surgery to replace the joint in his hip. He is married and employed at a chemical company. The doctor is concerned that he is about 20 pounds overweight. Before discharge from the hospital, what type of health care referrals might be appropriate in planning Mr. Wilson's care?

2. Mrs. Ramirez is a 42-year-old woman who is employed as an advertising agent for a large corporation. She travels 65% of the time. Her business requires her to have a physical examination every 2 years. During a recent "checkup," Mrs. Ramirez was found to have an elevated cholesterol and triglyceride level. Her blood pressure was 134/84 mm Hg, up from 2 years ago. The nurse who conducted the health history learned that Mrs. Ramirez eats "on the go" and only exercises when at home. She also smokes two packs of cigarettes a day. What level of health care did Mrs. Ramirez pursue?

3. Ms. Yim is a 65-year-old married woman who experienced a stroke 4 days ago. She has lost movement on her left side but is able to speak clearly. Mr. Rogers is a 60-year-old client who has been coming to the neighborhood clinic regularly for the last 5 years for ongoing monitoring of his diabetes. Which of these clients would benefit most from case management and why?

4. Don, the evening RN, is preparing to assess Mr. Sequera, who experienced a myocardial infarction 4 days ago and who will ambulate down the hall for the first time this evening, and Mrs. Lennox, a client newly admitted with gastrointestinal bleeding. Don finds that Mr. Sequera is resting comfortably and visiting with his daughter. He is anxious to start walking. Mrs. Lennox is very restless and experiencing discomfort from her nasogastric tube. The physician has ordered stool specimens to be collected. Which of these two clients should Don delegate to the nurse technician, Linda?

References

American Congress of Rehabilitation Medicine: *Guide to interdisciplinary practice in rehabilitation settings,* Skokie, Ill, 1992, The Congress.

American Nurses Association: *Standards of school nursing practice,* Kansas City, Mo, 1983, The Association.

American Nurses Association: *Nursing's agenda for health care reform,* Kansas City, Mo, 1991, The Association.

American Nurses Association: Position statement on registered nurse utilization of assistive personnel, *Am Nurse* 25(2):7, 1995.

AONE: The Consumer healthcare reform agenda, *Nurs Manage* 25(5):17, 1994.

Appleby C: Managed care's true values, *Hosp Health Netw* 70(8):20, 1996.

Aydelotte MK, Gregory MS: Nursing practice: innovative models. In *Nursing centers: meeting the demand for quality health care,* NLN Pub No. 21-2311, New York, 1992, National League for Nursing.

Bernstein SJ, Hilborne LH: Clinical indicators: the road to quality care? *J Comm J Qual Improv* 19(11):501, 1993.

Clemen-Stone S and others: *Comprehensive community health nursing,* ed 4, St. Louis, 1995, Mosby.

Clouten K, Weber R: Patient focused care . . . playing to win, *Nurs Manage* 25(2):34, 1994.

Curtin L: The heart of patient care, *Nurs Manage* 25(5):7, 1994.

Donabedian A: Evaluating the quality of medical care, *Milbank Memorial Fund Q* 44:166, 1966.

Ebersole P, Hess P: *Toward healthy aging: human needs and nursing response,* ed 4, St. Louis, 1994, Mosby.

Gerteis M and others: *Through the patient's eyes,* San Francisco, 1993, Jossey-Bass.

Gould R and others: Redesigning the RN and NA roles, *Nurs Manage* 27(2):37, 1996.

Green L: Think big, *Hosp Health Netw* 70(23):49, 1996.

Harrington C: Policy options for a national health care plan, *Nurs Outlook* 38(5):223, 1990.

Hospitals and Health Networks: 1997 guide: benchmarking under managed care, *Hosp Health Netw* 71(1):28, 1997.

Jamieson MK: Block nursing: practicing autonomous professional nursing in the community, *Nurs Health Care* 11(5):250, 1990.

Joint Commission on Accreditation of Healthcare Organizations: *Accreditation manual for hospitals,* Oakbrook Terrace, Ill, 1997, The Commission.

Kerr JCR: The Canadian health care system: overview and issues. In McCloskey JC, Grace HK, editors: *Current issues in nursing,* ed 5, St. Louis, 1997, Mosby.

Lueckenotte A: *Gerontologic nursing,* St. Louis, 1996, Mosby.

McCloskey JC, Grace HK: Change creates opportunities. In McCloskey JC, Grace HK, editors: *Current issues in nursing,* ed 4, St. Louis, 1994, Mosby.

McCourt A: *The specialty practice of rehabilitation nursing: a core curriculum,* ed 3, Skokie, Ill, 1993, The Rehabilitation Nursing Foundation of the Association of Rehabilitation Nurses.

Meyer H: The tide of times, *Hosp Health Netw* 70(8):34, 1996.

Montague J: Rural and primary care across the nation, *Hosp Health Netw* 68(8):60, 1994.

National Council of State Boards of Nursing, Inc: *Delegation: concepts and decision-making process,* Chicago, 1995, The Council.

Parkman CA: Delegation: are you doing it right? *Am J Nurs* 96(9):43, 1996.

Pender NJ: *Health promotion in nursing practice,* ed 3, St. Louis, 1996, Mosby.

Phillips DL, Steel JE: Factors influencing scope of practice in nursing centers, *J Prof Nurs* 10(2):84, 1994.

Riesch SK: Nursing centers: state of the art survey results. In *Nursing centers: meeting the demand for quality health care,* NLN Pub No. 21-2311, New York, 1992, National League for Nursing.

Scott CB, Moneyham L: Perceptions of senior residents about a community-based nursing center, *Image* 27(3):181, 1995.

Sharp N: Rural healthcare: new opportunities for nurses, *Nurs Manage* 22(3):22, 1991.

Shugars D, O'Neil E, Bader J, editors: *Health America: practitioners for 2005,* Durham, NC, 1991, The Pew Health Professions Commission.

Solovy A: Taming the tiger: the economics of health care reform, *Hosp Health Netw* 68(5):26, 1994.

Sovie M: Redesigning our future: whose responsibility is it? *Nurs Econ* 8(1):21, 1990.

Stahl D: Subacute care: the future of health care, *Nurs Manage* 25(10):34, 1994.

Streff MB: Third-party reimbursement issues for advanced practice nurses in the '90s. In McCloskey JC, Grace HK, editors: *Current issues in nursing,* ed 4, St. Louis, 1994, Mosby.

Terris M: Global budgeting and the control of hospital costs, *J Public Health Policy* 12(1):61, 1991.

Tonges MC: Work designs: sociotechnical systems for patient care delivery, *Nurs Manage* 23(1):27, 1992.

Vruwink M, Mitchell M: Improving quality of care: can managed care make a difference? In McCloskey JC, Grace HK, editors: *Current issues in nursing,* ed 5, St. Louis, 1997, Mosby.

Weiss S: Community health promotion demonstration programs: introduction. In Matarazzo JD and others, editors: *Behavioral health: a handbook of health enhancement and disease prevention,* New York, 1984, John Wiley & Sons.

Zander K: Quantifying, managing and improving quality, *New Definition* 7(2):1, 1992.

Zander K: Responsive restructuring, part IV: care management and case management, *New Definition* 9(2):1, 1994.

Nursing Management of Client Care

OBJECTIVES

Mastery of content in this chapter will enable the student to:

- Define the key terms listed.
- Differentiate between leadership and management.
- Discuss leadership and management styles.
- Explain when to use situational leadership styles in a given clinical situation.
- Describe the elements of decentralized decision making.
- Discuss the ways in which a nurse manager can support staff involvement in a decentralized decision-making model.
- Differentiate among types of nursing care delivery models.
- Discuss clinical care coordination skills in nursing practice.
- Explain a staff nurse's role in team communication.

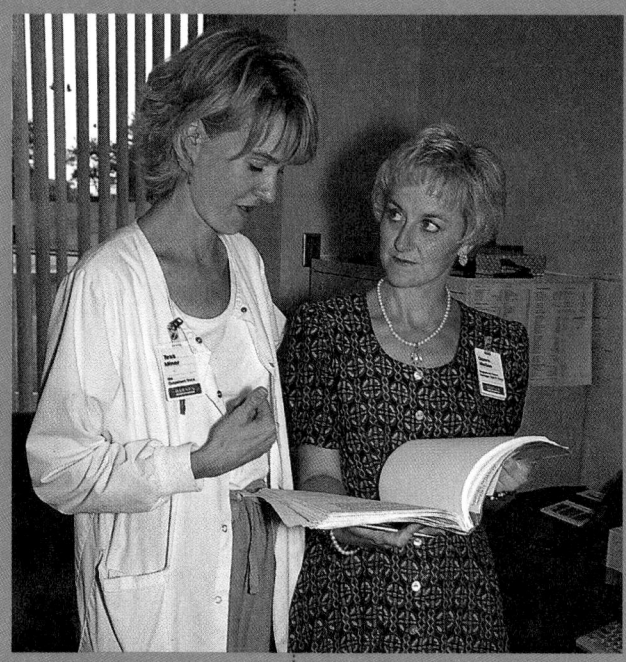

The delivery of nursing care within the health care system is a challenge because of the changes that are influencing health professionals, clients, and health care organizations. It is easy for a nurse to become frustrated in the midst of change, particularly if there is a sense that the quality of client care is being compromised. However, change offers opportunities. A nurse learns to take the initiative and become a leader when innovations in health care are being made and to make the decisions necessary to ensure clients receive excellent care.

Steven Covey in his book, *The Seven Habits of Highly Effective People* (1989), describes **proactivity** as the most basic habit of a highly effective person in any environment. Proactive individuals are value driven and make choices in their lives on the basis of the values they have selected. For example, nurses who choose the value of producing good-quality work always strive to make choices in daily work activities that result in better quality outcomes for their clients. Proactivity is more than taking initiative. It means that as human beings we are responsible for our own lives and the decisions that we make (Covey, 1989). If we allow others to influence our decisions and behavior, it is because we have chosen to let others have that effect.

Covey's description of proactivity is very useful as students of nursing consider the role they play in providing client care. Nurses become both managers and leaders. As managers of client care they assume responsibility and accountability for the direct care decisions that affect their clients. They seize the opportunities they have with each client contact to effectively problem solve and find solutions that improve the client's well-being. As leaders of client care, nurses collaborate with other members of the health care team to choose the programs and services that best meet the needs of clients and families. The professional nurse leads by example, creating a community of care whereby colleagues recognize the client-focused values that influence and guide decision making.

DEFINITIONS OF LEADERSHIP AND MANAGEMENT

Leadership is the use of one's skills to influence others to perform to the best of their ability (Dossett, 1992). It involves the art of getting someone to want to do something that another person considers important. Leadership is an interpersonal process that involves a relationship between followers and the person who is leading. It is more than simply being appointed to an important job or position. Effective leaders must be able to make people want to accomplish something and to therefore get the work done (Dossett, 1992). In the present health care environment, leadership is even more important, because nurses find themselves collaborating with members of all health care disciplines.

Management is closely related to leadership. The word **management** comes from a word meaning "hand." Managers handle the day-to-day operations of a work group to achieve a desired outcome. Management functions are summarized in Box 3-1. Managers are not automatically leaders. However, effective managers become leaders of people.

With changes in health care, management of a nursing unit or work group is becoming more complex. In addition to the common management functions, nurse managers have budgetary responsibilities, ensure appropriate staffing for each work shift, participate and lead agency committees, supervise ongoing quality improvement activities (see Chapter 9), and consult with medical staff and members of other disciplines regarding care delivery issues.

Successful organizations depend on good leaders and managers. The present health care environment requires nurses to manage clinical outcomes for clients and also to take a leadership role in meeting organizational objectives. To succeed in both roles, nurse managers are recognizing the importance of staff members playing a more active role in daily unit activities. For example, staff nurses are setting standards of care, deciding scheduling and staffing issues, and monitoring quality improvement outcomes. Health care settings are following a trend of fewer managers and more **self-directed work teams.** This makes the development of leadership and management skills of equal importance to developing clinical skills: through theory, application, and practice.

LEADERSHIP BEHAVIOR AND STYLE

A great deal has been written describing what makes an effective manager and leader. The characteristics of a leader have been found to be less important than what a leader chooses to do. Research has shown two major dimensions of leadership behavior: "initiating structure" and "consideration" (Dossett, 1992). *Initiating structure* refers to behavior in which a leader organizes and defines the work to be accomplished and establishes well-defined work patterns and channels of communication. For example, a nurse manager defines a philosophy of nursing practice for a nursing unit, selects a nursing care delivery model (e.g., **primary nursing**), determines staffing numbers, works with staff to develop standards of care for the client population, and sets expectations of how client needs and nursing interventions are clearly communicated among nursing staff members. The manager becomes a leader by setting a clear vision for an environment of nursing practice.

Box 3-1
Common Management Functions

Planning

Determining long- and short-term objectives of an institution or unit and the actions that must be taken to achieve these objectives.

Example: The nursing staff of a medical oncology unit established the following objective: improve clients' satisfaction with pain control. Actions taken to achieve the objective included implementation of an objective measure to assess clients' pain more accurately (see Chapter 33) and implementation of noninvasive pain relief measures.

Staffing

Selecting the personnel to carry out these actions and placing them in positions appropriate to their knowledge and skills.

Example: The manager of the nursing unit selected a staff committee to interview applicants for a new clinical nurse specialist position.

Organizing

Mobilizing human and material resources so institutional or unit objectives can be achieved.

Example: The staff development personnel from the hospital were called in to plan with the new nurse specialist and to assist in teaching classes on pain assessment for the medical oncology unit staff.

Directing

Motivating and leading personnel to carry out the actions needed to achieve the institution's or unit's objectives.

Example: The manager involved staff in selecting members for a nursing practice committee. The manager gave them the objective of communicating the new standards of care for pain management on the unit. The committee met weekly for the first month to review pain management literature for oncology clients and to share the information with all staff on the unit. Posters were displayed in the staff lounge. The nurse manager met with all staff to discuss ways in which new pain management interventions could best be incorporated into their practice.

Controlling

Comparing results with predetermined standards of performance and taking corrective action when performance does not meet standards.

Example: The practice committee established two outcome measures: client satisfaction with pain control and staff competency, which is measured on a test of knowledge of noninvasive pain control techniques. The manager set the expectation that staff would participate in additional training if competency levels were not met. Satisfaction results from all clients were reviewed weekly by the practice committee. If satisfaction results showed no improvement, the committee investigated causes and redesigned approaches.

Decision Making

Identifying a problem, searching for solutions, and selecting the alternative that best achieves the decision maker's objectives.

Example: Three months after staff had been trained and new practice guidelines for pain assessment had been implemented, the manager reviewed client records and found documentation of pain assessment to be inconsistently reported. The practice committee met with the manager to identify approaches that might improve the quality of documentation without adding unnecessary charting requirements.

Data from Gustafson D: The functions of a nurse manager in a health care setting. In Sullivan EJ, Decker PJ: Effective management in nursing, ed 3, Redwood City, Calif, 1992, Addison-Wesley.

Consideration refers to behavior that conveys mutual trust, respect, warmth, and rapport between manager and staff (Dossett, 1992). In the same example, the nurse manager meets regularly with the staff one-on-one and in small groups during practice committee and staff meetings. The manager welcomes input from staff on ways to improve the operations of the nursing unit. The manager deals with each employee fairly, based on the practice expectations set for the unit. Staff sense that they are treated as professionals and expected to work together to become an efficient work team. Nursing students can practice developing consideration in working with other nurses and health care providers in a clinical setting. Utilizing free time to assist others, seeking out the opinion of colleagues, listening to others' ideas and suggestions, and participating openly and noncritically in conferences are ways to establish considerate work behavior.

There are a variety of styles or approaches leaders use in an effort to be effective. **Leadership styles** are clusters of behaviors that characterize the manner in which a manager uses interpersonal behaviors to influence accomplishment of a work unit's goals (Dossett, 1992). The styles range from total control to extreme permissiveness.

Autocratic Style

The autocratic leader retains all authority and is primarily concerned with task accomplishment rather than interpersonal relationships. This type of leader assigns clearly defined tasks and establishes one-way communication with the work group. The autocratic leader is firm and dominating. Such a leader stresses prompt, orderly performance and uses power to pressure those who fail to follow expectations. Frequently staff do not enjoy working with an autocratic leader. The autocratic leader tends to make decisions alone.

The autocratic style of leadership can be appropriate in situations where most members of a work group are novices. This style meets the novice's need for guidance and structure during an orientation period. Eventually the autocratic style discourages creativity and innovation on the part of a work group. In situations in which immediate action is required and there is no time for group decisions, the autocratic leader is able to take quick action. Examples might include a crisis situation (e.g., cardiac arrest of a client) or an event that creates major disorder (e.g., a community disaster). Autocratic leaders often have the reputation of being able to get difficult assignments completed quickly and effectively.

Democratic Style

The democratic style is a people-centered approach that is primarily concerned with human relations and teamwork. Employees are given more control and participation in decision making for a work group. Democratic leaders facilitate goal accomplishment while stressing the self-worth of each individual employee. These leaders treat each staff member as an adult and expect the same in return. Criticism focuses on behaviors, not on personality, and is offered in an attempt to promote growth and development of staff.

The democratic style works best with mature employees who work well together as groups. This style sometimes does not work as well with ancillary staff, who may need more direction. The group decision-making process may be slow and frustrating to those who expect prompt action on an issue. Although this style may demand more of the leader, it is often valued for contributing to the growth and development of the staff. The results of the democratic leadership style in health care settings can be seen in **shared governance,** self-directed work teams, and quality improvement staff committees.

Laissez-Faire Style

The laissez-faire style is a "free run" or permissive style of leadership. This type of leader gives up control completely and chooses to avoid responsibility by delegating all decision making to the work group. The problem with this approach is that the leader fails to establish goals or policies and abstains from leading. The work group receives little or no direction. This style may be somewhat effective with a highly motivated, mature group of professionals. However, it seldom works well in health care settings because of the complexity of the environment.

···SITUATIONAL LEADERSHIP

Situational leadership theory takes into account the style of a leader, the maturity of the work group, and the situation at hand to form a comprehensive approach to management style. It is the situation itself, within any work setting, that is a major determinant of the extent to which leadership behaviors or characteristics influence the leader's effectiveness (Stogdill, 1974). Situational leadership theory argues that there is no single best leadership style but rather that the style used by the manager depends on the situation and maturity of the work group. The more managers adapt their leadership styles to work situations and the needs and abilities of staff, the more effective the managers will be.

Situational leadership identifies four typical styles for leaders. The leader may use all four styles at any one time, depending on the size of the work group, the maturity of the staff, and the situations the work group encounters. The four styles follow.

1. *Directing.* The leader provides specific instructions and supervises the accomplishment of tasks. There is high direction and low supportive behavior. Leaders give detailed instructions; state specific expectations; enforce rules and policies; and tell employees what to do, how to do it, and when to do it. This style applies with new employees, employees with repeated performance problems, and crisis work situations.
2. *Coaching.* The leader monitors the accomplishment of tasks while also explaining decisions, asking for feedback or suggestions, and recognizing good performance. There is high directive and high supportive behavior. Typically leader and staff have jointly developed a work plan.
3. *Supporting.* The leader supports the efforts of others, facilitates their goal accomplishment, and shares responsibility for decision making. There is high supportive and low directive behavior. The leader is willing to try new ideas of staff and uses **consensus decision making** to choose a course of action. The leader values growth and not perfection, collaboration and not competition (Cox, 1995).
4. *Delegating.* The leader gives the responsibility for decision making and problem solving to mature staff who have demonstrated their competence

(Hersey and Blanchard, 1988). There is low supportive and low directive behavior. The leaders recognize that there is more than one right way to do things and gives authority to staff that matches their level of responsibility.

The approach of gradually giving up control and giving increasing decision-making authority to staff is in keeping with modern management theory regarding staff **empowerment.** This means fostering the growth of others and facilitating their development so that they are less and less dependent on the leader. Staff become able to know when they can make decisions confidently on their own, such as intervening and resolving client and family complaints, dealing with unclear medical orders from a physician, or resolving conflicts between fellow staff nurses.

The cornerstone of situational leadership theory is the flexibility of the manager in adapting to the needs of the individual or work group. In a typical work setting the manager may be "directive" in dealing with staff who are in orientation, while acting as a "coach" for those on another shift who are more experienced but still need some guidance. The "supporting" style may be apparent as the manager works with a staff practice committee and assists members in solving a problem with another department. A manager who relies on seasoned staff nurses to monitor quality of care issues and to regularly report results of studies is using the "delegating" style to promote staff development. Obviously it is important to carefully assess developmental level or job maturity of staff in matching leadership style. The situational leadership style is growth producing for both manager and staff.

·········· BUILDING A NURSING TEAM ·····

Nurses are creative professionals who want to enjoy their work and achieve success in delivering the very best care to their clients (Trofino, 1996). They are also self-directed and if properly led and motivated can solve even the most complex problems. An empowering work environment is one that brings out the best in a professional, concentrating on effective client care systems (e.g., documentation systems, referral mechanisms, physician-nurse collaboration), supporting risk taking and innovation, focusing on results and rewards, and offering professional opportunities for growth and advancement.

It takes an excellent manager and an excellent staff to achieve such an enriching work environment. One of the first steps is establishing a vision for a nursing team. A vision is a shared image of a possible and desirable future state for an organization or work unit (Senge, 1990). It is a philosophy of how the work of a unit is managed (Gregory, 1995). A vision is derived from the personal visions each employee has for the work team (Box 3-2). In the case of a nursing unit, a shared vision

---

▪ **Box 3-2**

Developing a Vision for a Nursing Unit

What is the nursing unit's purpose or mission?
    Why do we exist?
    What makes us unique?
    What is unique about our clients?
How will staff work with clients and families?
    Place client and family needs first.
    Involve clients and families in all aspects of care.
    Make communication a priority.
What are the standards of the work unit?
    All staff will be competent.
    Each staff member is accountable for the care
      delivered to clients.
    Staff will work collaboratively with all members
      of the health care team.
Key values
    Create an environment of caring.
    Be self-motivated and self-managed.
    Support a learning environment.

---

is a pronouncement of a professional nursing staff's values and concerns for how clients should be viewed and cared for. Integral to this vision is the selection of a client care delivery model and management structure that support professional nursing practice.

Nursing Care Delivery Models

Since the time of Florence Nightingale, there have been a variety of nursing care delivery models. The essence of nursing rests in how nurses care for clients. Ideally the vision nurses establish for the care of clients should drive the selection of a care delivery model. Too often the scarcity of nursing resources and business initiatives from the health care organization influence the final decision. Care delivery should be effective in helping nurses achieve desirable outcomes for their clients. Key factors contributing to success are decision-making authority for direct care-giving nurses and effective methods of communicating with colleagues, physicians, and other health care providers (Duchene, 1992).

Total patient care. Total patient care delivery was the original care delivery model developed during Florence Nightingale's time. A registered nurse (RN) is responsible for all aspects of one or more client's care. The nurse works directly with the client, family, physician, and health care team members. The model typically has a shift-based focus. The same nurse does not necessarily care for the same client over time. Continuity of care from shift to shift or day to day can be a problem if staff do not clearly communicate client needs to one another.

Functional nursing. In the 1950s there was a shortage of nurses in the United States and **functional nursing** became the model of care. In this model, tasks are divided, with one nurse assuming responsibility for specific tasks, for example, hygiene and nursing therapies, whereas another nurse may assume responsibility for medication administration. Nurses tend to become highly competent with the tasks that are repeatedly assigned to them. The major disadvantages of functional nursing are problems with continuity, absence of a holistic view of clients, and the possibility that care becomes mechanical (Duchene, 1992). Functional nursing is task focused, not client focused. Communication is not always clear, because no one nurse is responsible for the overall care of the client.

Team nursing. **Team nursing** involves the delivery of nursing care by the staff of various educational levels. An RN leads a team composed of other RNs, LPNs, and nurse assistants or technicians. The team members provide direct client care to groups of clients, under the direction of the RN team leader. In this model, nurse assistants are given client assignments rather than nursing tasks. The role of the RN versus unlicensed assistive personnel may not be clearly defined.

The team leader coordinates team care by communicating with physicians and other health care personnel and resolving problems met by team members. The team leader also is responsible for coordinating each client's nursing plan of care. Limitations to the model include the lack of time the team leader can spend with clients. Depending on the mix of staff members, this may mean that clients see an RN infrequently. Risks exist if an RN is unable to make necessary client assessments and be involved in important clinical decision making. There also may be no attempt to assign the same nurse to the same client each day, potentially causing lack of continuity of care. An advantage of team nursing is the collaborative style that encourages each member of the team to help others.

Primary nursing. The primary nursing model of care delivery was developed with the aim of placing RNs at the bedside and improving the professional relationships among staff members (Manthey, 1980). The model became more popular in the 1970s and early 1980s as hospitals began to employ more RNs. Primary nursing is not a staffing model. The first primary nursing unit had fewer than 60% of RNs on staff (Manthey, 1980). Primary nursing is instead a model of care delivery whereby an RN assumes responsibility for a caseload of clients over time. Typically the RN selects the clients for his or her caseload and cares for the same clients during their hospitalization or stay in the health care setting. The RN assesses client needs, develops a care plan, and ensures that nursing interventions are delivered. In the absence of the primary nurse, associate nurses follow through with the care plan. If there are differences in opinion as to client needs, associates and primary nurses collaborate to redefine the plan as needed.

Primary nursing is one care delivery model designed to maintain continuity of care across shifts, days, or visits. It can be applied in any health care setting. Although primary nursing may require more professional staff, this does not mean that the model is more costly. Care consistently managed by a single professional can minimize delays in therapies, improve collaboration with other professionals, and enhance the client-nurse relationship.

Case management. Case management is a delivery of care approach that coordinates and links health care services to clients and their families (see Chapter 2). Case management involves a professional nurse maintaining responsibility for client care from admission to after discharge (Duchene, 1992). What is unique about case management is that clinicians, either as individuals or part of collaborative groups, oversee the management of case type–based care (e.g., clients with specific diagnoses) and are usually held accountable for some standard of cost management and quality. A case manager coordinates a client's acute care in the hospital, for example, and then follows the client once he or she is discharged home. Case managers may not provide direct care but instead collaborate with and supervise the care delivered by other staff members. The case manager frequently must oversee a caseload of clients with complex nursing and medical problems. Many organizations use CareMaps in a case management delivery system (see Chapter 2). CareMaps are multidisciplinary treatment plans designed for clients of a specific case type. The CareMap outlines the expected interventions and outcomes for a specific case type over a defined length of stay or number of health care visits. The case manager, along with members of the health care team, uses the CareMap to deliver timely interventions in a truly coordinated plan of care. CareMaps eliminate the guesswork in client care by having all members of the health care team work from the same plan.

Management Structure

There are three approaches to management structure in organizations. A **centralized management** structure usually has a single administrator leading the organization, with directors overseeing responsibilities for each department. An example might be a president of a hospital with directors managing nursing, the finance department, support departments (e.g., dietary, rehabilitation, pharmacy), and the service department (e.g., housekeeping, security, sterile processing). Typically decisions within a centralized structure are made by virtue of position in an organization. Decisions are made at the top, with minimal input from staff members. The nurse manager in a centralized structure might have little responsibility or accountability for the 24-hour operation of a nursing unit.

A **decentralized management** structure may in appearance be organized in the same manner as a centralized organization. However, the difference lies in how decisions are made. Decisions within a decentralized structure are made on the basis of knowledge (Cox, 1995). The individuals who are best informed about a particular problem or issue are involved in the decision-making process. For example, the nurse manager within a decentralized organization will likely have 24-hour accountability and responsibility for operations on a nursing unit. This includes staff, budget, and day-to-day management of client care. When issues pertaining to client care arise, staff nurses become the logical resource for problem resolution.

Another form of management structure is the matrix model. This model is becoming more common in large health care organizations that are reorganizing their hospitals into business units. As departments begin to merge, often staff members find themselves reporting to more than one manager. This matrix relationship can be confusing, especially if the employee reports to managers with different types of management styles.

Decentralized Decision Making

Decentralization within health care organizations has become very common. It is clear that progressive organizations achieve more when employees at all levels are actively involved. As a result the role of nurse manager has become critical in the management of effective nursing units or groups. The diverse responsibilities assumed by nursing managers are highlighted in Box 3-3.

To make decentralization work, managers must understand how to get decision making down to the lowest level possible. On a nursing unit, it is important for all staff members, RNs, licensed practical nurses (LPNs), nurse assistants, and unit secretaries to feel involved. Key elements to the decision making process are responsibility, authority, and accountability (Cox, 1995).

Responsibility refers to the duties and activities that an individual is employed to perform. A professional nurse's responsibilities in a given role are outlined in a job description describing the nurse's duties in client care and in participating as a member of the nursing unit. Responsibility reflects ownership; it must be allocated by the individual who oversees the employee and it must be accepted by the employee. For example, a primary nurse is responsible for completing a nursing assessment of all assigned clients and for developing a plan of care that addresses each of the client's nursing diagnoses (see Chapter 6). As the plan of care is delivered, the primary nurse is responsible for evaluating whether the plan is successful. This responsibility

---

Box 3-3
Responsibilities of the Nurse Manager

Assist staff in establishing annual goals for the unit and the systems needed to accomplish goals.
Monitor professional nursing standards of practice on the unit.
Develop an ongoing staff development plan, including one for new employees.
Recruit new employees (interview and hire).
Conduct routine staff evaluations.
Establish self as a role model for positive customer service (customers include clients, families, and other health care team members).
Submit staffing schedules for the unit.
Conduct regular client rounds and help to solve client or family complaints.
Establish and implement a quality improvement plan for the unit.
Review and recommend new equipment needs for the unit.
Conduct regular staff meetings.
Conduct rounds with physicians.
Establish and support necessary staff and interdisciplinary committees.

---

becomes a work ethic for the nurse in delivering excellent client care.

Authority refers to the right to act in areas where an individual has been given and accepts responsibility (Cox, 1995). For example, a primary nurse, managing a caseload of clients, may discover that members of the nursing team did not follow through on a discharge teaching plan for an assigned client. The primary nurse has the authority to consult with other nurses and to learn why recommendations on the plan of care were not followed and to choose appropriate teaching strategies that all members of the team will follow. The primary nurse has the final authority in selecting the best course of action for the client's care.

Accountability refers to individuals being answerable for their actions. It involves follow-up and a reflective analysis of one's decisions to evaluate their effectiveness (Cox, 1995). A primary nurse is accountable for his or her clients' outcomes. In the example above, the primary nurse is accountable for ensuring that the client learns the information necessary to improve self-care. By using authority in bringing the nursing team together, the primary nurse determines if collaboration was successful, if continuity in teaching occurred, and if the client and family were able to relate the information taught.

A successful decentralized nursing unit exercises the three elements of decision making on an ongoing basis.

An effective manager sets the same expectations for the staff in how decisions are made. Staff members must routinely meet to discuss and negotiate how to maintain an equality and balance in the elements. The staff must feel comfortable in expressing differences of opinion and challenging ways in which the team functions, while recognizing their own responsibility, authority, and accountability. Ultimately, decentralized decision making becomes a vehicle for realizing the unit's vision of what professional nursing care should be.

Supporting staff involvement. When a decentralized decision-making model exists on a nursing unit, regardless of setting, the results can be exciting. Staff members at all levels actively participate. Because the work environment promotes participation, all staff members benefit from the knowledge and skills of the entire work group. If the staff learns to value knowledge and the contributions of colleagues, better client care becomes an outcome. The nursing manager has the responsibility of nurturing and supporting staff involvement. A variety of approaches can be used.

1. *Establish nursing practice or problem-solving committees.* These groups are designed with a specific purpose, for example, reviewing standards of care on the unit, developing policy and procedure, resolving client satisfaction issues, or developing new documentation tools (Figure 3-1).

   The committees are typically chaired by a senior clinical staff member. Managers might not sit on the committee, but they receive regular reports of committee progress. The nature of work on the nursing unit determines committee membership. At times, members of other disciplines, for example, pharmacy, respiratory therapy, or clinical nutrition, might participate on practice committees.

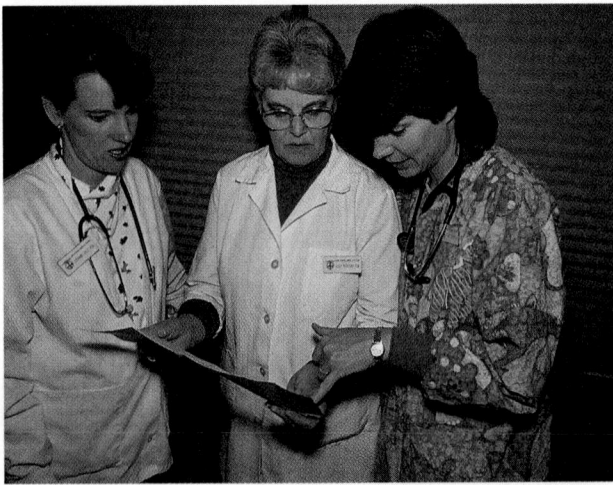

Figure 3-1.   Staff collaborating on practice issues.

2. *Nurse/physician collaborative practice.* The unit's delivery of care model influences how nurse and physician collaboration can best be fostered. If the unit practices team nursing, it is important for team leaders to regularly participate in physician rounds. If the unit practices primary nursing, the physician should communicate either with each primary nurse or the associate nurse who is assuming care for the client on that day. The manager avoids taking care of problems for the staff. Instead, staff members learn to keep physicians up to date on important information regarding their clients. Open communication is critical. Physicians can also be invited to attend practice committees when clinical problems are addressed and to present timely inservices on new medical procedures or research findings.

3. *Interdisciplinary collaboration.* The emphasis on efficiency in health care delivery has brought all members of the health care team together. The staff must recognize the importance of prompt referrals and timely communication. **Interdisciplinary** collaboration is fostered by including representatives of the various disciplines in practice projects, inservices, conferences, and staff meetings.

4. *Continuous quality improvement.* It is important for the staff to commit to quality care on their unit. Staff members learn to recognize when problems arise and try to seek solutions, rather than insisting on the status quo. Health care organizations are required to have continuous quality improvement programs (see Chapter 9). This means that staff members routinely receive information to review on quality of care issues, for example, client satisfaction, medication errors, and client outcomes such as infection rates or learning medication regimens. Staff members on quality improvement committees may become involved in a variety of activities: gathering data on quality measures, reviewing results and problem solving, making recommendations for change, and monitoring results of recommended changes.

5. *Staff communication.* Perhaps one of the manager's greatest challenges, especially if a work group is large, is communication with staff. It is difficult to ensure that all staff members receive the same message: the correct message. In the present health care environment, the staff can quickly become uneasy and distrusting if they fail to hear about planned changes on their unit. However, a manager cannot assume total responsibility for all communication. Instead, the manager can establish a variety of approaches to ensure information is communicated quickly and accurately to all staff members. For example, many managers distribute biweekly or monthly newsletters of ongoing unit or health care agency activities. Minutes of staff and practice

committee meetings should be posted in an accessible location for all staff members to read. When vital issues regarding the operations of the unit or the organization are to be discussed, the manager should conduct staff meetings. When the unit has practice or quality improvement committees, each member should be assigned responsibility to communicate directly to a select number of the staff. In that way all staff members are contacted and given the opportunity to comment.

6. *Staff education.* A professional nursing staff always grows in knowledge. It is impossible to remain knowledgeable of current medical and nursing practice trends without ongoing education. The nurse manager is responsible for giving staff members the necessary opportunities to remain competent in their practice. This involves planning in-services, sending the staff to professional conferences, and having members present case studies or practice issues during staff meetings.

Leadership skills for nursing students.

As nursing students become involved in clinical assignments with clients, it is important that they prepare themselves for leadership roles. This does not mean they have to quickly learn how to lead a team of nursing staff. Instead, they learn to become dependable and competent providers of client care. Just as is the case with the staff nurse, the nursing student has a responsibility for the care given to his or her clients and must assume accountability for that care. Even though the student has limited authority and consults with instructors and staff regarding decisions, the student must not avoid making decisions in client care. The student can learn to become a leader by making good clinical decisions, learning from mistakes and seeking guidance, collaborating closely with professional nurses, and striving to improve his or her performance during each client interaction.

There are certain leadership skills that the nursing student can learn to use, including clinical care coordination, team communication, delegation, and knowledge building.

Clinical care coordination. A student must learn to acquire the skills necessary to deliver client care in a timely and effective manner. In the beginning this might involve only one client but eventually will involve groups of clients. Clinical care coordination includes clinical decision making, priority setting, organizational skills, use of resources, time management, and evaluation.

When a nurse begins an assignment with a client, the first activity involves a focused but complete assessment of the client's condition that enables the nurse to make an accurate clinical decision as to the client's needs and required nursing therapies. This level of decision making is described in Unit 2. If the nurse fails to make accurate clinical judgments about a client, there can be undesirable outcomes. The client's condition might worsen or remain the same when the potential for improvement has been lost. An important lesson in organizational skills is to be thorough. The nurse must learn to attend to the client, look for any cues (obvious or subtle) that point to a pattern of findings, and direct the assessment to explore the pattern further. Accurate clinical decision making keeps the nurse focused on the proper course of action. A student nurse should never hesitate to ask for assistance when a client's assessment reveals a changing clinical condition.

As the nurse begins to make clinical judgments (including nursing diagnoses), a picture of the client's total needs begins to form. The nurse must then decide what client needs or problems need to be cared for first. If a client is experiencing extreme physiological difficulty, such as severe pain, vomiting, shortness of breath, hemorrhaging, or losing consciousness, the nurse's priority becomes clear. It becomes essential to act immediately to stabilize the client's condition. Similarly, psychological events such as reacting violently toward others or experiencing an anxiety attack also require immediate attention. If the client is in no acute distress, priority setting might be based on the client's basic needs. For example, a client who is immobilized in traction might report being uncomfortable from being in the same position. The nursing assistant arrives in the room to deliver a meal tray. Instead of immediately assisting the client with the meal, the nurse instead repositions the client and offers basic hygiene measures. Making the client comfortable first will likely enable him or her to become more interested in eating.

Priorities must also be made on the basis of client expectations. The nurse might have an excellent plan of care established, but if the client is resistant to certain therapies or disagrees with the nurse's approach, little success will be gained. Working closely with the client is important. The nurse shares the priorities defined with the client to establish a level of agreement and cooperation.

Implementing a plan of care requires the nurse to be efficient and well organized. A nurse learns to become efficient by combining various nursing activities, in other words, doing more than one thing at a time. For example, during medication administration or while obtaining a specimen, the nurse combines therapeutic communication skills, teaching interventions, and assessment and evaluation. The nurse always tries to establish and strengthen relationships with clients and uses any client contact as an opportunity to convey important information. The nurse always attends to the client's behaviors and responses to therapies to assess if any new problems are developing and to evaluate responses to interventions.

A well-organized nurse approaches any planned procedures by having all of the necessary equipment available and making sure the client is prepared. Being sure the client is comfortable and well informed increases the likelihood of the procedure going smoothly. Sometimes the nurse requires the assistance of colleagues to perform or complete a procedure. It is always wise to have the work area organized and preliminary steps completed before asking colleagues for assistance.

As the nurse attempts to deliver care based on established priorities, events may occur within the health care setting that can interfere with plans. For example, just as the nurse begins to provide morning hygiene for a hospitalized client, the x-ray technician enters to do a chest film. Once the x-ray film is completed, the phlebotomist arrives to draw a sample of blood. The nurse's priorities seem to conflict with the priorities of other health care personnel. It is important to always keep the client's needs as the center of attention. The client may have been experiencing symptoms earlier that required a chest film and lab work. In such a case it is important to be sure the diagnostic tests are completed. In another example, the client might be waiting to visit family and the chest film was a routine order from 2 days ago. The client's condition has since stabilized, and the x-ray technician is willing to return later to shoot the film. Attending to the client's hygiene and comfort so that family can visit is more of a priority at this time.

Another important aspect of clinical care coordination is appropriate use of resources. Resources in this case include members of the health care team. In any setting the administration of client care occurs more smoothly when staff work together. Students should never hesitate to have staff assist them, especially when there is the opportunity to make a procedure or activity more comfortable and safer for the client. For example, assistance in turning, positioning, and ambulating clients is frequently necessary when clients experience impaired mobility. Having a staff member assist with handling equipment and supplies during more complicated procedures such as catheter insertion or dressing change can help make procedures more efficient. This is an excellent way for students to learn how to work with unlicensed assistive personnel. There are also times when the student must recognize personal limitations and use professional resources for assistance. For example, the student may assess a client and find relevant clinical signs and symptoms but be unfamiliar with the underlying physical condition. Consulting with an RN leads to confirmation of findings and assurance that the proper course of action is taken for the client. Throughout a nurse's professional career there are always new experiences. A leader knows his or her own limitations and seeks professional colleagues for guidance and support.

Much of the stress experienced by nurses results from the perception that client needs must be met all at once (Gustafson and others, 1992). This is of course impossible, especially when the nurse is caring for more than one client. One way to manage this stress is through the use of time management skills. These skills involve learning how, where, and when to use time. Because the nurse has a limited amount of time with clients, it is essential to remain goal oriented and to use time wisely. The nurse learns early the importance of using client goals as a way to identify priorities. However, the nurse must also learn how to establish personal goals and time frames. For example, Ms. Arato is caring for two clients on a busy surgical nursing unit. One client underwent surgery the day before, whereas the second client is anticipating discharge tomorrow. Clearly the first client's goals center on restoring physiological function impaired as a result of the stress of surgery. The second client's goals center on adequate preparation to assume self-care at home. The nurse, in reviewing the therapies required for both clients, must learn how to organize her time so that the activities of care and client goals can be achieved. The nurse must anticipate when care will be interrupted for medication administration, any diagnostic testing, and planned therapies such as dressing changes and client ambulation. In addition, the nurse must be able to use time throughout the day to keep her charge nurse informed, document ongoing client care information, and consult with colleagues on care issues. Time management requires an ability to anticipate the day's activities, to combine activities when possible, to incorporate unexpected priorities, and to avoid interruption by nonessential activities. Box 3-4 summarizes principles of time management.

One of the most important aspects of clinical care coordination is that of evaluation (see Chapter 9). It is a mistake to think that evaluation occurs at the end of an activity. Evaluation is an ongoing process. Once a nurse assesses a client's needs and begins therapies directed at a specific problem area, the nurse should immediately evaluate if therapies are effective and the client's response. The process of evaluation compares actual client outcomes with those that are expected. When expected outcomes are not being met, evaluation reveals the need to continue current therapies for a longer period, revise approaches to care, or introduce new therapies.

Keeping a focus on evaluation of the client's progress lessens the chances of becoming distracted by the tasks of care. It is common to assume that staying focused on planned activities ensures that care is performed appropriately. However, task orientation does not ensure good client outcomes. The competent nurse learns that at the heart of good organizational skills is the constant inquiry into the client's condition and progress toward an improved level of health.

Team communication. As a part of a nursing team, each nurse is responsible for open, professional communication. Regardless of the setting, nurses learn that an enriching, professional environment is one in which staff members respect one another's ideas, share

---

Box 3-4
Time Management Principles

Goal Setting
Review the client's goals of care for the day and the goals you have for activities such as completing documentation, attending a client care conference, giving the staff report on time, or preparing medications for administration.

Time Analysis
Reflect on how you use your time. While working on a clinical area, keep track of how you use your time in different activities. This may provide valuable information to reveal how well organized you really are.

Priority Setting
Set the priorities that you have established for clients within set time frames. Determine the best time for activities such as conduct teaching sessions, planning ambulation, and providing times for rest.

Interruption Control
Everyone needs time to socialize or to discuss issues with colleagues. However, don't let this interrupt important client care activities. Use time during reports, meal breaks, or team meetings to the best advantage. Also, plan time to assist colleagues so that it complements your client care schedule.

Evaluation
At the end of each day, take time to think about how effectively time was used. If you are having difficulties, discuss them with an instructor or a more experienced staff member.

---

information, and keep one another informed. On a busy hospital unit this means keeping colleagues informed about clients with emerging problems, physicians who have been called for consultation, and unique approaches that solved a complex nursing problem. In a clinic setting it may mean sharing unusual diagnostic findings or conveying important information regarding a client's source of family support. One way of fostering good team communication is by setting expectations of one another. An efficient team knows they can count on all members when needs arise. Sharing expectations of what and when to communicate is a step toward establishing a strong work team.

Delegation. Chapter 2 covers the five rights of delegation and the appropriate ways to work collaboratively with unlicensed assistive personnel. The art of effective delegation is a skill nursing students need to observe and practice to improve their own manage-

ment skills. Delegation is the process of assigning part of one person's responsibility to another qualified person with their consent (Bernard and Walsh, 1995). One purpose of delegation is to improve efficiency. Asking a staff member to obtain an ordered specimen while the nurse attends to a client's pain medication request effectively prevents a delay in the client gaining pain relief. Delegation can also provide job enrichment. A nurse shows trust in colleagues by delegating tasks to them and showing staff members that they are important players in the delivery of care. It should be remembered that even though the delegation of a task transfers the responsibility and authority to another person, the delegator retains accountability for the delegated tasks. Box 3-5 lists important requirements for proper delegation.

Knowledge building. All professional nurses recognize the importance of pursuing knowledge to remain competent. A leader recognizes that there is always something new to learn. Opportunities for learning occur with each client interaction, each encounter with a professional colleague, and each meeting where health care professionals gather to discuss clinical care issues. There is always someone who has had different experiences and knowledge that you do not possess. Inservices, workshops, and college courses offer innovative and current information on the rapidly changing world of health care. To become a leader, a nurse actively pursues learning opportunities, both formal and informal, and learns to share knowledge with the professional colleagues he or she encounters.

Box 3-5
Requirements for Delegation

Determine the complexity of client needs or the nature of the work to be delegated.

Identify the staff member to whom tasks are to be delegated.

Determine that the work is consistent with the staff member's job description, level of competency, and normal duties.

Clearly communicate expectations and desired results using measurable terms; convey trust and sufficient authority.

Obtain the staff member's voluntary acceptance of the work request.

Keep communication lines open while giving direction, instruction, and supervision.

Compare actual results with expectations; give feedback, praise, and reward the staff member's efforts.

Modified from Wywialowski E: *Managing client care*, St. Louis, 1993, Mosby.

Key Terms

accountability
authority
centralized
  management
consensus decision
  making
decentralized
  management
empowerment
functional nursing
interdisciplinary

leadership
leadership styles
management
primary nursing
proactivity
responsibility
self-directed work team
shared governance
situational leadership
team nursing

▪ Key Concepts

Nurses should be proactive in assuming both managerial and leadership roles in providing client care.

To succeed as both a leader and manager it is important to encourage staff members to play a more active role in daily work activities.

A manager must set objectives for a work unit, ensure appropriate staffing, mobilize staff and institutional resources to achieve objectives, motivate staff members to carry out their work, set standards of performance, and make the right decisions to achieve objectives.

A leader initiates structure by organizing and defining the work to be accomplished and establishes well-defined work patterns and channels of communication.

Consideration conveys mutual trust, respect, and rapport between the manager and staff members.

Leadership style varies and is based on a manager's philosophy regarding how to lead people, which situations require staff direction, and the maturity level of each staff member.

Situational leadership involves four styles: directing, coaching, supporting, and delegating.

Empowering staff members brings out the best in a manager and allows him or her to concentrate on

effective client care systems, to support risk taking and innovation, and to focus on results and rewards.

Nursing care delivery models vary by the responsibility of the RN in coordinating care delivery and the roles that support staff play in providing care.

Critical to the success of decentralized decision making is making staff aware that they have the responsibility, authority, and accountability for the care they give and the decisions they make.

A nurse manager can foster decentralized decision making by establishing nursing practice committees, supporting nurse-physician and interdisciplinary collaboration, setting and implementing quality improvement plans, and maintaining timely staff communication.

Clinical care coordination involves accurate clinical decision making, establishing priorities, efficient organizational skills, appropriate use of resources and time management skills, and an ongoing evaluation of care activities.

Each member of a nursing work team is responsible for open, professional communication.

Delegation aims to improve work efficiency by assigning part of one person's work responsibilities to another qualified individual.

Critical Thinking Activities

1. Tina has worked on the general surgical unit for about 15 months. A client is transferred to the unit from the trauma intensive care unit. The client has had abdominal surgery for removal of a ruptured spleen and laceration of the liver. In addition, the client's left leg is suspended in traction for mobilization of a fracture. The surgeon arrives and finds Tina handling the traction incorrectly. Although Tina says she is unfamiliar with traction, the surgeon complains to the head nurse. If you were the head nurse, what approach to situational leadership would you use in this situation?

2. Mr. Tanaka is scheduled for surgery at 1 PM to repair torn ligaments in his knee. It is the first time he has had surgery. It is now 11:30 AM and the operating room (OR) has notified nursing that they will pick up Mr. Tanaka in 30 minutes. Mr. Lines enters the room to complete the preoperative checklist for Mr. Tanaka and to make final preparations for surgery. He finds the client moving about restlessly in bed and reluctant to talk. What should be Mr. Lines's priority in this situation: continue preparation for surgery, perform an assessment of the client, or call the OR to delay pick up?

3. Lisa is a student nurse assigned to two clients. She begins her afternoon by checking first on Mrs. Rhodes, a 49-year-old married school teacher who is being discharged in approximately 2 hours after a right lumpectomy that morning for cancer of the breast. She examines the surgical site and begins to take Mrs. Rhodes's blood pressure. The call light at the bedside comes on to let Lisa know that her second client, Mr. Sawyer, has finished lunch and wants to ambulate down the hall. Mr. Sawyer had surgery 2 days ago for acute appendicitis. Lisa tells Mrs. Rhodes that she will return in just a moment and leaves to check on Mr. Sawyer. When Lisa arrives in Mr. Sawyer's room, he tells her that he wants a pain medication. While preparing the medication, Lisa notices that Mrs. Rhodes's blood pressure should have been checked again 10 minutes ago. How might Lisa have managed her time more wisely?

References

Bernard L, Walsh M: *Leadership: the key to professionalization in nursing,* ed 2, St. Louis, 1995, Mosby.

Covey S: *The seven habits of highly effective people,* New York, 1989, Simon & Schuster.

Cox S: *Managing the workplace 2000,* seminar conducted at Barnes-Jewish Hospital, St. Louis, 1995.

Dossett D: Leadership skills. In Sullivan EJ, Decker PJ: *Effective management in nursing,* ed 3, Redwood City, Calif, 1992, Addison-Wesley.

Duchene P: Organizing care. In Sullivan EJ, Decker PJ: *Effective management in nursing,* ed 3, Redwood City, Calif, 1992, Addison-Wesley.

Gregory CS: Creating a vision for a nursing unit, *Nurs Manage* 26(1):38, 1995.

Gustafson D: The functions of a nurse manager in a health care setting. In Sullivan EJ, Decker PJ: *Effective management in nursing,* ed 3, Redwood City, Calif, 1992, Addison-Wesley.

Gustafson D and others: Stress and time management. In Sullivan EJ, Decker PJ: *Effective management in nursing,* ed 3, Redwood City, Calif, 1992, Addison-Wesley.

Hersey P, Blanchard K: *Management of organizational behavior: utilizing human resources,* ed 5, Englewood Cliffs, NJ, 1988, Prentice-Hall.

Manthey M: *The practice of primary nursing,* St. Louis, 1980, Mosby.

Senge PM: *The fifth discipline,* New York, 1990, Doubleday.

Stogdill RM: *Handbook of leadership: a survey of the literature,* New York, 1974, Free Press.

Trofino J: Vision: a professional model for nursing practice, *Nurs Manage* 27(3):43, 1996.

Wywialowski E: *Managing client care,* St. Louis, 1993, Mosby.

Critical Thinking in Nursing Practice

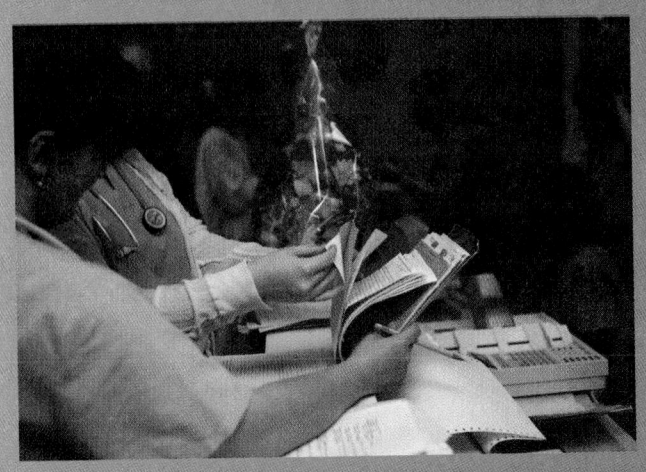

CHAPTER

4

Critical Thinking and Nursing Judgment

OBJECTIVES

Mastery of content in this chapter will enable the student to:

- Define the key terms listed.
- Discuss the nurse's responsibility in making clinical decisions.
- Describe the components of a critical thinking model for nursing judgment.
- Discuss critical thinking skills used in nursing practice.
- Explain the relationship between clinical experience and critical thinking.
- Discuss the effect attitudes for critical thinking have on clinical decision making.
- Explain how professional standards influence a nurse's clinical decisions.
- Discuss how reflection can improve knowledge of nursing.
- Discuss the relationship of the nursing process to critical thinking.
- Apply elements of a critical thinking model to a case study.

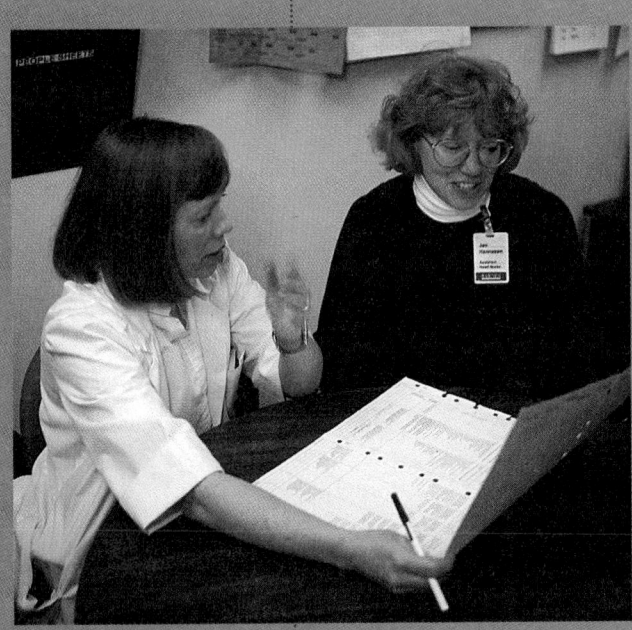

The professional nurse will encounter different clients with uniquely different types of health care problems. What is common to all clinical situations is the nurse's ability to think critically so that the client ultimately receives the very best in nursing care. Critical thinking cannot be learned overnight. It is a process that can only be acquired through hard work, commitment, and an active curiosity toward learning.

◼ Clinical Scenario

Mrs. Bryan is a widowed 78-year-old client who lives alone in a small rural community. Her daughter, Joyce, lives approximately 100 miles away in a large urban city. Mrs. Bryan has always been a very independent woman. She loves music, art, bird-watching, and cooking. Over the last year Mrs. Bryan's health has declined. She was diagnosed with stomach cancer over a year ago. Her condition cannot be treated with surgery. She comes to the community clinic at least monthly to see her physician for follow-up and recommendations for supportive care. As a result of her condition, Mrs. Bryan has had a 10-pound weight loss, and she reports a poor appetite and generalized weakness. She receives Meals on Wheels for lunch from a local church and frequently has dinner with a close friend who lives down the street. Mrs. Bryan's daughter wants her mother to move closer to her so that she can receive the appropriate care and attention she needs. This may mean that Mrs. Bryan will have to live in a nursing home, because Joyce has no room at home to care for her mother herself.

Inez Santiago is a 36-year-old married student nurse assigned to the community clinic Mrs. Bryan visits. Inez has two children and worked part-time as a schoolteacher while raising her children. Now that her children are older, Inez has chosen nursing as a career. When she first meets Mrs. Bryan, she finds the client to be friendly, alert, and happy to have a student. During their discussion, Inez and Mrs. Bryan discuss Mrs. Bryan's feelings about her health and the possibility of having to leave her home. Mrs. Bryan replies, "I love my home. I know Joyce knows what is best for me, but I cannot imagine never seeing my friends again."

CLINICAL DECISIONS IN NURSING PRACTICE

Nurses have the important responsibility of making accurate and appropriate clinical decisions. When given the responsibility to assist persons in maintaining, regaining, or improving their health, a nurse must be able to think critically to problem solve and find the best solution for a client's needs. Many clients have problems for which there are no textbook solutions. Their clinical symptoms, the information clients share about themselves, and the situation in which the nurse meets them do not automatically present the nurse with a clear picture of what actions should be taken. Nurses must learn how to make sense of what can be learned about a client by reflecting on previous knowledge and experience, identifying the nature of the client's problems, and se-

lecting the best solutions for improving the client's health. Over time, the nurse gains the expertise to test and refine nursing approaches, learn from successes and failures, and apply new knowledge (e.g., nursing research findings) that is appropriate to clients' needs. The ability to think critically is central to professional nursing practice.

Clients present to the nurse a wide variation of experiences, behaviors, social perspectives, values, and signs and symptoms of health alterations. To add to the complexity of clinical decisions, these variables can change while caring for a given client. In the presence of such variation it is the nurse who observes the client closely, examines ideas and **inferences** about client problems, considers scientific principles relating to the problems, recognizes the problems, and develops an approach to care. The nurse thinks creatively, seeks new knowledge as necessary, acts quickly when events change, and makes sound decisions that promote the client's well-being. No nursing action or interaction with a client is trivial or ordinary (Fox, 1980). Although the responsibility of making clinical decisions may seem frightening to a new student, it is what makes nursing a rewarding and challenging profession.

CRITICAL THINKING DEFINED

Thinking and learning are interrelated, lifelong processes (Chaffee, 1994). As a person selects a career path, it is important to become more aware and skilled in thinking. Over time, the knowledge and practical experiences gained help individuals to broaden their ability to make thoughtful observations and judgments.

Critical thinking is the active, organized, cognitive process used to carefully examine one's thinking and the thinking of others (Chaffee, 1994). It involves use of the mind in forming conclusions, making decisions, drawing inferences, and reflecting (Gordon, 1995). It means taking nothing for granted. A critical thinker identifies and challenges assumptions, considers what is important in a situation, imagines and explores alternatives, and thus makes informed decisions. When a nurse directs thinking toward understanding and assisting clients in finding solutions to their health problems, the process becomes purposeful and goal oriented.

The American Philosophical Association (APA) has recognized critical thinking to be purposeful and self-regulatory judgment that results in interpretation, analysis, evaluation, and inference (Facione, 1990). It is clear that critical thinking requires not only cognitive skills but also a person's disposition, or habit, to ask questions, to remain well informed, to be honest in facing personal biases, and always to be willing to reconsider and think clearly about issues (Facione, 1990). The APA identified core critical thinking skills that when applied to nursing are useful in showing the complex nature of clinical decision making (Table 4-1).

TABLE 4-1

Critical Thinking Skills Proposed by the American Philosophical Association

Skill	Description	Nursing Practice Applications
Interpretation	Categorization Decoding sentences Clarifying meaning	Be systematic in data collection. Look for patterns to categorize data (e.g., nursing diagnoses [see chapter 6]). Clarify any data you are uncertain about.
Analysis	Examining ideas Identifying arguments Analyzing arguments	Be open minded as you look at information about a client. Do not make careless assumptions. Do the data reveal what you believe is true, or are there other options?
Evaluation	Assessing claims Assessing arguments	Look at all situations from an objective view. Use criteria (e.g., expected outcomes) to determine results of any actions or interactions. Reflect on your own behavior.
Inference	Examining evidence Speculating or conjec- turing alternatives Making conclusions	Look at the meaning and significance of findings. Are there relationships between findings? Do the data about the client help you in seeing that a problem may exist?
Explanation	Stating results Justifying procedures Presenting arguments	Support your findings and conclusions. Use knowledge to select strategies you use in the care of clients.
Self-regulation	Self-examination Self-correction	Reflect on your experiences. Identify in what way you can improve your own performance. What will make you feel that you have been successful?

From Facione P: *Critical thinking: a statement of expert consensus for purposes of educational assessment and instruction. The Delphi report; research findings and recommendations prepared for the American Philosophical Association,* ERIC Doc No. ED 315-423, Washington, DC, 1990, ERIC.

Being able to apply all of these skills takes experience and the thoughtful consideration of the knowledge gained in the clinical care of clients.

The nurse who is a good critical thinker faces problems without forming a quick, single solution and instead is focused on the options for what to believe and do (Kataoka-Yahiro and Saylor, 1994). Learning to think creatively helps a nurse to care for clients as their advocate and to make better informed choices about their care. The nurse must be able to take in information, use recent and past memory, apply reason and logic, review data in a disciplined manner, and make decisions fairly and creatively.

▪ Clinical Scenario

Consider the situation involving Mrs. Bryan and Inez Santiago. Mrs. Bryan returns to the clinic with her friend. Inez observes the client's slow, deliberate movements, unsteady gait, and facial expression of fatigue. Drawing the preliminary conclusion that Mrs. Bryan is "tired" may result from Inez's experience with other clients or from having seen Mrs. Bryan the previous visit and witnessing that a change has occurred. When Mrs. Bryan provides more information on "feeling tired," Inez begins to consider the client's health status, observes for subtle signs of how Mrs. Bryan moves about or sits in the chair, and begins to ask the client focused questions. The questions may be direct, such as, "Tell me how you are feeling," "Have you been unable to sleep?" or "Are you having pain?" Measure-

ment of the client's pulse, blood pressure, and respiratory rate may offer further information about Mrs. Bryan's status. The process whereby Inez uses information to reason, make inferences as to the meaning and significance of findings, and form a mental picture of what is happening to Mrs. Bryan is called critical thinking.

Reflection

An important aspect of critical thinking is **reflection.** This is a process of thinking back or recalling an event to discover the meaning and purpose of that event (Miller and Babcock, 1996). In nursing, reflection involves thinking back on a client situation or experience to explore the information and other factors that influenced the handling of the situation (Boyd and Fales, 1983; Saylor, 1990). Reflection is necessary for self-evaluation and to make judgments about standards of practice. It is a process that helps make sense out of an experience and facilitates the incorporation of the experience into one's view of self as a professional (Baker, 1996). The nurse searches a mental data bank of knowledge and experience for the most likely explanation for each unique clinical problem (Saylor, 1990).

▪ Clinical Scenario

After spending the day at the clinic, Inez spends some time recalling her experience with Mrs. Bryan. In an attempt to learn more about Mrs. Bryan's feelings toward a nursing home, Inez had discussed the value of a nursing home as a safe environment. Mrs. Bryan immediately became less talkative. Inez reflects on why Mrs. Bryan's response concerned her; the client's willingness to participate in the discussion had changed. Perhaps her explanation was not the best approach if Mrs. Bryan had not yet accepted the idea of going to the nursing home. Asking open questions about Mrs. Bryan's feelings might have been more useful. For example, Inez might have asked, "Tell me what you think about your daughter's concerns for your safety." Inez thinks about how she will approach Mrs. Bryan differently during her next visit. Reflection allows Inez to be proactive and hopefully more effective.

. . . .

Engaging in reflection is very individualized (Miller and Babcock, 1996). Not everyone reflects in the same way. Some individuals make mental pictures of the information they contemplate, others prefer quiet thought, and some may prefer to reflect on new knowledge by discussing it with others. Learning to be reflective takes practice. A nurse who chooses to reflect on a clinical experience must be open to new information and be able to look at the client's perspective, as well as

---

| Box 4-1 |
| **Tips on Facilitating Reflection** |

When possible, work alongside another nurse colleague and discuss with one another what was done for a client, how the client responded, and whether the nursing care was effective.

Maintain a journal of your experiences with clients. Be sure to include the following elements: identification, description, significance, and implications (Baker, 1996). Telling a story and drawing a picture are two ways to identify the situation or experience you wish to reflect on. Describe in detail what you felt, thought, and did. Analyze the significance of the experience by considering feelings, thoughts, and possible meanings. Describe the implications of the experience in terms of your own clinical practice or self-perceptions as a learner. Refer to the journal often when you care for clients in similar situations.

Talk with peers who have observed your clinical work. Ask if their observations are the same as yours.

Keep all written care plans or clinical papers. Use them frequently as a resource.

Take time to reflect, both after having cared for a client and before caring for new clients with similar conditions.

Discuss your experiences with colleagues with whom you are comfortable and whose decisions you trust.

---

his or her own. Learning from experience with clients can create an "aha" feeling, because reflection reveals behavior significant to the nurse's professional development. The worth of reflection is evident in the actions that result from it (Dewey, 1933). Through reflection the nurse recognizes that the actions taken were either successful or unsuccessful. The next time a similar experience arises, the nurse uses approaches that were successful or revises an approach to ensure a successful outcome. Box 4-1 lists tips on how to improve reflection in practice.

Language

Another important aspect of critical thinking is the use of language. Thinking and language are closely related processes. The ability to use language is closely associated with the ability to think meaningfully (Miller and Babcock, 1996). To become a critical thinker, a nurse must be able to use language precisely and clearly. When language is sloppy (vague, inaccurate), it reflects similar thinking.

As nurses care for clients, it becomes important to not only communicate clearly with clients and families but to also be able to clearly communicate findings to other health professionals. When a nurse fails to use correct terminology and uses jargon or vague descriptions, communication is ineffective. This may become obvious if the client is unable to cooperate with nursing therapies or if members of the nursing team do not follow through on the nurse's recommendations. Critical thinking requires a framing of one's thoughts so that the focus and resultant message are clear. It helps to reflect on one's language and to consider whether what one communicates expresses an idea, position, or judgment precisely and clearly.

···LEVELS OF CRITICAL THINKING IN NURSING

As a nurse gains new knowledge and matures into a competent professional, the ability to think critically expands. Kataoka-Yahiro and Saylor (1994) identify three levels of critical thinking in nursing: basic, complex, and commitment.

In the basic level of critical thinking a learner trusts that experts have the right answers for every problem. Thinking tends to be concrete and based on a set of rules or principles. For example, a nurse uses an institution's procedures manual to confirm how to insert a Foley catheter. The nurse follows the procedure step-by-step without adjusting the procedure to meet a client's unique needs (e.g., positioning). For basic critical thinkers, answers to complex problems are either right or wrong, and one right answer usually exists for each problem. This is an early step in the development of reasoning ability and signifies that the individual has had limited experience in critical thinking (Kataoka-Yahiro and Saylor, 1994). Despite the tendency to be governed by others, a person learns to accept the diverse opinions and values of experts (e.g., instructors, staff nurse role models). Inexperience, weak competencies, and inflexible attitudes can restrict a person's ability to move to the next level of critical thinking.

In the complex level of critical thinking a person begins to detach from authorities and analyze and examine alternatives more independently. Kataoka-Yahiro and Saylor (1994) note that the nurse's best answer to a problem at this level is "It depends." The person's thinking abilities and initiative begin to change. A nurse realizes that alternative, perhaps conflicting, solutions do exist. In the case of Mrs. Bryan, there may be an option of letting Mrs. Bryan live with a close friend rather than having her placed in a nursing home. This would not meet Mrs. Bryan's daughter's desire to have her mother close by, but it would be an option to improve Mrs. Bryan's safety while maintaining her independence.

In complex critical thinking each solution has benefits and risks that the nurse weighs before making a final decision. There are options. Thinking can become more creative and innovative. There is a willingness to consider deviations from standard protocols or policies when complex situations develop. Nurses learn a variety of different approaches for the same therapy.

The third level of critical thinking is commitment. The individual anticipates the need to make choices without the assistance from others and then assumes accountability for them. At this level the nurse does more than just consider the complex alternatives a problem poses. At the commitment level the nurse chooses an action or belief based on the alternatives available and stands by it. Sometimes an action may be no action, or the nurse may choose to delay an action until a later time but does so as a result of experience and knowledge. Because the nurse assumes accountability for the decision, attention is given to the results of the decision and a determination of whether it was appropriate. Committed critical thinkers act in support of the client and in support of the professional beliefs that underlie the discipline of nursing.

CRITICAL THINKING COMPETENCIES

Critical thinking competencies are the cognitive processes a nurse uses to make judgments. There are three types of competencies: general critical thinking, specific critical thinking in clinical situations, and specific critical thinking in nursing (Kataoka-Yahiro and Saylor, 1994). General critical thinking processes include the **scientific method, problem solving,** and **decision making.** General critical thinking competencies are not unique to nursing but are used in other disciplines

and in nonclinical situations. Specific critical thinking competencies in clinical situations include **diagnostic reasoning,** clinical inferences, and clinical decision making. These competencies are used by physicians, social workers, nurses, and other health care professionals in deciding about the clinical care and support of clients. The specific critical thinking competency in nursing is the **nursing process.** The format for the nursing process is unique to nursing and offers one approach to critical thinking in clinical decision making.

Scientific Method

The scientific method is one approach to reasoning that is used in nursing, medicine, and a variety of other disciplines. It is a process that moves from observable facts of experience to reasonable explanations of those facts (Bandman and Bandman, 1995). It is an approach to seeking the truth or verification that a set of facts agrees with reality. Components of the scientific method are summarized in Table 4-2. Nurse researchers use the scientific method when testing research questions in nursing practice situations. For example, a nurse researcher might observe that clients in a hospice program often have difficulty communicating their feelings to family members. The nurse learns more about what causes this problem and considers the possibility that family members might have poor communication skills. The nurse asks the question, "Can family members who receive instruction on communication principles provide support to loved ones with a terminal illness?" The nurse might design a study that involves formal instruction on communication skills and uses a support group to help family members practice and apply the skills. Once the course is complete, the nurse may ask clients to interpret their feelings about communication with loved ones. The nurse hopes that results from the study will give other nurses working in hospice settings useful approaches for improving family communication. The scientific method is one formal way to approach a problem, plan a solution, test the solution, and come to a conclusion.

Problem Solving

Problem solving involves obtaining information and using information to reach acceptable solutions when there is a gap between what is occurring and what should be occurring. When a person starts to water the lawn and finds that the water is not flowing from the nozzle, a quick problem-solving approach involves looking for kinks in the hose. An example of problem solving in a clinical situation might involve a nurse entering a client's room and finding the client lying in a twisted manner. The nurse knows that the client underwent back surgery and is supposed to remain in straight anatomical alignment to avoid stress on the surgical area. The nurse suspects the client is having pain but instead learns through questioning that he or she is un-

TABLE 4-2
Steps of the Scientific Method

Step	Example in Practice
Identify the problem to be investigated.	Family members have difficulty communicating with a dying loved one.
Collect data about the problem.	Review previous studies about grieving families. Review literature on methods for improving communication. Talk with dying clients about feelings they think are important to communicate.
Formulate a hypothesis to explain the problem.	Family members who receive instruction on ways to communicate with dying loved ones will be perceived as more supportive by the dying family member.
Test the hypothesis through experimentation.	Include family members in a group session on communication approaches. Have the family members use the new approaches when communicating with their dying loved ones.
Evaluate the hypothesis.	Interview the clients to determine if they perceive family members to be more supportive.

comfortably cold. The nurse repositions the client and provides an additional blanket for warmth. When returning to the client's room 30 minutes later, the nurse finds the client asleep. The nurse obtained information that clarified the client's source of discomfort and tested a solution that was successful. Effective problem solving also involves the nurse evaluating the solution over time to be sure that it is still effective. The nurse returns to the client's room to evaluate whether the client remains comfortable. It may become necessary to try different options if the problem recurs. Having solved a problem in one situation allows the nurse to apply that knowledge to future client situations.

Decision Making

In decision making a person is faced with a problem or situation in which a choice must be made as to a course of action. Decision making is an end point of critical thinking that leads to problem resolution. For example, decision making occurs when a person decides on the choice of a physician. To make a decision an individual must recognize and define the problem or situation (need for a physician to provide medical care), assess all options (consider recommended physicians or choose one whose office is close to home), weigh each option against a set of criteria (experience, friendliness, reputation), test possible options (talk directly with the physicians), consider the consequences of the decision (examine pros and cons of selecting one physician over another), and then make a final decision. Although the set of criteria seems to follow a sequence of steps, decision making involves moving back and forth in considering all criteria. Utilization of such a process leads to a conclusion that is informed and supported by evidence and by reasons (Bandman and Bandman, 1995). Another example involves a nurse deciding on a choice of

dressings for a client with a surgical wound; several criteria are usually considered when selecting a dressing: location and size of wound, presence and type of drainage, and whether an infection is present. The nurse considers all available options of the dressing materials, which ones will be most effective given the client's wound status, and the extent to which the client will be mobile and applying stress to the dressing. The nurse may actually try different dressings over the course of a day before making the final choice. The nurse's ability to decide on the type of dressing is based on knowledge, experience, and an assessment of this particular client's unique needs. Utilization of all of this information increases the likelihood of a sound decision.

Diagnostic Reasoning and Inferences

As soon as a nurse receives information about a client in a particular clinical situation, diagnostic reasoning begins. It is a process that enables the nurse to assign meaning to the behaviors, physical signs, and reported client symptoms. Diagnostic reasoning is a series of clinical judgments made during and after data collection, resulting in an informal judgment or formal diagnosis (Carnevali and Thomas, 1993). An example of diagnostic reasoning involves the nurse who makes ongoing assessments on the basis of a client's known medical problem. Nurses do not make medical diagnoses, but they do monitor clients closely and compare signs and symptoms with those that are common to a diagnosis. This process assists in making clinical inferences or judgments about a client's progress. When certain symptoms present themselves, the nurse considers all variables influencing the client in addition to the medical diagnosis and then infers that the client is doing better or worse.

■ Clinical Scenario

In addition to stomach cancer, Mrs. Bryan had a myocardial infarction, "heart attack," just 10 months ago. She must periodically be monitored for possible chest pain, shortness of breath, and/or irregularity of vital signs (signs and symptoms of recurrent cardiac problems). If Mrs. Bryan has a regular heart rate, denies discomfort, and is breathing normally without difficulty Inez Santiago makes a diagnostic decision that the client's cardiac status is currently stable. The nurse must critically analyze changing clinical situations so that a client's status can immediately be determined. This allows the nurse to initiate appropriate therapies, such as activity restriction, so that the client's condition does not worsen. In addition, any diagnostic conclusions made by the nurse help the physician pinpoint the nature of a problem more quickly and select proper medical therapies.

Clinical Decision Making

When a nurse approaches a clinical problem, such as a client who has an injury to the skin or who is anxious about having surgery, a decision must be made in choosing the best approach for reaching a mutually desired goal. This may mean minimizing the severity of the problem or resolving the problem completely. The clinical decision-making process requires thoughtful reasoning so that the best options for the client are chosen on the basis of the client's condition and the priority of the problem. Nurses make clinical decisions all the time in an attempt to improve a client's health or to maintain ongoing wellness.

When making clinical decisions, the nurse first asks why a decision is necessary. For example, during a clinic visit Inez observes a bruised area of the skin over Mrs. Bryan's right hip. Mrs. Bryan describes it as a scrape that she received when she slipped on the edge of her bathtub. Inez must make a decision about the therapies that will promote healing and prevent further injury. Strader (1992) notes that criteria for decision making must be established so that the appropriate choices can be made. Criteria should include the following:

- What needs to be achieved (healing of the skin, a safe home environment)?
- What needs to be preserved (mobility, nutrition, comfort, safety)?
- What needs to be avoided (further tissue injury, infection, further falls)?

After considering each of the criteria, the nurse sets priorities as they relate to the client's situation (see Chapter 7). Because different clients bring different variables to a situation, an activity may be more of a priority in one situation and less of a priority in another. For example, if a client is physically dependent, unable to eat, and incontinent of urine, the nurse recognizes skin integrity as a greater priority than if the client was immobile but continent of urine and able to eat a normal diet. The nurse must not assume that a certain condition is an automatic priority. For example, a client who has surgery is anticipated to experience a certain level of pain, which often becomes a priority of nursing care. However, if the client is experiencing severe anxiety that heightens pain perception, it may become necessary to focus on ways to relieve the anxiety before pain-relief measures can be effective.

After determining the order of priority of the client's problems, the nurse chooses the nursing therapies most likely to relieve each problem. A wide range of choices may be available, from nurse-administered therapies to client self-care strategies. The nurse collaborates with the client and then selects, tests, and evaluates each approach. The nurse tries to anticipate what might go wrong and considers alternative approaches to minimize or prevent problems. For example, Inez will talk with Mrs. Bryan's daughter about having someone check the condition of Mrs. Bryan's bathroom to see if there are any obstacles creating a risk for falls. Based on the findings, Inez will make recommendations to Mrs. Bryan on ways to minimize any hazards or obstacles so that further injury is unlikely.

Nurses make decisions about individual clients, but they also make decisions about groups of clients. A nurse who works on a busy hospital unit is likely to care for several clients. The nurse uses criteria such as the clinical condition of the client, risks involved in treatment delays, and the clients' expectations of care to determine which clients have the greatest priorities for care. For example, a client who is having a sudden drop in blood pressure along with a change in consciousness requires the nurse's attention immediately as opposed to the client who needs to be assisted for a walk down the hallway. The nurse visits the client who has had no visitors and has recently been given a diagnosis of cancer before checking on the recovering surgical client whose family has just arrived. For nurses to be able to manage the wide variety of problems associated with groups of clients (Box 4-2), skillful, prioritized decision making is critical.

The Nursing Process as a Competency

Nurses who become good critical thinkers use the nursing process when making decisions about client care. The nursing process is a systematic approach that is used by nurses to gather client data, critically examine and analyze the client's data, identify the client's response to a health problem, design expected outcomes, take action, and then evaluate whether the action is effective. The format for the nursing process is unique to the discipline of nursing and provides a common language and process for nurses to "think through" clients' clinical problems (Kataoka-Yahiro and Saylor, 1994). The nursing process is a systematic and comprehensive approach for nursing care. An overview of the process is provided on p. 75.

THINKING AND LEARNING

Learning is a lifelong process. Our intellectual and emotional growth involve acquiring new knowledge and refining the ability to think, problem solve, and make judgments. To learn, one must be flexible and always open to new information. The science of nursing is growing rapidly, and there will always be new information for nurses to apply in practice. Learning and thinking are inseparable. Over time, as nurses have new experiences and apply the knowledge gained, they become better able to form assumptions, present ideas, and make valid conclusions.

A professional nurse must learn to think and to anticipate. This involves looking ahead and asking the following questions: What is a client's status? How might it change? How can nursing knowledge be applied to improve the client's condition? A nurse cannot allow thinking to become routine or standardized. Instead, a nurse learns to look beyond the obvious, recognizing that each client is unique. This does not mean that the nurse knows nothing about a client until having met him or her. A nurse's experience with other clients aids in recognizing patterns of behavior, seeing commonalities in signs and symptoms, and anticipating reactions to therapies. Thinking about those experiences enables the nurse to better anticipate client needs and recognize problems when they develop.

Nursing practice is always changing. As new knowledge becomes available, professional nurses must challenge traditional ways of doing things and discover those interventions that are most effective, have scientific relevance, and result in better client outcomes. The nurse's ability to think critically demonstrates a commitment to learning and enhances the ability to positively influence the nature of nursing practice.

	Box 4-2
	Clinical Decision Making for Groups of Clients

Identify the nursing and collaborative problems of each client.

Analyze clients' problems and decide which problems are most urgent on the basis of basic needs, the client's changing or unstable status, and problem complexity.

Consider the time it will take to care for clients whose problems are of high priority.

Decide how to combine activities to resolve more than one client problem at a time.

Consider how to involve the clients as decision makers and participants in care.

A CRITICAL THINKING MODEL

Models serve to explain concepts. Because critical thinking and clinical decision making are complex, a model can help to explain what is involved in making decisions and judgments about clients. Kataoka-Yahiro and Saylor (1994) have developed a model of critical thinking for nursing judgment based in part on previous work by Paul (1993), Glaser (1941), and Miller and Malcolm (1990) (Figure 4-1). The model defines the outcome of critical thinking as nursing judgment that is relevant to nursing problems in a variety of settings. According to the model, when a nurse enters into any clinical experience there are five components of critical thinking that lead the nurse to make the clinical judgments that are necessary for safe, effective nursing care (Box 4-3).

Specific Knowledge Base

The first component of critical thinking is the nurse's specific knowledge base. This varies according to the nurse's educational experience, including basic nursing education, continuing education courses, and additional college degrees that the nurse may pursue. A

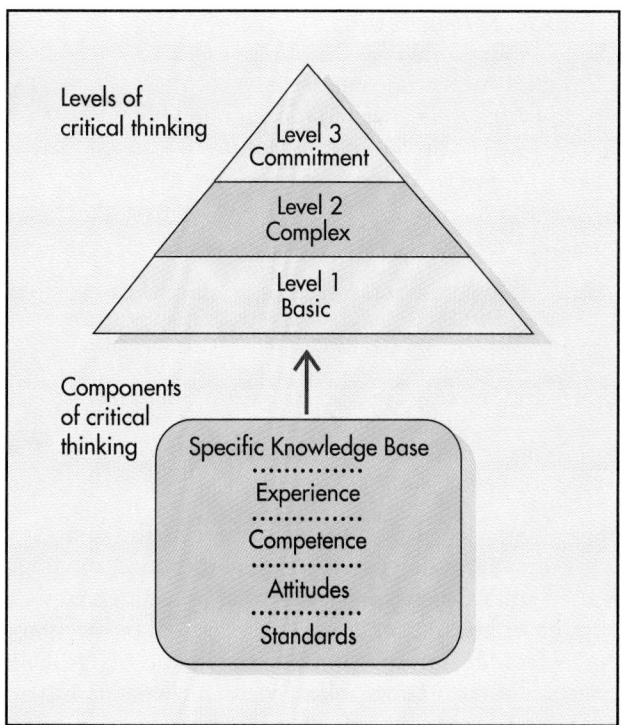

Figure 4-1. Critical thinking model for nursing judgment. (Redrawn from Kataoka-Yahiro M, Saylor C: A critical thinking model for nursing judgment, *J Nurs Educ* 33[8]: 351, 1994. Modified from Glaser, 1941; Miller and Malcolm, 1990; Paul, 1993; and Perry, 1970.)

Box 4-3
Components of Critical Thinking in Nursing

I.   Specific knowledge base in nursing
II. Experience in nursing
III. Critical thinking competencies
   A. General critical thinking competencies
   B. Specific critical thinking competencies in clinical situations
   C. Specific critical thinking competency in nursing
IV. Attitudes for critical thinking
   A. Confidence   G. Perseverance
   B. Independence   H. Creativity
   C. Fairness   I. Curiosity
   D. Responsibility   J. Integrity
   E. Risk taking   K. Humility
   F. Discipline
V.   Standards for critical thinking
   A. Intellectual standards
      1. Clear   9. Deep
      2. Precise   10. Broad
      3. Specific   11. Complete
      4. Accurate   12. Significant
      5. Relevant   13. Adequate
      6. Plausible   (for purpose)
      7. Consistent   14. Fair
      8. Logical
   B. Professional standards
      1. Ethical criteria for nursing judgment
      2. Criteria for evaluation
      3. Professional responsibility

Modified from Kataoka-Yahiro M, Saylor C: A critical thinking model for nursing judgment, J Nurs Educ 33(8):351, 1994.

Data from Paul R: The art of redesigning instruction. In Willsen J, Blinker AJA, editors: *Critical thinking: how to prepare students for a rapidly changing world*, Santa Rosa, Calif, 1993, Foundation for Critical Thinking.

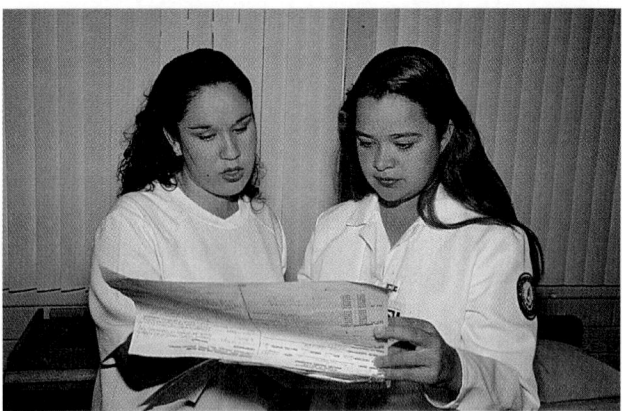

Figure 4-2. Student nurse in conversation with colleague.

nursing concepts, and communication principles. Although still a novice to nursing, her preparation and knowledge base will help her make the clinical decisions necessary to support Mrs. Bryan.

Experience

The second component of the critical thinking model is experience in nursing. Unless a nurse has the opportunity to practice and make decisions about client care, critical thinking in clinical decision making will not develop. A nurse learns from observing, sensing, talking with the client, and then reflecting actively on the experience. Clinical experience is the laboratory for testing nursing knowledge. The nurse will learn that "textbook" approaches lay important groundwork for practice but adaptations must be made to accommodate the setting, the unique qualities of the client, and the experience the nurse has gained from caring for previous clients. Benner (1984) notes that the expert nurse understands the context of a clinical situation, recognizes cues suggesting patterns, and interprets them as relevant or irrelevant. This level of competency comes only from experience. Perhaps the best lesson to be learned by a new nursing student is to value all client experiences. Each experience serves as a stepping stone to building new knowledge and stimulating innovative thinking.

Critical Thinking Competencies

The model for critical thinking includes the competencies discussed on p. 68. When the nurse is involved in the clinical care of clients, the competency utilized is the nursing process.

▪ Clinical Scenario

As Inez Santiago thinks about her clinical experiences with clients, she recognizes she still has a lot to learn. However, each client has provided her with valuable learning experiences. Specifically, she has been able to acquire good interviewing skills, she understands the importance of the family in

nurse's knowledge base includes information and theory from the basic sciences, humanities, and nursing. Nurses utilize their knowledge base in a different way from other health care disciplines in regard to how they think about client problems. The broad knowledge base gives the nurse a more holistic view of clients and their health care needs. The depth and extent of knowledge influence the nurse's ability to think critically about nursing problems (Figure 4-2). Referring to the clinical scenario, Inez Santiago previously earned a degree in education. She is just starting her third year of study in her nursing program. She has successfully completed courses in anatomy and physiology, introduction to

an individual's health, and she has learned the role nurses play as advocates for clients. Her time in the physical assessment laboratory and her first semester in a clinical area helped her to learn to be a watchful observer. Inez also knows that her previous experience as a teacher will help her apply educational principles in her nursing role.

Attitudes for Critical Thinking

The fourth component of the critical thinking model is attitudes. Paul (1993) has identified 11 attitudes that are central features of a critical thinker (see Box 4-3). These attitudes are the values that an individual must practice or show to be a successful critical thinker. Attitudes provide guidelines for how to approach a problem or decision-making situation. A person must have cognitive skills to think critically, but it is also important to ensure that these skills are used fairly and responsibly. Table 4-3 summarizes how critical thinking attitudes can be applied in nursing practice situations.

Confidence. To be confident is to feel certain in one's ability to accomplish a task or goal. Confidence grows with experience and a maturity in recognizing one's strengths and limitations. Critical thinkers have a realistic view of the knowledge and experience they bring to situations, a condition that promotes confidence. Clients recognize nurses who are confident in their decisions by the manner in which they speak and in the way they perform their responsibilities. Confidence builds trust between the nurse and client and is often instrumental in achieving client outcomes.

Thinking independently. As persons mature and gain new knowledge, they learn to consider a wide range of ideas and concepts before forming an opinion or making a judgment. This does not mean they discount other people's ideas. All sides of a given situation should be considered. However, a critical thinker does not accept another person's ideas without question. To think independently, one challenges the ways others

TABLE 4-3
Critical Thinking Attitudes and Applications in Nursing Practice

Critical Thinking Attitude	Application in Practice
Confidence	Learn how to introduce yourself to a client. Speak with conviction when you begin a treatment or procedure. Do not lead a client to think that you are uncertain of being able to perform care safely. Always be prepared before performing a nursing activity.
Thinking independently	Read the nursing literature, especially when there are different views on the same subject. Talk with colleagues and share ideas about nursing interventions.
Fairness	Listen to both sides in any discussion. If a client or family member complains about a colleague, listen to the story and then speak with the colleague as well. Weigh all facts.
Responsibility and authority	Ask for help if you are uncertain about an aspect of client care. Report any problems immediately. Follow standards of practice in your care.
Risk taking	If your knowledge causes you to question a physician's order, do so. Offer alternative approaches to nursing care when colleagues are having little success with clients.
Discipline	Be thorough in whatever you do. Use known criteria for activities such as assessment and evaluation. Take time to be thorough.
Perseverance	Be wary of an easy answer. If colleagues give you information about a client, and some fact seems to be missing, go clarify information or talk to the client directly. If problems of the same type continue to occur on a nursing division, bring colleagues together, look for a pattern, and find a solution.
Creativity	Look for different approaches if interventions are not working. A client may need a different positioning technique or a different instructional approach that will suit his or her unique needs.
Curiosity	Always ask "why." A clinical sign or symptom can indicate a variety of problems. Explore and learn more about the client so as to make the right clinical judgments.
Integrity	Recognize when your opinions may conflict with those of a client; review your position, and decide how best to proceed to reach mutually beneficial outcomes.
Humility	Recognize when you need more information to make a decision. When you are newly assigned to a clinical division and you are unfamiliar with the clients, ask to be oriented to the area. Ask RNs regularly assigned to the area for assistance. Read the professional journals regularly to keep updated on new approaches to care.

think and looks for rational and logical answers to problems. Independent thinking and reasoning are essential to the improvement and expansion of nursing practice.

Fairness. A critical thinker deals with situations in a just manner. This means that bias or prejudice does not enter into a decision. Fairness helps one to look at a situation objectively, analyzing all viewpoints, to understand the situation completely before arriving at a decision.

Responsibility and accountability. When caring for clients, a nurse has a responsibility to perform nursing care activities correctly based on standards of practice, the minimum level of performance accepted to ensure high-quality care. Part of a professional nurse's responsibility is remaining competent in performing nursing therapies and in making clinical decisions about clients. When a nurse intervenes for a client, he or she must be answerable or accountable for the results of any nursing actions. An accountable nurse is reliable and willing to recognize when nursing care is ineffective. Nurses demonstrate their responsibility and accountability in making decisions in response to a client's rights, needs, and interests. Ultimately the nurse assumes accountability for whatever decisions and resultant actions are made on the client's behalf.

Risk taking. When a person takes a risk in an action or decision, it often is perceived that a loss may be at stake. Driving 30 miles an hour over the speed limit is a risk that might result in injury to the driver and an unlucky pedestrian. However, risk taking does not have to cause injury. Risk taking can be desirable, particularly when the result is a positive outcome. A critical thinker is willing to take risks in trying different approaches to solving problems. The willingness to take risks often comes from experience with similar problems. In nursing, risk taking frequently results in client care innovations. Nurses in the past have taken risks in trying different approaches to skin and wound care, pulmonary hygiene, and pain management, to name a few. When taking a risk, the nurse considers all options, analyzes any potential danger to a client, and then acts in a well-reasoned, logical, and thoughtful manner.

Discipline. To be a good critical thinker one must use discipline. A disciplined thinker misses few details and follows an orderly approach when making decisions or taking action. Disciplined thinking does not lessen a person's creativity but instead ensures that any decision is made systematically with a comprehensive approach.

Perseverance. A critical thinker is determined to find effective solutions to client care problems. This is especially important when problems remain unresolved or when they reoccur. The nurse learns as much as possible about a problem, tries various approaches to care, and continues to seek additional resources until a successful approach is found. A critical thinker who perseveres is not satisfied with minimal effort. Achieving the highest level of quality in care is important.

Creativity. Creativity involves original thinking. This means finding solutions outside of standard, acceptable procedure. Miller and Babcock (1996) describe creativity as a great motivator that enables one to generate options and alternative approaches and to see the future. Often clients pose problems that require unique approaches. A client's clinical problems, social support systems, and living environment are just a few examples of factors that can make the simplest nursing procedure more complicated if the nurse does not consider a creative approach for the client's situation.

Curiosity. Probably the favorite question of a critical thinker is, "Why?" In any clinical situation, a nurse learns a great deal of information about a client. As the nurse analyzes client information, data patterns emerge that are not always clear. Having a sense of curiosity motivates the nurse to inquire further and to investigate a clinical situation so that all the information needed to make a decision is obtained.

Integrity. Critical thinkers question and test personal knowledge and beliefs as rigorously as they test the knowledge and beliefs of others. Personal integrity builds trust from peers and subordinates. A person of integrity is honest and willing to admit to any mistakes or inconsistencies in his or her own ideas and beliefs. Critical thinkers strive to adhere to high standards of practice even in the face of adversity.

Humility. It is important to admit to one's own limitations in knowledge and skill. Critical thinkers admit what they do not know and try to acquire the knowledge needed to make a proper decision. A client's safety and welfare may be at risk if a nurse is unable to admit to his or her inability to deal with a practice problem. The nurse must rethink a situation, pursue additional knowledge, and then use the information to form an opinion and draw a conclusion.

Standards for Critical Thinking

The fifth component of critical thinking includes intellectual and professional standards. Paul (1993) identified 14 intellectual standards (see Box 4-3) to be universal for critical thinking. When a nurse considers a client problem, it is important to apply standards such as preciseness, accuracy, and consistency to ensure that clinical decisions are sound. For example, when Inez tries to look at the extent of Mrs. Bryan's bruise, she seeks information from Mrs. Bryan and clarifies any confusing statements. Any measurements, such as the size of the bruise, and a description of its appearance are precisely made. The wound location is described in Mrs. Bryan's medical record using specific anatomical terms. Inez examines Mrs. Bryan further to ensure that her findings are accurate and that no other signs of injury, if present, can be found. The use of intellectual standards involves a rigorous approach to clinical practice and demonstrates that critical thinking cannot be done haphazardly.

Professional standards for critical thinking refer to ethical criteria for nursing judgments (see Chapter 11), criteria to be used for evaluation, and criteria for professional responsibility. Application of standards requires that nurses use critical thinking for the good of individuals or groups (Kataoka-Yahiro and Saylor, 1994). Standards also ensure that the highest level of quality is promoted. For example, Inez Santiago will be facing an ethical decision if Mrs. Bryan's daughter actively considers a nursing home for her mother. The decision must be made with Mrs. Bryan and her daughter involved so that the ethical standard of autonomy is met. This standard ensures client participation in decision making and support of the client's independence. Mrs. Bryan's feelings and ideas must be accepted, and she must have the support to make a well-informed decision about her future.

Critical thinking also requires the use of criteria for evaluation when clinical judgments are made. These criteria may be based on standards of care or practice developed by clinical agencies or professional organizations. The standards set the minimum requirements necessary to ensure quality of care. For example, CareMaps (see Chapter 2) used in managing the care of clients with designated medical diagnoses include both recommended interventions and outcomes that are used for evaluating the client's clinical progress. The outcomes provide evaluation criteria with which clinical staff can make sound and consistent judgments. Evaluation criteria also include norms established through research in nursing practice to be used when determining the clinical status of a client. Box 4-4 summarizes

---

Box 4-4
Examples of Evaluation Criteria

Character of pain: Onset, duration, location, severity, type or description of pain, precipitating factors, relieving factors, other related symptoms
Medication effectiveness: Change in physical signs or symptoms, development of side effects, extent of desired action
Client instruction: Client's ability to recount information learned, client's ability to perform learned skill correctly, client's success in adapting knowledge or skill in the home

---

types of evaluation criteria nurses commonly use in their daily practice.

NURSING PROCESS OVERVIEW

The nursing process is a critical thinking competency that allows nurses to make judgments and take actions based on reason. A process is a series of steps or components leading to achievement of a goal. The nursing process includes five steps: assessment, nursing diagnosis, planning, implementation, and evaluation (Figure 4-3). The three characteristics of a process are purpose, organization, and creativity (Bevis, 1978). Purpose is the goal or aim of the process. The nursing process is used to diagnose and treat human responses to health and illness (American Nurses Association, 1980). Organization is the series of steps or components needed to achieve the goal. The five steps of the process are dynamic but are inclusive of the clinical decision-making activities and clinical skills nurses use to help clients meet agreed-on outcomes for better health (Table 4-4). Creativity is characteristic of the nursing process, because the process is continually changing in response to a client's needs. For example, after a nurse has evaluated the results of nursing care and finds that the client has not improved, the nurse can reassess a client's condition to update data, redefine

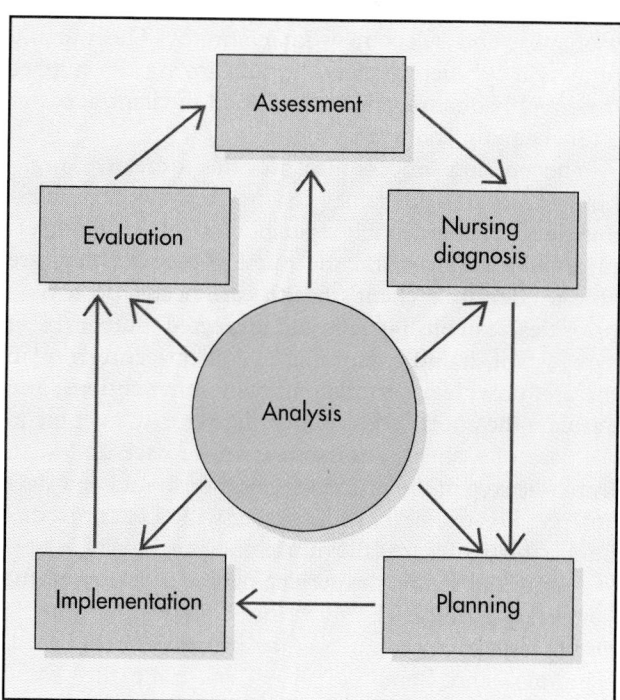

Figure 4-3. Five-step nursing process model. (Modified from Potter PA, Perry AG: *Fundamentals of nursing,* ed 4, St. Louis, 1997, Mosby.)

TABLE 4-4
Summary of Nursing Process

Component	Purpose	Steps
Assessment	To gather, verify, and communicate data about client so that database is established	1. Collecting nursing health history 2. Performing physical examination 3. Collecting laboratory data 4. Validating data 5. Clustering data 6. Documenting data
Nursing diagnosis	To identify health care needs of client, to formulate nursing diagnoses	1. Analyzing and interpreting data 2. Identifying client problems 3. Formulating nursing diagnoses 4. Documenting nursing diagnoses
Planning	To identify client's goals; to determine priorities of care, to determine expected outcomes, to design nursing strategies to achieve goals of care	1. Identifying client goals 2. Establishing expected outcomes 3. Selecting nursing actions 4. Delegating actions 5. Writing nursing care plan 6. Consulting
Implementation	To complete nursing actions necessary for accomplishing plan	1. Reassessing client 2. Reviewing and modifying existing care plan 3. Performing nursing actions
Evaluation	To determine extent to which goals of care have been achieved	1. Comparing client response to criteria 2. Analyzing reasons for results and conclusions 3. Modifying care plan

problems, and select new interventions. The nursing process is a blueprint for critical thinking that nurses use to individualize care and respond to client needs in a timely and responsible manner.

The nursing process also provides a creative, organized structure and framework for the delivery of nursing care, yet it is flexible enough to be used in all settings. When nurses use the nursing process, they are able to identify a client's health care needs, determine priorities, establish goals and expected outcomes of care, establish and communicate a client-centered plan of care, provide appropriate nursing interventions, and evaluate the effectiveness of nursing care. At any time in the care of a client, a nurse may move back and forth from one step of the process to another should new data emerge. For example, while sitting with a client to discuss a plan of care, the nurse may recognize a new symptom the client is experiencing and assess its status before continuing. The nurse must always be thinking and recognizing what step of the process is being used. Bandman and Bandman (1995) describe the whole nursing process as a series of means-ends relationships. The means are the nurse's accurate assessment, diagnosis, and treatment of the client, and the ends are the client's increased level of function and well-being.

⋯SYNTHESIS IN PRACTICE⋯⋯⋯⋯⋯⋯⋯⋯⋯

This chapter has provided a great deal of information about critical thinking and the clinical decision making in which nurses participate. How does it all fit together? How can one proceed to become a better critical thinker?

The critical thinking competency specific to nursing is the five-step nursing process: assessment, nursing diagnosis, planning (with outcome development), implementation, and evaluation. Each step is closely interrelated with the others. Gordon (1995) describes assessment and nursing diagnosis as essential for problem identification and planning, and intervention and evaluation as essential for problem solving. A nurse must be competent in the use of each step and at the same time be able to synthesize the components of critical thinking. A nurse's skill in problem identification and clinical problem solving is sometimes linear, sometimes branching when data from new programs are recognized, and at other times cyclical when the nurse must reassess and validate information (Yura and Walsh, 1988). The nurse is at the center of the decisional process and directs how the problem-solving process will proceed. As the nurse receives more data or recalls past knowledge, decisions are made as to whether to reassess a situation, proceed with a plan, revise a plan, or evaluate the results of care.

The nursing process is closely linked with critical thinking and reflective thought (Roberts and others, 1993). At every step of the way a competent nurse will synthesize the knowledge that applies to a clinical situation, reflect on previous experiences, and exercise the right attitudes and standards when using the nursing process to deliver safe and effective nursing care. For the purpose of students new to nursing, this text provides a model that reinforces the importance of critical thinking in nursing practice. Throughout the clinical chapters of this text, the components of critical thinking are synthesized into the five-step nursing process.

Remember, synthesis is ongoing. However, the text will have a section on synthesis built into the nursing process so that students will learn its importance. Let's look back to Mrs. Bryan and Inez Santiago one more time to show how synthesis of critical thinking and the nursing process works.

Assessment

Inez has scheduled a clinic appointment for Mrs. Bryan on a day when she knows that Mrs. Bryan's daughter is in town visiting. She has previously assessed Mrs. Bryan's physical condition (e.g., nutritional status, activity limitations, coordination and strength, condition of the skin, and respiratory and cardiac function). Although she has not fallen again, Mrs. Bryan is slow and deliberate as she walks into the clinic office. Inez knows how Mrs. Bryan feels about remaining independent and being able to stay in her home. Even though her physical condition has declined, Mrs. Bryan insists she can care for herself. Inez expands the assessment now to learn more about Mrs. Bryan's daughter, her concerns, her relationship with Mrs. Bryan, and the reasons for her wanting Mrs. Bryan to move. Inez learns that Mrs. Bryan and her daughter have a very good relationship. The two initially speak openly and listen to one another's feelings. However, when the topic of moving from home comes up, Mrs. Bryan becomes resentful. She acknowledges her daughter's concern but stresses that going to a nursing home would "kill her." She instead tells her daughter that she prefers to be able to stay in her home town, even if it means living with a nearby friend. The daughter is most concerned about her mother's safety, and she questions whether the friend is capable of caring for Mrs. Bryan properly. She seems uncertain about trusting her mother's friend. The friend is younger, reportedly healthy, and has offered to let Mrs. Bryan live with her.

Synthesis

(Knowledge) Inez has learned that family support is important to a client's well-being. If there is a way to find a solution that both Mrs. Bryan and her daughter can agree to, the outcome will likely be more positive. Inez has also read about home safety. She knows that certain conditions must be in place for a person to be able to move about freely within the home with minimal risk of injury. *(Experience)* After having seen Mrs. Bryan several times, Inez knows that Mrs. Bryan fears moving to a nursing home. Inez has also had the experience of caring for clients in a nursing home and has seen clients become depressed when separated from their home and family support. *(Attitudes)* Inez knows she cannot make a decision for Mrs. Bryan and her daughter. She must be fair and listen to the feelings and concerns of both individuals while working toward a creative solution that will meet the needs of both people. *(Standards)* Ethically, it is important to preserve Mrs. Bryan's autonomy. A decision must be made with her input and support.

Nursing Diagnosis

Inez reviews the information she has collected on Mrs. Bryan and her daughter. Mrs. Bryan has verbalized concern about having to leave her home. Joyce, the daughter, has verbalized concern that her mother will be at risk unless she moves to a nursing home. Joyce knows the neighbor is an option but has reservations about how living arrangements can be made. It is clear to Inez that Joyce cares very much for her mother. The daughter's concern over Mrs. Bryan's welfare is conflicting with Mrs. Bryan's desire for independence. After reviewing all assessment data, Inez sees a pattern in the information collected. Based on the guidelines of the North American Nursing Diagnosis Association (NANDA), Inez forms the following nursing diagnosis (see Chapter 6): *Decisional conflict related to threat over loss of independence.*

Planning

For the diagnosis of *decisional conflict,* Inez establishes a goal of "Client will make an informed choice regarding client's residence." Outcomes will include the following:

Client will choose place to reside.
Choice will be consistent with client's values.
Client and daughter will understand options for
    client's continued care.

Planned interventions will include the following:
    Plan a meeting with Mrs. Bryan, her daughter,
        and Mrs. Bryan's friend. Arrange a tour of the
        friend's home.
    Arrange a visit to the city where Mrs. Bryan's
        daughter lives, and have mother and daughter
        tour selected nursing homes.
    Have Mrs. Bryan identify features she feels are
        important to have in a living environment.
    Have the daughter and Mrs. Bryan plan time to-
        gether to make a decision.

▪ Implementation

Inez proceeds to arrange a visit to the clinic for Mrs. Bryan, Joyce, and Mrs. Bryan's neighbor. Inez also has her instructor attend so that some expert assistance is available. The visit is timed in the morning, when Mrs. Bryan feels most alert. Inez acts only as a mediator, being sure all participants discuss the issues most important to them. Before the meeting ends, Joyce agrees to visit the neighbor's home with her mother.

In planning the nursing home visits, Inez helps Mrs. Bryan pick features she believes are important to have in a living environment. Inez and Mrs. Bryan's daughter select two to three nursing homes that have the features Mrs. Bryan prefers.

A tour of the nursing homes is planned in the morning so that Mrs. Bryan will become less fatigued. Mrs. Bryan and her daughter make plans to discuss Mrs. Bryan's decision.

▪ Evaluation

Inez meets with Mrs. Bryan and her daughter to discuss their thoughts on the recent visits to the neighbor's home and the nursing homes. Together the three of them identify some criteria for a decision: safety, cleanliness, ability for Mrs. Bryan to remain independent with self-care, and availability of medical support.

Mrs. Bryan and her daughter agree that the neighbor's home appears safe and very clean. The neighbor is very independent and has offered to let Mrs. Bryan have a first-floor room as her bedroom. A small bath is adjacent to the room. The neighbor agrees to allow Mrs. Bryan's daughter to set up an alarm system in the home that will dial emergency medical services immediately if a problem arises. They decide to have Mrs. Bryan live with her friend for a 3-month trial period.

Inez will continue to care for Mrs. Bryan, assessing her client's situation and deciding when and if modifications are needed. The plan of care will be revised to ensure that Mrs. Bryan and her daughter take time over the next 3 months to evaluate how well things are going. Use of the nursing process coupled with strong critical thinking skills has helped Inez develop a workable and realistic plan of care for the Bryan family.

Key Terms

critical thinking	nursing process
decision making	problem solving
diagnostic reasoning	reflection
inferences	scientific method

▪ Key Concepts

Nurses learn how to make sense of what can be learned about clients by reflecting on previous knowledge and experience, identifying the nature of the client's problems, and selecting the best solutions for improving the client's health.

Critical thinking is the active, organized, cognitive process used to carefully examine one's thinking and the thinking of others.

Reflection requires a nurse to think back or recall an experience with a client and to explore the meaning and purpose of the event.

Reflection is a form of self-evaluation.

To become a critical thinker a nurse must be able to use language precisely and clearly.

The basic level of critical thinking is concrete and based on a set of rules or principles.

In complex critical thinking a person analyzes and examines alternatives more independently and takes initiative to solve problems.

In commitment a nurse chooses an action and remains accountable for it.

Decision making is an end point of critical thinking that leads to problem resolution.

Diagnostic reasoning is a series of clinical judgments about the meaning of clients' behaviors, physical signs, and reported symptoms that results in an informal judgment or diagnosis.

When making clinical decisions the nurse asks what needs to be achieved, preserved, and avoided.

A professional nurse learns to think and anticipate.

The five components of critical thinking include knowledge, experience, critical thinking competencies, attitudes, and standards.

A nurse learns through experience by observing, sensing, and talking with clients and then reflecting actively on the experience.

The attitudes for critical thinking are the values a person must practice to be a successful critical thinker.

The nursing process is a critical thinking competency specific to nursing.

Critical Thinking Activities

1. Put yourself in John's position as he completes a day on a busy medical nursing unit. John was involved with a medication error. At 10 AM that morning he had just completed a bed bath for one of his assigned clients. He next went to the medication room to prepare the medications for his four assigned clients. Just before John completed preparing the medications for administration, a nurse told him that Mr. Williams in Room 10 was requesting a pain medication. John saved some time and prepared the morphine 10 mg ordered for Mr. Williams. He gathered the medications he had prepared and went to Room 10 first, giving Mr. Lazar his ordered medications and then giving Mr. Williams the requested injection of morphine. After administering all of the medications, John gathered Mr. Williams' chart and discovered he had received morphine only 2 hours ago. The medication is to be given no sooner than every 4 hours. Within 15 minutes of giving the morphine, Mr. Williams' vital signs were stable. As a follow-up, John completed an incident report describing the medication error. Reflect on this experience while considering the errors that were made and describe what John might learn from the experience.

2. A staff nurse, Maria, tells the evening shift during report that no matter what she tries to do, she cannot get a client, Mrs. Lee, to do her postoperative exercises. Mrs. Lee had abdominal surgery just 24 hours ago. Maria reports, "The woman is just unwilling to do anything for herself. I have told her that she can develop pneumonia if she fails to cough routinely." What approach to problem solving might you take to understand Mrs. Lee's situation better?

3. Select a recently assigned client. Reflecting on your actions during that experience, prepare an outline that describes your plan of care for future clients with similar health care needs. As you complete the plan, consider these questions: What might you do differently? What might you do in the same way? How might you improve the client's participation in your plan?

References

American Nurses Association: *Nursing and social policy statement,* Kansas City, Mo, 1980, The Association.

Baker CR: Reflective learning: a teaching strategy for critical thinking, *J Nurs Educ* 35(1):19, 1996.

Bandman EL, Bandman B: *Critical thinking in nursing,* ed 2, Norwalk, Conn, 1995, Appleton & Lange.

Benner P: *From novice to expert,* Menlo Park, Calif, 1984, Addison Wesley.

Bevis EM: *Curriculum building in nursing: a process,* St. Louis, 1978, Mosby.

Boyd E, Fales A: Reflective learning: key to learning from experience, *J Hum Psychol* 23(2):99, 1983.

Carnevali DL, Thomas MD: *Diagnostic reasoning and treatment decision making in nursing,* Philadelphia, 1993, JB Lippincott.

Chaffee J: *Thinking critically,* ed 3, Boston, 1994, Houghton Mifflin.

Dewey J: How we think. In Regnery H: *Essays in experimental logic,* Chicago, 1933, University of Chicago.

Facione P: *Critical thinking: a statement of expert consensus for purposes of educational assessment and instruction. The Delphi report; research findings and recommendations prepared for the American Philosophical Association,* ERIC Doc No. ED 315-423, Washington, DC, 1990, ERIC.

Fox RC: The evolution of medical uncertainty, *Milbank Mem Fund Q Health Society* 58(1):1, 1980.

Glaser E: *An experiment in the development of critical thinking,* New York, 1941, Bureau of Publications, Teachers College, Columbia University.

Gordon M: *Nursing diagnosis: process and application,* ed 3, St. Louis, 1995, Mosby.

Kataoka-Yahiro M, Saylor C: A critical thinking model for nursing judgment, *J Nurs Educ* 33(8):351, 1994.

Miller M, Malcolm N: Critical thinking in the nursing curriculum, *Nurs Health Care* 11:67, 1990.

Miller MA, Babcock DE: *Critical thinking applied to nursing,* St. Louis, 1996, Mosby.

Paul R: The art of redesigning instruction. In Willsen J, Blinker AJA, editors: *Critical thinking: how to prepare students for a rapidly changing world,* Santa Rosa, Calif, 1993, Foundation for Critical Thinking.

Potter PA, Perry AG: *Fundamentals of nursing,* ed 4, St. Louis, 1997, Mosby.

Roberts JD and others: Problem solving in nursing practice: application, process, skill acquisition and measurement, *J Adv Nurs* 18:886, 1993.

Saylor CR: Reflection and professional education: art, science, and competency, *Nurs Educ* 15(2):8, 1990.

Strader M: Critical thinking. In Sullivan EJ, Decker PJ: *Effective management in nursing,* ed 3, Redwood City, Calif, 1992, Addison-Wesley Nursing.

Yura H, Walsh M: *The nursing process: assessing, planning, implementing, and evaluating,* ed 5, Norwalk, Conn, 1988, Appleton & Lange.

5

Nursing Assessment

OBJECTIVES

Mastery of content in this chapter will enable the student to:

- Define the key terms listed.
- Explain the interaction between critical thinking and data collection and data analysis.
- Discuss the purpose of nursing assessment.
- Describe the components of assessment.
- Explain the difference between comprehensive, problem-oriented, and focused assessments.
- Explain the role of client expectations in a nursing assessment.
- Differentiate between subjective and objective data.
- State the sources of data for assessment.
- Describe how to assess functional health patterns.
- State the purpose of a nursing history.
- State the purpose of a physical examination.
- Discuss the necessity for validating assessment data.
- Conduct and record a nursing assessment.

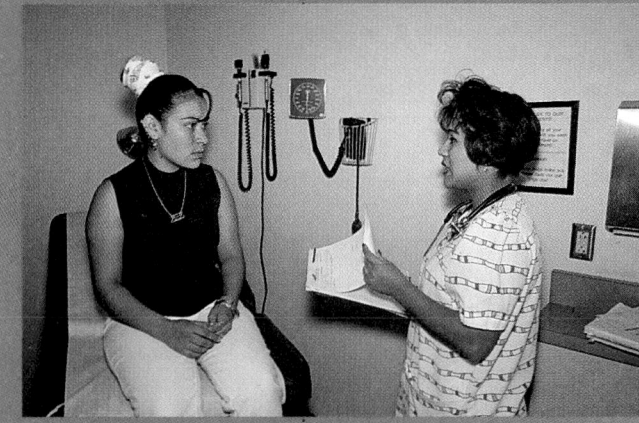

Nursing is unique because of its broad focus toward understanding and managing a person's health. A competent nurse must have an adequate knowledge base in physiology, pathophysiology, psychopathology, and medical treatment to safely perform prescribed treatments. For example, in the clinical scenario in Chapter 4, the physician may order a medication, such as a diuretic, for Mrs. Bryan's hypertension. The nurse must know the expected effect of the drug, the signs and symptoms of side effects, and the actions to take if problems occur. In this same example, the nurse must also have knowledge of therapeutic communication, know how the client's daily living activities affect health status, and principles of adult learning. In the delivery of competent, comprehensive nursing care, the nurse has two focuses for practice: as a primary care provider for the client and family and as a collaborator with other disciplines (Carpenito, 1997).

Mrs. Bryan's medical diagnosis of stomach cancer continues to affect her overall level of health and independence. However, it is the physiological, emotional, and lifestyle responses of Mrs. Bryan and her family to the diagnosis of stomach cancer and the associated health problems that change over time and provide the basis for the nursing assessment. The nurse critically thinks about the client and family and their response to these changes and performs focused assessments. To become expert in the practice of nursing, nurses and students need to remain open to changes in the client and family associated with the clinical situations they experience (Carnevali and Thomas, 1993).

A CRITICAL THINKING APPROACH TO ASSESSMENT

Our present health care system requires the nurse to solve problems accurately, thoroughly, and quickly. The nurse must be able to review information from a variety of sources and make critical judgments. During a nursing **assessment,** the nurse systematically collects, verifies, analyzes, and communicates data about a client. This phase of the **nursing process** includes two steps: collection and verification of data from a primary source (the client) and secondary sources (family, health professionals) and the analysis of that data as a basis for nursing diagnoses (Bandman and Bandman, 1995). The purpose of the assessment is to establish a **database** about the client's perceived needs, health problems and responses to these problems, related experiences, health practices, goals, values, lifestyle, and expectations from the health care system. The information contained in the database is the basis for developing nursing diagnoses and planning individualized nursing care, which is evaluated and refined as needed throughout the time the nurse cares for the client.

The assessment must be relevant pertaining to a particular health problem. The nurse uses critical thinking to determine what is relevant for the assessment database. For example, in an urgent care setting, it is not important to know a woman's childbirth history if she enters the facility because of a possible ankle fracture. In this situation the nurse would gather information regarding the injury; intensity, type, and location of pain; initial first aid measures; medication allergies; and perhaps when the client last ate. Nursing assessments are recorded on a variety of forms. In some settings, the nurse collects data on a standardized form, which is designed to collect targeted relevant data in a timely, efficient manner (Gordon, 1994). The assessment forms may be acute care based, in which the focus may be the monitoring of physical signs and symptoms that are associated with specific illnesses (Change and others, 1996). In a community setting the assessment focuses on the client's illness, the circle of family and friends, and the resources within the community (Bryans and McIntosh, 1996). Because of the variety of forms, the nurse must determine which is the most appropriate form to provide a comprehensive and accurate assessment database for the client's health care needs.

It is important that the nurse learn to think critically about what to assess. The independent judgment of when a question or measurement is appropriate is influenced by the nurse's clinical knowledge and experience and the client's response. When a nurse first encounters a client, there is an opportunity for a quick observational overview. This overview is usually based on the nurse's specialty practice or the treatment situation: a community health nurse assesses the neighborhood and the community of the client; an emergency room nurse uses the A-B-C (airway-breathing-circulation) approach; and a psychiatric nurse may focus on the client's orientation to reality, anxiety level, and violence potential (Carnevali and Thomas, 1993). The nurse continually assesses and interprets the cues from the client to know how in-depth the assessment should be. Assessing the client is a continuous dynamic process that should encourage the nurse to freely explore relevant client problems as they appear.

The initial overview of the client's situation allows the nurse to use key assessment data to respond to priorities, such as the onset of pain. It is important for the nurse to recognize that the client's situation can change at any time during assessment and that data collection must be accurate, relevant, and appropriate.

Carnevali and Thomas (1993) suggest two approaches to collecting more comprehensive data. One is through the use of a comprehensive database, such as Gordon's (1994) functional health patterns (Box 5-1). The **functional health pattern** assessment model provides a guide for an admission assessment and a database for deriving a broad range of nursing

Box 5-1
Typology of 11 Functional Health Patterns*

Health perception–health management pattern: Describes the client's perceived pattern of health and well-being and how health is managed

Nutritional-metabolic pattern: Describes the client's pattern of food and fluid consumption relative to metabolic need and pattern indicators of local nutrient supply

Elimination pattern: Describes patterns of excretory function (bowel, bladder, and skin)

Activity-exercise pattern: Describes patterns of exercise, activity, leisure, and recreation

Sleep-rest pattern: Describes patterns of sleep, rest, and relaxation

Cognitive-perceptual pattern: Describes sensory-perceptual and cognitive patterns

Self-perception–self-concept pattern: Describes the client's self-concept pattern and perceptions of self (e.g., self-conception/worth, body image, feeling state)

Role-relationship pattern: Describes the client's pattern of role engagements and relationships

Sexuality-reproductive pattern: Describes the client's patterns of satisfaction and dissatisfaction with sexuality pattern; describes reproductive pattern

Coping–stress-tolerance pattern: Describes the client's general coping pattern and the effectiveness of the pattern in terms of stress tolerance

Value-belief pattern: Describes patterns of values, beliefs (including spiritual), and goals that guide the client's choices or decisions

From Gordon M: *Nursing diagnosis: process and application,* ed 3, St. Louis, 1994, Mosby.

*The pattern areas were identified by the author in the mid-1970s to teach assessment and diagnosis at Boston College School of Nursing. Colleagues have suggested some minor changes in labels and content. Faye E. McCain's and Dorothy Smith's assessment concepts were particularly influential, as were the comments of clinical specialists and students who reviewed and tried out the categories in practice.

diagnoses (Gordon, 1993, 1994). For each of the 11 patterns the nurse assesses clients by organizing patterns of behavior and physiological responses that pertain to a functional health category. Thus this model directs the nurse's assessment to determine the client's level of function within each of the 11 patterns.

The second model to assessment is a problem-focused approach. The assessment begins with problematic areas, such as pain, and spreads out to relevant areas of the client's life. For example, a comprehensive pain assessment begins with a review of the nature of the pain itself and then broadens to categories such as the influence of pain on lifestyle, family relationships, and work habits.

Whatever approach is used, the nurse must systematically collect data, cluster cues of information, and begin to identify emerging patterns and potential problems. To do this well, a nurse critically anticipates, trying to stay one step ahead of the assessment. Once a question has been answered, an observation made, or diagnostic test results obtained, the nurse branches off to another series of questions to collect further, in-depth relevant data.

Organization of Data Collection

Accurate assessment makes it possible to identify accurate nursing diagnoses (see Chapter 6) and to devise appropriate goals, outcomes, and strategies for a client. Before the assessment is initiated, the nurse must organize the assessment process and determine which data must be collected. For example, during assessment it is important to consider the nurse-client interaction. What is the purpose of the interaction? Who will be involved? What knowledge does the nurse have about the situation? These factors influence the nurse's success in developing a relationship with the client and family, which assists in obtaining a purposeful and comprehensive assessment.

As a nurse conducts the assessment, there are many interactions, verbal and nonverbal, between the nurse and the client. In addition, the client presents physiological responses such as posturing, breathing patterns, and body movements that relay information to the nurse. The nurse must use all senses to accurately assess client signs, symptoms, and behaviors (Bandman and Bandman, 1995). The nurse continually asks more questions to gather more complete data. Inaccurate or incomplete data result in an incomplete plan of care for the client.

Data Collection

Data collection includes the nursing health history, physical examination, results of laboratory and diagnostic tests, and information from health care team members, the client's family, and significant others. Data collected during assessment should be descriptive, concise, and complete and should not include interpretative statements.

The **nursing health history** is obtained when the nurse interviews the client. To collect data from an interview, the nurse uses communication skills (see Chapter 13) to initiate the nurse-client relationship and progress through the three phases of an interview: orientation, working, and termination. The skills of inspection, palpation, percussion, and auscultation permit the nurse to collect data from the physical examination (see Chapter 24). Laboratory and diagnostic tests further validate the findings of the history and physical examination.

Client information is organized into subjective and objective data. **Subjective data** are clients' perceptions about their health problems. Only clients can provide this kind of information. For example, the presence of pain is a subjective finding. Only the client can provide information about its frequency, duration, location, and intensity. Subjective data usually include feelings of anxiety, physical discomfort, or mental stress. Subjective data are difficult to measure (McNaull and others, 1992). However, although only clients can provide subjective data relevant to these feelings, the nurse must be aware that these problems can result in physiological changes, which are identified through objective data collection.

Objective data are observations or measurements made by the nurse. Identifying the presence of a body rash is an example of observed objective data. The measurement of objective data is based on an accepted standard, such as a thermometer, on which the Fahrenheit or Celcius scale is the standard or unit of measure for body temperature. Measurements of a client's weight and blood pressure are additional examples of objective data.

For efficiency, the nurse should use a systematic "branching" technique during each phase of data collection (Milner and Collins, 1992). In branching, the nurse collects additional data in areas in which a dysfunction or abnormality appears to exist and abbreviates the assessment in areas in which no problem is apparent. For example, during the home visit, the nurse further assesses Mrs. Bryan's desire to remain independent and to stay in her own home along with Mrs. Bryan's level of physical functioning and comfort. During the assessment, the nurse obtains data from Mrs. Bryan's daughter regarding her fears for her mother's safety and ability to remain independent. To assist with collecting additional data, the nurse uses a branching technique to direct the assessment questions (Figure 5-1).

Subjective data

Interview and health history. The first step in establishing a database is to collect subjective information by interviewing the client. An **interview** is an organized conversation with the client to obtain the client's health history and current illness. The interview includes orientation, working, and termination phases. By doing the interview first, the nurse has an opportunity to do the following:

1. Introduce the client to the nurse as a staff member of an agency or hospital
2. Establish a therapeutic relationship with the client

3. Gain insight about the client's concerns and worries
4. Determine the client's goals and expectations of the health care delivery system
5. Obtain cues about which parts of the data collection phase require in-depth investigation (branching) (see Figure 5-1)

During the orientation phase of the interview, the nurse introduces himself or herself by name and position and states the purpose of the interview (Figure 5-2). The nurse then explains to the client why the data are being collected and assures the client that any information obtained will be used only by health care professionals who participate in the client's care. These courtesies lessen client anxieties about giving personal information to a stranger and enlist the client as a partner in health care management. Demographic data, as specified by the facility, are collected first. Because this information is the least personal, it helps to initiate development of the therapeutic relationship and to ease transition into the working portion of the interview.

The working part of the interview is designed to gather information pertinent to the client's health status. It should be focused and orderly and conducted in an unhurried manner. During the working part of the interview, the current illness, health history, and client expectations are investigated systematically. The general format for a nursing health history contains several basic components (Box 5-2).

The initial interview is normally the most extensive of all interviews. Major topics that should be covered include biographical data, progress of current illness, and health history. Ongoing interviews do not need to be as extensive; they update the client's status and are more focused toward changes in previously identified ongoing and new problems. Many aspects of the admission interview, such as demographic data, are omitted because they are already documented in the client's medical record.

If the client is hospitalized, the nurse caring for the client should conduct a brief ongoing interview at the beginning of each shift to validate any changes in status. In outpatient situations the nurse should ask the client for health status updates at every visit.

As in the other phases of the interview, termination requires skill on the part of the interviewer. Ideally the client should be given a clue that the interview is coming to an end. For example, the nurse may say, "There are just two more questions," or "We'll be finished in 5 to 6 minutes." With this method the client can maintain direct attention without being distracted by wondering about when the interview will end. This approach also gives the client an opportunity to ask any questions. When concluding the interview, the nurse summarizes the important points and asks the client whether the

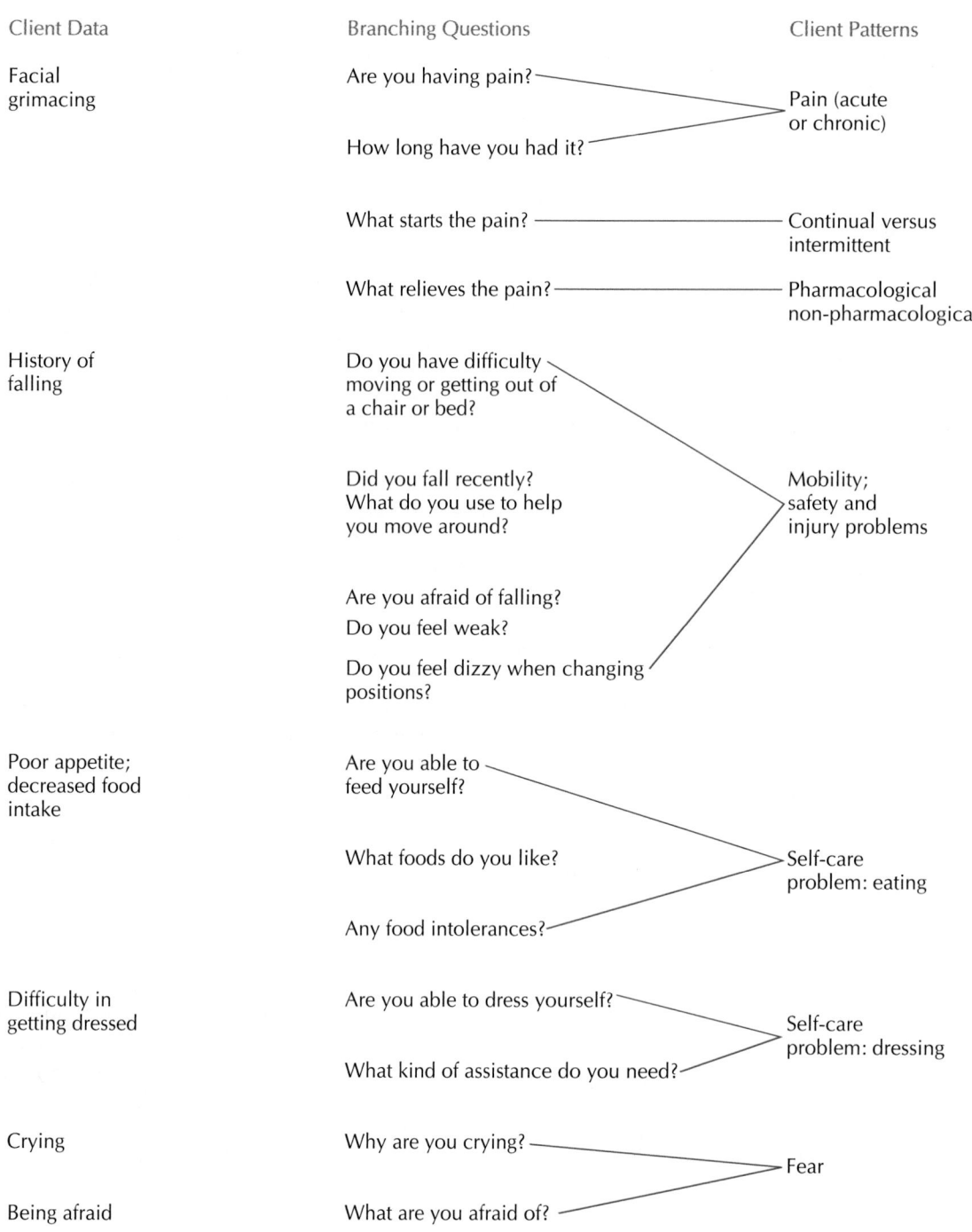

Figure 5-1. Example of branching logic for selecting assessment questions during home visit with Mrs. Bryan.

summary was accurate. Validation of the interview is essential because it allows the client to clarify or add information and may provide the nurse with information about the client's memory and attention span.

The nurse should be as organized during the last phase as in opening the interview. The interview is terminated in a friendly manner, with the nurse indicating when there will be additional contact.

Interviewing techniques. The manner in which the interview is conducted is just as important as the questions asked. Attention to environmental aspects and client comfort, as well as communication techniques (see Chapter 13), often ensures a successful interview. Nurses should remember that they are responsible for directing the flow of the interview so that adequate information is obtained and the client has the opportunity to contribute freely.

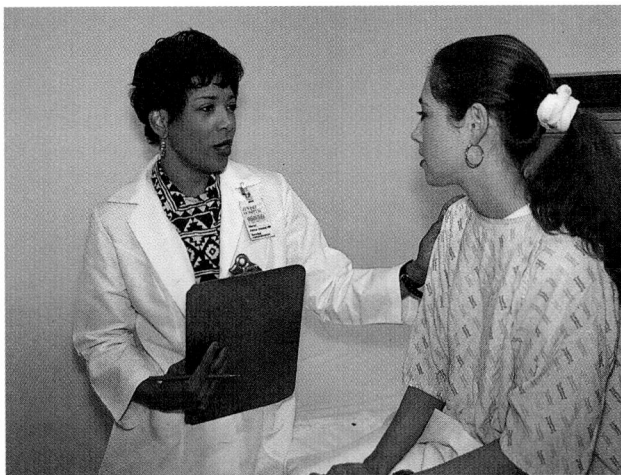

Figure 5-2. Nurse explains purpose of interview.

Environmental aspects include providing for privacy and eliminating distractions, unnecessary noise, and interruptions. The client is more likely to be candid if the interview is conducted privately, out of earshot of other clients, visitors, and staff. Privacy and quiet may be provided by going to an unoccupied room or drawing the curtains around the bed. Noise and distractions can be reduced by requesting that the television and radio remain off during the interview. Timing is important in avoiding interruptions. If possible, a 15- to 30-minute period should be set aside when no other activities are planned. The client should be made to feel relaxed and unhurried.

Before the interview is begun, the client should be comfortable. This includes adequate light, warmth, and positioning. If possible, the nurse should sit facing the client, to facilitate eye contact. During the interview, the nurse observes the client for signs of discomfort or fatigue.

Good communication starts with a nonjudgmental, interested, and caring attitude. This is conveyed nonverbally if the nurse and client are at approximately the same eye level. Throughout the interview many communication techniques should be used (Box 5-3). Initially, open-ended questions such as "Tell me about your pain" or "Describe the symptoms you've noticed" prevent stalls and provide the opportunity for the client to indicate major concerns. When more specific information about a topic is needed, closed questions serve best. "Why" questions must be avoided because they are often unanswerable and sometimes make the client defensive. Conducting the interview by only asking questions may make the client feel like a subject of interrogation. Other communication techniques such as making observations and clarifying should be interspersed throughout the interview to encourage the exchange of information. If the client is talkative, the nurse may need to refocus the interview when the client

strays from the topic. Summarization and validation are always used when concluding an interview. Active listening is important during the entire interview; it makes the nurse alert to unspoken cues and reinforces the therapeutic relationship.

Objective data. The remainder of the data collection process involves gathering observable information undistorted by client perceptions.

Physical examination. During **physical examination,** vital signs and other measurements are taken, and all body systems are examined. The examiner looks for abnormalities that may yield information about

---

Box 5-2
Basic Components for a Nursing Health History

Biographical information: Date of birth, sex, address, family members' names and addresses, marital status, religious preference and practices, occupation, source of health care, and insurance

Reasons for seeking health care: Goals of care, expectation of the services and care delivered, and expectations of the health care system

Present illness or health concern: Onset, symptoms, nature of symptoms (e.g., sudden or gradual), duration, precipitating factors, relief measures, and weight loss or gain

Health history: Prior illnesses throughout development, injuries and hospitalizations, surgeries, blood transfusions, allergies, immunizations, habits (e.g., smoking, caffeine intake, alcohol or drug abuse), prescribed and self-prescribed medications, work habits, relaxation activities, and sleep, exercise, and eating or nutritional patterns

Family history: Health status of the immediate family and living relatives, cause of death of relatives, and risk factor analyses for cancer, heart disease, diabetes mellitus, kidney disease, hypertension, or mental disorders

Environmental history: Hazards, pollutants, and physical safety

Psychosocial and cultural history: Primary language, cultural group, community resources, mood, attention span, and developmental stage

Review of systems: Head-to-toe review of all major body systems, as well as the client's knowledge of and compliance with health care (e.g., frequency of breast or testicular self-examination or last visual acuity examination)

Functional health patterns: Method for organizing assessment data based on function

Box 5-3
Strategies for Effective Communication

Silence is helpful for making observations and provides the client with time to organize thoughts and present complete information to the interviewer.

Attentive listening demonstrates interest in the client's needs, concerns, and problems. Listening can be facilitated by maintaining eye contact, remaining relaxed, and using appropriate touch techniques.

Conveying acceptance demonstrates the interviewer's willingness to listen to the client's beliefs, values, and practices without being judgmental.

Related questions are planned. When asking these questions, the nurse uses words and word patterns in the client's normal sociocultural context.

Paraphrasing provides an opportunity for the interviewer to validate information from the client without changing the meaning of the statement. Paraphrasing is the interviewer's formulation of what the client has said in more specific words.

Clarifying facilitates correct communication of information. It is achieved by asking the client to restate the information or by providing an example.

Focusing eliminates vagueness in communication, limits the area of discussion, and helps the interviewer direct attention to the pertinent aspects of a client's message.

Stating observations provides the client with feedback about how the interviewer observes behavior, action, facial expression, or activities.

Offering information allows the interviewer to clarify treatments, initiate health teaching, and identify and correct misconceptions.

Summarizing condenses the data into an organized review. It validates data because the client has the opportunity to confirm that they are correct. Summarizing indicates the end to a particular part of the interview.

---

past, present, and future health problems. Physical assessment is best begun in a nonthreatening manner. This is best accomplished by starting with the familiar procedure of taking vital signs (see Chapter 23).

Actual hands-on physical assessment should be conducted so that the client's anxiety is not aroused. The nurse should explain each step and continue talking throughout, explaining and asking about specific functions and discomforts. The nurse protects the client's privacy, dignity, and warmth; each body part is uncovered and re-covered in turn (see Chapter 24).

Physical assessment proceeds in an orderly sequence, using the four techniques of inspection, auscultation, palpation, and percussion (see Chapter 24). Inspection begins with the nurse's first contact with the client and continues throughout the history and physical examination. During inspection, the nurse visually examines the client's entire body for structure and function, paying particular attention to deviations or abnormalities. Auscultation is the process of listening to sounds produced by the body. A stethoscope is used to auscultate the cardiovascular, respiratory, and gastrointestinal systems. Palpation involves using the hands and sense of touch to detect tenderness, temperature, texture, vibration, pulsations, masses, and other changes in body integrity. The client should be instructed to let the nurse know when tenderness, pressure, or pain is experienced during palpation. The nurse should also closely observe the response to palpation for validation of the client's report. Percussion is the tapping of the body's surface to produce vibration and sound. The sounds indicate the density of the underlying tissue and thus detect the size and position of the organs. Percussion is most frequently used on the thorax for examining the heart, on the back for examining the lungs, and on the abdomen to assess abdominal integrity.

The initial physical assessment is the longest and most extensive part of assessment because it establishes a baseline of normal and abnormal findings. The abbreviated physical assessment focuses on those areas in which a dysfunction or abnormality was initially found and on those areas in which there was an initial assessment of potential dysfunction. As with the interview, familiarity with the client and previously documented information shortens and improves the process.

Observation of behavior. During the interview and physical examination, the nurse observes client behavior for level of function, consistency, and congruency. This information adds greater depth to the objective database.

The level of function includes physical, developmental, psychological, and social aspects. Observation of the level of function differs from the interview in that it is what the nurse sees the client doing, rather than what the client says he or she can do. Level of function differs from the physical assessment in that this is the degree of function at which the client is operating, rather than the greatest extent of function present determined by the hands-on physical examination.

Consistency refers to the degree to which the client operates at the same level of functioning (physical, developmental, psychological, and social) throughout the assessment and day by day. Any inconsistency is worthy of further data collection.

Congruency is the matching or agreement between two or more things. The client's statements should match mood and behavior. Subjective and objective data should generally agree. Incongruence indicates the need for further data collection.

Diagnostic and laboratory data. Another source of assessment data is the results of diagnostic and laboratory tests. These data can identify or verify alterations questioned or identified during the nursing health history and physical examination. For example, during the health history the client indicates recurrent upper respiratory tract infections and at present has a productive cough with brown sputum. On physical examination the nurse notes an elevated temperature, decreased right lower breath sounds, and dullness to percussion over the right lower lobe. The nurse may obtain a complete blood count to note for an elevated white blood cell count and a chest roentgenogram to determine the presence of a right lower lobe infiltrate. Clients may need to be taught how to collect and monitor some laboratory data in the home. This is especially true for clients with diabetes mellitus who need blood glucose monitoring (Figure 5-3). Both of these laboratory and diagnostic tests could be used to document the presence of right lower lobe pneumonia. These results include information about the response to illness and information about the effects of later treatment measures.

Laboratory data are compared with the established norms for a particular test, age-group, and gender (Box 5-4). These data are also valuable in helping to determine the degree to which medical and nursing interventions are successful. Diagnostic and laboratory test data are one more source of information the nurse uses in completing the assessment database.

Medical record. The **medical record** provides pertinent data about the client's medical history, laboratory tests, diagnostic studies, and the physician's proposed treatment plan. The data contained in the medical record are baseline information about the client's response to illness and information about the effects of later treatment measures. The nurse uses the chart as a resource for additional information and as a tool for checking the consistency and congruency of personal observations. All members of the health care team should be encouraged to read nursing notes because they provide an excellent means for validating assessment data and the client's response to treatment.

Other sources of data. Health care team members, families and significant others, and nursing and medical literature are important resources for completing the database.

Health care team members include physicians, nurses, and ancillary staff (see Chapter 10). Team members can provide data about the way the client interacts within the health care environment, reacts to information about diagnostic tests, and responds to visitors. Every team member who interacts with a client is a potential source of information and may provide invaluable insights into client behavior and needs.

The client's family, friends, and significant others know the client from a point of view unavailable to the health care team. They frequently provide background information essential to understanding the client's situation and responses. In cases of severe illness or emergency situations or when the client is an infant, a child, or mentally disabled, the family or significant others

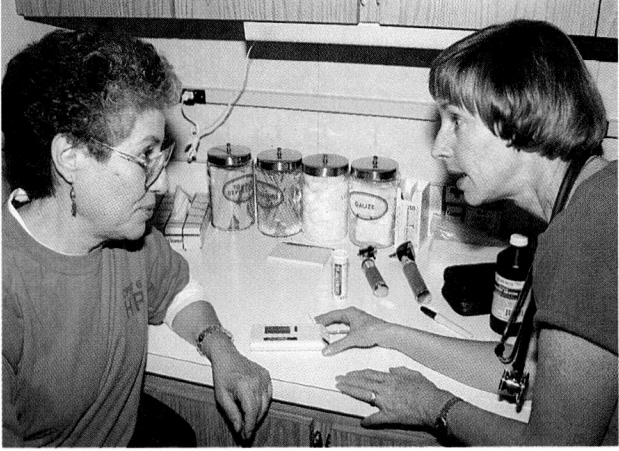

Figure 5-3. Nurse teaching client to do blood glucose monitoring. (Courtesy Phillip James Acker, Motorola, Inc.)

Box 5-4
Common Laboratory and Diagnostic Tests

Blood
Complete blood count (CBC)
Electrolyte tests: sequential multiple analyses—
    SMA_6, SMA_{12}
Arterial blood gas (ABG) analysis
Fasting blood sugar (FBS) test
Glucose tolerance test (GTT)

Urine
Urinalysis (UA)
Urine culture and sensitivity test

Radiological Examinations
Chest roentgenogram (CXR)
Upper gastrointestinal (UGI)
Lower gastrointestinal (LGI)
Scans: body, head, chest, and bone

Stool
Guaiac tests
Ova and parasites tests

Sputum
Culture and sensitivity test
Acid-fast bacilli (AFB) test
Cytology tests

Other
Electrocardiogram (ECG or EKG)
Stress test
Tuberculosis (TB) skin test

may be the only available source of data about health-illness patterns, current medications, allergies, and onset of illness.

A literature review about the client's illness helps to complete the database. The review increases the nurse's knowledge about the symptoms, treatment, and prognosis of a specific illness. The knowledgeable nurse researches information pertinent to assessment and planning.

CRITICAL THINKING APPROACH TO FORMULATING NURSING JUDGMENTS

To be useful, assessment data must refer to the intended purpose of nursing and relate to the client's health problems (Bandman and Bandman, 1995). The interrelationship between the purpose of nursing and the client's health care problems is the basis for nursing judgments. The nurse critically thinks about what type of information to collect, interprets the information to determine the presence of abnormal findings, conducts further observations to clarify information, and then identifies the client's problems in the form of nursing diagnoses (see Chapter 6).

Data Interpretation and Validation

After the subjective and objective data are gathered, the collected information must be validated to ensure its accuracy. **Validation** of each source of assessment data is obtained by comparing the data with another source. The client should be asked to validate the information obtained during the interview and health history. Any additions or corrections should be noted and added to the database. Findings concerning physical examination and observation of client behavior can be validated by comparing data in the medical record with consultation from another health team member, family member, or significant other. The nurse may consult current professional textbooks to confirm that collected data are consistent with the medical diagnosis.

During the home visit, Inez reviews the following information with both Mrs. Bryan and her daughter:

- Mrs. Bryan's need for independence and her fear of nursing home placement
- Her daughter's concerns and fears regarding her mother's safety and ability to care for herself

It is important to review these data with both the client and family. This serves two purposes. First, the data are validated as being correct. Second, such a review opens the door for gathering more information. Thus the nurse is continually analyzing and thinking about client data to make concise, accurate, and meaningful interpretations about the client's responses to health care problems. Critically thinking about client data enables the nurse to understand the problems more fully, to judge the extent of the problems more carefully, and to discover possible relationships between the problems. The nurse validates and verifies inferences by summarizing findings with the client or by comparing findings with another source or standard of measurement.

Data Clustering

After interpreting and validating the subjective and objective data, the nurse needs to organize the information into meaningful and usable clusters, keeping in mind the client's response to illness. The nurse uses professional knowledge to form the basis for sorting the data. During **data clustering,** the nurse organizes data and focuses attention on client functions needing support and assistance for recovery. Focused data clustering using a systems approach or functional health pattern approach assists the nurse in correctly classifying and organizing data, which ultimately provides the

---

> **Box 5-5**
> ## Focused Data Clustering
>
> **System-Oriented Format**
> *Integumentary System*
> Intact, flushed skin that is hot and dry to touch
> Dry oral mucosa, coated tongue, and cracked lips
>
> *Gastrointestinal System*
> Distended, firm abdomen that is tender to palpation in upper quadrants
> Decreased intake
> Twenty-pound weight loss
>
> *Medical Record*
> Hemoglobin: 10 g/dl
> Diagnosis of stomach cancer
>
> **Functional Health Pattern Format**
> *Activity and Exercise Pattern*
> Statement of increased fatigue when walking
> Demonstration of ability to perform activities of daily living (ADLs)
> Fatigued, dyspneic appearance when performing ADLs
>
> *Sleep and Rest Pattern*
> Report of difficulty in falling and remaining asleep
> Denial of use of sleeping aids
>
> *Medical Record*
> Previous history of decreased activity tolerance and poor sleeping 2 weeks before hospital admission for congestive heart failure
> Chest x-ray film showing pulmonary congestion

framework for developing individualized nursing diagnoses for the client (Box 5-5). Clustering also helps make documentation more concise and focused.

During data clustering, certain cues alert the nurse's thinking processes more than others (Gordon, 1994). These cues help to generate nursing diagnoses. As the nurse gains experience, the nurse more readily recognizes characteristics of the client's response to health problems, such as pain or altered mobility. This experience provides a foundation upon which more complicated clustering of data becomes recognizable.

Data Documentation

Data documentation is the last part of a complete assessment. A thorough and accurate documentation of facts is necessary when recording client data. If an item is not recorded, it is lost and unavailable to anyone researching the client's medical record. If specific information is not given, the reader is left with only general impressions.

The nurse is thorough for the client's benefit; thoroughness ensures that all information is available to those caring for the client's needs. Even information that does not seem to indicate an abnormality should be recorded. It may become important later, serving as baseline data for a change in status. A general rule of thumb is that if it was assessed, it should be recorded. The use of an admission assessment form that is integrated with client care outcome standards increases the accuracy, efficiency, and relevance in the documentation of assessment data (North and Serkes, 1996).

The nurse's professional competence and nursing license are protected by thoroughness. The nurse practice acts in all states and the American Nurses Association Social Policy Statement (1980, 1995) mandate accurate data collection and recording as independent functions essential to the role of the professional nurse. Thorough documentation visibly demonstrates professional competence and provides protection of the license by demonstrating that professional responsibilities were met (see Chapter 10).

Being factual is easy after it becomes a habit. The basic rule is to record all observations. When the nurse records data, attention should be paid to facts and effort should be made to be as descriptive as possible. Anything heard, seen, touched, or smelled should be reported exactly. The nurse should not generalize or form judgments too early. Conclusions about such observations become nursing diagnoses. Because of a familiarity with the signs and symptoms of a problem, the nurse often immediately assumes the existence of that problem. If the assumption is charted as data, the actual facts are lost. Because assessment includes the collection and documentation of subjective and objective client data, the nurse should make certain that the database is complete and factual before data clustering. Premature clustering can lead to inaccurate nursing diagnoses and ineffective care planning. In situations in which the client has just been admitted or when the client's status is changing rapidly, it is often better to collect and document the new data continually and to delay clustering.

■ Key Concepts

The nursing process is a method for organizing and delivering nursing care.

The purposes of the nursing process are to identify the client's health care needs, establish a nursing care plan, and complete nursing interventions designed to meet the needs.

The nursing process has five component steps: assessment, nursing diagnosis, planning, implementation, and evaluation.

Assessment is the collection, validation, sorting, and documentation of data about a client.

Sources of client data are the client interview and health history, physical examination, observation of client behavior, medical records, consultation with health team members and family or significant others, and professional literature.

The functional health pattern assessment model enables the nurse to collect data about the client's level of function in 1 or all 11 patterns.

Subjective data are the client's perceptions.

Objective data are observations or measurements by the data collector.

The interview comprises three phases: orientation, working, and termination.

Effective communication skills are essential to the client interview.

Physical examination requires the skills of inspection, auscultation, palpation, and percussion.

Data validation ensures accuracy of the assessment.

Data clustering organizes the assessed information into meaningful clusters for efficient documentation.

Thoroughness and factualness are essential to accurate data documentation.

Critical Thinking Activities

1. Develop examples of closed and open questions you would use to determine Mrs. Bryan's health care needs. Practice using them on a classmate, and compare the information you gather.
2. You greet Mrs. Jacob on your first home visit after her undergoing major abdominal surgery. You introduce yourself and explain your role and the physician's postoperative orders. What aspect of the interview has taken place? What will you do next?
3. Take the following narrative and identify subjective and objective data. Mr. Kantor is lying on his side, grimacing and rubbing his abdomen, moaning, and complaining of pain. His vital signs are as follows: blood pressure, 140/100 mm Hg; pulse, 120 beats per minute; respirations, 22 per minute. He is pale and diaphoretic, and his skin is warm to touch. Oral temperature is 102° F.

Key Terms

assessment
database
data clustering
data collection
data documentation
functional health
    patterns
health care team

interview
medical record
nursing health history
nursing process
objective data
physical examination
subjective data
validation

References

American Nurses Association: *Nursing: a social policy statement,* Washington, DC, 1980, The Association.

American Nurses Association: *Nursing: a social policy statement,* Washington, DC, 1995, The Association.

Bandman EI, Bandman B: *Critical thinking in nursing,* ed 2, Norwalk, Conn, 1995, Appleton & Lange.

Bryans A, McIntosh J: Decision making in community nursing: an analysis of the stages of decision making as they relate to community nursing, *J Adv Nurs* 24(1):24, 1996.

Carnevali DL, Thomas MD: *Diagnostic reasoning and treatment decision making in nursing,* Philadelphia, 1993, JB Lippincott.

Carpenito LJ: *Nursing diagnosis: application in clinical practice,* ed 7, Philadelphia, 1997, JB Lippincott.

Change BL and others: The validity of a nursing assessment and monitoring of signs and symptoms scale in ICU and non-ICU patients, *Am J Crit Care* 5(4):298, 1996.

Gordon M: *Manual of nursing diagnosis,* St. Louis, 1993, Mosby.

Gordon M: *Nursing diagnosis: process and application,* St. Louis, 1994, Mosby.

McNaull FW and others: A comparison of education methods to enhance nursing performance in pain assessment, *J Contin Educ Nurs* 23(6):267, 1992.

Milner EM, Collins MB: Tools to improve systematic client assessment in undergraduate nursing education, *J Nurs Educ* 31(4):186, 1992.

North SD, Serkes PC: Improving documentation of initial nursing assessment, *Nurs Manage* 27(4):30, 1996.

6

Nursing Diagnosis

OBJECTIVES

Mastery of content in this chapter will enable the student to:

- Define the key terms listed.
- Explain the relationship between the nursing diagnosis and the other components of the nursing process.
- Differentiate between medical and nursing diagnoses.
- List the steps of the nursing diagnostic process.
- Discuss the criteria for a nursing diagnosis.
- Identify the format for a nursing diagnosis.
- Describe the way in which defining characteristics and the etiological process individualize a nursing diagnosis.
- Discuss the advantages of nursing diagnoses for the client and nursing profession.
- Demonstrate the ability to prioritize a list of nursing diagnoses.
- Identify the common errors in the formulation of the nursing diagnostic statement.
- Explain how to correct an error in the nursing diagnostic statement.
- Formulate nursing diagnoses from a nursing assessment.

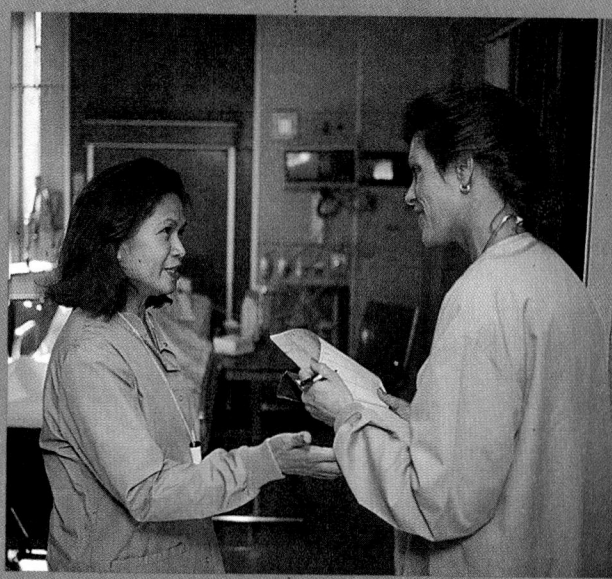

Nursing diagnosis, the second step of the nursing process, begins after assessment is complete. This step of the nursing process assigns meaning to the data collected and organized during assessment. The process of diagnosing is the culmination of the nurse's identification of specific client responses. These responses are then used as the basis for planning individualized nursing care (Collier and others, 1996). Data collected and sorted into clusters are analyzed to identify the client's responses to **health care problems.** Diagnosis means "to distinguish" or "to know." A **nursing diagnosis** is a clinical judgment about individual, family, or community responses to actual and potential health problems or life processes. Nursing diagnoses provide the basis for selection of interventions to achieve outcomes for which the nurse is accountable (North American Nursing Diagnosis Association [NANDA], 1996; Carpenito, 1995). A nursing diagnosis focuses on the client's actual or potential response to a health problem rather than on the physiological event or complication. The client's actual and potential responses are obtained from the assessment database and a review of literature, the client's past medical records, and consultation with other professionals, all of which are collected during assessment.

CRITICAL THINKING AND THE NURSING DIAGNOSTIC PROCESS

Critical thinking is a complex process (see Chapter 4). Its use in formulating a nursing diagnosis is essential.

As nursing care expands into a variety of health care settings, more aspects of critical thinking are required in diagnostic reasoning and judgment (Gordon, 1994).

Nursing diagnosis is the step of the nursing process that enables the nurse to individualize care for the client. During the diagnostic phase, the nurse uses scientific and nursing knowledge and experience to analyze and interpret data collected about the client. The nurse then identifies the client's health care problems and writes nursing diagnoses, which form the basis of a plan of care.

The use of standard formal nursing diagnostic statements endorsed by the North American Nursing Diagnosis Association **(NANDA)** serves several purposes (Box 6-1). Each diagnosis has a precise definition that gives all members of the health care team a clear understanding of the client's needs. Also, because the nursing diagnosis deals with the client's response to the illness or condition rather than the medical diagnosis, it distinguishes the nurse's role from the physician's role and helps the nurse to focus on the role of nursing.

Diagnostic Process

The **diagnostic process** consists of the decision-making steps that the nurse uses to develop a diagnostic statement (Carnevali and others, 1984; Liukkonen, 1992; Carnevali and Thomas, 1993). The nurse uses diagnostic reasoning, which uses critical thinking skills to formulate a nursing diagnosis or identify a collaborative problem (Collier and others, 1996). This process includes analysis and interpretation of data, identification of client needs, and formulation of nursing diagnoses

---

Box 6-1
NANDA-Approved Nursing Diagnoses 1997-1998

Activity intolerance	Communication, impaired verbal
Activity intolerance, risk for	Community coping, potential for enhanced
Adaptive capacity, decreased: intracranial	Community coping, ineffective
Adjustment, impaired	Confusion, acute
Airway clearance, ineffective	Confusion, chronic
Anxiety	Constipation
Aspiration, risk for	Constipation, colonic
Body image disturbance	Constipation, perceived
Body temperature, altered, risk for	Coping, defensive
Bowel incontinence	Coping, family: potential for growth
Breastfeeding, effective	Coping, ineffective family: compromised
Breastfeeding, ineffective	Coping, ineffective family: disabling
Breastfeeding, interrupted	Coping, ineffective individual
Breathing pattern, ineffective	Decisional conflict (specify)
Cardiac output, decreased	Denial, ineffective
Caregiver role strain	Diarrhea
Caregiver role strain, risk for	Disuse syndrome, risk for

From North American Nursing Diagnosis Association: *NANDA nursing diagnoses, 1997-1998*, Philadelphia, 1996, The Association.

Continued

Box 6-1
NANDA-Approved Nursing Diagnoses 1997-1998—cont'd

Diversional activity deficit
Dysreflexia
Energy field disturbance
Environmental interpretation syndrome, impaired
Family processes, altered: alcoholism
Family processes, altered
Fatigue
Fear
Fluid volume deficit
Fluid volume deficit, risk for
Fluid volume excess
Gas exchange, impaired
Grieving, anticipatory
Grieving, dysfunctional
Growth and development, altered
Health maintenance, altered
Health-seeking behaviors (specify)
Home maintenance management, impaired
Hopelessness
Hyperthermia
Hypothermia
Incontinence, functional
Incontinence, reflex
Incontinence, stress
Incontinence, total
Incontinence, urge
Infant behavior, disorganized
Infant behavior, disorganized: risk for
Infant behavior, organized: potential for enhanced
Infant feeding pattern, ineffective
Infection, risk for
Injury, perioperative positioning: risk for
Injury, risk for
Knowledge deficit (specify)
Loneliness, risk for
Management of therapeutic regimen, community: ineffective
Management of therapeutic regimen, families: ineffective
Management of therapeutic regimen, individual: effective
Management of therapeutic regimen, individuals: ineffective
Memory, impaired
Mobility, impaired physical
Noncompliance
Nutrition, altered: less than body requirements
Nutrition, altered: more than body requirements
Nutrition, altered: risk for more than body requirements
Oral mucous membrane, altered
Pain

Pain, chronic
Parent/infant/child attachment, altered: risk for
Parental role conflict
Parenting, altered
Parenting, altered, risk for
Peripheral neurovascular dysfunction, risk for
Personal identity disturbance
Poisoning, risk for
Post-trauma response
Powerlessness
Protection, altered
Rape-trauma syndrome
Rape-trauma syndrome: compound reaction
Rape-trauma syndrome: silent reaction
Relocation stress syndrome
Role performance, altered
Self-care deficit, bathing/hygiene
Self-care deficit, dressing/grooming
Self-care deficit, feeding
Self-care deficit, toileting
Self-esteem disturbance
Self-esteem, chronic low
Self-esteem, situational low
Self-mutilation, risk for
Sensory/perceptual alterations (specify) (visual, auditory, kinesthetic, gustatory, tactile, olfactory)
Sexual dysfunction
Sexuality patterns, altered
Skin integrity, impaired
Skin integrity, impaired, risk for
Sleep pattern disturbance
Social interaction, impaired
Social isolation
Spiritual distress (distress of the human spirit)
Spiritual well-being, potential for enhanced
Suffocation, risk for
Swallowing, impaired
Thermoregulation, ineffective
Thought processes, altered
Tissue integrity, impaired
Tissue perfusion, altered (specify type) (renal, cerebral, cardiopulmonary, gastrointestinal, peripheral)
Trauma, risk for
Unilateral neglect
Urinary elimination, altered
Urinary retention
Ventilation, inability to sustain spontaneous
Ventilatory weaning response, dysfunction (DVWR)
Violence, risk for: directed at others
Violence, risk for: self-directed

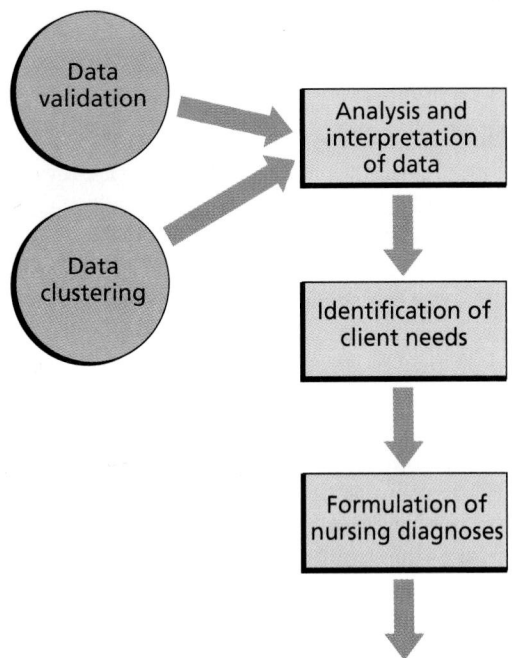

Figure 6-1.   Nursing diagnostic process.

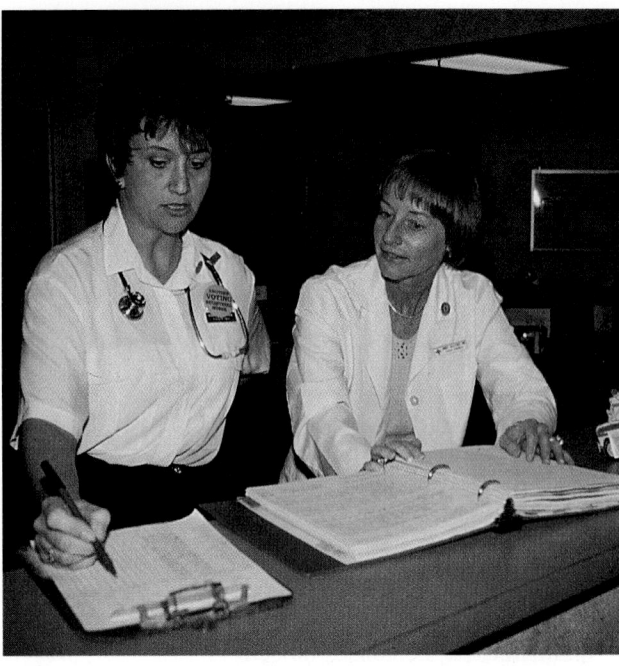

Figure 6-2.   Nurse analyzes ECG strip and other assessment data.

(Figure 6-1). Data validation and clustering follow assessment and lead to analysis and interpretation of data.

Analysis and Interpretation of Data

In the assessment phase, data are collected from a variety of sources, validated, and then sorted into clusters or categories (Figure 6-2). The database is continually revised to include changes in the client's physical and emotional status and the results of laboratory and diagnostic tests. Writing nursing diagnoses requires the nurse to draw from a knowledge and experience base, analyze and interpret data, apply diagnostic reasoning, and select the appropriate descriptor (diagnostic label) for the client need (Collier and others, 1996). It is important to review the assessment data to identify client needs and not to focus solely on the client's health problems. For example, a client with a diagnosis of *social isolation related to relocation into a retirement village* has a need to increase friends, social supports, and familiarity with new surroundings. Working with the client to resolve this nursing diagnosis may ultimately result in improving the client's independence and level of wellness and can avoid future health problems. When client needs and problems are identified, it is important for the nurse to remember that the formulation of nursing diagnoses is not solely the result of illness or physiological alterations.

Data analysis involves recognizing patterns or trends, comparing them with normal, healthful standards, and coming to a reasoned conclusion about the client's response (Box 6-2).

When looking for a pattern or trend, the nurse ex-

amines the clusters of data in the database. A cluster is a set of signs or symptoms that are grouped together in a logical order. Alone, these signs or symptoms cannot support a diagnostic label. However, when these signs are placed or clustered together as a group, the nurse is able to think about the relationship between and among these assessment findings. For example, in Chapter 5 Mrs. Bryan's assessment identified fatigue, decreased nutritional intake, weakness, and fear. Alone, these symptoms could be related to multiple nursing diagnoses, but when analyzing them together, the nurse begins to think about functional health patterns and the potential that Mrs. Bryan may not be able to safely live independently. When a relationship among these patterns is identified, a list of client-centered needs begins to emerge. The nurse groups together these clusters and patterns and looks for the presence of defining characteristics. **Defining characteristics** are the clinical criteria that support (validate) the presence of the diagnostic category. **Clinical criteria** are objective or subjective signs and symptoms, clusters of signs and symptoms, or risk factors (Carpenito, 1993, 1995). Multiple defining characteristics resulting from assessment data support the nursing diagnosis (Carpenito, 1995, 1997). Absence of these characteristics suggests that the proposed diagnosis should be rejected. Defining characteristics that either support or eliminate a particular diagnosis must be examined. Accuracy is achieved when all characteristics are evaluated, nonrelevant ones are eliminated, and relevant ones are confirmed (Collier and others, 1996) (Box 6-3).

Identification of a pattern is perhaps best demon-

Box 6-2
Example of Data Analysis

Recognize pattern (cluster of defining characteristics).
   20-lb weight loss
   Poor appetite
   Weakness
   Previous falls
Compare with normal standards.
   No weight loss
   Adequate nutritional intake
   No falls
Make a reasoned conclusion.
   Mobility and stability problems

Box 6-3
Characteristics of Accuracy of Nursing Diagnoses

The accuracy of a nursing diagnosis is relative to the interactive elements in a client situation.

The challenge of achieving high levels of accuracy ranges from simple to complex depending on the number of cues, types of cues, and characteristics of cues.

Accuracy includes the use of supporting and conflicting cues.

High degrees of accuracy of nursing diagnosis are the result of integrating all of the obtainable cues to make as precise a statement as possible.

The stringency of achieving accuracy is relative to the situation.

Low-accuracy diagnoses reflect one or more of the following characteristics:
   Use of unreliable or invalid cues
   Ignorance or misinterpretation of conflicting cues
   Lack of integration of relevant cues for other diagnoses
   Evidence that another diagnosis is more likely
   Lack of agreement with the client or other experts on the phenomena in question

From Lunney M: Accuracy of nursing diagnoses: concept development, *Nurs Diagnosis* 1:1, 1990. Reprinted with permission of Nursecom, Inc.

---

strated through the following example. Gray hair does not necessarily indicate that a person is an older adult. However, if gray hair, wrinkled skin, and age spots are clustered together, these characteristics increase the probability that the person is an older adult.

The identified pattern is then compared with data that are consistent with normal, healthful patterns. The nurse uses widely accepted norms, such as normal laboratory and diagnostic test values, and professional knowledge as the basis for comparison and judgment. When comparing patterns, the nurse judges whether the grouped signs and symptoms are normal for the client and whether they are within the range of healthful responses. Defining characteristics that are not within healthy norms are isolated and form the basis for **problem identification.**

Identification of Client Needs

As data are clustered, the nurse identifies emerging patterns of client needs. Identifying client needs enables the nurse to individualize the development of nursing diagnoses. When identifying client needs, the nurse considers all assessment data and focuses on the more relevant data. It may help the inexperienced nurse to think of this identification phase as the general health care need and the formulation of the nursing diagnosis as the specific health care need. Thus in describing the client's health care needs, the nurse moves from general to specific.

Formulation of the Nursing Diagnosis

Formulation of the nursing diagnosis results from identification of client needs. Once the assessment data are analyzed and interpreted, data are clustered into patterns and defining characteristics are identified, directing the nurse toward selection of appropriate nursing diagnoses.

NANDA has identified five types of nursing diagnoses. An **actual nursing diagnosis** is a judgment that is clinically validated by the presence of major defining characteristics. The presence of such a diagnosis indicates that sufficient assessment data are available to establish the nursing diagnosis (Collier and others, 1996).

A **risk nursing diagnosis** describes human responses to health conditions or life processes that may develop in a vulnerable individual, family, or community (NANDA, 1996). For example, an overweight client with a spinal cord injury is at *risk for impaired skin integrity.* The key assessment for this type of diagnosis is the data that support the client's vulnerability. Such data include physiological, psychosocial, familial, lifestyle, and environmental factors that increase the client's vulnerability to, or likelihood of developing, the condition.

A **possible nursing diagnosis** describes a suspected problem for which current, available data are insufficient for validation (Collier and others, 1996). This type of diagnosis, such as *fluid volume deficit,* has relevance because the nurse is directed to gather further data and relevant cues to confirm or eliminate the diagnosis. For example, a client has a history of nausea, vomiting, and diarrhea for 3 days. Further data about the client's overall level of health, age, skin turgor, intake and output, and analysis of laboratory data are needed before the nursing diagnosis can be validated. However, because of the symptoms listed earlier, *fluid volume deficit* is a possible nursing diagnosis.

Syndrome diagnosis is a diagnostic label given to a distinct cluster of nursing diagnoses that frequently go together and present a clinical picture (NANDA, 1996; Collier and others, 1996). This type of diagnosis is a useful and efficient way to describe a complex problem without documenting each component of the problem as a distinct nursing diagnosis. At present, NANDA (1996) has only approved three syndrome diagnoses. When writing these diagnoses, only the diagnostic label is used (Box 6-4).

A **wellness nursing diagnosis** is a clinical judgment about an individual, group, or community in transition from a specific level of wellness to a higher level of wellness (NANDA, 1996). This type of diagnosis is used when the client wishes to or has achieved an optimal level of health. For example, *family coping: potential for growth related to unexpected twins*. The nurse and the family unit work together to adapt to the stressors associated with twins and identify the family's strengths, resources, and needs. In doing so, the nurse incorporates the client's strength into a plan of care, with the outcome directed at an enhanced level of coping.

NURSING DIAGNOSIS STATEMENT

The nursing diagnosis statement is a way of communicating the client's health care needs. The statement itself is in a specific format, and the clinical findings from the assessment database must support the nursing diagnosis.

Nursing Diagnosis Format

The nursing diagnosis format (i.e., how the actual diagnosis is stated) flows from the diagnostic process. This format provides the beginning nurse with familiarity and rationale for the structure of a nursing diagnostic statement.

Throughout this text, nursing diagnoses are stated in a two-part format: the diagnostic label followed by a statement of related factors (Table 6-1) (Kim and others, 1997; NANDA, 1996). The diagnostic labels are categories approved by NANDA (see Box 6-1). The related factor is a condition or etiology that affects the client's actual or potential response to a health problem that can be changed by nursing interventions.

This two-part format is accepted by the majority of nursing leaders (Carpenito, 1995, 1997; Gordon, 1994). It assists the nurse in individualizing a client's nursing diagnoses and provides direction for selection of appropriate interventions. The nursing interventions are directed toward altering or resolving the etiological or related factors (McCloskey and Bulechek, 1992). This format supports the delivery of individualized nursing care for one client or a group of clients.

The nursing diagnosis is based on client needs and client response to health problems revealed in the nursing assessment. The diagnostic label is supported by defining characteristics present in the client's assessment database. The nursing diagnostic statement includes the diagnostic label (e.g., *risk for injury*) and its related factor (e.g., *related to confusion*). The diagnostic label is an actual or potential client response to health or illness. The **related factors** are etiological or other contributing conditions that have influenced the client's response (Carpenito, 1993, 1995).

The "related to" phrase identifies the etiology or cause of the problem. This is not a cause-and-effect statement; rather it indicates that the etiology con-

---

Box 6-4

Nursing Diagnoses for Clients With Disuse Syndrome

Constipation
Risk for infection
Risk for activity intolerance
Risk for injury
Impaired physical mobility
Altered thought processes
Body image disturbance
Powerlessness
Impaired tissue integrity

TABLE 6-1

NANDA Nursing Diagnosis Format

Diagnostic Statement	Related Factors
Constipation	Inadequate dietary fiber
	Effects of medications
	Inadequate fluid intake
	Decreased activity
Fatigue	Discomfort
	Excessive role demands
	Increased energy requirement
Impaired skin integrity	Fluid retention
	Excessive secretions
	Immobilization
	Altered circulation

tributes to or is associated with the problem (Figure 6-3). The inclusionary phrase "related to" requires the nurse to use critical thinking skills to individualize the nursing diagnosis and subsequent interventions (Table 6-2).

The **etiology** or cause of the nursing diagnosis must be within the domain of the nursing practice and a condition that responds to nursing interventions. Sometimes medical diagnoses are recorded as the etiology of the nursing diagnosis. This is incorrect. Nursing interventions cannot change a medical diagnosis. However, nursing interventions can be directed at behaviors or conditions that nurses can treat or manage. For example, the nursing diagnosis, *pain related to breast cancer,* is incorrect. Nursing actions cannot affect the medical diagnosis of breast cancer. Rewording the diagnosis to read *pain related to impaired skin integrity secondary to mastectomy incision* results in nursing interventions directed at reducing stress on the suture line and improving the client's comfort.

As the client's health status changes, nursing diagnoses are modified. For example, a client's pertinent assessment data may include the following: decreased dietary fiber and limited fluid intake, no bowel movement for 3 days, decreased bowel sounds, distention of the lower abdomen, hard fecal material extracted during

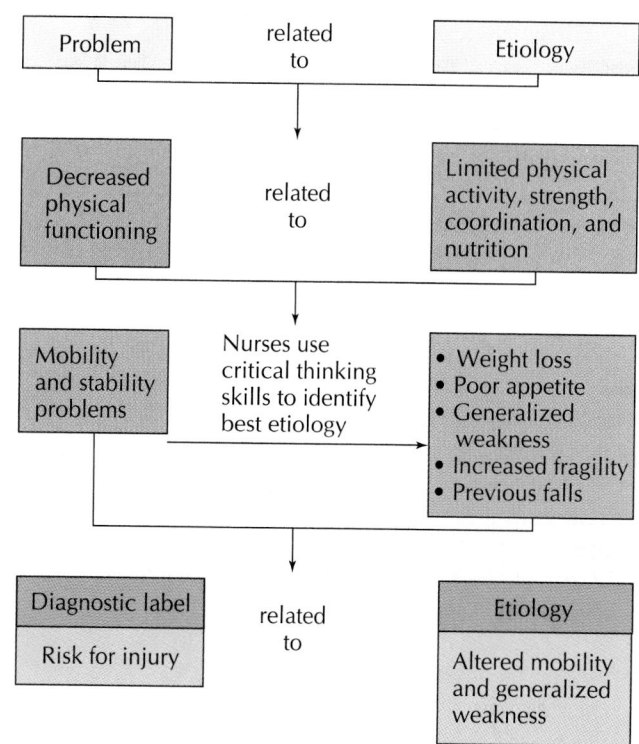

Figure 6-3. Relationship between diagnostic statement and format.

TABLE 6-2

Comparison of Interventions for Nursing Diagnoses With Different Etiologies

Nursing Diagnoses	Interventions
Client A	
Ineffective airway clearance related to obesity	Place client in high Fowler's position.
	Have client cough and deep breathe every 2 hours while awake.
	Start weight-reduction diet (1200 calories) to decrease obesity.
Feeding self-care deficit related to inability to bend arms secondary to bilateral arm casts	Encourage family to visit during meals.
	Be certain staff or family members are available to feed client.
	Provide high-calorie milkshakes with straw at 3 and 8 PM.
Anxiety related to social isolation secondary to protective isolation	Plan staffing patterns to include visits to client's room four times a day.
	Provide diversional activities.
Client B	
Ineffective airway clearance related to poor coughing technique	Teach client deep breathing and coughing.
	Splint client's abdominal incision during coughing.
Feeding self-care deficit related to inability to grasp feeding utensils	Provide large-handled eating utensils.
	Offer finger foods cut in large pieces for between-meal snacks: 10-2-8.
Social isolation related to effects of neighborhood	Provide client with phone numbers and location of local senior citizens' center.
	Draw client a map of neighborhood stores, restaurants, and libraries.

digital rectal examination, and a guaiac-negative stool specimen. The most appropriate nursing diagnosis is *constipation related to limited dietary fiber intake.*

Once the client's need is met or the health problem resolved, the nursing diagnosis no longer exists. In addition, as the client's physiological and emotional status changes, the health problem may remain relevant, but the etiology may change. Therefore the nurse must modify the nursing diagnoses or develop new nursing diagnoses as the client's needs and status change.

The modification of nursing diagnoses is ongoing. As the level of nursing care and level of wellness change, these changes are reflected in the statement of nursing diagnoses. Outdated nursing diagnoses do not accurately reflect the client's current needs.

Assessment Data and the Diagnostic Statement

Nursing assessment data must support the diagnostic label and the related factors. As nurses develop nursing diagnoses, they must ensure that the client's assessment data support the diagnostic label and etiology. It may help to identify assessment activities that produce specific kinds of data. For example, asking the client about the quality and perception of pain results in subjective data. However, palpating an area, which may elicit a grimace, provides objective information.

Box 6-5 contains an example summary of pertinent assessment data that may lead to the identification of an actual or potential health care problem. Table 6-3 demonstrates data clustering, identification of client need, and formulation of nursing diagnoses from the pertinent assessment data presented in Box 6-5.

Table 6-4 uses the three nursing diagnoses, *ineffective airway clearance, self-esteem disturbance,* and *ineffective individual coping,* to demonstrate the way that the defining characteristics and probable etiologies assist in the development of the total diagnostic label. The defining characteristics and relevant etiologies are from the text *Pocket Guide to Nursing Diagnoses* by Kim and others

---

Box 6-5

Summary of Mrs. Bryan's Relevant Assessment Data

Physical and Development
Poor appetite
Decreased food intake
Weight loss
Hemoglobin 10 g
Slight change in emphysema shown on chest x-ray film
Crackles in bilateral lung bases
Previous falls
Unsteady gait
Feels weak
Smoked for 20 years, 2 packs a day (40 pack-years)
Family history of stomach cancer
Family history of heart attack
Widowed for 4 years
Self-employed for 20 years
One adult daughter, 36 years old
Two grandchildren

Intellectual
Talkative
Knows diagnosis of stomach cancer
Good attention span

Emotional
Wants to remain independent
Fears nursing home placement
Conflict with daughter over need for autonomy

Social
Independent, lives alone
Active in her neighborhood
Supportive friend lives nearby

Spiritual
Methodist
Attends church weekly
Reads Bible daily

Box 6-6

Sources of Diagnostic Error

Collecting
Insufficient data
Too much data
Lack of knowledge or skill
Failure to generate multiple hypotheses

Interpreting
Inaccurate interpretation of cues
Failure to consider conflicting cues
Using an insufficient number of cues
Using unreliable or invalid data
Failure to consider cultural influences or developmental stage

Clustering
Insufficient cluster of cues
Premature or early closure
Incorrect clustering

Labeling
Wrong diagnostic label selected
Condition is a collaborative problem
Failure to validate nursing diagnosis with client
Failure to seek guidance

TABLE 6-3
Formulation of Nursing Diagnoses

Clustering Data	Identification of Client Need	Nursing Diagnosis Formulation
Weight loss Poor appetite Decreased hemoglobin	Excessive weight loss	Altered nutrition: less than body requirements related to poor nutritional intake
Decreased mobility Decreased stability Weight loss Poor appetite Previous falls Weakness Anemia, hemoglobin level of 10 g	Mobility and stability problems	Risk for injury related to altered mobility and generalized weakness
40 pack-year history of smoking Slight change of emphysema shown on chest x-ray film Crackles auscultated in lung fields	Risk for respiratory complications	Ineffective airway clearance related to generalized weakness
Weight loss Weakness	Change in body image	Self-esteem disturbance related to change in body image
Client's desire to remain independent Client's fear of nursing home placement Daughter's fear for her mother's comfort and safety	Conflict between mother and daughter regarding future care	Decisional conflict related to threat over loss of independence

TABLE 6-4
Defining Characteristics and Etiologies to Support Nursing Diagnoses

Defining Characteristics	Nursing Diagnoses	Etiologies ("related to")
Abnormal breath sounds Changes in rate or depth of respiration Cough Cyanosis Dyspnea Smoking history	Ineffective airway clearance	Decreased energy and/or fatigue Tracheobronchial infection, obstruction, secretion Pain
Verbal or nonverbal response to actual or perceived change in structure or function Missing or impaired body part, not looking at or touching body or body part Trauma to body Refusal to acknowledge change	Self-esteem disturbance	Biophysical (e.g., amputation or loss of function of extremity) Cognitive and/or perceptual (e.g., expressions of worthlessness and sorrow) Psychosocial (e.g., withdrawal behavior and excessive crying)
Verbalization of inability to cope Inability to meet role expectations Inability to problem solve Inability to meet basic needs Alteration in societal participation Destructive behavior Inappropriate use of defense mechanisms Verbal manipulation Change in usual communication patterns High rate of illness High rate of accidents	Ineffective individual coping	Situational crises (e.g., unexpected illness and financial difficulties) Maturational crises (e.g., marriage and parenthood)

(1997) and are derived from the NANDA classification. A complete list of the current NANDA classification of nursing diagnostic labels is in Box 6-1.

SOURCES OF DIAGNOSTIC ERRORS

Errors can occur in the diagnostic process. Such errors can occur during collecting, clustering, interpreting, and labeling data (see Box 6-6, p. 98). During data collection, care is needed to make sure that sufficient data are collected. When insufficient data exist, the nurse may fail to identify a problem. On the other hand, too much data may result in disorganized information, which may lead to confusion when identifying problems. The nurse must be skillful in the communication (see Chapter 13) and assessment processes (see Chapter 24). Lack of skill may lead to inappropriate and inaccurate data collection. Last, during the collection of data, the nurse needs to begin to make judgments regarding data interpretation and selection of the diagnostic label (Collier and others, 1996).

During data interpretation, care is taken to accurately interpret the findings from assessment. When analyzing cues, the nurse considers conflicting data. The nurse must also determine that sufficient cues are available to support the diagnostic label. Data must be reliable and valid. Therefore the nurse needs to determine that equipment used during assessment is functioning properly and that appropriate skills were used to assess the client's problems. Last, it is necessary to consider the client's developmental stage (see Chapter 20) and culture (see Chapter 18) when selecting diagnostic labels. What the nurse may incorrectly interpret as a deficit or abnormal finding may be entirely appropriate for the client's developmental state or cultural heritage.

Errors in data clustering occur when data are clustered prematurely, incorrectly, or not at all (Gordon, 1994). Premature closure of clustering occurs when the nurse makes the nursing diagnosis before all data have been grouped. Incorrect clustering occurs when the nurse tries to make the nursing diagnosis fit the signs and symptoms obtained. The nursing diagnosis should be derived from the data, not the other way around. An incorrect nursing diagnosis affects quality of care.

The last type of error that can occur is the manner in which the nursing diagnosis is stated. There are some common guidelines to reduce errors in the diagnostic statement itself. The nurse uses valid clustering of cues to select the appropriate diagnostic label and determines that the problem and etiology portions are within the scope of *nursing* to diagnose and treat. Concise wording ensures that collaborative resources from other disciplines are used appropriately. Because the client and family are often instrumental in supporting the

client's participation in the care plan, selected diagnoses should be validated and confirmed by them also.

Avoiding and Correcting Errors

Nursing diagnoses are easy to write if the nurse remembers that the problem portion of the statement is concerned with the client's response to the illness or condition and that the etiology portion must be within the scope of nursing to diagnose and treat (Box 6-7). The following suggestions should help the nurse avoid the most common errors in formulating nursing diagnoses accurately:

1. Identify the client's response, not the medical diagnosis (Carpenito, 1993, 1995). Because the medical diagnosis requires medical interventions, it is legally inadvisable to include it in the nursing diagnosis. The diagnosis, pain related to myocardial infarction, may be changed to *pain related to physical exertion*.
2. Identify a NANDA diagnostic statement rather than the symptom. Nursing diagnoses are derived from a cluster of defining characteristics; one symptom is insufficient for problem identification. For example, cough related to excessive mucus production should be written as *ineffective breathing pattern related to increased airway secretions*.
3. Identify a treatable etiology rather than a clinical sign or chronic problem. Nursing interventions are directed toward correcting the etiology of the problem. A diagnostic test or a chronic dysfunction is not an etiology or nursing intervention. Altered respiratory function related to abnormal arterial blood gases can be correctly stated as *altered*

Box 6-7
Avoiding Diagnostic Errors

Identify client's response to illness.
State a NANDA diagnostic statement.
Identify an etiology treatable by nursing.
Identify a client need associated with a treatment or test.
Identify client's response to equipment.
Identify client's, not nurse's, problem.
Identify client's problem, not interventions.
Identify client's problem, not goals.
Avoid prejudicial statements.
State the etiology legally.
Identify a problem and an etiology.
Identify only one client problem in a diagnostic statement.

peripheral tissue perfusion related to inadequate oxygen intake.

4. Identify the problem caused by the treatment or diagnostic study rather than the treatment or study itself. Clients experience many responses to diagnostic tests and medical treatment. These responses are the area of nursing concern. The diagnosis, cardiac catheterization related to angina, should be restated to read *anxiety related to lack of knowledge about cardiac catheterization.*

5. Identify the client response to the equipment rather than the equipment itself. Clients are often unfamiliar with medical technology. The diagnosis, anxiety related to cardiac monitor, can be changed to *knowledge deficit regarding the need for cardiac monitoring.*

6. Identify the client's problems rather than the nurse's problems. Nursing diagnoses are always client centered and form the basis for goal-directed care. Potential intravenous complications related to poor vascular access indicates a nursing problem in initiating and maintaining intravenous therapy. The diagnosis, *risk for infection related to presence of invasive lines,* properly centers attention on client needs.

7. Identify the client problem rather than the nursing intervention. Nursing interventions are planned to alleviate client problems. Failure to state a diagnostic label results in an inability to evaluate problem resolution. The statement, offer bedpan frequently because of altered elimination patterns, should be changed to identify the problem and etiology. *Diarrhea related to food intolerance* corrects the misstatement and allows proper implementation of the nursing process.

8. Identify the client problem rather than the goal. Goals are established in terms of client problems. If the problem is not identified, evaluation of problem resolution is difficult. Client needs high-protein diet related to potential alteration in nutrition should be changed to *altered nutrition: less than body requirements related to inadequate nutritional intake* to allow for planning to correct the etiology.

9. Make professional rather than prejudicial judgments. Nursing diagnoses are based on subjective and objective client data and should not include the nurse's personal beliefs and values. The nurse's judgment can be removed from risk for impaired skin integrity related to poor hygiene habits by changing the etiology to *lack of knowledge about perineal care.*

10. Avoid legally inadvisable statements (Carpenito, 1993, 1995). Statements that imply blame, negligence, or malpractice can result in litigation. The diagnosis, recurrent angina related to insufficient medication, implies inadequate prescription by the physician. Correct problem identification might read *pain related to improper use of medications.*

11. Identify the problem and etiology. Be careful to avoid a circular statement. Such statements are vague and give no direction to nursing care. Alteration in comfort related to pain can be changed to identify the client problem and the cause: *ineffective breathing pattern related to incisional pain.*

12. Identify only one client problem in the diagnostic statement. Every problem has different specific expected outcomes. Confusion during the planning step occurs when multiple problems are included in a nursing diagnosis. It is, however, permissible to include multiple etiologies contributing to one client problem. Pain and anxiety related to difficulty in ambulating should be restated as two nursing diagnoses, such as *impaired physical mobility related to pain in right knee* and *anxiety related to difficulty in ambulating.*

···NURSING DIAGNOSES VERSUS MEDICAL DIAGNOSES

Clients in all types of health care settings can have three types of diagnoses: nursing diagnoses, collaborative problems, and medical diagnoses. Nurses must recognize diagnoses that are independent and only require the domain of nursing and must know when the client's problems need collaborative interventions or interventions solely within the discipline of medicine. Such recognition ensures safe, efficient, appropriate care for clients within the health care delivery system.

A **medical diagnosis** is the identification of a disease condition based on a specific evaluation of physical signs, symptoms, history, diagnostic tests, and procedures. Physicians are licensed to treat diseases or pathological processes by performing surgery, prescribing medication, and ordering specific invasive and non-invasive therapies. Thus the focus of the medical diagnosis is the identification, treatment, and cure of the disease or pathological process.

A nursing diagnosis is a statement of a client's actual or potential response to a health problem that the nurse is licensed and competent to treat. It reflects the client's level of health or response to a disease or pathological process. Medical and nursing diagnoses are derived from the analysis of physiological, psychological, sociocultural, developmental, and spiritual dimensions of the client database (Figure 6-4).

The goals and objectives of a nursing diagnosis differ from those of a medical diagnosis. The goal of a nursing diagnosis is to identify actual and potential client responses, whereas the goals of a medical

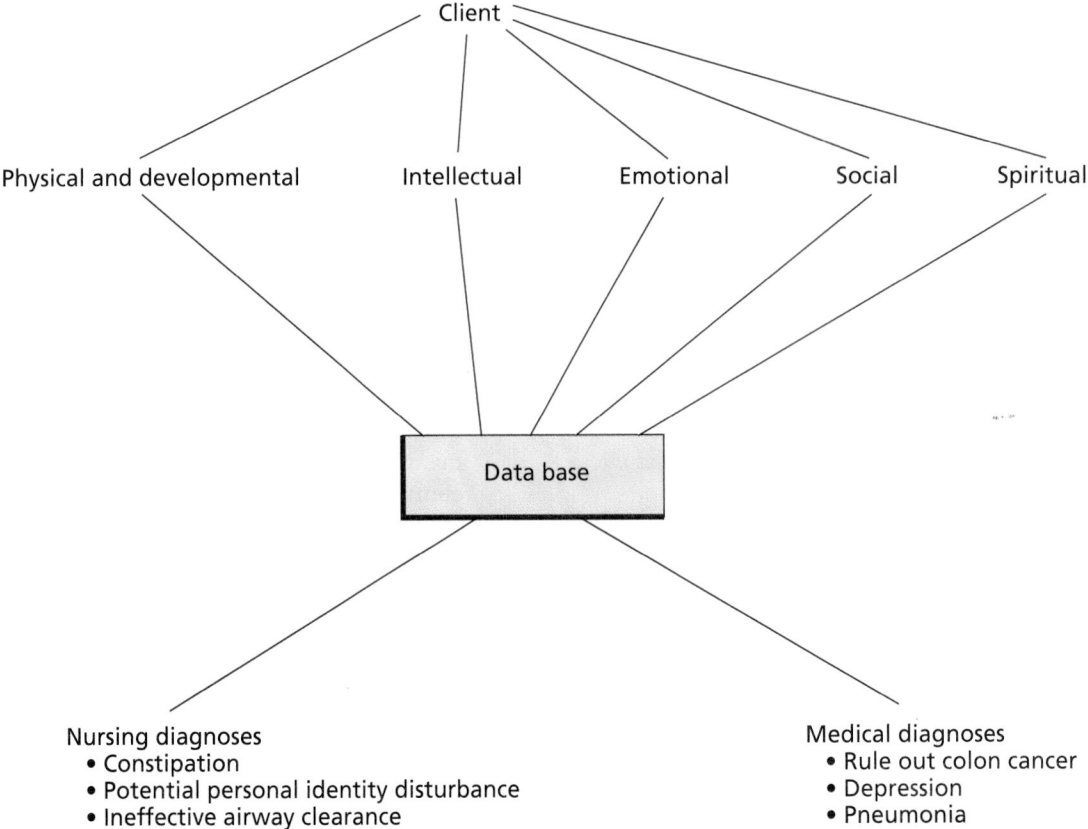

Figure 6-4. Comparison of nursing and medical diagnoses using same database.

diagnosis are to identify the cause of an illness or injury and design a treatment plan (Box 6-8).

The objective of a nursing diagnosis is development of an individualized plan of care so that the client and family can adapt to changes resulting from health problems. The objective of the medical diagnosis is to prescribe treatment. A medical diagnosis of appendicitis, for example, requires the physician to remove the infected appendix. After the appendectomy, the client may have a nursing diagnosis of *impaired physical mobility related to painful incision*. The nursing care would be directed at gradually increasing the client's mobility to preoperative levels by decreasing incisional pain.

···NURSING DIAGNOSES: APPLICATION TO CARE PLANNING

The use of nursing diagnoses is a mechanism for identifying the domain of nursing. The formulated nursing diagnoses provide direction for the planning process and the selection of nursing interventions to achieve the desired outcomes for the client. Thus expected outcomes are developed for each nursing diagnosis. The

---

| ▪ **Box 6-8** |
| **Comparison of Primary Goals: Nursing and Medicine** |

Nursing
Determines responses to health problems, level of wellness, and need for assistance
Provides physical care, emotional care, teaching, guidance, and counseling
Interventions aimed at assisting the client to meet own needs

Medicine
Determines cause of illness or injury
Provides medical treatments and surgery
Interventions aimed at preventing and curing injury or illness

From Lewis S and others: *Medical-surgical nursing: assessment and management of clinical problems,* ed 4, St. Louis, 1996, Mosby.

care plan (see Chapter 7) is a mechanism for demonstrating accountability (Carpenito, 1993, 1995, 1997). In addition, the nursing diagnoses and subsequent care plan assist in communicating to other professionals the client-centered problems through the nursing care plan, consultations, discharge planning, and client-care conferences (Zink, 1991).

Advantages

Nursing diagnoses are advantageous for the health care team, nurse, and client. Communication among nurses and other health care providers about a client's level of wellness, current needs, and discharge planning is facilitated by use of standardized NANDA-approved statements. As the list of client problems is modified, client progress becomes readily apparent and the health care team is able to effectively coordinate care. Nursing diagnoses provide a method to classify client responses to illnesses. Nursing research enables nurses to pair these client responses with specific nursing interventions and objectively measure improvements in nursing care.

The nurse benefits from the use of nursing diagnoses in two ways. Efficiency in client care is increased because the client's problems have been identified and the nurse can begin care to solve them. The nurse can then devote energies to ongoing assessment and organized problem resolution.

In addition, well-stated nursing diagnoses help to keep the nurse from straying into the realm of medical practice. Because nursing diagnoses identify responses to the medical illness or treatment, nursing care is directed specifically to actions within the standards of nursing practice. Nursing diagnoses individualized to specific health care needs result in consistent care. Nursing care is client centered, goal directed, and coordinated. The result is personalized care and effective problem resolution that promotes client and family function after discharge and return to the community.

Limitations of Nursing Diagnoses

Nursing diagnoses have limitations. Because of the continuous evolution of the phrasing and use of nursing diagnoses, the language can occasionally be wordy and contain jargon. This may limit the use of nursing diagnoses only to nursing professionals and result in confusion among other members of the health care team.

Priority Setting

Many methods can be used for **prioritization** of nursing diagnoses. One method for setting priorities reflects the biopsychosocial approach and involves looking for the most life-threatening problems, followed by problems that interfere with normal life functioning, and then those concerned with quality of life. A second method for priority setting is according to resource availability. By identifying priority nursing diagnoses, the nurse can best direct health care resources toward attaining client-centered goals (Carpenito, 1993, 1995). A final method of priority setting is by client preference. For example, a newly diagnosed diabetic may wish the nursing diagnosis *knowledge deficit regarding insulin self-administration* to have a higher priority than *knowledge deficit regarding use of a diabetic diet*. The nurse consults with the client, and, when possible, a collaborative agreement on the priority nursing diagnosis related to the client's desires for return to health and health maintenance is reached and potential problems are anticipated (Loomis and Conco, 1991).

Documentation

After analyzing assessment data, the nurse identifies the client's nursing diagnoses and decides how they should be listed on the care plan. In the clinical facility, nursing diagnoses are usually listed chronologically. When initiating the original care plan, the nurse should place the highest priority nursing diagnoses first. Thereafter, additional nursing diagnoses are added to the list. Each nursing diagnosis is dated at the time of entry. This documentation system and changes in the client's status eventually result in a list of nursing diagnoses that may not be in order of priority. When reviewing the list, the nurse must identify those nursing diagnoses with the greatest priority regardless of chronological order.

When completing a care plan class assignment, the student should list the identified nursing diagnoses in descending order of priority. Because school care plans are usually required only once for each client, the problems of ongoing identification and chronological listing of nursing diagnoses are bypassed.

Key Terms

actual nursing diagnosis	nursing diagnosis
clinical criteria	possible nursing diagnosis
data analysis	prioritization
defining characteristics	problem identification
diagnostic process	related factor
etiology	risk nursing diagnosis
health care problems	syndrome diagnosis
medical diagnosis	wellness nursing diagnosis
NANDA	

▪ Key Concepts

The statement of nursing diagnoses is the result of the diagnostic process.

The diagnostic process includes analysis and interpretation of data, identification of client and family needs, and formulation of the nursing diagnostic statement.

Nursing diagnoses state actual or potential problems in the client's health status.

Nursing diagnoses are written for the physical, developmental, intellectual, emotional, social, and spiritual dimensions of the client.

The problem and related factor portions of the nursing diagnostic statement must be within the domain of nursing to identify and treat.

Nursing diagnoses improve communication between nurses and other health professionals.

Nursing diagnoses result in efficient, high-quality care for the client.

Nursing diagnostic errors may lead to inadequate nursing care.

Nursing diagnostic errors can occur by omission or commission.

Nursing diagnostic errors can occur during assessment, data clustering, data analysis, or formulation of the diagnostic statement.

A correctly written nursing diagnosis contains a NANDA-approved diagnostic problem statement and a precise statement of the influencing factors contributing to the problem, connected by the phrase *related to*.

▪ Critical Thinking Activities

1. Describe the relationship of the nursing diagnosis step to the other steps of the nursing process.
2. During an assessment, the nurse notes that a client mentions an increase in the number of colds, sputum is thick and yellow, and an increase in shortness of breath. Which step of the diagnostic process is taking place?
3. These three nursing diagnoses are worded incorrectly. What is wrong? A. High risk of ineffective airway clearance due to pneumonia. B. Body disturbance due to anorexia nervosa. C. Fatigue and sleep disturbance related to interrupted sleep pattern.

References

Carnevali DL, Thomas MD: *Diagnostic reasoning and treatment decision making in nursing,* Philadelphia, 1993, JB Lippincott.

Carnevali DL and others: *Diagnostic reasoning in nursing,* Philadelphia, 1984, JB Lippincott.

Carpenito LJ: *Nursing diagnoses: application to clinical practice,* ed 5, Philadelphia, 1993, JB Lippincott

Carpenito LJ: *Nursing diagnoses: application to clinical practice,* ed 6, Philadelphia, 1995, JB Lippincott.

Carpenito LJ: *Nursing diagnoses: application to clinical practice,* ed 7, Philadelphia, 1997, JB Lippincott.

Collier IC and others: *Writing nursing diagnoses: a critical thinking approach,* St. Louis, 1996, Mosby.

Gordon M: *Nursing diagnosis: process and application,* ed 3, St. Louis, 1994, Mosby.

Kim MJ and others: *Pocket guide to nursing diagnoses,* ed 7, St. Louis, 1997, Mosby.

Lewis S and others: *Medical-surgical nursing: assessment and management of clinical problems,* ed 4, St. Louis, 1996, Mosby.

Liukkonen A: The nurse's decision-making process and the implementation of psychogeriatric nursing in a mental hospital, *J Adv Nurs* 17(3):356, 1992.

Loomis ME, Conco D: Patients' perceptions of health, chronic illness, and nursing diagnoses, *Nurs Diagnosis* 2(4):162, 1991.

Lunney M: Accuracy of nursing diagnoses: concept development, *Nurs Diagnosis* 1:12, 1990.

McCloskey JC, Bulechek GM: *Iowa intervention project: nursing interventions classification,* St. Louis, 1992, Mosby.

North American Nursing Diagnosis Association: *NANDA nursing diagnoses: definitions and classifications, 1995-1996,* Philadelphia, 1996, The Association.

Zink MR: Home care nurses' perception of standardized nursing diagnosis, *Home Healthcare Nurse* 9(6):27, 1991.

7

Planning for Nursing Care

OBJECTIVES

Mastery of content in this chapter will enable the student to:

- Define the key terms listed.
- Discuss the process of priority setting.
- Describe goal setting.
- List the seven guidelines of a written outcome statement.
- Discuss the difference between a goal and an expected outcome.
- Discuss the process of selecting nursing interventions.
- Define the three types of interventions.
- Discuss the differences among nurse-initiated, physician-initiated, and collaborative interventions.
- List the purposes of critical pathways.
- Describe the differences between care plans used in hospitals and community health settings.
- Describe the similarities and differences between nursing care plans and critical pathways.
- Develop a care plan from a nursing assessment.
- List the six steps involved in consultation.
- Discuss the consultation process.

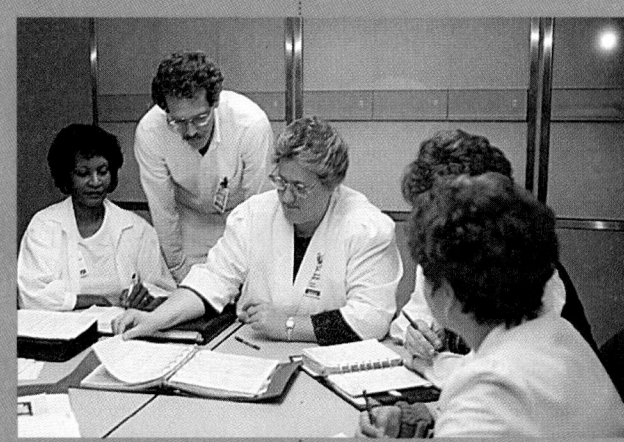

Nursing assessment and the formulation of nursing diagnoses initiate the planning step of the nursing process. **Planning** is a category of nursing behaviors in which client-centered goals are established and strategies are designed to achieve the goals. Planning requires the nurse to use deliberate decision-making and problem-solving skills to design nursing care for each client (Liukkonen, 1992). During planning, priorities are set, **goals** are determined, expected outcomes are developed, and a nursing care plan is formulated. In addition to collaborating with the client and family, the nurse consults with other members of the health care team, reviews pertinent literature, modifies care, and records relevant information about the client's health care needs and clinical management.

ESTABLISHING PRIORITIES

After formulating specific nursing diagnoses, the nurse establishes the priorities of the diagnoses by ranking them in order of importance. Priorities of care are established so that the nurse can best direct health care resources when a client has multiple problems or alterations (Carpenito, 1997).

Establishing priorities is not merely a matter of numbering the nursing diagnosis on the basis of severity or physiological importance. Rather, it is a method by which the nurse and the client mutually rank the diagnoses in order of importance based on the client's safety, desires, and needs.

Because clients have multiple nursing diagnoses, the nurse is not able to treat all of them when they are identified. The nurse selects mutually agreed-on priorities based on the urgency of the problem, the nature of the treatment indicated, and the interaction among the diagnoses (Gordon, 1994).

Priorities are classified as high, intermediate, or low (Table 7-1). Nursing diagnoses that, if untreated, could result in harm to the client or others have the highest priorities (Gordon and others, 1994). High priorities occur in both the psychological and the physiological dimensions. The nurse should avoid classifying only physiological nursing diagnoses as high priority.

Intermediate-priority nursing diagnoses involve the nonemergency, non–life-threatening needs of the client. Low-priority nursing diagnoses are client needs that may not be directly related to a specific illness or prognosis but may affect the client's future well-being.

Whenever possible, the client should be involved in priority setting. In some situations the client and nurse assign different priority rankings to the nursing diagnoses. If both place a different value on health care needs and treatments, these differences can be resolved through open communication. However, when the client's physiological and emotional needs are at stake, the nurse needs to assume primary responsibility for setting priorities.

CRITICAL THINKING AND ESTABLISHING GOALS AND EXPECTED OUTCOMES

Establishing goals and expected outcomes requires that the nurse critically evaluate the preestablished priorities, the urgency of the problems, and the resources of the client and the health care delivery system (Bandman and Bandman, 1995). Goals and expected outcomes are specific statements of client behaviors or responses that the nurse anticipates from nursing care. After assessing, diagnosing, and establishing priorities about the client's

---

TABLE 7-1
Priority Setting

Nursing Diagnoses	Rationale
High Priority	
Risk for ineffective individual coping related to anxiety about unknown medical diagnosis	Prompt intervention for anxiety will help client prepare for and cope with a diagnostic test, treatment, or diagnosis.
Risk for ineffective airway clearance after surgery related to abdominal incisional pain	Because of the risk of postoperative pulmonary complications, nurse will institute preventive client education early in nursing care.
Intermediate Priority	
Risk for altered nutrition: less than body requirements related to chronic diarrhea for 3 weeks	This nursing diagnosis does not affect client's immediate physiological or emotional status. Possible surgery will also assist nurse in resolving diagnosis.
Low Priority	
Knowledge deficit regarding smoking cessation programs	This nursing diagnosis reflects client's long-term needs.

health care needs, the nurse formulates goals and expected outcomes with the client for each nursing diagnosis (Gordon, 1994).

The purposes for writing goals and expected outcomes are twofold. First, goals and expected outcomes provide direction for the individualized nursing interventions. Second, the goals and outcomes are the focus of the nurses' evaluation to determine the effectivenes of the interventions.

In this text, the terms *goals* and *expected outcomes* are used to indicate anticipated client responses. Figure 7-1 illustrates the relationships between nursing diagnoses, goals and outcomes, and nursing interventions. Each goal and expected outcome statement must have a time frame for evaluation. The time element depends on the nature of the problem, etiology, overall condition of the client, and treatment setting.

Goals of Care

Individual nursing diagnoses and priority setting help determine the goals of care. The nursing diagnoses formulated are based on the client's response and perception of changes in level of wellness, activities of daily living, lifestyle patterns, and role performance. Because each person responds uniquely to a situation, the nursing diagnoses and client goals of health care are also unique. Bulechek and McCloskey (1985) define goals as "guideposts to the selection of nursing interventions and criteria in the evaluation of nursing interventions." Mutual goal setting involves the collaboration with the client to identify and prioritize care goals, then develop a plan to attain the goals (Bulechek and McCloskey, 1992a).

Role of the Client in Goal Setting

A **client-centered goal** is a specific and measurable objective designed to reflect the client's highest level of

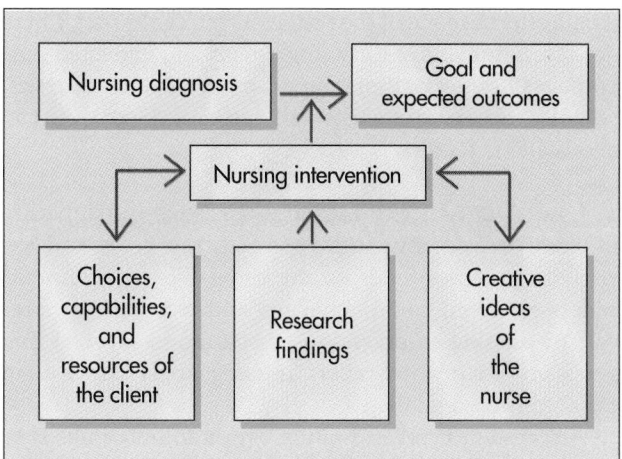

Figure 7-1. From diagnosis to outcome. (Redrawn from Gordon M: *Nursing diagnostic process and application,* ed 3, St. Louis, 1994, Mosby.)

wellness and independence in function. Whenever possible, client-centered goals are mutually set between the nurse and client.

When developing goals, the nurse also acts as an advocate for the client to ensure that the goals are realistic and to prevent further deterioration in either the level of wellness or of cognitive and physical functioning (Carpenito, 1995, 1997). When clients' cognitive and physical impairments are so severe that they cannot actively participate in goal setting, the nursing team acts in their behalf to develop client-centered goals. As the nurse practices, knowledge acquired through experience forms a basis for clinical decision making and goal setting (Miller and Babcock, 1996).

Goals should not only meet the immediate needs of the client but should also strive toward prevention and rehabilitation. Two types of goals, short-term goals and long-term goals, are developed for the client depending on the nature of the client's need or problems and the nature of the nursing services provided.

Short-term goals. A *short-term goal* is an objective that is expected to be achieved in a short time, usually less than a week (Alfaro, 1990; Carpenito, 1995, 1997). A short-term goal for a client with ineffective airway clearance, for example, may be "return of normal lung sounds within 2 days."

With the present health care system and shorter hospital stays, short-term goals are the direction for the immediate care plan.

Long-term goals. A *long-term goal* is an objective that is expected to be achieved over a longer period, usually over weeks or months (Carpenito, 1997). Long-term goals are appropriate for clients adapting to chronic illnesses who reside in long-term care facilities and for some clients in rehabilitation, mental health, ambulatory care, and community nursing settings (Carpenito, 1997). For example, a long-term goal for a client with an ineffective airway clearance may be to "remain free of upper respiratory infection for 6 months."

Goal setting establishes the framework for the nursing care plan. Table 7-2 shows the progression from nursing diagnoses to goals and expected outcomes, which are individualized to meet client needs. The first two nursing diagnoses are for the case study of Mrs. Byran, first introduced in Chapter 4. These goals often focus on prevention, rehabilitation, discharge, and health education. Through goals, the nurse is able to provide continuity of care and promote optimal use of time and resources.

Expected Outcomes

An **expected outcome** is the specific, step-by-step objective that leads to attainment of the goal and the resolution of the etiology for the nursing diagnosis (Table 7-2). An outcome is a measurable change of the

TABLE 7-2
Examples of Goal Setting With Expected Outcomes

Nursing Diagnoses	Goals	Expected Outcomes
Ineffective individual coping related to fear of negative prognosis	Client will openly discuss diagnosis.	Client will ask pertinent questions about diagnosis by 6/1. Client will express fears by 6/2. Client will identify at least two strategies for dealing with fears by 6/4.
Ineffective airway clearance related to incisional pain	Client's lungs will remain clear throughout postoperative period.	Client will turn, cough, and deep breathe every hour. Client achieves incentive spirometer goal of 90% every 2 hours. Client pain level remains ≤4 on a scale of 0-10.
Knowledge deficit regarding postoperative care at home related to inexperience	Client will state four postoperative risks before discharge.	Client drinks 2 to 3 L of fluid every day by 6/2. Client will name three signs of wound infection by 6/3. Client will demonstrate aseptic wound care by 6/3. Client will state home activity restrictions by 6/5.
Altered peripheral tissue perfusion related to postoperative venous status and risk for thrombophlebitis	Client will maintain adequate tissue perfusion by discharge.	Client performs active range-of-motion exercises every 2 hours while restricted to bed. Client's toes remain warm, dry with capillary refill of ≤2 seconds. Client increases ambulation by 50 feet every day.

client's status in response to nursing care (Carpenito, 1997; Gordon, 1994). **Outcomes** are the desired responses of a client's condition in the physiological, social, emotional, developmental, or spiritual dimensions. This change in condition is documented through observable or measurable client responses. The expected outcomes determine when a specific, client-centered goal has been met and later assist in evaluating the response to nursing care and resolution of the nursing diagnosis.

Expected outcomes have several functions. Projected before nursing actions are formulated, expected outcomes provide a direction for nursing activities (Gordon, 1987, 1994). They include observable client behaviors and measurable criteria for each goal. They also provide a projected time span for goal attainment and an opportunity to state any additional resources that may be required to achieve the goal, including additional equipment, personnel, or knowledge. Finally, the nurse uses expected outcomes as criteria to evaluate the effectiveness of nursing activities.

Expected outcomes are derived from short- and long-term client-centered goals and are based on nursing diagnoses developed during the second component of the nursing process (see Table 7-2). When writing expected outcomes, the nurse should ensure that the outcome statement is written in measurable behavioral terms. This allows the nurse to note specifically the behavior and the type of behavioral response expected for resolution of the problem. The expected outcome statements should be written sequentially, with given time frames. This provides the nurse with an order for the interventions, as well as a time reference for resolution of the problem.

Several expected outcomes are usually developed for each goal and nursing diagnosis. The rationale for the multiple expected outcomes is that few client problems can be resolved by one nursing action. In addition, the listing of the step-by-step expected outcomes gives the nurse practical guidance in planning interventions.

Guidelines for Writing Goals and Expected Outcomes

The goal should be written as a positive measure that indicates the absence of the problem (see Table 7-2). There are seven guidelines for writing goals and expected outcomes. These seven guidelines involve client-centered, singular, observable, measurable, time-limited, mutual, and realistic factors.

Client-centered factors. Because nursing care is directed from nursing diagnoses, the goals and expected outcomes focus on the client. These statements reflect expected client behaviors and responses as a result of nursing interventions. A common error is that goals are written to reflect nursing goals rather than client-centered goals.

A common error in writing expected outcomes is to write the statement as an intervention. The correct statement is, "Client will ambulate in the hall three times a day." A common error is to write, "Nursing assistant will ambulate client in the hall three times a day."

Singular factors. Each expected outcome statement should address only one behavioral response. This singularity provides a more precise method to evaluate client response to the nursing action. If the statement reads, "Client's lungs will be clear to auscultation and respiratory rate will be 22/min by 8/22," and the lungs are clear but the respiratory rate is 28/min after nursing actions, it is difficult to determine whether the expected outcome has been achieved. By splitting the statement into two parts, "Lungs will be clear to auscultation by 8/22" and "Respiratory rate will be 22/min by 8/22," the nurse can determine specifically that each outcome has been achieved.

Observable factors. The desired outcome of nursing care must be observable. Through observation, the nurse notes that the change has taken place. Observable changes can occur with changes in physiological findings or in the client's level of knowledge, comfort, or anxiety. The measurable results can be obtained by asking the client directly about the condition or by using assessment skills. Examples of outcomes involving assessment skills are, "Lungs will be clear on auscultation by 8/22" and "Wound drainage will be absent by 9/12."

Measurable factors. Goals and expected outcomes are written to give the nurse a standard against which to measure the client's response to nursing care. Examples of outcomes are "Body temperature will remain 98.6° F" and "Apical pulse will remain between 60 and 100 beats per min." A goal or an outcome that is stated in measurable terms allows the nurse to objectively quantify changes in the client's status.

Common mistakes are made when the nurse uses vague qualifiers such as "normal, acceptable, stable, or sufficient" in the expected outcome statement. Vague qualifiers have different meanings to different people. Using such terms results in guesswork in determining the client's response to care. Terms specifically describing quality, quantity, frequency, and weight allow the nurse to evaluate that the expected outcome was or was not achieved.

Time-limited factors. The time frame for each goal and expected outcome indicates when the expected response should occur. Time frames assist the nurse and client in determining that progress is being made at a reasonable rate. Time frames also promote accountability in the delivery and management of nursing care.

Time limits assist the nurse in keeping expected outcomes in order. When the date of evaluation arrives, the nurse assesses the client to determine whether that particular expected outcome has been reached. If the expected outcome is still appropriate for the client's care and has not yet been reached, another future evaluation date is set. If the expected outcome has been attained, the problem is considered resolved and is so noted on the appropriate documentation forms for the agency.

Mutual factors. Mutual setting of goals and expected outcomes ensures that the client and nurse agree on the direction and time limits of care. Mutual goal setting can increase the client's motivation and cooperation.

During this mutual setting of goals and outcomes, the nurse does not impose personal values on the client. However, the nurse must also be aware of client safety and basic human needs. Using experience and acquired knowledge, the nurse may need to direct some of the goals and expected outcomes to keep the client physically and emotionally stable and safe in the environment.

Realistic factors. Establishing realistic goals and expected outcomes can quickly provide the client and nurse with a sense of accomplishment. In turn, this sense of accomplishment can further increase the client's motivation and cooperation. When establishing realistic goals, the nurse, through assessment, must know the resources of the health care facility, family, and client; the client's physiological, emotional, cognitive, and sociocultural potential; and the costs associated with treatment and resources available to reach expected outcomes in a timely manner. Establishing goals and expected outcomes without thorough assessment of the client, environment, or resources can be frustrating to both the client and the nurse because the plan often contains unrealistic goals.

···CRITICAL THINKING AND DESIGNING NURSING INTERVENTIONS

Nursing interventions, therapies, or actions are selected after goals and expected outcomes are established. However, implementation of these interventions occurs during the implementation phase of the nursing process (see Chapter 8).

Choosing suitable nursing interventions is a decision-making process (Bulechek and McCloskey, 1987; Alfaro-LeFevre, 1995; Miller and Babcock, 1996). The nurse uses critical thinking to synthesize information from the assessment data, priority setting, knowledge, and experience to select interventions that will successfully meet the established goals and expected outcomes (Carnevali and Thomas, 1993). In addition, to initiate the intervention the nurse must be competent in three areas: (1) have knowledge of the **scientific rationale** for the intervention; (2) possess the necessary psychomotor and interpersonal skills; and (3) be able to function within a particular setting to use the available health care resources effectively (Bulechek and McCloskey, 1992b).

The method of intervention selection is always the same, but the types of interventions are individualized to the client's needs. Figure 7-1 on p. 107 illustrates the relationship of interventions to goals and expected outcomes.

Types of Interventions

McCloskey and Bulechek (1996) describe two categories of nursing interventions: nurse-initiated and physician-initiated. In addition, there are also collaborative interventions. The category selection is based on client needs. One client may require all three categories, whereas another client may need only nurse- and physician-initiated interventions.

Nurse-initiated interventions. Nurse-initiated interventions are the response of the nurse to the client's health care needs and nursing diagnoses. This type of intervention is "an autonomous action based on scientific rationale that is performed to benefit the client in a predicted way related to the nursing diagnosis and client centered goals" (McCloskey and Bulechek, 1996). Nurse-initiated interventions involve aspects of professional nursing practice encompassed by licensure and law. These interventions require no supervision or direction from others. For example, designing interventions for increasing a client's knowledge about adequate nutrition or activities of daily living related to hygiene are independent nursing actions.

In delineating the scope of nursing practice, the ANA (1980) listed 10 areas in nursing's domain (Box 7-1). This list, with the continuing work of NANDA, the

Nursing Intervention Classification (NIC) at the University of Iowa, and nurse researchers, clarifies and elaborates the realm of independent nursing practice.

Nurse-initiated interventions do not require a physician's order or an order from another professional. Physicians frequently include in their written orders the specifics of independent nursing interventions. However, according to the nurse practice acts in a majority of states, nursing actions pertaining to activities of daily living, health education, health promotion, and counseling are in the domain of nursing practice. These acts delineate the legal scope of the practice of nursing within the geographical boundaries of the jurisdiction (see Chapter 12).

Physician-initiated interventions. Physician-initiated interventions are based on the physician's response to a medical diagnosis. The nurse responds to the physician's written orders (McCloskey and Bulechek, 1996). Administering a medication, implementing an invasive procedure, changing a dressing, and preparing a client for diagnostic tests are examples of such interventions. It is not always within the legal practice of nursing for the nurse to prescribe and order these treatments, but it is within the practice of nursing for the nurse to complete such orders.

Each physician-initiated intervention involves specific nursing responsibilities and technical nursing knowledge. When administering medications, the nurse is responsible for knowing the classification of the drug, its physiological action, normal dosage, side effects, and nursing interventions related to its action or side effects (see Chapter 26). Nursing interventions associated with administering medication depend on the physician's written order.

▪ Clinical Scenario

Ms. Kline, RN, is caring for a preoperative client, Mrs. Wells, who has the following medication order: "Atropine sulfate, 0.4 mg intramuscular at 8 AM today." Ms. Kline recalls that atropine is an anticholinergic medication and that the desired preoperative effect is to control salivation, bronchial secretions, and rhinorrhea during surgical anesthesia. She consults a preprinted drug resource to determine that 0.4 mg is an appropriate preoperative dose. Ms. Kline prepares Mrs. Wells for the injection and tells Mrs. Wells to expect an increase in thirst caused by this medication. After administration of the drug, she observes the client for side effects such as flushing, tachycardia, restlessness, or disorientation, and she records in the client's medication administration record (MAR) that the drug has been administered.

With an invasive procedure or dressing changes, the nurse is responsible for knowing when the procedure is necessary, the clinical skills necessary to complete it, and its expected outcome and possible side effects; the nurse is also responsible for adequate preparation of the client and proper communication of the findings and results.

Box 7-1
Delineation of Nursing Practice

Self-care limitations
Impaired functioning in areas such as rest, sleep, ventilation, circulation, activity, nutrition, elimination, skin, or sexuality
Pain and discomfort
Emotional problems related to illness and treatment, life-threatening events, or daily experiences such as anxiety, loss, loneliness, or grief
Distortion of symbolic function, reflected in interpersonal and intellectual processes such as hallucinations
Deficiencies in decision making and the ability to make personal choices
Self-image changes required by health status
Dysfunctional perceptual orientations to health
Strains related to life processes such as birth, growth and development, and death
Problematic affiliative relationships

From American Nurses Association: *Nursing: a social policy statement*, Kansas City, Mo, 1980, The Association.

When a specific diagnostic or laboratory test is ordered by a physician, the nurse is responsible for scheduling the test, preparing the client, and knowing the normal findings and nursing implications associated with it.

Collaborative interventions. **Collaborative interventions** are therapies that require the knowledge, skill, and expertise of multiple health care professionals. For example, in the clinical scenario introduced in Chapter 4, Mrs. Bryan is a 78-year-old widow, living alone in a rural community. She has inoperable stomach cancer, and has just recently moved into the home of her friend. Mrs. Bryan's overall goal and health care need is to remain independent. Because of poor appetite and subsequent weight loss, she is very weak. She needs interventions from multiple health care professionals, as well as community resources. Inez Santiago, Mrs. Bryan's nurse, schedules a visit with a home health aide, an occupational therapist (OT), and a physical therapist (PT). During their visit, the OT and PT evaluate Mrs. Bryan's safety and tolerance for certain activities of daily living, modify the home to remove risks to safety, establish an exercise program, and develop a schedule of interventions to be completed by the home health aide. The weekly plan now includes one visit by the nurse, two visits from the home health aide, and one visit from the OT or PT, on alternating weeks. Thus in addition to Mrs. Bryan living with a friend, there is a total of four visits a week to Mrs. Byran's home. Her daughter is more accepting of her mother's recent move. The care for this client requires the coordination of collaborative interventions from multiple health care professionals all directed toward the long-term goal of maintaining Mrs. Bryan's independence and safety, as well as supporting her level of health.

Nurse-initiated, physician-initiated, and collaborative interventions require critical nursing judgment and decision making. When encountering physician-initiated or collaborative interventions, the nurse does not automatically implement the therapy but must determine whether it is appropriate for the client. Every nurse faces an inappropriate or incorrect order at some time. The nurse with a strong knowledge base will recognize the error and seek to correct it. The ability to recognize incorrect therapies is particularly important when administering medications or implementing procedures. An error can occur in writing the order or transcribing it to the Kardex or medication card. Clarifying an order is competent nursing practice, and it protects the client and members of the health care delivery system. The nurse carrying out an incorrect or inappropriate intervention is as much in error as the person who wrote or transcribed the original order and is liable for any complications resulting from the error. Chapter 19 explains legal issues affecting nursing practice.

Selection of interventions. The nurses uses clinical decision making skills when selecting nursing interventions. Specifically, the nurse considers six factors when choosing interventions for a client: (1) characteristics of the nursing diagnosis, (2) expected outcomes, (3) research base (nursing knowledge) for the intervention, (4) feasibility of the intervention, (5) acceptability to the client, and (6) competency of the nurse (Bulechek and McCloskey, 1987; McCloskey and Bulechek, 1996) (Box 7-2). To achieve this the nurse also reviews standardized care plans, textbooks, and nursing and related

---

Box 7-2
Choosing Nursing Interventions

Characteristics of the Nursing Diagnosis
Interventions must be directed toward altering the etiological factors or signs and symptoms associated with the diagnostic label.
Interventions may be directed toward altering or eliminating risk factors, which are associated with *"risk for"* nursing diagnoses.

Expected Outcomes
Outcomes are stated in measurable terms and used to evaluate the effectiveness of the interventions.

Research Base for the Intervention
Review clinical nursing research related to diagnostic label and client problem.
Review articles that describe the utilization of research findings in similar clinical situations and settings.

Feasibility of the Intervention
Interaction of nursing interventions with treatments being provided by other health professionals.
Cost: Is intervention both clinically effective and cost efficient?
Time: Are time and personnel resources well managed?

Acceptability to the Client
Treatment plan must be congruent with client's goals and health care values.
Mutually decided nursing goals.
Client must have required self-care abilities or have a person who can assist with health care.

Competency of the Nurse
Knowledgeable of scientific rationale for the intervention.
Possession of necessary psychosocial and psychomotor skill to complete interventions.
Ability to function within setting and effectively and efficiently use health care resources.

Modified from Bulechek GM, McCloskey JC: Nursing interventions: what they are and how to choose them, *Holistic Nurs Pract* 1(3):36, 1987.

health care literature and collaborates with other health care professionals. During deliberation, the nurse reviews client needs, priorities, and previous experiences to select nursing interventions that have the best potential for achieving the expected outcomes. As the nurse gains experience, selection of interventions becomes more efficient and experienced based (Benner, 1984).

Research of standardized care plans, textbooks, and nursing and related literature addresses usual problems and nursing actions for given conditions. Although they are written in general terms, the nurse may use these resources to acquire new knowledge. This knowledge then assists in the individualization of the intervention.

Collaboration completes the selection of interventions. Through collaboration the nurse is able to use the best resources to individualize the nursing actions to meet the expected outcomes. During collaboration the nurse includes the client to select suitable interventions. The collaboration process is discussed in a later section of this chapter.

The NIC project, developed at the University of Iowa, is a system to classify 336 direct care treatments that nurses perform (McCloskey and Bulechek, 1996). The purpose of the NIC is to provide standardization of language for nursing treatments that will facilitate communication and documentation of care among health care personnel (Carter and others, 1995). The classification is designed to be comprehensive, including independent and collaborative interventions, which cover all specialty areas (Carter and others, 1995).

The interventions were subdivided into six domains, which comprise the Taxonomy of Nursing Interventions. There are five major advantages of the taxonomy. First, the domains and classes help clinicians locate and select interventions appropriate to their clients. Second, the taxonomy helps in the design and revision of curricula for beginning and advanced nurses. Third, the structure of the taxonomy permits numerical coding, which can facilitate computer use and ease in analysis of data (Iowa Intervention Project [IIP], 1993). This feature assists in furthering nursing knowledge through nursing research (Carter and others, 1995). Fourth, the taxonomy can easily be expanded to include more interventions. Last, the taxonomy provides a mechanism to effectively determine the cost of nursing care (IIP, 1993; Carter and others, 1995).

Usually the nurse will have more interventions than are necessary to meet the desired outcome. Some are discarded as inappropriate, and others are adapted to the client's needs and abilities. As a result, the list of possible interventions is narrowed down to those suitable to the client (Redman, 1993). These interventions are then written on the nursing care plan.

NURSING CARE PLAN

One product of the planning component is the nursing care plan, which is based on assessment data, the client's nursing diagnoses, and priorities. Generally, nursing care plans involve the following areas: a nursing diagnostic statement, goals, expected outcomes, and specific nursing activities and interventions.

Purpose of Care Plans

The nursing care plan is a written guideline for client care. The care plan also coordinates nursing care, promotes continuity of care, and lists outcome criteria to be used in the evaluation of nursing care. In addition, the written care plan communicates to other nurses and health care professionals pertinent assessment data, a list of problems, and therapies. A written care plan decreases the risk of incomplete, incorrect, or inaccurate care.

The care plan is organized so that any nurse can quickly identify the nursing actions to be delivered. In hospitals, outpatient settings, and community-based settings, the client often receives care from more than one nurse, physician, allied health professional, and health technician. The written nursing care plan makes possible the coordination of nursing care, subspecialty consultations, and scheduling of diagnostic tests.

The care plan can also identify and coordinate resources used to deliver nursing care. The listing of specific equipment and supplies necessary for nursing actions is an economically efficient mechanism for selecting equipment. If all equipment and supplies are included in the care plan, the nurse's time is used more effectively in providing care as opposed to locating supplies.

The nursing care plan enhances the continuity of nursing care by listing specific nursing actions necessary to achieve the goals of care. These nursing activities can be carried out throughout the day and from day to day. A correctly formulated nursing care plan facilitates the continuity of care from one nurse to another. As a result, all nurses have the opportunity to deliver the same high quality care.

Written nursing care plans organize information exchanged by nurses in change-of-shift reports. Nurses focus these reports on nursing care and treatments delineated in care plans. At the end of nursing care, nurses discuss care plans with the next care givers. Thus all nurses are able to discuss current and pertinent information about the client's care plan.

The written care plan can also be adapted to the discharge needs of the client. Incorporating the goals of the care plan into discharge planning is particularly important for a client who will be undergoing long-term rehabilitation in the community. The adaptation of the care plan enhances the continuity of nursing care between nurses working in hospital settings and those working in community agencies.

Same-day surgeries and earlier discharges from hospitals require the nurse to begin planning discharge needs from the moment the client enters a health care agency. Mortensen and McMullin (1986) note that incomplete assessments and the absence of measurable outcome criteria extend client stays in short-term, 1-day surgical centers. Client stays were lengthened because there were no documented, measurable criteria for discharge readiness on the postoperative nursing care plan, resulting in confusion among all the health care professionals as to when the client could safely be discharged from the setting.

When developing an individualized care plan, the nurse involves the family and client. The family is a resource that can be used to help the client meet health goals. In addition, meeting some of the family's needs can improve the client's level of wellness.

The final component on the nursing care plan is the expected outcome criteria used in evaluation of care. Proper listing of the outcome criteria provides the nurse with objective statements that help determine whether the goals of care have been achieved.

The complete care plan is the blueprint for nursing action. It provides direction for implementation of the plan and a framework for evaluation of the client's response to nursing actions.

Care Plans in Various Settings

The structure of the nursing care plan varies from one health care setting to another. For example, the care plan used in a hospital is different from one used in a community health setting. The nursing care plan developed for the client returning home is usually based solely on long-term health needs. In addition, the client and family are more involved and assume more responsibility for care because the client is receiving nursing care in the home. Although the structure of the care plan varies depending on the setting, its overall purpose is to provide a written guideline for care so that the health care needs of the client and subsequent therapies are communicated among the health care team.

Institutional care plans. Institutional (staff) care plans are concise documents that become part of the client's medical record. Many hospitals use the Kardex nursing care plan. **Kardex** is a trade name for a card-filing system that allows quick reference to the particular needs of the client for certain aspects of nursing care. Each card is folded once. Information about medications, activity levels, level of self-care, diet, treatments, and procedures is usually included on the outside of the card. The nursing care plan is commonly placed on the inside (Figure 7-2). Each institution has its own format for the Kardex, but the basic information contained on it is universal. The care plan section of the Kardex also has institutional variations. One institution might use a three-column nursing care plan, which includes the problem, goal, and nursing action. Another institution may incorporate a four-column nursing care plan, which includes the nursing diagnosis, goal, nursing action, and evaluation. As the five-step nursing process has gained popularity, the nursing care plan on the Kardex in many hospitals has been revised to include the following components of the nursing process: assessment, nursing diagnosis, implementation, and evaluation (see Figure 7-2).

Computerized care plans. The use of computers and the need to efficiently organize the nurse's time have resulted in standardized care plans, which are forms created for a specific clinical problem (e.g., pain, immobility) that is commonly found in a clinical area (e.g., coronary care, abdominal surgery, postpartum, and same-day surgery units). Each care plan lists generalized nursing diagnoses, goals, outcome criteria, and interventions that can apply to specific clients.

After completing a nursing assessment, the nurse, using a computerized format, determines whether it should be used for that particular client. Even if the care plan is generally appropriate for a client, the nurse must add or delete information on the standardized form to individualize the plan for the client's needs. Failure to do so can result in incomplete and inaccurate care.

Computerized/standardized nursing care plans are a method to streamline and augment care planning, and they provide documentation for third-party reimbursement (Hirtzel-Trexler, 1994) (see Chapter 14). They are designed to incorporate current practice guidelines to achieve the desired client outcomes for a specific group of clients. In addition, these plans encourage the nurse to incorporate individual client care needs into the plan of care (Hirtzel-Trexler, 1994).

Student care plans. Nursing students learn to write and use a nursing care plan as part of their education. The student care plan is essential for learning the problem-solving technique, the nursing process, skills of written and verbal communication, and organizational skills needed for nursing care. Most important, by using the nursing care plan, students can learn to apply the knowledge gained from nursing and medical literature and the classroom to a practice situation.

The student care plan is often more elaborate than a care plan in a hospital or community health care agency, because its purpose is to teach the process of planning care. To learn the care-planning process, the student must progress in a step-by-step manner, beginning with assessment and ending with evaluation. Student care plans vary from one educational program to another and between beginning and more advanced students. Some educational institutions model the student care plan on the care plan used in the affiliated health care agency.

The only modification may be that the instructor requires the beginning student to include the scientific rationale for the nursing actions selected (Table 7-3). A scientific rationale is the reason that, based on supporting literature, a specific nursing action was chosen.

Medical Diagnosis and other pertinent medical information:				1083 13160 23-4

Medical Diagnosis and other pertinent medical information:

10/25 LBP c̄ RLE SCIATICA
10/26 LAMINECTOMY L4-L5 c̄ BONE GRAFT

1083 13160 23-4
SMITH, PHIL

Condition SATIS   PMH:
Allergies (Drugs, food, other) PCN, ASA, CODEINE   DM

Adm. Date 10/23 | Age 64 | Religion CATH | Mode of Travel
Service ORTHO | Doctor FORD | Resident KOWALSKI | Intern | Stamp Addressograph Plate Here

FREQUENTLY ORDERED ITEMS		Date	Specimens/Daily Lab	Date	Treatments
Temp.		10/25	ADM. BLOOD WORK	10/24	BR AND LOGROLL q 2°
Pulse & Resp. / 94°		10/25	UA c̄ MICRO		
BP		10/25	BS		
I & O 98°					
Weights					
Spot Checks					
Chest P.T.					
Incentive Spirometer					
P.T.					

ACTIVITIES	NUTRITION	Date	Diagnostic Procedures	
Ad lib	Diet REGULAR	10/25	MYELOGRAM	
Ambulate X 2			CT SCAN	
Chair				
BRP	Feedings	10/25	CXR	
Bedrest		10/25	EKG	
Bath Self				
Tub	Assist c̄ meals			
Shower	FLUID BALANCE			
Bed ✓	Force			
Assist.	D E N			
	Restrict			
	D E N			
Orderlies Needed				
Family:				

NURSING CARE PLAN

Date	Nursing Diagnosis	Expected Outcomes	Nursing Plan/Orders
10/26	ALTERED COMFORT, PAIN	1. Pt. REQUESTS FOR PAIN MED. DECREASES BY 10/30 2. Pt. RESPIRATORY EXPANSION ↑ BY 10/28	1. ENCOURAGE PATIENT TO SPLINT INCISION WHEN TURNING 2. INSTRUCT PATIENT IN RELAXATION EXERCISES
10/27	IMPAIRED PHYSICAL MOBILITY RELATED TO PAIN	1. Pt. INCREASES AMBULATION FROM BID TO QID OR GREATER 2. Pt. ASSUMES ADL BY 10/31	1. AMBULATE IN HALL c̄ PT 20 MINUTES AFTER ADMINISTRATION OF ANALGESIC 2. ENCOURAGE FAMILY TO WALK PATIENT 1. ALLOW Pt. EXTRA TIME TO DO SELF CARE FOR HYGIENE NEEDS

Discharge Planning: Destination: | Transportation: | Probable Date: | Referral Agencies | Appointment:
| | | Supplies:

Patient Name

Figure 7-2. Nursing care plan on a nursing Kardex.

Care plans for community-based settings.
Planning care for clients in community-based settings (e.g., clinics, community centers, client's home) involves using the same principles of nursing practice. However, in these settings the nurse must complete a more comprehensive community, home, and family assessment. In this setting the client/family unit is in equal partnership with health care professionals (Bond and others, 1994). Ultimately the client/family must be able to independently provide the majority of health care. The nurse designs a plan to (1) educate the client/family about the necessary care techniques, (2) teach the client/family how to integrate care within family activities, and (3) assist the client/family to gradually assume a greater percentage of care in graduated increments (Bond and others, 1994; Lund, 1994). Last, the plan is designed to include the evaluation of expected outcomes by nurses, clients, and families.

TABLE 7-3
Scientific Rationale for the Student Care Plan

Assessment	Goals	Implementation	Rationale	Expected Outcomes
Nursing diagnosis: Risk for impaired skin integrity related to immobility resulting from coma				
Definition: Risk for impaired skin integrity is the state in which an individual's skin is at risk of being adversely altered.★				
Fever: higher than 102° F for 72 hours Diaphoresis Incontinence of urine	Skin remains intact. Skin is free of pressure.	Turn client every 2 hours in following sequence: 8 AM—supine 10 AM—left side Noon—prone Repeat, beginning with supine position.	Critical time for skin tissue breakdown is between 1 and 2 hours of constant pressure.†	No skin breakdown is noted. Skin color, temperature, and capillary return are normal.
Decreased skin turgor No skin breakdown noted		Keep client's skin dry at all times.	Moisture increases maceration of skin and promotes bacterial growth.‡	Skin remains dry and intact. Skin turgor is improved.

★Data from Kim MJ, McFarland GK, McLane AM: *Pocket guide to nursing diagnoses,* ed 5, St. Louis, 1993, Mosby.
†Data from Bereck KH: *Nurs Clin North Am* 10(1):160, 1975.
‡Data from Kavchack-Keys MA: *Nurs* 77(7):60, 1977.

Critical Pathways

Critical pathways allow staff from all disciplines, such as medicine, nursing, and pharmacy, to develop integrated care plans for a projected length of stay or number of visits for clients with a specific case type (Figure 7-3). For example, the pathway in Figure 7-3 is for a lung transplant evaluation, which recommends on a day-by-day basis the client's activities, consults, procedures, and discharge planning activities, as well as educational topics expected for the client's progression through the transplantation process. The nurse and other health team members use the pathway to monitor a client's progress and as a documentation tool. Because of the arrival of managed care (see Chapter 2), documentation tools that integrate the standards of care for multiple disciplines are necessary. Critical pathways, also called CareMaps, meet this need, and charting by exception is frequently the method of choice (see Chapter 14). When using critical pathways to plan care, many other forms (e.g., the nursing care plan, flow sheets, nurse's notes) are eliminated, because all the pertinent components are included in the pathway format.

WRITING THE NURSING CARE PLAN

As an initial step in planning, the nurse assigns a priority to each nursing diagnosis. Priority can be based on Maslow's hierarchy of needs, urgent client physiological and safety needs, and important needs perceived by the client. The nursing diagnosis with the highest priority is the beginning point for the nursing care plan and is followed by other nursing diagnoses in order of assigned priority.

When using the five-column plan (Figure 7-4), in the assessment column (column 1) the nurse includes all data relevant to the corresponding nursing diagnosis (column 2). The nurse includes the previously developed goals in the next column (column 3). At this point the nurse begins to translate the short- and long-term goals into action plans that anticipate the needs of the client, coordinate nursing care, and use appropriate nursing measures.

The nurse writes the action plan in the implementation column (column 4) of the care plan. Each nursing action is written to include specific information necessary to accurately and consistently implement nursing care. It may help the beginning nurse to ask whether the plan answers the following questions:

1. What is the intervention?
2. When should each intervention be implemented? For how long?
3. How should the intervention be performed?
4. Who should be involved in each aspect of intervention?

In addition, the nurse should understand the reason for a specific intervention. Nonspecific nursing interventions result in incomplete or inaccurate nursing care, lack of continuity among care givers, and poor use of resources.

Common errors in writing nursing interventions include omissions regarding the action, frequency,

		CARE PATH®		
		501		
		LUNG TRANSPLANT EVALUATION		

BARNES

SERVICE	PHYSICIAN		
PRIMARY NURSE	PRIMARY NURSE		
DC DATE	ADM DATE	DATE OF SURGERY	**A-8**

Problem Number	PATIENT PROBLEMS / NURSING DIAGNOSES
#1	LACK OF KNOWLEDGE R/T LUNG TRANSPLANT EVALUATION EXPERIENCE
#2	DECREASE IN EXERCISE CAPACITY R/T IMPAIRED OXYGENATION/VENTILATION/DECONDITIONING
#3	POTENTIAL FOR ALTERATION IN COPING R/T SITUATIONAL CRISIS/TRANSITION
#4	POTENTIAL FOR ALTERATION IN FAMILY PROCESSES R/T SITUATIONAL CRISIS/TRANSITION
#5	POTENTIAL FOR ALTERATION IN NUTRITION R/T INAPPROPRIATE INTAKE/DYSPNEA
#6	IMPAIRED GAS EXCHANGE R/T ALVEOLAR-CAPILLARY MEMBRANE CHANGE/ALTERED BLOOD FLOW *IF APPROPRIATE

#	1 - 12	1 - 12	1 - 2, 6 - 8, 12	2, 10, 12	1
	ASSESSMENT / MONITORING	CONSULTS	PROCEDURES / TEST	TREATMENT	ACTIVITY
PRE ADMIT		Transplant office to preschedule following as needed for pt.: 2-D Echo, Quant. V-Q, Resting RVG, PFTs, MRI, Cardiac Cath, Chest CT, Transesophageal echocardiogram			
DAY 1	Braden scale Respiratory status Fall prevention Assess/individualize pt. problem list	Notify consults as per orders. Check with transplant P.A. for additional tests which may be needed. SMA 6 and 12, CBC, CMV, HSV, EBV, Vz titers, HbsAq, HbsAb, HIV, Hep. A, Hep. C titers, T & S, PT, PTT HLA (A,B,C,DR) Typing, incl. cytotoxic screen, u/a - routine & micro, CXR-AP & lat EKG	Apply skin tests 07 } Nursing, Pulm. Rehab., 08 } & H.O. 09 10 11 } 12 } Psychologist 13 14 } CDL 15 } 16 } PFTs } 17 } } Chaplain 18 } 19 Cardiology Consult 20	Appropriate bed surface for Braden scale O$_2$ • At rest • Activity CPT x1 x2 x3 x4 by Nursing, Physical Therapy, family Aerosols x1 x2 x3 x4 (Self)	Continue activity as done at home

SIGNATURE	INIT.	SIGNATURE	INIT.	SIGNATURE	INIT.

3100-45 (REV. 10/93)

Copyright 1993, Barnes Hospital - All Rights

501

Figure 7-3.   Critical pathway. (Courtesy Barnes-Jewish Hospital, St. Louis.)

Assessment	Nursing Diagnosis	Goals	Implementation	Evaluation
Weight loss: 15 lb in 10 days. Eats only 10% of meal due to feeling of fullness immediately after beginning meal.	Altered nutrition: less than body requirements related to sensation of fullness with meals.	Client will maintain weight during hospitalization. Client will eat 100% of meal by 2/4.	Weigh daily at 7 AM on scale #3. Small, frequent, high-calorie feedings at 08-10-12-14-16-18. Assist client to high Fowler's position for each meal.	Weight remains at 185 lb. Client consumes all food on meal tray.

Figure 7-4. Five-column nursing care plan.

TABLE 7-4

Frequent Errors in Writing Nursing Interventions

Type of Error	Incorrectly Stated Nursing Intervention	Correctly Stated Nursing Intervention
Failure to precisely or completely indicate nursing actions	Turn client every 2 hours.	Turn client every 2 hours, using the following schedule: 2 PM—right side / 8 AM—supine / 10 AM—left side / Noon—prone — Repeat at 4 PM and 2 AM
Failure to indicate frequency	Observe client cough and deep breathe.	Observe client cough and deep breath at 10 AM—2 PM—6 PM—10 PM
Failure to indicate quantity	Provide mouthwash to client every 2 hours while awake: 8-10-12-2-4-6-8-10.	Provide 50 ml of H_2O_2 mouthwash to client every 2 hours while awake: 8-10-12-2-4-6-8-10.
Failure to indicate method	Change client's dressing once a shift: 6 AM—2 PM—10 PM.	Replace client's dressing with Neosporin ointment to wound and two dry 4 × 4 dressings secured with hypoallergenic tape, once a shift: 2 PM—10 PM—6 AM.
Failure to indicate person to perform the action	Irrigate nasogastric (NG) tube every 2 hours (even) around the clock.	Irrigate NG tube every 2 hours (even) around the clock with 30 ml NS.

---

quantity, method, or person to perform them. These errors can occur if the nurse is unfamiliar with the planning process. Table 7-4 illustrates these types of errors by showing incorrect and correct statements of nursing interventions.

Column 5 of the nursing care plan contains the projected outcome criteria previously identified. Listing the criteria on the care plan gives a written estimation of when the goal of care has been achieved, thus indicating when a particular nursing diagnosis is no longer relevant to the client's plan of care.

···WRITING CRITICAL PATHWAYS

The writing of a critical pathway is a lengthy process, involving all members of a multidisciplinary health care team. Often it takes many weeks of research and review for a team to agree on the components of a critical pathway. Once developed, critical pathways become a case management tool, which delineates desired interventions and client outcomes within specific time frames (Windel, 1994). To write and use a critical pathway the nurse must understand each component of the nursing process (Zander and McGill, 1994). Critical pathways are multidisciplinary, outcome-based care plans.

Critical pathways not only delineate specific care but also provide a mechanism for timely revision of the plan of care (Zander, 1988). This method of care delivery reframes the work of nursing and other disciplines so that it is clear to the health care team and to the client and family (Zander, 1988; Zander and McGill, 1994). When writing a critical pathway, the team must be familiar with other pathways developed in the agency and the literature as it is related to a specific disease or surgical procedure. The pathway developed for a medical condition or procedure delineates related nursing diagnoses and the interventions to be administered by all health team members. Expected outcomes are developed during the planning phase, and a specific time interval for achieving the outcome is included. In addition, the critical pathway is written so that all members of the health care team can document delivery of care or changes in a client's status (see Chapter 14).

CONSULTING OTHER HEALTH CARE PROFESSIONALS

Consultation may occur at any step in the nursing process but is needed most often in the planning and intervention steps, because the nurse is more likely to identify a problem requiring additional knowledge or skills or a need to obtain community or agency resources. **Consultation** is a process in which a specialist's (such as a dietitian or clinical nurse specialist) help is sought to identify ways to handle problems in client management or problems related to the planning and implementation of programs. Consultation is based on the problem-solving approach, and the consultant is the stimulus for change.

Consultation completes the selection of interventions. Through consultation and collaboration the nurse is able to tap the best resources to individualize the nursing actions to meet the expected outcomes (Carpenito, 1997).

When to Consult
The need for consultation in nursing occurs when the nurse has identified a problem that cannot be solved using personal knowledge, skills, and resources. Consultation increases the nurse's knowledge about the problem and helps in learning skills and obtaining the resources needed to solve the problem. After the consultation the nurse may be able to resolve similar problems in the future.

Consultation is also used when the exact problem remains unclear. A consultant who is objectively entering a situation is often able to more clearly assess and identify the exact nature of the problem and determine whether it is client oriented, personnel oriented, or equipment oriented. An unbiased consultant can often objectively identify the problem and outline a method for resolving it.

How to Consult
The first step in the consultation process is identification of the general problem area, which provides the consultant with a starting point. Second, the consultation should be directed to the appropriate professional, who may be another nurse or another member of the health care team (Figure 7-5). A consultation requested of the wrong individual delays problem solving and diminishes the quality of care delivered to the client.

Third, the nurse provides the consultant with pertinent information about the problem area. Pertinent information includes a brief summary of the problem, methods used to resolve the problem, and outcome of those methods. Other resources may include the client's medical record and conversations with nurses, other members of the health team, and the client's family.

Fourth, the nurse should not bias consultants. Consultants are in the clinical setting to help identify and resolve a nursing problem, and biasing them can hinder problem resolution. Bias can be avoided by not overloading consultants with subjective and emotional conclusions about the client and problem.

Fifth, the nurse requesting consultation should be available to discuss the consultant's findings and recommendations. When a consultation is requested, the nurse provides a private, comfortable atmosphere in which the consultant and client can meet. However, this does not mean that the nurse leaves the environment. A common mistake is turning the whole problem over to the consultant. The consultant is not there to take over the problem but to assist the nurse in resolving it. When possible, the nurse requiring assistance should request

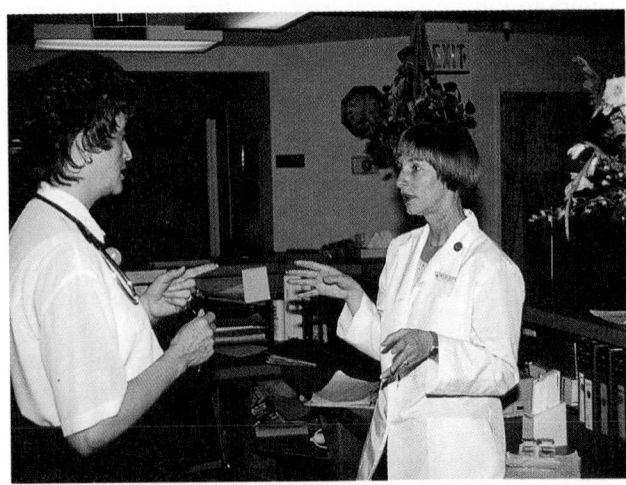

Figure 7-5. Consultation and planning care.

the consultation be arranged for a day when both the nurse and consultant are scheduled to work and during a time when distractions are minimal. Thus the consultant is available to the nurse, and the nurse is also available to the consultant.

Finally, the nurse incorporates the consultant's recommendations into the care plan. The success of the advice depends on the implementation of the problem-solving techniques suggested.

Key Terms

client-centered goals	Kardex
collaboration	nurse-initiated inter-
collaborative inter-	ventions
ventions	outcomes
consultation	physician-initiated
critical pathways	interventions
expected outcomes	planning
goals	scientific rationale

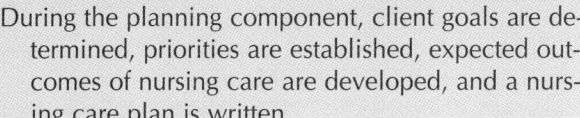

Key Concepts

During the planning component, client goals are determined, priorities are established, expected outcomes of nursing care are developed, and a nursing care plan is written.

Nursing care is planned and organized around specific nursing diagnoses, resulting in an individualized care plan.

When establishing priorities, the nurse ranks nursing diagnoses and goals in order of importance.

The nurse begins the nursing care plan by first addressing the nursing diagnoses that have the highest priority.

Goal setting establishes a framework for the care plan.

Using expected outcomes, the nurse evaluates the effectiveness of the care plan.

In general, care plans include the nursing diagnosis, goals, specific actions by the nurse, and expected outcomes.

The care plan is a written guideline for client care so that the care given can be quickly understood by all members of the health care team.

Critical pathways are multidisciplinary treatment plans that predict the interventions and outcomes to be met for selected clients over a projected length of stay.

Care plans and critical pathways increase communication among nurses and facilitate the continuity of care from one nurse to another and from one health care setting to another.

The planning of individualized care requires involvement of the client and family.

The care plan is a method for teaching students to apply knowledge gained from nursing and medical literature and the classroom in the practice setting.

Poorly written nursing care plans result in incomplete or inaccurate nursing care, lack of continuity among care givers, and poor use of resources.

Correctly written nursing interventions include specific information about the actions, frequency, quantity, method, and the person to perform them.

Nurse-initiated or independent nursing interventions can solve the client's problems without consultation or collaboration with physicians or other health care professionals.

Physician-initiated or dependent nursing interventions are completed with a physician's order but require nursing judgment or decision making.

Planning nursing care often involves consultation with other members of the health care team.

Critical Thinking Activities

1. How are goals and expected outcomes of nursing care linked to nursing diagnoses?
2. What criteria are used to determine expected outcomes for a given set of client-centered goals?
3. What information is necessary to plan nursing interventions for your clients? If you had nursing assistants, how would you plan those nursing strategies that could be delegated to these persons?

References

Alfaro R: *Application of nursing process: a step by step guide,* ed 2, Philadelphia, 1990, JB Lippincott.

Alfaro-LeFevre R: *Critical thinking in nursing: a practical approach,* Philadelphia, 1995, WB Saunders.

American Nurses Association: *Nursing: a social policy statement,* Kansas City, Mo, 1980, The Association.

Bandman EL, Bandman B: *Critical thinking in nursing,* ed 2, Norwalk, Conn, 1995, Appleton & Lange.

Benner P: *From novice to expert: excellence and power in clinical nursing practice,* Menlo Park, Calif, 1984, Addison-Wesley.

Bereck KH: *Nurs Clin North Am* 10(1):160, 1975.

Bond N and others: Family-centered care at home for families with children who are technology dependent, *Pediatr Nurs* 20:123, 1994.

Bulechek G, McCloskey J: *Nursing interventions: treatments for nursing diagnoses,* Philadelphia, 1985, WB Saunders.

Bulechek G, McCloskey J: *Nursing interventions: treatments for nursing diagnoses,* ed 2, Philadelphia, 1992a, WB Saunders.

Bulechek GM, McCloskey JC: Defining and validating nursing interventions, *Nurs Clin North Am* 27:289, 1992b.

Bulechek GM, McCloskey JC: Nursing interventions: What they are and how to choose them, *Holistic Nurs Pract* 1(3):36, 1987.

Carnevali DL, Thomas MD: *Diagnostic reasoning and treatment decision making in nursing,* Philadelphia, 1993, JB Lippincott.

Carpenito LJ: *Nursing diagnosis application to clinical practice,* ed 6, Philadelphia, 1995, JB Lippincott.

Carpenito LJ: *Nursing diagnosis application to clinical practice,* ed 7, Philadelphia, 1997, JB Lippincott.

Carter JH and others: Using the nursing interventions classification to implement Agency for Health Care Policy and Research guidelines, *J Nurs Care Qual* 9(2):76, 1995.

Gordon M: *Nursing diagnosis: process and application,* ed 2, New York, 1987, McGraw-Hill.

Gordon M: *Nursing diagnosis: process and application,* ed 3, St. Louis, 1994, Mosby.

Gordon M and others: *Clinical judgement: an integrated model, Adv Nurs Sci* 16:55, 1994.

Hirtzel-Trexler BJ: Commentary on practice guidelines: a standard whose time has come, *AONE Leadership Perspect* 2(2):22, 1994.

Iowa Intervention Project (IIP): The NIC taxonomy structure, *Image J Nurs Sch* 25:187, 1993.

Kavchack-Keys MA: *Nurs* 77(7):60, 1977.

Kim MJ and others: *Pocket guide to nursing diagnoses,* ed 5, St. Louis, 1993, Mosby.

Liukkonen A: The nurse's decision-making process and the implementation of psychogeriatric nursing in a mental hospital, *J Adv Nurs* 17(3):356, 1992.

Lund SM: Family-centered nurse coordinator—early childhood intervention: development and implementation of the CNS role, *Clin Nurs Spec* 8:109, 1994.

McCloskey JC, Bulechek GM: *Nursing interventions classification,* ed 2, St. Louis, 1996, Mosby.

Miller MA, Babcock DE: *Critical thinking applied to nursing,* St. Louis, 1996, Mosby.

Mortensen M, McMullin C: Discharge score for surgical outpatients, *Am J Nurs* 86:1347, 1986.

Redman BK: *The process of patient education,* ed 7, St. Louis, 1993, Mosby.

Windel PE: Critical pathways: an integrated documentation tool, *Nurs Manage* 25(9):80F, 1994.

Zander K: Nursing case management—resolving the DRG paradox, *Nurs Clin North Am* 23:503, 1988.

Zander K, McGill R: Critical and anticipated recovery paths: only the beginning, *Nurs Manage* 25(8):34, 1994.

Implementing Nursing Care

OBJECTIVES

Mastery of content in this chapter will enable the student to:

- Define the key terms listed.
- Discuss the relationship of implementation in the nursing process.
- Discuss the differences between protocols and standing orders.
- Describe the information-processing model for selecting nursing interventions.
- List and discuss the five steps of the implementation process.
- Select appropriate implementation methods for a client.

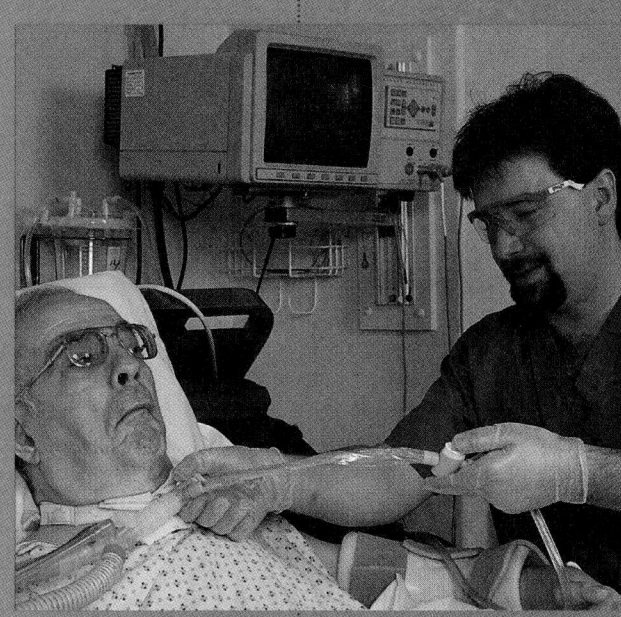

The delivery of nursing care is the focus of the implementation step of the nursing process. The purpose of implementation is to carry out the nursing care plan developed in the planning step of the nursing process.

Implementation describes a category of nursing behaviors in which the actions necessary for achieving the goals and expected outcomes of nursing care are initiated and completed. Implementation includes interventions for performing, assisting, or directing the performance of activities of daily living (ADLs); counseling and teaching the client or family; providing direct care; delegating, supervising, and evaluating the work of staff members; and recording and exchanging information relevant to the client's continued health care.

A **nursing intervention** is any action taken by the nurse to help the client move from a present state toward the health state described in the expected outcomes (Gordon, 1994). Implementation is a continuous process and interacts with the other components of the nursing process. To complete implementation effectively, the nurse must be knowledgeable about types of interventions and the implementation process.

TYPES OF NURSING INTERVENTIONS

Implementation is the step that puts the care plan into action. After the plan has been developed according to client needs and priorities, the nurse performs specific individualized nursing interventions, which include nurse-initiated, physician-initiated, and collaborative interventions (McCloskey and Bulechek, 1996) (see Chapter 7). In addition, nursing interventions may be entirely based on protocols and standing orders. A clear description of protocols and standing orders is necessary for safe nursing practice.

Protocols and Standing Orders

A **protocol** is a written plan specifying the procedures to be followed during an assessment or when providing treatment for a specific condition or nursing care problem. For example, nurses in advanced practice who provide primary care for clients in an outpatient setting follow treatment protocols. In such a setting, nurses assess clients and identify any abnormalities. The established protocol delineates the conditions that nurses are permitted to treat, such as controlled hypertension, and the recommended treatment plan, including therapies the nurse is permitted to administer, such as diet counseling, stress management, and prescriptions of antihypertensives.

A protocol can also be strictly within the framework of nursing such as a protocol for admission and discharge, pain management techniques (see Chapter 33), and cardiopulmonary resuscitation. Protocols are also used in multidisciplinary settings for diagnostic testing and physical, occupational, and speech therapies.

A **standing order** is a document containing orders for the conduct of routine therapies, monitoring guidelines, and/or diagnostic procedures for specific clients with identified clinical problems. The orders direct the conduct of client care in various clinical settings. Standing orders are approved and signed by the physician in charge of care before their implementation. They are commonly found in critical care settings and other specialized practice settings where clients' needs can change rapidly and require immediate attention. Standing orders are also common in the community health setting, in which the nurse encounters situations that do not permit immediate contact with a physician. Thus protocols and standing orders give the nurse the legal protection to intervene appropriately in the client's best interest.

Before implementing any therapy, including those included in protocols and standing orders, the nurse must use sound judgment in determining whether the intervention is correct and appropriate. Second, the nurse implementing any intervention has the responsibility to obtain correct theoretical knowledge and develop the clinical competencies necessary to perform the intervention. Nursing responsibility is equally great for all types of interventions.

CRITICAL THINKING IN IMPLEMENTING NURSING INTERVENTIONS

Nurses using the nursing process make two major types of decisions. During the diagnostic process, the nurse forms conclusions, makes decisions, and draws inferences about the client's assessment data and health care needs (Gordon, 1994; Miller and Babcock, 1996). The nurse then uses a methodological, systematic, research-based method to plan and select appropriate nursing interventions (Gordon, 1987, 1994; McCloskey and Bulechek, 1996).

The nurse must carefully select the interventions best suited to achieve expected outcomes and know how nurse-initiated, physician-initiated, and collaborative interventions differ. Several factors make decision making more difficult when choosing among nurse-initiated (independent) nursing interventions (Snyder, 1985; Snyder and others, 1996). One factor is the absence of objective data concerning the probable consequences of the interventions (Stewart and Archbold, 1993). Another factor is that nurse-initiated interventions are often not mutually exclusive. Frequently they must be administered with therapies in other disciplines. For example, the nurse may need to include relaxation, massage, and guided imagery techniques with prescribed analgesics for pain management (see Chapter 33). Lack of common intervention language can deter collaboration, development of research-based practice, and reimbursement for nursing services (Snyder and others, 1996).

Snyder (1985) proposes an information-processing model of decision making (Table 8-1). The objective of this model is to characterize the sequence of the thought process used by problem solvers. This model focuses on decisions that will be made rather than the ways that they are made. With the information-processing model, a student uses the following components of decision making when determining nursing interventions (Snyder, 1985):

1. Consider the set of all possible nursing actions.
2. List all possible consequences associated with each possible nursing action.
3. Determine the probability that each of the consequences will occur.
4. Make a judgment based on the value of that consequence to the client.

IMPLEMENTATION PROCESS

Adequate and thorough preparation before implementing the care plan ensures efficient and effective nursing care. There are five preparatory nursing activities: reassessing the client, reviewing and revising the care plan, organizing resources and care delivery, anticipating and preventing complications, and implementing nursing interventions.

Reassessing the Client

Assessment is a continuous process that occurs each time a nurse interacts with a client. When new data are gathered and a new client need is identified, the nurse modifies the care plan. During the initial phase of implementation, the nurse reassesses the client. This is a partial assessment and may focus on one dimension of the client, such as level of comfort, or on one system, such as the cardiovascular system. The reassessment provides a way to determine whether the proposed nursing action is appropriate for the client's level of wellness. For example, the nurse may have planned to ambulate a client following lunch; however, a reassessment reveals shortness of breath and increased fatigue, which require the client to return to bed.

Reviewing and Revising the Care Plan

Although the nursing care plan is developed according to the nursing diagnoses, changes in the client's status can require modification of planned nursing care. Before beginning care, the nurse reviews the plan and compares the established plan with current assessment data to validate stated nursing diagnoses and to determine whether the nursing interventions are still the most appropriate for the clinical situation. If the nurse determines that the client's status has changed and the nursing diagnoses and related nursing interventions are no longer appropriate, the nursing care plan should be modified (see Chapter 7).

TABLE 8-1

Information-Processing Model for Pain Related to Abdominal Incision Healing

Possible Actions	Possible Consequences Associated With Action	Probability of Consequence	Value of Consequence to Client
Teach relaxation exercises.	Client is able to control perception of pain.	Moderate	Ability to control perception and response to pain
	Pain is unrelieved.	Moderate	
	Pain increases.	Low	
Teach client use of controlled analgesia.	Client is able to control administration of analgesia within preset limits.	High	Ability of client to use analgesia to continuously relieve pain
	Pain is relieved.	High	
	Pain is unrelieved.	Moderate	
	Pain increases.	Low	
Administer narcotic analgesia every 4 hours.	Client is unable to control administration of analgesia.	High	Inability to control administration of analgesia
	Pain increases in intensity before nurse administers narcotic analgesia.	Moderate to high	Increase or decrease of pain perception based on
	Pain is relieved.	Moderate to high	blood levels of narcotic analgesia
	Client is confused after administration of narcotic analgesia.	Low to moderate	

Modified from Snyder M: *Independent nursing interventions,* New York, 1985, John Wiley & Sons.

Modification of the existing plan includes several steps (Table 8-2). First, data in the assessment column are revised to reflect the client's current status. New data entered in the care plan should be dated to inform the health care team when the change occurred.

Second, nursing diagnoses are revised. When the client's needs or problems change, some nursing diagnoses may no longer be relevant, and new nursing diagnoses are added.

Third, specific interventions are revised to correspond to the new nursing diagnoses and goals. The new implementation methods indicate the client's greater independence from or dependence on nursing. In addition, the revised implementation can include the client's specific needs for health care resources.

Finally, the nurse evaluates the client response to the nursing actions (see Chapter 9). If the client response is not consistent with the established expected outcomes, further revisions for the plan of care are needed. For example, in Chapter 4 the clinical scenario for Mrs. Bryan was introduced, and her plan of care required multiple collaborative interventions. As her fatigue and weight loss progressed, she became weaker and her nursing needs changed. Mrs. Bryan moved in with a friend, and more community, friends, and family resources were used to safely maintain Mrs. Bryan's independence.

Table 8-2 includes revisions for a care plan in an acute care setting. Mr. Brown is recovering from abdominal surgery, and as he progresses through a postoperative course, his nursing care needs change.

The nurse made modification in the care plan for one nursing diagnosis: risk for ineffective airway clearance after surgery related to pain of abdominal incision. On the second postoperative day, the nurse assessed Mr. Brown and noted decreased chest wall movements, crackles that were auscultated in the right lower lobes, and an elevated temperature (39° C). Mr. Brown had a standing order for a chest x-ray film, which was taken immediately and revealed the collapse of alveoli in the right lower lobe. The nursing diagnosis was revised to read *ineffective airway clearance related to decreased inspiratory effort secondary to pain of abdominal incision.* The

TABLE 8-2
Modified Nursing Care Plan for Mr. Brown

Assessment	Goals	Implementation	Evaluation
Nursing diagnosis: Risk for ineffective airway clearance after surgery related to pain of abdominal incision			
Definition: Risk for ineffective airway clearance after surgery is the state in which an individual is unable to clear secretions or obstructions from the respiratory tract to maintain airway patency.*			
Smoked two packs/day 20 years; chest x-ray film showing slight change of emphysema; crackles auscultated in lung field; scheduled for abdominal surgery	Client's airway remains patent by 7/1.	Demonstrate turn, cough, and deep breathing to client. Have client demonstrate turning, coughing, and deep breathing exercises.	Productive cough is produced. Airway is clear to auscultation.

Modified 24 Hours After Surgery

Nursing diagnosis: Ineffective airway clearance related to decreased inspiratory effort secondary to pain of abdominal incision

Assessment	Goals	Implementation	Evaluation
Decreased chest wall movements; crackles in base that do not clear with coughing; fever; tachypnea (7/1)	Client coughs productively by 7/2.	Administer chest physiotherapy to all lobes of the lung: 8-12-4-8-12-4. Ensure that Mr. Brown coughs and deep breathes every 2 hours around the clock.	Lung fields are clear on auscultation. Client becomes afebrile. Sputum is clear. Chest x-ray film demonstrates atelectasis resolving.
	Client's lungs are free of abnormal lung sounds 7/2.	Suction nasotracheal area every 2 hours if client is unable to cough productively. Teach client to splint incision with pillow before and during coughing.	Client does not report increased pain during coughing.

*Data from Kim MJ and others: *Pocket guide to nursing diagnoses,* ed 7, St. Louis, 1997, Mosby.

goal of maintaining a patent airway was still appropriate. Specific nursing interventions were developed to assist in achieving a patent airway.

Organizing Resources and Care Delivery

A facility's resources include equipment and skilled personnel. Organization of equipment and personnel makes efficient, skilled client care possible. After a plan of care is determined, the nurse prepares the necessary supplies and decides on the time and provider of care. Preparation for care delivery also involves preparing the environment and client for nursing intervention.

Equipment. Most nursing procedures, from bed making to client teaching, require some equipment or supplies. The nurse must analyze each planned intervention for needed items. Realistic interventions call for only those items available in the facility.

All necessary supplies should be gathered and put in a convenient location, usually where they will be used, before implementation. Extra supplies should be available in case of mishaps. Extra sterile gloves, for example, anticipate the possibility of a break in sterile technique. However, extra supplies should not be opened unless they are needed; this controls health care costs. The nurse also arranges the supplies in the order in which they will be used. After the procedure the nurse appropriately returns any unopened supplies.

Personnel. Nursing care delivery systems vary among facilities and must be considered when allocating resources. The system by which nursing is organized determines the way in which personnel are designated for client care delivery. The most common types of nursing delivery systems are functional, team, total client care, primary nursing, and case management (see Chapter 3).

Three categories of functions are inherent to professional nursing practice: direct client care, delegation, and coordination. These functions assume varying levels of importance, depending on the nursing system.

A functional nursing system divides client care into a series of tasks, each of which is delegated to the lowest level of personnel having the requisite skill and competence to complete the task. Each staff member then performs this same task for all clients on the unit. Thus the client is cared for by a number of people who concentrate on their own particular assignments.

A team nursing system is a method of care delivery in which a small group of personnel, supervised by a professional nurse, deliver care to a number of clients on each nursing shift. As the team leader on a specific shift, the nurse does not perform all direct care activity but is responsible for the client, care plan, and delivery of nursing care. The team leader delegates client care to team members, and coordinates the team's efforts. Cooperation and collaboration are hallmarks of good team nursing (Figure 8-1).

A total client care system has a registered nurse who is responsible for the total care of a number of clients throughout a shift. Client care is totally individualized; the nurse assigned to the client is responsible for direct client care, coordination with other departments for services, and contribution to the care plan. Direct client care is emphasized. When assigning clients, the unit manager should assign nurses to the same clients to ensure continuity of care. There is no delegation under this system; the nurse on each shift independently gives care and is responsible for the care plan during that time.

A primary nursing system has a primary nurse who is responsible for all aspects of a client's nursing care from admission to discharge. When the primary nurse is off duty, an associate nurse assumes care of the client. If a problem arises, the associate nurse confers directly or indirectly with the primary nurse, who retains full authority and responsibility for the client's nursing care plan.

Case management is an organized system for delivering health care to an individual client or a group of clients through an episode of illness. This system includes assessment and development of a plan of care, coordination of all services, referral, and follow-up usually assigned to one individual, commonly a registered nurse.

No matter what the nursing care delivery system, continuity of individualized care is a primary consideration when assigning and organizing personnel.

Environment. Environmental factors influence the delivery and reception of care. The surroundings in which nursing activities occur should be safe and conducive to the implementation of the therapy. Client

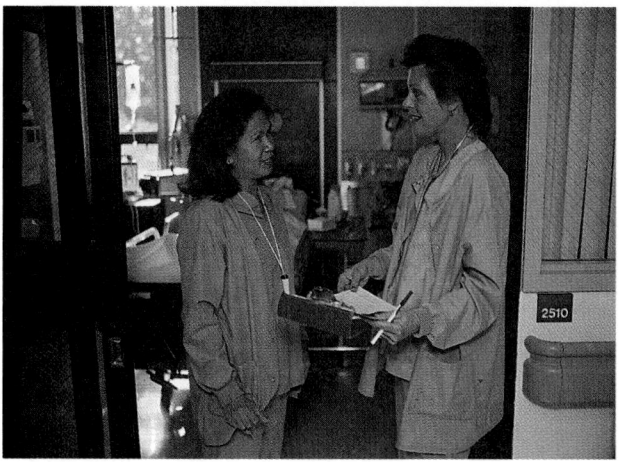

Figure 8-1. Collaboration with other health care providers results in effective interventions.

safety is always the first concern. If the client has sensory deficits or an alteration in level of consciousness, the environment must be arranged to prevent injury. Special rooms, rearrangement of furniture and equipment, rooms free of clutter, and provision for additional personnel are examples of creating safe surroundings.

The client benefits most from nursing interventions when surroundings are compatible with activities. Privacy promotes relaxation when body parts are exposed. Reducing distractions enhances learning opportunities. Provision of adequate warmth and lighting prevents intrusion of environmental factors.

Client.

Before beginning to perform interventions, the nurse should make the client as physically and psychologically comfortable as possible. Symptoms such as nausea, dizziness, or pain, for example, frequently interfere with a client's full concentration and cooperation. Comfort measures or medication for pain before initiating interventions enables the client to participate more fully. If client alertness is needed, the dose of pain medication should be sufficient to relieve discomfort but not impair mental faculties.

Even if symptoms are not a factor, the client should be made physically comfortable during interventions. Controlling environmental factors, positioning, and taking care of other physical needs should precede initiation of interventions. The nurse should also consider the client's level of endurance and plan only the amount of activity the client can comfortably tolerate.

Awareness of the client's psychosocial needs helps the nurse to create a favorable emotional climate. Some clients feel reassured by having a significant other present to lend encouragement and moral support. Other strategies include planning sufficient time or multiple opportunities for the client to work through and ventilate feelings and anxieties. Adequate preparation allows the client to obtain maximal benefit from each intervention.

Anticipating and Preventing Complications

Risks to the client arise from both illness and treatment. The nurse must identify these risks, evaluate the relative benefit of the treatment versus the risk, and initiate risk prevention measures.

Many client conditions place the client at risk for additional complications. For example, the client with preexisting chronic lung disease is at risk for developing pneumonia following abdominal surgery. The nurse's knowledge of pathophysiology helps in the early identification of complications that can occur. Scientific rationales for how certain interventions can prevent or minimize complications help the nurse to evaluate the usefulness of preventive measures. A confused client, for example, is at risk for pulmonary complications be-cause of extended periods of immobility. The nurse knows that getting the client out of bed will reduce this risk because mobility enables the client to breathe more deeply and expand the bases of the lungs. However, the nurse also realizes this activity poses a risk to the client's safety. Preventive safety measures may require remaining with the client while out of bed or having the family stay with the client to encourage deep breathing.

Some nursing procedures also pose risks for the client. The nurse needs to be aware of potential complications and institute precautionary measures. For instance, the client receiving feedings through a nasogastric tube is at risk for aspiration. The nurse should elevate the head of the bed and have pharyngeal suction equipment at the bedside before initiating the feedings.

Identifying areas of assistance.

Some nursing situations require the nurse to acquire assistance by seeking additional personnel, knowledge, and/or nursing skills. Before implementing care, the nurse evaluates the plan to determine the need for assistance and the type required.

Situations requiring additional personnel vary. For example, a nurse assigned to care for an overweight, immobilized client may need additional personnel to help to turn, transfer, and position the client. The nurse also needs to determine the number of additional personnel and when they are needed. The nurse must then discuss the need for assistance with potential resources.

Some nursing situations require additional knowledge and skills, as well as additional personnel. A nurse needs additional knowledge when administering a new medication or implementing a new procedure. Such information can be obtained from a hospital's formulary or procedure book. If the nurse still is uncertain about the new medication or procedure, other members of the health care team can be consulted.

Because of the continual growth of health care professions and related technology, a nurse may lack the skills to perform a new procedure. When this occurs, information about the procedure is obtained from the literature and the agency's procedures book. Next, all equipment necessary for the procedure is collected. Finally, another nurse who has completed the procedure correctly and safely provides assistance and guidance. The assistance can come from another staff nurse, a supervisor, an educator, or a nurse specialist. Requesting assistance occurs frequently in all types of nursing practice and is a learning process that continues throughout educational experiences and into professional development.

Implementing Nursing Interventions

The nurse uses nursing interventions to achieve the goals of care and selects from the following methods:

1. Performing, assisting, or directing the performance of ADLs

2. Counseling and teaching the client and family
3. Providing direct care
4. Delegating, supervising, and evaluating the work of other staff members
5. Recording and exchanging information relevant to the client's continued care

Nursing practice is composed of cognitive, interpersonal, and psychomotor (technical) skills. Each type of skill is needed to implement nursing interventions. The nurse is responsible for knowing when one intervention is preferred over another and for having the necessary theoretical knowledge and psychomotor skills to implement each. A later section introduces the general theoretical information for each method and refers to subsequent chapters that detail the necessary theoretical and psychomotor skills.

Cognitive skills. Cognitive skills involve nursing knowledge. The nurse must know the rationale for each therapeutic intervention, understand normal and abnormal physiological and psychological responses, be able to identify client learning and discharge needs, and recognize the client's health promotion and illness prevention needs.

Interpersonal skills. Interpersonal skills are essential to effective nursing action. The nurse must develop a trusting relationship and communicate clearly with the client, family, and other members of the health care team. Client teaching and counseling must be done to the level of the client's understanding. The nurse must also be sensitive to the client's emotional response to the illness and treatment. Proper use of interpersonal skills enables the nurse to be perceptive to the client's verbal and nonverbal communication (see Chapter 13).

Psychomotor skills. Psychomotor skills require the learner to integrate cognitive and motor activities, such as learning to give an injection. The learner must understand anatomy and pharmacology (cognitive) and the mechanics of preparing and giving an injection (motor). Psychomotor skills are needed to provide the direct care needs of clients such as changing a dressing, giving an injection, or suctioning a tracheostomy. The nurse has a professional responsibility to correctly complete these skills. Some of these skills may be new. If that is the case, the nurses assess their present level of competency and obtain the necessary resources to ensure that the client receives the treatment safely.

Communicating Nursing Interventions

Nursing interventions are written or communicated orally. When written, nursing interventions are incorporated into the nursing care plan and client's medical record. The care plan usually reflects nursing interventions. After the interventions are implemented, the nurse documents the interventions and the client's response to the treatment on the appropriate record (see Chapter 14). If there are any variations to an intervention, such as the number of repetitions of range of joint motion or the type of client education materials provided, the nurse documents the information to provide continuity of care. This information usually includes a brief description of the nursing assessment, the specific procedure, and the client's response.

Documenting a brief description of pertinent assessment findings and client response in the client's medical record validates the need for a continued nursing intervention. Writing the time and the details of the intervention documents that the procedure was completed.

Nursing interventions are also communicated orally from one nurse to another or to other health professionals. Nurses commonly communicate orally when changing shifts, transferring a client to another unit, or discharging a client to another health agency. Whether the nursing intervention is written or communicated orally, the language should be clear, concise, and to the point.

···IMPLEMENTATION METHODS

The nurse carries out the nursing care plan by using several implementation methods. For example, the client with the nursing diagnosis *impaired physical mobility related to bilateral arm casts* may require assistance in performing ADLs. The client with *ineffective individual coping related to fear of medical diagnosis* may require counseling as a method of nursing intervention. The client with a *knowledge deficit* needs client health education focusing on the area of need. The totally immobilized or disoriented client requires a variety of implementation methods while receiving total client care. Another method of implementation involves the supervision and evaluation of other members of the health care team.

For each nursing diagnosis, the nurse identifies appropriate interventions, each of which requires specific theoretical knowledge and clinical skills.

Assisting With Activities of Daily Living

Activities of daily living (ADLs) are activities usually performed in the course of a normal day. They include ambulating, eating, dressing, bathing, brushing the teeth, grooming, and toileting. Conditions resulting in the need for assistance with ADLs can be acute, chronic, temporary, permanent, or rehabilitative.

An acute disease is characterized by symptoms that are usually severe and that are present for a relatively short time, usually less than 6 months. An episode of acute disease results in recovery to a state of health and activity comparable to the state before the disease, passage into a chronic phase of the disease, or death. For example, the postoperative client who experiences no complications is often unable to independently complete all ADLs. While progressing through the postoperative period, the client gradually depends less on nurses for completing ADLs.

A chronic disease persists longer. Although the symptoms are usually less severe than those of the acute phase of the same disease, chronic disease may result in complete or partial disability. A client with partial paralysis after a cerebrovascular accident may have a chronic impairment requiring long-term assistance with ADLs.

The client's need for assistance with ADLs may be temporary, permanent, or rehabilitative. In the case of temporary assistance with ADLs, the client needs assistance during a specific period. A client with impaired mobility because of bilateral arm casts has a temporary need for assistance. After the casts are removed, the client will gradually assume full responsibility for ADLs. A client with a total self-care deficit related to an irreversible injury high in the cervical spinal cord has a permanent need for assistance. It is unrealistic for the nurse to plan a rehabilitation program with the goal that this client will be able to independently complete all ADLs. However, through restorative care, the client will learn new ways to perform ADLs, thus becoming more independent and better able to perform some self-care.

Through assessment the nurse collects data that verify the need for assistance with ADLs. As the nurse analyzes these data, nursing diagnoses are formed in relation to such assistance.

Counseling

Counseling is an implementation method that helps the client use a problem-solving process to recognize and manage stress and that facilitates interpersonal relationships among the client, family, and health care team. Nurses provide counseling to help the client accept actual or impending changes resulting from stress. Counseling involves the delivery of emotional, intellectual, spiritual, and psychological support. A client and family who need nursing counseling may have adjustment difficulties and are upset or frustrated but are not necessarily psychologically disabled. Clients having psychiatric diagnoses require therapy by nurses specializing in psychiatric nursing, or by social workers, psychiatrists, or psychologists.

Many counseling techniques are used to foster cognitive, behavioral, developmental, experiential, and emotional growth in clients (Box 8-1). Counseling encourages individuals to examine available alternatives and to decide which choices are useful and appropriate. When clients are able to examine alternatives, they can develop a sense of control and are able to better manage stress. To assist clients in need of counseling techniques, the nurse must be able to identify the need for counseling and possess communication skills to develop

---

> **Box 8-1**
> ### Examples of Counseling Strategies Used by Nurses
>
> Behavior modification
> Bereavement counseling
> Biofeedback
> Relaxation training
> Reality orientation
> Crisis intervention
> Guided imagery
> Play therapy

---

a therapeutic relationship (Sundeen and others, 1995).

Clients or families needing counseling include persons who must adjust to changes in lifestyle patterns, such as smoking cessation, weight reduction, or increasing activity. Clients coping with chronic or disabling diseases require counseling to help them adapt to changes in lifestyle or body image as the disease progresses. During life-threatening illnesses, clients and families need counseling to cope with the possibility of death.

Teaching

Counseling is closely aligned with teaching. Both involve using communication skills to effect a change in the client. However, with counseling the change results in the development of new attitudes and feelings, whereas in teaching the focus of change is intellectual growth or the acquisition of new knowledge or psychomotor skills (Redman, 1993).

Teaching is an implementation method used to present correct principles, procedures, and techniques of health care to clients and to inform clients about their health status (see Chapter 15). As a nursing responsibility, teaching is implemented in all health care settings, such as in acute care, home care, and community-based settings (Figure 8-2). The nurse is responsible for assessing the learning needs of clients and is accountable for the quality of education delivered.

The **teaching-learning process** is an interaction between the teacher and learner in which specific learning objectives are presented (Redman, 1993). This process provides the organizational structure and framework for client education. The teaching-learning process is much like the basic nursing process.

During assessment, the nurse determines the client's learning needs and readiness to learn. The nurse then interprets the data to formulate nursing diagnoses reflecting the identified needs. When planning, the nurse and client establish goals for learning. Implementation is the initiation of the teaching strategies designed to achieve the learning goal. Finally, evaluation measures

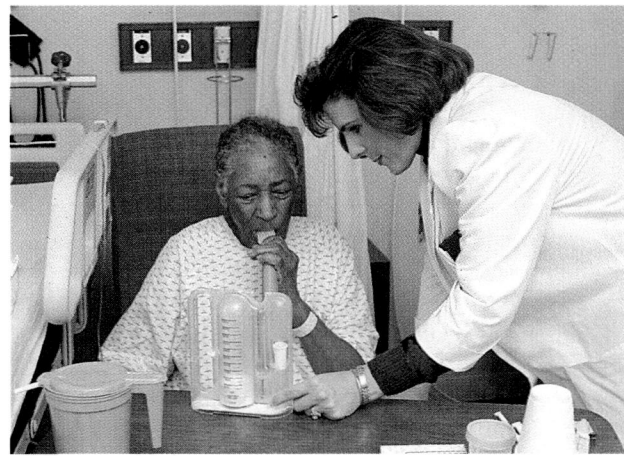

Figure 8-2. Explanations assist the client to safely and correctly use equipment.

the learning that has occurred. The purpose of the teaching-learning process is to develop and implement a teaching plan individualized for the client's needs, level of knowledge, and learning resources.

Providing Direct Care

To achieve therapeutic goals for the client, the nurse initiates direct care interventions to compensate for adverse reactions, uses precautionary and preventive measures in providing care, applies correct techniques in administering care and preparing the client for special procedures, and initiates lifesaving measures in emergency situations. The following sections briefly discuss the nursing interventions in these areas. The specific knowledge and skills needed to carry out these nursing procedures are detailed in subsequent chapters.

Compensation for adverse reactions. An **adverse reaction** is a harmful or unintended effect of a medication, diagnostic test, or therapeutic intervention. Adverse reactions can follow independent, dependent, or interdependent nursing interventions. Nursing actions that compensate for adverse reactions reduce or counteract the reaction. To intervene effectively, the nurse must have knowledge of the potential undesired effects. For example, when administering a medication, the nurse understands the known and potential side effects of the drug. After administration of the medication, the nurse evaluates the client for any adverse effects. The nurse should be aware of drugs that can counteract the side effects. For example, a client may have an unknown hypersensitivity to penicillin and may develop hives after three doses. The nurse records the reaction and stops further administration of the drug. The nurse also consults the physician's standing orders and administers diphenhydramine (Benadryl), an antihistamine (reduces allergic response) medication with antipruritic (anti-itch) properties.

When caring for a client who is undergoing or who has undergone a particular diagnostic test, the nurse must understand the test and any potential adverse effects. For example, a client has not had a bowel movement in 24 hours after a barium enema. Because a bowel impaction is a potential side effect of a barium enema, the nurse increases fluid intake and instructs the client to let the nursing personnel know when a bowel movement occurs.

◼ Clinical Scenario

Ms. Rice, registered nurse, assesses a stage I pressure ulcer on Mr. Blaskowitz's sacrum. She develops interventions designed to prevent further skin breakdown and promote wound healing. She obtains an order for an alternating air mattress and Tegaderm (film dressing). Ms. Rice also changes Mr. Allen's turning schedule from every 2 hours to every hour while awake and every 2 hours while asleep (10 PM to 7 AM). After the second day of treatment, Mr. Allen has stage I pressure ulcers on both heels; the sacral ulcer has also progressed to a stage III ulcer. To counteract the continued skin breakdown, the nurse discontinues the air mattress and obtains an order for the Clinitron bed, Tegaderm for the heel ulcers, and a hydrogel dressing for the sacral ulcer (see Chapter 38).

Although adverse effects are not common, they do occur. The nurse learns potential side effects, is able to recognize the presence of an adverse reaction, and is able to intervene accordingly.

Preventive measures. **Preventive nursing actions** are a category of nursing interventions that are directed at promoting health and preventing illness to avoid the need for acute or rehabilitative health care. Prevention includes assessment and promotion of the client's health potential, application of prescribed measures such as immunizations, health teaching, and early diagnosis and treatment.

In the case of a client who has a hypersensitivity to penicillin, the nurse can implement several preventive measures. The nurse indicates the penicillin allergy in the client's medical record, informs the client and family of the need for a Medic Alert bracelet, and teaches them actions they should take if the client is given penicillin again. The nurse also teaches the client and family that this is a potentially life-threatening allergy and provides a list of specific drugs to be avoided.

Preventive nursing actions are used to meet the therapeutic goals of the client. Through preventive actions the nurse is able to help the client attain the highest level of wellness.

Correct techniques in administering care and preparing a client for procedures. The administration of nursing care requires the nurse to be experienced in **techniques** used to perform specific procedures, such as administering medications, changing clients' dressings, or inserting Foley catheters. Client care, particularly in the home and hospital, involves many techniques. Every procedure the nurse does for the client is carried out by a specific method.

To carry out a procedure, the nurse must be knowledgeable about the procedure itself, the frequency, the steps, and the expected outcomes. In a hospital the nurse completes many procedures each day. Some of these procedures might be new, so before conducting a new procedure the nurse assesses personal competencies and determines the need for assistance, new knowledge, or new skills.

Lifesaving measures. A **lifesaving measure** is implemented when a client's physiological or psychological state is threatened. The purpose of the lifesaving measure is to restore physiological or psychological equilibrium. Such measures include administering emergency medications, instituting cardiopulmonary resuscitation, restraining a violent client, and obtaining immediate counseling from a crisis center for a severely anxious client.

The initiation of lifesaving measures is an essential component of nursing practice. As with any procedure, the nurse must be knowledgeable about the lifesaving procedure itself, the steps, and expected outcomes. If an inexperienced nurse encounters a situation requiring emergency measures, the proper nursing action may be to get an experienced professional.

Achieving the Goals of Care

The client's health care goals can be achieved by providing an environment conducive to meeting such goals; adjusting care in accordance with clients' expressed or implied needs; stimulating and motivating clients, thereby enabling them to achieve self-care and independence; and encouraging them to accept care or adhere to the treatment regimen. For each nursing intervention, the nurse and client work together to meet the mutually developed goals. With some interventions, the nurse assumes a more active role, and with others, the nurse assumes a more passive role.

Nurses can help create a health care environment conducive to achieving clients' goals. Ideally the nurse creates an environment that provides clients with adequate privacy for meeting basic needs and allows them to feel safe and free to interact with the health care team. An early step in establishing an appropriate environment is to orient clients and families to the health care agency. If it is a hospital, clients need to be oriented to their rooms, the health care team, and other clients. Clients in clinics should be oriented to clinic policies and procedures, the location of restrooms and cafeterias, and the health care team. When clients receive care in the home, the nurse should take time to acquaint clients and their families with the purposes and expectations of the home visits.

Whether clients are in the hospital, an outpatient

clinic, or a community setting, the nurse takes measures to provide privacy. Obviously clients need privacy to carry out activities of hygiene, grooming, and elimination. In addition, they need privacy to talk with families, friends, or members of the health care team. In an environment of privacy, clients may feel free to share concerns, ask questions about diagnosis and treatment, and resolve personal problems.

Nursing care and other therapeutic measures are designed to meet the client's needs. As a further aid in the attainment of health care goals, the nursing care plan should be flexible so the client is not placed into a fixed routine. Obviously the degree of flexibility depends on the nature of the need, the severity of the client's disability or illness, and the client's dependence on nursing care. However, even the smallest degree of flexibility, giving the client an opportunity to have some choice about the type or timing of nursing care, is valuable.

Clients with severe and chronic diseases should be encouraged to increase their levels of self-care and independence. To avoid discouraging clients, it is best to attempt to achieve this nursing goal gradually. The care plan is implemented so that clients successfully achieve one level of independence before attempting the next.

▪ Clinical Scenario

Mr. Porter is a 50-year-old executive, husband, and father of three teenagers. He is recovering from a severe myocardial infarction (heart attack). For the past 3 days, all of Mr. Porter's hygiene and grooming needs have been met by the nursing staff. One day, Mr. Porter expresses doubts of ever getting his energy back and being able to care for himself. That evening Mr. Martin, a student nurse, assesses Mr. Porter and develops a nursing care plan. One of the goals is that Mr. Porter will complete self-care within 1 week. With the help of his instructor, Mr. Martin implements the following nursing care plan, in various phases, which is designed to achieve the overall goal of independence:

Day 1   Wash face, shave, and comb hair; feed himself meals, wash face, shave, and comb hair
Day 2   Perform grooming activities and feed himself
Day 3   Shower and feed himself

Each day includes achievable tasks for Mr. Porter. Placing the tasks in sequential order serves the following purposes: (1) each task is developed with the knowledge that Mr. Porter can successfully complete the activity, (2) a sequence of successes motivates Mr. Porter to continue with the plan, and (3) the sequence is designed to gradually increase Mr. Porter's activity tolerance.

Clients with chronic diseases may need to adhere to many treatment modalities. **Client adherence** means that clients and families must invest time in carrying out the required home treatments. For example, a client with chronic obstructive pulmonary disease may need to spend several hours a day performing respiratory therapies designed to keep the airway open and maintain an acceptable level of wellness.

Some treatment plans include the need for the client and family to adjust to functional changes as a result of medications. For example, a client with high blood pressure being treated with atenolol (Tenormin) occasionally feels increasingly fatigued during the early stages of treatment. Another client with cancer who is undergoing chemotherapy may have changes in energy level and body image as a result of the medication.

Finally, adherence to treatment plans can require an increased financial investment by the client and family. For example, for a client who has cardiac disease, a two-story house may no longer be suitable because the client is unable to climb stairs without feeling short of breath. Thus the client and family may need to invest in a new house or have their present home modified.

Investments of time, money, and personal resources for a long period can be discouraging. The discouraged client may neglect the treatment regimen. After the client begins to reduce adherence to treatment, levels of wellness often decline.

Nurses are able to intervene and assist the client in adhering to a treatment plan. Adequate discharge planning and education of the client and family help promote a smooth transition from one health care setting to another or to the home. They also help increase the client's level of knowledge about the treatment plan. Counseling helps the client and family adapt to change resulting from the disease process or treatment. Continuity of care also provides a supportive professional who is familiar with the client's pattern of living, pattern of wellness, and treatment. In addition, reinforcing successes with the treatment plan encourages the client to maintain adherence to the regimen.

Delegating, Supervising, and Evaluating the Work of Other Staff Members

Depending on the system of health care delivery, the nurse who develops the care plan frequently does not perform all of the nursing interventions. Some activities must be delegated to other members of the health care team and coordinated by the nurse (see Chapter 2). Noninvasive and frequently repetitive interventions such as skin care, range-of-joint-motion exercises, ambulation, grooming, and hygiene measures are examples of care activities that can be assigned to a nursing assistant or a licensed practical nurse. The nurse assigning tasks is responsible for ensuring that each task is appropriately assigned and is completed according to the standard of care and that indirect care interventions are delegated to those personnel competent to provide the specific type of care (McCloskey and others, 1996).

Key Terms

activities of daily living (ADLs)
adverse reaction
client adherence
counseling
implementation
lifesaving measure
nursing intervention
preventive nursing actions
protocol
standing order
teaching
teaching-learning process
techniques

▪ Key Concepts

During implementation, the nurse carries out the nursing care plan developed in the planning component of the nursing process.

Preparation for implementation includes reassessing the client; reviewing, setting in order of priority, and modifying the care plan; identifying areas in which assistance is needed; organizing supplies and personnel; and preparing the client, family, and environment.

Implementation methods consist of assisting with ADLs, counseling and teaching, preventing adverse reactions, and compensating for adverse reactions.

Implementation methods require the nurse to use cognitive, interpersonal, and technical skills.

Assisting with ADLs is a nursing strategy that compensates for the client's self-care deficits until the client can resume normal activity.

Counseling helps the client to use problem solving to recognize and manage stress and facilitates interpersonal relationships among the client, family, significant others, and health care team.

Teaching is used to present correct principles, procedures, and techniques of health care to the client; to inform clients about their health status; and to refer the client and family to appropriate resources.

Nursing actions to achieve therapeutic goals include preventing adverse reactions, using correct techniques for administering care, preparing the client for procedures, and implementing lifesaving measures.

Delegating care to other personnel involves ensuring that the individuals are skilled in the tasks and evaluating that each task was completed according to the standard of care.

To complete any nursing procedure, the nurse must be knowledgeable about the procedure, the times it is needed, its steps, and its expected outcome.

Critical Thinking Activities

1. Mr. Clark is a 45-year-old man admitted with congestive heart failure. His lung sounds are clear; his blood pressure is 130/88 mm Hg, his pulse is 112 beats per minute, and his respirations are 24 per minute. His nursing history reveals that he does not consistently take all of his medications nor does he follow a low-sodium diet, which was designed to reduce fluid retention. List the specific types of interventions that you may select to assist in resolving Mr. Clark's present illness and prevent further complications. Include the type of intervention (e.g., nurse initiated, physician initiated, collaborative).

2. You are assigned to administer all medications. What measures will you take to reduce the incidence of an adverse reaction in clients receiving intravenous piggyback medications?

3. Mrs. Jones is a 240-pound comatose client. You assign your nursing assistant to provide skin and hygiene care. What type of help do you anticipate that the nurse assistant will need to provide safe care and reduce the risk of pressure ulcers in this client?

References

Gordon M: *Nursing diagnosis: process and application,* ed 2, New York, 1987, McGraw-Hill.

Gordon M: *Nursing diagnosis: process and application,* ed 3, St. Louis, 1994, Mosby.

Kim MJ and others: *Pocket guide to nursing diagnoses,* ed 7, St. Louis, 1997, Mosby.

McCloskey JC, Bulechek GM: *Nursing interventions classification (NIC),* ed 2, St. Louis, 1996, Mosby.

McCloskey JC and others: Nurses' use and delegation of indirect care interventions, *Nurs Econ* 14(1):22, 1996.

Miller MA, Babcock DE: *Critical thinking applied to nursing,* St. Louis, 1996, Mosby.

Redman BK: *The process of patient education,* ed 7, St. Louis, 1993, Mosby.

Snyder M: *Independent nursing interventions,* New York, 1985, John Wiley & Sons.

Snyder M and others: Defining nursing interventions, *Image J Nurs Sch* 28(2):137, 1996.

Stewart BJ, Archbold PG: Nursing intervention studies require outcome measures that are sensitive to change: part 2, *Res Nurs Health* 16:77, 1993.

Sundeen SJ et al: *Nurse-client interaction: implementing the nursing process,* ed 5, St. Louis, 1995, Mosby.

9

Evaluation

OBJECTIVES

Mastery of content in this chapter will enable the student to:

- Define the key terms listed.
- Explain the relationship between expected outcomes and goals of care.
- Explain how the step of evaluation involves critical thinking.
- Give examples of evaluation measures used to determine a client's progress toward outcomes.
- Evaluate nursing actions selected for a client.
- Describe how evaluation can lead to revision or modification of a plan of care.
- Explain the purpose of quality improvement (QI).
- Discuss the dimensions of performance that should be incorporated into an organization's quality improvement program.
- Describe the common features in models used for quality improvement.
- Describe the steps of the FOCUS-PDCA (Plan, Do, Check, Act) approach to quality improvement.

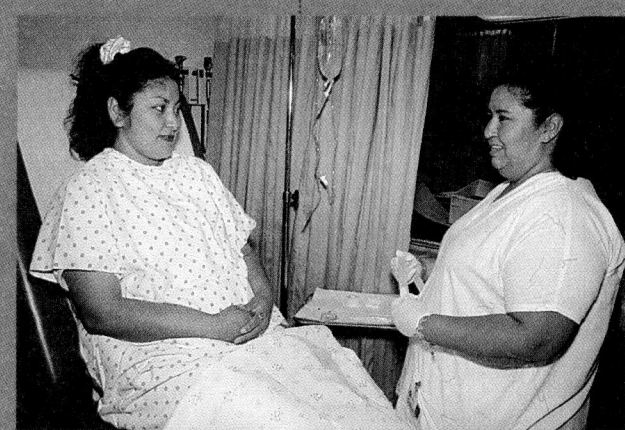

Nurses must be critical thinkers. The nursing process is a series of nursing actions based on and supported by clinical judgments. The previous chapters describe how the nurse uses critical thinking skills to gather client data, form nursing diagnoses, develop a plan of care, and implement the care plan.

Whenever a nurse delivers care and provides therapy, questions must be asked: "Was the therapy effective in improving the client's level of health or functional status?" "Did the client benefit?" It is important to evaluate whether each client reaches a level of wellness or recovery that the health care team and client established in the goals of care. The **evaluation** step of the nursing process measures the client's response to nursing actions and the client's progress toward achieving goals. Data are collected on an ongoing basis to measure changes in functioning, daily living, or in availability or use of external resources (Carnevali and Thomas, 1993). Evaluation occurs whenever the nurse has contact with a client. The emphasis is on client outcomes. The nurse evaluates whether the client's behaviors or responses reflect a reversal or improvement in a nursing diagnosis or maintenance of a healthy state. During evaluation, the nurse decides if the previous steps of the nursing process were effective in minimizing or resolving the client problems by examining the client's responses and comparing them with the behaviors stated in the previously established expected outcomes.

Another aspect of evaluation involves measurement of the quality of nursing care provided in a health care setting. Nurses evaluate each client's progress and recovery. However, that is not enough. A health care organization must be accountable and responsible for evaluating and improving how well nursing and other client care services are provided to all clients. The quality of health care delivery is a focus of the Joint Commission on Accreditation of Healthcare Organizations (JCAHO) and **professional standards review organizations (PSROs).** The JCAHO (1997) defines quality of care as the "degree to which health services for individuals and populations increase the likelihood of desired health outcomes and are consistent with current professional knowledge." Each health care professional must be competent, but to achieve quality care, an organization must have the right systems and processes to provide care that is appropriate and efficacious. There are always opportunities to improve because client care is complex, involving numerous variables. The larger an organization, the greater are the variables influencing how care is delivered. Nursing plays a key role in helping an organization find ways to improve the quality of client care. The emphasis is on client outcomes, professional practice, and the systems in which professionals practice.

CRITICAL THINKING SKILLS AND THE DYNAMICS OF EVALUATING NURSING CARE

While caring for clients, the nurse compares subjective and objective data gathered from the client, other nurses or care givers, and family to determine the degree of success in meeting expected outcomes established during planning. If outcomes are met, the overall goals for the client are also met. The nurse compares client behaviors and responses assessed before nursing interventions are delivered with behaviors and responses that occur after nursing care. The nurse applies knowledge about the client's condition, considers previous experience with similar clients, and reviews data from the assessed baseline to critically analyze if the client's condition is changing. Critical thinking directs the nurse to analyze the findings from evaluation. Is the client's condition improved? Can the client improve, or are there physical factors preventing recovery? To what degree does this client's motivation or willingness to pursue healthier behavior influence response to therapies?

Evaluation is the step in the nursing process whereby the nurse continually redirects nursing care to best meet client needs. For example, when evaluating a client for a change in vital signs, the nurse applies knowledge of disease processes and physiological responses to interpret whether a change has indeed occurred and whether the change is desirable. A client in acute pain may present an increased heart rate and increased muscular tension. The nurse knows this is a sympathetic nervous system response to painful stimuli. After administering a pain medication and repositioning the client, the nurse returns to evaluate if vital signs have returned either to a more acceptable level or to the client's baseline before pain. Positive evaluations occur when desired results are met, leading the nurse to conclude that the dosage of medication and nursing intervention effectively met the client's goal of improved comfort. Negative evaluations or undesired results indicate that the intervention was not effective in minimizing or resolving the actual problem or avoiding a potential problem, or that new data about the client's condition have altered the client's ability to meet the established outcome. As a result the nurse must change the care plan and try different therapies or a different approach in administering existing therapies.

This sequence of critically evaluating and revising therapies continues until problems are appropriately resolved. Outcomes must be realistic and adjusted on the basis of the client's prognosis and condition. The nurse must realize that evaluation is dynamic and ever changing, depending on the client's nursing diagnoses and condition. A client whose health status continuously changes requires more frequent evaluation. In addition, priority diagnoses are often evaluated first. For example, a nurse evaluates a client's acute *pain* before evaluating the status of *knowledge deficit*.

Goals

A goal specifies the behavior or response that indicates resolution of a nursing diagnosis or maintenance of a healthy state. It is a summary statement of what is to be accomplished when all expected outcomes have been met. Each nursing diagnosis in the client's care plan has a goal, and every goal has a time frame for evaluation. The nurse evaluates goals after comparing evaluative findings with all expected outcomes. When a goal has been accomplished, the nurse knows that interventions have been successful and that the client is progressing.

As hospital stays become shorter, many clients are discharged before all goals are met and all nursing diagnoses are resolved. When preparing a client for discharge, the nurse evaluates the status of each nursing diagnosis and writes an evaluative statement identifying the client's progress toward goal achievement and problem resolution. Appropriate revisions to the care plan are made for home or follow-up care (e.g., an extended-care facility). The nurse must clearly distinguish between goals that have been met and goals that require continued intervention. A home health nurse will probably revise interventions to adapt them to the client's home.

Expected Outcomes

Expected outcomes are the expected results of a goal-oriented process (see Chapter 7). They are statements of progressive, step-by-step responses or behaviors that the client needs to accomplish to achieve the goals of care. When outcomes are achieved, the related factors for a nursing diagnosis have been removed. For example, a client with a 2-cm pressure ulcer on the heel has a nursing diagnosis of *impaired skin integrity related to pressure of physical immobilization*. The goal of treatment is that the client will have intact skin on the heel. This will be accomplished by meeting the outcomes of "the skin lesion will be clean without drainage" and "showing evidence of healing through a gradual reduction in size, for example, 0.5-cm increments, and inflammation of the affected area on the heel." If the outcomes are met, the nurse has successfully eliminated pressure over the skin and used therapies that have healed the skin lesion. Expected outcomes have short time frames (depending on the health problem and health care setting) and in a home care or community-based setting may include as few as two intervention sessions (Hickey, 1991). To provide objective evaluation measurements, the outcomes are measurable, stated in behavioral terms, and have time frames for evaluation (see Chapter 7).

After a specified time or when all interventions in the plan of care have been completed, the nurse evaluates the client's ability to demonstrate the behavior or response stated in the outcomes. Evaluation of each expected outcome and its place in the sequence of care is essential. Failure to evaluate each expected outcome results in an inability to determine where the sequence faltered, that is, the nurse will not be able to revise and redirect the plan of care at the most appropriate time.

If the client achieves the expected outcome, the nurse either continues the care plan or discontinues interventions because the goal of care is met. If evaluation determines that the expected outcome was not met or only partially met, the nurse begins reassessment and revision of the care plan.

⋯ EVALUATION OF GOAL ACHIEVEMENT

The purpose of nursing care is to assist the client in minimizing or resolving actual health problems, preventing the occurrence of potential problems, and promoting the maintenance of a healthy state. Evaluation of the goals of care determines whether this purpose was accomplished. The nurse matches the client's behavior (e.g., self-administration of insulin or anxiety-free behavior) or physiological response (e.g., decrease in size of pressure ulcer or fall in body temperature) with the behavior or response specified in the goal. For example, during an initial assessment, a client may report acute abdominal pain, rate the pain 8 on a scale of 10 (see Chapter 33), and grimace or hold the abdomen during attempts to move in bed. This baseline is used by the nurse to identify the nursing diagnosis of *pain* and establish the goal, "client will perceive a reduction in pain within 48 hours." The nurse's evaluation determines if the outcomes that reflect goal accomplishment were met. Did the interventions of positioning, proper and timely administration of analgesics, and use of relaxation successfully reduce the client's pain? Outcomes may include, "client will verbalize pain at 3 on a scale of 10" and "client will position self without nonverbal signs of discomfort." After providing appropriate comfort measures, the nurse evaluates the client by measuring the subjective report of pain, observing facial expressions, and noting if the client initiates turning and repositioning. The new data or client responses are compared with outcome criteria to determine whether predicted changes have occurred (Table 9-1). To objectively evaluate the degree of success in achieving a goal, the nurse should use the following steps:

1. Examine the goal statement to identify the exact desired client behavior or response.
2. Assess the client for the presence of that behavior or response.
3. Compare the established outcome criteria with the behavior or response.

TABLE 9-1
Evaluation Measures to Determine the Success of Goals and Expected Outcomes

Goals	Evaluation Measures	Expected Outcomes
Client's pressure ulcer will demonstrate healing within 7 days.	Inspect color, condition, and location of pressure ulcer. Measure diameter of ulcer daily. Note odor and color of drainage from ulcer.	Erythema will be reduced in 2 days. Diameter of ulcer will decrease in 5 days. Ulcer will have no drainage in 2 days. Skin overlying ulcer will begin to close in 7 days.
Client will tolerate ambulation to end of hall by 11/20.	Palpate client's radial pulse before exercise. Palpate client's radial pulse 10 minutes after exercise. Assess respiratory rate during exercise. Observe client for dyspnea or breathlessness during exercise.	Pulse will remain below 110 beats per minute during exercise. Pulse rate will return to resting baseline within 10 minutes after exercise. Respiratory rate will remain within two breaths of client's baseline rate. Client will deny feeling of breathlessness.

TABLE 9-2
Examples of Objective Evaluation of Goal Achievement

Goals	Outcome Criteria	Client Responses	Evaluation Findings
Client will self-administer insulin by 12/18.	Client prepares insulin dosage in syringe by 12/17. Client demonstrates self-injection by 12/18.	Client prepared accurate dosage in syringe on 12/17. Client administered morning insulin dosage; self-injection was correctly performed on 12/18.	Client has progressed and achieved desired behavior.
Client's lungs will be free of secretions by 11/30.	Coughing will be nonproductive by 11/29. Lungs will be clear to auscultation by 11/30. Respirations will be 20 per minute by 11/30.	Client coughed frequently and productively on 11/29. Lungs were clear to auscultation on 11/30. Respirations were 18 per minute on 11/29.	Client will require continued therapy. Condition is improving.
Client will be able to perform self-care measures without discomfort in 2 days.	Client will verbalize pain at 3 on a scale of 10 within 2 days. Client will initiate bathing within 2 days.	Client reports severe right-sided abdominal pain at 5 on a scale of 10 while attempting bathing on day 2.	Client's condition still indicates a problem. Continued therapy with possibly new care measures is required.

4. Judge the degree of agreement between outcome criteria and the behavior or response.
5. If there is no agreement (or only partial agreement) between the outcome criteria and the behavior or response, what are the barriers? Why did they not agree?

There are different degrees of goal attainment. If the client's response matches or exceeds the outcome crite-ria, the goal is met. If the client's behavior begins to show changes but does not yet meet criteria set, the goal is partially met. If there is no progress, the goal is not met (Table 9-2). A clearly defined goal with specific outcomes is easily measured (see Chapter 7).

Evaluative Measures and Sources
Evaluative measures are simply the assessment skills and techniques used to collect data for evaluation. For

example, auscultation of lung sounds, observation of a client's skill performance, inspection of the skin, and inquiry regarding the severity of pain are all evaluative measures (Figure 9-1). In fact, they are the same as assessment measures, yet they are performed at a time during the care of a client when decisions are made as to the client's status and progress. The intent of assessment is to identify the existence of problems. The intent of evaluation is to determine if the nursing interventions have been effective in minimizing or resolving the problems, if the problems have worsened, or if the list of problems has changed.

The data collected during evaluation are critically analyzed and compared with expected outcomes to determine whether changes occurred. After caring for a client over a long period, the nurse is able to make subtle comparisons of responses and behaviors. Practice experience coupled with a nurse's scientific knowledge base are key to critical thinking. The accuracy of any evaluation improves when the nurse is familiar with the client's behavior and physiological status. Evaluation is also more accurate after the nurse has seen more than one client with a similar problem.

The primary source of data for evaluation is the client. However, the nurse may also use the family and other care givers. Documentation and reporting in the evaluation process are critical. Written nursing progress notes, assessment flow sheets, and information shared between nurses during change-of-shift reports (see Chapter 14) should communicate a client's progress toward meeting expected outcomes and goals for the nursing plan of care. If a client is cared for using a critical pathway or CareMap (see Chapter 14), the nurse and team members clearly know what outcomes are to be met for a given day (Figure 9-2). The CareMap as a documentation tool includes expected outcomes that the care team predicts will be met during the client's projected length of stay. The nurse and other team members refer to the outcomes on the CareMap on an

ongoing basis. If there is variance (unexpected outcomes or outcomes occurring at a different time than expected), the nurse reports these responses and revises the plan of care as needed. By having outcomes clearly documented either on a CareMap or other documentation form, the nurse and other health care providers clearly know what to evaluate for. All members of the health care team should have a sense of the client's progress. Each nurse summarizes data on an ongoing basis to ensure that the client is progressing to a better level of health.

CARE PLAN REVISION AND CRITICAL THINKING

As goals are evaluated, adjustments to the care plan are made as indicated. If a goal was successfully met, that portion of the care plan is considered resolved. Unmet and partially met goals require the nurse to reactivate the nursing process sequence. After a nurse reassesses a client, nursing diagnoses may be modified or added with appropriate goals, expected outcomes, and interventions established. At this time, the nurse also redefines priorities. Knowing how the client is progressing and how problems might resolve, stay the same, or worsen are important steps in critical thinking. The nurse's careful monitoring and early detection of problems are a client's first line of defense (Benner, 1984). Because changes in clients' status may be very subtle, evaluation must be client specific, based on a close familiarity with how clients behave, and take into account the client's physical status and reaction to care givers. Accurate evaluation leads to the appropriate revision of ineffective care plans and discontinuation of therapy that has been successful.

Discontinuing a Care Plan

After determining that expected outcomes and goals have been achieved, the nurse confirms this evaluation with the client. If both agree that the expected outcomes have been met, the nurse discontinues that care plan. For example, a client has the nursing diagnosis, *knowledge deficit regarding insulin therapy related to inexperience.* To achieve the ultimate goal of accurate client administration of insulin, the nurse establishes outcomes including, "Client will describe the purpose of insulin by 9/20," "Client will correctly prepare insulin in syringe by 9/20," and "Client will administer insulin injection independently by 9/22." The nurse discusses the information with the client and determines whether the client understands explanations and is comfortable with the information provided. In addition, the nurse will observe the client's preparation of the medication and actual self-injection. Once outcomes are met successfully it is unnecessary to teach additional information about insulin administration. The care plan for this

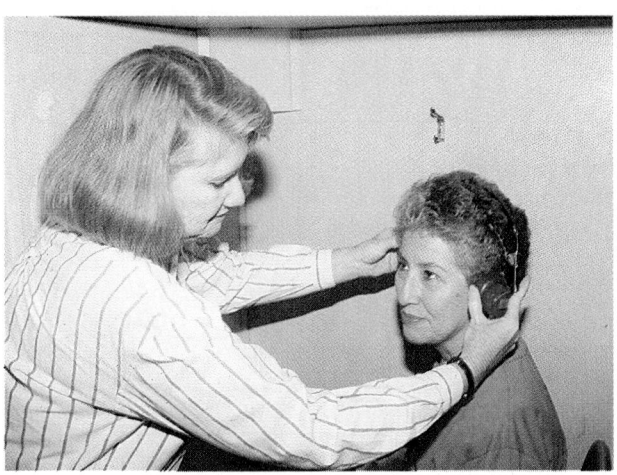

Figure 9-1. Nurse evaluates the client's hearing acuity. (Courtesy Philip James Acker, Motorola, Inc.)

SERVICE ORTHO_____ PHYSICIAN _____ CARE PATH 804
PRIMARY NURSE_____ ADM DATE _____
DC DATE _____

	PATIENT PROBLEMS/NURSING DIAGNOSIS
#1	Pain
#2	Impaired physical mobility
#3	Lack of knowledge
#4	High risk for injury

PROBLEM NUMBER		ED ADM DATE	MED CLEARANCE	DAY DOS	DAY POD 1
	ASSESSMENT MONITORING	Total Nursing Admission/Assessment Assess for hip or leg deformity Assess skin condition q shift NV status check	Assess NV status q 4o	Dressing D/I HMV patent to SS NV assessment q 1o x4 then q 2o to hip/LE Assess bowel sounds Assess lung sounds Assess abdominal distention Skin assessment q shift	Dressing D/I HMV patent to SS NV assessment q 2o Assess bowel sounds Assess lung sounds Assess abdominal distention Skin assessment q shift
	CONSULTS	Pre-Screening		Consults… P.T. O.T. S.W.	Initiate… P.T. O.T.
	PROCEDURE/ TEST	Admit labs CBC, 6, PT/PTT SMA 12, T & S UA with micro EKG CXR Hip x-ray Overhead frame Trapeze Advance 2000 bed	Medical clearance tests	X-ray post op m PAR/OU CBC, 6 post op in PAR	CBC, 6 Hgh/Hct > than transfuse
	TREATMENT	Traction (skeletal or Buck's 5lb) Foley cath Ice to hip prn I/O I.S. every 2o WA TCDB every 2o	Bucks tx I.S. every 2o Foley cath care	HMV I/O I.S. every 1o TCDB every 2o Foley cath care Check hip dressing	DC Foley cath I/O I.S. every 1o TCDB every 2o Check hip dressing
	ACTIVITY	Bedrest Turn 45o every 2o	Bedrest Turn 45o every 2o	Bedrest Turn every 2o	Chair BID MD to determine weight bearing status Stand with walker and P.T. Assist with ADL's
	MEDS/IVS	Heplock 20 gauge of > Prn analgesic LOC AAOC	PRN analgesics Flush HL every 8o IVF's stated after MN day before surgery	IVF's PCA Ancef x6 doses #1/#2	IVF to KVO PCA Ancef #3/4/5
	NUTRITION	Req. NPO after MN	Req. NPO after MN	Clear/full liquids	Advance to regular
	PATIENT/ FAMILY EDUCATION	Nursing Pre-op teaching Use of I.S. Traction Post-op routine Potential need for 730cu	Nursing Continue — pre-op post-op teaching	Reinforce pre-op Post-op teaching i.e., activity, I/O, I.S., PCA, diet	P.T./Nursing Wt bearing status Transfers OOB to chair
	DISCHARGE PLANNING	Nursing Assess condition at home Determine need for: Social Services P.T. O.T. Home Health **Pt./Family verbalizes understanding of Care Path. Plan of care has been mutually set with pt/family**	**High risk screening** Social Worker		Initiate P.T.
	PSYCHO-SOCIAL/ EMOTIONAL	Provide emotional support		Provide emotional support	Give positive feedback on activity
	VARIANCE				
	SIGNATURES				

Figure 9-2. Portion of total hip care path. (Courtesy Barnes-Jewish Hospital, St. Louis.)

nursing diagnosis can be documented as discontinued. This ensures that other nurses will not unnecessarily continue a care plan. Continuity of care assumes that care provided is relevant to client needs. Significant time is wasted when achieved goals are not communicated.

Modifying a Care Plan

When goals are not met, the nurse identifies the variables or factors that interfered with goal achievement. Usually a change in the client's condition, needs, or abilities makes alteration of the care plan necessary. For example, when teaching self-administration of insulin, the nurse discovers that the client has a literacy problem or a visual impairment that prevents the reading of insulin dosages on the syringe. As a result, original outcomes cannot be met. Thus the nurse uses new interventions and revises outcomes to meet the goal of care.

Lack of goal achievement may also result from an error in nursing judgment or failure to follow each step of the nursing process. Clients frequently have very complex problems. The nurse should always remember the possibility of overlooking or misjudging something. When there is failure to achieve a goal, no matter what the reason, the entire nursing process sequence is repeated to discover changes that need to be made to promote, maintain, or restore the client's health.

Reassessment. The nurse uses evaluation measures to determine the client's response to care. These evaluation measures require the nurse to use assessment skills to collect data about the client's status following the implementation step of the nursing process. The nurse reassesses all client factors relating to each nursing diagnosis and etiology. Reassessment requires the nurse to use critical thinking skills to compare data collected during evaluation with previously obtained information. Often a nurse applies intuition from previous experiences with other clients to direct the reassessment process. Day-by-day encounters over time with clients and families who have similar health problems give nurses a strong library of knowledge to use in anticipating client needs and planning care. For example, consider Mr. Landis, who has the nursing diagnosis *pain related to trauma of a surgical incision.* Two days after surgery the client continues to have a poor appetite despite the fact that there are no obvious surgical complications. If the client continues to have pain, the new nurse may associate loss of appetite with discomfort. However, the experienced nurse may recall a previous client who became depressed after surgery. After exploring the problem further, the nurse learns that Mr. Landis's family has not been visiting and the client is fearful of losing his job. For these reasons, the client simply has lost interest in eating. Although the client continues to have pain, a new priority may be *altered nutrition: less than body requirements related to loss of appetite.* As in the original assessment, data are collected from all available sources. Depending on the nurse's findings, it often becomes necessary to assess variables that were not covered on the initial assessment.

Reassessment ensures that the database is accurate and current. It may also reveal pieces of information that were previously overlooked and thus interfered with goal achievement. All new data are sorted, validated, and clustered to analyze and interpret differences from the original database. The nurse documents reassessment data to alert other nursing staff to the client's status.

Nursing diagnoses. After reassessment the nurse reevaluates all nursing diagnoses and determines whether the diagnostic statement continues to be valid or if it needs to be changed. The nurse asks whether the correct diagnosis was selected and whether it and the etiologic factor are current. The list of nursing diagnoses should then be revised to reflect the client's changed status. A new diagnosis may be made. If a previous diagnosis no longer accurately reflects the problem, it should be discontinued, and a modified statement entered. For example, if the nurse finds that a client with diabetes has a serious visual impairment, it may be unlikely that the client will be able to self-administer insulin. The nurse's assessment reveals that a family member is available as a resource. To develop a plan designed to educate an alternate care giver about the administration of insulin, the nurse then establishes a new diagnosis, *altered health maintenance related to inability to self-administer insulin secondary to visual impairment.*

A nurse's care is based on an accurate list of nursing diagnoses. Accuracy is more important than the number of diagnoses selected. As the client's condition changes, the diagnoses do too.

Goals and expected outcomes. When care plans are revised, the nurse reviews goals and expected outcomes for needed changes. Even the goals for unchanged nursing diagnoses should be examined for continued appropriateness. Determining that each goal and expected outcome is realistic for the problem, etiology, and time frame is particularly important. Unrealistic expected outcomes and time frames make goal achievement difficult.

The nurse clearly documents goals and expected outcomes for new or revised nursing diagnoses so that all team members are aware of the revised care plan. When the goal is still appropriate but has not yet been met, the nurse may change the evaluation date to allow more time. All goals and expected outcomes should be client centered, with realistic expectations for client achievement.

Interventions. The evaluation of interventions examines two factors: the appropriateness of the interventions selected and the correct application of the implementation process. The appropriateness of an intervention may be based on the **standard of care** for a client's health problem. If the client has a specific nursing diagnosis such as *ineffective airway clearance,* the standard of care established by a nursing department for this problem may include pain control measures with coughing or deep breathing exercises to help a client breathe more easily with a clear airway. The nurse reviews the standard of care to determine whether the right interventions have been chosen or if additional ones are required.

It may only be necessary to increase or decrease the frequency of interventions. The nurse uses judgment based on previous experience and the client's actual response to therapy. For example, if a client continues to have congested lung sounds, the nurse increases the frequency of coughing exercises to remove secretions.

During evaluation, the nurse may determine that some planned interventions are designed for an inappropriate level of nursing care. If the level of care needs to be changed, a different action verb, such as *assist* in place of *provide,* may be substituted. Sometimes the level of care is appropriate, but the interventions are unsuitable because of a change in the expected outcome. In this case the interventions should be discontinued and new ones planned.

During implementation, the nurse evaluates the client's response during and immediately after intervention. This is the beginning of the evaluation process. Evaluation must be integrated with ongoing nursing care activity. If the response is favorable, implementation continues. Reevaluation occurs when the intervention proves unsuccessful. The nurse then examines the other components of implementation such as client and environment preparation, anticipated complications, or use of personal or technical skills during care delivery (Hickey, 1991).

Changes in implementation should be guided by the nature of the client's unfavorable response. Consulting with other nurses may yield suggestions for improving the approach to care delivery. Senior nurses are often excellent resources because of their experience. Simply changing the care plan is not enough. The nurse must implement the new plan and reevaluate the client's response to the nursing actions. *Evaluation is continuous.*

Occasionally an error during care planning and delivery is discovered during evaluation. This should be anticipated. The nursing process is designed to be a systematic, problem-solving approach to individualized client care, but there is a wide array of variables for each client with a health care problem. Clients with the same health care problem are not treated the same. As a result, sometimes the nurse makes errors in judgment. The systematic use of evaluation provides a way for nurses to catch these errors in judgment. The nurse consistently incorporates evaluation into practice to minimize error and ensure that the most appropriate interventions are used.

Evaluation is the final step of the nursing process and provides a systematic method for analyzing the results of nursing care. In the absence of the evaluation step, the nurse is prevented from evaluating nursing practice and is unable to determine whether the outcomes of client care are beneficial. The consistent application of evaluation principles ensures that a client's care plan remains current and appropriate.

⋯QUALITY IMPROVEMENT ....

The evaluation of health care is a process used to determine the quality of care and service provided to clients. Each professional nurse is expected to evaluate his or her success in delivering effective nursing care. However, good client outcomes are a product of all individual actions and interactions that relate directly or indirectly to the care received by a client (Scoble and Hembrough, 1993). The outcomes of care are a measure of the performance of the entire health care team. For example, after surgery for a total hip repair, does the client regain functional mobility without severe pain and without complications such as wound infection? To achieve such results requires collaboration by nurses, physical therapists, physicians, dietitians, and perhaps even infection control specialists. More and more, emphasis is being placed on monitoring and evaluating the systems and processes that influence client care. This process is receiving more attention than ever before because of the increasing costs of health care.

Consumers are more interested today in the quality of health care because of rising costs and because they are more informed. Accrediting and regulatory agencies are attempting to set a uniform set of standards so that quality comparisons can be made across health care institutions (Health Care Advisory Board, 1994). There are wide variations in the quality of health care within and between institutions. High costs of care do not necessarily ensure high quality; therefore there is significant room for improvement within all health care organizations. The focus of quality improvement at one time was only on hospitals. Now even health care plans (see Chapter 2) are being asked to demonstrate quality because their coverage often restricts employers and consumers from choosing their provider of health care.

As health care institutions look for ways to differentiate themselves from other organizations, quality of care is the answer. Nursing has participated in the monitoring of quality for many years. For this reason, nurses are leading the efforts within organizations to better understand how to measure quality of care. The JCAHO (1996) defines **quality improvement (QI)** as an approach to the continuous study and improvement of the processes of providing health care services to meet the needs of clients and others. Staff within an organization work together in teams to identify what opportunities exist for improving care and what actions are necessary to achieve success. The purpose of quality improvement is not to retrospectively identify problems but to prospectively identify opportunities to improve the quality of care or service (Patton and Stanley, 1993). There are several dimensions of performance that a health care institution should include to have a comprehensive QI program (Box 9-1). Assessment of whether an organization is doing the right thing or doing the right thing well should be the focus of quality improvement activities.

Multidisciplinary Approach

Historically, most quality improvement efforts have been conducted by individual departments within health care organizations. For example, nursing, social service, pharmacy, and respiratory therapy would all have had individual QI plans. Clearly, all health care providers contribute to the outcomes of client care. Therefore it makes sense for staff, who are most familiar with client care activities, to collaborate on QI efforts. For example, if a team of staff identifies an opportunity to improve the timeliness and efficiency of the admission process to their unit, it makes sense to include nursing, admitting, transporters, pharmacy, and all other departments that make early contact with the client. A nursing plan alone will not improve the admission process as successfully as a multidisciplinary plan. To be successful the members of the team must share respect for one another's contributions to client care and be open to new ideas and change.

Quality Improvement Teams

In many health care organizations the units that provide client care have unit-based QI teams. In a unit-based program, members identify clinical priorities for a unit, monitor quality indicators, evaluate monitoring results, and recommend changes in service or practice. Unit-based teams are participative, decentralizing decision making and accountability for practice and placing them on the level of the staff. Ultimately an effective QI program leads to improved clinical practice, better participation by professional staff members, and increased sophistication of evaluation. It also achieves better outcomes for clients.

Many organizations also have organization-wide QI teams. These teams are composed of staff from all departments within a hospital. The problems these teams seek to solve usually affect processes that occur on all units within an organization. For example, the redesign of a client documentation system requires participation by all disciplines who enter information in the medical record. These organizational QI teams are usually given the responsibility to create innovations to improve the work of many health care professionals while also improving the quality of care provided.

Components of a QI Program

A well-organized QI program uses a systematic approach to improve processes throughout an organization. This ensures that everyone speaks the same language with regard to QI projects. The JCAHO's 10 steps to QI (Box 9-2) are incorporated within many health care organizations' programs. The 10 steps ensure a systematic approach for identifying opportunities to improve quality of care and to take appropriate action in resolving any problems. In addition to the JCAHO's 10 steps, there are numerous process improvement models to be found across the country (Table 9-3). All of the models have similar elements such as identification of a process or problem. Although they appear in the table to be linear, the processes are cyclical (Keill and Johnson, 1994). The models use a scientific approach to problem solving, similar to the

---

Box 9-1
Dimensions of Performance

Doing the Right Thing

Efficacy of a procedure or treatment (e.g., pain management, skin care) in relation to a client's condition. Does the procedure or treatment produce the desired result?

Appropriateness of a test, procedure, or service to meet the client's needs. Is the level of care given considered necessary (e.g., use of pulse oximetry instead of arterial blood gases)?

Doing the Right Thing Well

Availability of a needed test, procedure, treatment, or service to the client who needs it (e.g., appointment scheduling in clinics, access to emergency care)

Timeliness with which a needed test, procedure, treatment, or service is provided to the client (e.g., response time for stat x-ray, delays in operating room cases)

Effectiveness with which tests, procedures, treatments, and services are provided (e.g., success with established standard of care on a CareMap in meeting client outcomes)

Continuity of the services provided to the client with respect to other services, practitioners, and providers over time (e.g., prompt and appropriate referrals to home health; use of a teaching plan preadmission, during a hospital stay, and postadmission)

Safety of the client (and others) to whom the services are provided (e.g., use of physical restraints, use of Standard Precautions)

Efficiency with which services are provided, showing the relationship between outcomes and the resources used to deliver care (e.g., readmission rate to hospital, comparing client's functional status with the cost of providing care)

Respect and caring with which services are provided (e.g., client satisfaction ratings, informing clients about advance directives)

1. Establish responsibility and accountability for a QI program.
2. Define the scope of service for a clinical area.
3. Define the key aspects of service for the clinical area.
4. Develop quality indicators to monitor the outcomes and appropriateness of care delivered.
5. Establish thresholds for evaluation of indicators.
6. Collect and analyze data from monitoring activities.
7. Evaluate results of monitoring activities to determine the need for change in practice.
8. Resolve problems through development of action plans.
9. Reevaluate to determine if plan was successful.
10. Communicate QI results to the organization.

From Joint Commission on Accreditation of Healthcare Organizations: *1998 Accreditation manual for hospitals*, vol 1, *Standards*, Chicago, 1997, The Commission.

rector whose responsibilities include ensuring that nursing plays a key role in the organization's QI program. On nursing care areas, clinics, or within home health sections, a nurse manager is often responsible for supporting a unit-based program. That manager assists in bringing together the multidisciplinary team that conducts QI projects. Individual staff members are responsible for monitoring quality, making decisions about practice, and ensuring that quality care is administered.

Scope of service. Each nursing unit or practice area involved in the care of a select group of clients provides a well-defined set of services. An analysis of a unit's scope of service reveals the types of clients who receive nursing care and the types of processes involved in delivering care. An example might be a general medicine unit in an acute care hospital that cares for middle-age and older adult clients who have diabetes, heart failure, and gastrointestinal disorders. The unit is involved in processes including medication administration, diabetes education, referrals for cardiac diagnostic testing, and endoscopy. An understanding of the scope of service allows staff to focus on quality issues related to typical client groups.

Key aspects of service. The unit-based committee reviews activities or services considered most important in providing quality service to clients. Examples of key aspects of service on the medicine unit might include client education, postdiagnostic monitoring, and administration of intravenous therapy.

To identify the greatest opportunity for measuring quality, nurses categorize the key aspects of service by high volume, high risk, and problem areas. Aspects of care are high volume if over 50% of the unit's clients receive that service. An aspect of care is high risk if performing or omitting the activity could result in trauma

nursing process, that often requires returning to various steps in the model to evaluate and then reassess work that needs to be done. An organization may use the JCAHO's 10-step program to organize their QI program but use a QI model such as FOCUS-PDCA to structure problem analysis and resolution.

Responsibility for program. A Director for Quality Improvement can be found within each organization to assume responsibility for a QI program. Often the department of nursing has a director or assistant di-

---

TABLE 9-3
Models for Process Improvement

PRIDE	FOCUS-PDCA	FADE
Process—select one to improve	**F**ind process to improve	Focus on a problem
	Organize team that knows process	
Relevant dimensions of performance measurement	**C**larify current knowledge of process	**A**nalyze the problem
Interpret data and evaluate variance	**U**nderstand causes of process variation	
Design or redesign the process	**S**elect process improvement	
Execute the plan	PDCA: **P**lan	**D**evelop a plan
	Do	**E**xecute the plan
	Check	
	Act	
Improve—validate by remeasuring		

Modified from Keill P, Johnson T: Optimizing performance through process improvement, *J Nurs Care Qual* 9(1):1, 1994.

or death for the client or litigation or loss of license. Finally, problem-prone aspects of care are those that have the potential to produce problems for the client, staff, or institution (Patton and Stanley, 1993). This method for prioritizing helps the staff to focus on the most important care activities. In the example of the medicine unit, if a high volume of clients are diabetic and if the unit has seen a problem of readmissions resulting from poor glucose control, an opportunity may exist to improve client education and support.

Developing quality indicators.

A **quality indicator** is a quantitative measure of an important aspect of care that determines whether quality of service conforms to requirements. Examples might include percentage of clients who successfully self-administer insulin, incidence of wound infection, or percentage of serious medication errors. It is a standard of performance. The quality indicator is the focus for a QI project with the staff monitoring criteria that will show if an indicator is being met. There are three types of indicators: structure, process, and outcome.

Structure indicators evaluate the structure or systems for delivering care, for example, percentage of staff on nights, compliance in checking emergency cart contents, and nurses' attendance at required courses. **Process indicators** evaluate the manner in which care is delivered, for example, use of a pain assessment, recovery of clients from sedation, and client education methods. **Outcome indicators** evaluate the end result of care delivered (Patton and Stanley, 1993). They represent measurable changes in a client's status after receiving care, for example, the client's ability to administer insulin after instruction or the condition of the client's skin following use of a skin care protocol.

Processes of care are obviously closely related to outcomes and the structure in which a process of care occurs, enhances, or hinders the effectiveness of care (Donabedian, 1988). When a unit-based team selects an indicator for QI monitoring it is important that the indicator be relevant. It is often appropriate to measure a process as well as the anticipated outcome, to know if standards of care are being met. For example, the staff on the medicine unit may choose to measure the staff's success in implementing diabetes instruction early while measuring whether clients learn to administer insulin correctly. When a unit-based team sits together to select quality indicators for a QI project, it helps to ask which processes and related outcomes need improvement (Keill and Johnson, 1994). Processes to improve may include the following:

- A weak process that is causing problems (e.g., poor pain management for sickle cell clients)
- A stable process that is adequate but can benefit from improvement (e.g., waiting time for ambulatory surgery reduced to improve client satisfaction)

- A process linked to negative outcomes (e.g., education of newly diagnosed clients with diabetes with an incidence of readmission to the hospital for poor glucose control)

When staff analyze the processes that are high volume, high risk, and problem prone, the team selects indicators that are most relevant to improve.

Establishing thresholds for evaluation.

After selecting a quality indicator, staff members must determine ways to quantitatively measure the indicator. The occurrence of an indicator, or the percentage of times the indicator is observed (e.g., the number of clients who can successfully explain self-care instructions compared with the number instructed) is one common measure. The **threshold** is a standard for determining whether a problem exists. A measurement that falls below a threshold indicates a problem. For example, the staff may set a threshold that states 90% of the clients who receive instruction will correctly self-administer insulin. If after monitoring, the results show only 88% of clients correctly self-administer insulin, the threshold is not met. Staff members will then thoroughly review the factors interfering with successful client education. When QI is an ongoing process, staff continuously work to improve outcomes or performances by raising thresholds.

It is important to understand that almost all processes have variation. For example, consider the process of diabetic instruction and the associated outcome of clients administering insulin. Possible variations in this process and outcome might include time when teaching begins, the materials available for instruction, the number of staff who teach, and learner motivation. Setting a specific threshold, for example, clients score 90% on a diabetes skills test and staff complete instruction 100% of the time, may not be routinely achievable. The intent in any quality improvement program is to seek ways to continuously improve. This means to define the acceptable level of performance and allow for normal variability.

Data collection and analysis.

On unit-based committees, nurses and staff colleagues monitor criteria for each quality indicator for a predetermined number of clients or cases. Staff must collect meaningful information on a sufficient number of clients to allow accurate analysis of the appropriateness of care. In the example of diabetic instruction and insulin administration, staff might monitor criteria including use of recommended teaching materials, staff's compliance with teaching standards (e.g., topics and content), and each client's score on a return demonstration test. Additional criteria might include time when teaching begins, age of client, and client's experience with previous instruction. Collection of relevant data allows accurate analysis of potential problems with quality and their possible causes. For example, if diabetic clients perform poorly on their demonstration test, staff can analyze if standards are inconsistently met or if teaching is unnecessarily delayed. Learning ability may also differ between older adults and younger clients.

Evaluation of care.

Monitoring of quality indicators evaluates if specifically defined processes reach desired outcomes. If results exceed or meet a threshold or if performance is within the controls set for a process, no problem has been identified and the process is performing well. When thresholds for satisfactory care are not met or when performance is below the control limits set, staff must attempt to determine the cause of problems. For example, if clients who receive diabetic instruction are only able to score an average of 70% on a return demonstration test, staff must determine the reasons. This step requires nurses and colleagues to honestly review practice activities and look for opportunities to reinforce nursing care standards or improve practice.

This is a time when the team may choose to use one of the models for quality improvement. The **FOCUS-PDCA** model allows staff to find the aspect of the process to improve, organize an expert team who knows the process, clarify knowledge about the process, understand any sources of variation, and select an improvement or solution. A key requirement is to be sure the right experts are involved in reviewing the process. In the case of diabetic instruction, it is important to have dietitians, nursing staff, diabetes nurse specialists, educators, and pharmacists involved as part of the team. Many of these staff members might have been on the original QI committee. However, once a problem is identified, additional team members may be needed. The group uses the steps of FOCUS-PDCA to clarify the process used for client instruction, understand what sources of variation may be occurring, and recommend an approach to improve client learning through demonstration of injections.

Resolution of problems.

After evaluating factors contributing to quality problems, staff develop action plans to improve the process and expected outcomes. It is important to establish actions that will result in success. For example, the action of merely notifying staff that a problem exists is unlikely to change practice or improve outcomes. An action plan should be more direct. In FOCUS-PDCA staff *Plan* the action or improvement to make, *Do* or implement the change, *Check* or analyze results of the change, and then *Act* on the findings. For example, the team may discover that clients are not performing well with insulin administration because teaching is not being started as soon as the client learns that insulin will be a form of therapy. In addition, the staff is having difficulty acquiring teaching materials needed for instruction. In this case, the team recommends having the pharmacy send instructional materials when insulin is sent to the unit, and that a clinical pharmacist assist with instruction on insulin therapy. The staff nurses and nurse specialist develop a protocol that outlines specific content to teach daily until the client learns to administer injections. Collectively the team develops an innovative approach to teaching that is designed to get appropriate information to the client more quickly and efficiently so learning can take place.

Evaluation of improvement.

After implementing an action plan to improve quality of care, the staff must reevaluate the success of the plan. In the example, staff members repeat monitoring of the teaching process and the results of client testing to see if improvement has been made.

The change may be positive or negative. For example, if client test scores improve, the team has successfully improved outcomes. Similarly, if test scores show no improvement or even worsen, a new plan of action is needed. The QI process is similar to the nursing process. When desired outcomes (QI criteria) are not met, the staff reinstitutes the QI process.

Communication of results.

The results of QI activities must be communicated to staff in all appropriate organizational departments. If findings and results are not communicated, practice changes will likely not occur. Regular discussion of QI activities in staff meetings, distribution of QI newsletters or memos, and a mechanism for QI committee members to personally report to other colleagues are examples of communication strategies. Often a QI study reveals information that applies to other units or departments. In this case the organization must be responsible for responding to the problem with resources needed to make changes. Revision of policies and procedures, modification of standards of care, or implementation of system changes are examples of ways that an organization may respond.

The incorporation of a QI program within a health care setting benefits the client, professional staff, and institution. With a focus on client outcomes, QI activities lead to a selection of interventions that result in improved client care. Professional staff members learn from their own practice, identify opportunities to change practice, and gain greater satisfaction from improved client outcomes. An institution benefits from an improved level of care delivery that reduces excessive use of resources and improves client satisfaction.

Key Terms

evaluation	quality improvement
FOCUS-PDCA	(QI)
outcome indicators	quality indicator
process indicators	standard of care
professional standards	structure indicators
review organizations	threshold
(PSROs)	

■ Key Concepts

Evaluation determines a client's response to nursing actions and the extent to which goals of care have been met.

The nurse compares the client's response to nursing actions with expected outcomes established during planning.

Evaluation measures are assessment skills used to collect data to evaluate a client's care.

The nursing care plan is modified based on data obtained during evaluation.

As a result of evaluation, client priorities may change.

Expected outcomes are stated in behavioral terms to describe the desired effect of nursing actions.

Evaluation enables the nurse to determine the reason that the care plan was successful or unsuccessful.

For nurses to be accountable for their practice, they must know the outcomes of care.

Evaluation involves critical thinking because the nurse determines the optimal way to deliver nursing care.

Quality improvement is a disciplined approach to find ways to improve the processes and outcomes of health care.

The three types of quality indicators are structure, process, and outcome.

To successfully improve a process, all staff members who are familiar with the process need to be involved.

Establishing thresholds or statistical controls allows the staff to determine if changes to a process are successful.

■ Critical Thinking Activities

1. Mr. Vacaro has been visiting the clinic for over a month. He visits weekly for follow-up care for a chronic venous stasis ulcer of the left leg. The nurse's note at the time of his first visit contained the following information: "Ulcer with irregular margins, 4 cm wide by 5 cm long and approximately 0.5 cm deep, and foul-smelling purulent yellowish drainage. Only subcutaneous tissue visible. Brownish rust skin around ulcer. Zinc oxide and calamine gauze applied to ulcer. Ace bandage applied to gauze. Client instructed to return in 2 weeks." As the nurse caring for the client on the follow-up visit, what expected outcomes would you anticipate for the goal of "Wound will demonstrate healing within 4 weeks"? What evaluative measures would you use to determine if the wound is healing?

2. Mr. Chu is a 50-year-old man with chronic obstructive pulmonary disease (COPD) with hypoxemia, fatigue, and dyspnea. He is to be discharged with home oxygen at 2 liters. His primary nurse has identified the need to teach Mr. Chu about home oxygen. Mr Chu will likely be in the hospital for 2 more days. Explain why evaluation is important in this case example. How will the nurse's evaluation of Mr. Chu's learning influence the plan of care at discharge?

3. As a nurse on a general medicine unit you care for a number of clients who receive central line intravenous (IV) therapy. Over the last month, three clients have developed an infection at the line insertion site of their central IV lines. Develop a quality indicator and monitoring criteria to measure this clinical practice problem.

References

Benner P: *From novice to expert: excellence and power in clinical nursing practice,* Menlo Park, Calif, 1984, Addison-Wesley.

Carnevali DL, Thomas MD: *Diagnostic reasoning and treatment decision making in nursing,* Philadelphia, 1993, JB Lippincott.

Donabedian A: The quality of care: how can it be assessed? *JAMA* 260:1743, 1988.

Health Care Advisory Board: *Next generation of outcomes tracking: implications for health plans and systems,* vol 2, *Quality measures,* Washington, DC, 1994, The Advisory Board.

Hickey PW: *Nursing process handbook,* St. Louis, 1991, Mosby.

Joint Commission on Accreditation of Healthcare Organizations: *1998 Accreditation manual for hospitals,* vol 1, *Standards,* Chicago, 1997, The Commission.

Keill P, Johnson T: Optimizing performance through process improvement, *J Nurs Care Qual* 9(1):1, 1994.

Patton S, Stanley J: Bridging quality assurance and continuous quality improvement, *J Nurs Care Qual* 7(2):15, 1993.

Scoble KB, Hembrough B: Nursing clinical pertinence review: a step toward quality improvement, *J Nurs Care Qual* 7(2):52, 1993.

Professional Standards in Nursing Practice

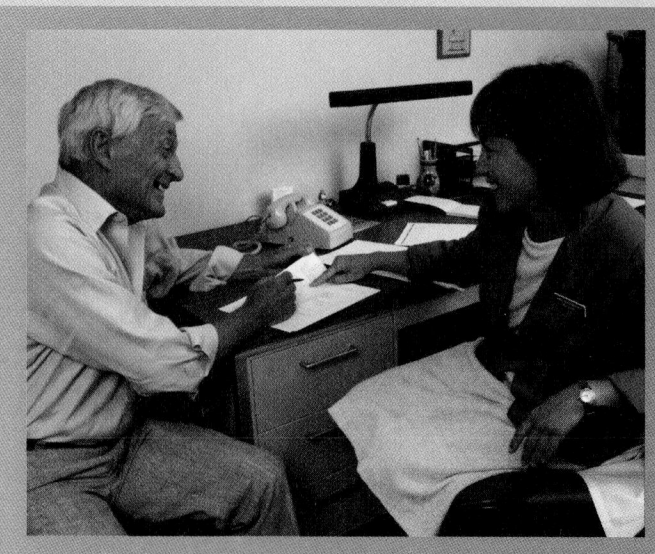

10

Professional Nursing Roles

OBJECTIVES

Mastery of content in this chapter will enable the student to:

- Define the key terms listed.
- List the characteristics of a profession.
- Define professional nursing and describe its evolution.
- Examine how the role of the professional nurse has evolved over time.
- List the skill set required for the professional nurse in the new health care environment.
- Describe the roles of the professional nurse.
- Examine career opportunities for the professional nurse.

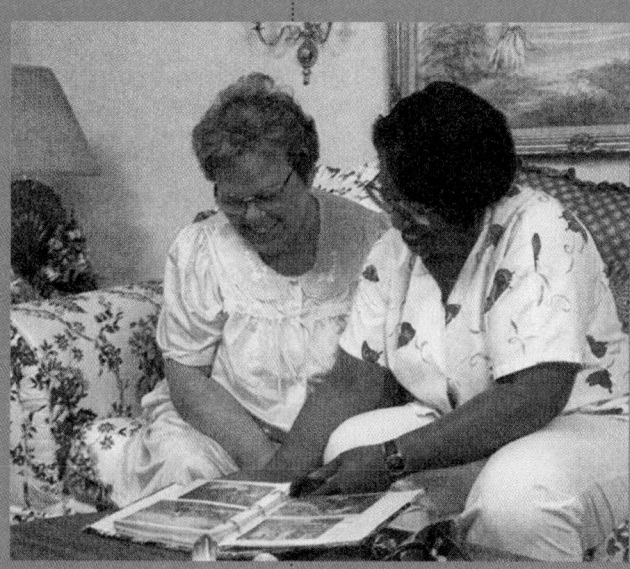

The nursing profession is evolving and is rooted in a basic education with a liberal, well-rounded foundation and extended education of its members. The basis for the profession is a theoretical body of information defining its skills, abilities, and norms. A professional nurse provides a specified service and follows a code of ethics for practice. Professional nurses have autonomy in decision making and practice. Criteria to assess a profession from a nonprofession include the presence of theory, relevance to basic social values, a training or educational period, motivation, autonomy, a sense of commitment, a sense of community, and a code of ethics (Bernhard and Walsh, 1995). Nursing has achieved professionalism in social values and a strong code of ethics. The priority areas for nursing to focus its development include education, entry level into practice and nursing research to develop a systematic body of nursing knowledge; theory, a single theoretical basis for practice; and commitment (Bernhard and Walsh, 1995).

The role of the professional nurse has evolved from the days of Florence Nightingale (1860) when nurses were expected to provide care, perform housekeeping duties, wash the linen, and prepare and serve the meals. Throughout history nurses have had many roles, including direct care provider, client advocate, teacher, counselor, and researcher. The evolution of nursing has brought us to one of the most exciting and challenging times in our history. There are many opportunities to shape the future of the nursing profession and nursing practice while we improve the quality of the lives of our clients and communities.

The uniqueness of nursing was its focus on the care of the client, the community, and society. Nurses not only provided for care of the sick but were also the first providers of primary health care. It is only in the last decade that our medical colleagues have come to understand health promotion and wellness as an integral part of health care. As nursing evolved in the nineteenth century, health promotion, wellness, and self-care were added to the traditional care and comfort of the sick. Nursing included keeping people healthy; assisting them to adapt to lifestyle changes resulting from illness or injury; promoting comfort measures; teaching and educating clients about their health and well-being; and striving to improve their quality of life and providing comfort, dignity, and respect at life's end. Virginia Henderson (1966) defined nursing in the following statement.

The unique function of the nurse is to assist the individual, sick or well, in the performance of those activities contributing to health, its recovery, or to a peaceful death that the client would perform unaided if he had the necessary strength, will or knowledge. And to do this in such a way as to help the client gain independence as rapidly as possible.

···EVOLUTION OF NURSING ROLES

Historical Perspective

Florence Nightingale, founder of modern nursing, wrote *Notes on Nursing: What It Is and What It Is Not* (Nightingale, 1860), which established the first nursing philosophy based on health maintenance and restoration. Her views on nursing were derived from her spiritual philosophy. She viewed nursing as a search for truth in finding answers to health care questions or discovering and using divine laws of healing in nursing practice (Macrae, 1995).

However, one has to look further back in history to identify the real beginnings of nursing. In early history, nursing was a community service provided to assist in preserving and protecting the family (Donahue, 1995). Nursing began as a desire to keep people healthy and provide comfort, care, and assurance to the sick. Nurses were caring for the sick, providing hygiene and comfort, as far back as the Middle Ages (1100-1200 AD). The nurse usually worked under the direction of a physician or, as in some ancient cultures, the religious leaders (Deloughery, 1995).

The Crusades expanded health care and nursing by developing nursing orders for men and establishing hospitals. Nursing grew out of societal needs. The bubonic plague stimulated formation of the Alexian Brothers to care for the victims, and other secular groups were formed to address specific health care needs (Box 10-1). After the Crusades, large cities developed, which led to overcrowding with inadequate ventilation, heating, cooling, sanitation, garbage collection, plumbing, water, and food preservation and a lack of elementary hygiene practice.

Woven throughout history is the nurse's role as midwife. Midwifery flourished during the Middle Ages. These women were accepted by medicine, nursing, and society to assist women in childbearing.

The Order of the Deaconesses is one of the earliest records of Christian nursing providing visiting nursing care. In 1663 St. Vicent de Paul founded the Sisters of Charity. They provided visiting nursing, caring for people in their homes, as well as hospitals, asylums, and poorhouses. The need for nurses and increased nursing responsibilities was the hallmark of the eighteenth century, mostly because of economic growth, development of cities and hospitals, smallpox epidemics, and the Revolutionary War. The Sisters of Charity were introduced in America in 1809, later changing their name to the Daughters of Charity (Donahue, 1995).

In 1853 Florence Nightingale went to study with the Sisters of Charity in Paris, France. After her training, she became the superintendent of the English General Hospitals in Turkey. Her influence and skills changed hygiene, sanitation, and nursing practice, resulting in a

Box 10-1
Milestones in Nursing History

300 AD   Entry of women into nursing.

1100-1200 AD   Formation of Hospital Brothers of St. Anthoney's.

Formation of the Brothers of Misericordia, Italy.

Formation of the Alexian Brothers.

1633   Sisters of Charity founded.

1809   Mother Elizabeth Seton introduced the Sisters of Charity into America, later known as the Daughters of Charity.

1836   Deaconess Institute of Kaiserwerth, Germany, was founded.

1846   Nightingale received the *Yearbook of the Institution of Deaconess at Kaiserwerth.*

1860   Establishment of the Nightingale Training School for Nurses at St. Thomas' Hospital in London, England.

1860   Florence Nightingale publishes *Notes on Nursing: What It Is and What It Is Not.*

1860-1865   Dorthea Lynde Dix served as superintendent of the Union Army female nurses.

Mary Ann Ball (Mother Bickerdyke) organized ambulance services, searched for wounded, and supervised nurses.

Harriett Tubman tended to soldiers and led over 300 slaves to freedom through the Underground Railroad Movement.

1874   First training school in Canada founded; St. Cahterine's, Ontario.

1882   United States ratified the American Red Cross founded by Clara Barton.

1884   Mary Agnes Snively assumed directorship of Toronto General Hospital.

1890   Establishment of the Nurses' Associated Alumni of the United States and Canada.

1893   First community health service for the poor, Henry Street Settlement.

1894   Isabel Hamptom Robb was the first superintendent of the Johns Hopkins Training School in Baltimore, Maryland.

1896   Nurses' Associated Alumnae of the United States and Canada (NAAUSC) founded.

1897   Initial discussion of nursing code of ethics.

1899   Canadian affiliation removed from NAAUSC.

1901   First university affiliated nursing program. Army Nurse Corps established.

1902   Sigma Theta Tau was formed by six student nurses from Indiana University.

1907   First professor of nursing, Mary Adelaide Nutting.

1908   Navy Nurse Corps established.

Canadian National Association of Trained Nurses (later changed to the Canadian Nurses Association, 1924) was founded.

1911   NAAUSC became the American Nurses Association (ANA).

1920   Graduate nurse midwifery programs established.

1923   Goldmark Report: Rockefeller Foundation–funded survey identified need for increased financial support to university-based schools of nursing.

1926   ANA Code of Ethics proposed.

1948   Brown Report: Dr. Esther Lucille Brown concluded that all nursing education programs should be affiliated with universities and have their own budgets. She recommended a broad academic education within a university and 2 years of nursing education focused on technical skills.

1949   Association of Operating Room Nurses formed.

1952   Dr. Mildred Montag established the associate degree nursing program.

Nursing Research, a journal reporting on the scientific investigations of nursing, was established.

1953   National League for Nursing (NLN), in collaboration with universities, developed graduate nursing education.

1960   Yale University School of Nursing defined nursing as a profession, interaction, and relationship between two human beings (Meleis, 1996).

1965   Jerome Lysaught directed the National Commission on Nursing and Nursing Education Report. Recommended that nursing roles and responsibilities be clarified in relation to other health care professionals and that increased financial support and career opportunities were needed to attract and retain nurses.

ANA position paper defined nursing.

1969   American Association of Critical Care Nurses (AACN) formed.

1975   Oncology Nursing Society formed.

NLN required theory-based curriculum for accreditation.

1985   ANA Code for Nurses with Interpretive Statements.

1996   The Pew Report.

1996   Institute of Medicine (IOM) Report.

40% reduction in the mortality rate over a 6-month period (Donahue, 1995).

Clara Barton and Harriett Tubman were very influential in the evolution of nursing and nursing practice during the Civil War (1861-1865). After the Civil War, nursing education programs developed using the Nightingale model. At the same time the first nursing organization, the NAAUSC, was formed by Mary Agnes Snively and Isabel Hamptom Robb.

Community nursing was started in the late nineteenth century through the efforts of Lillian Wald and Mary Brewster. They established the Henry Street Settlement (1893), which focused on the health care needs of the poor in New York City tenements. These nurses were some of the first to demonstrate **autonomy** in practice, dealing with situations that required quick and innovative **problem solving,** without the supervision or direction of a physician.

The 1900s saw a movement toward a scientific, researched-based defined body of nursing knowledge. Nurses began assuming advanced practice and expanded roles. In 1922 six student nurses at Indiana University School of Nursing founded Sigma Theta Tau, an organization dedicated to research, scholarship, and leadership in nursing. Between 1950 and 1980 nurses became more specialized, and advanced educational opportunities flourished. From 1980 to the present, nursing has continued to develop its scientific basis and theories and advanced its skill basis. As we move into the twenty-first century, nursing will continue to develop new and innovative roles, more clearly define its domain, and establish its uniqueness in providing service to society.

NURSING PRACTICE

Nursing practice was defined in 1980 by the ANA Congress for Nursing Practice as "the diagnosis and treatment of the human response to actual or potential health problems" (ANA, 1980). This is a much different definition than the one published by the ANA in 1955.

Nursing practice has evolved over the years in response to societal needs. It is unique in its focus on health promotion, maintenance, and continuing care. The 1965 ANA definition of nursing and the 1986 Canadian definition of nursing and standards of practice reflect this evolution (Box 10-2).

Theoretical Models of Nursing Practice

The strength of nursing practice lies in the diversity of its nurses and their experiences, commitment, and professionalism (Levine, 1995). There are a number of nursing theories. Levine (1995) supports multiple nursing theories, because there is no global theory of nursing that fits every situation. Nurses theorize about the nature of nursing practice; the principles on which nursing practice is based; and the goals, functions, and outcomes of nursing in society.

Conceptual and theoretical nursing models are used to provide knowledge to improve practice, guide research and curricula development, and identify the goals and domain of nursing practice. A **conceptual model** is a set of global or general ideas about the individuals, groups, populations, situations, or events of interest to a discipline. Theories are made up of concepts and propositions (e.g., the events and phenomena of the discipline) (Fawcett, 1992). The development of nursing science, conceptual models, and theory contributes to a sound basis for the practice of nursing (Chinn and Jacobs, 1995). The knowledge is designed to advance and support nursing practice and health care (Chinn and Jacobs, 1995) (Box 10-3).

Nursing theories provide nurses with goals for assessment, nursing diagnoses, and interventions; common ground for communication, professional autonomy, and accountability; and the future direction for nursing research, practice, education, and administration (Marriner-Tomey 1994; Chinn and Jacobs, 1995).

Definitions and theories of nursing can help the nursing student understand how the roles, actions, responsibilities, and outcomes of nurses and nursing practice are interconnected. Table 10-1 summarizes, in chronological order, concepts basic to selected nursing theories.

Nursing practice has many dimensions that contribute to its professional nature. These include standards of practice, the nursing process, educational preparation, nurse practice acts, delivery of care models, practice settings, and roles.

Box 10-2

1986 Canadian Definition of Nursing and Standards of Practice

The nursing profession exists in response to a need of society and holds ideals related to health throughout the life span. Nurses direct their energies toward the promotion, maintenance, and restoration of health; the prevention of illness; the alleviation of suffering; and the assurance of a peaceful death when life can no longer be sustained. Nurses value a holistic view and regard an individual as a biopsychosocial being who has the capacity to set goals and make decisions and who has the right and responsibility to make informed choices congruent with personal beliefs and values. Nursing, a dynamic and supportive profession guided by its code of ethics, is rooted in caring, a concept evident throughout its four fields of activity: practice, education, administration, and research.

TABLE 10-1
Summary of Nursing Theories

Theorist	Goal of Nursing	Framework for Practice
Nightingale (1860)	To facilitate "the body's reparative processes" by manipulating client's environment	Client's environment is manipulated to include appropriate noise, nutrition, hygiene, light, comfort, socialization, and hope.
Peplau (1952)	To develop interaction between nurse and client (Peplau, 1952)	Nursing is a significant, therapeutic, interpersonal process (Peplau, 1952). Nurses participate in structuring health care systems to facilitate natural ongoing tendency of humans to develop interpersonal relationships (Marriner-Tomey, 1994).
Henderson (1955)	To work interdependently with other health care workers (Marriner-Tomey, 1994), assisting client to gain independence as quickly as possible. To help client gain lacking strength	Nurses help client to perform Henderson's 14 basic needs.
Abdellah (1960)	To provide service to individuals, families, and society. To be kind and caring but also intelligent, competent, and technically well prepared to provide this service (Marriner-Tomey, 1994)	This theory involves Abdellah's 21 nursing problems (Abdellah and others, 1960).
Orlando (1961)	To respond to client's behavior in terms of immediate needs. To interact with client to meet immediate needs by identifying client behavior, reaction of nurse, and nursing action to be taken (Chinn and Jacobs, 1995)	Three elements, including client behavior, nurse reaction, and nurse action, compose nursing situation.
Hall (1962)	To provide care and comfort to client during disease process	The client is composed of the following overlapping parts: person (core), pathological state and treatment (cure), and body (care). Nurse is care giver (Marriner-Tomey, 1994; Chinn and Jacobs, 1995).
Wiedenbach (1964)	To assist individuals in overcoming obstacles that interfere with the ability to meet demands or needs brought about by condition, environment, situation, or time	Nursing practice is related to individuals who need help because of behavioral stimulus. Clinical nursing has the following components: philosophy, purpose, practice, and art (Chinn and Jacobs, 1995).
Levine (1966)	To use conservation activities aimed at optimal use of client's resources	This adaptation model of human as integral whole is based on "four conservation principles of nursing" (Levine, 1995).
Johnson (1968)	To reduce stress so that client can move more easily through recovery process	This basic needs framework focuses on seven categories of behavior. Individual's goal is to achieve behavioral balance and steady state by adjustment and adaptation to certain forces.
Rogers (1970)	To maintain and promote health, prevent illness, and care for and rehabilitate ill and disabled client through "humanistic science of nursing" (Rogers, 1970)	"Unitary man" evolves along life process. Client continuously changes and coexists with environment.
Orem (1971)	To care for and help client attain total self-care	This is self-care deficit theory. Nursing care becomes necessary when client is unable to fulfill biological, psychological, developmental, or social needs (Orem, 1985).

TABLE 10-1

Summary of Nursing Theories—cont'd

Theorist	Goal of Nursing	Framework for Practice
King (1971)	To use communication to help client reestablish positive adaptation to environment	Nursing process is defined as dynamic interpersonal process between nurse, client, and health care system.
Travelbee (1971)	To assist individual or family to prevent or cope with illness, regain health, find meaning in illness, or maintain maximal degree of health (Marriner-Tomey, 1994)	Interpersonal process is viewed as human-to-human relationship formed during illness and "experience of suffering."
Neuman (1972)	To assist individuals, families, and groups to attain and maintain maximal level of total wellness by purposeful interventions (Neuman, 1995)	Stress reduction is goal of systems model of nursing practice. Nursing actions are in primary, secondary, or tertiary level of prevention.
Patterson and Zderad (1976)	To respond to human needs and build humanistic nursing science (Chinn and Jacobs, 1995)	Humanistic nursing requires participants to be aware of their "uniqueness" and "commonality" with others (Chinn and Jacobs, 1995).
Leininger (1978)	To provide care consistent with nursing's emerging science and knowledge with caring as central focus (Chinn and Jacobs, 1995)	With this transcultural care theory, caring is the central and unifying domain for nursing knowledge and practice.
Roy (1979)	To identify types of demands placed on client, assess adaptation to demands, and help client adapt	This adaptation model is based on the physiological, psychological, sociological, and dependence-independence adaptive modes (Roy, 1989).
Watson (1979)	To promote health, restore client to health, and prevent illness (Marriner-Tomey, 1994)	This theory involves philosophy and science of caring; caring is interpersonal process comprising interventions that result in meeting human needs.
Parse (1981)	To focus on man as living unity and man's qualitative participation with health experience (nursing as science and art [Marriner-Tomey, 1994])	Man continually interacts with environment and participates in maintenance of health (Marriner-Tomey, 1994). Health is continual, open process rather than state of well-being or absence of disease (Marriner-Tomey, 1994; Chinn and Jacobs, 1995).

■ Box 10-3

Goals of Theoretical Nursing Models

Develop curricula for nursing education.

Establish criteria for measuring the quality of nursing care, education, and research.

Guide the development of nursing care delivery systems.

Provide knowledge to improve nursing administration, practice, education, and research.

Guide research to establish an empirical knowledge base for nursing.

Identify the domain and goals of nursing.

Standards of Practice

The evolution of nursing as an independent profession and a clearer definition of the domain of nursing have created a need for development of nursing practice standards. These standards provide guidelines for care and establish criteria by which the quality and competency of care can be evaluated. Standards of practice are developed and established by a strong scientific research base and the nurse clinical experts who provide nursing care to a select group of clients. **Standards of practice** provide clients with assurance that they are receiving high-quality nursing care, the nurses know how to provide the care, and there are measures to determine if the care meets the established standards and expected outcomes.

Standards of practice are developed both within organizations and externally by accrediting bodies such as the ANA or the Joint Commission on Accreditation of Healthcare Organizations (JCAHO). The ANA (Table 10-2) and the Canadian Nurses Association (CNA) have published standards of nursing performance or practice (Box 10-4).

Standards of Care

Standards of care define and describe competent levels of nursing care. These levels of care are demonstrated through the nursing process: assessment, diagnosis, outcome identification, planning, implementation, and evaluation (Table 10-3). The nursing process is the foundation of clinical decision making and includes all significant actions taken by nurses in providing care to all clients (ANA, 1991b). Within these standards are the nursing responsibilities for diversity, safety, education, health promotion, treatment, self-care, and planning for continuity of care (ANA, 1991b).

Nursing Education

Within nursing there are different levels of practice, some based on licensure and others on education and/or certification.

Basic preparation. Formal nursing education and training did not begin until the mid-nineteenth century. Diploma, hospital-based programs were the predominant educational path for nursing education between 1900 and 1935. Education and training focused on hygiene, activities of daily living, comfort, and assisting the physician with procedures.

In the early 1900s over 1800 diploma schools of nursing were in existence. By contrast, there were less than 100 baccalaureate nursing programs providing a generic nursing educational program. Affiliation of nursing education programs with a university was first accomplished in 1901 by Mary Adelaide Nutting, the first professor of nursing (1907). New York University developed the first doctoral nursing program in 1934.

By 1963 there were 32 graduate programs in nursing across the nation.

In 1952 the associate degree 2-year nursing education program was formed by Dr. Mildred Montag. Despite the rise in associate degree programs and baccalaureate programs, hospital-based diploma programs accounted for the primary education of nurses. By 1988 nurses graduating from diploma schools of nursing had declined to 9%, whereas 58% were prepared in associate degree programs and 33% in generic baccalaureate nursing programs; the number of doctoral programs in nursing had risen to 46.

Entry Into Practice

Entry level into practice in the United States can be at the associate degree level, diploma school, or baccalaureate level. Once students have completed their training, they take the National Council Licensure Examination for Registered Nurses (NCLEX-RN). In Canada a nurse may complete diploma programs associated with community colleges or hospitals, usually 2 years in length, or complete a bachelor of science in nursing (BScN). Canadian graduate nurses take the CNA Testing Service (CNATS) examination.

As nursing leaders continue to debate the entry into practice question, nursing education has seen a decline in the number of hospital-based diploma programs and more generic baccalaureate and RN completion programs. The associate degree program completes the core nursing curriculum in 2 years, preparing the student to sit for the examination. Many students choose this option for a variety of reasons and then complete the baccalaureate and/or master's in nursing later. The generic baccalaureate program offers the opportunity for a strong scientific background and more study in nursing theory, process, introduction to research, and skills for collaboration and coordination, preparing the nurse to assume leadership roles and a foundation for graduate education.

Graduate Nursing Education

Nurses are prepared at the graduate level to advance the practice of nursing through research, expanding nursing theory, and clinical excellence. The nurse in a graduate program has many career choices and opportunities. The nurse may choose an advanced clinical path, an administrative career, or an educator focus. Graduate preparation prepares the nurse for a career in research (doctoral in philosophy, PhD), advanced clinical focus (e.g., NP, CNS, CRNA, CNM [doctoral in nursing science, DNS]), or advanced education (doctoral in education, EdD).

Nurse Practice Acts

Each state in the United States and all Canadian provinces regulate the licensure and scope of nursing practice through **nurse practice acts.** The ANA defi-

---

Box 10-4
Canadian Nurses Association Standards for Nursing Practice

Nursing practice requires that a conceptual model(s) for nursing be the basis of practice.

Nursing practice requires the effective use of the nursing process.

Nursing practice requires that the helping relationship be the nature of the client-nurse interaction.

Nursing practice requires nurses to fulfill professional responsibilities.

Modified from Canadian Nurses Association: *A definition of nursing practice: standards for nursing practice,* Ottawa, 1986, The Association.

TABLE 10-2
ANA Standards of Professional Performance

Standard	Definition	Measurement Criteria
I: Quality of care	The nurse systematically evaluates the quality and effectiveness of nursing practice	Participation in quality of care activities Practice changes are the result of quality of care activities Quality of care activities are used to initiate changes throughout the health care delivery system
II: Performance appraisal	The nurse evaluates his or her own nursing practice in relation to professional practice standards and relevant statutes and regulations	Engages in performance appraisal on a regular basis Seeks constructive feedback Takes action to achieve goals identified during performance appraisal
III: Education	The nurse acquires and maintains current knowledge in nursing practice	Participates in ongoing educational activities related to clinical knowledge and professional issues Seeks experiences to maintain clinical skills Seeks knowledge and skills appropriate to the practice setting
IV: Collegiality	The nurse contributes to the professional development of peers, colleagues, and others	Shares knowledge and skills with colleagues and others Provides peers with constructive feedback regarding their practice Contributes to an environment that is conducive to clinical education of nursing students, as appropriate
V: Ethics	The nurse's decisions and actions on behalf of clients are determined in an ethical manner	Practice is guided by the *Code for Nurses* Maintains client confidentiality Acts as a client advocate Delivers care in a nonjudgmental and nondiscriminatory manner that is sensitive to client diversity Delivers care in a manner that preserves/protects client autonomy, dignity, and rights Seeks available resources to help formulate ethical decisions
VI: Collaboration	The nurse collaborates with the client, significant others, and health care providers in providing client care	Communicates with the client, significant others, and health care providers regarding client care and nursing's role in the provision of care Consults with health care providers for client care, as needed Makes referrals, including provisions for continuity of care, as needed

VII: Research	The nurse uses research findings in practice	Uses interventions substantiated by research as appropriate to the individual's position, education, and practice environment
		Participates in research activities as appropriate to the individual's position, education, and practice environment
		  Identification of clinical problems suitable for nursing research
		  Participation in data collection
		  Participation in a unit, organization, or community research committee or program
		  Sharing research activities with others
		  Conducting research
		  Critiquing research for application

VIII: Resource utilization	The nurse considers factors related to safety, effectiveness, and cost in planning and delivering client care	Evaluates factors related to safety, effectiveness, and cost when practice options would result in the same expected client outcome Assigns tasks or delegates care based on client needs and provider knowledge and skills Assists the client and significant others in identifying and securing appropriate services available to address health-related needs

Modified from American Nurses Association: *Standards of clinical practice*, Washington, DC, 1991b, The Association.

TABLE 10-3
ANA Standards of Care

Standard	Element
Assessment The nurse collects client health data.	The priority of data collection is determined by the client's immediate condition of needs. Pertinent data are collected using appropriate assessment techniques. Data collection involves the client, significant others, and health care providers when appropriate. The data collection process is systematic and ongoing. Relevant data are documented in a retrievable form.
Nursing Diagnosis The nurse analyzes the assessment data in determining diagnoses.	Diagnoses are derived from the assessment data. Diagnoses are validated with the client, significant others, and health care providers, when possible. Diagnoses are documented in a manner that facilitates the determination of expected outcomes and plan of care.
Outcome Identification The nurse identifies expected outcomes individualized to the client.	Outcomes are derived from the diagnoses. Outcomes are documented as measurable goals. Outcomes are mutually formulated with the client and health care providers, when possible. Outcomes are realistic in relation to client's present and potential capabilities. Outcomes are attainable in relation to resources available to the client. Outcomes include a time estimate for attainment. Outcomes provide direction for continuity of care.
Planning The nurse develops a plan of care that prescribes interventions to attain expected outcomes.	The plan is individualized to the client's condition or needs. The plan is developed with the client, significant others, and health care providers, when appropriate. The plan reflects current nursing practice. The plan is documented. The plan provides for continuity of care.
Implementation The nurse implements the interventions identified in the plan of care.	Interventions are consistent with the established plan of care. Interventions are implemented in a safe and appropriate manner. Interventions are documented.
Evaluation The nurse evaluates the client's progress toward attainment of outcomes.	Evaluation is systematic and ongoing. The client's responses to interventions are documented. The effectiveness of interventions is evaluated in relation to outcomes. Revisions in diagnoses, outcomes, and the plan of care are documented. The client, significant others, and health care providers are involved in the evaluation process, when appropriate.

Modified from American Nurses Association: *Standards of clinical practice,* Washington, DC, 1991b, The Association.

nition of nursing (1991b) is the basis for most practice acts. In many states the nurse practice acts have been revised to include expanded nursing roles and to differentiate between medical and nursing diagnosis and treatment.

Licensure

Each state regulates the practice of safe and competent nursing practice through the licensure process. Many states require evidence of continuing education for licensure (ANA, 1991a). This promotes ongoing education and the need to remain current with trends in nursing and health care.

Licensed practical nurse (LPN).

The **licensed practical nurse (LPN),** also known as the licensed vocational nurse (LVN), or in Canada, registered nurse's assistant (RNA), is trained in basic nursing skills and the provision of direct client care. Education usually includes a year of hospital and community college courses that focus on practical nurse education. After completion of the National Council Licensure Examination for Practical Nurses (NCLEX-PN), the LPN is licensed by the state. The LPN/LVN/RNA practices under the direction and supervision of a registered professional nurse. LPNs in many states have advanced skills training in care and initiation of intravenous fluids. LPNs practice in a variety of settings, including the hospital, ambulatory care, physician practice offices, and home care.

Registered professional nurse (RN).

The **registered professional nurse (RN)** is eligible to take the state licensing examination after completion of a program from an approved school of nursing. In the United States students usually take the examination in the state where they attended school, although they may take the exam in a state where they plan to practice. Once initial licensure is granted, the RN may request reciprocity for licensure in another state. Currently efforts are underway to establish mutual recognition for nurse licensure, meaning that once licensed, a nurse would be able to practice in other states as long as the state practice act is followed (National Council of State Boards of Nursing, 1997). In Canada the nursing program must be approved by the Provincial Board of Nursing in the province the student is seeking licensure.

NURSING ROLES

Nurses have many roles that will continue to change and evolve as the health care environment changes. The challenge will be to maintain the unique skills that define nursing. The roles of the nurse meet client and family needs; guide, assist, and teach the client and family; and provide an environment that facilitates client and family growth and development.

Direct Care Provider

As a **direct care provider** the nurse assists the client to regain health through the healing process. The nurse provides a holistic approach to care, including assisting the client/family in coping with the physical, emotional, social, and spiritual impacts of the illness. In **collaboration** with other health care providers and the client, the nurse develops a plan of care to address the client-identified care needs, as well as those identified by the professional team (Gerteis and others, 1993). Outcomes of care with intermediate goals are established to measure success and show progress of care.

Clinical decision making is an important aspect of providing direct care (Figure 10-1). The nursing process provides the template for clinical decision making. Critical thinking skills (see Chapter 4) are used to evaluate care options and potential client outcomes before interventions are implemented to ensure the most appropriate and cost-effective measures are used.

Excellent communication skills are needed to provide care, collaborate with other health care providers, and assist in decision making. The quality of communication is a critical factor in meeting client, family, and community needs (see Chapter 13).

Providing compassionate care and comfort is important in caring for clients. It is a traditional and historical role for nursing, one that has continued to be important

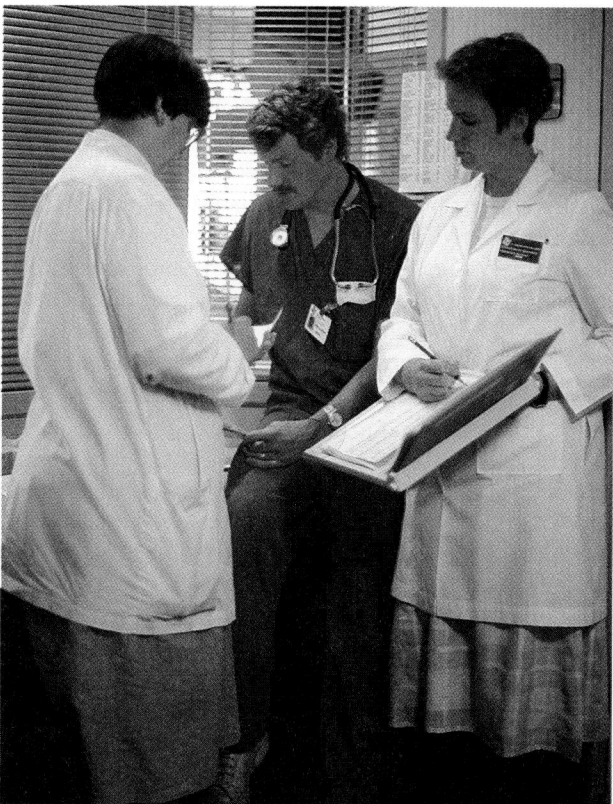

Figure 10-1. Decision making is at the core of nursing practice.

to nurses as roles evolve and expand. Nurses demonstrate their care and compassion by attending to the emotional and spiritual needs of the client, in addition to the client's physical and comfort needs. The nurse assists the client to reach therapeutic goals rather than emotional or physical dependence.

Each client has unique feelings, needs, values, and beliefs. It is critical for the nurse to separate his or her own feelings, values, beliefs, and needs from those of the client. The nurse must be nonjudgmental, accepting, and responsive to the client and family. Through education, influence, and collaboration with the client and family, the nurse is able to improve health and promote prevention and wellness.

Protector and Client Advocate

As **protector** the nurse helps maintain a safe environment for the client and takes steps to prevent injury and protect the client from possible adverse effects of diagnostic or treatment measures. Confirming that a client does not have a medication allergy or supplying an allergy alert bracelet to the client is an example of the protector role of the nurse.

In the role of **client advocate** the nurse protects clients' human and legal rights and provides assistance in asserting those rights if the need arises. For example, the nurse may assist the client in identifying new resources for home medical equipment supplies because of disputes with the original supplier.

Case Manager

In **case management** the nurse coordinates the activities of the other health care providers in collaboration with the direct care providers. The case manager is usually assigned to a specific population of clients and is usually not responsible for providing direct care. He or she collaborates with the other disciplines caring for the client, integrating all of the plans of care and client goals into a single, comprehensive, and coordinated experience for the client. The case manager focuses on moving the client through the health care environment, assisting with scheduling of tests and procedures, and interacting with various care providers and third-party payers. Many times case managers will follow a client across all settings, including ambulatory care and home care.

Client/Family Educator

Many nurses choose to focus their energies on providing client and family education. This may be in the acute care or ambulatory care setting. An example of this is the diabetic nurse educator. These nurses are experts in providing clients and their families with the information and skills necessary to manage their illness independently. These educators often arrange specific times to meet with the client and family for education. The nurse at the bedside plays an important role in reinforcing and validating information and skills the client and family have been taught.

This role is also part of the direct care provider responsibilities. The nurse uses every interaction with the client or family as an opportunity to provide information and education, providing a stepped progression to learning. In the acute care setting, education is focused on skills the client and family need to safely provide self-care from discharge to the next health care provider encounter. Clients are being discharged sicker than ever before and may still be in pain, groggy, or too worried and anxious about discharge to retain information.

⋯CAREER ROLES

Nurse Educator

The **nurse educator** primarily practices in schools of nursing and staff development departments of health care institutions. Faculty within schools of nursing usually have a clinical background and advanced skills in education. They are responsible for teaching nursing theory, clinical practice, and technical skills to prepare the student to take the licensure examination and assume the role of the nurse.

Staff development educators are nurses with a strong clinical background, advanced clinical skills, and expertise in teaching skills to staff. They develop and provide continuing education programs to meet the needs of the organization, the staff, and external requirements of the JCAHO and the Occupational Safety and Health Administration (OSHA). These may include nursing orientation; safety and infection control inservices; critical care education; cardiopulmonary resuscitation (CPR); and instruction about new procedures, products, or equipment.

Advanced Practice Nurse

The **advanced practice nurse (APN)** has a master's degree in nursing and expertise in a specialized area of practice (ANA, 1995). In almost all states, **certification** by an approved certifying body, such as the American Nurses Credentialing Center (ANCC), is required along with graduate education and advanced training in physical assessment, pharmacology, and clinical care. The ANA has many policy statements that define these roles and their scope of practice.

APNs include clinical nurse specialists, nurse practitioners, nurse midwives, and certified registered nurse anesthetists (Figure 10-2). An APN may specialize in the management of a specific population such as pediatrics or gerontology or a client population such as oncology or pulmonary.

In many states these individuals enter into collaborative agreements with physicians and are able to practice without direct physician supervision. In most states, APNs have prescriptive authority and are able to pre-

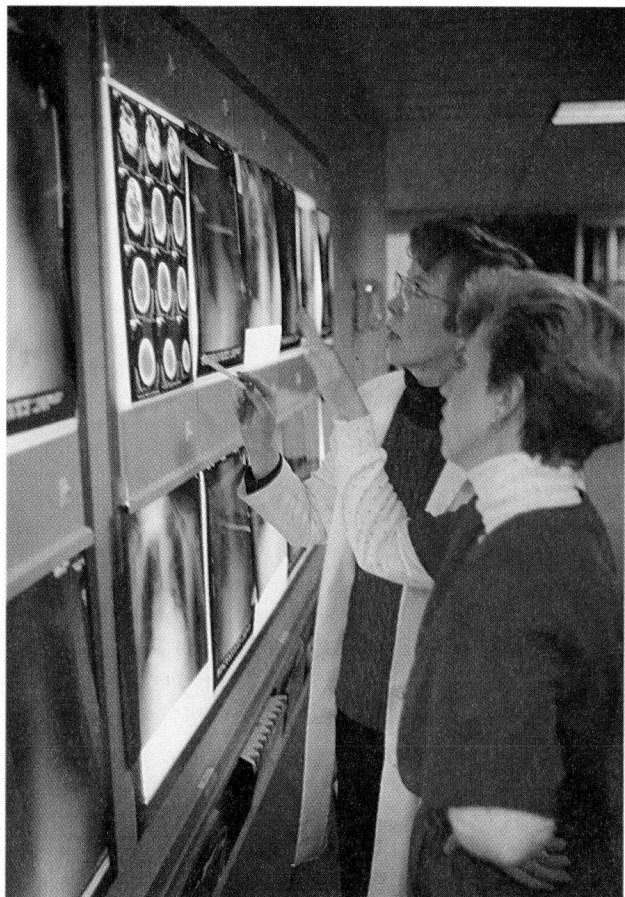

Figure 10-2. Nurse specialist consults on difficult client case.

scribe medications for clients. Some states also provide drug enforcement agency (DEA) numbers for the APN, who then can prescribe Schedule II drugs (narcotics). Each state is slightly different in its requirements for recognition as an APN.

Clinical nurse specialists (CNSs) are nurses prepared at the graduate level and who practice in a specialty area of nursing. The CNS functions as an expert clinician, educator, case manager, consultant, and researcher to plan or improve the quality of care provided to the client and family.

Nurse practitioners (NPs) are RNs with advanced education who focus their practice in primary care settings, such as ambulatory care, private practice, or community-based settings. A significant percentage of primary care encounters extend beyond the boundaries of medicine and demand the expertise of the nurse. The NP is able to establish a collaborative provider-client relationship.

The major nurse practitioner categories are adult, family, pediatric, obstetrics-gynecology, and geriatric NPs. An NP has the knowledge and skills necessary to detect and manage limited acute and chronic stable conditions. The NP's educational preparation includes

a practitioner program or a master's degree in nursing.

The idea of an acute care NP is being explored, mostly in the academic or university-based hospital. This is in response to the declining numbers of house officers and the additional requirements for residents and interns to spend more time in alternative care settings such as ambulatory and home care. These programs are just in the developmental stages.

Certified nurse midwives (CNMs) are RNs with advanced training in midwifery and are certified by the American College of Nurse-Midwives. Nurse midwives provide independent care for women during normal pregnancy, labor, and delivery, as well as newborn care. They may also provide routine gynecological services and family planning.

Certified registered nurse anesthetists (CRNAs) are nurses who have received advanced training in an accredited program in anesthesiology. They provide surgical anesthesia under the guidance and supervision of an anesthesiologist.

Nurse Administrator

A **nurse administrator** manages client care and specific nursing services within a health care agency. Positions range from middle management, such as the nurse manager or supervisor, to upper management, such as associate director, director, or vice president. Responsibilities include strategic planning, budgeting, staffing, employee selection and evaluation, and employee development. Middle management positions usually require a baccalaureate degree in nursing, and upper level positions require a master's degree.

Nurse Researcher

The **nurse researcher** is usually a doctorally prepared nurse who investigates problems to improve nursing care, further defines and expands the scope of nursing, or validates nursing care practices. The nurse researcher frequently enlists the assistance of staff nurses and CNSs to investigate nursing issues and quality improvement opportunities as they relate to client care and nursing practice.

▪▪▪PRACTICE SETTINGS

Traditionally the majority of nurses have practiced in the acute care hospital setting, although our history is rich in home care, primary care, and rehabilitative care. As health care reform moves into the twenty-first century, more and more of the care clients receive will be in an ambulatory care setting, home care, or short-term stay of less than 24 hours (see Chapter 2). The shift in where care is provided is driven by two factors: the rising cost of health care and the advances in technology. Clients who used to stay in the hospital 14 days after a multiple vessel coronary artery bypass graft (CABG) are now having minimally invasive surgery through a thorascope with a length of stay of 3 days and no intensive care unit (ICU) component. Clients are sent home with instructions to perform catheter care, manage the wound, and administer intravenous (IV) medications, skills previously reserved for the nurse caring for the client.

Acute Care, Skilled Care, and Extended Care Settings

The largest group of practicing nurses is those working in hospitals. Clients in hospitals require 24-hour care. The hospital may be acute care, long-term care, or rehabilitative care. Acute care hospitals have become more specialized and complex. The level of care provided in the hospital and extended care facilities is more complex. Clients are older, have more complex medical problems, and require more supportive therapies. Declining length of hospital stay is resulting in more clients needing continued care in the home setting or in extended care facilities. The hospital-based professional nurse is adept at providing early discharge planning and collaborative practice to meet the home care needs of clients (McEwen, 1994). Older adults with complex medical problems, functional impairments, and chronic illnesses have increased the number of long-term care facilities. The loss of the nuclear family and single parent families have contributed to the need to place older adults in these facilities, because many families are not able to assist the older adult with care needs.

Rehabilitative care facilities help clients adapt to changes in lifestyle related to their illness or injury. The goals of these institutions are to assist clients to achieve an optimal level of function and to teach families to help them reach that level.

Community-Based Settings

Community-based settings include ambulatory care, community health care centers, schools, occupational health settings, and home care. Care in these settings is focused on health promotion, health maintenance, education, screening, and long-term health management.

Nurses working in community-based centers often work more independently than those in institutional settings. In some settings, physicians are called in only when specific needs arise. Schools and college campuses also offer community health care for their students, focusing on disease prevention; health promotion; sex education; and nonemergent acute illness such as influenza, upper respiratory infections, or viruses.

Occupational health is provided in many large companies to serve the employees. Nursing care includes developing wellness programs, nonemergent treatment of acute illness, first aid, stabilization in emergencies (such as trauma or heart attack), and referrals to other health care professionals as necessary.

Home health care agencies provide nursing care for clients who are able to return home. The nurse provides skilled care, such as assessment and monitoring of medication, initiation and care of intravenous therapy, and respiratory treatments. The nurse must be skilled in assessment and in client and family education to enlist them in providing safe and effective care.

···THE HEALTH CARE TEAM·····················

The health care team is made up of four types of professionals: nurses, physicians, allied health professionals, and specialists (e.g., social workers) (Box 10-5).

Box 10-5
Other Health Care Team Members

Physician
A physician is a professional who has earned a degree of doctor of medicine or doctor of osteopathy and has passed a licensing examination. Most physicians specialize their practice of medicine. Nurses work closely with physicians under supervision or as collaborators.

Physician Assistant
Physician assistants have medical training and work under the direction of physicians in hospitals, clinics, and private offices (they do not practice in Canada).

Therapist
Therapists are licensed to assist in the examination and treatment of clients in special ways (i.e., as physical, occupational, or respiratory therapists). Their education varies but usually involves 4-year programs. Nurses collaborate with them and evaluate their work.

Pharmacist
Pharmacists are licensed to formulate and dispense drugs. They may have bachelor of science degrees or doctorates in pharmacology. Pharmacists provide valuable information to nurses about drugs and their use and effects.

Social Worker
Social workers are trained to counsel and refer clients to appropriate agencies. They have baccalaureate or master's degrees. Nurses work together with them to identify the best resources for the client, particularly when the client returns home.

Chaplain
Chaplains offer spiritual support and guidance to clients and their families. They may be employed by an agency or provided by a church in the community. A client may request a chaplain, or a nurse may refer the client to one.

Collaboration is the key to prevent fragmentation of the client's health care. The RN is most often responsible for coordinating and integrating services, because the RN has the opportunity to interact with each member of the health care team.

CHALLENGES FOR THE FUTURE

Nurses must now have a new set of skills for the roles of the future. In addition to the traditional skills of managing client care, providing direct care, and performing treatments and procedures, the new skill set is based on advanced communication techniques (see Chapter 13). The nurse must now be skilled in **delegation, team building, collaboration, coordination,** directing, problem solving, critical thinking, and conflict resolution.

Throughout the various roles described, a theme emerges: teamwork and collaboration. The nurse is an integral member of the health care team and must be able to work in a group, recognizing each health care team member's unique contribution to total client care. The nurse most often will be the team leader, responsible for delegating and directing unlicensed assistive personnel and other ancillary personnel. When delegating, the nurse must delegate the right task, to the right person, using the right communication techniques, and giving the right feedback in a timely manner (Parkman, 1996).

Unlicensed Assistive Personnel (UAP)

The use of **unlicensed assistive personnel (UAP)** is a new and often difficult concept to the nurse. Recent nursing education models have focused on the nurse as the central care giver, coordinator, and decision maker. The original impetus for implementing the UAP was the nursing shortage, to assist the RN in providing care (Krapohl and Larson, 1996). In the new health care model, nurses will be the coordinators, supervisors, key decision makers, planners, and critical thinkers. UAP will be there to assist the nurse in implementing the client plan of care.

UAP are trained and educated in either hospital-based programs or state programs, usually focusing on extended and continuing care. Many are undergraduate nursing students who are able to work as UAP, practicing and improving their basic care skills.

The Next Millennium

As the year 2000 approaches, roles for nurses will again evolve. The nurse of the future will need a different skill set to meet the challenges of new nursing roles in the changing health care environment. Nurses will have to know how to work smarter and must possess skills in collaboration, conflict resolution, problem solving, crit-

ical thinking, delegation, and team building. The professional nurse's role will move from primary direct care provider to coordinator, facilitator, director, and advocate. This role evolution almost parallels the changes seen in medical practice—from task- and technical-based skills to oversight and coordination skills. For many this will be a difficult time. Nurses value the client interaction and technical aspects of nursing. For the client, there will be some role confusion as traditional nursing roles and tasks are carried out by clinical support personnel such as LPNs, UAP, and other multi-skilled workers. Cross training and increasing generalization is the trend, rather than the specialization seen from 1950 to 1980.

The visionary nurse will be able to see the opportunities for growth, health promotion, wellness, and the advancement of nursing practice. We will be challenged to examine everything we do with clinical research to validate why it is done and how we might do it differently. Outcomes and quality will be the measures of success. Nurses more than ever will be partnering with physician colleagues and allied health professionals to provide a more global, holistic approach to care of our clients (Pew, 1995). Care will be less compartmentalized and more coordinated, with nursing leading the health care team. Clients are more aware of options, are more well read, and have access to the same types of information and research as we do. We are not returning to the past but are instead learning from days gone by, keeping the best, improving where there is opportunity, challenging the known, exploring the unknown, and advancing the practice and profession of nursing.

Key Terms

advanced practice nurse (APN)	direct care provider
autonomy	licensed practical nurse (LPN)
case management	nurse administrator
certification	nurse educator
certified nurse midwife (CNM)	nurse practice acts
certified registered nurse anesthetist (CRNA)	nurse practitioner (NP)
	nurse researcher
	problem solving
client advocate	protector
clinical nurse specialist (CNS)	registered professional nurse (RN)
collaboration	standards of care
conceptual model	standards of practice
coordination	team building
delegation	unlicensed assistive personnel (UAP)

▪ Key Concepts ▪▪

A professional nurse provides a specified service and follows a code of ethics for practice. Professional nurses have autonomy in decision making and practice.

Nursing practice was defined in 1980 by the ANA Congress for Nursing Practice as "the diagnosis and treatment of the human response to actual or potential health problems" (ANA, 1980).

Nursing practice has evolved over the years in response to societal needs. It is unique in its focus of health promotion, maintenance, and continuing care.

Conceptual and theoretical nursing models are used to provide knowledge to improve practice, guide research and curricula development, and identify the goals and domain of nursing practice.

A conceptual model is a set of global or general ideas about the individuals, groups, populations, situations, or events of interest to a discipline.

Nursing practice standards provide guidelines for care and establish criteria by which the quality and competency of care can be evaluated.

Standards of practice provide the client with assurance that they are receiving high-quality nursing care, the nurses know how to provide the care, and there are measures to determine if the care meets the established standards and expected outcomes.

Standards of care define and describe competent levels of nursing care. These levels of care are demonstrated through the nursing process: assessment, diagnosis, outcome identification, planning, implementation, and evaluation.

A license for a registered nurse is granted after the candidate has completed an accredited program and passed a national licensing examination (NCLEX).

Graduate nursing programs prepare clinical nurse specialists, nurse practitioners, educators, researchers, and administrators to improve nursing care, the advancement of nursing theory, and sciences.

The advanced practice nurse, which includes a clinical nurse specialist or nurse practitioner, has a master's degree in nursing and expertise in a specialized area of practice.

Continuing education programs help the nurse to remain current in skills, knowledge, and theory.

Each state in the United States and all Canadian provinces regulate the licensure and scope of nursing practice through nurse practice acts. In many states the nurse practice acts have been revised to include expanded nursing roles and to differentiate between medical and nursing diagnosis and treatment.

The roles and functions of the nurse include care giver, decision maker, client advocate, manager, rehabilitator, comforter, communicator, and teacher.

Employment positions can include staff nurse, educator, advanced practice nurse, researcher, and case manager.

The health care team is multidisciplinary and may include the physician, advanced practice nurse, physician assistant, physical therapist, occupational therapist, respiratory therapist, pharmacist, social worker, chaplain, and staff nurse.

Unlicensed assistive personnel are trained and educated in either hospital-based programs or state programs to assist the nurse in implementing the client plan of care.

▪ Critical Thinking Activities ▪▪

1. You are assigned eight surgical clients to care for on the day shift. Two clients are to have surgery today, one at 0800 and the other to follow. Three clients will be discharged by noon, and one is a fresh postop who had surgery during the night. Two clients are in admitting and are having procedures that will require overnight observation. You will have an LPN and a UAP to assist you with providing care. How will you utilize the personnel you will be working with to care for these clients? What tasks are appropriate to delegate to the UAP? How can you best utilize the LPN?

References

Abdellah FL and others: *Patient-centered approaches to nursing,* New York, 1960, Macmillan.

American Nurses Association: *Nursing: a social policy statement,* Washington, DC, 1980, The Association.

American Nurses Association: *Standards for continuing education in nursing,* Washington, DC, 1991a, The Association.

American Nurses Association: *Standards of clinical practice,* Washington, DC, 1991b, The Association.

American Nurses Association: *Nursing and social policy statement,* Washington, DC, 1995, The Association.

Bernhard LA, Walsh M: *Leadership: the key to the professionalization of nursing,* ed 3, St. Louis, 1995, Mosby.

Canadian Nurses Association: *A definition of nursing practice. Standards for nursing practice,* Ottawa, 1986, The Association.

Chinn PL, Jacobs MK: *Theory and nursing: a systematic approach,* ed 4, St. Louis, 1995, Mosby.

Deloughery C: *Issues and trends in nursing,* ed 2, St. Louis, 1995, Mosby.

Donahue MP: *Nursing: the finest art, an illustrated history,* St. Louis, 1995, Mosby.

Fawcett J: Contemporary conceptualization of nursing: philosophy or science? In Kikuchi J, Simmons H: *Philosophic inquiry in nursing,* Newbury Park, Calif, 1992, Sage.

Gerteis M and others, editors: *Through the patient's eyes,* San Francisco, 1993, Jossey-Bass.

Henderson V: *The nature of nursing,* New York, 1966, Macmillan.

Krapohl GL, Larson E: The impact of unlicensed assistive personnel on nursing care delivery, *Nurs Econ* 14:99, 1996.

Levine ME: The rhetoric of nursing theory, *Image J Nurs Sch* 27:11, 1995.

Macrae J: Nightingale's spiritual philosophy and its significance for modern nursing, *Image J Nurs Sch* 27:8, 1995.

Marriner-Tomey A: *Nursing theorists and their work,* ed 3, St. Louis, 1994, Mosby.

McEwen M: Promoting interdisciplinary collaboration, *Nurs Health Care* 15(6):304, 1994.

Meleis Al: *Theoretical nursing: development and progress,* ed 3, Philadelphia, 1996, Lippincott-Raven.

National Council of State Boards of Nursing: Boards of nursing adopt revolutional change for nurse regulation, *Issues* 18(3):1, 1997.

Neuman B: *The Neuman systems model,* ed 3, Norwalk, Conn, 1995, Appleton & Lange.

Nightingale F: *Notes on nursing: what it is and what it is not,* London, 1860, Harrison & Sons.

Orem DE: *Nursing: concepts of practice,* ed 3, New York, 1985, McGraw-Hill.

Parkman CA: Delegation: are you doing it right? *AJN* 96:43, 1996.

Peplau HE: *Interpersonal relations in nursing,* New York, 1952, Putnam.

Pew Health Professionals Commission: *Critical challenges: revitalizing the health profession for the twenty-first century,* San Francisco, Calif, 1995, USCF Center for the Health Professions.

Rogers ME: *An introduction to the theoretical basis of nursing,* Philadelphia, 1970, Davis.

Roy C: The Roy adaptation model. In Riehl JP, Roy C, editors: *Conceptual models for nursing practice,* ed 3, New York, 1989, Appleton-Century-Crofts.

Ethics and Values

OBJECTIVES

Mastery of content in this chapter will enable
the student to:

- Define the key terms listed.
- Describe and differentiate values, ethics, and
  morals.
- Discuss professionalism in nursing practice.
- Discuss accountability and responsibility as
  evident in nursing practice.
- Discuss client advocacy.
- Describe how values influence behavior and
  attitudes.
- Discuss how values are learned.
- Explain how personal and professional values
  interrelate.
- Describe the process of values clarification.
- Explain how values clarification strategies can
  be used to clarify nurses' professional values.
- Describe the role of ethics in nursing practice.
- Describe an ethic of care.
- Discuss the process used to analyze an ethical
  dilemma.
- Describe ethical conflicts experienced by nurses
  in different settings.

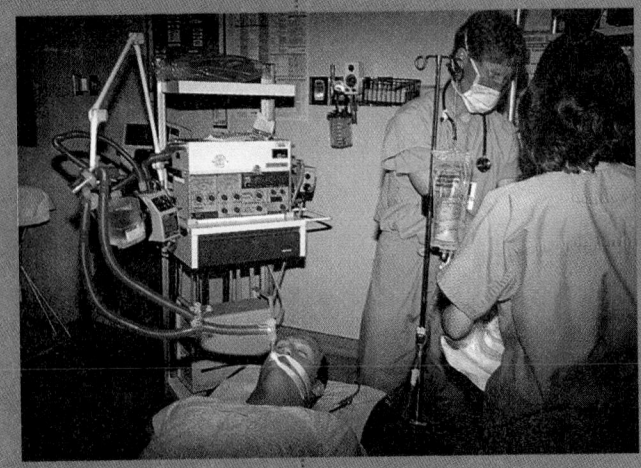

The nursing profession's domain of practice includes care during all aspects of health, sickness, personal life, and community life. These represent important and intimate aspects in the lives of others, and as a result the professional nurse assumes roles in which complex ethical situations often develop. Disagreement about certain decisions or practices may result in ethical dilemmas where the nurse, the client, or others in the health care team disagree about the best way to proceed. With the support of professional codes of practice and a commitment to critical thinking skills, the nurse contributes a vital and unique voice to the process of resolution.

The study of ethics has occupied the attention of civilization for thousands of years. Whenever human beings gather in community, they turn to concerns about right living. Whether one looks to the ancient Chinese philosophers, the dialogues of the ancient Greeks, or traces of Mayan and Aztec culture, one finds evidence of a fundamental human effort to define right and wrong behavior. In the United States the diversity of the origins of its citizens is reflected in the diversity of philosophical foundations for ethics. Judeo-Christian traditions characterize much of contemporary thought, action, and law in the United States. In Judeo-Christian belief, a fundamental respect for the individual and a commitment to sustain an ability to live in community with others constitute the foundation for guidance in daily life. The term **ethics,** then, refers to the consideration of standards of conduct or the study of philosophical ideals of right and wrong behavior (*American Heritage,* 1994).

BASIC DEFINITIONS

Ethical issues differ from legal issues. The term **law** refers to the codification of values that a community holds in common. The content of the law is determined by systems of government, and law is enforced by the same system (Harris, 1995). Breaking a law usually results in a public consequence. Although law and ethics both find a basis in commonly held values, they do not always cover all behaviors. The law tends to guide public behavior that will affect others and that will preserve community. Ethics has a broader base of interest and includes personal behavior and issues of character.

A **value** is a personal belief about the worth of a given idea, attitude, custom, or object that sets standards and influences behavior. The values an individual holds reflect cultural and societal influences, relationships with others, and personal needs. Both individual and community ethics are usually based on shared values.

People form values consciously and unconsciously through reasoning, observation, experience, and socialization. The formation of values is a continuous and lifelong process. Nurses undergo a socialization into the nursing profession, where the process of values formation continues. The process of **values clarification** is

useful for increasing awareness of the differences between one's own values and the values of others, especially client values. When values are known, stated, and positively affirmed, the client, nurse, or health care team is more capable of making objective decisions about health care.

The terms *ethics* and *morals* sometimes are used interchangeably. **Morals** usually refers to judgment about behavior, and ethics is the study of the ideals of right and wrong behavior. Although both morals and ethics evolve from social life, moral codes are more likely to reflect the character of the social setting from which they spring (Davis and Aroskar, 1991).

The study of **bioethics** represents a particular branch of ethics, namely, the study of ethics within the field of health care. Bioethics "narrows ethical inquiry to the moral 'oughts' of those who work in professional clinical practice, basic research, or the education of health professionals. Bioethics affects all health professionals and those who seek their knowledge and skills" (O'Neil, 1995).

The field of bioethics has become a prominent branch of the study of ethics, especially in the last 25 years. When kidney transplant technology was perfected in the early 1970s, the immediate ethical concern became the limited number of kidneys available compared with the greater number of clients in need of a transplant. The advent of advanced medical technologies requires society to face difficult ethical questions. Who should get what resources? What constitutes quality of life? Who should decide? In the study of bioethics, health care professionals agree to negotiate these difficult and important questions.

Nursing professionals play an increasingly important role in the study of bioethics. As O'Neil (1995) explains, "Only recently has nursing become an active participant in the interdisciplinary discussion of ethical practice. However, the focus now is a truly interdisciplinary effort by which professionals and society attempt to gain knowledge, guidelines, and agreement on these very complex issues."

Nurses participate in bioethical discourse in two distinct ways: as professionals, nurses construct a professional code of ethics that reflects and defines practice; and as colleagues in the practice of health care delivery, nurses develop a specific point of view for contribution to ethical discourse on client care issues.

PROFESSIONAL NURSING

Understanding the nature of nursing ethics begins with the concept of **professionalism.** The term *profession* refers to a group of people with specialized education, knowledge, and skills who serve a specific social need. To be a professional means that a person acquires specific skills and then agrees to practice those skills in accordance with standards that a community of practitioners agrees to uphold.

Chitty (1993) summarizes criteria for practitioners to meet to qualify as professionals:

1. A vital human service is provided to the society by the profession.
2. Professions possess a special body of knowledge that is continuously enlarged through research.
3. Practitioners are expected to be accountable and responsible.
4. The education of professionals takes place in institutions for higher education.
5. Practitioners have an independent function and control their own practice.
6. Professionals are committed to their work and are motivated by doing good.
7. A code of ethics guides professional decisions and conduct.
8. A professional organization oversees and supports standards of practice.

This list of criteria points to both values and ethics as necessary for professionalization. Through codes of ethics and the instillation of particular values, a profession fulfills its promises to society.

Professional nursing meets these criteria in a variety of ways. The nurse must complete education and training beyond high school. Research and education become a regular part of a nurse's career growth over time. A professional nurse agrees to care for the chronically and acutely ill and injured, to promote wellness, and to help people die peacefully. Society in return trusts that promise and relies on nurses to remain committed to their stated ideals. The values of care, accountability, responsibility, and advocacy provide the foundation for nursing practice. The code of ethics gives ethical guidance and establishes norms of behavior.

Codes of Ethics

A **code of ethics** is a set of **ethical principles** that are generally accepted by all members of a profession. A profession's ethical code is a collective statement about the group's expectations and standards of behavior. A useful code will be brief, yet detailed enough to offer clear guidance and attain widespread acceptance. Codes also serve as guidelines to assist nurses and other professional groups when conflict or disagreement arises about correct practice or behavior. The nursing profession has a code of ethics that sets forth ideals of conduct. These principles indicate factors that nurses consider when trying to determine proper conduct. Ethical codes also provide a common foundation for professional nurses' training. The American Nurses Association (ANA), the International Council of Nurses (ICN), and Canadian Nurses Association (CNA) have established widely accepted codes that the professional attempts to follow. Although these codes differ somewhat in specific emphasis, they reflect the same under-

---

Box 11-1
American Nurses Association
Code of Ethics

The nurse provides services with respect for human dignity and the uniqueness of the client unrestricted by considerations of social or economic status, personal attributes, or the nature of health problems.

The nurse safeguards the client's right to privacy by judiciously protecting information of a confidential nature.

The nurse acts to safeguard the client and the public when health care and safety are affected by the incompetent, unethical, or illegal practice of any person.

The nurse assumes responsibility and accountability for individual nursing judgments and actions.

The nurse maintains competence in nursing.

The nurse exercises informed judgment and uses individual competence and qualifications as criteria in seeking consultation, accepting responsibilities, and delegating nursing activities to others.

The nurse participates in activities that contribute to the ongoing development of the profession's body of knowledge.

The nurse participates in the profession's efforts to implement and improve standards of nursing.

The nurse participates in the profession's efforts to establish and maintain conditions of employment conducive to high-quality nursing care.

The nurse participates in the profession's effort to protect the public from misinformation and misrepresentation and to maintain the integrity of nursing.

The nurse collaborates with members of the health professions and other citizens in promoting community and national efforts to meet the health needs of the public.

From American Nurses Association: *Code for nurses with interpretive statements,* Kansas City, Mo, 1985, The Association.

---

lying principles (see Boxes 11-1 to 11-3). These fundamental principles include responsibility, accountability, and advocacy. Nurses agree to responsibility for specific actions and accountability for the consequences. To practice responsibly, nurses also agree to maintain competence in their practice and to utilize competence in the application of judgment. In addition, nurses establish guidelines for the role of client advocate. ▪

Box 11-2
Canadian Nurses Association Code of Ethics

Values

Health and Well-being

Nurses value health and well-being and assist persons to achieve their optimum level of health in situations of normal health, illness, injury, or in the process of dying.

Choice

Nurses respect and promote the autonomy of clients and help them to express their health needs and values and to obtain appropriate information and services.

Dignity

Nurses value and advocate the dignity and self-respect of human beings.

Confidentiality

Nurses safeguard the trust of clients so that information learned in the context of a professional relationship is shared outside the health care team only with the client's permission or as legally required.

Fairness

Nurses apply and promote principles of equity and fairness to assist clients in receiving unbiased treatment and a share of health services and resources proportionate to their needs.

Accountability

Nurses act in a manner consistent with their professional responsibilities and standards of practice.

Practice Environments Conducive to Safe, Competent, and Ethical Care

Nurses advocate practice environments that have the organizational and human support systems and the resource allocations necessary for safe, competent, and ethical nursing care.

Reprinted with permission from Canadian Nurses Association: *Code of ethics for registered nurses,* Ottawa, 1997, The Association.

Responsibility, accountability, competence, and judgment. A nurse assumes responsibility and accountability for all nursing care delivered. **Responsibility** refers to the execution of duties associated with a nurse's particular role (ANA, 1985). The term refers to the characteristics of reliability and dependability. When administering a medication, for example, a nurse is responsible for assessing the client's need for the drug, for giving it safely and correctly, and for evaluating the response to it. By agreeing to responsibility, the nurse gains trust from clients, colleagues, and society.

A responsible nurse is competent in knowledge and skills and ethically executes duties within the guidelines of the profession. **Competence** refers to a specific range of skills necessary to perform a task (*American Heritage,* 1994). Regulations that guide the maintenance of competence vary from state to state, but the fundamental agreement to practice with competence is contained in the nursing code of ethics. For example, the reliable nurse ensures knowledge about a drug before administration of it. The nurse understands unusual responses to medications, and the client is able

to trust that medications offered by the nurse are safe. The nurse agrees to measure responses to medications accurately and appropriately. The ability to make decisions based on this measure depends on the nurse's commitment to practice good judgment. **Judgment** refers to the ability to form an opinion or draw sound conclusions (*American Heritage,* 1994). The nurse begins to learn the skill of judging in nursing school and then adds to the skill and improves the skill over time, throughout the lifetime of the career. Finally, the nurse agrees to document findings clearly in the appropriate location. Colleagues rely on the documentation and trust its accuracy.

When nurses perform care, they must be accountable. **Accountability** refers to the ability to answer for one's own actions. A nurse is accountable to self most of all. In addition, the nurse also must balance accountability to the client, the profession, the employing institution, and society (Potter and Perry, 1997). For example, a nurse may know that a client who will be discharged soon remains confused about how to self-administer insulin. The action that a nurse takes in

Box 11-3
International Council of Nurses Code for Nurses

The fundamental responsibility of the nurse is four-fold: to promote health, to prevent illness, to restore health, and to alleviate suffering.

The need for nursing is universal. Inherent in nursing is respect for life, dignity, and rights of man. It is unrestricted by considerations of nationality, race, creed, color, age, sex, politics, or social status.

Nurses render health services to the individual, the family, and the community and coordinate their services with those of related groups.

Nurses and People

The nurse's primary responsibility is to those people who require nursing care.

The nurse, in providing care, promotes an environment in which the values, customs, and spiritual beliefs of the individual are respected.

The nurse holds in confidence personal information and uses judgment in sharing this information.

Nurses and Practice

The nurse carries personal responsibility for nursing practice and for maintaining competence by continual learning. The nurse maintains the highest standards of nursing care possible within the reality of a specific situation.

The nurse uses judgment in relation to individual competence when accepting and delegating responsibilities.

The nurse when acting in a professional capacity should at all times maintain standards of personal conduct which reflect credit upon the profession.

Nurses and Society

The nurse shares with other citizens the responsibility for initiating and supporting action to meet the health and social needs of the public.

Nurses and Co-workers

The nurse sustains a cooperative relationship with co-workers in nursing and other fields. The nurse takes appropriate action to safeguard the individual when his care is endangered by a co-worker or any other person.

Nurses and the Profession

The nurse plays the major role in determining and implementing desirable standards of nursing practice and nursing education.

The nurse is active in developing a core of professional knowledge.

The nurse, acting through the professional organization, participates in establishing and maintaining equitable social and economic working conditions in nursing.

From International Council of Nurses: *ICN code for nurses: ethical concepts applied to nursing,* Geneva, 1973, Imprimeries Populaires.

response to this situation will be guided by the professional commitment to accountability. The client, the employing institution, and society rely on the good judgment of the nurse and trust that the nurse will take action in response to this situation. The nurse may request more hospitalization to provide further teaching or arrange home care to continue teaching at home. The goal is the prevention of injury to the client. The principle that guides the nurse is accountability.

To remain accountable to society, the profession of nursing agrees to evaluate its practices and actions and to take action to preserve nursing excellence. The following activities promote the principles of professional accountability in nursing practice:

1. Evaluation of new professional practices and reassessment of existing ones

2. Maintenance of standards of health care
3. Facilitation of personal reflection, ethical thought, and personal growth
4. Provision of a basis for ethical decision making

Advocacy. Advocacy involves giving clients the information they need to make decisions and then supporting those decisions. It also implies that caretakers will strive to understand and then to articulate a client's point of view. Within the health care system, a multidisciplinary team of health care providers participates in the delivery of care, and all team members strive to advocate for the client. Nurses are an important and unique part of that team. Nurses usually come to know clients through regular assessments, while administering difficult or uncomfortable procedures, and while teaching new skills and preparing for discharge or home care. These activities expose nurses to important aspects of a client's ability to cope, learn, and heal. These aspects may be less well known by other professionals on the health care team. The nurse's ability to document, articulate, and contribute this knowledge to the team who cares for the client constitutes an essential aspect of nurses' advocacy for the client.

Basic Standards of Ethics in Health Care

Practitioners of health care delivery agree to a basic set of ethical standards that influence and guide professional practice and decision making. The language used in these standards recurs throughout the field and is common to all professions in health care. Nurses find these standards especially useful because they promote and define the nature of autonomy and advocacy (Table 11-1).

Autonomy refers to a person's independence. As a standard in bioethics, autonomy represents an agreement to respect the client's right to determine a course of action. Respect for the client's autonomy is fundamental to the practice of health care. It serves to justify the inclusion of clients in all aspects of decision making regarding care. The agreement to respect autonomy represents the recognition that clients are "in charge of their own destiny in matters of health and illness" (O'Neil, 1995). The purpose of the preoperative consent, for example, is the assurance in writing that the health care team respects the client's independence by obtaining permission to proceed. The consent process implies that a client may refuse treatment, and in most cases, the health care team must agree to abide by the client's refusal. Health care professionals agree to abide by a standard of respect for the client's autonomy.

Justice refers to the standard of fairness. Health care professionals often use this standard when facing the difficult issues of limited resources. Health care providers agree to strive for justice in health care. What constitutes a fair distribution of resources may not always be clear. For example, approximately three times more candidates are on a waiting list for liver transplants than the United States has livers available for transplant. The just distribution of available organs can be difficult to determine. In the United States, criteria set by a national multidisciplinary committee strive for fairness by ranking recipients according to need, rather than resorting to selling organs for profit or distributing them by lottery.

Fidelity refers to the agreement to keep promises. The standard justifies the reluctance to abandon clients, even when disagreement arises about decisions that a client may make. The standard of fidelity also

---

TABLE 11-1
Principles of Health Care Ethics

Definitions	Nursing Implications
Autonomy Independence; self-determination; self-reliance	Display respect for all persons; support client's right to informed consent; autonomy is truly exercised when members of the health care team agree to the importance of autonomy.
Justice Fairness or equity	Ensure fair allocation of resources such as nursing care to all clients; determine the order in which clients should be treated (e.g., clients at greatest risk are treated first).
Fidelity Faithfulness; striving to keep promises	Keep promises made to clients, families, and other professionals; avoid abandonment of clients, even when client goals differ from health care provider goals.
Beneficence Actively seeking benefits; promotion of good	Promote actions that benefit clients; seek benefits that provide the least harm; consider client's best interest above self-interest.
Nonmaleficence Actively seeking to do no harm	Avoid deliberate harm, risk of harm, and harm that occurs during performance of nursing actions; seek to do the least harm if benefits must result in some harm.

promotes an obligation to follow through with the care offered to clients. For example, if the nurse assesses a client for pain and then offers a plan to manage the pain, the standard of fidelity encourages the nurse to do the best in keeping the promise to improve the client's comfort.

The standard of **beneficence** promotes taking positive, active steps to help others. It encourages the urge to do good for the client and helps to guide difficult decisions where the benefits of a treatment may be challenged by risks to the client's well-being or dignity. A child's immunization may cause discomfort during administration, but the benefits of protection from disease, both for the individual and for society, outweigh the temporary discomforts. The agreement to act with beneficence also requires that the best interest of the client remains more important than self-interest. For example, a nurse will not simply practice in obedience to medical orders but will act thoughtfully to understand client needs and then work actively to help meet those needs.

Nonmaleficence refers to the fundamental agreement to do no harm. It is closely related to the standard of beneficence. The health care professional tries to balance, to the best of one's abilities, the risks and benefits of a plan of care while striving to do the least harm possible. This standard is often helpful in guiding discussions about new or controversial technologies. For example, a new bone marrow transplant procedure may promise a chance at cure, but the long-term prognosis may be uncertain, or the procedure may require long periods of pain or suffering. These risks should be considered in relationship to the potential good that may come of the procedure. The standard of nonmaleficence promotes a continuing effort to consider the potential for harm even when it may be necessary to promote health.

one's own values and then to assess and speak for the values of clients provides the foundation for the nurse's ability to adhere to a professional code of ethics.

Values

A value is a personal belief about the worth of a given idea, attitude, custom, or object that sets standards that influence behavior. If persons hold a particular value, they have personally chosen, interpreted, justified, and preferred that value over others. Louis Raths pioneered values clarification as an approach to an individual's appraisal of values (Raths and others, 1979). Valuing involves the following actions: choosing, prizing, and acting (Box 11-4).

The values an individual holds reflect cultural and societal influences, relationships with others, and personal needs. Values vary among people and develop and change over time. Understanding one's own value system and assessing the value systems of others may help reduce conflict during decision making.

Uustal (1992) summarizes elements often found in discussions about values. Valuing has cognitive, selective, affective, and action components. The act of valuing begins with a thoughtful process to consider all the options or perhaps with a list of the possible different ways to value. The next step involves selecting a value and identifying it as one to embrace or support. A part of this choosing may involve the act of prioritizing, or recognizing that a particular value may have more or less value than others. Making a choice requires the acknowledgment that feelings or emotional responses play a role in the decision to choose a certain value. Finally, a personally held value implies a willingness to take action to support, promote, or express the choice.

DEVELOPING A PERSONAL POINT OF VIEW AS A NURSE

The nursing profession promotes the practice of reliable care, by responsible and accountable nurses, in a way that promotes healing and comfort in concert with other members of the health care team. To practice nursing that meets these high standards, the individual nurse will benefit from a clear understanding of values. Personal values influence the development of one's point of view, including one's ethical point of view. When differences of opinion arise for professionals or between professionals and a client, an **ethical dilemma** may develop. An ethical dilemma exists when the right thing to do is not clear or when members of the health care team cannot agree on the right thing to do. Most ethical dilemmas require the negotiation of differing values. The ability to clarify and articulate

---

Box 11-4
The Three Actions of Values Clarification

Choosing one's beliefs and behaviors
   Choosing from alternatives
   Choosing freely
   Considering all consequences
Prizing one's beliefs and behaviors
   Prizing and cherishing the choice
   Publicly affirming the choice
Acting on one's beliefs
   Making the choice part of one's behavior
   Acting with a pattern of consistency and repetition

Modified from Raths LE and others: *Values and teaching*, ed 2, Columbus, Ohio, 1979, Merrill.

Values Formation

People acquire values in many ways. An understanding of values begins in earliest childhood and is influenced by the way a child is raised. Children develop through different stages of cognitive and emotional growth. The classic works of Piaget (1932), Kohlberg (1981), and Gilligan (1982) provide descriptions of this intricate process. Basically, as children become more complex cognitively, they become more capable of complex emotional behavior as well. Since a fundamental part of values formation involves the ability to identify strong feelings and to act on them, the acquiring of values depends in large part on experiences within the family.

The character of parenting influences how children form values as adults. In some cultures, children may be prized and indulged until they reach school age and then must face more rigorous discipline as they enter school and the world outside the family. In other cultures, children may be raised according to strict gender expectations. For example, girls assume household duties early in their lives, and boys acquire more physical or labor-related skills. In still others, children are raised quite separately from adult activities, in communal settings with less exposure to adult socialization or patterning opportunities. These variations in child rearing result in variations in values and variations in adult behavior. The fundamental urge to love and nurture children takes on many different expressions and produces many different kinds of value systems with which we must contend, as individuals and as professionals.

Once children begin to experience life outside the family, they experience a broad range of influences on values formation. Religious institutions are often charged with the primary responsibility for teaching and enforcing values. Schools, governments, and other social institutions also play a role. The nature of the role depends to a large degree on the nature of the institution. Religions with a strict code of behavior might teach the value of obedience, while religions that focus on helping the poor might focus on the value of charity. A young person who begins to learn about other religions might experience conflict over these differences. Institutional lessons may undergo change from one generation to another. A basic task of the young adult is the identification of values within the context of the community. Over time, an individual acquires values by choosing some that are strongly held in the community and perhaps discarding or transforming others.

Finally, individual experience influences what we come to value. A person who suffers much loss early in life, of a parent or sibling, may grow to value certain things very differently than someone whose life has been free of suffering. A person whose employment has been menial may form certain values that reflect experience of a lack of dignity in the workplace. An appreciation of the source of these differences may promote respectful and effective communication. Within health care, nurses and other providers agree to respect the wide variety of value systems that clients may hold and to try to understand how these differences affect client health and wellness.

Values Clarification

To better articulate one's point of view, it will be helpful to clarify one's own values. One's values constitute an important part of the way one sees the world and influence how a person interprets confusing or conflicting information. As individuals mature and experience new situations, their values change. It would be unusual if any one value remained the primary motivating factor throughout a person's life. Value changes may involve a reordering of values or the replacement of old values with new ones. As a result of changing values, a person may modify attitudes and behavior. The willingness to change shows a healthy attitude toward life and the ability to adapt to new experiences.

To adopt new values, a person must first be aware of existing values and how those values affect behavior. Yet individuals do not suddenly become aware of their values, and many are unable to define their values clearly and meaningfully. To achieve awareness of personal values, it may be helpful to practice the process of values clarification. This is a process of self-discovery that helps a person gain insight into values. It is not a set of rules designed to interfere with conscientious decision making, and it does not suggest that a specific set of values should be accepted by all persons. The exercise "Strategies for Values Clarification" represents one way to help identify one's own values (Box 11-5). A person clarifying values learns to make choices when alternatives are presented and determines whether choices are carefully made. The result of values clarification is greater self-awareness and personal insight.

Cultural values are those adopted as a result of the social setting in which a person lives. Cultural values vary according to the community and the needs of the community. **Ethnocentrism** refers to the belief that one's own culture is superior (Deloughery, 1995). As Deloughery explains, the nurse who holds this belief "may assess and plan intervention for the client, as well as evaluate the effectiveness of what was done, based on personal perceptions and values, without taking into account the perceptions and beliefs of the client." The "Cultural Values Exercise" (Box 11-6) illustrates the wide varieties of cultural values that affect perception of health care issues.

By understanding their own point of view, nurses will become better prepared to understand a client's values and the values of other members of the health care team. The ultimate test of a value system lies in its ability to guide individuals through dissent or confusion. The technologies of contemporary medicine often create ethical dilemmas, where competing points of view leave members of the health care team or the team and

Box 11-5
Strategies for Values Clarification

Sentence Completion

Complete the following sentences. Use them to examine your feelings and values.

I feel I succeed in caring for a client when . . .

A client has a right to . . .

I wish my clinical supervisor would . . .

Physicians and nurses work together best when . . .

I fail in caring for a client if I cannot . . .

The most difficult client is one who . . .

Health Value Scale

Below you will find 10 values listed in alphabetical order. Arrange the values in order of their importance as guiding principles in your life. Study the list carefully and choose the value that is most important to you. Write the number "1" in the space to the left of that value. Write the number "2" for the value that ranks second in importance. Continue in the same manner for the remaining values until you have included all ranks. Each value will have a different rank.

____ A comfortable life (a prosperous life)

____ An exciting life (a stimulating, active life)

____ A sense of accomplishment (lasting contribution)

____ Freedom (independence, free choice)

____ Happiness (contentedness)

____ Health (physical and mental well-being)

____ Inner harmony (freedom from inner conflict)

____ Pleasure (an enjoyable, leisurely life)

____ Self-respect (self-esteem)

____ Social recognition (respect, admiration)

Modified from Uustal DB: *Am J Nurs* 78:2058, 1978.

Box 11-6
Cultural Values Exercise

If persons from a variety of cultures were given this questionnaire, some would strongly agree with the beliefs listed on the left and others would strongly agree with the opposite viewpoint listed on the right. Circle 1 if you strongly agree or 2 if you moderately agree with the statement on the left. Circle 3 if you moderately agree or 4 if you strongly agree with the statement on the right.

1. Preparing for the future is an important activity and reflects maturity.	1 2 3 4	Life has a predestined course. The individual should follow that course.
2. Vague answers are dishonest and confusing.	1 2 3 4	Vague answers are sometimes preferred because they avoid embarrassment and confrontation.
3. Punctuality and efficiency are characteristics of a person who is both intelligent and concerned.	1 2 3 4	Punctuality is not as important as maintaining a relaxed atmosphere, enjoying the moment, and being with family and friends.
4. When in severe pain, it is important to remain strong and not to complain too much.	1 2 3 4	When in severe pain, it is better to talk about the discomfort and express frustration.
5. It is self-centered and unwise to accept a gift from someone you do not know well.	1 2 3 4	It is an insult to refuse a gift when it is offered.
6. Addressing someone by their first name shows friendliness.	1 2 3 4	Addressing someone by their first name is disrespectful.
7. Direct questions are usually the best way to gain information.	1 2 3 4	Direct questioning is rude and could cause embarrassment.
8. Direct eye contact shows interest.	1 2 3 4	Direct eye contact is intrusive.
9. Ultimately, the independence of the individual must come before the needs of the family.	1 2 3 4	The needs of the individual are always less important than the needs of the family.

Modified from Renwick GW, Rhinesmith SH: *An exercise in cultural analysis for managers*, Chicago, 1995, Intercultural Press. Reprinted with permission of Intercultural Press, Yarmouth, Maine.

the client in conflict. Values clarification plays a significant role in the resolution of these dilemmas. In addition, nurses strengthen their ability to advocate for a client when nurses are able to identify personal values and then accurately identify the values of the client.

Once the nurse has mastered the skill of clarifying personal values, it will be possible to turn to the client and apply similar practices that enhance the nurse's ability to construct and implement health care interventions. Values clarification can promote a consciousness-raising through which clients gain an awareness of personal priorities, identify ambiguities in values, and resolve major conflicts between values and behavior. The nurse may help the client clarify the meaning and significance of values and emotions. The goal of values clarification with a client is effective nurse-client communication. As the client becomes more willing to express problems and feelings, the nurse can better establish an individualized plan of care. The nurse who learns about client values and needs can devise a successful plan of care to promote well-being.

A useful method for values clarification with a client is structured communication. Simple strategies that promote the process of sharing feelings can be quite effective. For example, responding to a client by repeating the client's sentence as a question ("You wish you could be at home?") will encourage the client to elaborate. Avoiding questions that can be answered with a yes or no encourages the client to answer in greater detail. Rather than "Do you exercise regularly?" the nurse might ask, "What kind of activities do you do when not at work or at home?"

The character of a nurse's response to a client can motivate the client to examine personal thoughts and actions. When the nurse makes a clarifying response, it should be brief and nonjudgmental. For example, when talking with a client who exercises rarely, the nurse might say, "I see. So, what is your understanding of the purpose of exercise?" An effective clarifying response encourages the client to think about personal values after the exchange is over without imposing one's own values onto the client's. In this way, the nurse respects client self-direction and avoids inappropriately introducing personal values into the conversation. Although values clarification can occur in any setting, it is often most successful when the nurse has contact with the client over several occasions.

In summary, values clarification plays a critical role in communication between people. Especially when the topic concerns issues of health, personal habits, and quality of life, all participants in a discussion will benefit by a clarity of personal values. The nurse who understands personal values will more fairly and accurately articulate personal opinion on important issues. The nurse better serves the needs of clients, especially when values differ. The respect demonstrated for clients' differences and the skill used in helping a client clarify values promote a nurse's ability to teach and to heal.

ETHICS IN NURSING PRACTICE

Ethics concerns itself with what people see as good and in that sense flows from values. Values clarification is not a substitute for ethics, however. Ethics is a disciplined reflection on good conduct, character, and motives. It also seeks to settle claims of what constitutes the "good" or valuable among people with differences. It strives to go beyond personal preferences and to establish standards on which individuals, professions, and societies agree.

As O'Neil (1995) discusses, the traditional philosophies of ethics tend to be highly abstract and theoretical. The difficult situations with which health care providers struggle require more concrete strategies. Still, the traditional theories provide a strong foundation for bioethics. These perspectives overlap in some areas and compete in others. It is important to acquire a basic understanding of these perspectives because many health care providers use the language from one or another of these perspectives. In addition, it is important for an individual to be aware of the different perspectives as they relate to one's own values.

Deontology, a traditional theory of ethics, proposes a system of ethics that is perhaps most familiar to practitioners in health care. It proposes to define actions as right or wrong based on their "right-making characteristics such as fidelity to promises, truthfulness, and justice" (Beauchamp and Childress, 1989). It locates the essence of right or wrong in these principles, as opposed to looking to consequences of actions to determine rightness or wrongness. The conventional use of ethical terms such as justice, autonomy, and beneficence (see Table 11-1 on p. 169) constitutes the practice of deontology.

Deontology proposes that we determine the presence or absence of each of these principles in an individual situation as a guide for determination of right action. If an act is just, respects autonomy, and provides good, then the act will be ethical. Difficulty arises when a person must choose between conflicting principles, which is often the case in health care ethical dilemmas, or when people use conflicting definitions of the principles.

Utilitarianism describes another ethical theory. A utilitarian ethic proposes that the value of something is determined by its usefulness. The greatest good for the greatest number of people constitutes the guiding principle for all action in this system. As with deontology, this theory relies on the application of certain principles, namely, measures of "good" and "greatest." The fundamental difference between utilitarianism and deontology is in the focus on consequences or outcomes. Utilitarianism measures the effect that an act will have; deontology looks to the pure presence of principle. A difficulty arises with utilitarianism when individuals have conflicting definitions of "greatest good."

A growing body of writing in health care ethics has focused on a **feminist ethic.** A strong foundation for feminist ethics grew out of the changes in society that occurred as more women entered the workplace during the last century. New approaches to old problems and identification of new problems to solve have come to light (Sherwin, 1992). For example, until the early

1980s, conventional teachings held that the highest stages of moral development tend to be more commonly reached by men than by women (Kohlberg, 1981). For Kohlberg, moral development occurs in measurable, predictable stages. The most complex stage incorporates a sense of justice, and by Kohlberg's measure, young girls do not reach this sense as often as young boys. Research that disputed these findings surfaced during the 1980s. In this research Carol Gilligan (1982) proposes that Kohlberg's tools to measure moral development were gender biased. Gilligan describes a theory of moral development that attempts to accommodate gender differences. Specifically, she concludes that young girls tend to pay attention to community and to individual circumstances, and young boys tend to process dilemmas through ideals or principles determined abstractly.

Feminist ethics proposes that an inequality of attention to women can be remedied by routinely asking how bioethical decisions will affect women (Sherwin, 1992). For example, in a discussion regarding the ethics of fetal surgery (surgical intervention before birth of the child), feminist ethics would propose that the effect of the intervention on the mother is paramount and would hold the mother's autonomy higher than the autonomy of the fetus.

The **ethics of care** represents an important development in the field of bioethics. This ethical theory explores issues of nursing, gender, ethics, and ethical dilemmas. Its supporters pay special attention to the nursing point of view and nursing practice (Fry, 1989). As Leininger (1988) has written, care is the "central and unifying domain for the body of knowledge and practices in nursing." Its principles apply to all members of a health care community, not just nurses.

The word **care** derives from an old English term, *caru,* meaning "sorrow" or "troubled state of mind" (*American Heritage,* 1994). Contemporary use generally implies feeling concern or interest in one who has sorrow or perhaps even sharing that concern to the point of becoming sorrowful oneself as a show of support. A variation from that meaning suggests taking care of in the sense of providing for or protecting against trouble.

Is it caring to place a disabled relative in an extended care facility? Should the indigent be cared for? If so, how? Is a shortened hospital stay an expression of caring? How, and for whom? An ethic of care tries to place ethical discourse at the level where these activities of relationship are located, rather than in an intellectual or purely analytical discussion. Leaders in the field of the ethics of care find in nursing a natural ally. Nurses base their work in caring: for the client, for the client's family, and for the maintenance of the institutions that provide the services. Ethics of care suggest that ethical dilemmas will be solved by attention to relationships, by attention to particular narratives, and by the examination and promotion of any fundamental act of caring.

This attention to relationship distinguishes the ethics of care from other ethical view points because it refrains from applying universal principles that are purely intellectual or analytical processes (Watson, 1994).

How to Process an Ethical Dilemma

Ethical problems can be distressing for both clients and care givers. Controversy is the very nature of ethical deliberations, and few people like conflict. To overcome controversy and determine a course of action, ethical issues are processed carefully and deliberately. Participants refrain from making decisions solely on an emotional level while preserving the free expression of feelings. As discussed previously, however, an ethical outcome is not obtained by considering only what people want and feel. A pattern or guide for thinking through ethical conflicts or dilemmas is very helpful.

Most health care institutions utilize an ethics committee to process ethical dilemmas. These committees are generally multidisciplinary and include representatives who are nurses, as well as representatives from other disciplines. Some institutions, especially hospitals, may maintain a council specifically for nurses. These councils serve to educate nurses and others about the ethical process. They may also assume responsibility for policies that guide nursing practice in the care of clients near the end of life. An ethics committee can be especially helpful for the nurse who feels powerless or confused in the presence of an ethical dilemma. Access to an ethics committee or council provides an important resource for the nurse who identifies an ethical conflict or dilemma.

Whether an ethical dilemma is resolved, however, in a committee setting, at the bedside, or in a family conference, the nurse applies a careful, critical processing of the dilemma. Resolving an ethical dilemma is similar to the nursing process because it requires deliberate, systematic thinking (Miller and Babcock, 1996).

The first step guides the nurse to determine if the problem is an ethical one. Not all problems are ethical in nature. The nurse learns to distinguish ethical problems from questions of procedure, legality, or medical diagnosis. To distinguish an ethical problem from other problems, Curtin and Flaherty (1982) recommend that the nurse decide whether the problem has one or more of the following characteristics:

1. It cannot be resolved solely through a review of scientific data. To make this determination, it is necessary to gather detailed information about the situation from medical records, health care literature, or consultation with colleagues or with the client and family. What at first appears to be a dilemma may resolve on learning, for example, that a review of a diagnostic procedure reveals a different prognosis.
2. It is perplexing. One cannot easily think logically or make a decision about the problem, or the nurse

may disagree with a decision that others are making, and the difference of opinion is perplexing.

3. The answer to the problem will have a profound relevance for several areas of human concern.

A part of gathering information includes an examination of one's own values as they relate to the issues. The distinction between personal opinion and the facts of the case or the opinions of others is essential for resolution to proceed. To clarify the true ethical issues in any situation, a nurse needs to be aware of personal responses. People come to different conclusions about the

same situation with no malice intended toward other people. Remembering this will help the nurse be an effective arbitrator in conversation.

On review of relevant information and review of one's own values, a clear statement of the problem, in language that all concerned people can understand, lays the groundwork for the negotiations that follow. Discussions are more likely to remain focused and constructive when all parties agree on the statement of the dilemma. These discussions are next facilitated by listing possible courses of action as they occur to the group. Possibilities may occur at any time during deliberations. After alternatives are considered, persons in an ethical conflict come to a point of resolution or agreement, and action is taken. Decisions are made that can be evaluated in an ongoing manner (Box 11-7).

Documentation of the ethical process can take a variety of forms. Whenever the process involves a family conference or results in a change in the management plan, the process should be documented in the medical record. Some institutions may use a formal consultation format whenever a request for discussion comes to the ethics committee. If the ethical dilemma does not directly affect client care, however, documentation may occur by means of minutes from a meeting or in a memorandum to affected parties. In the following clinical scenario, the nursing concerns and the family conferences would be recorded in the medical record and in nursing flow sheets.

Box 11-7
How to Process an Ethical Dilemma

Step 1. Is this an ethical dilemma?
If a review of scientific data does not resolve the question, the question is perplexing, and the answer will have profound relevance for several areas of human concern, then an ethical dilemma may exist.

Step 2. Gather all the information relevant to the case.
To be sure it is a true dilemma, it will be important to review all pertinent information. Occasionally, an overlooked fact may provide quick resolution. At this point, client, family, institutional, and social perspectives are important sources of relevant information.

Step 3. Examine and determine one's own values on the issues.
Values clarification provides a foundation for clarity and for confidence during discussions that will be necessary for resolution of a dilemma.

Step 4. Articulate the problem.
A clear, simple statement of the dilemma may not always be easy, but it is essential for the next step to take place.

Step 5. Consider possible courses of action.
To respect all sides of an issue, it is helpful to list potential actions, especially when the list will reflect opinions that conflict.

Step 6. Negotiate the outcome.
Sometimes courses of action that seem unlikely at the beginning of the process take on new possibility as they are put to rational and respectful consideration. Negotiation requires a confidence in one's own point of view and a deep respect for the opinions of others.

Step 7. Evaluate the action.

▪ Clinical Scenario

On your unit, a young 35-year-old woman has been hospitalized in the final stages of a struggle with brain cancer. She is a single mother with two young children at home. Although she has been treated by both conventional and some experimental regimens, the tumor continues to grow, and the medical team has agreed that further treatment would be futile. You have cared for this client during past admissions, and during an especially open discussion, she expressed wishes to explore "do not resuscitate" (DNR) orders. During the current admission, her primary physician is out of town. The attending physician does not know the client personally, but he has spent time with her. He has reviewed the clinical data and agrees that the client is entering the terminal stages of her disease. In his opinion, however, he believes that the client is not ready to discuss end of life issues. In fact, he states that on offering the option to discuss DNR, the client declined. You have asked him to convene a family conference to discuss DNR orders, but he refuses to do so because, in his opinion, the client is not ready to participate.

Step 1: Is this an ethical dilemma?
The distinction between an ethical dilemma and a question of legality or procedure begins with a review of scientific data. What may at first appear to be a question of ethics may be resolved by clarifying one's knowledge base about clinical facts. A review of policy and procedure or standards of care may explain legal obligations that determine a course of action, regardless of personal opinion. If the question remains perplexing

and the answer will have profound relevance for several areas of human concern, then an ethical dilemma may exist.

The clinical scenario meets the criteria for an ethical dilemma. Further review of scientific data will probably not contribute to a resolution of the dilemma, but it is important to review the data carefully to make this determination. The disagreement does not revolve around whether the client is in a terminally ill state, so further clinical information will not change the basic question: should the client have an opportunity to discuss DNR orders at this time? The question is perplexing. Basically, two professional team members disagree on an assessment of a client's readiness to confront the very difficult issues around dying. The answer to the question "Is this client ready to discuss end of life?" has important human implications. If she is not ready, then raising the issues may cause anguish and fear in the client and her family. If she is ready and the team avoids discussion, she may suffer unnecessarily in silence. If she is very close to death, then the lack of a DNR order will require the application of cardiopulmonary resuscitation (CPR) in a futile situation. As a nurse, you know that CPR can cause pain. If applied in a situation where further life is unlikely, then CPR could prolong suffering and reduce dignity.

Step 2: "Gather" all the information relevant to the case.

Because resolutions to dilemmas may arise from unlikely sources, it is helpful to incorporate as much knowledge as possible, at every step of the process. At this point, the information could include looking at laboratory and test results, the clinical state of the client in question, and perhaps current literature about the diagnosis or condition of the client. It may include careful investigation into the psychosocial concerns of the client and of the client's significant others. A client's religious, cultural, and family orientation are part of the nurse's assessment.

In this case you obtain all of the clinical information pertinent to the question. It may be helpful to determine if the client retains most cognitive functions, even though her brain tumor is aggressive. You review the chart and discuss this aspect with the physician, and you agree that she is fully competent but definitely afraid and overwhelmed by the prognosis. The dilemma exists because two professionals do not agree on a client's state of mind; thus it may be helpful to reassess the client or even to request that an independent person assess the client's readiness to discuss end of life issues. Sometimes family members or significant other people in the client's life will hold important clues to a client's psychological state of mind.

Step 3: Examine and determine one's own values on the issues.

This step is important for all participants in the discussion. It is at this stage that the nurse and others must practice values clarification and try to differentiate between one's own values and the values of the client and other team members. Part of the goal is the accurate formation of one's own opinion. An equally essential part of the goal is the establishment of respect for others' opinions.

At this point you stop to reflect on your own values. You realize that your own religious practices would not prohibit you from deciding to forego further treatment if you were in the client's condition. You also realize that you do not yet have family members who rely on you, like children or elderly parents. This client's religious practices are perhaps more strictly constructed than your own. Her religion discourages actions that diminish life in any way, and you realize that she may have come to see a DNR order as giving up or as "acting like God." In addition, you understand that the attending physician has not had time to know this client like her own physician or like you have. You continue to feel, however, that the client would be capable of a discussion, in spite of her statements to the physician. In fact you feel she would benefit from a discussion because the combination of an unfamiliar care giver and declining physical health may have silenced her, but her fears and concerns persist.

Step 4: Articulate the problem.

Once all of the relevant information has been gathered, then accurate definition of the problem may proceed. It is helpful to try to state the problem in a few sentences. Also, by waiting until this point to articulate the problem, it may be possible to separate feelings from facts. The team may determine that the dilemma exists at the level of interpretation of the facts, rather than at the level of competing philosophies. By agreeing to a statement of the problem, the group can proceed with discussion in a focused way.

Here, the problem seems to be this: Should this client discuss DNR at this time? What are the benefits and what constitute risks of a DNR order at this time?

Step 5: Consider possible courses of action.

Once you have asked the basic question, other questions and possible courses of action arise: Should you initiate a discussion with the client independently of the physician? Would you act outside your professional domain if you facilitated a DNR order? What if your assessment were incorrect; would you contribute not to the dignity but to the distress of the client? The answers to these questions may be elusive because they depend on an understanding of client feelings that are not necessarily obvious. Even if legally the nurse cannot actually write a DNR order, this fact does not relieve the nurse of troubling questions because the ability to influence a physician's or client's decision regarding DNR remains.

Step 6: Negotiate the outcome.

This step represents the most important and delicate part of the process. During these negotiations, the nurse has an obligation to speak for the nursing point of view. The nurse's point of view, by definition, represents a unique contribution to the discussion. The nurse often will contribute essential information about a client and the things that are revealed by the more intimate contact that a nurse has with a client.

All members of the team will participate in the discussion until some agreement is reached. Often, participants may leave the discussion disappointed or even opposed to the decision. But in a successful discussion, all members will have agreed on an action or decision that can be implemented and whose outcomes can be measured. In the best of circumstances, participants discover a course of action that meets criteria for acceptance by all.

The discussion focuses on the disagreement between your assessment and the physician's regarding the client's readiness to discuss end of life issues. The principles invoked during the discussion include beneficence and nonmaleficence: which plan would constitute providing the most good for this client—a DNR order or no order? A separate question addresses the client's point of view: would a discussion with the client promote well-being or promote anguish? The principle of autonomy reveals that a troublesome question remains: does the client want something different from what she is expressing?

With several members of the health care team present, the discussion proceeds. You present your point of view. You continue to sense that the client is ready to discuss but that she may be reluctant to trust the circumstances of this admission. But you also respect the attending physician and his analysis and continue to harbor concerns that the client, for whatever reasons, may have experienced a change of mind between the last admission and this one. In the end, the team proposes the following: a formal meeting with the client, where you, the attending physician, and a supportive family member are all present. You support this proposal with the argument that this planned setting would provide the maximum atmosphere of trust for this client. Team members agree to keep the discussion open-ended and exploratory. You suggest that rather than asking if the client wants a DNR, perhaps the team could wait for her to bring up the issue. In this way the team could be assured of her consent and willingness to participate in the discussion.

Step 7: Evaluate the action.
At the meeting, the client in fact opens up. She expresses relief at the chance to explore her options and feelings. Pain management issues are clarified. She wants to discuss a DNR order but requests a visit from her priest before making a final decision.

POTENTIAL ETHICAL PROBLEMS IN NURSING

Nursing care contributes to all aspects of health care. Independent roles for nurses emerge in almost every health care setting (see Chapter 2). In any practice setting, a nurse may be confronted with ethical issues unique to that practice. The following sections describe examples of ethical dilemmas in these different practices and suggest critical thinking skills that help guide nursing interventions.

Ambulatory Care Settings
The nurse in the ambulatory care setting is especially concerned with the social and environmental factors in health and wellness. The implementation of an effective plan of care often depends on factors that are difficult or impossible to control, such as personal habits, poverty, or access to care. For example, a nurse may explain the importance of regular Pap smears, and the client may be well motivated, but lack of community resources to provide the Pap smear or lack of resources to pay for it will prevent the client from following through.

Step 1: Is this an ethical dilemma?
Cancer prevention for women clients depends in part on regular Pap smears. Yet this client cannot obtain one. Not only is this situation perplexing for the client and the nurse, but also the solution would have profound relevance.

Step 2: Gather all the information relevant to the case.
An investigation into the client's community resources, a search into other communities for their solutions to similar situations, and perhaps even a review of nursing literature might offer ideas for a solution to this problem. The nurse might also look to the client and her personal resources to see if the client herself is able to contribute to the solution.

Step 3: Examine and determine one's own values on the issues.
What does the nurse feel are the obligations to this client? What does the nurse feel are obligations to the community? Perhaps the nurse is very busy with a personal life and other job responsibilities, and the follow-through on this project might diminish time available for other worthy activities. Or the nurse may determine that an investment of expertise into this project would be valuable.

Step 4: Articulate the problem.
What are the nurse's obligations to this client and to her community? How can the nurse practice fidelity to the client?

Step 5: Consider possible courses of action.
The nurse may decide to pursue the establishment of better community resources for this client and others like her. The nurse may seek out others, such as community leaders or social workers, who could recruit resources to help this client. The client herself might have ideas on the location for support, such as other family members or civic groups.

Step 6: Negotiate the outcome.
In this case a part of the negotiation would include a determination of the best use of the nurse's time, taking into consideration the implications for all parts of the nurse's personal and professional life and obligations to this client and her community.

Step 7: Evaluate the action.
The successful resolution will include obtaining the Pap smear for the client.

Acute Care/Managed Care Settings
In the acute care setting, managed care systems place a growing emphasis on decreasing hospitalization days. To safely accomplish a shorter hospitalization, a great deal of teaching and discharge planning falls to the bedside nurse. An ethical dilemma arises when the nurse determines that the client and the client's family have not mastered a skill needed to provide safe care in the home, yet their insurance will not cover further days in the hospital.

Step 1: Is this an ethical dilemma?
The situation is perplexing because it seems that

whether the client remains in the hospital or not, the consequences will be dire. A safe and affordable solution to this dilemma would have relevance for the client and for the acute care setting.

Step 2: Gather all the information relevant to the case.

Who pays for this client's care, and who in this setting is responsible for negotiating with payers? What is the prognosis for this client, and how long will home care be necessary? What might be the financial impact of unsafe care in the home? How much longer does the nurse estimate the client will need to learn the home care? Can a home care service provide the care and continued teaching?

Step 3: Examine and determine one's own values on the issues.

The nurse may have had very positive or very negative experiences with managed care in the past. It would be important to separate personal responses in the past from this situation. The professional evaluation of the client's readiness for discharge will play a critical role in the negotiations, so opinion must be clear-headed.

Step 4: Articulate the problem.

What resources will provide the safest AND most cost-effective care for this client? How can the nurse protect the principle of beneficence for this client and yet remain accountable to the hospital and to the managed care plan?

Step 5: Consider possible courses of action.

The nurse could take time to educate administrators and physicians about the lack of knowledge for this client. The nurse could construct a proposal for solution by investigating the location and quality of home care services. From the client, the nurse might learn more about family resources.

Step 6: Negotiate the outcome.

Working with social workers, physicians, and admission and utilization review personnel may help to devise a safe plan for discharge. Certainly, working within the guidelines of the managed care plan will be essential for success. In addition, the client may respond to the dilemma by identification of other family members or community resources that might facilitate a safe discharge. At the very least, the nurse can ensure that the physician and others become aware of the potential for unsafe conditions after discharge.

Step 7: Evaluate the action.

The nature of the outcome will depend on the path that the nurse is able to pursue in an effort to protect this client during and after discharge.

Restorative Care Settings

Working with the chronically ill or disabled client places the nurse in contact with decisions about quality of life, such as the client's ability to maintain independence and functional status (Tilden and others, 1996). The determination of measures of quality represents a relatively new field of study. For example, a stroke victim who is profoundly disabled may begin to suffer from aspiration problems during feedings. Would a gastrostomy tube serve to prevent aspiration, or would it represent a surgical intervention that would prolong suffering?

Step 1: Is this an ethical dilemma?

A review of scientific data will not help clarify the risks and benefits of this decision. Scientific data could help to predict improved nutrition and improved safety for this client, but it does not help to address the ethical issues about quality of life. The nurse may be perplexed, as is the family, about the right decision. A decision that felt "right" to all parties would have profound relevance for this dilemma and might influence similar clinical situations in a positive way.

Step 2: Gather all the information relevant to the case.

What is the prognosis for this client, to the best of the health care team's ability to determine it? What are the surgical risks to placement of the gastrostomy tube? What is the medical risk of aspiration pneumonia in this client? How is aspiration pneumonia treated? Would pneumonia and the treatment represent an uncomfortable experience for the client?

Step 3: Examine and determine one's own values on the issues.

The nurse might explore personal feelings about the quality of this client's life. Is the client able to express an opinion? If yes, the nurse will probably have personal opinions about the competence of the client. These opinions are important to articulate. How does the nurse feel about the competence of the family members and significant others? If a decision were made with which the nurse disagrees, it might be important to consider whether one could still participate in the care of the client. Could one advocate for a position that was in conflict with one's own values?

Step 4: Articulate the problem.

Will a gastrostomy tube improve the quality of this client's life, or will a gastrostomy tube prolong suffering? How can the team best respect this client's autonomy?

Step 5: Consider possible courses of action.

The gastrostomy tube could be placed. Perhaps a nasogastric tube could be placed while the more difficult ethical issues are explored with the client and the client's family. The client or the client's significant others could elect to decline a gastrostomy tube.

Step 6: Negotiate the outcome.
If the client is competent and an adult, the client's decision will determine the outcome. If not, then the health care team will have to rely on family members, significant others, or even legal documents that identify legal guardians to make the decision. In this last case the decision may be more difficult to obtain. The nurse's role in the negotiations would include the contribution of the nursing perspective on quality of life for this individual.

Step 7: Evaluate the action.
Regardless of the decision in this case, it would be possible to reverse the decision if conditions or feelings changed. Continuing discussion with the client and the family or significant others would ensure a satisfactory conclusion to this dilemma.

Multidisciplinary Collaboration

As new technologies introduce improved outcomes for many diseases, these technologies may also require collaboration of several disciplines. Not only will different subspecialties be involved but also social workers, psychologists, physical therapists, and others (Figure 11-1). Disagreement about prognosis or plan of care often evolves. The role of the nurse may include advocating for the client's point of view or coordinating communication between teams. The nurse may also disagree with a plan of care. For example, a client with a brain tumor may have medical providers from oncology, neurology, neurosurgery, and radiology. The nurse may care for a client for whom conventional therapy has not controlled the tumor growth. One specialty may wish to proceed with experimental therapy; another specialty may not. Perhaps the nurse feels the experimental therapy would prolong suffering.

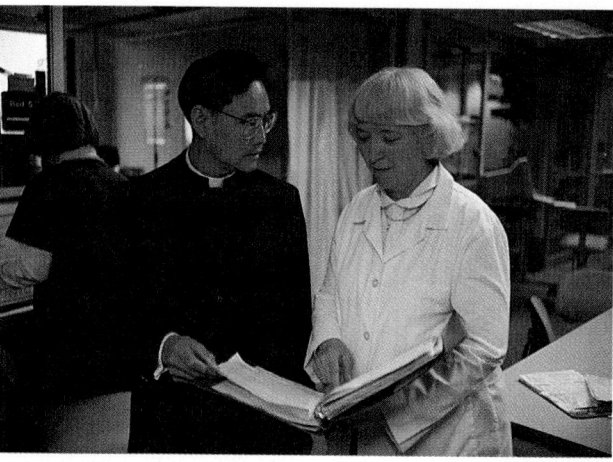

Figure 11-1. Nurses collaborate with other professionals in making ethical decisions.

Step 1: Is this an ethical dilemma?
The client is confused and unable to exercise true autonomy. Because the team that cares for this client is multidisciplinary, a decision must come from consensus, and consensus seems impossible. Further review of the scientific literature will not change the opinion of any of the medical providers. The situation is perplexing because both options seem to have merit. In addition, the client's point of view is difficult to determine because the client has access only to information from the physicians who disagree. The solution will have relevance for this client's condition. It may also provide guidance for similar clinical situations.

Step 2: Gather all the information relevant to the case.
Perhaps the best way to begin would be to request a team conference. An important piece of information includes the current clinical condition of the client. Nursing assessment of this condition is critical to the discussion.

Step 3: Examine and determine one's own values on the issues.
What is the nursing opinion on the prognosis of this client? If one were in the condition of the client, what would one's personal decision be? How does the answer to this questions differ from the client's answer? This last question is perhaps most important. When the nurse presents a point of view at a conference, it will be essential to differentiate between one's personal point of view and the client's point of view.

Step 4: Articulate the problem.
What plan of care will provide the best quality of life for this client? Who will make this decision?

Step 5: Consider possible courses of action.
The client might decide to receive experimental therapy, even after learning of the suffering that the nurse predicts. The client might decline experimental therapy. The team might determine that the prognosis is poor regardless of further therapy and relieve the client of a need to make a decision.

Step 6: Negotiate the outcome.
Once the team has reached consensus, then the client and the client's family will be better able to make an informed decision. The nurse is best positioned to emphasize the confusion that the client suffers so that the team members will be motivated to negotiate differences. The nurse may also provide a neutral voice that can organize a discussion between medical teams that are in conflict. The nurse's own point of view, however, is equally important. If in one's personal opinion further treatment might constitute prolonged suffering, then the conference between caregivers will be an effective place to negotiate and discuss this position.

Step 7: Evaluate the action.
The outcome could be considered successful if the client's autonomy receives respect while the health care team practices nonmaleficence or keeps a commitment to do the least harm. Even if team members continue to disagree about the correct course of action, a general sense of resolution remains the goal.

Cultural Sensitivity

The professional standards of justice and beneficence require respect for cultural differences in the health care setting, regardless of personal opinion or feeling (Davis and Koenig, 1996). Occasionally a nurse may face a challenging situation where cultural differences present an ethical dilemma. For example, a 15-year-old girl is admitted for management of her leukemia. The nurse notes that the client's religious beliefs do not allow her to receive blood transfusions, yet her condition will soon require a blood transfusion to prevent dire consequences. Her parents share her religious convictions but would be willing to compromise. The client is refusing to compromise.

Step 1: Is this an ethical dilemma?
Further review of the clinical situation will not change the dilemma. Scientific data will not affect the strong feelings of the client or of her parents. The case is perplexing because respecting the client's autonomy will conflict with the health care team's wish to do no harm. The resolution of this dilemma will be difficult and will have a profound relevance for several areas of concern, including the life of the client.

Step 2: Gather all the information relevant to the case.
How soon must the transfusion be administered? What are the legal definitions of "minor" in your state? Has the family agreed to transfusions in the past, and if so, what was the mechanism for reaching a compromise? What are the specific religious constraints against blood transfusions that affect this case? Is the client competent? Is she fully aware of the consequences of her decision to refuse the transfusion?

Step 3: Examine and determine one's own values on the issues.
How does one feel about this client's religious beliefs? How close or distant are the client's beliefs from one's personal beliefs? What is one's personal opinion on the rights of minors to determine their medical course?

Step 4: Articulate the problem.
A client, who is a minor, will refuse a lifesaving transfusion on the grounds of religious belief. If she is forced to receive the transfusion, she will consider herself violated in the eyes of her God. If she does not receive the transfusion, she will probably not survive.

Step 5: Consider possible courses of action.
The client could be forced to receive a transfusion, requiring restraints or use of physical force. The client's wishes could be respected. The client and the client's family could be encouraged to explore this dilemma with the guidance of a religious leader from their faith.

Step 6: Negotiate the outcome.
In this case the nurse's contribution could consist of accurate documentation of the client's state of mind. A client care conference with the client and the client's family would be necessary. If the medical team decides to insist on the transfusion, then a court order would be sought. As advocate for the client, even in the face of personal disagreement, the nurse would ensure that the client's voice was fairly represented to the judge.

Step 7: Evaluate the action.
The outcome will depend on the ability of the conference members to reach consensus. The goal will be the balancing of respect for autonomy with the principle of beneficence.

Delegation

Most health care systems utilize a team approach to nursing care. The team includes assistants, licensed and some unlicensed, who work with a registered nurse leader. The registered nurse will use delegation skills and the guidance of legal statutes to determine and assign work to assistants. Occasionally this collaboration may present ethical dilemmas to the nurse. The dilemmas may be especially troubling because the nurse leader is accountable for the actions of the team members. Furthermore, the issues may not always be associated directly with client care issues, but with behavior and work habits. For example, an unlicensed assistant who is basically a reliable team member performs her work in a timely and accurate manner. But the nurse notices that the assistant spends most of her time with one client, ignoring the special needs of others.

Step 1: Is this an ethical dilemma?
Technically this situation constitutes a personnel issue rather than an ethical dilemma. Still, professional standards of beneficence and justice suggest that care for clients be equally distributed. Because the assistant's behavior is otherwise meeting expectations, the situation is perplexing. A solution could have relevance for her work with others.

Step 2: Gather all information relevant to the situation.
If other nurses work with this assistant, how do they describe their relationship with her? What is her job description officially? What was her training for this position? Who is her supervisor? How do clients describe her care? How does the law hold the nurse ac-

countable for the actions of others on the health care team?

Step 3: Examine and determine one's own values on the issue.
What is one's personal opinions about the team approach to nursing? Has the nurse leader had training in delegation skills or supervision skills? How does the assistant's behavior impact one's own work responsibilities?

Step 4: Articulate the problem.
Is this assistant working in an inappropriate way? If yes, who is responsible for correcting the behavior?

Step 5: Consider possible courses of action.
The nurse could meet privately with the assistant to confer about the reasons for the assistant's behavior and determine resolutions. The nurse could refer the situation to a supervisor. The nurse could devise classes on caring for all assistants.

Step 6: Negotiate the outcome.
The nurse might first confer with the nursing supervisor. As health care systems move through rapid changes, it is helpful to stay informed about institutional policies, and it is important to seek guidance from colleagues. What does the law dictate in regard to accountability for client care? The ability to advocate for nursing standards, especially an ethic of care, will

remain a professional obligation. The recognition and articulation of an ethical dilemma begin the process.

Step 7: Evaluate the action.
The outcome to this dilemma might be measured best by monitoring client satisfaction.

To resolve an ethical problem, the nurse refers to a systematic process to understand the nature of the problem and to plan a responsible course of action. Although ethical dilemmas may present challenging problems, the nurse offers a unique and valuable voice to the process of resolution.

Key Terms

accountability	ethnocentrism
advocacy	feminist ethic
autonomy	fidelity
beneficence	judgment
bioethics	justice
care	law
code of ethics	morals
competence	nonmaleficence
cultural values	professionalism
deontology	responsibility
ethical dilemma	utilitarianism
ethical principles	value
ethics of care	values clarification
ethics	

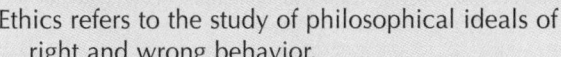

■ Key Concepts

Ethics refers to the study of philosophical ideals of right and wrong behavior.

A code of ethics provides a foundation for professional nursing.

Professional nursing promotes accountability, responsibility, and advocacy.

An ethical nurse maintains competence in practice and assumes responsibility for nursing judgments.

The primary functions of advocacy are to inform and to support.

Professional nurses have a commitment to clients, the profession, and society to provide high-quality health care.

Basic standards of ethics in health care include autonomy, justice, fidelity, beneficence, and non-maleficence.

A nurse's ethics grow from personal values.

People develop ethically just as they do physically, emotionally, and spiritually.

A child acquires values by observing behaviors that prove successful or productive for others.

A child acquires values from parents, other family members, school, religious institutions, and other social institutions.

Values clarification helps a nurse to explore personal values and feelings and to decide how to act on personal beliefs.

Values clarification promotes effective reasoning and decision making.

A nurse guided by an ethic of care will be sympathetic and able to take action on behalf of another.

Ethical problems arise from differences in values, changing professional roles, technological advances, and uncertainty in decision making.

A standard process for thinking through ethical dilemmas helps nurses resolve difficult situations.

Critical thinking is an essential part of processing ethical dilemmas.

Ethical dilemmas in nursing may occur in any segment of the health care delivery system.

The nurse's point of view provides a unique and valuable voice in the resolution of ethical dilemmas.

Critical Thinking Activities

1. Complete the "Cultural Values Exercise" (see Box 11-6) with your classmates or with members of another class of professionals. Compare the answers, and discuss the differences.

2. You are caring for a 17-year-old client who has been admitted for treatment of sickle cell crisis. She needs fluid management and comfort management. Even though she is receiving narcotics around the clock, she continues to complain of pain. She also complains about her roommate, the food, and the intravenous therapy. She comes from a community far from the hospital, and her mother cannot visit every day. She has an older brother who has been convicted of possession of illegal drugs. Discuss your approach to this client. Rank her needs. What is your priority action, based on what you know so far? Examine and describe your opinions about pain, pain management, and addiction.

3. You are a clinic nurse in a small community clinic. A 45-year-old male client has been coming to the clinic for several years for treatment and support of his acquired immunodeficiency syndrome

(AIDS). During recent months, he has lost his long-term companion to AIDS. In addition, both his parents died many years ago. His clinical condition has deteriorated. His vision is failing, his nutritional status is difficult to maintain, and he has been hospitalized three times in the past 3 months for pneumonia. He asks for your help in planning his suicide. Discuss your response to his request. Begin by an examination of your personal feelings about suicide. Include a discussion about your understanding of AIDS: where it comes from, who gets the disease and why, and what your feelings and opinions are about people with AIDS. Construct your response keeping in mind the ethical principles of fidelity, autonomy, beneficence, and nonmaleficence. Because all of these principles collide in this example, it will be necessary to rank them according to your feelings and then according to how you imagine the client would rank them. For the sake of this discussion, it is illegal in your state for nurses to prescribe medicines. What are your possible courses of action?

References

American Heritage Dictionary, ed 3, Boston, 1994, Houghton Mifflin.

American Nurses Association: *Code for nurses with interpretative statements,* Kansas City, Mo, 1985, The Association.

Beauchamp T, Childress J: *Principles of biomedical ethics,* ed 3, New York, 1989, Oxford University Press.

Canadian Nurses Association: *Code of ethics for registered nurses,* Ottawa, 1997, The Association.

Chitty K: *Professional nursing: concepts and challenges,* Philadelphia, 1993, WB Saunders.

Curtin L, Flaherty MJ: *Nursing ethics: theories and pragmatics,* Bowie, Md, 1982, Brady.

Davis A, Aroskar M: *Ethical dilemmas and nursing practice,* Norwalk, Conn, 1991, Appleton & Lange.

Davis AJ, Koenig BA: A question of policy: bioethics in a multicultural society, *Nurs Policy Forum* 2(1):7, 1996.

Deloughery G: *Issues and trends in nursing,* ed 2, St. Louis, 1995, Mosby.

Fry ST: The role of caring in a theory of nursing ethics, *Hypatia* 4(2):88, 1989.

Gilligan C: *In a different voice,* Cambridge, Mass, 1982, Harvard University Press.

Harris CH: Legal aspects of nursing. In Deloughery G: *Issues and trends in nursing,* ed 2, St. Louis, 1995, Mosby.

International Council of Nurses: *ICN code for nurses: ethical concepts applied to nursing,* Geneva, 1973, Imprimeries Populaires.

Kohlberg L: *Essays on moral development,* vols I-III, San Francisco, 1981, Harper & Row.

Leininger M: *Caring: an essential human need,* Detroit, 1988, Wayne State University Press.

Miller MA, Babcock DE: *Critical thinking applied to nursing,* St. Louis, 1996, Mosby.

O'Neil J: Ethical decision making and the role of nursing. In Deloughery G: *Issues and trends in nursing,* ed 2, St. Louis, 1995, Mosby.

Piaget J: *The moral development of the child,* New York, 1932, The Free Press.

Potter P, Perry A: *Fundamentals of nursing: concepts, process, and practice,* ed 4, St. Louis, 1997, Mosby.

Raths LE, Harmin M, Simon SB: *Values and teaching,* ed 2, Columbus, Ohio, 1979, Merrill.

Renwick GW, Rhinesmith SH: *An exercise in cultural analysis for managers,* Chicago, 1995, Intercultural Press.

Sherwin S: *No longer patient: feminist ethics and health care,* Philadelphia, 1992, Temple University Press.

Tilden V and others: Decisions about life-sustaining treatment, *Arch Intern Med* 155:633, 1996.

Uustal D: *Values and ethics in nursing: from theory to practice,* ed 4, East Greenwich, RI, 1992, Educational Resources in Nursing & Holistic Health.

Uustal DB: *Am J Nurs* 78:2058, 1978.

Watson J, editor: *Applying art and science of human caring,* New York, 1994, National League of Nursing Press.

12

Legal Concepts in Nursing Practice

OBJECTIVES

Mastery of content in this chapter will enable the student to:

- Define the key terms listed.
- Explain the legal concepts that apply to nurses.
- Give examples of legal issues that arise in nursing practice.
- Describe the legal responsibilities and obligations of nurses.
- Understand the concept of negligence.
- List sources for standards of care for nurses.
- Define the legal aspects of nurse-client, nurse-physician, and nurse-employer relationships.

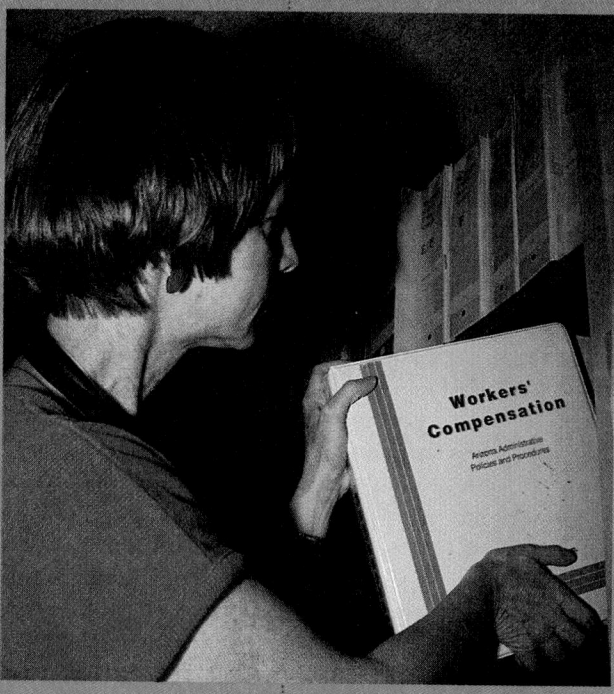

Nurses must have an understanding of the law and how it affects nursing practice. Many legal issues arise that require the nurse to use critical thinking abilities to practice safe nursing care. Safe nursing care includes an understanding of the legal boundaries within which nurses must function.

Laws are changing constantly to reflect changes in society and changes in the delivery of health care. Nurses should be aware that state laws vary widely across the country. A nurse should know the law in his or her own state, know the rules and regulations of state **regulatory agencies,** and consult his or her employing institution's attorney for specific questions.

LEGAL LIMITS OF NURSING

Professional nurses should understand the legal limits or standards that affect nursing practice. An understanding of the law coupled with sound judgment should ensure safe and appropriate nursing care.

Sources of Law

Nursing practice is subject to statutory law, regulatory law, and common law. **Statutory law** is created by elected legislative bodies such as the U.S. Congress and state legislatures. An example of a federal statute is the Americans With Disabilities Act (ADA), which protects the rights of handicapped individuals (ADA, 1995). Examples of state statutes are the Nurse Practice Acts found in all 50 states. Regulatory law or administrative law is created by administrative bodies such as state boards of nursing when they pass rules and regulations. An example of regulatory law is the duty to report incompetent or unethical nursing behavior to the state board. **Common law** is created by judicial decisions made in courts when individual legal cases are decided. An example of common law is **informed consent** and the client's right to refuse treatment.

Statutes are either criminal or civil. **Criminal laws** prevent harm to society and provide punishment for crimes (Black, 1990). The violation of a criminal statute is classified as a felony or a misdemeanor. A **felony** is a serious offense that has a penalty of imprisonment for greater than a year or possibly even death. A **misdemeanor** is a less serious **crime** that has a penalty of a fine or imprisonment for less than a year. An example of criminal conduct for nurses would be misuse of a controlled substance.

Civil laws protect private rights. These laws protect the rights of individuals and encourage fairness within our society. For example, the state statutes that create a cause of action for wrongful death protect an individual's right to health care that meets the standard of care. Wrongful death statutes specifically state which family members can sue, the time within which the suit must be filed, and the specific damages that may be claimed, such as loss of services and funeral and burial bills. The violation of a civil statute results in the payment of money damages.

A **tort** is a private or civil wrong or injury for which the court provides a remedy in the form of money damages (Black, 1990). A tort is committed against a person or property. Torts are classified as intentional or unintentional. *Intentional torts* are willful acts that violate another person's rights. Examples of intentional torts are assault, battery, defamation, invasion of privacy, false imprisonment, and fraud. Unintentional torts include negligence. **Negligence** is the failure to use care that a reasonable person would use under similar circumstances. It is simply carelessness or conduct that falls below the standard of care. Malpractice is one example of negligence. **Malpractice** is defined as professional misconduct or unreasonable lack of skill (Black, 1990).

Intentional torts

Assault. **Assault** is any intentional threat to bring about harmful or offensive contact. No actual contact is necessary. The law protects clients who are afraid of harmful contact. It is an assault for a nurse to threaten to give a client an injection or to threaten to restrain a client for an x-ray procedure when the client has refused consent. The key issue is the client's consent. In a lawsuit where assault is alleged, the client's consent would bar the claim of assault against a nurse.

Battery. **Battery** is any intentional touching without consent. The contact can be harmful to the client and cause an injury or it can be merely offensive to the client's personal dignity. A battery always includes an assault, which is why the two terms *assault and battery* are commonly combined. In the example of a nurse threatening to give a client an injection without the client's consent, if the nurse actually gives the injection, it is considered a battery. A battery can also result if the health care provider performs a procedure that exceeds the client's consent. For example, if the client gives consent for an appendectomy and the physician performs a tonsillectomy, a battery has occurred. Once again the key issue is the client's consent.

In some situations consent is implied. For example, if a client gets into a wheelchair or transfers to a stretcher after being advised that it is time to be taken for an x-ray procedure, the client has given implied consent to the procedure. If the client learns that an x-ray film of the head instead of the foot is to be taken, and the client refuses to have the x-ray film taken, the consent has been revoked or withdrawn.

Invasion of privacy. The tort of **invasion of privacy** protects the client's right to be free from unwanted intrusion into his or her private affairs. The four types of invasion of privacy torts are intrusion upon seclusion, appropriation of name or likeness, publication of private or embarrassing facts, and publicity placing one in a false light (Prosser and Keeton, 1988).

Clients are entitled to confidential health care. For example, in a classic case, reporters published photographs of a female client in her hospital room without her consent. A claim for invasion of privacy was upheld. This case is an example of intrusion upon seclusion or publication of private embarrassing facts (*Barber v. Time Magazine,* 1942).

Another form of invasion of privacy is the release of a client's medical information to an unauthorized person such as a member of the press or the client's employer. A client's medical information is confidential. It should be shared with health care providers for the purpose of medical treatment only.

The nurse should not disclose the client's confidential medical information without the client's consent. For example, a nurse should respect a wish not to inform the client's family of a terminal illness. Similarly, a nurse should not assume that a client's spouse or family members know all of the client's history, particularly with respect to private issues such as mental illness, medications, pregnancy, abortion, birth control, or sexually transmitted diseases.

An individual's right to privacy may conflict with the public's right to know. In one case, a married couple was filmed by a television crew while attending a hospital function regarding the success of the in vitro fertilization program in which they participated. The couple had previously told no one but their immediate family that they were involved in the in vitro program and had been assured that there would be no publicity or public exposure. After the newscast they were subjected to phone calls and embarrassing questions. The couple filed a lawsuit. The court held that the husband and wife stated a claim for invasion of privacy and that even though the in vitro program may have been of public interest, the identity of the plaintiffs was a private matter (*Y.G. v. Jewish Hospital,* 1990).

Many states, through their respective public health departments, require that certain infectious or communicable diseases be reported. Sometimes the client is a public figure whose physical condition is considered newsworthy (Prosser and Keeton, 1988). There are also cases in which information is given out about a scientific discovery or a major medical breakthrough, as with the first heart transplant case or the first artificial heart recipient. If an event falls into any of these categories, information should be channeled through the public relations department of the institution to ensure that invasion of privacy does not occur. The nurse should not independently attempt to decide the legality of disclosing information.

Defamation of character. Defamation of character is the publication of false statements that result in damage to a person's reputation (Box 12-1). The statements must be published with malice in the case of a public official or public figure. Malice means that the person publishing the information knows it is false and

---

Box 12-1
Defamation of Character

1. Publication—verbal or in writing
2. Defamatory statement of fact—damaging to reputation
3. About the plaintiff—which is false
4. Published with the requisite degree of fault
   Actual malice—for public figures or public officials
   Negligence—for private figures
5. Damages resulting from the defamation

---

publishes it anyway or that it is published with reckless disregard as to the truth or falsity of the statement. If the statement is presented orally, it is called **slander.** If the statement is made in writing, it is called **libel.** For example, if a nurse tells people erroneously that a client has venereal disease and the disclosure affects the client's business, the nurse could be held liable for slander.

Unintentional torts

Negligence and malpractice. Negligence is conduct that falls below the standard of care. The **standard of care** is established by law for the protection of others against an unreasonably great risk of harm (Black, 1990). For example, if a driver of a car acts unreasonably in failing to stop at a stop sign, it is negligence. In general, courts define negligence in car accident cases and other negligence cases as the failure to use that degree of care that an ordinarily careful and prudent person would use under the same or similar circumstances (Missouri Approved Instructions [MAI], 1991a).

Malpractice is one type of negligence, called *professional negligence.* Nursing malpractice results when nursing care falls below the standard of care. If nurses give care that does not meet appropriate standards, they may be held liable for negligence (Box 12-2). Negligence may involve failing to check a client's arm band and then administering medication to the wrong client. Negligence may also involve administering a medication to a client even though it has been documented that the client has an allergy to that medication. In general, courts define nursing negligence as the failure to use that degree of skill or learning ordinarily used under the same or similar circumstances by the members of the nurses' profession (MAI, 1991b).

Nurses have been involved in several common negligent acts including the following:

1. Medication errors that result in injury to clients
2. Intravenous therapy errors resulting in infiltrations or phlebitis

Proof of Malpractice

In a malpractice suit against a nurse, the client must prove the following:

1. The nurse (defendant) owed a duty to the client (plaintiff). (The **plaintiff** is the person bringing the lawsuit and the **defendant** is the person being sued.)
2. The nurse did not carry out that duty or breached the duty.
3. The client was injured.
4. The client's injury was caused by the nurse's failure to carry out his or her duty.

3. Burns to clients caused by equipment, bathing, or spills of hot liquids and foods
4. Falls resulting in injury to clients
5. Failure to use aseptic technique where required
6. Errors in sponge, instrument, or needle counts in surgical cases
7. Failure to give a report, or giving an incomplete report, to an oncoming shift
8. Failure to adequately monitor a client's condition
9. Failure to notify a physician of a significant change in a client's status

The best way for nurses to avoid being liable for negligence is to follow standards of care, give competent health care, communicate with other health care providers, document assessments, interventions, and evaluations fully, and develop empathetic rapport with the client. Poor client relations are leading causes of lawsuits (Rutherford, 1994; Ladebauche, 1995). A client who believes that the nurse performed duties correctly and was concerned with his or her welfare is unlikely to initiate a lawsuit. In addition, if a nurse is brought into a lawsuit, careful, complete, and thorough documentation is one of the best defenses. Nurses should also know the current nursing literature in their areas of practice. They should know and follow the policies and procedures of the institution in which they work. Nurses should be sensitive to common sources of client injury, such as falls and medication errors. Finally, nurses must communicate with the client, explain the tests and treatment to be performed, and listen to the client's concerns about the treatment. Any significant changes in the client's condition must be reported to the physician and documented in the chart.

Malpractice insurance. Malpractice insurance provides for a defense when a nurse is sued for medical malpractice. This includes the payment of a judgment or settlement and the payment of attorney's fees. Nurses employed by health care institutions generally are covered by that institution's insurance and do not need to purchase any supplemental insurance, unless the nurse plans to practice nursing outside of the employing institution. The employing institution's insurance, however, only covers nurses while working within the scope of their employment. A nurse who is called on by neighbors and friends to provide nursing care on a volunteer basis would not be covered by the hospital's policy if a neighbor or friend filed suit.

•••STANDARDS OF CARE

The standards of care are the legal guidelines for the safe and appropriate practice of nursing. Nursing standards of care are defined in the Nurse Practice Acts and State Board of Nursing of each state, state and federal hospital licensing laws, professional and specialty organization standards, and in the written policies and procedures of the employing institution. There is also a body of law referred to as *case law* or *common law,* which consists of prior court rulings that affect nursing practice.

The **Nurse Practice Acts** of each state define the scope of nursing practice and expanded nursing roles, set educational requirements for nurses, and distinguish between nursing practice and medical practice. There are also rules and regulations enacted by the State Board of Nursing that define the practice of nursing more specifically. For example, a state board may develop a rule regarding intravenous therapy.

Professional organizations are another source for defining the standards of care. The American Nurses Association (ANA) has developed standards for nursing practice, policy statements, and similar resolutions. The standards delineate the scope, function, and role of the nurse and establish clinical practice standards. For example, the standards for Community Health Nursing Practice include data collection, diagnosis, planning, treatment, and evaluation. The Joint Commission on Accreditation of Healthcare Organizations (JCAHO) requires that accredited hospitals fulfill certain standards with regard to nursing such as having written policies and procedures. Nursing specialty organizations also define standards of care for nurses to be certified in specialty areas such as the operating room or critical care areas. These standards of care also determine whether nurses are acting appropriately when performing their duties.

The written policies and procedures of the employing institution define the standards of care at that institution. These policies are usually quite specific and are set forth in policy and procedure manuals found on most nursing units. For example, a policy and procedure outlining the steps that should be taken when changing a dressing or administering medication gives specific information for nurses to perform these tasks. It is important that nurses know the policies and procedures because the same standard of care must be used by all nurses in the health care institution (Autonberry, 1995).

In a malpractice lawsuit, a nursing expert is called to testify about the standards of nursing care as applied to the facts in the lawsuit. Nurse experts must base their opinions on existing standards of practice established by Nurse Practice Acts, professional organizations, institutional policies and procedures, federal and state hospital licensing laws, standards of the JCAHO, job descriptions, and current nursing literature (Ladebauche, 1995). Some hospitals are also now using procedural textbooks to outline the institution's general policies and procedures.

The standards of care are used by the jury to determine whether the nurse has acted as would any reasonable nurse with the same level of education and experience, and in the same or similar circumstances. Specialized nurses such as nurse anesthetists, intensive care nurses, certified nurse midwives, or operating room nurses are held to standards of care and skill exercised by those in the same specialty as defined by applicable standards. Since the jury is not familiar with nursing practice, an expert is necessary for the client to establish negligence. In most cases the defendant hospital or defendant nurse also has a nursing expert testify as to the standard of care and to the appropriateness of the defendant's actions. At the time of trial, the standard of care is what the nurse experts testify that standard to be and ultimately what the jury believes (Carroll, 1996).

One of the first and most important cases to discuss a nurse's liability was *Darling v. Charleston Community Memorial Hospital*. The verdict in the case, decided by the Illinois Supreme Court in 1966, has been adopted by almost every state. It involved an 18-year-old man with a fractured leg. When a cast was applied to the leg, the physician placed insufficient padding under the plaster. The man's toes became swollen and discolored, and he had decreased sensation in them. He complained to the nursing staff many times. Although the nurses recognized the symptoms as signs of impaired circulation, they failed to notify their supervisor that the physician did not respond to their calls or the client's needs. During the next 4 days, gangrene developed, and the man's leg had to be amputated. The physician in the emergency room was liable for applying the cast incorrectly. The nursing staff was also liable because it had not adhered to the standards of care for monitoring and reporting the client's symptoms (*Darling v. Charleston Community Memorial Hospital*, 1966).

The best way for nurses to keep up with the current legal issues affecting nursing practice is to read the nursing literature in their practice area. Current nursing literature deals with the changing obligations and standards of care for nurses, explains pertinent state and federal laws, and keeps the nurse up to date on any new rules or regulations and case law.

GOOD SAMARITAN LAWS

Nurses may act as Good Samaritans by providing emergency assistance at an accident scene. **Good Samaritan laws** have been enacted in almost every state to encourage health care professionals to assist in emergency situations. These laws limit liability and offer legal immunity for nurses who help at the scene of an accident. They also provide that a nurse can assist a minor in an emergency at the scene of an accident or competitive sports event before obtaining the parent's consent. If a nurse stops at the scene of an automobile accident and gives appropriate emergency care such as applying pressure to stop hemorrhage, the nurse is acting within accepted standards, even though proper equipment was not available. If the client subsequently develops complications as a result of the nurse's actions, the nurse is immune from liability as long as he or she acted without gross negligence.

LICENSURE

All registered nurses are licensed by the Board of Nursing of the state in which they practice. Most states require a number of educational credits and a passing score on a licensing examination to obtain a nursing license. Licensure permits nurses to offer special skills and knowledge to the public, and it also provides legal guidelines for protection of the public. All states use the National Council Licensure Examinations (NCLEX) for registered nurses.

A nurse's license can be suspended or revoked by the Board of Nursing if the nurse's conduct violates provisions of the licensing statute. For example, nurses who perform illegal acts such as selling or taking controlled substances jeopardize their license status. Because a license is considered a property right, due process must be followed before a license can be suspended or revoked. Due process means that the nurse must be notified of the charges and a hearing must be conducted so that the nurse can present evidence to defend against the charges. The hearings are not conducted in court but are usually heard by the State Board of Nursing. Some states provide for judicial review of such cases in court if the nurse has tried all other forms of appeal.

LEGAL RELATIONSHIPS IN NURSING PRACTICE

The professional nurse has a relationship with the client, with other nurses and health care providers, with the physician, and with the employer. Liability issues can arise in any of these relationships. A Patient's Bill of Rights, adopted by the American Hospital Association, is an unofficial statement of guidelines related to nurse-client interaction (Box 12-3).

Box 12-3
A Patient's Bill of Rights

INTRODUCTION

Effective health care requires collaboration between patients and physicians and other health care professionals. Open and honest communication, respect for personal and professional values, and sensitivity to differences are integral to optimal patient care. As the setting for the provision of health services, hospitals must provide a foundation for understanding and respecting the rights and responsibilities of patients, their families, physicians, and other caregivers. Hospitals must ensure a health care ethic that respects the role of patients in decision making about treatment choices and other aspects of their care. Hospitals must be sensitive to cultural, racial, linguistic, religious, age, gender, and other differences, as well as the needs of persons with disabilities.

The American Hospital Association presents *A Patient's Bill of Rights* with the expectation that it will contribute to more effective patient care and be supported by the hospital on behalf of the institution, its medical staff, employees, and patients. The American Hospital Association encourages health care institutions to tailor this bill of rights to their patient community by translating and/or simplifying the language of this bill of rights as may be necessary to ensure that patients and their families understand their rights and responsibilities.

BILL OF RIGHTS*

1. The patient has the right to considerate and respectful care.

2. The patient has the right to and is encouraged to obtain from physicians and other direct caregivers relevant, current, and understandable information concerning diagnosis, treatment and prognosis.

    Except in emergencies when the patient lacks decision-making capacity and the need for treatment is urgent, the patient is entitled to the opportunity to discuss and request information related to the specific procedures and/or treatments, the risks involved, the possible length of recuperation, and the medically reasonable alternatives and their accompanying risks and benefits.

    Patients have the right to know the identity of physicians, nurses, and others involved in their care, as well as when those involved are students, residents, or other trainees. The patient also has the right to know the immediate and long-term financial implications of treatment choices, insofar as they are known.

3. The patient has the right to make decisions about the plan of care prior to and during the course of treatment and to refuse a recommended treatment or plan of care to the extent permitted by law and hospital policy and to be informed of the medical consequences of this action. In case of such refusal, the patient is entitled to other appropriate care and services that the hospital provides or transfer to another hospital. The hospital should notify patients of any policy that might affect patient choice within the institution.

4. The patient has the right to have an advance directive (such as living will, health care proxy, or durable power of attorney for health care) concerning treatment or designating a surrogate decision maker with the expectation that the hospital will honor the intent of that directive to the extent permitted by law and hospital policy.

    Health care institutions must advise patients of their rights under state law and hospital policy to make informed medical choices, ask if the patient has an advance directive, and include that information in patient records. The patient has the right to timely information about hospital policy that may limit its ability to implement fully a legally valid advance directive.

5. The patient has the right to every consideration of privacy. Case discussion, consultation, examination, and treatment should be conducted so as to protect each patient's privacy.

6. The patient has the right to expect that all communications and records pertaining to his/her care will be treated as confidential by the hospital, except in cases such as suspected abuse and public health hazards when reporting is permitted or required by law. The patient has the right to expect that the hospital will emphasize the confidentiality of this information when it releases it to any other parties entitled to review information in these records.

7. The patient has the right to review the records pertaining to his/her medical care and to have the information explained or interpreted as necessary, except when restricted by law.

*These rights can be exercised on the patient's behalf by a designated surrogate or proxy decision maker if the patient lacks decision-making capacity, is legally incompetent, or is a minor.

Box 12-3
A Patient's Bill of Rights—cont'd

8. The patient has the right to expect that, within its capacity and policies, a hospital will make reasonable response to the request of a patient for appropriate and medically indicated care and services. The hospital must provide evaluation, services, and/or referral as indicated by the urgency of the case. When medically appropriate and legally permissible, or when a patient has so requested, a patient may be transferred to another facility. The institution to which the patient is to be transferred must first have accepted the patient for transfer. The patient must also have the benefit of complete information and explanation concerning the need for, risks, benefits, and alternatives to such a transfer.

9. The patient has the right to ask and be informed of the existence of business relationships among the hospital, educational institutions, other health care providers, or payers that may influence the patient's treatment and care.

10. The patient has the right to consent to or decline to participate in proposed research studies or human experimentation affecting care and treatment or requiring direct patient involvement, and to have those studies fully explained prior to consent. A patient who declines to participate in research or experimentation is entitled to the most effective care that the hospital can otherwise provide.

11. The patient has the right to expect reasonable continuity of care when appropriate and to be informed by physicians and other caregivers of available and realistic patient care options when hospital care is no longer appropriate.

12. The patient has the right to be informed of hospital policies and practices that relate to patient care, treatment, and responsibilities. The patient has the right to be informed of available resources for resolving disputes, grievances, and conflicts, such as ethics committees, patient representatives, or other mechanisms available in the institution. The patient has the right to be informed of the hospital's charges for services and available payment methods.

The collaborative nature of health care requires that patients, or their families/surrogates, partici-

pate in their care. The effectiveness of care and patient satisfaction with the course of treatment depend, in part, on the patient fulfilling certain responsibilities. Patients are responsible for providing information about past illnesses, hospitalizations, medications, and other matters related to health status. To participate effectively in decision making, patients must be encouraged to take responsibility for requesting additional information or clarification about their health status or treatment when they do not fully understand information and instructions. Patients are also responsible for ensuring that the health care institution has a copy of their written advance directive if they have one. Patients are responsible for informing their physicians and other caregivers if they anticipate problems in following prescribed treatment.

Patients should also be aware of the hospital's obligation to be reasonably efficient and equitable in providing care to other patients and the community. The hospital's rules and regulations are designed to help the hospital meet this obligation. Patients and their families are responsible for making reasonable accommodations to the needs of the hospital, other patients, medical staff, and hospital employees. Patients are responsible for providing necessary information for insurance claims and for working with the hospital to make payment arrangements, when necessary.

A person's health depends on much more than health care services. Patients are responsible for recognizing the impact of their life-style on their personal health.

CONCLUSION
Hospitals have many functions to perform, including the enhancement of health status, health promotion, and the prevention and treatment of injury and disease; the immediate and ongoing care and rehabilitation of patients; the education of health professionals, patients, and the community; and research. All these activities must be conducted with an overriding concern for the values and dignity of patients.

Student Nurses

Student nurses are responsible for all of their actions that cause harm to clients. When a client is injured as a direct result of the student nurse's actions, the liability for the incorrect action may be shared by the student, instructor, assigned staff nurse, and hospital or health care facility. Even though the student nurse is not considered an employee of the hospital or health care facility, the institution should monitor the acts of the nursing student. Faculty members are usually responsible for instructing and observing students, but in some situations the staff nurses may share these responsibilities. Student nurses should never be assigned to tasks for which they are unprepared and should be carefully supervised by instructors as they learn new procedures. Every nursing school should provide clear definitions of responsibility. During the clinical rotation, the student nurse is generally covered by the hospital's medical malpractice insurance; however, the student nurse should always inquire as to the specific coverage.

Sometimes student nurses are employed as nursing assistants or nurse's aides when they are not attending classes. During the time a student works as an employee of a health care facility, the student should perform only tasks that appear in a job description for a nurse's aide or nursing assistant. For example, even if a student has learned to administer intramuscular medications in class, this task may not be performed by a nurse's aide. When a student is working at a health care facility, he or she is probably covered by the institution's insurance. Any time that a student nurse is employed, he or she should always inquire about malpractice insurance coverage.

Physician Orders

The physician is responsible for directing the medical treatment of a client. The nurse is obligated to follow the physician's order unless it is believed that the order is in error, violates hospital policy, or would be detrimental to clients (Squadroni, 1994). Therefore all orders must be assessed, and if one is determined to be erroneous or harmful, further clarification from the physician is necessary (Figure 12-1).

If the physician confirms the order, but the nurse still believes it is inappropriate, the supervising nurse is informed. The nurse should not perform the physician's order if there is a risk that harm will come to the client. A written memorandum to the supervisor detailing the events in chronological order and the reasons for refusing to carry out the order should protect the nurse from disciplinary action. The supervising nurse should help resolve the questionable order. If the questionable order is carried out, the nurse may be legally responsible for harm suffered by the client.

All physician orders should be in writing. They should all be dated and timed appropriately. The nurse must make sure that the orders are transcribed cor-

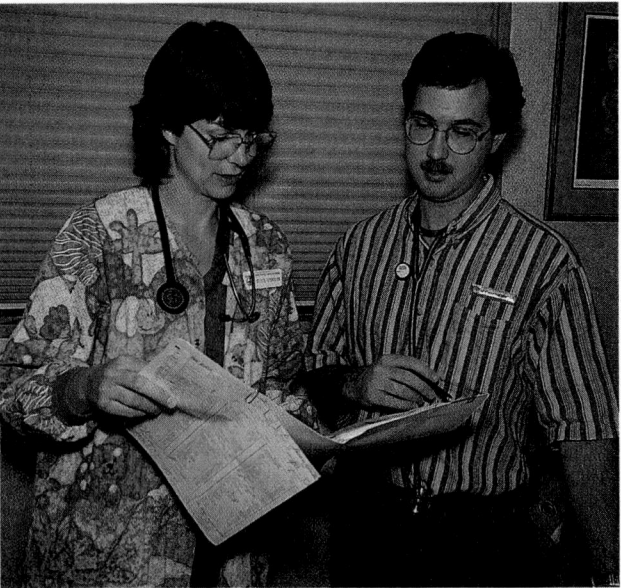

Figure 12-1. If an order creates questions, the nurse clarifies it with the physician.

rectly. Verbal orders or telephone orders are not recommended because they leave possibilities for error. If a verbal order or telephone order is necessary, as in an emergency, it should be written and signed by the physician as soon as possible, usually within 24 hours (JCAHO, 1995).

In the event that a physician has documented in the progress notes that the client is deteriorating and the decision not to administer cardiopulmonary resuscitation has been made by the physician and client, the physician should write a "no code" or "do not resuscitate" (DNR) order. Many times the decision regarding lifesaving treatment is in writing in the client's living will or durable power of attorney. If the client is competent, the order should be discussed with the client. If the client is not able to make health care decisions, the order should be discussed with the health care surrogate. A "no code" or DNR order should be written, not given verbally. Physicians should regularly review DNR orders in case the client's condition warrants a change. The nurse should be familiar with the institution's policies and procedures concerning DNR orders. Physicians can list all specifics of DNR orders pursuant to the client's living will or health care surrogate. For example, a physician may order vasopressor and fluid management to maintain a client's blood pressure but specifically state no chest compression or intubation for cardiac arrhythmias or respiratory arrest.

Consent

A signed consent form is required for all routine treatment, hazardous procedures such as surgery, some treatment programs such as chemotherapy, and research involving clients (JCAHO, 1995). A client signs general consent forms when admitted to the hospital or other health care facility. Separate special consent forms must be signed by the client or a representative before specialized procedures are performed.

State statutes provide the designation of individuals who are legally able to give consent to medical treatment. In general, those who may consent to medical treatment include the following:

I. Adults
   A. Any competent individual 18 years of age or older for himself or herself
   B. Any parent for his or her unemancipated minor
   C. Any guardian for his or her ward
   D. Any adult for the treatment of his or her minor brother or sister (if an emergency and parents are not present)
   E. Any grandparent for a minor grandchild (if an emergency and parents are not present)
II. Minors
   A. For his or her child and any child in his or her legal custody
   B. For himself or herself in the following situations:
      1. Lawfully married or a parent (emancipated)
      2. Pregnancy (excluding abortions)
      3. Venereal disease
      4. Drug or substance abuse
   C. Unemancipated minors may not consent to abortions without one of the following:
      1. Consent of one parent
      2. Self-consent being granted by court order
      3. Consent specifically given by a court

If a client is deaf, illiterate, or speaks a foreign language, an interpreter should be available to explain the terms of consent. A client under the effects of a sedative is not able to clearly understand the implications of an invasive procedure. Every effort should be made to assist the client in making an informed choice.

Nurses must be sensitive to the cultural issues of consent. The nurse must understand the way in which clients and their families communicate and make important decisions. It is essential for nurses to understand the various cultures with which they interact. The cultural beliefs and values of the client may be very different from those of the nurse. It is important for nurses not to impose their own cultural values on the client. Insensitivity and stereotyping of different ethnic groups is of equal concern. A conscious awareness of the different values and beliefs held by various cultures is essential for sensitive nursing care.

Informed consent.
Informed consent is a person's agreement to allow something to happen, such as surgery, based on a full disclosure of risks, benefits, alternatives, and consequences of refusal (Black, 1990). Informed consent not only requires that a person be given all relevant information required to reach a decision regarding treatment but also requires that the person be capable of understanding the relevant information and does, in fact, give consent. One who performs a procedure on a client without informed consent may be found civilly liable for committing battery.

The following factors must be verified for a consent to be valid (Prosser and Keeton, 1988):

1. The person giving the consent must be mentally and physically competent and be legally an adult (usually over 18 years of age or emancipated).
2. The consent must be given voluntarily; no forceful measures may be used to obtain it.
3. The person giving the consent must thoroughly understand the procedure, its risks and benefits, and alternative procedures.
4. The person giving consent has a right to have all questions answered satisfactorily and confirm his or her understanding of the treatment to be given.

Informed consent is part of the physician-client relationship. Because nurses do not perform surgery or direct medical procedures, obtaining clients' informed consent does not fall within the nursing duty. Even though the nurse assumes the responsibility for witnessing the client's signature on the consent form, the nurse does not legally assume the duty of obtaining informed consent. When nurses provide consent forms for clients to sign, the clients should be asked if they understand the procedures for which consent is being given. If clients deny understanding or the nurse suspects they do not understand, the nurse must notify the physician or nursing supervisor and must make certain that clients are informed before signing. Some consent forms also have a line for the physician to sign after explaining the risks and alternatives to a client. Such a form is helpful in a court case when a client alleges that consent was not informed. A client refusing surgery or other medical treatment must be informed about any harmful consequences of refusal. If the client persists in refusing the treatment, this rejection should be written, signed, and witnessed.

If a client participates in an experimental treatment program or submits to the use of experimental drugs or treatments, an even more detailed and stringently regulated informed consent form is used. The Food and Drug Administration (FDA) and an organization's institutional review board (IRB) review the information in the consent form for research involving human subjects. The client may always withdraw from the experiment at any time.

Parents are usually the legal guardians of pediatric clients, and therefore they are the persons who must sign consent forms for treatment. If the parents are divorced, the parent with legal custody must give consent. Occasionally a parent or guardian refuses treatment for a child. In those cases the court may intervene on the child's behalf.

In some instances obtaining informed consent is difficult. If, for example, the client is unconscious, consent must be obtained from a person legally authorized to give consent on the client's behalf. Other surrogate decision makers may have legally been delegated this authority through special process of attorney documents or through court guardianship procedures. If a person has been declared legally incompetent in a judicial proceeding, consent must be obtained from the person's legal guardian (Coker and Johns, 1994). In emergency situations, if it is impossible to obtain consent from the client or an authorized person, the procedure required to benefit the client or save a life may be undertaken without liability for failure to obtain consent. In such cases the law assumes the client would wish to be treated.

Psychiatric clients must also give consent. They retain the right to refuse treatment until a court has legally determined that they are incompetent to decide for themselves.

Death and Dying

Nurses must know their legal responsibilities concerning death and dying. Nurses must document all events that occur when the dying client is in their care. The statutory definition of death states that death occurs when there is total and irreversible cessation of all brain function, despite function of other body organs. One reason for the development of the definition is to facilitate recovery of organs for transplantation. Even though the client may be considered "brain dead," other organs may be healthy for donation. This definition is also useful when there is a question of whether to continue life support.

Consent for an autopsy must have been given previously by the decedent or by a close family member at the time of the decedent's death. In many states there is an order of priority for the giving of consent for autopsies, such as (1) decedent, in writing; (2) durable power of attorney; (3) surviving spouse; and (4) surviving child, parent, brother, or sister in the order named. The death is to be reported and investigated by the coroner when there are reasonable grounds to believe that the person died as a result of violence, homicide, suicide, accident, or death occurring in any unusual or suspicious manner. The coroner must also be notified when a client's death is unforeseen and sudden and the client has not been seen by a physician in over 36 hours.

There are legal issues associated with caring for clients who are terminally ill, severely debilitated, or in a persistent vegetative state (permanently comatose). Active **euthanasia** involves an intentional act such as administering a lethal drug dose to cause death. This is considered homicide, a crime. Passive euthanasia involves the lack of action that ultimately results in the death of a client. For example, by withholding food and nutrition at the request of the client, the nurse is po-

tentially participating in passive euthanasia. The doctrine of informed consent ensures that the client has the right to refuse treatment. Withholding of food and nutrition has been upheld in court cases that support the client's right to refuse treatment (Daly, 1995).

Suicide is the taking of one's own life. Helping a person to commit suicide has come to be known as "assisted suicide." The American Nurses Association's (ANA) position statement on assisted suicide defines assisted suicide as making a means of suicide (e.g., pills or a weapon) available to a client with knowledge of the client's intention to commit suicide (Price and Murphy, 1995). The ANA believes that the nurse should not participate in assisted suicide. The ANA also differentiates active euthanasia from assisted suicide. In assisted suicide someone makes the means of death available but does not act as the direct agent of death (ANA, 1994).

Nurses are legally obligated to treat a deceased person's remains with dignity and care. Wrong handling could cause emotional harm to survivors. In one case, for example, survivors sued when a mislabeling of bodies led to an Orthodox Jewish person being prepared for a Roman Catholic funeral and a Roman Catholic person being prepared for an Orthodox Jewish burial (Schiller, 1977).

Organ and Tissue Donation

Consent must be obtained before a client's body, tissues, or organs can be donated for medical use. In some states the client can sign the back of his or her driver's license in the presence of witnesses indicating consent to having his or her body donated. Consent is valid unless the license is revoked, canceled, or suspended, and consent has to be given each time the license is renewed. State laws provide whether a nurse may witness the consent of an individual donating his or her body, organs, or tissues for medical use. Nurses should be aware of the policies and procedures of the employing institution and the state laws when they are asked to serve as a witness for a person who is giving consent for organ donation.

In most states there is a law requiring that at the time of death a qualified health care provider must ask the client's family members to consider organ or tissue donation (National Organ Transplant Act, Public Law 98-507, 1984). These laws came about because of the shortage of organs for transplantation. The physician who certifies death shall not be involved in removal or transplant of organs. The National Organ Transplant Act prohibits selling or purchasing of organs and regulates this area of medical and nursing practice. Organ and tissue donation remains voluntary. Consent forms are available for this purpose.

Advance Directives

The nurse will find that many clients have **living wills** or powers of attorney identifying health care surrogates

(Weiler, 1995). The Patient Self-Determination Act (42 CFR 417, 1992) requires health care institutions to inquire whether an advance directive such as a living will has been created. The nurse should be familiar with the institution's policies and procedures that comply with the Act because the nurse may be asked to provide information about these documents or inform clients about how they can obtain legal assistance.

Living wills are documents instructing physicians to withhold or withdraw life-sustaining procedures in clients whose death is imminent. Health care surrogates are individuals named by the client to make health care decisions for the client if and when the client becomes incapacitated. Each state providing for living wills has its own requirements for executing them, but generally two witnesses, neither of whom can be a relative or the physician, are needed when the client signs the documents. Health care surrogate statutes are sometimes referred to as *durable powers of attorney*. These documents must be legally prepared with the appropriate witnessing of the client's signature.

Contracts and Employment Agreements

A contract is an agreement between two or more persons that creates an obligation to do something (Black, 1990). The agreement can be in writing or oral. An oral contract is as legally binding as a written one, but it may be more difficult to prove. A breach of contract occurs if either party fails to carry out agreed obligations. Even though nurses usually do not have a written contract, the employee handbook manuals that describe the nurse's responsibilities may be interpreted as the written form of agreement between the employing institution and the nurse.

By accepting a job, a nurse enters into an agreement with an employer. The nurse will perform professional duties competently, adhering to the policies and procedures of the institution. In return the employer not only pays for services but also furnishes the facilities and equipment in proper working order to enable the nurse to provide efficient and competent care. Nurses should become aware of the state law related to firing for cause or no cause dismissal in the state in which they work.

Employment discrimination. Employers may be subject to legal consequences depending on their employee practices. Title VII, a federal statute, prohibits employment discrimination on the basis of race, color, creed, gender, or national origin (Title VII, 1964). This law prevents the employer from firing, hiring, or promoting an individual on the basis of those "protected classes." Subtle discrimination is also prohibited by Title VII. Lack of promotions or objective assignments for minorities may be suspect (Blouin and Brent, 1995). If

an employee is discriminated against, the employee should file a claim with the Equal Employment Opportunity Commission (EEOC). The EEOC then investigates the charge of discrimination. Based on the EEOC's findings, the employee may be able to file suit against the employer.

⋯MINIMIZING LIABILITY

Short Staffing

During nursing shortages, staff downsizing periods, and cost containment, the issue of inadequate staffing may arise. The JCAHO requires institutions to have guidelines for the number of staff needed to care for clients. These are referred to as *staffing ratios*. Legal problems may arise if there are not enough professional nurses to provide competent care. Liability issues occur if the client is injured as a result of negligent care by any personnel (Blouin and Brent, 1995). The registered nurse (RN) is always responsible for performing the nursing process. Even though the nurse may delegate care to assistive personnel, the RN may be responsible for client outcome (Barter and Furmidge, 1994).

If a nurse is assigned to care for more clients than is reasonable for safe care, nurses should notify the nursing supervisor. If nurses are required to accept the assignments, they should document this information in writing and provide the document to nursing administrators. Although documentation does not relieve nurses of responsibility if clients suffer harm because of inattention, it shows that the nurse attempted to act appropriately. Whenever a nurse documents information about short staffing, a copy of the document should be kept by the nurse. Nurses should not walk out when staffing is inadequate because a charge of abandonment could be made. It is important to know the institution's policies and procedures on how to handle inadequate staffing before such a situation arises. The institution is ultimately responsible for staffing the hospital so that safe care can be provided (Fiesta, 1994).

Floating

Nurses are sometimes required to "float" from the area in which they normally practice to other nursing units. Nurses who float should inform the supervisor of any lack of experience in caring for the types of clients on the new nursing unit. They should also request and be given orientation to the unit. Nurses floated to a unit are held to the same standard of care as nurses who regularly work in that area. A supervisor can be held liable if a staff nurse is assigned a client that he or she cannot safely care for. In one case the court noted that if employers are going to float nurses out of their usual work area of practice, then the employers should provide training and education to prepare the nurses to work in the other areas (Winkelman, 1992).

CONFIDENTIAL INCIDENT REPORT

NOT PART OF MEDICAL RECORD—DO NOT COPY OR RELEASE. This report is prepared in anticipation of litigation for the purpose of securing legal advice on potential claims and to facilitate the prompt intervention and management of such claims by the hospital's attorneys and risk manager. This report and the information contained herein is priviliged.

Dept. #	Incident Date	Incident Time _____ a.m. _____ p.m.	Person Involved ____ Patient ____ Visitor
Sex ___ Male ___ Female	**Age**	**Condition Prior to Incident** ___ Alert & Oriented ___ Other: _____	

\# _____
Use addressograph plate or list full name, address and date of birth.

BRIEF DESCRIPTION OF INCIDENT & LOCATION: _____
_____
_____
_____
_____

MEDICATION ☐

____ Dosage
____ Route
____ Omission
____ Duplication
____ Transcription
____ IV Rate
____ IV Infiltration
____ Patient Identification
____ Adverse Reaction to
    Medication/Contrast Media
____ Different Medication/IV Fluid
____ Time Administered
____ Discontinued/Unordered
____ Missing/Stolen
____ Protocol Not Followed
____ Equipment Failure/Malfunction
____ Other _____

Medication(s) Involved:
_____
_____
_____

FALL ☐

____ From Bed With Rails Up Full
____ From Bed With Rails Down x _____
____ From Bedside Commode
____ From Chair/Equipment
____ Going To/From Bathroom
____ While Walking or Standing
____ On Stairs/Ramp
____ Assisted/Lowered to Floor
____ Fainting/Dizziness
____ Slip/Twist (Other than fall)
____ Unknown

Fall Risk Assessment _____

Describe Footwear: _____
_____

Describe Surface: _____
_____

Other: _____
_____

	YES	NO
Out of Bed Privileges	____	____
Up With Assistance	____	____
Call Light Within Reach	____	____
Call Light Used	____	____
Bed Alarm On	____	____
Sitter on Duty	____	____
Family Notified of Fall	____	____
Protective Device Used	____	____

(Check Type)
    ____ Posey ____ Wrist
    ____ Other_____

On Medication	____	____

(Check Types)
    ____ Hypnotics
    ____ Narcotics, I, II
    ____ Diuretic
    ____ Antihypertensive
    ____ Psycotropic
    ____ Antianxiety
    ____ Antidepressant

OTHER ☐

NATURE OF INJURY
____ No Apparent Injury ____ Puncture ____ Abrasion ____ Property ____ Other *(describe)*
____ Redness/Edema ____ Contusion/Hematoma ____ Laceration/Skin Tear ____ Burn   Damaged/ _____
____ Numbness ____ Sprain/Strain/Soreness ____ Fracture/Dislocation ____ Hives   Lost _____

ASSESSMENT OF CONDITION   V.S.: B/P_____ T_____ P_____ R_____
Other _____
_____

Physician Notified: ____ Yes _____ *(Time/Date)* ____ No   Orders Received: ____ Yes ____ No ____ N/A
To Emergency Department: ____ Yes ____ No ____ Care Refused   **Assessment**
X-Ray Taken: ____ Yes ____ No   Results: _____   **Performed By:** _____

WITNESSES
(List Names & Addresses,
Unknown or None)   _____   _____
  _____   _____

EQUIPMENT INVOLVED   ____ YES ____ NO   If **Yes**, list: Type: _____   Manufacturer: _____
Serial No.: _____   Hospital ID No.: _____   Present Location: _____

Report Prepared By *(Name and Title):* _____   **Report Date:** _____

FORM-01

Figure 12-2. ▪ Confidential Incident Report.

Incident Reports

An **incident report** is prepared by a nurse when anything unusual happens that could potentially cause harm to a client, or when the nurse makes an error. For example, an incident report should be prepared whenever the nurse administers an incorrect medication or when a client suffers a fall in the hospital. Most institutions provide specific forms for this purpose (Figure 12-2). The nurse should objectively record the details of the incident and any statements made by the client. An example of the nurse's documentation is as follows: "Mrs. Jones found lying on floor on right side. Abrasion on right forehead. Client stated, 'I fell and hit my head.'" The nurse should contact the physician to examine the client. After examining the client, the physician should document the incident and report any untoward effects caused by the incident. Subjective assumptions and statements assigning blame should not be included on the incident report.

Incident reports are not a part of the client's medical record. The reports are generally not admissible in a court of law and in some jurisdictions are considered privileged. The nurse should know an institution's policies and procedures. Incident reports should also be prepared if there is any injury to an employee or a visitor.

Incident reports are used by employing institutions for quality improvement and risk management. By reviewing incident reports, administrators can determine areas of client risk (Figure 12-3). For example, if a certain kind of problem has occurred repeatedly, such as pressure ulcers, educational methods can be used to help prevent the problem in the future. In addition, the insurance carrier for a hospital or other institution relies on incident reports to assess liability and possible future claims. Incident reports supplement quality improvement programs to ensure provision of high-quality care.

Risk Management

Risk management is a system of ensuring appropriate nursing care. All nurses should be risk managers. The steps involved in risk management include identifying possible risks, analyzing them, acting to reduce the risks, and evaluating the steps taken. One tool used in risk management is the incident report.

For nurses in practice, the underlying rationale for quality improvement and risk management programs is the highest possible quality of care. Some insurance companies, medical and nursing organizations, and the JCAHO require the use of quality improvement and risk management procedures (JCAHO, 1995).

Risk management also requires good documentation. The nurse's documentation can be the nurse's memory of what actually was done for a client and can serve as proof that the nurse acted reasonably and safely. Documentation should be thorough, accurate, and performed in a timely manner (see Chapter 14). To protect the nurse and the client, the nurse should document the care given and the details associated with it (Eggland, 1995). Charting "physician notified" may be insufficient if at the time the nurse is being questioned about the lawsuit, he or she does not recall what facts were told to the physician. When a lawsuit is filed, very often the nurse's notes are the first thing reviewed by an attorney. The nurse's assessments and the reporting of significant changes in the assessments are very important factors in defending a lawsuit.

Reporting Obligations

Nurses are required to report to the appropriate authorities situations such as child, spousal, or older adult abuse; rape; gunshot wounds; attempted suicide; or certain communicable diseases. For example, if a nurse examines a sexually abused child in the emergency department, it is the nurse's responsibility to report that information to the Division of Family Services. The nurse may also be required to report unsafe or impaired professionals. Because information that must be reported varies among states, the nurse should become familiar with the appropriate statutes.

···LEGAL ISSUES IN NURSING PRACTICE

The nurse must be aware of changes in the laws that affect nursing practice and the delivery of the client's care. Certain areas of the law such as the administration of narcotics have remained constant, whereas the issues of abortion and human immunodeficiency virus (HIV) are changing and will change in the future.

Controlled Substances

In 1970 the Comprehensive Drug Abuse Prevention and Control Act was passed in the United States. It controls substances such as narcotics, depressants, stimulants, and hallucinogens. The Act regulates hospital distribution systems. Nurses may administer controlled substances only under the direction of a licensed

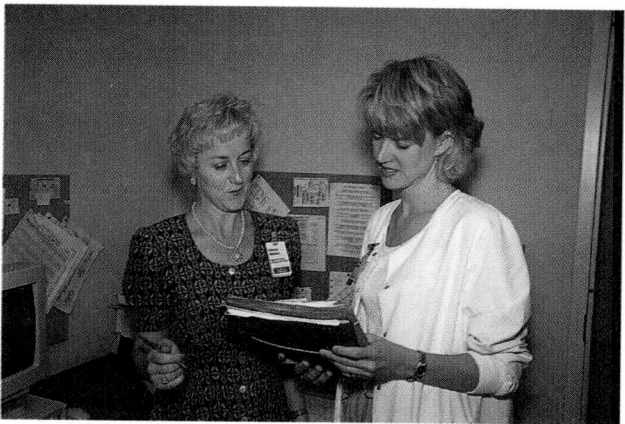

Figure 12-3. Nurses discussing an incident report.

physician. (Some states allow advance practice nurses to prescribe controlled substances.)

Controlled substances should be kept securely locked, and only authorized personnel should have access to them (see Chapter 26). Precise records must be maintained regarding the dispensing and storage of controlled substances. Criminal penalties for misuse of controlled substances exist. There have been cases in which physicians have illegally prescribed and dispensed controlled substances, and if nurses employed by such physicians fail to report these activities, they may be legally accountable for aiding and abetting the physicians.

Acquired Immunodeficiency Syndrome

Acquired immunodeficiency syndrome (AIDS) is found in clients in virtually every segment of nursing practice, from clients with AIDS on medical-surgical units, to mothers and infants in perinatal units, to pediatric clients with hemophilia. The nurse utilizes Standard Precautions when caring for all clients (see Chapter 25). The nurse has the responsibility to safeguard himself or herself and others from exposure to infectious material. Therefore items or areas contaminated with body fluids must be appropriately handled, discarded, and/or decontaminated.

The ADA discusses the rights of disabled people and is the most extensive law on how employers must treat HIV-infected clients and health care workers (ADA, 1995). Persons with infectious diseases are protected under the handicapped and disabilities laws. Co-workers who refuse to work with HIV-infected people can leave companies open to indirect charges of discrimination if the employer does not monitor the work environment.

Issues of disclosure, privacy, and confidentiality are an important concern when working with HIV- or AIDS-infected clients or peers. Several cases have held that the health care provider may be obligated to disclose the fact that he or she is infected with HIV. The ADA regulations protect the privacy of infected people by giving individuals the opportunity to decide whether to disclose their disability.

Health care workers are not required to be tested for HIV as a condition of employment. If a health care worker is contaminated by a client whose HIV status is unknown, the health care worker cannot check the client's blood for HIV without the client's consent. The statute provides that the client must be provided "consultation" before being tested for HIV and during the reporting of the test result.

Abortion Issues

In 1973 in the case of *Roe v. Wade*, the U.S. Supreme Court ruled that there is a fundamental right to privacy, which includes a woman's decision to have an abortion. The court ruled that during the first trimester a woman could end her pregnancy without state regulation because the risk of natural mortality from abortion is less than with normal childbirth. During the second trimester the state has an interest in protecting maternal health and the state may enforce regulations regarding the person performing the abortion and the abortion facility. By the third trimester, when the fetus becomes viable, the state's interest is to protect the fetus, so the state can therefore prohibit abortion except when necessary to save the mother.

In 1989 in the case of *Webster v. Reproductive Health Services*, the court substantially narrowed the *Roe v. Wade* case. States may require viability tests before conducting abortions if the fetus is thought to be over 28 weeks' gestational age. States may also require a minor's parental consent or a judicial decision that the minor is mature and can self-consent.

In the case of *Planned Parenthood of Southeastern Pennsylvania v. Casey*, informed consent was upheld in that the physician must present the woman with a description of the nature of the abortion procedure, the health risk related to abortion and childbirth, the probable gestational age of the fetus, and the availability of state-published material about medical assistance, adoption agencies, and child support from the father. The court also upheld a mandatory 24-hour waiting period between when the materials are provided to the client and when the abortion is performed. An emancipated minor must get informed consent of one parent or a judicial determination that the minor is mature and can give her own informed consent.

···LEGAL ISSUES IN NURSING SPECIALTIES

Within every specialty of nursing there are legal issues that affect nursing practice. Some of the more common legal issues follow.

Nursing of Children

Every state with child abuse legislation requires that suspected child abuse or neglect be reported. Health care professionals such as nurses are mandated to report suspected cases. To encourage reports of suspected cases, states provide legal immunity for the reporter if the report is made in good faith. Health care professionals who do not report suspected child abuse or neglect may be held liable for civil or criminal legal action.

As in all areas of nursing practice, negligence involving pediatric clients is possible, and the nurse is responsible for preventing a child in his or her care from accidentally coming to harm. Cribs, which sometimes have a restraining device over the top, are designed to keep infants and toddlers from climbing out of bed and injuring themselves. All poisonous substances and sharp objects should be kept out of the reach of small children. When possible, small children should be kept under constant watch to minimize opportunities for accidental harm.

Medical-Surgical Nursing

Many hospitals and long-term care facilities are considered to be "restraint free." Adults who are disoriented or confused, however, may require some form of restraining device to prevent accidental self-injury. Standards of care, laws, and regulations concerning the use of restraints and supervision required apply to nursing practice with medical-surgical and other clients. In the general hospital and long-term care settings, the most frequent indications for restraints are as follows: (1) risk of injury to self (falls) or others, (2) interference with treatment, and (3) disruptive or disturbing behavior (Ortiz-Pruitt, 1995). The FDA has set forth guidelines for the use of restraints (FDA, 1992). Side rails and bed alarms are available on most hospital beds for use with adult clients. The nurse must know when and how to use restraints correctly. A physician's order including the purpose for the restraint is required to physically restrain a client. Orders for a restraint are limited to 24 hours. After a client is restrained, the nurse is required to make frequent client assessments and to periodically release restraints (see Chapter 28). A client who falls out of bed and becomes injured or who suffers injury from improper restraint application may bring a lawsuit against the nurses and the institution.

Critical Care Nursing

Critical care nurses require special training and ongoing in-service education with regard to advanced client monitoring and management of critical illness. The staffing ratio in an intensive care setting should be one nurse for each client, depending on the severity of the clients' conditions. The JCAHO recommends these ratios because of the intensity of care required by such clients (JCAHO, 1995). These clients usually require careful observation and assessment of their conditions, and treatments, procedures, and medications. If a nurse is assigned to three or four intensive care clients, is unable to give appropriate care, and a client suffers harm, the nurse is liable for accepting the client assignment.

Potential legal problems for critical care nurses are associated with the use of electronic monitoring devices. No monitor is totally reliable, and the nurse must not completely depend on it. Therefore the nurse's continual assessment of a client is necessary to help document the accuracy of electronic monitoring. There may also be electrical hazards to the nurse and the client. The equipment should be checked routinely by biomedical engineers to ensure that it is in proper working order and to make sure that a client will not receive an electrical shock.

Operating Room Nursing

Sponge, needle, and instrument counts are routine standards in the operating room (OR) to prevent lawsuits. Even though the physician inserts sponges and instruments into the surgical wound, the physician relies on the nurse's counts at the end of the procedure. Generally, when the chart records a correct sponge count and the client suffers an injury because of a retained sponge, the hospital is liable because the nurse charted a correct count when it was not correct.

Every piece of equipment must be carefully used to prevent injury to the client. Laser equipment has created the potential for burns and other tissue injuries (Merriman, 1995). There can also be liability for nurses because of incorrect positioning or insufficient padding placed when positioning the client.

Psychiatric Nursing

A client can be admitted to a psychiatric unit involuntarily or on a voluntary basis. A petition for involuntary detention must be filed with the court within 96 hours of the client's initial detention. A hearing must be conducted within 2 days of the filing of the involuntary petition. If the judge determines that the client is a danger to himself or others, the judge will grant the involuntary detention and the client can be detained for 21 more days for psychiatric treatment.

Potentially suicidal clients are admitted to psychiatric units. If the client's history and medical records indicate suicidal tendencies, the client must be kept under supervision. Lawsuits result from clients' attempts at suicide within the hospital. The allegations in the lawsuits are that the health care provider failed to provide adequate supervision and failed to safeguard the facilities. Documentation of precautions against suicide is essential.

Home Health Care Nursing

With the increased focus on managed care, hospital stays are much shorter, and as a result many clients may be discharged from the acute care setting at an earlier time in their disease process and still require nursing care (Fiesta, 1995). Nursing care may range from assistance with daily living activities to ventilator care. The nurse has greater responsibility and autonomy in the home. Home health care, however, differs from the acute care setting because in the hospital setting, hospital personnel and physicians are available to assess client changes. In the home the nurse must know when to call in the supervisor or the physician. Nurses must know the policies and procedures of the employing institution, particularly with respect to chain of command, equipment failure, and informed consent (Sullivan, 1994). Chain of command generally means that the nurse must know the hierarchy of supervisors and physicians to report to if problems arise. Most of all nurses must be sure to document their assessments and interventions so that any claim of inadequate or improper care can be defended.

Key Terms

assault	defendant	invasion of privacy	Nurse Practice Acts
battery	euthanasia	libel	plaintiff
civil law	felony	living wills	regulatory agencies
common law	Good Samaritan laws	malpractice	slander
crime	incident report	malpractice insurance	standard of care
criminal law	informed consent	misdemeanor	statutory law
defamation of character		negligence	tort

■ Key Concepts ■

With the increased emphasis on client rights, a nurse in practice must understand legal obligations and responsibilities to clients.

Under the law the practicing nurse must follow standards of care, which originate in Nurse Practice Acts, the guidelines of professional organizations, and written policies and procedures of employing institutions.

Nurses are responsible for performing procedures correctly and exercising professional judgment when they carry out physician orders.

All clients are entitled to confidential health care and freedom from unauthorized release of information.

A nurse can be found liable for malpractice if the following are established: (1) the nurse (defendant) owed a duty to the client (plaintiff), (2) the nurse did not carry out that duty or breached that duty, (3) the client was injured, and (4) the client's injury was caused by the nurse's failure to carry out that duty.

Informed consent must meet the following criteria: (1) the person giving consent must be competent and of legal age; (2) the consent must be given voluntarily; (3) the person giving consent must thoroughly understand the procedure, its risks and benefits, and alternative procedures; and (4) the person giving consent has a right to have all questions answered satisfactorily.

The nurse is obligated to follow the physician's order unless he or she believes the order is in error, violates hospital policy, or could be detrimental to the client, in which case the nurse must make a formal report explaining the refusal.

The nurse must file an incident report in any unusual situation that could potentially cause harm to a client; such reports are also used for quality assurance and risk management.

A legal definition of death aids in determining when it is appropriate to pursue organ or tissue donation.

The nurse must be aware of changes in the law that affect nursing practice, including the changing areas of AIDS and abortion.

■ Critical Thinking Activities

1. Mrs. Smith is an 80-year-old client with a fractured hip. Dr. Jones writes a pain medication order for Mrs. Smith that reads: "Morphine sulfate 50 mg IM every 6 hours." You transcribe that order and note that 50 mg of morphine is an extremely large dose. In fact, you know that the normal dose of morphine is less than 10 mg. What risk do you face if you follow the doctor's order? What should you do? If you cannot get Dr. Jones on the phone, can you give a smaller dose of morphine?

2. Mrs. Brown is expecting her first baby. She and her husband have arrived at the labor and delivery suite. You have a copy of Mrs. Brown's prenatal record, which indicates that she has had two elective abortions. When you are filling out the history on the labor and delivery record, Mrs. Brown states in the presence of her husband that this is her first and only pregnancy. How should the nurse handle the situation? What is the nurse's legal obligation regarding confidentiality of the

Critical Thinking Activities—cont'd

client's previous elective abortions? What is the nurse's legal responsibility for sharing the client's pregnancy information with her husband?

3. Mr. Adams is hospitalized for congestive heart failure. He is occasionally confused and tries to get out of bed without assistance. The physician orders side rails up at all times and to restrain the client if necessary. While you are bathing Mr. Adams you remove the restraint and put the side rails down. When you run out of the room for a second

to get another washcloth, Mr. Adams falls out of bed and fractures his hip. Identify the elements of negligence and use this scenario to apply those elements.

4. Miss Smith, a 16-year-old, brings her newborn baby to the hospital emergency department with a high fever. The physician wants to perform a lumbar puncture on the baby and advises Miss Smith of the risks involved. Since Miss Smith is a minor, who can sign the consent form for the baby?

References

American Nurses Association: Position statement on assisted suicide, Unpublished, 1994.

Autonberry D: Risk management and non-employed nurses, *Nurs Manage* 26(9):70, 1995.

Barter M, Furmidge M: Unlicensed assistive personnel, *JONA* 14(4):36, 1994.

Black HC: *Black's law dictionary,* ed 6, St. Paul, Minn, 1990, West Publishing.

Blouin A, Brent N: Unlicensed assistive personnel: legal considerations, *JONA* 25(11):7, 1995.

Carroll M: Nursing malpractice and corporate negligence, *J Nurs Law* 3(3):53, 1996.

Coker L, Johns A: Guardianship for elders: process and issues, *J Gerontol Nurs* 20(12):25, 1994.

Daly B: Withholding nutrition and hydration revisited, *Nurs Manage* 26(5):30, 1995.

Eggland E: Charting tips: avoiding incomplete charting, *Nurs 95* p 73, October 1995.

Fiesta J: Staffing implications: a legal update, *Nurs Manage* 25(6):34, 1994.

Fiesta J: Home care liability, part 1, *Nurs Manage* 26(11):24, 1995.

Joint Commission on Accreditation of Healthcare Organizations: *Accreditation manual for hospitals,* Chicago, 1995, The Commission.

Ladebauche P: Limiting liability to avoid malpractice litigation, *MCN Am J Matern Child Nurs* 20:243, 1995.

Merriman J: How have changes in health care affected perioperative nurses' liability, *AORN J* 61(1):258, 1995.

Missouri Approved Instructions, section 11.02, 1991a.

Missouri Approved Instructions, section 11.06, 1991b.

Ortiz-Pruitt J: Physical restraint of critically ill patients: a human issue, *Crit Care Nurs Clin North Am* 7(2):363, 1995.

Price D, Murphy P: Assisted suicide: new ANA policy reflects difficulty of issue, *J Nurs Law* 2(2):53, 1995.

Prosser W, Keeton W: *Prosser and Keeton on the law of torts,* ed 5, St. Paul, Minn, 1988, West Publishing.

Rutherford M: Legally speaking: small patients, big legal risks, *RN* 57:51, September 1994.

Squadroni T: Following hospital policy: a legal risk? *Nurs 94* 24:26, May 1994.

Sullivan G: Legally speaking: home care: more autonomy, more legal risks, *RN* 57:63, May 1994.

U.S. Food and Drug Administration, Department of Health and Human Services: *FDA safety alert,* Rockville, Md, 1992, The Department.

Weiler K: Ethical dilemmas that evolve into legal issues, *J Gerontolog Nurs* 21(5):47, 1995.

Statutes and cases

Americans with Disabilities Act, 42 USC section 12101 et seq, 1995.

National Organ Transplant Act, Public Law 98-507, October 19, 1984.

Patient Self Determination Act, 42 CFR 417, 1992.

Title VII of the Civil Rights Act of 1964, 42 USC 2000e-2 et seq.

National Organ Transplant Act, Public Law 98-507, 1984.

Barber v Time Magazine, 159 SW2d 291 (1942).

Darling v Charleston Community Memorial Hospital, 33 Ill 2d 326 (1966), 200 NE 2d 149, 211 NE 2d 253.

Planned Parenthood of Southeast Pennsylvania v Casey, 505 U.S. 883 (1992).

Roe v Wade, 410 U.S.113 (1973).

In Re: Schiller, 148 NJ Super 168 (1977).

Webster v Reproductive Health Services, 492 U.S. 490 (1989).

Winkelman v Beloit Memorial Hospital, 484 NW 2d 211 (Wi 1992).

YG v Jewish Hospital, 795 SW2d 488 (Mo App 1990).

13

Communication

OBJECTIVES

Mastery of content in this chapter will enable the student to:

- Define key terms related to communication.
- Describe aspects of critical thinking that are important to the communication process.
- Identify challenging situations that require careful communication decision making.
- Describe the elements of the communication process.
- Describe the three levels of communication and their uses in nursing.
- Differentiate aspects of verbal and nonverbal communication.
- Identify features and expected outcomes of the nurse-client helping relationship.
- List nursing focus areas within each phase of a therapeutic nurse-client helping relationship.
- Describe behaviors and techniques that affect communication.
- Explain the focus of communication within each phase of the nursing process.
- Discuss effective communication for clients of varying developmental levels.
- Identify client health states or responses that contribute to impaired communication.
- Explain techniques used to assist clients with special communication needs.

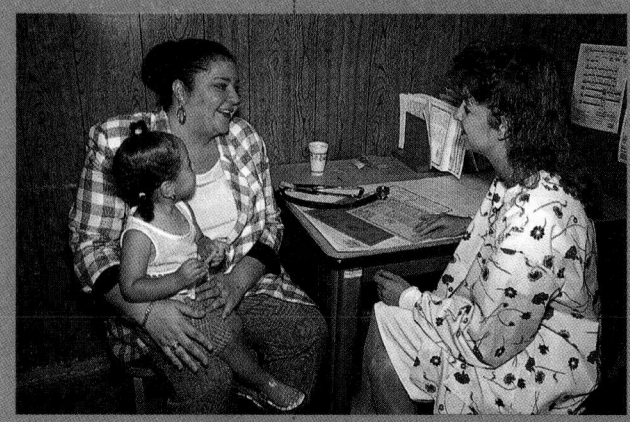

Communication is the process of transmitting messages and interpreting meaning (Wilson and others, 1995). It is basic to all human interaction and permeates all of nursing practice. As an important nursing skill, communication competency is acquired through study and application. Nurses exchange information and establish and maintain interpersonal relationships with many persons in the course of their work, including clients and their loved ones, nurse colleagues, physicians, case managers, assistive personnel, health team members, nursing students, nursing faculty, and members of the public. Principles and techniques of effective communication facilitate relationships within the entire sphere of the nurse's interactions and help the nurse meet legal, ethical, and clinical standards of practice.

At the core of nursing are the caring relationships formed between the nurse and those affected by the nurse's practice. Watson (1985) has identified the "carative factors" that manifest this human-to-human caring as instilling faith and hope, cultivating sensitivity to self and to others, developing a helping-trust relationship, promoting and accepting the expression of positive and negative feelings, using scientific problem solving for decision making, promoting interpersonal teaching-learning, providing a supportive environment, assisting with gratification of human needs, and allowing for spiritual forces and phenomena. These aspects of caring within interpersonal relationships are intimately connected to the nurse's ability to communicate effectively.

Nurses use nonverbal, verbal, and technological skills to communicate in both personal and impersonal situations. Nurses send and receive information through many different channels, including in person, in writing, over the telephone, through fax and electronic mail, and through the Internet. Communication in all these modes is an ongoing, dynamic, and often complex process.

CRITICAL THINKING AND COMMUNICATION

Critical thinking skills enhance the communication process. The nurse must be able to *interpret* messages received from others, *analyze* their content, *make inferences* about their meaning, *evaluate* their effect, *explain* the rationale for communication techniques used, and *self-examine* personal communication skills (Creasia and Parker, 1996). Other aspects of critical thinking identified in the American Philosophical Association's Delphi Report (1990) also facilitate effective communication. Being *inquisitive* is important, because the desire to know more about a person or understand a situation motivates the nurse to communicate. Being *systematic* is necessary, because good communicators tend to seek and provide information in an organized, focused, and

diligent way. Being *analytical* helps the nurse examine communication for congruency between verbal and nonverbal behavior, identify recurrent themes, and examine the impact of the communication on its expected outcomes. Being a *truth seeker* is essential to understand or to clarify the true meaning of what is being communicated. Being *open minded* helps the nurse enter into a situation without preconceived ideas about the nature of the communication. Being *self-confident* is crucial, because the nurse who conveys confidence and comfort while communicating can more readily establish interpersonal helping-trust relationships and convey competence in the professional role. Being *mature* is important, because the helping relationship requires the ability to first meet the needs of the other person.

It is challenging to understand human communication within interpersonal relationships. Each person's perceptions of others are influenced by a multitude of factors, including one's own cultural conditioning, educational background, and personal experience (Knapp and Vangelisti, 1996). Critical thinking can help the nurse overcome **perceptual biases**, which are human tendencies that interfere with accurately perceiving and interpreting messages from others. People naturally tend to assume that others are like themselves and that everyone else would think, feel, act, react, and behave as they would in similar circumstances. People tend to see what they expect to see, to form unshakable first impressions, and to notice negative characteristics more readily than positive characteristics (Griffin, 1994). By thinking critically about their own communication patterns, nurses learn to control these tendencies and become more effective in their interpersonal relationships.

THE POWER OF COMMUNICATION

Like any therapeutic agent, the nurse's communication can result in both harm and good. Every nuance of posture, every small expression and gesture, every word chosen, and every phrase uttered can hurt or heal and affect others through the messages they send. Even techniques intended to be therapeutic can have unexpected negative effects, and nontherapeutic techniques can at times bring comfort and achieve goals. Failure to communicate leads to serious problems, increases liability, and threatens professional credibility. Inappropriate or missing communication frequently causes many "glitches" in the health care system with added cost to the client and agency. Communication must be respected for its potential power and not misused to manipulate, bully, or coerce others. At its best, good communication empowers others and enables people to know themselves and to make their own choices (Beebe and others, 1996).

DECISION MAKING AND COMMUNICATION

The nature of the communication process requires that nurses constantly make decisions about what, when, where, why, and how to convey messages to others. Benner (1984) has stated that the nurse's decision making always takes place within a specific context, so each situation will have individual features that influence the nature of the decisions made. Effective communication techniques can be easily learned, but their application is more difficult. Deciding which techniques best fit each unique nursing scenario is challenging. Throughout this chapter, examples are provided to guide the learner in the use of a variety of effective communication techniques. Situations that challenge the nurse's decision-making skills and call for careful use of therapeutic techniques often involve persons such as those described in Box 13-1. Because the best way to acquire

skill is through guided practice, it is useful for students to discuss and role play these scenarios before encountering them in the clinical setting. Consider that clients, family, nurse colleagues, assistive personnel, physicians, or other health team members might be involved, and decide which communication techniques might be most effective in each situation.

BASIC ELEMENTS OF THE COMMUNICATION PROCESS

The basic elements of the communication process are shown in Figure 13-1. Although this model oversimplifies a very complex process, it helps the nurse identify its essential components. In everyday conversation, people rarely analyze the meaning of every gesture or word. When communicating in the professional role, the nurse must be aware of each aspect so that interactions can be purposeful and effective.

The **referent** motivates one person to communicate with another. In a health care environment, sights, sounds, odors, time schedules, messages, objects, emotions, sensations, perceptions, ideas, and other cues initiate communication between the nurse and others. Considering the referent during an interaction helps the sender develop and organize the message.

The **sender** is the person who delivers the message. The roles of sender and receiver change back and forth as two persons interact.

The **message** is the verbal and nonverbal information expressed by the sender. The most effective message is clear, organized, and expressed in a manner familiar to the receiver.

Box 13-1
Challenging Communication Situations

The *silent, withdrawn* person who does not express any feelings or needs

The *sad, depressed* person who has slow mental and motor responses

The *angry, hostile* person who does not listen to explanations

The *sullen, uncooperative* person who resents being asked to do something

The *talkative, lonely* person who wants someone with him or her all the time

The *demanding* person who wants someone to wait on him or her or meet his or her requests

The *ranting and raving* person who blames nursing staff unfairly

The *sensory impaired* person who cannot hear or see well

The *verbally impaired* person who cannot articulate words

The *gossiping, catty* person who violates confidentiality and stirs up trouble

The *bitter, complaining* person who is negative about everything

The *mentally handicapped* person who is frightened and distrustful

The *confused, disoriented* person who is bewildered and uncooperative

The *anxious, nervous* person who cannot cope with what is happening

The *grieving, crying* person who has had a major loss

The *unresponsive, comatose* person who cannot communicate at all

---

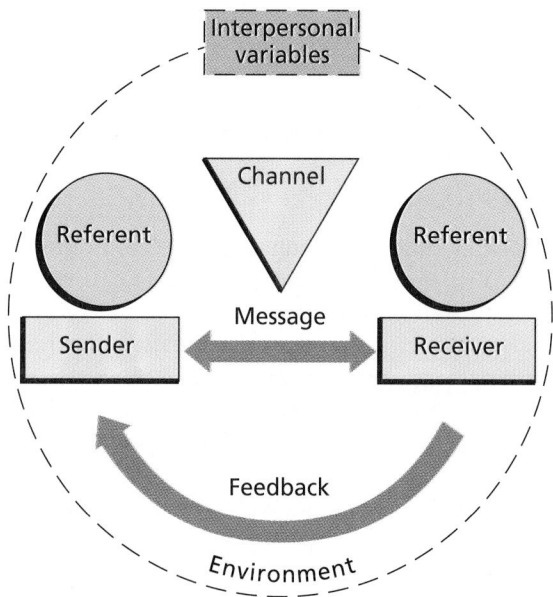

Figure 13-1. Communication as active process between sender and receiver.

The **channel** is the means of conveying and receiving the message through visual, auditory, and tactile senses. The sender's facial expression conveys a visual message, spoken words travel through auditory channels, and placing a hand on another person uses the channel of touch. Usually, the more channels the sender uses to convey a message, the more clearly it will be received.

The **receiver** is the person to whom the message is sent. The message then acts as one of the receiver's referents, prompting a response. The more the sender and receiver have in common and the closer the relationship, the more likely the receiver will accurately perceive the sender's meaning and respond appropriately.

The **environment** is the physical and emotional atmosphere in which the interaction takes place. For effective communication, the environment should be comfortable and suited to participants' needs. The more positive an environment the sender and receiver can create, the more successful the exchange.

The **feedback** is the message returned to the original sender by the receiver. Feedback indicates whether the meaning of the sender's message was understood. The nurse's intent to communicate is not enough to ensure accurate reception of a message. The nurse must seek verbal and nonverbal feedback from the receiver to be sure the message has been understood.

Levels of Communication

There are three levels of communication, each with important uses in nursing. **Intrapersonal communication** is a powerful form of communication that occurs within an individual. Intrapersonal communication is also called *self-talk, self-verbalization, self-instruction, inner thought,* and *inner dialogue* (Balzer-Riley, 1996). People "talk to themselves" by forming thoughts internally, and these thoughts strongly influence perceptions, feelings, behavior, and self-concept. Nurses should be aware of the nature and content of their thinking and try to replace negative, self-defeating thoughts with positive assertions. Positive self-talk can be used as a tool to improve one's health and self-esteem. In forms such as imagery or meditation, it can be used to enhance coping and reduce stress. Self-instruction can provide a mental rehearsal for difficult tasks or situations so individuals can deal with them more effectively. During interactions, participants engage in both intrapersonal and interpersonal or public communication.

Interpersonal communication is interaction that occurs between two people or within a small group. It refers to nonverbal and verbal behavior within a social context and includes all symbols and cues used to give and receive meaning. Because messages received may be different from messages intended, meaning must be validated, or mutually negotiated, between participants. Interpersonal communication is thus an act of sharing. Desired outcomes of effective interpersonal communication include idea sharing, problem solving, expression of feelings, decision making, goal accomplishment, team building, and personal growth.

Public communication is the interaction of one individual with large groups of people. Nurses often have opportunities to speak with groups of clients or consumers about health-related topics. Public communication requires special adaptations in eye contact, posture, gestures, voice inflection, and use of media materials to communicate messages effectively. Desired outcomes of public communication include increasing the public's knowledge about health-related topics, health issues, and other issues important to the nursing profession.

FORMS OF COMMUNICATION

Messages are conveyed verbally and nonverbally, concretely, and symbolically. People express themselves through language, movements, gestures, voice inflection, facial expressions, and use of space. Many forms of communication merge to create meaning in the sender's message.

Verbal Communication

Verbal communication involves the spoken or written word. Verbal **language** is a code that conveys specific meaning as words are combined. The most important aspects of verbal communication are discussed in the following sections.

Vocabulary. Communication is unsuccessful if the receiver cannot translate the sender's words and phrases. Nurses work with persons of various cultures who speak many different languages. Those who speak the nurse's language may use subcultural variations of certain words (e.g., the word *dinner* may mean a midday meal to one person and the last meal of the day to another). Medical jargon may sound like a foreign language to clients unfamiliar with the health care setting. A child's vocabulary is much more limited than an adult's, and children may use special words to describe bodily functions or a favorite blanket or toy. Adolescents often use words in unique ways that are unfamiliar to adults.

Denotative and connotative meaning. A single word can have several meanings. The **denotative meaning** is shared by individuals who use a common language. The word *baseball* has the same meaning for all individuals who speak English, but the word *code* denotes cardiac arrest primarily to health care providers. The **connotative meaning** is the shade or interpretation of a word's meaning influenced by the thoughts, feelings, or ideas people have about the word. Families who are told a loved one is in serious condition may believe that death is near, but to nurses the term *serious* may simply describe the nature of the illness. Nurses should carefully select words that cannot be easily misinterpreted, especially when explaining a client's medical condition or therapy.

Pacing. Verbal communication is more successful when expressed at an appropriate speed or pace. Talking rapidly, using awkward pauses, or speaking slowly and deliberately can convey an unintended message. Consider the following exchange:

Client: "Do you know if the doctor found anything wrong?"

Nurse: "No . . . but I'm sure if he did . . . he would have come to explain things to you. (then very rapidly) Now let's get back to where we were."

The long pauses and rapid shift to another subject may give the impression that the nurse is hiding the truth. The nurse should speak slowly enough to enunciate clearly, and pauses should be used to accentuate or stress a particular point, giving the listener time to digest and comprehend the meaning of the speaker's words. Pacing is improved by thinking before speaking.

Intonation. Tone of voice dramatically affects a message's meaning, and emotions directly influence tone of voice. Depending on the intonation, even a simple question or statement can express enthusiasm, anger, or concern. Nurses must be aware of their intonation to avoid sending unintended messages. If the client interprets a nurse's message as uncaring or condescending, further communication may be inhibited. A client's intonation often provides information about his or her emotional state or energy level.

Clarity and brevity. Effective communication is simple, short, and to the point. Fewer words result in less confusion. Phrases such as "you know" or "OK?" at the end of every sentence detract from a message's clarity. Giving examples also helps clarify messages for the receiver. Brevity is achieved by using short sentences and words that express an idea simply and directly.

Timing and relevance. Timing is critical in communication. Even though a message is clear, poor timing can prevent it from being effective. For example, the nurse should not begin routine teaching when a client is in severe pain or emotional distress. Often the best time for interaction is when a client expresses an interest in communicating. Messages are also more effective if they are relevant. When a client is facing emergency surgery, discussing the risks of smoking is less relevant than explaining perioperative procedures.

Nonverbal Communication
Nonverbal communication includes messages sent through the language of the body, without using words.

Nonverbal forms of communication include facial expressions; vocal cues; eye contact; gestures; posture; touch; odor; physical appearance; dress; silence; and the use of space, time, and objects (Yerby and others, 1995). Nonverbal communication often accurately reveals true feelings, because one has less control over nonverbal reactions. A client who says he feels fine but grimaces with each movement and holds his body rigidly is probably in pain. Nonverbal cues add meaning to verbal communication and help the nurse judge the reliability of verbal messages.

Perceiving and interpreting nonverbal cues require concentration and sensitivity to others. Because nonverbal messages are usually more subtle than verbal messages, becoming an astute observer of nonverbal behavior takes practice. Nurses must try to be sure their nonverbal and verbal messages match. Conflict arising from a mismatch can threaten the nurse-client relationship. The nurse who says a client is getting better but wears an expression of doubt will not relieve the client's anxiety.

Metacommunication is the deeper "message within a message." It conveys the sender's attitude toward himself or herself and the message, as well as his or her attitudes, feelings, and intentions toward the receiver. Metacommunication can be an explicit statement or an implicit, nonverbal demonstration of feelings. For example, the client who has had facial reconstructive surgery tells the nurse, "This scar doesn't look as bad as I thought it would," but is teary eyed and appears apprehensive. Based on this metacommunication, the nurse knows that further exploration of the client's feelings and concerns is indicated.

Personal appearance. A person's appearance is one of the first things noticed during an encounter. Physical characteristics, manner of dress and grooming, and jewelry are indicators of well-being, personality, social status, occupation, religion, culture, and self-concept. First impressions are largely based on appearance, and the nurse's physical appearance influences the client's perception of care. Nurses today wear uniforms, scrubsuits, laboratory coats, business suits, and street clothes as practice roles dictate. Although the traditional white uniform does not reflect the nurse's abilities, it may take longer to establish trust if the nurse differs from the client's preconceived image.

Posture and gait. The way people sit, stand, and move is a form of self-expression. Posture and gait reflect emotions, self-concept, and health status. An erect posture and a quick, purposeful gait communicate a sense of well-being and assuredness. A slumped posture and slow, shuffling gait may indicate depression or fatigue. Leaning forward conveys attention. Leaning backward in a more relaxed manner may show less interest or indicate caution.

Facial expression. The face is the most expressive part of the body, adding overt and subtle cues that impart meaning to messages. The face reveals emotions such as surprise, fear, anger, disgust, happiness, and sadness. The sender's facial expressions often become the basis for important judgments by the receiver, although because of the diversity in facial expressions, meaning may be misunderstood. Facial expressions may reveal, contradict, or suppress true emotions. People are often unaware of the messages their expressions convey. When facial expressions are unclear, verbal feedback should be sought to be sure of the sender's intent. For example, a client who frowns after receiving information may be confused, angry, disapproving, or simply concentrating on a reply. The nurse might say, "I notice you're frowning," and encourage further clarification of the client's response.

Nurses are watched closely by clients. Consider the impact a nurse's facial expression might have on a client who asks, "Am I going to die?" The slightest change in the eyes, lips, or face can reveal the nurse's true feelings. Although it is difficult to control all facial expressions, the nurse should try to avoid showing overt shock, disgust, dismay, or other distressing reactions in the client's presence.

Eye contact. Eye contact signals a readiness to communicate. By maintaining eye contact during conversation, those involved communicate respect for one another and a willingness to listen. Eye contact also allows one to closely observe another. Lack of eye contact may indicate anxiety, defensiveness, discomfort, or lack of confidence in communicating. Some cultures, such as Asian and Indochinese, Native American, and Appalachian, consider eye contact to be intrusive, threatening, or harmful and minimize its use.

Eye movements communicate feelings and emotions. Wide eyes express frankness, terror, and naivete. Downward glances show modesty. Raised upper eyelids reveal displeasure, and a constant stare may be associated with hatred or coldness. Looking down on a person establishes authority, whereas interacting at the same eye level indicates equality in the relationship. The nurse appears less dominant and less threatening when interacting at the client's eye level. Rising to the same eye level of an angry person helps establish the nurse's autonomy.

Gestures. A salute, a thumbs-up, and a tapping foot are types of gestures. Hands and feet emphasize, punctuate, and clarify the spoken word. Gestures alone carry specific meanings, or they may create messages with other communication cues. A finger pointed toward a person may communicate several meanings, but when accompanied by a frown and a stern tone of voice, the gesture becomes a sign of accusation or threat.

Sounds. Sighs, moans, groans, sobs, and other sounds also communicate feelings and thoughts. Combined with other nonverbal communication, sounds help send clear messages. Sounds can be interpreted in several ways; moaning can convey pleasure or suffering, and crying can communicate happiness, sadness, or anger. The nurse must validate such nonverbal messages with the client to interpret them accurately.

Territoriality and space. Territoriality is the need to gain, maintain, and defend one's exclusive right to space. *Territory* can be separated and made visible to others, such as a fence around a yard, a towel on the beach, or a bed in a hospital room. *Personal space* is invisible, individual, and travels with the person. During interpersonal interaction, people consciously maintain varying distances between themselves, depending on the nature of the relationship and situation. When personal space becomes threatened, people respond defensively and communicate less effectively. Examples of nursing actions within the four zones of personal space are listed in Box 13-2.

Nurses must frequently move into clients' territory and personal space because of the nature of care giving. The nurse must convey confidence, gentleness, and respect for privacy, especially when actions require intimate contact. As the distance between them becomes greater, the client and nurse may feel less threatened or constrained. Communication in groups is generally less threatening, because an intimate sharing of thoughts and feelings is less likely.

Symbolic Communication

Good communication requires awareness of verbal and nonverbal symbolism used by others. **Symbolic communication** is the use of an image, object, or action to represent something else and to help convey meaning, which is established by the symbol's association, resemblance, or conventional or personal use. For example, if a Native American client says that managing his or her diabetes is like "going into battle," during diabetic teaching the nurse can use words like *planning strategies*, *defending against*, being *brave and vigilant*, and so forth (Huttlinger and others, 1992). Comfort measures such as plumping and turning pillows, offering cold cloths, and giving sips of clear liquids during nausea may symbolize the parenting received by clients when they were sick as young children and can powerfully convey a nurse's care and concern. Art and music are additional forms of symbolic communication that may be used by the nurse to enhance understanding and promote healing. Dreams, drawings, metaphorical language, and even the symptoms of illness are all symbolic forms of self-expression that have rich messages for health care providers (Seigel, 1989).

Box 13-2
Nursing Actions Within the Zones of Personal Space and Touch

Zones of Personal Space
Intimate Zone (0 to 18 inches)
Holding a crying infant
Performing physical assessment
Bathing, grooming, dressing, feeding, and toileting a client
Changing a client's dressing

Personal Zone (18 inches to 4 feet)
Sitting at a client's bedside
Taking the client's nursing history
Teaching an individual client
Exchanging information at change-of-shift

Social Zone (4 to 12 feet)
Making rounds with a physician
Sitting at the head of a conference table
Teaching a class for clients with diabetes
Conducting a family support group

Public Zone (12 feet and greater)
Speaking at a community forum
Testifying at a legislative hearing
Lecturing to a class of students

Zones of Touch
Social Zone (permission not needed)
Hands
Arms
Shoulders
Back

Consent Zone (permission needed)
Mouth
Wrists
Feet

Vulnerable Zone (special care needed)
Face
Neck
Front of body

Intimate Zone (great sensitivity needed)
Genitalia

Box 13-3
Contextual Factors Influencing Communication

Psychophysiological Context
The *internal factors* influencing communication:
    Physiological status
    Emotional status
    Growth and development status
    Unmet needs
    Attitudes, values, and beliefs
    Perceptions and personality
    Self-concept and self-esteem

Relational Context
The *nature of the relationship* between the participants:
    Social, helping, or working relationship
    Level of trust between participants
    Level of self-disclosure between participants
    Shared history of participants
    Balance of power and control

Situational Context
The *reason for* the communication:
    Information exchange
    Goal achievement
    Problem resolution
    Expression of feelings

Environmental Context
The *physical surroundings* in which communication takes place:
    Degree of privacy
    Degree of comfort and safety
    Noise level
    Presence of distractions

Cultural Context
The *sociocultural elements* that affect the interaction:
    Educational level of participants
    Language and self-expression patterns
    Customs and expectations

FACTORS INFLUENCING COMMUNICATION

Situations have several contextual aspects that influence the nature of communication and interpersonal relationships (Beebe and others, 1996). These include the participants' physical and emotional status, the nature of their relationship, their environment, the situation prompting communication, and the sociocultural elements present. The many factors influencing communication within these contexts are described in Box 13-3. Awareness of these factors helps the nurse make sound decisions during the communication process.

The following scenario illustrates how the nurse might use these concepts in interpersonal communication with a client.

Mrs. Geraldine (Gerry) Crocker enters Memorial Hospital's outpatient chemotherapy room, a pleasant, cheerful setting made warm and inviting with comfortable couches, a television set, and plenty of reading materials. The reason she is here is to receive her first round of chemotherapy from the RN on duty, Ruth Marks. Because she and Ruth have a shared history (Ruth cared for Mrs. Crocker after her mastectomy), they greet each other by first name and Ruth asks about her family. Gerry's German Catholic cultural background gives her a need to bear things in a stoic manner, so Ruth asks about her comfort and tells her how important it is to inform the nurse if she feels any symptoms during the treatment. Ruth senses Gerry's feelings about being here; because she seems anxious, Ruth helps her relax by using gentle humor and carefully explaining each step of the chemotherapy procedure. Gerry has a hopeful attitude about the drugs, which Ruth reinforces with positive affirmations. Gerry has a high school education, so Ruth uses the unit's informational pamphlets while teaching. Ruth sees that Gerry is yawning frequently and thus encourages her to meet her physical need for rest by taking a nap during the infusion, which interrupts further conversation.

Developmental factors also influence communication. Communication techniques can be adapted to the special needs of infants, toddlers and preschoolers, children, and adolescents (see Chapter 20). Communication with older adults involves adapting to any special needs resulting from sensory, motor, or cognitive impairments that may be present and remaining sensitive to the frail older adult's need for time and patience during communication.

THE NURSE-CLIENT HELPING RELATIONSHIP

Helping relationships are created through the nurse's application of scientific knowledge, understanding of human behavior and communication, and commitment to caring. Helping relationships are the foundation of clinical nursing practice; they are an essential element in every setting, with every client, and in every situation (Edelman and Mandle, 1994). In such relationships, the nurse assumes the role of professional helper and comes to know the client as an individual who has unique health needs, human responses, and patterns of living. The relationship is built through **therapeutic communication**, which is interpersonal communication that promotes a psychological climate that facilitates positive change, growth, and healing. "The nurse's therapeutic use of communication is the mechanism by which clients can achieve successful outcomes to the problems currently preventing them from achieving optimum health" (Fortinash and Holoday-Worret, 1996). There is an explicit time frame, a goal-directed approach, and a high expectation of confidentiality. The nurse establishes, directs, and takes responsibility for the interaction, and the client's needs take priority over the nurse's needs.

A helping relationship between nurse and client does not just happen—it is created with care and skill, and it is built on the client's trust in the nurse. Through ther-

apeutic communication the nurse develops a relationship with the client to fulfill several purposes. Nurse theorist Imogene King (1971) calls the nurse-client relationship "learning experiences whereby two people interact to face an immediate health problem, to share, if possible, in resolving it, and to discover ways to adapt to the situation." Clients are helped to clarify needs and goals, solve problems, cope with situational or maturational crises, clarify and strengthen values, reduce stress and anxiety, and gain insight and self-understanding (Edelman and Mandle, 1994). Creating this therapeutic environment depends on the nurse's ability to communicate, to provide comfort, and to help the client meet his or her needs. Comforting strategies used by nurses include gentle humor, physical comfort measures, emotionally supportive statements, and comforting and connecting touch. Nurses provide information, support clients' active decision making, and offer opportunities for clients to engage in social exchange. These comforting strategies demonstrate the nurse's caring and depend on the nurse's skill in communication and relationship building (Bottorff and others, 1995).

Many nursing situations, especially those in community and home health settings, require the nurse to form helping relationships with entire families. The same principles that guide one-to-one helping relationships are also applied when the client is a family unit. Communication within families requires additional understanding of the complexities of family dynamics, needs, and relationships.

The nurse-client relationship is characterized by a natural progression of four goal-directed phases that often begin before the nurse meets the client and continue until the care giving relationship ends. From the *preinteraction* period, through the *orientation* and *working* phases, and during the *termination* phase, the nurse and client work together to achieve positive health outcomes in a relationship built on the client's trust and the nurse's caring. These phases and their significant features are described more fully in Box 13-4.

NURSE–HEALTH TEAM MEMBER RELATIONSHIPS

Nurses are members of a larger health care community and often function in roles that require interaction with multiple health team members. Many elements of the nurse-client helping relationship are also applied in these collegial relationships, which are focused on accomplishing the work and goals of the clinical setting. Communication in such relationships may be geared toward team building, facilitating the group process, collaboration, consultation, delegation, supervision, leadership, and management.

Social, informational, and therapeutic interactions

Box 13-4
Phases of the Helping Relationship

Preinteraction Phase

Before meeting the client, the nurse:

Reviews available data, including the medical and nursing history

Talks to other care givers who may have information about the client

Anticipates health concerns or issues that may arise

Identifies a location and setting that will foster comfortable, private interaction

Plans enough time for the initial interaction

Orientation Phase

When the nurse and client meet and get to know one another, the nurse:

Sets the tone for the relationship by adopting a warm, empathetic, caring manner

Recognizes that the initial relationship may be superficial, uncertain, and tentative

Expects the client to test the nurse's competence and commitment

Closely observes the client and expects to be closely observed by the client

Begins to make inferences and form judgments about client messages and behaviors

Assesses the client's health status

Prioritizes client problems and identifies client goals

Clarifies the client's and nurse's roles

Forms contracts with the client to specify who will do what

Lets the client know when to expect the relationship to be terminated

Working Phase

When the nurse and client work together to solve problems and accomplish goals, the nurse:

Encourages and helps the client to express feelings about his or her health

Encourages and helps the client with self-exploration

Provides information needed to understand and change behavior

Encourages and helps the client to set goals

Takes actions to meet the goals set with the client

Uses therapeutic communication skills to facilitate successful interactions

Uses appropriate self-disclosure and confrontation

Termination Phase

During the ending of the relationship, the nurse:

Reminds the client that termination is near

Evaluates goal achievement with the client

Reminisces about the relationship with the client

Separates from the client by relinquishing responsibility for his or her care

Achieves a smooth transition for the client to other care givers as needed

---

are all needed among the nurse and health team members to build morale, accomplish goals, and strengthen relationships within the work setting. Everyone has interpersonal needs for inclusion, such as feeling accepted, wanted, and a part of the group; identity; privacy; power and control; and affection (Stewart and Logan, 1993; Wilson and others, 1995). Nurses need friendship, support, guidance, and encouragement from one another to cope with the many stressors imposed by the nursing role, and they must extend the same caring communication used with clients to build positive relationships with colleagues and co-workers.

COMMUNICATION WITHIN CARING RELATIONSHIPS

Principles and guidelines for using effective communication techniques can strengthen all caring relationships established within the professional role. Caring and helping relationships are manifested by the qualities and behaviors explained in the following sections of the text. Examples of nurses using both effective and in-

effective techniques are integrated throughout each section, as are suggestions for improving ineffective responses. Although some of the techniques may seem artificial or unnatural at first, the nurse's skill and comfort will increase with practice and experience, and tremendous satisfaction will result as therapeutic relationships and outcomes are achieved.

Professionalism

The nurse's verbal and nonverbal behavior greatly influence the helping relationship. The client's acceptance of the nurse as a professional often depends on the manner in which the nurse presents a professional and caring image. Professional appearance, demeanor, and behavior are important in establishing the nurse's trustworthiness and competence. They communicate that the nurse has assumed the professional helping role, is clinically skilled, and is focused on the client rather than the self. Nothing harms nursing's image like inappropriate appearance and behavior in those who hold a professional role. Consider the level of trust one might feel while being cared for by each of the following nurses.

Annie Robbins is late for her shift. She left her stethoscope and note pad at home. She is chewing gum, she has a large chunky necklace and long dangling hair, and her underwear is visible beneath her uniform. She is wearing heavy makeup and perfume, has long painted fingernails, and there is smoke on her breath and clothing. She giggles, talks loudly, uses slang, rolls her eyes, sulks, grimaces, writes vital signs on the skin of her hand, and reacts to problems by blaming others and behaving immaturely.

Allie Roberts is admired and respected for her professionalism. She is on time, organized, and well prepared and equipped for the responsibilities of her nursing role. She is clean, neat, well-groomed, appropriately dressed, and scent- and odor-free. Her behavior reflects warmth, friendliness, confidence, and competence. She speaks in a clear well-modulated voice, uses good grammar, listens to others, helps and supports teammates, communicates effectively, and handles problems in a mature manner.

Courtesy

Common courtesy is important to the nursing role. It conveys respect for others and oneself. Courtesy techniques include saying hello and goodbye, knocking on doors before entering, introducing oneself and stating one's purpose, addressing people by name, saying "please" and "thank you" to team members, and apologizing for inadvertently making an error or causing someone distress—all are integral parts of good professional communication. Being discourteous causes the nurse to be perceived as rude, crude, or insensitive. It sets up barriers between the nurse and client and causes friction among team members.

Self-introduction is especially important. The nurse's failure to give a name, indicate RN status, or acknowledge the client can create uncertainty about the interaction and conveys an impersonal lack of commitment or caring. Making eye contact and smiling at another, rather than ignoring them, gives recognition. Acknowledging others by name evidences the nurse's respect for human dignity and for the uniqueness of the other person. Because using last names conveys respect in most cultures, nurses usually begin initial interactions by using the client's last name. The nurse should ask others how they would like to be addressed and let them know personal preference as well. Using first names is appropriate for infants, young children, confused or unconscious clients, and close team members.

Avoid terms of endearment. Calling the client "honey," "dear," "Grandpa," or "sweetheart" rather than by a personal name is inappropriate. Most people are offended by such casual familiarity from care givers.

Avoid referring to clients by diagnosis, room number, or other attribute. Referring to clients by attributes rather than their names is demeaning and sends the message that the nurse does not care enough about the person to know him or her as an individual.

Confidentiality

It is essential that the nurse safeguard the client's right to privacy by carefully protecting information of a confidential nature. This is accomplished by reassuring the person that information will be kept private and then keeping that promise. It is often tempting to share exciting or shocking information or to share information with those who are genuinely interested and concerned, but that temptation must be resisted. In situations where the nurse is obligated to report information to others, the client should be told in advance if at all possible.

Client: "What's wrong with my roommate? She seems so sick."

Nurse: "I know you're concerned about Mrs. Hoover, but I can't share any personal information about a client without his or her permission."

Avoid violating confidentiality. Sharing personal information or gossiping about others violates both nursing's ethical code and practice standards. It sends the message that the nurse cannot be trusted and damages interpersonal relationships.

Trust

Being trustworthy means helping others without doubt or question when help is needed. To foster trust the nurse communicates warmth and caring and demonstrates consistency, reliability, honesty, and competence. Trusting another person involves risk and vulnerability, but it also fosters open, therapeutic communication and enhances the expression of feelings, thoughts, and needs. Without trust, a nurse-client relationship rarely progresses beyond social interaction and superficial care.

Being untrustworthy or dishonest seriously undermines relationships. Knowingly withholding key information, lying, or distorting the truth violates both legal and ethical standards of practice.

Nurse, lying to a client who asked why his 24-hour urine collection was being repeated: "The lab wants us to repeat the test, because their machine broke down during the analysis and they need a fresh specimen."

A better response would be, "I'm sorry, Mr. Gottleib. One of the staff didn't save some of your urine by mistake. We will make every effort to make sure it is all saved this time."

Availability

Availability means being present for the other person when needed. By expressing a willingness to be available, even though the other person may not verbalize such a need, the nurse shows a caring attitude. Offering oneself is a communication technique used to convey the nurse's willingness to listen, talk, be available, or be physically present with another person.

Do not avoid others. Going out of one's way to avoid contact with another person communicates the nurse's unwillingness to face discomfort or resolve conflict. Clients often sense when they are being avoided, and negative behavior may escalate as a result.

Avoid task orientation.

A nurse who is *task oriented* makes the task or technical procedure the entire focus of the interaction with the client, missing opportunities to assess the client, explore concerns, allay anxiety, demonstrate empathy, integrate client teaching, and involve the client in care. Task-oriented nurses are often perceived as cold, uncaring, and unapproachable. When students first perform technical skills, it is difficult to integrate therapeutic communication because of the need to focus on the procedure. In time, nurses learn to integrate communication with high-visibility tasks and accomplish several goals simultaneously. Consider the quality of care given in each of the following scenarios.

Nurse A silently enters the client's room: "It's time for your pain shot."

Client, Mr. Stewart, is mildly startled and grimaces as he turns toward the nurse. As he starts to ask a question, Nurse A quickly reaches for his arm, gives the injection, then leaves.

Nurse B, calling the client's name as she enters the room: "Mr. Stewart, I have your pain medication. Are you feeling as uncomfortable as you look?"

Client: "Yes, my back feels like a knife went through it. Will the pain ever go away?"

Nurse B lays syringe down and sits next to the client: "It's normal to have severe pain the first few days after surgery. This medicine should help a lot. Let me give you the shot, then I'll show you how to move more carefully in bed so the pain won't get worse. Also, if you have more breakthrough pain, I will call the doctor to see about adjusting your medicine."

EMPATHY

Empathy is the ability to understand and accept another person's reality, to accurately perceive feelings, and to communicate this understanding to the other. Balzer-Riley (1996) states that "when clients or colleagues are hurting, confused, troubled, anxious, alienated, terrified, doubtful of self-worth, or uncertain as to identity, then understanding is called for." Such empathetic understanding requires the nurse to be both sensitive and imaginative, especially if the nurse has not had similar experiences. Although nurses cannot be empathetic in all situations, it is an important goal to strive for—a key to unlocking concern and communicating emotional support for others.

Empathy statements reflect an understanding of what has been communicated. They are highly effective, because they tell the person that the nurse heard both the feeling and the factual content of the communication. Empathy statements are neutral and nonjudgmental. They can be used to establish trust in very difficult situations.

Nurse to client who has received bad news: "That must have been a difficult thing to hear."

Nurse to family member: "It sounds like you're really afraid of what might happen to your husband."

Sympathy

Sympathy is concern, sorrow, or pity felt by the nurse for the client, in which the nurse personally identifies with the client's needs. Sympathy is a subjective look at another person's world that prevents a clear perspective of all sides of the issues confronting that person. Sharing sympathy with another feels good, creates a bond, and minimizes differences. Although sympathy is a compassionate response to another's situation, it is not as therapeutic as empathy because the nurse's own emotional issues can prevent effective problem solving and impair good judgment. Stuart and Sundeen (1995) explain that sympathy can cause problems in a helping relationship, because helpers who share the client's needs may be unable to help the client select realistic solutions for problems and may assume the client's feelings are similar to their own.

Nurse to client who is grieving an amputation: "I'm so sorry about your amputation. I know just how you feel."

A better response would be, "I can imagine how hard it might be to lose a leg."

Listening and Responding

Active listening means listening attentively with the whole person—mind, body, and spirit. It includes listening for main and supportive ideas; acknowledging and responding; giving appropriate feedback; and paying attention to the other person's total communication, including the content, the intent, and the feelings expressed (Berko and others, 1997). Attentive listening allows a person to better understand the entire message being communicated and is an excellent way to build trust. In many situations, a person's primary need is simply for someone to listen.

To listen attentively, the nurse faces the client at a distance of about 3 feet, removes physical barriers between them, maintains eye contact, assumes a relaxed posture, leans forward slightly, and nods in acknowledgment to give feedback and encouragement as the client speaks.

Provide information.

Giving information, whether factual information or professional advice, provides the other person with data needed for decision making. It helps reduce anxiety and meet client needs for safety and security. When offering suggestions, the nurse should stress that the client has the right to make decisions about options so that client autonomy is maintained. The partnership between the client and health care provider is enhanced when information is understood and the meaning of commonly used medical words and abbreviations is made clear (Anspaugh and others, 1994). Information should be given in direct, understandable terms in lay language, and medical terms should be translated for the client.

Nurse: "Mr. Valdez, this new medicine is called Lanoxin. It acts as a cardiotonic and antidysrhythmic—that means it will help your heart have a stronger and more regular beat."

Paraphrase communication. *Paraphrasing* is a communication technique in which the sender's message is restated in the receiver's own words. It is used to send feedback that information has been accurately received.

Clarify communication. *Clarifying* is a communication technique used to convey active listening. It is used to validate whether the message was interpreted correctly. The nurse can try to restate an unclear or ambiguous message or ask the other person to restate it, explain further, or give an example of what was meant.

Focus communication. *Focusing* is a communication technique that directs conversation to a specific topic or issue when a discussion becomes vague or ill defined, limiting the area to which the sender can respond. It is useful when the sender rambles or introduces many unrelated topics in the same conversation.

Summarize communication. *Summarizing* is a communication technique that serves as a concise review of main ideas from a discussion. It can bring a sense of satisfaction and closure to an individual conversation, or it can be used during the termination phase of a nurse-client relationship. By reviewing a conversation, the participants focus on key issues and can add additional relevant information as needed.

Nurse to client: "We've talked about what to expect when you go home and the self-care you'll need to do, and you feel like you're ready, but you still need to make arrangements for a leave of absence from work."
  Client to nurse: "Yes, and I also have to fill out workman's compensation papers."

Use appropriate self-disclosure. *Self-disclosure* is a communication technique used during the working phase of a helping relationship. Self-disclosures are personal statements about the nurse, intentionally revealed to the other person for the purposes of modeling and educating, fostering a therapeutic alliance, validating reality, and encouraging autonomy (Stuart and Sundeen, 1995). Self-disclosures should be relevant, appropriate, made to benefit the client and not the nurse, and used sparingly so that the client remains the focus of the interaction.

Avoid inattentive listening. Fidgeting, breaking eye contact, daydreaming during conversation, and "pseudo listening"—pretending to listen when one really is not—convey the message that what the sender has to say is not important. These behaviors inhibit conversation and undermine trust.

Nurse looks at watch and taps foot impatiently, gazing out the window as client talks.

Avoid medical jargon. Medical jargon or unfamiliar words can cause confusion and anxiety and should be avoided or translated for the client. Even a much-used phrase such as "I'm going to take your vital signs" can be frightening to a child.

Nurse to client: "Sit up while your lungs are auscultated."
  A better response would be, "Let me help you sit up while I listen to your lungs."
  Nurse to young child: "Do you need to urinate?"
  A better response would be, "Do you need to use the potty?"

Avoid giving personal opinions. When the nurse gives a personal opinion, it takes decision making away from the client. The problem and its solution belong to the client rather than the nurse. Personal opinion differs from professional advice, which can be given in the form of information about options that are available.

Client: "I don't know how much longer I'll be able to take care of my husband. I just don't know what to do."
  Nurse: "If I were you, I'd put my husband in a nursing home."
  A better response would be, "Sounds like that's a difficult decision. Let's talk about what choices are available for someone like your husband who needs a lot of care."

Avoid prying. Asking personal questions that are not relevant to the situation, simply to satisfy the nurse's curiosity, is inappropriate. Such questions are nosy, invasive, and unnecessary. If clients wish to share private information, they will.

Avoid changing the subject. Changing the subject when the sender is trying to communicate is rude and shows a lack of empathy. It tends to block further communication, and the sender may then withhold important messages or fail to openly express feelings. If changing the subject is necessary, the nurse should explain why.

Client: "I really miss my kids. I cry every time I think of them."
  Nurse: "Dr. Marcus will be here in a minute to take out your chest tube."
  A better response would be, "It must be hard to be apart from your children. Maybe we can talk about it after Dr. Marcus takes out your chest tube."

Avoid clichés. A *cliché* is a stereotyped comment that tends to gloss over the other person's feelings. It can cause the sender to believe that the nurse is not taking his or her concerns seriously or is giving an automatic response.

Acceptance and Respect

Conveying acceptance is one of the most important aspects of therapeutic communication. The need to be nonjudgmental is emphasized in the American Nurses Association's *Code of Ethics* (1985), which states that the nurse provides services unrestricted by considerations of social or economic status, personal attributes, or the nature of the problem. Acceptance is a willingness to hear a message or to acknowledge feelings. It does not mean that the nurse agrees with the other person or approves of his or her decisions or actions. Acceptance can be demonstrated through giving positive feedback, making sure verbal and nonverbal cues match, using touch, using empathy statements, restating what has been implied, and avoiding arguments.

Appropriate confrontation. *Confrontation* is a communication technique sometimes used after trust has been established or during the working phase of a nurse-client relationship. In confrontation, the nurse makes the client aware of inconsistencies in behavior or thoughts that interfere with self-understanding. The technique helps clients recognize growth or deal with important issues and works by helping the client become more aware of incongruence in feelings, attitudes, beliefs, and behaviors (Stuart and Sundeen, 1995).

Asking for explanations. Asking "why" may imply an accusation and can result in resentment, insecurity, and mistrust. If additional information is needed, it is best to phrase a question to avoid using "why."

Avoid approval or disapproval. Nurses must not impose their own attitudes, values, beliefs, and moral standards on others while in the professional helping role. Other people have the right to be themselves and make their own decisions. Judgmental responses by the nurse often contain terms like "should," "ought," "good," "bad," "right," or "wrong."

Likewise, agreeing or disagreeing sends the subtle message that the nurse has the right to make value judgments about client decisions. The nurse can convey agreement or disagreement by helping the other person anticipate the consequences of decisions.

Avoid arguing. Challenging or arguing against someone's perceptions denies that they are real and valid to the sender. These behaviors imply that the other person is lying, misinformed, or uneducated. The skillful nurse can present information or present reality in a way that avoids argument.

Avoid being defensive. Defensiveness in the face of criticism implies the sender has no right to an opinion. The sender's concerns may be ignored when the nurse focuses on the need for self-defense, defense of the health care team, or defense of others.

Silence

It takes time and experience to become comfortable with silence. Most people have a natural tendency to fill empty spaces with words, but sometimes what those spaces really need is time for the nurse and the sender to observe one another, to sort out feelings, to think how to say things, and to consider what has been communicated. Interrupting a meaningful silence is just as rude as interrupting conversation. Silence may be especially therapeutic during times of profound sadness, deep thought, or grief.

Mrs. Hartz, who is dying of renal failure, has just voiced feelings of deep grief about having to leave her family and friends behind. The nurse sits quietly while they both wipe away tears, think about love and loss, and appreciate the sharing that is taking place between them.

Hope and Encouragement

Nurses recognize that hope is essential for healing and learn to communicate a "sense of possibility" to others (Benner, 1984). Encouragement and positive feedback are important in fostering hope and self-confidence and for helping people achieve their potential and reach their goals. The nurse can give hope and encouragement by commenting on the positive aspects of the other person's behavior, performance, or response. Hope can also be strengthened by sharing a vision of the future and reminding others of their resources and strengths.

Avoid false reassurance. Offering false reassurance can do more harm than good. Although it might be intended kindly and help the nurse avoid the sender's distress, it tends to block conversation and discourages further expression of feelings.

Client: "I don't think I'm going to beat this lupus."
   Nurse: "Don't worry, I'm sure everything will be all right."
   A better response would be, "Go on...tell me more about what you're thinking," or "What's it like to feel that way?"

Socializing

Socializing is an important component of the nurse's communication. It is a good way to get to know one another and to help people relax. It is easy, superficial, and not deeply personal, whereas therapeutic interactions are often more intense, difficult, demanding, and uncomfortable. Nurses may use social conversation at the beginning of an interaction to make connections and help the client feel comfortable in sharing feelings and concerns. A friendly, informal, and warm communication style helps establish trust.

Nurse: "It certainly is a lovely day, Mrs. Spier."

Client: "Yes, isn't it? If I were home and feeling better, I'd be planting my garden."

Nurse: "You're a gardener? What types of plants do you grow?"

Client: "Oh, a little of everything. I like some tomatoes, lettuce, radishes, and maybe some squash."

Avoid inappropriate socializing. When the nurse never gets beyond social conversation to talk about issues or concerns impacting the client's health, social conversation is excessive and inappropriate. It is also inappropriate if the time and place call for a more serious approach.

Assertiveness and Autonomy

Assertive communication is a type of communication based on a philosophy of protecting individual rights and responsibilities. It includes the ability to be self-directive in acting to accomplish goals and advocate for others. Assertive responses promote self-esteem and uphold personal and professional rights. They are characterized by feelings of security, competence, power, positivity, and professionalism. Assertive statements are the best way to get messages across without resorting to sarcasm, whining, anger, blaming, or manipulation. Assertive responses are good tools for dealing with criticism, change, negative conditions in personal or professional life, and conflict or stress in relationships.

Assertive responses often contain "I" messages, such as "I want," "I need," "I think," or "I feel." Simple assertive messages are usually stated in three parts, referencing the nurse, the other individual's behavior, and its impact.

The nurse can state a more complex assertive message by using the ASSERT formula: Describe the *Action* that prompted the need for the message; express a *Subjective* interpretation of the action; express *Sensations* related to the action; indicate the *Effects* of the action; make a *Request* of the other person; and *Tell* one's intentions if the request is not met (Berko and others, 1997).

Nurse to supervisor: "When you say I'm not performing well, that sounds serious. I feel surprised and confused, because I had a sense that I was doing a good job. Please give me some examples of what you mean. If there are none, I'll discuss this evaluation with the director of nursing."

Avoid passive responses. Passive responses are those that avoid issues or conflict. They are characterized by feelings of sadness, depression, anxiety, and hopelessness.

Nurse to co-worker, hopelessly: "I guess there's nothing we can do about it."

Nurse to spouse during argument: "Whatever you say."

A better response would be, "What can we do to make things better?"

Avoid aggressive responses. Aggressive responses are those that provoke confrontation at the other person's expense. They are characterized by feelings of anger, frustration, resentment, and stress.

Avoid triangulation. **Triangulation** is complaining to a third party rather than confronting the problem or expressing concerns directly to the source. It lowers team morale and is often contagious.

Nurse to nurse, about co-worker: "Janice makes me so mad. She never gets all her work done, then expects me to cover for her. I'm sick and tired of it."

A better response would be, "Janice, when you left that new admission for me, I couldn't get all my work done. I was really angry and frustrated because it's happened three times this week."

Humor

Humor has been defined as a coping strategy based on an individual's cognitive appraisal of a stimulus, which results in behavior such as smiling, laughing, or feelings of amusement that lessen emotional distress (Simon, cited in Wooten, 1993). According to Wooten, humor can help promote well-being by changing perspective, releasing tension, and giving a feeling of superiority or mastery. Laughter can be good "medicine" when nurses use humor to help clients adjust to stress imposed by illness. Wooten notes that laughter helps to relieve stress-related tension and pain by decreasing serum cortisol levels, increasing immune system activity, and stimulating endorphin release from the hypothalamus. Humor can increase the nurse's effectiveness in providing emotional support to clients and can humanize the illness experience. Laughter provides both a psychological and physical release for both nurse and client. Humor can help others to interact more openly and comfortably and can make the nurse's own humanity more apparent.

Wooten (1993) advises that nurses should establish professional competency and caring before using humor, take care of the client's comfort and security needs first, and test receptivity to humor with small, safe doses. Wooten also suggests avoiding sexual, religious, or ethnic humor. Using gentle humor, or "hoping humor," can be accomplished through telling jokes, sharing humorous incidents or situations, using props (such as giving an angry client a squirt gun), and using puns. Nurses should realize that humor can backfire; not everyone will appreciate a humorous approach because of negative moods, stress, or physical discomfort.

Avoid inappropriate humor. A kind of dark, negative humor is sometimes used after difficult or traumatic situations as a way to survive intact and defuse unbearable tension and stress. This "coping humor" has a high potential for being misinterpreted as callous or uncaring by those not involved in the situation. For example, nursing students are sometimes offended and wonder how nurses can laugh and joke after unsuccessful resuscitation efforts. When nurses use "coping humor" within earshot of clients or their loved ones, extreme emotional distress can result.

Touch

Touch is one of the nurse's most potent forms of communication. It is an integral part of human behavior; from the moment of birth until death, people need to be touched and to touch others (Rousalato, 1996b). Nurses are privileged to experience more of this intimate form of personal contact than almost any other professional. Many messages such as affection, emotional support, encouragement, tenderness, and personal attention are conveyed through touch (Bottorff, 1993). Comfort touch is especially important for vulnerable clients who are experiencing severe illness with its accompanying physical and emotional losses (Butts and Janes, 1995). Research has shown that nurses use nonprocedural touch with clients to get their attention, to arouse them from sleep, to begin a nursing intervention, to add emphasis to explanations, to make requests, to comfort, to emphasize or point things out, to tease, to thank, and to reprimand (Rousalato, 1996a). Touch is a basic communication technique that can often convey understanding better than words or gestures. Therapeutic touch is a special form of alternative touch therapy used by nurses to achieve health assessment, pain reduction, and relaxation by influencing a client's energy fields. Learning therapeutic touch involves knowing how to meditate, acquiring experimental knowledge of energy fields, and practicing with guidance from specially trained advanced practice nurses (Edelman and Mandle, 1994).

Because much of what nurses do involves touching, nurses must learn to use it wisely. The zones of touch (Rousalato, 1996a) are described in Box 13-2. Touch delivered in the social or consent zones is less anxiety producing than touch delivered in the vulnerable or intimate zones. Seed (1995) discovered that students may initially find giving intimate care to be stressful, especially when caring for clients of the opposite gender, and that students learn to cope with intimate contact by changing their perception of the situation. Similarly, the client who is ill and dependent must permit closer physical contact than is normally tolerated and may be uncomfortable with touch. Nurses should remain sensitive to their own responses and to clients' feelings. Shying away from touch or refusing to hold the nurse's hand during an episode of pain means the client is probably uncomfortable with being touched.

Avoid inappropriate touch. Touch may be perceived negatively when it is given without consent; used within a hostile or nontrusting relationship; and delivered to a vulnerable, intimate, or painful area of the body. The nurse's touch should never be angry, rough, violent, overly stimulating, threatening, overly tentative, sexual, or unnecessarily painful.

The nurse takes Mr. Ackerman's face between her hands and turns his head so he is forced to make eye contact.

A better response would be to reposition herself in front of the client and gently touch his hand while speaking his name.

Cultural Sensitivity

Cultural sensitivity in communication means understanding that persons of different cultures use different degrees of eye contact, personal space, gestures, loudness of voice, pace of speech, touch, silence, and meaning of language (Davidhizar and Giger, 1994; Grossman, 1994; Nance, 1995). It means making a conscious effort not to interpret messages through the nurse's own cultural perspective, instead considering the communication within the context of the other individual's background (see Chapter 18). Consider the cultural sensitivity demonstrated by the nurse in the following example (Jambunathan and Stewart, 1995).

Carrie Barton is caring for Huan Mi, a young female refugee from Vietnam's Hmong delta who has just delivered a small baby boy. Carrie understands that childbirth in different cultures is treated as a traumatic life crisis and a time of vulnerability for the mother and infant. She knows that Ms. Huan's lack of prenatal care was related to the woman's fear of miscarriage if touched by doctors or nurses, and she is careful in her use of touch to communicate with Ms. Huan. She especially avoids touching her on the head, which is perceived as very dangerous. Carrie did not try to argue with Ms. Huan when she refused an episiotomy, because she preferred to tear and heal naturally. She also respected Ms. Huan's decision that having the baby circumcised would be "unnatural." When teaching her about birth control, Carrie was aware that Ms. Huan might have difficulties practicing the techniques because of male/female role expectations. She was careful in how she sought feedback about Ms. Huan's understanding of the information, recognizing that Asian persons often agree with the speaker to be polite rather than to indicate agreement or understanding.

Avoid cultural insensitivity. Cultural insensitivity in communication takes many forms, including making fun of another's culture, ethnicity, language, or dress; telling culture- or ethnic-denigrating jokes; stereotyping; patronizing; and incorrectly interpreting culturally based behavior. It also includes behaving in ways that offend the cultural practices of others.

Gender Sensitivity

Gender influences how we think, act, feel, and communicate. *Gender sensitivity* in communication means recognizing the differences in male and female communication patterns. Males grow up using communication to achieve goals, establish individual status and authority, and compete for attention and power. Females grow up using communication to build connections with others; include others; and cooperate with, respond to, show interest in, and support others. Men typically prefer to talk about topics that do not expose personal feelings, whereas women enjoy discussing feelings and personal issues. Men find closeness in doing, and women find closeness in dialogue (Wood, 1996). Men tend to speak directly when giving criticism or orders. Women speak indirectly, couching criticism and commands in praise or vagueness to avoid causing offense or hurt feelings. A male nurse might say to his colleague, "Help me turn Jeremy." A female nurse might say, "Jeremy needs to be turned," expecting her colleague to understand the implied request for help. Men use more banter, teasing, and playful "put-downs." They sometimes hesitate to ask questions for fear of appearing unknowledgeable, whereas women ask questions to elicit information. Men usually want others to know of their accomplishments; women may tend to downplay their achievements (Beebe and others, 1996). Research has shown that gender differences also influence the way male and female nurses use silence, touch, and humor in their practice (Perry, 1996).

Avoid gender insensitivity. Gender-insensitive communication means that a nurse of one gender misinterprets or reacts to messages differently than they were intended by the other gender. It also includes conversation with sexual innuendos, gender-denigrating jokes, male-female stereotyping, and so forth.

COMMUNICATION WITHIN THE NURSING PROCESS

The communication skills presented in the previous sections are integrated throughout the nursing process as nurses collaborate with clients and health team members to achieve goals. The nurse constantly uses communication skills to gather, analyze, and transmit information and to accomplish the work of each phase. Although the nursing process is a reliable framework for delivering comprehensive client care, it will not work well unless the nurse masters the art of effective interpersonal communication.

Communication techniques used within the nursing process are also applied during the problem-solving process with team members (Box 13-5). Whether the nurse is assessing a client or gathering data about the nature of a quality management problem, the same information-seeking techniques are used. Encouraging goal setting, suggesting collaboration, and facilitating evaluation are essential aspects of working with clients within the nursing process. They are also used with team members to resolve problems or accomplish goals within the clinical setting that are not directly related to client care. A few techniques deserve special mention because of their importance in the nursing and problem-solving processes.

Assessment

The assessment of a client's communication ability involves activities that systematically collect data; orga-

---

Box 13-5
Communication Through the Nursing Process

Assessment
Interviewing and history taking
Physical examination (use of visual, auditory, and tactile channels)
Observation of nonverbal behavior
Review of medical records, literature, diagnostic tests

Nursing Diagnosis
Written analysis of assessment findings
Discussion of health care needs and priorities with client and family

Planning
Written care plans
Health team planning sessions
Discussions with client and family to determine methods of implementation
Making referrals

Implementation
Discussion with other health professionals
Health teaching
Provision of therapeutic support
Contact with other health resources
Record of client's progress in care plan and nurse's notes

Evaluation
Acquisition of verbal and nonverbal feedback
Written results of expected outcomes
Update of written care plan
Explanation of revisions to client

---

nize the data collected; and document the information that has been obtained from the client, family, and significant others. This is the first step in establishing a beneficial nurse-client relationship and the rapport needed for good communication.

Information gathering

Seek information. Seeking information, or asking questions, is an essential skill used during assessment. Asking relevant questions allows the nurse to gather data about the client or problem situation. *Focused questions* are used to elicit more information about a particular subject. A focused question that is open ended, such as, "What is your usual sleep pattern?" cannot be answered with a yes/no or one-word response. A closed question, such as, "How many hours of sleep do you average each night?", requires a more specific answer.

Do not overuse information seeking. Overuse of information seeking as a therapeutic communication technique can be dehumanizing, because informational interactions do not allow the nurse or client to establish a more meaningful relationship or deal with important emotional issues. It may be a way for the nurse to ignore uncomfortable areas in favor of more comfortable, neutral topics.

Client, worried: "I don't know what to do about my daughter; her tantrums are driving me crazy. The doctor thinks she might be either hyperactive or mentally retarded."

Nurse: "What's your daughter's name?" or "How long has she been having tantrums?"

A better response yielding more assessment data would be, "You sound worried about this. Tell me what happens when your daughter has a tantrum."

Physical and psychological barriers to communication. A client may suffer physical or psychological alterations that impair communication. To speak spontaneously and clearly, a person must have an intact respiratory system, normal oral and nasal cavities, and a functioning speech center. Normal reception of language requires an intact auditory system. The nurse assesses a child's ability to communicate, including the observation of sounds, gestures, and vocabulary. When an adult develops hearing problems, the ability to receive and understand messages is impaired. The medical history and physical assessment provide clues to the client's physical ability to communicate (Table 13-1).

The nurse should also consider whether clients are taking medications that impair speech or impair the ability to understand the message (e.g., antidepressants, neuroleptics, sedatives). The nurse should be familiar with common side effects of such medications.

Some psychological illnesses such as psychosis or depression influence the ability to communicate. The client may demonstrate flight of ideas, constant verbalization of the same words or phrases, or a loose association of ideas. The nurse must isolate psychological causes of speech problems from possible neurological causes.

▪ Nursing Diagnosis

The inability to communicate effectively influences a client's ability to express needs or react to the environment. After collecting assessment data the nurse clusters pertinent defining characteristics for patterns and problems. Success in accurately identifying the client's communication problem will ensure the formulation of an accurate nursing diagnosis (see nursing diagnoses box). The related factor should focus on the cause of the communication disorder so that appropriate nursing interventions are selected.

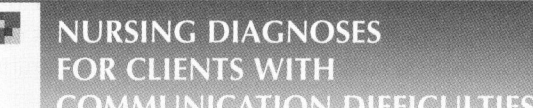

> **NURSING DIAGNOSES FOR CLIENTS WITH COMMUNICATION DIFFICULTIES**
>
> Communication, impaired verbal
> Social interaction, impaired
> Coping, family: potential for growth
> Coping, ineffective family: compromised
> Coping, ineffective individual
> Powerlessness

Impaired verbal communication is the nursing diagnostic label used to describe the client who has limited or no ability to communicate verbally. This diagnosis is useful for a wide variety of clients with special problems and needs related to communication. It is defined as "the state in which an individual experiences a decreased or absent ability to use or understand language in human interaction" (Kim and others, 1995).

▪ Planning

As the nurse uses assessment data to formulate and support nursing diagnoses, the focus becomes directed to the appropriate actions that will effectively assist in addressing the identified problem or need. In planning, the nurse will begin to establish goals and expected outcomes of care and determine specific nursing interventions to assist in dealing with the client's communication difficulties. Consideration must be given to interventions and communication techniques appropriate for the client's age, cultural beliefs, and practices. Whenever possible, the nurse collaborates with the client, family, friends, other health care team members,

TABLE 13-1 **Assessment of Physical Communication Barriers**	
Speech and Language Mechanisms	Alterations Affecting Speech
Respiratory system	Extreme dyspnea (shortness of Breath)
	Artificial airways: endotracheal tube or tracheostomy
	Laryngectomy (surgical removal of larynx)
Oral and nasal cavities	Cleft palate
	Loose-fitting dentures
	Neurological disease affecting articulation (parkinsonism)
Speech center	Aphasia related to cerebrovascular accident (stroke) or brain tumor
Auditory system	Conduction or nerve deafness

and the discharge planning team. Often the family can suggest ways that foster communication with the client. Goals of care established with the client and nurse should be mutually set. The importance of collaboration allows the opportunity for all health care team members to have knowledge of the techniques that will best promote the client's ability to communicate.

Success in promoting a client's ability to communicate depends not only on the client's participation in goal setting but also on the nurse's style of communication and the ability to establish a therapeutic relationship. Therapeutic communication skills enable the nurse to perceive, react to, and respect the client's uniqueness.

Collaboration

Encourage collaboration. Collaboration is especially useful during the planning and intervention phases of the nursing or problem-solving process. Collaboration among the nurse, client, and family care givers is especially important. Davidhizar and Rexroth (1994) cite that such collaboration can provide support to the family and client, increase the care giver's understanding, increase compliance, increase the nurse's understanding, reinforce teaching, decrease manipulative behavior, promote communication among family members, and facilitate positive client-family relationships.

Collaboration can be encouraged by asking others for input and suggestions about what should be done to reach goals. It gives others the opportunity to express themselves and strengthens problem-solving ability.

Do not avoid collaboration. When nurses fail to collaborate with clients, the nursing process becomes a lopsided effort with little chance of success. When health team members fail to collaborate with one another, clients are denied the expertise that can make a crucial difference in health outcomes. It is selfish and egotistical for nurses to believe in their ability to meet a client's total health needs without assistance from others. The Clinical Scenario for Miss O'Hara includes a special focus on creating a plan of care for the client with impaired verbal communication.

■ Clinical Scenario

Betty O'Hara, a 56-year-old secretary, is on the progressive care unit recovering from a stroke. Her brain responded to the decrease in circulation by losing the ability to form words, a condition known as expressive aphasia. Miss O'Hara is alert and follows directions but makes only inarticulate sounds when she tries to speak. Because the stroke also affected her right side, her handwriting is slow and nearly illegible. She appeared anxious and frustrated with efforts to communicate at first, and she has now stopped making any effort to talk and seems withdrawn and discouraged.

Bill Pelham has just been assigned as Miss O'Hara's nurse. From assessing data in her medical record, he knows that she has had a cerebrovascular accident and is unable to name objects or speak intelligibly. From the nurse's notes, he knows that she has appeared withdrawn and depressed and makes little effort to communicate. From this data, he has made the nursing diagnosis of impaired verbal communication related to decreased cerebral perfusion and possible hopelessness. He knows that a speech therapist will be in to see her later today, and he plans to establish trust with Miss O'Hara and talk with her about her nursing diagnosis. As Bill enters her room, he pulls the curtain for privacy and turns down the TV to minimize environmental distractions while they communicate.

"Miss O'Hara? My name is Bill Pelham. I'll be one of your nurses while you're on the PCU." (He extends his left hand for her to shake and watches her closely to see whether she seems to understand. She reaches to shake his hand, and he knows she can interpret nonverbal gestures.)

"I understand you had a stroke that left you unable to talk." (Bill knows that using short sentences and incorporating "yes" or "no" questions will be less frustrating for his client.)

She nods her head, and Bill knows she understands verbal communication as well.

"We call this impaired verbal communication. In your case, it's because the part of your brain that forms speech was affected. Now, other parts of your brain will have to learn to take over and do that job."

Miss O'Hara gives him a skeptical look.

"I've worked here a long time, and I've known many people who regained all or part of their speech."

She turns her head away from him.

"You know, people communicate so much without words! Just now, I think you told me you don't believe this will be true for you. Is that right?" (Bill knows that interpreting nonverbal behavior and seeking validation are very important for the client with expressive aphasia.)

She looks back and nods again.

"You're not feeling very hopeful right now, maybe because no one has helped you with this problem yet . . . (pause) . . . Have you ever known anyone with a broken hip? They have to work really hard to walk again, but with therapy, most do. I believe the same can be true for you, if we set some goals and try to reach them."

She seems to be thinking this over, so Bill is quiet a moment.

"Norma Lee, our speech therapist, will be seeing you later today and that will help a lot. In the meantime, I'd like our first goal to be that you let me know by your facial expressions and gestures whether I'm interpreting your messages correctly. Is it a deal?"

Miss O'Hara gives him a lopsided smile and an "OK" sign with her thumb and forefinger.

"Until you regain some speech, we need to figure out the best method to tell us what you need. I'll name some things first. When I go back over the list, you nod when you hear the one that sounds best." (Bill has Miss O'Hara's full attention now.)

"We could use, one, flash cards with pictures of different objects and emotions. Two, a magic slate for you to write on. Three, a picture board with pictures to point to. Four, a toy computer for you to type on. Five, a letter board for you to spell with. . . . Now I'll name them again, and you tell me what you'd like to try." (He names the methods, and Miss O'Hara nods at "picture board.") Bill is happy, because he's made initial progress toward restoring communication for Miss O'Hara.

He knows that the next step will be for her to practice vocalization, then slowly learn to form words again. A few days later, Bill talks with Miss O'Hara about her progress.

"Miss O'Hara, you're doing so much better now in communicating. The board is working well for basic things. Your face has more expression in it, and I think you trust us enough to let us know when you're mad or frustrated, too."

(She shrugs as if to say, "What else can I do?")

"I asked Norma Lee what the nurses could do to help you with your speech. She said to encourage you to name what you're pointing to, and to practice your vowels. Can we use those as your two new goals?"

(She looks down, and tears come to her eyes.)

Bill, gently: "What's wrong?"

(She looks up and makes a circle with her forefinger by the side of her head.)

"You're afraid people will think you're crazy if they hear you trying to talk?"

(She nods, embarrassed, then makes an unintelligible sound as if to demonstrate.)

"That sounds to me like a lady who's working hard to get something she wants. I hope you can be as proud of yourself as other people will be, for having the courage to make those sounds. They have to come before clear speech, there's no way around it."

(She thinks this over, then points to the board and says, "Wahh.") Bill grins and hands her a glass of water. He thinks about her nursing diagnosis, mentally removes hopelessness as an etiology, and adds the new goals to her plan of care. He communicates to the staff that she is very sensitive about practicing speech in front of others, and he plans to give her as much privacy as possible. He wonders whether a visit from another client who has overcome aphasia might help, and he plans to ask Miss O'Hara whether she would agree. He notes that positive feedback and encouragement have worked well, and he experiences a sense of hope that his client's impaired verbal communication will diminish daily.

▪   ▪   ▪   ▪   ▪   ▪   ▪

▪ Implementation

There are many altered health states and human responses that contribute to impaired communication. Examples include the infant whose self-expression is limited to crying, body movement, and facial expression; the person who receives messages through fewer channels because of hearing or visual impairment; the person who cannot understand or form words because of a stroke or late-stage Alzheimer's disease; the person with autism or schizophrenia who responds to internal stimuli and misinterprets external stimuli; the person who does not speak or understand English; the client with learning disabilities and limited vocal skills who uses gaze and body orientation to display a readiness to communicate; and the unresponsive or heavily sedated person who cannot send or receive verbal messages.

The client who cannot communicate effectively will have difficulty expressing needs and responding appropriately to the environment. Interacting with persons who have conditions that impair communication requires special thought and sensitivity. Such persons benefit greatly when the nurse adapts communication techniques to their unique circumstances (Box 13-6). There are many communication aids available to encourage, enhance, restore, or substitute for verbal communication. The nurse's actions are directed at meeting the goals and expected outcomes identified in the plan of care. For example, the nurse caring for a client with impaired verbal communication related to cultural differences may provide a table of simple words in the client's language to meet the expected outcome that the client will communicate basic needs to the nursing staff. The nurses use the table to help the client communicate needs such as food, water, toileting, rest, sleep, pain relief, and so forth. The nurse also needs to collaborate with other team members who can help design the best communication strategies. A speech therapist can help the client with aphasia, an interpreter (translator) may be needed for the client who speaks a foreign language, and a psychiatric nurse specialist might help an angry or highly anxious client to communicate.

Good communication will improve the quality of the client's interpersonal relationships and well-being; it is a very important aspect of holistic health. If the client uses ineffective communication techniques that interfere with coping or interpersonal relationships, the nurse should intervene to help the client send, receive, and interpret messages more effectively. Nurses can serve as communication role models and teachers to help such persons express their needs, feelings, and concerns; develop social interaction skills; communicate thoughts and feelings clearly so needs can be met; interpret messages sent from others; and increase feelings of autonomy and assertiveness. Methods such as role playing can allow clients to practice situations in which they have difficulty communicating.

Providing alternative communication methods. Clients with physical communication barriers (e.g., those with a laryngectomy or endotracheal tube) may be unable to speak, or the clarity of speech may be so poor that alternative methods of communication are needed (see Box 13-6). For these clients the nurse should provide simple communication methods. Anything complicated can be frustrating and make communication more difficult. The nurse should be patient as the client tries to communicate. The client must be able to physically use the method the nurse provides (e.g., communication boards, pencil and pad). A client who is unable to speak can be at risk for injury unless personal needs can be quickly communicated.

Communicating with children. Communication with a child requires special considerations so the nurse can develop a working relationship with the child and family. The nurse receives much information about a child from parents. Because contact between parent and child is usually close, the information communicated by parents can be assumed to be reliable, although some parents may exaggerate. If the client is a

Box 13-6
Communicating With Clients Having Special Needs

Clients With Difficulty Hearing

Avoid shouting.

Use simple sentences.

Punctuate speech with facial expressions and gestures.

Clients With Difficulty Seeing

Communicate verbally before touching the client.

Orient the client to sounds in the environment.

Inform the client when the conversation is over and when you are leaving the room.

Clients Who Are Mute or Cannot Speak Clearly

Place sign by unit call system to answer call light in person.

Listen attentively, be patient, and do not interrupt.

Do not finish clients' sentences for them.

Ask simple questions that require "yes" or "no" answers.

Allow time for understanding and responses.

Use visual cues (e.g., words, pictures, objects) when possible.

Allow only one person to speak at a time.

Do not shout or speak too loudly.

Encourage the client to converse.

Let the client know if you do not understand.

Use communication aids as needed:

  Pad and felt-tipped pen or magic slate

  Flash cards

  Communication board with words, letters, or pictures denoting basic needs

  Computer toy ("speak and spell" type)

  Call bells or alarms

  Sign language

  Use of eye blinks or movement of fingers for simple responses ("yes" or "no")

Clients Who Are Cognitively Impaired

Reduce environmental distractions while conversing.

Get the client's attention before speaking.

Use simple sentences and avoid long explanations.

Avoid shifting from subject to subject.

Ask one question at a time.

Allow time for the client to respond.

Include family and friends in conversations, especially in subjects known to the client.

Clients Who Are Unresponsive

Call the client by name during interactions.

Communicate both verbally and by touch.

Speak to the client as though he or she could hear.

Explain all procedures and sensations.

Clients Who Do Not Speak English

Speak to the client in a normal tone of voice (shouting may be interpreted as anger).

Establish a method for the client to signal the desire to communicate (call light or bell).

Provide an interpreter (translator) as needed:

  Use a person familiar with the client's culture and with biomedicine if possible.

  Allow plenty of time for the interpreter to transmit messages.

  Communicate directly to the client and family rather than the interpreter.

  Ask one question at a time.

  Avoid making comments to the interpreter about the client or family (they may understand some English).

Develop a communication board, pictures, or cards using words translated into English for the client to make basic requests (e.g., pain medication, water, elimination).

Have a dictionary (English/Spanish and so forth) available if the client can read.

---

young child, it helps to offer the child toys or materials so the parent can give full attention to the nurse. The nurse gives periodic attention to infants and younger children as they play to make them participants. An older child can be actively involved in communication. To communicate effectively with children, the nurse must understand the influence of development on language and thought processes. Both factors affect the way a child communicates and the manner in which the nurse can successfully engage a child in an interaction (see Chapter 20).

Children, particularly the young, are especially responsive to nonverbal messages. Sudden movements or threatening gestures can frighten a child. The nurse walking into an examination room with a broad grin and animated hand movements will likely inhibit the formation of a relationship with a child. The nurse should remain calm and gentle. It helps to let the child make the first move in interpersonal contacts. A quiet, friendly, confident tone of voice is best when interacting with a child. Children do not like people to stare at them. Adults looking down on them make them feel vulnerable. While communicating with a young child, the nurse should meet the child at eye level. The child feels helpless in most situations involving health care personnel.

When it is necessary to give explanations or directions, the nurse uses simple, direct language. The nurse must be honest. Deceiving a child into thinking a painful procedure is painless will only make the child angry. To minimize fear and anxiety immediately before a procedure begins, a child should always be told what to expect.

Drawing and play are two effective ways of communicating with young children (Figure 13-2). Drawing allows the child to communicate nonverbally (by making the drawing) and verbally (by explaining the picture). The nurse can use a child's drawing as a basis for beginning a conversation.

Communicating with older adult clients.
Because of sensory disturbances and motor disabilities, older adults often have communication problems. Sensory alterations prevent them from receiving messages clearly. Motor disturbances such as dysarthria interfere with speech clarity. Many older adults adapt to sensory losses (see Chapter 38) and can learn to communicate effectively. When obvious deficits exist, the nurse maximizes existing motor and sensory function so the client can communicate more effectively (see Box 13-6 on p. 219).

Ebersole and Hess (1994) indicate that older adults may suffer from other sensory deprivations (elimination of order or meaning and restricting the environment to dull monotony) and sensory overload (Box 13-7). The nurse identifies these challenges and works with the client to enhance effective communication.

Evaluation

Client care. Evaluating whether communication has been therapeutic is determined by the client's progress or lack of progress toward goals and expected outcomes. The nurse evaluates if nursing interventions met established outcomes to determine if goals were achieved. If so, interventions were effective. For example, the nurse delivering care to the client with *impaired*

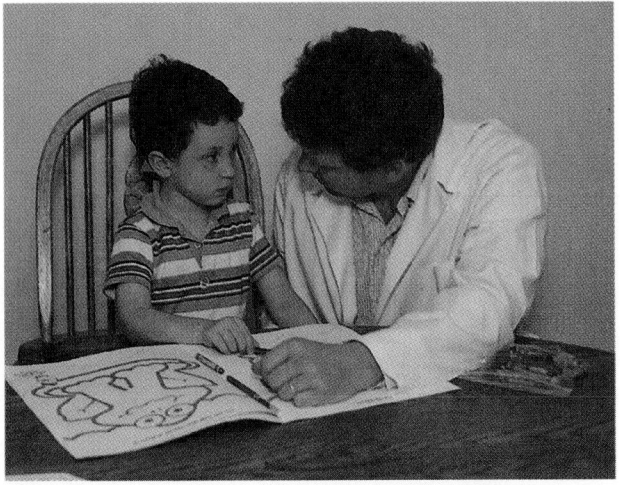

Figure 13-2.   Drawing helps children communicate.

verbal communication related to cerebral dysfunction may have established the goal of the client being able to communicate basic needs (e.g., water, food, toileting). The outcome would then be that the client uses a communication board to request water, food, and assistance with toileting. While caring for the client, the nurse observes whether the client uses the communication board easily and effectively. Was the client able to communicate basic needs with the staff, and thus were the needs met? The nurse might question the client about whether needs were adequately met. If the goal was met, interventions were appropriate for the client. If not, the plan of care should be modified to achieve the goal and outcome. This modification process is ongoing and continues until the time of discharge.

For clients with actual communication alterations, a variety of approaches can be used to evaluate the success of the plan of care. Goals, outcomes, and corresponding evaluative measures for the problem of impaired communication should include client's expectations.

Client expectations. Reviewing the client's expectations of care and determining if these expectations were achieved are also an important part of the evaluation process. This aspect of evaluation can be encouraged by asking clients and their families for input about

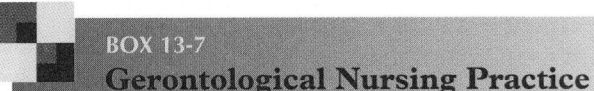

BOX 13-7
Gerontological Nursing Practice

In dealing with impaired communications with older adults, the primary goal is to establish a reliable communication system that is easily understood by all health care team members because nursing care of the older adult is ideally delivered by an interdisciplinary model. Communication with older adults requires special attention. The nurse must be aware of the physical, psychological, and social changes of aging.

The nurse can utilize the following interventions to assist with impaired communication with older adults:

- During conversation, maintain a quiet environment that is free from background noise.
- Avoid shifting from subject to subject; allow time for conversation.
- Be an attentive listener. Use explorative questions to facilitate conversation (e.g., "How do you feel?").
- Avoid long sentences to explain the subject. Try to keep it short, simple, and to the point.
- Allow the older adult the opportunity to reminisce. Reminiscing has therapeutic properties that increase the sense of well-being.
- If you are experiencing problems understanding the client (e.g., dysarthria), let the client know and facilitate methods that help the client speak more clearly. The nurse may need to consult with a speech therapist.
- Include the client's family and friends in conversations, particularly in known subjects to the client.
- Be aware of cultural differences among clients.

goal achievement, factors that affected outcomes, and suggestions for changes that might be made in the plan of care.

Nurse to client: "You wanted to increase your weight. Let's look at what you've accomplished so far with your goal of increasing your calorie intake."

Nurse to client: "Since your calorie intake hasn't increased as much as we would like, let's figure out what's preventing that from happening."

Nurse to client: "John, did it help your appetite to brush your teeth and get up in a chair before eating?"

Avoiding client input into evaluation and its resultant care plan modification leads to a task-oriented approach rather than a critical thinking, client-centered approach to nursing. It denies the client's right to see the total picture of care and to be involved in all phases of the nursing process.

Key Terms

active listening	message
assertive communication	metacommunication
channel	nonverbal communication
communication	perceptual biases
connotative meaning	public communication
denotative meaning	receiver
empathy	referent
environment	sender
feedback	symbolic communication
humor	sympathy
interpersonal communication	therapeutic communication
intrapersonal communication	triangulation
language	verbal communication

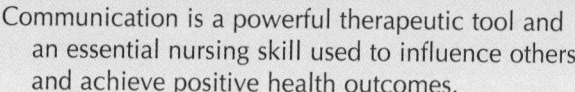

■ Key Concepts

Communication is a powerful therapeutic tool and an essential nursing skill used to influence others and achieve positive health outcomes.

Critical thinking facilitates communication through creative inquiry, focused self-awareness and awareness of others, purposeful analysis, and control of perceptual biases.

Nurses consider many contexts and factors influencing communication when making decisions about what, when, where, how, why, and with whom to communicate.

Communication is most effective when the receiver and sender accurately perceive the meaning of one another's messages.

Message transmission is influenced by the sender's and receiver's physical and developmental status, perceptions, values, emotions, knowledge, sociocultural background, roles, and environment.

Effective verbal communication requires appropriate intonation, clear and concise phrasing, proper pacing of statements, and proper timing and relevance of a message.

Effective nonverbal communication complements and strengthens the message conveyed by verbal communication so that the receiver is less likely to misinterpret the message.

Nurses use intrapersonal, interpersonal, and public interaction to achieve positive change and health goals.

Helping relationships are strengthened when the nurse demonstrates caring by establishing trust, empathy, autonomy, confidentiality, and professional competence.

Effective communication techniques are facilitative and tend to encourage the other person to openly express ideas, feelings, or concerns.

Ineffective communication techniques are inhibiting and tend to block the other person's willingness to openly express ideas, feelings, or concerns.

The nurse must blend social and informational interactions with therapeutic communication techniques so that others can explore feelings and manage health issues.

Methods that facilitate communication with children include sitting at eye level; interacting with parents; using simple, direct language; and incorporating play activities.

Older adult clients with sensory, motor, or cognitive impairments require the adaptation of communication techniques to compensate for their loss of function and special needs.

Clients with impaired verbal communication require special consideration and alterations in communication techniques to facilitate the sending, receiving, and interpreting of messages.

Desired outcomes for clients with impaired verbal communication include increased satisfaction with interpersonal interactions, the ability to send and receive clear messages, and attending to and accurately interpreting verbal and nonverbal cues.

Critical Thinking Activities

1. Walter Jordan is a 34 year old brought to the emergency room with crushing chest pain, shortness of breath, and exercise intolerance. His wife is at his side, in tears, moaning, "He's dying." What factors influencing communication are present in this scenario, and how would they affect the nurse's communication?

2. The nurse takes Mrs. Jordan's arm to escort her to the waiting room. She reacts angrily, wrenching her arm out of the nurse's grasp. What should the nurse do now?

3. The couple's child, a 4-year-old boy, is in the emergency room. His eyes are wide open, his skin is pale, and his eyes are tearing. How would you explain to him what is happening with his father?

4. The Jordans' 16-year-old daughter is pacing and picking at her nails. Construct a way to establish a helping-trust relationship with her.

5. The nurse notices Emily, a team member, going into the bathroom in tears. How can the nurse offer help without invading privacy?

References

American Nurses Association: *Code of ethics with interpretive statements,* Kansas City, Mo, 1985, ANA.

American Philosophical Association: *Critical thinking: a statement of expert consensus for purposes of educational assessment and instruction. The Delphi report: research findings and recommendations prepared for the committee of pre-college philosophy,* Washington, DC, 1990, ERIC.

Anspaugh DJ and others: *Wellness concepts and application,* ed 2, St. Louis, 1994, Mosby.

Balzer-Riley JW: *Communications in nursing,* ed 3, St. Louis, 1996, Mosby.

Beebe SA and others: *Interpersonal communication: relating to others,* Boston, 1996, Allyn & Bacon.

Benner P: *From novice to expert: excellence and power in clinical nursing practice,* Menlo Park, Calif, 1984, Addison-Wesley.

Berko MR and others: *Connecting: a culture-sensitive approach to interpersonal communication competency,* ed 2, Philadelphia, 1997, Harcourt Brace.

Bottorff JL: The use and meaning of touch in caring for patients with cancer, *Oncol Nurs Forum* 20(10):1531, 1993.

Bottorff JL and others: Comforting: exploring the work of cancer nurses, *J Adv Nurs* 22(6):1077, 1995.

Butts JB, Janes S: Transcending the latex barrier: the therapeutics of comfort touch in patients with acquired immunodeficiency syndrome, *Holistic Nurs Pract* 10(1):61, 1995.

Creasia JL, Parker P: *Conceptual foundations of professional nursing practice,* St. Louis, 1996, Mosby.

Davidhizar R, Giger JN: When your patient is silent, *J Adv Nurs* 20(4):703, 1994.

Davidhizar R, Rexroth R: The benefits of triad communication in home health care, *Rehabil Nurs* 19(6):352, 1994.

Ebersole P, Hess P: *Toward a healthy aging: human needs and nursing response,* ed 4, St. Louis, 1994, Mosby.

Edelman CL, Mandle CL: *Health promotion throughout the lifespan,* St. Louis, 1994, Mosby.

Fortinash KM, Holoday-Worret PA: *Psychiatric mental health nursing,* St. Louis, 1996, Mosby.

Griffin E: *A first look at communication theory,* ed 2, New York, 1994, McGraw Hill.

Grossman D: Enhancing your "cultural competence," *Am J Nurs* 94(7):58, 1994.

Huttlinger K and others: "Doing battle": a metaphorical analysis of diabetes mellitus among Navajo people, *Am J Occup Ther* 46(8):706, 1992.

Jambunathan J, Stewart S: Hmong women in Wisconsin: what are their concerns in pregnancy and childbirth? *Birth* 22(4):204, 1995.

Kim MJ and others: *Pocket guide to nursing diagnoses,* ed 6, St. Louis, 1995, Mosby.

King I: *Toward a theory for nursing,* New York, 1971, John Wiley & Sons.

Knapp ML, Vangelisti AL: *Interpersonal communication and human relationships,* ed 3, Boston, 1996, Allyn & Bacon.

Nance TA: Intercultural communication: finding common ground, *J Obstet Gynecol Neonatal Nurs* 24(3):249, 1995.

Perry B: Influence of nurse gender on the use of silence, touch, and humor, *Int J Palliative Nurs* 2(1):7, 1996.

Rousalato P: Non-necessary touch in the nursing care of elderly people, *J Adv Nurs* 23(5):904, 1996a.

Rousalato P: The right to touch and be touched, *Nurs Ethics* 3(2):165, 1996b.

Seed A: Crossing the boundaries—experiences of neophyte nurses, *J Adv Nurs* 21(6):1136, 1995.

Seigel BS: *Peace, love and healing,* New York, 1989, Harper & Row.

Stewart J, Logan C: *Together: communicating interpersonally,* ed 4, New York, 1993, McGraw Hill.

Stuart GW, Sundeen SJ: *Principles and practice of psychiatric nursing,* ed 5, St. Louis, 1995, Mosby.

Watson J: *Nursing: human science and health care,* Norwalk, 1985, Appleton-Century-Crofts.

Wilson GL and others: *Interpersonal communication,* ed 4, Madison, 1995, Brown & Benchmark.

Wood JT: *Gendered relationships,* Mountain View, Calif., 1996, Mayfield.

Wooten P: Jest for the health of it! making humor work, *J Nurs Jocularity* 3:(4)40, 1993.

Yerby J and others: *Understanding family communication,* ed 2, Scottsdale, Ariz, 1995, Gorsuch Scarisbrick.

Documentation and Reporting

OBJECTIVES

Mastery of content in this chapter will enable the student to:

- Define the key terms listed.
- Describe multidisciplinary communication within the health care team.
- Identify purposes of health care records.
- Discuss legal guidelines for recording.
- Identify ways to maintain confidentiality of records and reports.
- Describe six guidelines for quality documentation and reporting.
- Describe different methods used in documentation.
- Describe case management and critical paths as related to documentation.
- Identify common record-keeping forms.
- Discuss advantages and disadvantages of standardized documentation forms.
- Identify elements to include when documenting discharge plans.
- Identify computerized applications for documentation.
- Describe the purpose of change-of-shift reports.
- Explain documentation relating to telephone use.

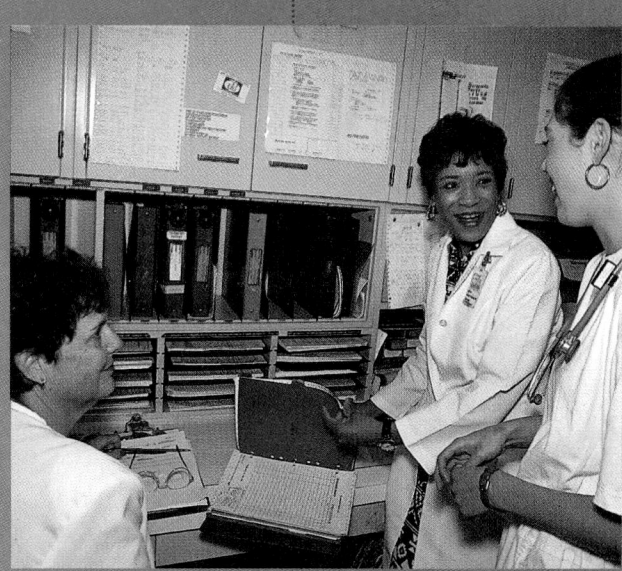

Documentation is a vital aspect of nursing practice. Over time, the format and quality of documentation have evolved with a focus that continues to have a positive impact on client care. At present, one of the most challenging issues in nursing is how to document quality client care within the constraints imposed by regulations, resources, and finances. Nursing documentation has become increasingly important because of fiscal and legal requirements in determining the cost of client care. Regulations require health care institutions to monitor and evaluate the quality and appropriateness of client care. Such monitoring requires a thorough review of the documentation in a client's medical record.

Accreditation agencies such as the Joint Commission on Accreditation of Healthcare Organizations (JCAHO) specify guidelines for the type of information in and the format for documentation. Under the prospective payment system, hospitals are reimbursed a set dollar amount by Medicare for each **diagnosis-related group (DRG)** (see Chapter 2). All interventions performed for a client should be documented in the medical record (e.g., assessments, administration of medications, changing dressings). If the documentation is incomplete, a health care institution may not be reimbursed for its costs.

The health care environment creates many challenges for accurately documenting and reporting the care delivered to clients. The quality of care deserved by clients, the standards of regulatory agencies, the reimbursement structure in the health care system, and the legal guidelines for nursing practice make documentation and reporting two of the most important functions of a nurse. Any information about a client's care should be communicated with careful thought. All members of the health care team depend on recorded and reported information. Accurate information ensures continuity and quality of care.

MULTIDISCIPLINARY COMMUNICATION WITHIN THE HEALTH CARE TEAM

Client care requires proficient communication among members of the health care team. The quality of client care depends on the care givers' ability to communicate with one another. Care givers use a variety of ways to exchange information about clients. The nurse is held accountable for the accuracy of documentation entered into the client's record.

Reports are oral, written, or audiotape exchanges of information shared between care givers in a number of ways. After completing a work shift, nurses give a verbal report to nurses on the next shift. A pharmacist may call a nursing unit to clarify a written prescription on a client's medications for the day. The laboratory submits a written report describing the results of diagnostic tests for inclusion in the permanent medical record.

A **record** is a permanent written communication that documents information relevant to a client's health care management (e.g., a clinic record or chart). After each home visit, clinic visit, or consultation, information about the client's health care is recorded. With each successive visit, the record is available to the physician and other members of the health care team. It is a continuing account of the client's health care status and needs.

Another way that information is communicated is through discussions among team members. Discussions may be informal or formal. They allow a review of information so that problems are identified and solutions are recommended. A formal discussion, for example, is a discharge planning conference in a restorative care unit. The members of all disciplines (e.g., nursing, social work, medicine, physical therapy) meet to discuss the client's progress toward established discharge goals.

Consultations are another form of discussion whereby one professional care giver gives formal advice about client care. For example, a family nurse practitioner confers with a staff nurse about the best choice of nonmedicinal therapies for controlling chronic back pain. Another example of a consultation is when a staff nurse consults with a dietitian in the selection of the best diet therapy for a client with a diagnosis of diabetes. Consultations should be documented in a client's permanent record so that all care givers can benefit and plan care accordingly.

··DOCUMENTATION

Documentation is important in health care. Many types of records are used to convey information about the client's health status and care. **Documentation** is defined as anything written or printed that is a record or proof of activities. Good documentation reflects the quality of care and evidence of each health care team member's accountability in giving care. Although each agency uses a different record format, all records contain basically the same information (Box 14-1).

Purpose of Records

The record is a valuable source of data used by all members of the health care team. Its purposes include communication, legal documentation, financial billing, education, assessment, research, and auditing and monitoring.

Communication. The record is a means by which health care team members communicate client needs and contributions to the client's care, including individual therapies, client and family education, and use of referrals for discharge planning. The record explains measures needed for continuity and consistency of care. The record provides additional data to identify and support nursing diagnoses and plan appropriate interventions. The record also includes the client's re-

General Information Contained in a Medical Record

Client identification and demographic data
Informed consent for treatment and procedures
Admission nursing history
Nursing diagnoses or problems
Nursing or multidisciplinary care plan
Record of nursing care treatment and evaluation
Medical history
Medical diagnoses
Therapeutic orders
Medical and health discipline's progress notes
Reports of physical examinations
Reports of diagnostic studies
Summary of operative procedures
Discharge plan and summary

sponses to interventions and consequent modifications in the plan of care.

Legal documentation. The client's record is a legal document, and contents of the record document the level of care provided for a client. A record that is thorough and accurate is one of the best defenses for legal claims associated with health care. Clients have the right to review their records, and each institution has policies for controlling the manner in which records are shared.

Recording should not become merely routine or superficial, and the nurse must understand the legal implications of documentation. Malpractice litigation has shown four common communication problem areas caused by inadequate documentation: (1) not charting the correct time when events occurred, (2) failing to record verbal orders or have them signed, (3) charting actions in advance, and (4) documenting incorrect data (Martin, 1994). Table 14-1 lists legal guidelines for recording.

Financial billing. The patient care record is a document that shows the extent to which health care agencies should be reimbursed for services. DRGs have become the basis for establishing reimbursement for client care. Effective nursing documentation can verify the client care provided to justify the reimbursement to health care agencies.

Education. A client's record contains a variety of information (e.g., medical and nursing diagnoses, signs and symptoms of disease, successful and unsuccessful therapies, diagnostic findings, client behaviors). An ef-

fective way to learn the nature of an illness and the client's response to the illness is to read the client care record. Patterns of information can be identified in clients with similar medical problems. Health care team members can learn patterns and be able to anticipate the type of care a client may require.

Assessment. Information from the record adds to the nurse's observations and assessment. The record provides data that nurses use to identify and support nursing diagnoses and plan proper interventions for care. The initial admission nursing assessment, for example, is in the record. Thus it is unnecessary for the nurse to collect information that is already available unless there is reason to believe that the information is inaccurate. Previous nursing progress notes detail the nurse's findings at the time of assessment. Before caring for any client, the nurse refers to the client care record for new and relevant assessment findings. The nurse is able to enter a client's room, anticipate the status of the client, and then conduct a holistic assessment of the client. The documentation allows the nurse to note changes from previous assessment findings.

Research. Statistical data can be gathered from client records. Examples are the frequency of clinical disorders, complications, use of specific medical and nursing therapies, recoveries from illnesses, and mortality. Records are a valuable resource for describing client populations. A nurse may use a client's records during a research study to collect information that describes the client's health problem. For example, if nurses suspect that early extubation decreases the complications in post–cardiac surgery clients, the client records could be examined to evaluate that supposition.

Auditing and monitoring. A regular review of information in client records gives a basis for evaluation of the quality and appropriateness of client care. The JCAHO requires hospitals to establish quality-improvement programs to conduct objective, ongoing reviews of client care. The JCAHO has standards for the types of information found in the client's record. Discharge planning and client education are both evaluated by JCAHO standards.

The JCAHO asks institutions to establish standards for quality care. Nurses monitor or review records throughout the year determining whether quality-improvement standards are met. One method of reviewing is the critical pathway, which is often used in case management. It provides an excellent method of organizing an evaluation process while documenting (Smith, 1996). Deficiencies identified during monitoring are shared with all members of the nursing staff so that corrections in policy or practice can be made. Quality-improvement programs keep nurses informed of standards of nursing practice to maintain excellence in nursing care (see Chapter 9).

TABLE 14-1
Legal Guidelines for Recording

Guideline	Rationale	Correct Action
Do not erase, apply correction fluid, or completely obliterate errors made while recording.	Charting becomes illegible. It may appear as though you were attempting to hide information or deface record.	Draw single line through error, write word *error* above it, and sign your name or initials. Then record note correctly.
Do not write retaliatory or critical comments about client or care by other health care professionals.	Statements can be used as evidence for nonprofessional behavior or poor quality of care.	Enter only objective descriptions of client's behavior. Client comments should be quoted.
Correct all errors promptly.	Errors in recording can lead to errors in treatment.	Avoid rushing to complete charting. Be sure information is accurate.
Record only facts.	Record must be accurate and reliable.	Be certain entry is factual. Do not speculate, guess, or assume.
Do not leave blank spaces in nurse's notes.	Another person can add incorrect information in space.	Chart consecutively, line by line. If space is left, draw line horizontally through it and sign your name at end. Do not indent left margin.
Record all entries legibly and in ink.	Illegible entries can be misinterpreted, causing errors and lawsuits. Ink cannot be erased. Records are photocopied and stored on microfilm.	Never erase entries or use correction fluid, and never use pencil.
If order is questioned, record that clarification was sought.	If you perform order known to be incorrect, you are just as liable for prosecution as physician.	Do not record "physician made error." Instead chart that "Dr. Smith was called to clarify order for—."
Chart only for yourself.	You are accountable for information you enter into chart.	Never chart for someone else (exception: if care giver has left unit for day and calls with information).
Avoid using generalized, empty phrases such as "status unchanged" or "had good day."	Specific information about client's condition or case can be accidentally deleted if information is too generalized.	Use complete, concise descriptions of care.
Begin each entry with complete date, time, and end with your signature and title.	This ensures that correct sequence of events is recorded. Signature documents who is accountable for care delivered.	Do not wait until end of shift to record important changes that occurred several hours earlier. Be sure to sign each entry.

GUIDELINES FOR QUALITY DOCUMENTATION AND REPORTING

The nurse is responsible for ensuring that all information needed for nursing care is documented. Six important guidelines must be followed for quality recording and reporting: factual basis, accuracy, completeness, currentness, organization, and confidentiality.

Factual Basis
Information documented about clients and their care must be factual. A record should contain descriptive, objective information about what a nurse sees, hears, feels, and smells (Gulanick and others, 1994). Objective data are defined as data that are measured and observed. In a problem-oriented medical record (POMR), an entry describing objective data is labeled with an *O*. The nurse should avoid words such as *appears, seems,* or *apparently* because they lead to conclusions that cannot be supported by objective information.

The nurse should also document subjective information, but only when it is supported by facts. Documentation should clearly explain the nurse's observations of the client's behaviors and not interpret those observations. Subjective data are defined as the verbalizations of the client and in the POMR are labeled with an *S.* Subjective information can be written with quotation marks and in that instance would use the client's own words. For example, "I am hurting and would like something for pain" is factual and acceptable. The nurse can then add any objective findings that more clearly describe the client's pain, such as an increased blood pressure and pulse rate. It would also be acceptable not to use quotation marks when the client's words are paraphrased by the nurse.

Accuracy

A client's record must be accurate so that precise documentation is sustained. The nurse records descriptions such as "Client voided 450 ml clear urine" rather than "Voided an adequate amount." Using precise measurements ensures accuracy in determining whether a client's condition has changed. Using an institution's accepted abbreviations, symbols, and system of measurement ensures that all staff members will use the same language in their documentation. To avoid misunderstandings, write out any abbreviations that may be confusing (e.g., od [once daily] can be interpreted to mean OD [right eye]).

Correct spelling increases the accuracy of documentation and benefits client care. Terms can easily be confused or misinterpreted (e.g., *accept* and *except, dysphagia* and *dysphasia*). Medications such as digitoxin and digoxin must be spelled carefully or a client may receive the wrong medication.

An accurate entry in a client chart reflects observations and client care during a given time frame. Nurses may include observations reported to another care giver and interventions performed by someone else, for example, "Client suctioned by J. Hill, RN. Case manager, R. Frazier, RN, notified of change in secretions."

JCAHO standards (1995) require that "all entries in medical records are dated and authenticated, and a method is established to identify the authors of entries." Therefore any descriptive entry in a client's record ends with the care giver's full name and status, such as "Adria Thompson, RN." Nicknames are not used. A nursing student should enter the full name, student nurse abbreviation, and educational institution, such as "Marianne Gonzales, SN [student nurse], OHSU [Oregon Health Sciences University]." The abbreviation for *student nurse* may be regionally different, being either *NS,* which stands for *nursing student,* or *SN,* which stands for *student nurse.* The signature holds a nurse accountable for information recorded.

Completeness

The information within a recorded entry or report should be complete, concise, and thorough. When reports are incomplete, communication is compromised, and nurses are unable to prove specific care was provided. Concise information is easy to understand, and clear, succinct wording makes interpretation easier. An example of completeness in a nursing entry is as follows:

0845 Client verbalizes continuous throbbing pain localized along the lateral aspect of left fractured femur, beginning 10 minutes ago. Pain is increased with movement of the leg, which is elevated in balanced suspension traction. Pin sites remain dry with no signs of warmth or rubor; pedal pulses equal bilaterally; B/P = 132/74, T = 37, P = 92, R = 18. Morphine 10 mg IM given for pain. Sue Jacobs, RN.

Currentness

Timely entries are essential in the client's concurrent care (JCAHO, 1995). Delays in documentation can result in serious omissions and untimely delays in client care. Activities or findings to communicate at the time of occurrence include the following:

1. Vital signs
2. Administration of medications and treatments
3. Preparation for diagnostic tests or surgery
4. Change in client status
5. Admission, transfer, discharge, or death of client
6. Treatment for sudden changes in client status
7. Client response to intervention

Routine activities such as daily hygiene measures do not need to be charted immediately. This information is often included in flow sheets. In addition, writing anecdotal notes at the time of an event helps ensure accuracy. Many agencies use military time, a 24-hour system that uses digit numbers to indicate morning, afternoon, and evening times. Table 14-2 gives examples of military and corresponding civilian times.

Organization

The nurse communicates information in a logical format or order. Health care team members understand information better when it is given in the order in which it occurred. For example, an organized note describes the client's pain, the nurse's assessment, and interventions in a logical order of occurrence. The disorganized

TABLE 14-2
Comparison of Military and Civilian Times

Military	Civilian
0100	1:00 AM
0200	2:00 AM
0245	2:45 AM
1200	Noon
1440	2:40 PM
1700	5:00 PM
2400	Midnight
0001	12:01 AM

note is fragmented and does not clearly explain what happened first. Poorly organized notes can lead to confusion about whether proper care was given. To illustrate, the following is an example of a disorganized nursing note: "Client requesting pain medication. His family is visiting, and his abdominal dressing is dry and intact. Breath sounds clear upon auscultation, and he states he feels better today than he did yesterday. Tess Evans, RN." The nurse's documentation is unclear and confusing in regard to the assessment findings.

Confidentiality

Nurses should not disclose clients' status to other clients or to staff not involved in their care. Nurses are legally and ethically obligated to keep information about clients confidential. Only staff members directly involved in care have legitimate access to the records. Nurses and other health care professionals may have reason to use records for data gathering, research, or continuing education. These uses are not breaks in confidentiality if the records are used as specified and permission is granted from hospital internal review boards.

METHODS OF RECORDING

The documentation system selected by a nursing service should reflect the philosophy of the department and the way nursing care is implemented. Professional charting proves what the nurse has done and communicates the client's status and progress. Because the nursing process shapes a nurse's approach, effective documentation reflects the nursing process.

It is challenging to create a record-keeping system that ensures optimal communication and yet simplifies the charting process. The JCAHO (1995) requires documentation of nursing diagnoses or problems within the context of the nursing process, as well as evidence of client and family teaching and discharge planning. If more than one discipline regularly cares for a client, the JCAHO also expects evidence of a multidisciplinary plan of care. There are many differences in the methods used by health care institutions to organize information. For example, a nursing department may use a framework such as Gordon's functional health patterns (Gordon, 1995). This is a documentation system that uses nursing diagnoses and health patterns in care plans and other forms.

Narrative Documentation

Narrative documentation is the traditional method for nursing care records. It is the use of a storylike format to document information specific to client conditions and nursing care. There is no single "correct" order in which to chart client events. Consequently, nurses chart in varying formats in their use of narrative documentation.

Currently, narrative charting is seldom the primary method of documentation and is being replaced by other formats (e.g., SOAP, PIE, focus). Narrative charting is easy to use in emergency situations where a simple chronological order is needed. However, narrative documentation is seen as the least desirable form of charting in most nursing settings. Among the disadvantages of the narrative style are its likelihood of being subjective, the lack of organized structure, and the lack of analysis and critical decision making on the part of the nurse.

Problem-Oriented Medical Records

The **problem-oriented medical record** (POMR) is a structured method of documentation that places emphasis on the client's problems. The method corresponds to the nursing process and facilitates communication of client needs. Data are organized by problem or diagnosis. Ideally, each member of the health care team contributes to a single list of identified client problems. The POMR is composed of the following: database, problem list, care plan, and progress notes.

Database. The database contains all available assessment information pertaining to the client. This section is the foundation for identifying client problems and planning care. The database should remain active and current, and revisions should be made as new data are available.

Problem list. The problem list is developed after the data are analyzed. The problems are listed in chronological order to serve as an organizing guide for the client's care. New problems are added as they are identified. After a problem has been resolved, the date is recorded, and a line is drawn through the problem and its number. A problem may be well defined, such as a specific NANDA-approved nursing diagnosis.

Care plan. The care plan is developed for each problem by the disciplines involved in the client's care. Nurses document the plan of care in a variety of formats. Generally, these plans of care include nursing diagnoses, expected outcomes, and interventions.

Progress notes. Progress notes are used by health care team members to monitor and record the progress of a client's problems. Narrative notes, flow sheets, and discharge summaries are forms used to document the client's progress.

SOAP documentation. SOAP is an acronym for the POMR method of documentation as follows:

S: Subjective data (verbalizations of the client)
O: Objective data (data that are measured and observed)
A: Assessment (diagnosis based on the data)
P: Plan (what the care giver plans to do)

An *I* and *E* are sometimes added (e.g., SOAPIE) in various institutions. The *I* stands for *intervention,* and the *E* represents *evaluation.* The logic for SOAP(IE) notes is similar to that of the nursing process. Data are collected about each of the client's problems, a conclusion is made, and a care plan is developed. Each SOAP note is numbered and titled according to the problem on the list it addresses.

PIE documentation. The **PIE** documentation format is similar to SOAP charting in its problem-oriented nature. However, it differs from the SOAP method in that PIE charting has a nursing origin, whereas SOAP originated from the medical model. PIE is an acronym for *problem, interventions, evaluation* as follows:

P: Problem or nursing diagnosis applicable to client
I: Interventions or actions taken
E: Evaluation of the outcomes of nursing interventions

This format simplifies documentation by unifying the care plan and progress notes into a complete record. The PIE format differs from SOAP because the narrative note does not include assessment information. Daily assessment data appear instead on special flow sheets, thus preventing duplication of information. The PIE notes can be numbered or labeled according to the client's problems. Resolved problems are dropped from daily documentation after the nurse's review.

Source Records

In a **source record** the client's chart is organized so that each discipline (e.g., nursing, medicine, social work, respiratory therapy) has a separate section in which to record data. Unlike in the POMR, the information is not organized by client problems. The advantage of a source record is that care givers can easily locate the proper section of the record in which to make entries. Components of a source record are summarized in Table 14-3.

A disadvantage of source records is fragmented data. Information is well organized but not according to the client's problems. Details about a particular problem may be distributed throughout the record. For example, in the case of a wound infection, the nurse describes the appearance of the wound in the nurse's notes. The physician notes in a separate section the progress of the wound's healing and the proposed course of therapy. The results of tests measuring growth of bacteria from the wound can be found in the laboratory test section. Thus any data relevant to a single problem may be difficult to locate.

TABLE 14-3
Organization of Traditional Source Record

Sections	Contents
Admission sheet	Specific demographic data about client: legal name, identification number, sex, age, birth date, marital status, occupation and employer, health insurance, nearest relative to notify in an emergency, religious preference, name of attending physician, date and time of admission
Physician's order sheet	Record of physician's orders for treatment and medications, with date, time, and physician's signature
Nurse's admission assessment	Summary of nursing history and physical examination
Graphic sheet and flow sheet	Record of repeated observations and measurements such as vital signs, daily weights, and intake and output
Medical history and examination	Results of initial examination performed by physician, including findings, family history, confirmed diagnoses, and medical plan of care
Nurses' notes	Narrative record of nursing process: assessment, nursing diagnosis, planning, implementation, and evaluation of care
Medication records	Accurate documentation of all medications administered to client: date, time, dose, route, and nurse's signature
Physician's progress notes	Ongoing record of client's progress and response to medical therapy and review of disease process
Health care discipline's records	Entries made into record by all health-related disciplines: radiology, social work, and laboratories
Discharge summary	Summary of client's condition, progress, prognosis, rehabilitation, and teaching needs at time of dismissal from hospital or health care agency

In the source record the nurse charts a narrative description of nursing care delivered. In a hospital, entries are made in the client's record during each shift of duty. If a client is seen in a clinic or at home, the nurse documents the care provided during each visit or telephone contact. The nurse's description summarizes important observations relating to the client's condition, nursing care, and evaluation of response.

Charting by Exception

Charting by exception (CBE) is an innovative approach to streamline documentation. Charting by exception reduces repetition and time spent in charting. It is a shorthand method for documenting normal findings and routine care based on clearly defined standards of practice and predetermined criteria for nursing assessments and interventions. A nurse need only document significant findings or exceptions to the predefined norms. In other words, the nurse writes a longhand note only when the standardized statement on the form is not met. Assessments are standardized on forms so that all care givers evaluate and document findings consistently. The assumption with charting by exception is that all standards are met with a normal or expected response unless otherwise documented. When nurses see entries in the chart, they know that something out of the ordinary has been observed or occurred. For that reason, when changes in a client's condition have developed, it is easy to track them.

Focus Charting

Focus charting allows the documentation of any client situation. Each entry includes data, actions, and client response **(DAR)** for the particular client situation (Table 14-4). Focus charting moves away from charting only problems and does not label client concerns as "problems." In addition, focus charting does not require the use of formalized nursing diagnoses. This allows for greater flexibility in client documentation. Examples of focus charting include a sign or symptom, a condition, a nursing diagnosis, a behavior, a significant event, or an acute change in a client's condition.

Case Management Plan and Critical Pathways

The case management model of delivering care incorporates a multidisciplinary approach to documenting client care (Tahan and Cesta, 1995). The standardized plan of care is summarized into **critical pathways** within a **case management plan.** Case management plans are one- to two-page multidisciplinary integrated care plans for the problems, key interventions, and expected outcomes of the client with a specific disease or condition (see Figure 14-1 on pp. 232-233). The nurse and other health care team members use the critical pathway to monitor the client's progress during client care. All care givers use one critical pathway as a monitoring and documentation tool. Critical pathways incorporated into documentation tools can be developed to eliminate other nursing forms and thus reduce duplication and the amount of charting (Lavin and Enright, 1996).

The critical pathways are used on each shift of care to direct and monitor the flow of client care. The critical pathways define client-focused outcomes and specify those interventions necessary for a given day of care. Due to the nature of human response, there are **variances** in the client outcomes as the client deviates from the critical path plan. These variances refer to either positive or negative changes, depending on the clinical situation (Tahan and Cesta, 1995). A positive variance occurs when a client progresses more rapidly than the case management plan expected (e.g., a nasogastric tube may be discontinued a day early). A negative variance occurs when the activities on the clinical pathway are not completed as predicted or the client does not meet the expected outcomes. An example of a negative variance is the addition of oxygen therapy and oximetry for a postoperative client experiencing pulmonary problems. A variance analysis is necessary to review the data

TABLE 14-4			
Examples of Focus Charting			
Date	Time	Focus	Data, Actions, Client Response (DAR)
6/20/96	8:20 AM	Hypotension	D—BP in left arm 90/60; client's skin diaphoretic; client responds to name.
			A—Client placed in Trendelenburg position; IV fluid rate increased to 100 ml/hr per protocol; Dr. Arkin notified.
			R—Client remains responsive; BP in left arm 94/68, 3 min after increasing fluids. S. Wilson, RN
6/30/96	4:20 PM	Pain	D—Twisting in bed; grimacing with movement; states has sharp lower back pain.
			A—Morphine sulfate 10 mg IM given.
			R—Verbalized relief within 15 minutes; lying quietly. T. Newson, RN

TABLE 14-5
Example of Variance Documentation in Open Text Format

A 76-year-old client is on a surgical unit 1 day after cholecystectomy. He is beginning to have an elevated temperature, his breath sounds are decreased bilaterally in the bases of both lobes of the lungs, and he is slightly confused. The following is an example of the variance documentation for this client.

Date/Time	Variance	Reason	Comments/Plan
9/23/95 10:00 AM	Decreased breath sounds	Decreased respiratory rate due to incisional pain	Administer oxygen 2 L per physician's protocol
	Elevated temperature	Bilateral consolidation of secretions in bases of both lung lobes	Place continuous pulse oximetry on client; monitor vital signs every hour
	Mental confusion	Decreased oxygenation	Frequently assess client's cerebellar function

for trends and developing and implementing an action plan to respond to the identified client problems (Table 14-5). Deviations from the case management plan can be classified into operational-, community-, practitioner-, or client-caused variances. The nurse's responsibility is to determine why the problem arose and to "correct" the client change (variance) or to justify the actions taken to manage the critical path deviation (Iyer and Camp, 1995).

As the use of critical pathways is refined, the ultimate beneficiary is the client. More accuracy of predicted outcomes will evolve, and variations in client progress will be more easily determined (Sowell and Meadows, 1994). This will potentiate the proactive nature of client care. In addition, there are advantages of multidisciplinary involvement in the plans and interventions for the client (Box 14-2).

Box 14-2
Benefits of Case Management and Critical Pathways

Continuity of care is more easily communicated.
Novice health care providers are given a structure within which to provide care.
Clients are integral to the planning process.
The entire health care team is involved in all phases of client care.
Discharge planning and teaching begin very early in the client care process.
A more creative critical decision–making process is encouraged, which leads to better client outcomes.

Common Record-Keeping Forms
The client chart comprises a variety of forms to make documentation easy, quick, and comprehensive. Duplication within the record should be avoided.

Admission nursing history forms. Admission nursing history forms provide baseline data for later comparisons with changes in the client's condition. The form allows the admitting nurse to make a thorough assessment (e.g., biographical data, holistic assessment, review of health risk factors) and to identify relevant nursing diagnoses or problems for the client's care pathway. Each institution designs nursing history forms based on its standards of practice and philosophy of nursing care. Figure 14-2 on p. 234 is an example of an admission nursing history form.

Graphic sheets and flow sheets. Flow sheets allow documentation of certain routine observations or specific measurements made repeatedly. It is unnecessary to chart a narrative note each time a drug or bath is given. The flow sheets are a quicker and more efficient way to record information. Figure 14-3 on p. 235 is an example of a nursing assessment flow sheet.

The only time the nurse includes information from a flow sheet in other nursing documentation is when a significant change results. For example, if a client's blood pressure becomes dangerously high, the nurse may record the pressure and the medication administered to lower the pressure in the progress note. Subsequent evaluation of the client's blood pressure and additional interventions are included. Flow sheets provide a quick and easy reference for assessing changes in a client's status. Critical care units commonly use flow sheets for many types of data. Flow sheets are part of the permanent record.

BARNES		CARE PATH® 405 MULTIPLE SCLEROSIS EXACERBATION			1

SERVICE **NEUROLOGY** PHYSICIAN

PRIMARY NURSE   PRIMARY NURSE

DC DATE   ADM DATE   DATE OF SURGERY   **A-8**

Problem Number	PATIENT PROBLEMS / NURSING DIAGNOSES
#1	SELF CARE DEFICIT R/T MUSCLE WEAKNESS, PAIN, COORDINATION OR PARALYSIS
#2	IMPAIRED PHYSICAL MOBILITY R/T MUSCLE WEAKNESS
#3	ALTERATION IN ELIMINATION R/T NEUROMUSCULAR IMPAIRMENT
#4	LACK OF KNOWLEDGE R/T UNFAMILIARITY WITH TREATMENT AND DISEASE PROCESS

* IF APPROPRIATE

DATE	#	1, 2 ASSESSMENT / MONITORING	1, 2 CONSULTS	3 PROCEDURES / TEST	1, 2, 3 TREATMENT	1 ACTIVITY
	DAY 1	Assess for fall prevention Assess for skin breakdown Assess neuro status and information processing Assess urinary elimination Assess bowel function VS q shift with NC Notify House Officer for Temp ≥ 37.9 Malaise, change in bladder habits, weakness Monitor VS q 30 min. during 1st dose of Solumedrol infusion. House Officer to remain with pt. for 1st 15 min. of infusion.	Physical Therapy evaluation *Occupational Therapy *Social Work *Pastoral Care *Speech-communication and swallow	EKG prior to 1st dose of Solumedrol and after 1st dose completed *MRI *LP Straight cath for PVR *Straight cath q 6 hrs. Guaiac all stools Notify House Officer if + on guaiac Monitor blood glucose 2 hrs. after Solumedrol Notify House Officer if ≥ 250 I & O	Urinalysis	Up with assist Out of bed in chair at least TID for ½ hr. periods
	DAY 2	Assess for fall prevention Assess for skin breakdown Assess neuro status and information processing Assess urinary elimination Assess bowel function Notify House Officer if no BM after 48 hrs. VS routine with NC Notify House Officer for Temp ≥ 37.9 Malaise, change in bladder habits, weakness **Skin remains intact** **Pt. maintains bowel function** **Pt. remains free of injury**	Evaluation completed Frequency of tx and pain established Social Work-Consult Occupational Therapy to address functional performance *Foot care nurse if indicated	Speech-Functional communication established Bedside swallow evaluation completed within 24 hrs. **Stool remains guaiac negative**		
		SIGNATURE	INIT.	SIGNATURE	INIT.	SIGNATURE	INIT.

405

Figure 14-1. Portion of critical path for multiple sclerosis exacerbation. (Courtesy Barnes-Jewish Hospital, St. Louis.)

| | | | | | 2 |

BARNES

CARE PATH® 405
MULTIPLE SCLEROSIS
EXACERBATION

CNS	DIETARY	RT
HOME HEALTH	OT	OTHER
PT	SW	OTHER

A-8

Problem Number	PATIENT PROBLEMS / NURSING DIAGNOSES

1, 2, 3	2	4	1, 2, 3, 4	1, 2, 4	INITIALS (SEE KEY AT BOTTOM)		
MEDS / IVS	NUTRITION	PATIENT / FAMILY EDUCATION	DISCHARGE PLANNING	PSYCHOSOCIAL/ EMOTIONAL/ SPIRITUAL NEEDS			
IV-Hep lock flush q shift with NS Solumedrol 250mg/100cc NS q 6 hrs.-given over ½-1 hr. times 12-30 doses Zantac 150 mg PO BID Oscal 500 mg with Vit. D - 1 tab BID Docusate Sodium 100 mg q hs Mylanta 30cc PO pc and hs Dalmane 15-30 mg or Restoril 15-30 mg q hs	*Low sodium Advance diet as tolerated Maintain hydration	Orient to unit Provide information on Solumedrol therapy **Pt. verbalizes understanding of Solumedrol Protocol and IV Therapy**	**Pt./family understands goal of therapy. Pt./family verbalizes understanding of disease process. Pt./family understands safety needs. Pt./family verbalizes understanding of care path. Plan of care has been mutually set with pt./family.**	*Social Work for crises intervention *Pastoral Care- emotional and spiritual			
Evaluate time schedule for Solumedrol to minimize sleep interruption	**Pt. caloric needs met body weight maintained. Pt. adequate fluid intake of 3,000/day.**		Social Work- consult with nursing, MD, and therapists to assess pt. needs. Social Work assessment completed.	Pastoral Care- Pt./family support needs assessed. **Social Work- high risk screening form completed.**			
SIGNATURE	INIT.	SIGNATURE	INIT.	SIGNATURE	INIT.		

Figure 14-1, cont'd   Critical path for multiple sclerosis exacerbation.

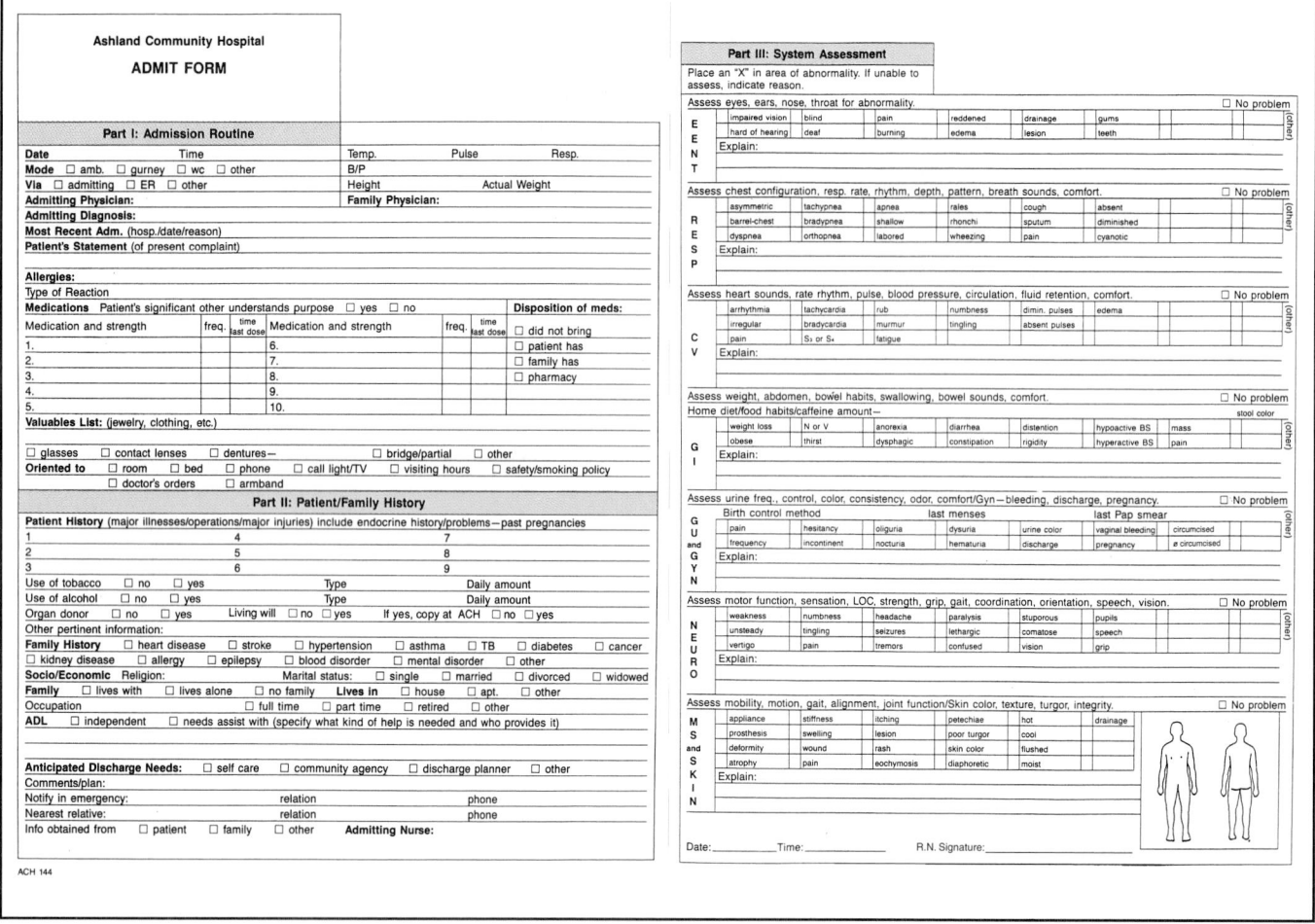

Figure 14-2.   Admission form. (Courtesy Ashland Community Hospital, Ashland, Ore.)

Kardex and client care summary. Nursing information needed for the daily care of a client is readily accessible in a nursing **Kardex.** This is a flip-over card file usually kept at the nurse's station. It often has two parts: an activity and treatment section and a nursing care plan section. The Kardex contains information concerning the client's current ongoing plan of care. The updated information in the Kardex eliminates the need for the nurse to refer continually to the client's chart. Many hospitals now have computerized systems that provide this same information in the form of a client care summary. This is printed for each client during each shift. Data are automatically updated as orders are entered and as nursing decisions are made. Information commonly found in the Kardex or client care summary includes the following:

1. Basic demographic data (name, age, sex)
2. Primary medical diagnosis
3. Current physician's orders to be implemented with the client (e.g., diet, activity, vital signs, medications, diagnostic tests)

4. A nursing care plan
5. Nursing orders or nursing interventions (e.g., intake and output, positioning, comfort measures, teaching)
6. Scheduled tests and procedures
7. Safety precautions used in the client's care
8. Factors related to activities of daily living

Twenty-four-hour client care records and acuity charting forms. Consolidation of the nursing records into a system that accommodates a 24-hour period is often utilized. According to Addy-Keller and McElwaney (1993), a 24-hour record-keeping system is essential in the elimination of unnecessary record-keeping forms. Accurate assessment information and documentation of activities of daily living are more easily obtained with 24-hour notations. In addition, 24-hour client care records often utilize flow sheets and checklists to further enhance efficiency.

Twenty-four-hour client care records are also foundational for an **acuity charting** system. Acuity charting requires staff to document their interventions and

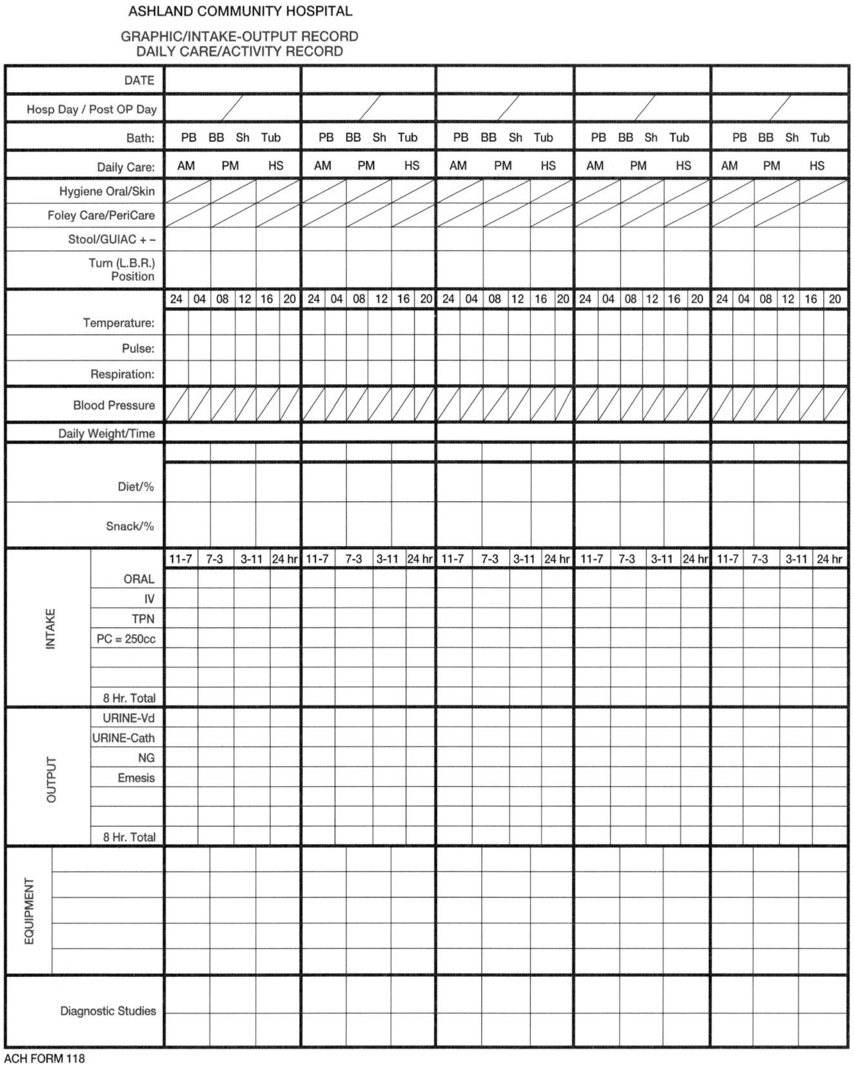

ASHLAND COMMUNITY HOSPITAL
GRAPHIC/INTAKE-OUTPUT RECORD
DAILY CARE/ACTIVITY RECORD

DATE					
Hosp Day / Post OP Day					
Bath:	PB BB Sh Tub	PB BB Sh Tub	PB BB Sh Tub	PB BB Sh Tub	PB BB Sh Tub
Daily Care:	AM PM HS	AM PM HS	AM PM HS	AM PM HS	AM PM HS
Hygiene Oral/Skin					
Foley Care/PeriCare					
Stool/GUIAC + −					
Turn (L.B.R.) Position					
	24 04 08 12 16 20	24 04 08 12 16 20	24 04 08 12 16 20	24 04 08 12 16 20	24 04 08 12 16 20
Temperature:					
Pulse:					
Respiration:					
Blood Pressure					
Daily Weight/Time					
Diet/%					
Snack/%					
	11-7 7-3 3-11 24 hr	11-7 7-3 3-11 24 hr	11-7 7-3 3-11 24 hr	11-7 7-3 3-11 24 hr	11-7 7-3 3-11 24 hr
INTAKE — ORAL					
IV					
TPN					
PC = 250cc					
8 Hr. Total					
OUTPUT — URINE-Vd					
URINE-Cath					
NG					
Emesis					
8 Hr. Total					
EQUIPMENT					
Diagnostic Studies					

ACH FORM 118

Figure 14-3. Nursing assessment flow sheet. (Courtesy Ashland Community Hospital, Ashland, Ore.)

thereby obtain an overall level of acuity for each client. The acuity level determined by the nursing care allows clients to be rated in comparison to one another. For example, an acuity system might rate clients from 1 to 5 (1 is high, 5 is low). A client returning from surgery with multisystem problems is an acuity level 1. On the same continuum, another client awaiting discharge after a very successful recovery from surgery is an acuity level 5. Staffing patterns can then be determined by examining the acuity levels of the clients on a particular nursing unit. The client to staff ratios depend on a composite gathering of data in regard to the 24-hour interventions necessary for implementing care.

Standardized care plans. Many institutions use **standardized care plans** to make documentation more efficient for nurses. The plans, based on the institution's standards of nursing practice, are preprinted estab-lished guidelines used to care for clients with similar health problems. After a nursing assessment is completed, the staff nurse identifies the standard care plans appropriate for the client. The care plans are placed in the client's record. Modifications can be made to individualize nursing activities. Most standardized plans also allow the nurse to insert specific desired outcomes and the dates when these outcomes should be achieved.

Standardized care plans are generally prepared by a group of expert clinicians, which results in sophisticated plans. Standard care plans also educate nurses about the nursing care of a client with a particular nursing diagnosis (Coenen and others, 1996). These standards can be useful for quality improvement audits.

Controversy exists over the use of standardized care plans. The major disadvantage is the risk that they inhibit nurses' identification of unique, individualized interventions for clients. A second disadvantage is the need to formally update the plans routinely to ensure that content is current and appropriate. When standardized care plans are used in a health care facility, the nurse remains responsible for an individualized approach to care. Standardized care plans are not meant to replace the nurse's professional judgment and decision making.

Discharge summary forms. Much emphasis is placed on preparing a client for a timely discharge from a health care institution (Ebert and Bethel, 1996). Ideally, discharge planning begins at admission and in some cases even before admission, as is necessary with same-day surgery admissions and childbirth. Nurses continue discharge planning as the client's condition changes. Clients and family should be involved in the discharge planning process.

A discharge summary form provides important information pertaining to the client's continued health care after discharge (Lowenstein and Hoff, 1994). The reason for hospitalization, significant findings, client's status, and any specific teaching plan is given to the client and/or family (JCAHO, 1995). Discharge summary forms (Figure 14-4) make the summary concise and instructive. Many forms include a copy that is given to a client, family member, or home health care nurse. Home health care agencies or extended nursing care facilities can also benefit from receiving information on the summary forms (Box 14-3) to ensure better continuity of care.

Home Health Care Documentation

The overriding challenge in the current home health care environment is to enhance quality within constraints imposed by limited resources (Adams and Biggerstaff, 1995). In addition, the home health care business continues to grow as the growing proportions of older adults require an ever increasing use of home care services. Medicare has specific guidelines for establishing eligibility for home care reimbursement. In the fulfillment of these Medicare guidelines, documentation by home health care nurses has become the largest problem area: 50% of the nursing time is spent in documentation (Braunstein, 1993). Documentation in the home care system has different implications than in other areas of nursing. The primary difference is the

DATE	TIME	Temp	Pulse	Resp	B/P	Admitted From:
Wt.	Ht.				L / R	

Reason for Admission | Emergency Contact
Allergies & Reactions
Medications taken at home (include over the counter)
Meds Taken Today?
Past medical/surgical history: Hx TB Yes No Uncertain Hx Positive Skin Test Yes No Uncertain Hx Hepatitis Yes No
Teaching Needs?
Orientation to Unit Yes No (Safety precaution letter / call light & TV control / valuables / bed operation & lights / telephone / visiting hours / closet & table)

Physical Aids Used (circle) None	With Patient on Admission	
Cane / crutches / walker / wheel chair / Prosthesis	Yes	No
Glasses / contacts	Yes	No
Hearing Aid	Yes	No
Dentures: Full Upper Lower	Yes	No
Partial Upper Lower	Yes	No

Valuables: Bedside Home Safe | Diet at Home?
Tobacco Use: Yes No Amount Alcohol Use: Yes No Amount Street Drug Use: Yes No Amount
Usual Physical Problems (circle / brief explanation) None Urination ______ Bowels Walking Eating

ASSESSMENT (Document Abnormalities)

SKIN: WNL = Warm, dry, intact, IV 0 phlebitis, incision clean ☐ WNL ☐ ABNORMAL (explain)
GI: WNL = Abdomen soft, nondistended, nontender ☐ WNL ☐ ABNORMAL (explain) LAST BM ______
NEURO: WNL = Alert, oriented, PERL, MAE, grips equal and strong ☐ WNL ☐ ABNORMAL (explain)
GU: WNL = Continent of clear yellow urine ☐ WNL ☐ ABNORMAL (explain) ☐ FOLEY ☐ SUPRA PUBIC
CARDIOVASCULAR: WNL = apical pulse reg, & pedal pulses, 0 edema ☐ WNL ☐ ABNORMAL (explain)
MUSCULOSKELETAL: Swelling, Deformities of Spine & Extremities, Gait, Need for Prosthesis ☐ WNL ☐ ABNORMAL (explain)
PULMONARY: WNL = Respirations regular, unlabored, breathsounds clear bilat. ☐ WNL ☐ ABNORMAL (explain)
I.V.? YES NO TYPE / SITE:
COMMENTS: ______

DATE: TIME: RN: LPN ______
INCLUDES COMPLETION OF SIDE 2 (ADMISSION) CNA ______
N-29 (REV. 6/95)

ROGUE VALLEY MEDICAL CENTER
a member of Asante health system
NURSING ADMISSION/DISCHARGE DATA

FALL PRECAUTION CHECKLIST: **(IF ANY RISK FACTORS - INITIATE FALL ALERT)**
- ☐ Confused/disoriented
- ☐ Unsteady on feet
- ☐ Weakness/lethargy (can be secondary to anemia/bleeding/ fluid deficit/malnutrition/recent surgery, etc.)
- ☐ Takes meds affecting mentation
- ☐ Psychological problems that affect mobility
- ☐ Utilizes any device to assist with mobility (cane, walker, brace or other prosthesis)
- ☐ History of previous falls/syncope
- ☐ History of drug/alcohol abuse
- ☐ Other physical disabilities that impair mobility
- ☐ Needs frequent assistance for elimination activities
- ☐ NO FALL RISK

Before admission Patient lived: Alone With Family With other Help Foster Home at Extended Care Facility Other
Anticipated discharge destination: Home Rehabilitation Extended Care Facility Foster Home Other
Are You worried about taking care of yourself when you go home? Yes No
Help needed after discharge? Yes No Unknown at this time Agency
Anticipated Available Help: Spouse Family Other None
Family / significant other to include in teaching: None Yes Who
DISCHARGE PLANNING: ☐ LEVEL I - home independent ☐ LEVEL II - home with equipment ☐ LEVEL III - home with nursing or rehab visits ☐ LEVEL IV - not returning to home or previous place of residence
Social Service Referral: Yes No Financial / Home Health / Personal Request in Computer Yes No
Previously seen by any community agency? No Yes Which one?
Would you like me to contact anyone regarding your spiritual needs: Yes No
Who Contacted? ______ Date ______

DISCHARGE DATA

Date: Time: Mode: Car Medical Van Ambulance Other
ACCOMPANIED BY: Self Family Friends Other
DISCHARGED TO: Home Foster Care ECF Rehab Other Facility AMA Expired Other
MOBILITY STATUS: Ambulatory Ambulatory With Assist Crutches / Walker Wheelchair Stretcher
MENTAL STATUS: Alert Oriented Lethargic Confused
ACTIVITY LEVEL: Independent Needs Assistance Total Care
Note changes in patient since shift assessment. None
Document changes
DC INST. Written CCP
RN:

Figure 14-4. Discharge summary form. (Courtesy Rogue Valley Medical Center, Medford, Ore.)

Box 14-3

Information for Clients Discharged to Home Health Care or Extended Care Facilities

Use clear concise descriptions in client's own language.

Provide step-by-step description of how to perform a procedure (e.g., home medication administration). Reinforce explanation with printed instructions.

Identify precautions to follow when performing self-care or administering medications.

Review signs and symptoms of complications that should be reported to physician.

List names and phone numbers of health care providers and community resources that the client can contact.

Box 14-4

Multidisciplinary Example of Health Care Team Working Together

A home health care agency in a five-county region addressed the need to provide quality documentation in its services. A task force of clinical nurse specialists, clinicians, and an education director analyzed the nursing care plan system and identified seven specific goals to guide the new system: (1) improve quality of care, (2) maintain and expand concept of nursing diagnosis, (3) integrate physician's plan of treatment and nursing plan, (4) measure client outcomes, (5) interface data entry functions, (6) reduce documentation time, and (7) develop outcome standards for the program. The task force elected to use the NANDA taxonomy and developed a concise, operational, and visually appealing nursing plan that integrated the physician's plan with the nursing plan. The revised system exhibits positive benefits of relevance of the nursing plan to client care needs, decreased duplication of documentation, comprehensive record keeping (e.g., physicians, nurses, and others), an enhanced continuity of care, and a severe reduction in care plan development. The increased ease of use and a broader inclusion of members of the health care team make this revised documentation system a positive new method of record keeping.

---

nature of the home setting, which dictates that the majority of care is witnessed by a narrower scope of persons (i.e., client, family, direct health care provider). This situation demands that the documentation be accurate and complete so that the entire health care team has a valid means of identifying what care is rendered in the home. Home health care requires that the entire health care team work closely together (Box 14-4). In addition, the documentation is both the quality control and the justification for reimbursement from Medicare, Medicaid, or private insurance companies. Nurses must document all of their services for payment (e.g., direct skilled care, client instructions, skilled observation, evaluation visits) (JCAHO, 1995). The chart forms are similar to those used in other settings but are somewhat more detailed and greater in number. The nurse is the pivotal person in the documentation of the delivery of home health care.

Delivery of home health care is changing with advancements in technology. The nurse can communicate and even assess client needs via modem linkages. The future continues to hold solutions for nursing care in the home via "distance learning." Likewise, documentation has unique problems because of this changing mode of health care delivery.

Long-Term Care Documentation

There is an ever increasing number of older adults requiring care in long-term health care facilities. The acuity of conditions in these persons continues to escalate as geriatric clients develop more disabilities commensurate with their age. Nursing personnel often face challenges much different from those in the acute care setting. These differences require a significantly different basis for nursing documentation (Iyer and Camp,

1995). For example, outside agencies are instrumental in determining the standards and policies for documentation in long-term health care.

Long-term care documentation supports a multidisciplinary approach in the assessment (referred to as a minimum data set) and planning process (referred to as resident assessment protocols) of the clients. Communication among such health care providers as nurses, social workers, recreational therapists, and dietitians is essential in the regulated documentation process. The fiscal support for long-term care residents hinges on the justification of nursing care as demonstrated in sound documentation of the services rendered.

Computerized Documentation

Computers are used in health care facilities in a variety of ways. The technology that exists is virtually unlimited, and the future holds incredible potential for the continuing impact of computerization in the health care delivery system. Nurses have traditionally been the primary users of the health care computerized systems. Supplies, equipment, stock medications, and diagnostic testing are examples of services linking nurses to computers. However, with regulatory bodies and the legal system requiring increased documentation, nurses must be encouraged and allowed to use computerized recording to enhance their professional productivity (Pabst and others, 1996).

There are many benefits to computerized documentation. The new documentation systems that are now available can relieve nurses of repetitive clerical and monitoring tasks and increase the time available for direct client care. Software programs allow nurses to enter specific assessment data quickly, and the information is automatically transferred to different reports. Computers also help reduce errors (e.g., legibility better than handwritten notations), standardize nursing care plans, increase nursing satisfaction and productivity, and document all facets of client care (Johnson and Martin, 1996). Another benefit to computerized documentation is the enhancement of quality-improvement activities. Meeting JACHO outcome standards is easier with computerized documentation because of the standardized nature of care planning on the computer.

Computerized documentation will potentially change drastically with the increased use of new technological **nursing interfaces.** Typical **user interfaces** (e.g., keyboard, monitor) require typing and result in data entry errors. The increasingly prevalent **graphic user interfaces** (e.g., trackball, touch pads, mouse, icons) are not well suited for the large volumes of data necessary in nursing documentation. Therefore in the future, nursing will potentially use either pen-based or voice recognition computers in documentation. A notebook-sized computer with handwriting recognition capabilities would allow nurses to document with an ease and flexibility not possible in the current systems. In addition, **automated speech recognition** (ASR) or voice recognition technology also allows nursing documentation to expand to a new horizon of capabilities. The expansive nature of the developed **Internet** to be a resource to nurses in their documentation is also an important aspect of computerized documentation. Networking among other health care institutions, libraries, and seemingly unlimited resources continues to increase the knowledge base for nurses as they document in client records (Simpson, 1995). Although it is still in its developmental phases, **virtual reality** (a virtual environment is a computer-simulated world that changes in response to a person's actions) may also play a role in the future of computerized documentation. For example, nurses could potentially practice advanced cardiac life support skills and document the results of the scenario in the virtual reality simulation (McConnell, 1996).

Another form of computerized documentation is a complete **computer-based client record** (CCR) as a futuristic trend for client records. The CCR is a comprehensive system that utilizes many components of data collection and makes use of a broad scope of computerization capabilities. The new CCR has a much broader scope than the current charting systems and has a greater role in the utility of client care and in clinical decision making. The CCR allows the nurse to have an instrumental role in this new form of documentation.

Nurses must also know the legal risks of computerized documentation. Computers increase access to information by almost everyone. Consequently, the American Nurses Association, the American Medical Record Association, and the Canadian Nurses Association developed guidelines for safe computer charting (Charting Tips, 1993):

1. The password that is used to enter and sign off computer files should not be shared with another care giver. (Note: a good system requires frequent changes in personal passwords to prevent unauthorized persons from accessing and tampering with records.)
2. Never leave the computer terminal unattended after being logged on.
3. Follow the correct protocol for correcting errors. To correct an error after storage, mark the entry "mistaken entry," add the correct information, and date and initial the entry. If you record information in the wrong chart, write "mistaken entry—wrong chart," and sign off.
4. Make sure that stored records have backup files—an important safety check. If you inadvertently delete part of the permanent record, type an explanation into the computer file with the date, time, and your initials, and submit an explanation in writing to your manager.
5. Don't leave information about a client displayed on a monitor where others may see it. Keep a log that accounts for every copy of a computerized file that you've generated from the system.
6. Follow the agency's confidentiality procedures for documenting sensitive material, such as a diagnosis or HIV infection.

Finally, printouts of computerized records should be protected. Shredding of printouts and the logging of the number of copies generated by each care giver are ways to minimize duplicate records and protect the confidentiality of clients.

⋯REPORTING

Information about clients is exchanged among health care team members, clients, and family members. Reports offer a summary of activities or observations seen, performed, or heard. Common types of reports given by nurses include change-of-shift reports, telephone reports, transfer reports, and incident reports.

Change-of-Shift Report

The **change-of-shift report** occurs 2 or 3 times a day in all types of nursing units. At the end of each shift, nurses report information about their assigned clients to nurses working on the next shift. The purpose of the report is to provide better continuity of care among nurses who are caring for a client. If one nurse finds a certain position increases a client's breathing difficulties, it is important that the information be relayed to the next nurse caring for the client so that breathing enhancement interventions can be optimized. A complete report establishes the nurse's accountability in ensuring that client care is uninterrupted.

Change-of-shift reports are given orally in person, by audiotape recordings, or during rounds at the client's bedside. Oral reports are given in person, with staff members from both shifts participating. Audiotaped reports may be done before the end of the shift, which can increase efficiency and minimize social interactions. An opportunity for a last-minute update on events that occur after taping and for clarification when there are questions is essential. Reports given in person or during rounds permit nurses to obtain immediate feedback when questions are raised about a client's care. When nurses make rounds, the client and family members also have the opportunity to participate in any decisions. The nurse giving the report ensures the client's privacy by speaking in a low voice to prevent others from overhearing.

The change-of-shift report should be given quickly and efficiently. A good report provides a baseline for comparisons and indicates the kind of care to be anticipated for the next shift. An organized and concise approach helps nurses set goals and anticipate client needs and lessens the chance of important information being overlooked. An example format is as follows: background information, primary problem, nursing diagnoses, interventions, and family involvement. It is especially important to report any recent changes or priority situations concerning the client's condition. Box 14-5 is an example of a change-of-shift report.

When giving a report, the nurse discusses the client or family in a professional manner. It may be necessary to describe interactions in behavioral terms. A good report is objective, and the content of the report should be pertinent to the client's health care. Value-laden terms do not establish good working relationships. The nurse should avoid using such judgmental labels as "uncooperative," "difficult," or "bad" when describing client behaviors. Any derogatory statements overheard by the client could lead to a lawsuit against the nurse. Staff members may unintentionally form a prejudicial opinion about the client.

Telephone Reports and Orders

Telephone reports. Health care team members frequently talk to one another by telephone. Information in a telephone report should be permanently documented in written form if significant events or changes in a client's condition have occurred. Thus the persons involved with a telephone report should ensure that the information is clear, accurate, and concise. To document a phone call, the nurse includes when the call was made,

---

> ### Box 14-5
> ### Sample Taped Change-of-Shift Report
>
> In room 238b is Diane Langhorn, a 42-year-old patient of Dr. Rayne's who was admitted with exacerbation of ulcerative colitis. Her main problems are:
> Abdominal pain: She has had no pain or cramping for the last 12 hours.
> Diarrhea related to bowel inflammation: She has had no diarrhea or bloody stools for 24 hours. She had a brown formed stool this morning. We need one more stool to test for occult blood.
> Altered nutritional intake, less than body requirements: Ms. Langhorn is on clear liquids and is receiving IV therapy. If she has no further diarrhea, her diet will be advanced in the morning. Her daily weight has been stable at 110 lb for 24 hours. The dietitian has visited her to provide diet instruction.
>
> Modified from Mosher C, Bontomasi R: How to improve your shift report, *Am J Nurs* 96(8):13, 1996.

---

who made it (if other than the writer of the information), who was called, to whom information was given, what information was given, and what information was received (Figure 14-5). An example follows: "At 2030, called laboratory; J. Ignacio, technician, reported Mr. Abernathy's potassium at 5.9. D. Markle, RN."

Telephone orders (TOs). A telephone order involves a physician's stating a prescribed therapy over the phone to a registered nurse. Clarifying messages is important when a nurse accepts a physician's orders over the telephone. The order must be verified by repeating it clearly and precisely. Then the nurse writes the order on the physician's order sheet in the client's permanent record and signs it. An example follows: "10/16/96: 0815, ketorolac 30 mg IM q6 hours for incisional pain. T.O. Dr. Knight/J. Woods, RN." The physician later verifies the telephone order legally by signing it within a set time (e.g., 24 hours). Telephone orders are frequently given at night or during an emergency. Telephone orders should be used only when absolutely necessary and not for the sake of convenience. Box 14-6 provides guidelines that the nurse can use to prevent errors in receiving telephone orders.

Transfer Reports

Clients frequently transfer from one unit to another to receive different levels of care. For example, clients transfer from intensive care units to general nursing units after the level of care no longer requires intense monitoring. A **transfer report** involves communication of information about clients from the nurse on the

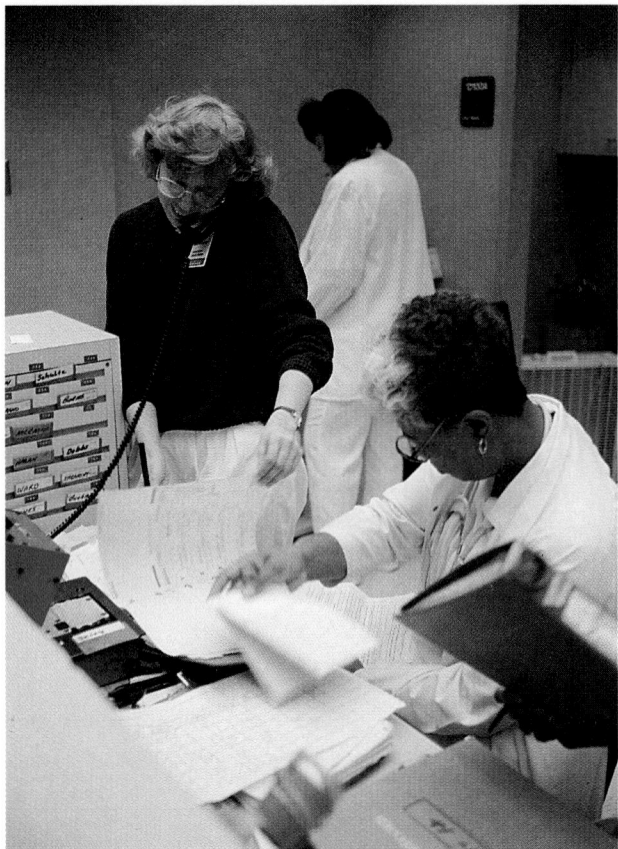

Figure 14-5.   Telephone reports require the nurse's attention to ensure accurate information is conveyed.

Box 14-6

Telephone Order Guidelines

If the physician sounds hurried over the phone, use clarification questions to avoid misunderstandings.

Clearly determine the client's name, room number, and diagnosis.

Repeat any prescribed orders back to the physician.

Write a telephone order to include date and time given; name of client, nurse, and physician; and the complete order.

Follow agency policies; some institutions require telephone (and verbal) orders to be reviewed and signed by two nurses.

Have the physician cosign the order within the time frame required by the institution (usually 24 hours).

sending unit to the nurse on the receiving unit. Transfer reports may be given by phone or in person. When giving a transfer report, nurses include the following information:

1. Client's name, age, primary physician, and medical diagnosis
2. Summary of medical progress up to the time of transfer
3. Current health status (physical and psychosocial)
4. Current nursing diagnoses or problems and care plan
5. Any critical assessments or interventions to be completed shortly after transfer (helps receiving nurse to establish priorities of care)
6. Need for any special equipment

After the sending nurse completes the transfer report, the receiving nurse should have time to ask any questions about the client's status.

Incident Reports

An incident is any event not consistent with the routine operation of a health care unit or routine care of a client.

Examples include client falls, needle-stick injuries, a visitor becoming ill, and medication errors. When something that could have caused or did cause injury occurs, the nurse files an **incident report** (e.g., unusual occurrence form, medication discrepancy form). This is a method of documentation for the institution and not part of the medical record. However, when the incident involves a client, the nurse documents in the medical record an objective description of what was observed. The nurse also records in the medical record any follow-up care given. Incident reports are an important part of a unit's quality-improvement program (Figure 14-6). Incidents should trigger an investigation of the circumstances involved and the changes needed to prevent recurrences. This could include educational programs, revised policies and procedures, improved equipment, or changes in client delivery systems (Gobis, 1994).

When an incident occurs, the nurse involved objectively documents the details in the incident report. A number of crucial elements must be described, including the date and time, how the nurse found the client, witness information, assessment of the client's injury, actions taken, and follow-up notations. An incident report should be concise and accurate, reporting exactly what the nurse observes and administers in the way of care (Box 14-7). Parisi (1994) states that an incident report for a medication error should include the following: (1) an accurate and concise description of the medication error, (2) relevant information, without making excuses for the error, and (3) any adverse reactions the client has experienced.

Nurses usually become involved in client-related incidents at some point in their careers. They must understand the purpose of incident reports and the correct way to report information.

DO NOT COPY
OREGON HEALTH SCIENCES UNIVERSITY
UNIVERSITY HOSPITAL & CLINICS

QA&I CONFIDENTIAL INCIDENT REPORT

Unit No.

Name

Birthdate

Complete immediately for every incident and send to the Quality Management Medical Director/Medical Services Director, MBS.

INCIDENT INVOLVES: (Check all involved)

Patient ☐   Visitor ☐   Other ☐   Medical Device ☐

Address (if
pertinent) _____

Diagnosis (if
patient) _____

Location of Incident
(unit, rm)_____ Date _____ Hour_____

Involved Medical Device:
    Device description _____

    Identifier   (Manufacturers' Model #, Serial # or Clinical Engineering #.

                    _____ / _____ / _____

Involved Medical or_____
Nursing Personnel Names

Were Witnesses Present _____
(List names if pertinent)

Description of Incident incl. immediate action taken _____
(Use back if necessary)

Bed High	☐
Bed Low	☐
Rails Up	☐
Rails Down	☐
Restraints	☐
Activity Orders:	
Bed Rest	☐
Limited	☐
BRP	☐

To Whom was Incident Reported _____

Signature of Person Reporting _____

Physical Findings and Diagnosis

Supervisor's Report and Final Action Taken

_____
Supervisor or Physician's Signature

Figure 14-6.   Incident report. (Courtesy Oregon Health Sciences University Hospitals and Clinics, Portland, Ore.)

Box 14-7
Guidelines for Completing an Incident Report

1. The nurse who witnessed the incident or who found the client at the time of the incident should file the report.
2. The nurse describes specifically what happened in concise, objective terms.
3. The nurse does not interpret or attempt to explain the cause of the incident.
4. The nurse describes objectively the client's condition when the incident was discovered.
5. Any measures taken by the nurse, other nurses, or physicians at the time of the incident are reported.
6. No nurse is blamed in an incident report.
7. The report is submitted as soon as possible to the appropriate administrator.
8. The nurse should never make a photocopy of the incident report for a personal file because the copy could be subpoenaed in court.

Key Terms

accreditation
acuity charting
automated speech recognition
case management plan
change-of-shift report
charting by exception (CBE)
computer-based client records
consultations
critical pathways
DAR
diagnosis-related group (DRG)
documentation
flow sheets
focus charting

graphic user interface
incident report
Internet
Kardex
nursing interface
PIE
problem-oriented medical record
record
reports
SOAP
source record
standardized care plans
transfer report
user interface
variance
virtual reality

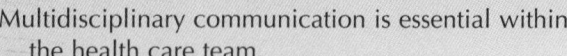

▪ Key Concepts

Multidisciplinary communication is essential within the health care team.

A client's health care record is written documentation of the care received.

The client care record is a legal document and requires information describing exactly the care delivered to a client.

The medical record is a client's bill or financial record that serves as the basis for reimbursement to hospitals.

A nurse's signature on an entry in a record designates accountability for the contents of that entry.

Accurate record keeping requires an objective interpretation of data with precise measurements, correct spelling, and proper use of abbreviations.

Any change in a client's condition warrants immediate documentation to keep a record current.

All information pertaining to a client's health care management that is gathered by examination, observation, conversation, or treatment is confidential.

Problem-oriented medical records are organized by the client's health care problems.

There are advantages and disadvantages to the different formats for charting (e.g., focus, charting by exception, POMR).

Critical pathways are instrumental in the evolving documentation methods that focus on client outcomes.

There are a variety of record-keeping forms used in client documentation (e.g., admission nursing history forms, flow sheets, Kardex).

Medicare guidelines for establishing a client's home care reimbursement are the basis for documentation by home health nurses.

Long-term care documentation is multidisciplinary and closely linked with fiscal requirements of outside agencies.

Computerized information systems provide information about clients in an organized and easily accessible fashion.

The major purpose of the change-of-shift report is to maintain continuity of care.

Rounds allow nurses to perform needed assessments, evaluate clients' progress, and determine the best interventions for a client's needs.

When information pertinent to care is communicated by telephone, the information must be verified.

Incident reports objectively describe any event not consistent with the routine care of a client.

Critical Thinking Activities

1. Obtain a client care record in a nursing setting, and find examples that follow guidelines for good documentation of the following: factual basis, accuracy, completeness, currentness, organization, and confidentiality.
2. Personally observe a change-of-shift report at a health care facility, and critique it in a clinical conference.
3. Document client care performed in the clinical setting using two of the following formats: charting by exception, narrative documentation, focus charting, and SOAP charting.
4. Participate in a client interview, and separate observations into objective versus subjective data.

References

Adams C, Biggerstaff N: Reduced resource utilization through standardized outcome-focused care plans, *J Nurs Adm* 25(10):43, 1995.

Addy-Keller J, McElwaney E: A new documentation tool, *Nurs Manage* 24(11):46, 1993.

Braunstein M: The electronic patient records solution, *Caring* 12(7):23, 1993.

Charting Tips: Computer charting: minimizing legal risks, *Nurs 93* 23(5):86, 1993.

Coenen A and others: Using nursing diagnoses to explain utilization in a community nursing center, *Res Nurs Health* 19(3):441, 1996.

Ebert V, Bethel S: Mission accomplished: a system for discharge planning, *Nurs Manage* 27(8):27, 1996.

Gobis L: Demystifying incident reports, *Am J Nurs* 94(4):16, 1994.

Gordon M: *Manual of nursing diagnosis: 1995–1996,* St. Louis, 1995, Mosby.

Gulanick M and others: *Nursing care plans: nursing diagnosis and intervention,* ed 3, St. Louis, 1994, Mosby.

Iyer P, Camp NH: *Nursing documentation: a nursing process approach,* St. Louis, 1995, Mosby.

Johnson D, Martin K: Preparing for electronic documentation, *Nurs Manage* 27(7):43, 1996.

Joint Commission on Accreditation of Healthcare Organizations, *Standards for the accreditation of home care,* Chicago, 1995, The Commission.

Lavin J, Enright B: Charting with managed care in mind, *RN* 59(8):47, 1996.

Lowenstein A, Hoff P: Discharge planning: a study of nursing staff involvement, *J Nurs Adm* 24(4):45, 1994.

Martin F: Documentation tips: to help you stay out of court, *Nurs 94* 24(6):30, 1994.

McConnell E: The future of technology in critical care, *Crit Care Nurse* 16(3):12, 1996.

Mosher C, Bontomasi R: How to improve your shift report, *Am J Nurs* 96(8):13, 1996.

Pabst M and others: The impact of computerized documentation on nurse's use of time, *Comput Nurs* 14(1):25, 1996.

Parisi S: What to do after a med error, *Nurs 94* 24(6):24, 1994.

Smith A: Chart reviews made simple, *Nurs Manage* 27(8):33, 1996.

Simpson R: Getting wired for success, *Nurs Adm Q* 19(4):89, 1995.

Sowell R, Meadows T: An integrated case management model: developing standards, evaluation, and outcome criteria, *J Nurs Adm* 18(2):24, 1994.

Tahan H, Cesta T: Evaluating the effectiveness of case management plans, *J Nurs Adm* 25(9):58, 1995.

15

Client Education

OBJECTIVES

Mastery of content in this chapter will enable the student to:

- Define the key terms listed.
- Identify a client's health promotion and health restoration needs.
- Describe the similarities and differences between teaching and learning.
- Identify the purposes of client education.
- Compare the communication and teaching processes.
- Describe the domains of learning.
- Differentiate factors that determine readiness to learn from those that determine ability to learn.
- Compare the nursing and teaching processes.
- Write learning objectives for a teaching plan.
- Describe the characteristics of a good learning environment.
- Identify the principles of effective teaching.
- Describe ways to adapt teaching for clients with different learning needs.
- Describe ways to incorporate teaching with routine nursing care.
- Identify the methods for evaluating learning.

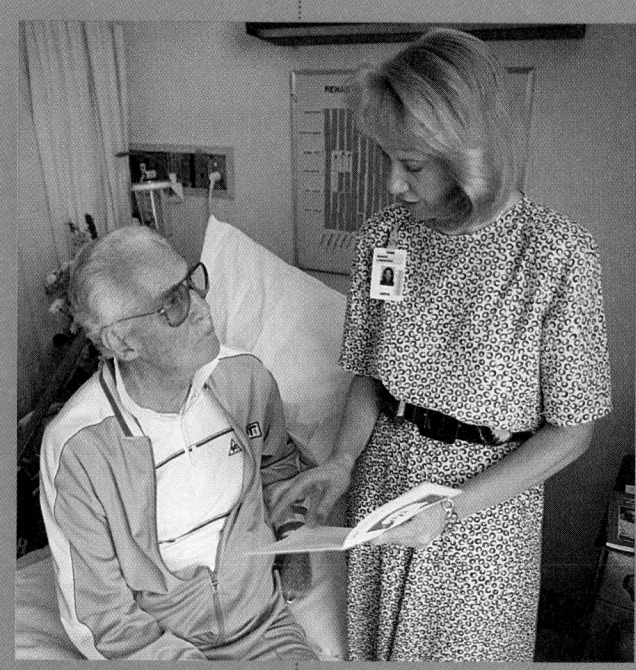

Client education has become one of the most important roles of nurses working in any health care setting. Shorter hospital stays, increased demands on nurses' time, and the need to give seriously ill clients concise, meaningful information as soon as possible emphasize the importance of quality client education (London, 1995). As nurses try to find the best way to educate clients, the general public has become more assertive in seeking knowledge and understanding of their health and the resources available within the health care system (Visser and Herbert, 1994). Providing clients with needed information for self-care is necessary to ensure continuity of care from the hospital to the home (Bostrom and others, 1994). The significance of client education is enhanced because of the client's right to know and to be informed about diagnosis, prognosis, treatments, and risks. A well-designed, comprehensive teaching plan that fits a client's learning needs can reduce health care costs, improve the quality of care, and help clients to gain optimum wellness and increased independence.

STANDARDS FOR CLIENT EDUCATION

Accrediting agencies in the United States and Canada set guidelines for providing client education in health care institutions (American Association of Diabetes Educators, 1992; Barnes, 1993). The guidelines ensure that clients and their families receive information necessary to maintain the client's optimal level of health. In the United States the Joint Commission on Accreditation of Healthcare Organizations (JCAHO) (1997) describes nine standards for client and family education (Box 15-1).

The successful accomplishment of these standards depends on participation of all health care professionals. Evidence of successful client education is noted in the client's medical record.

PURPOSES OF CLIENT TEACHING

Nursing's Agenda for Health Care Reform (ANA, 1991) recommends restructuring the health care system and focusing on wellness and care rather than on illness and cure. The emphasis is on maintaining health. Clients now know more about health and want to be involved in health maintenance. Nursing needs to provide education so that clients receive information about care in more convenient and familiar places (e.g., church or schools) (ANA, 1991). Comprehensive client education includes three important purposes, each involving a separate phase of health care.

Box 15-1
JCAHO Client and Family Education Standards

The client's learning needs, abilities, preferences, and readiness to learn are assessed.

The assessment considers cultural and religious practices, emotional barriers, desire and motivation to learn, physical and cognitive limitations, language barriers, and the financial implications of care choices.

When called for by the age of the client and the length of stay, the hospital assesses and provides for client's academic education needs.

Clients are educated about the safe and effective use of medication, according to law and their needs.

Clients are educated about the safe and effective use of medical equipment.

Clients are educated about potential drug-food interactions, and are provided counseling on nutrition and modified diets.

Clients are educated about rehabilitation techniques to help them adapt or function more independently in their environment.

Clients are informed about access to additional resources in the community.

Clients are informed about when and how to obtain any further treatment they may need.

Modified from Joint Commission on Accreditation of Healthcare Organizations: *Accreditation manual of hospitals,* Chicago, 1997, The Commission.

Maintenance and Promotion of Health and Illness Prevention

The public has become more health conscious. Participation in fitness clubs, diet programs, regular exercise activities, and health-screening programs are examples of ways people pay attention to their health. The nurse is a visible, competent resource for clients intent on improving physical and psychological well-being. In the school, home, clinic, or workplace the nurse provides clients with information and skills that allow them to assume healthier behaviors (Box 15-2). For example, in childbearing classes, nurses teach expectant parents about physical and psychological changes in the woman and about fetal development. After learning about normal childbearing, the mother is more likely to eat healthy foods, engage in physical exercise, and avoid substances that might harm the fetus. Promoting healthful behavior through education increases self-esteem by allowing clients to assume more responsibility for health. When clients become more health conscious,

---

Box 15-2
Topics for Health Education

**Health Maintenance and Promotion
and Illness Prevention**

First aid
Avoidance of risk factors (smoking, alcohol)
Growth and development
Hygiene
Immunizations
Prenatal care and normal childbearing
Nutrition
Exercise
Safety (in home and hospital)
Screening (blood pressure, vision, cholesterol level)

Restoration of Health

Client's disease or condition
    Anatomy and physiology of body system affected
    Cause of disease
    Origin of symptoms
    Expected effects on other body systems
    Prognosis
    Limitations on function
    Rationale for treatment
    Medications

Tests and therapies
Nursing measures
Surgical intervention
Expected duration of care
Hospital or clinic environment
Hospital or clinic staff
Long-term care
Methods for client participation in care

Coping With Impaired Function

Home care
    Medications
    Diet
    Activity
    Self-help devices
Rehabilitation of remaining function
    Physical therapy
    Occupational therapy
    Speech therapy
Prevention of complications
    Knowledge of risk factors
    Implications of noncompliance with therapy
    Environmental alterations

---

they are more likely to seek early diagnosis of health problems (Redman, 1997).

Restoration of Health

Injured or ill clients need information or skills that will help them regain improved levels of health (see Box 15-2). Clients recovering from the initial stress of illness or injury and adapting to the changes that result, seek information about their conditions. However, clients who find it difficult to adapt to illness may become passive and uninterested in learning. The nurse learns to identify clients' willingness to learn and helps motivate interest.

The family is a vital part of a client's return to health and may need to know as much as the client. If the nurse excludes the family from a client's teaching plan, conflicts may arise. For example, if the family does not understand a client's need to regain independent function, their efforts may cause the client to become unnecessarily dependent and slow the client's recovery. The nurse should not assume the family should be involved and must first assess the client-family relationship.

Coping With Impaired Functioning

Not all clients fully recover from illness or injury. Many must learn to cope with permanent health changes.

New knowledge and skills are often needed for clients to continue activities of daily living (see Box 15-2). For example, the client whose ability to speak is lost after surgery of the larynx learns new ways of communicating, and the client with severe heart disease learns to avoid physical activities that might cause further heart damage.

In the case of serious disability, the client's family role may change. Family members thus need to be understanding and accepting. The family's ability to provide support results from education, which begins as soon as the client's needs are identified and the family displays a willingness to help. The nurse teaches family members to assist clients with health care management. This includes, for example, giving medications and baths and applying dressings. Families of clients with alcoholism, mental retardation, or drug dependence also learn to adapt to the additional emotional effects of these chronic conditions.

A nurse learns to recognize the information to teach to clients at different levels of wellness by assessing clients' needs and abilities. Learning occurs when information is practical and useful to the learner. Comparing the desired level of health with the actual state enables the nurse to plan effective teaching programs.

TEACHING AND LEARNING

It is impossible to separate **teaching** from **learning.** Teaching is an interactive process that promotes learning. It consists of a conscious and deliberate set of actions that helps individuals gain new knowledge or perform new skills (Redman, 1997). A teacher provides information that prompts the learner to engage in activities that lead to a desired change. For example, when a nurse demonstrates application of an elastic bandage, the client is able to see the skill and then demonstrate self-application.

Learning is the acquisition of new knowledge or skills through reinforced practice and experience. A client with diabetes demonstrates the technique for preparing insulin in a syringe. Preoperatively, a surgical client discusses ways to relieve postoperative pain. Generally, teaching and learning begin when a person identifies a need for knowing or acquiring an ability to do something. Teaching is most effective when it responds to a learner's needs. The teacher identifies these needs by asking questions and determining the learner's interests. Interpersonal communication is essential for successful teaching.

Role of the Nurse in Teaching and Learning

Clients and their families often ask nurses for health information. If they do not, then the need for teaching may not be obvious. The nurse should try to anticipate clients' needs for information based on their physical conditions or treatment plans. The nurse needs to teach information that clients and their families need and are likely to use. The nurse clarifies information provided by physicians and becomes the primary source of information for adjusting to health problems.

To be an effective educator, the nurse must engage the client in learning and not merely pass on facts. The nurse must carefully determine what clients need to know and find the time when they are ready to learn. Hayslip (1995) noted three ultimate client outcomes that are the result of effective client education: (1) attaining realistic or desired health status; (2) empowering clients toward active participation in their plan of care; and (3) achieving optimal rehabilitation levels.

When nurses value client education and are able to implement it, clients can become better prepared to assume health care responsibilities. The relationship between client education and favorable client outcomes is an important nursing research issue.

TEACHING AS COMMUNICATION

The teaching process closely parallels the communication process (see Chapter 13). Effective teaching depends, in part, on effective interpersonal communication. A teacher applies each element of the communication process while giving information to learners. Thus the teacher and student become involved in a teaching process that increases the student's knowledge and skills.

The steps of the teaching process can be compared with those of the communication process (Table 15-1). In teaching, the referent is the need to provide the client with information. The client may request information, or the nurse may perceive a need for information. The nurse then identifies specific learning objectives. A **learning objective** describes what the learner will be able to do after successful instruction.

The nurse is the sender who wants to convey a message to the client. The nurse promotes learning by communicating in a language recognized by the learner. Many intrapersonal variables influence the nurse's style and approach. Attitudes, values, emotions, and knowledge influence the way the nurse sends messages. Past experiences with teaching help the nurse to choose the best way to present information.

The message or content to be taught is delivered clearly and precisely. The nurse organizes information in a logical sequence so that the client will more easily understand the skills or ideas. Each lesson progresses from the simple to the more complex skills or ideas (Houston and Haire-Joshu, 1996).

The nurse may use a variety of ways to present teaching content. All the senses are channels for presenting information. The auditory channel is the simplest, as in a lecture or discussion. The learning process becomes more active and stimulating, however, when several sensory channels are used together.

The receiver in the teaching-learning process is the learner. Intrapersonal variables affect a client's motivation and ability to learn. Clients are ready to learn when they express a desire to do so and are more likely to receive the message when they understand the content. Language, attitudes, anxiety, and values influence the ability to understand a message. The ability to learn depends on emotional and physical health, education, stage of development, and previous knowledge.

An effective teacher provides a mechanism for evaluating the success of a teaching plan. **Return demonstration** is a good form of feedback. The learner restates the received information or demonstrates learned skills, which allows the teacher to assess the success of learning.

DOMAINS OF LEARNING

Learning occurs in the cognitive (understanding), affective (values), and psychomotor (motor skills) domains. Any topic to be learned may involve all domains or only one. The nurse often works with clients who need to learn in each domain. For example, a client with diabetes needs to learn how diabetes affects the

TABLE 15-1
Comparison of Terms Used in Teaching and Communication

Communication	Teaching
Referent	
Idea that initiates reason for communication	Perceived need to provide person with information, establishment of relevant learning objectives by teacher
Sender	
Person who conveys message to another	Teacher who performs activities aimed at assisting other person to learn
Intrapersonal Variables (Sender)	
Knowledge, values, emotions, and sociocultural influences that affect sender's thoughts	Teacher's philosophy of education (based on learning therapy), knowledge of teaching content, teaching approach, experiences in teaching, emotions and values
Message	
Information expressed or transmitted by sender	Content or information taught
Channels	
Methods used to transmit message (visual, auditory, touch)	Methods used to present content (visual and auditory materials, touch, taste, smell)
Receiver	
Person to whom message is transmitted	Learner
Intrapersonal Variables (Receiver)	
Knowledge, values, emotions, and sociocultural influences that affect receiver's thoughts	Willingness and ability to learn (physical and emotional health, education, experience, developmental level)
Feedback	
Information revealing that true meaning of message was received	Determination of whether learning objectives were achieved

body and methods to control blood sugar levels (cognitive domain) and to accept the chronic nature of the disease (affective domain). In addition, many clients with diabetes must also learn to administer daily insulin injections (psychomotor domain). The characteristics of learning within each domain affect the teaching and evaluation methods the nurse selects.

Cognitive learning includes all intellectual behaviors such as the acquisition of knowledge, comprehension (ability to understand), application (using abstract ideas in concrete situations), analysis (relating ideas in an organized way), synthesis (recognizing parts of information as a whole), and evaluation (judging the worth of a body of information).

Affective learning deals with the expression of feelings related to attitudes, opinions, or values. The learner receives the information, responds to the information and the teacher, values the worth of the teacher and the information, organizes values, and characterizes by acting and responding with a consistent value system.

Psychomotor learning involves acquiring skills that require the integration of mental and muscular ac-

tivity such as the ability to walk, use an eating utensil, or climb stairs. The learner perceives objects or information through sensory organs. Then the learner demonstrates readiness to take an action through mental, physical, and emotional acts. The teacher guides the learner's response, leading to the confidence to perform the desired behavior in gradually more complex ways. Adaptation is the next step, involving responses to changes and problems. This results in origination, which involves creating new patterns of behavior.

Teaching the client a specific behavior often involves incorporating behaviors from all three learning domains. A client being taught the proper method of giving an injection must first understand the reasons injections are needed and then must know the proper location for administering the injection and the importance of using sterile technique (cognitive). The techniques of locating an acceptable area on the skin and introducing the needle use the senses of touch and vision (psychomotor). In addition, the client must be willing to accept the need for injections and must overcome any fear of or distaste for injections (affective).

BASIC LEARNING PRINCIPLES

To teach effectively and efficiently, the nurse must first understand how people learn. Learning depends on the motivation to learn, the ability to learn, and the learning environment. **Motivation** addresses a person's desire to learn (Redman, 1997). Previous knowledge, attitudes, and sociocultural factors influence motivation.

The ability to learn depends on physical and cognitive attributes, developmental level, physical wellness, and intellectual thought processes. The environment also affects the ability to learn. The nurse must manipulate environmental conditions to facilitate learning.

Motivation to Learn

Attentional set. An **attentional set** is the mental state that allows the learner to focus on and comprehend the material. People often use mental pictures to visualize ideas. While a teacher explains how to give support to a dying client, students might envision themselves grasping the fragile hand of a dying person. Before learning anything, students must give attention to, or concentrate on, the information to be learned. Physical discomfort, anxiety, and environmental distractions can influence the ability to attend. Any physical condition that impairs the ability to concentrate (e.g., pain, fatigue, or hunger) interferes with learning. Therefore the nurse determines the client's level of comfort and energy before beginning a teaching plan and ensures that the client is comfortable. Verbal and nonverbal cues can also reveal that a client is not ready to learn.

Anxiety may increase or decrease the ability of a person to pay attention. Anxiety is uneasiness or uncertainty resulting from anticipating a threat or danger. When faced with change or the need to act differently, a person feels anxious. Learning requires a change in behavior and thus produces anxiety. A mild level of anxiety may motivate learning. However, a high level of anxiety prevents learning from taking place. It incapacitates a person, creating an inability to attend to anything other than to relieve the anxiety.

Motivation. Motivation is an internal impulse (e.g., an idea, an emotion, a physical need) that causes a person to take action. If a person does not want to learn, it is unlikely that learning will occur. Social, task mastery, and physical motives stimulate a person to learn. Social motives are a need for connection, social approval, or self-esteem. Task mastery motives are based on needs such as achievement and competence. After a person succeeds at a task, the person is usually motivated to achieve more.

Often client motives are physical. A client with a physical change in function may be motivated to learn strategies to help adapt to the functional change. Teaching strategies reflect the relative importance of each kind of physical motive. A client with a lower limb amputation will most likely be motivated to learn to ambulate with a prosthesis.

A client's view of health may not be congruent with the nurse's view of health. A client with lung disease may continue to smoke. An obese client may worsen a heart condition by refusing to follow a low-fat diet. Information and client education are not sufficient as motivators alone. No therapy will have an effect unless a client is motivated by the belief that health is important. The trend in health care is to treat clients in their own homes after they recover from the acute phase of illness. Such treatment can be successful only if clients adhere to the prescribed course of therapy. However, the client may not perceive health or the therapy to be of value. The nurse must assess the client's view of health, motivation to learn, and what the client needs to know to adhere to the prescribed therapy.

Health beliefs. A client's **health beliefs** can be powerful motivators, and they are influenced by a number of variables (see Chapter 1). Although this model may help the nurse in developing a client's education program, it has limitations when used with adolescents because it does not account for peer group influence or the emotional and cognitive level of adolescents (Hiltabiddle, 1996).

Knowledge of a client's health beliefs helps to determine the factors that will motivate learning. However, there is no standard method for motivating a person with a given health belief. Health teaching often involves changing attitudes and values that cannot be altered by teaching facts. Therefore the nurse gives attention to ideas or beliefs that motivate a person to learn and applies the motivating factor to the teaching plan. For example, when a client is a busy executive with high blood pressure, the nurse can use the following factors to motivate the client to learn new health habits: the client's desire to succeed and the concern that illness will impair work. To facilitate more successful teaching, the motivating factor should be stressed and encouraged for several months after the initial teaching intervention (Elford and others, 1994).

Psychosocial adaptation to illness. A temporary or permanent loss of health is difficult for clients to accept. The process of grieving gives clients time to adapt psychologically to the emotional and physical implications of illness. The stages of grieving (see Chapter 21) also encompass a series of responses clients experience during illness. People experience these stages at different rates and sequences.

Readiness to learn is significantly related to the stage of grieving (Table 15-2). When unwilling or unable to accept the reality of illness, clients cannot learn. However, properly timed teaching can facilitate adjustment to illness or disability.

TABLE 15-2

Relationship Between Psychosocial Adaptation to Illness and Learning

Stage	Client's Behavior	Learning Implications	Rationale
Denial or disbelief	Client avoids discussion of illness ("There's nothing wrong with me"), withdraws from others, and disregards physical restrictions. Client suppresses and distorts information that has not been presented clearly.	Provide support, empathy, and careful explanations of all procedures while they are being done. Let client know you are available for discussion. Explain situation to family. Teach in present tense (explain current therapy).	Client is not prepared to deal with problem. Any attempt to convince or tell client about illness will result in further anger or withdrawal. Provide only information client pursues or absolutely requires.
Anger	Client blames and complains and often directs anger toward nurse.	Do not argue with client, but listen to concerns. Teach in present tense. Reassure family of client's normality.	Client needs opportunity to express feelings and anger. Client is still not prepared to face future.
Bargaining	Client offers to live better life in exchange for promise of better health ("If God lets me live, I promise to be more careful").	Continue to introduce only reality. Teach only in present tense.	Client is still unwilling to accept limitations.
Resolution	Client begins to express emotions openly, realizes that illness has created changes, and begins to ask questions.	Encourage expression of feelings. Begin to share information needed for future, and set aside formal times for discussion.	Client begins to perceive need for assistance and is ready to accept responsibility for learning.
Acceptance	Client recognizes reality of condition, actively pursues information, and strives for independence.	Focus teaching on future skills and knowledge required. Continue to teach about present occurrences. Involve family in teaching information for discharge.	Client is more easily motivated to learn. Acceptance of illness reflects willingness to deal with its implications.

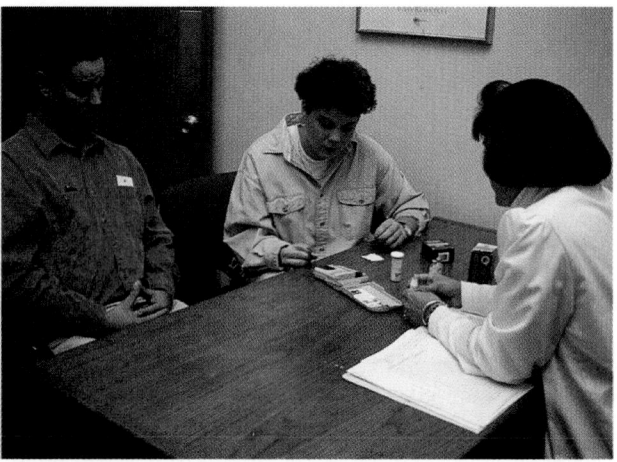

Figure 15-1. Nurse instructing a client with a glucose meter. (Courtesy Steve Frazier, Barnes-Jewish Hospital, St. Louis.)

The nurse identifies the client's stage of grieving on the basis of typically displayed behaviors. When the client enters the stage of acceptance, which is compatible with learning, the nurse introduces a teaching plan. Continuous assessment of the client's behaviors determines the stages of grieving. Teaching continues as long as the client remains in a stage conducive to learning.

Active participation. A client's involvement in learning implies an eagerness to acquire knowledge or skills and improves the opportunity for the client to make decisions during teaching sessions. For example, a client with diabetes learns to monitor blood glucose levels to gain control of the disease. The nurse assists the client in choosing a blood glucose meter and adapting a monitoring system and schedule to personal lifestyle patterns (Figure 15-1).

Box 15-3
Teaching Methods Based on Client's Developmental Capacity

Infant

Keep routines (feeding, bathing) consistent.
Hold infant firmly while smiling and speaking softly to convey sense of trust.
Have infant touch different textures (soft fabric, hard plastic).

Toddler

Use play to teach procedure or activity (handling examination equipment, applying bandage to doll).
Offer picture books that describe story of children in hospital or clinic.
Use simple words such as *cut* instead of *laceration* to promote understanding.

Preschooler

Use role playing, imitation, and play to make it fun for preschoolers to learn.
Encourage questions and offer explanations. Use simple explanations and demonstrations.
Encourage children to learn together through pictures and short stories of how to perform hygiene.

School-Age Child

Teach psychomotor skills needed to maintain health. (Complicated skills, such as learning to use a syringe, may take considerable practice.)
Offer opportunities to discuss health problems and answer questions.

Adolescent

Help adolescent learn about feelings and need for self-expression.
Use teaching as collaborative activity.
Allow adolescents to make decisions about health and health promotion (safety, sex education, substance abuse).
Use problem solving to help adolescents make choices.

Young or Middle Adult

Encourage participation in teaching plan by setting mutual goals.
Encourage independent learning.
Offer information so that adult can understand effects of health problem.

Older Adult

Teach when client is alert and rested.
Involve adult in discussion or activity.
Focus on wellness and the person's strength.
Use approaches that enhance sensorially impaired client's reception of stimuli (see Chapter 39).
Keep teaching sessions short.

Ability to Learn

Developmental capability. Cognitive development influences the ability to learn. A nurse can be a competent teacher, but if the client's intellectual abilities are not considered, teaching is unsuccessful. For example, sometimes a nurse shares teaching booklets and brochures and then discovers that the client cannot read (Estey and others, 1994). Learning, like developmental growth, is an evolving process. The nurse must know the client's level of knowledge and intellectual skills before beginning a teaching plan. For example, reading a thermometer or measuring liquid or solid food portions requires the ability to perform math calculations. Reading a medication label or instructions in a teaching booklet requires reading and comprehension skills, and learning to regulate insulin dosages requires problem-solving skills. Following directions when performing self-care in accordance with limitations requires comprehension and application skills.

A requisite level of maturation and cognitive development must exist before an individual is capable of learning new information. It is wrong to assume that a client has a certain level of knowledge; instead, the nurse should assess the client's level of knowledge. Learning occurs more readily when new information complements existing knowledge.

Age-group. Age reflects the developmental capability for learning and learning behaviors that can be acquired (Box 15-3). Without proper biological, motor, language, and personal-social development, many types of learning cannot take place (see Chapter 20). Learning occurs when behavior changes as a result of experience or growth (Wong, 1995).

Physical capability. The ability to learn often depends on a person's level of physical development and overall physical health. To learn psychomotor skills, a client must have the necessary level of strength, coordination, and sensory acuity. For example, it would be useless to teach a client to transfer from a bed to a wheelchair if the client has insufficient upper body strength. An older adult cannot learn to apply an elastic bandage with poor eyesight or the inability to grasp the bandage tightly. Therefore the nurse should not overestimate the client's physical development. The following physical attributes are required to learn psychomotor skills:

1. Size (height and weight match the task to be performed or the equipment to be used [e.g., crutch walking])
2. Strength (ability of the client to follow strenuous exercise program)
3. Coordination (dexterity needed for complicated motor skills such as using utensils or changing a bandage)
4. Sensory acuity (visual, auditory, tactile, gustatory, and olfactory: sensory resources needed to receive and respond to messages taught)

Any condition that depletes a person's energy will also impair the ability to learn. A client who spends a morning undergoing a rigorous schedule of diagnostic studies is unlikely to be capable of the effort needed for any learning discussion. When an illness becomes aggravated by complications such as a high fever or respiratory difficulty, teaching should be postponed. After working with a client, the nurse can assess the energy level by noting the client's willingness to communicate, amount of activity initiated, and responsiveness toward questions. The nurse may halt teaching temporarily if the client needs rest. The nurse achieves greater teaching success when the client is an active participant in learning (Northern and others, 1995).

Learning Environment

Factors in the physical environment where teaching takes place make learning a pleasant or difficult experience. The nurse chooses a setting that helps the client to focus attention on the learning task. The number of persons being taught, need for privacy, room temperature, room lighting, noise, room ventilation, and room furniture are important when choosing the setting.

The ideal environment for promoting learning is a room that is well lit and has good ventilation, appropriate furniture, and a comfortable temperature (Figure 15-2). A darkened room interferes with the client's ability to watch the nurse's actions, especially when demonstrating a skill or using visual aids such as posters or pamphlets. A room that is too cold, hot, or stuffy will make the client too uncomfortable to attend to the nurse's activities. Comfortable furniture helps to eliminate distractions such as the need to change position or shift body weight.

It is also important to choose a quiet setting that offers privacy and where interruptions are infrequent. If the client desires, family members might share in discussions. However, the client may be reluctant to dis-

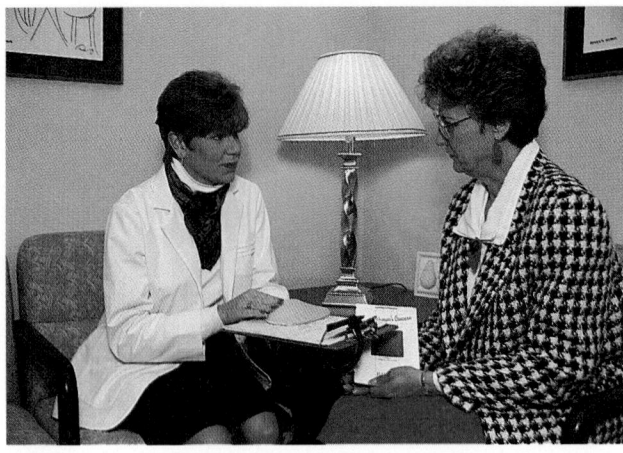

Figure 15-2. Choosing comfortable, pleasant environments enhances the learning experience. This nurse is explaining the breast self-examination procedure to the client.

cuss the nature of the illness when other persons, even family members, are in the room.

Teaching a group of clients requires a room that allows all persons to be seated comfortably and within hearing distance of the teacher. The size of the room should not overwhelm the group, tempting participants to sit outside the group along the perimeter. Arranging the group to allow participants to observe one another further enhances learning. More effective communication occurs as learners observe others' verbal and nonverbal interactions.

⋯ INTEGRATING THE NURSING AND TEACHING PROCESSES ⋯

A relationship exists between the nursing and teaching processes. During the nursing process, assessment reveals the client's health care needs. The nursing diagnoses identified are unique to the client's situation. A care plan is individualized, appropriate interventions are implemented, and evaluation determines the level of success in meeting goals of care.

While diagnosing a client's health care problems, the nurse may identify the need for education. When education becomes a part of the care plan, the teaching process begins. Like the nursing process, the teaching process requires assessment; in this case it requires analyzing the client's need, motivation, and ability to learn (Table 15-3). A diagnostic statement specifies the information or skills the client requires. The nurse sets specific learning objectives and implements the teaching plan using teaching and learning principles to ensure that the client acquires knowledge and skills. Finally, the teaching process requires an evaluation of learning based on learning objectives.

The nursing and teaching processes are not the

TABLE 15-3
Comparison of the Nursing and Teaching Processes

Basic Steps	Nursing Process	Teaching Process
Assessment	Collect data about client's physical, psychological, social, cultural, developmental, and spiritual needs from client, family, diagnostic tests, medical record, nursing history, and literature.	Gather data about client's learning needs, motivation, ability to learn, and teaching resources from client, family, learning environment, medical record, nursing history, and literature.
Nursing diagnosis	Identify appropriate nursing diagnoses.	Identify client's learning needs on basis of three domains of learning.
Planning	Develop individualized care plan. Set diagnosis priorities based on client's immediate needs. Collaborate with client on care plan.	Establish learning objectives, stated in behavioral terms. Identify priorities regarding learning needs. Collaborate with client on teaching plan. Identify type of teaching method to use.
Implementation	Perform nursing care therapies. Include client as active participant in care. Involve family in care as appropriate.	Implement teaching methods. Actively involve client in learning activities. Include family participation as appropriate.
Evaluation	Identify success in meeting desired outcomes and goals of nursing care.	Determine outcomes of teaching-learning process. Measure client's ability to achieve learning objectives. Reteach as needed.

same. The nursing process requires assessment of all sources of data to determine a client's total health care needs. The teaching process focuses on the client's learning needs and willingness and capability to learn.

▪ Assessment

Success in teaching a client requires the nurse to assess all factors influencing relevant content, the client's ability and willingness to learn, and the resources for instruction. The client's learning needs determine the choice of teaching content.

Learning needs. The nurse and client determine the information critical for the client to learn, which determines the choice of teaching content. Questions such as "What do you believe is important for you to know to adequately care for yourself?" allow the client to be an active participant in planning self-care. Learning needs change depending on where the client is in the recovery process. Assessment is thus an ongoing activity. An effective assessment is the basis by which instruction can be individualized to each client (Redman, 1997). Some examples of key areas of assessment are (1) questions raised by the client or family about health issues; (2) the client's level of understanding of current health status, implications of illness, types of therapy, and prognosis; (3) information or skills needed to perform self-care; (4) experiences that influence the client's need to learn; and (5) information necessary for family members to support the client's needs.

Motivation to learn. Nurses use several tools to assess the client's motivation to learn. In the absence of such tools the nurse can ask questions that define the client's motivation. These questions help to determine whether the client is prepared and willing to learn. They include asking the client about learning behaviors, health beliefs, attitudes about health care providers, knowledge of information to be learned, physical symptoms that interfere with learning (e.g., fatigue, pain, dizziness), sociocultural background, and learning-style preference.

Ability to learn. The nurse determines the client's physical and cognitive levels. Many factors can impair the ability to learn. The nurse needs to assess the client's physical strength and coordination, any sensory deficits, the client's reading and developmental level (see Box 15-3), and the client's level of cognitive functioning (see Chapter 24). For example, does the client possess the fine motor skills necessary to manipulate a syringe or perform a dressing change? Can the client see and hear adequately to absorb written and verbal instructions? Is the client able to perform the calculations necessary to administer a medication such as insulin?

Teaching environment. The environment for a teaching session must be conducive to learning. The nurse assesses for distractions, noise, the client's comfort level, and the availability of rooms and equipment.

In the home setting, lighting, space, and equipment availability are especially important to assess.

Resources for learning.
A client may require the support of family members or significant others. Are family members present at teaching sessions? Do they appear interested and ask pertinent questions? The nurse must assess the readiness of family and friends to learn any information necessary to help care for the client, as well as family perceptions and understanding of the client's illness, the client's willingness to involve family members in care, the family's willingness to help provide care, resources available in the home (e.g., a magnifier needed to see the markings on a syringe), and needed teaching tools. The nurse should ensure that available teaching resources such as brochures, audiovisual materials, and posters are available when needed and that the most appropriate teaching tool for the client's needs and ability to learn is selected. Written materials should be assessed for reading level. There are computer programs designed to facilitate this task. Also, organizations such as a literacy council can be of great assistance.

Cultural issues must be explored because there is a dearth of culturally sensitive teaching resources (Wilson, 1996). Are brochures written in the client's native language? What is the client's role in the family and how is this illness perceived culturally? What significance do medications have in the client's culture, and are alternative therapies used?

The assessment phase brings the scope of a teaching plan into focus. A thorough assessment helps the nurse choose the best teaching methods and ensures a more individualized approach toward client education.

▪ Nursing Diagnosis

After assessing information related to the client's ability and need to learn, the nurse interprets the data to form diagnoses that reflect the client's specific learning needs (see nursing diagnoses box). This ensures that teaching will be goal directed and individualized. If a client has several learning needs, nursing diagnoses allow for priority setting.

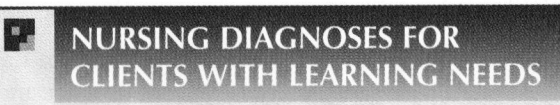

NURSING DIAGNOSES FOR CLIENTS WITH LEARNING NEEDS

Health maintenance, altered
Knowledge deficit (affective)
Knowledge deficit (cognitive)
Knowledge deficit (psychomotor)
Management of therapeutic regimen, individuals: ineffective
Noncompliance (with medications)
Self-care deficit, bathing/hygiene

Several nursing diagnoses apply to learning needs. Each diagnostic statement describes the specific type of learning need and its cause. Classifying diagnoses by the three learning domains helps the nurse focus specifically on the subject matter and teaching methods.

Some health care problems can be managed or eliminated through education. In these situations the related factor of the diagnostic statement is *knowledge deficit*. For example, a client may have difficulty interacting socially because of a lack of effective communication skills, or a self-care deficit may exist because of an inadequate knowledge base.

Some nursing diagnoses also indicate that teaching may be inappropriate. The nurse may identify conditions that can cause barriers to effective learning (e.g., pain, activity intolerance). In these cases the nurse delays teaching until the nursing diagnosis is resolved or the health problem is controlled.

▪ Planning

After determining nursing diagnoses that identify a client's learning needs, the nurse develops a teaching plan, including goals and expected outcomes, and involves the client in selecting learning experiences. Expected outcomes guide the choice of teaching strategies and approaches with a client. Client participation ensures a more relevant and meaningful plan (see care plan).

A learning objective identifies the expected outcome of a planned learning experience and helps establish priorities for learning. Objectives are short term (relating to the client's immediate learning needs) or long term (relating to the acquisition of the knowledge and skills that are needed to permanently adapt to a health problem). The nurse and client develop learning objectives together. Each objective is a statement of a single behavior that identifies the client's ability to do something after a learning experience. The objective contains an active verb describing what the learner will do after the objective is met, such as perform a crutch gait, administer an injection, or identify drug doses. The verb should have few interpretations and be stated in terms of how the client is to demonstrate learning, rather than what or how the teacher is to teach (Redman, 1997).

Behavioral objectives are measurable and observable, indicating how learning is evidenced (e.g., to perform the three-point crutch gait). If content is missing, the objective cannot guide teaching and learning. The precise behaviors and content set the standard for feedback that reflects learning and forms the basis for evaluation of the teaching plan.

An objective is more precise when it also describes the conditions or timing under which the behavior occurs. Conditions or time frames should be realistic and designed for the learner's needs. It helps to consider the conditions under which the client or family will typically perform the learned behavior (e.g., to walk from bedroom to bath using crutches).

◼ SAMPLE NURSING CARE PLAN

Assessment

The nurse's assessment reveals that Mrs. Schulte is 5 feet, 1 inch tall and weighs 164 pounds. Her blood sugar levels in the clinic are repeatedly elevated, indicating poor glucose control. Mrs. Schulte is to take an oral hypoglycemic medication every morning, monitor her blood glucose levels twice a day, follow a 1500-calorie diet, and walk for 20 minutes 3 to 4 times per week.

When discussing Mrs. Schulte's condition with her, Ms. Sommers learns that her client **knows only that diabetes is "a touch of bad sugar." The client does not understand** the cellular **action of insulin or the interplay of diet, exercise, medication, and blood glucose monitoring in blood glucose control.** Mrs. Schulte has never seen a nutritionist and is **unaware of how her obesity affects her diabetes.** She admits to not adhering to her meal plan, refuses to exercise, and **does not monitor her blood glucose levels.** Mrs. Schulte does take her diabetes medication as prescribed but is **unaware of its mechanism of action or side effects** (knowledge deficit).

Ms. Sommers is concerned that if Mrs. Schulte has a history of not adhering to the treatment plan, she may not benefit from a teaching plan. However, she learns that Mrs. Schulte has an interest in learning more because she **asks the nurse several questions** (readiness to learn).

The client is **unfamiliar with many of the terms** Ms. Sommers uses to describe diabetes (cognitive capability).

Mrs. Schulte is married to an employed laborer and has four children, one of whom is 18 years of age and still lives at home. Mrs. Schulte does all of the cooking for her family and has never seen a nutritionist for dietary counseling. When asked if Mr. Schulte could be present at a teaching session, Mrs. Schulte says "Yes, he will come if I ask him to" (family support).

Ms. Sommers reserves a conference room for the first teaching session. She arranges to use a short videotape on general facts of diabetes. She then locates pamphlets on diabetes medications (teaching resources).

Nursing Diagnosis

Assessment reveals a number of diagnoses as follows:
Knowledge deficit: (cognitive) regarding illness related to:
Poor understanding of pathophysiology of diabetes
Poor understanding of components of diabetes therapy
Knowledge deficit: (psychomotor) regarding blood glucose monitoring related to:
Inexperience with blood glucose self-monitoring skills

Planning

On the basis of the diagnoses, Ms. Sommers and Mrs. Schulte set mutually agreed-on learning objectives. After proper instruction Mrs. Schulte will be able to accomplish the following:

1. Develop a 1500-calorie diabetic meal plan for 1 week.
2. Monitor blood glucose levels independently, 2 times per day.
3. Describe the action and side effects of her diabetes medication.
4. Lose 2 pounds in 1 month.

The nurse does not plan to cover all topics in one teaching session. Mrs. Schulte agrees to have her husband attend to learn about diabetes and the treatment program. Mrs. Schulte also agrees to follow up after the initial session with a nutritionist. The nurse and client agree to hold the initial session on Thursday morning, when Mr. Schulte does not work.

Continued

SAMPLE NURSING CARE PLAN—cont'd

Implementation

Ms. Sommers begins the session by getting to know Mr. Schulte and observing how he and his wife interact. She recognizes that Mr. Schulte is interested in helping his wife. The client and her husband are attentive and responsive to Ms. Sommer's questions.

The nurse shows the film to give Mr. and Mrs. Schulte a thorough introduction to diabetes. After the film the nurse and her clients discuss aspects of the film relevant to Mrs. Schulte's condition, and the nurse answers the couple's questions. Ms. Sommers discusses the diabetes medication and its side effects. She also explains how obesity affects diabetes control and Mrs. Schulte's need to see a nutritionist. The nurse asks questions designed to help Mr. Schulte gain an understanding of the long-term impact of his wife's disease. Throughout the discussion Ms. Sommers uses simple terms to explain key concepts. When the Schultes show confusion, Ms. Sommers clarifies information with illustrations on the blackboard.

Ms. Sommers uses the remaining class time to demonstrate blood glucose self-monitoring with a glucose meter. This type of teaching gets Mr. and Mrs. Schulte actively involved. The nurse demonstrates the cleaning and operation of the meter. She has Mr. and Mrs. Schulte each perform a return demonstration of these procedures. She then explains the appropriate blood/glucose target ranges and the proper procedure for recording blood glucose levels.

Evaluation

The nurse asks the Schultes to briefly explain the nature of diabetes. After viewing the film they are able to give a simple but complete description of the action of insulin and the treatment components of diabetes. Ms. Sommers understands that it is easy to forget information that is not reinforced. She gives Mr. and Mrs. Schulte a pamphlet to review before the next class and asks them to write down any questions they might have.

It is too early to evaluate Mrs. Schulte's adherence to the diabetic diet or her weight loss. However, she is to see the nutritionist within the week.

Mrs. Schulte is to bring her blood glucose meter and record book to the next visit so that Ms. Sommers can evaluate her adherence to her glucose monitoring schedule. Mrs. Schulte is to perform the glucose monitoring herself, relying on Mr. Schulte for assistance and support only if needed. Thus the nurse has begun a constructive teaching plan that will enable Mrs. Schulte and her husband to cope more effectively with her disease. As the teaching process continues, Ms. Sommers will work with Mr. and Mrs. Schulte to reach all the objectives based on the nursing diagnoses.

Defining characteristics are shown in bold type.

Criteria for acceptable performance set a standard by which achievement is measured. A teacher sets criteria on the basis of a desired level of accuracy, success, or satisfaction. For example, a client undergoing therapy for a fractured leg will walk on crutches to the end of the hall within 3 days. Criteria are more acceptable when established by the teacher and learner. However, the nurse serves as a resource in setting the minimal criteria for success. Criteria on which the client and nurse agree help to define the expected behaviors and the quality of performance. The client also uses these criteria for self-evaluation, which is a powerful motivator of behavior.

After formulating objectives, the nurse and client work to establish a teaching plan. During planning the nurse integrates basic teaching principles and develops and prioritizes a well-timed, organized teaching plan.

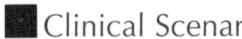
Clinical Scenario

Mrs. Schulte is a 58-year-old woman seen in the clinic for the treatment of type II (non–insulin-dependent) diabetes. She has had diabetes for 2 years and repeatedly returns to the clinic as a result of difficulty in following the prescribed therapy. The nurse, Ms. Sommers, decides that Mrs. Schulte might benefit from a teaching program directed toward improving her ability to cope with diabetes and increasing her self-management skills. Ms. Sommers has worked with diabetic clients in the past. Her experience leads her to use teaching strategies that were successful with other clients.

Integrating basic teaching principles. Teaching priorities should reflect the priorities of the nursing diagnoses. Teaching, or instruction, is the process of leading someone to learn. When developing a teaching plan, the nurse considers principles that improve its effectiveness. The realm of teaching deals with the teacher's behavior, the reason teachers behave the way they do, and effects of their behavior on learners. There is no single correct way to teach because each learning situation determines the best way to teach. The principles of teaching are, in effect, techniques that incorporate the principles of learning.

Setting priorities. Priorities for teaching are based on nursing diagnoses and the learning objectives established for the client. A client's learning needs must be set in order of priority to conserve the client's and nurse's time and energy. For example, a client with a permanent leg injury has a knowledge deficit regarding the nature of the injury and its implications and the types of skills needed to resume a normal life at home. The client will benefit most from first learning about the injury and the resultant physical changes to aid in coping with the disability. Then self-care skills necessary at home can be introduced.

Timing. When is the right time to teach? When a client first enters a clinic or hospital? At discharge? At home? Each may be appropriate because clients continue to have learning needs and opportunities as long as they stay in the health care system. The nurse determines the client's readiness to learn. Timing can be difficult because emphasis is placed on a client's early discharge from a hospital. For example, it may take several days after surgery for a client to become free of discomfort so that attention can be given to learning. By the time the client feels ready to learn, discharge may already be scheduled. The nurse should plan teaching activities for a time when the client is most attentive, receptive, and alert. Many hospitals provide information to clients before admission. The client's activities should be organized to provide time for rest and teaching-learning interactions.

The length of teaching sessions also influences learning ability. Prolonged sessions cause clients to lose concentration and attentiveness, especially older adult clients. Frequent sessions lasting 20 to 30 minutes are more easily tolerated and retain the client's interest in the material. The nurse can assess a client's loss of concentration by observing for nonverbal cues such as poor eye contact or slumped posture. After loss of concen-

tration is noted, the session should be stopped. However, teaching sessions should not be too brief. The client needs time to comprehend the information and to give feedback.

Teaching sessions should be held frequently enough to document the client's learning. The frequency of sessions depends on the learner's abilities and the complexity of the material. Intervals between teaching sessions should not be so long that the client might forget information. For clients discharged from a hospital, home health nurses must reinforce learning or arrangements must be made for telephone or outpatient educational follow-up.

Organizing teaching material. A good teacher gives careful consideration to the order of information presented. An outline of content helps to organize information into a logical sequence. Material should progress from simple to complex ideas because a person must learn simple facts and concepts before learning how to make associations or complex interpretations of ideas. For example, to teach a client with diabetes how to calculate a 1200-calorie diet, the nurse first teaches the client about calories, proteins, and carbohydrates and then uses simple mathematical problems to help the client learn to calculate amounts.

The nurse begins any instruction with essential content and completes the teaching session with informative but less critical content (London, 1995). It helps to provide verbal instruction over time, in small amounts (Burke and Dunbar-Jacob, 1995). Repetition reinforces learning. A concise summary of key topics will help the learner to know the most important information.

Maintaining learner attention and participation. Active participation is a key to learning. Persons learn better when more than one of the body's senses is stimulated. Audiovisual aids and role playing are good teaching strategies. By actively experiencing a learning event, the person is more likely to retain the knowledge gained.

A teacher's actions can also increase learner attention and interest. When conducting a discussion with a learner, the teacher should stay active by changing tone and intensity of voice, making eye contact, and using gestures that accentuate key points of discussion. An effective teacher often uses as much energy as the learner, talking and moving among a group rather than remaining stationary behind a lectern or table. A learner remains interested in a teacher who is actively enthusiastic about the subject under discussion.

Building on existing knowledge. A client learns best on the basis of preexisting cognitive abilities and knowledge. Thus a teacher is more effective by presenting information that builds on a learner's existing knowledge. For example, when teaching a client about care after a heart attack, the nurse should determine whether the client has had experience with a family member requiring such care. The key is assessing the

Box 15-4
Teaching Methods

Cognitive

Discussion (one-on-one or group)

May involve nurse and client or nurse with several clients

Promotes active participation and focuses on topics of interest to client

Allows peer support

Enhances application and analysis of new information

Lecture

Is more formal method of instruction because it is controlled by teacher

Helps learner acquire new knowledge and gain comprehension

Question-and-answer session

Is designed specifically to address client's concerns

Assists client in applying knowledge

Role play, discovery

Allows client to actively apply knowledge in controlled situation

Promotes synthesis of information and problem solving

Independent project (computer-assisted instruction), field experience

Allows client to assume responsibility for completing learning activities at own pace

Promotes analysis, synthesis, and evaluation of new information and skills

Affective

Role play

Allows expression of values, feelings, and attitudes

Discussion (group)

Allows client to acquire support from others in group

Permits client to learn from other experiences

Promotes responding, valuing, and organization

Discussion (one-on-one)

Allows discussion of personal, sensitive topics of interest or concern

Psychomotor

Demonstration

Provides presentation of procedures or skills by nurse

Permits client to incorporate modeling of nurse's behavior

Allows nurse to control questioning during demonstration

Practice

Gives client opportunity to perform skills using equipment

Provides repetition

Return demonstration

Permits client to perform skill as nurse observes

Is excellent source of feedback and reinforcement

Independent project, game

Requires teaching method that promotes adaptation and origination of psychomotor learning

Permits learner to use new skills

---

learner's level of knowledge by finding out how much is known about the topic.

Selection of teaching methods. During planning the nurse chooses appropriate teaching methods and encourages the client to offer suggestions. A teaching method is the way that the teacher delivers information and is based on the client's learning needs (Box 15-4). For example, a client with a psychomotor deficit learns best through demonstration and supervised practice. The client masters skills by handling equipment and practicing manual skills. Discussions, question-and-answer sessions, and formal lectures are effective methods for promoting cognitive learning. Clients with intellectual deficits are given the opportunity to explore new ideas, recognize new relationships, and apply knowledge to their unique needs. A highly effective method

for stimulating affective learning is group discussion. The method should complement the client's needs, and more than one method may be used for instruction.

Writing teaching plans. In all health care settings, nurses develop written teaching plans for use by colleagues in a variety of disciplines. In the past, client education was often solely hospital based. Now the domain includes a variety of settings (such as the home, clinic, physician's office, or rehabilitation center) and several professions (such as physicians, pharmacists, physical therapists, and home health care nurses) to provide information to the client (Visser and Herbert, 1994). Often, however, one nurse is primarily responsible for developing the initial teaching plan.

The teaching plan may be lengthy or concise and includes topics for instruction, teaching resources (e.g., equipment, booklets), recommendations for involving family, and objectives. The setting may influence the complexity of the plan, with a home health care teaching plan proving to be more extensive in scope than an acute care setting plan because more teaching time is available in the home setting. No matter what the length, the teaching plan should provide continuity of instruction, especially when several nurses or disciplines are collaborating in educating the client.

▪ Implementation

Implementation of a teaching plan (see clinical scenario) involves applying all teaching and learning principles. Implementation involves believing that each interaction with a client is an opportunity to teach. The nurse maximizes opportunities for effective learning and creates an active learning environment.

Teaching approaches. A nurse's approach in teaching is different from teaching methods. Some situations require the teacher to be directive. Others may require a nondirective approach. An effective teacher concentrates on the task and uses teaching approaches according to client needs. A client's learning needs may change over time; therefore the nurse must be aware of the need to modify teaching approaches.

Telling. The telling approach is useful when limited information must be taught (e.g., when preparing the client for an emergent diagnostic procedure). When this approach is used, the nurse outlines the task to be done by the client and gives explicit instructions. There is no time for feedback with this method.

Selling. The selling approach uses two-way communication. The nurse paces instruction based on the client's response. Specific feedback is given to the client who shows success at learning. For example, the client learns a step-by-step procedure for changing a dressing. The nurse uses information from the client to adapt the teaching approach.

Participating. The participating approach involves the nurse and client in setting objectives and participating in the learning process together. The client helps decide content, and the nurse guides and counsels the client. For example, a client with diabetes works with the nurse to plan a menu or self-administer insulin. In this method there is opportunity for discussion, feedback, and revision of the teaching plan.

Entrusting. The entrusting approach provides the client the opportunity to manage self-care. The client accepts responsibilities and performs the tasks well. The nurse observes the client's progress. For example, for a diabetic client who has correctly administered injections for 3 months, the nurse instructs the client about a new prescribed dose of insulin and allows the client to perform the injection.

Reinforcing. The principle of **reinforcement** applies to the process of learning; however, the teacher must often be the source of reinforcement. Reinforcement is using a stimulus that increases the probability of a response. A learner who receives reinforcement before or after a desired learning behavior will likely repeat the behavior. Feedback is a common form of reinforcement.

Reinforcers are positive or negative. Positive reinforcement such as a smile or praise and approval produces the desired responses. Negative reinforcement such as frowning or complaining produces the desired behavior when the reinforcers are removed. People usually respond better to positive reinforcement.

Three types of reinforcers are social, material, and activity. When a nurse works with a client, most reinforcers are social (e.g., smiles, compliments, words of encouragement, physical contact), which are used to acknowledge a learned behavior. Examples of material reinforcers are food, toys, and music. These work best with young children. Activity reinforcers rely on the principle that a person is motivated to engage in an activity if promised that, after its completion, the opportunity to engage in more desirable activity will be available. For example, a client will more likely perform a painful exercise if given the chance to take a nap afterward.

Choosing an appropriate reinforcer involves careful thought and attention to individual preferences. Reinforcers should never be used as threats. Reinforcement is not always effective with every client.

Incorporating teaching with nursing care. Many nurses find that they can teach more effectively while delivering nursing care. An informal, unstructured style relies on the positive therapeutic relationship between nurse and client, which fosters a spontaneity in the teaching-learning process. This does not suggest that teaching should occur without a formal plan. When the nurse follows a teaching plan informally, the client feels less pressure to perform and learning becomes more of a shared activity. Teaching during routine care is efficient and cost effective (Figure 15-3).

Instructional methods. Instructional methods chosen depend on the client's learning needs, the time available for teaching, the setting, the resources available, and the nurse's own comfort level with teaching. There are a variety of appropriate methods (see Box 15-4). Skilled teachers are flexible and combine more than one method into a teaching plan.

One-on-one discussion. When teaching a client at the bedside, in a physician's office, or in the home, the nurse directly shares information through one-on-one discussion. Information is provided informally, allowing the client to ask questions or share concerns. Various teaching aids can be used during the discussion, depending on the client's learning needs.

Group instruction. A nurse uses group instruction with clients or families because groups offer an economical way to teach a number of clients at one time, and often the experience of being part of a group may provide the support necessary for clients to meet learning

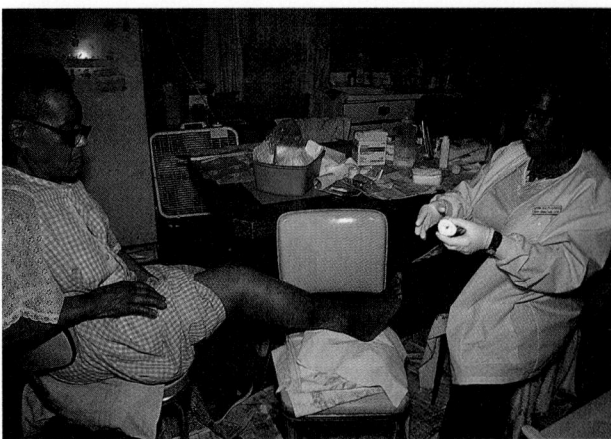

Figure 15-3. Nurse teaching a client about care in the home setting.

objectives (Redman, 1997). Group instruction often involves both lecture and discussion. Lectures are highly structured and are efficient in helping groups of clients learn standard content about a subject. After hearing information from a lecture, learners need the opportunity to share ideas and seek clarification. Group discussions allow clients and families to learn from each other as they review common experiences (Redman, 1997).

Preparatory instruction. Clients frequently face unfamiliar tests or procedures that create anxiety. Providing information about procedures helps clients form realistic images of what to anticipate. When the experience matches expectations, the client is more likely to attend to the nurse's future explanations. A nurse gains respect when preparatory explanations prove useful. The following are guidelines for giving preparatory explanations:

1. Physical sensations during the procedure are described but not evaluated. For example, when drawing a blood specimen, the nurse explains that the client will feel a sticking sensation as the needle punctures the skin.
2. The cause of the sensation is described, preventing misinterpretation of the experience. For example, the nurse explains that a needle insertion burns because alcohol used to cleanse the skin enters the puncture site.
3. Clients are prepared only for aspects of the experience that have commonly been noticed by other clients. For example, the nurse explains that it is normal for a tight tourniquet to cause a person's hand to tingle and feel numb.

The client finds comfort in knowing what to expect. When the nurse's descriptions accurately portray the actual experience, the client is able to cope more effectively with the stress from procedures and therapies.

Demonstrations. Demonstrations are useful methods for teaching psychomotor skills. An effective demonstration requires advance planning, including the following:

1. Ensure that the learner can easily see the demonstration by positioning the learner to provide a clear view of the skill being performed.
2. Review the rationale and steps of the procedure.
3. Assemble and organize equipment.
4. Perform each step in sequence while analyzing the knowledge and skills involved.
5. Determine when explanations need to be given, considering the client's learning needs.
6. Judge the proper speed and timing of the demonstration, based on the client's cognitive abilities and anxiety level.

The nurse demonstrates a procedure or skill in the same order in which the client will perform it. In addition, the nurse encourages the client to ask questions so that each step is clearly understood. To enable the client to easily observe each step of the procedure, demonstrations should be performed slowly, avoiding a hurried approach. The nurse gives an opportunity to practice the procedure under supervision after the client has practiced handling equipment. Ultimately the client demonstrates the procedure independently to ensure acquisition of the skill. This demonstration should occur under the same conditions that the client will experience at home.

Analogies. Learning occurs when a teacher translates complex language or ideas into words or concepts that the client understands. In addition, the client benefits by integrating new information into daily routines. **Analogies** supplement verbal instruction with familiar images that make complex information more real and understandable (Redman, 1997). For example, comparing arterial blood pressure to the flow of water through a hose is an analogy that might be useful when explaining hypertension to a client. When using analogies, the nurse must be familiar with the concept; be aware of the client's background, experience, and culture; and keep the analogy simple and clear.

Role playing. The nurse uses role play for teaching ideas and attitudes. An example might include teaching family care givers better ways of communicating with older adult parents. The technique involves rehearsing a desired behavior, and as a result, clients are taught required skills and feel more confident in performing them independently.

Discovery. Discovery is a useful technique for teaching problem solving, application, and independent thinking. During individual or group discussion, the nurse may pose a problem or situation pertaining to the client's learning needs for clients to solve. For example, clients with heart disease may be asked to plan a meal low in cholesterol.

Speaking the client's language. It is important to use words a client can understand. The nurse should define unfamiliar medical or nursing terms and offer them consistently throughout a teaching session. Medical jargon can be confusing.

In a classic study, Byrne and Edeani (1984) found that clients understood fewer medical words than health professionals predicted. The problem of **functional illiteracy** is also real. Approximately 25 million Americans are functionally illiterate or unable to read above a fifth-grade level, and 45 million are considered marginally illiterate or unable to use written information to get their everyday needs met (Fain, 1994). Years of schooling do not appear to be accurate indicators of reading ability (Miller and Bodie, 1994) and American Indians, blacks, and Hispanics have the highest rates of illiteracy (Fain, 1994).

To compound the problem, the readability of health education material has been found to range from elementary school level to college level (Owen and others, 1993; Wilson, 1996), even though studies have shown that clients are more apt to understand information prepared at a fifth-grade level (Estey and others, 1994). Thus it appears that written health information available to a client often exceeds the client's reading ability.

The nurse must address literacy problems by using simple terminology to enhance the client's understanding. Frequently asking clients for feedback determines whether clients comprehend and provides a time for repeated review of procedures. Teaching materials should be written on a fifth-grade level with attention given to short words and sentences, large type, and simple format.

Cultural variables. Health education materials also often fail to recognize cultural beliefs, values, language, perceptions, and attitudes held by clients and families (Wilson, 1996). The nurse must be aware of the client's cultural background, beliefs, and ability to understand instructions developed outside of the native language (Box 15-5). Cultural diversity is widespread and poses a great challenge to the nurse attempting to provide culturally sensitive health care. When educating clients of different ethnic groups, the nurse should do the following:

1. Become aware of each culture's distinctive aspects (Trask, 1995).
2. Collaborate with other nurses and educators to assist in dealing with cultural diversity.
3. Enlist the help of people in the cultural group to share values and beliefs.
4. Use input and experiences of ethnic nurses in providing care to members of their community (Bernal, 1993).

Special needs of children and older adults.
A nurse's choice of instructional methods and applica-

> ▪ **Box 15-5**
> **Cultural Aspects of Care**
>
> The community health nurse assessed the need to provide acquired immunodeficiency syndrome (AIDS) education to the three teenage sons in a Mexican-American family in her caseload. Substance abuse (alcohol and drug addiction) is higher among Hispanics than among other groups, largely because of machismo, a cultural view that drinking and drug use demonstrate strength and masculinity. In addition, some Hispanics share needles and syringes to administer vitamins, medications, or contraceptives purchased in Mexico.
>
> In providing health education to this family, the nurse relied on the interpretation of true cultural machismo in which Hispanic men take responsibility for their families and protect them from harm. Using this cultural value, the nurse encouraged these young Hispanic men to protect their loved ones from the threat of diseases such as AIDS. The nurse also discussed appropriate methods of contraception and proper medication and vitamin administration.
>
> From Caudle P: Providing culturally sensitive health care to Hispanic clients, *Nurse Pract* 18(12):40, 1993.

tion of teaching-learning principles may be based on a client's age. Children, adults, and older adults learn differently. The nurse adapts teaching strategies to each learner.

Children pass through several developmental stages (see Chapter 20). In each stage, children acquire new cognitive and psychomotor abilities that respond to different types of learning. Parental input and participation are needed in planning health education for children.

Older adults experience numerous physical and psychological changes as they age. These changes can create barriers to learning. Sensory changes require teaching methods that enhance the client's functioning. Research shows that older adults learn and remember effectively if the learning is paced properly and the material is relevant to the learner's needs and abilities (Deakins, 1994; Dellasega and others, 1994). Educational strategies for gerontological nursing practice are highlighted in Box 15-6.

▪ Evaluation

Client education is not complete until the nurse evaluates the outcomes of the teaching-learning process. Did the client learn what was intended? The nurse evaluates success by observing the client's performance of each expected behavior. Success depends on the client's ability to meet the established performance criteria.

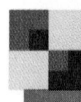

Gerontological Nursing Practice

- Use a slow pace of presentation.
- Give information in short frequent sessions.
- Repeat information frequently.
- Reinforce teaching with audiovisual material, written exercises, and practice.
- Use examples.
- Allow more time for learners to express themselves, demonstrate learning, and ask questions.
- Establish reachable short-term goals.
- Apply teaching to present situations.
- Base new information on clients' previous level of learning.

Modified from Deakins D: Teaching elderly patients about diabetes, *Am J Nurs* 94(4):38, 1994.

Return demonstrations, use of questions, observation of client behaviors, role playing, and discussions can be used to evaluate clients. For example, the client who will use a three-point crutch gait while walking to the end of the hall must demonstrate the actual crutch-walking technique. A client who is to identify five signs and symptoms of a heart attack must be able to do so when questioned or during a discussion of the disease.

If evaluation indicates a knowledge or skill deficit, the nurse repeats or modifies the teaching plan. Alternative teaching methods often help to clarify information or strengthen skills that the client was unable to comprehend or perform originally.

Evaluation may also reveal new learning needs or new factors that may interfere with the client's ability to learn. The nurse reassesses those factors to update the teaching plan and make it relevant to client needs. Like the nursing process, the teaching process is continuous and ever changing.

··· DOCUMENTATION OF CLIENT TEACHING

Because client teaching often occurs informally between nurse and client (e.g., during medication administration, physical examination), it is difficult to document client education consistently. Nurses often fail to take the time to write down information they have taught. However, because a nurse is legally responsible for providing accurate and timely information to clients, quality documentation is essential. Casey (1995) suggests the following for documenting client education:

1. *Specific content.* Specifically describe subject matter so that other nurses can follow up and reinforce teaching (e.g., "insulin injection demonstrated," "explained side effects of Inderal"). Avoid generalizations such as "medications taught" that leave staff uninformed about what content has been taught.
2. *Evaluation of learning.* Document evidence of learning (e.g., a return demonstration, the attempt to evaluate learning). This informs staff about the client's progress and determines material that still needs to be taught.
3. *Method of teaching.* Describe teaching methods used. Knowing methods used in instruction (e.g., demonstrations, discussion) helps staff to follow up more efficiently or offer alternative teaching methods if learning does not occur. When resources such as pamphlets or audiovisual materials are used, the nurse documents it in the client's record. Many institutions have special forms that allow easy documentation. For instance, teaching flow sheets (Figure 15-4) are excellent records that document the plan, implementation, and evaluation of client teaching (Snyder, 1996).

Key Terms

affective learning	learning objective
analogies	motivation
attentional set	psychomotor learning
cognitive learning	reinforcement
functional illiteracy	return demonstration
health beliefs	teaching
learning	

GOOD CARE HOSPITAL	*John Doe*
DIABETIC INSTRUCTION RECORD	*123 Main St.*
	Anywhere, USA
TI = Teaching Initiated D/V = Demonstrates/Verbalizes Understanding FI = Family Included	ADDRESSOGRAPH PLATE

ASSESSMENT

1. Highest level of formalized education attained *– 11th Grade*
2. Vision *– Glasses required for reading*
3. Literacy *– Able to read and explain information in teaching booklet*
4. Identified barriers to learning *– None noted –; client and wife receptive and interested in teaching*

	DATE AND INITIAL			COMMENTS
	TI	D/V	FI	
A. DISEASE OVERVIEW 1. Definition of diabetes	P.L. 3/28/98	R.K. 3/29/98	P.L. 3/28/98	
2. Long-term complications (microvascular/macrovascular/ neuropathy)	P.L. 3/28/98	R.K. 3/29/98	P.L. 3/28/98	
3. 3 Factors of control (diet, exercise, medication)	P.L. 3/28/98	R.K. 3/29/98	P.L. 3/28/98	
B. NUTRITION 1. Type (Diet) *1800 cal ADA*	C.S. 3/29/98		C.S. 3/29/98	
Snack times *4:00 PM/8:00 PM*	3/29/98	C.S.	3/29/98	C.S.
2. Meal timing *8:00 AM/12N/6:00 PM*	3/29/98	C.S.	3/29/98	C.S.
3. Food types to avoid (fried fatty foods, simple sugars)				
4. Importance of weight control				
C. EXERCISE/ACTIVITY 1. Type				
2. Frequency				
3. Duration				
4. Effects on blood sugar control and insulin utilization				
D. MEDICATION 1. Name/dosage				
2. Oral agent				
a. When to take				
b. Action of medication				
3. Insulin				
a. Action, kinds, storage				
b. Preparation, administration				
c. Site selection/rotation				

SIGNATURES FOR INITIALS

PL - Patricia L, RN   *CS - Catherine S, RD*

RK - Rebecca K, RN

Figure 15-4. Documentation tool for client teaching. (Courtesy Barnes-Jewish Hospital, St. Louis.)

▪ Key Concepts ▪

In the present health care system, there is greater emphasis on providing quality health education.

The nurse must ensure that clients, families, and communities receive information needed to maintain optimal health.

Health education is aimed at the promotion, restoration, and maintenance of health.

Teaching is most effective when it is responsive to the learner's needs.

Teaching is a form of interpersonal communication, with teacher and student actively involved in a process that increases the student's knowledge and skills.

Teaching a client a specific behavior can involve incorporation of behaviors from all three learning domains.

The client's ability to attend to the learning process depends on physical comfort and anxiety level and the presence of environmental distraction.

A person's health beliefs influence the willingness to gain the knowledge and skills necessary to maintain health.

Clients of different age-groups require different teaching strategies as a result of developmental capabilities.

Presentation of teaching content should progress from simple to more complex ideas.

The client should be an active participant in a teaching plan, agreeing to the plan, helping to choose instructional methods, and recommending times for instruction.

A combination of teaching methods improves the learner's attentiveness and involvement.

A teacher is more effective when presenting information that builds on a learner's existing knowledge.

Teaching methodologies should match the client's learning need.

Learning objectives describe what a person is to learn in behavioral terms.

A nurse evaluates a client's learning by observing the performance of expected learning behaviors under desired conditions.

▪ Critical Thinking Activities

1. Mr. Clifford is a 75-year-old widower diagnosed with uncontrolled type II diabetes mellitus, now requiring insulin injection. He is hard of hearing, has poor eyesight, and lives alone, although he has a daughter who lives nearby. Mr. Clifford has the dexterity necessary to manipulate a syringe. Design a teaching plan, including appropriate resources and modifications for Mr. Clifford to monitor his blood glucose and administer his insulin.

2. Mr. Taylor, who is 53 years of age, has a cast on his right leg after repair of a fractured ankle. He is to begin crutch walking tomorrow and must learn about cast care. You ask Mr. Taylor to read the cast care pamphlet and discuss its content with you. You discover that he is unable to read and comprehend the information in the brochure. Describe

the interventions you would employ in developing a teaching plan for this client.

3. Mrs. Sanchez, a 38-year-old woman, is scheduled for a breast biopsy. Her mother and sister have a history of breast cancer. They are both in remission and in their sixth and seventh year, respectively, after initial diagnosis. Mrs. Sanchez has never had surgery. She is nervous and "scared of the diagnosis." List your teaching priorities for this client.

4. Joey Carter is a 4-year-old boy recently diagnosed with asthma. He, along with his parents, is being taught to use an inhaled and nebulized bronchodilator. Describe teaching methods that are effective with a preschool-age child.

References

American Association of Diabetes Educators: The scope of practice for diabetes educators and the standards of practice for diabetes educators, *Diabetes Educator* 18(1):52, 1992.

American Nurses Association: *Nursing's agenda for health care reform,* Kansas City, Mo, 1991, The Association.

Barnes L: Patient education standards, *MCN Am J Matern Child Nurs* 18(1):45, 1993.

Bernal H: A model for delivering culture-relevant care in the community, *Public Health Nurs* 10(4):228, 1993.

Bostrom J and others: Learning needs of hospitalized and recently discharged patients, *Patient Educ Counsel* 23(2):83, 1994.

Burke L, Dunbar-Jacob J: Adherence to medication, diet, and activity recommendations: from assessment to maintenance, *J Cardiovasc Nurs* 9(2):62, 1995.

Byrne T, Edeani D: Knowledge of medical terminology among hospitalized patients, *Nurs Res* 33(3):178, 1984.

Casey F: Documenting patient education: a literature review, *J Continuing Educ Nurs* 26(6):257, 1995.

Caudle P: Providing culturally sensitive health care to Hispanic clients, *Nurse Pract* 18(12):40, 1993.

Deakins D: Teaching elderly patients about diabetes, *Am J Nurs* 94(4):38, 1994.

Dellasega C and others: Nursing process: teaching elderly clients, *J Gerontol Nurs* 20(1):331, 1994.

Elford R and others: A practical approach to lifestyle counseling in primary care, *Patient Educ Counsel* 24(2):175, 1994.

Estey A and others: Patient's understanding of health information: a multi-hospital comparison, *Patient Educ Counsel* 24(1):73, 1994.

Fain J: When your patient can't read, *Am J Nurs* 94(5):16B, 1994.

Hayslip D: Nurse's role in achieving patient outcomes: educator's role, *ANNA J* 22(2):132, 1995.

Hiltabiddle S: Adolescent condom use, the health belief model, and the prevention of sexually transmitted disease, *JOGNN* 25(1):61, 1996.

Houston C, Haire-Joshu: Application of health behavior models to promote behavior change. In *Management of diabetes mellitus: perspective of care across the life span,* ed 2, St. Louis, 1996, Mosby.

Joint Commission on Accreditation of Healthcare Organizations: *Accreditation manual of hospitals,* Chicago, 1997, The Commission.

London F: Teach your patients faster and better, *Nurs 95* 25(8):68, 1995.

Miller B, Bodie M: Determination of reading comprehension level for effective patient health-education materials, *Nurs Res* 43(2):118, 1994.

Northen J and others: Involvement of adult rehabilitation patients in setting occupational therapy goals, *Am J Occup Ther* 49(3):214, 1995.

Owen P and others: Reading, readability, and patient education materials, *Cardiovasc Nurs* 29(2):9, 1993.

Redman B: *The practice of patient education,* ed 8, St. Louis, 1997, Mosby.

Snyder B: An easy way to document patient ed, *RN* 59(3):43, 1996.

Trask K: The challenges of teaching universal precautions to multicultural, diverse patients and their family members, *J Intravenous Nurs* 18(65):532, 1995.

Visser A, Herbert C: Beyond the hospital: the role of public information campaigns, general practitioners, pharmacists, laypersons and patient associations in patient education and counseling, *Patient Educ Counsel* 24(2):97, 1994.

Wilson F: Patient education materials nurses use in community health, *West J Nurs Res* 18(2):195, 1996.

Wong D: *Whaley and Wong's nursing care of infants and children,* ed 5, St. Louis, 1995, Mosby.

Psychosocial Basis for Nursing Practice

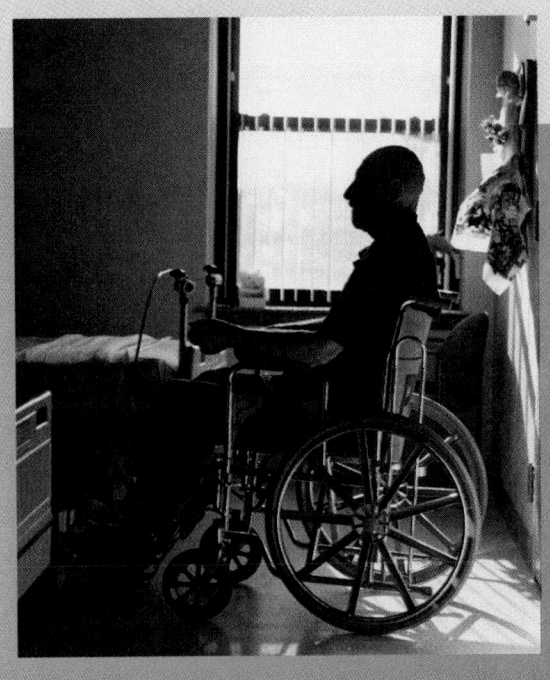

UNIT

4

CHAPTER

16

Self-Concept and Sexuality

OBJECTIVES

Mastery of content in this chapter will enable the student to:

- Define the key terms listed.
- Discuss factors that influence the following components of self-concept: body image, self-esteem, roles, and identity.
- Identify stressors that affect each of the four components of self-concept.
- Discuss ways in which the nurse's self-concept and nursing activities can affect the client's self-concept.
- Discuss the nurse's role in maintaining or enhancing a client's sexual health.
- Define sexuality as a component of personality.
- Describe key concepts of sexual development during infancy, childhood, adolescence, and adulthood.
- Apply the nursing process to assess, diagnose, plan, implement, and evaluate interventions to promote a client's self-concept and sexual health.

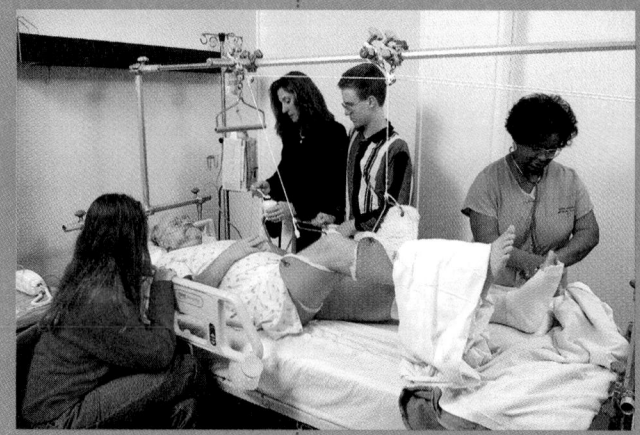

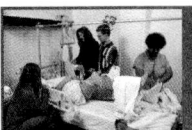

Case Study

John Finch is a 46-year-old white male who was admitted to the hospital 2 days ago after a motor vehicle accident. He is married and has two teenage children. He was involved in a single vehicle accident when his car skidded on ice. He sustained crushing injuries to both of his lower legs. He was transferred to the orthopedic unit from a rural hospital near his home. Surgery was performed on admission, and an external fixation device was applied to his right leg. He is scheduled for an open reduction and internal fixation of his left tibia in the morning. This surgery will include performing a skin graft over the injury site. Because of the extent of his injuries, there are questions regarding how functional his lower extremities will be in the future; the surgeon has mentioned the possibility of amputation. There is concern on the part of the surgeon in performing the surgery, because Mr. Finch is a Jehovah's Witness and has refused any blood products. His hemoglobin is currently 10.8. The surgery consent has been signed. A progress note indicates his physicians have talked with him repeatedly about the danger of blood loss and questioned his refusal of blood products. Mr. Finch has remained firm regarding no administration of blood products. He has clearly told his health care providers of his religious beliefs and his faith in his beliefs. The unit staff have expressed concern among themselves regarding his decision. Mr. Finch has consistently been polite to the staff. Since admission, he has experienced considerable pain and required frequent administration of morphine to control his pain. Repositioning often causes pain. When he is moved during daily care, he has very specific requests regarding how he wants to be turned and positioned. Because of the pain and the extent of his injuries, Mr. Finch is immobile and unable to engage in most of his personal care.

Mia Kendal is a 28-year-old freshman nursing student assigned to care for Mr. Finch. Mia is married and working part-time as a certified nursing assistant at a local long-term care facility while in school. She worked as a CNA for 7 months before beginning nursing school. She has had personal experience with orthopedic injuries, because she was in a skiing accident several years ago and suffered a fractured femur that required surgery (open reduction and internal fixation).

Changes in health status often result in stressors that affect a person's self-concept and sexuality. Such stressors influence a person's ability to interact with others and to function effectively. The nurse's knowledge of self-concept and sexuality can aid in identifying stressors that affect the client and promote effective planning to support the client's growth and adaptation to change.

⋯ SELF-CONCEPT

Nursing Knowledge Base

The self is one of the most important aspects of human experience, yet it is one of the most difficult to define. How people see themselves affects how they care for themselves both physically and emotionally. If a person has a poor self-concept, the person will often have difficulty caring for himself or herself in a way that supports physical and emotional health.

A person's **self-concept** represents a subjective sense of the self. It is a complex integration of conscious and unconscious feelings, attitudes, and perceptions. The self-concept is a frame of reference affecting behaviors and relationships with others.

Development of self-concept. The development of a self-concept is a complex process involving many variables. Erikson's (1963) psychosocial theory of development is helpful in understanding the key tasks individuals face at various stages of development. Erikson describes eight stages, which end with senescence. Each stage builds on the tasks of the former stage. In each stage of development, an individual faces certain tasks that, if not positively completed, may negatively influence self-concept and lead to difficulty in subsequent stages. For a discussion of each stage and its related task, see Chapter 20.

The nurse can use Erikson's theory to identify the stage of psychosocial development a client is likely to be experiencing, assess if the client is in that particular stage, and determine how the client is negotiating the task(s) of that particular stage (Box 16-1). Awareness of the client's developmental stage aids in knowing what may be important to the person in that particular stage of development.

A relatively new dimension in the area of self-concept is the field of gender differences. Formerly, females fell short on measures of maturity that had been developed by male theorists. For example, Erikson places identity versus role confusion before intimacy versus isolation. Carol Gilligan (1982) believes that women develop identity in the context of developing intimate relationships. Rather than being delayed in their development, women are seen as developing differently. Females are socialized in American culture to value caring as the highest form of development; males are socialized to value justice and fairness (Gilligan, 1982). These gender difference can result in misunderstandings between men and women and influence self-concept.

Components of self-concept.
A person's self-concept involves body image, self-esteem, roles, and identity. Each aspect develops from birth onward and reflects the changes that take place throughout life. Although they will be considered as separate aspects, they overlap and are interrelated.

Box 16-1

Erickson's Developmental Tasks and Key Areas Relating to Self-Concept

Trust Versus Mistrust (Birth to 1 yr)
Relationship to care giver

Autonomy Versus Doubt and Shame (1 to 3 yrs)
Success in gaining control of bodily functioning (including dressing, feeding, talking, walking)
Beginning independence

Initiative Versus Guilt (3 to 6 yrs)
Trying out new things
Imagination
Using language more effectively to meet needs

Industry Versus Inferiority (6 to 12 yrs)
Achieving recognition for skills and accomplishments in "the world"
Involved in school and group activities with peers

Identity Versus Role Confusion (Puberty to 18 to 21 yrs)
Continued involvement with peers (important to be a part of peer group)
Experiencing body changes associated with puberty
Exploring relationships with those found sexually attractive
Beginning to consider vocation/career

Intimacy Versus Isolation (18 to 21 to 40 yrs)
Forming and maintaining intimate relationships with significant other(s) and family
Forming relationships with peers at work

Generativity Versus Self-Absorption (40 to 65 yrs)
Reconsideration of life direction and goals
Consideration of changing appearance and functioning as ages
Broadening circle of concern to include the future of the community and/or world

Ego Integrity Versus Despair (65 to Death)
Examining life and satisfaction with "contributions"
Interest in "nurturing" the next generation

The body is the container for the self. **Body image** is the component of self-concept that involves experiences and attitudes related to the body, including appearance, perceptions regarding masculinity and femininity, physical abilities, and capabilities (Drench, 1994). Cultural and societal norms have a bearing on what each person considers an acceptable body (Figure 16-1). If a person's body deviates markedly from cultural norms, body image and thus self-concept may be negatively affected. Concerns regarding body image are often most pronounced during adolescence and aging.

Because of the multifaceted components of body image, people generally adapt slowly to physical changes. For example, it may take someone who has chosen to lose a great deal of weight a long time to incorporate the thin self into the self-concept. Formerly obese people may tell you there is still a "fat person" inside.

Self-esteem is our emotional evaluation of our self-worth. Self-esteem is influenced both by our own evaluation of our worth and the evaluation of others. Thus an individual's self-esteem is heavily influenced by the love and approval received as an infant and child. When love and approval are not given, the child frequently incorporates a low sense of self-esteem. A child's developing self-esteem is also related to how the child evaluates himself or herself at school and within the family. Adults are also influenced by the evaluation of significant others. Thus successful experiences in one's world tend to promote positive self-esteem.

Another factor that influences self-concept is the life roles a person plays. A **role** is a set of behaviors that have been sanctioned by the family, community, and culture as appropriate in particular situations. A person's role, such as student, nurse, or parent, will influence how the person sees himself or herself. A person's perception of personal performance in a role will influence self-esteem.

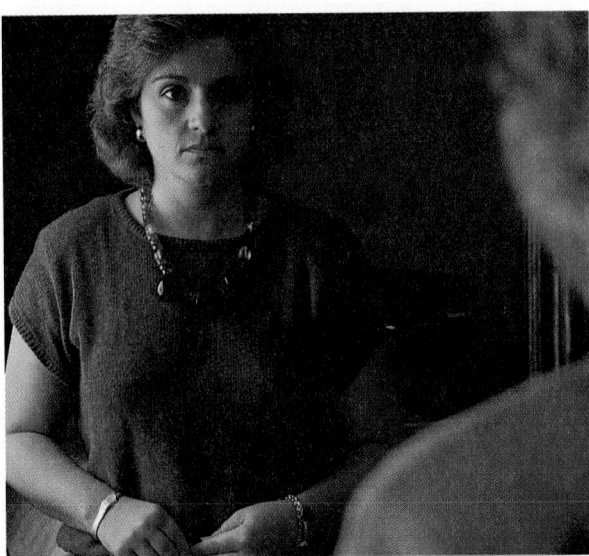

Figure 16-1.   A person's appearance influences identity.

The fourth component of self-concept is **identity.** The word is derived from the Latin word *idem,* which means "the same." Identity involves the persistent individuality and sameness of a person over time and in various circumstances. It implies a consciousness of being oneself, distinct and separate from others. This element of self-concept is what might lead a person to say, "I'm a fighter," because this is the way the person perceives himself or herself facing life circumstances over time. Another person may identify strongly with a life role, such as teacher. Another may identify with a negative self-esteem and identify himself or herself as a loser.

Stressors affecting self-concept. A self-concept stressor is any factor or change, whether real or perceived, that threatens body image, self-esteem, performance of roles, or sense of identity (Figure 16-2). The response to various self-concept stressors is as unique as the individual experiencing the stress. A person's perception of the situation is the most important factor determining his or her response. For example, a man who has had a heart attack may perceive that this means he will no longer be able to be the aggressive businessman he has prided himself as being. This perception of what the heart attack will mean could lead to depression. Another man could see his heart attack as a message to

slow down and enjoy his life. This perception could lead to gratitude to have a chance to change his life and make more time for the things he values.

Body-image stressors. When the body changes in appearance or function, the body image may be affected. The significance of a loss of function or a change in appearance is affected by the individual's perception of the alteration (e.g., if a woman considers her breasts key to her femininity, a mastectomy could negatively affect her body image) and the relative importance of body image in the individual's self-concept. The greater the importance of body image, the greater the threat that a change in body image may alter the perception of self.

Self-esteem stressors. Persons with high self-esteem are generally happier and more able to cope with demands and stressors than persons with low self-esteem (Gibson, 1980). Persons with low self-esteem tend to feel unloved and often experience depression and anxiety. Illness, surgery, or accidents that interrupt or change life patterns may decrease the feeling of self-esteem. Chronic illnesses such as diabetes, arthritis, and cardiac dysfunction may require changes in lifestyle and job performance to impact self-esteem.

Role stressors. Throughout life, a person undergoes many role changes. For example, when a woman has

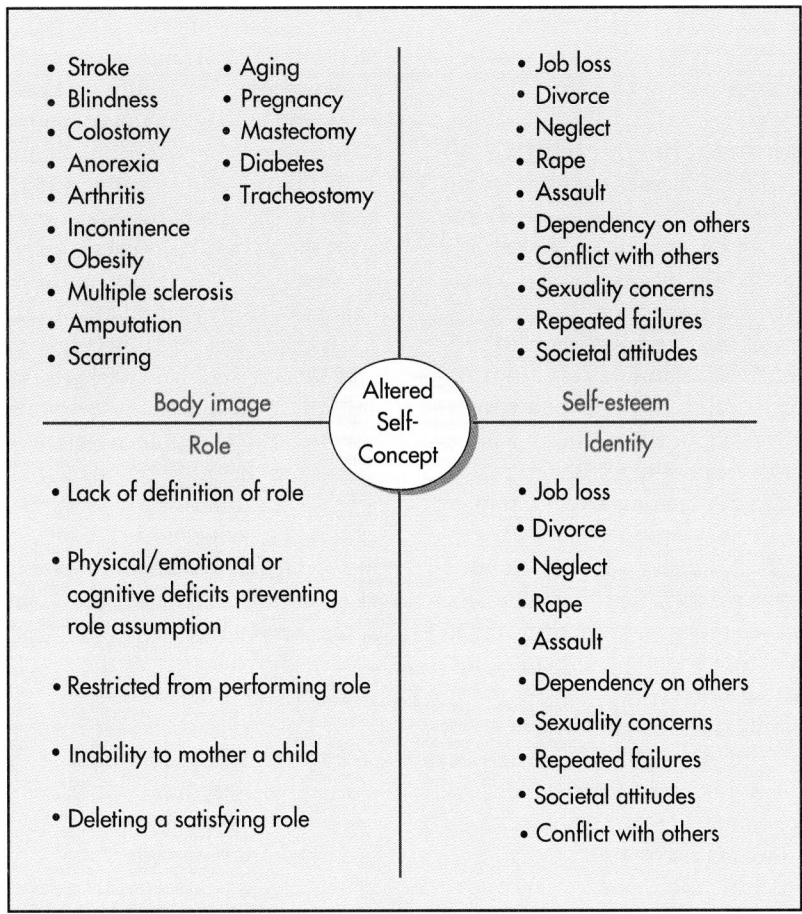

Figure 16-2. Examples of stressors that can affect a person's self-concept.

a child, she becomes a mother. The new role of mother will entail many changes in behavior if the woman is to be successful in her new role. Change within the same role and the adoption of new roles require the incorporation of new expectations and standards for behavior. Certain chronic illnesses can alter a person's ability to carry out various roles, which may affect self-esteem and identity.

Identity stressors. Identity is closely tied to physical appearance and ability. As physical appearance or abilities to carry out life activities change, individuals are often faced with significant stress in terms of their identity.

Although identity is challenged throughout the life span, adolescence is one of the critical periods for identity stress. Adolescence is a time of change, insecurity, and anxiety. The changes in body and emotion, peer pressure, and the unclear role of adolescents in our society cause much anxiety. An adult generally has a more stable identity and a more firmly held image of self. Once the identity is stable, the adult can better weather stressors such as marriage, divorce, menopause, aging, and retirement.

Retirement can result in numerous changes that lead to stress regarding identity. With retirement, numerous roles change and financial resources are often reduced. Another frequent identity stressor to the older adult is the death of a spouse. With a spouse's death, the surviving spouse may come to realize that much of his or her identity has come from the role of husband or wife and the loss of this role impacts the person's sense of identity.

How the nurse can influence a client's self-concept. The nurse is in a key role to positively influence a client's self-concept. Often the nurse is the first health care provider to see the client. Verbal and nonverbal behaviors that convey sincere interest and acceptance can have a profound impact on the client. In addition, the nurse's recognition and inclusion of self-concept issues and problems in planning care from the onset of client contact can significantly affect outcomes. For example, a nurse working with a client who is scheduled for a mastectomy can contact Reach to Recovery (a support group for mastectomy clients) to plan to have another woman who has experienced a mastectomy visit the client after surgery. Seeing another woman who has undergone a mastectomy can allow the client to realize that she can still be an attractive woman who is able to do what she wants to in her life, thus positively influencing her self-concept.

The manner in which the nurse responds to a client who has experienced a change in body appearance, such as a mastectomy or ostomy, sets the stage for how the person comes to see himself or herself. The client with a change in body functioning or appearance is often extremely sensitive to the nurse's verbal and nonverbal responses. The nurse's positive and matter-of-fact approach to caring for the wound can serve as a model for both the client and family for acceptance of any body changes.

To provide meaningful, effective care that enhances a person's self-concept, the nurse must understand the significant components of each person's self-concept. There are general nursing measures that can be supportive of most clients' self-concept, such as being recognized as a worthwhile person and building a trusting relationship in which the client can comfortably discuss his or her concerns. There are also measures a nurse can implement that are specific to a particular individual, for example, supporting a client's use of alternative healing techniques or methods of spiritual expression.

⋯CRITICAL THINKING IN CLIENT CARE

Synthesis

As the nurse assumes care for a client, synthesis of factors comprising critical thinking ensures good clinical decisions. When a client's self-concept is threatened, the nurse must utilize knowledge of factors affecting self-concept and previous experience to provide a quality approach to care.

Knowledge. In considering the various aspects of a client's self-concept, knowledge of how various medications and chronic pain influence functioning and thinking may be helpful. Many medications have actions and side effects that can influence a client's sense of identity. In considering clients who might have alterations in self-concept, the nurse should be particularly alert to the client who is experiencing chronic pain. Chronic pain predisposes a person to decreased ability to function, irritability, and decreased sleep. These changes can negatively affect self-concept.

Another area of knowledge for the nurse to consider is the client's cultural background. The importance persons place on such things as appearance, performance in a role, and acceptance by others can be influenced culturally. In addition, personal space promotes self-identity by offering opportunities for a person's self-expression (Giger and Davidhizar, 1995). Some cultures are comfortable with intimate space, whereas others find close contact offensive (see Chapter 18). The personal space over which a person has jurisdiction often becomes an extension of the self and a reflection of personality and interests (Giger and Davidhizar, 1995).

Experience. Throughout life, all individuals, including nurses, have experience with self-concept issues. The nurse can use personal memories of changes in appearance or times when the ability to carry out usual roles was affected by a temporary illness or an accident to aid in empathizing with clients who are experiencing stressors to their self-concept. Past experiences with clients who have undergone changes in self-concept or experienced self-concept stressors can provide useful insight in how to work effectively with a current client.

Attitudes. A useful attitude for the nurse to employ when caring for clients with threats to self-concept is one of independence. If the nurse accepts other professionals' assessments and conclusions regarding a client without personally considering and thinking through the situation, the nurse may miss important data and fail to implement interventions that could be useful in helping the client move toward a higher level of functioning. For example, if a nurse hears several health care providers talking about a client's lack of progress and relating it to a lack of motivation, the nurse could fail to explore the resources the client sees as being available. The client may be unaware that there are resources within the community to provide support. Approaching the client with an attitude of independence and the intention of performing an appropriate assessment of the situation allows the nurse to see options that might not otherwise be evident.

An issue related to independence is the existence of biases regarding a particular group. Nurses often develop and internalize the attitudes and perspectives of those with whom they interact. This can lead to biases and stereotypical perceptions of groups of people such as those of a particular culture, sexual orientation, or belief system. Awareness of the possibility of biases can promote examination of one's underlying attitudes and beliefs, thus helping to eliminate unconscious operation of biases in interacting with a particular individual.

Standards. There are several codes of professional conduct for nurses, but each reflects a commitment to the principle of respect for client autonomy. Autonomy relates to individuals having the freedom to choose their own life plan and ways of being moral. Supporting clients' autonomy to make choices and live their lives in keeping with their values and beliefs supports the development and maintenance of a strong and positive self-concept.

NURSING PROCESS

Assessment

The nursing assessment should focus on each component of self-concept, behaviors suggestive of an altered self-concept (Box 16-2), actual and potential self-concept stressors, and coping patterns. Much of the data regarding self-concept are most effectively gathered through observation of clients' nonverbal behavior and paying attention to the content of clients' conversations rather than through direct questioning. Notice the manner in which individuals talk about the people in

---

Box 16-2

Behaviors Suggestive of Altered Self-Concept

Avoidance of eye contact
Overly apologetic
Hesitant speech
Overly critical
Excessive anger
Frequent or inappropriate crying
Puts self down
Excessively dependent
Hesitant to express views or opinions
Lack of interest in what is happening
Passive attitude
Difficulty in making choices
Slumped posture
Unkempt appearance

---

their lives. This can provide clues to both stressful and supportive relationships and to key roles. Utilize knowledge of Erikson's developmental stages (see Box 16-1) to determine what areas are likely to be important to the client, and inquire about these aspects of the person's life. For example, you might ask a 44 year old about his or her family and job. These are areas that are likely to be central to the lives of individuals at this age. The individual's discussion of these areas will likely provide data related to role performance, identity, self-esteem, stressors, and coping patterns. At times, specific questions may be useful (Table 16-1).

The nursing assessment should also include consideration of previous coping behaviors; the nature, number, and intensity of the stressors; and the client's internal and external resources. Knowledge of how a client has dealt with stressors in the past can provide insight into the client's style of coping. Not all issues are addressed in the same way by clients, but many times one uses a familiar coping pattern for newly encountered stressors. Exploring resources and strengths, such as helpful significant others, can be important in formulating a realistic and effective plan. Also helpful in planning is to determine how the client sees the situation. What is viewed as a crisis by one client may be seen as less significant by another client. For example, one client might express great fear and distress over needing to have a colonoscopy and biopsy, whereas another client may see the need for the diagnostic testing as a manageable outgrowth of growing older and take the attitude that "If there is something to be concerned about, I'll know soon enough."

Client expectations. Also important in assessing self-concept are the client's expectations. Asking the client how he or she believes interventions will make a

TABLE 16-1

Examples of Self-Concept Assessment Questions

Questions From the Nurse	Typical Responses That Indicate Low Self-Esteem
Identity "If I did not know you, how would you describe yourself to me?"	Answers that are derogatory about oneself (e.g., "I'm not much good," "I don't matter," or "I'm too skinny, fat, ugly").
Body Image "Is there something about your body you'd change? If so, what is it?"	It is normal for people to make comments about specific attributes, such as "My nose is too long" or "My thighs are too fat." If the answer focuses on many items, this is not healthy. Answers that indicate marked divergence from what the person is are also cause for concern, such as "I would weigh 150 pounds less" or "I would not be Hispanic." These responses indicate great discomfort.
Self-Esteem "How do you feel about yourself?" "Are you accomplishing what you want in your life so far?"	Statements of not liking oneself or not achieving what one had hoped are cause for concern. Verbalizing hopelessness or helplessness indicates distress of the self.
Roles "Do you feel you've been able to be a (mother, daughter, wife, husband, father, son) in your family, in the way you wanted to be?"	Feelings of dissatisfaction in the role are distressing to the self-concept.

difference in the problem can provide useful information regarding the client's expectations and an opportunity to discuss the client's goals. For example, a nurse working with a client who is experiencing anxiety related to an upcoming diagnostic study might ask the client about his or her expectations of the relaxation exercise they have been practicing together. The client's response will provide the nurse with valuable information about the client's beliefs and attitudes regarding the efficacy and appropriateness of the interventions.

Cultural variables. When assessing self-concept the nurse needs to be attuned to the client's cultural background. Individuals are socialized into a particular cultural heritage. Cultural heritage can influence each of the aspects of self-concept. The behaviors expected in various roles can differ from culture to culture. What is viewed as attractive in terms of body appearance varies between cultures. Cultural beliefs regarding what is attractive will influence a person's body image and self-esteem. Identity will be influenced by characteristics that are valued in a particular culture. See Chapter 18 for a more detailed discussion of cultural heritage and guidance in assessing individuals from different cultures.

Successful critical thinking requires a synthesis of knowledge, experience, information gathered from clients, and critical thinking attitudes and standards. Clinical judgments require the nurse to anticipate what information is needed, to analyze the data, and to then make decisions regarding client care. The client expects competent and informed care. Mia incorporates previous knowledge and experience in providing care for Mr. Finch.

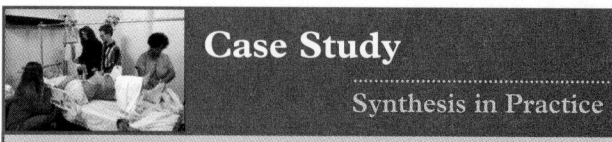

Case Study

Synthesis in Practice

As Mia prepares to care for Mr. Finch, she recalls what she has learned about self-concept. She recognizes that his accident and resulting injuries are likely to be significant stressors in regard to his self-concept. Being in the hospital and his dependence on the staff for personal care threaten his sense of independence. His inability to work for the next several months and the questions about his returning to preaccident mobility affect his ability to carry out his occupation as a plumber. His role of provider for his family is threatened, as is his role of an "able-bodied man." Recognizing the significance of these changes and their possible influence on his self-concept, Mia plans to explore with Mr. Finch what it is like for him being in the hospital and if he is thinking, at this juncture, about finances and work.

Mia remembers that after her own accident, her initial concerns were with her pain and surgery. It was not until several days after surgery that she began to consider the impact her changed mobility would have on her life. This knowledge will guide her in knowing that assessing Mr. Finch's current concerns is important. It may be some time before he begins to consider the impact of his accident on other aspects of his life.

When Mia is reading Mr. Finch's chart before meeting him, she overhears two staff members talking about Mr. Finch and his "pickiness" about positioning. They are expressing their distress at how long it takes to complete his care because of his specific requests in regard to his personal hygiene and positioning. In hearing these comments, Mia realizes that the staff may not be aware of the extent of Mr. Finch's pain and how his requests for care in movement might be related to his pain or to fear of further injury. Mia hears the comments but recognizes that she will make her own independent assessment of his status and needs. She recognizes that if she allows others' attitudes to influence her view of Mr. Finch, she will be less likely to develop a therapeutic relationship or be able to effectively support him in coping with his current situation.

As Mia reads the surgeon's progress notes relating to Mr. Finch's upcoming surgery and his repeated refusals to accept blood products, she recognizes an issue of autonomy. She will be alert to the responses of others to his decision. She will also be alert for an opportunity to explore with him what it has been like to make choices based on his beliefs when others have repeatedly asked him to make different choices.

Nursing Diagnosis

In analyzing data regarding a client's self-concept, the nurse reviews data in terms of the four primary areas of body image, role, self-esteem, and identity. Threats to any of these areas may result in a nursing diagnosis. Making nursing diagnoses in the realm of self-concept is complex.

Often, isolated data could be defining characteristics for more than one nursing diagnosis. For example, a client might express feelings of regret and inadequacy. These are defining characteristics for both *anxiety* and *situational low self-esteem*. To make the most appropriate nursing diagnosis, the nurse must be open to seeing the possibilities of both nursing diagnoses. In fact, the awareness that the client is demonstrating defining characteristics of more than one nursing diagnosis can guide the nurse in gathering specific data to differentiate the underlying problem.

To further assess the possibility of anxiety, the nurse might consider the following defining characteristics of anxiety: Is the person experiencing increased muscle tension, shakiness, a sense of being "rattled," or restlessness? These symptoms would suggest *anxiety* as the more appropriate diagnosis. On the other hand, if the person expresses a predominantly negative self-appraisal, evaluation of self as unable to handle situations or events, and difficulty making decisions, these characteristics would suggest the more appropriate nursing diagnosis to be *situational low self-esteem*.

To further aid the nurse in differentiating between these two diagnoses, information regarding recent events in the person's life and how the person has viewed himself or herself in the past would provide insight into the most appropriate nursing diagnosis. In this example, the two nursing diagnoses are closely related. The person might have several defining characteristics from each diagnosis, but as additional data are gathered, usually the most appropriate or predominant nursing diagnosis becomes evident. If this is not the case, the nurse can consider consultation with or referral to other nurse colleagues or a mental health professional to help identify the priority problem.

It is also important that the nurse have sufficient data to correctly identify the factors contributing to the nursing diagnosis. These factors will be reflected in the *"related to"* component of the nursing diagnostic statement. If a thorough database is not gathered before formulating the nursing diagnosis, diagnostic errors are likely. For example, a nurse was working with a 62-year-old woman who was admitted because of chronic back pain. The client demonstrated signs of anxiety (inattentiveness, frequent startling), and the client reported she did not sleep well and had a diminished appetite. The nurse knew that the client had undergone diagnostic testing to rule out cancer as the cause of the back pain. The nurse made the following nursing diagnosis: *anxiety related to possibility of cancer*. The nurse later learned that the woman was anxious because her grandson had been in a serious motor vehicle accident and was in intensive care. This example illustrates the danger in making a diagnosis without sufficient data. The nursing diagnoses box on p. 276 summarizes diagnoses that may apply to clients with self-concept alterations.

Planning

Realistic planning to enhance and support a client's self-concept is based on assessment data and client input regarding his or her perception of the problem and

NURSING DIAGNOSES FOR CLIENTS WITH ALTERATIONS IN SELF-CONCEPT

Adjustment, impaired
Anxiety
Body image disturbance
Coping, ineffective individual
Fear
Parental role conflict
Parenting, altered
Personal identity disturbance
Powerlessness
Rape-trauma syndrome
Role performance, altered
Self-esteem disturbance
Self-esteem, situational
Social interaction, impaired
Spiritual distress (distress of the human spirit)
Violence, risk for: self-directed

contributing factors. For interventions to be effective, the interventions must be acceptable to the client and realistic within the context of the client, setting, and community resources.

The first step in effective planning is the development of goals and outcome criteria. To formulate a goal, consider a realistic resolution of the nursing diagnosis for this particular person. Consultation with the client can facilitate the development of realistic goals and outcome criteria. Other sources that can provide valuable input and guidance in planning are consultation with family, other health care providers, and community resources. Once the goal has been formulated, consider how the clues that alerted you to the problem would change if the problem was diminished. Allow these changes to be reflected in the outcome criteria (see care plan). Another example is a client who is diagnosed with *situational low self-esteem related to recent job loss.* The defining characteristics she demonstrates are verbalizing that she just cannot seem to do anything right these days and expression of shame about losing her job. The nurse formulates the goal that the client's

CASE STUDY NURSING CARE PLAN

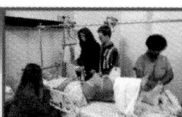

Alterations in Self-Concept

Assessment

Mia learns from Mr. Finch's chart that he was transferred from his local hospital 70 miles away to the acute care center. The transfer was made because of the extent of his injuries and the need for specialized orthopedic treatment. He has been in essentially good health up until the time of the accident.

When Mia first goes in to meet Mr. Finch, she finds he makes eye contact and answers her questions, but his **answers are brief** and to the point, without elaboration. As Mia spends more time with Mr. Finch, his eye contact increases but the answers to her questions remain brief. He is **restless** and **shifts frequently in the bed.** Mr. Finch tells Mia that before the accident he had a near ideal life. He describes his family as a source of pleasure and satisfaction. He tells her briefly about a recent trip the family took and the adventures of the two teenagers. He describes his work as OK. He states, "Fixing pipes is not the most exciting thing in the world, but it pays the bills and I know how to do it."

In gathering the nursing history, Mia learns that Mr. Finch has had **trouble sleeping** since admission. He says that in addition to the pain, there is **too much to think about.** Specifically, he says, "You know, they may not be able to save my legs."

In reviewing the flow sheets since admission, Mia notes that Mr. Finch's **appetite has been recorded as poor and he usually only eats one quarter to one half of his meals.**

Nursing Diagnosis

Anxiety related to pain, uncertainty of outcome of upcoming surgery, and treatment of injuries.

Defining characteristics are shown in bold type.

CASE STUDY NURSING CARE PLAN—cont'd

Planning

Goal

Client's anxiety will be diminished within 1 week.

Expected Outcomes

Client will state that his anxiety/worry is less within 3 days.

Client will discuss his concerns openly with a staff person within 3 days.

Client will report having slept for 4 consecutive hours during the night within 1 week.

Client will report an increased appetite and will eat at least three quarters of his meals within 1 week.

Implementation

Steps

1. Help the client to define his level of anxiety (use the terminology the client is comfortable with; e.g., worried, nervous).
2. Explore coping skills the client has used in the past. Encourage and support adaptive coping skills used in the past.
3. Encourage the client to express concerns verbally.

4. Decrease the number of new stressors (e.g., answer client's call bell promptly, explain procedures, decrease unnecessary noise).
5. Treat pain before it becomes moderate to severe.
6. Teach the client progressive relaxation techniques.

Rationale

Anxiety is highly individualized, and different clients manifest anxiety in varying degrees.

Most clients have developed effective coping skills during their lives. Supporting these coping skills in currently stressful situations can aid adaptation.

Verbalizing a concern can allow the client to be more objective about what is happening.

The number of stressors affects the stress experience (Sundeen and others, 1994).

Pain is a stressor that can increase anxiety.

Relaxation is psychophysiologically in opposition to anxiety. Relaxation is energy conserving and nurturing (Sundeen and others, 1994).

Evaluation

Explore with the client his current level of anxiety.

Ask the client how he slept the night before.

Inquire regarding the client's appetite, and monitor the amount of food eaten from meal trays.

Explore with the client his concerns, and note areas he discusses.

Observe nonverbal clues regarding eye contact and degree of restlessness during discussion.

---

self-esteem will improve within 1 week. Appropriate outcome criteria might be that the client discusses areas of her life where she is functioning well and voices a recognition that losing her job is not reflective of her worth as a person.

▪ Implementation

Once the goals and outcome criteria have been developed, the nurse selects nursing interventions that help move the client toward the goal of care. Effective nursing interventions are based on the client's nursing diagnosis and etiological factors that contributed to the problem. Standardized care plans can provide valuable guidance in selecting nursing interventions. A standardized care plan should be tailored to the individual client. Individualization is facilitated by considering the related factors of the nursing diagnosis. Developing interventions that influence the etiological factors can decrease the problem reflected in the nursing diagnosis.

Health promotion. The nurse may have the opportunity to work with clients to help them develop healthy lifestyle measures that contribute to a healthy self-concept. Measures that support adaptation to stress, such as sound nutrition and regular exercise within the client's capabilities; measures that facilitate adequate sleep and rest; and stress-reducing practices all contribute to a healthy self-concept. Nurses are in a unique position to identify lifestyle practices that put a person's self-concept at risk or are suggestive of altered self-concepts. A client may have been admitted to an acute care facility for treatment of a multiple fracture resulting from a motor vehicle accident. In gathering the nursing history, the nurse may learn of lifestyle practices such as too little rest, a large number of life changes occurring simultaneously, or excessive use of alcohol, which either are suggestive of self-concept disturbances or put the person at risk for self-concept disturbances. The nurse in this situation has the opportunity to talk with the client to determine how he or she sees the various lifestyle elements, to facilitate the client seeing the behavior as potentially problematic, and to make appropriate referrals or provide needed health teaching.

Acute care. In the acute care setting, the nurse is likely to encounter clients who are experiencing threats to their self-concept. Clients may be faced with the need to adapt to an altered body image as a result of surgery or other physical change. Often a visit by someone who has experienced similar changes and adapted to them is helpful. The timing of such a visit is important. The nurse must be sensitive to the client's level of acceptance of the change. Forcing confrontation with the change before the client is ready could delay the person's acceptance. Signs that a person may be receptive to such a visit would be the client asking questions related to how to manage a particular aspect of what has happened or looking at the changed area.

Restorative care. Often in a long-term nurse-client relationship in a home health or restorative care environment, a nurse has the opportunity to work with a client to reach the goal of attaining a more positive self-concept. Interventions designed to help a client reach the goal of adapting to changes in self-concept or attaining a positive self-concept are based on the premise that the client first develops insight and self-awareness concerning problems and stressors and then acts to solve the problems and cope with the stressors. This approach, outlined by Stuart and Sundeen (1995), involves the following levels of intervention: expanded self-awareness, self-exploration, self-evaluation, planning realistic goals, and commitment to action (Table 16-2). Interventions proceed in a stepwise manner to promote increasing awareness and facilitate effective problem solving.

Increasing the client's self-awareness is achieved through establishing a trusting relationship that allows the client to openly explore feelings. Open exploration can make the situation less threatening for the client and encourages behaviors that expand self-awareness.

Encouraging the client's self-exploration is achieved by accepting the client's feelings and thoughts, by helping the client to clarify interactions with others, and by being empathetic. The nurse encourages self-expression and stresses the client's self-responsibility.

Assisting the client in self-evaluation involves helping the client to define problems clearly and identifying positive and negative coping mechanisms. The nurse works closely with the client to help analyze adaptive and maladaptive responses, contrast different alternatives, and discuss outcomes.

Assisting the client to establish realistic goals involves helping the client to identify alternative solutions and develop realistic goals based on them. This facilitates real change and encourages further goal-setting behaviors. The nurse designs opportunities that result in success, reinforces the client's skills and strengths, and assists the client in obtaining needed assistance.

Assisting the client to commit to decisions and actions to achieve goals involves teaching the client to move away from ineffective coping mechanisms and develop successful coping strategies. Supporting client attempts at health promotion is essential, because with each success another attempt can be made. Supporting adaptive, flexible coping is central to promoting a positive self-concept.

Clients who experience threats to or alterations in self-concept often benefit from collaboration with mental health and community resources to promote increased awareness. Knowledge of available community resources, such as counseling and peer support groups, allows the nurse to make appropriate referrals.

▪ Evaluation

Client care. Evaluating the effectiveness of nursing interventions is aided by the earlier formulation of goals and outcome criteria. If realistic individual goals and outcome criteria were developed, the nurse can reassess the client to see if he or she has attained the changes that were desired. Key indicators of self-concept can be the client's nonverbal behaviors. For example, a client who has had difficulty making eye contact may demonstrate a more positive self-concept by making more frequent eye contact during conversation. Patterns of interacting can also reflect changes in self-concept. For example, a client who has been hesitant to express his or her views may more readily offer opinions and ideas as self-esteem increases.

Client expectations. If the nurse has developed a good rapport with the client, the client may well be able to share how things are going from his or her perspective. The nurse may be able to facilitate this sharing by initiating a review of what has happened over time. This offers the nurse the opportunity to share perceptions and encourages the client to consider and voice how he or she has experienced any changes.

TABLE 16-2
Levels of Nursing Interventions for Self-Concept Disturbance

Principle	Rationale	Nursing Actions
Goal: Expand Client's Self-Awareness		
Work with resources client possesses.	Some resources, such as self-control and self-perception, are needed as foundations for later nursing care.	Confirm identity. Provide support measures to reduce anxiety. Approach client in an undemanding way. Accept and attempt to clarify any verbal or non-verbal communication. Prevent client isolation. Help establish simple routine. Help set limits on inappropriate behavior. Orient client to reality. Reinforce appropriate behavior. Gradually increase activities and tasks that provide positive experiences. Assist in personal hygiene and grooming. Encourage client to care for self.
Maximize client's participation in therapeutic relationship.	Mutuality is necessary for client to assume ultimate responsibility for behavior and coping responses.	Gradually increase client's participation in decisions that affect care. Convey that client is a responsible individual.
Goal: Encourage Client's Self-Exploration		
Show interest in and accept client's feelings and thoughts.	When nurse shows interest in and accepts client's feelings and thoughts, the nurse helps client to do so also.	Attend to and encourage client's expression of emotions, beliefs, behavior, and thoughts—verbally, nonverbally, symbolically, or directly. Use therapeutic communication skills and empathetic responses. Note use of logical and illogical thinking and reported and observed emotional responses.
Help client clarify self-concept and relationships to others through self-disclosure.	Self-disclosure and understanding self-perceptions are prerequisites to bringing about future change; this may, in itself, reduce anxiety.	Elicit client's perceptions of strengths and weaknesses. Help describe ideal self. Identify self-criticisms. Help describe how client perceives relationships to other people and events.
Be aware and have control of your own feelings.	Self-awareness allows nurse to model authentic behavior.	Be open to your own feelings. Accept your positive and negative feelings. Practice therapeutic use of self: share your feelings with client, describe how another might have felt, and mirror your perception of client's feelings.
Respond empathetically, not sympathetically, emphasizing that power to change lies with client.	Sympathy can reinforce client's self-pity; rather, nurse should communicate that client's life situation is subject to one's own control.	Use empathetic responses and monitor yourself for feelings of sympathy or pity. Reaffirm that client is not helpless or powerless when dealing with problems. Convey verbally and behaviorally that client is responsible for behavior, including choice of maladaptive or adaptive coping responses. Discuss with client scope of choices, areas of strength, and coping resources available.

Modified from Stuart GW, Sundeen SJ: *Principles and practice of psychiatric nursing*, ed 5, St. Louis, 1995, Mosby.

Continued

TABLE 16-2

Levels of Nursing Interventions for Self-Concept Disturbance—cont'd

Principle	Rationale	Nursing Actions
Goal: Assist Client in Self-Evaluation		
Help client to clearly define problem.	Only after problem is accurately defined can alternative choices be proposed.	Identify relevant stressors with client and ask for appraisal of them. Clarify that client's beliefs influence feelings and behaviors. Mutually identify faulty beliefs, misperceptions, distortions, delusions, and unrealistic goals. Mutually identify areas of strength. Place concepts of success and failure in proper perspective. Explore use of coping resources.
Explore client's adaptive and maladaptive coping responses to problem.	Examination of client's choices made during coping will help define successful and unsuccessful responses.	Describe how coping responses are chosen and have positive and negative consequences. Contrast adaptive and maladaptive responses. Mutually identify disadvantages of client's maladaptive coping responses. Mutually identify advantages or "payoffs" of client's maladaptive coping responses.
Goal: Assist Client in Forming Realistic Goals		
Help client identify alternative solutions.	Only when all possible alternatives have been evaluated can change be effected.	Help client understand that one can only change oneself, not others. If client holds inconsistent perceptions, show that the following can change: beliefs or ideals to bring them closer to reality, and environment to make it consistent with beliefs. If self-concept is not consistent with behavior, client can change the following: behavior to conform to self-concept, beliefs underlying self-concept to include behavior, and self-ideal. Mutually review use of coping resources.
Help client conceptualize realistic goals.	Goal setting that includes clear definition of expected change is necessary.	Encourage client to form personal (not nurse's) goals. Mutually discuss emotional and practical consequences of each goal. Help client define concrete change to be made. Encourage client to enter new experiences for growth potential. Use role modeling and role playing when appropriate.
Goal: Assist Client in Becoming Committed to Decision and in Achieving Goals		
Help client take necessary action to change maladaptive coping responses and maintain adaptive ones.	Ultimate objective in promoting client's insight is to replace maladaptive coping responses with more adaptive ones.	Provide opportunity for success. Reinforce strengths, skills, and healthy aspects of client's personality. Assist client in gaining assistance (e.g., vocational, financial, social services). Use family and groups to enhance client's self-esteem. Allow client sufficient time to change. Provide support and positive reinforcement to maintain progress.

TABLE 16-2
Levels of Nursing Interventions for Self-Concept Disturbance—cont'd

Principle	Rationale	Nursing Actions
Goal: Assist Client in Acknowledging Goals Achieved and Evaluating Those Not Achieved		
Help client to purposefully review achievements and explore reasons for any problems or setbacks.	Reinforcement of gains made in strengthening self-concept will motivate continued change.	Mutually review progress made. Affirm achievements with client and family or significant others. Evaluate what contributed most to success. Help client discuss feelings regarding goals not achieved.
Goal: Assist Client to Re-Form Plan for Achieving Goals		
Support client in reviewing goals.	Insight gained from attempts to change will support further progress.	Review with client the need for further self-evaluation. Encourage client to continue those experiences that were successful.
Identify alternatives not tried previously	Different approaches may be necessary to achieve desired outcomes.	Explore how new coping resources can be applied to continued change. Redefine changes in adaptive behaviors to be made. Continue to reinforce strengths and successes.

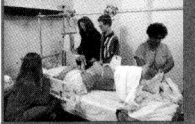

Case Study
Evaluation

Mia is absent from the acute care hospital for 2 weeks. When she returns, she is again assigned to care for Mr. Finch. Since she last cared for him, he has undergone two surgeries, the surgery that was scheduled for the day after she was there and another surgery to do a second graft when the first did not take. Mr. Finch is glad to see her. He tells her that he is in a "much better place" now than when they first met. The second skin graft is not doing well, and the surgeons have talked with Mr. Finch about further surgery. He is questioning whether further surgery to save his right leg is reasonable. The prognosis for functioning of the leg even if it heals is not good. He tells Mia he thinks that if further surgery is required he will choose an amputation. He says, "You know, I now can see I'll be OK even if they have to amputate my leg. If I had it to do over again, I would have made that choice when

they did the second surgery. But it took me awhile to realize that I will not have the same functioning in my legs regardless of what they do. And I can live without my leg." As he relates what had happened over the last 2 weeks and the upcoming plans to transfer him to a hospital near his home, his speech is animated and he makes frequent eye contact. During the course of the day, Mia notices that his restlessness has decreased. He reports that his appetite has returned, and he ate all of both his breakfast and his lunch. He also reports that he has become more accustomed to the hospital and is sleeping most of the night.

Documentation Note
Mia documents Mr. Finch's progress toward the goal as follows:

Client's anxiety has decreased, as evidenced by his statement that he is in a "much better place" now than when he was first admitted. Client reports sleeping most of the night and eating all of his last two meals. He is more open in discussing his condition and prognosis, and he is less restless.

SEXUALITY

Sexuality involves the whole person. Sexuality includes a person's sense of femaleness or maleness. Sexuality involves biological, psychological, sociological, spiritual, and cultural dimensions of the person's being. In addition, sexuality influences values, attitudes, behaviors, and relationships with others, including the need to be emotionally close (MacLaren, 1995).

Because of the all-encompassing nature of sexuality it is appropriate for nurses to consider sexual health. The intimacy of the nurse-client relationship, whether it is involved in providing physical care or discussing the impact of a recent diagnosis, provides a unique opportunity for discussing sexual concerns.

Scientific Knowledge Base

Sexual development. As a person grows and develops, so does his or her sexuality. Each stage of development brings changes in sexual functioning, sexual focus, and sexual relating.

Infancy. At birth, the infant is identified as female or male. Psychologically the infant is developing trust (Erikson, 1963). Trust in self involves exploration and experimentation to define body limits, actions and responses, and pleasant from unpleasant sensations. Exploration includes the discovery of self-soothing behaviors such as touching the genital area. Parental response to these exploratory behaviors can set the tone for the child's sexual development. Parents should be encouraged to accept the infant's exploratory behavior as a normal part of development.

Preschool. The child from age 1 to 5 or 6 continues to solidify the sense of **gender identity** and to differentiate socially defined, gender-appropriate behaviors. This learning process occurs in the course of normal adult-child interactions, from the toys given to the child to clothing worn, games played, and responses encouraged. Children also observe adult behavior, begin to imitate actions of the same-sex parent, and maintain or modify behavior based on parental feedback.

Body exploration continues at this age, and the child may extend exploration to others. Children may role play games of doctor or mommy and daddy and explore each other's bodies in various stages of undress. Nurses can teach parents that this is a normal aspect of sexual development. Rather than responding with shock or punishment, care givers can respond by redirecting play.

Childhood. Children from 6 to 10 years of age, or prepuberty, expand their horizons from home to include school and the community. Learning and reinforcement of gender-appropriate behavior come from parents and teachers but more significantly from the peer group. Children in this age group will probably continue self-stimulating behavior. Teaching children the difference between behaviors that are culturally acceptable in public and those that need to be private is appropriate. The behavior of masturbation is an example.

Children at this age continue to have questions about sex. They may assert their independence by testing the limits of appropriate behavior by using "dirty words" or telling jokes with sexual connotations while watching adult reaction. Limit testing is a normal and important part of developing a sense of independence. Parents can be taught to respond by setting limits on unacceptable behaviors.

Children have a desire and need for privacy. As the child moves toward puberty, he or she will experience an increased sense of modesty and need for privacy. This need for privacy should be honored.

Puberty and adolescence. The onset of puberty in girls is usually signaled by development of the breasts. This process, which in part is controlled by heredity, may begin as early as age 8 and may not be complete until the late teen years. The age of menarche varies widely but usually occurs at about 12 years of age.

Ejaculation in boys does not occur until the sex organs begin to mature, around the age of 12 or 14. Ejaculation may first occur during sleep (nocturnal emission). This may be interpreted as an episode of bed-wetting and even in knowledgeable boys can be very embarrassing.

The emotional changes during puberty and adolescence are as dramatic as the physical ones. Same-sex peers remain influential in defining appropriate behavior, but the task of establishing relationships with the opposite sex begins.

The adolescent is faced with many decisions and thus needs accurate information on topics such as body changes, sexual relationships and activity, sexually transmitted diseases (STDs), and pregnancy.

Many American adolescents are sexually active. A survey by the Alan Guttmacher Institute (1994) revealed that by age 16, 42% of teenagers have had sexual intercourse and by age 18, 71% have had sexual intercourse. A substantial number of these teenagers do not protect themselves from pregnancy or STDs. The dynamics of sexual risk taking are not fully understood, but consistencies have been noted across studies linking drug and alcohol use and unsafe sexual practices (Keller and others, 1996).

If not recognized earlier, this may be the age of identifying a same-sex sexual orientation. Many adolescents will have at least one homosexual experience with an individual or in a group. Adolescents may fear that this experience defines their total sexuality as homosexual. Many individuals continue with a strictly heterosexual orientation after such experiences. However, some teens may recognize their preference as distinctly homosexual. This can be a frightening and confusing recognition for the adolescent and family and may require a great deal of support.

Adulthood. The adult has gained physical maturation but is continuing to explore and define emotional maturation in relationships. Sexual health has been defined as "the integration of the somatic, emotional, intellectual, and social aspects of sexual being, in ways that are positively enriching and that enhance personality, communication, and love" (World Health Organization, 1975). People can be sexually healthy in numerous ways. Sexual activity is often defined as a basic need, but sexual desire can be channeled into other forms of intimacy throughout a lifetime.

All sexually active adults, as they develop intimate relationships, should learn techniques of stimulation and sexual response that are satisfying to themselves and their sexual partners. Some adults may need information or therapy to achieve mutually satisfying sexual relationships.

Older adulthood. The capacity for sexuality is life-long (Figure 16-3). Theoretically, people can engage in sex as far into old age as they choose. The best indicator for continued sexual satisfaction with aging is a regularly active sex life during adulthood and into later life (Masters and others, 1992). Older people may face health concerns and societal attitudes that may make it difficult for them to continue sexual activity. Although declining physical abilities may make sex as they knew it painful or impossible, with sympathetic intervention they can experiment with and learn alternative ways of sexual expression. For example, older adults who experience joint dysfunction may find greater comfort in a side-lying position during intercourse. Research has consistently shown that many older adults remain sexually active and value this expression (Johnson, 1996).

Sexual orientation. **Sexual orientation** is a clear, persistent sexual preference for persons of one sex. Human sexual attraction is on a continuum between heterosexual and homosexual orientations. Based on Kinsey's studies (1948, 1953), most people cluster toward the heterosexual end of the continuum; a smaller percentage are at the homosexual (gay or lesbian) end. Other individuals are bisexual. Sell and others (1995) report on a nationally representative sample which found that 20.8% of males and 17.8% of females in the United States report either homosexual behavior or homosexual attraction since age 15. Examination of

homosexual behavior separately found that 6.2% of males and 3.6% of females in the United States reported having had sexual contact with someone of the same sex in the previous 5 years. Gays or lesbians may keep their sexual orientation hidden or be more open about their sexual preference. The process of "coming out" involves self-acknowledgement, self-acceptance, and self-disclosure (Alexander and LaRosa, 1994). "Coming out" can be particularly difficult because of **homophobia,** an irrational fear of homosexuality, displayed by some individuals.

Sexual response cycle. Kaplan (1979) identified three phases of the **sexual response cycle:** desire, arousal, and orgasm. These phases are the result of vasocongestion and myotonia, the basic physiological responses of sexual arousal. In women, this reaction leads to vaginal lubrication, tumescence of the clitoris and labia minora and majora, and engorgement of the outer third of the vagina (orgasmic platform). In men, vasocongestion leads to erection of the penis. **Myotonia,** or neuromuscular tension, gradually increases throughout the body during the excitement and plateau phases. Myotonia peaks during orgasm, resulting in involuntary contractions of the female vagina and the male vas deferens and urethra. Women and men may experience contractions of the arm and leg muscles, facial muscles, and gluteal muscles. After orgasm, vasocongestion and myotonia return to prearousal levels. The phases described are not absolute. Female and male response patterns are similar.

Contraception. At present, there are numerous contraceptive options available to sexually active couples. Some methods do not require a prescription, whereas other methods do require intervention by a health care provider. Nonprescription contraceptive methods include abstinence, timing of intercourse in regard to the menstrual cycle, and various barrier methods. Abstinence from sexual intercourse is 100% effective. Barrier methods include over-the-counter spermicidal products such as creams, jellies, foams, and sponges that are placed into the vagina before intercourse to create a spermicide barrier between the uterus and ejaculated sperm. A "rubber" or condom is a thin latex sheath that fits over the penis. Condoms provide a barrier against all STDs. Vaginal spermicides and condoms are most effective when instructions are carefully followed; their combined use has been found to be more effective in preventing pregnancy than the use of either alone. Effectiveness varies with each method and with the consistency of use. The percentage of women experiencing an accidental pregnancy using these nonprescription methods ranges from 3% to 36% (Hatcher and others, 1994).

Contraceptive methods based on the menstrual cycle include the rhythm method, basal body temperature, cervical mucus, and fertility awareness method. These

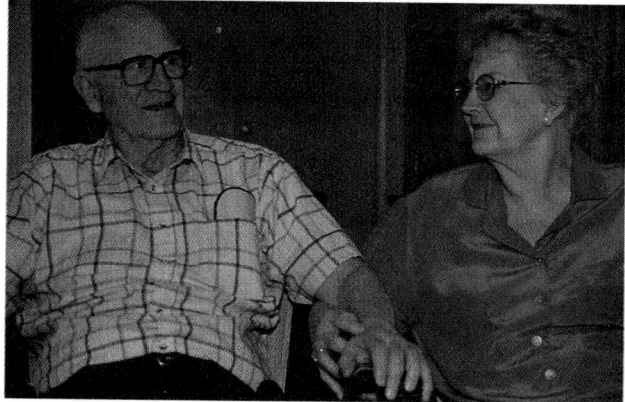

Figure 16-3. Sexuality is important across the life span.

methods require the female to understand the reproductive cycle of her body and be aware of the subtle signs and signals her body gives during the cycle. These methods also require abstinence from sexual intercourse during designated fertile periods. The failure rate for these methods during the first year of use is 20% (Hatcher and others, 1994).

Additional nonprescription methods that clients may use include withdrawal and douching. Neither of these methods offers significant protection against an unwanted pregnancy.

Contraception methods that require the intervention of a health care provider include hormonal contraception, the intrauterine device (IUD), the diaphragm or cervical cap, and sterilization. Hormonal contraception is available in several forms, including oral contraceptive pills, intramuscular injection, subdermal implant, and IUDs that contain progesterone. Hormonal contraception alters the hormonal environment to prevent ovulation and thicken cervical mucus. IUDs are plastic devices inserted by a health care provider into the uterus through the cervical opening. They vary in shape and may contain copper or may be impregnated with progesterone. The diaphragm is a round, rubber dome that has a flexible spring around the edge. It must be used with a contraceptive cream or jelly and is inserted in the vagina so that it provides a contraceptive barrier over the cervical opening. The cervical cap functions like the diaphragm; however, it covers only the cervix. It may be left in place longer and may be perceived as more comfortable than the diaphragm. Effectiveness rates are reported as follows: oral contraceptives 97% to 99.9%, IUD from 98% to 99.9%, diaphragm from 88% to 94%, and cervical cap from 64% to 91% (Hatcher and others, 1994).

Sterilization is the most effective contraception method other than abstinence. It should be considered permanent. Female sterilization, or tubal ligation, involves cutting, tying, or otherwise ligating the fallopian tubes. In male sterilization, or vasectomy, the vas deferens that carries the sperm away from the testicles is cut and tied.

Sexually transmitted disease.
At present, STDs are epidemic, with the highest prevalence being among teens and young adults (Youngkin, 1995). Acquired immunodeficiency syndrome (AIDS) continues to receive wide public attention; however, other STDs also need to be considered. Prevalent STDs include syphilis, gonorrhea, chlamydia, genital warts, the human papillomavirus (HPV), and herpes simplex virus (HSV) type II.

Nursing Knowledge Base

Decisional issues.
Issues relating to sexuality are significant for most people. Nurses encounter clients who are making decisions or working with issues related to sexuality on a regular basis. Understanding some of the decisions and issues clients may be facing can increase the nurse's effectiveness in assisting clients to reach their maximum level of health in the area of sexuality.

Contraception.
The decisions that women and men make regarding contraception have far-reaching effects on their lives. A pregnancy either planned or unplanned significantly affects the life of the pregnant woman and often the father and other family members. Effects are physical, interpersonal, social, financial, and societal. The use of effective contraception is multifaceted and is not completely understood. One national survey of low-income women who had had an abortion found that 58% of the women reported using some form of contraception when they became pregnant (Forrest and Frost, 1996). This finding suggests that the use of contraception does not necessarily mean effective contraception. Effective contraception involves factors relating to the sexually active couple, the method of contraception, the consistency of use, and the compliance with the requirements of the particular contraceptive method. Personal characteristics that have been identified as positively influencing contraceptive use include motivation to avoid unintended pregnancy, ability to plan, comfort with sexuality, and previous contraceptive use (Beckman and Harvey, 1996).

Abortion.
Abortion remains an issue that stimulates heated discussions. Reasons for selecting an abortion vary and may include a decision to terminate an untimely pregnancy or a choice to abort a fetus known to have a defect incompatible with life. The woman and her partner who have chosen an abortion may experience a sense of loss, grief, and/or guilt. Guilt may surface immediately or may be more covert and manifest by sexual dysfunction or inappropriate perceptions.

STD prevention.
Safe sex is a term used to describe responsible sexual behavior aimed at preventing the spread of STDs, including AIDS. Responsible sexual behavior includes knowing one's sexual partner, being able to openly discuss sexual and drug use behaviors with the partner, and using protective devices.

Alterations in sexual health

Infertility.
A group with special needs is adults who want to conceive but cannot. Infertility is defined as the inability to conceive after 1 year of unprotected intercourse. A couple who desires to conceive but cannot may experience a sense of failure and may feel that their bodies are somehow defective.

Sexual abuse.
Sexual abuse is widespread in our society. Abuse crosses all socioeconomic and ethnic groups. The abuser may not fit any classic description. It is estimated that from one fourth to one half of all females experience some type of sexual abuse by the age of 18 (Guidry, 1995; Bohn and Holz, 1996). Most often this abuse is at the hands of an intimate partner or

family member. Abuse may begin, continue, or even intensify during pregnancy. Sexual abuse is also an issue for males. Studies indicate that one in six young boys has experienced at least one sexually abusive incident before reaching adulthood (Guidry, 1995). Sexual abuse has far-ranging effects on physical and psychological functioning. Women who have been sexually abused are disproportionately frequent users of health care resources (Bohn and Holz, 1996).

When abuse is recognized, support should be mobilized for the victim and the family. All family members may require therapy to promote healthy interactions and relationships.

Personal and emotional conflicts. Ideally, sex is a natural, spontaneous act that passes easily through a number of recognizable physiological stages and culminates in one or more orgasms. In reality, this sequence of events is more the exception than the rule. Nurses encounter clients who have problems with one or more of the stages of sexual behavior, including the feeling of wanting sex, the physiological processes and emotions of having sex, and the feelings experienced after sex.

Sexual dysfunction. The causes of **sexual dysfunction** may be physiological or psychological. Sometimes the cause of a dysfunction cannot be identified or is a combination of several factors. Common chronic illnesses that can contribute to sexual dysfunction include diabetes mellitus, kidney disease, alcoholism, neurological disorders, hormone deficiencies, multiple sclerosis, and vascular insufficiency. Medication side effects can also contribute to sexual dysfunction (Box 16-3).

CRITICAL THINKING

Synthesis

A client's sexuality is complex and interrelated with the person's self-concept and physical and emotional health. Critical thinking by the nurse considers all variables affecting a client's sexuality. Reflection on personal and professional experiences as a nurse enables the nurse to provide appropriate interventions for the client's care.

Box 16-3
Drug Categories That May Contribute to Sexual Dysfunction

Antihypertensives	Ethyl alcohol (ETOH)
Antidepressants	Barbiturates
Antihistamines	Diuretics
Antispasmodics	Narcotics
Sedatives and tranquilizers	

Knowledge. As the nurse considers the sexuality of clients, knowledge regarding sexual development, sexual orientation, sexual response cycle, STDs, contraception, alterations in sexual health, and the decisional issues that clients frequently face in regard to their sexuality is useful. Also helpful is knowledge regarding self-concept. A person's body image will affect how he or she interacts with actual and potential sexual partners. A person's self-esteem will influence how he or she perceives personal attractiveness and thus affect how the person interacts with others. If the person perceives himself or herself as attractive, the person will interact more openly and spontaneously, thus inviting a relationship. If the person has low self-esteem, he or she will be less relaxed and less open to relating.

Experience. The nurse's own sexuality and sexual experience can provide a valuable resource for understanding a client's experiences. In addition, the nurse's own sexual experiences can add to understanding about what a first sexual encounter may have been like or what it is like to broach the topic of STDs before intercourse. In addition to personal experience related to sexuality, nurses can use what they have learned through working with other clients as they assess and work with current clients.

Attitudes. In approaching clients about their sexuality and sexual functioning, an attitude of risk taking can be helpful. Certainly for novice nurses, it can be unnerving to inquire about another person's sexual functioning. The nurse may have a fear that the client will not appreciate being asked about sexuality and sexual practices. The nurse's willingness to risk asking a client about sexual issues can move the nurse to a place of greater comfort in discussing sexuality. With experience the nurse will come to recognize that many clients welcome the opportunity to talk about their sexuality. When clients are experiencing difficulty in sexual relating, they often are appreciative of the nurse opening the subject area. Once the topic is broached, the client can express concerns and explore possible ways to proceed in seeking some resolution to the problem.

Standards. Ethical standards may come into play when one is faced with caring for a client whose sexual practices and values differ from one's own. The American Nurses Association *Code of Ethics* (1985) states, "The nurse provides services with respect for human dignity and the uniqueness of the client, unrestricted by considerations of social or economic status, personal attributes, or the nature of health problems."

Another place that ethical standards come into play in regard to sexuality is in the reporting of STDs. An element in both the ANA *Code of Ethics* (1985) and the International Council of Nurses *Code for Nurses* (1973) is the protection of the public. This involves reporting certain diseases and/or incidents of abuse to the appropriate health officials so that follow-up can be instituted. Most states mandate a report to a social service agency if abuse is suspected.

·················
NURSING PROCESS ·····························

▪ Assessment

Sexuality involves physical, psychological, social, and cultural variables. The nurse must assess all relevant factors to determine a client's sexual well-being.

Many nurses find that they are uncomfortable talking about sexuality with clients. To increase comfort in discussing sexuality, the nurse should build a sound knowledge base, including understanding of healthy sexuality and the most common sexual dysfunctions. Also important is personal assessment of comfort level when discussing sexuality. Realizing that the nursing role in addressing sexual concerns can encompass assessment, providing information, and referral can decrease the pressure of feeling as though the nurse must have all the answers to a client's questions or problems.

Sexual health history. Every complete nursing history, whether taken in a clinic or hospital, should include a few questions related to sexual functioning to determine whether the client has any sexual concerns. An opening statement such as "Sex is an important part of life and can be affected by our health status" or "To better understand your health, it is useful to know if you have concerns about your sexual function" is a good example to use. Other questions for adults may include the following:

1. How do you feel about the sexual aspect of your life?
2. How has your illness, medication, or impending surgery affected your sex life?
3. It is not unusual for people with your condition to experience some sexual problems. What has been your experience?

Also significant to explore, while gathering the sexual history for sexually active clients, is the client's use of contraception and safe sex practices. Adolescents may best respond to a question such as, "Many adolescents have questions about STDs or whether their bodies are developing at the right rate. Do you have any questions about sex?"

Factors influencing sexual function. In gathering a sexual history the nurse should consider physical, functional, relationship, lifestyle, and self-esteem factors that may influence sexual functioning. Sexual desire and function may be influenced, positively or negatively, by a variety of physical factors. For example, sexual intercourse may result in pain or discomfort from arthritis, angina, endometriosis, or lack of vaginal lubrication. Sexual performance can be altered by neuropathies, vascular deficiencies, and hormonal alter-

ations. Even imagining that sex may hurt, such as post-partum or postoperatively, can lessen sexual desire. The nurse learns to what extent these physical factors affect sexual performance.

Medications may affect sexual desire (see Box 16-3). Ingestion of alcohol or drugs may cloud judgment and contribute to ill-considered acts that may lead to STDs or pregnancy. The nurse gathers a complete history of any medications or illicit drugs the client is taking. It may also become appropriate, when counseling is being offered, to assess the same for the client's partner.

Perceptions of self may lead to personal and emotional conflict involving sexuality. Lower self-esteem can negatively influence sexual functioning. Communication skills play a critical role in the partner's sexual compatibility. The nurse tries to learn how the client feels about his or her sexuality and the ability to perform sexually. Ask clients if they feel comfortable when they are relating to their partner and whether there is an openness in the interaction.

There are a variety of normal changes associated with aging that can affect sexual function. Females experience a reduction in vaginal secretions, and the vagina becomes shorter and does not expand as well to accommodate the penis (Lueckenotte, 1996). Orgasmic contractions are fewer and may be accompanied by painful uterine contractions. In males, the penis may not become firm as quickly and may not be as firm as at a younger age. Ejaculation can take longer to achieve and may be shorter in duration, and erection often diminishes more quickly. The nurse's assessment includes a history of past sexual experiences, perceptions, and difficulties.

Sexual dysfunction. The nurse should be alert for sexual dysfunction. Considering the nature of physical problems, medications, and the factors addressed thus far, the nurse can identify clients who may be at risk for sexual dysfunction.

Also relevant, in light of the prevalence of domestic violence and sexual abuse, is consideration of sexual abuse. The nurse should be alert to clues that may suggest abuse (Box 16-4). In addition, observing the interaction between a woman and her partner may provide additional clues. Controlling behaviors such as speaking for the woman or belittling her are suggestive of emotional and perhaps physical or sexual abuse (Bohn and Holz, 1996). If the nurse suspects abuse, the client should be interviewed privately. It is unusual for a client to admit to problems of abuse with the sexual partner present during the interview. Some of the following questions may be useful: "Are you in a relationship in which someone is hurting you?" or "Have you ever been forced to have sex when you didn't want to?" These questions avoid using the emotionally laden and sometimes confusing terms of *abuse* or *rape*. If questions related to abuse are asked, the nurse ensures the client's confidentiality so that the client can safely discuss experiences or concerns.

Box 16-4

Signs and Symptoms That May Indicate Current Sexual Abuse or a History of Sexual Abuse

Bruises
Lacerations
Abrasions
Burns
Frequent visits to health care providers
Vague symptoms
Headaches
Gastrointestinal problems
Eating disorders
Abdominal pain
Vaginal pain
Dysmenorrhea
Premenstrual syndrome
Sleep pattern disturbances
Nightmares
Repetitive dreams
Insomnia
Depression
Anxiety
Fear
Decreased self-esteem
Difficulty developing trust
Difficulties with intimate relationships
Substance abuse

Modified from Bohn D, Holz K: Sequelae of abuse: health effects of childhood sexual abuse, domestic battering, and rape, *J Nurse Midwifery* 41(6):442, 1996.

NURSING DIAGNOSES FOR CLIENTS WITH ALTERATIONS IN SEXUALITY

Body image disturbance
Decisional conflict
Knowledge deficit regarding STD prevention
Rape-trauma syndrome
Self-esteem disturbance
Sexual dysfunction
Sexuality patterns, altered

Client expectations. As in the case of any client assessment, it is important to understand the client's expectations regarding care. Questions such as, "What do you expect from us in the way we perform your care?" or "In what way can we make your care best meet your needs?" give the client the opportunity to express any desires. When nursing care involves consideration of the client's sexuality, the need for sensitivity, confidentiality, and understanding are likely client expectations.

Nursing Diagnosis

Possible nursing diagnoses related to sexual functioning are listed in the nursing diagnoses box. Clues that signal a possible diagnosis related to sexuality include surgery of reproductive organs or changes in appearance, chronic fatigue or pain, past or current physical abuse, chronic illness, and developmental milestones such as puberty or menopause. Interventions are contingent on selecting the correct related factors.

As with making any nursing diagnosis, the process of making a nursing diagnosis regarding sexuality is often one of clarification with the client to establish that the nursing diagnosis defining characteristics exist and that the client perceives a problem or difficulty with regard to sexuality. Determining the etiological or contributing factors is important. Inclusion of all relevant contributing factors can help to focus effective planning. For example, the nursing diagnosis *altered sexuality pattern related to acceptance of recent mastectomy* might be appropriate for a woman who has recently undergone a mastectomy. Further expanding the *"related to"* section to include more about how the mastectomy is affecting sexuality would be helpful. Altered sexuality could be related to postoperative pain or fear of pain, fear of diminished attractiveness, and/or difficulty in moving. The approaches to each of these etiological factors would be slightly different.

Planning

When developing a plan of care the nurse should involve the client and, with permission, the sex partner. For planning to be effective, the client must be involved in setting goals and outcome criteria. For example, for the nursing diagnosis *altered sexuality pattern related to recent mastectomy and fear of pain* the nurse might explore with the client how she would envision a satisfactory recovery after her mastectomy. This would give the client the opportunity to share, for example, that she would like to return to her presurgical sexual relationship with her partner, which would entail feeling comfortable having her remaining breast caressed and being able to comfortably engage in intercourse one to two times per week.

Planning in the area of sexuality may include referrals to a clinical psychologist, social worker, or sex therapist. Sexual conflict in marriage or trauma over past sexual assault or incest may require intensive treatment with mental health professionals or a certified sex therapist.

Implementation

The nurse's role includes the promotion of sexual health as a component of overall wellness. The nurse can promote sexual health by helping clients gain insight into their problems and explore methods to deal with them effectively.

Health promotion. Exploring a person's sexuality and being able to provide useful sex education require good communication skills. The environment and timing should be structured to provide privacy, uninterrupted time, and client comfort. For example, when discussing contraception methods with a woman, the nurse provides comfortable chairs in an office rather than discussing this in the examination room when the client is only partially clothed.

Topics of education vary (Box 16-5). Education may offer explanation of normal developmental changes; for example, the nurse might talk to a school-age child about the appearance of pubic hair or a 60-year-old man regarding the normalcy of delayed ejaculation. Details of physiological changes resulting from illness or treatment effects should be provided as a part of general health care. This gives clients permission to raise questions or concerns regarding personal functioning. Box 16-6 summarizes special considerations for the older adult.

Discussions of healthy sex should always include contraception when talking with clients who are capable of having children. The discussion may include desire for children, usual sexual practices, and acceptable methods of contraception. Factors to consider when educating clients about contraceptives include scheduling or frequency of sex, comfort with genital touching, and comfort with interruption of sexual acts. All methods of contraception should be reviewed to provide necessary information for an informed client choice. The best method is the one the client will use consistently.

Individuals having more than one sex partner or whose partner has other sexual experiences need to learn more about safe sex practices. As discussed earlier, information should be provided on STD transmission and symptoms, use of condoms, and risky sexual activities (e.g., anal sex). Safe sex may also consider the client's emotional risks within a relationship. Role play may be a useful educational tool so that the client can learn to say "No" or negotiate with a partner to use a condom.

Nursing interventions that address client alterations in sexual patterns or sexual dysfunction raise awareness, assist clarification of issues or concerns, and provide information. Nurses should recognize when a client's needs exceed their expertise. Referral to a sexual counselor may be necessary.

Acute care. Illness and surgery can be significant situational stressors. Clients may experience major physical changes, the effects of drugs or treatments, and the emotional stress of prognosis and future limited function. Sexuality, as a component of personality, may be affected by all aspects of illness (physical and psychological). The nurse should never assume that sexual functioning is not a concern merely because of an individual's age or severity of prognosis. After concerns are assessed and identified, they can be addressed in the context of the person's value system. When a client experiences physical limitations to sexually performing, the nurse might suggest therapies such as planning sexual activity when the client is rested, experimenting with positions that are more comfortable, encouraging partners to give one another more time to achieve arousal, and encouraging the use of foreplay to increase sexual arousal. For example, a client experiencing joint pain may appreciate a discussion of how the side-lying position can be effective in intercourse. Use of fantasy or a sense of playfulness may add new romance or stimulation to a long-term relationship.

BOX 16-5

Client Teaching for Promoting Sexual Function

- Refrain from drinking alcohol 1 to 2 hours before sexual activity.
- Encourage partners to discuss what types of intimate behavior provide the most sexual stimulation and satisfaction.
- Explain options available for contraception.
- Discuss side effects of medications that commonly alter sexual function and response.
- For a client with cardiac dysfunction, encourage use of the usual position during intercourse and selection of a time of day when the client feels rested.
- Explain that safe sex involves the following practices: avoidance of multiple or anonymous partners, prostitutes, and other people with multiple sex partners; avoidance of sexual contact with a person who has a genital discharge, genital warts, herpes, other suspicious lesions, or a medical diagnosis of human immunodeficiency virus (HIV) or hepatitis B; avoidance of oral/anal sex; avoidance of genital contact with oral sores; and use of latex condoms and diaphragms along with spermicides.

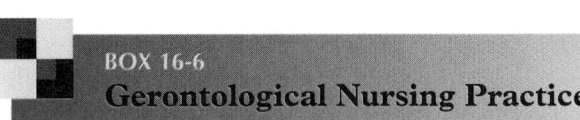

BOX 16-6
Gerontological Nursing Practice

- Females may benefit from use of an artificial water-based lubricant during intercourse.
- Alternative positions for intercourse (e.g., side-lying, lying on a bed with legs over the side) may decrease discomfort during intercourse.
- A longer period of foreplay helps the male to achieve penile firmness.
- Conserve strength by not working hard at the beginning of intercourse, so as to avoid tiring before climax.
- Resume foreplay or use time for touching and talking so as to achieve a second orgasm.

From Lueckenotte A: *Gerontologic nursing,* St. Louis, 1996, Mosby.

Restorative care. In the home environment it is important to assist clients in creating an environment comfortable for sexual activity. This may involve making recommendations for ways to rearrange the client's bedroom to accommodate any limitations the client might have. For example, wheelchair-bound clients may prefer being able to move the chair close up to the side of the bed at an angle that allows the partner to assume a coital position more easily. Clients and partners need to know how to accommodate barriers such as Foley catheters or drainage tubes that may make coital positioning difficult.

In the long-term care setting, facilities should make proper arrangements for privacy during an older client's sexual experience (Lueckenotte, 1996). The ideal situation is to set up a pleasant room that can be used for a variety of activities but may also be reserved by the older adult for private visits with a spouse or partner. In most settings, this may not be possible, so the next option is to use the client's room while making other arrangements for the client's roommate. Although privacy of clients is important, clients should not be allowed to be alone in a situation in which they may injure themselves (Lueckenotte, 1996).

▪ Evaluation

Client care. The nurse will review goals and outcome criteria that were developed during the planning process and determine if they have been met. In addition, the nurse will also want to consider the overall status of the identified problems or nursing diagnoses. This will require a follow-up discussion with the client to determine if the level of satisfaction with sexual performance or sexual function has improved. Sometimes the goal and outcome criteria may have been achieved but sexual functioning is still not ideal. The nurse should then consider what other steps might be appropriate.

Client expectations. In evaluating care provided to clients with sexual alterations or those in need of sexual health education, the nurse must determine if the client's expectations are met. After determining the progress in care, the nurse asks if the client perceives the nurse as being effective and supportive. Again it is important for the nurse to remain aware of any personal limitations in being able to counsel the client. Referrals to other health care providers may still be necessary.

Key Terms

body image	self-concept
gender identity	self-esteem
homophobia	sexual dysfunction
identity	sexual orientation
myotonia	sexual response cycle
role	sexuality

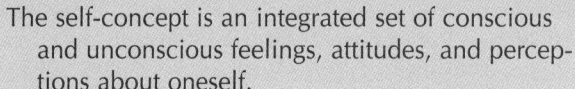

▪ Key Concepts

The self-concept is an integrated set of conscious and unconscious feelings, attitudes, and perceptions about oneself.

Components of self-concept are body image, self-esteem, roles, and identity.

Roles are learned through socialization; they involve the expectations of others about behavior in particular positions (e.g., family member, employee).

The nurse should be aware of how his or her self-concept and nursing actions can affect a client's self-concept.

Sexuality is related to all dimensions of health; therefore sexual concerns or problems should be addressed as a part of nursing care.

Attitudes toward sexuality vary widely and are influenced by spirituality, society's values, the media, family, and other factors. A nurse should not judge a client's sexual preferences and needs.

Sexual development begins in infancy and involves some kind of sexual behavior or growth in all developmental stages.

Sexual health involves physical and psychosocial aspects and contributes to an individual's sense of self-worth and positive interpersonal relationships.

A client's sexuality is affected by development and life changes, ethical decisional issues, fertility, personal and emotional conflicts, illness, and hospitalization; the nurse helps the client adapt to situations and maintain healthy sexuality.

Critical Thinking Activities

1. Jack Fisher is a 28-year-old manager of a local food store. He comes to his primary care provider for blood work before his upcoming marriage. The nurse knows Mr. Fisher because he has been coming to the clinic for minor health issues over the past 4 years. In talking with Mr. Fisher, the nurse learns that this is his first marriage, the woman he is marrying has a 3-year-old son, and although he has spent a good deal of time with his fianceé's 3-year-old son he has not lived in a household with young children since his own childhood. The nurse recognizes that Mr. Fisher will be undergoing several role changes related to his upcoming marriage. What new roles will he likely be taking on? How might the nurse explore with Mr. Fisher his readiness to assume new roles and his awareness of the possible stress of taking on new roles?

2. Mrs. Smith, a 48-year-old married woman, is scheduled for a hysterectomy tomorrow. She expresses concern regarding whether this is the right choice. What issues may be influencing Mrs. Smith? How do you proceed with her care?

3. Mr. Jackson is 65 years old and is admitted with postdiabetic ketoacidosis. During his stay you notice great intimacy (hand holding, kissing, massage, affectionate names) expressed between Mr. and Mrs. Jackson. How might you approach the topic of sexuality? What is relevant information to provide regarding age and disease state?

4. Mrs. Jones has given birth to her third child. In assisting her with activities of daily living you notice bruises on her neck and both arms. Mr. Jones seems to be in constant attendance and very resistant to leaving the room. You suspect that some form of domestic abuse may be occurring. How do you approach validating this suspicion without putting Mrs. Jones at risk? What referrals, education, and support materials can you provide Mrs. Jones during this brief 24-hour stay? What are your further obligations?

References

Alan Guttmacher Institute: *Sex and America's teenagers,* New York, 1994, Author.

Alexander LL, LaRosa JH: *New dimensions in women's health,* Boston, Mass, 1994, Jones & Bartlett.

American Nurses Association: *Code for nurses with interpretive statements,* Kansas City, Mo, 1985, The Association.

Beckman LJ, Harvey SM: Factors affecting the consistent use of barrier methods of contraception, *Obstet Gynecol,* 88(10):65S, 1996.

Bohn D, Holz K: Sequelae of abuse: health effects of childhood sexual abuse, domestic battering, and rape, *J Nurse Midwifery* 41(6):442, 1996.

Drench M: Changes in body image secondary to disease and injury, *Rehabil Nurs* 19(1):31, 1994.

Erikson EH: *Childhood and society,* ed 2, New York, 1963, WW Norton.

Forrest JD, Frost JJ: The family planning attitudes and experiences of low-income women, *Fam Plann Perspect* 28(11-12):246, 1996.

Gibson DE: Reminiscence, self-esteem, and self-other satisfaction in adult male alcoholics, *J Psychiatr Nurs* 18(7), 1980.

Giger JN, Davidhizar RE: *Transcultural nursing: assessment and intervention,* St. Louis, 1995, Mosby.

Gilligan C: *In a different voice,* Cambridge, Mass, 1982, Harvard University Press.

Guidry HM: Childhood sexual abuse: role of the family physician, *Am Fam Physician* 51(2):407, 1995.

Hatcher RA and others: *Contraceptive technology,* New York, 1994, Irvington.

International Council of Nurses: *ICN code for nurses: ethical concepts applied to nursing,* Geneva, 1973, Imprimeries Poplaires.

Johnson B: Older adults and sexuality: a multidimensional perspective, *J Gerontol Nurs* 22(2):6, 1996.

Kaplan J: *Disorders of sexual desire,* New York, 1979, Simon & Schuster.

Keller M and others: Adolescents' views of sexual decision-making, *Image J Nurs Sch* 28(2):125, 1996.

Kinsey AC and others: *Sexual behavior in the human male,* Philadelphia, 1948, WB Saunders.

Kinsey AC and others: *Sexual behavior in the human female,* Philadelphia, 1953, WB Saunders.

Lueckenotte L: *Gerontologic nursing,* St. Louis, 1996, Mosby.

MacLaren A: Primary care for women: comprehensive sexual health assessment, *J Nurse Midwifery* 40(2):104, 1995.

Masters W and others: *Human sexuality,* Boston, 1992, Little, Brown.

Sell RL and others: The prevalence of homosexual behavior and attraction in the United States, the United Kingdom and France: results of national population-based samples, *Arch Sex Behav* 24(6):235, 1995.

Stuart GW, Sundeen SJ: *Principles and practice of psychiatric nursing,* ed 5, St. Louis, 1995, Mosby.

Sundeen S and others: *Nurse-client interaction,* ed 5, St. Louis, 1994, Mosby.

World Health Organization: *Education and treatment in human sexuality: the training of health professionals,* WHO Tech Rep Ser, 572, Geneva, 1975, The Organization.

Youngkin E: Sexually transmitted diseases: current and emerging concerns, *J Obstet Gynecol Neonatal Nurs* 24(8):743, 1995.

17

Spiritual Health

OBJECTIVES

Mastery of content in this chapter will enable the student to:

- Define the key terms listed.
- Describe the relationship between faith, hope, and spiritual well-being.
- Compare and contrast the concepts of religion and spirituality.
- Discuss the relationship of spirituality to an individual's total being.
- Perform an initial assessment of a client's spiritual well-being.
- Discuss nursing interventions designed to promote spiritual health.
- Evaluate attainment of spiritual health.

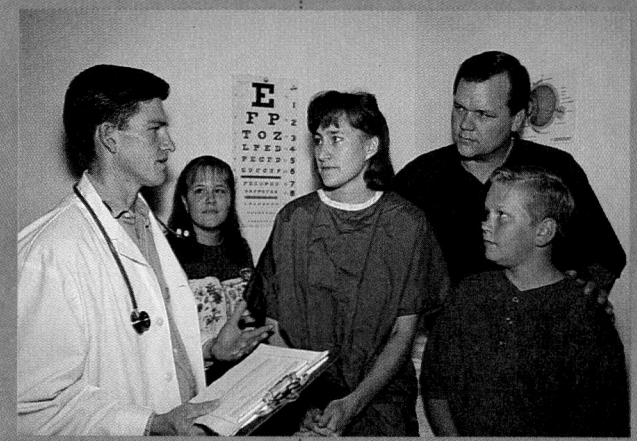

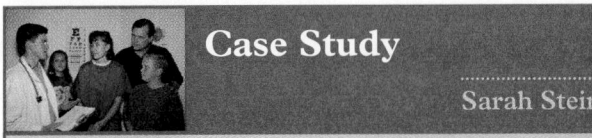

Case Study

Sarah Stein

Sarah Stein is a 48-year-old college professor, diagnosed 3 months ago with breast cancer. She is married to Joe, an insurance salesman, and is the mother of two children: Valerie, who is 16 years of age, and Peter, who is 12. Surgeons removed Sarah's cancerous tumor and two involved lymph nodes. Lymphatic involvement increases the risk that the cancer might spread. Sarah has completed a course of radiation and now visits the local cancer clinic with her husband 3 times a week for a course of chemotherapy. She has received instruction from one of the clinic nurses about the side effects of chemotherapy. Both Sarah and Joe discuss their concern for their children. Their son is preparing for his Bar Mitzvah, which is only 6 months away. Sarah hopes to attend the ceremony but worries about how she will feel. Valerie, their daughter, has been showing behavioral outbursts since her mother's illness.

Jeff is a 36-year-old, married student nurse assigned to the oncology clinic. One of the clinic case managers, who serves as Jeff's preceptor, assigns Jeff to follow Sarah during her clinic visits. Jeff is in his last semester at school and hopes to get a position in the clinic after graduation. Sarah's experience is significant for Jeff because he has children in the same age-group and wonders how they might react to their mother being ill.

During one of their clinic visits, Sarah and Joe spend some time discussing ways to manage chemotherapy side effects with Jeff. Jeff has noticed that Sarah and Joe appear very calm and relaxed when discussing cancer therapy. Joe explains, "What happens will happen, but we both have a lot of faith in God." Sarah responds, "Even though I know I have cancer, I hope to be able to attend my son's Bar Mitzvah next year. Joe is my support, and together I know we will make it."

A person's health depends on a balance of physical, psychological, sociological, cultural, developmental, and spiritual variables. This **holistic** view of health is the focus and heart of nursing practice. Holism encourages nurses to constantly look for factors and relations that affect the complexity of health and illness. Recently nurse researchers, pastoral care professionals, physicians, social workers, and others have proposed that spirituality has special importance as the integrating theme that unifies all aspects of an individual's health. **Spirituality** and **spiritual well-being** are terms often used interchangeably. Haase and colleagues (1992) note that spirituality is a basic quality of all humans. Spiritual well-being has been described as an integrating aspect of human wholeness, characterized by meaning and hope (Clark and others, 1991). Nursing requires skills in spiritual care to support clients as they identify and explore what is meaningful in their lives and find ways to cope with the impact of illness and the ongoing stressors of life. Appropriate spiritual care requires openness and acceptance so that the nurse's personal beliefs and religious views are not forced on the client. Gaining skill in spiritual care enhances nurses' abilities to establish strong, caring relationships with their clients.

SCIENTIFIC KNOWLEDGE BASE

Recently health care research has begun to show the association between spirituality and health. There may be beneficial health outcomes when an individual is able to engage his or her beliefs in a higher power and sense a source of strength or support. Turner and Clancy (1986) studied clients with chronic low back pain and found that increased use of praying and hoping was related to decreased pain intensity. Prayer is frequently used as a method of coping and is effective in minimizing physical stressors. Remen (1988) suggests that healing is not a matter of mechanism but rather a work of spirit. Research has shown, for example, that meditation is successful in treating chronic pain, insomnia, anxiety, and depression (Culligan, 1996).

The relationship between spirituality and healing is not completely understood. However, it is the individual's intrinsic spirit that seems to be the factor in healing. When clients are given a placebo (sugar pill) instead of a prescribed medication, often they improve, not because of the sugar pill but because of their faith in the doctor who prescribed it. The placebo phenomenon shows that healing can take place because of believing.

New research is showing a link between spirit, mind, and body. An individual's beliefs and expectations can and do have effects on the person's physical well-being (Coe, 1997). Many of these effects may be tied to hormonal and neurological function. Relaxation training and guided imagery, for example, have been shown to improve individuals' immune function (Kiecolt-Glaser and others, 1985). A person's inner beliefs and convictions can become powerful resources for healing. A nurse will be more successful in helping clients achieve desirable health outcomes after learning to support clients and families spiritually, as well as mentally and physically.

······· # NURSING KNOWLEDGE BASE····

Concepts in Spiritual Health

To provide meaningful and supportive spiritual care, it is important for a nurse to understand the concepts that are at the foundation of spiritual health. The need for meaning in life runs deep within each person. The concepts of **faith, hope,** spiritual well-being, and religion give direction in understanding the view each individual has of life and its value.

Faith. The concept of faith has two uses described in the literature. The first use pertains to a relationship with a divinity, higher power, authority, or spirit that incorporates a reasoning faith (belief) and a trusting faith (action) (Benner, 1985). The reasoning faith deals with an individual's belief and confidence in something for which there is no proof. It is an acceptance of what our reasoning cannot reach. Sometimes it involves a belief in a higher power, spirit guide, God, or Allah (Fryback, 1993). However, faith also might be the manner in which a person chooses to live life. Faith in this sense enables action. For example, a person might believe that having a positive outlook on life is the best way to achieve life's goals. The belief that comes with faith involves transcendence, or an awareness of that which cannot be seen or known in ordinary physical ways (Reed, 1987). It gives purpose and meaning to an individual's life. A trusting faith deals with the inner resources that allow an individual to act. For example, cancer clients who have faith in a positive outlook on life might pursue more knowledge about their disease and continue to pursue daily activities rather than resign themselves to the disease's symptoms. Fryback (1993) studied clients diagnosed with HIV and found faith to be an inner power that enabled clients to act, to go on with life, and to gain a sense of freedom from their illness.

Faith is also defined as a cultural or institutional religion, such as Judaism, Buddhism, Islam, or Christianity (Benner, 1985). Many clients practice a faith or belief in the doctrines and expressions of a specific religion or sect, such as the Lutheran church within Christianity or the Orthodox Jewish faith. A person's religious faith influences the manner in which he or she exercises a faith of belief and action. For example, a member of the Buddhist faith believes in the Four Noble Truths taught by Buddha: life is suffering, suffering is caused by desire, suffering can be eliminated by eliminating desire, and to eliminate desire, one must follow an eightfold path (Giger and Davidhizar, 1995). The eightfold path includes right understanding, purpose, speech, conduct, vocation, effort, thinking, and meditation. The Buddhist turns inward, holding faith in the importance of self-control, versus the faith of Christians, who look to the teachings of God to provide enlightenment and direction in life.

Hope. When a person has the attitude of something to live for and look forward to, hope is present. Miller and Powers (1988) describe hope as a multidimensional concept consisting of anticipation of a continued good, an improvement, or the lessening of something unpleasant. Hope is energizing, giving individuals a motivation to achieve and the resources to use toward that achievement. Nowotny (1989) notes that hope can be found in all aspects of life as a force that helps individuals cope with life stressors (Box 17-1). Hope is an invaluable personal resource whenever someone is faced with a loss (see Chapter 21) or a challenge that seems difficult to achieve. Hope has purpose and direction and gives reason for being (Post-White and others, 1996).

In studies with cancer clients, having hope has been found to help individuals find meaning in their illness (O'Connor and others, 1990; Fryback, 1993). When clients with cancer face uncomfortable symptoms, increasing disability, or the fear of death, hope enables them to face the discomforts of their disease and continue to value living as fully as possible.

Spiritual well-being. Spiritual well-being is a concept that is unique to each individual. Individuals' definitions of their own spirituality are influenced by their culture, development, life experiences, beliefs, and ideas about life. An individual's spirituality or spiritual well-being enables the person to love, have faith and hope, seek meaning in life, and to nurture relationships with others. Spirituality offers a sense of connectedness

---

Box 17-1
The Concept of Hope

Hope is future oriented. An individual imagines what is not yet seen.

Hope usually includes active involvement by the individual. Involvement might include goal setting, caring, planning, or praying.

Hope comes from within a person (though its locus or center might be outside the person, as in God or "medicine") and is related to trust.

That which is hoped for is seen by the person as truly possible. Hope is more than a desire or wish.

Hope relates to or involves other people or a higher being. This can include thoughts, feelings, and actions that involve others.

The outcome of hope is important to the individual. The expectation is often a future outcome that has meaning to the individual.

Modified from Nowotny ML: Assessment of hope in patients with cancer: development of an instrument, *Oncol Nurs Forum* 16(1):57, 1989.

intrapersonally (connected within oneself), interpersonally (connected with others and the environment), and transpersonally (connected with the unseen, God, or a higher power). Hungelmann and others (1996) describe spiritual well-being as a sense of harmonious interconnectedness between self, others and/or nature, and an Ultimate Other that exists throughout and beyond time and space. There are two important characteristics of spiritual well-being about which most authors agree: (1) it is a unifying theme in our lives, and (2) it is a state of being.

From a holistic perspective, spiritual well-being unifies the various dimensions that make up an individual (Figure 17-1). Clark and others (1991) stress how spirituality spreads throughout all other dimensions in life, whether a person acknowledges or develops it. Spirituality is the glue that can help keep all other aspects of a person's life together.

Religion. Many times nurses have difficulty differentiating spirituality from religion. Religion is commonly associated with the "state of doing" or a specific system of practices associated with a particular denomination, sect, or form of worship. Emblen (1992) defines religion as a system of organized beliefs and worship that a person practices to outwardly express his or her spirituality. Religion serves different purposes in people's lives. For some, religion is a set of rules and rituals used to worship a Supreme Being. For others, religion is a way of life providing nourishment and a connectedness to all of life. In this latter context, religion is more directly associated with spiritual well-being.

When providing spiritual care to clients, it is important to understand the differences between religion and spirituality. Religious care is helping clients maintain their faithfulness to their belief systems and worship practices. Spiritual care is helping people maintain personal relationships and a relationship to a higher being or life force, to identify meaning and purpose in life, and to hopefully look beyond the present (Aldridge, 1993).

Spiritual Health

Spiritual health is achieved when a person finds a balance between his or her life values, goals, and belief systems and their relationship within himself or herself and with others. Throughout life an individual may grow more spiritual, becoming increasingly aware of the meaning, purpose, and values of life. In times of stress, illness, recovery, or loss a person may turn to previous ways of responding or adjusting to a situation. Often these coping styles lie within the person's spiritual beliefs.

Spirituality begins as children learn about themselves and their relationships with others. Many adults experience spiritual growth by entering into lifelong relationships. An ability to care meaningfully for others and the self is evidence of a healthy spirituality. Older adults often turn to important relationships and the giving of themselves to others as spiritual tasks.

Spiritual Problems

When illness, loss, grief, or a major life change affects a person, spiritual resources either help the person move to recovery or spiritual needs and concerns develop. **Spiritual distress** is the disruption of an individual's "life principle," which fills the person's entire being and transcends or exceeds biological and psychosocial nature (Kim and others, 1997). A catastrophic illness, for example, can upset a person's spiritual well-being sufficiently to cause doubt and loss of faith. Spiritual distress may cause the person to feel alone or even abandoned by resources that at one time were very nurturing. Individuals may question their spiritual values, raising questions about their whole way of life, purpose for living, and source of meaning. Spiritual distress also occurs when there is conflict between a person's beliefs and prescribed health regimens or the inability to practice usual rituals.

Acute illness. Sudden, unexpected illness that poses both an immediate and a long-term threat to a client's life, health, and/or well-being can create significant spiritual distress. For example, the 40-year-old man who has a stroke and the 20-year-old who is injured in a motor vehicle accident both face crises that may threaten their spiritual health. The illness or injury creates an unanticipated scramble to integrate and cope with new realities (e.g., disability). A person looks for ways to remain faithful to his or her beliefs and value systems. Often conflicts can develop around a person's beliefs and the meaning of life. Anger is not uncom-

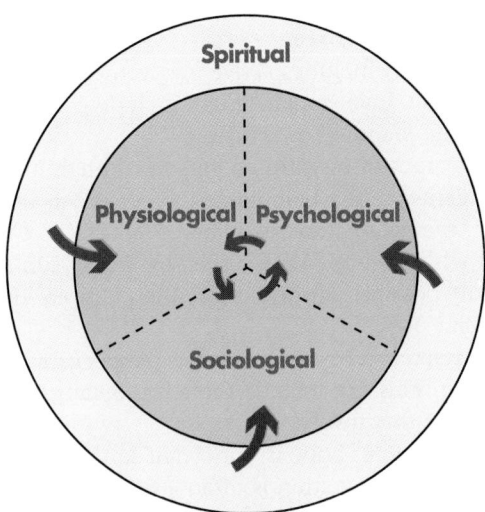

Figure 17-1. The spiritual dimension: the unifying approach. (Modified from Farran CJ and others: Development of a model for spiritual assessment and intervention, *J Religion Health* 28[3]:185, 1989.)

mon, and clients may express it against God, their families, themselves, or the nurse. The strength of a client's spirituality influences how he or she copes with sudden illness and how quickly he or she can move to recovery. Yim (1996) has developed a spiritual healing critical pathway for coronary artery bypass clients. His research has shown that knowledge of a person's spiritual well-being can be used to maximize a client's recovery. Hope and the ability to speak about life values and gain meaning from illness influence a client's ability to recover from heart surgery. The pathway identifies where clients are in their spiritual recovery and recommends appropriate interventions that help clients find purpose and worth in order to move forward and recover.

Chronic illness. Persons with chronic illness often suffer debilitating symptoms that change their lifestyles. Independence can be threatened, causing fear, anxiety, and an overall dispiritedness (Figure 17-2). Dependence on others for routine self-care measures can create a feeling of powerlessness. A person may feel a loss of a sense of purpose in life that affects the inner strength needed to deal with alterations in functioning. A person's spirituality can be a significant factor in how he or she adapts to the changes resulting from chronic illness. Successfully adapting to those changes can strengthen a person spiritually. A reevaluation of life may occur. Those who are able to engage and use their spiritual resources have a much better chance to reestablish a self-identity and live to their potential.

Terminal illness. Terminal illness commonly causes fear of physical pain, isolation, the unknown, dying, and the threat to integrity (Turner and others, 1995). Clients may have an uncertainty about what death means and thus be susceptible to spiritual dis-

tress. There are also clients who have a spiritual sense of peace that enables them to face death without fear.

Individuals experiencing a terminal illness often find themselves reviewing their life and questioning its meaning. Common questions asked include, "Why is this happening to me" or "What have I done?" Family and friends can be affected just as much as the client. Terminal illness causes members of the family to ask important questions about its meaning and how it will affect their relationship with the client (see Chapter 21).

Fryback (1993) conducted a study to learn how people with a terminal illness describe health. Clients in the study identified the following three domains of health: mental-emotional, spiritual, and physical (Figure 17-3). The spiritual domain was seen as essential for health and included having a relationship with a higher power, recognizing mortality, and striving for self-actualization. Although many of the participants in the study either attended church or stated a desire to do so, others found that spirituality was not dependent on a religion or church. They associated health with belief in a higher power that gave them faith and the ability to love (Fryback, 1993). The study revealed that when terminally ill clients have a perception of being unhealthy, it is not due to the disease but to being unable to live their lives fully and do the things they desire.

Near-death experience. Nurses may encounter clients who have had a near-death experience (NDE).

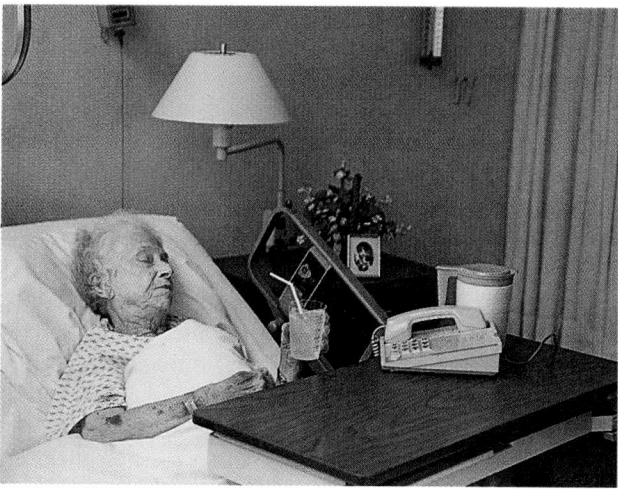

Figure 17-2. Dispiritedness can affect a person's adjustment to illness.

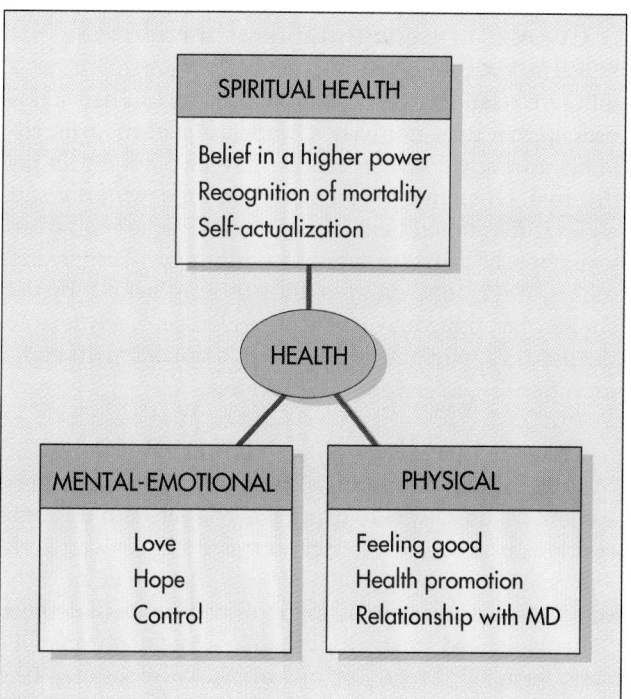

Figure 17-3. Domains of health based on perceptions of terminally ill clients. (Modified from Fryback PB: Health for people with a terminal diagnosis, *Nurs Sci Q* 6(3):147, 1993.)

An NDE has been identified as a psychological phenomenon of people who have either been close to clinical death or have recovered after being declared dead. It is not associated with a mental disorder (Basford, 1990). Persons who experience an NDE after cardiopulmonary arrest, for example, often tell the same story of feeling themselves rising above their bodies and watching care givers initiate lifesaving measures. Most individuals describe passing through a tunnel to a bright light, encountering people who preceded them in death, and feeling an inner tranquility and peace. Instead of moving toward the light, they learn it is not time for them to die and they return to life.

Clients who have an NDE are often reluctant to discuss it, thinking family or care givers will not understand. Isolation and depression can occur. However, individuals experiencing an NDE who can discuss it with family or care givers find openness to the power of the experience as it is reported. They consistently report positive aftereffects, including a positive attitude and spiritual development (Turner and others, 1995). After a client has survived cardiopulmonary arrest, it is important for the nurse to remain open and give the client a chance to explore what happened.

Religious Problems

A client's religious problems can affect his or her spirituality. Interruptions or changes to customary religious practices may affect the structure or support that religion contributes to the person's sense of well-being.

Change in denominational membership or religious conversion.

Marrying a person from a different religious background or moving to a new community that does not have a branch of a particular religious group will create, at least initially, loss for an individual. Of course, it can also open up new options. If a loss is felt, the individual experiences separation from a previously valued religious community (Turner and others, 1995). The extent of the loss is influenced by the choice the individual had in the change, how flexible the person's religious expression is, and what faith communities the individual is able to find.

Loss or questioning of faith.

Faith is a way of relating to self, community, and a higher power. A person often finds a way to express his or her faith through religious practices. Faith develops over time, along with a person's spiritual growth. Persons who are at an early stage of development of their faith or who find their faith challenged by an event such as acute or chronic illness, terminal disease, or loss of a loved one, may become vulnerable to loss of or doubt about their faith (Turner and others, 1995). This can also occur when a person is shunned by his or her religious community (e.g., a Jehovah's Witness who elects to have surgery requiring a blood transfusion or a traditionally religious person who is diagnosed with HIV) or when the person seriously questions the position his or her religious denomination takes on a public issue (e.g., abortion, euthanasia). A loss or questioning of faith can cause serious guilt and a sense of loneliness, even when it can lead to a more mature faith and stronger convictions.

CRITICAL THINKING IN CLIENT CARE

Synthesis

Benner (1984) has described the helping role as an important domain of nursing practice. Clients look to nurses for a different kind of help than that sought from other health care professionals. Expert nurses acquire the ability to anticipate the personal issues affecting clients' abilities to receive and seek help, including their spiritual well-being. Critical thinking knowledge and skills are used to enhance clients' spiritual well-being and health and to assist those in need of help and support in engaging their own spirituality for healing and recovery. Throughout the application of the nursing process, the nurse applies knowledge, experience, attitudes, and standards in providing appropriate spiritual care.

Knowledge. The provision of appropriate spiritual care requires the nurse to use knowledge about a client's faith and belief systems. A client's faith history may reveal the individual's beliefs toward life, health, and a Supreme Being or state of mind. In addition, knowledge of good communication principles (see Chapter 13) must be applied for nurses to establish a therapeutic trust with clients. An individual's spiritual beliefs are very personal and relational. Nurses who are able to convey caring and openness to individuals, their spiritual beliefs, and how their beliefs operate in their lives will be more successful in promoting honest discussion.

When caring for clients with terminal illness, knowledge of loss and grief dynamics (see Chapter 21) is important. A person's reaction to loss is in part a function of the grief response. However, the individual's spiritual resources also influence the manner in which the loss is accepted and managed. Another area of knowledge that is important to consider while providing spiritual care is that of family dynamics (see Chapter 19). For many individuals, their spiritual health is often integrated with the relationships between family members. Nurses should be familiar with theory and principles of family systems and understand the role family plays for a particular client.

A final area of knowledge for the nurse to reflect on is his or her own spiritual beliefs and values. The nurse must differentiate personal spirituality from that of the client. This becomes important during the delivery of care when the nurse must be able to help engage a client spiritually rather than try to exercise personal spiritual convictions. Nurses must be clear and firm about their own faith to keep it from coloring their perceptions or understanding of the faith of the client and family.

Finally, a sound understanding of ethics and values (see Chapter 11) is also essential to provide spiritual care. A person's values or beliefs about the worth of a given idea, attitude, or custom are linked to the individual's spiritual well-being. Application of ethical principles ensures respect for a client's spiritual and religious convictions.

Experience. Recognizing that spirituality is more than religion, nurses need to consider personal views and philosophies about life and reflect on whether their own spirituality can be beneficial in assisting clients. If a nurse senses a personal faith and hope regarding life, it is likely that he or she will be better able to help clients. Previous experiences with dying clients or clients who have experienced significant losses can provide lessons in how to help clients face difficult challenges and to offer support to family and friends.

Attitudes. A nurse should not presume to know how a client might react to illness or loss. Humility becomes very important, particularly when caring for clients from diverse cultural and/or religious backgrounds. The nurse must recognize any limitations in knowledge about a client's spiritual beliefs and religious practices and be willing to pursue the knowledge needed to provide appropriate, individualized care.

Standards. A good critical thinker exercises completeness and significance when making decisions about clients' spiritual needs. The nature of a person's spirituality can be complex. It is important for the nurse to conduct a complete assessment of the client's spiritual beliefs and resources. Assumptions must be avoided regarding the client's religion and what beliefs may or may not be best for another. Significance as a standard of critical thinking in this case means that the nurse has explored issues most meaningful to the client and that are most likely to affect his or her spiritual well-being.

NURSING PROCESS

Application of the nursing process from the perspective of a client's spiritual needs is not simple. It goes beyond assessing a client's religious practices and rituals. Understanding a client's spirituality and then appropriately identifying the level of support and resources needed requires a new, broader perspective. Heliker (1992) describes the importance of shared community and compassion. *Compassion* comes from the Latin words *pati* and *cum,* meaning "to suffer with." *Commu-*

nity is derived from the Latin word meaning "fellowship." To be compassionate is to "enter into places of pain, to share in brokenness with other human beings" (Heliker, 1992). To practice compassion as a nurse requires awareness of the very human tie between clients and a healing community. The nurse must remove from the assessment and plan any personal biases or misconceptions. The nurse must be willing to share and discover another person's meaning and purpose in life, sickness, and health. A nurse learns to look beyond a personal view when establishing a client relationship. This means identifying the common values that make us human and respecting the commitments and values that make humans unique. Love, trust, hope, forgiveness, meaning, and community are spiritual needs we all have (Carson, 1989). Learning to share these needs helps the nurse find a way to give clients spiritual care and support.

Another important aspect of spiritual care is recognizing that a client does not have to have a spiritual problem. Clients bring certain spiritual resources that the nurse can engage as resources to help them assume healthier lives, recover from illness, or face impending death. Supporting and recognizing the positive side of a client's spirituality goes a long way in delivering effective, individualized nursing care.

▣ Assessment

A nurse's ability to gain a reliable picture of a client's spiritual dimension may be limited by the setting in which the nurse practices. This is true if nurses have limited contact with clients or fail to build therapeutic relationships with them. But once a trusting relationship with a client is established, the nurse and client reach a point of learning together, and spiritual caring can occur. The nurse must learn to consciously integrate an attitude of spiritual care into the nursing process. The assessment should focus on aspects of spirituality most likely to be influenced by life experiences, events, and questions in the case of illness and hospitalization. Even conducting an assessment can be therapeutic because it conveys a level of caring and support. The nurse who understands the overall approach to spiritual assessment can enter into thoughtful discussions with the client and gain a greater awareness of the personal resources an individual brings to a situation. These resources ought to be incorporated into an effective plan of care.

A spiritual well-being screening tool. The JAREL spiritual well-being scale (Figure 17-4) was developed by nurse researchers to provide nurses and other health care professionals with a simple tool for assessing a client's spiritual well-being (Hungelmann and others, 1996). The tool was developed for clients from Christian, non-Christian, and atheist belief systems. Items on the tool comprise three key dimensions: the faith/belief

DIRECTIONS: PLEASE CIRCLE THE CHOICE THAT **BEST** DESCRIBES HOW MUCH YOU AGREE WITH EACH STATEMENT. CIRCLE
ONLY **ONE** ANSWER FOR EACH STATEMENT. THERE IS NO RIGHT OR WRONG ANSWER.

		Strongly Agree	Moderately Agree	Agree	Disagree	Moderately Disagree	Strongly Disagree
1.	Prayer is an important part of my life.	SA	MA	A	D	MD	SD
2.	I believe I have spiritual well-being.	SA	MA	A	D	MD	SD
3.	As I grow older, I find myself more tolerant of others' beliefs.	SA	MA	A	D	MD	SD
4.	I find meaning and purpose in my life.	SA	MA	A	D	MD	SD
5.	I feel there is a close relationship between my spiritual beliefs and what I do.	SA	MA	A	D	MD	SD
6.	I believe in an afterlife.	SA	MA	A	D	MD	SD
7.	When I am sick I have less spiritual well-being.	SA	MA	A	D	MD	SD
8.	I believe in a supreme power.	SA	MA	A	D	MD	SD
9.	I am able to receive and give love to others.	SA	MA	A	D	MD	SD
10.	I am satisfied with my life.	SA	MA	A	D	MD	SD
11.	I set goals for myself.	SA	MA	A	D	MD	SD
12.	God has little meaning in my life.	SA	MA	A	D	MD	SD
13.	I am satisfied with the way I am using my abilities.	SA	MA	A	D	MD	SD
14.	Prayer does not help me in making decisions.	SA	MA	A	D	MD	SD
15.	I am able to appreciate differences in others.	SA	MA	A	D	MD	SD
16.	I am pretty well put together.	SA	MA	A	D	MD	SD
17.	I prefer that others make decisions for me.	SA	MA	A	D	MD	SD
18.	I find it hard to forgive others.	SA	MA	A	D	MD	SD
19.	I accept my life situations.	SA	MA	A	D	MD	SD
20.	Belief in a supreme being has no part in my life.	SA	MA	A	D	MD	SD
21.	I cannot accept change in my life.	SA	MA	A	D	MD	SD

Figure 17-4.   JAREL spiritual well-being scale. (Copyright 1987 by Hungelmann J, Kenkel-Rossi E, Klassen L, Stollenwerk R, Marquette University College of Nursing, Milwaukee, Wis. 53201.)

dimension, life/self-responsibility, and life-satisfaction/self-actualization. The tool is simple to use, requiring clients to rate their level of agreement with each item along a five-point scale (strongly agree to strongly disagree). For clients with visual or literacy problems, the nurse can read the items and record the client's response. If the client's score on any item, group of items, or a particular dimension is low, it may indicate an area to explore further (Hungelmann and others, 1996).

The tool helps the nurse explore with a client any perceptions or concerns he or she might have. For example, if a client disagrees about accepting life situations, the nurse needs to spend time understanding how illness is being accepted and managed by the client. Whether a nurse uses a tool like the JAREL scale or directs an assessment with questions that are based on principles of spirituality, it is important to not impose personal value systems on the client. This is particularly true when the client's values and beliefs are similar to those of the nurse, as it can then become very easy to make false assumptions.

Faith/belief.   Each individual has some source of authority and guidance in his or her life. The authority can be a Supreme Being, a code of conduct, a specific religious leader, family or friends, oneself, or a combination of sources. Faith in an authority provides a sense of confidence that guides a person in exercising beliefs and experiencing growth. Knowing a client's source of faith and guidance can direct interaction with him or her. The nurse can assess a person's faith in an authority by asking, "To what or whom do you look for guidance in life?"

The nurse must determine if the client has a religious source of guidance that conflicts with medical treatment plans. This can seriously affect the options nurses and other health care providers can offer clients. For example, if a client looks to the Jehovah's Witnesses as a source of authority, blood products cannot be accepted as a form of treatment. Members of the Christian Science faith often refuse any medical intervention, believing that their faith will heal them.

It is also important to understand a client's philosophy of life. Asking the client, "Describe for me what is most important in your life," or "Tell me what gives your life meaning or purpose" may help to assess what is the basis of the client's belief system regarding meaning and purpose in life. This information reveals the client's spiritual focus and may help to reflect the impact illness, loss, or disability has on the person's life. Depending on a client's religious practices, views about health and the response to illness may influence how nurses provide support (Table 17-1).

Life satisfaction. Spiritual well-being seems to be tied to a person's satisfaction with life and what he or she has accomplished (Hungelmann and others, 1996). When an individual is satisfied with life and the manner in which he or she is using his or her abilities, there is more energy available to deal with new difficulties and to resolve problems. A sense of satisfaction with life and self gives an individual resources to live for the moment, face difficulties directly, and remain motivated to deal with adversity. Satisfaction with someone or something has been found by Haase and others (1992) to be associated with acceptance. Acceptance is the process of resolving issues within oneself or dealing with life experiences and is closely tied to hope and spirituality. A nurse can assess a client's satisfaction with life by asking, "How happy or satisfied are you with your life" or "Tell me to what extent you feel satisfied with what you have accomplished in life."

Fellowship and community. Fellowship is one kind of relationship an individual can have with other persons (Farran and others, 1989), including immediate family, close friends, associates at work or school, fellow members of a church, and neighbors. More specifically, this includes the extent of the community of shared faith between clients and their support networks. The nurse can ask, "With whom do you have a bond or find the greatest source of support in times of difficulty?" When a client knows that others of similar faith care, they can become a source for hope.

The nurse's holistic assessment explores the extent and nature or quality of a person's support networks and their relationship with the client. It is unwise to assume that a given network offers the kind of support a client desires. For example, calling the client's clergy to request a visit might be inappropriate if the client finds little support or fellowship from the individual. Does the client have one significant fellowship or several? What is the level of support received from the community? How does the community express feelings of concern? Do they visit, say prayers, or support the client's immediate family? The nurse needs to learn whether openness exists between the client and those persons with whom a fellowship has formed.

TABLE 17-1

Religious Beliefs About Health

Religion	Health Care Beliefs	Response to Illness
Hinduism	Accepts modern medical science	Illness is caused by past sins Prolonging life is discouraged
Sikhism	Accepts modern medical science	Females to be examined by females Removing the undergarment will cause great distress
Buddhism	Accepts modern medical science	May refuse treatment on Holy Days Nonhuman spirits invading the body cause illness May want a Buddhist priest May permit withdrawal of life support Does not practice euthanasia
Shinto	Accepts modern medical treatments along with ancient traditions	Will not allow treatments that "appear" to injure the body
Islam	Must be able to practice the Five Pillars of Islam (see p. 300) May have a fatalistic view of health	Uses faith healing Family members are a comfort Group prayer is strengthening May permit withdrawal of life support Does not practice euthanasia
Judaism	Believes in the sanctity of life God and medicine must have a balance Observance of the Sabbath is important May refuse treatments on the Sabbath	Visiting the sick is an obligation Is obligated to seek care Euthanasia is forbidden Life supports are discouraged
Christianity	Accepts modern medical science	Uses prayer, faith healing Appreciates visits from clergy Some will use laying on of hands Holy Communion is commonly used

Ritual and practice. One of the easiest areas to assess about a client's spirituality is the use of rituals and practice. Rituals include participation in a religious group or private worship, prayer, sacraments such as baptism or communion, fasting, singing, icons, meditating, scripture reading, and making offerings or sacrifices. Different religions have established various rituals for certain life events (Table 17-2). The nurse examines whether a client's usual rituals or practices have been interrupted as a result of illness or hospitalization. A ritual can provide a client with structure and support during difficult times. Often clients may request the ability to practice rituals during hospitalization. For example, Muslims practice the "Five Pillars of Islam," with the second pillar requiring a person to pray 5 times a day while facing east (toward Mecca, the holy city of Islam).

Vocation. Individuals express their spirituality daily in life routines, work, play, and relationships (Farran and others, 1989). Spirituality can be used in their vocation in life and be part of their identity. The nurse determines if illness or hospitalization has altered the person's ability to express his or her spirituality. Expression of spirituality may include showing an appreciation for life in the variety of things people do, living in the mo-

ment and not worrying about tomorrow, appreciating nature, expressing love toward others, and being productive. The nurse assesses whether the client loses the ability to express a sense of relatedness to something greater than the self (Fryback, 1992). Questions might include, "Has your illness affected the way you live your life spiritually" or "Has your illness affected your ability to express what's important in life for you?" If illness or loss prevents an individual from exercising his or her spirituality, the nurse must understand the implications psychologically, socially, and spiritually and find ways to offer guidance and support.

Client expectations. Before completing an assessment of a client's spiritual well-being, it is important to understand what, if anything, the client expects from care givers. If the client senses the nurse's compassion, an expectation might involve maintaining a trusting and open relationship. In addition, it might be important that the client perceives care givers to be accepting of his or her religious practices or rituals. Asking the client what expectations are held of care givers can be very beneficial in establishing a strong nurse-client partnership.

TABLE 17-2
Religious Rituals Related to Birth and Death

Religion	Birth Rituals	Death Rituals
Hinduism	No special rituals	The dying may want to lie on the floor A priest will tie a thread around the neck or wrist (*do not remove*) A priest will pour water in the client's mouth Family will wash the body before cremation
Sikhism	Allow mother and child to remain together	The deceased will need the five Ks: *Kesh,* uncut hair; *Kangra,* wooden comb; *Kara,* wrist band; *Kirpan,* sword; *Kach,* shorts
Buddhism	No special rituals Baptism later in childhood	A priest should be called Last rites and chanting at bedside Burial or cremation is acceptable
Shinto	No special rituals	All jewelry should be removed, and the body washed and dressed in a white kimono and straw shoes
Islam	A prayer is said into the infant's ear	The dying must confess their sins The body is washed and wrapped in white cloth The head is turned toward right shoulder The body faces east, toward Mecca A prayer called *Kalima* is said
Judaism	Circumcision on day 8 for Orthodox and Conservative Jews	Body is washed by burial society and someone needs to remain with the body for Orthodox and Conservative Jews
Christianity	Rituals vary Many baptize	Rituals vary greatly among groups Many give last rites or Communion Prefers burial to cremation
Church of Jesus Christ of Latter-Day Saints (Mormon)	Baptism by immersion	Many give last rites or Communion Prefers burial to cremation

Successful critical thinking requires a synthesis of knowledge, experience, information gathered from clients, and critical thinking attitudes and standards. Clinical judgments require the nurse to anticipate what information is needed, analyze the data, and then make decisions regarding client care. The client expects competent and informed care. Jeff incorporates previous knowledge and experience in providing care for Sarah Stein.

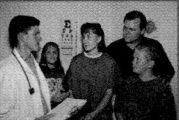

Case Study

Synthesis in Practice

Jeff has anticipated the next visit by Sarah and Joe Stein to the clinic. He has spent time learning more about Sarah's disease and treatment plan so that he can better explain what to expect as chemotherapy progresses. Jeff recognizes that Joe usually comes to the clinic with Sarah and has been described by her as a strong source of support. However, Jeff does not know enough about the couple's relationship and wants to explore this further. The role of family members in providing support, particularly with regard to decision making, is important for Jeff to understand before a plan of care can be developed. In reviewing information about loss and grieving, Jeff recognizes that Sarah shows acceptance of her disease since she is able to discuss cancer and the plan for treatment. Jeff knows that as clients begin to accept the fact of being diagnosed with a life-threatening disease, it is important to offer opportunities to share feelings and begin to provide time to discuss future plans.

Jeff's previous experience with clients with cancer has taught him that when clients express hope, they seem to be able to move forward and cope with the challenges of their disease. During the last clinic visit, Sarah expressed an intermediate hope, in being able to attend her son's Bar Mitzvah. Jeff reflected on that experience and thinks that Sarah and Joe may have a strong sense of spiritual well-being that will help them cope with cancer. Further assessment will be necessary.

Jeff wants to be complete in assessing Sarah and Joe's level of spiritual health. Jeff is Lutheran and is not well informed about the couple's religion, Judaism. However, he knows that the Jewish sense of community is very strong and that it is important to learn more about how members of the Stein's temple or synagogue play a role in offering support to the family. Jeff recognizes that spiritual well-being is more complex than simply religion. He spends time reflecting on his own value and belief systems so that he can remain open and receptive to understanding the spiritual belief systems that Sarah and Joe possess.

Nursing Diagnosis

When reviewing a spiritual assessment, the nurse considers the client's current health status from a holistic perspective. Nurses care for clients in a variety of settings and during times of health and illness. During events such as birth, illness, pain, daily life activities, and death, individuals have experiences that create options. These options are linked to a person's spirituality (Farran and others, 1989). Some options, such as the acceptance of a disability, help clients learn to better understand life. Other options, such as choosing a form of treatment, result in a person merely maintaining his or her spiritual focus. Finally, there are options such as recognizing a spouse's illness to be terminal, that alter a person's functioning, resulting in an inability to find meaning in life events, with loss of hope. To support clients, the nurse focuses not only on the alterations in functioning, but also on the options that provide hope and encouragement during times of illness.

As a nurse identifies the diagnoses for a client, it is important to recognize the significance that spirituality has for all types of health problems. Almost any nursing diagnosis has implications for a client's spirituality. *Pain, anxiety,* and *self-care deficit* are examples of common nursing diagnoses that require the nurse to incorporate spiritual care principles (see nursing diagnosis box).

There are two nursing diagnoses accepted by the North American Nursing Diagnosis Association (NANDA) that pertain to spirituality. *Potential for enhanced spiritual well-being* is based on defining characteristics that show a pattern of well-being and the interconnectedness that comes from inner faith and hope (Kim and others, 1997). When the nurse's assessment reveals that the client has inner strength through hope and faith, believes in a higher power or unifying force, and has a defined purpose and meaning in life, *spiritual well-being* is a likely diagnosis. The presence of this state shows the client has potential resources to draw on when faced with other nursing diagnoses such as *chronic pain, fatigue, sensory/perceptual alterations,* or *body image disturbance.* Since the client may not know how to engage the resources to cope with health problems, the nurse offers support in exploring options.

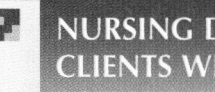

NURSING DIAGNOSES FOR CLIENTS WITH NEED FOR SPIRITUAL SUPPORT

Anxiety
Coping, family: potential for growth
Coping, ineffective individual
Family processes, altered
Grieving, dysfunctional
Hopelessness
Self-esteem disturbance
Spiritual distress
Spiritual well-being, potential for enhanced

The nursing diagnosis of *spiritual distress* creates a different clinical picture. Defining characteristics may reveal patterns that reflect a person's dispiritedness, for example, expressing concern with the meaning of life and belief systems, anger toward God, verbalizing conflicts about personal beliefs, or asking for spiritual assistance. Defining characteristics must be validated and clarified with the client before a diagnosis and plan of care are made. Each diagnosis must have an accurate related factor so that resulting interventions can be purposeful and goal directed.

▪ Planning

When the nurse and client identify that a client has spiritual needs, it is important for both to collaborate closely on a plan of care. Compassion and caring must clearly be communicated between the nurse and client. This begins with a well-designed assessment, but the nurse-client relationship must continue to be based on caring and trust for interventions to be effective. Communication will be an integrated theme for whatever nursing interventions are chosen. The personal nature of spirituality requires the client to be able to speak openly with the nurse and recognize the nurse's interest in his or her needs.

Significant others, such as spouses, siblings, parents, and friends, need to be involved, as appropriate, to lend support. This means that the nurse learns from the assessment which individuals or groups have formed a relationship with the client. These individuals may become involved in all levels of the nurse's plan. The client's support network may assist in giving physical care, providing emotional comfort, and sharing spiritual support.

In a hospital setting, one of the best resources to use in planning a client's spiritual care is the hospital's pastoral care department. A health care chaplain has special expertise in dealing with the spiritual problems confronted by clients. These professionals should be part of the health care team, lending insight as to how and when to best support clients and families.

If the client participates in a formal religion, members of the clergy or members of the church, temple, mosque, or synagogue may need to be involved in the plan of care. Depending on the client's health status and needs, part of the plan will involve a continuation of appropriate religious rituals. The nurse must make sure that any icons or religious materials such as scriptures or a prayer book are available (see care plan).

In establishing a plan of care, there are several goals for spiritual caregiving:

1. The client will sense a feeling of trust in care givers.
2. The client will improve personal harmony and connections with members of his or her support system.
3. The client's personal quest for meaning and self-awareness will be enhanced.

In the case of terminal illness or serious loss, spiritual care can be a priority, supporting those resources clients require to deal with physical and psychological problems. The nurse collaborates with the client in setting realistic outcomes for supporting or restoring spiritual well-being. Examples of outcomes for the goal of achieving a personal quest for meaning and self-awareness might include the following:

1. Client will express feelings regarding illness and its implications for life goals.
2. Client will discuss meaning of health in his or her life.

▪ Implementation

If a client experiences spiritual distress or has a health problem that requires the client to use spiritual resources, a compassionate and understanding relationship between the nurse and client is necessary. Both the client and nurse must feel free to let go and discover together the meaning illness or loss poses for the client and the impact it has on the meaning and purpose of life. Achieving this level of understanding with a client enables the nurse to deliver care in a sensitive, creative, and appropriate manner.

Health promotion. Spiritual care should be a central theme in promoting an individual's overall well-being. Spirituality is one personal resource that affects the balance between health and illness. The nurse who applies spiritual care practices in all aspects of nursing care shows a respect for the person's entire being.

Establishing presence. Clients have reported that the presence of nurses and their care-giving activities contributes to a sense of well-being and provides hope for recovery (Clark and others, 1991). Behaviors that establish the nurse's presence include giving attention, answering questions, listening, and having a positive and encouraging (but realistic) attitude. The ability to establish presence is part of the art of nursing. It is not simply being in the same room with a client performing procedures or sharing technical information with a client. Benner (1984) clarifies that presence involves "being with" a client versus "doing for" a client. Presence is being able to offer a closeness with the client: physically, psychologically, and spiritually.

A nurse can convey a caring presence in a variety of subtle ways: working with a client to slowly and cautiously move from the bedside to a chair, carefully repositioning a client without causing pain, and willingly involving family in discussions about the client's health. Providing a soothing and supportive touch, displaying self-confidence, and taking time with a client as therapies are administered also help to establish presence. The client who seeks health care may be experiencing an illness that threatens loss of control and looks for someone to offer direction and competent care. The nurse's artful use of hands, encouraging words of sup-

CASE STUDY NURSING CARE PLAN

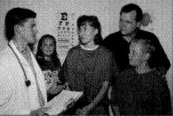

Spirituality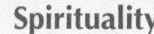

Assessment

Sarah has been told her prognosis is promising, although treatment will be needed to prevent spread of her disease. Sarah expresses a **connectedness with her God,** "I do not feel alone, God is with me. I have a better appreciation of each day God gives me and I believe God will help me see my son's Bar Mitzvah." Sarah and Joe **attend synagogue regularly and hope** to continue doing so even during the chemotherapy. Jeff learns that Joe encourages Sarah and has been trying to arrange work so that he can take her to the clinic. This means that since their mother's illness, he has less time in the evening to spend with the children. In the past, Joe and Sarah have always had discussions with the children during mealtime, but this has been difficult. **Members of their synagogue have offered support** by taking Sarah to the clinic if Joe is unable.

Sarah worries about her children. During the last month she has spent less time with Valerie and Peter because of her cancer treatments and resultant fatigue. Peter is having some difficulty with studying for the Bar Mitzvah. He is also doing poorly in school. Valerie has recently expressed concern that her mother might die. Both children reportedly have been acting angrily toward their parents. Before Sarah's illness the children were very **close to their parents and shared their faith in God.**

Nursing Diagnosis

Potential for enhanced spiritual well-being, related to renewed appreciation of life after cancer diagnosis.

Planning

Goal

Client will restore connectedness with children (within 2 months).

Expected Outcomes

Client, husband, and children will discuss client's beliefs about the future and her hope of having the cancer cured (to be met in 2 weeks).

Client will report son and daughter's ability to discuss fears with mother (to be met in 4 weeks).

Implementation

Steps

1. Plan a conference late in afternoon at cancer clinic where children can attend to hear discussion of mother's progress.

2. Encourage client to discuss with family the meaning life now has for her after being diagnosed with breast cancer.

3. Recommend use of story telling to reminisce with family about experiences that were positive and representative of mutual support.

4. Encourage client and husband to focus a discussion with children on their fears about mother's well-being.

Rationale

Ensures children will have accurate perception of mother's clinical condition and course.

Situations seen from the individual's point of view will enhance understanding and sensitivity on the part of the family.

Story telling allows a pattern to emerge that describes client's way of life filled with meaning. Helps family understand need for mutual love and support (Heliker, 1992).

Gives children opportunity to discuss their primary concerns and to clarify their roles as part of the family.

Evaluation

Have client and husband report on outcomes of discussions with children.

Observe interactions between parents and children.

Ask client to describe feelings she has when communicating with children about cancer.

Defining characteristics are shown in bold type.

port, and calm and decisive approach establish a presence that builds trust and well-being.

Trust is fundamental to any relationship. The attitude a nurse conveys when first interacting with a client sets the tone for all conversations (see Chapter 13). Listening to the meaning of what a client says is most important. It involves paying attention to the person's words, tone of voice, and entering his or her frame of reference. By observing expressions and body language of the client, the nurse can find cues to help assist the client in exploring ways to achieve inner peace, take action, or do whatever a situation demands (Hungelmann and others, 1996). Emblen and Halstead (1993) found in their research that nurses listening to clients was the option clients preferred when spiritual care was provided.

Supporting a healing relationship. An expert nurse looks beyond isolated client problems and recognizes the broader picture of a client's needs. This involves having a holistic view of client care. For example, the nurse does not just look at a client's back pain as a problem to solve with quick remedies but rather how the pain influences the client's ability to function and achieve goals established in life. A holistic view enables the nurse to establish a helping role. Within a helping role, nurses learn to establish healing relationships (Benner, 1984). There are three steps evident when a healing relationship develops between the nurse and client:

1. Mobilizing hope for the nurse and for the client
2. Finding an interpretation or understanding of the illness, pain, anxiety, or other stressful emotion that is acceptable to the client
3. Assisting the client to use social, emotional, or spiritual resources (Benner, 1985)

Central to a healing relationship is mobilizing the client's hope. Hope motivates people with strategies to face challenges in life. The nurse can help a client find things to hope for. A client newly diagnosed with diabetes might hope to learn how to manage the disease so as to continue a productive and satisfying way of life. A terminally ill client may hope to attend a daughter's graduation and live each day to the fullest.

Hope has both short- and long-term implications in a client's care. From a long-term perspective, hope gives individuals motivation to carry on with life's responsibilities. In the short-term view, hope provides an incentive for constructive coping with obstacles and for finding ways to realize the object of hope (Dufault and Martocchio, 1985). Hope is future oriented and helps a client work toward recovery. To help clients achieve hope, the nurse and client work together to find an explanation of the situation that is acceptable to both. Then the nurse helps the client realistically exercise hope. This might include supporting a client's positive attitude toward life or a desire to be informed and to make decisions.

To further support a healing relationship the nurse must remain aware of the client's spiritual resources and needs. It is always important for a client to be able to express and exercise his or her beliefs and to find spiritual comfort. When illness or treatment create confusion or uncertainty for the client, the nurse must recognize the possible effect this can have on a client's well-being. How can spiritual resources be used and strengthened? Having a clear sense of what illness may hold for an individual helps the person to apply all resources toward recovery.

Prayer. The act of prayer gives an individual the opportunity to renew personal faith and belief in a higher being in a specific, focused way that may be highly ritualized and formal or quite spontaneous and informal. Prayer has been shown to be an effective coping resource for physical and psychological symptoms. Clients may pray in private or pursue opportunities for group prayer with family, friends, or clergy. The nurse can be supportive of prayer by giving the client privacy if desired, learning if the client wishes to have the nurse participate, and by suggesting prayer when it is known to be a coping resource for the client. If prayer is not suitable for a client, an alternative may be to read from a book selected by the client or from poetry or inspirational texts.

Acute care. Within an acute care setting, clients experience multiple stressors that threaten to overwhelm their coping resources. Support and enhancement of a client's spiritual well-being can be a challenge when the focus of health care seems to be one of treatment and cure rather than care. The nurse works closely with the client to maximize resources known to support his or her spirituality.

Support systems. Use of support systems is, of course, important in any health care setting. Clark and others (1991) found that support systems provided clients with the greatest sense of well-being during hospitalization. Support systems serve as a human link connecting the client, the nurse, and the client's lifestyle before an illness. Part of the client's care-giving environment is the regular presence of family and friends viewed by the client as supportive. The nurse plans care with the client and the client's support network to promote the interpersonal bonding that is needed for recovery. The support system is a source of faith and hope, and it becomes an important resource in conducting the religious rituals on which a client relies.

When it is known that clients depend on family and friends for support, the nurse encourages them to visit the client regularly. The nurse's encouragement to family to be themselves during visits can facilitate the family's ability to provide the spiritual comfort that they are capable of sharing. Often illness and the treatment environment produce unknowns that intimidate family members and friends. The nurse helps the family feel welcome and uses their support and presence to promote the client's healing. Including family members in prayer, for example, is a thoughtful gesture if it is appropriate to the client's religion, and if family members are comfortable participating. Encouraging the family to bring meaningful religious symbols to the client's bedside can offer significant spiritual support.

Other important resources to clients are spiritual advisors and members of the clergy. Many hospitals have pastoral care departments that assist in notifying community clergy of their congregant's admission. If not, the nurse should ask if clients desire to have their clergy notified of their hospitalization. All clergy should be made welcome on nursing units. When requested by clients or families, the nurse should keep clergy informed of any physical, psychosocial, or spiritual concerns affecting the client. The nurse shows respect for clients' spiritual values and needs by willingly cooperating with others giving spiritual care and by facilitating the administration of sacraments, rites, and rituals.

Providing privacy for the client and clergy is a thoughtful and sensitive gesture. The nurse determines the proper routine in a client's religion by asking the clergy, family, or client. Often a client within the hospital may want to discuss spiritual concerns in the evening or late at night, when support services such as clergy and social services are unavailable. The nurse can help to meet the client's needs by careful, skilled, and active listening.

Diet therapies. Food and nutrition are important aspects of nursing care. Food is also an important component of some religious observances (Table 17-3). As with many aspects of a particular culture or religion, food and the rituals surrounding the preparation and serving of food can be important to a person's spirituality. The nurse can integrate the client's dietary preferences into daily care. This requires consultation with the health care institution's dietitian. In the event that a hospital or other health care agency cannot prepare food in the preferred way, the family may be asked to bring meals fitting into any dietary restrictions posed by the client's condition.

Supporting rituals. Nurses can become especially active in their clients' spiritual care by supporting clients' participation in church services, visitations by members of a worship group, and use of rituals. Arrangements may need to be made with pastoral care staff for the client and family to receive the sacraments. Personal care of the client should be planned to allow time for religious readings, spiritual visitations, or attendance at religious services. Some churches and synagogues offer audiotapes of their services for those members who cannot attend in person. Family members can plan a prayer session or an organized reading of scriptures on a regular basis. Clergy will routinely offer to make home visits for persons unable to attend religious services. Taped meditations, religious music, and televised religious services provide another effective option. The nurse should be respectful of icons, medals, prayer rugs, or crosses that clients bring to a health setting to be sure they are not accidentally lost or misplaced.

TABLE 17-3
Religious Dietary Regulations Affecting Health Care

Religion	Dietary Practices
Hinduism	Some sects are vegetarians. The belief is not to kill *any* living creature.
Buddhism	Some are vegetarians, and many will not use alcohol or tobacco and may hesitate to use drugs. Many will fast on Holy Days.
Islam	Eating pork and consuming alcohol are prohibited. Fasting is done during the month of Ramadan.
Judaism	Some observe the kosher dietary restrictions of avoiding pork and shellfish and not preparing and eating milk and meat at the same time.
Christianity	Some Baptists, Evangelicals, and Pentecostals discourage the use of alcohol, caffeine, and tobacco. Some Roman Catholics may fast during Lent, Ash Wednesday, Good Friday, and 1 hour before receiving communion.
Jehovah's Witnesses	Members may avoid food prepared with or containing blood.
Mormonism	Members abstain from alcohol, caffeine, and tobacco.
Baha'i	Members abstain from alcohol, caffeine, and tobacco.

▪ Evaluation

Client care. Attainment of spiritual health is a lifelong goal. Clients will experience the need to clarify values (see Chapter 11), reshape philosophies, and live those experiences that help to shape purpose in life. The nurse conducts a plan of therapy for the client's spiritual health while always evaluating whether planned outcomes and goals were achieved. The nurse compares the client's level of spiritual health with the behaviors and perceptions noted in the nursing assessment (see case study). For example, if the nurse's assessment finds the client losing hope, the follow-up evaluation involves a discussion with the client to determine if the client has regained an attitude of something to live for. Family and friends with whom the client seeks to have fellowship can be a useful source of evaluative information. Successful outcomes should reveal the client developing an increased or restored sense of connectedness with family, maintaining, reviewing, or reforming a sense of purpose in life and, for some, a confidence and trust in a Supreme Being or higher power.

For clients with a serious or terminal illness, evaluation focuses on the goal of helping the client retain faith and hope or express openly the uncertainties life poses. The nurse evaluates how the client is accepting the illness and whether hope has enabled the client to recognize individual mortality and focus on living for each day. Fryback (1993) found that the terminally ill, regardless of whether they followed a formal religion, held a belief in a higher power, which gave them a sense that God was with them and they were not alone. The nurse must not assume all clients have such faith. However, the nurse's support aims to help clients accept their destiny and to be at peace.

Client expectations. The nurse evaluates whether client expectations of the nurse and health care team were met. Evaluating spiritual care requires determining if the client's spiritual practices were respected and if the quality of the nurse-client relationship was supportive. Both the client and family should be able to relate if opportunities were offered for religious rituals. With respect to the nurse-client relationship, does the client express trust and confidence in the nurse? Is the client able to discuss those things important to him or her? Taking time to ask the client to reflect on the quality of the nurse-client relationship is time well spent. Asking the client, "Have I helped you to become comfortable in saying what you feel is important to you spiritually," will determine whether an effective healing relationship was developed.

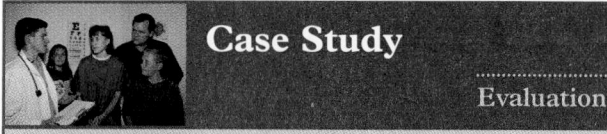

Case Study
Evaluation

Sarah returns to the clinic the week after establishing the plan with Jeff. A member of the synagogue accompanies Sarah because Joe is out of town on a business trip. Jeff wants to evaluate whether Sarah has begun to spend time with the children to discuss the effect her experience has had on them. Jeff asks, "Tell me, Mrs. Stein, have you had a chance yet to try any of the approaches we talked about last week to give the kids a chance to talk about their feelings? If so, what were the results?" Sarah reports, "Yes, Joe and I spent a couple of hours Saturday evening talking about what all of this means. It was during a time when we have always tried to be together as a family, and the kids seemed to appreciate it. They asked many questions. They are looking forward to coming to the clinic Thursday. I hope this will help them settle down a bit and feel less frightened." Jeff also determines that Sarah has spoken with close friends from her church and they plan to visit her this week. The client also is going to see the physical therapist today.

In an effort to evaluate if Sarah's expectations were met, Jeff asks, "Do you believe we have helped you so far with your concerns about your children? Your faith is strong, and it is my hope you have felt comfortable in talking about your worries." Sarah replies, "The best thing you have done is listen and recognize how important my family is to me. Your suggestions have helped so far; I am encouraged by them."

Documentation Note
The client visited the clinic for her third week of chemotherapy. She denies nausea but is complaining of some soreness in the mouth and a loss of hair. She asks questions readily and has made an appointment with the physical therapist as recommended. She has expressed hope that her children will feel less frightened over the diagnosis. The children will be attending the next clinic visit.

Key Terms

faith	**spiritual distress**
holistic	**spirituality**
hope	**spiritual well-being**

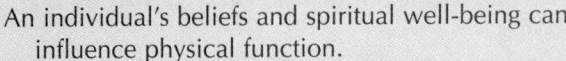

Key Concepts

An individual's beliefs and spiritual well-being can influence physical function.

Spiritual well-being is an integrating aspect of human wholeness.

Faith and hope are closely linked to a person's spiritual well-being, providing an inner strength for dealing with illness and disability.

Religion is a system of organized beliefs that a person practices to outwardly express his or her spirituality.

Acute and chronic illness, terminal illness, and near-death experiences pose spiritual problems for individuals.

The provision of appropriate spiritual care requires the nurse to critically apply knowledge from principles related to cultural care, loss and grief, and therapeutic communication.

Learning to practice compassion helps a nurse to discover a client's life values and meaning.

Fellowship with other persons can be a source of hope for a client.

Clients often have spiritual strengths that the nurse can use as resources to help them assume healthier lives.

Interruptions or changes to customary religious practices may affect the support that religion contributes to a person's well-being.

Common religious rituals include private worship, prayer, singing, use of a rosary, and scripture reading.

The personal nature of spirituality requires open communication and the establishment of trust between nurse and client.

Establishing presence involves giving attention, answering questions, having an encouraging attitude, and conveying a sense of trust.

Part of a client's care-giving environment can be the regular presence of family, friends, and spiritual advisors.

Critical Thinking Activities

1. Mr. Bruns is a terminally ill client suffering from AIDS. He has sensed abandonment by friends and even family as his disease has progressed. The nurse finds him crying, "Oh, I feel that God has left my life." How might the nurse offer him spiritual support?

2. Norma Lee is a 72-year-old woman with advanced glaucoma. Recently her close friend and neighbor, who assisted in administering her eyedrops, died. The friend also regularly attended church with Ms. Lee. The registered nurse (RN) from the home health agency is visiting to evaluate Ms. Lee for home health aid services. How might the nurse help Ms. Lee continue exercising her religious rituals?

3. Jim Tenant is a 30-year-old construction worker who is visiting the community health clinic for a routine physical examination that is part of his health insurance screening. The physician explains that he wants Jim to receive a tetanus injection to guard against infection that could be acquired during an industrial accident. Jim is a member of the Christian Science faith and refuses the immunization. What would be your course of action?

References

Aldridge D: Is there evidence for spiritual healing? *Adv J Mind-Body Health* 9(4):4, 1993.

Basford TK: *Near death experience: an annotated bibliography,* New York, 1990, Garland.

Benner DG: *Baker encyclopedia of psychology,* Grand Rapids, Mich, 1985, Baker Book House.

Benner P: From novice to expert, Menlo Park, Calif, 1984, Addison-Wesley.

Carson V: *Spiritual dimensions of nursing practice,* Philadelphia, 1989, WB Saunders.

Clark CC and others: Spirituality: integral to quality care, *Holistic Nurs Pract* 5(3):67, 1991.

Coe RM: The magic of science and the science of magic: an essay on the process of healing, *J Health Soc Behav* 38(3):1, 1997.

Culligan K: Spirituality and healing in medicine, *America,* p 17, August 31, 1996.

Dufault K, Martocchio BC: Hope: its spheres and dimensions, *Nurs Clin North Am* 20(2):379, 1985.

Emblen JD: Religion and spirituality defined according to current use in nursing literature, *J Prof Nurs* 8(1):41, 1992.

Emblen JD, Halstead L: Spiritual needs and interventions: comparing the views of patients, nurses, and chaplains, *Clin Nurs Specialist* 7(4):175, 1993.

Farran CJ and others: Development of a model for spiritual assessment and intervention, *J Religion Health* 28(3):185, 1989.

Fryback PB: Health for people with a terminal diagnosis, *Nurs Sci Q* 6(3):147, 1993.

Giger JN, Davidhizar RE: *Transcultural nursing: assessment and intervention,* ed 2, St. Louis, 1995, Mosby.

Haase JE and others: Simultaneous concept analysis of spiritual perspective, hope, acceptance, and self-transcendence, *Image J Nurs Sch* 24(2):141, 1992.

Heliker D: Reevaluation of a nursing diagnosis: spiritual distress, *Nurs Forum* 27(4):15, 1992.

Hungelmann J and others: Focus on spiritual well-being: harmonious interconnectedness of mind-body-spirit—use of the JAREL spiritual well-being scale, *Geriatric Nurs* 17(6):262, 1996.

Kiecolt-Glaser JK and others: Psychosocial enhancement of immunocompetence in a geriatric population, *Health Psychol* 4:25, 1985.

Kim MJ and others: *Pocket guide to nursing diagnoses,* ed 7, St. Louis, 1997, Mosby.

Miller JF, Powers MJ: Development of an instrument to measure hope, *Nurs Res* 37(1):6, 1988.

Nowotny ML: Assessment of hope in patients with cancer: development of an instrument, *Oncol Nurs Forum* 16(1):57, 1989.

O'Connor AP and others: Understanding the cancer patient's search for meaning, *Cancer Nurs* 13:167, 1990.

Post-White J and others: Hope, spirituality, sense of coherence, and quality of life in patients with cancer, *Oncol Nurs Forum* 23(10):1571, 1996.

Reed PG: Spirituality and well-being in terminally ill hospitalized adults, *Res Nurs Health* 10:335, 1987.

Remen RN: Spirit: resource for healing, *Noetic Sci Rev,* p 61, Autumn 1988.

Turner JA, Clancy S: Strategies for coping with chronic low back pain: relationship to pain and disability, *Pain* 24:355, 1986.

Turner RP and others: Religious or spiritual problem: a culturally sensitive diagnostic category in the DSM-IV, *J Nerv Ment Dis* 183(7):435, 1995.

Yim RJR, VandeCreek L: Unbinding grief and life's losses for thriving recovery after open heart surgery, *Caregiver J* 12(2):8, 1996.

18

Cultural Care in Nursing

OBJECTIVES

Mastery of content in this chapter will enable the student to:

- Define the key terms listed.
- Describe ways in which demographic factors and culture influence an individual and family.
- Describe the interrelated components of cultural care.
- Describe the relationship of sociocultural background to health and illness beliefs and practices.
- Describe the Health Traditions model.
- Describe the cultural phenomena that affect health.
- Compare concepts of traditional and modern health and illness beliefs and practices.
- List examples of traditional health and illness beliefs and practices from selected ethnic groups.
- Describe communication and economic sociocultural barriers to health care.
- Perform a cultural assessment using heritage consistency, cultural phenomena, and the Health Traditions model.
- List potential nursing diagnoses related to a client's ethnocultural background.
- Design nursing interventions appropriate to a client's ethnocultural background.

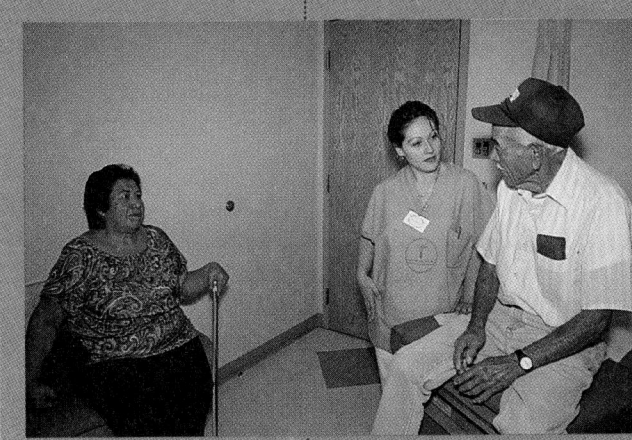

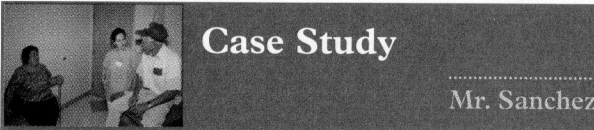

Case Study

Mr. Sanchez

Mr. Sanchez is a 60-year-old man who is coming to the community health center for the first time and is complaining of a deep cough, fatigue, and weight loss. He is diagnosed with bronchitis and possible adult onset diabetes mellitus. Mr. Sanchez has lived in the United States 5 years, but this is the first time he has sought medical assistance. He is a Spanish-speaking field laborer who is a legal immigrant but not an American citizen. He has no health insurance and does not receive any welfare assistance. He lives with his wife and two grandchildren. Their food is mainly a Spanish-Mexican type of diet, with very few fruits or vegetables and a lot of rice and starches. Initially he is given a bottle of antibiotics and is instructed in English to take one pill 4 times a day.

Alice Walters is a sophomore nursing student assigned to the community health center. She is 31 years of age, Anglo-American, single, and neither speaks nor understands Spanish. The interpreter is unavailable and there is no one to assist her. She warmly greets Mr. Sanchez and mimes the English instructions, but she does not think that Mr. Sanchez truly understands the instructions regarding the medications or when he should return to the clinic. At this point Alice is worried and fears that unless she is able to intervene in a manner that Mr. Sanchez will understand, he will not take his medications correctly or return for next week's follow-up visit. He is to have blood work evaluated regarding the diabetes and the status of his bronchitis. Alice is aware of the cultural and language differences and quickly identifies these as challenges to providing competent care for this client.

As we enter the twenty-first century, nurses are perched on the cutting edge of enormous demographic, social, and cultural change. Many of these changes will play a dramatic role in the delivery of nursing care to a given client and family. Knowledge about cultures provides a practice framework for broadening nurses' understanding of health-related beliefs, practices, and issues that are part of the experiences of people from diverse cultural backgrounds. In addition, such information provides the nurse the opportunity to explore, understand, and learn from the background of clients and fellow workers, including their unique perspectives on health and health care, as well as their perspective on community and social issues. With a basic knowledge and understanding of culture, the nurse can appreciate the total diversity of our society (Figure 18-1).

···SCIENTIFIC KNOWLEDGE BASE

A person's cultural background primarily involves internal standards of behavior and shared values and attitudes. The standards of a given group, however, are not clearly defined or expressed and vary among and between group members (Figure 18-2). Many members of a given group do not follow all behaviors and standards, and others assume that all people share the same behaviors, values, and attitudes. There are certain demographic, immigration, and heritage issues that affect nursing care.

Demographic Issues

It is predicted that in the United States the percentage of people of European origin, which was 80.3% in 1990 (U.S. Bureau of the Census, 1991), will be only 54% by the year 2020 (Hodgkinson, 1988). The natural population changes within the United States—the combination of aging and low birth rates among the European majority and of youth and high reproductive rates among Asians, African Americans, Hispanics, and Native Americans—are shifting the population, and people of color are an **"emerging majority."** Nurses must be aware of this demographic reality so they can address the future nursing care needs of the changing population. A nurse must have a basic understanding of and sensitivity to the unique culturally diverse health and illness beliefs and practices found among populations in the United States and Canada.

Immigration Issues

Since 1970, more than 30 million foreign citizens and their descendants have been added to the population of this country. In fact, since 1990 nearly 1 million people a year have immigrated. This massive legal demographic change has resulted in some major social issues, such as increased poverty, lower wages, increased illiteracy in the English language, and increased unfair labor practices (Beck, 1996). This rapid influx is causing stress on the health care system in general and on nursing practice in particular.

Heritage Consistency

One theory for analyzing belief systems is through the "melting pot" theory, whereby people have been **acculturated** and **assimilated** into the dominant culture through schools, television, radio, and motion pictures (McLemore, 1980). Another theory is **heritage consistency,** which looks at acculturation as a continuum. Using this theory, the nurse analyzes not only the degree to which a person identifies with the dominant culture but also how that client identifies with their traditional culture. It is possible to assess health beliefs by determining a person's ties to traditional beliefs by the stage of acculturation.

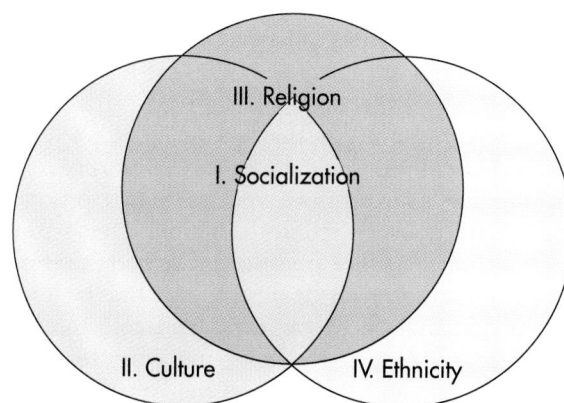

I. Socialization — Extended family
                   Place reared
                   Visits home
                   Raised with extended family
                   Name

II. Culture   — Extended family
                   Participation in folk ways
                   Language

III. Religion   — Extended family
                   Church membership and
                     participation
                   Historic beliefs

IV. Ethnicity   — Extended family
                   Residence in ethnic community
                   Participation in folk ways
                   Socialization with members of same
                     ethnic group
                   Identification as ethnic American

Figure 18-1.   Model of heritage consistency. (From Spector R: *Cultural diversity in health and illness,* ed 3, Norwalk, Conn, 1991, Appleton & Lange.)

Heritage consistency was developed to assess and counsel Native American alcoholics within a cultural context. It describes "the degree to which one's lifestyle reflects his/her tribal culture" (Estes and Zitzow, 1980). The theory has now been expanded in an attempt to study the degree to which any person's lifestyle reflects the traditional culture, whether it is European, Asian, African, or Spanish. For the same person, some aspects of lifestyle may reflect cultural heritage, whereas other aspects are inconsistent with that heritage because the person has undergone acculturation (Spector, 1993, 1996).

The degree of heritage consistency is evaluated by determining the importance of culture, ethnicity, and religion to a person, although it is difficult to isolate the specific aspects of these factors that shape a person's worldview. These variables intertwine in the socialization of the person. When religion is discussed, culture and ethnicity must also be included. It is possible to describe and compare diverse health and illness beliefs and practices within North American society.

Culture. **Culture** is the socially inherited characteristics of a group of people that are transmitted from one generation to the next (Fejos, 1959). These include worldview, values, beliefs, and patterns of social conduct. In addition, culture is learned and serves as the framework of our individuality, personhood, and social relationships. Culture occurs simultaneously in a person's cognitive and behavioral development (Bohannan, 1992). Culture shapes a person's way of experiencing health and illness. Such beliefs are an integral part of life.

Ethnicity. **Ethnicity** is a cultural group's sense of identification associated with its common social and cul-

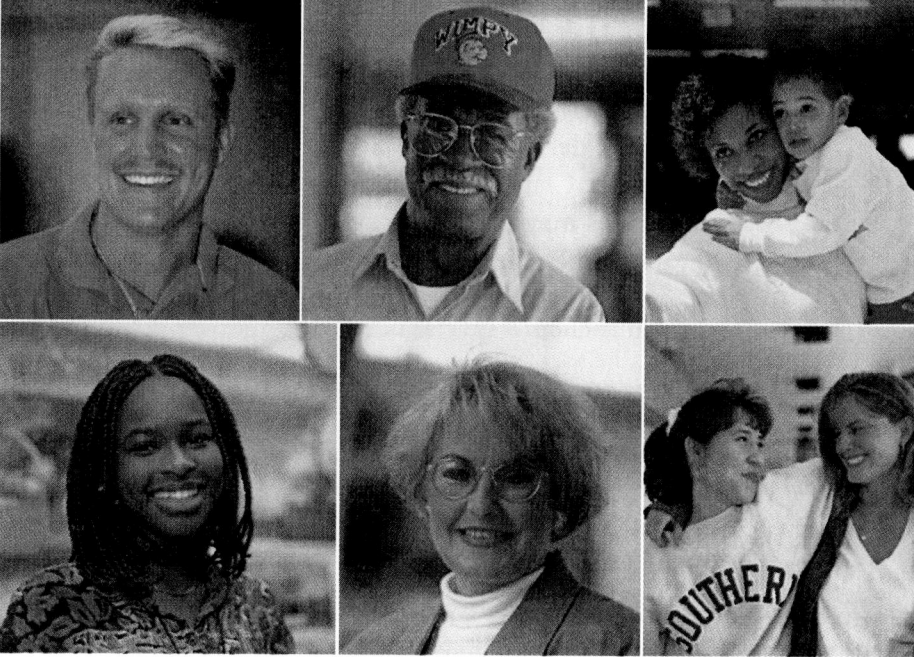

Figure 18-2.   Ethnic and cultural diversity makes home care challenging and rewarding. (From Birchenall J, Streight E: *Mosby's textbook for the home care aide,* St. Louis, 1997, Mosby-Lifeline.)

tural heritage. It is the characteristics a group may have in common. These characteristics include nationality, race, language, religious faith, food preferences, and folklore and many traits relevant to physical appearance. There are more than 106 ethnic groups and 170 Native American tribes in North America (Thernstrom, 1980).

Religion. **Religion** is the belief in a divine or superhuman power or powers to be obeyed and worshiped as the creator(s) and ruler(s) of the universe (see Chapter 17). Ethical values and religion, a system of beliefs and practices, further clarify ethnicity (Abramson, 1980) by providing a frame of reference and perspective within which to organize information. The major religions in North America are Protestant, Catholic, Jewish, Eastern Orthodox, Muslim, Hindu, Baha'i, and Buddhist (Eck, 1995). Countless religious beliefs and practices are related to health and illness.

Socialization. **Socialization** is the process of learning a culture. Initially, young children are socialized into the culture of their families. Later, they attend schools, where a great deal of socialization into the dominant culture takes place. The adult person is socialized into adult and occupational roles.

Heritage consistency occurs on an ever-changing continuum. This concept does not stereotype or diagnose. Rather it is a way to understand a client's or family's sociocultural background and how it creates a framework within which the client can view and interpret life events. The client may interpret events through a traditional or modern viewpoint.

Ethnocultural Groups in North America

The populations of the United States and Canada consist largely of the descendants of immigrants. The only true natives are American Indians, Aleut, and Eskimos because they settled here thousands of years before the Europeans, Asians, Hispanics, and African Americans. People have come to North America from every nation in the world and continue to immigrate in large numbers.

Table 18-1 presents an overview of the nationalities of the North American population and themes of traditional ethnocultural health and illness beliefs and practices. The range of health beliefs is infinite, and there are differences within and between groups. However, some recognizable commonalities exist. The nurse must remember that it is important to constantly assess and communicate with clients to clarify their beliefs about health and illness.

Traditional health beliefs. A person's beliefs about health and illness and the causes and treatments of illness are that person's health beliefs. Modern beliefs are "established, scientific" health beliefs, for example, that bacteria or viruses cause communicable diseases and antibiotics are effective treatment for bacterial infections.

A person who thinks that the "evil eye" or "envy" is the cause of illness and that disease is best treated by removing the "source of evil or envy" has traditional beliefs. A religious or ethnic background may produce these beliefs. Another traditional theme is that of balance; for example, the Chinese believe that factors such as yin (feminine, negative, dark, and cold forces) and yang (masculine, positive, light, and warm forces) must be in balance, and the Spanish believe that "hot" and "cold" must be balanced.

Traditional health practices. Health practices are actions one performs to prevent or treat illness. Modern health practices are recognized by contemporary health care workers as established scientific ways of preventing illness (e.g., immunizations) and treating illness (e.g., medication, surgery). Traditional health practices are those in which a person wears amulets to ward off "evil," eats select foods to prevent illness, and uses folk medicine or healers to treat illness.

Traditional remedies. The admitted use of a folk or **traditional approach** to care is increasing, and the practice may be observed among people from all walks of life and cultural and ethnic backgrounds. Among people who are heritage consistent, this is not a new practice; many of the remedies have been used and passed on for generations. The pharmaceutical properties of vegetation—plants, roots, stems, flowers, seeds, and herbs—have been studied, tested, catalogued, and used for many centuries. Many of these plants are used by specific communities; others cross ethnic-community lines and are used geographically. These remedies are generally purchased in special stores or markets that serve the members of the community, or they may be purchased in the person's country of origin. Frequently the active ingredients of these traditional remedies are unknown. When clients do not adhere to a pharmacological regimen, an effort must be made to determine whether they are taking traditional remedies. If a nurse believes a client is taking these remedies, the nurse must make an effort to determine the active ingredients of the remedy. These ingredients can often be antagonistic or synergistic to the prescribed medications. When this is the situation, the medication may have no effect or a severe overdose may occur. Figure 18-3 presents an array of available remedies from African, Asian, European, Native American, and Hispanic sources.

African Americans. Bangles in the folk tradition are silver bracelets worn by people originating in the West Indies. They are open to let out evil and closed to prevent evil from entering the body. They are worn from infancy, but as the child grows, they are replaced with larger bracelets. These bracelets tend to tarnish

TABLE 18-1

Cultural Groups: Examples of Health Beliefs, Health Practices, Illness Beliefs, Illness Practices, and Traditional Remedies

Origin	Health Beliefs	Health Practices	Illness Beliefs	Illness Practices	Traditional Remedies
Asian American China Hawaii Philippines Korea Japan Southeast Asia 　Laos 　Cambodia 　Vietnam	Balance of yin and yang	Prevent imbalances of yin and yang and changes in climate	Imbalance of yin and yang	Restore balance of yin and yang; use herbal remedies and acupuncture	*Huo li jian mei su* *Jen shen lu jung wan* Ginseng root Tiger balm White flower
African Americans West coast of Africa (as slaves) Many African countries West Indian islands Dominican Republic Haiti Jamaica	Harmony with nature	Prevent disharmony; respect cleanliness and religion; avoid sick people	Disharmony	Use folk remedies and healers	Bangles Talisman Asafoetida Voodoo candles
European England France Germany Other European countries	Physical and emotional well-being; feeling OK	Respect proper nutrition, exercise, cleanliness, faith in God	Absence of well-being; feeling bad	Use home remedies, liniments, poultices, and medical care	Amulets Syrup of Black Draught Father John's Medicine Swamp root *Olbas*
NAI/AN (North American Indians/Alaska Natives) 170 Native American tribes Western part of United States Reservations Tribal homelands	Living in harmony with nature	Respect nature; avoid evil spirits	Disharmony with nature	Use medicine man and traditional herbal remedies	Masks Sweet grass Thunderbird Sand paintings
Spanish and Central American Spain Cuba Central and South America Mexico Puerto Rico	Reward for good behavior; balance of "hot and cold" humors	Wear amulets; use proper diet to maintain balance of "hot and cold"; pray	Punishment for wrong-doing; imbalance of hot and cold	Restore body's balance; use folk healers and remedies	Amulets: *Mano Negro* Special soaps Candles Manzanilla Anise

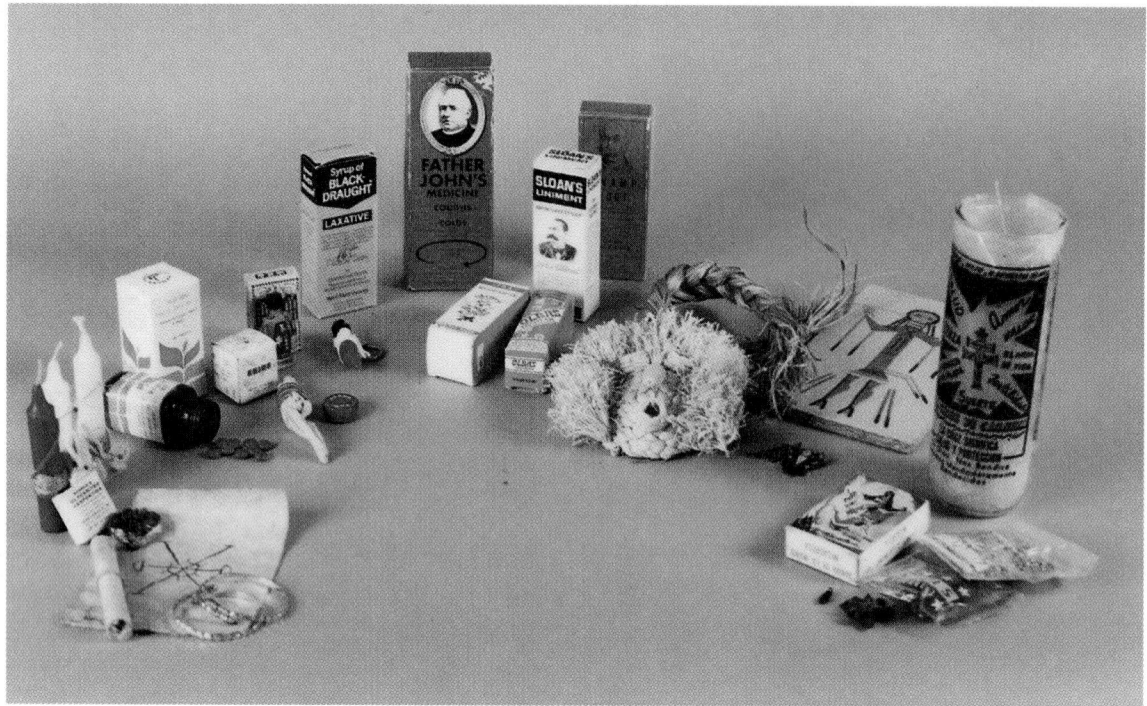

Figure 18-3. A variety of remedies are used by many cultural groups in the United States. (Photo by Lucy Rozier, Boston College Audio Visual Services, Boston College, Chestnut Hill, Mass.)

and leave a black ring on the skin when a child becomes ill. When this occurs, the parent knows that the child must rest, improve the diet, and be wary of any other sources of harm. Some individuals wear several bangles; when they move, the bracelets jingle to frighten away evil spirits. Many people believe that they are extremely vulnerable to evil, even to death, when such bracelets are removed. Nurses must realize that the child and parents experience a great deal of anxiety when these bracelets are removed.

Talismans are sacred pieces of parchment believed to protect the wearer from all illness when worn on a string around the waist or carried in a pocket. Asafoetida is a foul-smelling, gummy substance from a plant resin that is worn to ward off colds and evil. It is known as "the incense of the devil." Voodoo candles are said to have a peculiar spiritualistic character and are used for sacred rituals and rites. Their colors are significant; for example, pink corresponds to love, white to peace, and blue to success and protection from harm.

Asian Americans. *Huo li jian mei su* are small, brown, round pills taken twice a day for prevention of senility, relief of fatigue, and maintenance of youth, health, and beauty. *Jen shen lu jung wan* is a brown liquid used as a general tonic to brace the whole system or as an aid to improve digestion; it may be taken before elective surgery. Tiger balm is a clear, smooth salve used for temporary relief of minor aches and pains. White flower is a colorless liquid used to treat colds, influenza, headache, and coughs.

Ginseng root is the most famous of Chinese medicines. It has universal medicinal usage and is used to "build the blood," especially after childbirth. The legend states that the more the root looks like the human form, the more effective it is. Ginseng is also native to the United States, where it is used as a restorative tonic.

European Americans. An example of an amulet is the *Malocchio*, an Italian horn worn with the *Gobo*, a hunchbacked man, to ward off the "evil eye." The *Gobo* is holding a horseshoe for luck in his left hand and is pointing the first and fourth digits of his right hand to ward off the evil spirit.

Syrup of Black Draught is used as an "over-the-counter" laxative. Father John's Medicine is a medicine used for colds and coughs since 1855. Sloan's Liniment aids in the temporary relief of minor pains from arthritis and other ailments. Swamp root is a liquid used as a diuretic. *Olbas* and *Magentropfen* are medicines purchased in Germany to treat sore throats and lack of appetite.

Native Americans. Masks are worn to hide from the devil or evil spirits. Sweet grass is burned as a rite of purification by the medicine man. The thunderbird is an amulet worn for good luck and protection. Sand painting is executed by the Navajo medicine man to guide the diagnosis of an ailment.

Hispanic. *Mano Negro* (Puerto Rican) is an amulet, a black hand in the shape of a fist with a coral bead on top, that is pinned on a baby's shirt to protect it from evil. *Jabon de la Mano Milagrosa* is a soap used to cleanse and protect a person. Candles are burned to ward off evil. Manzanilla is an herb taken as a tea; it is used to treat stomach and intestinal pain, uterine cramps, anxiety, and insomnia. Anise is a star-shaped seed used to treat painful gas, upset stomach, colic, and anorexia and to increase breast milk.

Traditional health healers. In the traditional context, **healing** is the restoration of the person to a state of health. Within a community, there are specific people who have the power to heal. The healer may be a man or woman and is most often a person thought to have received the gift of healing from a divine source.

In many instances a person who is heritage consistent may consult a traditional healer before, instead of, or concurrent with the use of a Western health care provider. The relationship between the person and healer is quite often much closer than that of the person and the health care professional. The healer understands the problem within a cultural context, speaks the same language, and shares a similar worldview. The following are some examples of traditional healers:

1. Medicine man: the traditional healer of Native Americans
2. *Senora:* a Puerto Rican woman knowledgeable in the treatment of illness
3. *Esperitista:* a person who possesses more sophisticated skills than the *Senora*
4. *Curandero:* a person with a God-given ability to heal using a religious approach
5. *Partera:* a Mexican American midwife
6. Root-worker: an African American who is able to determine the cause of an illness and the treatment

The nurse must remember that traditional healers have been a part of human cultures for as long as they have existed. The methods used to heal have been developed over generations by trial and error, with religious beliefs and social circumstances contributing to the methods. The effective methods have been preserved and adapted to meet the needs of the time. There are several differences between the modern health care provider and the traditional healer; Table 18-2 compares the two.

⋯NURSING KNOWLEDGE BASE⋯⋯⋯⋯⋯⋯⋯

Health and illness beliefs and practices vary among ethnic groups. These differences occur not only among groups but also among the nurse, client, and family. In addition to these health and illness beliefs and practices, the nurse must be sensitive to other factors, such as communication, physiological susceptibility to disease, and emotional and mental health differences, to practice safely and effectively.

Cultural Phenomena Affecting Health

Six major phenomena have been identified by Giger and Davidhizar (1995) as having an impact on health, and their manifestations vary both within and between cultural groups.

Time orientation. Time may be viewed in the present, past, or future. People who are future oriented have long-range goals; this is the orientation of the dominant culture. Other people are oriented more to the present than the future and are less concerned about planning ahead. The concept of time is not

TABLE 18-2	
Comparisons: Traditional Healer Versus Physician	

Traditional Healer	Health Care Provider
Maintains an informal, friendly, effective relationship with the entire family	Business-like and formal, dealing primarily with the client
Comes to the house day or night	Client must go to the physician's office or clinic; home visits are rarely, if ever, made
Consults with head of house, creates a mood of awe, talks to all family members, is not authoritarian, has social rapport, builds expectation of cure	Deals primarily with the ill person, may address only person's illness, authoritarian manner can create fear
Less expensive than the physician	More expensive than the healer
Has ties to the "world of the sacred"; has rapport with the symbolic, spiritual, creative, or holy force	Primarily secular; pays less attention to the religious beliefs of a client or meanings of an illness
Shares the worldview of the client; that is, speaks the same language, lives in the same neighborhood or in similar socioeconomic conditions, may know the same people, understands the lifestyle of the client	Generally does not share the worldview of the client; that is, may not speak the same language, may not live in the same neighborhood or in the same socioeconomic conditions; may not understand the lifestyle of the client

Modified from Spector RE: *Cultural diversity in health and illness,* ed 4, Stamford, Conn, 1996, Appleton & Lange.

formed by wearing a watch or following the calendar but rather by the needs of the client, for example, eating when hungry, going someplace as the occasion arises versus eating dinner at 6:00 PM, and making plans to go places.

A nurse who has an ethnocentric attitude toward time may find it difficult to understand and plan care for clients with a different **time orientation.** For example, certain cultural groups see a value in taking steps early to prevent the occurrence of illness in the future. Other cultural groups may see little value in planning for the future and thus fail to make appointments or try to stop habits that place them at risk for disease. This time orientation difference may become important in health care measures such as long-term planning and explanations about when medications should be taken. Table 18-3 provides examples of time orientation found among people from several cultures.

Personal space and territoriality. Personal space involves a person's set of behaviors and attitudes toward the space around the self. **Territoriality** is an attitude toward an area a person has claimed and defends or reacts emotionally about when another person

TABLE 18-3

Cross-Cultural Examples of Selected Phenomena Affecting Cultural Care

Nations of Origin	Time Orientation	Space	Communication
Asian China Hawaii Philippines Korea Japan Southeast Asia Laos Cambodia Vietnam	Present	Noncontact	National and local languages Cantonese Tagalog Korean Haragei* French and national languages
African West Coast (as slaves) Many African countries West Indian Islands Dominican Republic Haiti Jamaica	Present over future	Close personal space	National languages Dialect Creole Spanish French
European Germany England Italy Ireland Other European countries	Future over present	Noncontact people Aloof Distant Southern countries— closer contact and touch	National languages Many learn English immediately
NAI/AN† 170 North American tribes Aluets Eskimoes	Present	Space is very important and has no boundaries	Tribal languages Use of silence and body language
Hispanic Spain and Portugal Cuba Mexico Central and South America	Present	Tactile relationships Touch Handshakes Embracing Values physical presence	Spanish and Portuguese primary languages Native languages and dialects

Modified from Spector R: Culture, ethnicity, and nursing. In Potter P, Perry A: *Fundamentals of nursing,* ed 4, St. Louis, 1997, Mosby.
Haragei, the Japanese art or practice of using nonverbal communication. (From Matsumoto M: *The unspoken way,* Tokyo, 1988, Kodansha International.)
†*NAI/AN,* North American Indian/Alaska Native.

enters it. Personal space involves a person's set of behaviors and attitudes toward the space around the self. Territoriality and personal space are influenced by culture, and thus different ethnic groups have varying norms related to the use of space.

Staff members and other clients frequently encroach on a client's territory in the hospital. The client's territory includes the room, bed, closet, and belongings. The nurse should try to respect the client's territory as much as possible, especially when performing nursing procedures. Even routine procedures should be explained to all clients to indicate to them that the nurse respects their belief, values, and cultural differences.

Personal space is involved in many nursing activities, and the nurse should be sensitive about the client's attitudes toward space. For example, certain nursing measures involve touching clients, an action that may be threatening to members of certain cultural groups. Standards of behavior vary also in terms of who, male or female, can touch the client and where. The meaning of personal space also varies among cultures. Hall (1963) studied the meaning of space and identified the following zones:

1. Intimate zone (up to 1½ feet)
2. Personal distance (1½ to 4 feet)
3. Social distance (4 to 12 feet)
4. Public distance (12 feet or more)

Use of personal space varies among individuals and ethnic groups. The modesty practiced by members of some groups may prevent members from seeking preventive health care. For example, women who are shy about physical exposure may avoid being examined by male physicians. In some cultures the exposure of a woman's body to a man is prohibited; in others, men are not allowed to be touched by women.

Communication. Communication is an integral part of culture because culture can be called a **meta-communication system.** Communication, like culture, influences and reflects how feelings are expressed and what verbal and nonverbal languages mean. Nurses must be sensitive to several factors related to communication. These include both nonverbal and verbal communication, language, space, and time (Table 18-4).

Language differences are possibly the most important factor when providing nursing care to ethnic group clients because these differences can affect all stages of the nursing process. Clear and effective communication is important when dealing with any client and is crucial if language differences create a cultural barrier (Box 18-1). If the client and nurse do not speak the same language, a translator is necessary. More often, however, the client speaks the nurse's language with limited ability or uses language with denotative or connotative meanings different from the nurse's meanings. For example, a client with limited language ability might know customary greetings

---

Box 18-1

Suggestions for Communicating With Clients Who Speak Other Languages

Respect clients as individuals, regardless of differences in language skills and values. Avoid judging clients' intellectual abilities or emotional states on the basis of how they use language.

Avoid treating emerging majority group members differently from other clients because such "special" treatment may be interpreted as patronizing.

Take care not to assume that clients are angry, aggressive, or hostile if they speak more loudly or emotionally than most European Americans.

Use titles such as "Mr." or "Ms." unless you have established a first-name basis for the relationship.

Never attempt to use ethnic dialects with clients. This may be interpreted as making fun of clients or as condescension.

Avoid attempting to impress clients by saying you have friends of the same ethnic or racial background.

Be attentive to clients' nonverbal communications, which can help to clarify seemingly confusing verbal communications.

Make use of ethnic group preferences when giving care. Involve the extended family in communication, for example, or focus on oral rather than written teaching methods.

Explain medical and nursing terms in simple, everyday words, and be sure that clients truly understand.

If you do not understand what a client is saying, ask for clarification. Do not let embarrassment at not understanding lead to the risks of misinformation.

---

such as "How are you?" or "Hello" but not understand health terms such as "inflammation" or "temperature" that are usually understood by lay persons in the dominant cultural group. Failure to communicate effectively with the client not only may cause unnecessary and costly delays in diagnosis and treatment but also may lead to tragic consequences.

Nurses need the ability to communicate with clients limited in the use of the nurse's language because when deprived of the most common medium of interaction with clients (the spoken word), nurses often become frustrated and ineffective in interventions. Some nurses avoid clients with whom they cannot communicate. Unfortunately, this creates a vicious circle of cultural

TABLE 18-4

Examples of Spoken Languages, Nonverbal Communication, Literacy Skills, and Greetings That May Be Observed Among Selected Cultural Groups

Group	Spoken Language	Nonverbal Communication	Literacy Skills	Greetings
American Indians	Most people speak English; 150 indigenous languages continue to be spoken	Avoid eye contact to show respect	At least 56% of the people are high school graduates	Light touch handshake
Arab Americans	Arabic; different dialects	Expressive, warm, other-oriented; traditional women may avoid eye contact	Inquire if able to read and understand written English	Greet using title; shake hands; smile warmly; eye contact may be helpful
Black/African Americans	English; some dialects Ebonics or Black English	Silence may indicate a lack of trust of care giver	Inquire as to schooling completed	Address as Mr., Mrs., or professional title; handshake appropriate
Cambodians Khmer	Khmer	Inappropriate to touch heads without permission; silence; eye contact not made	Older adults may not read Khmer or English; young may read English	Sompeah—both palms brought together and pointed up
Central Americans	Spanish and dialects	Nonverbal gestures used	Many people do not read	Friendly and outgoing
Chinese Americans	Cantonese, Mandarin, and dialects	Eye contact avoided with strangers	Ability to read English varies	Address people as Mr./Mrs.; use of first names is disrespectful
Cubans	Castilian Spanish	Outgoing; eye contact expected	High degree of literacy in Spanish and English	Only formal with initial meeting; handshake common
Ethiopians	Amharic, Tigrigna, and Oromigna	Polite; reserved; little eye contact	Many people are able to read some English	Hugging, touching, kissing among family and friends; handshake and often bowing
Haitians	French and Creole	Avoid eye contact	Many people do not read or write	Polite and respectful greeting is a handshake
Japanese Americans	Japanese and English	Quiet and polite	Read both Japanese and English	Formal handshake and/or small bow
Koreans	Korean	Touching considered disrespectful; direct eye contact infrequent	Elders may not read English	Use Mr. or Mrs.; bow is common
Mexican Americans	Spanish or English; many people are bilingual	Respeto (respect); direct eye contact avoided	Diversity in reading skills; many people read Spanish but not English	Handshake used
Puerto Ricans	Spanish and English	Respect and affectionate; eye contact avoided	Depends on years of education	Handshake; hugs among friends
Russians	Russian and other languages	Eye contact used	Many immigrants read English	Use Mr., Mrs., or professional title
Vietnamese	Vietnamese, French, and Chinese	Gentle touch; avoid eye contact to show respect	Many people do not read English	Use Mr./Mrs. with last name mentioned first; older people may smile and bow

Modified from Lipson J and others: Culture and nursing care: a pocket guide, San Francisco, 1996, University of San Francisco Press.

misunderstandings between the nurse and client. All too often, the nurse might behave toward the client in ways that could be misconstrued by the client (e.g., shouting, focusing on the task instead of the client, doing things for the client without speaking) or use body language (e.g., arms folded across the chest) that might be read by the client as anger or hostility.

Language differences can be overcome, however. Differences in denotative and connotative meanings may exist between members of two cultures, causing miscommunication. The health institution must provide an interpreter. Medical terms must be clearly explained to all clients. Hospital jargon (e.g., "force fluids") or abbreviations (e.g., qid) should be eliminated. Another linguistic block to communication between ethnic groups comes from differences in connotative meanings for certain words, even when the denotative meanings are the same. For example, the word *hospital* may mean a facility for health care to one client, but it may represent death or a threat to life for another.

By giving special attention to the communication process, nurses can overcome language barriers. Observing nonverbal behaviors, for example, can help to clarify a client's communication, although nonverbal communication is also influenced by culture. Nurses can also learn to phrase questions and statements to elicit information from clients whose ethnic background shapes their response.

Social organization.
The social organization includes cultural aspects such as the family unit, gender roles and behavior, and social-group organizations (religious or ethnic) with which identification takes place.

Attitudes toward the family. Chapters in this book discuss the importance of involving the client's family or significant others in all stages of the nursing process. The nurse should encourage visits from members of the extended family, which can remind the client of home and thus lessen the effects of isolation and shock from hospitalization. When planning home care, the family plays a vital role in providing the necessary follow-up and long-term care.

Gender roles. The accepted norms for traditional gender role behaviors vary among cultures. Certain roles for men and certain roles for women may be stressed. For example, in matriarchal cultures, the wife or mother is responsible for many family decisions, including when to seek health care. When providing family health care and involving family members in the client's care, the nurse needs to know variables in gender role behaviors to understand the client's behaviors.

Understanding multicultural behavioral differences is also crucial when the nurse provides client care involving emotional and social dimensions. Family and gender role behavior patterns vary among cultural groups; however, the nurse must be aware of such variations when involving the family in care.

Social organizations. There are countless social organizations of both a religious and/or ethnic nature within the community that may be called on in a time of need to assist people. For example, Parish Nursing is becoming a nursing service that is offered in several faith communities around the country, and many fraternal organizations are willing to assist families when home care services, such as meals, are needed. Nursing must be increasingly aware of these resources.

Physiological differences.
Countless differences regarding susceptibility to disease, dermatological conditions, and food and eating habits exist among ethnic groups. The nurse should assess the family history carefully.

Susceptibility to disease. Because of genetic or lifestyle differences, some ethnic groups are more susceptible to certain diseases than others. In general, ethnic groups with lower socioeconomic status are more susceptible to acquired diseases and conditions such as malnutrition and infections. Box 18-2 lists selected diseases and the ethnic groups with high occurrences.

Dermatological conditions. For all ethnic groups, skin color is an important factor in physiological assessment, but assessment of skin color depends more on the individual than on racial or genetic factors because individuals within a race vary widely in skin color. Color changes in dark-skinned clients must be determined

---

Box 18-2
Examples of High Morbidity Incidence Among Selected Cultural Groups

Asian American

Liver cancer	Hypertension
Stomach cancer	Parasites
Coccidioidomycosis	

African American

Cancer of the esophagus	Hypertension
Stomach cancer	Sickle cell anemia
Coccidioidomycosis	

European

Breast cancer
Thalassemia

NAI/AN (North American Indians/Alaska Natives)

Accidents	Diabetes mellitus
Heart disease	Lung cancer
Cirrhosis of the liver	

Spanish and Central American

Diabetes mellitus
Parasites
Coccidioidomycosis

differently from those in whites. For instance, in a dark-skinned person, pallor is the absence of the underlying red tones that normally give brown and black skin its glow. The skin of a black person with pallor will appear ashen gray, and an individual with brown skin will become yellow brown (Geiger and Davidizhar, 1995).

Food and eating habits. Food and eating habits vary widely among cultural groups, but these customs usually carry emotional and social significance. Therefore it helps for nurses to have a general understanding of the food habits of ethnic clients. In many cases, family members can be permitted to bring special foods to hospitalized clients unhappy about hospital food. When teaching a client about dietary requirements related to specific illnesses, the nurse should be sensitive to cultural meanings of eating and food preferences.

Nurses should also be aware of their own cultural values related to food and eating because these values influence their attitudes toward eating, including determinations about the best foods, preferable methods of preparation, appropriate times for eating, and ways in which illness affects these factors. Nurses can be aware of a client's differences only when they identify their own cultural values related to food.

Psychological differences.
Differences may exist between the nurse's expectations and the client's perceptions of emotional and mental health and emotional expression and reactions to pain.

Emotional and mental health. People from all cultural groups undergo emotional and mental stresses and conflicts. An additional stressor, however, is the prejudice and discrimination by the dominant group toward members of other ethnic groups. Clients may form defense mechanisms for relating to others from the dominant culture. The following patterns of behavior are linked to these defense mechanisms: acceptance, aggression, obsessive sensitivity, efforts of ego enhancement, self-hatred, and assimilation. A person might use more than one of these mechanisms when attempting to cope with a situation.

Acceptance occurs when group members accommodate themselves to the prejudice of the dominant group. This apparently good-natured behavior can block genuine communication and often causes a client to accept unpleasant symptoms and situations without alerting a nurse.

Aggression occurs when group members strike out with hostile acts against members of the dominant group. Sullenness and stubbornness are effective ways of expressing frustration with the nurse. When interacting with members of the dominant group, the person may be hypersensitive to signs of bigotry. Clients who detect bigotry may fail to seek health care because of prejudices seen in health care workers.

As a defense mechanism, a person may also seek to enhance self-concept through ego enhancement. An ex-

ample might involve clients who request a private duty nurse for their personal care.

Acceptance of the dominant group's evaluation might also lead a person to develop unconscious self-hatred, usually accompanied by ambivalent feelings of inferiority. For example, clients may be quick to criticize behaviors of their own family during visitation in the hospital.

Another reaction of a person is assimilation. In this case the person acquires behaviors or attitudes similar to the dominant culture.

Reactions to pain. To determine a client's emotional state, the nurse needs to understand how patterns of emotional expression vary among ethnic groups. Reaction to pain is influenced by cultural background, and it is important for the nurse to objectively evaluate pain. To do so, nurses should be aware that their own attitudes about pain are culturally influenced (see Chapter 33). Table 18-5 illustrates responses to pain that may be observed among selected cultural groups.

Environmental control.
Environmental control is the ability of members of a particular cultural group to plan activities that control nature or direct environmental factors. Included are the complex systems of traditional health and illness beliefs, the practices of folk medicine, and the use of traditional healers. These beliefs and practices play a vital role in the response that a given person, family, or community may have in respect to the health care system and form the line to the health traditions.

Health Traditions Model
The Health Traditions model (Table 18-6) describes the traditions related to the maintenance, protection, and restoration of physical, mental, and spiritual health in a nine-dimensional interrelated fabric. To understand health traditions, health must be defined as a balance of the person, both within one's being—physical, mental, and spiritual—and within the outside environment—natural, familial and communal, and metaphysical. Health traditions are the beliefs and practices the persons or family may have to maintain, protect, and restore their health. The **health maintenance** beliefs and practices include daily health-related activities (e.g., diet, exercise, rest, clothing). **Health protection** beliefs and practices include the use of special health-related activities, such as food taboos, special exercise, seasonal activities, and protective items worn daily. **Health restoration** beliefs and practices are activities that may include necessary diet changes, rest, and special clothing. The health maintenance, protection, and restoration beliefs and practices that may be found among people from different ethnocultural backgrounds are infinite. There are individual differences both within and between given groups. Figure 18-4 illustrates symbols for each category

TABLE 18-5
Responses to Pain That May Be Observed Among Selected Cultural Groups

Group	Pain Responses
American Indians	Often undertreated because pain may be referred to in general terms such as, "I do not feel good"; may complain to a close relative, who may then tell the nurse
Arab Americans	Often very expressive about pain with family members; believe injections are more effective than pills
Black/African Americans	May openly and publicly express pain but may avoid medication
Brazilians	Generally low pain threshold; men may be less tolerant of pain than women; may moan, cry, or scream
Cambodians	Stoic with pain; prefer injections; may massage with Tiger Balm or practice cupping to suck pain from body
Central Americans	May be viewed as a necessary part of life or consequence of "misconduct"; acceptable to moan or cry
Chinese Americans	May not complain of pain but show nonverbal clues
Colombians	Women may express more pain than men; may use heat or cold to control pain
Cubans	Acceptable to express feeling of pain
Ethiopians	Stoic; high pain threshold; very general about symptoms
Filipinos	Often stoic; do not like injections; prefer oral medications
Haitians	Low pain threshold; may be verbal about experience
Hmong	May take a lot of pain medications; opium traditionally grown and used to relieve pain
Japanese Americans	Can be stoic in expression of pain; some people have a high pain threshold; others fear addiction and do not take medication
Koreans	May be stoic; prefer oral or IV medications; injections considered invasive
Mexican Americans	Tend not to complain of pain
Puerto Ricans	May be loud and outspoken in expressing pain; herbal teas may be used to manage pain
Russians	High pain threshold; may be stoic
Vietnamese	May be stoic; will not voluntarily request pain medication

Modified from Lipson J and others: *Culture and nursing care: a pocket guide,* San Francisco, 1996, University of San Francisco Press.

TABLE 18-6
Health Traditions Model

	Body	Mind	Spirit
Maintain health	Traditional clothing, traditional diet, traditional activities	Concentration, social and family supports, hobbies	Religious worship, prayer, meditation
Protect health	Special foods and diets; symbolic clothing	Avoidance of those who cause illness; family and community activities	Religious customs, superstitions, amulets and talismans, candles
Restore health	Homeopathic remedies, liniments, herbal teas, special foods, massage	Relaxation, exorcism, *curanderos* and other traditional healers, nerve teas	Religious rituals, special prayers, changing names, meditation, traditional healings, exorcism

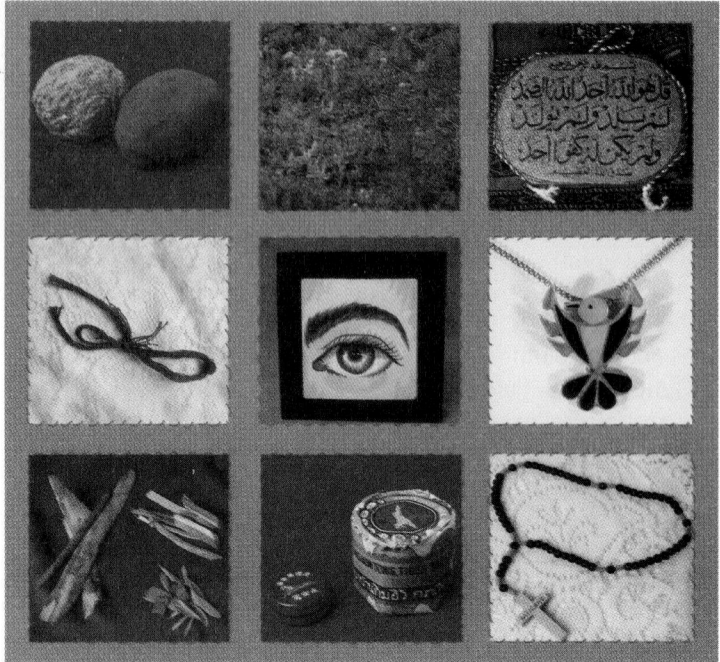

Figure 18-4.   Health Traditions model. **Row 1,** Thousand-year eggs (China): foods that may be eaten daily to maintain physical health. Nature: enjoyment of nature may be a universal way of maintaining mental health. Islamic Prayer (East Jerusalem): may be a way of maintaining spiritual health. **Row 2,** Red String (Tomb of Rachel in Bethlehem, Israel): worn to protect physical health. Eye (Cuba): hung in the home to protect the mental health of the household. Thunderbird (Hopi Nation): worn for spiritual health protection. **Row 3,** Herbal Remedy (Africa): herbs used in preparations to restore health. Tiger Balm (Singapore): massage may be a way of restoring mental health. Rosary Beads (Italy): prayer and meditation may be used to restore spiritual health. (Courtesy © Spector Collection. Photographs, Stephen Vedder, Assistant Director, Photography Production Service, Boston College Audiovisual Department, Chestnut Hill, Mass. Graphics, Sarah Bastille, Boston College Audiovisual Department, Chestnut Hill, Mass.)

from a wide range of traditions. In the Health Traditions model, each symbolic panel represents an image or an example of an object from various ethnocultural heritages. The rows are health maintenance, protection, and restoration. The columns represent physical, mental, and spiritual health.

CRITICAL THINKING AND CULTURAL CARE

Synthesis

A broad range of health and illness beliefs exists among cultural groups in North America. Many of these beliefs have roots in the cultural, ethnic, religious, or social background of a person, family, or community. When people anticipate, fear, or experience an illness or crisis, they may use a modern approach, the present-day beliefs and practices of the providers within the American, or Western, health care delivery system. Some clients may wish to use a traditional approach, ancient ethno-

cultural or religious beliefs and practices regarding illness prevention or healing that have been handed down through generations. The nurse applies a critical thinking approach to understanding a client's cultural orientation and preferences. Synthesis of critical thinking factors will enable the nurse to provide more culturally sensitive care.

Knowledge. For a nurse to provide care for a client of a different cultural or ethnic background, effective intercultural communication must take place. The demographic profile of the North American population is changing rapidly, and the need for intercultural awareness and understanding is escalating. Because nurses deal with clients on a one-to-one basis, they must interact and relate to all peoples. Nurses must bring knowledge of their client's culture, their own culture, and cultural biases into the nurse-client relationship. When health care diverts away from the client's cultural beliefs and practices, there is a risk of the client's not completing his health care plan. Care that is sensitive to the client's culture is care that is individualized and complete.

Experience. Nurses also come from diverse ethnic, cultural, and religious backgrounds, and rapport is established when nurses are able to convey to the client and family that they are aware of and sensitive to their unique health and illness beliefs and practices. This rapport facilitates the delivery of safe and effective multicultural nursing care.

Attitude. A person's cultural background primarily involves internal standards of behavior and shared values and attitudes. To meet individual cultural care needs, the nurse can independently and creatively modify the client's plan of care (e.g., environment, hygiene, prescribed diet) to blend health care and cultural priorities. When modifying care the nurse is responsible for the delivery of competent, individualized care. A nurse's attitude toward culture can be value laden and biased. Becoming aware of one's own biases and gaining knowledge of other cultures enable the nurse to begin to develop an attitude in which the client's culture and health care beliefs, values, and practices are respected and incorporated into the plan of care.

Standards. When providing family health care and involving family members in the client's care, the nurse needs to know variables in age and gender role behaviors to understand the client's behaviors. The standards of a given group, however, are not clearly defined or expressed and vary among and between group members. Implementing culturally sensitive care requires the nurse to integrate the client's cultural practices into the plan of care. In doing so, the nurse uses critical thinking skills to identify which cultural standards and practices are important to the client and therefore should not be altered. Likewise, the nurse is also able to determine which standards may be adopted. Finally, understanding standards related to multicultural behavioral differences is crucial when the nurse provides client care involving emotional and social dimensions.

CULTURAL CARE AND THE NURSING PROCESS

When caring for clients, the nurse uses the nursing process. Because nurses are frequently from a cultural group other than that of the client, they must consider their client's cultural values, behaviors, and attitudes during all stages of the nursing process. The initial assessment nurses must make is that of their own heritage and health traditions. This process enables them to view their personal traditions, the nursing actions they have learned, and their clients' beliefs in a wider way, and in so doing they will observe both similarities and differences of health beliefs and practices.

▪ Assessment

There must be an awareness of one's own ethnocultural heritage, both as a person and as a nurse. In addition, an awareness and sensitivity must be developed to the health beliefs and practices of a client's heritage. This awareness and sensitivity can be developed through careful assessment of a client's heritage and cultural beliefs. Box 18-3 describes the factors that must be explored during a multicultural nursing assessment.

Box 18-3
Multicultural Nursing Assessment

Cultural

What customs and values of the client may influence health behaviors and the provision of care?

Could the client's communication process or language affect the provision of care? How?

What health care beliefs and practices of the client may influence acceptance of and response to illness?

Could nutritional variables and preferences or restrictions affect the provision of care?

Sociological

Could the client's economic status affect the provision of care?

Could educational status affect the provision of care?

How does the client's social network affect the provision of care?

What family structural variables may influence the provision of care?

Are community support systems available, and do they help to fight against institutional racism?

Psychological

Could self-concept and identity factors affect the provision of care?

What are the client's defense mechanisms, and are they adaptive or maladaptive?

Could religious or cultural considerations affect the provision of care?

Biological and Physiological

Does the nurse need to take racial or anatomical characteristics or factors into account when providing care?

Do growth and development patterns influence physical assessment findings?

What variations in physical features and body systems are present?

Are there any culturally specific diseases to note? Are there any diseases to which the client has increased (decreased) resistance?

Data gathered relating to providing care for a particular client are divided into the following three assessment steps: (1) heritage assessment, (2) background assessment relating to the cultural phenomena, and (3) health traditions assessment. Not all areas apply to all ethnic groups or to all individuals within a group; the nurse addresses the applicability of each factor for each client. This information can be gathered with standard nursing history data during the interview.

Heritage assessment.
The **heritage assessment** data include the client's age, ethnic origin, race, place of birth, religion, and identification with a given heritage. An assessment tool (Box 18-4) of the factors constituting heritage consistency and some sample questions is helpful when gathering these data. By using such a tool, the nurse can determine the degree to which clients identify with their heritage. Clients who deeply identify with a traditional heritage are more likely to maintain the traditional health beliefs and practices of the group.

Cultural phenomena.
Data related to **cultural phenomena** are gathered to discover relocation trends,

---

Box 18-4
Heritage Assessment

Childhood development occurred in the country of origin or in an immigrant neighborhood of like ethnic group.
>   Where were you born?
>   Where did you grow up?
>   What was your neighborhood like?
>   Are your parents from the same or different ethnic and religious or racial background?

Extended family members encourage participation in traditional religious or cultural activities.
>   Do you and your family celebrate holidays and festivals together at home and in the community?
>   Do you participate in other church or fraternal events with family members?

Client and family members frequently visit the country of origin or the "old neighborhood."
>   How often do you return to the neighborhood in which you grew up?

Client's and family members' homes are within an "ethnic" community.
>   What ethnic group or groups live in your neighborhood?

Client and family members participate in ethnic cultural events such as religious festivals or holidays, sometimes with singing, dancing, and national costumes.
>   Do you now participate in ethnic or religious events?

Client was reared in an extended family setting.
>   Who lived in your home when you were young?
>   Did you live with grandparents, aunts, uncles, and cousins?
>   What are the present circumstances?

Client and family members maintain regular contact with the extended family.
>   How often do you visit family members?

Do you keep in close contact with those at a distance?

Family name has not been "Americanized."
>   What was your family's name when it immigrated?
>   Have the members kept or changed their name?

Client was educated in a parochial (nonpublic) school with a religious or ethnic philosophy similar to the family's background.
>   Where did you go to school?
>   What kind of a school is it?

Client and family members engage primarily in social activities with others of the same ethnic or religious background.
>   What are the ethnic and religious backgrounds of your friends?
>   Are they from your same ethnic or religious background?

Client and family members have a knowledge of the culture and language of origin.
>   Have you studied the history of the people from the nation from which you originate?
>   Do you speak your native language?
>   What language did you learn first?
>   What language do you speak at home?

Client and family members possess elements of personal pride about their heritage.
>   How do you identify yourself?
>   With which group, if parents are from the different groups?

Client and family members incorporate elements of historical beliefs and practices into the present philosophy.
>   What is your history?
>   What can you tell me about your specific health and illness beliefs?

habits and customs, valued behaviors, cultural sanctions and restrictions, language, and communication process. Social data include economic status, educational status, social networks, family support networks, community support systems, and the influence of institutional racism. Nurses who are practicing in a setting where clients come from cultures that are not their own should be knowledgeable in this information and seek resources to assist in learning about their clients' cultures. Table 18-7 describes the information that may be gathered and the etiquette necessary for this phase of the assessment.

Health traditions.
The **health traditions** data include health and healing beliefs and practices, nutritional variables, and food practices. The assessment questions for this phase of the assessment are found in Table 18-8.

Client expectations.
When discussing health beliefs and practices as they stem from a cultural, ethnic,

and religious framework, the nurse needs to be sensitive to the client expectations. The range of health and illness definitions, beliefs, and practices is infinite, and there are differences within and between groups. However, some recognizable commonalities exist. The nurse must remember that it is important to constantly assess and communicate with clients to clarify their beliefs about health and illness.

Additional data.
Psychological data include self-concept and identity factors, cognitive and behavioral processes, religious influences, and psychological-cultural responses to stress and illness. Biological and physiological data include racial and physical findings, growth and development patterns, variations in body systems, diseases more prevalent in an ethnic group, and diseases to which an ethnic group might be more resistant. The nurse must be aware of cultural variations that can affect both the timing and type of nursing care provided.

TABLE 18-7
Selected Examples of Cultural Care Etiquette as Related to the Cultural Phenomena

Time	Visiting	Inform client when you are coming.
	Being on time	Avoid surprises.
		Explain your expectations about time.
		Ask clients from other regions and cultures what they expect.
	Taboo times	Be familiar with the times and meanings of client's ethnic and religious holidays.
Space	Body language and distances	Know cultural and/or religious customs regarding contact and touch with others from many perspectives.
Communication	Greetings	Know the proper forms of address for people from a given culture and the ways by which people welcome one another.
		Know when touch, such as an embrace or handshake, is expected and when physical contact is prohibited.
	Gestures	Gestures do not have universal meaning—what is acceptable to one cultural group is taboo with another.
	Smiling	Smiles may be indicative of friendliness to some and taboo to others.
	Eye contact	Avoiding eye contact may be a sign of respect.
Social organization	Holidays	Know what dates are important and why, whether or not to give gifts, what to wear to special events, and what the customs and beliefs are.
	Special events Births Weddings Funerals	Know how the event is celebrated, meaning of colors used for gifts, and expected rituals at home or religious services.
Biological variations	Food customs	Know what can be eaten for certain events, what foods may be eaten together or are forbidden, and what and how utensils are used.
Environmental control	Health practices and remedies	Know what the general health traditions are for a given client, and question observations for validity.

Modified from Dresser N: *Multicultural manners*, New York, 1996, John Wiley & Sons.

Successful critical thinking requires a synthesis of knowledge, experience, information gathered from clients, and critical thinking attitudes and standards. Clinical judgments require the nurse to anticipate what information is needed, to analyze the data, and then to make decisions regarding client care. The client expects competent and informed care. Alice incorporates previous knowledge and experience in providing care for Mr. Sanchez.

NURSING DIAGNOSES FOR CLIENTS WITH CULTURALLY RELATED HEALTH PROBLEMS

Communication, impaired verbal
Coping, family: potential for growth
Coping, ineffective family: compromised
Health maintenance, altered
Noncompliance
Social interaction, impaired
Spiritual distress

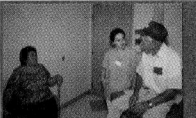

Case Study

Synthesis in Practice

Alice is able to apply cultural care principles that she has learned from experience and a review of the literature. She knows that the community health clinic is a public facility, and Mr. Sanchez is able to obtain his care and medication either free or at a low cost. However, Alice's fear that Mr. Sanchez may not take his medications is well-founded. First, he does not understand the English language, and up to this point in time the directions have been provided in only English and mime. Second, in reviewing traditional beliefs and practices of a culture, Alice remembers that it is common practice for Mr. Sanchez's culture to use roots and herbs in the treatment of illnesses. Alice collaborates with the pharmacist, who then consults a Spanish-speaking herbalist, and together they provide Mr. Sanchez with comprehensive instructions for taking his antibiotic.

◼ Nursing Diagnosis

Nursing diagnoses for an ethnic client are the same as those for any client; however, there are diagnoses specifically related to cultural differences. A diagnosis might involve problem areas during the client's interaction with the health care delivery system or the principal complaint for which the client is seeking health care (see nursing diagnoses box). When determining nursing diagnoses for a client, the nurse should be as specific as possible when identifying cultural variables so individualized interventions can be planned.

The nurse also identifies clusters of defining characteristics that support the diagnostic label. For example, the nurse may diagnose impaired verbal communication related to language differences. The nurse verifies certain assessment data such as the client's inability to speak the dominant language, the client's frustration in not making needs known, and the client's ability to speak only in the native language. The related factor must be accurate to ensure that the correct interventions are used.

◼ Planning

When establishing the goals and expected outcomes of care and planning interventions, the nurse again considers cultural variables. The extended family should be involved in care, for example, if the family is the client's strongest support group. When a goal of nursing care is to incorporate cultural beliefs and practices into the client's care plan, achievement of realistic outcomes of care is enhanced. This is especially important if interventions will eventually be directed toward changing the client's behavior. When cultural factors influence the planning of care, the client and key family members must become active participants in the plan.

As with all other needs, the client's cultural needs must be included when establishing the goal and expected outcomes of care. For example, the newly diagnosed diabetic client may need to know that his diet modification can be coordinated with cultural food preferences. To creatively blend a client's cultural food preferences with a 1500-calorie diet may take creative multidisciplinary planning, coordination, and collaboration among nursing, nutritionists, physicians, community support groups, and the client/family (see care plan).

◼ Implementation

Health promotion. Knowing the client's cultural health beliefs and practices enables the nurse to develop interventions aimed at promoting optimal health of the client. Designing a total health promotion program that includes the traditional practices of diet, exercise, traditional remedies, and folk medicine can assist in maintaining wellness in our culturally diverse clients. These practices can also optimize the client's level of wellness in the presence of a chronic illness.

Communication and open-mindedness are keys to successful interventions with clients. In almost all cases the nurse will be able to adapt nursing interventions to avoid cultural conflicts after the client understands that the nurse maintains respect for ethnicity and individuality.

TABLE 18-8

Assessment Guide: Methods to Maintain, Protect, and Restore Health

	Physical	Mental	Spiritual
Maintain health	Are there special clothes you must wear at certain times of the day, week, year? Are there special foods you must eat at certain times? Do you have any dietary restrictions? Are there any foods that you cannot eat?	What do you do for activities, such as reading, sports, and games? Do you have hobbies? Do you visit family often? Do you visit friends often?	Are you active in church or other communal activities? Do you pray or meditate?
Protect health	Are there foods that you cannot eat together? Are there special foods that you must eat? Are there any types of clothing that you are not allowed to wear?	Are there people or situations that you have been taught to avoid? Do you take extraordinary precautions under certain circumstances? Do you take time for yourself?	Do you observe religious customs? Do you wear any amulets or hang them in your home? Do you have any practices, such as always opening the window when you sleep? Do you have any other practices to protect yourself from "harm"?
Restore health	What kinds of medicines do you take before you see a doctor or nurse? Are there herbs that you take? Are there special treatments that you use?	Do you know of any specific practices your mother or grandmother may use to relax? Do you know how big problems can be cared for in your community? Do you drink special teas to help you unwind or relax? Do you know of any healers?	Do you know of any religious rituals that help to restore health? Do you meditate? Did you ever go to a healing service? Do you know about exorcism?

Modified from Spector RE: *Guide to heritage assessment and health traditions,* Stamford, Conn, 1996, Appleton & Lange.

Acute care. Client education and effective communication are important interventions when a client's ethnic or cultural heritage is a factor in the plan of care. An explanation of all aspects of care ensures a client's understanding of the therapeutic plan. If a client's language skills inhibit communication, the nurse may use interpreters, word signs, or charts. Nurses may have to alter usual ways of interacting with clients to avoid offending or alienating a client and family members with different attitudes toward social interaction and etiquette. For example, a client who is modest and self-conscious about the body will need psychological preparation before some procedures and tests.

In the acute care setting and other settings as well, clients from different cultures may have different responses to pain (see Table 18-5, p. 321). As a result, the pain management plan for these clients also differs. Clients from some cultures need the presence of the family and extended family to be comfortable and decrease pain. As a result, flexible visiting hours are needed in the plan of care.

Clients from other cultures may have a reluctance to use blood and blood products. If such a client is scheduled for invasive surgery, these concerns need to be addressed before the procedure. In some cases the client may need to accept the blood product. In other cases the surgeon may need to modify the procedure.

Likewise clients from some cultures may have an aversion to observing their wounds from surgery or trauma. If this is the case, incorporate these variances into the plan of care. In some cases it may never be necessary for a client to observe or care for a wound. A relative may do that activity.

The acute care setting can be modified to accommodate dietary, activity, and religious practices for the culturally diverse client. It is important, however, to understand different cultures and their practices so that the care is individualized for the client.

Restorative care. In the restorative care setting, some cultures depend heavily on the family and extended family to provide ongoing care. If this is so, the

CASE STUDY NURSING CARE PLAN

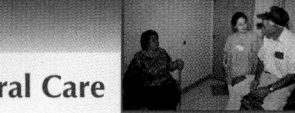

Cultural Care

Assessment

Mr. Sanchez's bronchitis is resolved. But he does have adult-onset, non–insulin-dependent diabetes mellitus. He is placed on an 1800-calorie diet with an oral hypoglycemic agent. His total carbohydrate intake should be between 55% and 60%. On Mr. Sanchez's first return clinic visit, Alice notices that his **carbohydrate intake is about 75% with a total caloric intake of 2000 calories/day and his glucose for that visit was 200 mg/dl,** showing poor glucose control. Mr. Sanchez and his wife both have **difficulty understanding the diet,** although they were given the English/Spanish version. Alice knows that this client is not due back into the clinic for another month. However, she has developed a plan of care and set up a midmonth follow-up visit to occur when the Spanish-speaking interpreter is available. An overriding goal of care is to keep Mr. Sanchez's diabetes under control and in so doing try to avoid insulin injections.

Nursing Diagnosis

Altered health maintenance related to cultural and language differences.

Planning

Goal

Maintain an 1800-calorie ADA diet with appropriate carbohydrate, protein, and fat balance.

Expected Outcomes

Blood glucose remains 90 to 120 mg/dl.

Twenty-four-hour diet recall confirms appropriate food group selection.

Client/wife correctly measures blood glucose.

Client/wife asks questions regarding client's care.

Implementation

Steps	**Rationale**
1. Obtain English/Spanish ADA food guide.	Guide is in client's native language, with simple menus and colorful examples. This increases client's knowledge and comfort in making diet changes.
2. In 2 weeks have client and family come to meet with interpreter.	Two weeks gives clients an opportunity to use the food guide. Since they will have questions, having an interpreter available will increase the opportunity of both nurse and clients to ask questions and clarify diet management.
3. Demonstrate to client/wife how to measure blood glucose. Provide time for return demonstration for each clinic visit.	Demonstration shows client how to use the equipment. Return demonstration documents learning.

Evaluation

Observe client's serum glucose log since last clinic visit.

Ask client for diet recall for last 24 hours.

Observe client/wife measure serum glucose.

Ask client/wife to describe how they are managing integrating the diet into their daily lives.

Defining characteristics are shown in bold type.

discharge plan needs to incorporate these resources. In addition, home care services need to be coordinated to include the family care provider. In the extended care setting, the agency needs to know about the family or extended family, what type and amount of care they wish to do, and the timing of such care.

The client and family should be involved in all aspects of the care. This should occur in every case, even if nursing care cannot be modified because of the client's condition. Discussing with the client and family any cultural questions related to care ensures individualization of interventions because the client will understand the way cultural variables relate to health beliefs and practices.

Evaluation

Client care. The nurse evaluates the results of nursing care, determining the extent to which the goals of care have been met. Evaluation continues throughout the nursing process and should include clear feedback from the client and family. Clear, concise communication is critical to evaluate the progress of the client's care fairly.

Nurses should evaluate their attitudes toward multicultural nursing care. Some nurses may believe that they should treat all clients the same and simply act naturally, but this attitude fails to acknowledge that cultural differences exist and that there is no "natural" human behavior. The nurse cannot act the same with all clients and still hope to deliver effective, individualized, holistic care. Sometimes inexperienced nurses are so self-conscious about cultural differences and so afraid of making a mistake that they impede the nursing process by not asking questions about areas of difference or by asking so many questions that they seem to pry into the client's personal life.

Self-evaluation can help the nurse to become more comfortable when providing care to clients. To determine whether goals that incorporate cultural needs are met, the nurse uses specific evaluative measures. The nurse should consider the following questions:

1. Am I open to understanding ways in which the client's values differ from mine?
2. Have I given sufficient attention to communicating with the client with limited language skills?
3. Have I successfully involved the client's family in the nursing process?
4. Am I incorporating the client's traditional beliefs and practices into nursing therapies?
5. Is my therapeutic relationship with the client respectful, regardless of cultural differences?

Client expectations. It is important to determine to what level the client's expectations of care were achieved. In regard to cultural aspects of care, the nurse would want to know if the plan of care was able to be incorporated into the client's daily life and whether the client was satisfied with the care. Did the client expect more diversity in the diet or activities of the care plan? Did the client feel that his or her cultural needs were even considered? Each client is unique and has individual expectations. When the client represents another culture, the expectations differ. Blending these expectations into a plan of care increases the client's understanding of and hopefully adherence to the plan of care.

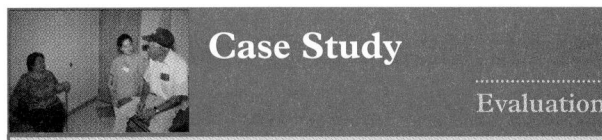

Case Study

Evaluation

It has been 6 months since Mr. Sanchez was diagnosed with diabetes mellitus. His blood glucose levels are still elevated (160 to 180 mg/dl), but they are steadily coming down. The frustration for Mr. Sanchez and his wife is decreasing because they have adjusted to the diet. Through their interactions with the interpreter, the Sanchezes have become more knowledgeable regarding the care regimen, and Alice has become more knowledgeable regarding Mexican American culture. The interpreter assisted Alice in finding other Mexican American clients who also have diabetes mellitus. These clients worked with Mr. Sanchez and his wife to adapt their cultural dietary preferences into the American Diabetes Association (ADA) 1800-calorie diet. Both the client and his wife believe that once they were able to adjust the diet toward their food preferences, it became easier to manage the care. The last two serum glucose levels were in the 160 mg/dl range, and these coincided with the adaptation of the diabetic diet toward the client's cultural diet preferences. Both the client and his wife refer to the English/Spanish guide for ideas and clarifications.

Documentation Note

Blood glucose 170 mg/dl. Client reports that he is feeling better and has more energy. Both client and wife are attending social gatherings with other people who are on an ADA diet; they find this very helpful in meal preparation. Twenty-four-hour diet recall demonstrates that Mr. Sanchez is improving in his ability to follow the prescribed diet. Scheduled a follow-up clinic phone call for 1 month, return appointment in 2 months.

Key Terms

acculturation	health traditions
assimilation	heritage assessment
cultural phenomena	heritage consistency
culture	metacommunication
emerging majority	system
ethnicity	religion
healing	socialization
health maintenance	territoriality
health protection	time orientation
health restoration	traditional approach

▪ Key Concepts

Cultural background and heritage consistency affect health in all dimensions; therefore the nurse should consider the client's background when planning care.

Many ethnic groups in North America retain the traditional heritage of their original culture.

The way in which traditional beliefs influence behaviors, attitudes, and values depends on many factors and thus is not the same for different members of a cultural group.

Stereotyping ethnic group members can lead to mistaken assumptions about a client and family.

Cultural groups vary widely in health and illness beliefs and practices; areas of verbal and nonverbal communication; time orientation; use of personal space and territoriality; susceptibility to disease; emotional and mental health; emotional expression and pain reactions; gender role behaviors; and attitudes toward the family.

Before assessing the heritage and cultural background of a client, nurses should assess personal influences of their own culture.

The nursing diagnosis for a traditional client should include problems involving the effects of cultural conflict.

The planning and implementation of nursing interventions should be adapted as much as possible to the client's cultural background.

Critical Thinking Activities

1. Discuss the problems that ethnic stereotyping and ethnocentrism may cause for the nurse. Suggest some ways nurses can learn to recognize such tendencies in themselves.

2. Discuss modifications in the health care system that can discourage members of ethnic and cultural groups to access and continue with health care programs.

3. Discuss the different illnesses and their susceptibility in different ethnic and cultural groups.

References

Abramson HE: Religion. In Thermstrom S, editor: *The Harvard encyclopedia of American ethnic groups,* Cambridge, Mass, 1980, Harvard University Press.

Beck R: *The case against immigration,* New York, 1996, WW Norton.

Bohannon P: *We, the alien,* Prospects Heights, Ill, 1992, Waveland Press.

Dresser N: *Multicultural manners,* New York, 1996, John Wiley & Sons.

Eck D: *World religions in Boston,* Cambridge, Mass, 1995, Harvard University Press.

Estes G, Zitzow D: Heritage consistency as a consideration in counseling Native Americans. Paper presented at the convention of the National Indian Education Association, Dallas, 1980.

Fejos P: Man, magic, and medicine. In Goldstone I, editor: *Medicine and anthropology,* New York, 1959, International Universities Press.

Giger JN, Davidhizar RE: *Transcultural nursing intervention,* ed 2, St. Louis, 1995, Mosby.

Hall ET: Proxemics: the study of man's spatial relations. In Goldstein I, editor: *Man's image in medicine and anthropology,* New York, 1963, International Universities Press.

Hodgkinson H: The changing demographics of minority populations and their effects on American higher education: trends, projections, and larger implications. Address delivered at the conference on Developing Multi-Cultural Leadership for the Twenty-First Century, Boston, June 15, 1988, Boston College.

Lipson J, and others: *Culture & nursing care: a pocket guide,* San Francisco, 1996, San Francisco Press.

McLemore SD: *Racial and ethnic relations in America,* Newton, Mass, 1980, Allyn & Bacon.

Spector RE: Culture, ethnicity, and nursing. In Potter PA, Perry AG: *Fundamentals of nursing,* ed 4, St. Louis, 1997, Mosby.

Spector RE: *Cultural diversity in health and illness,* ed 4, Stamford, Conn, 1996, Appleton & Lange.

Spector RE: *Guide to heritage assessment and health traditions,* Stamford, Conn, 1996, Appleton & Lange.

Thernstrom S, editor: *The Harvard encyclopedia of American ethnic groups,* Cambridge, Mass, 1980, Harvard University Press.

U.S. Bureau of the Census: *Current population reports, 1990 census of population and housing, summary population and housing characteristics, United States,* Washington, DC, 1991, U.S. Government Printing Office.

Family Context in Nursing

OBJECTIVES

Mastery of content in this chapter will enable the student to:

- Define the key terms listed.
- Examine current trends in the American family.
- Evaluate common family forms and their health implications.
- Assess the way family structure and pattern of functioning affect the health of family members and the family as a whole.
- Compare family as context to family as client and explain the way these perspectives influence nursing practice.
- Utilize the nursing process to provide for the health care needs of the family.
- Interpret both external and internal factors that promote family health.

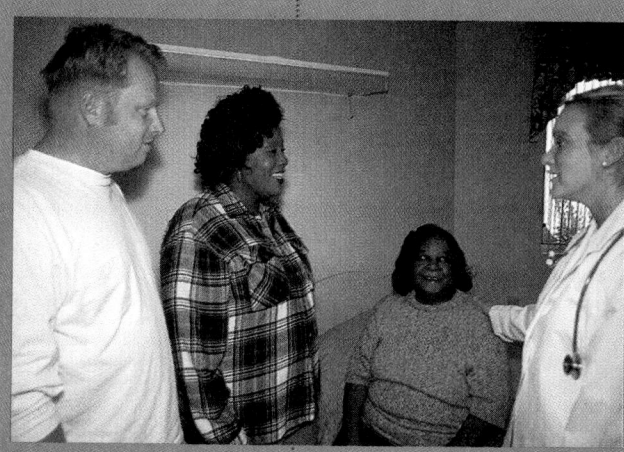

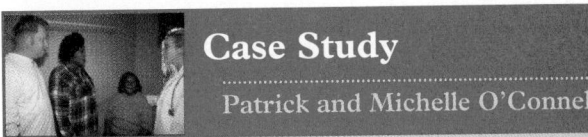

Case Study

Patrick and Michelle O'Connell

Patrick and Michelle O'Connell have been married 9 years and live in Auburn, Maine. Patrick is 38 years old, and after being employed by the state in the Department of Public Safety for the past 8 years, he has recently learned that he is in danger of being laid off in the next round of cuts. Patrick has been diagnosed with borderline hypertension and admits his stress level is an 8 on a scale of 1 to 10. He enjoys watching TV, playing war games on the computer, and playing with the family's pet dogs and cats. The family's health insurance is provided through Patrick's job. Michelle is 32 years old, is employed part-time as a receptionist at a building supply company, and attends nursing school. They are a child-free couple by choice. Michelle received a diagnosis of cervical cancer 3 months after their wedding, however, and had a vaginal hysterectomy 2 years ago. Michelle has been very worried about their financial problems and her grandmother's health problems, and she fears needing to work full-time. She describes herself as spiritual and attends church occasionally.

Michelle plays the role of keeping the couple connected to their extended families. Because each of their parents divorced and either have since remarried or are cohabitating, they have four sets of parents and 28 step-, half, and whole brothers and sisters between them. Michelle manages the household duties and finances, works, and goes to school. She is the oldest daughter in her family and is the only one of the siblings to keep in contact with her grandmother, Lois. Michelle has learned from the visiting nurse that Lois's condition has worsened—she is becoming more forgetful and less tolerant of physical activity related to severe cardiac myopathy. Michelle worries about what she can do from 2 hours away geographically. Lois needs continuous support, and for Lois to move in with her, Michelle would have to rid the house of pets, which Lois is allergic to, and her home would require major renovations to accommodate her 80-year-old grandmother.

Bethany, age 28, is the nursing student assigned to Lois in her community health rotation. She sees Lois living alone in a clean mobile home in a nice park. She understands that Lois has been widowed 17 years and that she receives Social Security and has Medicare. However, she cannot afford supplemental insurance to pay for her medications. Bethany is concerned about Lois's financial situation, especially in light of the fact the visiting nurse has said Lois may need different living arrangements.

Major changes have occurred in the concept and structure of the family, but it is clear that the family remains the central institution in American society. The current general assumption is that although the family is in transition and may look very different from the family of the 1950s, this concept of family is here to stay. Although contemporary families have their share of problems and challenges, they are characterized by three important attributes: durability, resiliency, and diversity.

Family durability is the term for the intrafamilial system of support and structure that may extend beyond the walls of the household. The players may change, the parents may remarry, the children may or may not leave home as adults, but the "family" is considered to transcend long periods and inevitable lifestyle changes.

Family resiliency is the ability to cope with expected and unexpected stressors. The family's ability to adapt to role changes, developmental milestones, and crises shows resilience. The goal of the family is not only to survive "the challenge" but also to thrive and grow as a result of the newly gained knowledge.

Family diversity is the attention to uniqueness. Some families will be experiencing marriage for the first time and having children in later life, when others are grandparents at the same age. Every person within this familial unit has specific needs, strengths, and important developmental considerations. It is our job as nurses to first understand the make-up (configuration), structure, function, and coping capacity of the family and then see how we might build on their relative strengths to overcome their weaknesses.

⋯ SCIENTIFIC KNOWLEDGE BASE

Concept of Family

Family evokes a visual image of adults and children living together in a satisfying, harmonious manner. Families are, however, as diverse as the individuals that compose them, and clients have deeply ingrained values about their families that deserve respect. Thus the nurse must think of family as defined by each individual. In other words, the nurse can think of the **family** as a set of relationships that the client identifies as family or as a network of individuals who influence each other's lives whether there are actual biological or legal ties.

Family Forms

Family forms are patterns of people considered by family members to be included in the family. Although all families have some things in common, each family form has unique problems and strengths. The nurse needs to have an open mind about what constitutes a family so that potential resources and concerns are not overlooked. Several family forms are displayed in Box 19-1.

Box 19-1
Family Forms

Nuclear Family
This family consists of husband and wife (and perhaps one or more children).

Extended Family
This family includes relatives (aunts, uncles, grandparents, and cousins) in addition to the nuclear family.

Single-Parent Family
This family is formed when one parent leaves the nuclear family because of death, divorce, or desertion or when a single person decides to have or adopt a child.

Blended Family
This family is formed when parents bring unrelated children from prior or foster parenting relationships into a new joint living situation.

Alternate Patterns of Relationships
These relationships include multi-adult households, "skip-generation" families (grandparents caring for grandchildren), communal groups with children, "non–families" (adults living alone), cohabitating partners, and homosexual couples.

Current trends and new family forms. Families are smaller today. People are marrying later, women are delaying childbirth, and couples are choosing to have fewer children or none at all. Divorce rates have tripled since the 1950s, and although the rate appears to have stabilized, it is estimated that 60% of marriages will end in divorce (U.S. Bureau of the Census, 1997).

Adolescent pregnancy is an ever-increasing concern. The majority of these adolescents continue to live with their families. A teen pregnancy tends to have long-term consequences for the mother and often severely stresses family relationships and resources. Teen fathers have stressors placed on them as well when their partner becomes pregnant. As a result, both of these adolescents are often struggling with the normal tasks of development and identity but now are also forced to accept responsibility that they may not be ready for physically, emotionally, socially, and/or financially.

Although unable to marry by law in many states, homosexual couples define their relationship in family terms. Approximately half of all gay male couples live together, compared with three fourths of lesbian couples. Homosexuals have become more open about their sexual preference and more vocal about their legal rights.

The fastest-growing age-group is 65 years and older. For the first time in history, the average American has more living parents than children, and children are more likely to have living grandparents and even great-grandparents. This "graying" of America has affected the family life cycle, perhaps most significantly for middle-age adults. Seven million American households now contain an individual who is helping an older adult with household management or personal care (Fink, 1995). This generation is finding that they must balance the needs of their offspring and the needs of their aging parents, sometimes at the expense of their own well-being and resources. Caring for a frail or chronically ill relative is a primary concern for a growing number of families.

Factors influencing family forms. Families face many challenges including changing structures and roles in the changing economic status of society. It is important to note the lack of parental supervision, role modeling, and positive interaction with caring adults if single parents are working or dual-income families are spending so much time on the job. In addition to family challenges related to divorce and the aging of its older members, there are three additional trends that social scientists identify as threats or concerns facing the family: (1) changing economic status (e.g., declining family income, lack of access to health care, growing hunger and homelessness), (2) family violence, and (3) acquired immunodeficiency syndrome (AIDS).

Making ends meet is a daily concern for many people because of the declining economic status of families. Even though two-income families have become the norm, real family income has not increased since 1973. Families at the lower end of the income scale have been particularly affected, and single-parent families are especially vulnerable. According to the Children's Defense Fund, 40% of all children in young families were living in poverty in 1990 (Clemen-Stone and others, 1995). Forty percent of all children lacked employer health coverage in 1990, and only about 25% of all infants were born to mothers who received early prenatal care.

The statistics regarding family violence are even more disturbing. Clemen-Stone and others (1995) state the following pair of staggering statistics: 2.7 million children were reported abused or neglected in 1991, up from 1.1 million in the preceding 11 years, and in the 4 years between 1986 and 1990, the need for foster care increased by almost 50%. The inflicting of emotional and physical pain on family members occurs in more than half of all households in the United States; approximately 50 million people are victimized each year. Emotional, physical, and sexual abuse occurs toward spouses, children, older adults, and across all social classes. The cause of family violence is complex and multidimensional. Factors associated with violence include stress, poverty, social isolation, psychopathology, and the cycle of violence—the intergenerational transmission of violence.

The statistics regarding human immunodeficiency virus (HIV) are becoming more alarming every day. It is estimated that in 1992 between 1 and 1.5 million people in the United States were infected with HIV. Finding that a family member is HIV-positive is devastating not only for the individual but also for the family. As with all terminal illnesses, caring for an ill family member is emotionally and financially devastating. Unfortunately, a diagnosis of HIV often carries the additional burdens of guilt, social stigma, and isolation that affect all family members.

Structure and function. Each family has a unique structure and way of functioning. Structure and function are closely related and continually interact with one another. **Family structure** is based on organization (i.e., the ongoing membership of the family and the pattern of relationships). Relationships can be numerous and complex. For example, a woman's relationships may include wife-husband, mother-son, and mother-daughter and employee-boss, boss-employee, and work colleague-colleague, each with different demands, roles, and expectations.

Although the definitions of structure vary, the nurse asks the following questions: "Who is included in the family?" "Who performs which tasks?" and "Who makes which decisions?" Structure may enhance or detract from the family's ability to respond to the expected and unexpected stressors of daily life. Very rigid or very flexible structures can threaten the functioning of the family. A rigid structure specifically dictates persons permitted to accomplish a task and may also limit the number of persons outside the immediate family allowed to assume these tasks. For example, the mother might be considered the only acceptable person to provide emotional support for the children and/or to perform all of the household chores. The husband may be the only acceptable person to provide financial support, maintain the vehicles, do the yard work, and/or do all of the home repairs. A change in the health status of the person responsible for a task places a burden on the family because no other person is available or considered acceptable to assume that task. An extremely open structure can also present problems for the family. Stability that otherwise leads to automatic action during a crisis or rapid change is often absent.

Friedman (1992) describes functioning as "what the family does." **Family functioning** involves the processes used by the family to achieve its goals. These processes include communication among family members, goal setting, conflict resolution, nurturing, and use of internal and external resources. The reproductive, sexual, economic, and educational goals once considered central family goals no longer apply to all families. Although many families pursue these goals at various times during their development, the provision of psychological support remains an important goal throughout the life span.

Developmental stages. Families, like individuals, change and grow over time. Although families are far from identical to one another, they have a basic pattern and similarity in experiences resulting in predictable stages. Each of these developmental stages has its own challenges, needs, and resources and includes tasks that need to be completed before the family can successfully move on to the next stage (Table 19-1).

Family and health. Family health influences family functioning, and family functioning, in turn, influences its own and society's perceptions of its health. When the family satisfactorily meets its goals through adequate functioning, its members tend to feel positive about themselves and their family. Conversely, when they do not meet goals, families view themselves as ineffective. Constant stress resulting from inadequate functioning can also adversely affect an individual family member's health. Constant stress may disrupt cardiovascular function, blood pressure, and circulating neuroendocrine substances, and these disruptions may cause poor health (see Chapter 21). Maladaptive behaviors within the family have a negative impact on the health of members and the overall ability of the family to meet its goals. A lack of communication or poor communication inhibits the family's ability to make decisions and solve problems. Good health may not be highly valued by the client and by the family, and in fact, detrimental practices may be accepted. In some cases a family member may provide mixed messages about health. For example, a parent may continue to smoke while telling children that smoking is bad for them. Family environment is crucial because health behavior reinforced in early life has a strong influence on later health practices.

The crisis-proof or effective family is able to integrate the need for stability with the need for growth and change and has a flexible structure allowing adaptable performance of tasks and acceptance of help from outside the family unit. Recently, health promotion research has started to focus on the stress-moderating effect of "hardiness" as a factor that contributes to long-term health. Danielson and others (1993) define **family hardiness** as "the internal strengths and durability of the family unit, characterized by a sense of control over the outcome of life events and hardships, a view of change as beneficial and growth-producing, and as an active rather than passive orientation in responding to stressful life events."

⋯NURSING KNOWLEDGE BASE

To begin work with families, nurses must have not only a scientific knowledge base in family theory but also an adequate knowledge base in family nursing. Because nurses must apply these concepts of family theory in

TABLE 19-1
Stages of the Family Life Cycle

Family Life Cycle Stage	Emotional Process of Transition: Key Principles	Changes in Family Status Required to Proceed Developmentally
Between families: unattached young adult	Accepting parent-offspring separation	Differentiation of self in relation to family of origin Development of intimate peer relationships Establishment of self in work
Joining of families through marriage: newly married couple	Commitment to new system	Formation of marital system Realignment of relationships with extended families and friends to include spouse
Family with young children	Accepting new generation of members into system	Adjusting marital system to make space for children Taking on parenting roles Realignment of relationships with extended family to include parenting and grandparenting roles
Family with adolescents	Increasing flexibility of family boundaries to include children's independence	Shifting of parent-child relationships to permit adolescents to move into and out of system Refocus on midlife marital and career issues Beginning shift toward concerns for older generation
Launching children and moving on	Accepting multitude of exits from and entries into family system	Renegotiation of marital system as dyad Development of adult-to-adult relationships between grown children and their parents Realignment of relationships to include in-laws and grandchildren Dealing with disabilities and death of parents (grandparents)
Family in later life	Accepting shifting of generational roles	Maintaining own or couple functioning and interests in the face of physiological decline; exploration of new familial and social role options Support for more central role for middle generation Making room in system for wisdom and experience of older adults; supporting older generation without overfunctioning for them Dealing with loss of spouse, siblings, and other peers, and preparation for own death; life review and integration

From McGoldrick M, Carter E: The stages of the family life cycle. In Henslin J, editor: *Marriage and family in a changing society,* New York, 1985, Free Press; in Walsh F: *Normal family processes,* New York, 1982, Guilford Press.

nursing practice, they must consider how the concepts interact to affect the care that is delivered to the family. Family nursing is the focus of the future across all practice settings and is emphasized in all health care environments.

Family Nursing: Family as Environment and as Client

The goal of the family nurse is to help the family and its individual members reach and maintain maximum health in any given situation. Bradley (1996) examines the shift of health care focus from the individual to the family. With earlier discharges and technological ad-

vances, the informal care delivery system assumes the greatest role in providing care and support to clients (Lyman, 1995). The nurse must always be aware that clients are affected by their families whether members are present and that clients, in turn, affect their families. A family nursing focus includes both **family as context** and **family as client** (Figure 19-1). Although theoretical and practical distinctions can be made between the two approaches, they are not necessarily mutually exclusive. Both approaches recognize that a nursing intervention for one member influences all members and affects family functioning. Friedman (1992) and Robinson (1995) believe a person should not be thought of as *either* an individual *or* a family member

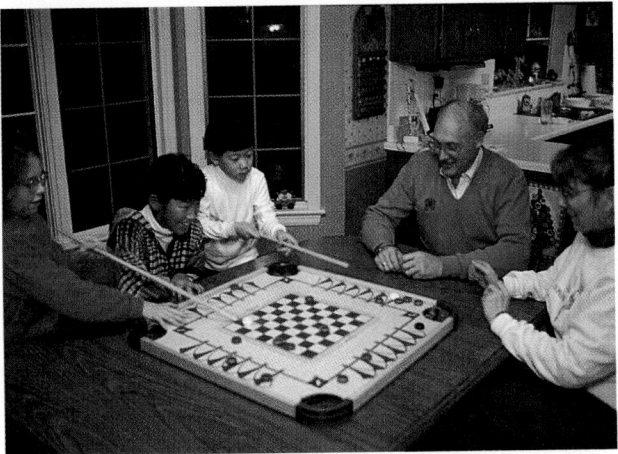

Figure 19-1.   Observing family interactions assists in understanding family functioning.

but *both* (now called the **family as system**). The family is viewed as an irreducible whole that is not understood by knowledge of individual members (Newby, 1996). In utilizing this theoretical framework, nurses can consider the family to be in a state of change that is innovative and continuous. In more simple language, it means nurses must try to understand that the family is more complex than simply a combination of individual members.

Family as context. With family as context the primary focus is the health and development of an individual member existing within a specific environment. Although the nursing process concentrates on the individual's health status, the nurse assesses the extent to which the family provides for the individual's basic needs. Families provide more than just material essentials, so their ability to help the client meet psychological needs and strive for optimal health must also be considered.

Family as client. With this approach the family is the primary focus of nursing care. Family patterns and processes are studied. The nursing process concentrates on the extent to which these patterns and processes are consistent with reaching and maintaining family and individual health.

CRITICAL THINKING IN CLIENT CARE

Critical thinking is crucial in the care of clients and their families. The elements of critical thinking require synthesis and ongoing evaluation of the family. The care of a family as a client is an ongoing mutually acceptable relationship, not just a product or care plan tool for

nurses to follow like a cookbook recipe. There is ongoing thought, analysis, and reflection required to meet the goals and needs of the clients and their families as nurses attempt to elevate them to their highest possible functional level or toward a dignified death.

Synthesis

The scientific knowledge and family nursing knowledge bases enable nurses to identify the needs of both clients and their families. The nurse assesses the family as context, family as client, family systems theory, family life-cycle perspective, family structure, family functioning, and family health. Nurses combine knowledge about the family and their functioning with nursing knowledge of holistic practice, including the biological, psychological, sociological, spiritual, and cultural dimensions of analysis.

Knowledge. The health and functioning of each member in the family to some degree depends on the health of the other levels of the family system. Nurses draw on knowledge from growth and development, psychology, basic and social sciences, and the family life-cycle perspective. When a family is in a transitional phase of the life-cycle perspective (e.g., birth of a first child) and there is an additional stressor to the family unit (e.g., chronic illness), it creates a quantum leap of anxiety within the family system. Illness and its treatment affect each family member and the family functioning.

Experience. Past experience in a related situation often helps us to problem solve. We all draw on life experience even if we are not able to draw on nursing knowledge. Experiences with our own family members enable nurses to design family-centered care. We remember how illness may have brought family members closer together because they all shared duties, roles, and responsibilities. Past life experience can be used to enhance problem solving in current situations. Application of experience-related information needs to be considered carefully because no two families are alike.

Nurses use a variety of techniques, among them problem solving, critical thinking, and the nursing process, to provide individualized nursing care. Textbooks offer suggestions and demonstrate skills, but ultimately it is the nurse interacting with the client who must assess, diagnose, plan, implement, and evaluate whether an intervention is effective in this particular case. No two clients and families are the same, but there is value in sharing experience and transferring learning from one situation to the next, rather than "reinventing the wheel" if an idea works.

Attitudes. Demonstrating an open mind, creativity, perseverance, and risk taking, the nurse can identify the client's needs and begin to solve the problems. Respect for the client's family structure and function, beliefs, values, and expectations enables nurses to develop a comprehensive, multidisciplinary plan *in partnership with* the client and family.

Standards. Nurses must use applicable nursing content area standards (e.g., obstetrical, gerontological) plus delivery area standards (e.g., home health, acute care, long-term care) and ethical and professional standards when providing care to the family. Because a portion of family-centered nursing may be provided in community-based, clinic, or restorative care settings, as well as in the acute care setting, information about the family must be kept confidential, and documentation of pertinent information must be accurate, consistent, and accountable.

NURSING PROCESS FOR THE FAMILY

The nursing process is the same whether the focus is family as client or family as context. It is also the same as that used with individuals.

Assessment

Family assessment is an essential component of the nursing process. Box 19-2 can be used as an assessment tool. There are many family assessment forms available. Although the family as a whole differs from individual members, the measure of family health must be more than a summation of the health of all members. Areas included in family assessment are the form, structure, and function of the family; its developmental stage; and its progress toward or accomplishment of developmental tasks. Cultural background is an important variable when assessing the family because race and ethnicity have an impact on structure and function and influence health beliefs and values. The nurse begins assessment by considering the attitudes of family members and the client toward family. The nurse also incorporates family needs into the nursing process. To determine the family form and membership, the nurse can ask the client "Whom do you consider your family?" or "With whom do you share strong emotional feelings?" If the client is unable to express a concept of family, the nurse can ask with whom the client lives, spends time, and shares confidences and then ask the client to validate this observation: "Do you consider this person to be family or like family to you?" To further assess the family structure, the nurse can ask questions that determine the power structure and patterning of roles and tasks, for example, "How are the tasks divided in your family?" "Who does the laundry?" "Who mows the lawn?" and "Who decides on where to go on vacation?" Because a moderately flexible structure is generally most beneficial to the family, nursing interventions therefore may involve

modulating the family patterns away from extremely rigid or flexible structures if either extreme causes problems related to the health of an individual or the family as a whole. In general, however, the nurse attempts to work within the family structure when providing care and does not attempt to change the structure.

The nurse assesses family functions such as the ability to provide emotional support for members, the ability to cope with their current health problem or situation, the appropriateness of their goal setting, and progress toward achievement of tasks of the developmental stage. Although families' goals vary, measures of family health care must be flexible. The nurse also assesses whether the family can provide and allocate sufficient economic resources and if their social network is extensive enough to provide support.

Client expectations. Families, like individual clients, have certain expectations for care. The family may expect to be consulted as a whole unit when discussing care of their loved one, or the family may wish to have a designated decision maker. The family may expect the health care system to meet all of their needs, not only those related to health issues. When meeting the family's expectations, the nurse should be clear whether the family is the client and receiver of care or whether the family member is the client and receiver of care. Determining these expectations early in the assessment can avoid problems resulting from misunderstandings in the future.

Successful critical thinking requires a synthesis of knowledge, experience, information gathered from clients, and critical thinking attitudes and standards. Clinical judgments require the nurse to anticipate what information is needed, analyze the data, and then make decisions regarding client care. The client and family expect competent and informed care. Bethany incorporates previous knowledge and experience in providing care for Patrick, Michelle, and Michelle's grandmother, Lois.

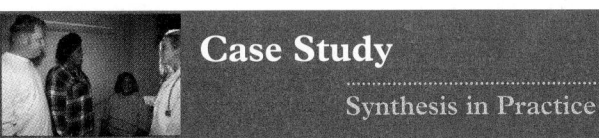

Case Study
Synthesis in Practice

Bethany assesses Lois's social belonging, health care, and basic physiological needs. She analyzes the role strain on Michelle and how this affects her relationship with Patrick. She operates under the ethical principle of beneficence and tries to do the most good for the most people in this case. She understands that Lois wants to stay in her home, and Michelle wants Lois to do what will make her happiest. Patrick wants Michelle to do whatever will not aggravate Michelle's stress level or force her to quit

Continued

Box 19-2
Assessment Tool

The family assessment tool is used when the beginning student interviews family members and observes family interaction. It is a guideline only and is not meant to be all inclusive. The student must also ensure that individual health histories accompany this assessment.

Family Form and Structure

Names of adults   Ages

_____

Relationship _____
                                    (Single, married, divorced, separated, cohabiting)

Names of children   Ages

_____

_____

_____

Others living in home (include age, sex, relationship) _____

_____

Cultural background (include pertinent health beliefs, child-rearing practices, related health concerns)

_____

Developmental stage _____

Progress toward accomplishment of developmental tasks _____

Concerns related to developmental stage _____

Resources

Significant relatives and friends not occupying immediate residence _____

Strengths and coping skills _____

How does the family obtain health services? _____

Membership in community groups (e.g., church affiliation) _____

Education (formal and informal) _____

Finances (ability to meet current and future needs) _____

Family Patterns

Persons working outside the home _____

Type of work _____ Number of hours _____

Satisfaction with work _____

How are the housekeeping tasks accomplished? _____

Are family members satisfied with the way tasks are divided? _____

How are child-rearing responsibilities divided? _____

Who makes the major decisions in the family? _____

Who makes day-to-day decisions? _____

Are family members satisfied with the way decisions are made? _____

Family Function

Goals

Long term _____

Short term _____

Individual family member's goals _____

Are individual and family goals appropriate, considering their current health problem and status? _____

How are individual family members and the family as a whole coping with their current health problem and status?

_____

Communication

Do husband and wife communicate regularly and effectively with each other? _____

Are family members able to communicate openly and honestly with each other? _____

Is conflict openly expressed and discussed? _____

Do family members respect one another's point of view? _____

Do family members offer emotional support to each other? _____

Continued from p. 337

school, because they may soon have to depend on more income from her.

If the family is viewed as context, the nurse focuses on the client as an individual. Bethany assesses Patrick's knowledge of high-sodium foods, strategies for reducing the number of high-sodium foods in the diet, realistic opportunities to reduce the number and extent of perceived stressors in work and family environments, and knowledge and skill in stress management such as relaxation or biofeedback techniques.

If the family is viewed as client, Bethany assesses the family's current dietary patterns and their desire and resources for changing the patterns. The nurse determines the demands placed on the hypertensive client and the family. The family's capabilities to support the hypertensive member's development and use of stress management are also assessed.

Nursing Diagnosis

Nursing assessment results in clustering pertinent data that support the nursing diagnosis and identifying cases in which functioning is inadequate or deficient and intervention is needed. The nursing diagnosis may include the family's health needs, current and potential health problems, level of wellness, or a combination of the above. In addition, the diagnostic statement should indicate possible causes and etiologies.

The nursing diagnosis often focuses on the family's ability to cope with their current situation, whether it is an acute illness, an anticipated developmental transition, or negative behaviors that are threatening short-term or long-term health (see nursing diagnoses box). Appropriate use of internal and external resources can allow the family to cope with day-to-day challenges and with unexpected occurrences that threaten health and equilibrium. Coping strategies can be adaptive or maladaptive. During times of acute illness the family can become extremely distressed and focuses solely on the ill member, neglecting the needs of the other family members. The needs of other family members can be easily overlooked unless the nurse consistently employs a family nursing perspective. The diagnosis of *risk for care-giver role strain*, for example, should always be considered a possibility when long-term care of a family member is necessary.

Nursing diagnosis involves a database about the family and the nurse's identification and evaluation of potential stressors that pose a threat to the stability of the family unit (Berkey and Hanson, 1993). Identifying the correct related factor or factors is essential to choosing the appropriate plan of action.

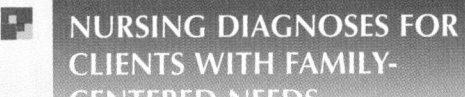

NURSING DIAGNOSES FOR CLIENTS WITH FAMILY-CENTERED NEEDS

Caregiver role strain, risk for
Coping, family: potential for growth
Coping, ineffective family: compromised
Coping, ineffective family: disabling
Family processes, altered
Parenting, altered
Parental role conflict
Role performance, altered
Spiritual well-being, potential for enhanced
Violence, risk for: directed at others

Planning

After nursing diagnoses are developed, the next step is to plan care with the family. Nursing practice may be enhanced by a family-focused approach (St. John and Rolls, 1996). Planning includes goal setting, identification of potential internal and external resources, choosing effective approaches, and setting priorities. It is imperative that the plan of care be clearly understood and agreed on by the family. Goal setting must be mutual, and the goals must be concrete, realistic, compatible with the developmental stage, and acceptable to the family.

Collaboration with family members is an essential component during this stage (Figure 19-2). A positive collaborative relationship is based on mutual respect and trust (Danielson and others, 1993) and is facilitated by allowing the family to feel as "in control" as possible. For example, offering alternative actions and

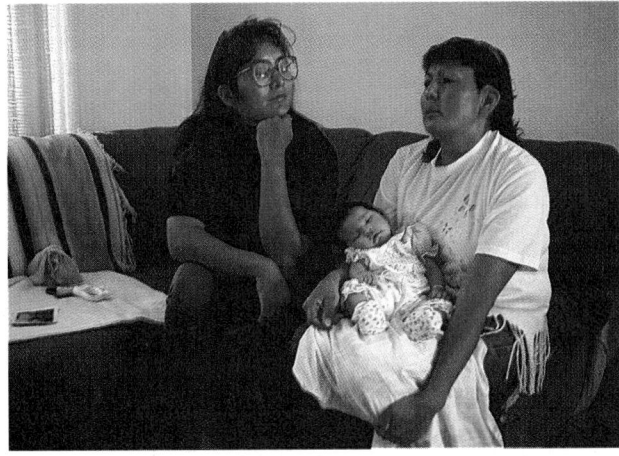

Figure 19-2. Family members assisting one another in caring for a newborn. (Photo by Michael S. Clement, MD, Mesa, Ariz.)

asking family members for their own ideas and suggestions can reduce feelings of powerlessness. Collaboration also extends to other health care professionals. As Danielson and others (1993) point out, it is impossible to be all things to all families. Collaborating with other disciplines and utilizing good delegation skills increases the likelihood of a comprehensive care plan and can provide for continuity of care. Using other disciplines is particularly important for discharge planning because referrals are often necessary to ensure that long-term goals will be attained.

CASE STUDY NURSING CARE PLAN

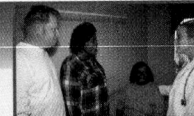

Ineffective Family Coping: Compromised

Assessment
Patrick and Michelle are **care givers to Michelle's grandmother,** Lois, who has severe cardiac myopathy, which causes less oxygen flow to the brain and muscles, creating her forgetfulness, fatigue, and fear-producing angina episodes.

Patrick also needs assistance in altering his diet and **developing stress management techniques** to help him cope with his borderline hypertension, which is thought to be related to high sodium intake, **a stressful job,** and continuing expectations by his family for participation in their activities.

Nursing Diagnosis
Ineffective family coping: compromised related to husband's inadequate understanding of his stress management's impact on primary care giver, Michelle.

Planning

Goals

Husband will gain improved understanding of stress and adaptive management techniques (5/1).

Husband will accept wife's household role limitations (3/30).

Husband will accept non–family member help if needed (3/30).

Expected Outcomes

Husband will be able to identify and perform a share of household activities (4/30).

Husband will not demonstrate impatient behavior (if tasks are not done at home) while she performs some care-giving activities (3/27).

Husband will be comfortable with help non–family member can give with household roles (3/27).

Implementation

Steps

1. Discuss with Patrick effects of stress and reasons it occurs, and provide reading material designed for family members of clients with stress and its effect on families.

2. Provide list of support groups for Patrick and care giver support groups for Michelle.

3. Consult with Patrick and Michelle to establish a list of community resources, friends, and volunteers to assist with care-giver tasks and household activities.

Rationale

Accurate information will assist husband in interpreting wife's limitations.

Group support allows care giver to share experiences, stresses, and coping methods.

Provides a potential list of family resources. Having a list available can provide family with the security of a "backup" system.

Evaluation
Ask husband to describe household activities he will be able to perform and activities that will require assistance from wife.

Observe husband interacting with wife during home visit for signs of frustration and violent temper that may impede Michelle's functioning and her caregiving activities for Lois.

Observe effectiveness of combined efforts of husband and wife, and determine if they are sufficient. If not, consider suggesting non–family member assistance.

Defining characteristics are shown in bold type.

Goals for a care plan that incorporates a family approach may include those that view the family as client or the family as context or a combination of the two. The client situation and availability of family members dictate the type of goals that are feasible. A broad goal could be "The family functions at its optimal level," with the expected outcome being "communication between family members is appropriate, direct, and clear." Family members are able to confront and resolve conflict in a healthy way. *The broader the goals, however, the less measurable and practical they become.* For examples of specific goals for the case study, see the care plan box.

Implementation

After goals and actions have been defined, implementation begins. Interventions are strategies that help families adjust goals or are the processes by which the family attains them. Family interventions include nursing actions that increase members' abilities in a certain area, remove barriers to health care, and do things that the family cannot do for themselves. The nurse guides family members in problem solving and provides practical service and concrete aid. One of the roles the nurse will need to adopt is that of educator. Providing accurate health information about diagnosis and prognosis helps the care giver not to "blame" the client and to interpret behavior correctly. Care givers are not born with the knowledge of how to be care givers, and older adults are not born with the knowledge of how to accept dependency (Box 19-3).

Health promotion. As part of the implementation phase, health promotion is always included. This encourages clients and families to reach their optimum level of wellness.

Identifying attributes that contribute to healthy and resilient families has been a focus of ongoing research for at least three decades. "Strong" families that adapt to expected transitions and unexpected crises and change tend to be characterized by clear communication, problem-solving skills, a commitment to each other and to the family unit, and a sense of cohesiveness and spirituality. Prevention programs aimed at enhancing or developing these attributes are available for families and children in many communities (Thomas, 1994). The nurse needs to be aware of family-oriented offerings so that clients can be referred as needed. Often, health promotion behaviors that the nurse needs to encourage are tied to the developmental stage of the family, for example, effective prenatal care for the childbearing family and adherence to immunization schedules for the child-rearing family (Box 19-4).

One approach for meeting goals and promoting health is the use of family strengths. Families are not accustomed to looking at their own system as one that has inherent positive components. The nurse can help the family become aware of its own unique strengths, thereby increasing its potentials and capabilities. Family strengths include clear communication, adaptability, healthy child-rearing practices, support and nurturing among family members, active community participation, and the use of crisis for growth. The nurse can help the family focus on its strengths instead of its problems and weaknesses (see care plan box).

Challenges for family nursing. Delegation in the management of nursing care activities can become a challenge in family nursing. Often nurses are trying to make an impact on family health by delegating duties to family members or to other members of the health care team. For example, the nurse helps family members learn how to provide certain types of procedures to care for an ill family member. With earlier discharge and more complex family needs at time of discharge, planning for discharge begins with the initiation of care by the registered nurse.

Multidisciplinary collaboration from registered dietitians, wound care specialty nurses, clinical nurse

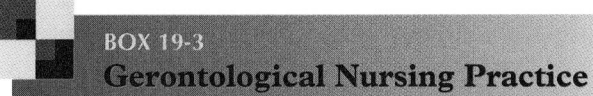

BOX 19-3
Gerontological Nursing Practice

- The nurse must consider care-giver strain; care givers are usually either spouses, who may also be an older adult and may have declining physical stamina, or middle-age children, who often have other responsibilities.
- Later-life families may have a different social network than younger families because friends and same-generation family members may have died or been ill themselves. The nurse may need to look for social support within the community and church affiliation.
- Greater physical health impairment increases the risk of the older adult's depression.
- As in the other stages of life, members of later-life families need to be working on developmental tasks (see Chapter 20).

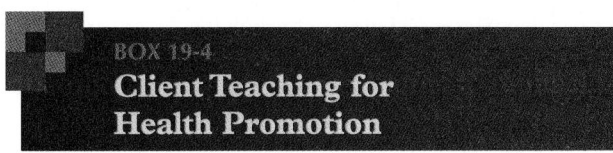

BOX 19-4
Client Teaching for Health Promotion

- Instruct client and family members about medication, treatment, and future appointments.
- Provide specific strategies for modification in family's nutritional, exercise, and coping patterns.
- Provide new parents with immunization schedules and community resources for obtaining necessary immunization.
- Contact national organizations for resources, publications, and low-cost membership for parents (e.g., Children's Defense Fund, Family Resource Coalition).

specialists, clergy or spiritual healers, physical therapy, and/or occupational therapy can all help better meet the needs of families. Cost management, regardless of practice setting, is becoming an ever important issue requiring more efficient use of resources. These resources are often personnel. Collaboration is becoming a key component within cost management.

Cultural sensitivity (see Chapter 18) in family nursing requires recognizing not only the diverse ethnic, cultural, and religious backgrounds of nurses dealing with the clients but also the differences and similarities even within the same family. Different-age family members may ascribe to different folk remedies, health care beliefs, and religious influences. Using effective and respectful communication techniques enables the nurse to determine the family's strengths and areas for potential problems.

Acute care.

The family is becoming more of the focus and nursing will need to take more of a role in emphasizing family and client needs within the context of health care delivery in a managed care environment. Nurses need to be ever mindful of the early discharge states, paired with the increasing numbers of people within the household now being employed outside the home. These factors are challenges to the nurse to prepare family members to assist with health care or to locate appropriate community resources. Often when family members assume the role of care giver, they may lose support from significant others. The nurse must be sure that families are willing to assume care responsibilities.

Restorative care.

Family nurses emphasize approaches used in maintaining clients' functional abilities. These include trying to seek home health nurses to allow clients to remain in their homes after an acute injury, surgery, or illness. It may also entail looking into ways in which nurses can better the lives of chronically ill individuals and their families. Nurses assess clients' strengths and areas of concern and then emphasize their strengths so they may be used to help overcome their weaknesses. Clients with diabetes (a chronic condition) can learn to feel very much in control of their diet, exercise, medication regimen, and overall family/social lifestyle and thus "feel" healthy.

▪ Evaluation

Client care. When the client's family functions as context, evaluation focuses on attainment of client needs. Thus evaluation is client centered, although nursing measures may have involved assisting the client to adapt to the family environment. The response of the client is compared with predetermined outcomes.

When the family receives care while functioning as the client, the measure of family health must be more than a summation of the health of all family members. For example, the family's attainment of family developmental tasks may be a useful criterion. The nurse evaluates the family's change in functioning and their satisfaction with the new level of functioning.

Evaluation is an ongoing process. Goals and interventions are modified as needed. Evaluation must come not only from the nurse but also from the client's and family's perspectives. The goals are constantly evaluated by both to see that the health care team is meeting the expectations of family members, as well as family members meeting the expectations of the health care team.

Client care. The nurse uses critical thinking skills and clinical decision making to evaluate the client's responses to interventions. Often the client and/or family doesn't know how care could be delivered differently or better. They may think the pain medication doesn't work at all; however, an adjustment in scheduling may be all that is required. They may not be as trusting, or they may want to be a "good patient" and not complain. So the Cambodian client may not eat at all or may select a very limited menu that doesn't provide all the nutrients the client needs to heal well.

It is this constant evaluation of the client's response to care provided, both verbally and nonverbally, that determines future implementation strategies. Each client and family is so unique. Family nursing requires the use of therapeutic communication skills, scientific and family nursing knowledge, critical thinking skills, knowledge of oneself, and extensive learning about the clients and their families.

Client expectations. It is important to obtain the family's perspective of the care: how the care was delivered, how it was planned, whether it was delivered to satisfy them, whether it worked to attain those mutually planned goals, and if not, what they think was needed instead. With a truly trusting relationship between client and nurse, this information can be obtained to create an even more positive atmosphere. This evaluation is requested throughout the care planning to modify or adjust care delivery techniques (e.g., how soon the home health nurse was able to make a visit, adequacy of comfort measures, timeliness of care) or even to adjust care delivery personnel (e.g., sending a dietitian who is familiar with Cambodian cuisine rather than the dietary technician who tries to get the client to select foods on a ready-made list for meal planning).

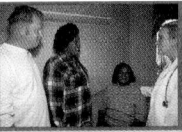

Case Study

Bethany visits Lois periodically throughout the semester and checks to see how the family's short-term goals are coming along regarding Patrick's stress management program. She also checks to see how Lois's short-term and long-term goals are being fulfilled regarding her care in the home, activity tolerance, forgetfulness, loneliness, and financial worries. Bethany assesses Michelle's stress level with school, home, and long-distance planning around her grandmother's needs. To assess Michelle and Patrick, she may request that a family meeting be arranged once a month. This ongoing evaluation requires frequent input from the care givers working with Lois in the home, the primary nurse who knows the family best, the family members themselves, the health care provider who is involved, and the chaplain, social worker, nutritionist, and physical and/or occupational therapist who are involved. This is not always an easy thing to accomplish. The nurse dealing with the family, whether in the hospital or home setting, is the invisible glue that holds things together. The nurse is the true coordinator and evaluator of care provided, and Bethany knows this.

Bethany learns through the course of the semester that Patrick has been able to begin implementing some of the more positive coping strategies he has learned. He is also able to help Michelle around the house with some of the laundry, cooking, and dishes every other night and has even begun to learn the finances. When he realized how important his help has become to everyone in the family, he felt more needed and wanted to help. Michelle has more free time to concentrate on her studies every other night so she can "hurry through school to get a better job to help their financial future plans," as she and Patrick have wanted. One day a week and every other weekend she spends with Lois to observe her grandmother's condition, help to plan her care, ease Lois's loneliness, and reduce the number of paid nursing care hours per week.

Bethany had discussed the long-term goals of including the community in Lois's care, and though it was not easy to implement, she later learned from the primary nurse that the plan is working. Lois has a political candidate to back, and every Tuesday afternoon for 2 hours she stuffs envelopes and visits with other volunteers working on the campaign. She goes to the Salvation Army Senior Enrichment Program every Monday morning for bingo and lunch. Her church auxiliary meets Wednesday mornings for 2 hours at her home, and the quilting/sewing circle has begun meeting on Friday mornings for 2 hours there as well. This creative use of resources within the community disperses Lois's care among home health aides for morning care/baths and afternoon care. A registered nurse visits for 1 hour per week, a hospice volunteer takes Lois to the Senior Enrichment Program on Mondays, Lois receives Meals-on-Wheels a couple of days per week, and a clergyman visits once per week. Lois has regional transportation for those times when Michelle or the volunteer is unavailable, and she receives paid CNAs from a local agency for overnights. In addition, Lois sees the physician once per month. The CNA overnight service is used during the week, and the cost is divided among all the family members who live too far away to help with Lois's care. Michelle has found family members willing to take turns caring for Lois during the weekends that Michelle stays with Patrick.

Documentation Note

Patrick and Michelle are participating in family meetings; both report that sitting down together helps them deal with the stress of their jobs, school, and the care of Lois. Michelle feels that she and Patrick are partners in the work of the family. The overnight care of Lois by the CNA has helped relieve some of the stress. Both Patrick and Michelle know that Lois will eventually need nursing home care and have begun looking at agencies together.

Key Terms

family	family as system
family form	family functioning
family hardiness	family health
family as client	family structure
family as context	

▪ Key Concepts ▪▪

The family has a significant impact on the lives of its members.

Family members mutually influence one another's health beliefs, practices, and status.

Because the concept of family is highly individualized, the nurse should base care on the client's attitude toward family rather than on an inflexible definition of it.

Specific family forms tend to have typical family health problems with which the nurse should be familiar.

The family's structure and functioning significantly influence its health and ability to respond to health problems.

The nurse can view the family as an important context for the individual family member, can view the family unit as the client, or both. The approach for any family depends in part on the situation.

Measures of family health involve more than a summation of an individual members' health.

The family's health is influenced by their social class, economic stability, and racial and ethnic background.

Critical Thinking Activities

1. Imagine one of your clients is a young child with a contagious illness. List some suggestions you might give the parents to deal with the care of the child and to provide a positive family life for the client's siblings. How would your approach differ if the child was from a single-parent family?

2. Think of the family in which you grew up. Describe the values and attitudes you learned in this environment and the influence they may have on how you view your client's family and health practices.

References

Berkey KM, Hanson SM: *Family assessment and intervention,* St. Louis, 1993, Mosby.

Bradley SF: Processes in the creation and diffusion of nursing knowledge: an examination of the developing concept of family-centered care, *J Adv Nurs* 23(4):722, 1996.

Clemen-Stone S and others: *Family-centered approach to community health nursing practice,* St. Louis, 1995, Mosby.

Danielson DB and others: *Family, health and illness,* St. Louis, 1993, Mosby.

Fink SV: The influence of family resources and family demands on the strains and well-being of caregiving families, *Nurs Res* 44(3):139, 1995.

Friedman MM: *Family nursing: theory and assessment,* ed 2, New York, 1992, Appleton-Century-Crofts.

Lyman MJ: Supporting one another: the nature of family work when a young adult has cancer, *J Adv Nurs* 22(1):116, 1995.

McGoldrick M, Carter E: The stages of the family life cycle. In Henslin J, editor: *Marriage and family in a changing society,* New York, 1985, Free Press; in Walsh F: *Normal family processes,* New York, 1982, Guilford Press.

Newby NM: Chronic illness and the family life-cycle, *J Adv Nurs* 23(4):786, 1996.

Robinson CA: Beyond dichotomies in the nursing of persons and families, *Image J Nurs Sch* 27(2):116, 1995.

St. John W, Rolls C: Teaching family nursing: strategies and experiences, *J Adv Nurs* 23(1):91, 1996.

Thomas HS: Conceptual underpinnings of the family support movement, *J Pediatr Health Care* 8(2):57, 1994.

U.S. Bureau of the Census: *Statistical abstracts of the United States: 1996,* ed 116, Washington DC, 1997, U.S. Government Printing Office.

CHAPTER

20

Growth and Development

OBJECTIVES

Mastery of content in this chapter will enable the student to:

- Define the key terms listed.
- Compare the frameworks for growth and development as described by major developmental theorists.
- Describe the growth and development changes that occur in individuals from conception through old age.
- Identify factors that can facilitate or interfere with normal growth and development of individuals at each stage of life.
- Specify the physical and psychosocial health concerns of infants, children, adolescents, and adults.
- Use knowledge of growth and development to enhance nursing assessments, interventions, and evaluation of individuals across the life span.
- Identify specific nursing interventions for the health promotion of clients across the life span.
- Use critical judgment to determine appropriate teaching topics for individual clients across the life span.

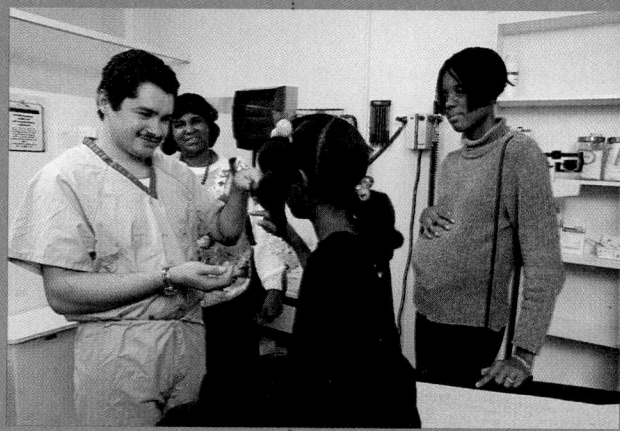

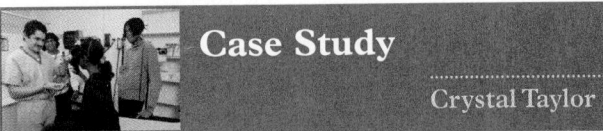

Case Study

Crystal Taylor

Crystal Taylor, a 25-year-old black young adult, is the single parent of 2½-year-old Zachary and 5½-year-old Monica and is in the sixth month of a current pregnancy. She lives with her 44-year-old mother and 15-year-old brother. Crystal's 68-year-old maternal grandmother and uncle live next door and often help care for Zachary and Monica. Crystal's family has used the city clinic for years, and she now brings her children to the neighborhood clinic for their health care. Today she has brought Monica to the clinic for her checkup before beginning school.

Louis Ruiz is a 28-year-old student assigned to the clinic, where he is to select a family to follow throughout the semester. Louis, who is married and has a 4-year-old son who attends day care, was a medical technician in the army for 4 years. The clinic is Louis' first clinical experience as a student nurse, and he is eager to become involved in health promotion activities but also anxious about his new role as a professional nurse.

Nursing promotes the health of individuals of all ages. This requires the nurse to have a strong knowledge base of developmental changes that occur in persons across the life span. A clear understanding of normal or expected growth and behavior allows the nurse to detect deviations and promote normal development. Viewing clients from a developmental perspective assists the nurse to provide care in a manner that takes into consideration the unique needs and level of development of each individual.

SCIENTIFIC KNOWLEDGE BASE

Growth and Development Theory

The terms *growth* and *development* are often referred to as a unit that expresses the sum of numerous changes that take place throughout the individual's lifetime (Wong, 1995). **Growth** is the measurable (quantitative) aspect of an individual's increase in physical dimensions as a result of an increase in cell number. Indicators of growth include changes in height, weight, teeth, skeletal structures, and sexual characteristics. **Development** is the behavioral (qualitative) aspect of an individual's adaptation to the environment. Behaviors that indicate development are increased functioning capacity such as occurs in learning to walk and talk.

Maturation is the genetically determined biological plan for growth and development. Physical growth and motor development are a function of maturation. Examples of age-related behaviors that follow a specific sequence are sitting, walking, and reading, which are a result of maturation. Children cannot be taught these behaviors until their bodies are physiologically ready, yet environmental forces can hasten or prolong this hereditary timetable. Babies who are carried on their mother's back or hip will be slower to crawl than those who have regular playtime on the floor and are encouraged to crawl.

A **critical period of development** refers to a specific time period when the environment has its greatest effect on a specific aspect of development of the individual (Papalia and Olds, 1995). This concept is true during both intrauterine and extrauterine periods of life and can be applied to both psychological and physical aspects of development. An example of a critical period in psychological development would be related to language development before puberty. Young children may learn to speak a foreign language without an accent, whereas those beyond puberty may speak quite fluently but retain an accent.

Major Factors Influencing Growth and Development

The human being is a complex, open system influenced by natural forces from within and by external forces from the environment. Interaction between these forces affects development. In general, natural factors provide potential for development such as height and intelligence, whereas external factors provide opportunities for achieving potential or not fulfilling genetic potential (Table 20-1). The most influential forces of nature are heredity and temperament. Family and peer relationships are the primary external forces (Figure 20-1).

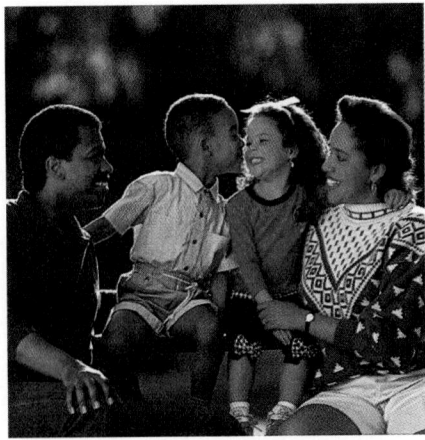

Figure 20-1. Family relationships are an influential factor. (From Wong DL: *Whaley and Wong's nursing care of infants and children,* ed 5, St. Louis, 1995, Mosby.)

TABLE 20-1
Major Factors Influencing Growth and Development

Factors	Relevant Influences
Forces of Nature	
Heredity	Genetic endowment determines sex, race, hair and eye color, physical growth, stature, and to some extent psychological uniqueness.
Temperament	Temperament is the characteristic psychological mood with which the child is born and includes behavioral styles of easy, slow-to-warm, and difficult. It influences interactions between the individual and environment.
External Forces	
Family	Family purpose is to protect and nurture its members.
	Family functions include means for survival, security, assistance with emotional and social development, assistance with maintenance of relationships, instruction about society and world, and assistance in learning roles and behaviors.
	Family influences through its values, beliefs, customs, and specific patterns of interaction and communication.
Peer group	Peer group provides new and different learning environment.
	Peer group provides different patterns and structures of interaction and communication, necessitating different style of behavior.
	Functions of peer group include allowing individual to learn about success and failure; to validate and challenge thoughts, feelings, and concepts; to receive acceptance, support, and rejection as unique person apart from family; and to achieve group purposes by meeting demands, pressures, and expectations.
Life experiences	Life experiences and learning processes allow individual to develop by applying what has been learned to what needs to be learned.
Health environment	Level of health affects individual's responsiveness to environment and responsiveness of others to the individual.
Prenatal health	Preconception (e.g., genetic and chromosomal factors, maternal age, health) and postconception (e.g., nutrition, weight gain, use of tobacco and alcohol, medical problems, use of prenatal services) factors affect fetal growth and development.
Nutrition	Growth is regulated by dietary factors. Adequacy of nutrients influences whether and how physiological needs, as well as subsequent growth and development needs, are met.
Rest, sleep, and exercise	Balance between rest or sleep and exercise is essential to rejuvenating body. Disturbances diminish growth, whereas equilibrium reinforces physiological and psychological health.
State of health	Illness or injury potentially hampers growth and development. Nature and duration of health problem influence its impact. Prolonged injury or illness may leave one unable to cope and respond to demands and tasks of developmental stages.
Living environment	Growth and development are affected by season, climate, home life, and socioeconomic status.

Theories of Human Development

Research into human growth and development has led to a number of developmental theories that vary in the way humans are viewed and in the aspect of development emphasized. Some theories view development as a continuous process, moving from the simple to the more complex. Others consider it as discontinuous, with alternating periods of relative equilibrium and disequilibrium. To communicate effectively with other health professionals when providing coordinated health care, the nurse must be familiar with the common theories of growth and development. No single framework addresses all developmental concerns.

Freud's psychosexual theory. Sigmund Freud (1856-1930), in his classic psychoanalytical theory, suggested that the personality is firmly formed early in life as children deal with conflicts between their inborn biological, sexually related urges and the requirements of society. He proposed that every individual passes through five stages of psychosexual development before reaching maturity (Table 20-2).

TABLE 20-2	
Freud's Psychosexual Developmental Theory	
Stages and Ages	**Characteristics of Stages**
Oral-sensory (birth to 12-18 mo) (infancy)	Activities involving mouth such as sucking, biting, and chewing are chief source of pleasure.
Anal-muscular (12-18 mo to 3 yr) (toddlerhood)	Sensual gratification is derived from retention and expulsion of feces. Smearing is common activity.
Phallic-locomotion (3-6 yr) (preschool)	Manipulation of genitalia results in pleasurable sensations. Masturbation begins, and sexual curiosity becomes evident.
Latency (6 yr to puberty) (school-age)	This is a tranquil period when Freud believed sexual drives were dormant; however, the child may engage in erogenous activities with same-sex peers.
Genital (puberty through adulthood) (adolescence and adulthood)	Genitalia become the center of sexual tension and pleasure. Sexual hormone production stimulates development of heterosexual relationships.

Erikson's psychosocial development theory.

Erikson (1902-1994) described eight stages of personality development across the life span (1963) (Table 20-3). Each stage involves a psychosocial crisis or task to master. The individual's personality that develops is a reflection of the way in which each crisis was resolved. Mastery of the conflict or crisis at each stage requires balancing a positive trait and a corresponding negative one. Although the positive trait should predominate, some degree of the negative one is also needed. Successful resolution of each crisis allows a strength or virtue of the personality to develop.

Piaget's theory of cognitive development.

The theory of Jean Piaget (1896-1980) helps us to understand the structure of the mind and how thinking develops during the first 15 years of life. He views cognitive development as the combined result of the development of the brain and nervous system and of experiences.

Piaget views the development of the mind as occurring through adaptation to the environment via assimilation and accommodation. **Assimilation** is the process by which a person incorporates new experiences into existing cognitive structures (schema) and thus adapts experiences for repeated use. For example, the toddler seeing a horse for the first time fits it into the current scheme of four-legged animals and calls it a "doggie." The experience and the environment are thus adapted by the child. **Accommodation** is the process of responding to the environment through new activity and thinking and changing the existing schema or developing a new schema to deal with the new information. For example, the toddler whose parent consistently corrected him when he called a horse a "doggie" accommodates and forms a new schema for horses. The child thus changes to fit the experience and the environment. The combination of these two processes al-

lows the individual to organize the world by ordering and classifying experiences, which results in adaptation.

Piaget identifies four distinct stages of cognitive development that evolve through the process of maturation as a natural unfolding of the child's intellectual abilities occurs. Each of these stages with their substages is summarized in Table 20-4.

Maslow's theory of human needs.

Abraham Maslow (1908-1970), a humanistic psychologist, developed a theory of human needs from his study of individuals without physical or mental illness. He described a hierarchy of needs that motivate human behavior that is often depicted as a pyramid composed of five levels (Table 20-5). When the most basic needs for hunger, thirst, and so on have been fulfilled, the person strives to satisfy those needs for safety and security on the next highest level. The highest level, self-actualization, the realization of one's potential, is easily interfered with by disturbances at lower levels. This humanistic theory has made a valuable contribution to understanding human development through its positive viewpoint and recognition of needs that motivate all humans. It has been criticized for not differentiating needs according to ages.

Kohlberg's theory of moral development.

According to Kohlberg (1964, 1969), moral development is one component of psychosocial development. It involves the reasons an individual makes a decision about right and wrong behavior within the culture. Moral development depends on the child's ability to accept social responsibility and to integrate personal principles of justice and fairness. In addition, the child's knowledge of right and wrong and behavioral expression of this knowledge must be founded on respect and regard for the integrity and rights of others. Cognitive development underlies the progression of a person's

TABLE 20-3
Erikson's Psychosocial Developmental Theory

Stages and Ages	Characteristics of Stages
Trust versus mistrust (birth to 1 yr) (infancy) Mode: taking in and getting Virtue: hope	Care giver's satisfaction of infant's basic needs for food and sucking, warmth and comfort, and love and security in consistent and sensitive manner results in trust.
Autonomy versus doubt and shame (1-3 yr) (toddlerhood) Mode: holding on and letting go Virtue: will	Child develops beginning independence while gaining control over bodily functions of undressing and dressing, walking, talking, feeding self, and toileting. Self-control begins.
Initiative versus guilt (3-6 yr) (preschool) Mode: intrusive attack and conquest Virtue: purpose	Child develops initiative when planning and trying out new things. Behavior of child is characterized as vigorous, imaginative, and intrusive. Conscience and identification with same-sex parent develop.
Industry versus inferiority (6-12 yr to puberty) (school-age) Mode: doing and producing Virtue: competence	Child wins recognition by demonstration of skill and production of things and develops self-esteem through achievements. Child is greatly influenced by teachers and school.
Identity versus role confusion or diffusion (puberty to 18-21 yr) (adolescence) Virtue: fidelity	Individual develops integrated sense of "self." Peers have major influence over behavior. Major decision is to determine vocational goal.
Intimacy versus isolation (18-21 to 40 yr) (young adulthood) Mode: loving Virtue: love	Task is to develop close and sharing relationships with others, which may include sexual partner.
Generativity versus self-absorption or stagnation (40-65 yr) (middle adulthood) Mode: nurturing Virtue: care	Mature adult is concerned with establishing and guiding next generation. Adult looks beyond self and expresses concern for future of world in general.
Ego integrity versus despair (65 yr to death) (older adulthood) Mode: acceptance Virtue: wisdom	Older adult can look back with sense of satisfaction and acceptance of life and death.

morality from level to level. Kohlberg theorized that these stages occur in the same order regardless of culture, although individuals differ as to how quickly and how far they progress through these stages (Table 20-6).

Adult theories. Robert Peck (1955) identified seven psychological developments as important to healthful adaptation and successful aging of the adult. Critical adjustments for middle age involve a shift from physical prowess to mental and emotional flexibility. Critical adjustments for later life require individuals to move beyond concerns with work, physical well-being, and mere existence to a broader view of one's purpose in life. These adjustments include the following:

1. Valuing wisdom versus valuing physical powers; ability to make the best choices in life
2. Socializing versus sexualizing in human relationships; valuing friends as companions rather than primarily as sex objects
3. Emotional flexibility versus emotional impoverishment; ability to shift emotional investment from one person to another and from one activity to another becomes crucial
4. Mental flexibility versus mental rigidity; ability to continue to seek new answers and not be closed to new ideas or "set in one's ways"
5. Broader self-definition versus preoccupation with work roles; exploring new interests and pride in other attributes after retirement

TABLE 20-4
Piaget's Cognitive Developmental Theory

Stages and Ages	Characteristics of Stages
Sensorimotor (birth to 2 yr)	Child learns about world through sensory and motor activities.
Reflex activities (birth to 1 mo)	Child exercises inborn reflexes and gains some control over them.
Primary circular reactions (1-4 mo)	Infant repeats pleasurable actions that first occur by chance. Activities focus on body of infant; coordination begins.
Secondary circular reactions (4-8 mo)	Child attempts to reproduce interesting, pleasant events in environment. Interest goes beyond body.
Coordination of secondary schemas (8-12 mo)	Child puts together skills used earlier to reach goal in new situation.
Tertiary circular reactions (12-18 mo) ("trial and error")	Child actively explores world and varies actions to see novelty of object, event, or situation. Trial and error are used to problem solve.
Invention of new means through mental combinations (18-24 mo) ("representation")	Toddler begins creating mental images and thus can devise new ways to deal with environment. Child begins to think about events without resorting to action.
Preoperational (2-7 yr)	Child develops representational system and uses symbols such as words to represent people, places, and objects.
Preconceptual (2-4 yr)	Child is primarily egocentric. Perceptual-bound and transductive thinking begin; child is animistic.
Intuitive (4-7 yr)	Child begins to figure things out but cannot explain them rationally. Child is unable to consider parts as composing the whole.
Concrete operations (7-11 yr)	Ability to understand law of conservation results in logical thought patterns and mental operations such as reversibility, decentering, seriation, transformation, classification of two or more attributes, and inductive and deductive reasoning.
Formal operations (develops 11-15 yr, used throughout life)	Ability to think in abstract manner develops, and scientific reasoning emerges. Initially, thought is rigid, but it becomes adaptable and flexible.

TABLE 20-5
Maslow's Theory of Human Needs

Needs	Characteristics
Physiological needs	Physiological needs include food, beverages, and sleep.
Safety needs	Satisfying safety needs allows the individual to feel safe and secure.
Belongingness and love needs	Belongingness allows the individual to affiliate with and be accepted by others.
Esteem needs	Esteem allows the individual to gain approval of others and helps to promote own self-esteem.
Self-actualization	Self-fulfillment potential is recognized.

6. Transcendence of the body versus preoccupation with the body; focusing on relationships and activities that do not demand perfect health
7. Transcendence of the ego versus preoccupation with the ego; moving beyond concern with oneself and one's present life to acceptance of one's achievements and certainty of death

Many researchers have been critical of the theory of Peck because his studies did not include women. Carol Gilligan (1982) compared male and female personality development and highlighted the differences. She identified attachment within relationships as the most important factor in successful female development. Females learn to value relationships and become interdependent at an earlier age. According to Gilligan

TABLE 20-6
Kohlberg's Theory of Moral Development

Stages and Ages	Characteristics of Stages
Premoral level (birth to 9 yr)	There is little awareness of what is socially acceptable moral behavior. Control is external.
Punishment and obedience orientation (birth to 6 yr)	Rules of others are followed to avoid punishment.
Naively egoistic orientation (6-9 yr)	Child conforms to rules out of self-interest; child reasons that reward or favor will be earned.
Conventional morality (9-13 yr)	Efforts are made to please other persons. Control is becoming internal.
"Good boy, nice girl" (9-10 yr)	Desire to please and help others is foremost. Child conforms to avoid rejection.
Authority maintaining morality	Child does duty to avoid criticism by authorities.
Postconventional level of morality (13 yr to death)	Individual attains true morality. Conduct control is internal.
Contractual and legalistic orientation	Individual selects moral principles by which to live and obeys laws.
Universal ethical-principle orientation	Individual behaves in a way that respects dignity of all.

(1982), women struggle with the issues of care and responsibility. As women progress toward adulthood, the moral dilemma changes from how to exercise their rights without interfering in the rights of others to "how to lead a moral life," which includes obligations to themselves, their families, and people in general.

⋯⋯⋯NURSING KNOWLEDGE BASE⋯

Nursing practice based on an understanding of the growth and development of individuals is organized and directed at helping clients and their families adapt to changing internal and external conditions. The nurse who has developed a strong body of knowledge about growth and development has good insight regarding how individuals may perceive an event or behave in response to a given situation at a particular age or stage of life. Development at each stage of life will be further examined, and health concerns will be addressed.

Conception and Fetal Development
From the moment of conception, human development proceeds rapidly. The ovum and sperm each carry half the genetic material that guides biochemical processes essential to the developing organism. Abnormalities in the genes or chromosomes can alter health. Other health problems, such as fetal alcohol syndrome, result from environmental factors (e.g., the mother's diet).

Physical development. Intrauterine life generally lasts 9 calendar or 10 lunar months. The organism's life begins when the ovum is penetrated by one sperm.

The first **trimester** is the first 3 calendar months. After implantation the fetal cells continue to differentiate and develop into essential organ systems. These processes occur at different rates and times. Because several organ systems are developing during the same time, disruption of one system is often associated with disruption of others.

The second trimester is the period from the third to the sixth prenatal months of life. Some organ systems continue basic development during this time, and the functional capabilities of others are refined. By the end of the second trimester most organ systems are complete and can function. The fetus weighs about 0.7 kg (1½ pounds) and is approximately 30 cm (12 inches) long.

During the last 3 months of intrauterine life, the fetus grows to approximately 50 cm (19 to 20 inches) in length. Subcutaneous fat is stored, and weight increases to approximately 3.2 to 3.4 kg (7 to 7½ pounds). The skin thickens, lanugo begins to disappear, and the fetal body becomes rounder and fuller. A tremendous spurt in brain growth begins during this trimester and lasts well into the first few years of life. The central nervous system has established its total number of neurons and connections between neurons, and myelination of nerve fibers progresses rapidly. Damage to the central nervous system during the third trimester can potentially alter later, higher-level cognitive functions. Exposure to noxious agents and the absence of essential nutrients are the most common causes of damage during this trimester. The nurse can teach the woman about these factors in prenatal education. At the end of the third trimester the normal fetus is physically able to make the transition from intrauterine to extrauterine life.

Cognitive and psychosocial development.

Relationships between prenatal events and cognitive development are difficult to establish. However, periods of diminished oxygen (hypoxia) during fetal life are associated with deficits in later cognitive functioning. Some research shows an association between severely inadequate prenatal nutrition and subsequent lower brain weight, head circumference, and specific cognitive abilities.

Little is known about the relationship between prenatal experiences and the child's later psychosocial development.

Health promotion.

Before implantation the embryo is relatively safe from the external environment. However, the organism is sensitive to changes in the environment of the fallopian tube and uterus through which it travels. With implantation the embryo is connected to the larger maternal environment via the placenta. Materials essential for healthy growth and development (oxygen and nutrients) are received, and waste products and carbon dioxide are excreted. Because the placenta is extremely porous, **teratogens** (agents capable of having adverse effects on the fetus) such as viruses, drugs, alcohol, and environmental pollutants can also pass from mother to fetus. The fetal effect of these harmful agents depends on the developmental stage in which exposure takes place. Some teratogens produce defects only if the fetus is exposed to the agent at a critical time when the vulnerable organ is developing. One such teratogen is the rubella or measles virus, which can cause spontaneous abortion; stillbirth; or defects of the eyes, ears, and heart, primarily when exposure is in the first trimester.

Many drugs are teratogenic during the period of rapid organ growth in the first trimester. Barbiturates, alcohol, anticonvulsants, and anticoagulants are associated with fetal abnormalities. The benefits of prescribed medications must be weighed against potentially harmful fetal effects. In addition, there is evidence that mothers who smoke deliver infants with lower birth weights than nonsmoking mothers.

Nurses should explore lifestyle changes that can help women abstain from tobacco, alcohol, and drugs not only during pregnancy but also while planning for pregnancy. Preconception counseling is a growing trend in health care. The goal is to facilitate an optimal outcome for mother, fetus, and significant others, and this can be achieved with good prenatal care. Many mothers under the age of 15 years have had little or no **prenatal care.** Health guidance during pregnancy should include nutrient requirements, balanced rest and activity, and stress management.

Transition from intrauterine to extrauterine life.

The transition from intrauterine to extrauterine life at birth requires rapid changes in the **neonate.** The nurse assesses the neonate's ability to make these changes and intervenes as needed to ensure success. Gestational age, exposure to depressant drugs before or during labor, and the neonate's own behavioral style influence adjustment to the external environment. The initial nursing assessment includes physical and psychosocial elements. The nurse assesses the neonate's current functioning, supports transition, and provides opportunities for parents and child to develop close emotional ties.

Because the nurse's first concern is the physiological functioning of the neonate's major organ systems, an immediate assessment of the neonate's condition is performed. Care is then directed toward maintaining an open airway, stabilizing body temperature, and protecting the neonate from infection and injury.

Neonate

The neonatal period is the first 28 days of life. The nurse performs a more comprehensive assessment as soon as the neonate's physiological functioning is stable, generally within a few hours after birth. The length, weight, head circumference, temperature, pulse, and respirations are measured, and general appearance, body functions, sensory capabilities, and responsiveness are observed. The nurse also coordinates screening tests and other laboratory tests as indicated by the neonate's state of health. Blood tests, such as those for hypothyroidism and phenylketonuria (PKU), are eventually performed on all neonates and allow early detection and treatment.

Physical development.

The newborn's physical functioning is primarily reflexive, and stabilization of major organ systems is the body's primary task. The average full-term newborn weighs 3450 g (about $7\frac{1}{2}$ pounds), is 50 cm (20 inches) in length, and has a head circumference of 34 cm ($13\frac{1}{2}$ inches). Growth grids demonstrate that males are slightly taller and heavier than females from birth until females begin accelerated skeletal growth just before puberty (Wong, 1995).

Normal physical characteristics include the continued presence of lanugo on the skin of the back; cyanosis of the hands and feet (acrocyanosis), especially during activity; and a soft, protuberant abdomen. Skin color varies according to racial and genetic heritage and gradually darkens during infancy. Molding, or overlapping of the soft skull bones, is common during birth. The bones readjust in a few weeks, producing a more rounded appearance. Suture lines and fontanelles are palpable between the unfused skull bones. The anterior (diamond-shaped) and posterior (triangular-shaped) fontanelles are usually palpable at birth and will feel almost flat and soft when the neonate is at rest. Normal behavioral characteristics of the newborn include periods of sucking, crying, sleeping, and activity. Movements are generally sporadic, but they are symmetrical and involve all extremities. Newborns respond to sensory stimuli, particularly the care giver's face, voice, and touch.

Cognitive and psychosocial development.
Early cognitive development begins with innate behaviors, reflexes, and sensory functions. During this time newborns initiate reflex activities, add new objects into behavior, and accommodate these behaviors to achieve their desires. For example, neonates learn to turn to the nipple. Newborns can focus on objects 8 to 10 inches (20 to 25 cm) from their faces and respond to auditory stimuli. Therefore parents should be taught the importance of talking to their babies and providing appropriate visual stimuli.

Whether infant crying leads to refined language is debatable. However, crying elicits a response and care givers discriminate among cry patterns. Crying therefore has significance to newborns and parents. For neonates, crying is a means of communication. They cry for a reason, although at times this reason is difficult to determine. Crying may be frustrating for parents if they cannot see an apparent cause. With the nurse's help, parents can learn to define their infant's cry patterns and take appropriate action.

Health promotion.
During the first month of life, parents and newborns normally develop a strong bond that grows to a deep attachment. Feeding, hygiene, comfort measures, and brief periods of play are interactive experiences that provide a foundation from which later attachments form.

Parental concerns during the neonatal period most frequently center around the baby's crying, feeding, eliminating, and sleeping behaviors. Box 20-1 contains topics that most parents have questions about and would like to discuss with the nurse. Not all new parents are aware of the newborn's immature immune system and may need information about how to protect the baby from infection (i.e., not taking infant to church/grocery store until at least 4 weeks old).

Since 1992 the American Academy of Pediatrics has recommended that for sleeping, infants be placed on their back or propped on their side and not placed on thick bedding, sheepskins, waterbeds, or cushions. These measures have been associated with a decreased incidence of Sudden Infant Death Syndrome (SIDS) (Herda, 1992). Nurses assist parents to attain the knowledge and skills required to foster the newborn's physical, psychosocial, and cognitive well-being and development.

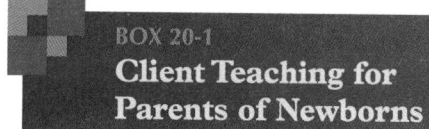

BOX 20-1
Client Teaching for Parents of Newborns

- Selection of a crib with slats less than 2³/₈ inches apart and crib rails as high as possible
- No pillows in baby's crib
- Expected physiological newborn behaviors
- Variability of behavioral cycles (sleep-awake states)
- Importance of not positioning newborn on stomach for sleep
- Principles and techniques for feeding method chosen
- Appropriate stimulation techniques and support for parents' attempts to provide sensory stimulation to the newborn
- Feeding patterns and behaviors
- Care measures, including hygiene, dressing, comfort
- Not to expose newborn to drafts or cool air during bathing process
- Protective measures, including asepsis, safety, CPR, thermoregulation
- Cleansing of umbilical cord stump with alcohol until it falls off
- Signs and symptoms of the newborn requiring evaluation by a health care professional
- Recommended health care guidance

Acute care.
If the newborn or the parents experience health complications after the birth, bonding may be compromised. Neonatal behavioral cues may be weak or absent. Care and care giving are less mutually satisfying. A tired, ill parent may have difficulty interpreting cues and responding to the newborn. Neonates who have congenital anomalies, who are too weak to be responsive to parental cues, or who require special care need supportive nursing measures. For example, infants born with heart defects may tire easily during feeding. They may rest frequently after several bursts of sucking and may awaken hungry after 1½ hours. Parents who do not understand the physiological reason for the behavior may think the infant is being fussy or that they are inadequate as parents. The attachment process is not enhanced and may even be hindered without nursing intervention.

Infant
Growth and development are more rapid during the first 12 months of life than they will ever be again. The infant depends completely on caretakers to provide for basic needs of food and sucking, warmth and comfort, love and security, and sensory stimulation.

Physical development.
Typically infants double their birth weight by 5 months and triple it by 12 months. Their length increases about 1 inch per

month during the first 6 months and then ½ inch per month to the end of their first year. These rates are greatly influenced by nutrition and genetic inheritance. Charts, called *growth grids,* provide average age- and sex-related measurements for head circumference, height, and weight. Health team members participating in infant assessments can evaluate their progress. Muscular development makes possible the rapid motor advancements identified in Table 20-7. Play provides opportunities for the infant to develop many motor skills. Rattles, plastic stacking rings, and wooden blocks are just a few examples of toys that promote fine motor development of the hands and fingers (Figure 20-2).

The quality and quantity of nutrition influence the infant's growth and development. Breast feeding is recommended for infants, because human milk contains an appropriate balance of protein, fat, and carbohydrate essential for growth during the first few months and immunoreactive proteins that help protect against infection. Commercially prepared formulas fortified with vitamins and minerals are also acceptable. The nurse supports the parents' choice of feeding method and helps them feed their infant successfully.

Cognitive and psychosocial development.

Infants learn through gross and fine movement and the use of their senses. Developing motor skills and increasing mobility expand an infant's environment and, with developing visual and auditory skills, enhance cognitive development. For these reasons Piaget (1952) identified the first period of cognitive development as the **sensorimotor period.** The infant progresses from responding through reflex activity to symbolic behavior during the first 2 years. The characteristics of the first four subphases of this period that occur during the first year are described in Table 20-4.

Speech is an important part of cognition that begins to develop during the first year. Infants proceed from crying, cooing, and laughing to imitating sounds, comprehending the meaning of simple commands, and repeating words with knowledge of their meaning. By 1 year of age, infants not only recognize their own

---

TABLE 20-7
Milestones in Infant and Toddler Development

Age	Gross Motor	Fine Motor
3 months	Lifts head 90 degrees when prone Sits with support	Grasps and briefly holds objects and takes them to mouth
6 months	Rolls completely over Good head control in sitting position Crawls on abdomen with arms	Uses palm grasp with fingers encircling object Transfers cube from hand to hand
9 months	Attains sitting position independently Creeps on all four extremities Pulls self to standing position	Crude thumb-finger pincer grasp Bangs hand-held cubes together
12 months	Walks holding onto walls and furniture (cruising) Stands alone Takes one or two independent steps	Places tiny object (e.g., raisin) into container Makes marks with crayon
15 months	Walks alone Stoops and recovers	Scribbles with crayon Builds tower of two cubes Drinks from cup
18 months	Runs Walks up steps with help Kicks ball forward	Builds tower of four cubes Removes garment Uses spoon and fork
24 months	Walks up steps alone Throws ball overhand	Builds tower of six cubes Puts on clothing Turns doorknob
30 months	Jumps Stands on one foot	Builds tower of eight cubes Washes and dries hands
36 months	Balances on one foot for 1 second Walks up and down steps easily	Puts on T-shirt Unbuttons buttons

Modified from Frankenburg WK and others: The Denver II: a major revision and restandardization of the Denver Developmental Screening Test, *Pediatrics* 89(1):91, 1992.

names but also have two- or three-word vocabularies. The nurse can promote language development by encouraging parents to name objects on which the infant's attention is focused.

During the first year, infants begin to differentiate themselves from others as separate beings capable of acting on their own. Infants at 2 to 3 months of age begin to smile responsively rather than reflexively. They also begin to recognize differences in people as their sensory and cognitive capabilities improve. Between 6 and 8 months of age most infants begin to differentiate a stranger from a familiar person and respond differently to the two. Close **attachment** to the primary care givers, most often parents, is usually established by this age. Infants seek out these persons for support and comfort during times of stress. Finally, the ability to distinguish self from others allows infants to interact and socialize more within their environment. They primarily engage in solitary play but are capable of participating in simple games such as pat-a-cake and peek-a-boo. According to Erikson (1963), infants develop a sense of trust when their parents or other caretakers are sensitive and consistently reliable in meeting their basic needs when expressed. Parents who meet the infant's needs at their own convenience or not at all allow the sense of mistrust to develop. Nurses can encourage parents to feed their infants on demand and smile and talk to them during feedings.

Health promotion. In addition to those health promotion activities regarding feeding, crying, eliminating, and sleeping for the newborn, new health promotion activities for the 1- to 12-month-old infant are often related to dentition, immunizations, and safety.

The first tooth to erupt is usually one of the lower central incisors at the average age of 7 months. Most babies have six teeth by their first birthday (Behrman and others, 1996). The use of a frozen teething ring and

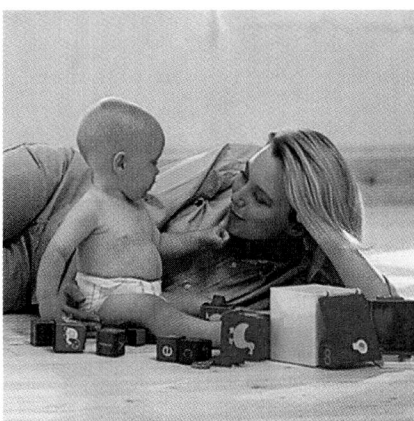

Figure 20-2. Playing with blocks helps to develop infant's motor skills. (From Wong DL: *Whaley and Wong's nursing care of infants and children,* ed 5, St. Louis, 1995, Mosby.)

medication to numb the gums is helpful to comfort the irritable infant during teething episodes. Tooth decay can be prevented by providing adequate fluoride through formula or otherwise, cleaning inside the baby's mouth at least once a day with a wet washcloth, and not allowing the baby to take the bottle to bed (VonBurg and others, 1995).

The use of immunizations has resulted in a dramatic decline of infectious diseases over the past 50 years. More recently, complacency and fears regarding side effects of vaccines have resulted in inadequate immunization of children under 2 years. Nurses play a major role in assisting community organizations to promote immunizations and eradicate preventable childhood disease. Chapter 25 outlines the recommended childhood immunization schedule.

Infants' quickly developing motor skills increase their mobility and their ability to place all types of objects in their mouths. Infants need constant supervision when not sleeping in their cribs. Nurses need to help parents raise their level of awareness regarding potential hazards in their homes. Common accidents during infancy include automobile accidents, aspiration, burns, drowning, falls, poisoning, and suffocation (Box 20-2).

Acute care. When infant hospitalization is required, it is important for parents to provide most of the infant's routine daily care to avoid disruption of the attachment process. Whenever this is impossible, an attempt should be made to limit the number of care givers who have contact with the infant and to follow the parents' directions for care, thus fostering the

---

BOX 20-2
Client Teaching for Parents of Infants

- Keeping crib away from radiators, the blast of air ducts, and cords from drapes or blinds
- Expected growth and developmental norms
- Play activities to stimulate gross and fine motor development
- Techniques to encourage development of language
- Readiness for weaning from breast or bottle to cup
- Addition of solid foods and other fluids
- Need for immunizations
- Safety measures related to use of approved car seats, falls, drowning, and use of mouth to explore everything in environment
- Development of attachment, stranger awareness, and separation anxiety
- Use of voice, eyes, and facial gestures as disciplinary measures
- Signs of illness, measures for assessment (temperature taking), and appropriate action
- Criteria to use when choosing day care

infant's continuing development of trust. The nurse assesses the availability and appropriateness of experiences contributing to psychosocial development. Hospitalized infants may have difficulty establishing physical boundaries because of repeated bodily intrusions and painful sensations. Limiting these negative experiences and providing pleasurable sensations support early psychosocial development.

Infants need opportunities to use and develop the senses. Nurses evaluate the appropriateness and adequacy of these opportunities. For example, ill or hospitalized infants may lack the energy to interact with their environments, thereby slowing cognitive development. On the other hand, continuous stimulation can overwhelm and confuse infants. Stimulation activities should be selected according to the infant's age, energy level, and temperament.

Toddler

The toddler period ranges from the time when children begin to walk independently until they walk and run with ease, which is approximately from 12 to 36 months of age. A toddler is characterized by increasing independence bolstered by greater physical mobility and cognitive abilities. Toddlers are increasingly aware of their abilities to control and are pleased with their successful efforts with this new skill. Unsuccessful attempts at control may result in undesirable behaviors and temper tantrums. Parents need support in finding ways to set consistent, firm limits for a toddler while also promoting the child's independence.

Physical development. The rapid development of motor skills allows the child to participate in self-care activities such as feeding, dressing, and toileting. Toddlers walk in an upright position with a broad-stanced gait, bowed legs, protuberant abdomen, and arms flung out to the sides for balance. Soon the child begins to navigate stairs, run, jump, stand on one foot for several seconds, and kick a ball. Most toddlers can ride a tricycle, climb ladders, and run well by their third birthday. Fine motor capabilities move from scribbling spontaneously to drawing circles and crosses accurately. Improved mobility, the ability to undress, and development of sphincter control allow toilet training if the toddler has the necessary cognitive abilities.

The cardiopulmonary system becomes stable in the toddler years. The heart and respiratory rates slow. The blood pressure rises slightly. The rate of increase in weight and height slows. By 2 years of age the child weighs four times the birth weight. Height during toddlerhood increases 3 to 5 inches a year, mainly as a result of increases in leg length.

Cognitive and psychosocial development. According to Piaget (1952), toddlers' completion of the development of **object permanence** (recognition that an object or person out of sight still exists), their ability to remember events, and their beginning ability to put thoughts into words at about 24 months of age signal their transition from the sensorimotor stage to the preoperational stage. Toddlers recognize they are separate beings from their mothers, but they are unable to assume the view of another because their thoughts have an **egocentric** focus. The toddler becomes increasingly capable of using symbols to represent objects and persons; this is demonstrated when children imitate the behavior of others (e.g., shaving like daddy).

Because moral development is closely associated with cognitive ability, the moral development of toddlers is only beginning and is also egocentric. Toddlers do not understand concepts of right and wrong. However, they do grasp that some behaviors bring pleasant results (positive reinforcement) and others elicit unpleasant results (negative reinforcement). Parents who are consistent in their responses to toddlers' behaviors help them learn what is culturally acceptable or unacceptable.

Toddlers are generally able to speak in short sentences, and common questions they ask are, "Who's that?" and "What's that?" By 36 months of age, the toddler has a beginning mastery of speech.

According to Erikson (1963), a sense of autonomy emerges during toddlerhood. Toddlers are moving out to explore their immediate environment; they continue to return at periodic intervals for encouragement and the emotional support of parents (called *refueling*). Toddlers, who are just learning what belongs to them, are possessive of their toys and are often heard to say, "That's mine!" They begin to learn that sharing is a desirable behavior when they offer parents toys to hold and the parents express pleasure. Play, although frequently solitary in nature, begins to include **parallel play,** playing beside another child with a similar toy or object but not actively interacting through their play. Gradually play begins to include the exchanging or sharing of objects when playing beside another toddler engaged in a similar activity. An example of this **associative play** would be sharing a shovel, bucket, or truck with a playmate when playing in a sandpile.

Health promotion. Slower growth rates are accompanied by a decrease in caloric needs and a smaller food intake. Confirming the child's pattern of growth with charts can be reassuring to parents concerned about their toddler's decreased appetite (physiological anorexia). Parents are encouraged to offer a variety of nutritious foods, in reasonable servings, for mealtime and snacks. Special dietary considerations must be made for the toddler who is ill, is going to have surgery, or is on a vegetarian diet. Finger foods allow the toddler to be independent and "eat on the run." Toilet training is a major task of toddlerhood. The success of toilet training is based on three primary factors: physical ability to control anal and urethral sphincters (after the child learns to walk), child's ability to recognize urge and communicate it to parent, and the desire to please the parent by holding on and letting go at appropriate times. The average age for achieving control is 2 years for daytime and 3 years for nighttime control; girls usually toilet train earlier than boys (Bloom and others, 1993).

This is a good time for parents to demonstrate positive health habits, because children often mimic parents' health care practices. Most toddlers will brush their teeth frequently as a play activity but still need mom or dad to brush them at least once, preferably just before bedtime. Toddlers should make their first visit to the dentist by 18 months of age to get acquainted with the environment and checking of teeth when nothing painful or invasive is necessary (Behrman and others, 1996).

The natural curiosity and the mobility of the toddler, without good reasoning abilities, makes him or her an accident waiting to happen. Parents talk of "child proofing" their homes, which means putting anything and everything that could be dangerous to the child out of reach and preferably out of sight also. Toddlers seem to want to put everything into their mouths (e.g., bugs, bleach, electrical cords) or place their hands, feet, or entire bodies into dangerous sites (e.g., electrical outlets, clothes dryers, tubs with very hot water, pools). They need constant supervision unless they are in a totally child-proofed area such as their bed. Toddlers have little awareness of physical safety, and accidents continue to be the leading cause of death and injury in this age group. The most common accidents are burns, drowning, falls, motor vehicle accidents, and poisoning (Behrman and others, 1996). Nurses can often help parents anticipate the safety needs of their toddlers and make appropriate suggestions (Box 20-3).

Acute care. Whenever toddlers are hospitalized, the nurse works with the child life worker to assist other health team members to adjust their approaches to those appropriate for toddlers. These approaches should reflect an understanding of the toddler's developmental needs, which include the following:

1. Minimizing separation anxiety
2. Establishing trust
3. Reducing fear
4. Minimizing physical discomfort
5. Setting limits
6. Providing accurate knowledge
7. Fostering normal growth and development
8. Incorporating play and diversional activity into care

The nurse uses the responses of children and their parents to determine their specific care (Box 20-4). Being separated from one's family in an unfamiliar envi-

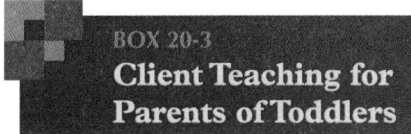

BOX 20-3

Client Teaching for Parents of Toddlers

- Expected growth and developmental norms
- Play activities to stimulate gross and fine motor development (e.g., push/pull, nesting toys)
- Physiological anorexia; good nutritional habits and feeding of self
- Techniques to encourage development of language
- Readiness and appropriate methods for toilet training
- Need for autonomy and setting limits on behavior
- Need to set limits and provide firm, gentle discipline to resolve negativism and temper tantrums
- Continued separation anxiety and development of ritualism
- Safety measures including child proofing the home environment (e.g., storage of cleaning products and medication, use of car seats, selection of appropriate safe toys, pool and water precautions, outdoor play, placing plants out of reach and getting rid of poisonous ones)
- Keeping electrical cords out of reach and covering unused electrical outlets
- Blocking stairways and balconies and not leaving infant unsupervised near water
- Not leaving iron on ironing board
- Continued need for immunizations and developmental assessments

ronment when not feeling well is a great stress for a young child to experience. Parents are more likely to remain with their young child when the nurse and members of the health care team create a comfortable environment for them. If a significant caretaker does not remain with the toddler, it is especially important that one nurse assume responsibility for providing the toddler with consistent and appropriate care. Limiting the number of strange caretakers will help establish trust and reduce separation anxiety for the toddler. During times of stress or illness children often return to behaviors of an earlier time that provide them comfort and security. This **regression** of behavior is often disturbing to parents, and they need reassurance of the normalcy of this behavior and that the child will return to more mature behavior patterns when the stressful situation is resolved.

Toddlers cannot clearly identify where pain is felt and often find anything that causes pressure to be intrusive or extremely painful. Nurses can reduce physical discomfort by keeping periods of restraint or immobility to a minimum. A soft voice, physical contact, and a security item can also comfort the child. Opportunity for play stimulates all aspects of development. Play activities that promote walking, talking, and use of hands and fingers (e.g., push/pull toys, large balls, picture books, stack toys) are especially useful for toddlers.

Box 20-4
Fostering Normal Growth and Development in the Ill Child

Accept regressive behavior and teach parents how to handle regressive behavior with a firm, kind, consistent approach.

Encourage participation in self-care activities such as bathing, dressing, and feeding. Incorporate usual activities of daily living into hospital care.

Provide intermittent auditory and visual stimulation by such activities as rides in a wheelchair or wagon, playing records or tapes from home, and reading stories.

Provide opportunities for social interaction with other children in a playroom, and encourage sibling visits.

Provide toys and play equipment that promote development of fine and gross motor activities.

Provide favorite toys from home.

Encourage development of new vocabulary by learning names for hospital items and personnel.

Explain routines, procedures, and therapies in age-appropriate language.

Encourage participation in assessment and procedures, allowing the child to make choices when possible.

Discuss the effects of hospitalization on growth and development with parents and other team members. Explain how they can help children regain and attain optimal levels of growth and development.

TABLE 20-8
Motor Development in the Preschool Child

Age	Gross Motor	Fine Motor
3-4 years	Balances on each foot 2 seconds Hops Rides tricycle	Copies circle Dresses without help
4-5 years	Balances on each foot 5 seconds Descends steps with alternating feet	Copies cross Draws person (3 parts) Brushes teeth without help Prepares own cereal
5-6 years	Balances on each foot 6 seconds Heel-to-toe walk Skip	Copies square and triangle Ties shoelaces Draws person (10 parts)

Modified from Frankenburg WK and others: The Denver II: a major revision and restandardization of the Denver Developmental Screening Test, *Pediatrics* 89(1):91, 1992; and Wong DL: *Whaley and Wong's nursing care of infants and children,* ed 5, St. Louis, 1995, Mosby.

Preschool Child

Early childhood is a period between the ages of 3 and 6 years when children refine the mastery of their bodies and eagerly await the beginning of formal education. Many parents find this age group more enjoyable than toddlerhood because children are more cooperative, can share thoughts with greater accuracy, and can interact and communicate more effectively. Physical development continues to slow, whereas cognitive and psychosocial development accelerate.

Physical development. Several aspects of physical development stabilize in the preschool years. Heart and respiratory rates decrease only slightly to approximately 90 beats and 22 to 24 breaths per minute. Blood pressure rises slightly to an average of 95/58 mm Hg. Weight increases about 5 pounds per year, making the average weight about 42 pounds (6 times the birth weight) by age 5. Height increases 2 to 3 inches (5 to 7.5 cm) per year. Birth length is generally doubled by age 4, making the average height 42 inches. The elon-

gation of the legs results in the preschooler's more slender appearance.

Large and fine muscle coordination improves as shown in Table 20-8. Preschoolers run well, walk up and down steps with ease, and learn to hop. By their sixth birthday they can usually skip and throw and catch balls. Improving fine motor skills allows intricate manipulations such as printing letters and numbers. Children, especially those with chronic illness, need opportunities to learn and practice these skills. Nursing care of healthy and ill children includes assessing the availability of these opportunities.

Cognitive and psychosocial development. Three year olds' stage of cognition is characterized by **perceptual bound thinking,** in which children judge persons, objects, and events by their outward appearance or what seems to be (Piaget, 1952). For example, they prefer having two nickels over a dime because it appears to be more. The continued egocentricity of early thinking makes it difficult to suggest acceptable alternatives to the preschooler. When they are hungry they expect others also to be hungry, and they think they must eat now! With maturation, the child becomes more able to take the view of another and is capable of improved social interactions.

Around 4 years of age, the intuitive phase of **preoperational thought** develops. Preschoolers can increasingly solve problems intuitively on the basis of one aspect of a situation. For example, they can classify objects according to size or color but not both, and they can ask questions such as, "Why do they call it the thirty-first day of the month instead of the thirty-last?" They also have a great sense of imagination. Their tall tales may be misinterpreted by adults as lying when they are actually presenting reality from their perspective. Their imagination also contributes to the development of fears, the greatest of which in this age group is the fear of bodily harm. It may be manifested as fear of various animals, the dark, or of procedures such as having their blood pressure measured.

Early causal thinking is evident in preschoolers' thoughts (reasoning occurs from one particular to another). If two events are related in time or space, children link them causally. The hospitalized child, for example, may reason, "I cried last night and that's why the nurse gave me the shot." As children near age 5, they begin to use or can be taught to use rules to understand causation. They then begin to reason from the general to the particular.

Preschoolers begin to identify with the same-sex parent and learn appropriate male and female roles. They enjoy mimicking that parent's behavior and often want to do the activities that parent is doing, from putting on a tie like dad to putting on make-up when mom does.

The preschooler's moral development expands to include a beginning understanding of behaviors considered socially right or wrong. The child continues to be motivated, however, by the wish to avoid punishment or the desire to obtain a reward. The preschooler is better able than the toddler to identify behaviors that elicit rewards or punishment and begins to label these behaviors as right or wrong.

Preschoolers' vocabularies increase rapidly. By 5 years of age children use more than 2000 words, and questions expand to "Why?" and "How come?" They identify colors and body parts and define familiar objects. Language is more social and they begin to talk on the phone, rather than just listen as they did earlier. The child may confuse phonetically similar words such as "die" and "dye." Because of this limitation and a literal interpretation of words, the preschooler may misunderstand things. The nurse should avoid such words and assess comprehension of explanations when preparing children for procedures.

Preschoolers continue to rely heavily on the support of parents or primary care givers for security but increasingly venture out to initiate contact with other children and adults.

Play becomes more socially interactive during the preschool period. Most 3 year olds are able to play with one other child in a cooperative manner, where there is organization and division of responsibility. Their play plans often assign roles (e.g., "You be the mama and I'll be the baby."). By age 4, children play in groups of three or four, and by age 5 the group has a temporary leader for each activity with pretend (sociodramatic) play becoming more dominant. With play, children learn sex role identification; express questions, fears, anger, and frustration; and develop skills in solving problems and interacting with others. Nurses can use play as an effective tool for learning about children's feelings and preparing them for procedures, hospitalizations, and surgery.

Health promotion. The most common nutritional deficiencies in children under 6 years of age are vitamins A and C and iron. Ingestion of large amounts of carbohydrates and fats from junk foods may result in overweight and undernourishment. It is recommended that they have 3 to 5 servings of vegetables and 2 to 4 servings of fruit per day. Nurses should encourage parents to role model good eating habits and offer their children a varied diet that prevents deficiencies and excesses. The earlier and more frequently children see particular foods, the more likely they will choose to eat them (Stephens and others, 1996). Children enjoy helping prepare healthy snacks such as fruit slices, carrot sticks, celery stuffed with peanut butter, and popcorn.

Preschoolers require role modeling and instruction to develop good hygiene measures such as brushing their teeth after meals and sugary snacks, covering their mouths and nose when coughing or sneezing, keeping their fingers out of their nose and eyes, and washing their hands before eating and after using the toilet. Little girls need to learn to wipe from front to back to prevent fecal bacteria from entering the urinary tract.

Preschoolers begin to ask questions about sex. It is best to find out what the child thinks, then give simple, brief, and honest answers. A little bit of information often satisfies the child's curiosity, and too much information may be overwhelming or confusing.

Accidents are the major cause of mortality for this age group, and motor vehicle accidents (usually as a pedestrian) are the major cause of death. Emphasis is placed on education for safety and potential hazards (Box 20-5). This is a good time for children to learn what to do in case of fire, safety regulations for crossing the street, the necessity of riding in the back seat of the car, and how to get help when someone is hurt.

Acute care. Hospitalization of preschoolers is stressful, but their beginning abilities to reason and understand make it less so than for the toddler. They continue to need the same developmental considerations that were discussed for the toddler. Although preschoolers have developed object permanence and recognize their parents still exist when out of sight, most tolerate only short absences without becoming distressed. Parents should be encouraged to tell the child when they are leaving and when they will return in terms the child can understand (e.g., after lunch). The

BOX 20-5
Client Teaching for Parents of Preschool Children

- Expected growth parameters and developmental tasks
- Encouraging parents to support their child's sense of initiative and recognizing they will be unable to complete all activities begun
- Nutritional requirements for optimal growth
- Methods to stimulate continued progress in the development of motor skills, language, cognitive skills, and social skills
- Signs of common childhood communicable diseases and measures to reduce their risk and spread
- Criteria to use when evaluating preschool education programs
- Teaching methods used to help preschoolers learn about their health, including nutrition, exercise, and rest
- Safety measures and education related to motor vehicles, tricycles, and fire
- Increased sexual curiosity and need for use of correct anatomical terminology
- Child abuse, including how to protect children, identify signs of abuse, and know community agencies available for assistance
- Great sense of imagination and development of fears, particularly in regard to bodily harm
- Development of conscience

nurse should be present when they leave to provide distraction and support. Parents should understand that protest is normal and demonstrates a strong parent-child relationship.

It is common for preschoolers to fear not only abandonment but also bodily harm. Strategies for reducing their fears are allowing the child to sit up for assessments and procedures when possible, demonstrating procedures on another person or doll, allowing the child to see and handle equipment, encouraging parents to be present, allowing the child to assist with a procedure as appropriate, and leaving the room door open at night if the child requests it. Simple and factual information is especially important to this age group because of their great sense of imagination.

Preschoolers can point to the painful area but have difficulty describing it or discussing it. Their response to pain is often exaggerated by the fear and anxiety it arouses and they may perceive it as a punishment for a misdeed or "bad" thought. Just like toddlers, restraint and being forced to lie down threaten their sense of control and thus should be kept to a minimum. Preschoolers can better cooperate with procedures such as blood pressure measurement and venipuncture if they are comforted, allowed to participate and to make acceptable choices, and given medication for pain when appropriate. Nurses should use a developmentally ap-

propriate pain assessment tool to determine effectiveness of pain-relief measures (see Chapter 33).

All areas of growth and development are promoted through approaching the child at an age-appropriate level. Play not only allows the child to develop motor, cognitive, and social skills but also allows the child to work out fears, release frustrations, and meet stimulation needs. Play is the "work of the child" and brings a sense of normalcy to the strange and sometimes seemingly hostile environment and allows the preschooler to focus attention on pleasurable experiences.

School-Age Child

During the "middle years" of childhood (ages 6 to 12), the foundation for adult roles in work, recreation, and social interaction is laid. Great developmental strides are made in physical, cognitive, and psychosocial skills. Children become "better" at things. For example, they can run faster and farther as proficiency and endurance develop.

The school or educational experience expands the child's world and is a transition from a life of relatively free play to a life of structured play, learning, and work. The school and home influence growth and development. For optimal development to occur, the child must learn to cope with the rules and expectations of school and peers. Parents should learn to allow their child to make decisions, accept responsibility, and learn from life's experiences.

Physical development. The rate of growth during these early school years is slower than at any time since birth but continues steadily. Growth accelerates at different times for different children. Height increases approximately 2 inches (5 cm) per year. Weight, which is more variable, increases by 4 to 7 pounds per year and often doubles during this period. Muscle tissue represents an increased percentage of the body weight. Children lose their babylike contours and appear slimmer as leg length increases in proportion to height and fat decreases, changing its distribution pattern (Wong, 1995).

School gives children the opportunity to compare themselves with other children of the same age. Boys are slightly taller and heavier than girls during these early school years. Approximately 2 years before puberty, school-agers experience a rapid acceleration in skeletal growth; girls, who reach puberty first, begin to surpass boys in height and weight, which often causes embarrassment to both sexes. These changes may begin as early as 9 years of age in girls and 12 years of age in boys. Regular measurement of height and weight will reveal any deviations that should be further evaluated by a member of the medical team.

School-age children become more graceful as they gain increasing control over their bodies (Figure 20-3). Strength doubles, and large muscle coordination im-

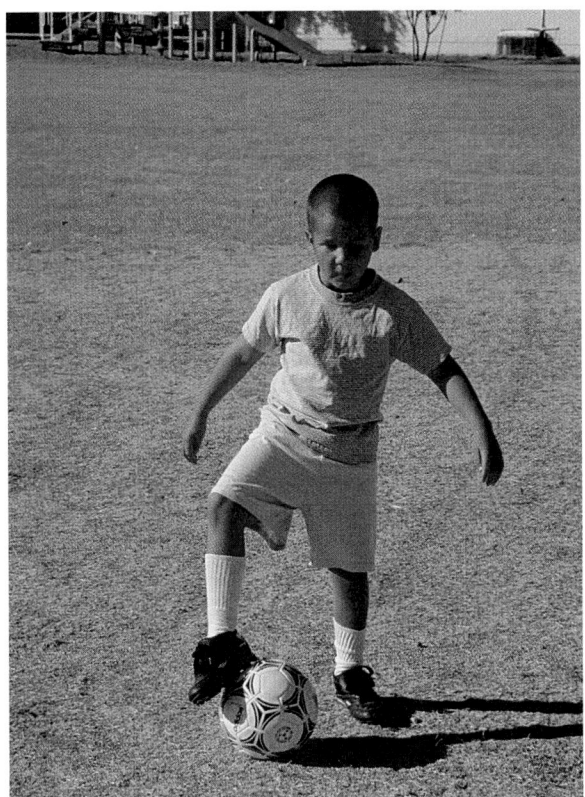

Figure 20-3. Coordination improves in school-age children as they gain control over their bodies.

proves. Participation in the basic gross motor skills of running, jumping, balancing, throwing, and catching refines neuromuscular function and skills. Evidence of fine motor coordination improvement is that most 6-year-old children can easily hold a pencil and print letters and words. By age 12 the child can make detailed drawings and write sentences in script. Assessment of neurological development is often based on fine motor coordination. Teachers often ask school nurses to conduct fine motor assessment of children with questionable ability. Nurses need to know the items that constitute normal fine motor functioning and should refer the child with deviations for more comprehensive assessments. Independence in the self-care activities of basic hygienic measures and dressing is facilitated by these advances in fine motor capabilities (Table 20-9).

These middle childhood years are often referred to as the "age of the loose tooth," because all of the primary teeth are lost during this period. The secondary teeth are much larger in proportion and are often referred to as "tombstone teeth." Regular dental visits will validate if children are brushing their teeth with regularity and good technique. The dentist will also be able to assess if the child has a sufficient source of fluoride. Children should learn to take pride in good dental hygiene.

Eye shape, which is altered as a result of skeletal growth, usually results in 20/20 visual acuity. Myopia is

not an uncommon development in later childhood and can be suspected when the child holds objects very close for clear vision. Auditory perception is fully developed, and children are able to identify very fine differences in sound and pitch of voices. Screening for vision and hearing problems is easier in school-agers and results are more reliable because they can more fully understand and cooperate with test directions.

Cognitive development. Cognitive changes provide the school-age child with the ability to think logically about the here and now but not about abstraction. The thoughts of school-agers are no longer dominated by their perceptions, and thus their ability to understand the world greatly expands. Around 7 years of age, children enter Piaget's stage of **concrete operations,** in which they are able to use symbols to carry out operations (mental activities) in thought rather than in action. They begin to use logical thought processes and concrete materials (e.g., objects, people, events they can touch and see).

Children in this stage are much less egocentric than younger children and develop the ability to decenter (concentrate on more than one aspect of a situation). They also develop reversibility (ability to trace a line of thinking back to its origin). This is seen in their comprehension that ice is frozen water, which can be changed back to water and then to steam when heated. Both of these cognitive skills allow the child to use **conservation** (the ability to recognize that the amount or quantity of a substance remains the same even when its shape or appearance changes). By age 7 or 8, the child can place objects in order according to their increasing or decreasing size **(seriation).** This ability to seriate is seen when the child arranges pencils from the longest to the shortest or vice versa. The mental process of classification becomes more complex as the child develops the ability to separate objects into groups according to more than one aspect or quality (e.g., shape, color, size). During the school-age years, children also refine their understanding of spatial relationships.

Middle childhood youngsters can use their newly developed cognitive skills to solve problems. Middle school-agers who are good problem solvers demonstrate a positive attitude. They see the problem can be solved with persistence, a concern for accuracy, and the ability to avoid guessing while searching for facts. Problem solving can be improved by helping children to define the problem and its nature, plan their solution carefully, and evaluate their plan and the solution. Nurses can use these strategies to help school-agers assume responsibility for their general health and understand an illness and its treatment.

Language growth is so rapid it is no longer possible to match age with language achievements. The average 6-year-old child has a vocabulary of 8000 words that quickly expands with exposure to peers, adults, and

TABLE 20-9
Motor Development in the School-Age Child

6-7 Years	8-10 Years	11-12 Years
Fine Motor Skills		
Uses knife to butter bread and learns to cut tender meat.	Uses knife and fork simultaneously.	Learns to peel apples and potatoes.
Cuts, folds, and pastes paper.	Learns to thread needle and tie knot.	Sews simple garments on machine.
Prints with pencil.	Uses hammer, saw, and screwdriver.	Builds simple objects like birdhouse.
Draws man with 12-16 details.	Becomes proficient at writing cursive.	Enjoys using decorative script.
Copies triangle at 6 years and diamond by 7 years.	Uses symbols in drawing (e.g., bird, star).	Begins to use creative and artistic talents.
Colors within lines of picture.	Builds simple models of cars and planes and does simple hand-crafts.	Builds complex models of cars and planes and does complex hand-crafts.
Needs assistance to clean teeth thoroughly.	Learns to play jacks and marbles.	Learns to play musical instrument.
	Can learn to floss teeth effectively and be independent in tooth care.	Becomes proficient in caring for teeth with braces and other appliances.
Gross Motor Skills		
Remains in constant motion.	Can catch, throw (70 feet), and hit baseball.	Can do standing broad jump of 5 feet.
Moves more cautiously at 7 years than at 6 years.	Engages in alternate rhythmic hopping in 2-2, 2-3, or 3-3 pattern.	Can do standing high jump of 3 feet.
Hops and jumps into small squares.	Engages in complex styles of skipping rope accompanied by verbal jingles.	Plays games involving simultaneous use of two or more complex motor skills such as roller skating, ice hockey, or dance skating.
Learns to roller skate, skip rope, ride a bicycle, and swim.		
Self-Care		
Takes bath without supervision.	Learns to clean bathroom after bath.	Dusts, vacuums, and straightens own room.
Often returns to finger feeding.	Enjoys fixing own snacks and sack lunch.	Learns to cook simply prepared foods.
Learns to brush and comb hair in acceptable fashion without help.	Learns to part hair and insert hair ribbons and barrettes.	Washes, dries, and fixes own hair in braids, curls, and ponytails.
Puts on most clothes but may need assistance with shirttails, sashes, and final adjustments.	Dresses self completely and can help younger siblings with clothes.	Learns to sort, wash, dry, and press own clothing.
	Can make own bed.	Learns to care for fingernails and toenails.

reading materials. These children are less bound by the restrictions of their family's language, and by the end of this period their language is similar to adults.

Psychosocial development. Erikson's developmental task for these middle years is the development of a sense of industry versus inferiority. As children begin to move away from their family and into the world of school, there are many opportunities for them to gain a sense of competence as they learn reading, writing, and other academic skills; to follow the rules of a new authority person; and to compete and cooperate with peers in play and work. The recognition that a child receives at home for achievements also bolsters the child's developing self-esteem and provides reason to put forth further good efforts. Children's success in work and

play leads to an increasing sense of independence and a need to participate in any decisions that involve them. As children move through these middle years of childhood they are confronted with a number of stressors too numerous to list; however, an attempt is made to summarize them in Table 20-10. It is important for parents and nurses to help children develop positive coping behaviors and feel successful about dealing with a particular stress.

The school-age child prefers same-sex peers to opposite-sex peers. In general, girls and boys view the opposite sex negatively. Peer influence becomes diverse during this stage. Conformity is evidenced in mannerisms, clothing styles, and speech patterns that are reinforced and influenced by peer contact.

Many researchers believe school-agers have a great

TABLE 20-10

Potential School-Related Stressors

Stressor	Nursing Intervention
Meeting teacher's behavioral expectations	Encourage parents to share information with teachers that will help them understand the child better
	Encourage unhurried communication about school expectations, events
Maintaining self-concept	Be positive on daily basis to foster child's success
Separation; school adjustment	Assist child in identifying physical set-up of school and daily routines
Testing out new ideas	Encourage originality by helping children make their own projects from discarded or other available materials
Integrating peer values into behavior	Reinforce positive peer activities and interactions
Assuming responsibility for own learning	Encourage use of problem solving by child
Meeting cognitive requirements	Demonstrate interest in what child is learning
	Take advantage of situations that support and reinforce school learning
	Provide well-lit study area that is free of interruptions
	Share an interest in reading
Behavioral standard development	Promote good conduct through praise and example
Participation in school events	Assist parent in realizing need for extracurricular activities
	Assist child to select activity in which he or she is likely to be successful

Modified from Wong DL: *Whaley and Wong's nursing care of infants and children,* ed 5, St. Louis, 1995, Mosby.

deal of interest in their sexuality and engage in sex play and masturbation. Children hide it, however, because of adult disapproval. During the school-age years children also begin to develop a moral code. Between 6 and 9 years of age they recognize and label behaviors as right or wrong, good or bad. This labeling is influenced by their family and culture. Gradually children apply these labels to personal behavior based on the pleasurable or unpleasurable results of an action.

Health promotion. Accidents and injuries are major health problems affecting school-age children and are the causative factor in 51% of deaths in this age group. Motor vehicle accidents, followed by drownings, fires, burns, and firearms are the most frequent fatal accidents. Other major causes of accidents involve recreational activity and equipment, most frequently involving bicycles, swings, skateboards, and contact sports (Edelman and Mandle, 1994). Parents should encourage school-agers to assume some responsibility for their own safety by establishing rules and acting as good role models (Box 20-6). A good health education program will help children learn about their bodies and how their actions influence their health.

The control of childhood obesity is a significant factor in avoiding elevated levels of blood pressure and blood cholesterol (Williams, 1993). Helping the child

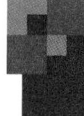

BOX 20-6

Client Teaching for School-Agers and Their Parents

- Expected growth parameters and developmental tasks including the middle childhood growth spurt and puberty
- Measures to enhance adjustment to school and reduce school-related stressors
- Promotion of child's sense of industry through opportunities for achievement
- Influence and importance of peers as they learn to follow rules and be competitive
- Development and expression of sexuality, including sex play (i.e., masturbation)
- Encourage parents to teach and model safety practices
- Recreational safety including helmets for sports, bicycling, and skateboarding
- Substance abuse (tobacco, alcohol, drugs), including dangers, signs of use, and available community agency support
- Measures to facilitate development of cognitive skills (reading out loud, appropriate use of television, family discussions regarding school performance and homework) and decision-making skills, including weighing the consequences of actions taken
- Responsibility for health promoting activities, including nutrition, exercise, and safety

who is obese is a difficult task and must involve the entire family changing eating patterns and increasing their level of physical activity on a regular basis (Edelman and Mandle, 1994).

Blood pressure elevation in childhood is the single best predictor of adult hypertension. This recognition has reinforced the significance of making blood pressure measurement a part of every routine assessment of the child, which should occur yearly (Purath, 1995). Measurement on at least three separate occasions with the appropriate size cuff and in a relaxed situation should be made before concluding that the child's blood pressure is elevated and needs further medical attention. Daily exercise and maintaining normal body weight are important both as interventions and prevention.

Reducing the risk of osteoporosis and skeletal fractures in later life has placed new emphasis on the role of calcium in building strong bones during childhood and adolescence. Many children today fail to meet the recommended calcium intake levels. Those who are predisposed to osteoporosis are girls and female teens, children low in weight or with prolonged poor nutrition, and children with various chronic disease states such as chronic renal disease. Nurses can educate families about the benefits of consuming foods rich in calcium.

Acute care. School-agers usually tolerate the absence of their parents better than the younger child because of their reasoning abilities. Although they understand their parents often need to be elsewhere, they want and expect daily visits and intervening phone calls. The items school-agers often bring from home such as their own pillow and favorite books, board games, and hand-held computer games give them a sense of security and independence. Honesty, factual information, and interest in their concerns are helpful in establishing a trusting relationship with this age group. The hospital is an interesting and almost enjoyable experience for many children during middle childhood.

School-agers can usually pinpoint their pain, describe it with moderate assistance, and may attempt to explain its cause. They may use play to cope with their pain or withdraw in an attempt to deal with their discomfort. They are usually aware that they can receive medication for pain but may not ask for it until the pain is intense. They are quick to learn to use a scale to assess their discomfort. Although children in this age group are less likely to regress than younger children, it does occur.

School-agers' fears associated with health care include being stuck with needles, taking bad-tasting medicine, invasive procedures, being forced to lie down, and being subjected to the unknown. These fears can be minimized by giving them choices and some control over difficult situations.

Most school-agers are eager learners who gain much

satisfaction from learning to find their various pulses, read a thermometer, or operate the blood pressure machine during hospitalization. Many school-agers can assist in checking their urine for sugar or protein or learn to do their own finger-sticks for blood samples. School-agers who become ill are often threatened by a loss of their recently developed independence by needing to use a bedpan, having help with bathing, bed rest, or having someone else select their menu. Care givers can allow them to gain some control over these situations by activities such as giving them some responsibility for keeping a record of their intake and output, marking their menu, doing part or all of their bath, and allowing them to choose their own diversional activities.

Preadolescent

At present, children experience more emotional and social pressures than youngsters 30 years ago. As a result, children 10 to 12 years of age are now having experiences that were once unique to 13- and 14-year-old youths. This transitional period between childhood and adolescence is often referred to as **preadolescence.** Others refer to this period as late childhood, early adolescence, pubescence, and transescence. Physically it refers to the beginning of the second skeletal growth spurt, when the physical changes such as the development of pubic hair and female breasts begin. Children also become more social, and their behavioral patterns become much less predictable.

Adolescent

Adolescence is the transition from childhood to adulthood, usually between 13 and 18 years of age but sometimes extending until graduation from college. The term *adolescence* refers to the psychological maturation of the individual, whereas *puberty* refers to the point when reproduction is possible. This period is characterized by a steady progression of physical, social, cognitive, psychological, and moral changes. The adaptations required by these changes push adolescents to develop individualized coping mechanisms and styles of behaviors, which they will continue to use or adapt throughout life. Most teenagers successfully meet the challenges of this period.

During this stage of development an adolescent must establish an identity, make major decisions regarding life and a vocation, develop and refine adult cognitive skills, and establish a code of morality by which all of these tasks are ordered. The nurse's understanding of adolescents' developmental tasks provides a unique perspective for helping teenagers and their parents anticipate and cope with the stresses of adolescence.

Physical development. Although timing varies greatly, physical changes occur rapidly during adolescence. Sexual maturation occurs with the development of primary and secondary sexual characteristics. Primary characteristics are physical and hormonal changes necessary for reproduction. Secondary characteristics externally differentiate males from females.

Height and weight increases accelerate during the prepubertal growth spurt. The growth spurt for girls generally begins between 8 and 14 years of age, with height increases of 2 to 8 inches (5 to 20 cm) and weight increases of 15 to 55 pounds. The male growth spurt usually takes place between 10 and 16 years of age, with height increases of approximately 4 to 12 inches (10 to 30 cm) and weight increases of 15 to 65 pounds.

Girls attain 90% to 95% of their adult height by **menarche** (the onset of menstruation) and reach their full height by 16 to 17 years of age. Boys continue to grow taller until 18 to 20 years of age. Fat is redistributed into adult proportions as height and weight increase, and gradually the adolescent torso takes on an adult appearance.

Adolescents are sensitive about physical changes that make them different from peers. Thus they are generally interested in the normal pattern of growth, as well as in their personal growth curves.

Puberty. A wide variation exists between the sexes and within the same sex as to when the physical changes of **puberty** begin. The sequence of pubertal growth changes is the same in most individuals (Table 20-11). Ranges of normal should be used when assessing progress of growth. As with increases in height and weight, the pattern of sexual changes is more significant than their time of onset. Large deviations from normal time frames require attention.

Visible and invisible changes take place during puberty as a result of hormonal change. The hypothalamus begins to produce gonadotropin-releasing factors that signal the pituitary to secrete gonadotropic hormones. Gonadotropic hormones stimulate the ovarian cells to produce estrogen and the testicular cells to produce testosterone. These hormones contribute to the development of secondary sex characteristics such as pubic hair growth and voice changes and play an essential role in reproduction (see Chapter 16).

Cognitive development. The adolescent's intellectual abilities usually reach Piaget's formal operations, which is marked by the capacity for abstract thought. The individual can now think beyond the present to consider the infinite possibilities of the future (hypothesize), use logical reasoning to solve complex verbal problems, and rationalize. Young persons must have sufficient neurological development to reach this stage and still may not do so if they are not encouraged culturally and educationally (Papalia and Olds, 1995). Cognitive abilities and performance vary greatly among adolescents, and an individual may perform at different cognitive levels in different situations based on past experiences and formal education.

Language development is fairly complete by adolescence, although vocabulary continues to expand. The

---

TABLE 20-11
Average Sequence of Physiological Changes in Adolescence

Age Range for Girls	Characteristics	Age Range for Boys
8-14½ (peak: 12)	Beginning of skeletal growth spurt	10½-16
8-13	Beginning of breast development	
	Enlargement of testes and scrotal sac	10-13½
8-14	Appearance of straight, pigmented pubic hair, which gradually becomes curly	10-15
	Early voice changes (cracks)	11-14½
	Enlargement of penis and prostate gland	11-14½
10½-15½ (average: 12¼)	Menarche	
	Spermatogenesis (ejaculation of sperm)	11-17
11-18	Ovulation and completion of breast development	
	Appearance of downy facial hair	12-17
10-16	Appearance of axillary (underarm) hair and increased output of oil and sweat-producing glands, which may lead to acne	12-17
10-18	Widening and deepening of female pelvis, with deposition of subcutaneous fat that gives rounded appearance to body	
	Increase in shoulder width	11-21
	Deepening of voice, appearance of coarse and pigmented facial hair, and appearance of chest hair	16-21

primary focus becomes developing diverse communication skills that can be used effectively in many situations and refined later in life. Adolescents need to communicate thoughts, feelings, and facts to peers, parents, teachers, and other persons of authority. The skills used in these diverse communication situations are varied.

Developing moral judgment depends on cognitive and communication skills and peer interaction. Moral development, begun in early childhood, matures. Adolescents learn to understand that rules are cooperative agreements that can be changed to fit the situation, rather than absolutes. Adolescents learn to apply rules by using their own judgment rather than simply to avoid punishment as in the earlier years. They judge themselves by internalized ideals, which often leads to conflict between personal and group values. Group values become less significant in later adolescence. Not all adolescents attain the same level of moral development, but the progression through the stages of moral development follows a similar sequence for all individuals.

Psychosocial development. The search for personal identity is the major task of adolescent psychosocial development. Teenagers must establish close peer relationships or remain socially isolated. Erikson (1968) sees identity (or role) confusion as the prime danger of this stage. Teenagers must become emotionally independent from their parents and yet retain family ties. They also need to develop their own ethical systems based on personal values. Teenagers must make choices about vocation, future education, and lifestyle. The various components of total identity evolve from the accomplishment of these tasks and comprise an adult personal identity unique to the individual.

Achievement of sexual identity is enhanced by the physical changes of puberty. These changes encourage the development of masculine and feminine behaviors. If these physical changes involve deviations, the person has more difficulty developing a comfortable sexual identity. Adolescents depend on these physical clues because they want assurance of maleness or femaleness and because they do not wish to be different from peers. Sexual identity is also influenced by cultural attitudes, expectations of sex role behavior, and available role models. The masculine and feminine behaviors teenagers see and the expectations they perceive for behaving as a man or woman affect how they express sexuality. Adolescents master age-appropriate sexuality when they feel comfortable with sexual behaviors, choices, and relationships (Figure 20-4).

Adolescents seek a group identity because they need approval, support, and acceptance. The strong need for group identity seems to conflict at times with the search for personal identity. It is as though adolescents require close bonds with peers so they can later redefine themselves against this group identity.

The movement toward stronger peer relationships is

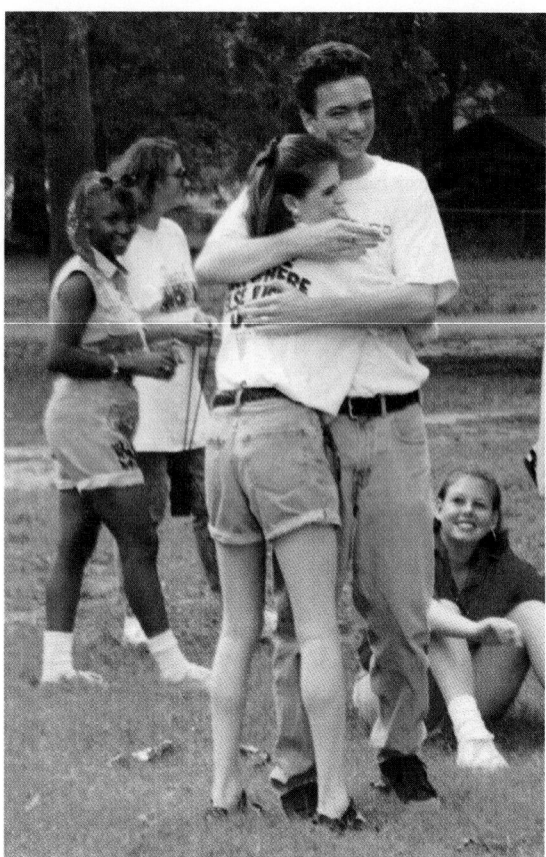

Figure 20-4. Heterosexual relationships are an important part of adolescence. (From Wong DL: *Whaley and Wong's nursing care of infants and children,* ed 5, St. Louis, 1995, Mosby.)

contrasted with the movement away from parents. Some adolescents and families have more difficulty during these years than others. The differences can result from the number, extent, and nature of the movements from periods of independence to relative dependence. Adolescents need to make choices, act independently, and experience the consequences of their actions. This testing is best done against a firm, supportive family foundation. Nurses can provide support by assisting families to consider ways appropriate for them to foster the independence of the adolescent.

Health promotion. A component of personal identity is perception of health. Healthy adolescents evaluate their own health according to feelings of well-being, ability to function normally, and absence of symptoms. Health problems causing severe or long-term alteration of these factors may permanently alter self-identity. Nurses can assist adolescents to take responsibility for their own health status and practices (Box 20-7).

The major causes of mortality in the adolescent age period are injuries, homicide, and suicide, which ac-

BOX 20-7

Client Teaching for Adolescents and Their Parents

- Clear, reasonable limits for acceptable behavior and consequences for breaking the rules
- Automobile safety, including driver's education course; use of seat belts; risks to self and others associated with drinking, drugs, and driving; use of helmet by bicyclists and motorcyclists
- Awareness of warning signs of depression and suicide, alternatives to suicide, and methods to deal with a suicidal peer
- Dealing with peer pressure, school-related stressors, anger, and violent feelings through decision-making skills, conflict resolution, and positive coping strategies
- Prevention of unintentional injuries (e.g., classes on use of firearms, danger of swimming alone or under the influence of alcohol or drugs)
- Sexual experimentation and measures to prevent STDs and pregnancy, including abstinence, transmission of infection, symptoms of disease, prophylactic measures, and community organizations that provide assistance
- Allowing increasing independence within limits of safety and well-being
- Providing privacy and unconditional love
- Listening to and respecting the adolescent's viewpoint

count for 75% of their deaths (Wong, 1995). Motor and other vehicular accidents, pregnancy, sexually transmitted diseases (STDs), and substance abuse are major causes of morbidity; mental disorders, chronic illness, eating disorders, and oral health problems are other causes.

Females are more likely to have eating disorders and emotional distress, and males are more often involved in vehicular accidents (Millstein and others, 1993; Bearinger and Blum, 1994). Black and American-Indian males have higher risk of early death than any other cultural group. Deaths during late adolescence are more violent, greater in number, and more than twice as common in males as females. Homicide is the most frequent cause of death among older black adolescents, whereas vehicular accidents are the leading cause of death among white males. The Youth Risk Behavior Surveillance Study conducted by the CDC (USDHHS, 1995) identifies the following adolescent behaviors that contribute to unintentional injuries:

1. White male students (22.6%) were significantly more likely than white females (11.5%) to rarely or never use safety belts; this behavior was reported significantly more often by black students (30%) than white (17.3%) or Hispanic students (19.5%).

2. Among students who rode motorcycles, 40% rarely or never wore a motorcycle helmet; this behavior was most prevalent among Hispanics.
3. Almost 93% of these students rarely or never wore a bicycle helmet; this was reported most frequently by black males.
4. Approximately one third of students surveyed nationwide reported having ridden with a driver who had been drinking alcohol.
5. Nearly one quarter of students nationwide had carried a weapon, males more frequently than females; black males and females reported a higher incidence than whites.

Health services for adolescents must be readily available, affordable, and approachable if parents and communities expect teens to use them. School-based programs, where instituted, have been well used by adolescents. Health care workers must be skilled in interviewing adolescents and identifying those most at risk. Health promotion activities to be successful must actively involve teenagers at all times. The involvement of teens in organizations that promote responsible behaviors such as Drug Abuse Resistance Education (DARE) and Students Against Drunk Driving (SADD) is a key element. Through their efforts in the school and community, nurses can make a contribution in meeting the Healthy People 2000 objectives (USDHHS, 1992).

Substance abuse is a major concern to those who work with teenagers. All adolescents are at risk for experimental or recreational substance use. The nurse can identify those at risk, educate them to prevent accidents related to substance abuse, and counsel those in rehabilitation.

Suicide is the third leading cause of death in persons between 15 and 24 years of age and the second leading cause of death for white males in this age group (USDHHS, 1992). Depression and social isolation commonly precede a suicide attempt, but suicide most likely results from a combination of several factors. Nurses should be alert to the following warning signs, which often occur for at least 1 month before a suicide attempt (Papalia and Olds, 1995).

1. Decrease in school performance
2. Withdrawal from family and friends
3. Drug or alcohol abuse
4. Personality changes such as boredom, anger, apathy, anxiety, panic, and neglect of appearance
5. Appetite and sleep disturbances
6. Talking about death, the hereafter, or suicide
7. Giving away prized possessions

Immediate referrals to mental health professionals should be made when assessment suggests an adolescent may be considering suicide. Guidance can help focus on the positive aspects of life and strengthen coping abilities.

Another area of concern is the formation of healthy habits for daily living. Emphasis on regular exercise, sleep, nutrition, and stress-reduction habits is important. The nurse must recognize the value of these habits and help adolescents identify ways to incorporate them into their lifestyle.

Sexual experimentation is common among adolescents. Peer pressure, physiological and emotional changes, and societal expectations contribute to heterosexual and homosexual relations. More than 50% of adolescent students have had sexual intercourse during their lifetime (CDC, 1991), and two thirds of these sexually active teenagers are inconsistent in their use of safe sex. Even after going to a health clinic, only a small percent use birth control pills correctly all the time (Papalia and Olds, 1995). Consequently STDs and teenage pregnancy are major problems for many adolescents.

Each year in the United States there are over 12 million cases of STDs, and two thirds of them occur in persons under 25 years of age (Donovan, 1993). This high degree of incidence requires sexually active adolescents to be screened regularly for STDs (see Chapter 16).

The United States has one of the highest rates of teenage pregnancy in the world. According to the Children's Defense Fund, 1.1 million teenage females became pregnant in 1993. Not quite half of them had their babies; 40% had abortions and 13% miscarried. About 68% of these births occurred outside of marriage, and a high number were born to minority or disadvantaged mothers. These young mothers often cannot manage this responsibility, and their children often enter the state's foster care system. Adolescent mothers, and to a lesser degree fathers, face many social, educational, and economic problems as a result of pregnancy. Nurses can counsel teenagers concerning appropriate measures to use to avoid pregnancy. If pregnancy does occur, the nurse can guide teens in decision making and help them to obtain assistance.

Acute care. Hospitalization imposes rules and separates adolescents from their usual support system, restricts their independence, and threatens their personal identity. Adolescents who are forced into dependency or have their need for privacy ignored may respond with frustration, anger, or self-assertion. Although most hospitals allow peers to visit, some adolescents will isolate themselves until they can compete on an equal basis with peers. The telephone is often the lifeline between adolescents and their friends and helps them maintain their place in their social group. Many adolescents welcome peer visitors, and hospitals often allow the client to go to a lounge or cafeteria with them.

Adolescents who are engaged in emancipating themselves from their parents usually do well with intermittent visiting but expect some type of daily contact.

Some will request their parent remain with them throughout the hospitalization and others will not object to it, demonstrating that they also experience regression with the stress of illness. Nurses who address the client rather than the parents during the assessment process and show respect for adolescents' concerns usually establish a trusting relationship with them. Adolescents want nurses who will not "talk down" to them but relate to them at their level and understand their language. Nurses need to provide clear expectations for the behavior of adolescents during hospitalization and explain the reasons for these limits if the client asks. Once the nurse has the respect of the adolescent, it is possible to teach about the illness, positive health care practices, and treatment.

Adolescents can usually describe their pain with minimal assistance, pinpoint its location, and often explain its cause. They are usually aware of the medication they receive for pain and like to be in control of when it is given. Many of them are able to use distraction and relaxation techniques to decrease their discomfort.

Young Adult

Setting the age limits for the young adult period is an even more arbitrary affair than for other age spans. The beginning of this life phase is determined more by the acceptance of adult responsibilities for one's own maintenance than it is by a specific age. Somewhere between the age of 18 and 21, most adults complete the basic education or training they need to enter their chosen occupation, attain employment, set up their own living arrangements, and select a significant other. These changes in their lifestyle are recognized by others as the entrance into adulthood. The completion of this period is usually recognized as 40 years.

Young adults have reached physical maturity, have achieved the highest level of cognitive ability according to Piaget, and are expected to exhibit a high degree of psychosocial maturity. Personal traits suggesting maturity include acceptance of one's own strengths and weaknesses, acceptance of (but not necessarily approval of) the behavior of others, accountability and responsibility for one's own behavior, respect for others, open mindedness, tolerance for ambiguity, decision-making skills, emotional stability, use of positive mechanisms to cope with stress, and ability to delay immediate gratification of needs to reach a goal. Many adults recognize that they are continuously in the process of becoming more mature in their behavior.

Physical development. Young adults usually complete their physical growth by the age of 20. They are usually at their peak of health and less commonly experience severe illnesses compared with older adults. Although physical changes associated with aging have begun, the effects are not great enough to be noticed or require attention (Lewis and others, 1996).

Cognitive development. Rational thinking habits and flexibility of thought increase steadily through the adult years. Formal and informal educational experiences, general life experiences, and occupational opportunities dramatically increase conceptual, problem-solving, and motor skills. A rich, stimulating environment for the growing and maturing adult encourages the development of full creative potential.

An understanding of how adults learn assists the nurse in developing teaching plans for them. Adults come to the teaching-learning situation with a background of unique life experiences. Therefore the nurse should view adults as unique individuals. Their compliance with regimens such as medications, treatments, or lifestyle changes involves a decision-making process. The nurse should present as much information as the adult needs to make decisions about the prescribed course of treatment.

Psychosocial development. The emotional health of young adults is related to their ability to effectively address personal and social tasks. According to developmental theorists, certain patterns or trends are relatively predictable. Once young adults have begun to work in their chosen area, they have more time and energy to select a mate (if they have not already done so) and develop a greater sense of intimacy. Many will choose to marry, but an increasing number of young adults are choosing to remain single. Many want to be free to actively seek further education and/or pursue their career. Others choose to live with persons of the same or opposite sex and share living arrangements, and others are gay or lesbian and may be very committed life partners.

Identifying preferred occupational areas is a major task of young adults. When individuals know their skills, talents, and personality characteristics, occupational choices are easier and they are generally more satisfied with their choices. In the young and middle adult years, job satisfaction has been found to be a major factor in achievement and responsibility.

The developmental tasks of young adults are potentially filled with stressful situations. Most young adults have the physical and emotional resources and support systems to meet the many challenges, tasks, and responsibilities they face. During a psychosocial assessment, the nurse can assess for 10 hallmarks of emotional health (Box 20-8) that indicate successful maturation in this developmental stage. Nurses can often assist young adults to develop time-management skills or to mobilize their resources and support system, especially when one of their immediate family members is ill or hospitalized.

Health promotion. Health teaching and health counseling are often directed at assisting clients to improve their health habits. Understanding the dynamics

---

> **Box 20-8**
> ## Hallmarks of Emotional Health
>
> A sense of meaning and direction in life
> Successful negotiation through transitions
> Absence of feelings of being cheated or disappointed by life
> Attainment of several long-term goals
> Satisfaction with personal growth and development
> When in a stable intimate relationship, feelings of mutual love for partner; when single, satisfaction with social interactions
> Satisfaction with friendships
> Generally cheerful attitude
> Ability to view self realistically
> No unrealistic fears
>
> Modified from Stanhope M, Lancaster J: *Community health nursing: process and practice for promoting health,* ed 3, St. Louis, 1992, Mosby.

of behavior and habits will assist the nurse in designing interventions that will help the client develop or reinforce health promoting behaviors. To help clients form positive health habits, the nurse becomes a teacher and facilitator. The nurse cannot change clients' habits but can raise their level of knowledge regarding the potential impact of behavior on health. Clients have control of and are responsible for their own behaviors. The nurse can explain psychological principles of changing habits, offer information about health risks, and provide positive reinforcement of health-directed behaviors and decisions. Barriers to change, such as lack of knowledge or motivation, must be minimized or eliminated to bring about change.

Young adults are generally active and have no major health problems. However, their fast-paced lifestyles may put them at risk for illnesses or disabilities during their middle or older adult years. People have considerable control over their health and longevity. If people choose to follow the following seven recommendations they will maximize their potential for good health and a long life (Breslow and Breslow, 1993; Papalia and Olds, 1995).

1. Eat for health.
2. Exercise regularly.
3. Use your seat belt.
4. Do not smoke.
5. Do not drink alcohol to excess.
6. Avoid abuse or misuse of drugs and other substances.
7. Lead a healthy sexual life.

Violence is the greatest cause of mortality and morbidity among young adults. The USDHHS (1995) reported that the death rates per 100,000 population in 1992 for 25 to 44 year olds was 17.1% for motor vehicle accidents, 14.3% for homicide, and 14.8% for suicide.

Occupational risk factors may be a concern for the young adult. Certain work environments result in exposure to airborne particles, which may cause lung diseases and cancer (see Chapter 30). Cancers resulting from occupational exposures may involve a variety of organs. Young adults need to become aware of the dangers in their environment and take measures to protect themselves.

Poor adherence to routine screening schedules can put the client at risk for severe illnesses because of failed early detection. Clients should be encouraged to perform monthly breast self-examination (BSE), testicular self-examination (TSE), and regular genital self-examination (see Chapter 24). Women should be informed of the benefits and suggested schedule for routine mammography, and men should be informed about the need for regular prostate gland examinations.

Family stressors can occur at any time. Family life has peaks, when everyone in the family works together, and valleys, when everyone appears to pull apart. Situational stressors occur during events such as births, deaths, illnesses, marriages, divorces, and job losses.

The psychosocial assessment allows the nurse to identify areas of particular stress for the young adult. After identifying these stressors, the client and nurse can work together to modify the stress response. Chapter 22 reviews specific interventions for stress reduction.

Community health programs for young adults are designed to prevent illness, promote health, and detect disease in the early stages. Nurses can contribute to community health by actively planning screening and teaching programs. Family planning, birthing, and parenting skills are program topics in which adults are often interested. Health screening is a good opportunity for the nurse to perform assessment and provide health teaching and health counseling.

Acute care.
Many young adults do not experience hospitalization, but when they do it is often threatening because it interferes with their employment and fulfillment of family responsibilities. Scheduled hospitalizations allow adults to effectively plan to meet the needs of their families and expectations of their employment. Unanticipated hospitalizations often cause chaos for adults and all those directly involved in their lives. If they do not have a strong support system, they may welcome the nurse's help to establish priorities and mobilize their resources. Adults are often impatient with the time and energy requirements that a chronic health problem may require for good management. Support groups can often help clients deal with these challenges.

Middle-Age Adult
Middle adulthood usually refers to those years between 40 and 65 and is often described as that period when one

has both grown children and elderly parents (Papalia and Olds, 1995). Personal and career achievements have often already been experienced, along with socioeconomic stability. Using leisure time in satisfying and creative ways is a challenge that, if met satisfactorily, will enable middle adults to prepare for retirement.

Physical changes.
Accepting and adjusting to the physiological changes of middle age is one of the major developmental tasks of this age period (Havighurst, 1972). Because middle adulthood spans 25 years, many of the physical changes described may not occur until later in the developmental period. Middle-age adults use much energy to adapt self-concept and body image to physiological realities and changes in physical appearance. Table 20-12 summarizes these expected physical changes.

Climacteric is a term used to describe the decline of reproductive capacity and accompanying changes brought about by the decrease in sexual hormones. Men and women are affected differently. Males begin to experience decreased fertility, but they can continue to father children. **Menopause,** when a woman stops ovulating and menstruating, occurs only when 12 months have passed since the last menstrual flow (Lewis and others, 1996). The female's ability to bear children comes to an end. Women usually have a change in the amount and frequency of flow several years before menopause occurs. The average age of menopause is 51 years, but the usual range varies between 45 and 55 years of age.

Cognitive development.
Changes in the cognitive function of middle adults are few except during illness or trauma. Performance on intelligence tests indicates increases in some areas, particularly verbal abilities and tasks involving stored knowledge. Although middle-age adults may perform more slowly and not be as adept at solving new or unusual problems, the ability to solve practical problems based on experience peaks at midlife because of the ability to think integratively (Papalia and Olds, 1995).

Psychosocial development.
According to Erikson (1968), the primary developmental task of the middle adult years is to achieve generativity, which is the willingness to establish and guide the next generation and care for others. Many find particular joy in assisting their children and other young people to become productive and responsible adults. During this period adult children often begin to help older adult parents. Individuals have the time and interest to become more involved in their church, charitable activities, politics, fundraising, and other voluntary activities that bring them satisfaction. The opposing developmental trait, stagnation, occurs when people become preoccupied with themselves or self-indulgent or through inactivity become bored, withdrawn, and isolated. Short stagnant

TABLE 20-12

Physiological Changes in the Middle-Age Adult

Body System	Findings
Integument	Intact condition
	Appropriate distribution of pigmentation
	Slow, progressive decrease in skin turgor
	Graying and loss of hair
Head and neck	Symmetry of scalp, skull, and face
Eyes	Visual acuity by Snellen chart that is less than 20/50
	Loss of accommodation of lens to focus light on near objects
	Pupillary reaction to light and accommodation
	Normal visual fields and extraocular movements
	Normal retinal structures
Ears	Normal auditory structures; acuity of high-pitched sounds may decline
Nose, sinuses, and throat	Patent nares and intact sinuses, mouth, and pharynx
	Location of trachea at midline
	Nonpalpable lateral thyroid lobes
Thorax and lungs	Increased anteroposterior diameter
	Respiratory rate 16-20 breaths per minute and regular
	Normal tactile fremitus, resonance, and breath sounds
Heart and vascular system	Normal heart sounds
	Point of maximal impulse: at fifth intercostal space in midclavicular line and 2 cm or less in diameter
	Vital signs
	Temperature: 36.7°-37.6° C (97°-99.6° F)
	Pulse: 60-100 (conditioned athlete ≈ 50)
	Blood pressure: 95-140/60-90 mm Hg
	All pulses palpable
Breasts	Decreased size resulting from decreased muscle mass
	Normal nipples
Abdomen	No tenderness or organomegaly
	Decreased strength of abdominal muscles
Female reproductive system	Change in menstrual cycle and in duration and quality of menstrual flow
	"Hot flashes"
	Change in cervical mucosa
Male reproductive system	Normal penis and scrotum
	Prostatic enlargement in some individuals
Musculoskeletal system	Decreased muscle mass
	Decreased range of joint motion
Neurological system	Appropriate effect, appearance, and behavior
	Lucidity and appropriate level of cognitive ability
	Intact cranial nerves
	Adequate motor and sensory responses

periods allow one to gather energy for the next project, but prolonged stagnation may result in destructive behavior toward children and the community.

Expected changes in the middle adult may involve expected events such as children moving away from home or unexpected events such as a marital separation or the death of a spouse or parent. These changes may result in stress that can affect the middle adult's overall level of health.

Career changes may occur by choice or as a result of changes in the workplace or society as a whole. In recent decades, middle adults more often change occupations because they find themselves less satisfied with their present employment. In some cases, technological advances or changes in the direction of industry force middle adults to change work situations. Such changes, especially when unanticipated, may result in stress that affects family relationships, self-concept, and financial security for the later years.

Marital changes that may occur during middle age include death of a spouse, separation, divorce, and the choice of remarrying or remaining single. A widowed, separated, or divorced client goes through a period of loss and grief during which it is necessary to adapt to the change in marital status. If the single middle adult decides to marry, the stressors of marriage are similar to those for the young adult. In addition, the couple may have to cope with the social expectations and pressures related to middle-age marriage.

The departure of the last child from the home of the middle-age parents may be a stressor. Many parents welcome freedom from child-rearing responsibilities, whereas others feel lonely or without direction. Parents may need to reassess relationships, resolve conflicts, and plan for the future.

The increasing life span in the United States and Canada has led to increased numbers of older adults in the population. Therefore greater numbers of middle-age adults must address the personal and social issues confronting their aging parents. Adult children frequently assume partial or total care-giving responsibilities for their older parents. This means adult children assist with personal care, housekeeping, financial, transportation, and medical care management tasks. The burden placed on adult care givers is increased if they are also employed and continuing to raise children. The middle-age adult and the older adult parent may have conflicting relationship priorities. The older adult may desire to remain independent, while the adult child strives to protect the parent. Negotiations and compromises are useful in defining and resolving such problems.

Health promotion.
Because middle-agers experience physiological changes and face certain health realities, their perceptions of health and health behaviors are often important factors in maintaining health. At present, individuals are more prone to stress-related illnesses such as heart attacks, hypertension, migraine headaches, backache, arthritis, cancer, and autoimmune diseases.

The leading causes of death in persons between the ages of 45 and 64 years are heart disease, cancer (primarily lung, breast, and colorectal), stroke, accidental injuries, and chronic obstructive pulmonary diseases. Females' risk for coronary heart disease increases with middle age, particularly after menopause. One in nine women from age 45 to 64 has some form of heart disease or stroke, and one in six men has heart or blood vessel disease.

Middle-age adults should continue the same seven recommended health practices that were outlined in the young adult section. Additional considerations for the middle-ager include the following:

- Women should have a screening mammogram at age 40 and every 1 to 2 years thereafter until age 50, when an annual mammogram is recommended (ACS, 1997).
- A proctosigmoidoscopic examination for colorectal cancer should be done at 3- to 5-year intervals after the age of 50, provided negative exams have been recorded for 2 consecutive years.
- Annual stool guaiac testing should be done over the age of 50.
- Annual digital examination of the rectum should be performed over the age of 40 (American Cancer Society, 1997).
- Women should get between 1000 and 1500 mg of calcium a day and sufficient vitamin D to facilitate calcium absorption (to prevent osteoporosis).
- Middle-age adults should recognize that obesity is more of a threat during middle age.

When middle adults seek health care, the nurse focuses on goals of positive health behaviors and wellness to evaluate health behaviors, lifestyle, and environment. Middle adults are more interested in health promotion activities than in previous decades. Exercise and fitness clubs, for example, give adults the opportunity to participate in many physical activities. Attention to risk factors that can be altered to improve the client's health can add years and quality to the client's life.

Acute care.
Middle-agers hold the same family and occupational concerns regarding hospitalization as do young adults. There may be less stress because of the security of employment or because the children who are still at home are usually old enough to care for themselves. However, those who are underinsured are faced with serious financial threats. Middle-age adults are at risk for a decline in their physical health. The American Cancer Society (1997) reports that most cancer cases affect adults middle-age or older. Chronic health problems such as sickle cell anemia, arthritis, asthma, diabetes, and lung disease require ongoing medical care and may require brief hospitalizations. The middle-age adult is usually interested in his or her health and desires to be informed. The family can be an important resource in helping the individual cope with any health problems. It is important for the nurse to understand the significance health has for an individual so that appropriate support can be provided in helping clients make choices and take action to improve their health.

Older Adult
Most older adults are physically active, intelligent, and socially engaging (Figure 20-5). Extended life spans allow many older adults to enjoy their retirement by pursuing interests that they previously had little time for. The percentage of Americans 65 years or older has more than tripled since 1900 and is expected to continue to rise until at least 2050.

Older adulthood traditionally begins after retire-

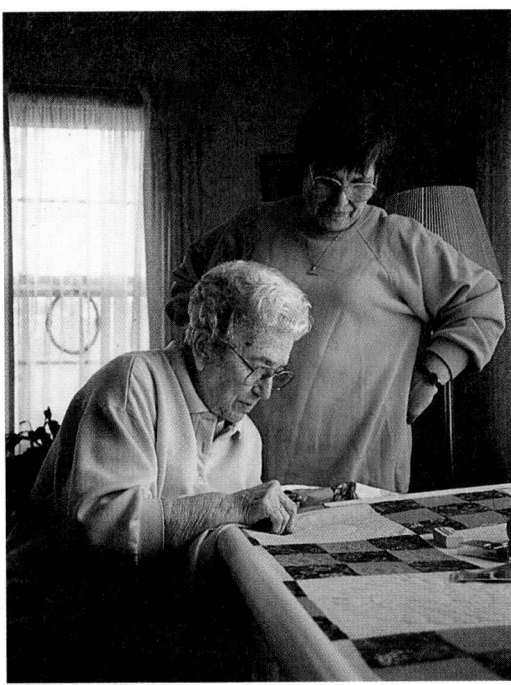

Figure 20-5.   Quilting keeps this older adult active.

ment, but the time when people retire varies greatly. Some people retire at 50 and others work into their eighties and nineties. It is not unusual for those who write about older adults to divide them into the "young old" who are vital, vigorous, and active and the "old old" who are frail and infirm. The fastest growing subset is the nearly 3 million people over the age of 85, whose growth rate is nearly three times that of the overall older adult population (Lueckenotte, 1996).

Geriatrics is the branch of health care dealing with the physiology and psychology of aging and with the diagnosis and treatment of diseases affecting older adults. **Gerontology** is the study of all aspects of the aging process and its consequences.

Nursing care of older adults poses special challenges because of diversity in clients' physical, cognitive, and psychosocial health. Older adults vary in level of function and productivity. Before making a health assessment, the nurse should be aware of the normal expected findings of physical and psychosocial assessment for an older adult and should consider the normal changes of aging.

Physical development. The older adult must adjust to the physical changes of aging. These changes are not associated with a disease state but are the normal changes anticipated with aging. The physiological changes that occur with advancing age vary with each client. Table 20-13 describes the general types of physiological changes that can be expected with older adults. Some are visible to the eye, and others are not.

They occur in all persons but take place at different rates and depend on accompanying circumstances in an individual's life. The nurse assessing the older adult client should also consider the potential for sensory changes that may influence data gathering.

Cognitive development. Older adults often remain alert and highly perceptive until the time of their death. Nevertheless, the misconception that older adults always have cognitive impairments and suffer from memory loss and confusion persists. Because cognitive impairment can occur in this age group, nurses must be aware of the nature and type of these impairments.

Intelligence testing in late adulthood seems to indicate that fluid intelligence, the ability to solve new problems, declines during late adulthood, but crystallized intelligence, based on learning and experience, may increase or at least is maintained. Practical thinking, specialized knowledge and skills, and wisdom continue to increase although the mechanics of intelligence often decline. Certain aspects of short-term memory (e.g., numbers) decrease with age, but visual memory, which allows a person to remember how to read, remains strong. Long-term memory for newly learned information decreases significantly with age, but recall for distant experiences and procedural experiences (e.g., driving) does not seem to be affected in the later years of life. Both intelligence and memory vary greatly among individuals. Many people incorrectly believe that older adults have little if any ability to learn. As a result, health care professionals often fail to provide appropriate health education opportunities for older adult clients. Most older people who want and need to learn new skills and information can do so when it is presented more slowly over a longer period. Continuing mental activity is considered essential to keep older adults alert, and older people do benefit from memory training (Papalia and Olds, 1995).

Dementia is a broad category of disorders that affect older adults' memory and cognitive function. Vocational and interpersonal functioning is also altered (Lueckenotte, 1996). Clients experience memory impairment, disturbed language (aphasia), impaired motor activity (apraxia), and the inability to recognize objects (agnosia). Certain forms of dementia are acute and treatable. Early recognition is thus important, requiring the nurse to make thorough observations of client behavior, neurological function (see Chapter 24), and laboratory diagnostic studies. Family and friends can be valuable resources in detecting behavioral changes.

Alzheimer's disease is a progressive form of dementia that usually ends in death after a period of 5 to 8 years. The disease progresses in three stages: an early stage involving memory loss; a middle stage involving loss of language skills and motor function; and the final

TABLE 20-13
Normal Physical Changes of Aging

System	Normal Findings
Integumentary	
Skin color	Brown age spots and spotty pigmentation in areas exposed to sun; pallor even in absence of anemia
Moisture	Dry, scaly
Temperature	Extremities cooler; perspiration decreased
Texture	Decreased elasticity; wrinkles; folding, sagging
Fat distribution	Decreased on extremities; increased on abdomen
Hair	Thinning and graying on scalp; axillary and pubic hair and hair on extremities may be decreased; facial hair in men decreased; chin and upper lip hair may be present in women
Nails	Decreased growth rate
Head and neck	
Head	Nasal and facial bones sharp and angular; loss of eyebrow hair in women; men's eyebrows become bushier
Eyes	Decreased visual acuity; decreased accommodation; reduced adaptation to darkness; sensitivity to glare
Ears	Decreased pitch discrimination; diminished light reflex; diminished hearing acuity
Nose and sinuses	Increased nasal hair; decreased sense of smell
Mouth and pharynx	Use of bridges or dentures; decreased sense of taste; atrophy of papillae of lateral edges of tongue; occasionally change in voice pitch
Neck	Thyroid gland nodular; slight tracheal deviation resulting from muscle atrophy
Thorax and lungs	Increased anterior-posterior diameter; increased chest rigidity; increased respiratory rate with decreased lung expansion
Heart and vascular	Significant increase in systolic pressure with slight increase in diastolic pressure; peripheral pulses easily palpated; pedal pulses weaker and lower extremities colder, especially at night; orthostatic hypertension common
Breasts	Diminished breast tissue; pendulous, flabby condition
Gastrointestinal	Decreased salivary secretions, which make swallowing more difficult; decreased peristalsis; decreased production of digestive enzymes; hydrochloric acid, pepsin, and pancreatic enzymes, leading to indigestion and constipation
Reproductive	
Female	Decreased estrogen; decreased uterine size; decreased secretions; atrophy of epithelial lining of the vagina; vaginal dryness
Male	Decreased testosterone; decreased sperm count; decreased testicular size
Urinary	Decreased renal filtration and renal efficiency; subsequent loss of protein from kidney; nocturia
Female	Urgency and stress incontinence from decrease in perineal muscle tone
Male	Frequent urination resulting from prostatic enlargement
Musculoskeletal	Decreased muscle mass and strength; bone demineralization (more pronounced in women); shortening of trunk from intervertebral space narrowing; decreased joint mobility; decreased range of joint motion; kyphosis (usually in women); slowed reaction time
Neurological	Decreased rate of voluntary or automatic reflexes; decreased ability to respond to multiple stimuli; insomnia; shorter sleeping periods

Modified from Ebersole P, Hess P: *Toward healthy aging: human needs and nursing response,* ed 4, St. Louis, 1994, Mosby.

stage involving incontinence, inability to ambulate, and a complete loss of language skills (Brady, 1993).

Alzheimer's disease affects the brain parenchyma. The diagnosis is made by excluding other possible causes of the client's symptoms (e.g., psychiatric disorder, brain tumor, degenerative neurological disease). The mental and physical changes that these clients experience increase their risk of injury. The stress experienced by family and friends is extensive, particularly for those assuming care for the Alzheimer's victim.

Nursing management of clients with Alzheimer's disease is complex. Detwiler (1993) outlines four goals in planning nursing care for Alzheimer's clients: prevent acceleration of symptoms, preserve the client's dignity, promote health and independent functioning as much as possible, and preserve the family's unity.

Long-term abuse of alcohol and drugs can also affect cognitive functioning. The incidence of identified alcohol abuse in older adults is currently less than 10% of that population, but it is expected to rise in the near future as more middle-agers who are accustomed to the use of alcohol enter late adulthood (Thibault and Maly, 1993).

Psychosocial development. The older adult must adapt to many psychosocial changes that occur with aging. Among the more common transitions that occur with aging include retirement, volunteerism, and loss of spousal roles (Ebersole and Hess, 1994). There are also many older adults who have experienced occupational success and spend their later years forming independent businesses (e.g., consulting, travel agencies, sales). Despite the changes that occur, the older adult has the potential for developing new and fulfilling life patterns.

Retirement. Most older adults desire to work as long as they are physically able (Ebersole and Hess, 1994). The time a person chooses to retire is often based on type of work, status achieved, and length of time employed. When a client describes retirement it is important to know whether the individual is fully retired, partially retired, or retired from one position to assume another.

Ebersole and Hess (1994) note that retirement is no longer just a few years of rest before death. Instead, retirement represents a developmental stage that may occupy 30 years of one's life. It may also represent a highly productive and fulfilling period of life.

The nurse can help clients and their families prepare for retirement by gathering information as to why the client is considering retirement and giving **anticipatory guidance** related to retirement issues. Counseling of older adults may focus on the following six issues. First, what provisions have the client and family made for retirement income? The incomes of most older adults are fixed or do not rise as quickly as inflation increases. Older adults need resources to adequately meet housing, food, clothing, and health care expenses. Second, what postretirement activities are available? It is important to assess clients' abilities, skills, and interests. The older adult must also learn to acquire new activities and interests to maintain the quality of life. People vary in their ability to adjust to new circumstances brought on by aging. Persons who have not acquired social and communication skills and who then need to make new social contacts will have more difficulty in adjusting. Third, what living arrangements may be needed? Many older adults decide to relocate into smaller living quarters for easier maintenance. Fourth, what preparations have been made for family role changes? Sharing of household tasks and spending more time with grandchildren or doing community work are options. Fifth, what provisions have been made to meet health care needs? With increasing health care costs, this can be a serious concern. Sixth, how will the retired person attend to legal affairs? Older adults should understand the importance of estate planning.

Volunteerism. Thirty-five percent of the population age 65 and older are engaged in some type of volunteer work (Ebersole and Hess, 1994). This includes offering assistance for religious and charitable organizations and government and community service programs.

Death. The majority of older adults experience death of spouses, friends, and in some cases children. These losses require individuals to go through a process of grieving (see Chapter 21). Losing a partner that one has lived with for many years in a satisfying relationship is like losing one's self (Ebersole and Hess, 1994). For many older adults the grief associated with loss of a spouse can last for many years. Experiencing the grieving process requires support from family, nurses, and other health professionals.

The nurse can lend support by showing warmth and caring to help the client feel he or she is not alone. Helping the client understand the normal process of grief is important (see Chapter 21). The family can also serve as a resource, learning how to give support appropriately. When older adults meet new partners, the nurse might become a resource in helping clients discuss their sexuality and need for therapy. Because loss of a spouse means the assumption of new roles, widowers might benefit from homemaking classes; widows might benefit from learning about financial management. The nurse connects the client to self-help groups for widows and widowers.

A common misconception is that death of an older adult is always a blessing and the culmination of a full and rich life. Many dying older adults still have life goals and are not emotionally prepared to die. **Reminiscence,** or *life review,* is a technique that may facilitate the individual's preparation for the end of life on earth. It is an adaptive function of older adults that allows them to recall the past for the purpose of assigning new meaning to past experiences. Reminiscence is the natural way older adults revive their past in an attempt to establish order and meaning and to reconcile conflicts and disappointments as they prepare for death (Butler, 1963). Nurses can support reminiscence by sharing some of their own conflicts or ambivalence so as to encourage clients to participate in the process (Ebersole and Hess, 1994). It takes time to help clients truly explore how they feel. The sharing of personal memories requires both nurse and client to trust one another. The nurse must be patient and recognize it can take several weeks or months for a client to review past hopes and future expectations.

Aloneness and loneliness. With advancing age, more people live alone. This is particularly common for older, white women (Ebersole and Hess, 1994). The growing percentage of unmarried individuals, the likelihood of widowhood for women, and the support of families in allowing older adults to maintain their independence all contribute to more individuals living by themselves. However, living alone is not equivalent to the feeling of loneliness. A person can be surrounded by others yet still feel lonely. Ebersole and Hess (1994) define loneliness as an affective state of longing and emptiness, whereas being alone is to be solitary, apart from others, and undisturbed. Many clients choose to

be alone or isolated simply because of the desire to gain privacy or an opportunity for self-reflection and creativity. Loneliness on the other hand can be a passive and painful emotion, influenced by psychological, economic, sociological, and physiological factors (Figure 20-6).

It is important for the nurse to understand the differences between aloneness and loneliness and to be able to recognize which condition is affecting a client. Too often the two concepts are confused. When a nurse notices a client spending time alone it is important to share observations with the client and to determine why the client chooses privacy. The client may desire to be left alone to have time to think about existing concerns or thoughts about an illness. It may be necessary to help the client find more time for privacy and to find ways to minimize disturbances (especially for the hospitalized client).

Sexuality. Many misconceptions exist concerning the sexuality of older adults. They are often thought to be without sexual desire for a variety of reasons. In reality, the older adult still experiences sexual drive and activity, although these may be altered because of physiological changes, sociocultural expectations, health problems, and medications.

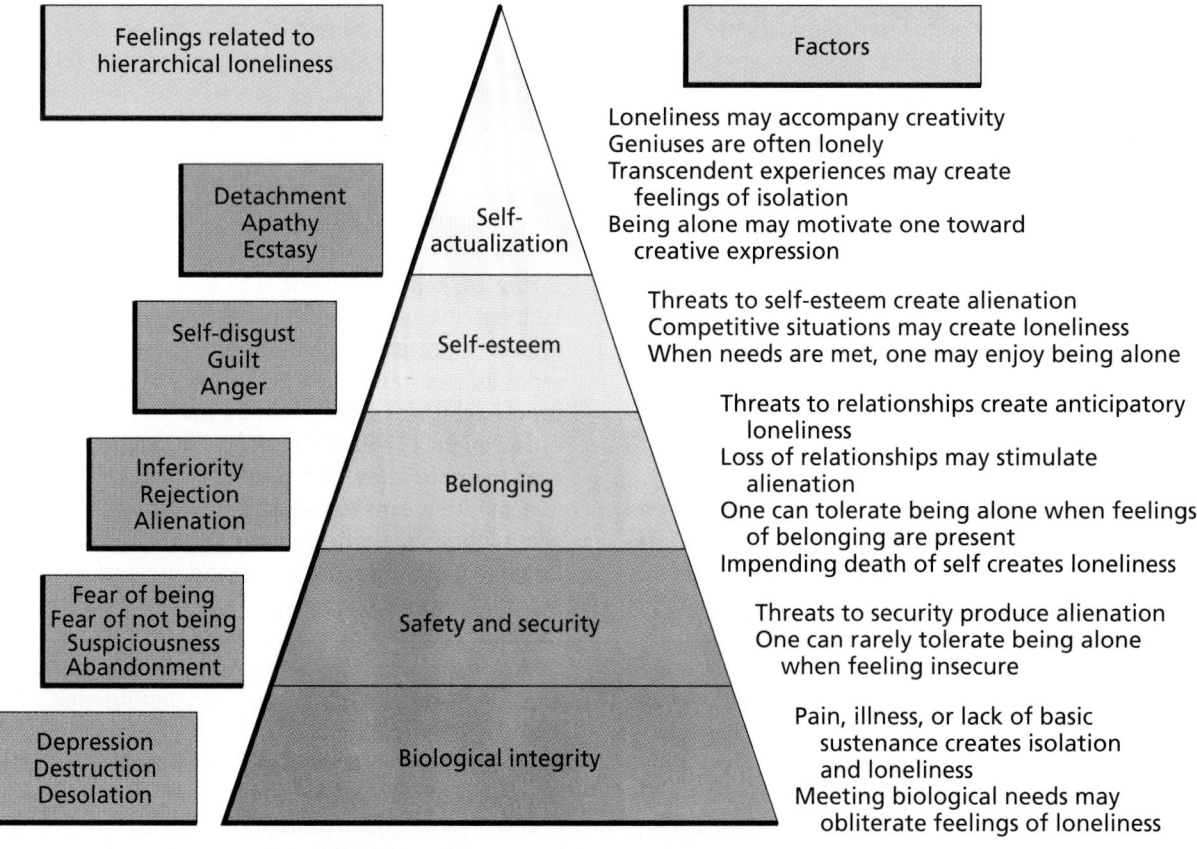

Figure 20-6. Loneliness in relation to Maslow's hierarchy of needs. (Modified from Ebersole P, Hess P: *Toward healthy aging: human needs and nursing response,* ed 3, St. Louis, 1990, Mosby.)

When caring for the older adult, the nurse must help the client maintain sexual health. Sexual relationships can provide love, intimacy, and physical stimulation, all of which add quality to the adult's life and are motivating factors for improved health behaviors. Nurses and society in general are often uncomfortable discussing sexual needs of older clients. To help older adults achieve or maintain sexual health, nurses must understand the physical changes in sexual response. The knowledge of sexual changes described in Table 20-14 enables the nurse to educate the older adult client about changes to expect in sexual functioning. It is important for older adults to know if they have been prescribed drugs that may interfere with sexual activity. Physicians should attempt to prescribe drugs without sexual side effects if clients request it.

Housing and environment. Changes in social roles, family responsibilities, and health status influence the older client's choice of living arrangements. An older adult may need to change living arrangements because of the death of a spouse or a change in health sta-

tus. A change in an older client's living arrangements may require an extended period of adjustment during which assistance and support will be needed from health care professionals and the client's family.

Housing and the environment as a whole are important, because they can have a major impact on the health of the older adult. Nurses are often asked to help clients and their families determine appropriate living arrangements. It is important for the nurse to assess clients' activity level, financial status, access to public transportation and community activities, environmental hazards, and support systems. For example, certain physical problems would make it difficult to live on the second floor or have laundry facilities in the basement. Because falls commonly occur in older adulthood, care givers should use preventive measures to decrease their incidence. Making changes in the house environment to reduce the client's fear of falling can be helpful. Physical assessment of older adults may reveal risk factors that predispose to falls, such as neuropathy of the feet, severe joint problems, abnormal gait, changes in

TABLE 20-14
Physical Changes in Sexual Response in the Older Adult

Female	Male
Excitation	
Diminished vaginal lubrication (1 to 3 minutes may be required for adequate amounts to appear)	Less intense and slower erection (but can be maintained longer without ejaculation)
Diminished flattening and separation of labia majora	Less vasocongestion of scrotal sac
Disappearance of elevation of labia majora	Less pronounced elevation and congestion of testicles
Decreased vasocongestion of labia minora	Decreased muscle tension
Decreased elastic expansion of vagina (depth and breadth)	
Decreased muscle tension	
Plateau	
Decreased capacity for vasocongestion	Nipple erection and sexual flush less often
Decreased areolar engorgement	Decrease or absence of secretory activity (lubrication) by Cowper's gland before ejaculation
Labial color change less evident	
Decreased secretions of Bartholin's glands	
Orgasm	
Fewer contractions of orgasmic platform	Fewer penile contractions
Rectal sphincter contractions with severe tension only	Fewer rectal sphincter contractions
	Decreased force of ejaculation with decreased amount of semen (if long ejaculation, seepage of semen occurs)
Resolution	
Observably slower subsidence of nipple erection	Slow subsidence of vasocongestion of nipples and scrotum
Quicker subsidence of vasocongestion of clitoris and orgasmic platform	Loss of erection and descent of testicles shortly after ejaculation
	Refractory time extended (time before another erection ranges from several to 24 hours or longer)

Modified from Ebersole P, Hess P: *Toward healthy aging: human needs and nursing response,* ed 4, St. Louis, 1994, Mosby.

posture, poor vision, loss of muscle control, and affected memory. Changes that provide a safer environment for older adults to live in include rails along outside steps, colored step strips, safety rails in tubs and showers, toilets with elevated seats and grab bars, and brightly lit living quarters. The environment can support or hinder physical and social functioning, enhance or drain the individual's energy, and complement or tax existing physical changes such as vision and hearing. Housing arrangements for older adults should also provide them with ample privacy and a variety of opportunities to socialize.

Health promotion. The possibility of an individual being reasonably healthy and fit in later life often depends on the person's lifestyle. Older adults should continue the same seven recommended health practices that were introduced in the young adult section. Some older adults will need encouragement to maintain a pattern of physical exercise and activity. It is not too late for an older person to begin an exercise program; however, older adults should have a complete physical examination, which usually includes a stress cardiogram or stress test. Assessment of activity tolerance will help the nurse and client plan a program that meets physical needs while allowing for physical impairments.

In addition to maintaining an intake of 1000 to 1500 mg of calcium and vitamin D, older individuals need greater amounts of vitamins A and C. Total caloric intake usually declines in response to decreases in metabolic rate and physical activity. Nutritional needs of the older adult are further discussed in Chapter 34.

Older adults particularly value good health. A state of wellness provides energy, vitality, and a zest for life. The nurse often practices in health maintenance programs that promote the older adult's wellness. Senior citizens' centers, churches, schools, shopping malls, supermarkets, libraries, and hospital lobbies can be used as sites for screening programs and to present information to older adults on specific health topics (Box 20-9).

Most older adults are in good health; however, chronic medical conditions increase dramatically with age and sometimes cause disability. In 1994 nearly half of all adults age 65 and older reported some limitation of activity as a result of a chronic health problem (Lueckenotte, 1996). The effect of a particular chronic health problem on mobility and independence depends greatly on the individual. Most older adults are capable of taking charge of their lives and assume responsibility for preventing disability. Coronary artery disease (CAD) remains the leading cause of death in those 65 years of age or older (Edelman and Mandle, 1994). Hypertension contributes to both strokes and heart attacks (see Chapter 23). Blacks are at greater risk than whites, and men are at greater risk than women. The relationship between hypertension and CAD (including myocardial infarction, congestive heart failure, periph-

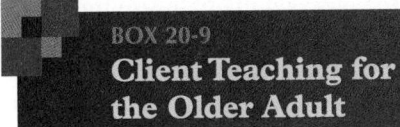

BOX 20-9

Client Teaching for the Older Adult

- Inform client about preretirement planning, to ease the transition from a full-time work schedule.
- Discuss housing alternatives to help the older adult make a decision regarding the sale of the home, relocation to another area of the country, or retirement communities.
- Instruct client about health maintenance programs, such as exercise activities, that are designed to increase exercise tolerance, flexibility, and socialization.
- Teach client that the need for annual influenza immunizations increases, especially with chronic illness.
- Teach client about safe and appropriate administration of prescribed drugs: purpose; effect; possible other prescription, over-the-counter, or dietary interactions; and reportable side effects.
- Instruct client regarding environmental safety issues (e.g., home lighting, floor coverings, stairs, shoes, electrical cords) to reduce the risk of falling.
- Discuss changes in sleep patterns with age and methods to promote adequate rest and energy.
- Instruct client about nutritional aspects related to disease (e.g., a low-fat diet with hypertension, the need for a balanced diet with reduced total calories because of aging changes and lower energy expenditures).
- Teach an individual exercise program based on an assessment of the client's overall health status and lifestyle.

eral vascular disease, and stroke) is well documented (Stammer and others, 1993). Lifestyle modifications including weight reduction; adequate physical activity; salt restriction (6 g/day); limiting alcohol intake; reducing dietary saturated fat and cholesterol; adequate intake of potassium, calcium, and magnesium; and smoking cessation will lower the blood pressure and reduce the incidence of CAD (Lueckenotte, 1996).

Malignant neoplasms are the second most common cause of death among older adults. Sixty percent of all cancer occurs after the age of 60, and cancer affects 1 in 10 persons 70 years of age or older. The organs most commonly affected are the lung, prostate, colon, rectum, pancreas, bladder, skin, breast, and uterus (American Cancer Society, 1997). Early detection and treatment are important. Older adults should continue the cancer screenings recommended for the middle-age adult. The nurse can also develop programs to decrease the older adult's risk for cancer, including encouraging smoking cessation, teaching clients to perform breast self-examinations (see Chapter 24), encouraging clients to have routine Pap smears, cautioning clients about risks for skin cancer, and educating clients about the warning signs of other forms of cancer.

Sensory impairments such as changes in vision, hearing, taste, and smell are common in the older adult. These changes are frequently the result of the normal aging process. The nurse can aid the older adult in identifying resources to help correct visual and auditory problems (see Chapter 39). The sense of touch usually remains strong. Older adults who often become victims of social isolation are often deprived of touching and holding, which convey affection and friendliness. The touch of nurses and all care givers who work with older adults can serve to provide sensory stimulation; reduce anxiety; relieve physiological and emotional pain; orient the person to reality; and provide comfort, particularly during the dying process.

Dental problems are common in older adults. They can lead to changes in taste and a decrease in nutritional intake. Because of missing teeth or poorly fitting dentures, older adults may restrict their diet to soft foods. The nurse can help prevent dental and gum disease through health education. In addition to teaching the older adult to maintain routine dental care, the nurse can teach specific measures to reduce the risk of gum disease. The nurse can help the client with ill-fitting dentures or other dental problems by identifying resources in the community that provide dental services to older adults at reduced rates.

As a group, adults over 65 years of age are the greatest users of prescription drugs. Many drugs may interact with one another, potentiating or negating the effect of another drug. Some drugs cause confusion; affect balance; cause dizziness, nausea, or vomiting; or promote constipation or urinary frequency. Polypharmacy, the prescription, use, or administration of more medications than are indicated clinically, is a common problem of older adults. The combined use of multiple drugs can cause serious untoward effects.

Health care services. A variety of health care services are available to the population. Chapter 2 outlines a variety of services such as day care centers and respite care used frequently by older adults and their families. Home health care services and homemaker services prevent or delay institutionalization for older adults who need assistance with self-care and activities of daily living.

The hospice is a community resource for the terminally ill. A hospice can be an independent unit within the community or may be contained within an institutional setting. The hospice program focuses on meeting the needs of the dying client and the family (see Chapter 21). Hospice programs do not institute life-support or other measures to prolong the life of the terminally ill.

Situations of declining health, decreased physical and human resources, and increased dependence may necessitate the older adult's institutionalization in a long-term care facility. Such a facility provides extended residential, intermediate, or skilled nursing care, medical care, and personal and psychosocial services. The decision for institutional care is not easy to make, and the family requires a great deal of support. In addition, the family may need the nurse's help in locating the proper facility to meet the needs of the client. When possible, the facility chosen should be close to the client's and family's home to provide accessibility for visits.

Acute care. Hospitalization of older adults is often disturbing to them, because the environment and routines are very different from those they are accustomed to. Even those who are able to live independently with some assistance from their families may become temporarily disoriented by the strange surroundings of a hospital. The nurse should monitor the client for confusion and encourage frequent visitation by family members.

The nurse can use reality orientation techniques to help reorient the older adult who has been disoriented by a change in environment, surgery, illness, or emotional stress. **Reality orientation** is a communication modality used for making the client aware of time, place, and person. The major purposes of reality orientation include restoring clients' sense of reality; improving their level of awareness; promoting socialization; elevating clients to a maximal level of independent functioning; and minimizing confusion, disorientation, and physical regression. Environmental changes within a hospital, such as the bright lights and lack of windows in intensive care and the noise from nearby roommates, often lead to disorientation and confusion. The client's environment and the nursing personnel are constantly changing in the hospital, and the immediate environment is unstable, making coping and adaptation difficult. The problem is compounded, for example, by tranquilizers, sleeping pills, anesthesia, pain, and the physiological changes of illness. Nurses and other health team members should anticipate disorientation and confusion as a consequence when older adults are hospitalized, and incorporate reality orientation interventions into their care. These interventions are based on seven principles. Consistent use of the techniques of reality orientation helps to reorient older adults to their surroundings.

When an older adult is hospitalized or has an acute or chronic illness, the related physical dependence makes it difficult for the person to maintain a positive body image. The nurse has a direct influence on the older adult client's appearance. The nurse must consider the importance of maintaining a pleasant appearance and presenting a socially acceptable image.

CRITICAL THINKING IN CLIENT CARE

Knowledge. Before beginning the assessment of an individual, students should review the developmental theories, outlined earlier, that relate to their clients. Students should recognize that familiarity with physical developmental milestones, psychosocial developmental crises, cognitive development, and health concerns for each age group is essential if they are going to be effective in assisting clients to attain optimal health.

Another important area of knowledge to consider when caring for a client's developmental needs is that of cultural diversity. The nurse must explore the cultural variations in family roles and relationships as they influence an individual's development, to have a clear understanding of client needs.

Experience. Nurses who are parents or have been involved in the teaching of children will be aware that the thinking abilities of individuals of different ages will differ and it will be necessary to change one's approach to gain their cooperation. Previous experiences with individuals of various ages through family or other relationships will make it easier for the nurse to determine appropriate or inappropriate behaviors and health concerns related to that age group.

Attitudes. Humility is an important attitude for the nurse to apply when collecting data about a client's developmental history. It is easy to form opinions about clients' developmental needs on the basis of developmental theory and related psychosocial principles. However, as is the case in any nursing situation, the nurse must not assume knowing what the client's needs are without gathering a clear picture of a client's physical and psychosocial health concerns. Often information about the client's health practices will reflect the client's cultural background, which may be very different from that of the nurse.

Creativity is a valuable critical thinking attitude when the nurse conducts an assessment of an infant or child. Often the nurse must incorporate play or other activities into the assessment to better visualize the child's physical developmental capacities.

Standards. Critical thinking standards help ensure that the right decisions are made. When developing a plan of care that incorporates growth and development principles and approaches, the nurse strives to apply the intellectual standards of relevance and completeness. It is important to not employ a developmental approach that does not fit with the client's level of maturation. For example, having a preschooler attempt a motor skill that is not within his or her ability would be irrelevant and inappropriate for promoting developmental enrichment. When selecting a plan of care, the nurse is complete in using psychosocial, cognitive, and physical approaches that complement and strengthen the client's developmental abilities.

The nurse will also use professional standards when providing care to clients of various age groups. For example, when supporting parents' health promotion practices it is important to refer to standards for immunizations. These standards help to determine not only the required immunizations for certain age groups but also the parents' success in ensuring a child is immunized. Similarly, there are a variety of standards established for health screening of adult age groups. These standards are used by the nurse during health education efforts.

⋯ NURSING PROCESS ⋯⋯⋯⋯⋯⋯⋯⋯⋯⋯

▣ Assessment

Nursing assessment of individuals across the life span requires the nurse to be familiar with the physiological, cognitive, and psychosocial changes that occur during each stage of development and the health concerns for each age group. A number of assessment tools have been developed to facilitate concise but comprehensive data collection for individuals of various ages. During the health history, physical assessment, and developmental assessment, the nurse also observes the interactions between the individual and any present family member. Data gathered will provide information regarding the client's lifestyle, level of functioning, family relationships, health concerns, and health promotion activities.

Throughout life, illness and hospitalization are stressful experiences. The ability of individuals to cope is affected by their level of development, their coping skills, their previous experiences with illness and hospitalization, the seriousness of the diagnosis, the degree to which the illness interferes with their activities of daily living and their lifestyle, and the availability of a support system. The nurse's assessment should demonstrate an awareness of specific client concerns at various stages of life.

Client expectations. During an assessment it is important to determine what clients and/or their families expect from the care giver. At the beginning of a home visit the nurse might ask, "What do you think is most important for us to accomplish today?" or when preparing to leave, the nurse might ask, "Have we met your expectations for this visit?" In the outpatient setting one might ask what expectation(s) the client and/or family have for the visit. In the hospital setting it is wise to determine if and how family members wish to participate in the care of the client and how members of the health team can be most helpful to them. The client's primary nurse should begin each day with a brief assessment to determine any change in condition and the client's perceptions of the care received.

⋯⋯⋯⋯⋯⋯⋯⋯⋯⋯⋯⋯

Successful critical thinking requires a synthesis of knowledge, experience, information gathered from clients, and critical thinking attitudes and standards. Clinical judgments require the nurse to anticipate what information is needed, analyze the data, and then make decisions regarding client care. The client expects competent and informed care. In the case study, Louis incorporates previous knowledge and experience in providing care for Crystal Taylor.

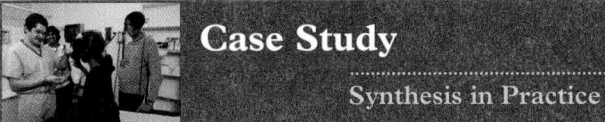

Case Study

Synthesis in Practice

Louis Ruiz, a 28-year-old nursing student, has selected 25-year-old Crystal Taylor and her family to follow throughout this semester of his nursing program. As he prepares to begin an assessment, he focuses on 5½-year-old Monica, who has been brought by her mother, Crystal, to the clinic for a checkup before beginning school. Louis will recall the physical, psychosocial, and cognitive developmental characteristics that are typical of the older preschool child and prepare to use this information as a basis for his observations. Louis will engage Monica in play activities with dolls to ensure that observations of her physical abilities are relevant and complete. He is also interested in any concerns Crystal has regarding Monica's health. In preparation for doing anticipatory guidance with Monica and her mother he reviews types of accidents common among her age group and appropriate health promotion activities. He is also interested in observing the quality of the interaction between Monica and her mother and assessing how Crystal copes with being a single parent.

As the parent of a 4 year old, Louis knows the importance of immunizations in keeping children free of many contagious diseases with serious consequences, and he is aware that children are not admitted to school without the completion of certain immunizations. His own child has made him very conscious of the great fear young children have for bodily harm and the fact that Monica may have difficulty cooperating with an injection. He recalls the approach he has used to help his own son cooperate with and recover from the discomfort of an injection. Louis refers to the standards for immunizations that are updated twice yearly by the American Academy of Pediatricians, the American Academy of Family Physicians, and the CDC to determine Monica's immunization needs. Louis knows that the key to his having a positive effect on the practice of health promotion activities by Crystal Taylor's family members is the development of trust through positive interactions.

Louis's nursing instructors have informed him that he is responsible for encouraging health promotion activities among his clients. Louis recognizes that *Healthy People 2000: National Health Promotion and Disease Prevention Objectives* can be a guide for choos-

ing health promotion activities for Crystal's family (see Chapter 1). Louis knows he must be accepting of Ms. Taylor as a single parent and assess the resources she has to support health promotion in her family. Understanding that Crystal likely has some definite ideas about parenting and health promotion will ensure that Louis is complete in assessing client needs and in offering appropriate suggestions to support Crystal and her family.

◼ Nursing Diagnosis

Nursing assessment of the client reveals clusters of data from the nursing history, physical examination, and developmental assessment. These data include defining characteristics, which the nurse analyzes through critical thinking to select the nursing diagnoses that apply. Accuracy is important, because the defining characteristics help to differentiate the nursing diagnosis that applies to the clinical situation. For example, *parental role conflict* and *altered parenting* are two distinctly different nursing diagnoses. The nurse must carefully review all information before selecting the nursing diagnosis applicable to the client and family's needs. Defining characteristics for the nursing diagnosis of *altered sexuality patterns* would include factors such as difficulties or limitations in sexual functioning, expressions of concern about sexuality, and inappropriate verbal and nonverbal sexual behavior. The nursing diagnoses box on p. 382 contains examples of nursing diagnoses for clients with problems related to developmental factors.

The second part of the nursing diagnostic statement states suspected causes or related factors for the client's response to the health problem. Revealed in the assessment data, the related factors allow the nurse to target specific interventions toward the client's diagnosis. For example, the nursing diagnosis of *altered sexuality patterns* might be related to the stress of an impaired relationship with a significant other, fear of pregnancy, or lack of a significant other. The related factors are different, and each would require different nursing strategies.

◼ Planning

During the planning phase of the nursing process, the nurse formulates a plan of care that is directed toward the identified nursing diagnoses for the client. Chosen nursing diagnoses are addressed in order of priority, with the most pressing problems receiving immediate attention. Prioritizing of nursing diagnoses is based on such factors as the nature of the problem (e.g., whether it is life threatening, interferes with activities of daily living, affects level of comfort) and the degree of importance attributed to the problem by the client or family. Maslow's theory of human needs is helpful as a guide

---

▪ NURSING DIAGNOSES FOR CLIENTS ACROSS THE LIFE SPAN

Adjustment, impaired
Body image disturbance
Breastfeeding, effective
Breastfeeding, ineffective
Caregiver role strain
Caregiver role strain, risk for
Coping, family: potential for growth
Coping, ineffective family: compromised
Coping, ineffective family: disabling
Coping, ineffective individual
Decisional conflict
Family processes, altered
Grieving, dysfunctional
Growth and development, altered
Health-seeking behaviors
Infant feeding pattern, ineffective
Injury, risk for
Parental role conflict
Parenting, altered
Parenting, altered, risk for
Poisoning, risk for
Sexual dysfunction
Sexuality patterns, altered
Social interaction, impaired
Social isolation

---

when arranging nursing diagnoses in order of priority.

The plan addresses each identified nursing diagnosis by determining goals, client outcomes, and interventions for the alleviation or resolution of the diagnosis. Collaboration with clients and their families is essential when determining goals and outcomes. Clients' degree of participation in planning depends on their developmental status, as well as physiological and psychological condition. For example, because young children may be unable to articulate feelings and needs, their parents must become involved in establishing goals. The participation of clients and their families in this process will increase their motivation for achievement of identified goals and outcomes.

The goal for each nursing diagnosis identifies a specific and measurable client behavior that is realistic and reflects the client's highest level of wellness and independence in function. An example might include "Client acquires healthy psychosocial behavior within 3 months." Long-term goals are usually achieved over weeks or months, and short-term goals are usually expected to be met within days or weeks. Expected outcomes are individual client behaviors that demonstrate the resolution of the etiological factors of the nursing

diagnosis statement and the attainment of goals. An example of an outcome is "Client participates in health promotion activities within 6 weeks." See the care plan for detailed examples of goals and outcomes.

Discharge planning should begin at time of admission to the hospital, because length of stay is usually very brief. Effective planning involves the health care team, the client, and the client's support system. Nursing interventions should be individualized for the client and modified accordingly for home- or hospital-based nursing care. Needed referrals to community agencies should be made to coincide with the client's arrival home.

▪ Implementation

Developmental interventions are performed by nurses, the client, and the family or significant others. The nurse strives to keep clients and their families as active in this process as possible. Interventions are designed to be appropriate for both the client's developmental level and the client's unique needs and thus support and promote normal developmental processes. Collaboration with a variety of health team members facilitates the provision of optimal care for clients.

Earlier in this chapter, nursing strategies for health promotion and acute care were discussed for each age group. Restorative care measures for older adults were also outlined. Students can refer to each of the developmental age groups for specific interventions regarding age-related health concerns. It is important to remember that a client's developmental needs should be incorporated into any plan of care, regardless of the nature of the client's health problem. Whether the client has serious physiological alterations or merely is seeking health promotion information, developmental care considerations ensure a more individualized and thorough nursing approach.

▪ Evaluation

Client care. During evaluation the nurse measures the client's progress and the degree to which the planned interventions were effective in meeting the expected outcomes and goals of care (see case study). The nurse evaluates the client's behavioral response to the interventions and thus determines the success or failure of the nursing action. This might include observing family members interact, having the client describe health promotion habits, or visiting the home to see if suggestions for improving child safety were followed. Both the nurse and the client and/or family evaluate if the expected outcomes were met in the manner anticipated. When outcomes are not met, a review must determine if they are realistic, if the interventions are appropriate, or if there is a need to modify an approach. Ongoing evaluation is necessary to ensure that progress toward defined goals is achieved.

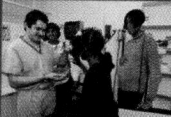

CASE STUDY NURSING CARE PLAN

Health-Seeking Behaviors

Assessment

Louis' physical assessment reveals that Monica's weight of 45 pounds places her between the 50th and 75th percentiles, and her height of 46 inches places her on the 75th percentile for age 5½ years on the growth grid. In comparison with her 2½ year old brother, she appears thinner with longer legs. She has a gap-toothed grin from the loss of a front tooth. Monica is able to do all of the items for a 6 year old on the Denver II (Denver Developmental Screening Test). This includes the gross motor skill of balancing on each foot for 6 seconds; the language ability to define seven words such as house and banana; the fine motor skill of copying a square; and the reported personal/social skills of brushing teeth and dressing without assistance, preparing her own cereal, and playing a board game. It was also noted that she does not squint or hold the story book at an unusual distance from her eyes. She enjoys showing and telling Louis about the pictures she is coloring and often giggles. **Her mother reports that Monica is very protective of and bossy with her brother, and she always wants to sit on Crystal's lap when she is holding Zachary.** Crystal denies that Monica has ever been involved in any accident that required a visit to the doctor, but **she did say she had found Monica playing with her father's cigarette lighter one day.** Crystal reports that Monica rides a tricycle with ease but has no experience with a bicycle.

When Louis inquires, Crystal tells him that she is feeling tired but well during this pregnancy and that she has been told she is doing well during her prenatal clinic appointments. **Crystal wants to be sure that Zachary and Monica have all their health care up to date before the baby comes, because she knows the baby will keep her busy and she wants them to be healthy.** Louis asks Crystal how she plans to prepare Monica and Zachary for the new sibling. She tells him that other than informing them of the event, she hasn't done anything in particular. Monica did ask her mother why she was getting so fat, and Crystal told her that she has a baby brother or sister growing in a special place inside her tummy. She is expecting that Monica will soon want to know how the baby will get out, but so far she has not asked. **Crystal asks Louis what suggestions he has for preparing her children for the arrival of the new baby.**

Nursing Diagnosis

Health-seeking behaviors related to a lack of knowledge regarding age-related health promotion activities (Ackley and Ladwid, 1997).

Planning

Goal

Crystal will become more knowledgeable about health concerns related to her children's ages within the next 3 months.

Expected Outcomes

Crystal will begin to discuss the safety needs of her children with all other family members who participate in their care before her next clinic visit.

Crystal will talk to other family care givers and Monica about protecting Monica from the danger of playing with fire before the next clinic visit.

Crystal will begin to prepare Monica and Zachary for the birth of a sibling before the next clinic visit.

Crystal will make sure her children keep appointments for well-baby/child checkups and receive appropriate immunizations.

Defining characteristics are shown in bold type.

Continued

CASE STUDY NURSING CARE PLAN—cont'd

Implementation

Steps	Rationale
1. Louis will provide Crystal with handouts that describe safety measures according to age of child.	Handouts provide initial information and allow for a quick review of information whenever needed (Wong, 1995).
2. Louis will discuss with Crystal measures to decrease Monica's risk for playing with fire.	Adults must remember to keep potentially hazardous items out of reach of children; a lighter, like a match, is an adult tool (Wong, 1995).
3. Louis will provide Crystal with a list of books about preparing children for a new sibling.	The list will assist Crystal to find these books in a bookstore or at the local library.
4. Louis will encourage Crystal to write appointment dates for well-child checkups on a pocket calendar she carries in her purse and to keep a copy of her children's immunization records with the calendar.	Placement of all appointments and records in one central area makes them available for reference whenever needed.

Evaluation

Ask Crystal to report on success of holding a discussion about child safety with the family.

Ask Monica to talk about the arrival of a new baby in the family.

Observe Monica during the next clinic visit to see if she continues to play with the lighter.

Client expectations. Nurse-client relationships are often long-term when a developmental plan of care is implemented. The nurse must always remember to determine if the client's expectations of care are continuing to be met. Over time the client's expectations can change. To add to the complexity of evaluation, expectations may be varied when family members are involved. Basic to understanding the client and family members' expectations is trust. When the nurse and client have established trust it becomes easier on a frequent basis to evaluate how the nurse-client relationship is proceeding and whether the client senses his or her health care needs are being adequately and professionally addressed.

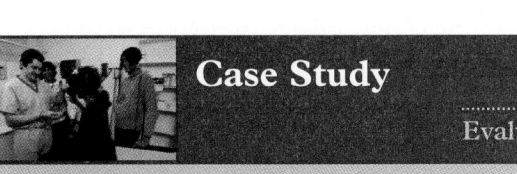

Case Study

Evaluation

Louis sees Crystal 1 month later when she returns to the clinic for a scheduled prenatal visit. She has left the children at home with their grandmother. As she waits to see her primary care giver Louis takes the opportunity to evaluate the progress she has made in meeting expected outcomes. Louis asks Crystal if she has been able to find any of the list of books he had given her about preparing young children for the birth of a sibling. Crystal reports that the librarian helped her locate two books, one appropriate for her toddler and the other one for Monica. She adds that the children loved the books and want her to read them every night at bedtime. Louis asks her if she thinks the content of the books was the kind of information she wanted to share with her children, and she replies that they explained childbirth so simply it really made it easy for her to talk about the new baby with both children.

During the previous clinic visit, Louis had also given Crystal pamphlets that described important safety measures for infants and young children. He asks her if she has discussed any of this information with any family members. Crystal tells him that her mother and grandmother have looked at the pamphlets and have told her it is a big responsibility to watch those two grandchildren and that they are very hard to keep up with. She also reports that they have all talked to Monica about not playing with candles, matches, or lighters. She tells Louis about the evening news on TV talking about a child who hid in her bedroom playing with a lighter and caught herself and the mattress on fire and almost died. The story seemed to scare Monica, and they talked about what young children should do if anything caught fire around them. She says Monica has often brought up the situation and asked what happened to the little girl on TV.

Crystal asks Louis if he will be there for her next prenatal appointment, and he tells her that he plans to be. He asks if there is anything in particular that she would like to talk about next time, and Crystal replies, "Just tell me how I can manage a new baby and my other two at the same time!" Before leaving, Crystal agains tells Louis she likes having him be with her at each clinic visit and that he has given her helpful information. Louis is satisfied that they are developing a good relationship and that he has assisted her in developing her knowledge base for managing health promotion activities for her children.

Documentation Note

After the primary care giver has documented Crystal's prenatal visit, Louis adds the following documentation in Crystal's clinic chart:

"While waiting for primary care giver, client reports that she has begun to prepare her two children for the birth of a new sibling through reading books and talking about the event. States she has shared safety measures for children, particularly in regard to fire, with family care givers. Has requested additional information pertaining to child rearing; will assess further during next visit."

Key Terms

accommodation	menarche
adolescence	menopause
Alzheimer's disease	menstrual cycle
anticipatory guidance	neonate
Apgar score	nocturnal enuresis
assimilation	object permanence
associative play	parallel play
attachment	perceptual bound
bonding	thinking
climacteric	preadolescence
concrete operations	prenatal care
conservation	preoperational thought
critical period of devel-	puberty
opment	reality orientation
dementia	regression
development	reminiscence
egocentric	sensorimotor period
fertilization	seriation
geriatrics	teratogens
gerontology	trimester
growth	zygote
maturation	

■ Key Concepts

Growth and development are orderly, predictable, interdependent processes that continue throughout the life span.

Growth is most rapid during the prenatal and infancy stages and continues to slow until the second skeletal growth spurt announces that puberty is approaching.

People progress through similar stages of growth and development but at an individual pace and with individual behaviors.

Theories of growth and development provide nurses with a framework for understanding the behavior of individuals.

Erikson identified psychosocial developmental crises for each stage of life that must be resolved in a positive manner to achieve optimal emotional health.

Piaget identified how the individual's cognitive development changes and progresses through the various stages of life.

Cognitive abilities develop from birth through adolescence and continue to mature during young and middle adulthood. Older adults can still learn new skills if given sufficient time and support.

Physiological, cognitive, and psychosocial development continue across the life span, and the nurse must be familiar with normal expectations (including developmental milestones) to determine potential problems and promote normal development.

Accidental injuries are the major cause of death in individuals between 1 and 25 years of age, and their prevention should be a focus of many health promotion activities.

Continued

■ Key Concepts—cont'd

Immunizations across the life span help individuals develop their protection against infections.

The nurse educates clients about their changing health needs across the life span and health promotion activities and provides support for their development of healthy lifestyles.

Young adults have few health problems but need to develop positive health habits to avoid many health problems in middle and late adulthood.

The health concerns of the middle adult commonly involve hormonal changes, stress-related ill-

nesses, screening for health problems, and adoption of positive health habits.

The health concerns of older adults are commonly related to their ability to continue to care for themselves and any health problems they have.

Individuals can begin to assume some responsibility for their own health care during the middle years of childhood and continue it across the life span unless they experience a severe loss of physical or cognitive abilities.

■ Critical Thinking Activities

1. Zachary at 2½ years of age is admitted to the hospital with a second-degree burn on the palm of his right hand. He grabbed the barrel of his mother's curling iron, which was plugged in and sitting on the bathroom counter. What measures can the nursing staff take to increase his sense of security and promote his sense of autonomy?

2. Monica, 5½ years old, is having a checkup in preparation for beginning school. The nurse needs to perform a number of procedures, which Monica may perceive as threatening because of their intrusive or invasive nature (e.g., measure her blood pressure, check her throat, look in her ears). What nursing approaches will be most likely to gain her cooperation?

3. Crystal is concerned that her 15-year-old brother may soon become sexually active and wants to be sure that he knows the risks involved and how

to protect himself from STDs (including AIDS) and from becoming a father before he is ready for the responsibility. As a nurse, how would you advise her?

4. Crystal's 44-year-old mother began having very short, minimal-flow menstrual periods several months ago and has not had a period for 2 months. She tells the nurse during her checkup that she thinks she is experiencing an early menopause and does not need to use birth control any longer. What information should the nurse give her?

5. Crystal's 40-year-old uncle has felt healthy and has not been to the neighborhood health clinic for a number of years. Since he has entered middle age, Crystal has convinced him to go to the clinic for a checkup. What should the assessment of the middle-age male include?

References

Ackley BJ, Ladwid GB: *Nursing diagnosis handbook,* ed 3, St. Louis, 1997, Mosby.

American Cancer Society: *Cancer facts and figures—1997,* Atlanta, Ga, 1997, The Society.

Bearinger L, Blum R: Adolescent health care. In Wallace H and others, editors: *Maternal and child health practices,* ed 4, Oakland, Calif, 1994, Third Party Publishing.

Behrman RE and others: *Nelson textbook of pediatrics,* ed 15, Philadelphia, 1996, WB Saunders.

Bloom DA and others: Toilet habits and continence in children: an opportunity sampling in search of normal parameters, *J Urol* 149(5):1087, 1993.

Brady PF: Mental health of the aging. In Johnson B, editor: *Psychiatric-mental health nursing: adaptation and growth,* ed 3, Philadelphia, 1993, JB Lippincott.

Breslow L, Breslow N: Health practices and disability: some evidence from Alameda County, *Prev Med* 22(1):86, 1993.

Butler R: Life review: an interpretation of reminiscence in the aged, *Psychiatry* 26:65, 1963.

Centers for Disease Control and Prevention: Survey: teen health and sex habits, Atlanta, 1991, The Centers.

Children's Defense Fund: *Birth to teens,* CDF Reports, 0276-6531, 1993.

Detwiler CS: Organic mental disorders. In Johnson B, editor: *Psychiatric-mental health nursing: adaptation and growth,* ed 3, Philadelphia, 1993, JB Lippincott.

Donovan P: *Testing positive: sexual transmitted diseases and the public health response,* New York, 1993, Alan Guttmacher Institute.

Ebersole P, Hess P: *Toward healthy aging: human needs and nursing response,* ed 3, St. Louis, 1990, Mosby.

Ebersole P, Hess P: *Toward healthy aging: human needs and nursing response,* ed 4, St. Louis, 1994, Mosby.

Edelman CL, Mandle CL: *Health promotion throughout the lifespan,* ed 3, St. Louis, 1994, Mosby.

Erikson E: *Childhood and society,* ed 2, New York, 1963, WW Norton.

Erikson E: *Identity: youth and crisis,* New York, 1968, WW Norton.

Frankenburg WK and others: The Denver II: a major revision and restandardization of the DDST, *Pediatrics* 89(1):91, 1992.

Gilligan C: *In a different voice,* Cambridge, Mass, 1982, Harvard University Press.

Havighurst RJ: Successful aging. In Williams RH and others, editors: *Process of aging,* vol 1, New York, 1972, Atherton Press.

Herda JA: Nursing interventions aimed at reducing risks of SIDS, *Pediatr Nurs* 18(5):531, 1992.

Kohlberg L: Development of moral character and moral ideology. In Hoffman ML, Hoffman LNW, editors: *Review of child development research,* vol 1, New York, 1964, Russell Sage Foundation.

Kohlberg L: Stages and sequence: the cognitive-developmental approach to socialization. In Goslin DA, editor: *Handbook of socialization theory and research,* Chicago, 1969, Rand McNally.

Lewis SM and others: *Medical/surgical nursing: assessment and management of clinical problems,* ed 4, St. Louis, 1996, Mosby.

Lueckenotte AG: *Gerontologic nursing,* St. Louis, 1996, Mosby.

Millstein S and others: Adolescent health promotion: rationale, goals, and objectives. In Millstein S and others, editors: *Promoting the health of adolescents: new directions for 21st century,* New York, 1993, Oxford University Press.

Papalia DE, Olds SW: *Human development,* ed 6, St. Louis, 1995, McGraw-Hill.

Peck RC: Psychological developments in the second half of life. In Anderson JE, editor: *Psychological aspects of aging,* Washington, DC, 1955, American Psychological Association.

Piaget J: *The origins of intelligence in children,* New York, 1952, International University Press.

Purath J: Pediatric hypertension: assessment and management, *Pediatr Nurs* 21(2):173, 1995.

Stammer J and others: Blood pressure, systolic and diastolic, and cardiovascular risks, *Arch Intern Med* 153(5):598, 1993.

Stanhope M, Lancaster J: *Community health nursing: process and practice for promoting health,* ed 3, St. Louis, 1992, Mosby.

Stanhope M, Lancaster J: *Community health nursing: process and practice for promoting health,* ed 4, St. Louis, 1996, Mosby.

Stephens D and others: Subclinical vitamin A deficiency: a potentially unrecognized problem in the U.S., *Pediatr Nurs* 22(5):377, 1996.

Thibault JM, Maly RC: Recognition and treatment of substance abuse in the elderly, *Prim Care* 20(1):155, 1993.

U.S. Bureau of the Census: *Statistical abstract of the United States,* ed 113, Washington, DC, 1993, The Bureau.

USDHHS, PHS: *Healthy people 2000: national health promotion and disease prevention objectives,* Boston, 1992, Jones & Bartlett.

USDHS, PHS: *Monthly vital statistics report: advance report of final mortality statistics,* 1992, 43(6), supplement, Hyattsville, Md, 1995, Centers for Disease Control and Prevention, National Center for Health Statistics.

VonBurg MM and others: Baby bottle tooth decay: a concern for all mothers, *Pediatr Nurs* 21(6):515, 1995.

Williams SR: *Nutrition and diet therapy,* ed 7, 1993, Mosby.

Wong DL: *Whaley and Wong's nursing care of infants and children,* ed 5, St. Louis, 1995, Mosby.

21

Loss and Grief

OBJECTIVES

Mastery of content in this chapter will enable the student to:

- Define the key terms listed.
- Identify the nurse's role in assisting clients with problems related to loss, death, and grief.
- Describe and compare the phases of grieving from Kübler-Ross, Bowlby, and Worden.
- List and discuss five basic categories of loss.
- Describe six dimensions of hope.
- Describe characteristics of a person experiencing grief.
- Discuss variables that influence a person's response to grief.
- Develop a care plan for a client or family experiencing grief.
- Describe effective therapeutic communication interventions for grieving clients.
- Select interventions aimed at maintaining a dying client's independence and self-esteem.
- Describe how the nurse provides comfort to a dying client.
- Explain ways for the nurse to assist a family in caring for a dying client.
- Describe the procedure for care of the body after death.
- Discuss the nurse's own loss experience as it influences care of grieving clients.
- Identify two ways nurses can meet their own needs related to loss.

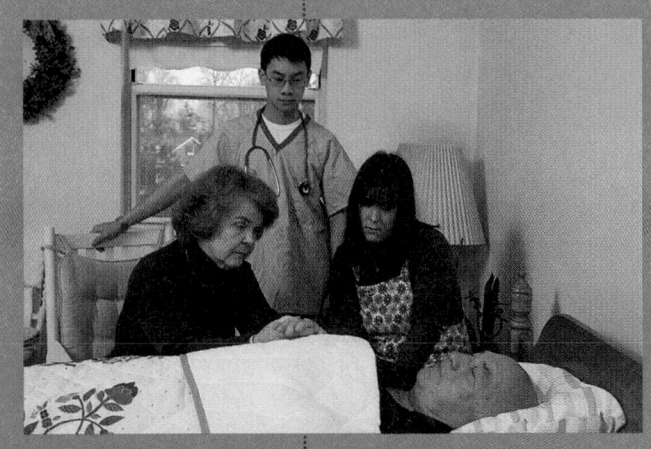

Case Study

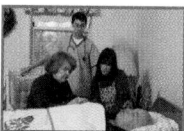

The Holloway Family

Mr. Holloway is a 73-year-old man with a history of colon cancer diagnosed 18 months ago and treated with surgery and chemotherapy. As a result of surgery he has experienced incontinence and chronic diarrhea. Chemotherapy has been associated with oral ulcers and loss of appetite. He was recently admitted to the hospital for evaluation and treatment of severe anemia and dehydration. When diagnostic studies completed at the time of hospitalization identified widespread metastases to his liver and lungs, his oncologist decided to stop all chemotherapy. Medical treatment included pain management, blood replacement, and rehydration. The discharge plan is for Mr. Holloway to be given comfort care at home through the hospital's hospice program.

Living in the household with Mr. Holloway are his wife of 53 years and their only child, a single daughter who is 38 years old. Mr. Holloway's daughter has taken a leave of absence from her teaching job and moved back home to help care for him during his final illness. His wife, however, is unwilling to accept that he is near death. She continues to insist, "If he would only eat right, take vitamins, and go to a gym, he would regain his strength and recover." Mr. Holloway's wife and daughter argue often about how best to help him. He in turn becomes very angry with them and screams at them both to stop fighting. At other times he is very withdrawn and tearful. The Holloways have few ties to the community and very limited social support. The health care team is concerned about how they will cope now that Mr. Holloway is ready for discharge.

Peter Wong is a 22-year-old nursing student in his last year of education, completing a rotation in community health. He considers himself fortunate to have never lost a family member to death and has never been assigned to care for a terminally ill client. When he learns that he will be providing home health care for Mr. Holloway and his family, he becomes very anxious. He feels unprepared to intervene effectively with all of the sadness and conflict in the Holloway household. He is also personally fearful of death and worried that Mr. Holloway might die while he is actually providing care. He is not sure that he would be able to cope if such a thing were to happen, and he believes he does not have enough experience to help the family with their grief. He wonders if he is the "right" student for this family. His anxiety is so great that he asks his instructor to change his assignment and give him another case instead, but his instructor refuses, telling him that this will be a good opportunity for him to learn.

Loss and grief are experiences that affect not only the client and the client's family but also the nurse. In part, the intense emotion associated with grief is precipitated by very real, concrete losses, such as the death of a family member, amputation of a body part, or diminished capacity to function. However, feelings of grief and sadness are also triggered by the awareness that we as individuals are ultimately powerless to prevent death and are alone at the moment of death. Most nurses enter the profession with the intent of helping clients recover from illness and move toward health-promoting self-care. It is frightening therefore to be confronted with the reality that knowledge, skill, and technology cannot always come together to result in cure. In providing care for clients who are at the end of their life, the nurse is reminded that it is possible to intervene in a way that brings comfort to clients and families, even when hope for cure is gone. Providing the client and family with an environment that supports completion of the essential tasks of bringing closure to life and relationships becomes the goal of nursing.

⋯NURSING KNOWLEDGE BASE
Concepts of Loss, Death, Grief, and Nursing

Most nurses interact daily with clients and families experiencing loss and grief. While caring for clients and their families, nurses also experience personal loss as client-family-nurse relationships end through transfer, discharge, recovery, or death. Many nurses find that it is easy to relieve physical symptoms associated with illness and death but difficult to become involved in a meaningful interpersonal relationship to support a person who is suffering or dying. Personal feelings, values, and experiences influence the extent to which nurses can support clients and families during loss or death. Self-assessment, the exploration of personal attitudes, feelings, and values, is necessary before nurses can use sensitive, therapeutic approaches with others.

A person experiences **loss** in the absence of an object, person, body part or function, or emotion or idea that was formerly present (Table 21-1). Losses may be actual or perceived. An **actual loss** is easily identified, such as in the case of an aging adult who is aware of increased forgetfulness and disorientation associated with early Alzheimer's disease or a woman who has a mastectomy. A **perceived loss** is less obvious, such as the loss of confidence or in the case of a woman who delivers a male child instead of the female that she preferred. Perceived losses are easily overlooked or misunderstood, yet the process of grief in these instances follows the same sequencing and progression as losses that are considered "real." Loss may also be maturational, situational, or both. The client may experience **maturational loss** (loss resulting from normal life transitions,

TABLE 21-1
Types of Loss

Definition	Implications of Loss
Loss of external objects (e.g., loss, misplacement, deterioration, theft, destruction by natural causes)	Extent of grieving depends on object's value, sentiment attached to it, and its usefulness.
Loss of a known environment (e.g., moving from a neighborhood, hospitalization, a new job, moving out of ICU)	Loss occurs through maturational or situational events and through injury or illness. Loneliness or newness of unfamiliar setting threatens self-esteem and makes grieving difficult.
Loss of a significant other (e.g., being promoted, moving, or running away; loss of a family member, friend, trusted nurse, acquaintance, or animal companion)	Significant other typically fulfills another person's need for psychological safety, love and belonging, and self-esteem.
Loss of an aspect of self (e.g., body part, psychological or physiological function)	Illness, injury, or developmental changes result in loss of aspect of self that causes grief and permanent changes in body image and self-concept.
Loss of life (e.g., death of family member, friend, or acquaintance, own death)	Loss of life creates grief for those left behind. Person facing death often fears pain, loss of control, and dependency on others.

such as parents feeling sadness when their youngest child marries and moves away from home) or **situational loss** (loss occurring in response to a specific external event, such as moving to an unfamiliar city). Keeping in mind that every person will respond to loss differently, the nurse must assess the special meaning that loss has for a client and its effect on the client's health status.

The type of loss and the perception of the loss influence the degree of grief experienced. Each individual responds to loss differently. It is often incorrectly assumed that the loss of an object or animal would not generate the same stress as loss of a loved one. However, the value that the individual places on the lost object determines the emotional response to separation. The death of a pet that has been a constant companion would likely cause more sadness for a person than the loss of a distant relative not seen for years.

Hospitalization and chronic illness or disability are special circumstances that have multiple associated losses. When persons are hospitalized, they lose their privacy, control over their bodies and their daily routines, much of their modesty, and any illusions they may have had regarding their personal indestructibility. Chronic or debilitating illness may also result in financial strain. Furthermore, long-term illness may require occupational change, threaten independence and self-reliance, and force alterations in lifestyle. Even a brief illness or hospitalization requires temporary shifts in family role functioning, but chronic or debilitating illness may pose a major threat to the stability of relationships.

Death represents the ultimate loss. Although death is part of the continuum of life and as such a universal

and inevitable part of the human experience, it is a mystical event that very often generates great fear and anxiety. Death ends the relationships that bind families and individuals together and separates people from the physical presence of persons who have influenced their lives. Even in the presence of strong religious beliefs, such as faith in God and an afterlife, facing death is often difficult for the dying person, as well as for the person's family, friends, and care givers. When a person becomes terminally ill, people close to them are reminded of their own mortality. Feelings of guilt, anger, and fear can cause family members and care givers to withdraw at a time when the dying person needs love, reassurance, and support. The way in which individuals approach dying will be influenced by their fundamental beliefs and values, their personality structure, and the quality of the emotional supports that are available to them.

Grieving Process

Loss requires adaptation through the **grieving process.** The terms *grief, mourning,* and *bereavement* are often used interchangeably to describe this process of healing, but there are subtle differences among these terms that make them distinct from each other. **Bereavement** is the state of thought, feeling, and activity that follows loss. It includes grief and mourning. **Grief** is the personal, individual experience of loss. It is a form of sorrow that follows the perception or anticipation of a loss of anything or anyone who is important or valued. Grief is demonstrated through responses that often include feelings of helplessness, loneliness, hopelessness, sadness, guilt, and anger. These same feelings and behaviors can occur when individuals face their own death.

Grief occurs not only in the persons experiencing the loss but also in family or friends. **Mourning** is the process that follows a loss and includes working through grief. There is no one "right" way to grieve and no simple "magic formula" to speed grief resolution or diminish its intensity. It is also significant that as a process, mourning is not linear. It does not proceed in sequential stages that can be precisely predicted. Rather, an individual will move back and forth across phases of mourning many times, possibly extending over a period of several years, before the process is eventually completed. Numerous authors have attempted to conceptualize the process of grief resolution, but three theorists are especially known for their work in the study of grief, loss, and bereavement: Kübler-Ross (1969), Bowlby (1980), and Worden (1991).

Kübler-Ross' stages of dying. The framework provided by Kübler-Ross (1969) is behavior oriented and includes five stages (Table 21-2). In the denial stage, the individual acts as though nothing has happened and may refuse to believe or understand that a loss has occurred. In the anger stage, the individual resists the loss and may strike out at everyone and everything in the environment. In the bargaining stage, there is postponement of the reality of the loss; the individual may try to deal in a subtle or overt way to prevent the loss from occurring. The depression stage occurs when the loss is realized and the full impact of its significance is apparent; the grieving person may feel overwhelmingly lonely and withdraw from interpersonal interactions. In the fifth stage, acceptance, the individual finally accepts the loss.

Although Kübler-Ross has conceptualized these stages as sequential, in reality there is some movement back and forth between stages. For example, persons diagnosed with a life-threatening cancer and treated with chemotherapy may experience a period of remission during which they believe that they never had the disease in the first place and may discontinue treatment as a result. If and when their symptoms recur, they may start the process of letting go and accepting the reality of their situation all over again.

Bowlby's four phases of mourning. Bowlby's attachment theory (1980) forms a foundation for his work on separation and loss. He describes attachment as an instinctive behavior that leads to the development of affectional bonds between a child and the primary care giver. These bonds are present and active throughout the life cycle and are later generalized to other persons with whom individuals form close relationships. Attachment behavior helps to ensure our survival because it keeps us in close contact with persons who can offer us protection and support.

Bowlby describes four phases of mourning (see Table 21-2) but cautions that they are not clear-cut. An individual may move back and forth between any two of these phases in the process of responding to the loss. The first phase, the phase of numbing, may last from a few hours to a week or more and may be interrupted by periods of extremely intense emotion or panic. The bereaved person may describe this phase as feeling "stunned," "dreamlike," or "unreal." The second phase is one of yearning and searching for the lost person. At this time the reality of the loss arouses emotional outbursts of tearful sobbing and acute distress in most persons but may also be experienced less openly as an intense yearning for the one who is lost. This phase may last for months or years. The third phase is characterized by disorganization and despair. An individual in this phase engages in an endless examination of how and why the loss occurred, with anger at anyone who might have been responsible. Gradually this examination gives way to an acceptance that the loss is permanent. Finally, in the phase of reorganization, which may require a year or more, the bereaved person begins to accept unaccustomed roles, acquire new skills, resume some social life, and build new relationships.

Worden's four tasks of mourning. Worden's task approach (1991) (see Table 21-2) implies that persons who mourn can be actively involved in helping themselves and can be assisted and influenced by outside intervention.

- Task I: *To accept the reality of the loss.* Even when a death has been expected, there is always some period of disbelief and surprise that the event has really happened. This task involves all the

TABLE 21-2
The Grief Process

Kübler-Ross' Five Stages of Dying	Bowlby's Four Phases of Mourning	Worden's Four Tasks of Mourning
Denial	Numbing	Accepting the reality of loss
Anger	Yearning and searching	
Bargaining		
Depression	Disorganization and despair	Working through the pain of grief
	Reorganization	Adjusting to the environment without the deceased
Acceptance		Emotionally relocating the deceased and moving on with life

processes required to accept that the person is gone and will not return.

▪ Task II: *To work through the pain of grief.* Even though people respond to loss differently, it is not possible to experience a loss and work through grief without emotional pain. Those individuals who deny or shut off the pain prolong their grief or may have what is referred to as **complicated bereavement.**

▪ Task III: *To adjust to the environment in which the deceased is missing.* The realization of the full impact of the loss is usually not felt for at least 3 months. At this point many visitors and friends stop calling often, and the person is left to ponder the full impact of loneliness that characterizes life without the deceased. People completing this task must take on roles formerly filled by the deceased, including some tasks that they never fully appreciated.

▪ Task IV: *To emotionally relocate the deceased and move on with life.* The goal of this task is not to forget the deceased or give up the relationship with the deceased but to have the deceased take a new, less prominent place in a person's emotional life. This is often the most difficult task to complete because people fear that if they make other attachments they will forget their loved one or somehow become disloyal. This stage is complete when the bereaved person realizes that it is possible to love other people without loving the deceased person less.

Worden's tasks of mourning usually require a minimum of four seasons (one full year). This time frame is often very helpful to persons who mourn because it seems to make instinctive sense.

Anticipatory grief.

Anticipatory grief refers to the process of disengaging or "letting go" that occurs before the actual loss or death has occurred. Once a person or family receives a terminal diagnosis, they begin the process of saying good-bye, concluding life affairs, and "getting their business in order."

When the actual process of dying is extended for a very long time, persons in the client's family may exhibit very few symptoms of grief when the death finally occurs. This seeming absence of grief symptoms may result because the family has been engaged in a slow grief process over time. By the time the actual moment of death arrives, much of the denial, numbness, and tearfulness may have already been experienced.

There are risks involved in anticipatory grieving. One is that family members may withdraw emotionally from the dying client too soon, leaving the client with no emotional support as death draws near. There may also be complications if a person who was thought to be near death survives. Family members may then have problems emotionally reconnecting and may even be resentful that the person has lived past the life expectancy.

Special circumstances that affect grief resolution.

Although no experience of grief is easy, some deaths occur under conditions that complicate the process of coming to terms with the loss and moving on with life (Table 21-3). Most often these special circumstances are ones that deprive the family of social support or cause the family to be isolated in some way.

Complicated bereavement.

Abnormal grief reactions are those in which one of the factors affecting grieving interferes with the normal progression of mourning. In these cases, grief appears to "go wrong" and loss never resolves, threatening a person's relationships with others. Abnormal grief takes on different forms, manifesting itself as one of the following:

▪ Chronic grief: There is active, acute mourning that never resolves but extends for many years without remission. Persons in this state often verbalize that they cannot "get past it" and move on.

▪ Delayed grief: Active grieving is held back, only to resurface later, usually in response to a very trivial upset or loss. For example, a woman may only grieve for several days or weeks following the death of her spouse, only to become hysterically upset and sad a year later when she loses her car keys. The extreme sadness she feels in response to this "little loss" is really a delayed response to the death of her husband.

▪ Exaggerated grief: These persons become so overwhelmed by grief that they cannot function at all. This may surface as panic attacks, the development of phobic behavior, or the development of alcoholism or substance abuse to self-medicate one's feelings.

▪ Masked grief: Symptoms develop that the person does not recognize as being grief related. Very often this is a physical symptom or complaint (e.g., alteration in eating or sleeping).

Application of grief theory to other types of loss.

Although grief theories are directed to the way individuals cope with the death of a loved one, each of these theories can just as easily be applied to other losses. They have equal relevance when describing the way persons who are given a terminal diagnosis respond and process the reality that their own time of death is very near. They also apply to the way individuals and families respond to the loss of body function or to disability. In these instances a person will also need to progress through stages of mourning for lost independence and possibly for the loss of body integrity and body image. Persons with these types of losses progress through the same phases, stages, or tasks of mourning.

TABLE 21-3
Special Circumstances That Affect Grief Resolution

Special Circumstance	Complicating Factors That Affect Grieving
Suicide	Social stigma surrounds suicide and results in shame
	Survivors fear rejection and lack of social and religious support
	Survivors may become obsessed with their failure to "see the signs"
	Survivor guilt, sometimes projected as blaming
	Anger toward the person who has died
	Survivor ambivalence about feelings of anger and shame
Sudden/unexpected death	Preoccupation with the final hours or minutes before death
Accidental	"Unfinished business," such as things left unsaid or undone
Homicidal (or violent)	Guilt feelings ("If only I had not let him go to the party, he would still be alive")
Sudden illness (such as	Involvement of law authorities such as the police, coroner
myocardial infarction)	Obsessive need to understand or know "why" this has happened
Infant, neonatal, or child death	Involvement of the legal system in investigation of events such as sudden infant death syndrome
	Need to know and understand reasons for death (feelings of responsibility)
	Crises of religious faith ("Why would a good God do this?")
	"Unnatural" for child to die before parents
Miscarriage	Social isolation: no one may have known the woman was pregnant
	Sense of "unreality" due to no birth certificate, no death certificate, no name
	Absence of funeral rituals with which to validate the infant's life
AIDS	Social isolation
	Multiple losses (for both families and care givers)
	Prolonged illness and disability (also fear of contagion)
	Untimely (early) deaths during peak creative, productive years

Their emotional pain is just as real and intense as that experienced by those whose loved one has died.

Grieving in the Context of Human Development

Erik Erikson (1982) reviewed the developmental pathways that characterize human growth (see Chapter 20). He proposed a series of eight psychosocial stages that define the problems and crises that must be resolved in the process of moving from infancy through adulthood. Where individuals are along this continuum will determine their ability to understand the certainty of death and cope with disability. Although people generally pass through these stages sequentially, when faced with radical, life-altering disability or impending death, many people seem to move ahead and engage in the type of life review that typically occurs in old age. This process of life review includes reflecting on the events that have shaped an individual's lifetime and evaluating the merits, value, and fulfilled purpose of one's life. A successful review process will enable the person approaching death to say good-bye to significant relationships, to finish personal business, to make arrangements for possessions or dispose of personal belongings, and to reflect on a life well lived. This self-examination and process of letting go of life's attachments is seen even in older children and adolescents when they know that their remaining life span is short.

The way in which an individual perceives a loss and responds to it with grief and mourning will be heavily influenced by many factors (Box 21-1). It is of critical importance, however, that the nurse recognize that the grief process takes place in the context of basic growth and development. Persons of differing ages and stages of development will manifest differing and unique symptoms of grief and bereavement.

Hope

Hope is a multidimensional, changing life force, characterized by a confident yet uncertain expectation of achieving a future goal, and is essential to life (Poncar, 1994). Hope is not a single act but a complex series of thoughts, feelings, and actions that change often. Clients dealing with loss and the families of these clients may experience different dimensions of hope and can be supported by nurses as they work to maintain hope (Table 21-4).

Hafen and others (1996) discuss the healing power of hope. By definition the existence and maintenance of hope depend on having strong relationships and a sense of emotional connectedness to other persons. Nurses

Box 21-1
Factors Influencing a Grief Reaction

Age
Infant

It is assumed that infants are not able to understand concepts of loss and death until they are able to recognize familiar persons or form an attachment to a care giver. After trust forms with parents, even temporary loss can cause anxiety.

Toddler

Self-centeredness and confusion of fact and fantasy prevent an understanding of death. Toddlers feel anxiety over loss of objects and separation from parents.

Preschooler

Preschoolers perceive death as a kind of sleep or temporary absence. Unfamiliarity with the concept of time prevents understanding the finality of death. Toddlers may react to less significant loss (e.g., a pet) with more outward grief.

School-age Child

School-age children experience grief over the loss of a body part or function. They associate misdeeds with causing death and may feel guilty about the loss of significant others. They equate death with destruction.

Adolescent

Adolescents usually feel acute grief over the loss of a body part or function. They fear peer rejection. Teenagers have an adult comprehension of the concept of death but are the least likely of any age-group to accept the loss of life because of the developmental task of establishing identity and purpose in life.

Young Adult

Young adults relate loss to its significance for status, roles, and lifestyle. The loss of economic well-being, divorce, or health causes much grief. The concept of death is greatly influenced by religious and cultural beliefs.

Middle-age Adult

Middle-age adults usually begin to reexamine life and are sensitive to physical changes. The loss of others poses a significant threat to lifestyle. They consider how death will occur.

Older Adult

Older adults experience anticipatory grief because of aging and the possible loss of capabilities for self-care. They often fear loss of independence. Acceptance of

death depends on many personal factors. They may fear events surrounding death more than death itself.

Cultural and Spiritual Beliefs
Cultural

Values, attitudes, beliefs, and customs influence reactions to loss, grief, and death. Each individual is influenced by them in many ways. Chapter 18 explores aspects of culture and ethnic background.

Spiritual

Spiritual reactions include practices, rites, and rituals involving loss and grieving. Some people turn to religion for solace and support. Loss can sometimes cause internal conflicts about spiritual values and the meaning of life.

Sex Roles
Men

It is often socially and culturally more difficult for men to express grief openly because they are expected to be strong and supportive.

Women

It is often socially and culturally more acceptable for women to express grief openly because they are expected to need support.

Socioeconomic Status
All Levels

The family's financial resources often determine options.

Social Support

The support that clients receive is based on their value to the members of the social system and the manner and circumstances of their loss.

Nature of Loss
Circumstances

Sudden, unanticipated death frequently leads to slower resolution from grief. Deaths by violence are generally more difficult to accept.

Dying Person's Grief

The intensity and rate of grieving are influenced by the time between clients' first awareness that they will die and the moment of death. In intensive care units, death is frequently sudden, and clients and family have little time for grief.

Box 21-1
Factors Influencing a Grief Reaction—cont'd

Nature of Relationships

Spouse

Impact of the death of a spouse is usually greater than that of the death of a parent because of the effect on lifestyle. The loss of a sexual partner threatens perception of sexuality and desire for sex. It can be difficult to establish new friendships.

Child

The death of a child is generally perceived as premature. Parents often feel guilt and blame.

Significant Other

The death of a significant other involves many needs for the survivor, including a need for support and a need to express emotions.

Goals

The more goals a person has, the more likely the person will be able to adapt to a loss of only one goal. The more central to one's life the goal is, the more intense the grief.

TABLE 21-4
Interventions to Help Maintain Hope

Dimension of Hope	Possible Intervention or Strategy to Support Hope
Affective	Showing empathetic understanding of the client's and family members' strengths, such as patience and courage
Cognitive	Offering information about the illness and correcting misinformation, thus clarifying or modifying the client's and family's perceptions
Behavioral	Assisting the client to use personal resources and make use of external supports to better balance the need for independence with healthy interdependence and dependence
Affiliative, valued	Fostering relationships that will support the client's feelings of being
Temporal	Attending to the client's experience of time, focusing on short-term goals as life expectancy diminishes
Contextual	Encouraging development of achievable goals, reminiscing, and factors that influence hope, such as religious belief or deriving meaning from suffering

---

and other health professionals may provide that personal link that is essential to hope. The client and family often interpret the nurse's involvement as indicating that the client's life is worthwhile and has purpose. This view is essential to maintaining hope. Hope also depends on the ability to maintain goals, yet hope does not necessarily relate to the anticipation of or wish for cure. Hope may be directed toward reaching a goal of death with dignity, freedom from pain, or in contact with loved ones. In the face of certain death or disability, the nurse may need to help the client and family establish or revise goals so that they are attainable (Nowotny, 1991). For example, instead of encouraging a client to plan weeks or months in advance, the nurse may help the client develop goals for one day or hour at a time.

···CRITICAL THINKING IN CLIENT CARE

Synthesis

The process of providing client care demands that the nurse integrate a wide range of knowledge and experience to develop a plan for intervention that is as unique as the client. Although there are general guidelines and established rationales for intervening in particular ways to manage health care deficits, all clients have their own special way of relating to family, the community, and the nurse. Each client enters the health care environment at a different developmental, spiritual, and cultural place, bringing expectations for care that are unique. The skilled nurse will be able to consider all of these factors, blending assessment data together to establish a comprehensive plan of care that meets the needs of the client as a whole person.

Knowledge.
As the nurse approaches a client and family experiencing loss, there will be much information to consider and integrate in the process of completing a comprehensive nursing assessment. It will be necessary to have a clear understanding of the exact nature of the loss (death, disability, or loss of function), how the client and family perceive the loss, and how the loss will impact their lives. The nurse's knowledge of communication principles will help in establishing a good working relationship with the client and family. A baseline knowledge of pathophysiology, treatment alternatives, and medications used in management of a disease state is essential when the nurse is caring for clients who face a loss associated with an illness.

Beyond this fundamental knowledge, the nurse must also understand that the client and the disease do not exist in isolation. Rather, they are part of a complex family system and have connections to the greater community. The expert nurse knows that the family is truly the unit for intervention.

Experience.
Although some nurses may have never experienced the death of a family member, every nurse has known loss at some time during life. Perhaps the nurse has experienced the death of a pet during childhood. In a more symbolic way, the nurse may remember what it was like to suffer personal embarrassment by failing a critical course or test and feel the associated loss of confidence or position of respect. The reality is that no one ever experiences loss in exactly the same way as another person, so that even if nurses have experienced losses that seem "just like" the loss the client is experiencing, the truth is that their perceptions and emotions are likely to have been quite different.

Attitudes.
Risk taking, self-confidence, and humility are key attitudes that will affect the nurse's ability to make accurate judgments and assessments of clients experiencing grief. Many nurses are very anxious about caring for clients who grieve. They feel uncomfortable when clients cry, feel helpless to "make it all better," and are uncertain of what to say that will be of benefit and comfort. Being with a client or family who are sad requires a personal risk. It requires nurses to tolerate their own discomfort in the interest of being supportive of the client.

Self-confidence goes hand in hand with risk taking. The nurse who is confident understands that in the absence of something "to do" or something "to say," what the client and family need most is the personal connection with someone who cares. The nurse who silently shares a moment of sadness with a client or family communicates this caring and sends a message that the client's feelings and emotions are respected and accepted.

Finally, humility is critical to providing excellence in nursing care. Clients know that the nurse cannot possibly understand everything about their family, but they are often very willing to explain their own thinking, their personal family belief systems, and their thoughts about death, dying, and such spiritual matters as afterlife. The nurse with humility will put aside personal assumptions of how loss might be interpreted by the client and be open to hearing and understanding the client's unique view and interpretation of events.

Standards.
Clients facing death have the right to some self-determination in their final days. There are now such documents as living wills in which individuals can state their wishes regarding life support, organ donation (Box 21-2), and other considerations regarding their death. Other documents such as the Dying Patient's Bill of Rights (Box 21-3) are honored at hospitals and posted in prominent areas. In addition, the nurse has the moral responsibility to support clients in the exercise of their personal faith or spirituality as death approaches (see Chapter 17). This may mean obtaining consultation from pastoral care, social workers or psychologists or obtaining referrals to grief groups or other community agencies such as hospice that can provide needed support.

Nurses are ethically bound to provide the best quality care to clients at all times. They must be diligent and sensitive in maintaining the physical integrity of the client, preserving the client's modesty and dignity, administering medications and other comfort care designed to minimize pain and discomfort, and guarding confidentiality.

⋯NURSING PROCESS

◼ Assessment

In approaching a client who has experienced a loss, it is important for the nurse to begin with an open mind and an accepting attitude. Because there is no single "right" way to grieve and because all persons grieve in their

---

Box 21-2
Tissues and Organs Used for Transplant

Nonvital Tissues	Vital Organs*
Corneas	Heart
Skin	Liver
Long bones	Lungs
Middle ear bones	Kidneys
	Pancreas

*These organs are recovered after a client is pronounced clinically dead or brain dead; circulatory and ventilatory support is maintained to perfuse the organs before removal.

own way, preconceived ideas about how a client or family might feel are, more often than not, likely to be wrong. The assessment must begin with an exploration of the unique meaning of the loss for the client. Adequate information must be gathered before accurate conclusions and diagnoses can be made.

Assessment of the client and family begins by exploring the meaning of loss to them. The nurse interviews the client and family, observes their responses and behaviors, and uses open communication, emphasizing listening skills. The nurse should be alert for nonverbal cues. Initial impressions are validated with the client and family so that nursing diagnoses and effective interventions can be developed.

The nurse must assess not how the client *should be* reacting but how the client *is* reacting. Sequences of behavior or phases may occur in order, they may be skipped, or they may recur. Many variables affect grief. Assessment of these variables gives the nurse a broad database from which to individualize care.

Grief behaviors. Assessment of the client and family includes consideration of the stages of grief. By observing behavior, the nurse can make an assessment regarding the effects of loss. The nurse carefully assesses the existence of unique individual, family, and situational characteristics such as the relationship of spouses or events leading to the loss. It may be possible on the basis of careful observations and nurse-client interactions to predict the nature of grief resolution.

No two people grieve in exactly the same way, but most persons who grieve have at least some outward signs and symptoms that are associated with grief. These signs fall into several categories, including feelings, physical sensations, cognitions or thought patterns, and behavior patterns (Table 21-5). The purpose in observing and noting these signs and symptoms of grief is not to specifically document a stage or phase of mourning but rather to guide interventions and evaluate outcomes.

The experience of loss takes place in a social context.

Box 21-3
The Dying Person's Bill of Rights

I have the right to be treated as a living human being until I die.

I have the right to maintain a sense of hopefulness, however changing its focus may be.

I have the right to be cared for by those who can maintain a sense of hopefulness, however changing this might be.

I have the right to express my feelings and emotions about my approaching death in my own way.

I have the right to participate in decisions concerning my care.

I have the right to expect continuing medical and nursing attention even though "cure" goals must be changed to "comfort" goals.

I have the right not to die alone.

I have the right to be free from pain.

I have the right to have my questions answered honestly.

I have the right not to be deceived.

I have the right to have help from and for my family in accepting my death.

I have the right to die in peace and dignity.

I have the right to retain my individuality and not be judged for my decisions that may be contrary to beliefs of others.

I have the right to discuss and enlarge my religious and/or spiritual experiences, whatever these may mean to others.

I have the right to expect that the sanctity of the human body will be respected after death.

I have the right to be cared for by caring, sensitive, knowledgeable people who will attempt to understand my needs and will be able to gain some satisfaction in helping me face my death.

From Barbus AJ: The dying person's bill of rights, *Am J Nurs* 75:99, 1975.

TABLE 21-5
Symptoms of Normal Grief

Feelings	Physical Sensations
Sadness	Hollowness in the stomach
Anger	Tightness in the chest
Guilt or self-reproach	Tightness in the throat
Anxiety	Oversensitivity to noise
Loneliness	Sense of depersonalization
Fatigue	("Nothing seems real")
Helplessness	Feeling short of breath
Shock/numbness	Muscle weakness
(lack of feeling)	Lack of energy
Yearning	Dry mouth
Emancipation/relief	
	Behaviors
Cognitions	Sleep disturbances
(Thought Patterns)	Appetite disturbances
Disbelief	Absentminded behavior
Confusion	Dreams of the deceased
Preoccupation about	Sighing
the deceased	Crying
Sense of the presence	Carrying objects that be-
of the deceased	longed to the deceased
Hallucinations	
Hopelessness	
("I'll never be	
OK again")	

In the case of a family experiencing a death, the family begins to reorganize itself as soon as the client is no longer able to fulfill the same number and types of roles. When a person is disabled or loses some vital aspect of themselves, both the client and family undergo a similar reorganization, realigning roles and responsibilities to meet the new demands. The nurse assesses the entire family's response to loss, recognizing that family members may be dealing with different aspects of grief than the client.

Client expectations.

As part of the assessment, the nurse must take time to determine the client's expectations for nursing care. The client's perceptions and expectations will enter into the way the nurse prioritizes diagnoses. For example, if clients perceive that their level of pain and discomfort is severe, they will be less attentive to the treatment plan. If clients perceive pain as their major problem, the nurse will do well to consider this perception and make pain relief a high priority. Once the client perceives less discomfort, greater attention can then be given, for example, to discussing the meaning of a loss. In this case, if the nurse fails to consider the client's needs, it is likely that efforts to help the client accept a loss will fall short of the goal.

Similarly, the nurse should include an opportunity for the family to explain how they perceive the role of the nurse and what their goals are for the nurse's involvement with them. This part of the assessment process gives the opportunity for misunderstandings to be clarified. For example, if the family thinks that the nurse will change the client's prescription for pain medication, the nurse can clarify that this is not within the scope of practice and suggest alternative means for having the client's needs met, such as having the client or family member call the physician to discuss it. Taking time to determine what clients and their families expect and desire from nursing helps to ensure that a comprehensive plan is developed that will meet the client's and family's needs.

Nurses' experience with grief.

As part of the assessment process, nurses need to monitor their own emotional well-being, a process of self-reflection that is also part of critical thinking behavior central to successful nursing care. When working with families experiencing grief, the nurse must be aware of how much personal sadness is related to the client and how much is related to unresolved experiences from the past. Although it is not wrong to have personal feelings and emotions, it is rarely if ever appropriate to discuss one's personal family situation with the client. To do so would put the client in the position of comforting and supporting the nurse, and this role reversal is *never* appropriate in a professional relationship. Part of the professional responsibility of the nurse is to know when there is a need to get away from the situation and take care of oneself.

Successful critical thinking requires a synthesis of knowledge, experience, information gathered from clients, and critical thinking attitudes and standards. Clinical judgments require the nurse to anticipate what information is needed, analyze the data, and then make decisions regarding client care. Peter incorporates previous knowledge and experience in providing care for Mr. Holloway.

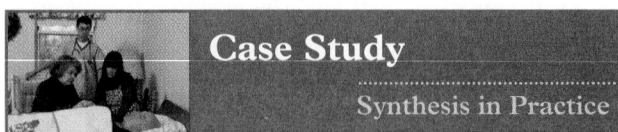

Case Study
Synthesis in Practice

As Peter Wong prepares to meet the Holloway family for the first time, he goes through a mental review of all of the information that will be essential to making an accurate assessment. He has read extensively about colon cancer and has tried to anticipate key symptoms to look for in a client who has metastases to the lungs and liver. He will attempt to be sensitive to any embarrassment Mr. Holloway might feel about his incontinence. He also remembers that all family members are experiencing grief in their own way, and roles and responsibilities for all of them are shifting. Mr. Holloway is facing his own death and has become very dependent. Regardless of Mrs. Holloway's seeming denial, she is being forced to assume new responsibilities as her husband's health deteriorates. Mr. Holloway's daughter has already given up her home and job to care for her father. The stress of Mr. Holloway's condition may be exaggerated by the conflict between these two women as the needs of the family change.

Peter has no past experience with death, but he has cared for critically ill clients. Humility and the willingness to take risks will be key attitudes to have in working with this family. If they ask him what he knows about death, he can honestly tell them that he thinks it must be very difficult to live through so many stresses. He will ask them to discuss their perceptions and feelings with him, and he will try to understand their feelings and accept them. If family members cry or are upset, he will try to show confidence that he knows he does not need to "fix" things. He just needs to be there to share their sadness. If they ask questions he cannot answer, he will have the humility to admit that he does not know and will try to obtain the information for them or put them in contact with someone who can help.

Peter will be especially careful to attend to Mr. Holloway's complaints of pain and discomfort and teach family members how to position him and medicate him when no nurses are in the home. He will respect Mr. Holloway's privacy, modesty, and need for dignity, especially in the face of medical problems such as incontinence. At school and at hospice, he will take care to protect confidentiality.

While he works with the family, he will facilitate discussion of important subjects such as preparation for death and will be sensitive to Mr. Holloway's need and desire to discuss his wishes regarding his death.

Nursing Diagnosis

After thorough and thoughtful data collection, the nurse identifies nursing diagnoses applicable to the client's clinical situation. Clustering of client or family behaviors, actual or potential losses, and data involving the loss leads to an individualized nursing diagnosis (see nursing diagnoses box).

The mere presence of one or two defining characteristics is usually insufficient to make an accurate diagnosis. The nurse should be vigilant and consider competing diagnoses. For example, if a client who is dying manifests an increase in crying or tearfulness, displays of anger, and frequent nightmares, this could signal the possibility of several nursing diagnoses because these characteristics are common to more than one diagnosis. Possibilities include *pain, ineffective individual coping,* and *spiritual distress.* Until the nurse examines all of the available data and inquires about the presence of other behaviors and symptoms, it will not be possible to determine with any accuracy a correct diagnosis.

The nurse must identify the appropriate related factor for a diagnosis. For example, *dysfunctional grieving related to loss of physical function* will require different interventions than *dysfunctional grieving related to the loss of a job.* Clarification of the related factor will ensure that appropriate interventions are selected for the client's care.

For the client who is seriously ill, several nursing diagnoses may apply. It is not possible to address all of these complex problems simultaneously. On any given day or at any one time, two or three problem areas will demand the attention of the nurse. These priorities will shift based on the client's condition and will constantly be reworked.

NURSING DIAGNOSES FOR CLIENTS WITH LOSS, DEATH, AND GRIEF

Adjustment, impaired
Coping, ineffective family: compromised
Family processes, altered
Grieving, anticipatory
Hopelessness
Nutrition, altered: less than body requirements
Self-esteem, situational low
Sleep pattern disturbance
Social isolation
Spiritual distress
Spiritual well-being, potential for enhanced

In addition to a diagnosis related directly to grief, the nurse may also diagnose other health problems common to grieving, such as *anxiety* or *altered nutrition.* In these situations the nurse's interventions must focus on supporting or resolving grief before the problems are solved. For example, simply improving the nutritional value and variety of available foods will do little to improve nutritional status if the client continues to have loss of appetite related to severe depression.

Planning

Grieving is the natural response to loss and has a therapeutic value. Nursing care is planned to meet the physical, emotional, developmental, and spiritual needs of grieving clients and their family. Nurses support clients' self-esteem by asking for their opinions and wishes regarding care. Nurses encourage families to make decisions *with* the client, not *for* the client. This helps clients maintain autonomy and feelings of control for as long as possible. The nurse develops a plan of care that is based on nursing diagnoses and designed to meet goals set with the client (see care plan).

Goals for a client dealing with loss might include adjusting to grief, accepting the reality of the loss, regaining a sense of self-esteem, and renewing normal activities in relationships. Expected outcomes are established to help gauge the client's progress in meeting each goal. For example, a client who has the diagnosis *situational low self-esteem related to impending job loss* might have the goal of care "to regain former positive self-esteem" (Kim and others, 1997). Outcomes established for the client might include "increases confidence in handling job situation" or "increases ability to problem solve and take action." Again, the family can become a partner in supporting goal achievement.

In developing a comprehensive plan, the nurse should access other professionals within the health care team and in the greater community as resources for helping clients deal with loss and grief. Clients may have concerns about financial matters or the making or revision of a will. Clients who express these concerns to the nurse can be referred to Legal Aid or to private attorneys. The nurse contributes to client well-being by suggesting intervention from other professionals or by providing resources. Utilization of these external resources is then incorporated into the plan of care. Each client and family should be treated as unique, with recognition that their needs, fears, hopes, expectations, and concerns will change throughout the illness.

Implementation

Health promotion. Although a return to full functioning will not be an expected outcome for a terminally ill client or even a person who experiences significant disability or other loss of function, there is always the goal of enabling the client to return to *optimal* physical and emotional functioning. This does not

CASE STUDY NURSING CARE PLAN

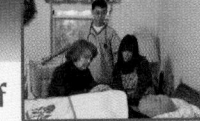

Loss and Grief

Assessment

During Peter's home visit, he finds Mr. Holloway appearing to be in reasonably good physical condition 1 week after discharge. His appetite has improved, and his mouth ulcers have disappeared. He continues to have bowel incontinence, however, and he has become very unsteady while walking. One night he fell while attempting to get out of bed and badly bruised his face. Peter finds Mr. Holloway easy to talk with and very receptive to Peter's questions. Mr. Holloway is easily moved to tears when talking about his situation, yet he becomes more relaxed when talking with Peter about memories of his younger years. He confides that his wife **disappears for hours every day** and **does not seem to realize how ill her husband really is.** Mr. Holloway states, "I know this is very **hard for her to accept,** but I also know I need her help." When asked about his daughter, Mr. Holloway reports that she appears tired and has not been sleeping well. "I think she feels as though she doesn't know what to do."

During Peter's visit, Mrs. Holloway comes into the room. She begins to **describe plans for their summer vacation, still 9 months away.** She avoids Peter's question about what she and her daughter have done to deal with Mr. Holloway's symptoms. Instead she suggests that her husband might benefit from "getting some exercise and eating a more balanced diet." Peter asks to talk with Mrs. Holloway alone for a few minutes. During this time, Mrs. Holloway begins to cry and voices her **fear of being unable to support her husband** appropriately. Mrs. Holloway states, "**I still can't believe this is happening to us.**" She collects her thoughts and asks Peter what the family should do; both she and her daughter want to be more helpful.

Nursing Diagnosis

Compromised ineffective family coping related to stress of impending death of father/husband

Planning

Goal

Client and family understand client's terminal condition and its implications within 1 month.

Family assumes care-giving tasks within 1 week.

Expected Outcomes

Wife and daughter participate in home visits with home health nurse within 3 days.

Client and family set short-term goals together for Mr. Holloway within 1 week.

Wife and daughter will assist with husband's hygiene and safety care within 1 week.

Wife and daughter will identify support resources to use within 1 week.

Mr. Holloway will begin the process of life review, sharing his thoughts with his family within 2 days.

Implementation

Steps

1. Involve Mrs. Holloway and daughter in discussion between home health nurse and Mr. Holloway, focusing instruction on symptom management.

2. Offer time for Mrs. Holloway and daughter to ask questions and discuss course of cancer.

Rationale

The family unit is the "client" and unit of care (Rando, 1984). Even with a poor prognosis, quality of life can be improved through discussion and planning for possible problems (Poncar, 1994).

Clarifying expectations better prepares individuals to face changes that will develop as cancer progresses.

Defining characteristics are shown in bold type.

CASE STUDY NURSING CARE PLAN—cont'd

Implementation—cont'd

Steps	Rationale
3. Explain to family that setting easily achievable goals helps foster hope. Enlist their help to establish goals for the next week.	Restructuring goals to be more short-term and achievable is a means of supporting and sustaining hope in terminally ill clients (Nowotny, 1991).
4. Provide family with names and phone numbers of support groups such as those provided by the hospice and the Cancer Society.	Accessing social support helps to facilitate grief and reduce anxiety and feelings of loneliness (Worden, 1991).
5. Discuss with Mrs. Holloway and daughter the value of reminiscence as part of looking back and evaluating life and its meaning.	Life review is a normal developmental task that needs to be supported as life nears its end (Erikson, 1982). Engaging in this process will help move the family along the process of anticipatory grieving (Worden, 1991).

Evaluation

During home visit, observe Mrs. Holloway and daughter's behavior and level of involvement in care.

Review with family the goals they have established.

Two weeks after family instruction, ask family to discuss if any problems exist in providing care to Mr. Holloway.

Ask family about their progress in locating a support group and about their plans to attend.

Discuss the family's degree of participation in the life review and reminiscence with Mr. Holloway. Evaluate if he becomes less dependent on the nurse to fulfill this role as his family becomes more involved in sharing.

---

mean that the client and family will not experience sadness or other disturbing emotions, but that they will adapt and cope effectively with the stressors in their life. In this sense the nurse is always working to promote "health." A variety of techniques and interventions are intended to assist clients to function optimally under severe stress, make effective decisions regarding their care, and cope with disappointment, frustration, and other emotions that are caused by their illness.

Therapeutic communication. Nursing care of the grieving client and family begins with trying to understand the significance of the loss to them. It is important that the nurse use effective communication skills to assist both client and family (see Chapter 13). At times this will be a relatively easy process because clients and families will be searching for someone to listen. At other times this may be difficult, such as if the client or family are unwilling to express their feelings or are in shock or denial. In either situation nurses will gain the most accurate information and be better able to understand the client's own personal experience if they use therapeutic communication techniques. The nurse will observe the visible response to the loss and then attempt to identify each person's strengths in dealing with it. Nurses use body language, such as sitting down to talk, to indicate that they have time to listen to the family. Allowing adequate time with the client and family promotes open communication, and providing a private location makes discussion of emotional subjects more comfortable.

The nurse's words and actions convey acceptance of the client's and family's grief reactions. For example, if a client begins to cry, the nurse quietly remains ready to offer support, rather than abandoning the client when comfort needs are the greatest. Acknowledging grief through touching the client and expressing concern may evoke the client's trust. Clients have differing needs regarding touch. It is important to be sensitive to the client's reactions to closeness and touch. In some instances it is appropriate to ask clients and family how they feel about touch. Comments such as "Would a hug help right now?" or "Would it help to have my hand to hold on to?" allow the client or family member to indicate a preference. When touch is used, it needs to be brief.

If a client chooses not to share feelings or concerns, the nurse conveys a willingness to be available when needed. When the nurse is reassuring and respects the client's needs and expressed preference for privacy, a therapeutic relationship may evolve. Sometimes clients need to begin resolving the grief before they can discuss the loss.

It is also important to recognize clients' normal styles of dealing with difficult situations. If they do not normally talk about their feelings, they are unlikely to discuss feelings regarding loss. When considering reactions to loss, the nurse is alert to the possibility of expressions of denial, anger, depression, or guilt. Nurses need to understand their own personal feelings before encouraging clients' expression of anger. The nurse remains supportive by letting the client and family know that feelings such as anger are normal. For example, the nurse might say, "You are obviously upset. I just want to let you know I'm available to talk if you'd like." It is important for the nurse to avoid erecting barriers to communication (see Chapter 13) by denying the client's grief, providing false reassurance, or avoiding discussion of the problem.

No topic that a dying client wishes to discuss should be avoided. Clients will be more likely to discuss impending death with a person willing to listen. When the nurse senses clients' desire to begin a discussion, it is important to let clients discuss their concerns. The nurse should respond to questions as honestly and positively as possible without giving false reassurance and should seek to support a client and family's therapeutic hope (see Table 21-4).

Eight principles that facilitate effective mourning. Worden (1991) lists eight general principles as a guide to facilitating the process of uncomplicated grief. These principles or guidelines are equally effective when applied to persons who are mourning a death and to persons who are grieving an important loss of self, such as through disability or chronic illness.

▪ *Help the client accept that the loss is real.* Discussing how the loss or illness occurred or was discovered, when, under what circumstances, who told them about it, and other similar topics helps to make the event more real and put it in perspective.

▪ *Encourage the expression of feelings.* Sometimes people defend themselves against emotions by discussing things in a very detached way. Encouraging and providing an opportunity to express emotions are important.

▪ *Support efforts to live without the deceased person or in the face of disability.* Using a problem-solving approach is often very helpful. Have clients or family make a list of their problems, help them prioritize them, and then lead them step-by-step through a discussion of how they might tackle each one. Encourage them to make use of family members, community resources, or others who can help them.

▪ *Encourage establishment of new relationships.* Many people will fear that in doing so they will be disloyal to the person who has died. They will need reassurance that new relationships do not mean that they are replacing the person who has died.

▪ *Allow time to grieve.* It is common to have "anniversary reactions" around the time of the loss in subsequent years. Some people worry that they are going crazy when sadness or other signs of grief recur after a period of relative calm.

▪ *Interpret "normal" behavior.* Being distractible, having difficulty with sleep or concentration, and thinking that they have heard the deceased person's voice or felt pain in a lost body part are common after a loss. These symptoms do not mean that they are "losing their mind" or becoming ill in some other way.

▪ *Provide continuing support.* Clients and their families may need to talk and may look to the nurse for support for many months or years following a loss. If the nurse has occasion to see the client or family after an extended time, it is appropriate to inquire about how they are managing and coping. This provides the opportunity for them to talk if needed.

▪ *Be alert for signs of ineffective coping.* Be aware of coping mechanisms that may be harmful, such as alcohol or other substance abuse, including overuse of over-the-counter medications such as sleep aids. Even these classes of drugs can be overused.

Maintenance of self-esteem and sense of dignity. Nursing interventions focus on promoting the client's sense of identity, dignity, and self-esteem. The nurse can help by listening, responding quickly and positively to requests, maintaining confidentiality and privacy, and providing comfort and support. The quality and quantity of time spent with the client are important in creating a therapeutic environment. Measures that provide comfort and support should be implemented in a caring, unhurried manner to reinforce the client's feelings of self-worth and dignity and to decrease the fear of rejection, isolation, and the sense of hopelessness. **Dignity** is the person's ability to maintain a self-concept as a person of value. Disabilities experienced by the client may threaten dignity, especially when care givers take control of the client's life. Taking away the client's right to make decisions about care fosters hopelessness and feelings of despair. The nurse can maintain and promote dignity and self-esteem by giving attention to the client's appearance. Cleanliness, a lack of body odors, attractive clothing, and personal grooming are some ways to promote a sense of worth. It is important for the nurse, who assumes management of the client's body functions, to show an attitude of respect, even when the client becomes very dependent.

Acute care

The nurse's role in providing terminal care. The nurse has special responsibilities in the care of clients who are very near death. These expand on interventions previously discussed and require sensitivity to the fact that as a client approaches death there are many friends who feel a need to pay their final respects and offer comfort to the family. It is often difficult to find the balance between encouraging social support and limiting demands that hinder rest and privacy.

Promotion of comfort. Comfort for a dying client includes pain control and control of symptoms of disease or therapies (Table 21-6). Fear of pain is common in many clients and may heighten perception of discomfort. The nurse assesses the character of the client's pain and carefully individualizes interventions (see Chapter 33). Once a dying client gains pain relief, more energy is available to maintain quality life activities. Personal hygiene is also a routine part of keeping the terminally ill comfortable. The client eventually depends on the nurse or family for basic needs.

Maintenance of independence. Most dying clients gain satisfaction from being independent as long as possible. When a client becomes physically unable to perform self-care, the nurse still encourages participation and decision making to give a sense of control.

Prevention of loneliness and isolation. To prevent loneliness and sensory deprivation, the nurse intervenes to improve the quality of the client's immediate environment. Dying clients should not be routinely placed in private rooms in out-of-the-way locations. Clients feel a sense of involvement when sharing a room and watching the nurse's activities. The client can then also share conversation and companionship with roommates and visitors. When the client dies, however, the nurse should give attention to the client's roommate because watching a person die or being in the room when a person dies can be frightening.

Perhaps the most important factor in preventing loneliness is visits by family members or significant others. If several family members visit, it may be necessary to provide a private room. Older adults often become particularly lonely at night and may feel more secure if someone stays at the bedside during the night. Nurses should allow visitors to remain with dying clients at any time if the client wants them. The nurse should know how to contact family members at any time if the client requests a visit or if the client's condition worsens.

Providing a soothing environment. Rooms should be well lit, attractively decorated, and offer a stimulating view. Pictures, cherished objects, cards or letters from family members, and live plants and flowers create an environment that is more familiar and comforting than that found in a typical health care setting.

The nurse cares for the client's bodily needs, helping to provide comfort and eliminating unpleasant odors. This may require long intervals of time with the client. The nurse has the responsibility to stay with dying clients when needed and to show concern and compassion.

Promotion of spiritual comfort. Providing a client with spiritual comfort means much more than asking clergy to visit (see Chapter 17). The nurse must support the client in the expression of a philosophy of life. As death approaches, clients often seek comfort by analyzing values and beliefs related to life and death. Dying clients seek to find purpose and meaning to life before surrendering to death. Dying clients often feel guilty if they perceive their life as unfulfilled. Therefore clients will often ask for forgiveness from God, a higher power, and/or people around them. In many religious traditions, there are special blessings or rituals intended for use with persons who are very sick or dying, and it is important for family members to know the appropriate

---

TABLE 21-6

Promoting Comfort in the Terminally Ill Client

Symptoms	Characteristics or Causes	Nursing Implications
Pain	Pain can be acute or chronic.	Individualize pharmacological therapies for each client. Administer narcotic analgesics on a regular schedule to prevent pain recurrence (see Chapter 33).★
	Pain from progressive cancer is usually chronic and constant.	Cutaneous stimulation, including application of heat and cold, massage, pressure, or vibration, relieves pain of muscle tension or spasm.★ Relaxation and guided imagery relieve pain through distraction. Oral route for narcotics is preferred, but choose route with fewest risks and greatest benefit.★ Introduce psychosocial intervention early.

★Data from Jacox A and others: Management of cancer pain, *Clinical Practice Guideline No. 9*, AHCPR Publication No. 94-0592, Rockville, Md, Agency for Health Care and Policy Research, Public Health Service, U.S. Department of Health and Human Services, March 1994.

Continued

TABLE 21-6

Promoting Comfort in the Terminally Ill Client—cont'd

Symptoms	Characteristics or Causes	Nursing Implications
Discomfort	Any source of physical irritation may worsen pain.	Provide thorough skin care including daily baths, lubrication of skin, and dry, clean bed linens to reduce irritants.
	As client approaches death, mouth remains open, tongue becomes dry and edematous, and lips become dry and cracked.	Provide oral care at least every 2 to 4 hours. Use soft toothbrushes or foam swabs for frequent mouth care. Apply a light film of petroleum jelly to lips and tongue (see Chapter 29).
	Blinking reflexes diminish near death, causing drying of cornea.	Eye care removes crusts from eyelid margins. Artificial tears reduce corneal drying.
Nausea and vomiting	Nausea and vomiting result from disease process (e.g., gastric cancer), complications (e.g., bowel obstruction), or medications.	Confer with physician about changing medications when possible. Administer antiemetics before meals. Bowel decompression with a nasogastric tube may relieve obstruction. Give mouth care and quickly clean up emesis.
Fatigue	Metabolic demands of a cancerous tumor cause weakness and fatigue.	Help client to identify valued or desired tasks; then help client to conserve energy for only those tasks. Promote frequent rest periods in a quiet environment.
	Exhaustion phase of the general adaptation syndrome causes energy depletion.	Time and pace nursing care activities.
Constipation	Narcotic medications and immobility slow peristalsis. Lack of bulk in diet or reduced fluid intake may occur with appetite changes. Constipation can add to discomfort.	Give preventive care, which is most effective: increase fluid intake; include bran, whole grain products, and fresh vegetables in diet; encourage exercise. Administer prophylactic stool softeners. Assess for fecal impaction.
Diarrhea	Results from disease process (e.g., colon cancer) and complications of treatment or medications.	Confer with physician to change medication if possible. Provide low-residue diet.
Urinary incontinence	Incontinence results from progressive disease (e.g., involvement of spinal cord, reduced level of consciousness).	Protect skin from irritation or breakdown. Indwelling urinary catheter or condom catheters may be used.
Inadequate nutrition	Nausea and vomiting can decrease appetite.	Serve smaller portions and bland foods, which may be more palatable.
	Depression from grieving may cause anorexia.	Allow home-cooked meals, which may be preferred by client and gives the family a chance to participate.
Dehydration	As disease progresses, client is less willing or able to maintain oral fluid intake.	Remove factors causing decreased intake; give antiemetics, apply topical analgesics to oral lesions. Reduce discomfort from dehydration; give mouth care minimum of every 4 hours; offer ice chips or moist cloth to lips.
Ineffective breathing patterns	Causes include disease progression involving lung tissue capacity, pneumonia, and pulmonary edema. Clients may also be severely anemic, causing reduced oxygen-carrying capacity.	Position upright to improve breathing capacity. Administer supplemental oxygen as ordered. Administer bronchodilator as ordered. Narcotics can suppress cough and ease breathing and apprehension. Suction secretions from mouth and nose.

time for administration of such rites. Prayer should not be used as a means to avoid the client or the dying process or as a substitute for the discussion of feelings. Prayer is an appropriate intervention when the client or family requests it. At no time should nurses attempt to "convert" clients to religion or impose their own religious beliefs on clients. When clients seek clergy, the nurse can help make necessary arrangements and arrange privacy when clergy visit. If clients do not have their own minister, priest, or rabbi but request to speak with someone about spiritual concerns, the nurse makes referrals, using the hospital chaplain as a resource.

Box 21-4
Suggestions for Involving the Family in the Care of a Dying Client

Assist in planning a visitation schedule for family members to prevent client and family from becoming fatigued.

Allow young children to visit a dying parent when the client is able to communicate.

Be willing to listen to family complaints about the client's care, as well as positive or negative feelings about the client.

Help family members learn to interact with the dying person (e.g., using attentive listening, avoiding false reassurances, conducting conversations about normal family activities or problems).

When the family becomes fatigued with care activities, relieve them from their duties so they can acquire needed rest and support. Refer them to resources for meals and lodging.

Support grieving between client and family. Provide privacy when preferred. Do not discourage open expression of grief between family and client.

Provide information daily with regard to the client's condition. Prepare the family for sudden changes in appearance and behavior.

Communicate news of impending death when the family is together if possible. Members can provide support for one another. Convey the news in a private area and be willing to stay with the family.

At the time of death, help the family to stay in communication with the dying person through short visits, caring silence, touch, and telling the client of their love for him or her.

After death, assist the family with decision making such as selection of a mortician, transportation of family members, and collection of the client's belongings.

Support for the grieving family. Nurses support family members through the dying and death of the client and simultaneously encourage support of the client. Suggestions for involving the family in the care of the dying client are included in Box 21-4 and Box 21-5. Nursing care of the dying client assumes that the entire family is the unit of care (Rando, 1984).

Special considerations for children. A child's reaction to and understanding of death and dying depend on the developmental stage of the child, parental values and beliefs, culture, and religious orientation. The nurse helps children to develop positive attitudes toward death by first counseling parents regarding a child's age-specific understanding of death and the normal reactions of a child to death (Wong, 1995). Parents may use "small deaths"—of a pet, for example—to help children become familiar and comfortable with a loss.

When death in a family occurs, parents often try to shield children from the loss. They fear the child will not be able to cope with the grief. However, allowing children to feel emotions prepares them for more traumatic experiences later in life (Wong, 1995). The child's developmental level determines the amount and type of detailed information that need to be discussed with the child.

When a child is dying, parents and siblings can feel considerable anger and resentment. The death of a child is usually seen as unfair. Parents may prefer to withhold information about the illness from the dying child. It is believed that even young children, however, can perceive that something is wrong with them because of the changes in behavior they see in parents. Nursing implications include planning the child's care with parents to determine the level of participation they desire. A nurse should not attempt to assume a parental

---

BOX 21-5
Client Teaching for the Dying Client's Family

- Describe and demonstrate feeding techniques and selection of foods to facilitate ease of chewing and swallowing.
- Demonstrate bathing, mouth care, and other hygiene measures, and allow family to perform return demonstration.
- Show video on simple transfer techniques to prevent injury to themselves and the client; help family to practice.
- Describe ways the family can promote the client's comfort, such as frequent rest periods and repositioning.
- Teach family to recognize signs and symptoms to expect as the client approaches death and information on whom to call in an emergency.
- Discuss ways to support the dying person and listen to needs and fears.
- Solicit questions from family and provide information as needed.

role or relinquish important nursing responsibilities (Wong, 1995). Parents and children need to know specifics about the plan of therapy and the normalcy of their reaction to the loss. It is common for friends and relatives to avoid contact with the dying child and family because of fear over the child's illness. Parents must decide whether they wish to maintain contact with significant others. Such a resource can prove valuable.

Hospice care. **Hospice** care is an alternative for terminally ill clients. It is not a facility but a concept for family-centered care designed to assist the terminally ill to be comfortable and maintain a satisfactory lifestyle until death. A hospice program emphasizes **palliative** treatment and the control of symptoms rather than curative treatment of disease (Aroskar, 1985). The client and family participate in care. Client care is well coordinated between the home and inpatient setting. Efforts are directed at keeping the client at home as much as possible. The family becomes the care giver, administering medication and treatment, whereas the interdisciplinary team provides psychological and physical resources needed for family support.

Care after death. The nurse who has cared for a client is often the best person to provide postmortem care because of the nurse-client relationship. The client's body should be cared for with dignity and sensitivity. After death, the body undergoes many physical changes. The body should be cared for as soon as possible after death to prevent tissue damage or disfigurement of body parts.

Every hospital has its own policies and procedures for preparation of the body, but in general the following practices are observed. The nurse prepares the body by making it look as natural and comfortable as possible. If it is placed in a supine position with arms at the sides, palms down, or across the abdomen, a mortician can better prepare the body for internment. The nurse places a small pillow or folded towel under the head to prevent discoloration from blood pooling. The eyelids usually remain closed if gently held down for a few seconds. The nurse inserts the client's dentures to maintain normal facial features. The nurse washes soiled body parts, dresses the body in a clean gown, combs or brushes the hair, and covers the body to the shoulders with clean linen. Hospital policy will dictate if tubes can be removed at this time.

After the body has been cleaned and extraneous equipment, dirty linens, and extra supplies have been removed from the room, the nurse offers the family the opportunity to view the body and, if they desire, to have a few private moments with the deceased person. It may help to suggest that this is an opportunity to say "good-bye," especially if they were not present at the time of death. If the family hesitates, the nurse gives them time to think about it. If they decide not to view the body, the nurse accepts their decision without judgment. If the family decides to view the body, they are assured

that they need not be alone and that the nurse will accompany them or will request whomever they would like. The nurse removes jewelry and presents it and other valuables to the family or allows the family to remove the jewelry themselves. The nurse spends time assisting the grieving family and offers to contact other support services such as social services and a spiritual adviser. The family has become the client.

After the family leaves the room, the nurse places tags containing name and other information on the client's wrist and ankle or toe. A rolled-up towel under the chin helps to keep the mouth closed. Most shroud kits or body bags contain absorbent pads that are placed under the perineal and rectal area to collect oozing feces or urine from relaxed sphincter muscles. The gown is removed, and the body is wrapped completely in either a body bag or shroud, a large rectangular piece of plastic or cotton material (Figure 21-1). Another identification tag is placed on the bag or shroud. If the client had a known transmissible infection, special labeling may be used to alert those who move and store the remains. The body is then transported to the morgue, or the mortician picks it up from the client's room. Although methods for transporting the body through hallways vary among institutions, the nurse should be certain that this procedure is as unobtrusive as possible. Such action protects the privacy of the deceased and respects the needs of other clients.

Nursing personnel are also responsible for disposition of the deceased's personal belongings and noting this in the medical record. The nurse can check with the client's family about taking the belongings or ensure that the belongings are transported with the deceased. If the family or friends have left, the supervisor is usually contacted.

Documentation of all of the events surrounding death is important to avoid misunderstandings and to clarify

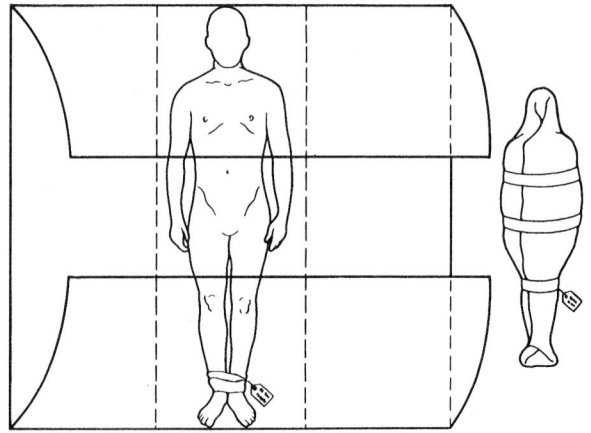

Figure 21-1. Be sure the shroud completely encircles all body parts. (From Elkin MK and others: *Nursing interventions and clinical skills,* St. Louis, 1996, Mosby.)

the final events in a person's life. Often family members are distressed and have little recollection of the exact time of death, decisions about the disposition of personal effects, or when certain family members were called or notified of the death. The nurse's note should reflect time of death, the name of the person who pronounced the client dead, preparation of the body, stipulation of what equipment (such as tubing or packing) was left in place, what possessions were given to the family, what possessions were left with the client, what funeral home was notified, and time of removal to the hospital morgue. Complete and accurate documentation offers a summary of activities that can become the focus of a legal or risk management review in the future.

Self-care for the nurse. When a nurse has cared for a client for weeks, months, or years, as is sometimes the case, it is possible to have deep personal feelings of loss and sadness for the family when the client dies. In these instances some nurses cope with their grief by attending the viewing at the mortuary or attending the funeral service. Once again, under these circumstances nurses should be clear that they are doing these things as part of their own grief process. When nurses experience multiple losses and fail to adequately process them, they can experience bereavement overload. They experience frustration, anger, guilt, sadness, helplessness, anxiety, depression, and feelings of being overwhelmed. Nurses need to develop personal support systems that allow time away from the care-giving setting and provide opportunities to share feelings. They should use stress management techniques to restore energy.

◼ Evaluation

Client care. Because nurses work in a wide variety of clinical settings, they are likely to encounter clients and families at every phase of their response to grief. This demands awareness of signs and symptoms of grief, even when clients are not specifically seeking care for symptoms directly related to grief and loss. These same signs and symptoms serve as criteria to evaluate whether a client is able to deal with a loss and progress through the grief process.

To determine the effectiveness of nursing interventions in meeting the goals of care, the nurse uses evaluative measures to identify actual behavioral outcomes. Actual behaviors are compared with expected outcomes to determine the client's health status and the need for revising the plan of care. Consider the goal for a terminally ill client and family to participate in the process of life review as a part of their terminal illness grief process. The nurse will evaluate the outcome of care by asking the client to describe the activities used to review important events in the client's life. If the client participated in activities such as the review of family photos, the nurse will evaluate further whether the activity

helped the client and family in preparing for the client's eventual death.

Client expectations. Nurses need to maintain open and ongoing communication with clients regarding their evaluation of nursing care. It should be expected that clients who have developed a good relationship with the nurse will feel comfortable in discussing their perceptions of "how things are going." When clients give feedback or suggestions to the nurse, the nurse should consider this a sign of a satisfactory relationship. Such suggestions indicate that the client and family perceive the nurse as someone they can approach with their concerns and from whom they can expect assistance. Once the client has identified new approaches or problems to be addressed, the plan of care can be revised to meet these emerging needs. Similarly, the nurse can be encouraged by feedback that indicates that planned interventions have helped move the client toward the achievement of important goals.

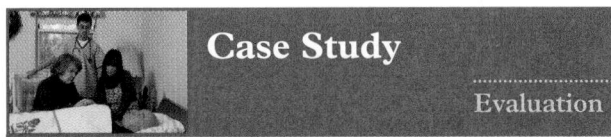

Case Study

Evaluation

One week after discussing his proposed interventions with the Holloway family, Peter is pleased to observe that, when he arrives for his visit, Mrs. Holloway is at home, helping Mr. Holloway with his bath. She explains that her daughter is "out taking a break, reading a book in the park." Mrs. Holloway has obtained a walker from the hospital supply store, and Mr. Holloway states that he feels much more secure when he uses it and is less fearful of walking. Mr. Holloway explains that he and his daughter have enjoyed looking through old photo albums together, and in the last day or two Mrs. Holloway has "wanted to join in the fun, too." They are enjoying their time as a family. Mrs. Holloway and her daughter have decided to "rotate" with each other at night, taking shifts watching over Mr. Holloway in case he needs anything. Now that they have agreed on this system, both are sleeping better, with less worry.

Documentation Note

Peter enters the following note on the client's chart at the home health agency: "Client reports that he is now using walker to ambulate in the home. States he feels much more secure. Observed in use of walker. Grip strong, posture erect, and gait steady with support. Wife now more engaged in direct care giving and in direct interpersonal interaction with client. Wife and daughter working together to provide care and ensure adequate rest for each other by taking "shifts" to monitor client during the night. Daugh-

Continued

ter out of the home during visit, but mood of both client and wife very positive, cheerful. Bath in progress at time of visit. Skin condition observed to be clear, without redness, tenderness, or evidence of tissue breakdown. Client and family independently report that pain management at this time is satisfactory. Client complains of recurrent right side pain every 3 to 4 hours, rapidly relieved with current pain medication. Is sleeping at night, waking only once for pain meds. Vital signs: T 98.0, pulse 68, resp. 18, BP 110/60. Plan is to continue supportive care and current medication management."

Key Terms

actual loss	hope
anticipatory grief	hospice
bereavement	loss
complicated	maturational loss
bereavement	mourning
death	palliative
dignity	perceived loss
grief	situational loss
grieving process	

■ Key Concepts

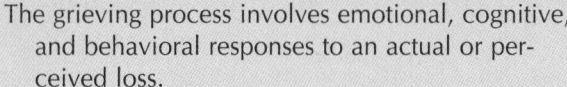

The grieving process involves emotional, cognitive, and behavioral responses to an actual or perceived loss.

Individuals experience different aspects of the grieving process at different times.

Dying may lead to a grief response similar to that with other kinds of losses.

A nurse's support of a client's hope can help promote an effective grieving process associated with a loss.

The individual's reaction to loss is influenced by many factors, including developmental stage, beliefs, roles, culture, relationships, and socioeconomic status.

The process of mourning is often considered to be composed of "stages" or "phases," yet in reality these phases are not sequential, and the client may move back and forth along a continuum of grief.

Assessment of the grieving client considers behavioral characteristics that suggest the client's stage of grieving.

Grief resolution is a process that should be expected to take a year or more, with "anniversary reactions" common for several years following the loss.

Nursing diagnoses focus on the type of grief experienced by clients or health-related problems common to grieving clients.

Therapeutic communication is an important nursing intervention to assist the grieving and dying client in coping with loss.

Nursing care of the grieving and dying client should promote the client's sense of identity, dignity, and self-esteem.

Nursing care of the terminally ill focuses on promoting comfort and improving the quality of remaining life.

As death approaches, a client should review and analyze values and beliefs pertinent to the meaning of life and death.

A nurse must assess whether family members are willing to be involved in a dying client's care before using them as resources.

Evaluation must also include the client's appraisal of the effectiveness of intervention. Clients and families are partners in care planning and delivery.

Care after death involves caring for the body with dignity and sensitivity.

The evaluation of nursing care for the grieving and dying client is ongoing and is based on identifiable behavioral changes through the grieving process.

The nurse's own loss history influences responses to client losses.

Nurses who work with critically or terminally ill clients experience loss and grief.

Critical Thinking Activities

1. Kim Harbor, a 29-year-old diagnosed with breast cancer following what was anticipated to be a benign cyst removal, has become very withdrawn and threatens to sign herself out of the hospital against medical advice (AMA). She refuses to have any further surgery, stating that to lose a breast would be the "end of life anyway, so why bother?" Describe how you would approach Kim and what you think you need to assess.

2. Mr. Hightower, an 84-year-old single (never married) man, has been admitted for the third time for complaints of dizziness, numbness and tingling in his fingers, and difficulty breathing. He tells the emergency department physician that he thinks he has a brain tumor. His tests continue to reveal no physical cause for the symptoms, and once he is admitted to the hospital his symptoms resolve within a matter of hours. A review of the chart indicates that he lost his 17-year-old cat to bone cancer 2 months ago. What do you think is happening, and how would you approach Mr. Hightower?

3. Harvey is in the final phase of his terminal illness. It is clear he will die soon. He has no family in this state but is very involved with his church, and his minister visits often. His minister asks if it would be appropriate for members of the church to keep a vigil at the bedside until Harvey dies. The medical resident who is following the case has written an order that reads "Family visitors only." Identify three needs that Harvey is likely to be experiencing as he approaches the end of life. Discuss what nursing interventions would be most appropriate.

References

Aroskar MA: Access to hospice-ethical dimensions, *Nurs Clin North Am* 20:299, 1985.

Barbus AJ: The dying person's bill of rights, *Am J Nurs* 75:99, 1975.

Bowlby J: *Attachment and loss,* vol III, *Loss, sadness and depression,* New York, 1980, Basic Books.

Erikson E: *Childhood and society,* New York, 1982, Norton.

Hafen BQ and others: *Mind/body health,* Boston, 1996, Allyn & Bacon.

Kim MJ and others: *Pocket guide to nursing diagnoses,* St. Louis, 1997, Mosby.

Kübler-Ross E: *On death and dying,* New York, 1969, Macmillan.

Nowotny M: Every tomorrow a vision of hope, *J Psychosoc Oncol* 9(3):117, 1991.

Poncar PJ: Inspiring hope in the oncology patient, *J Psychosoc Nurs* 32(1):33, 1994.

Rando TA: *Grief, dying and death,* Champaign, Ill, 1984, Research Press.

Wong DL: *Whaley & Wong's nursing care of infants and children,* ed 5, St. Louis, 1995, Mosby.

Worden, JW. *Grief counseling and grief therapy,* New York, 1991, Springer.

CHAPTER

22

Stress and Adaptation

OBJECTIVES

Mastery of content in this chapter will enable
the student to:

- Define the key terms listed.
- Describe the three phases of the general
  adaptation syndrome.
- Discuss task-oriented behaviors that are
  responses to stress.
- Discuss the most common ego-defense
  mechanisms that are responses to stress.
- Discuss the integration of stress theory in
  nursing theory.
- Describe a multimodal method of assessing the
  stress and anxiety that are manifested in
  cognition and behavior.
- Describe effective ways of coping with stress
  and anxiety.
- Discuss the effects of prolonged stress.
- Conduct a nursing assessment of a client under
  stress.
- Describe stress management techniques
  beneficial for coping with stress.
- Discuss the process of crisis intervention.
- List nursing diagnoses related to stress.
- Develop a nursing care plan for clients
  experiencing stress.
- Discuss how stress in the workplace can affect
  the nurse.

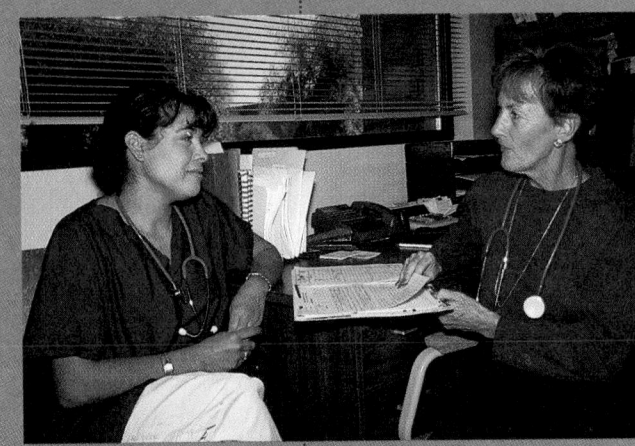

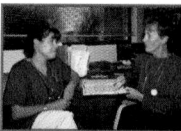

Case Study

Rhonda Bennett, RN

Rhonda Bennett is a 35-year-old married mother of three children who has worked for City Hospital since her graduation from a 2-year nursing program 15 years ago. She began her professional career on a general medical unit and through the years has earned a reputation as a skilled clinician and compassionate care giver. She presently is the nurse manager on the evening shift in the medical intensive care unit and has always described herself as "the happiest employee at City Hospital."

Rhonda's family life is also of great importance to her. She is a Girl Scout leader and "soccer team mom." Until last year she also enjoyed playing tennis with her husband, who was self-employed as a contractor. Within the past year, however, he has had several hospitalizations related to severe diabetes, and, following recent amputation of both legs below the knee, he is unemployed. He is depressed that he will require extensive physical therapy to adapt to the use of prosthetic devices as well as occupational retraining before he can return to any form of work. In an effort to help her husband overcome his depression and make progress in rehabilitation, Rhonda has reduced her community involvement, attempted to spend any free time working with him, and taken on all available overtime. Because of Rhonda's employment, the Bennetts have been able to maintain their home and standard of living.

After a year of declining profitability, however, City Hospital has announced a "major restructuring" effort. Based on comments that the administration has made, Rhonda knows that she will almost certainly lose her job. Yet she feels overwhelmed by the burden of being breadwinner, mother, wife, and nurse to her family. At this stage in her life she wishes that someone could take care of *her*. She has tried to "put on a face" of confidence, but every day it is becoming harder to keep going. She feels defeated and hopeless, has no energy, and is having difficulty organizing her thoughts. Her boss has noticed that Rhonda often complains of severe headaches and has become especially concerned since Rhonda tearfully confided to her that she cannot sleep and therefore has begun drinking at night to help herself "unwind." Because of these behaviors, Rhonda has been referred to the hospital's Employee Health Office. This department has been charged with the duty of helping employees cope with the stresses associated with being laid off.

Becky Howard is the nurse in the Employee Health Office who has been assigned to do prelimi-nary screening and crisis intervention with staff members who will be laid off. She herself has a bachelor's degree in nursing and extensive experience working both in acute care hospitals and on a crisis intervention telephone "hot line." She is a 52-year-old divorced mother of four children and has been hired by City Hospital on a temporary basis to help manage the employee response to restructuring and layoffs.

Stress is a universal part of the human experience and is necessary for survival. It affects every person regardless of age, gender, race, economic condition, or educational level. **Stress** evolves out of life events and experiences, stimulates our thinking processes, and helps maintain a basal level of autonomic arousal. Persons who experience no stress at all for even short periods of time report high levels of boredom and a lack of purpose and direction. In contrast, mildly elevated levels of stress are associated with increased attentiveness and engagement with others. Thus mild levels of stress actually add pleasure to life and can serve to make us more aware of and responsive to hazards to survival.

In common terminology, stress is most often associated with negative, troublesome circumstances such as death, divorce, or job loss (distress), but in reality stress is also linked with positive, happy life changes such as birth, vacation, or graduation (eustress) (Holmes and Rahe, 1967). Stress, then, is a topic of interest to all of us. It is of importance in nursing not only so that professionals can recognize stress in clients and families and intervene effectively but also because the professional nurse is affected by stressful events that occur in the course of clinical practice. Nurses must be able to recognize in their own lives the signs and symptoms of stress and be knowledgeable about stress management techniques to aid personal coping in themselves as well as in clients and their families.

···SCIENTIFIC KNOWLEDGE BASE

Overview of the stress response. Research has documented that the human response to **stressors** is multifaceted and complex, placing demands on physiological processes as well as emotional coping. The amount of physical and psychological energy required and the effectiveness of the attempt to adapt depend on many factors, as detailed in Box 22-1.

There are two forms of physiological response to stress. These include the local adaptation syndrome and the general adaptation syndrome (Figure 22-1). Using assessment skills, the nurse can determine which type of response an individual is experiencing.

Box 22-1
Factors Influencing the Response to Stressors

Intensity

Minimal, severe, or somewhere in between. The greater the perceived magnitude of the stressor, the greater the stress response.

Scope

The pervasiveness with which a stressor impacts a person's total being. The greater the scope of a stressor, the greater the stress response.

Duration

The length of time the person is exposed to the stressor. The greater the duration, the greater the stress response.

Number and Nature of Other Stressors Present

Multiple stressors experienced simultaneously or a succession of single stressors with no opportunity for the person to rest and regroup results in a greater stress response.

Predictability

Being able to anticipate the occurrence of an event, even if one cannot control it, generally results in a reduced experience of stress.

Level of Personal Control

Believing that we have control over an unpleasant experience, even if that control is never exercised or the belief is erroneous, lessens the level of associated stress and anxiety.

Feelings of Competence

Greater self-confidence in one's ability to manage a stressful event results in less tension and anxiety.

Cognitive Appraisal

The greater the personal meaning of an event, the greater the stress associated with it. Thus the same event may cause differing levels of stress in different people.

Availability of Social Supports

The emotional concern and support of other people reduce the negative effects of stressful events.

Local adaptation syndrome. The **local adaptation syndrome** is a response of body tissue, an organ, or a part of the body to the stress of trauma, illness, or other physiological change. All forms of the local adaptation syndrome share similar characteristics. The response is localized (not involving entire body systems) and short-term.

The **reflex pain response,** for example, is a localized reaction of the central nervous system to the stimulus of pain (see Chapter 33) and serves to protect tissue from further damage. An example would be a person's unconscious reflex of removing a hand from a hot surface.

Another local adaptation syndrome, the **inflammatory response,** is adaptive in that it serves to prevent the spread of infection and promotes wound healing (see Chapter 38). This response is stimulated by trauma or infection and may produce localized pain, swelling, heat, redness, and changes in functioning. These changes occur in three phases. The first involves changes in cells and the circulatory system. When trauma occurs, there is an initial narrowing of blood vessels at the site of injury to control bleeding. This narrowing occurs only when trauma causes a break in the skin and underlying blood vessels. Then histamine is re-

leased at the site, increasing blood flow to the area and the number of white blood cells to combat infection. The release of kinins, which increase capillary permeability to permit the flow of proteins, fluid, and leukocytes to the site, occurs almost simultaneously with the release of histamine. At this point the localized blood flow decreases, keeping leukocytes in the area of injury to fight infection.

The second phase of the inflammatory response involves the release of exudate from the wound. Exudate is a combination of fluid, cells, and other substances produced in the area of injury. The type and amount vary from injury to injury and person to person. Exudate is usually released at the site of injury, which may be a cut, laceration, or surgical incision.

The last phase is the repair of tissue by regeneration or scar formation. Regeneration replaces damaged cells by identical or similar cells. Scar formation replaces original tissue but is not functional. The inflammatory response indicates the body is adapting to a local injury.

General adaptation syndrome. The **general adaptation syndrome** is a physiological response of the whole body to stress and involves several body systems, mainly the autonomic nervous system and the endocrine system (Table 22-1). It can be triggered by any

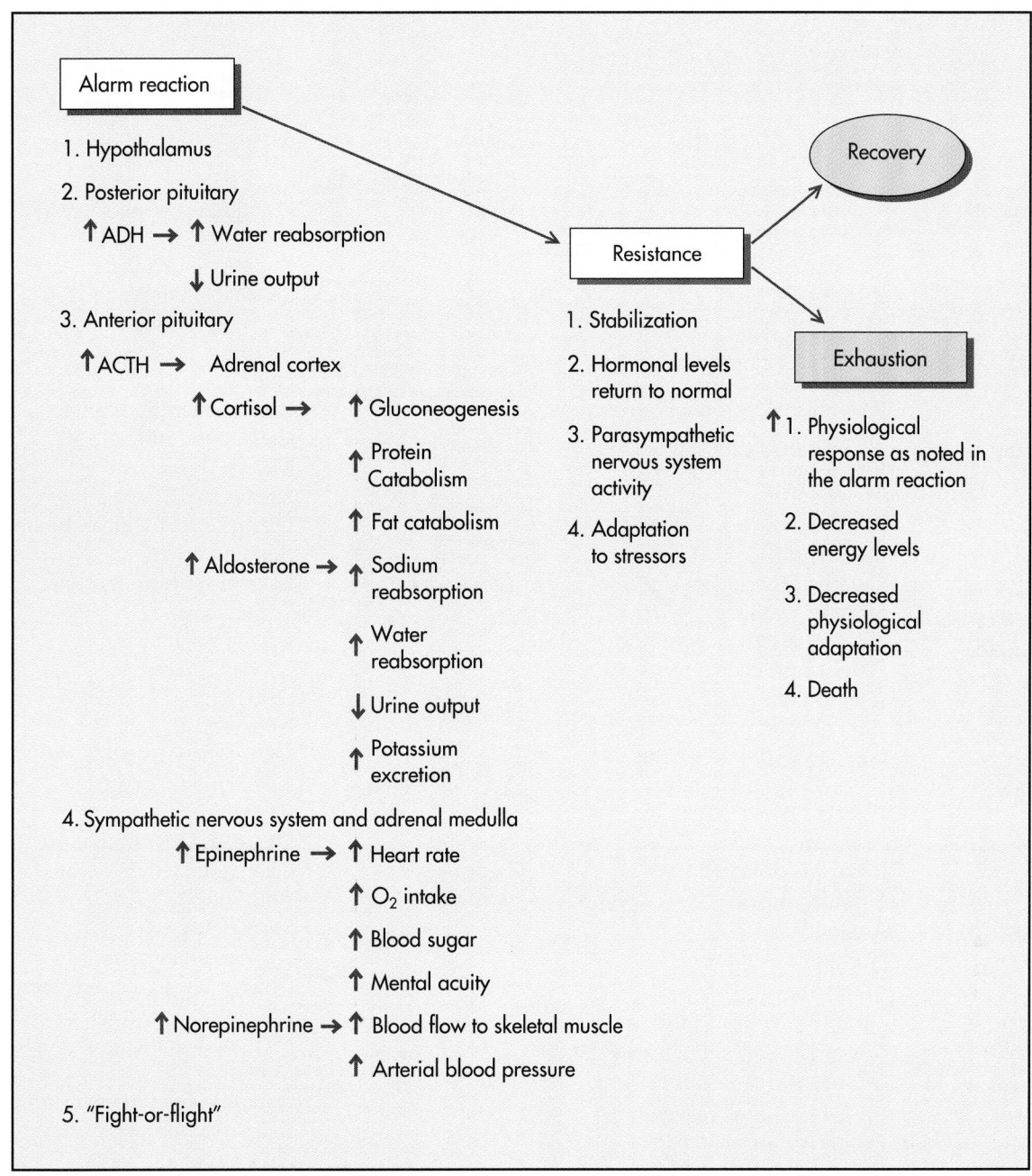

Figure 22-1. General adaptation syndrome. (From Potter PA, Perry AG: *Fundamentals of nursing: concepts, process, and practice,* ed 4, St. Louis, 1997, Mosby).

event, either physical, psychological, or both, that results in an actual or perceived threat to the viability of the organism.

The general adaptation syndrome consists of three stages: the alarm reaction, the resistance stage, and the exhaustion stage (see Figure 22-1). Although everyone generally goes through all three stages, the duration and effectiveness of each stage vary from person to person.

The **alarm reaction** is the mobilization of the defense mechanisms of the body and mind to cope with the stressor. Hormone levels rise to increase blood vol-

ume and thereby prepare the person to act. Increased blood sugar levels make energy available for adaptation. Rising levels of epinephrine and norepinephrine result in increased heart rate, increased blood flow to muscles, increased oxygen intake, and greater mental alertness. In addition, the pupils of the eyes dilate to produce a greater visual field, and other changes occur to prepare the person to act (Figure 22-2). This massive change in all body systems prepares an individual to choose to flee or to remain and fight the stressor. This total physiologic response to stress has come to be known as the

TABLE 22-1
Indicators of Stress

System	Assessment Findings	System	Assessment Findings
Physical		**Psychological—cont'd**	
Cardiovascular	Tightness of chest	Cognitive—	Orientation to past instead of
	Increased heart rate	cont'd	present
	Elevated blood pressure		Decreased creativity
Respiratory	Breathing difficulty		Slower thinking, reactions
	Tachypnea		Learning difficulties
Neuroendocrine	Headaches, migraines		Apathy
	Fatigue, exhaustion		Confusion
	Insomnia, sleep disturbances		Lower attention span
	Feeling uncoordinated		Calculation difficulties
	Restlessness, hyperactivity		Memory problems
	Tremors (lips, hands)		Distressing dreams
	Profuse sweating (palms)		Disruption of logical thinking
	Dry mouth		Blaming others
Gastrointestinal/	Cold hands and feet	Emotional	Lack of motivation to get up in the
genitourinary	Urinary frequency		morning
	Nausea, diarrhea, vomiting		Crying tendencies
	Weight gain or loss of more		Lack of interest
	than 10 pounds		Irritability
	Change in appetite		Isolation
	Gastrointestinal bleeding		Diminished initiative
Diagnostic	Blood in stools/vomitus		Negative thinking
	Elevated blood sugar		Worrying
Musculoskeletal	Backaches, muscle aches		Decreased involvement with others
	Bruxism (clenched jaw)	Behavioral/	Change in activity level
	Slumped posture	lifestyle	Withdrawal
Reproductive	Amenorrhea		Suspiciousness
	Failure to ovulate		Change in communication
	Impotency in men		Change in interactions with others
	Loss of libido		Increased or decreased food intake
Immunological	Frequent or prolonged colds/flu		Increased smoking or alcohol
Psychological			intake
Cognitive	Forgetfulness/preoccupation		Over vigilance to environment
	Denial		Excessive humor or silence
	Increased fantasy life		No exercise
	Poor concentration		Type A personality
	Inattention to detail		

fight-or-flight response and may last from 1 minute to many hours. If the stressor poses an extreme threat to life or remains for a long time, the person progresses to the second stage, resistance.

During the **resistance stage** the body stabilizes, and hormone levels, heart rate, blood pressure, and cardiac output return to normal. During this stage the person attempts to adapt to the stressor. If the stress can be resolved, the body repairs any damage that may have occurred. However, if the stressor remains, as in continued blood loss, debilitating disease, or long-term severe

mental illness, and the person is unable to adapt, the person enters the third stage, exhaustion.

The **exhaustion stage** occurs when the body can no longer resist the effects of the stressor and when the energy necessary to maintain adaptation is depleted. The physiological response is intensified, but the person's energy level is compromised, and adaptation to the stressor diminishes. The body is unable to defend itself against the impact of the event, physiological regulation diminishes, and, if the stress continues, death may result.

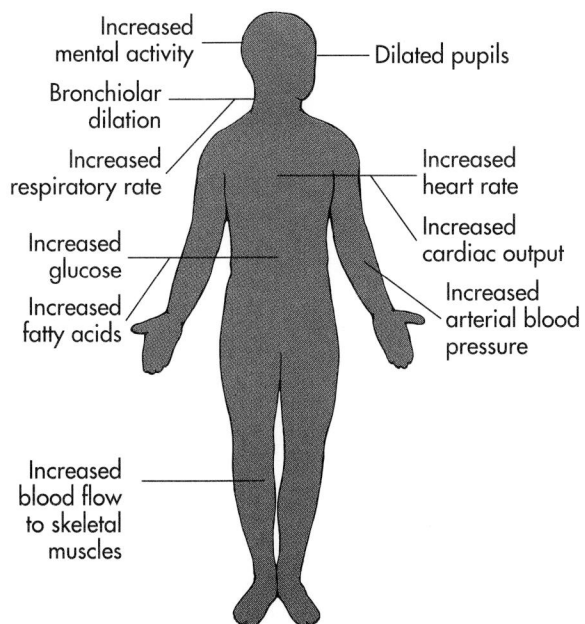

Increased mental activity

Dilated pupils

Bronchiolar dilation

Increased respiratory rate

Increased heart rate

Increased cardiac output

Increased glucose

Increased fatty acids

Increased arterial blood pressure

Increased blood flow to skeletal muscles

Figure 22-2. Fight-or-flight response. (From Potter PA, Perry AG: *Fundamentals of nursing: concepts, process, and practice,* ed 4, St. Louis, 1997, Mosby).

Although the general adaptation syndrome serves as the foundation for our understanding of the body's response to stressful events, these physiological processes take place in the context of the unique developmental and psychosocial variables of an individual and will by definition vary from person to person.

NURSING KNOWLEDGE BASE

Stress has been the object of study and the focus of scholarly thought across many disciplines. The central role of stress as a potential factor in disease development has been recognized by multiple nursing theorists. Symptoms or behaviors that are manifestations of stress often require nursing intervention. In the social sciences, particularly psychology, the effects of stress and the mind-body connection have been widely studied. Much scholarly effort has been devoted to researching ways of coping. When considered together with biomedical research, this body of knowledge becomes the scientific rationale that drives nursing interventions.

Nursing Theory and the Role of Stress

Betty Neuman (1972) theorizes that all persons experience multiple known stressors, each of which has a differing potential to disturb equilibrium. Stressors may be intrapersonal, occurring within the person; interpersonal, occurring as a result of relationships between individuals; or extrapersonal variables (such as finances) that impinge on the person from life circumstances. According to Neuman, every person has developed a set of

responses to stress that constitute their "normal line of defense." This line of defense helps to maintain health and wellness. However, when physiological, psychological, sociocultural, or developmental influences are unable to buffer stress, then the normal line of defense is broken, and disease can result. Nursing as a profession is concerned with all of the variables that influence a person's response to stress. At the primary level of prevention, the nurse uses knowledge to identify possible risk factors associated with stress in the client and to intervene appropriately to modify stress and prevent illness. At the secondary level of prevention, the nurse identifies symptoms of illness through the assessment process, prioritizes interventions, and carries out a plan of treatment. At the tertiary level of prevention, nursing supports adaptive processes involved in healing, moving the client back to wellness and the primary level of disease prevention. Neuman's model of nursing is dynamic, assessing on multiple levels the relationship of persons to stressors in the environment.

Sister Calista Roy (1980), in her adaptation model, defines the concept of "client" as including the family and greater community, as well as the individual. This conceptualization has proved to be particularly useful as nursing has increasingly moved out of hospital settings and into the communities in which clients live. According to Roy, the goal of nursing is to use the nursing process to support a person's adaptation to alterations (stressors) in the environment. This adaptation takes place in each of four modes: physiological, self-concept, role, and interdependence on others.

Orem's (1985) self-care theory has as its central concept the notion of self-care agency. Agency is an individual's ability to initiate and sustain activities that will nurture health as well as have sufficient knowledge and understanding to promote health. Implied in this concept of self-care is the need for persons to be aware of stressors in their environment (both internal and external) and to proactively respond in a way that supports health-promoting balance. Nursing activities function in this model until clients are able to act on their own behalf. In these and other nursing models and theories, the role of the nurse is central to restoring the delicate life balance that has been threatened or disrupted by stress.

Developmental, Psychological, Sociocultural, and Spiritual Factors

There are a number of factors governing the way an individual perceives threats to the integrity of the self and moves to adapt effectively in response to stress. These include the individual's developmental level, cognitive appraisal, existence of defense mechanisms, mastery of other coping strategies, and the presence of social support. In addition, such variables as social class, cultural influences, and belief in God or a higher power will

TABLE 22-2
Defense Mechanisms

Defense	Definition	Normal Use	Patient Example
Repression	Unconscious and involuntary forgetting of painful ideas, events, and conflicts	A car accident victim is unable to remember details of the impact but was aware at the time.	Mrs. Young, a victim of incest, does not know why she has always hated her uncle.
Denial	Unconscious refusal to admit an unacceptable idea or behavior	A nursing student refuses to admit that she is flunking out of school despite Fs in two courses.	Mr. Davis, who is alcohol dependent, states that he can control his drinking.
Suppression	Voluntary exclusion from awareness of anxiety-producing feelings, ideas, and situations	A student states, "I cannot think about my wedding tonight. I have to study."	Michelle states to the nurse that she is not ready to talk about her recent divorce.
Rationalization	Attempts to make or prove that one's feelings or behaviors are justifiable	A student states, "I got a C on the test because the teacher asked poor questions."	Mr. Jones, a paranoid schizophrenic, states that he cannot go to work because he is afraid of his co-workers instead of admitting that he is mentally ill.
Intellectualization	Using only logical explanations without feelings or an affective component	A wife states to her husband that a dented car fender is much better than a completely wrecked car and garage door.	Mrs. Mann talks about her son's death and bout with cancer as being mercifully short without showing any signs of sadness.
Identification	A conscious or unconscious attempt to model oneself after a respected person	When a little girl dresses up like her mother to play house, she tries to talk and act like her mother.	Sheila states to the nurse, "When I get out of the hospital, I want to be a nurse just like you."
Introjection	Unconsciously incorporating wishes, values, attitudes of others as if they were your own	While her mother is gone, a young girl disciplines her brother just like her mother would.	Without realizing it, a patient talks and acts like his therapist, analyzing other patients.
Compensation	Covering up for a weakness by overemphasizing or making up a desirable trait	An academically weak high school student becomes a star in the school play.	A schizophrenic patient who is unable to talk to other patients becomes known for his expressive poetry.
Reaction formation	A conscious behavior that is the opposite of an unconscious feeling	An older brother who dislikes his younger brother sends him gifts for every holiday.	Miss Marla, who unconsciously hates her mother, continuously tells staff how wonderful her mother is.
Displacement	Discharging pent-up feelings to a less threatening object	A husband comes home and yells at his wife after a bad day at work.	Mrs. Faust screams at another patient after being told by her psychiatrist that she cannot have a weekend pass.
Projection	Blaming someone else for one's difficulties or placing one's unethical desires on someone else	A teenager comes home late from a date and states that her friend did not bring her home on time.	Katrina states that she used marijuana while on pass because her boyfriend made her smoke it.

Modified from Keltner NL and others: *Psychiatric nursing,* ed 2, St. Louis, 1995, Mosby.

TABLE 22-2
Defense Mechanisms—cont'd

Defense	Definition	Normal Use	Patient Example
Conversion	The unconscious expression of intrapsychic conflict symbolically through physical symptoms	A student awakens with a migraine the morning of a final examination and feels too ill to take it. She does not realize that 1 hour of cramming left her unprepared.	Mr. Jenson suddenly develops impotence after his wife discovers he is having an affair with his secretary.
Undoing	Doing something to counteract or make up for a transgression or wrongdoing	After spanking her son, a mother bakes his favorite cookies.	After eating another patient's cookies, Mrs. Donnelly apologizes to the patients, cleans the refrigerator, and labels everyone's snack with their names.
Dissociation	The unconscious separation of painful feelings and emotions from an unacceptable idea, situation, or object	A young wife talks about her husband's extensive gambling debts as if they were nothing to be concerned about.	A patient tells the nurse that when she was sexually molested as a child, she felt as if she were outside of her body watching what was happening without feeling anything.

influence both the person's perception of events and the body's response to stress.

Developmental factors. Erikson (1963) discusses in great detail the psychosocial stages common to human development (see Chapter 20). From his research it is known that there are optimal times in the course of growth for persons to master critical tasks and build essential relationships. Prolonged stress can interrupt or slow passage through any of these stages, leading to a developmental crisis. Such a crisis can occur at any point in life if circumstances prevent a person from mastering the tasks of a particular stage.

Similarly, Piaget (1952) discusses the normal progression of the human thought process throughout the life span. In responding to stressors, the stage of a person's cognitive development will affect the ability to conceptualize the nature of the threat and effectively problem solve. For example, a young child develops trust through the experience of receiving unconditional love and protection from harm. If this same child is severely injured in a car crash in which his mother is killed, there is risk for developmental crisis.

Psychological factors. Psychological adaptive behaviors, also referred to as "coping mechanisms," are learned through experience and are used to manage stress. **Coping mechanisms** can be either constructive or destructive. Constructive behaviors help an individual meet the challenge of resolving the conflict causing stress. For example, a woman experiencing anxiety about her new parenting role can use constructive behavior if she actively reads books about infant development and attends an educational and support group for new parents. Destructive behaviors do not help a person to cope with a stressor and may result in further physical or emotional harm. To continue the previous example, if the woman responds to parenting stress by drinking alcohol beginning in the early morning and continuing throughout the day, she is engaging in destructive behavior. This pattern of drinking alcohol impairs her judgment, potentially placing both the mother and child in danger, and ultimately threatening the health of both.

Coping mechanisms can be **task-oriented behaviors,** involving the use of direct problem-solving techniques to cope with the threats, or they can be **defense mechanisms,** which regulate emotional distress and thus protect a person from anxiety and stress (Table 22-2). Defense mechanisms are often misunderstood. Many people make the mistake of regarding them as always harmful or indicative of psychological weakness. In reality, defense mechanisms can be quite healthy and occur naturally in response to stress or illness. They only become an unhealthy means of coping if they totally distort reality so that the person is immobilized in dealing with problems, resulting in even greater harm.

The following are examples of adaptive defense mechanisms. In a psychologically stressful situation, such as the sudden death of a spouse, use of **suppression** may allow a new widow to methodically notify her children of their father's death and make necessary arrangements for his funeral. In this case, deferring the full expression of emotion until critical decisions have been made is healthy. It allows the new widow to function until the presence of supportive persons makes the expression of emotion "safe." In another example, **regressive behavior** such as staying in bed and assuming a dependency role during hospitalization may promote rest and conserve the body's energy (Grainger, 1989).

Maladaptive use of defense mechanisms would include an instance in which a person uses **denial** to avoid the psychologically painful reality of a cancer diagnosis. Denial is an unconscious refusal to admit an unacceptable idea. In this example, if the presence of cancer is denied and no treatment initiated, death will be the likely result.

The types of adaptive behaviors that a person uses are related to the cognitive appraisal process. **Cognitive appraisal** relates to the extent to which individuals perceive a stressful situation as a challenge or an obstacle that exceeds their capacity to cope (Lazarus and Folkman, 1984). The way an individual perceives a situation, including the personal meaning of the event, is perhaps the most significant factor in determining the nature of the response. Situations and events that are perceived as challenges are less likely to evoke extreme stress or anxiety than are situations that are interpreted as exceeding the individual's capacity to cope. The client's appraisal of stressors is influenced by beliefs, values, and the extent to which social support is available. Very often a major goal of nursing is to help the client view life events as challenges that can be mastered using existing or new strategies or by making effective use of situational and social supports.

Sociocultural influences. No person lives in total isolation. All live as members of communities that share many elements of a common culture. Social networks may include family members, co-workers, and peers. These groups may provide formal or informal psychological support to assist a person in adapting to stress. Cultural groups can have a major influence on health behaviors (see Chapter 18). Poverty is also a critical factor that limits the access of many people to health care and delays intervention. All of these influences must be considered when assessing a client's health-related behaviors and symptoms of illness. The nurse must be open to differing views of health care and flexible in working within a client's health belief system and culture.

Spiritual considerations. Every person also has some belief system that helps to explain the relationship of events and the ultimate purpose of life. These belief systems are taught within the framework of the family, evolve over time, and may be tied either directly to religion or may exist outside formal membership in a religious group. The experience of severe stress may cause a reevaluation of previously unquestioned, fundamental belief systems (see Chapter 17).

In the face of massive stress, persons who have never had cause to question their faith may express doubt in the goodness of a supreme being or higher power or may struggle with the meaning and purpose of life. Other individuals who have never believed in God may suddenly experience a need to pray. The nurse needs to respect the spiritual beliefs of others, accept their personal struggles as healthy and adaptive, and be aware of these complex issues during the process of nursing assessment.

Mind-Body Interaction

Health care professionals have become increasingly aware of the relationship between psychological stress and medical illness, frequently called the **mind-body interaction.** It is often debatable which comes first, stress or illness. The reality, however, is that the relationships between stress and illness are very complex. Stress can have effects that are directly causative of disease, or stress may be a response to illness and medical treatments. Thus their association is often unclear. Multiple studies have shown that there is at least an association between stress and disease (Newberry and others, 1991).

The more intense and the longer the stressful situation, the higher the risk for a negative health outcome (Stanford, 1994). Mild stress situations, such as sitting in a traffic jam, do not usually produce long-lasting physiological damage. Such incidents are usually short-term and isolated and are unlikely to increase the risk of illness unless a person experiences them continually. Moderate stress, as is experienced during a case of the flu, may last from several hours to a number of days. These situations can be significant because they increase the risk of more serious physical illness in a person with a compromised immune system. Severe stress, such as that resulting from continual marital disagreements or long-term physical illness, may last several weeks to several years. Even in instances where stress is not the primary causative factor in the development of disease or illness, it is generally recognized that stress can intensify illness and slow the process of healing.

⋯CRITICAL THINKING IN CLIENT CARE

Synthesis

In approaching the care of the client or family, many factors will influence the nurse. Each person, client as well as nurse, brings to the health care setting a unique background of personal life experience. Although this individual perspective is rarely openly discussed, it affects every health care encounter. Both the nurse and client have preexisting ideas about health and wellness in addition to past experiences with the health care system. Building on this base of past experience are the nurse's professional knowledge and attitudes. To provide the best care, the nurse must take into consideration all of these factors, assessing the client as a whole person.

Knowledge. The nurse who is working with clients and families must consider all factors that relate to the experience of stress and illness. It is important to have a clear understanding of how clients perceive stressors, and what meaning events or illnesses have for them in their personal lives. The nurse must recognize that even a "small" or medically insignificant event, such as the death of an elderly person's pet or a fractured ankle in a 17-year-old on the night before the prom, can be highly stressful or even emotionally devastating under certain circumstances. What is of critical importance is how clients understand and emotionally interpret their experience. Assessment of developmental factors, culture, previously used coping mechanisms, spiritual concerns, and the availability of social supports is also essential. All of these things will form the context in which the nurse can evaluate the physical symptoms and physiological processes associated with stressors, illness, and disease.

The nurse's ability to assist clients experiencing stress will depend on application of good therapeutic communication skills (see Chapter 13). Knowledge of approaches that reduce the client's anxiety and help to build trust between the nurse and client is essential.

Experience. While the experience of stressful events is common to all persons, all persons do not interpret or respond to stressful events in the same way. What is perceived as extremely stressful to one person may be only mildly stressful to another. This is true for illnesses as well as emotional trauma or pressure. The skilled nurse is most concerned with understanding the client's unique perspective. The nurse must view every person as an individual, recognizing that no two people are exactly alike. Experience with clients helps the nurse to recognize responses to stress; however, being open to "seeing things through the client's eyes" will enable the nurse to gain an understanding of viewpoints that are unfamiliar or different. The nurse must recognize, however, that to respect a client's perspective does not mean that the nurse must accept or embrace those same viewpoints or beliefs. Nevertheless, understanding the client's position enables the nurse to intervene more effectively.

Attitudes. Critical attitudes that will affect the nurse's ability to work with clients experiencing stress or manifesting symptoms of stress include confidence,

independence, humility, and curiosity. The nurse must be confident in the belief that stress can be effectively managed. Clients who are overwhelmed and perceive events as being beyond their capacity to cope will rely on the nurse as an expert. Clients will respect the advice and counsel of the nurse and gain confidence from the nurse's belief in their ability to move past the stressful event or illness. Independence is important in seeking out agencies, individuals, or support services that can assist clients and their families in coping effectively with stress or illness. Clients overwhelmed by life events are often unable, at least initially, to act on their own behalf and require either direct intervention or guidance from the nurse. Humility is an essential attitude through which nurses are reminded that they cannot understand the client's perspective entirely. Effort must be made to have clients explain their unique viewpoint and situation. Closely tied to humility is curiosity. The curious nurse will be alert to signs and symptoms of the stress response and will take the time to inquire about the presence of possible symptoms that the client may have neglected or forgotten to report. Curiosity is also tied to keen observation, driving the nurse to take time for comprehensive assessment with every client.

Standards. Clients are prone to all forms of stress. In order for the nurse to make sound clinical decisions, intellectual standards must be applied. To understand the true impact of stress, the nurse's assessment must be relevant. The nurse must be able to clearly and precisely understand a client's perception of the stress and focus on factors significant to the client's well-being. In addition, the nurse will select interventions that are logically adapted to the client's needs so the stress of therapy is minimized.

···NURSING PROCESS

▪ Assessment

The nursing assessment for clients experiencing stress involves collection of subjective and objective information. To gather useful and relevant subjective information the nurse needs to have established a therapeutic nurse-client relationship. The likelihood of a client sharing personal and sensitive information about those aspects of life causing stress is poor unless the client trusts the nurse as a competent professional. In addition, it will be helpful for the nurse to anticipate and apply a critical thinking attitude while observing and analyzing client behaviors that provide important objective assessment data.

Subjective findings. The interview helps the nurse gather information about the health status of the client from the client's perspective and begin the process of developing a trusting relationship with the client. The interview is an opportunity to evaluate such critical variables as mental status, developmental level, current cognitive appraisal of stressors, spiritual and cultural beliefs, and the existence of support systems. The interview is the primary means of identifying critical information related to the health history, including any present symptoms of illness. As in all interactions with the client, the nurse must respect the confidentiality and sensitivity of the information shared. The nurse should choose a private, comfortable environment conducive to sharing sensitive details of stressful events. Box 22-2 lists suggestions for collecting subjective assessment data related to stress and adaptation. A nurse should be cautioned to use sensitivity and judgment when phrasing the questions and to use only those that are pertinent to the specific situation.

Objective findings.
Objective findings related to the assessment of stress and adaptation include direct observation by the nurse of client behavior, direct physical examination, and data available from the medical record and supplemental documents.

Physical examination (see Chapter 24) data include basic vital signs as well as purposive observation for findings (e.g. client behavior, body movements) that would suggest that a stress-induced response has been activated. In addition, the nurse will examine body systems for evidence of stress-related illness. For example, an abdominal assessment can help rule out the presence of gastrointestinal disturbances.

Certain components of the mental status examina-tion can be integrated into the physical examination, whereas other elements must be administered separately. While conducting the interview and health history, the nurse can observe client appearance, affect, and general presentation, deciding whether these behaviors are appropriate or inappropriate to the existing situation. Discussions with the client and family can clarify whether the observed behaviors, such as the presence of certain defense mechanisms, are typical for the client or represent a change from baseline. Box 22-3 describes in detail the critical observations that are included in an evaluation of mental status. A more formal review of the client's mental status may be made by using the mini-mental status examination (see Chapter 24).

Client expectations.
An essential part of any assessment includes consideration of client expectations. In planning care for a client experiencing stress, it is important to understand the meaning the event has for the client and the ways in which stress is affecting the client's life. As part of the assessment, the nurse should set aside time to allow the client to express priorities for coping with stress. For example, in the case of a woman who has just been told that a breast mass was identified on a routine mammogram, it would be important for the nurse to know what the client wants and needs most from nursing. Although some persons in this situation might identify their need for information about biopsy or mastectomy as their personal priority, other women might need guidance and support in discussing how to

---

Box 22-2
Sample Interview Questions for Gathering Subjective Data

1. In your own words, what has been the most stressful thing for you during this hospitalization?
2. When you have experienced stress in the past, how did you solve the stress?
   a. Sought out reasons for those feelings
   b. Blamed others
   c. Withdrew from family, friends, or co-workers
   d. Talked with others (spouse, clergy, friends, support groups)
   e. Used distraction
      (1) Examples of positive distractors (music, exercise, relaxation techniques)
      (2) Examples of negative distractors (alcohol and drug usage, smoking, changes in eating habits)
3. Describe any stress-related problems for which you have been treated in the past.
4. Describe any recent major life changes (within the last year) related to any of the following:
   a. Health (physical and mental)
   b. Family
   c. Lifestyle habits
   d. Changes in daily activities (eating, sleeping, getting up to go to work)
   e. Supportive network
   f. Work (Do you enjoy your work?)
   g. Financial/legal problems
   h. Recent losses or trauma
5. Can you rate how stressful these major life changes have been on a scale of 1 to 10 (from least stressful to most stressful)?
6. How many people are you responsible for (older adult parents, children, other dependents)?
7. Tell me how you spend your leisure time. Are these activities done alone or with a group of friends?
8. How often do you take vacations or mental health days off?

Box 22-3
Select Components of Assessment of Mental Status

Mental Status Examination
Appearance

Dress, grooming, hygiene, cosmetics, apparent age, posture, facial expression

Behavior/Activity

Hypoactivity or hyperactivity, rigid, relaxed, restless or agitated motor movements, gait and coordination, facial grimacing, gestures, mannerisms, passive, combative, bizarre

Attitude

Interactions with the interviewer: cooperative, resistive, friendly, hostile, ingratiating

Mood and Affect

Mood (intensity, depth, duration): sad, fearful, depressed, angry, anxious, ambivalent, happy, ecstatic, grandiose
Affect (intensity, depth, duration): appropriate, apathetic, constricted, blunted, flat, labile, euphoric, bizarre

Perceptions

Hallucinations, illusions, depersonalization

Thoughts

Form and content: logical vs. illogical, loose associations, flight of ideas, autistic, blocking, broadcasting, delusions, abstract vs. concrete

Sensorium/Cognition

Levels of consciousness, orientation, attention span, recent and remote memory, concentration; ability to comprehend and process information; intelligence

Judgment

Ability to assess and evaluate situations, make rational decisions, understand consequences of behavior, and take responsibility for actions

Insight

Ability to perceive and understand the cause and nature of own and others' situations

Reliability

Interviewer's impression that individual reported information accurately and completely

Psychosocial Criteria
Stressors

Internal: psychiatric or medical illness, perceived loss, such as loss of self-concept/self-esteem
External: actual loss, e.g., death of a loved one, divorce, lack of support systems, job or financial loss, retirement, dysfunctional family system

Coping Skills

Use of functional adaptive coping mechanisms and techniques, management of activities of daily living

Relationships

Attainment and maintenance of satisfying, interpersonal relationships congruent with developmental stage

---

share the news with family members. Gaining an understanding of client expectations does not mean that the nurse will exclude certain types of care that are important simply because a client does not identify them as needs. However, by inquiring about client expectations and priorities, the nurse is better able to ensure that *all* client needs will be met.

....

Successful critical thinking requires a synthesis of knowledge, experience, information gathered from clients, and critical thinking attitudes and standards. Clinical judgments require the nurse to anticipate what information is needed, to analyze the data, and then to make decisions regarding client

care. The client expects competent and informed care. Becky Howard incorporates previous knowledge and experience in providing care for Rhonda.

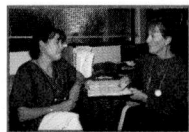

Case Study
Synthesis in Practice

Becky talked briefly over the phone with Rhonda to set up her appointment. She learns that Rhonda is concerned about losing her job since she is now the sole breadwinner for her family. She also learns about

Continued

Mr. Bennett's recent illness and the effect it is having on Rhonda's overall well-being. Becky has also talked with Rhonda's manager and knows that Rhonda has been having headaches and difficulty concentrating when making decisions. Becky sets aside some time to plan for her meeting with Rhonda.

Becky takes time to reflect on other employees she has recently seen in the Employee Health Office. Many of the registered nurses have had physical complaints of stress including headaches, sleep disorders, changes in eating habits, and exacerbations of existing medical problems. Becky knows she wants to be thorough in assessing the types of problems Rhonda has been experiencing. Previous experience with other employees also has taught Becky the importance of learning about the employee's family and the type of support it offers.

After talking with Rhonda on the phone, Becky detects a great deal of anxiety but also some anger. Becky knows it is important to build trust with Rhonda as quickly as possible. As a single parent, Becky can identify with Rhonda's crisis of being the sole financial support for the family. Yet Becky decides not to tell her life history to Rhonda because it is important to recognize that no two persons have exactly the same experience. Becky wants to demonstrate an attitude of humility as she reminds herself that Rhonda's perspective of life will be unique. Becky plans to allow Rhonda time to fully describe her feelings and to listen carefully to the message being conveyed. Becky wants to be able to work closely with Rhonda and establish priorities that are realistic for her to achieve.

Finally, Becky can identify with Rhonda's job concerns. As a staff member of the employee assistance program, Becky's role is to be the employee's advocate while at the same time trying to help the employee return as a productive member of the workforce. Keeping Rhonda's concerns confidential will be important. It will be Rhonda's choice as to whether she will choose to discuss her visits with her manager.

▪ Nursing Diagnosis

Nursing diagnoses must be supported by actual assessment data (see nursing diagnoses box). When existing data regarding stress are not apparent, relevant risk factors and client circumstances along with anticipated changes or needs should prompt the nurse to consider potential nursing diagnoses. It is possible that there may be many nursing diagnoses related to stress and the adaptation response. This is because stress may reveal itself through illness or physical/somatic complaints as well as through behavioral responses. Therefore there

---

▪ NURSING DIAGNOSES FOR CLIENTS WITH STRESS

Activity intolerance
Anxiety
Coping, ineffective family: compromised or disabling
Coping, ineffective individual
Fatigue
Fear
Growth and development, altered
Hopelessness
Injury, risk for
Powerlessness
Self-esteem disturbance
Sleep pattern disturbance
Spiritual distress

---

may be diagnoses that address more physiological states (e.g., *altered nutrition: less than/more than body requirements*) and those that address the psychological response to stress (e.g., *ineffective individual coping*).

The nurse must also be aware that many nursing diagnoses share similar defining characteristics. Therefore the nurse must carefully complete a comprehensive, accurate assessment of the client. For example, disturbances in sleep patterns may signal the presence of a *sleep pattern disturbance* diagnosis or may represent but one of a greater set of symptoms that would be defining for a diagnosis of *rape-trauma syndrome*. If the nurse made an incorrect *sleep pattern disturbance* diagnosis based on insufficient data, then the planned interventions would most likely be insufficient to provide competent, effective care to the survivor of a rape.

For any given nursing diagnosis, there can be several associated factors. For example, based on assessment data, an adult male athlete hospitalized with multiple pelvic and limb fractures following an auto accident may be given a nursing diagnosis of *powerlessness*. In this instance, powerlessness may be related to both loss of ability to care for his own bodily needs, such as toileting, as well as fear that he will not be able to again participate in athletics. Recognizing the appropriate "related to" factor will indicate what type of nursing interventions are likely to be most effective.

Equally important as making the correct nursing diagnosis is the process of prioritization. To continue the example of the athlete with multiple fractures, in the early stages of his hospitalization, when his condition was most critical, the diagnosis of *powerlessness* might well have been of much less immediate importance than a diagnosis of *risk for fluid volume deficit related to bleeding*. Although both diagnoses would have been valid and both appropriate to the experience of stress and adaptation, the priority for nursing intervention during the early hours of hospitalization would almost certainly be restoration of physiological homeostasis.

Planning

Once nursing diagnoses are made and prioritized, the nurse develops a plan of care individualized for the client (see care plan). The plan should focus not only on ways to directly minimize stress but also on how to assist the client in using coping resources that are most realistic and appropriate to the client's needs. Ideally, the client and nurse work together in partnership to develop realistic goals, some of which may take time to achieve. Although some goals are easily anticipated, others are not so universal.

The nurse should also make a determination as to the involvement of other professionals in the plan of care. When clients have nursing diagnoses related to stress, there are times when the scope of nursing practice is insufficient to meet all of the client's needs. Collaboration and consultation may be needed with physical and occupational therapists, dietitians, or pastoral care professionals. Clients experiencing stress from medical conditions or psychiatric disorders will often require consultation of psychiatrists, psychologists, psychiatric social workers, or nurses who have advanced degrees in mental health nursing. Such a multi-disciplinary approach to care is often most effective in addressing the holistic needs of the client. The nurse's role is to recognize the need for collaboration and consultation, inform the client about potential resources, and make arrangements for interventions (e.g., consultations, group sessions) as needed.

If both client and nurse are involved in making goals together, there is a greater likelihood that the goals will be achieved. The client should also assist in setting time frames when possible. If the client's stress is at a level that affects decision-making ability, the nurse may set the initial goal and time line and then revise accordingly as the client's level of participation increases. An example of a goal for a client experiencing stress is "Client will assume self-care practices within 1 week."

Expected outcomes establish measurable behaviors that serve to indicate the client's progress toward the goals of care. Examples of outcomes for this goal is "Client will identify changes in behavior and poor hygiene practices as reflective of stress within 2 days" and "Client will initiate hair and nail grooming in 5 days."

Implementation

Stress is an inevitable life experience and must be anticipated in planning care for clients of all ages. Intervention strategies must be selected based on the client's

---

CASE STUDY NURSING CARE PLAN

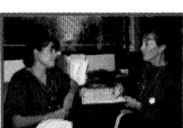

Stress and Individual Coping

Assessment

When Becky Howard first meets Rhonda, she is immediately struck by Rhonda's appearance. She observes Rhonda showing signs of being nervous, **frequently licking her lips, picking at her fingernails, and being easily startled.** Rhonda's **vital signs show changes in response to stress:** pulse 120, respirations 24, blood pressure 168/84. Rhonda appears thin and pale and reports that she has **lost 15 pounds in the last 3 months.** Her appetite has been poor, and she has stopped cooking meals, instead picking up fast food for her family at night. She also reports **difficulty in falling and remaining asleep at night.** In discussing her situation, including both fear of losing her job and being unable to support her family, Rhonda **uses poor eye contact** and then **bursts into tears and expresses feelings of being overwhelmed.** Rhonda admits to having started **drinking at night to help herself "unwind."** During the discussion, Rhonda also talks about **feelings of shame and embarrassment.** She has always been the one to care for other people, and she is ashamed that she cannot "get a grip" on her own life. She cannot easily accept herself in a "client" role and **thinks of herself as a failure for not coping better.** Rhonda has high expectations of herself as a wife, mother, and nurse.

Nursing Diagnosis

Ineffective individual coping related to threatened job loss and multiple family stresses and responsibilities.

Defining characteristics are shown in bold type.

Continued

CASE STUDY NURSING CARE PLAN—cont'd

Planning

Goal

Client will reestablish normal pattern of sleeping and eating within 2 weeks.

Client will demonstrate coping strategies in relation to threat of job loss and family security within 1 month.

Client will establish career plan within 6 weeks.

Expected Outcomes

Client will return to normal sleep pattern, requiring less than 1 hour to fall asleep and staying asleep all night.

Client will have three meals a day, joining family during evening meals within 1 week.

Client will participate in a support group offered by the counselor at the employee assistance program in 1 week.

Client will begin to verbally express feelings of loss and powerlessness in an environment that is both supportive and "safe" in 2 weeks.

Client will set time frame to pursue employment opportunities in 2 weeks.

Implementation

Steps

1. Set mutually agreed on appointment at employee assistance program clinic with client two times a week. Provide a private place where client can discuss feelings and express normal range of emotion.

2. Provide information on cost-free counseling and support groups. Encourage participation with possibility of including husband.

3. Instruct client on avoiding alcohol and caffeine in the evening. Recommend return to usual sleep preparation habits used before sleep disturbance.

4. Refer for medical consultation for possible use of antidepressants, and assess for suicide potential.

5. Teach relaxation techniques for stress reduction, general calming, and sleep enhancement.

6. Have client plan a meal schedule with husband; include ordering out and preparation of meals at home. Have client plan smaller "mini-meals" during times when her work schedule is most stressful. Stress the importance of selecting foods the family enjoys.

7. Have client begin to prepare a resume and gather ads listing job placements.

Rationale

Being able to express intimate fears and concerns to someone who is nonjudgmental and supportive assists individuals in gaining understanding of their own problems.

Support groups provide common bond with other clients because stressors are similar and potential solutions are more realistic. Support groups provide a social outlet for a realistic cure for loneliness and social isolation (Newberry and others, 1991).

Caffeine, alcohol, and disruption of sleep habits have insomnia-producing effects.

Client symptoms may indicate depression, requiring more intense medical therapy.

Performing relaxation exercises has a recuperative effect that normalizes physical, mental, and emotional processes (Davis and others, 1988).

Setting regular meal schedule with husband as a support will lessen stress of responsibility on client. Persons are better able to deal with stress if they slow eating to savor food, eat smaller "mini-meals" more frequently, and avoid heavy meals (Williams, 1993).

Establishing a career plan helps client look to future and reinforces own self-worth.

Evaluation

Ask client to report over the course of a week ability to fall asleep and hours slept per night.

Weigh client regularly and ask for a report on food intake over a week's time.

Observe personal hygiene, attitude toward therapy, and expressions of despair.

Continue to assess for suicide potential or other signs of worsening depression.

Discuss with client her perceptions of counseling and support group in terms of meeting her needs for support and assistance with problem solving.

Have client present revised resume for review and job interview selections.

unique characteristics as these pertain to level of health, motivation, sources of support, and prior coping experiences.

Health promotion.

In an ideal world, all persons would anticipate the effects of stress in daily life and engage in regular, health-promoting activities to counter the effects of stress. Health-enhancing habits can reduce the impact of stress on physical and mental health. These commonsense approaches often provide a sound basis for effective, low-stress living. They include regular exercise, good nutrition and diet, adequate rest, interactions with persons who constitute a support system, and effective time management. Nurses are in a position to educate clients and families about the importance of health promotion and to engage in primary prevention (Box 22-4).

Regular exercise. A regular exercise program improves muscle tone and posture, controls weight, reduces tension, and promotes relaxation. In addition, exercise reduces the risk of cardiovascular disease and improves cardiopulmonary functioning (Figure 22-3).

Clients who have a history of a chronic illness, who are at risk for developing an illness, or who are older than 35 years of age should begin a physical exercise program only after discussing the plan with a physician. In general, for a fitness program to have positive physical effects, a person should exercise at least 3 times a week for 30 to 40 minutes.

Nutrition and diet. Nutrition and exercise are closely related. Diet provides the body with fuel for activity, whereas exercise improves circulation and the delivery of nutrients to body tissues. Everyone is encouraged to maintain a normal weight, according to standard ranges for sex, age, and body build. In addition to avoiding overeating or undereating, the nutritional quality of food is also important. Too much caffeine, salt, fat, or sugar or deficiencies in vitamins, minerals, and nutrients can upset the body's metabolic functioning and intensify the negative effects of stress. Chapter 34 reviews dietary goals for health promotion.

Rest. An established, habitual pattern of sufficient rest and sleep is also important to stress management. Persons who are well rested are better able to cope, focus attention, and apply problem-solving strategies to better manage stress. Chapter 32 reviews therapies designed to promote rest and sleep.

Support systems. A support system of family, friends, and colleagues who will listen, offer advice, and provide emotional support benefits a client experiencing stress. There are many support groups available to individuals such as those sponsored by the American Heart Association, the American Cancer Society, local hospitals and churches, and mental health organizations.

Time management. A person who uses time efficiently generally experiences less stress related to social, family, and job activities. Time management techniques include developing lists of tasks to be performed in order of priority, for example, those tasks that require immediate attention, those that are important and can be delayed, and those tasks that are routine and can be accomplished when time becomes available. In many cases, setting priorities helps individuals identify tasks that are not necessary or perhaps can even be delegated to someone else. Time management also involves learning to say "no" to potential disruptions and some requested tasks. Persons must learn to recognize that they cannot perform every request made by others and taking care of oneself involves establishing a realistic daily schedule.

Acute care

Crisis intervention. By definition, a crisis is a state of intense emotional upset or disequilibrium that is a turning point in the life of a person or family. Usually precipitated by an unexpected event, a crisis is self-limiting, resolved within a period of approximately 6 weeks. Because a crisis is an event of such magnitude as to be called a turning point, without intervention this resolution may leave the person or family functioning

---

BOX 22-4
Client Teaching for Stress

- Mild stress can be useful and productive.
- Mild anxiety can enhance motivation on a daily basis.
- Teach client to recognize signs of stress (e.g., change in sleep and appetite, reliance on alcohol to create a sense of calm, mood swings and behavior changes).
- Have client participate in stress reduction strategies appropriate to individual (e.g., reading, walking, planning time with friends, playing with a pet).

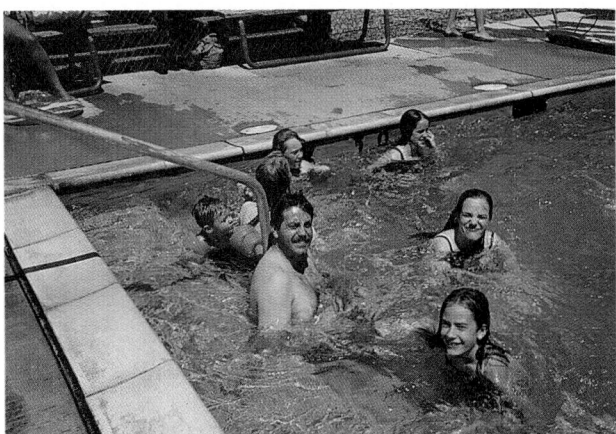

Figure 22-3. A regular exercise program reduces tension and promotes relaxation. (Courtesy of Michael S. Clement, MD, Mesa, Arizona).

less effectively than they were before the crisis. Crisis states result in extreme stress, disrupted communication patterns, reduced effectiveness of support systems, and ineffective coping.

Although stressful experiences occur frequently during the life span, a crisis results when the usual and customary methods of coping are inadequate to reduce stress and maintain equilibrium or homeostasis. In a crisis the usual attempts at adaptation fail, and biological, psychological, and behavioral disorganization results. The stress-crisis sequence follows the following paradigm, known as the ABCX formula (Hill, 1965):

A	$\leftrightarrow$	B	
Stressor event	(interacts with)	Crisis-meeting resources	$\leftrightarrow$

C	$\rightarrow$	X
Meaning/ interpretation of the event	(producing)	CRISIS

Because an individual's or family's usual coping strategies are ineffective in managing the stress of the precipitating event, the use of new coping mechanisms is required. This experience, which forces the use of unfamiliar strategies, can result either in a heightened awareness of previously unrecognized strengths and resources or in deterioration in functioning. Thus a crisis is often referred to as a situation of both danger and opportunity. Some persons or families will emerge from a crisis state functioning more effectively, whereas others may find themselves weakened, and still others completely dysfunctional.

Persons experiencing crisis may describe their feelings and emotions in one or more of the following ways that constitute a classic profile of disequilibrium (Parad and Parad, 1990):

- Bewilderment—"I never felt this way before."
- Danger—"I feel so scared. Something terrible is going to happen."
- Confusion—"I can't think straight; my mind isn't working right."
- Impasse—"I'm stuck. Nothing I do seems to work."
- Desperation—"I've got to do something!"
- Apathy—"I really don't care. I can't win."
- Helplessness—"I can't do this on my own. I need help."
- Urgency—"I need help now."
- Discomfort—"I feel miserable, restless, unsettled."

Crises typically fall into one of two broad categories: maturational and situational (Parad and Parad, 1990; Aguilera, 1998). **Maturational crises,** sometimes referred to as **developmental crises,** are those associated with normal and expected phases of growth and development. Although these life changes are expected, they nonetheless require individuals to make significant changes in the way they relate to others and society. These new demands are often uncomfortable and cause significant distress. For example, a young adult who must accept the challenge of obtaining a job, working steadily, and assuming responsibility for debts, rent, car payments, and relationships with a mate may experience a significant crisis when the implications of these responsibilities become real. Similarly, older adults who approach retirement may experience a crisis in needing to organize time differently and in facing the reality that they have entered the last major phase of their adult life.

Situational crises occur in response to an event as "minor" as a job change or as catastrophic as a natural disaster such as a flood or fire. The meaning that an individual attributes to an event determines, in large part, whether a crisis will result. For example, a person who loses a job that pays a low wage and is very unpleasant may be very relieved to be out of an unhappy situation. In contrast, if that same person were to lose a job that provided great satisfaction and an excellent salary, job loss could be perceived as devastating. Further complicating the experience of stressful events is the reality that such experiences do not take place in isolation. Thus it is not simply the loss of a job, for example, that might be at risk but also the potential loss of status, place of residence, or relationships with friends. One stressful event sets in motion a series of responses that may be sufficient in themselves to cause a crisis, depending on whether they are perceived as either positive or negative. Therefore in a crisis situation, although there is usually only one precipitating event, a person may be experiencing many simultaneous changes at once. Attempting to address the full complexity of issues involved in a crisis can feel overwhelming and very frightening. Nurses are often the professionals to whom clients and family members turn in times of crisis.

Crisis intervention is a therapeutic approach that addresses the immediate urgent need for stress reduction. The goal is to restore the client as quickly as possible to the precrisis level of functioning or to a level of functioning that is improved over the precrisis level. Crisis intervention differs from traditional psychotherapy in that it focuses only on the present situation or problem and is very limited in time (from one to six sessions). Furthermore, although psychotherapists involved in longer therapeutic relationships with clients are often nondirective, the nurse or therapist involved in the process of crisis intervention typically takes a very active role.

Steps in crisis intervention. After determining that a crisis exists, the nurse plans and implements measures to help resolve it. Resolution depends on the client's realistic perception of the stressful event, having adequate support, and using appropriate coping mechanisms.

Typically there are four phases or steps in crisis intervention:

Step 1: Assessment of the client and the problem
The nurse obtains an accurate description of the precipitating event, gains an understanding of the meaning of the event in the life of the client, and reviews all of the strategies that the client has attempted to use in an effort to respond to the crisis. The precipitating event most often occurs within a 2-week period before an individual seeks help but may have occurred as recently as hours before the nurse is contacted. This level of assessment typically takes place at the first meeting.

Step 2: Planning the intervention
After the nurse has explored with the client all of the coping mechanisms the client has employed successfully in the past and identified possible support persons or resources that can be used to help resolve the current situation the nurse plans the intervention. The nurse also seeks to help the client identify personal strengths and explore new ways of coping.

Step 3: Implementing the intervention
This phase may involve helping the client gain an understanding of the crisis, providing an opportunity for the client to express feelings and emotions in a safe environment, encouraging the client to use methods of coping that have been successful in the past but have not been used in this situation, and encouraging the person in crisis to make contact with available social supports. Implementing the crisis intervention may require more than one meeting with the client. If an initial suggestion is less than fully successful, alternative strategies may be attempted.

Step 4: Reflecting on the resolution of the crisis and engaging in anticipatory planning
These are key steps to ensuring that in subsequent stressful situations the client will be able to cope effectively. In this phase the nurse helps the client remember and focus on the actions that were most effective in resolving the crisis and discusses with the client ways in which similar strategies can be mobilized in the future. This final step of retrospective review is important in helping clients gain perspective on their progress and to help them appreciate the new skills and strategies that they have successfully employed.

The steps in crisis intervention are easily incorporated within the context of nursing care and fall within the scope of nursing. In the event that the nurse determines that a client is so distressed by the crisis situation that the client has become suicidal or homicidal, it is appropriate to seek immediate consultation and referral of the client to a psychiatrist who can manage this complex level of care.

Stress management in the workplace. Rapid changes in society, health care technology, health care knowledge, and the nursing profession can place stress on nurses. Job stress is individually perceived but is dependent on individual personality and hardiness, health status, previous experience with stress, and coping mechanisms. Burnout, a state of cumulative stress manifested through negative feelings, high absenteeism, and reduced productivity, occurs as a result of chronic stress. Nurses also frequently encounter traumatic and unexpected critical incidents that can be overwhelming and can exhaust the usual coping strategies (Clark and Friedman, 1992).

Many employers offer critical incident stress debriefings to help nurses respond to unusually upsetting events such as the death of a child or a major disaster. These debriefings are most often structured group meetings that emphasize ventilating emotions and other reactions to a critical event (Mitchell and Bray, 1990).

Increasingly common are employee assistance programs through which nurses can access free, short-term counseling services with contracted counselors or therapists. Nurses can reduce both personal and work-related stresses by using the stress management techniques they teach to clients.

Additionally, nurses can use the following problem-solving approach to reduce stress and resolve conflict in their personal and professional life:

1. Define the stress-related problem.
2. Generate a list of alternative solutions that can be used to resolve the problem.
3. Analyze the positive and negative consequences associated with implementing each alternative solution.
4. Select the best alternative solution that has the probability of a successful outcome (resolving the problem).
5. Implement the alternative solution.
6. Evaluate the effectiveness of the solution.
7. If the alternative solution does not achieve a successful outcome, select another alternative and begin the process over again.

Restorative care. When clients are handling stress ineffectively, the nurse is often the first to identify or address this behavior. The nurse can help clients make lifestyle changes that will support health restoration such as a more healthful approach to diet, exercise, and stress management. Other more sophisticated techniques for stress reduction (e.g., biofeedback or hypnosis) require experiential training and should be implemented by experienced nurses or other providers. Many of these activities are well within the scope of practice of the nurse.

Guided imagery and visualization. Guided imagery is based on the belief that a person can significantly reduce stress with imagination. Guided imagery is a relaxed state in which a person actively uses imagination in a way that allows visualization of a soothing, peaceful setting. Typically the image created or suggested uses many sensory words to engage the mind and offer distraction and relaxation (see Chapter 33).

Progressive muscle relaxation. In the presence of anxiety-provoking thoughts and events, a common physiological symptom is muscle tension. Physiological tension will be diminished through a systematic approach to releasing tension in major muscle groups. Typically a relaxed state is achieved through deep chest breathing, and then the client is directed to alternately tighten and relax muscles in specific groupings (see Chapter 33).

Music or art therapy. For some individuals music can be beneficial in relaxation. It can be used as an intervention to lessen the stress response and therefore decrease the anxiety level. Music can be a distraction from the stressor or it may act directly on the limbic system through increased production of endorphins. Music should be carefully selected because it can trigger many different emotions and memories. It is imperative for the nurse to work in partnership with the client to select the best music to achieve the goals of intervention, which always include keeping the client safe and comfortable. Art is also very therapeutic, as it provides a nonverbal means of expressing emotions and feelings. Even persons who are not "artistic" can benefit from painting, drawing, or working with clay.

Humor. The ability to laugh at oneself when faced with situations that are unpleasant and out of one's control reduces stress. Examples of using humor include sharing embarrassing situations, telling jokes, playing noncompetitive games, or using amusing video- and audiotapes. The energizing effects of humor can also be stabilizing for the nurse (Busman, 1991).

Assertiveness training. Unresolved conflicts cause stress. The ability to resolve conflict with others through assertiveness training is important for reducing stress. When used effectively, these skills can empower clients to feel more in control of their life and experience. Assertiveness training is not synonymous with aggression. Rather it is a skill for helping individuals communicate effectively regarding their needs and desires.

Journal writing. For many people, keeping a private, personal journal provides a therapeutic outlet for stress, and it is well within the realm of nursing to suggest journal keeping to clients experiencing difficult situations. In a private journal, clients can express a full range of emotion and vent their honest feelings without hurting anyone's feelings and without concern for how they might appear to others.

◼ Evaluation

Client care. Evaluation of the goals and expected outcomes of care will let the nurse know if nursing interventions were effective and if the client is progressing in regard to coping with stress. The nurse will review the behaviorally stated, measurable goals and will assess whether the client has met the criteria for success as stated in the outcomes. If the nursing interventions have not been effective in helping the client achieve targeted goals, the nurse must reevaluate the strategies implemented and revise the plan of care in light of the client's current health status.

Evaluation of the client experiencing stress will involve observation of client behaviors, focused and deliberate discussions with clients, and reports from family members. It is important to remember that coping with stress can take time. If the nurse is in a setting where contact with a client must end before resolution of goals has been achieved, it is important to refer clients to appropriate resources so that progress is not delayed or interrupted.

Client expectations. Nurses must maintain ongoing communication with their clients regarding the plan of care. Clients under stress often experience feelings of powerlessness, vulnerability, and loss of control. The nurse can help to reduce these feelings by actively involving clients and families in the process of problem identification (assessment), prioritizing, and goal setting and evaluation. Involving clients in these processes gives them an opportunity to direct their energy in a positive way and moves them toward taking greater responsibility for health maintenance and promotion.

Engaging the client as a partner in health care sets the stage for open communication. In such an environment the client can feel more freedom to give important feedback to the nurse about interventions that are successful and can help the nurse better understand why some interventions fail to meet the established goals.

An essential part of the evaluation process is collaborating with clients to determine if their own expectations from nursing have been met. Any revision in the plan of care must then include steps to address client expectations.

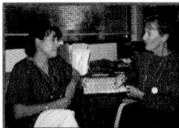

Case Study

Three weeks after their initial discussion, Rhonda makes her routine appointment at the Employee Health Office to see Becky. Becky is relieved to see that Rhonda is less anxious and looking better. Her blood pressure is 140/82 and pulse is 88. Her weight reflects a gain of 3 pounds since her last visit. The nervous behaviors previously assessed are no longer present. Rhonda is taking an antidepressant that her physician has prescribed and is reportedly sleeping through the night. She admits to Becky that she tried the relaxation exercises but initially had trouble concentrating. She feels further instruction might be useful. Feeling less drained, Rhonda has begun to make progress on her career planning. She has enlisted her husband to help scan the papers for open nursing positions in the area and to assist her in mailing out resumes and keeping her calendar clear for potential interviews. She has withdrawn temporarily from her Girl Scout and "soccer mom" duties to reduce the demands on her time. As a result, her dilemma has become known among other mothers, and many have offered to help drive her husband to his therapy ses-

sions or to provide casseroles for the family to eat. Rhonda has now accepted this help by reminding herself that it will only be needed on a temporary basis. Furthermore, Rhonda and her husband are going together to a family support group meeting held every week at his rehabilitation facility. She is finding the encouragement of that group to be of benefit to her and an important addition to her individual counseling sessions with her employee assistance program counselor. Although the Bennett family has not yet found full resolution for their stress, they are making progress toward achievable, short-term goals.

Documentation Note

Client reports feelings of increased hopefulness and return to normal sleep and eating patterns. She is taking Zoloft, 100 mg daily, as prescribed by her personal physician, Dr. Smith, and is returning to see him for follow-up in 1 week. Is attending weekly counseling with Dr. Moody and also a rehab support group with husband. Blood pressure today is 140/82, P 88. Weight gain of 3 pounds in last 3 weeks. Has requested more instruction with relaxation techniques. Recommended use of music to help relaxation process. Continue to follow present plan and return for follow-up in 2 weeks.

Key Terms

adaptation
alarm reaction
cognitive appraisal
coping mechanisms
crisis intervention
defense mechanisms

denial
developmental crises
exhaustion stage
fight-or-flight response
general adaptation
 syndrome
inflammatory response

local adaptation
 syndrome
maturational crises
mind-body interaction
reflex pain response
regressive behavior

resistance stage
situational crises
stress
stressor
suppression
task-oriented behaviors

▪ Key Concepts ▪

Stress is a physiological or psychological tension that can affect a person.

Stressors are events, situations, or other stimuli an individual may encounter in the internal or external environment.

Stressors necessitate change or adaptation so a state of equilibrium can be maintained.

Adaptation is the process through which a person changes in response to stress.

Physiological adaptation is the body's attempt to maintain optimal functioning.

The physiological responses to stress are the local and the general adaptation syndromes.

Psychological responses to stress include task-oriented behaviors and ego-defense mechanisms.

Stress has an impact on the onset, course, and outcome of illness.

Prolonged stress decreases the ability to adapt to the stress.

Stress management techniques include health-enhancing habits, crisis intervention, and methods of reducing job stress.

▪ Critical Thinking Activities ▪

1. You are caring for a 30-year-old single mother who has recently received a diagnosis of metastatic breast cancer. She is the sole provider for three young children (all under 7 years of age). Discuss the various stressors that will need to be considered when writing an appropriate discharge plan.

2. A client comes to the emergency room with complaints of dizziness, which are not related to any physical finding on examination. During the health history the client reports that her life is very stressful and she is barely coping. She finalized her divorce 3 months ago, is working 32 hours per week, and is attending college. Her ex-husband recently lost his job and can no longer pay child support. Finally, she tearfully confesses that she thinks she might be pregnant but does not want her ex-husband to know. Develop nursing diagnoses related to this situation.

3. An older adult woman is admitted to the hospital with a fractured hip. Prior to her injury she lived with her husband, who suffers from advancing Alzheimer's disease. While she is hospitalized, he is staying with a niece who lives 100 miles away, but this cannot be a permanent situation because her niece is also in frail health. The client has no children who can help her when she returns home. She is concerned not only about who will care for her after she is discharged but also about her husband. What approach would be the best to take in establishing goals for treatment?

References

Aguilera DC: *Crisis intervention: theory and methodology,* ed 8, St. Louis, 1998, Mosby.

Busman K: Humor in therapy for the mentally ill, *J Psychosoc Nurs Ment Health Serv* 29:15, 1991.

Clark M, Friedman D: Pulling together: building a community debriefing team, *J Psychosoc Nurs Ment Health Serv* 30(7):27, 1992.

Davis M and others: *The relaxation and stress reduction workbook,* Oakland, Calif, 1988, New Harbinger Publications.

Erikson EH: *Childhood and society,* New York, Norton, 1963.

Grainger R: The patient with anxiety. In Lewis S and others, editors: *Manual of psychosocial nursing interventions: promoting mental health in medical-surgical settings,* Philadelphia, 1989, WB Saunders.

Hill R: Generic features of families under stress. In Parad HJ, editor: *Crisis intervention: selected readings,* New York, 1965, Family Service Association of America.

Holmes TH, Rahe RH: The social readjustment rating scale, *J Psychosom Res* 11:213, 1967.

Keltner NL and others: *Psychiatric nursing,* ed 2, St. Louis, 1995, Mosby.

Lazarus RS, Folkman S: *Stress, appraisal and coping,* New York, 1984, Springer.

Mitchell J, Bray G: *Emergency services stress: guidelines for preserving the health and careers of emergency services personnel,* Englewood Cliffs, NJ, 1990, Prentice-Hall.

Neuman, B: A model for teaching total person approach to patient problems, *Nurs Res* 21(3):264, 1972.

Newberry B and others: *A holistic conceptualization of stress and disease,* New York, 1991, AMS Press.

Orem DE: *Nursing concepts of practice,* New York, 1985, McGraw-Hill.

Parad HJ, Parad LG: *Crisis intervention: book 2,* Milwaukee, 1990, Family Service America.

Piaget J: *The origins of intelligence in children,* New York, 1952, International Universities Press.

Potter PA, Perry AG: *Fundamentals of nursing: Concepts, process, and practice,* ed 4, St. Louis, 1997, Mosby.

Roy C: The Roy adaptation model. In Riehl, JP, Roy C, editors: *Conceptual models for nursing practice,* New York, 1980, Appleton-Century-Crofts.

Stanford GC: The stress response to trauma and critical illness, *Crit Care Nurs Clin North Am* 6(4):693, 1994.

Williams SR: *Nutrition and diet therapy,* ed 7, St. Louis, 1993, Mosby.

Scientific Basis for Nursing Practice

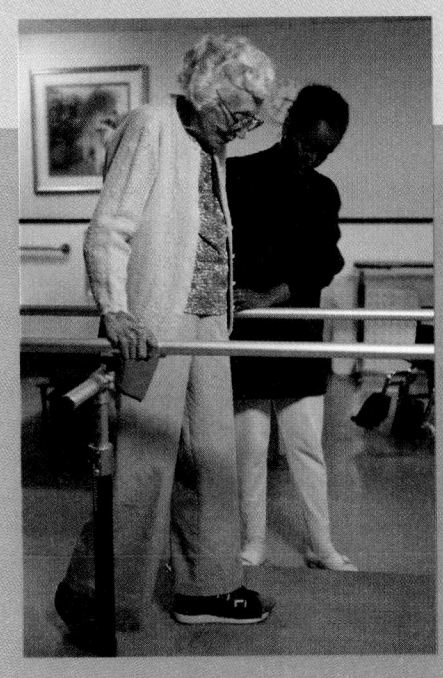

UNIT

5

Vital Signs

OBJECTIVES

Mastery of content in this chapter will enable the student to:

- Define the key terms listed.
- Explain the principles and mechanisms of thermoregulation.
- Describe nursing measures that promote heat loss and heat conservation.
- Discuss physiological changes associated with fever.
- Accurately assess body temperature.
- Accurately assess pulse, respirations, oxygen saturation, blood pressure, and central venous pressure.
- Describe factors that cause variations in body temperature, pulse, oxygen saturation, respirations, blood pressure, and central venous pressure.
- Identify ranges of acceptable vital sign values for an adult, child, and infant.
- Explain variations in technique used to assess an infant's, child's, and adult's vital signs.
- Appropriately delegate vital sign measurement to unlicensed assistive personnel.

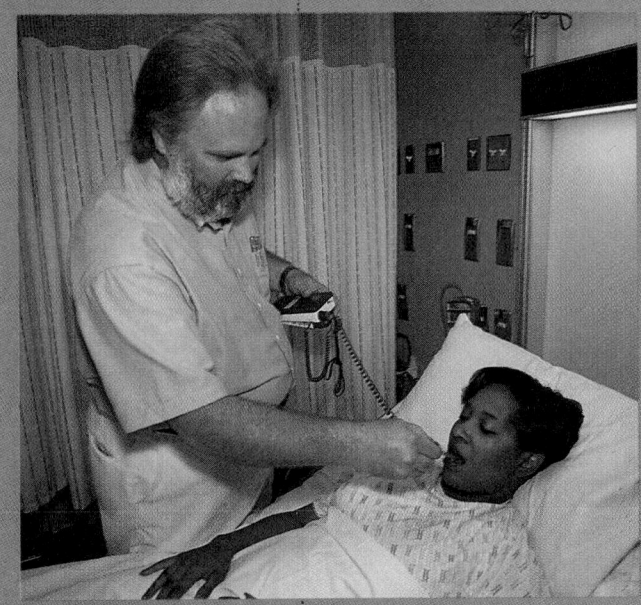

The cardinal **vital signs** are temperature, pulse, respiration, blood pressure, and oxygen saturation. Many factors such as the temperature of the environment, physical exertion, and the effects of illness cause vital signs to change, sometimes outside the acceptable range. Measurement of vital signs provides data to determine a client's usual state of health (baseline data) and response to physical and psychological stress and medical and nursing therapy. A change in vital signs can indicate a change in physiological functioning. An alteration in vital signs may signal the need for medical or nursing intervention.

Vital signs are a quick and efficient way of monitoring a client's condition or identifying problems and evaluating the client's response to intervention. The basic skills required to measure vital signs are simple but should not be taken for granted. Vital signs and other physiological measurements are the basis for clinical problem solving.

GUIDELINES FOR TAKING VITAL SIGNS

The nurse assesses vital signs whenever a client enters a health care agency. Vital signs are included in a complete physical assessment (see Chapter 24) or obtained individually to assess a client's condition. The client's needs and condition determine when, where, how, and by whom vital signs are measured. The nurse must be able to measure vital signs correctly, understand and interpret the values, communicate findings appropriately, and begin interventions as needed. The following guidelines help the nurse incorporate vital sign measurement into nursing practice:

1. The nurse caring for the client is responsible for vital sign measurement. Measurement of selected vital signs may be delegated to unlicensed assistive personnel. However, the nurse must analyze the vital signs to interpret their significance and make decisions about interventions.
2. Equipment should be functional and appropriate to ensure accurate findings.
3. Equipment should be selected based on the client's condition and characteristics (e.g., an adult-size blood pressure cuff is not used for a child).
4. The nurse knows the client's usual range of vital signs. A client's usual values may differ from the standard range for that age or physical state. The client's usual values serve as a baseline for comparison with findings taken later.
5. The nurse knows the client's medical history, therapies, and prescribed medications. Some illnesses or treatments cause predictable vital sign changes.
6. The nurse controls or minimizes environmental factors that may affect vital signs. Measuring the

pulse after the client exercises may yield a value that is not a true indicator of the client's condition.
7. The nurse uses an organized, systematic approach when measuring vital signs.
8. Based on the client's condition, the nurse collaborates with the physician to decide the frequency of vital sign assessment. In the hospital the physician orders a minimum frequency of vital sign measurements for each client. After surgery or treatment intervention, vital signs are measured frequently to detect complications. As a client's physical condition worsens, it may be necessary to monitor vital signs as often as every 5 to 10 minutes. The nurse may use vital sign assessment to determine indications for medication administration. The physician may order certain cardiac drugs to be given only within a range of pulse or blood pressure values. Outside of the hospital, vital sign assessment occurs whenever the client seeks care from a health care provider. In either environment the nurse is responsible for judging whether more frequent assessments are needed (Box 23-1).
9. The nurse analyzes the results of vital sign measurement. Vital signs are not interpreted in isolation. The nurse must also know other physical signs or symptoms and be aware of the client's ongoing health status.
10. The nurse verifies and communicates significant changes in vital signs. Baseline measurements allow a nurse to identify changes in vital signs.

Box 23-1
When to Take Vital Signs

When the client is admitted to a health care facility
In a hospital on a routine schedule according to a physician's order or hospital standards of practice
Before and after a surgical procedure
Before and after an invasive diagnostic procedure
Before, during, and after a transfusion of blood products
Before and after the administration of medications that affect cardiovascular, respiratory, and temperature-control function
When the client's general physical condition changes (as with loss of consciousness or increased intensity of pain)
Before and after nursing interventions influencing a vital sign (e.g., before a client previously on bed rest ambulates, before a client performs range-of-motion exercises)
When the client reports nonspecific symptoms of physical distress (e.g., feeling "funny" or "different")

When vital signs appear abnormal, it may help to have another nurse or a physician repeat the measurement. The nurse informs the physician of abnormal vital signs and documents and reports vital sign changes to nurses working the next shift.

BODY TEMPERATURE

The body temperature is the difference between the amount of heat produced by body processes and the amount of heat lost to the external environment.

Heat produced − Heat lost = Body temperature

Despite extremes in environmental conditions and physical activity, temperature-control mechanisms of human beings keep the body's core temperature or temperature of deep tissues relatively constant (Figure 23-1). However, surface temperature fluctuates, depending on blood flow to the skin and the amount of heat lost to the external environment. Because of these surface temperature fluctuations, the acceptable temperature of human beings ranges from 36° C to 38° C (96.8° F to 100.4° F). The body's tissues and cells function best within this relatively narrow temperature range. For healthy young adults the average oral temperature is 37° C (98.6° F). In clinical practice, nurses learn the temperature range of individual clients. No single temperature is normal for all people.

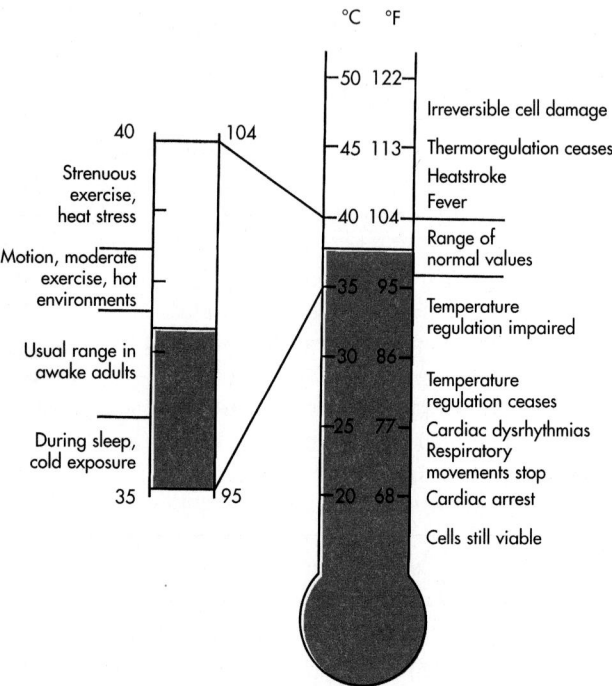

Figure 23-1. Ranges of normal temperature values and physiological consequences of abnormal body temperature. (From Thibodeau GA, Patton KT: *Anatomy and physiology,* ed 3, St. Louis, 1996, Mosby.)

The measurement of body temperature is aimed at obtaining a representative average temperature of core body tissues. Average normal temperatures vary depending on the measurement site. Sites reflecting **core temperature,** such as the pulmonary artery are more reliable indicators of body temperature than sites reflecting surface temperature. The pulmonary artery offers accurate readings because of the blood mix from all regions of the body. The pulmonary artery temperature is the standard against which all other sites are judged for accuracy.

Body Temperature Regulation

Body temperature is precisely regulated by physiological and behavioral mechanisms. For the body temperature to stay constant and within an acceptable range, the relationship between heat production and heat loss must be maintained.

Neural and vascular control. The hypothalamus, located between the cerebral hemispheres of the brain, controls body temperature. A comfortable temperature is the "set point" at which a heating system operates. In the home a fall in environmental temperature activates the furnace, whereas a rise in temperature shuts the system off. The hypothalamus senses minor changes in body temperature. The anterior hypothalamus controls heat loss, and the posterior hypothalamus controls heat production.

When nerve cells in the hypothalamus become heated beyond the set point, impulses are sent out to reduce body temperature. Compensatory mechanisms to induce heat loss include sweating, **vasodilation** (widening of blood vessels), and inhibition of heat production. If the hypothalamus senses the body's temperature lower than set point, signals are sent out to increase heat production by muscle shivering or heat conservation by **vasoconstriction** (narrowing of surface blood vessels). Disease or trauma to the hypothalamus or spinal cord, which carries hypothalamic messages, can cause serious alterations in temperature control.

Heat production. **Thermoregulation** requires the normal function of the heat production processes. Heat is produced as a by-product of metabolism. As metabolism increases, additional heat is produced. When metabolism decreases, less heat is produced. Heat production occurs during rest, voluntary movements, involuntary shivering, and **nonshivering thermogenesis.**

1. Basal metabolism accounts for the heat produced by the body at absolute rest. The average **basal metabolic rate (BMR)** depends on the body surface area.
2. Voluntary movements such as muscular activity during exercise require additional energy. The

metabolic rate can increase up to 2000 times normal during activity. Heat production can increase up to 50 times normal.

3. Shivering is an involuntary body response to temperature differences in the body. The skeletal muscle movement during shivering requires significant energy. Shivering can increase heat production to four to five times normal.

4. Nonshivering thermogenesis occurs primarily in neonates. Because neonates cannot shiver, a limited amount of vascular brown adipose tissue present at birth can be metabolized for heat production.

Heat loss. Heat loss and heat production occur simultaneously. The skin's structure and exposure to the environment result in constant, normal heat loss through radiation, conduction, convection, and evaporation.

Radiation is the transfer of heat between two objects without physical contact. Heat radiates from the skin to any surrounding cooler object. Up to 85% of the human body's surface area radiates heat to the environment.

Conduction is the transfer of heat from one object to another with direct contact. When the warm skin touches a cooler object, heat is lost until their temperatures are similar. Heat conducts through solids, gases, and liquids. Conduction normally accounts for a small amount of heat loss. The nurse increases conductive heat loss when applying an ice pack or bathing a client with cool water. Applying several layers of clothing reduces conductive loss. The body gains heat by conduction when contact is made with materials warmer than skin temperature.

Convection is the transfer of heat away by air movement. An electric fan promotes heat loss through convection. Convective heat loss increases when moistened skin comes into contact with slightly moving air.

Evaporation is the transfer of heat energy when a liquid is changed to a gas. The body continuously loses heat by evaporation. About 600 to 900 ml of water a day evaporates from the skin and lungs, resulting in water and heat loss. By regulating perspiration or sweating, the body promotes additional evaporative heat loss. **Diaphoresis** is visual perspiration of the forehead and upper thorax. When diaphoresis occurs, the body temperature is reduced.

Behavioral control. Humans take actions to maintain a comfortable body temperature. When the environmental temperature falls, a person can add clothing, move to a warmer place, raise the thermostat setting on a furnace, increase muscular activity by running in place, or sit with arms and legs tightly wrapped together. In contrast, when the temperature becomes hot, a person can remove clothing, stop activity, lower the thermostat setting on an air conditioner, seek a cooler place, or take a cool shower.

Temperature Alterations
Changes in body temperature outside the normal range affect the set point. These changes can be related to excess heat production, heat loss, minimal heat production, or any combination of these alterations. The nature of the change affects the type of clinical problems a client experiences.

Fever. Pyrexia, or **fever,** occurs because heat loss mechanisms are unable to keep pace with excess heat production, resulting in an abnormal rise in body temperature. The level at which a fever threatens health is often a source of disagreement among health care providers. A fever is usually not harmful if it stays below 39° C (102° F). A single temperature reading may not indicate a fever. In addition to physical signs and symptoms of infection, a fever determination is based on several temperature readings at different times of the day compared with the usual value for that person at that time.

A true fever results from an alteration in the hypothalamic set point. Substances that trigger the immune system or **pyrogens** stimulate the release of hormones in an effort to promote the body's defense against infection. These hormones also trigger the hypothalamus to raise the set point, inducing a febrile episode. To meet the new set point, the body produces and conserves heat. Several hours may pass before the body temperature reaches the new set point. During this period the person experiences chills, shivers, and feels cold, even though the body temperature is rising. The chill phase resolves when the new set point, a higher temperature, is achieved. In the plateau phase the chills subside and the person feels warm and dry. If the set point has been "over shot" or the pyrogens are removed, the third phase of a **febrile** episode occurs. The skin becomes warm and flushed because of vasodilation. Diaphoresis assists in evaporative heat loss. When the fever "breaks," the client becomes **afebrile.**

Fever, or **pyrexia,** is an important defense mechanism. Mild temperature elevations up to 39° C (102° F) enhance the body's immune system by stimulating white blood cell production. Increased temperature reduces the concentration of iron in the blood plasma, suppressing the growth of bacteria. Fever also fights viral infections by stimulating interferon, the body's natural virus-fighting substance.

Fevers also serve a diagnostic purpose. Fever patterns differ depending on the causative pyrogen (Box 23-2). The duration and degree of fever depend on the pyrogen's strength and the ability of the individual to respond. The term *fever of unknown origin* (FUO) refers to a fever whose etiology (cause) cannot be determined.

Hyperthermia. An elevated body temperature related to the body's inability to promote heat loss or reduce heat production is **hyperthermia.** Any disease or

Box 23-2
Patterns of Fever

Sustained	A constant body temperature continuously above 38° C (100.4° F) that demonstrates little fluctuation.
Intermittent	Fever spikes interspersed with usual temperature levels. Temperature returns to acceptable value at least once in 24 hours.
Remittent	Fever spikes and falls without a return to normal temperature levels.
Relapsing	Periods of febrile episodes interspersed with acceptable temperature values. Febrile episodes and periods of normothermia may be longer than 24 hours.

TABLE 23-1
Classification of Hypothermia

	C	F
Mild	33.1°–36°	91.5°–96.8°
Moderate	30.1°–33°	86.1°–91.4°
Severe	27°–30°	80.6°–86.0°
Profound	<27°	<80.6°

trauma to the hypothalamus can impair heat loss mechanisms. **Malignant hyperthermia** is a hereditary condition of uncontrolled heat production. Malignant hyperthermia occurs when susceptible persons receive certain anesthetic drugs.

Prolonged exposure to the sun or high environmental temperatures can overwhelm the body's heat loss mechanisms. Heat also depresses hypothalamic function. These conditions cause **heat stroke,** a dangerous heat emergency. Signs and symptoms of heat stroke include giddiness, confusion, delirium, excess thirst, nausea, muscle cramps, visual disturbances, and even incontinence. The most important sign of heat stroke is hot, dry skin.

Hypothermia. Heat loss during prolonged exposure to cold overwhelms the body's ability to produce heat, causing **hypothermia.** Hypothermia is classified by core temperature measurements (Table 23-1). It can be accidental or intentional.

Accidental hypothermia develops gradually and may go unnoticed for several hours. The hypothermic client suffers uncontrolled shivering, loss of memory, depression, and poor judgment. As the body temperature falls below 34.4° C (94° F), heart and respiratory rates and blood pressure fall.

NURSING PROCESS AND THERMOREGULATION

Knowledge of body temperature physiology helps a nurse to assess the client's response to temperature alterations and to intervene safely.

Assessment

Sites. There are several sites for measuring core and surface body temperature. The core temperatures of the pulmonary artery, esophagus, and urinary bladder are often used in intensive care settings. These measurements require the use of continuous invasive devices placed in body cavities or organs. The temperature devices obtain accurate readings quickly and continually display readings on an electronic monitor.

Intermittent measurements are obtained from the routinely used invasive sites of the tympanic membrane, mouth, rectum, and axilla. Noninvasive special chemically prepared thermometer patches can also be applied to the skin.

To ensure accurate temperature readings, each site must be measured correctly (Skill 23-1). The temperature obtained varies depending on the site used but should be between 36.0° C (96.8° F) and 38.0° C (100.4° F). Rectal temperatures are usually 0.5° C (0.9° F) higher than oral temperatures. Axillary temperatures are usually 0.5° C (0.9° F) lower than oral temperatures. Each of the common temperature measurement sites has advantages and disadvantages (Table 23-2). The nurse chooses the safest and most accurate site for the client. The same site should be used when repeated measurements are necessary.

Thermometers. The three types of thermometers used for measuring body temperature are mercury-in-glass, electronic, and disposable. Each device measures temperature in either the **centigrade** or **Fahrenheit** scale. Electronic thermometers allow the nurse to convert scales by activating a switch. When it is necessary to convert temperature readings, the following formulas can be used:

1. To convert Fahrenheit to centigrade, subtract 32 from the Fahrenheit reading and multiply the result by 5/9.

   Example: (104° F − 32° F) × 5/9 = 40° C

Delegation Considerations

The skill of temperature measurement can be delegated to unlicensed assistive personnel.

- Inform care giver of appropriate route and device to measure temperature.
- Inform and observe care giver performing proper positioning of clients for rectal temperature measurement.
- Inform care giver of factors that can falsely raise or lower temperature.

Equipment

- Appropriate thermometer
- Soft tissue
- Lubricant (for rectal measurements only)
- Pen, pencil, vital sign flow sheet or record form
- Disposable gloves, plastic thermometer sleeve or disposable probe cover

STEPS	RATIONALE
1. Assess for signs and symptoms of temperature alterations and for factors that influence body temperature.	Physical signs and symptoms may indicate abnormal temperature. Nurse can accurately assess nature of variations.
2. Determine any previous activity that would interfere with accuracy of temperature measurement. When taking oral temperature, wait 20 to 30 minutes before measuring temperature if client has smoked or ingested hot or cold liquids or foods.	Smoking and hot or cold substances can cause false temperature readings in oral cavity.
3. Determine appropriate site and measurement device to be used.	Chosen on basis of preferred site for temperature measurement (see Table 23-2).
4. Explain way temperature will be taken and importance of maintaining proper position until reading is complete.	Clients are often curious about such measurements and should be cautioned against prematurely removing thermometer to read results.
5. Wash hands.	Reduces transmission of microorganisms.
6. Assist client in assuming comfortable position that provides easy access to mouth.	Ensures comfort and accuracy of temperature reading.
7. Obtain temperature reading.	
A. Oral temperature measurement with glass thermometer:	
(1) Apply disposable gloves.	Maintains standard precautions when exposed to items soiled with body fluids (e.g., saliva).
(2) Hold end (if color-coded, tip will be blue) of glass thermometer with fingertips.	Reduces contamination of thermometer bulb.
(3) Read mercury level while gently rotating thermometer at eye level (see illustration). If mercury is above desired level, grasp tip of thermometer securely, stand away from solid objects, and sharply flick wrist downward. Continue shaking until reading is below 35.5° C (96° F).	Mercury should be below 35.5° C (96° F). Thermometer reading must be below client's actual temperature before use. Brisk shaking lowers mercury level in glass tube.

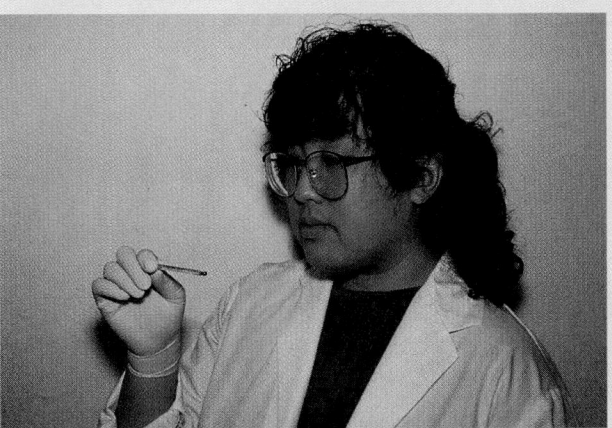

Step 7A(3)

STEPS	RATIONALE
(4) Insert thermometer into plastic sleeve cover.	Protects from contact with saliva.
(5) Ask client to open mouth and gently place thermometer under tongue in posterior sublingual pocket lateral to center of lower jaw (see illustration).	Heat from superficial blood vessels in sublingual pocket produces temperature reading.
(6) Ask client to hold thermometer with lips closed. Caution against biting down on thermometer.	Maintains proper position of thermometer during recording. Breakage of thermometer may injure mucosa and cause mercury poisoning.
(7) Leave thermometer in place for 3 minutes or according to agency policy.	Studies vary as to proper length of time for recording. Holtzclaw (1992) recommends 3 minutes.
(8) Carefully remove thermometer, remove and discard plastic sleeve cover in appropriate receptacle, and read at eye level. Gently rotate until scale appears.	Prevents cross contamination. Ensures accurate reading.
(9) Cleanse any additional secretions on thermometer by wiping with clean soft tissue. Wipe in rotating fashion from fingers toward bulb. Dispose of tissue in appropriate receptacle. Store thermometer in appropriate protective storage container.	Avoids contact of microorganisms with nurse's hands. Wipe from area of least contamination to area of most contamination. Glass thermometers should not be shared between clients unless terminal disinfection is performed between each measurement. Protective storage container prevents breakage and reduces risks of mercury spill.
(10) Remove and dispose of gloves in appropriate receptacle. Wash hands.	Reduces transmission of microorganisms.
B. Oral temperature measurement with electronic thermometer:	
(1) Apply disposable gloves (optional).	Use of oral probe cover, which can be removed without physical contact, minimizes need to wear gloves.
(2) Remove thermometer pack from charging unit. Attach oral probe (blue tip) to thermometer unit. Grasp top of stem, being careful not to apply pressure to ejection button.	Charging provides battery power. Ejection button releases plastic cover from probe.

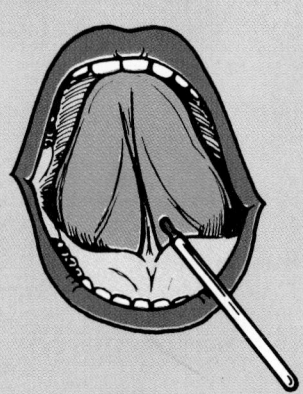

Step 7A(5)

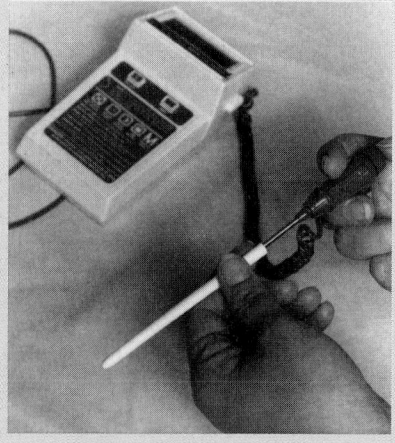

Step 7B(3)

STEPS	RATIONALE
(3) Slide disposable plastic probe cover over thermometer probe until it locks in place (see illustration).	Soft plastic cover will not break in client's mouth and prevents transmission of microorganisms between clients.
(4) Ask client to open mouth; then gently place thermometer probe under tongue in posterior sublingual pocket lateral to center of lower jaw.	Heat from superficial blood vessels in sublingual pocket produces temperature reading. With electronic thermometer, temperatures in right and left posterior sublingual pocket are significantly higher than in area under front of tongue.
(5) Ask client to hold thermometer probe with lips closed.	Maintains proper position of thermometer during recording.
(6) Leave thermometer probe in place until audible signal occurs and client's temperature appears on digital display; remove thermometer probe from under client's tongue.	Probe must stay in place until signal occurs to ensure accurate reading.
(7) Push ejection button on thermometer stem to discard plastic probe cover into appropriate receptacle.	Reduces transmission of microorganisms.
(8) Return thermometer stem to storage well of recording unit.	Protects probe from damage. Automatically causes digital reading to disappear.
(9) If gloves worn, remove and dispose in appropriate receptacle. Wash hands.	Reduces transmission of microorganisms.
(10) Return thermometer to charger.	Maintains battery charge.
C. Rectal temperature measurement with glass thermometer:	
(1) Draw curtain around bed and/or close room door. Assist client to Sims' position with upper leg flexed. Move aside bed linen to expose only anal area. Keep client's upper body and lower extremities covered with sheet or blanket.	Maintains client's privacy, minimizes embarrassment, and promotes comfort. Exposes anal area for correct thermometer placement.
(2) Apply disposable gloves.	Maintains standard precautions when exposed to items soiled with body fluids (e.g., feces).
(3) Hold end (if color-coded, tip will be red) of glass thermometer with fingertips.	Reduces contamination of thermometer bulb.
(4) Read mercury level while gently rotating thermometer at eye level. If mercury is above desired level, grasp tip of thermometer securely, stand away from solid objects, and sharply flick wrist downward. Continue shaking until reading is below 35.5° C (96° F).	Mercury should be below 35.5° C (96° F). Thermometer reading must be below client's actual temperature before use. Brisk shaking lowers mercury level in glass tube.
(5) Insert thermometer into plastic sleeve cover.	Protects from contact with feces.
(6) Squeeze liberal portion of lubricant on tissue. Dip thermometer's blunt end into lubricant, covering 2.5 to 3.5 cm (1 to 1½ inches) for adult.	Lubrication minimizes trauma to rectal mucosa during insertion. Tissue avoids contamination of remaining lubricant in container.
(7) With nondominant hand, separate client's buttocks to expose anus. Ask client to breathe slowly and relax.	Fully exposes anus for thermometer insertion. Relaxes anal sphincter for easier thermometer insertion.

Continued

Measuring Body Temperature

STEPS	RATIONALE
(8) Gently insert thermometer into anus in direction of umbilicus 3.5 cm (1½ inches) for adult. Do not force thermometer.	Ensures adequate exposure against blood vessels in rectal wall.
(9) If resistance is felt during insertion, withdraw thermometer immediately. Never force thermometer.	Prevents trauma to mucosa. Glass thermometers can break.

CRITICAL DECISION POINT

If thermometer cannot be adequately inserted into rectum, remove thermometer and consider alternative method for obtaining temperature.

STEPS	RATIONALE
(10) Hold thermometer in place for 2 minutes or according to agency policy.	Prevents injury to client. Studies vary as to proper length of time for recording. Holtzclaw (1992) recommends 2 minutes.
(11) Carefully remove thermometer, remove and discard plastic sleeve cover in appropriate receptacle, and wipe off any remaining secretions with clean tissue. Wipe in rotating fashion from fingers toward bulb. Dispose of tissue in appropriate receptacle.	Prevents cross contamination. Wipe from area of least contamination to area of most contamination.
(12) Read thermometer at eye level. Gently rotate until scale appears.	Ensures accurate reading.
(13) Wipe client's anal area with soft tissue to remove lubricant or feces and discard tissue. Assist client in assuming a comfortable position.	Provides for comfort and hygiene.
(14) Store thermometer in appropriate protective storage container.	Glass thermometers should not be shared between clients unless terminal disinfection is performed between each measurement. Protective storage container prevents breakage and reduces risks of mercury spill.
(15) Remove and dispose of gloves in appropriate receptacle. Wash hands.	Reduces transmission of microorganisms.
D. Rectal temperature measurement with electronic thermometer:	
(1) Follow steps C(1) and C(2).	
(2) Remove thermometer pack from charging unit. Attach rectal probe (red tip) to thermometer unit. Grasp top of stem, being careful not to apply pressure to ejection button.	Charging provides battery power. Ejection button releases plastic cover from probe.
(3) Slide disposable plastic probe cover over thermometer probe until it locks in place.	Probe cover prevents transmission of microorganisms between clients.
(4) Continue as for C(6), (7), (8), and (9).	
(5) Leave thermometer probe in place (see illustration) until audible signal occurs and client's temperature appears on digital display; remove thermometer probe from anus.	Probe must stay in place until signal occurs to ensure accurate reading.

STEPS   **RATIONALE**

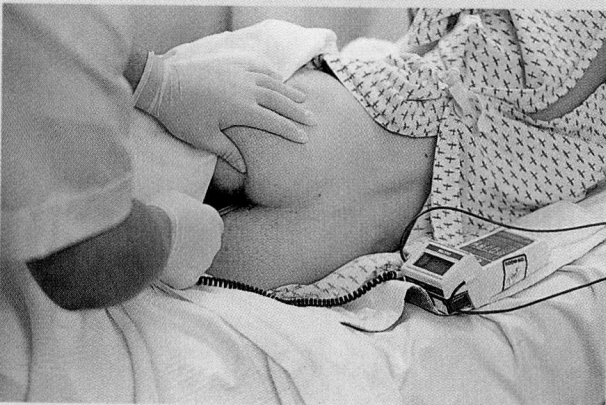

Step 7D(5)

(6) Push ejection button on thermometer stem to discard plastic probe cover into appropriate receptacle.

Reduces transmission of microorganisms.

(7) Return thermometer stem to storage well of recording unit.

Protects probe from damage. Automatically causes digital reading to disappear.

(8) Wipe client's anal area with soft tissue to remove lubricant or feces and discard tissue. Assist client in assuming a comfortable position.

Provides for comfort and hygiene.

(9) Remove and dispose of gloves in appropriate receptable. Wash hands.

Reduces transmission of microorganisms.

(10) Return thermometer to charger.

Maintains battery charge.

E. **Axillary temperature measurement with glass themometer:**

(1) Wash hands.

Reduces transmission of microorganisms.

(2) Draw curtain around bed and/or close door

Provides privacy and minimizes embarrassment.

(3) Assist client to supine or sitting position.

Provides easy access to axilla.

(4) Move clothing or gown away from shoulder and arm.

Exposes axilla.

(5) Prepare glass thermometer following Steps 7A(2), (3).

Mercury must be below client's temperature level before insertion.

(6) Insert thermometer into center of axilla, lower arm over thermometer, and place arm across chest (see illustrations).

Maintains proper position of thermometer against blood vessels in axilla.

Continued

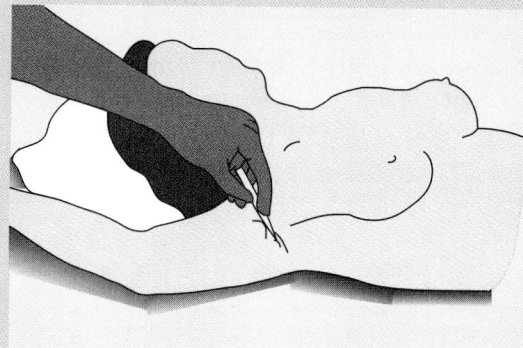

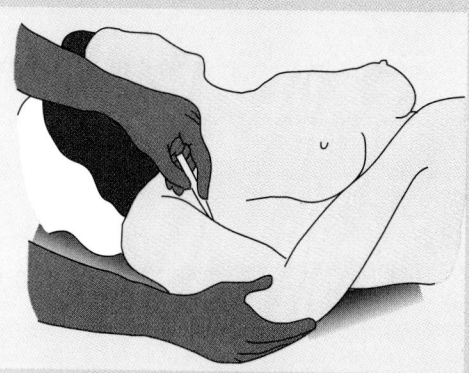

Step 7E(6)

Skill 23-1—cont'd
Measuring Body Temperature

STEPS	RATIONALE
(7) Hold thermometer in place for 3 minutes or according to agency policy.	Studies as to proper length of time for recording vary. They concluded that changes after 3 minutes had little clinical significance.
(8) Remove thermometer, remove plastic sleeve, and wipe off remaining secretions with tissue. Wipe in rotating fashion from fingers toward bulb. Dispose of sleeve and tissue in appropriate receptacle.	Avoids nurse's contact with microorganisms. Wipe from area of least contamination to area of most contamination.
(9) Read thermometer at eye level.	Ensures accurate reading.
(10) Inform client of reading.	Promotes participation in care and understanding of health status.
(11) Store thermometer at bedside in protective storage container.	Glass thermometers should not be shared between clients unless terminal disinfection is performed between each measurement. Storage container prevents breakage and reduces risk of mercury spill.
(12) Assist client in replacing clothing or gown.	Restores sense of well-being.
(13) Wash hands.	Reduces transmission of microorganisms.

F. **Axillary temperature measurement with electronic thermometer:**

STEPS	RATIONALE
(1) Position client lying supine or sitting.	Provides easy access to axilla.
(2) Move clothing or gown away from shoulder and arm.	Provides optimal exposure of axilla.
(3) Remove thermometer pack from charging unit. Be sure oral probe (blue tip) is attached to thermometer unit. Grasp top of stem, being careful not to apply pressure to ejection button.	Ejection button releases plastic cover from probe.
(4) Slide disposable plastic probe cover over thermometer probe until it locks in place.	Soft plastic cover prevents transmission of microorganisms between clients.
(5) Raise client's arm away from torso, inspect for skin lesion and excessive perspiration. Insert probe into center of axilla, lower arm over probe, and place arm across chest.	Maintains proper position of probe against blood vessels in axilla.
(6) Leave probe in place until audible signal occurs and temperature appears on digital display.	Probe must stay in place until signal occurs to ensure accurate reading.
(7) Remove probe from axilla.	
(8) Push ejection button on probe to discard plastic probe cover into appropriate receptacle.	Reduces transmission of microorganisms.
(9) Return probe to storage well of recording unit.	Protects probe from damage. Automatically causes digital reading to disappear.
(10) Assist client in assuming a comfortable position.	Restores comfort and promotes privacy.
(11) Wash hands.	Reduces transmission of microorganisms.

STEPS	RATIONALE
G. Tympanic membrane temperature with electronic thermometer:	
(1) Assist client in assuming comfortable position with head turned toward side, away from nurse.	Ensures comfort and exposes auditory canal for accurate temperature measurement.
(2) Remove thermometer handheld unit from charging base, being careful not to apply pressure to ejection button.	Base provides battery power. Removal of handheld unit from base prepares it to measure temperature. Ejection button releases plastic cover from probe.
(3) Slide disposable speculum cover over otoscopelike tip until it locks into place.	Soft plastic probe cover prevents transmission of microorganisms between clients.
(4) Insert speculum into ear canal following manufacturer's instructions for tympanic probe positioning (see illustration):	Correct positioning of the probe with respect to ear canal ensures accurate readings. The ear tug straightens the external auditory canal, allowing maximum exposure of the tympanic membrane.
(a) Pull ear pinna upward and back for adult.	Some manufacturers recommend movement of the speculum tip in a figure-eight pattern that allows the sensor to detect maximum tympanic membrane
(b) Move thermometer in a figure-eight pattern.	heat radiation. Gentle pressure seals ear canal from ambient air temperature.
(c) Fit probe snug into canal and do not move.	
(d) Point toward nose.	

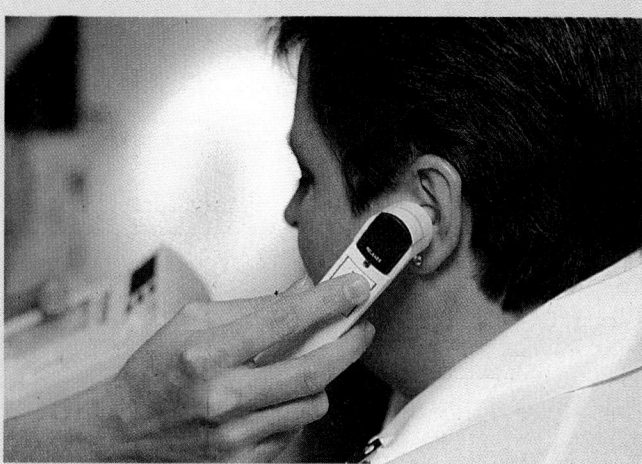

Step 7G(4)

STEPS	RATIONALE
(5) Depress scan button on handheld unit. Leave thermometer probe in place until audible signal occurs and client's temperature appears on digital display.	Depression of scan button causes infrared energy to be detected. Probe must stay in place until signal occurs to ensure accurate reading.
(6) Carefully remove speculum from auditory meatus.	
(7) Push ejection button on handheld unit to discard plastic probe cover into appropriate receptacle.	Reduces transmission of microorganisms. Automatically causes digital reading to disappear.
(8) Return handheld unit to charging base.	Protects probe from damage.
(9) Assist client in assuming a comfortable position.	Restores comfort and sense of well-being.
(10) Wash hands.	Reduces transmission of microorganisms.

Continued

Skill 23-1—cont'd
Measuring Body Temperature

STEPS	RATIONALE
8. Discuss findings with client as needed.	Promotes participation in care and understanding of health status.
9. If temperature is assessed for the first time, establish temperature as baseline if it is within normal range.	Used to compare future temperature measurements.
10. Compare temperature reading with client's previous baseline and normal temperature range for client's age group.	Normal body temperature fluctuates within narrow range; comparison reveals presence of abnormality. Improper placement or movement of thermometer can cause inaccuracies. Second measurement confirms initial findings of abnormal body temperature.

Recording and Reporting

▪ Record temperature in nurses' notes or vital sign flow sheet. Measurement of temperature after administration of specific therapies should be documented in narrative form in nurses' notes.
▪ Report abnormal findings to nurse in charge or physician.

Home Care Considerations

▪ Assess temperature and ventilation of client's environment to determine existence of any environmental condition that may influence outcome of client's temperature.
▪ Assess safe storage of mercury-in-glass thermometers to protect from breakage and mercury spills.

2. To convert centigrade to Fahrenheit, multiply the centigrade reading by 9/5 and add 32 to the product.

Example: (9/5 × 40° C) + 32 = 104° F

Glass thermometers. The mercury-in-glass thermometer is the most familiar. It is a glass tube sealed at one end, with a mercury-filled bulb at the other. Exposure of the bulb to heat causes the mercury to expand and rise in the enclosed tube. The length of the thermometer is marked with Fahrenheit or centigrade calibrations.

Three types of glass thermometers are the oral, the stubby, and the rectal (Figure 23-2). The oral thermometer is slender, allowing for greater exposure of the bulb against the blood vessels in the mouth. An oral thermometer usually has a blue tip. The stubby thermometer is shorter and thicker than the oral type. It can be used to measure temperature at any site. The rectal thermometer has a blunt end designed to prevent trauma to rectal tissues during insertion. It is usually recognized by a red tip.

The time delay to obtain readings and the easy breakability are disadvantages of mercury-in-glass thermometers. Mercury is a hazardous material if it is not properly contained. Do not touch spilled mercury droplets. Contact the agency's environmental services

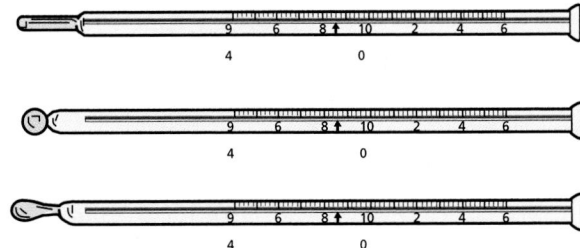

Figure 23-2. Comparison of oral, stubby, and rectal thermometers *(top to bottom).*

department or safety officer for the procedure in the event of a mercury spill.

Electronic thermometer. The electronic thermometer consists of a rechargeable battery-powered display unit, a thin wire cord, and a temperature-processing probe covered by a disposable plastic sheath (Figure 23-3). One form of electronic thermometer uses a pencil-like probe. Separate nonbreakable probes are available for oral and rectal use. The oral probe can also be used for axillary temperature measurement. Within 20 to 50 seconds of insertion, a reading appears on the display unit. A sound signals when the peak temperature reading has been measured.

Another form of electronic thermometer is used ex-

TABLE 23-2
Advantages and Disadvantages of Select Temperature Measurement Sites and Methods

Tympanic Membrane Sensor
Advantages
Easily accessible site
Minimal client repositioning required
Provides accurate core reading
Very rapid measurement (2 to 5 seconds)
Can be obtained without disturbing or waking client
Eardrum close to hypothalamus; sensitive to core
    temperature changes

Disadvantages
Hearing aids must be removed before measurement
Should not be used with clients who have had surgery of the
    ear or tympanic membrane
Requires disposable probe cover
Expensive

Electronic Thermometer
Advantages
Plastic sheath unbreakable; ideal for children
Quick readings

Disadvantages
May be less accurate by axillary route

Rectum
Advantages
Argued to be more reliable when oral temperature cannot be
    obtained

Disadvantages
May lag behind core temperature during rapid temperature
    changes
Should not be used with clients who have had rectal surgery,
    a rectal disorder, bleeding tendencies, and heart disease
Requires positioning and may be source of client em-
    barrassment and anxiety
Risk of body fluid exposure
Requires lubrication
Contraindicated in newborns

Oral
Advantages
Accessible—requires no position change
Comfortable for client
Provides accurate surface temperature reading
Indicates rapid change in core temperature

Disadvantages
Affected by ingestion of fluids or foods, smoke,
    and oxygen delivery (Neff and others, 1992)
Should not be used with clients who have had oral
    surgery, trauma, history of epilepsy, or shaking
    chills
Should not be used with infants, small children, or
    confused, unconscious, or uncooperative clients
Risk of body fluid exposure

Axilla
Advantages
Safe and noninvasive
Can be used with newborns and uncooperative
    clients

Disadvantages
Long measurement time
Requires continuous positioning by nurse
Measurement lags behind core temperature dur-
    ing rapid temperature changes
Requires exposure of thorax

Skin
Advantages
Inexpensive
Provides continuous reading
Safe and noninvasive

Disadvantages
Lags behind other sites during temperature
    changes, especially during hyperthermia
Diaphoresis or sweat can impair adhesion

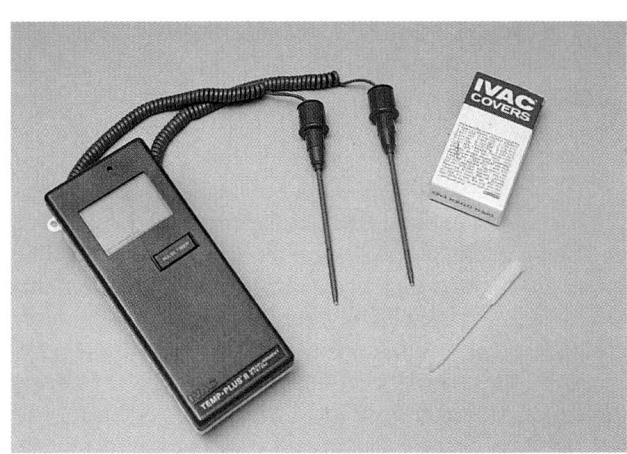

Figure 23-3. Electronic thermometer used for oral, rectal, or axillary measurements.

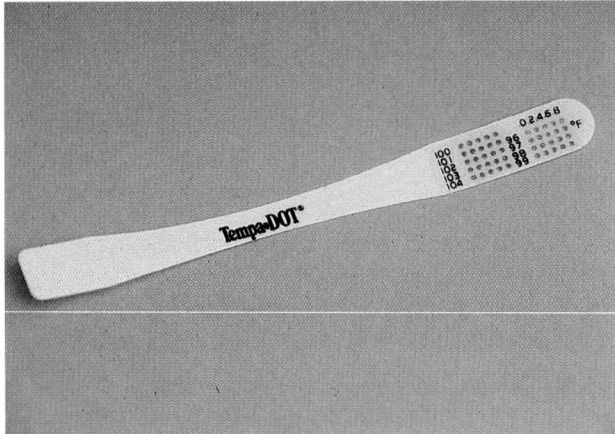

Figure 23-4. Disposable, single-use thermometer strip.

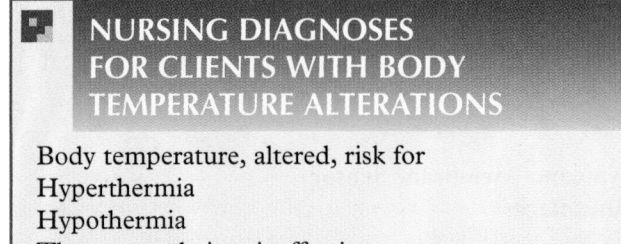

NURSING DIAGNOSES FOR CLIENTS WITH BODY TEMPERATURE ALTERATIONS

Body temperature, altered, risk for
Hyperthermia
Hypothermia
Thermoregulation, ineffective

clusively for tympanic temperature measurement. An otoscope-like speculum with an infrared sensor tip detects heat radiated from the tympanic membrane. Within 2 to 5 seconds of placement in the auditory canal, a reading appears on the display unit. A sound signals when the peak temperature reading has been measured.

Disposable thermometers. Disposable, single-use thermometers are thin strips of plastic with chemically impregnated paper. They are used for measurement of oral or axillary temperatures, particularly in children (Figure 23-4). They are inserted the same way as an oral thermometer and used only once. Chemical dots on the thermometer change color to reflect the temperature reading. Only 45 seconds are needed to record a temperature.

Another form of disposable thermometer is a temperature-sensitive patch or tape. Applied to the forehead or abdomen, the patch changes color at different temperatures.

Nursing Diagnosis

After assessment, the nurse reviews all of the available data and looks for patterns and trends that are suggestive of a health problem relating to temperature alteration (see nursing diagnoses box). For example, an increase in body temperature, flushed skin, skin that is warm to touch, and tachycardia are defining characteristics for the diagnosis of *hyperthermia*. The nurse will validate findings to ensure the accuracy of the diagnosis. A colleague may be asked to repeat the temperature measurement, or the nurse may discuss the symptoms with the client.

Once a diagnosis is determined, the nurse must determine the factor that likely caused the client's health problem. The related factor allows the nurse to select appropriate nursing interventions. In the example of *hyperthermia*, the related factor of vigorous activity will result in much different interventions than the related factor of infectious process.

Planning

The plan of care (see care plan) depends on the nurse's assessment of the client's perception and acceptance of the body temperature alteration. It also depends on the extent to which the client's internal compensatory mechanisms and behaviors have adjusted to the temperature alteration. The client must actively participate in choosing therapies for the care plan.

Priorities of care must be set with regard to the extent the temperature alteration affects a client. Safety is a top priority.

Implementation

Health promotion. Health promotion for clients at risk of altered body temperature is directed toward promoting balance between heat production and heat loss. Client activity, temperature of the environment, and clothing are all considered. The nurse teaches clients to avoid strenuous exercise in hot, humid weather; to drink fluids such as clear fruit juices before, during, and after exercise; to wear light, loose-fitting, light-colored clothing; to avoid exercising in areas with poor ventilation; to wear a protective covering over the head when outdoors; and to expose themselves to hot climates gradually.

Prevention is the key for clients at risk for hypothermia. Prevention involves educating clients, family members, and friends. Clients most at risk include the very young and the very old and persons debilitated by trauma, stroke, diabetes, drug or alcohol intoxication, sepsis, and Raynaud's disease. Mentally ill or handicapped clients may fall victim to hypothermia because they are unaware of the dangers of cold conditions. Persons without adequate home heating, shelter, diet, or clothing are also at risk.

Acute care

Hyperthermia. Treatment for an elevated temperature depends on the fever's cause, any adverse effects, and the strength, intensity, and duration of the fever. The nurse plays a key role in assessing fever and implementing reducing strategies. The physician may try to determine the cause of the fever by isolating the causative pyrogen. The nurse obtains necessary culture specimens for laboratory analysis, such as urine, blood, sputum, and wound sites. The physician will order antibiotics to be

▣ SAMPLE NURSING CARE PLAN

Assessment

Mr. Coburn is a 45-year-old school teacher who arrives at the outpatient clinic with the complaint of malaise. His skin is **warm and dry to touch.** His face is **flushed** and he appears to have **labored breathing.** He admits to smoking one pack of cigarettes per day and recently began expectorating yellow-green sputum. Vital signs obtained are: BP RA 116/62, LA 114/64; right radial **pulse 128,** regular and bounding; **RR 26;** SpO$_2$ 98% on room air; tympanic **temperature 39.2° C (102.6° F).**

Nursing Diagnosis

Hyperthermia related to infectious process.

Planning

Goals	**Expected Outcomes**
Client will regain normal range of body temperature within next 24 hours.	Body temperature will decline at least 1° C (1.8° F) within next 8 hours.
Client will attain sense of comfort and rest within next 48 hours.	Client will verbalize increased satisfaction with rest and sleep pattern.
	Client will report increase in energy level within next 3 days.
Fluid and electrolyte balance will be maintained during next 3 days.	Intake will equal output within next 24 hours.
	No evidence of postural hypotension during ambulation.

Implementation

Steps	**Rationale**
1. Instruct client to reduce external coverings and keep clothing and bed linen dry.	Promotes heat loss through conduction and convection.
2. Instruct client to monitor temperature at home and administer acetaminophen every 4 hours as ordered for temperature over 39° C (102° F).	Antipyretics reduce set point.
3. Instruct client to limit physical activity and increase frequency of rest periods over next 2 days.	Activity and stress increase metabolic rate, contributing to heat production.
4. Instruct client to increase oral fluids of choice.	Fluids lost through insensible water loss require replacement.

Evaluation

During ambulatory center follow-up phone call, ask client to identify temperature and describe energy level.

Defining characteristics are shown in bold type.

---

given after the cultures have been obtained. Antibiotics destroy pyrogenic bacteria and eliminate the body's stimulus for fever. The nurse administers antibiotics promptly (Box 23-3).

The objective of fever therapy is to increase heat loss, reduce heat production, and prevent complications. Nonpharmacological therapy for fever uses methods that increase heat loss by evaporation, conduction, convection, or radiation.

Nursing measures to enhance body cooling must avoid stimulating shivering. Shivering is counterproductive because of the heat produced by muscle activity.

Antipyretics are drugs that reduce fever. Nonsteroi-

dal drugs such as acetaminophen, salicylates, indomethacin, ibuprofen, and ketoralac reduce fever by increasing heat loss. Corticosteroids reduce heat production by interfering with the hypothalamus response. These drugs mask signs of infection by suppressing the immune system. Corticosteroids are not used to treat a fever. However, the nurse must be aware of their effect on suppressing the ability of the client to develop a fever in response to a pyrogen.

Heat stroke. First aid treatment for victims of heat stroke includes moving the client to a cooler environment, reducing clothing covering the body, placing wet towels over the skin, and using oscillating fans to

Box 23-3
Nursing Measures for Clients With a Fever

Assessment

Obtain core temperature during each phase of febrile episode.
Assess for contributing factors such as dehydration, infection, or environmental temperature.
Identify physiological response to temperature.
Obtain all vital signs.
Observe skin color.
Assess skin temperature.
Observe for shivering and diaphoresis.
Assess client comfort and well-being.
Determine phase of fever—chill, plateau, fever break.

Interventions (Unless Contraindicated)

Obtain blood cultures when ordered. Blood specimens are obtained to coincide with temperature spikes when the antigen-producing organism is most prevalent.
Initiate therapies to minimize heat production: reduce the frequency of activities that increase oxygen demand such as excessive turning and ambulation; allow rest periods; limit physical activity.

Initiate therapies to maximize heat loss: reduce external covering on client's body to promote heat loss through radiation and conduction; keep clothing and bed linen dry to increase heat loss through conduction and convection.
Initiate therapies to meet requirements for increased metabolic rate: provide supplemental oxygen therapy as ordered to improve oxygen delivery to body cells; provide measures to stimulate appetite, and offer well-balanced meals; provide fluids (at least 3 L/day for a client with normal cardiac and renal function) to replace fluids lost through insensible water loss and sweating.
Initiate therapies to promote client comfort: encourage oral hygiene because oral mucous membranes dry easily from dehydration; control temperature of the environment without inducing shivering.
Identify onset and duration of febrile episode phases: examine previous temperature measurements for trends.
Initiate health teaching as indicated.

increase convective heat loss. Emergency medical treatment may include hypothermia blankets, intravenous fluids, and irrigating the stomach and lower bowel with cool solutions.

Hypothermia. The priority treatment for hypothermia is to prevent a further decrease in body temperature. The nurse removes wet clothes, replaces them with dry ones, and wraps the client in blankets. In emergencies away from a health care setting, the client lies under blankets next to a warm person. A conscious client benefits from drinking hot liquids such as soup. Keeping the head covered, placing the client near a fire or in a warm room, or placing heating pads next to areas of the body (head and neck) that lose heat the quickest helps.

Restorative care. The nurse educates the client regarding the importance of taking and continuing any antibiotics as directed until the course of treatment is completed. Children and older adults are especially at risk for fluid volume deficit because they can quickly lose large amounts of fluids in proportion to their body weight. Identifying preferred fluids and encouraging oral fluid intake is an important nursing intervention.

Evaluation

All nursing interventions are evaluated by comparing the client's actual response with the outcomes of the

care plan. This reveals whether goals of care have been met. After any intervention the nurse measures the client's temperature to evaluate for change. In addition, the nurse uses other evaluative measures such as palpation of the skin and assessment of pulse and respirations. If therapies are effective, body temperature will return to an acceptable range, other vital signs will stabilize, and the client will report a sense of comfort.

···PULSE

Blood flows through the body in a continuous circuit. Electrical impulses from the sinoatrial (SA) node travel through heart muscle to stimulate cardiac contraction. Approximately 60 to 70 ml of blood enters the aorta with each contraction (**stroke volume [SV]**). The pulse is the palpable bounding of the blood flow in a peripheral artery. It can be felt as a tap when palpating an artery lightly against underlying bone or muscle. The number of pulsing sensations occurring in 1 minute is the pulse rate.

The volume of blood pumped by the heart during 1 minute is the **cardiac output (CO),** the product of heart rate and the ventricle's stroke volume (see Chapter 30). The cause of an abnormally slow, rapid, or irregular pulse may ultimately alter cardiac output. Although cardiac output depends on heart rate, a change in heart rate alone does not alter cardiac output.

The nurse assesses the heart's ability to meet the body's demands for cardiac output by palpating a peripheral pulse or by using a stethoscope to listen to heart sounds (apical rate).

Locating the Peripheral Pulse

Any artery can be assessed for pulse rate, but the radial and carotid arteries are easily palpated peripheral pulse sites. When a client's condition suddenly deteriorates, the carotid site is the best for finding a pulse quickly.

The radial and apical locations are the most common sites for pulse rate assessment. They are used by persons learning to monitor their own heart rates (e.g., athletes). If the radial pulse is abnormal, difficult to palpate, or inaccessible because of a dressing or cast, the apical pulse is assessed. When a client takes a medication that affects the heart rate, the apical pulse provides a more accurate assessment of heart rate. Table 23-3 summarizes pulse sites and criteria for measurement. Skill 23-2 outlines radial and apical pulse rate assessment.

Stethoscope

When assessing the apical rate, the nurse uses a stethoscope (Figure 23-5). The four major parts of the stethoscope are the earpieces, binaurals, tubing, and chestpiece.

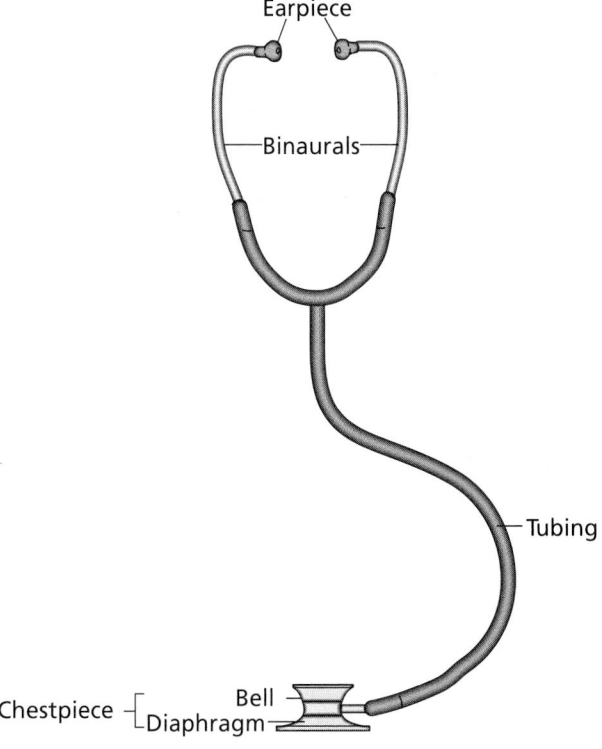

Figure 23-5. Parts of a stethoscope.

TABLE 23-3
Pulse Sites

Site	Location	Assessment Criteria
Temporal	Over temporal bone of head, above and lateral to eye	Easily accessible site used to assess pulse in children
Carotid	Along medial edge of sternocleido-mastoid muscle in neck	Easily accessible site used during physiological shock or cardiac arrest when other sites are not palpable
Apical	Fourth to fifth intercostal space at left midclavicular line	Site used to auscultate for heart sounds; site used for infants and young children
Brachial	Groove between biceps and triceps muscles at antecubital fossa	Site used to assess status of circulation to lower arm; site used to assess pulse rate; site used to auscultate blood pressure
Radial	Radial or thumb side of forearm at wrist	Common site used to assess character of pulse peripherally and assess status of circulation to hand
Ulnar	Ulnar side of forearm at wrist	Site used to assess status of circulation to hand, using the Allen test
Femoral	Below inguinal ligament, midway between symphysis pubis and anterior superior iliac spine	Site used to assess character of pulse during physiological shock or cardiac arrest when other pulses are not palpable; used to assess status of circulation to leg
Popliteal	Behind knee in popliteal fossa	Site used to assess status of circulation to lower leg
Posterior tibial	Inner side of ankle, below medial malleolus	Site used to assess status of circulation to foot
Dorsalis pedis	Along top of foot, between extension tendons of great and first toe	Site used to assess status of circulation to foot

Assessing the Radial and Apical Pulses

Delegation Considerations
The skill of pulse measurement can be delegated to unlicensed assistive personnel.
▪ Inform care giver of appropriate client position when obtaining apical pulse measurement.
▪ Inform care giver of appropriate duration of apical pulse count.
▪ Any abnormalities should be reported and reconfirmed by the nurse.

Equipment
▪ Stethoscope (apical pulse only)
▪ Wristwatch with second hand or digital display
▪ Pen, pencil, vital sign flow sheet, or record form
▪ Alcohol swab

STEPS	RATIONALE
1. Determine need to assess radial or apical pulse: a. Note risk factors for alterations in apical pulse.	Certain conditions place clients at risk for pulse alterations. Heart rhythm can be affected by heart disease, cardiac dysrhythmias, onset of sudden chest pain or acute pain from any site, invasive cardiovascular diagnostic tests, surgery, sudden infusion of large volume of IV fluid, internal or external hemorrhage, and administration of medications that alter heart function.
b. Assess for signs and symptoms of altered SV and CO such as dyspnea, fatigue, chest pain, orthopnea, syncope, palpitations (person's unpleasant awareness of heartbeat), jugular venous distention, edema of dependent body parts, cyanosis or pallor of skin.	Physical signs and symptoms may indicate alteration in cardiac function.
2. Assess for factors that normally influence apical pulse rate and rhythm:	Allows nurse to accurately assess presence and significance of pulse alterations.
a. Age	Normal pulse rates change with age (Table 23-4).
b. Exercise	Physical activity requires an increase in CO that is met by an increased HR and SV.
c. Position changes	Heart rate increases temporarily when changing from lying to sitting or standing position.

The plastic or rubber earpieces should fit snugly and comfortably in the nurse's ears. The binaurals should be angled and strong enough that the earpieces stay firmly in the ears without causing discomfort. To ensure the best reception of sound, the earpieces follow the contour of the ear canal, pointing toward the face when the stethoscope is in place.

The polyvinyl tubing should be flexible and 30 to 40 cm (12 to 18 inches) in length. Longer tubing decreases the transmission of sound waves. The tubing should be thick walled and moderately rigid to eliminate transmission of environmental noise and prevent the tubing from kinking, which distorts sound wave

TABLE 23-4
Acceptable Ranges of Heart Rate for Age

Age	Heart Rate (beats/min)
Infants	120-160/min
Toddlers	90-140/min
Preschoolers	80-110/min
School agers	75-100/min
Adolescent	60-90/min
Adult	60-100/min

Modified from Hazinski MF: Children are different. In Hazinski MF, editor: *Nursing care of the critically ill child*, St. Louis, 1984, Mosby; and Kinney MR and others: *AACN's clinical reference for critical care nursing*, ed 3, St. Louis, 1993, Mosby.

STEPS	RATIONALE
d. Medications	Antidysrhythmics, sympathomimetics, and cardiotonics affect rate and rhythm of pulse; large doses of narcotic analgesics can slow HR; general anesthetics slow HR; central nervous system stimulants such as caffeine can increase HR.
e. Temperature	Fever or exposure to warm environments increases HR; HR declines with hypothermia.
f. Emotional stress, anxiety, fear	Results in stimulation of the sympathetic nervous system, which increases HR.
3. Determine previous baseline apical rate (if available) from client's record.	Allows nurse to assess for change in condition. Provides comparison with future apical pulse measurements.
4. Explain that pulse or heart rate is to be assessed. Encourage client to relax and not speak.	Activity and anxiety can elevate heart rate. Client's voice interferes with nurse's ability to hear sound when apical pulse is measured.
5. Wash hands.	Reduces transmission of microorganisms.
6. If necessary, draw curtain around bed and/or close door.	Maintains privacy.
7. Obtain pulse measurement.	
A. Radial Pulse:	
(1) Assist client to assume a supine or sitting position.	Provides easy access to pulse sites.
(2) If supine, place client's forearm straight alongside or across lower chest or upper abdomen with wrist extended straight (see illustration). If sitting, bend client's elbow 90 degrees and support lower arm on chair or on nurse's arm. Slightly extend wrist with palm down.	Relaxed position of lower arm and extension of wrist permits full exposure of artery to palpation.
(3) Place tips of first two fingers of hand over groove along radial or thumb side of client's inner wrist (see illustration).	Fingertips are most sensitive parts of hand to palpate arterial pulsation. Nurse's thumb has pulsation that may interfere with accuracy.

Continued

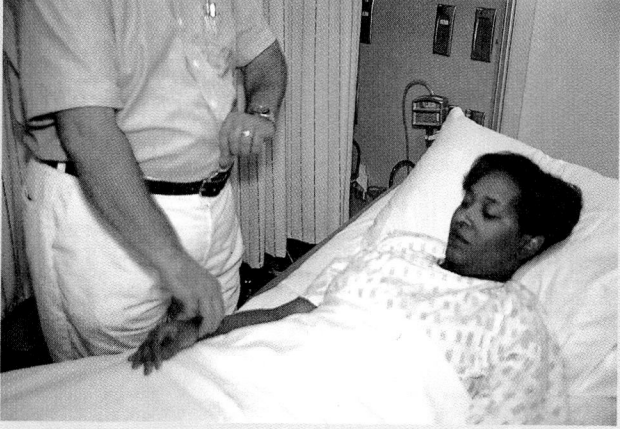

Step 7A(2)

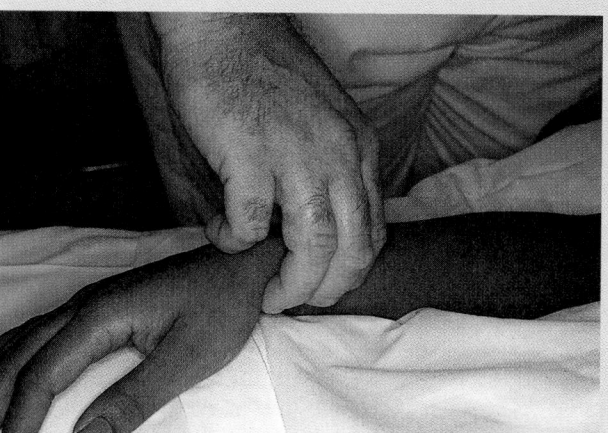

Step 7A(3)

Skill 23-2—cont'd
Assessing the Radial and Apical Pulses

STEPS	RATIONALE
(4) Lightly compress against radius, obliterate pulse initially, and then relax pressure so pulse becomes easily palpable.	Pulse is more accurately assessed with moderate pressure. Too much pressure occludes pulse and impairs blood flow.
(5) Determine strength of pulse. Note whether thrust of vessel against fingertips is bounding, strong, weak, or thready.	Strength reflects volume of blood ejected against arterial wall with each heart contraction.
(6) After pulse can be felt regularly, look at watch's second hand and begin to count rate: when sweep hand hits number on dial, start counting with zero, then one, two, and so on.	Rate is determined accurately only after nurse is assured pulse can be palpated. Timing begins with zero. Count of one is first beat palpated after timing begins.
(7) If pulse is regular, count rate for 30 seconds and multiply total by 2.	A 30-second count is accurate for rapid, slow, or regular pulse rates.
(8) If pulse is irregular, count rate for 60 seconds. Assess frequency and pattern of irregularity.	Inefficient contraction of heart fails to transmit pulse wave, interfering with CO, resulting in irregular pulse. Longer time ensures accurate count.

CRITICAL DECISION POINT

If pulse is irregular, assess for pulse deficit. Count apical pulse (Step 7B) while colleague counts radial pulse. Begin apical pulse count out loud to simultaneously assess pulses.

B. Apical Pulse:	
(1) Assist client to supine or sitting position. Move aside bed linen and gown to expose sternum and left side of chest.	Exposes portion of chest wall for selection of auscultatory site.
(2) Locate anatomical landmarks to identify the point of maximal impulse (PMI), also called the apical impulse. Heart is located behind and to left of sternum with base at top and apex at bottom. Find angle of Louis just below suprasternal notch between sternal body and manubrium; can be felt as a bony prominence. Slip fingers down each side of angle to find second intercostal space (ICS). Carefully move fingers down left side of sternum to fifth ICS and laterally to the left midclavicular line (MCL). A light tap felt within an area 1 to 2 cm (½ to 1 inch) of the PMI is reflected from the apex of the heart.	Use of anatomical landmarks allows correct placement of stethoscope over apex of heart, enhancing ability to hear heart sounds clearly. If unable to palpate the PMI, reposition client on left side. In the presence of serious heart disease, the PMI may be located to the left of the MCL or at the sixth ICS.
(3) Place diaphragm of stethoscope in palm of hand for 5 to 10 seconds.	Warming of metal or plastic diaphragm prevents client from being startled and promotes comfort.
(4) Place diaphragm of stethoscope over PMI at the fifth ICS, at left MCL, and auscultate for normal S_1 and S_2 heart sounds (heard as "lub dub") (see illustration).	Allow stethoscope tubing to extend straight without kinks that would distort sound transmission. Normal sounds S_1 and S_2 are high pitched and best heard with the diaphragm.

STEPS	RATIONALE
(5) When S₁ and S₂ are heard with regularity, use watch's second hand and begin to count rate: when sweep hand hits number on dial, start counting with zero, then one, two, and so on.	Apical rate is determined accurately only after nurse is able to auscultate sounds clearly. Timing begins with zero. Count of one is first sound auscultated after timing begins.
(6) If apical rate is regular, count for 30 seconds and multiply by 2.	Regular apical rate can be assessed within 30 seconds.
(7) If heart rate is irregular or client is receiving cardiovascular medication, count for 1 minute (60 seconds).	Irregular rate is more accurately assessed when measured over longer interval.
(8) Note regularity of any **dysrhythmia** (S₁ and S₂ occuring early or later after previous sequence of sounds; for example, every third or every fourth beat is skipped).	Regular occurrence of dysrhythmia within 1 minute may indicate inefficient contraction of heart and alteration in cardiac output.
(9) Replace client's gown and bed linen; assist client in returning to comfortable position.	Restores comfort and promotes sense of well-being.
(10) Clean earpieces and diaphragm of stethoscope with alcohol swab as needed (optional).	Controls transmission of microorganisms when nurses share stethoscope.
8. Discuss findings with client as needed.	Promotes participation in care and understanding of health status.
9. Wash hands.	Reduces transmission of microorganisms.
10. Compare readings with previous baseline and/or acceptable range of heart rate for client's age (see Table 23-4).	Evaluates for change in condition and alterations.
11. Compare peripheral pulse rate with apical rate and note discrepancy.	Differences between measurements indicate pulse deficit and may warn of cardiovascular compromise. Abnormalities may require therapy.
12. Compare radial pulse equality and note discrepancy.	Differences between radial arteries indicate compromised peripheral vascular system.
13. Correlate pulse rate with data obtained from blood pressure and related signs and symptoms (palpitations, dizziness).	Pulse rate and blood pressure are interrelated.

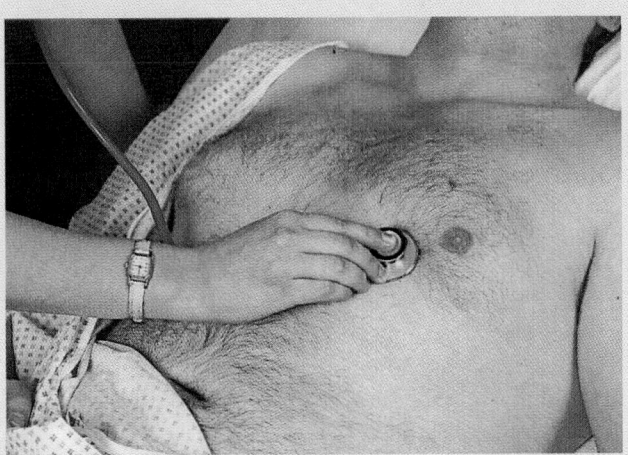

Step 7B(4)

Recording and Reporting

▪ Record pulse rate with assessment site in nurses' notes or vital signs flow sheet. Measurement of pulse rate after administration of specific therapies should be documented in narrative form in nurses' notes.

▪ Report abnormal findings to nurse in charge or physician.

Home Care Considerations

▪ Assess home environment to determine room that will afford quiet environment for auscultating apical rate.

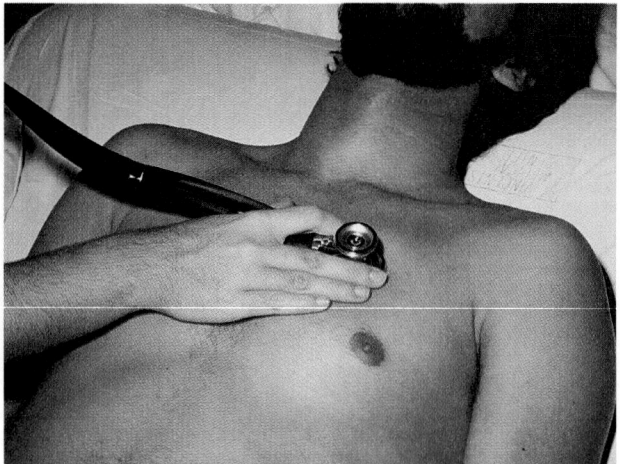

Figure 23-6. Positioning the diaphragm of the stethoscope.

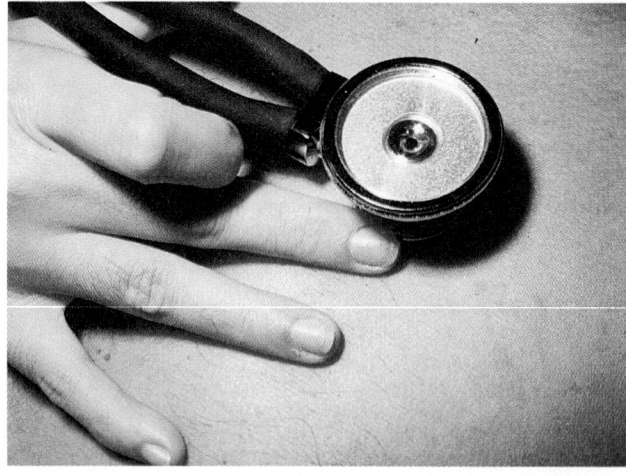

Figure 23-7. Positioning the bell of the stethoscope.

transmission. Stethoscopes can have single or dual tubes.

The chestpiece consists of a bell and a diaphragm. The diaphragm is the circular, flat-surfaced portion of the chestpiece covered with a thin plastic disk. It transmits high-pitched sounds created by the high velocity movement of air and blood. Bowel, lung, and heart sounds are auscultated using the diaphragm. The nurse positions the diaphragm to make a tight seal against the client's skin (Figure 23-6). Enough pressure is exerted to leave a temporary red ring on the client's skin when the diaphragm is removed.

The bell is the bowl-shaped chestpiece usually surrounded by a rubber ring. The ring avoids chilling the client with cold metal when placed on the skin. The bell transmits low-pitched sounds created by the low-velocity movement of blood. Heart and vascular sounds are auscultated using the bell. The nurse applies the bell lightly, resting the chestpiece on the skin (Figure 23-7). Compressing the bell against the skin reduces low-pitched sound amplification and creates a "diaphragm of skin." The bell and diaphragm are rotated into position on the chestpiece, depending on which part the nurse chooses to use. The size of the stethoscope chestpiece varies from small, used for infants and young children, to large. The nurse determines the appropriate size chestpiece by assessing the surface area to be auscultated.

Assessment of Pulse

Pulse rate. Before measuring a pulse, the nurse reviews the client's baseline rate for comparison (see Table 23-4 on p. 452). When assessing the pulse, the nurse must consider the variety of factors influencing pulse rate (Table 23-5). A combination of these factors may cause significant changes. If the nurse detects an abnormal rate while palpating a peripheral pulse, the next step is to assess the apical rate. The apical rate requires

auscultation of the heart sounds, which provides a more accurate assessment of cardiac contraction.

The nurse assesses the **apical pulse** by listening for heart sounds (see Chapter 24). The nurse tries to identify the first and second heart sounds (S_1 and S_2). At normal slow rates, S_1 is low pitched and dull in quality, sounding like a "lub." S_2 is a higher pitched and shorter sound and creates the sound "dub." Each set of "lub-dub" is counted as one heartbeat. Using the diaphragm or bell of the stethoscope, the nurse counts the number of "lub-dubs" occurring in 1 minute.

Peripheral and apical pulse rate assessment may reveal variations in heart rate. Two common abnormalities in pulse rate are **tachycardia** and **bradycardia.** Tachycardia is an abnormally elevated heart rate, above 100 beats per minute in adults. Bradycardia is a slow rate, below 60 beats per minute in adults.

Pulse rhythm. Normally a regular interval of time occurs between each pulse or heartbeat. An interval interrupted by an early or late beat or a missed beat indicates an abnormal rhythm or dysrhythmia. A dysrhythmia may alter cardiac output, particularly if it occurs repetitively. The nurse identifies a dysrhythmia by palpating an interruption in successive pulse waves or auscultating an interruption between heart sounds. If a dysrhythmia is present, the regularity of its occurrence should be assessed. Dysrhythmias may be described as regularly irregular or irregularly irregular. The physician may order additional tests to evaluate the occurrence of dysrhythmias (see Chapter 30).

An inefficient contraction of the heart that fails to transmit a pulse wave to the peripheral pulse site creates a **pulse deficit.** To assess a pulse deficit the nurse and a colleague assess radial and apical rates simultaneously and then compare rates. The difference between the apical and radial pulse rates is the pulse deficit. Pulse deficits are frequently associated with dysrhythmias.

TABLE 23-5

Factors Influencing Pulse Rates

Factor	Increase Pulse Rate	Decrease Pulse Rate
Exercise	Short-term exercise	Long-term exercise conditions the heart, resulting in lower rate at rest and quicker return to resting level after exercise
Temperature	Fever and heat	Hypothermia
Emotions	Acute pain and anxiety increase sympathetic stimulation, affecting heart rate	Unrelieved severe pain increases parasympathetic stimulation, affecting heart rate; relaxation
Drugs	Positive chronotropic drugs such as atropine	Negative chronotropic drugs such as digitalis
Hemorrhage	Loss of blood increases sympathetic stimulation	
Postural changes	Standing or sitting	Lying down
Pulmonary conditions	Diseases causing poor oxygenation	

Strength and equality. The strength or amplitude of a pulse reflects the volume of blood ejected against the arterial wall with each heart contraction and the condition of the arterial vascular system leading to the pulse site. Normally the pulse strength remains the same with each heartbeat. The nurse assesses both radial pulses to compare the characteristics of each. A pulse in one arm may be unequal in strength or absent in many disease states. Pulse strength may be graded or described as strong, weak, thready, or bounding. Evaluating pulse strength and equality is included during assessment of the vascular system (see Chapter 30).

BLOOD PRESSURE

Systemic or arterial blood pressure, the blood pressure in the system of arteries in the body, is a good indicator of cardiovascular health. Blood pressure is the lateral force on the walls of an artery created by the pulsing blood under pressure from the heart. Blood flows throughout the circulatory system because of pressure changes, moving from an area of high pressure to an area of low pressure. The heart's contraction ejects blood under high pressure into the aorta. The peak of maximum pressure when ejection occurs is the **systolic** blood pressure. When the heart relaxes, the blood remaining in the arteries exerts a minimum or **diastolic** pressure. Diastolic pressure is the lowest pressure exerted against the arterial walls at all times.

The standard unit for measuring blood pressure is millimeters of mercury (mm Hg). The measurement indicates the height to which the blood pressure can raise a column of mercury. Blood pressure is recorded as a ratio with the systolic reading before the diastolic

(e.g., 120/80). The difference between systolic and diastolic pressure is the **pulse pressure.** For a blood pressure of 120/80, the pulse pressure is 40.

Physiology of Arterial Blood Pressure

Blood pressure reflects the interrelationships of cardiac output, peripheral vascular resistance, blood volume, blood viscosity, and artery elasticity.

Cardiac output. A person's cardiac output is the volume of blood pumped by the heart (stroke volume) during 1 minute (heart rate):

$$CO = HR \times SV$$

The blood pressure (BP) depends on the cardiac output (CO) and peripheral vascular resistance (R):

$$BP = CO \times R$$

When volume increases in an enclosed space, such as a blood vessel, the pressure in that space rises. Thus as cardiac output increases, more blood is pumped against arterial walls, causing the blood pressure to rise. Cardiac output can increase as a result of greater heart muscle contractility, an increase in heart rate, or an increase in blood volume.

Peripheral resistance. Blood circulates through a network of arteries, arterioles, capillaries, venules, and veins. Arteries and arterioles are surrounded by smooth muscle that contracts or relaxes to change the diameter of the lumen. The size of arteries and arterioles changes to adjust blood flow to the needs of local tissues. For example, when more blood is needed by a major organ, the peripheral arteries constrict, decreasing their supply of blood. More blood becomes available to the major organ because of the resistance change in the peripheral arteries. Peripheral vascular resistance is the resistance to blood flow determined by the tone of vascular musculature and diameter of blood vessels. The smaller the lumen of a vessel, the greater peripheral vascular resistance to blood flow. As resistance rises, arterial blood pressure rises. As vessels dilate and resistance falls, blood pressure drops.

Blood volume. The volume of blood circulating within the vascular system affects blood pressure. Most adults have a constant circulating blood volume of 5000 ml. However, if volume increases, more pressure is exerted against arterial walls. For example, the rapid, uncontrolled infusion of intravenous fluids ele-

vates blood pressure. When circulating blood volume falls, as in the case of hemorrhage or dehydration, blood pressure falls.

Viscosity. The thickness or viscosity of blood affects the ease with which blood flows through small vessels. The hematocrit, or percentage of red blood cells in the blood, determines blood viscosity. When the hematocrit rises and blood flow slows, arterial blood pressure increases. The heart must contract more forcefully to move the viscous blood through the circulatory system.

Elasticity. Normally the walls of an artery are elastic and easily stretched. As pressure within the arteries increases, the diameter of vessel walls increases to accommodate the pressure change. Arterial distensibility

---

Box 23-4
Factors Influencing Blood Pressure

Age

Blood pressure tends to rise with advancing age:

Age	Arterial Pressure (mm Hg)
Newborn (3000 g [6.6 1b])	40 (mean)
1 month	85/54
1 year	95/65
6 years	105/65
10-13 years	110/65
14-17 years	120/75
Middle adult	120/80
Older adult	140-160/80-90

Level of a child's or adolescent's blood pressure is assessed with respect to body size and age. Larger children have higher blood pressures than smaller children of the same age. Older adults have a rise in systolic pressure related to decreased elasticity.

Stress

Anxiety, fear, and pain can initially increase blood pressure because of increased heart rate, increased cardiac output, and increased peripheral vascular resistance. (If the stressor is not relieved, the blood pressure falls.)

Gender

There is no clinically significant difference in blood pressure levels between boys and girls.

After puberty, males have higher readings.

With menopause, women tend to have higher levels of blood pressure than men of the same age.

Race

The incidence of hypertension is greater in blacks than whites because of genetic and environmental influences.

Daily Variation

Variations may include a lower blood pressure during sleep, highest blood pressure in the afternoon, a fall in the evening, and a rise beginning at 4 to 6 AM.

Medications

Some medications directly or indirectly affect blood pressure. Antihypertensive medications including diuretics, β-adrenergic blockers, vasodilators, ACE inhibitors, and calcium-channel blockers lower blood pressure. Narcotic analgesics can lower blood pressure. Vasoconstrictors and intravenous fluids such as normal saline can increase blood pressure.

Activity

Older adults often experience a 5 to 10 mm Hg fall in blood pressure about 1 hour after eating.

Blood pressure can be reduced for several hours after a period of vigorous exercise.

Data from Pickering TG: *Lancet* 344(8914):31, 1994; Thomas SA, DeKeyser F: *Annu Rev Nurs Res* 14:3, 1996; and from Task Force on Blood Pressure Control in Children: *Pediatrics* 79:1, 1987.

prevents wide fluctuations in blood pressure. When arterial elasticity is reduced there is greater resistance to blood flow. As a result, when the heart ejects its stroke volume, the vessels no longer yield to pressure. Instead, a given volume of blood is forced through the rigid arteries and the systemic blood pressure rises. Systolic pressure is more significantly elevated than diastolic pressure as a result of reduced arterial elasticity.

Blood Pressure Variations

Blood pressure is continually influenced by many factors during the day. A single blood pressure measurement cannot adequately reflect a client's blood pressure. Blood pressure trends, not individual measurements, guide nursing interventions. Understanding the factors that influence blood pressure ensures a more accurate interpretation of blood pressure readings. Box 23-4 summarizes factors affecting blood pressure.

Hypertension. The most common alteration in blood pressure is **hypertension,** an often asymptomatic disorder characterized by persistently elevated blood pressure. The diagnosis of hypertension in adults is made when an average of two or more diastolic readings on at least two subsequent visits is 90 mm Hg or higher or when the average of two or more systolic readings on at least two subsequent visits is consistently higher than 140 mm Hg. Categories of hypertension have been developed and determine medical intervention (Table 23-6).

One elevated blood pressure measurement does not qualify as a diagnosis of hypertension. However, if the nurse assesses a high reading during the first blood pressure measurement (e.g., 150/90 mm Hg), the client should be encouraged to return for another checkup at least within 2 months (Table 23-7).

Persons with a family history of hypertension are at significant risk. Obesity, cigarette smoking, heavy alco-

---

TABLE 23-6

Classification of Blood Pressure for Adults Age 18 Years and Older*

Category	Systolic (mm Hg)	Diastolic (mm Hg)
Normal†	<130	<85
High normal	130-139	85-89
Hypertension‡		
STAGE 1 (Mild)	140-159	90-99
STAGE 2 (Moderate)	160-179	100-109
STAGE 3 (Severe)	180-209	110-119
STAGE 4 (Very Severe)	≥210	≥120

Modified from National High Blood Pressure Education Program; National Heart, Lung and Blood Institute; National Institutes of Health: *The fifth report of the Joint National Committee on Detection, Evaluation and Treatment of High Blood Pressure,* NIH Pub No. 93-1088, Bethesda, Md, NIH, January 1993.

*Not taking antihypertensive drugs and not acutely ill. When systolic and diastolic pressures fall into different categories, the higher category should be selected to classify the individual's blood pressure status. For instance, 160/92 mm Hg should be classified as Stage 2, and 180/120 mm Hg should be classified as Stage 4. Isolated systolic hypertension (ISH) is defined as SBP ≥140 mm Hg and DBP < 90 mm Hg and staged appropriately (e.g., 170/85 mm Hg is defined as Stage 2 ISH).

†Optimal blood pressure with respect to cardiovascular risk is SBP < 120 mm Hg and DBP < 80 mm Hg. However, unusually low readings should be evaluated for clinical significance.

‡Based on the average of two or more readings taken at each of two or more visits following an initial screening.

Note: In addition to classifying stages of hypertension based on average blood pressure levels, the clinician should specify presence or absence of target-organ disease and additional risk factors. For example, a client with diabetes and a blood pressure of 142/94 mm Hg plus left ventricular hypertrophy should be classified as "Stage 1 hypertension with target-organ disease (left ventricular hypertrophy) and with another major risk factor (diabetes)." The specificity is important for risk classification and management.

TABLE 23-7

Recommendations for Follow-up Based on Initial Set of Blood Pressure Measurements for Adults Age 18 and Older

Initial Screening Blood Pressure (mm Hg)*		
Systolic	Diastolic	Follow-up Recommended†
<130	<85	Recheck in 2 years
130-139	85-89	Recheck in 1 year ‡
140-159	90-99	Confirm within 2 months
160-179	100-109	Evaluate or refer to source of care within 1 month
180-209	110-119	Evaluate or refer to source of care within 1 week
≥210	≥120	Evaluate or refer to source of care immediately

From National High Blood Pressure Education Program; National Heart, Lung and Blood Institute; National Institutes of Health: *The fifth report of the Joint National Committee on Detection, Evaluation and Treatment of High Blood Pressure,* NIH Pub No-93-1088, Bethesda, Md, NIH, January 1993.

*If the systolic and diastolic categories are different, follow recommendations for the shorter time follow-up (e.g., 160/85 mm Hg should be evaluated or referred to source of care within 1 month).

†The scheduling of follow-up should be modified by reliable information about past blood pressure measurements, other cardiovascular risk factors, or target-organ disease.

‡Consider providing advice about lifestyle modifications (see Chapter 22).

hol consumption, high blood cholesterol levels, and continued exposure to stress are also linked to hypertension.

Hypotension. Hypotension is considered present when the systolic blood pressure falls to 90 mm Hg or below. Although some adults have low blood pressure normally, hypotension is an abnormal finding. Hypotension occurs when arteries dilate, the peripheral vascular resistance decreases, the circulating blood volume decreases, or the heart fails to provide adequate cardiac output. Signs and symptoms associated with hypotension include pallor, skin mottling, clamminess, confusion, dizziness, chest pain, increased heart rate, and decreased urine output. Hypotension is life threatening and is reported to the physician immediately.

Assessment of Blood Pressure

Arterial blood pressure may be measured either directly (invasively) or indirectly (noninvasively). The direct method requires the insertion of a thin catheter into an artery. The more common noninvasive method requires use of the **sphygmomanometer** and stethoscope. The nurse measures blood pressure indirectly by auscultation or palpation. Auscultation is the most widely used technique (Skill 23-3).

Blood pressure equipment. Before assessing blood pressure the nurse must be comfortable in using a sphygmomanometer and stethoscope. A sphygmomanometer includes a pressure manometer, an occlusive cuff that encloses an inflatable rubber bladder, and a pressure bulb with a release valve to inflate the cuff. The two types of sphygmomanometers are the aneroid and the mercury (Figure 23-8). The aneroid manometer has a glass-enclosed circular gauge containing a needle that registers millimeter calibrations. A metal bellows within the gauge expands and collapses in response to pressure variations in the inflated cuff.

Aneroid manometers have the advantages of being lightweight, portable, and compact. Because metal parts in the aneroid model are subject to temperature expansion or contraction, the aneroid instrument is less reliable than the mercury type. Aneroid sphygmomanometers require biomedical calibration at routine intervals to verify their accuracy.

Mercury manometers are more accurate than aneroid manometers. Repeated calibrations are not necessary. The mercury manometer is an upright tube containing mercury. Pressure created by the inflation of the compression cuff moves the column of mercury upward against the force of gravity. Millimeter calibrations mark the height of the mercury column. To ensure accurate readings, the mercury column should fall freely as pressure is released and should always be at zero when the cuff is deflated. Mercury manometers may be wall mounted or portable. Accurate readings are obtained by looking at the meniscus of the mercury at eye level.

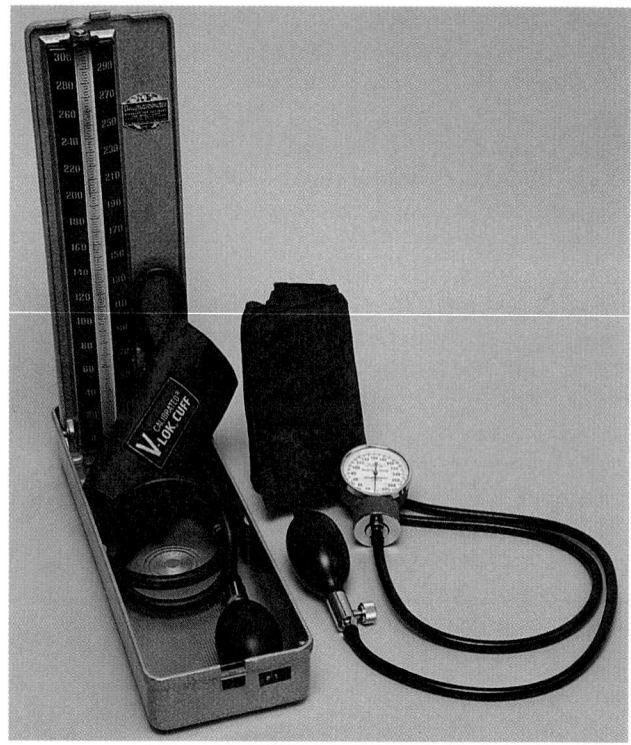

Figure 23-8. Sphygmomanometers.

Looking up or down at the mercury results in distorted readings.

Cloth or disposable vinyl compression cuffs used with the sphygmomanometer come in several sizes. The size selected is proportional to the circumference of the limb being assessed. Ideally, the width of the cuff should be 40% of the circumference (or 20% wider than the diameter) of the midpoint of the limb on which the cuff is to be used. The bladder, enclosed by the cuff, should encircle at least 80% of the arm of an adult and the entire arm of a child (Perloff and others, 1993). The lower edge of the cuff should be above the antecubital fossa, allowing room for placement of the stethoscope. An improperly fitting cuff causes inaccurate blood pressure measurement.

Auscultation. The best environment for blood pressure measurement by auscultation is a quiet room at a comfortable temperature. Although the client may lie or stand, sitting is the preferred position. The client's position should be the same during each blood pressure measurement to permit a meaningful comparison of values. Before assessment the nurse should attempt to control factors responsible for artificially high readings such as pain, anxiety, or exertion.

In some clients, however, blood pressure changes with position. The nurse may compare sitting and standing blood pressure readings to determine whether a change occurs. **Orthostatic** or **postural hypotension**

Measuring Blood Pressure (BP)

Delegation Considerations

The skill of blood pressure measurement can be delegated to unlicensed assistive personnel.

- Inform care giver of appropriate client position when obtaining blood pressure measurement.
- Inform care giver if client has alterations affecting the appropriate limb for blood pressure measurement.
- Inform care giver of appropriate size blood pressure cuff for designated extremity.

- Inform care giver if client is at risk for orthostatic hypotension and how to measure.

Equipment

- Mercury or aneroid sphygmomanometer
- Cloth or disposable vinyl pressure cuff of appropriate size for client's extremity
- Stethoscope
- Alcohol swab
- Pen, pencil, vital sign flow sheet or record form

STEPS	RATIONALE
1. Determine need to assess client's BP: a. Note risk factors for alteration in BP.	Certain conditions place clients at risk for BP alteration: history of cardiovascular disease, renal disease, diabetes, circulatory shock (hypovolemic, septic, cardiogenic, or neurogenic), acute or chronic pain, rapid IV infusion of fluids or blood products, increased intracranial pressure, postoperative conditions, toxemia of pregnancy.
b. Observe for signs and symptoms of BP alterations: (1) High BP (hypertension) is often asymptomatic until pressure is very high. Assess for headache (usually occipital), flushing of face, nosebleed, and fatigue in older adults. (2) Low BP (hypotension) is associated with dizziness; mental confusion; restlessness; pale, dusky, or cyanotic skin and mucous membranes; cool, mottled skin over extremities.	Physical signs and symptoms may indicate alterations in BP.
2. Determine best site for BP assessment. Avoid applying cuff to extremity when: intravenous fluids infusing; an arteriovenous shunt or fistula is present; breast or axillary surgery has been performed on that side; extremity has been traumatized, diseased, or requires a cast or bulky bandage. The lower extremities may be used when the brachial arteries are inaccessible.	Inappropriate site selection may result in poor amplification of sounds, causing inaccurate readings. Application of pressure from inflated bladder temporarily impairs blood flow and can further compromise circulation in extremity that already has impaired blood flow.
3. Determine previous baseline BP (if available) from client's record.	Allows nurse to assess for change in condition. Provides comparison with future BP measurements.
4. Encourage client to avoid exercise and smoking for 30 minutes before assessment of BP.	Exercise and smoking can cause false elevations in BP.
5. Have client assume sitting or lying position. Be sure room is warm, quiet, and relaxing.	Maintains client's comfort during measurement. The client's perceptions that the physical or interpersonal environment is stressful affect the BP measurement (Thomas and others, 1993).
6. Explain to client that BP is to be assessed and have client rest at least 5 minutes before measurement. Ask client not to speak when BP is being measured.	Reduces anxiety that can falsely elevate readings. Blood pressure readings taken at different times can be objectively compared when assessed with client at rest. Talking to a client when the BP is being assessed increases readings 10% to 40% (Thomas and DeKeyser, 1996).

Continued

Skill 23-3—cont'd
Measuring Blood Pressure (BP)

STEPS	RATIONALE
7. Obtain blood pressure.	
A. Ausculation method:	
(1) Wash hands.	Reduces transmission of microorganisms.
(2) With client sitting or lying, position client's forearm, supported if needed, with palm turned up (see illustration).	If arm is unsupported, client may perform isometric exercise that can increase diastolic pressure 10%. Placement of arm above the level of the heart causes false low reading.
(3) Expose upper arm fully by removing constricting clothing.	Ensures proper cuff application.
(4) Palpate brachial artery (see illustration). Position cuff 2.5 cm (1 inch) above site of brachial pulsation (antecubital space). Center bladder of cuff above artery (see illustration). With cuff fully deflated, wrap cuff evenly and snugly around upper arm (see illustration).	Inflating bladder directly over brachial artery ensures proper pressure is applied during inflation. Loose-fitting cuff causes false high readings.

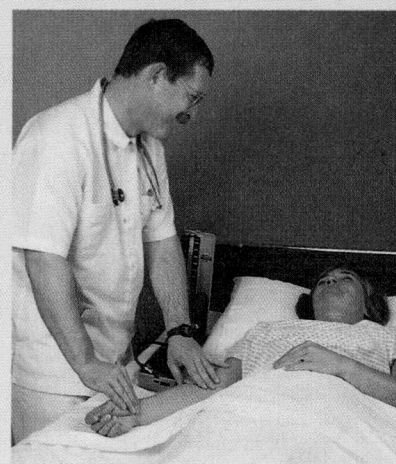

Step 7A(2)

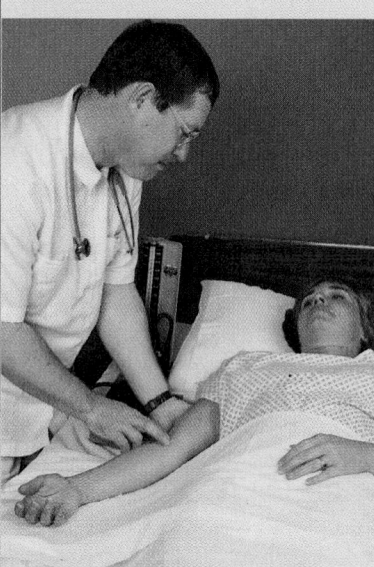
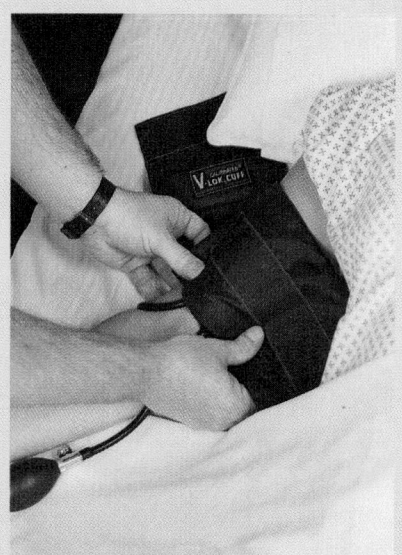
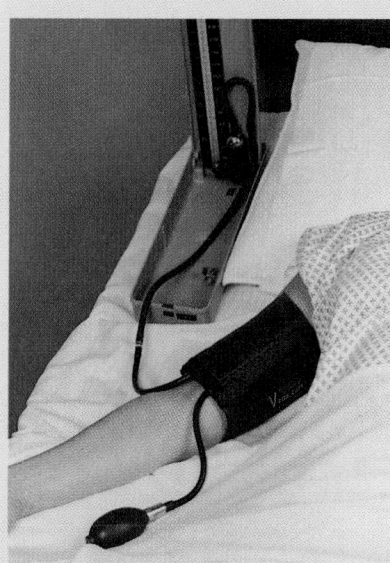

Step 7A(4)

STEPS	RATIONALE
(5) Position manometer vertically at eye level. Observer should be no farther than 1 m (approximately 1 yard) away.	Accurate readings are obtained by looking at the meniscus of the mercury at eye level. The meniscus is the point where the crescent-shaped top of the mercury column aligns with the manometer scale. Looking up or down at the mercury results in distorted readings.
(6) Palpate brachial or radial artery with fingertips of one hand while inflating cuff rapidly to pressure 30 mm Hg above point at which pulse disappears. Slowly deflate cuff and note point when pulse reappears.	Identifies approximate systolic pressure and determines maximal inflation point for accurate reading. Prevents auscultatory gap. If unable to palpate artery because of weakened pulse, an ultrasonic stethoscope can be used (see Chapter 24).
(7) Deflate cuff fully and wait 30 seconds.	Prevents venous congestion and false high readings.
(8) Place stethoscope earpieces in ears and be sure sounds are clear, not muffled.	Each earpiece should follow angle of ear canal to facilitate hearing.
(9) Relocate brachial artery and place bell or diaphragm chestpiece of stethoscope over it. Do not allow chestpiece to touch cuff or clothing (see illustration).	Proper stethoscope placement ensures optimal sound reception. Stethoscope improperly positioned causes muffled sounds that often result in false low systolic and false high diastolic readings.
(10) Close valve of pressure bulb clockwise until tight.	Tightening of valve prevents air leak during inflation.
(11) Inflate cuff to 30 mm Hg above palpated systolic pressure (see illustration).	Ensures accurate measurement of systolic pressure.
(12) Slowly release valve and allow mercury to fall at rate of 2 to 3 mm Hg/sec.	Too rapid or slow a decline in mercury level can cause inaccurate readings.
(13) Note point on manometer when first clear sound is heard.	First Korotkoff sound indicates systolic pressure.
(14) Continue to deflate cuff, noting point at which muffled or dampened sound appears.	Fourth Korotkoff sound involves distinct muffling of sounds and is recommended as indication of diastolic pressure in children (Perloff and others, 1993).

Continued

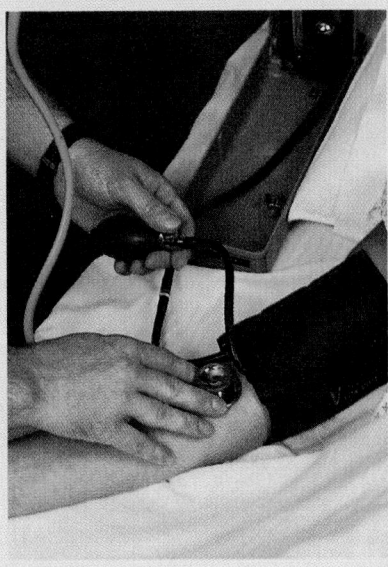

Step 7A(9)

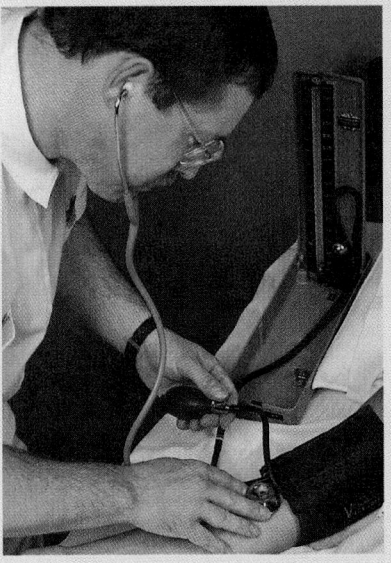

Step 7A(11)

Skill 23-3—cont'd
Measuring Blood Pressure (BP)

STEPS	RATIONALE
(15) Continue to deflate cuff gradually, noting point at which sound disappears in adults. Note pressure to nearest 2 mm Hg.	Beginning of the fifth Korotkoff sound is recommended by American Heart Association as indication of diastolic pressure in adults (Perloff and others, 1993).
(16) Deflate cuff rapidly and completely. Remove cuff from client's arm unless measurement must be repeated.	Continuous cuff inflation causes arterial occlusion, resulting in numbness and tingling of client's arm.
(17) If this is first assessment of client, repeat procedure on other arm.	Comparison of BP in both arms detects circulatory problems. (Normal difference of 5 to 10 mm Hg exists between arms.)
8. Assist client in returning to comfortable position and cover upper arm if previously clothed.	Restores comfort and promotes sense of well-being.
9. Discuss findings with client as needed.	Promotes participation in care and understanding of health status.
10. Wash hands.	Reduces transmission of microorganisms.
11. Compare reading with previous baseline and/or acceptable value of blood pressure for client's age.	Evaluates for change in condition and alterations.
12. Compare blood pressure in both arms.	Arm with higher pressure should be used for subsequent assessments unless contraindicated.
13. Correlate blood pressure with data obtained from pulse assessment and related cardiovascular signs and symptoms.	Blood pressure and heart rate are interrelated.

Recording and Reporting
- Inform client of value and need for periodic reassessment.
- Record blood pressure in nurses' notes or vital sign flow sheet. Measurement of blood pressure after administration of specific therapies should be documented in narrative form in nurses' notes.
- Report abnormal findings to nurse in charge or physician.

Home Care Considerations
- Assess home noise level to determine room that will provide quietest environment for assessing BP.
- Consider electronic blood pressure cuff for home if client has hearing difficulties and if client has sufficient financial resources.

is the lowering of blood pressure when the client moves from a sitting to a standing position. Dizziness, lightheadedness, and even syncope (fainting) are frequent findings associated with orthostatic hypotension. Orthostatic hypotension may be a symptom of fluid volume deficit or inadequate neurovascular control.

Antihypertensive medications may cause orthostatic blood pressure changes. Blood pressure should always be measured before administering such medications. When recording orthostatic blood pressure measurements, the nurse records the client's position in addition to the blood pressure measurement. For example: 140/80 supine, 132/72 sitting, 108/60 standing. The

readings are obtained 1 to 3 minutes after the client changes position.

During the initial assessment the nurse should obtain and record the blood pressure in both arms. Normally there is a difference of 5 to 10 mm Hg between the arms. In subsequent assessments the blood pressure should be measured in the arm with the higher pressure. Pressure differences greater than 10 mm Hg indicate problems in the arm with the lower pressure.

Indirect measurement of arterial blood pressure works on a basic principle of pressure. Blood flows freely through an artery until an inflated cuff applies pressure to tissues and causes the artery to collapse. After the cuff pressure is released, the point at which blood flow returns and sound appears through auscultation is the systolic pressure.

Korotkoff, a Russian surgeon, first described the sounds heard over an artery during cuff deflation in 1905. The first **Korotkoff sound** is a clear, rhythmical tapping corresponding to the pulse rate that gradually increases in intensity. Onset of the sound corresponds to the systolic pressure. A murmur or swishing sound appears as the cuff continues to deflate, the second Korotkoff sound. As the artery distends, there is a turbulence in blood flow. The third Korotkoff sound is a crisper and more intense tapping. The fourth Korotkoff sound becomes muffled and low pitched as the cuff is further deflated. Cuff pressure falls below the pressure within the vessel walls; this sound is the diastolic pressure in infants and children. The fifth Korotkoff sound is an absence of sound; in adolescents and adults, this sound corresponds with the diastolic pressure (Figure 23-9).

The American Heart Association (Joint National Committee, 1993) recommends recording two numbers for a blood pressure measurement: the point on the manometer when the first sound is heard for systolic and the point on the manometer when the fifth sound is heard for diastolic. Some institutions recommend recording the point when the fourth sound is heard as well, especially for clients with hypertension. The numbers are divided by slashed lines (e.g., 120/80, 120/100/80), and the arm used to measure the blood pressure is noted (e.g., RA 130/70).

Many decisions and nursing interventions about a client's health care are made on the basis of blood pressure findings. The importance of obtaining an accurate blood pressure cannot be overemphasized. There are several possibilities for error if the auscultation procedure is not followed correctly (Table 23-8). When the nurse is unsure of a reading, a colleague should reassess the blood pressure.

Assessment in children. The Task Force on Blood Pressure Control in Children (1987) recommends that all children 3 years of age through adolescence should have blood pressures checked at least yearly. Blood pressure in children changes with growth and development. The nurse can help parents to understand the importance of this routine screening to detect children who may be at risk for hypertension. The measurement of blood pressure in infants and children is difficult for several reasons.

1. Different arm size requires careful and appropriate cuff size selection.
2. Readings are difficult to obtain in restless or anxious infants and children.
3. Placing stethoscope too firmly on the antecubital fossa can cause errors in auscultation sounds.

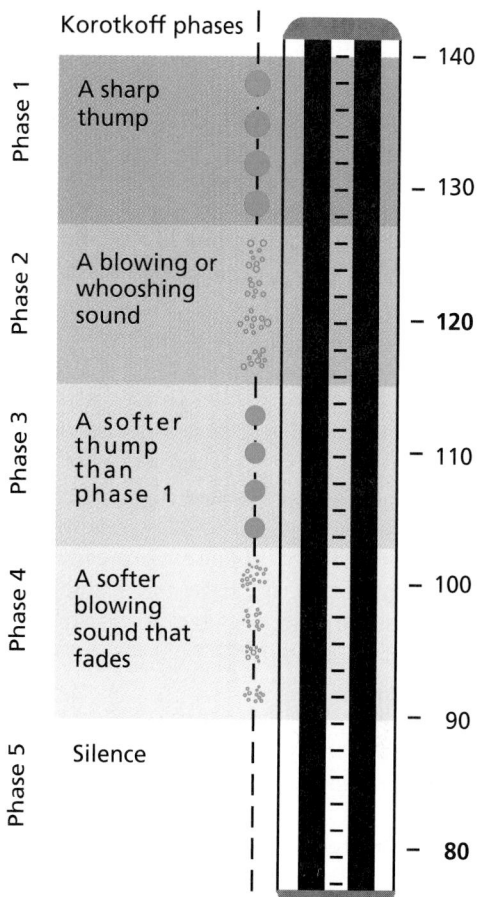

Figure 23-9. The sounds auscultated during blood pressure measurement can be differentiated into five Korotkoff phases. In this example, the blood pressure is 140/90.

4. Korotkoff sounds are difficult to hear in children because of low frequency and amplitude.

The same auscultation method used with adults is appropriate for children. An infant or child under 5 years of age should lie supine with the arms supported at heart level. Older children may sit. It is important to have the child relaxed and calm. A delay of at least 15 minutes before taking a reading is recommended to allow the child to recover from recent activity or apprehension. Those 15 minutes can be used for other quiet nursing activities. It may help to have a parent nearby. The nurse should prepare the child for the blood pressure cuff's unusual sensation during inflation. Most children understand the analogy of a "tight hug on your arm" and will be more cooperative.

Ultrasonic stethoscope. If a nurse is unable to auscultate sounds because of a weakened arterial pulse, an ultrasonic stethoscope can be used (see Chapter 24). This stethoscope allows the nurse to hear low-frequency systolic sounds and is commonly used when

TABLE 23-8
Common Mistakes in Blood Pressure Assessment

Error	Effect
Bladder or cuff too wide	False low reading
Bladder or cuff too narrow	False high reading
Cuff wrapped too loosely or unevenly	False high reading
Deflating cuff too slowly	False high diastolic reading
Deflating cuff too quickly	False low systolic and false high diastolic reading
Arm below heart level	False high reading
Arm above heart level	False low reading
Arm not supported	False high reading
Stethoscope that fits poorly or impairment of the examiner's hearing, causing sounds to be muffled	False low systolic and false high diastolic reading
Stethoscope applied too firmly against antecubital fossa	False low diastolic reading
Inflating too slowly	False high diastolic reading
Repeating assessments too quickly	False low systolic reading
Inaccurate inflation level	Inaccurate interpretation of systolic and diastolic readings
Multiple examiners using different Korotkoff sounds for diastolic readings	False high systolic and low diastolic reading

Box 23-5
Procedural Guidelines for Palpating the Systolic Blood Pressure

1. Apply blood pressure cuff to the upper arm in the same manner as the auscultation method.
2. Palpate the radial artery.
3. Inflate blood pressure cuff 30 mm Hg above the point at which the radial pulse can no longer be palpated.
4. Release valve and allow mercury to fall 2 mm Hg per second.
5. As soon as the radial pulse is palpable, note the manometer reading.

measuring the blood pressure of infants and children, and low blood pressure in adults.

Palpation. Indirect measurement of blood pressure by palpation is useful for clients whose arterial pulsations are too weak to create Korotkoff sounds. Severe blood loss and weakened heart contractility are examples of conditions that result in blood pressures too low to auscultate accurately. Only the systolic blood pressure can be assessed by palpation (Box 23-5). The diastolic pressure is difficult to determine by palpation. A subtle change in sensation, usually in the form of a thin, snapping vibration, marks the diastolic level. When the palpation technique is used, the systolic value and the manner in which it was measured are recorded (e.g., RA 78/-, palpated).

The palpation technique is used along with auscultation in some instances. In some hypertensive clients, the sounds usually heard over the brachial artery when the cuff pressure is high disappear as pressure is reduced and then reappear at a lower level. This temporary disappearance of sound is the **auscultatory gap.** It typically occurs between the first and second Korotkoff sounds. The gap in sound may cover a range of 40 mm Hg and thus may cause an underestimation of systolic pressure or overestimation of diastolic pressure. The examiner must be certain to inflate the cuff high enough to hear the true systolic pressure before the auscultatory gap. Palpation of the radial artery helps to determine how high to inflate the cuff. The examiner inflates the cuff 30 mm Hg above the pressure at which the radial pulse was palpated. The range of pressures in which the auscultatory gap occurs is recorded (e.g., "BP RA 180/94 with an auscultatory gap from 180 to 160").

Assessment of lower extremities. Dressings, casts, intravenous catheters, or arteriovenous fistulas or shunts can make the upper extremities inaccessible. Blood pressure must then be measured in the lower extremities. Comparing upper extremity blood pressure with that in the legs is also necessary for clients with certain cardiac and blood pressure abnormalities. The popliteal artery, palpable behind the knee in the popliteal space, is the site for auscultation. The cuff is positioned with the bladder over the posterior aspect of the midthigh. The cuff must be wide and long enough to allow for the larger girth of the thigh. Placing the client in a prone position is best. If such a position is impossible, the client should be asked to flex the knee slightly for easier access to the artery. The procedure is identical to brachial artery auscultation. Systolic pressure in the legs is usually higher by 10 to 40 mm Hg than in the brachial artery, but the diastolic pressure is the same.

Automatic blood pressure devices. Electronic devices are available that can determine blood pressure automatically. Once the blood pressure cuff is applied, the nurse can program the device to obtain and record blood pressure readings at preset intervals.

The advantages of automatic devices are the ease of use and efficiency when repeated or frequent measurements are indicated. The ability to use a stethoscope is not required. However, automatic devices are more sensitive to outside interference and are susceptible to error. Indirect measurements obtained from automated devices may not yield equivalent readings from those obtained with the traditional auscultatory method (Jones and others, 1996). Using the same technique consistently avoids errors introduced by variability in equipment.

RESPIRATION

Respiration is the mechanism the body uses to exchange gases between the atmosphere and the blood and the cells. Respiration involves three processes: **ventilation** (the mechanical movement of gases into and out of the lungs), **diffusion** (the movement of oxygen [O_2] and carbon dioxide [CO_2] between the alveoli and the red blood cells), and **perfusion** (the distribution of red blood cells to and from the pulmonary capillaries). Analyzing respiratory efficiency requires integrating assessment data from all three processes. Ventilation is assessed by determining respiratory rate, depth, and rhythm. Diffusion and perfusion can be assessed by determining oxygen saturation.

Assessment of Ventilation

Adults normally breathe in a smooth, uninterrupted pattern of 12 to 20 breaths per minute. Ventilation is regulated by levels of CO_2 and O_2 in the arterial blood. The most important factor in the control of ventilation is the level of CO_2 in the arterial blood. Excessive CO_2 or **hypercarbia** causes the respiratory control system in the brain to increase rate and depth of breathing. The increased ventilatory effort removes excess CO_2 by increasing exhalation. However, hypercarbia is chronic in clients with chronic lung disease. In these clients the constantly elevated CO_2 level fails to increase the rate and depth of breathing. **Hypoxemia,** also present in these clients, becomes the stimulus to increase ventilation. Hypoxemia, or low levels of arterial O_2, is detected by chemoreceptors in the carotid artery and aorta. If arterial oxygen levels fall, these receptors signal the brain to increase the rate and depth of ventilation. Hypoxemia helps to control ventilation in clients with chronic lung disease. Because low levels of arterial O_2 provide the stimulus that allows the client with chronic lung disease to breathe, administration of high oxygen levels can be fatal.

The normal rate and depth of ventilation, **eupnea,** is interrupted by sighing. The sigh, a prolonged deeper breath, is a protective physiological mechanism for expanding small airways and alveoli not ventilated during a normal breath.

The accurate assessment of ventilation depends on the nurse's recognition of normal thoracic and abdominal movements. During quiet breathing the chest wall gently rises and falls. Contraction of the intercostal muscles between the ribs or contraction of the muscles in the neck and shoulders, the accessory muscles of breathing, is not visible. During normal quiet breathing, diaphragmatic movement causes the abdominal cavity to rise and fall slowly.

When breathing requires greater effort, the intercostal and accessory muscles work actively to move air in and out. The shoulders may rise and fall, and the accessory muscles of ventilation in the neck visibly contract. Diaphragmatic movement becomes less noticeable as costal breathing increases.

Measurement of Respirations

Respirations are the easiest of all vital signs to assess, but they are often the most haphazardly measured. A nurse must not estimate respirations. Accurate measurement requires observation and palpation of chest wall movement.

A sudden change in the character of respirations may be important. Because respiration is tied to the function of numerous body systems, the nurse must consider all variables when changes occur. For example, a drop in respirations occurring in a client after head trauma may signify injury to the brainstem.

When assessing a client's respirations, the nurse should keep in mind the client's usual ventilatory rate and pattern, the influence any disease or illness has on respiratory function, the relationship between respiratory and cardiovascular function, and the influence of therapies on respirations. Box 23-6 summarizes factors influencing respirations. The objective measurement of respirations includes the rate and depth of breathing and the rhythm of ventilatory movements (Skill 23-4).

Respiratory rate. The nurse observes a full inspiration and expiration when counting ventilation or respiration rate. The respiratory rate varies with age (Table 23-9). A respiratory rate lower than acceptable limits is **bradypnea,** whereas a rate over acceptable limits is **tachypnea.** A respiratory monitoring device that aids the nurse's assessment is the apnea monitor. This noninvasive device uses leads attached to the client's chest wall to sense movement. The absence of chest wall movement is interpreted by the monitor as **apnea** and triggers an alarm. Apnea monitoring is used frequently with infants in the hospital and at home to observe for prolonged apneic events.

Box 23-6
Factors Influencing Character of Respirations

Exercise

Exercise increases rate and depth to meet the body's need for additional oxygen and to rid the body of CO_2.

Acute Pain

Pain alters rate and rhythm of respirations, breathing becomes shallow.

Client may inhibit or splint chest wall movement when pain is in area of chest or abdomen.

Anxiety

Anxiety increases rate and depth as a result of sympathetic stimulation.

Smoking

Chronic smoking changes the lung's airways, resulting in increased rate of respirations at rest when not smoking.

Body Position

A straight, erect posture promotes full chest expansion.

A stooped or slumped position impairs ventilatory movement.

Lying flat prevents full chest expansion.

Medications

Narcotic analgesics, general anesthetics, and sedative hypnotics depress rate and depth.

Amphetamines and cocaine may increase rate and depth.

Bronchodilators slow rate by causing airway dilation.

Neurological Injury

Injury to the brainstem impairs the respiratory center and inhibits respiratory rate and rhythm.

Hemoglobin Function

Decreased hemoglobin levels (anemia) reduce oxygen-carrying capacity of the blood, which increases respiratory rate.

Increased altitude lowers the amount of saturated hemoglobin, which increases respiratory rate and depth.

Abnormal blood cell function (e.g., sickle cell disease) reduces ability of hemoglobin to carry oxygen, which increases respiratory rate and depth.

TABLE 23-9
Acceptable Range of Respiratory Rates for Age

Age	Rate
Newborn	35-40
Infant (6 months)	30-50
Toddler (2 years)	25-32
Child	20-30
Adolescent	16-19
Adult	12-20

Ventilatory depth. The depth of respirations is assessed by observing the degree of excursion or movement in the chest wall. The nurse subjectively describes ventilatory movements as deep, normal, or shallow. A deep respiration involves a full expansion of the lungs with full exhalation. Respirations are shallow when only a small quantity of air passes through the lungs and ventilatory movement is difficult to see. More objective techniques are used if the nurse observes that chest excursion is unusually shallow (see Chapter 24). Table 23-10 summarizes types of respiratory alterations.

Ventilatory rhythm. With normal breathing a regular interval occurs after each respiratory cycle. Infants tend to breathe less regularly. The young child may breathe slowly for a few seconds and then suddenly breathe more rapidly. While assessing respirations, the nurse estimates the interval after each respiratory cycle. Respiration is regular or irregular in rhythm.

Measurement of Arterial Oxygen Saturation

A pulse oximeter permits the indirect measurement of oxygen saturation for the client's vital sign database (Skill 23-5). The pulse oximeter is a probe with a light-emitting diode (LED) and photosensor connected by cable to an oximeter (Figure 23-10). The LED emits light, which oxygenated and deoxygenated hemoglobin molecules absorb differently. The photosensor detects the light-absorbing differences between each type of hemoglobin and the oximeter calculates pulse saturation (SpO_2). SpO_2 is a reliable estimate of SaO_2.

Text continued on p. 475

Assessing Respirations

Delegation Considerations
The skill of respiration measurement can be delegated to unlicensed assistive personnel.
- Inform care giver of appropriate client position when obtaining respirations.
- Inform care giver of appropriate duration of respiratory rate count.

- Inform care givers if client is at risk for increased or decreased respiratory rate and instruct them to inform nurse of any changes.

Equipment
- Wristwatch with second hand or digital display
- Pen, pencil, vital sign flow sheet or record form

STEPS	RATIONALE
1. Determine need to assess client's respirations: a. Note risk factors for respiratory alterations.	Certain conditions place client at risk for alterations in ventilation detected by changes in respiratory rate, depth, and rhythm. Fever, pain, anxiety, diseases of chest wall or muscles, constrictive chest or abdominal dressings, gastric distention, chronic pulmonary disease (emphysema, bronchitis, asthma), traumatic injury to chest wall with or without collapse of underlying lung tissue, presence of a chest tube, respiratory infection (pneumonia, acute bronchitis), pulmonary edema and emboli, head injury with damage to brainstem, and anemia can result in respiratory alteration.
b. Assess for signs and symptoms of respiratory alterations such as bluish or cyanotic appearance of nail beds, lips, mucous membranes, and skin; restlessness, irritability, confusion, reduced level of consciousness; pain during inspiration; labored or difficult breathing; adventitious breath sounds (Chapter 30), inability to breathe spontaneously; thick, frothy, blood-tinged, or copious sputum produced on coughing.	Physical signs and symptoms may indicate alterations in respiratory status related to ventilation.

2. Assess pertinent laboratory values:
   a. Arterial blood gases (ABGs): normal ABGs (values may vary slightly within institutions):
     pH 7.35-7.45
     PaCO$_2$ 35-45
     PaO$_2$ 80-100
     SaO$_2$ 94%-98%
	Arterial blood gases measure arterial blood pH, partial pressure of O$_2$ and CO$_2$, and arterial O$_2$ saturation, which reflects client's oxygenation status.

b. Pulse oximetry (SpO$_2$): normal SpO$_2$ 90%-100%: 85%-89% may be acceptable for certain chronic disease conditions; less than 85% is abnormal (see Skill 23-5).	SpO$_2$ less than 85% is often accompanied by changes in respiratory rate, depth, and rhythm.

c. Complete blood count (CBC): normal CBC for adults (values may vary within institutions):
     (1) Hemoglobin: 14 to 18 g/100 ml, males; 12 to 16 g/100 ml, females.
     (2) Hematocrit: 40% to 54%, males; 38% to 47%, females.
     (3) Red blood cell count: 4.6 to 6.2 million/μl, males; 4.2 to 5.4 million/μl, females.
	Complete blood count measures red blood cell count, volume of red blood cells, and concentration of hemoglobin, which reflects client's capacity to carry O$_2$.

Continued

Skill 23-4—cont'd
Assessing Respirations

STEPS	RATIONALE
3. Determine previous baseline respiratory rate (if available) from client's record.	Allows nurse to assess for change in condition. Provides comparison with future respiratory measurements.
4. Be sure client is in comfortable position, preferably sitting or lying with the head of the bed elevated 45 to 60 degrees.	Sitting erect promotes full ventilatory movement.

CRITICAL DECISION POINT

Clients with difficulty breathing (dyspnea) such as those with congestive heart failure or abdominal ascites or in late stages of pregnancy should be assessed in the position of greatest comfort. Repositioning may increase the work of breathing, which will increase respiratory rate.

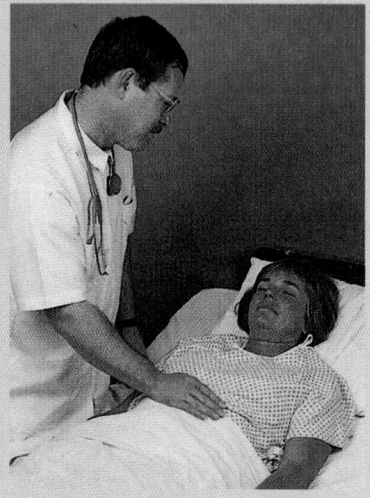

Step 7

5. Draw curtain around bed and/or close door. Wash hands.	Maintains privacy. Prevents transmission of microorganisms.
6. Be sure client's chest is visible. If necessary, move bed linen or gown.	Ensures clear view of chest wall and abdominal movements.
7. Place client's arm in relaxed position across the abdomen or lower chest, or place nurse's hand directly over client's upper abdomen (see illustration).	A similar position used during pulse assessment allows respiratory rate assessment to be inconspicuous. Client's or nurse's hand rises and falls during respiratory cycle.
8. Observe complete respiratory cycle (one inspiration and one expiration).	Rate is accurately determined only after nurse has viewed respiratory cycle.
9. After cycle is observed, look at watch's second hand and begin to count rate: when sweep hand hits number on dial, begin time frame, counting one with first full respiratory cycle.	Timing begins with count of one. Respirations occur more slowly than pulse; thus timing does not begin with zero.
10. If rhythm is regular, count number of respirations in 30 seconds and multiply by 2. If rhythm is irregular, less than 12, or greater than 20, count for 1 full minute.	Respiratory rate is equivalent to number of respirations per minute. Suspected irregularities require assessment for at least 1 minute.

CRITICAL DECISION POINT

Respiratory rate less than 12 or greater than 20 requires further assessment (Chapter 24) and may require immediate intervention.

STEPS	RATIONALE
11. Note depth of respirations, subjectively assessed by observing degree of chest wall movement while counting rate. Nurse can also objectively assess depth by palpating chest wall excursion (Chapter 24) after rate has been counted. Depth is shallow, normal, or deep.	Character of ventilatory movement may reveal specific disease state restricting volume of air from moving into and out of the lungs.
12. Note rhythm of ventilatory cycle. Normal breathing is regular and uninterrupted. Sighing should not be confused with abnormal rhythm.	Character of ventilations can reveal specific types of alterations.
13. Replace bed linen and client's gown.	Restores comfort and promotes sense of well-being.
14. Wash hands.	Reduces transmission of microorganisms.
15. Discuss findings with client as needed.	Promotes participation in care and understanding of health status.
16. If respirations are assessed for the first time, establish rate, rhythm, and depth as baseline if within normal range.	Used to compare future respiratory assessment.
17. Compare respirations with client's previous baseline and normal rate, rhythm, and depth.	Allows nurse to assess for changes in client's condition and for presence of respiratory alterations.

Recording and Reporting

▪ Record respiratory rate and character in nurses' notes or vital sign flow sheet. Indicate type and amount of oxygen therapy if used by client during assessment. Measurement of respiratory rate after administration of specific therapies should be documented in narrative form in nurses' notes.

▪ Report abnormal findings to nurse in charge or physician.

Home Care Considerations

▪ Assess for environmental factors in the home that may influence client's respiratory rate such as second-hand smoke, poor ventilation, or gas fumes.

TABLE 23-10
Alterations in Breathing Pattern

Alteration	Description	Alteration	Description
Bradypnea	Rate of breathing is regular but abnormally slow (less than 12 breaths/min).	Cheyne-Stokes respiration	Respiratory rate and depth are irregular, characterized by alternating periods of apnea and hyperventilation. Respiratory cycle begins with slow, shallow breaths that gradually increase to abnormal rate and depth. The pattern reverses, breathing slows and becomes shallow, climaxing in apnea before respiration resumes.
Tachypnea	Rate of breathing is regular but abnormally rapid (greater than 20 breaths/min).		
Hyperpnea	Respirations are increased in depth. Occurs normally during exercise.		
Apnea	Respirations cease for several seconds. Persistent cessation results in respiratory arrest.		
Hyperventilation	Rate and depth of respirations increases. Hypocarbia may occur.	Kussmaul respiration	Respirations are abnormally deep but regular.
Hypoventilation	Respiratory rate is abnormally low, and depth of ventilation may be depressed. Hypercarbia may occur.	Biot's respiration	Respirations are abnormally shallow for two to three breaths followed by irregular period of apnea.

Measuring Oxygen Saturation (Pulse Oximetry)

Delegation Considerations

The skill of oxygen saturation measurement can be delegated to unlicensed assistive personnel.

- Inform care giver of appropriate sensor site for measurement of oxygen saturation.
- Inform care giver to notify nurse immediately about abnormal findings.

Equipment

- Oximeter
- Oximeter probe appropriate for client and recommended by manufacturer
- Acetone or nail polish remover
- Pen, pencil, vital sign flow sheet or record form

STEPS	RATIONALE
1. Determine need to measure client's oxygen saturation:	
a. Note risk factors for alteration of oxygen saturation.	Certain conditions place clients at risk for decreased oxygen saturation: acute or chronic compromised respiratory function, recovery from general anesthesia or conscious sedation, or traumatic injury to chest wall with or without collapse of underlying lung tissue.
b. Assess for signs and symptoms of alterations in oxygen saturation such as altered respiratory rate, depth, or rhythm; adventitious breath sounds (Chapter 24); cyanotic appearance of nail beds, lips, mucous membranes, and skin; restlessness, irritability, confusion; reduced level of consciousness; labored or difficulty breathing.	Physical signs and symptoms may indicate abnormal oxygen saturation.
2. Assess for factors that normally influence measurement of SpO_2 such as oxygen therapy, hemoglobin level, and temperature.	Allows nurse to accurately assess oxygen saturation variations. Peripheral vasoconstriction related to hypothermia can interfere with SpO_2 determination.
3. Assess site most appropriate for sensor probe placement (e.g., bridge of nose, ear, fingernail bed). Site must have adequate local circulation and be free of moisture.	Sensor requires pulsating vascular bed to identify hemoglobin molecules that absorb emitted light. Changes in SpO_2 are reflected in the circulation of finger capillary bed within 30 seconds and the capillary bed of earlobe within 5 to 10 seconds. Moisture impedes ability of sensor to detect SpO_2 levels.
4. Determine previous baseline SpO_2 (if available) from client's record.	Allows nurse to assess for change in condition. Provides comparison with future SpO_2 measurements.
5. Explain purpose of procedure to client and how oxygen saturation will be measured.	Promotes client cooperation and increases compliance.
6. Wash hands.	Reduces transmission of microorganisms.
7. Position client comfortably. If finger is chosen as monitoring site, support lower arm.	Ensures probe positioning and decreases motion interference with signal.
8. Instruct client to breathe normally.	Prevents large fluctuations in respiratory rate and depth and possible changes in SpO_2.
9. If finger is to be used, remove any fingernail polish with acetone from digit to be assessed.	Ensures accurate readings. Opaque coatings decrease light transmission; nail polish containing blue pigment can absorb light emissions and falsely alter saturation.

STEPS	RATIONALE
10. Attach sensor probe to finger, ear, or bridge of nose (see Figure 23-10).	Select sensor site based on peripheral circulation and extremity temperature. Peripheral vasoconstriction can alter SpO_2.

CRITICAL DECISION POINT

Do not attach probe to finger, ear, or bridge of nose if area is edematous or skin integrity is compromised. Do not attach probe to fingers that are hypothermic. Select ear or bridge of nose if client has a history of peripheral vascular disease.

11. Turn on oximeter by activating power. Observe pulse waveform/intensity display and audible beep. Correlate oximeter pulse rate with client's radial pulse. Differences require reevaluation of oximeter probe placement and may require reassessment of pulse rates.	Pulse waveform/intensity display enables detection of valid pulse or presence of interfering signal. Pitch of audible beep is proportional to SpO_2 value. Double checking pulse rate ensures oximeter accuracy.
12. Leave probe in place until oximeter readout reaches constant value and pulse display reaches full strength during each cardiac cycle. Read SpO_2 on digital display.	Reading may take 10 to 30 seconds depending on site selected.
13. Discuss findings with client as needed.	Promotes participation in care and understanding of health status.
14. Remove probe and turn oximeter power off.	Batteries can be depleted if oximeter is left on.
15. Assist client in returning to comfortable position.	Restores comfort and promotes sense of well-being.
16. Wash hands.	Reduces transmission of microorganisms.
17. Compare SpO_2 readings with client baseline and acceptable values.	Comparison reveals presence of abnormality.
18. Correlate SpO_2 with SaO_2 obtained from arterial blood gas measurements (see Chapter 30) if available.	Documents reliability of noninvasive assessment.
19. Correlate SpO_2 reading with data obtained from respiratory rate, depth, and rhythm assessment (see Skill 23-4).	Measurements assessing ventilation, perfusion, and diffusion are interrelated.

Recording and Reporting
- Record SpO_2 value on nurses' notes or vital sign flow sheet indicating type and amount of oxygen therapy used by client during assessment. Also record any signs and symptoms of oxygen desaturation in narrative form in nurses' notes. Measurement of SpO_2 after administration of specific therapies should be documented in narrative form in nurses' notes.
- Report abnormal findings to nurse in charge or physician. Assessment of oxygen saturation after ad-ministration of specific therapies should be documented in narrative form in nurses' notes.
- Record in nurses' notes client's use of continuous or intermittent pulse oximetry. Documents use of equipment for third-party payers.

Home Care Considerations
- Pulse oximetry is used in home care to noninvasively monitor oxygen therapy or changes in oxygen therapy.

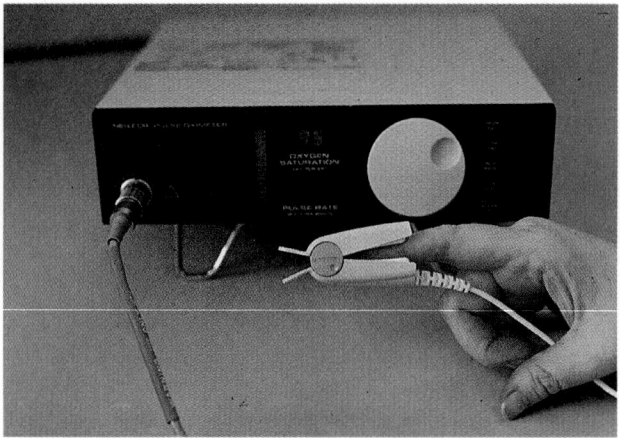

Figure 23-10. Pulse oximeter.

Box 23-7
Factors Affecting Determination of Pulse Oxygen Saturation (SpO$_2$)

Interference With Light Transmission

Outside light sources can interfere with the oximeter's ability to process reflected light.

Jaundice may interfere with the oximeter's ability to process reflected light.

Intravascular dyes (methylene blue) absorb light similar to deoxyhemoglobin and artificially lower saturation.

Reduction of Arterial Pulsations

Peripheral vascular disease can reduce pulse volume.

Vasoconstriction decreases peripheral pulse volume.

Low cardiac output and hypotension decrease blood flow to peripheral arteries.

Peripheral edema can obscure arterial pulsation.

BOX 23-8
Client Teaching for Vital Sign Assessment

Temperature

▪ Identify client's ability to initiate preventive health measures and recognize alteration in body temperature. Educate clients and family members about measures to prevent body temperature alterations.
▪ Teach clients risk factors for hypothermia and frostbite: fatigue; malnutrition; hypoxemia; cold, wet clothing; alcohol intoxication.
▪ Teach clients risk factors for heat stroke: strenuous exercise in hot, humid weather; tight-fitting clothing in hot environments; exercising in poorly ventilated areas; sudden exposures to hot climates; poor fluid intake before, during, and after exercise.
▪ Teach clients the importance of taking and continuing antibiotics as directed until course of treatment is completed.

Pulse Rate

▪ Clients taking certain prescribed cardiac medications should learn to assess their own pulse rates to detect side effects of medications. Clients undergoing cardiac rehabilitation should learn to assess their own pulse rates to determine their response to exercise.

Blood Pressure

▪ Teach client risk factors for hypertension. Persons with family history of hypertension are at significant risk. Obesity, cigarette smoking, heavy alcohol consumption, high blood cholesterol and triglyceride levels, and continued exposure to stress are factors linked to hypertension (Joint National Committee on Detection, Evaluation, and Treatment of High Blood Pressure, 1993).

▪ Clients with hypertension should learn about their BP values, long-term follow-up care and therapy, the usual lack of symptoms, therapy's ability to control but not cure, and benefits of a consistently followed treatment plan.
▪ Instruct clients on the importance of appropriate size blood pressure cuff for home use.
▪ Instruct primary care giver to take BP at same time each day and after client has had a brief rest. Take BP sitting or lying down, use same position and arm each time pressure is taken.
▪ Instruct primary care giver that if it is difficult to hear the pressure, it may be that the cuff is too loose, not big enough, or too narrow; the stethoscope is not over arterial pulse; cuff was deflated too quickly or too slowly; or cuff was not pumped high enough for systolic readings.

Respirations

▪ Clients who demonstrate decreased ventilation may benefit from being taught deep-breathing and coughing exercises (see Chapter 30).
▪ Instruct family member to contact home care nurse or physician if unusual fluctuations in respiratory rate occur.
▪ Teach client signs and symptoms of hypoxemia: headache, somnolence, confusion, dusky color, shortness of breath, dyspnea.
▪ Teach client effect of high-risk behaviors such as cigarette smoking on oxygen saturation.

The measurement of SpO_2 is affected by factors that affect light transmission or peripheral arterial pulsations. An awareness of these factors allows the nurse to interpret abnormal SpO_2 measurements accurately (Box 23-7). SpO_2 can be measured intermittently or continuously. Continuous SpO_2 monitoring is used to assess ongoing therapies. Alarm limits can be programmed to alert the nurse if the SpO_2 drops to an unacceptable level.

CLIENT TEACHING AND VITAL SIGN MEASUREMENT

The emphasis on health promotion and health maintenance, as well as early discharge from hospital settings, has resulted in an increase in the need for clients and their families to monitor vital signs in the home. Teaching considerations affect all vital sign measurements and should be incorporated within the client's plan of care (Box 23-8).

When considering how to teach clients and their families about vital sign measurements, the client's age is an important factor. With the increased older adult population, there is an increased need for care givers to be aware of changes from normal vital sign values that are unique to older adults. Box 23-9 identifies some of these variations unique to the older adult.

RECORDING VITAL SIGNS

Specific graphic flow sheets exist for recording vital signs (see Chapter 14). The nurse identifies and uses the agency's policy for recording vital signs. In a community-based setting, the vital signs may be recorded on the progress notes for that particular clinic or home visit. However, in acute care and some restorative care settings a graphic flow sheet is used.

Clients whose care is facilitated through a critical path may have their vital signs listed as outcomes. When a vital sign is above or below the expected value, a note is written to explain when the difference exists.

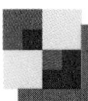

BOX 23-9
Gerontological Nursing Practice

Temperature
- The temperature of older adults is at the lower end of the normal temperature range, 36° C (96.8° F).
- Temperatures considered within normal range may reflect a fever in an older adult.
- Older adults are very sensitive to slight changes in temperature (Lueckenotte, 1996).
- Environmental temperature plays a greater role in older adults because their thermoregulatory systems are not as efficient (Lueckenotte, 1996).
- A decrease in sweat gland reactivity in the older adult results in a higher threshold for sweating at high temperature, which can lead to hyperthermia and heatstroke (Burke and Walsh, 1997).
- With aging, a loss of subcutaneous fat reduces the insulating capacity of the skin; older men are at especially high risk for hypothermia (Burke and Walsh, 1997).

Pulse Rate
- It is often difficult to palpate the pulse of an older adult or obese client. A Doppler device will provide a more accurate reading.
- The older adult has a decreased heart rate at rest (Lueckenotte, 1996).
- Once elevated, the pulse rate of an older adult takes longer to return to normal resting rate (Wold, 1993).
- When assessing elderly women with sagging breasts, the breast tissue is gently lifted and the stethoscope placed at the fifth ICS or the lower edge of the breast.
- Heart sounds may be muffled or difficult to hear in the elderly because of an increase in air space in the lungs.

Blood Pressure
- Older adults, especially the frail elderly, have lost upper arm mass, requiring special attention to selection of BP cuff size.
- An older adult's BP range is normally 140 to 160/80 to 90.
- Older adults have an increase in systolic pressure related to decreased vessel elasticity. The diastolic pressure remains the same, resulting in a wider pulse pressure (Lueckenotte, 1996).
- Older adults are instructed to change position slowly and wait after each change to avoid postural hypotension and prevent injuries.

Respirations
- Aging causes ossification of costal cartilage and downward slant of ribs, resulting in a more rigid rib cage, which reduces chest wall expansion. Kyphosis and scoliosis that can occur in older adults may also restrict chest expansion and decrease tidal volume (Lueckenotte, 1996).
- Older adults may depend more on accessory abdominal muscles during respiration than on weakened thoracic muscles (Burke and Walsh, 1997).
- Decreased efficiency of respiratory muscles results in breathlessness at low exercise levels (Lueckenotte, 1996).
- Responses to hypercapnia and hypoxia are reduced 50% in older adults as compared with the young (Timiras, 1994), limiting the ability of older adults to respond to hypoxia with respiratory changes.
- Identifying an acceptable pulse oximeter probe site may be difficult on older adults because of the likelihood of peripheral vascular disease, decreased cardiac output, cold induced vasoconstriction, and anemia.

Key Terms

afebrile	core temperature	hypotension	pulse pressure
antipyretic	diaphoresis	hypothermia	pyrexia
apical pulse	diastolic	hypoxemia	pyrogens
apnea	diffusion	Korotkoff sound	sphygmomanometer
auscultatory gap	dysrhythmia	malignant hyper-	stroke volume (SV)
basal metabolic rate	eupnea	thermia	systolic
(BMR)	Fahrenheit	nonshivering thermo-	tachycardia
bradycardia	febrile	genesis	tachypnea
bradypnea	fever	orthostatic hypotension	thermoregulation
cardiac output (CO)	heat stroke	oxygen saturation	vasoconstriction
centigrade	hypercarbia	perfusion	vasodilation
central venous pres-	hypertension	postural hypotension	ventilation
sure (CVP)	hyperthermia	pulse deficit	vital signs

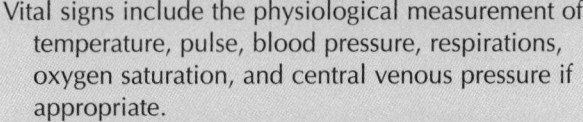

Key Concepts

Vital signs include the physiological measurement of temperature, pulse, blood pressure, respirations, oxygen saturation, and central venous pressure if appropriate.

Vital signs are measured as part of a complete physical examination or in a review of a client's condition.

The nurse assesses vital sign changes with other physical assessment findings using clinical judgment to determine measurement frequency.

Knowledge of the factors influencing vital signs assists the nurse in determining and evaluating abnormal values.

Vital signs provide a basis for evaluating response to nursing interventions.

Vital signs are best measured when the client is inactive and the environment is controlled for comfort.

The nurse assists the client in maintaining body temperature by initiating interventions that promote heat loss, production, or conservation.

A fever is one of the body's normal defense mechanisms.

The tympanic route is the most accessible and acceptable site for core temperature measurement.

To assess cardiac function, pulse rate and rhythm are most easily measured using the radial or apical pulses.

Respiratory assessment includes determining the effectiveness of ventilation, perfusion, and diffusion.

Assessment of respirations involves observing ventilatory movements throughout the respiratory cycle.

Oxygen saturation is influenced by variables affecting ventilation, perfusion, and diffusion.

Several hemodynamic variables contribute to blood pressure determination.

Hypertension is diagnosed only after an average of readings made during two or more subsequent visits reveals an elevated blood pressure.

Errors in blood pressure measurement can be made by selecting and applying the cuff improperly.

Circulating blood volume, venous return to the heart, and heart function contribute to central venous pressure.

Changes in one vital sign can influence characteristics of the other vital signs.

Critical Thinking Activities

1. A 68-year-old widowed woman has been referred to the hypertension clinic held by the Visiting Nurses Association. During her first visit, you are assigned to do an admission assessment. She reports that her primary care physician told her that her blood pressure was 164/94. You obtain a blood pressure of 148/86. What further data are required to analyze the discrepancy of blood pressure findings? How would you explain the difference to the client? Develop a plan for the health promotion of this new client.

2. A 23-year-old, black college athlete is brought to the emergency room after collapsing during a basketball game. He is awake and oriented but complains of being dizzy and sweaty. He is 6 feet 6 inches tall and weighs 105 kg. He states that just before he passed out he felt his "chest beating like a drum." List the vital signs to be obtained from this client in order of priority. What signs and symptoms would indicate orthostatic hypotension?

3. A 78-year-old retired coal miner is admitted to the surgical floor after a left pneumonectomy for carcinoma of the lung. An IV is present in his right forearm. He complains of shortness of breath and pain. During report the post anesthesia care unit (PACU) nurse states that his preoperative SpO_2 was 95% and in the immediate postoperative period SpO_2 was 92% on 4 L O_2 via nasal cannula. What are the most effective methods for obtaining this client's vital signs? What is the priority nursing diagnosis for this client? Explain the difference between the SpO_2 readings.

4. During a home visit, the client requests that you "take a look at" her 4-year-old son. The child has been quietly lying on the couch watching television for the past 30 minutes of your visit. You note flushed skin that is warm and dry to the touch. Skin lesions indicative of chicken pox are present on his face and torso. Vital signs are apical rate 126, regular; BP RA 90/52; RR 28; tympanic temperature 103° F (39.3° C). Which vital signs are outside acceptable limits? What is the likely cause of the alteration in vital signs? Provide three nursing diagnoses to be included in the plan of care.

References

Banasik J, Broderson M: The effect of lateral position on CVP, *Heart Lung* 23:296, 1991.

Burke MM, Walsh MB: *Gerontologic nursing*, St. Louis, 1997, Mosby.

Hazinski MF, editor: *Nursing care of the critically ill child*, St. Louis, 1984, Mosby.

Holtzclaw B: The febrile response in critical care: state of the science, *Heart Lung* 21(5):482, 1992.

Joint National Committee on Detection, Evaluation, and Treatment of High Blood Pressure: *The fifth report of the Joint National Committee on Detection, Evaluation, and Treatment of High Blood Pressure*, NIH Pub No. 93-1088, Bethesda, Md, January 1993, NIH.

Jones D and others: A comparison of two noninvasive methods of blood pressure measurement in the triage area, *J Emerg Nurs* 22:111, 1996.

Kinney MR and others: *AACN's clinical reference for critical care nursing*, ed 3, St. Louis, 1993, Mosby.

Lueckenotte AG: *Gerontologic nursing*, St. Louis, 1996, Mosby.

Neff J and others: Effect of respiratory rate, respiratory depth, and open versus closed mouth breathing on sublingual temperature, *Res Nur Health* 12:195, 1992.

Perloff D and others: Human blood pressure determination by sphygmomanometry, *Circulation* 88:2460, 1993.

Pickering TC: *Lancet* 344(8914):31, 1994.

Task Force on Blood Pressure Control in Children: Report of second task force on blood pressure control in children—1987, *Pediatrics* 79:1, 1987.

Thibodeau GA, Patton KT: *Anatomy and physiology*, ed 3, St. Louis, 1996, Mosby.

Thomas SA, DeKeyser R: Blood pressure, *Annu Rev Nurs Res* 14:3, 1996.

Thomas SA and others: Nursing blood pressure research, 1980-1990: a bio-psychosocial perspective, *Image J Nurs Sch* 25(2):157, 1993.

Timiras PS: *Physiological basis of aging and geriatrics*, ed 2, Boca Raton, Fla, 1994, CRC Press.

Wold G: *Basic geriatric nursing*, St. Louis, 1993, Mosby.

24

Health Assessment and Physical Examination

OBJECTIVES

Mastery of content in this chapter will enable the student to:

- Define the key terms listed.
- Discuss the purposes of physical examination.
- Describe the techniques used with each physical assessment skill.
- Discuss the importance of understanding cultural diversity as it influences the approach to health assessment.
- Describe the proper position for the client during each phase of a physical examination.
- List techniques used to prepare a client physically and psychologically before and during an examination.
- Describe interview techniques used to enhance communication during history taking.
- Make environmental preparations before an examination.
- Identify information to collect from the nursing history before an examination.
- Discuss normal physical findings in a young and middle-age adult compared with an older adult.
- Discuss ways to incorporate health teaching into the examination process.
- Use physical assessment skills during routine nursing care.
- Conduct assessments in an organized and proper fashion.
- Describe physical measurements made in assessing each body system.
- Identify self-screening examinations commonly performed by clients.
- Document findings on a physical examination form.

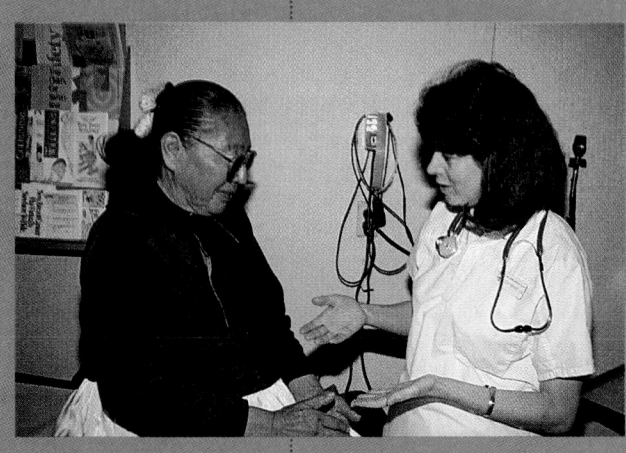

Nurses work in many settings, seeking information about clients' health status. The nurse conducts health assessments at health fairs, clinics, in physicians' offices, in a client's home, or in hospitals. Health screenings focus on a specific physical problem. If a screening determines that a client has a risk for a disease, the client is referred for a more complete physical examination. A complete health assessment involves a health history and behavioral and physical examination. The health history involves a lengthy client interview to gather subjective data about the client's condition. A physical examination is a head-to-toe review of each body system that offers objective information about the client. In contrast, a health screening helps to determine whether a person has a high probability of having a characteristic for a disease. For example, blood pressure screenings detect the risk for high blood pressure.

The nurse uses physical assessment skills during an examination to make clinical judgments. The client's condition and response affect the extent of the examination. The accuracy of the nurse's assessment influences the choice of therapies a client receives and the evaluation of response to those therapies. Continuity of health care improves when the nurse makes ongoing objective and comprehensive assessments.

PURPOSES OF PHYSICAL EXAMINATION

An examination should be designed for the client's needs. If a client is acutely ill, the nurse may assess only the involved body systems. A more comprehensive examination is conducted when the client feels more at ease, and the nurse then learns about the client's total health status. A complete physical examination is performed for routine screening to promote wellness behaviors and preventive health care measures; to determine eligibility for health insurance, military service, or a new job; and to admit a client to a hospital setting or long-term care facility.

The nurse uses physical examination to do the following:

1. Gather baseline data about the client's health status.
2. Supplement, confirm, or refute data obtained in the nursing history.
3. Confirm and identify nursing diagnoses.
4. Make clinical judgments about a client's changing health status and management.
5. Evaluate the physiological outcomes of care.

Gathering a Database

The nurse initially gathers thorough and detailed information about the client's health status from the client's health history (see Chapter 5). However, a client may

be unaware of a physical problem, so a thorough assessment of physical status is necessary. Even if a history is complete, physical examination may reveal information that refutes, confirms, or supplements the existing database. One assessment finding usually cannot conclusively reveal the nature of an abnormality. A complete assessment is needed for a definitive diagnosis. The nurse groups significant findings into patterns of data that reveal actual or at-risk nursing diagnoses. Each abnormal finding also directs the nurse to gather additional information. Information gathered during an initial physical examination provides a baseline of the client's functional abilities. The baseline is not the normal range of physical findings but is the pattern of findings identified when the client was first assessed. This baseline is used as a comparison for future assessment findings.

CULTURAL SENSITIVITY

As is the case with any other aspect of nursing, a physical examination must be performed with the nurse respecting the cultural differences of clients. How members of different cultures behave can influence their willingness to assume responsibility for their health and their tendency to seek professional health care. This is important for the nurse to remember before attempting to conduct a physical examination. A client's health beliefs, use of alternative therapies, nutritional habits, relationships with family, and comfort with the nurse's physical closeness must be considered during examination and history taking.

It is extremely important for nurses to remain culturally aware and to avoid stereotyping on the basis of gender or race. There is a sharp difference between distinguishing cultural characteristics and distinguishing physical characteristics. It is important for nurses to learn common disorders of those ethnic populations within the nurse's community. For example, Navajo Indians often have ear anomalies, Polynesians often suffer clubfoot, and many blacks experience sickle cell disease. Similarly, it is important to know variations in physical characteristics, such as in the skin and musculoskeletal system, that are related to cultural variables. Recognition of cultural diversity helps the nurse respect a client's uniqueness and provide higher-quality care.

INTEGRATION OF PHYSICAL EXAMINATION WITH NURSING CARE

An examination should be integrated into routine care. For example, the nurse can assess the condition of body parts during a bed bath. The nurse observes a client's gait and muscle strength while assisting with ambulation down a hallway. This practice makes more efficient use of time. The nurse also learns that physical assessment should become automatic when the nurse and client interact. The result is the nurse's ability to gather more comprehensive and relevant assessment findings.

SKILLS OF PHYSICAL ASSESSMENT

The five skills of physical assessment—inspection, palpation, percussion, auscultation, and olfaction—are used in a comprehensive examination.

Inspection

Inspection is the use of vision, hearing, and smell to detect normal characteristics or significant physical signs of body parts and function. It helps to know normal physical characteristics before trying to distinguish abnormal findings. It is also important to know normal characteristics of clients of different ages. Experience is needed to recognize normal variations among clients. Inspection is a simple technique, but it is often underused. The quality of an inspection depends on the nurse's willingness to spend time to be thorough and systematic. If hurried, a nurse may overlook significant findings or make incorrect conclusions. To inspect body parts accurately, the nurse follows certain principles:

1. Make sure good lighting is available.
2. Position and expose body parts so that all surfaces can be viewed.
3. Inspect each area for size, shape, color, symmetry, position, and abnormalities.
4. If possible, compare each area inspected with the same area on the opposite side of the body.
5. Use additional light (e.g., a penlight) to inspect body cavities.
6. Do not hurry inspection. Pay attention to detail.

After inspection of a body part, findings may indicate the need for further examination. Palpation is often used with or after visual inspection.

Palpation

Further assessment of body parts is made through **palpation,** which involves use of the hands to touch body parts to make sensitive measurements of specific physical signs. Palpation is used to examine all accessible parts of the body. For example, the skin is palpated for temperature, moisture, texture, turgor, tenderness, and thickness. Organs such as the liver are palpated for size, shape, tenderness, and absence of masses. The nurse uses different parts of the hand to detect characteristics such as texture, temperature, and perception of movement.

The client should be relaxed and comfortable, because muscle tension during palpation impairs effective assessment. Requesting a client to take slow, deep breaths enhances muscle relaxation. Placing arms along the side of the body will decrease abdominal rigidity. Tender areas are palpated last. The nurse asks the client to point out the more sensitive areas and notes any nonverbal signs of discomfort.

The client appreciates warm hands, short fingernails, and a gentle approach. The nurse applies palpation slowly, gently, and deliberately. Light palpation of structures such as the abdomen determines areas of tenderness (Figure 24-1, *A*). The nurse's hand is placed on the part to be examined and depressed about 1 cm (½ inch). Tender areas are examined further for potentially serious abnormalities. The sensation of touch is best preserved with light, intermittent pressure. Heavy, prolonged pressure causes loss of sensitivity in the nurse's hand.

After light palpation, deeper palpation is used to examine the condition of organs such as those in the abdomen (Figure 24-1, *B*). The nurse depresses the area being examined approximately 2 to 4 cm (1 to 2 inches) (Seidel and others, 1995). Caution is the rule. A nursing student should not attempt deep palpation without clinical supervision to avoid injuring a client. Deep palpation may be applied with one hand or both hands

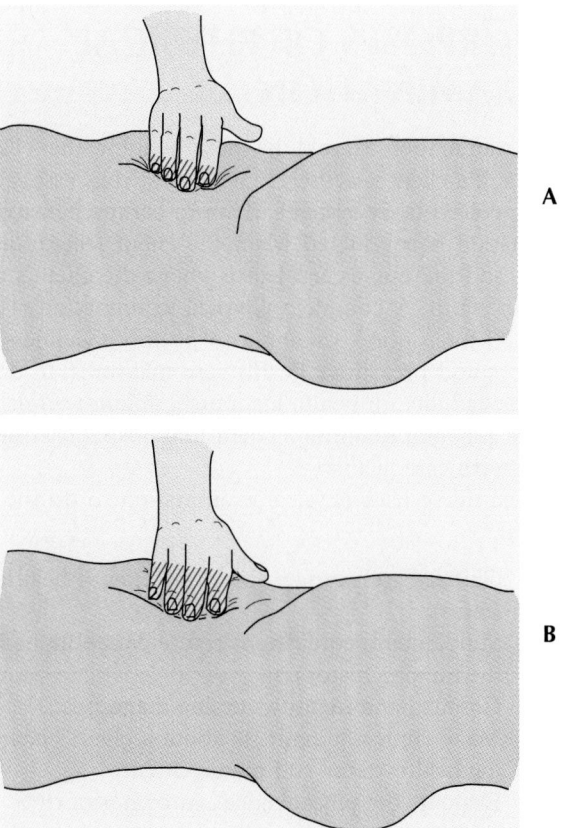

Figure 24-1. **A,** During light palpation, gentle pressure against underlying skin and tissues can detect areas of irregularity and tenderness. **B,** During deep palpation, nurse depresses tissue to assess condition of underlying organs.

(bimanually). When the nurse uses bimanual palpation, one hand (sensing hand) is relaxed and placed lightly over the client's skin. The other hand (active hand) applies pressure to the sensing hand. The lower hand does not exert pressure directly and thus retains the sensitivity needed to detect organ characteristics.

The most sensitive parts of the hand, the pads of the fingertips, are used to assess texture, shape, size, consistency, and pulsation (Figure 24-2, *A*). Temperature is best measured using the dorsum or back of the hand and fingers (Figure 24-2, *B*) where the examiner's skin is thinnest. The palm of the hand (Figure 24-2, *C*) is more sensitive to vibration. The nurse measures position, consistency, and turgor by lightly grasping the body part with the fingertips (Figure 24-2, *D*).

The nurse must not palpate without considering the client's condition. For example, if the client has a fractured rib, extra care is used to locate the painful area. A vital artery is not palpated with pressure that obstructs blood flow. The nurse also considers the body area being palpated and the reason for using palpation and must be able to discriminate and interpret the significance of what is sensed.

Percussion

Percussion involves tapping the body with the fingertips to produce a vibration that travels through body tissues. The character of the sound determines the location, size, and density of underlying structures to verify abnormalities assessed by palpation and auscultation.

This vibration is transmitted through the body tissues, and the character of the sound heard depends on the density of the underlying tissue. By knowing the way various densities influence sound, the nurse can locate organs or masses, map their boundaries, and determine their size. An abnormal sound suggests a mass or substance such as air or fluid within an organ or body cavity. The skill of percussion requires dexterity.

Direct percussion involves striking the body surface directly with one or two fingers. Indirect percussion is performed by placing the middle finger of the nondominant hand (called the pleximeter) firmly against the body surface (Figure 24-3). With palm and fingers remaining off the skin, the tip of the middle finger of the dominant hand (plexor) strikes the base of the distal joint of the pleximeter. The examiner uses a quick, light stroke with the plexor finger, keeping the forearm stationary. The wrist must remain relaxed to deliver the proper blow. If the blow is not sharp, if the pleximeter is held loosely, or if the palm rests on the body surface, the sound is dampened or softened. This prevents transmission of sound to underlying structures. The same force must be applied to each area so that an accurate comparison of sounds can be made. A light, quick blow usually produces the clearest sounds.

Percussion produces five types of sounds: tympany, resonance, hyperresonance, dullness, and flatness. Each sound is typically created by certain types of underlying tissues and is judged by its intensity, pitch, duration, and quality (Table 24-1).

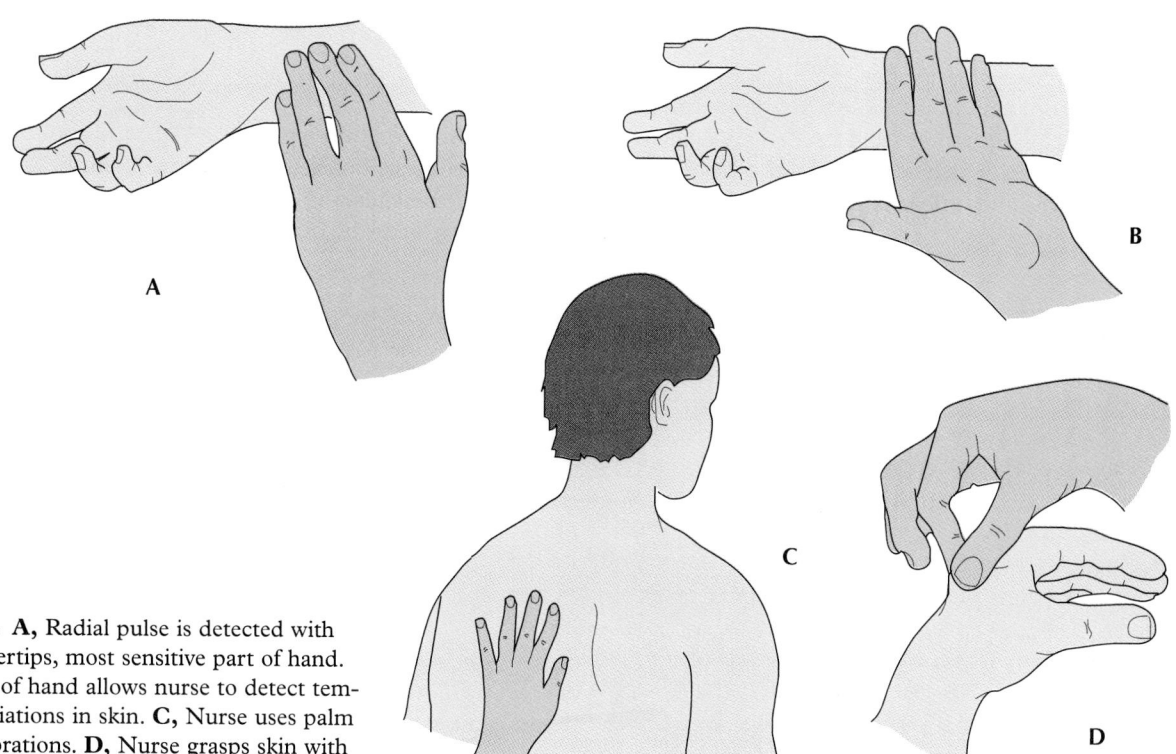

Figure 24-2. A, Radial pulse is detected with pads of fingertips, most sensitive part of hand. **B,** Dorsum of hand allows nurse to detect temperature variations in skin. **C,** Nurse uses palm to detect vibrations. **D,** Nurse grasps skin with fingertips to assess turgor.

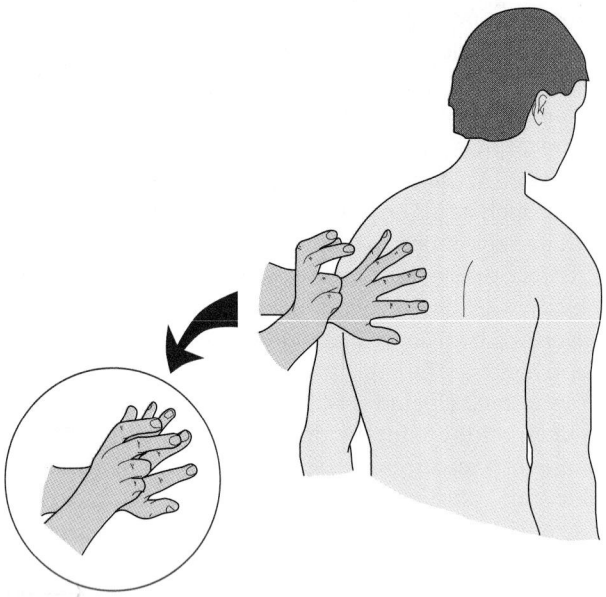

Figure 24-3. To perform indirect percussion, nurse places middle finger of nondominant hand against body's surface. Tip of middle finger of dominant hand strikes top of middle finger of nondominant hand.

Auscultation

Auscultation is listening to sounds created in body organs to detect variations from normal. Some sounds can be heard with the unassisted ear, although most sounds can be heard only through a stethoscope. A student must first become familiar with the normal sounds created by the cardiovascular, respiratory, and gastrointestinal systems. Abnormal sounds can be recognized only after learning normal variations. The nurse becomes more successful in auscultation by knowing the types of sounds arising from each body structure and the location in which they can most easily be heard. Likewise, the nurse learns the areas that normally do not emit sounds.

To auscultate correctly, the nurse needs to hear well, have a good stethoscope, and know how to use the stethoscope properly. Nurses with hearing disorders should use stethoscopes with greater sound amplification or ask colleagues to check findings through auscultation. Always place the stethoscope on naked skin, because clothing obscures sound.

Chapter 23 describes the parts of the acoustic stethoscope and the general use of the bell and diaphragm. The bell is best for low-pitched sounds such as vascular and certain heart sounds, and the diaphragm is best for high-pitched sounds such as bowel and lung sounds.

A nurse must be familiar with the stethoscope before attempting to use it with a client. It helps to practice using the stethoscope with a friend. Extraneous sounds created by movement of the tubing or chestpiece can interfere with auscultation of body organ sounds. By deliberately producing these sounds, the nurse can learn to recognize and disregard them during the actual examination (Box 24-1). Through auscultation, the nurse notes the following characteristics of sounds:

1. Frequency, or the number of sound wave cycles generated per second by a vibrating object. The higher the frequency, the higher the pitch of a sound and vice versa.
2. Loudness, or the amplitude of a sound wave. Auscultated sounds are described as *loud* or *soft*.
3. Quality, or the sounds of similar frequency and loudness from different sources. Terms such as *blowing* or *gurgling* describe the quality of sound.
4. Duration, or the length of time sound vibrations last. The duration of sound is short, medium, or long. Layers of soft tissue dampen the duration of sounds from deep internal organs.

Auscultation requires concentration and practice. The nurse considers the part of the body auscultated and the causes of the sounds. For example, the sounds heard over the abdomen are caused by intestinal peri-

TABLE 24-1
Sounds Produced by Percussion

Sound	Intensity	Pitch	Duration	Quality	Anatomical Finding
Tympany	Loud	High	Moderate	Drumlike	Enclosed, air-containing space; gastric air bubble, puffed-out cheek
Resonance	Moderate to loud	Low	Long	Hollow	Normal lung
Hyperresonance	Very loud	Very low	Longer than resonance	Booming	Emphysematous lung
Dullness	Soft to moderate	High	Moderate	Thudlike	Liver
Flatness	Soft	High	Short	Flat	Muscle

stalsis. The nurse identifies where the sound is best heard and how the sound is heard normally. Peristalsis is heard over all four abdominal quadrants as intermittent "tinkling" sounds. After understanding the cause and character of normal auscultated sounds, it becomes easier to recognize abnormal sounds and their origins.

Olfaction

While assessing a client, the nurse should be familiar with the nature and source of body odors (Table 24-2). Olfaction helps to detect abnormalities not recognized by other means. For example, a client's cast should not have a sweet, heavy, thick odor indicative of an

---

Box 24-1
Exercises to Increase Familiarity With the Stethoscope

Ensure that the earpieces follow the contour of the ear canals. Learn what fit is best for you by comparing amplification of sounds with the earpieces in both directions.

Place the earpieces in your ears with the tips of the earpieces turned toward the face. Lightly blow into the diaphragm. Again place the earpieces in your ears, this time with the ends turned toward the back of the head. Lightly blow into the diaphragm. After you have learned the right fit for the loudest amplification, wear the stethoscope the same way each time.

Put on the stethoscope and lightly blow into the diaphragm. If the sound is barely audible, lightly blow into the bell. Sound is carried through only one part of the chestpiece at a time. If the sound is greatly amplified through the diaphragm, the diaphragm is in position for use. If the sound is

barely audible through the diaphragm, the bell is in position for use. Rotation of the diaphragm and bell places the chestpiece in the desired position. Leave the diaphragm in position for the next exercise.

Place the diaphragm over the anterior part of your chest. Ask a friend to speak in a normal conversational tone. Environmental noise seriously detracts from hearing the noise created by body organs. When a stethoscope is used, the client and the examiner should remain quiet.

Put the stethoscope on and gently tap the tubing. It is often difficult to avoid stretching or movement of the stethoscope's tubing. The examiner should be in a position so that the tubing hangs free. Moving or touching the tubing creates extraneous sounds.

TABLE 24-2
Assessment of Characteristic Odors

Odor	Site or Source	Potential Causes
Alcohol	Oral cavity	Ingestion of alcohol
Ammonia	Urine	Urinary tract infection, renal failure
Body odor	Skin, particularly in areas where body parts rub together (e.g., under arms and breasts)	Poor hygiene, excess perspiration (hyperhidrosis), foul-smelling perspiration (bromidrosis)
Feces	Wound site	Wound abscess
	Vomitus	Bowel obstruction
	Rectal area	Fecal incontinence
Foul-smelling stools in infant	Stool	Malabsorption syndrome
Halitosis	Oral cavity	Poor dental and oral hygiene, gum disease
Sweet, fruity ketones	Oral cavity	Diabetic acidosis
Stale urine	Skin	Uremic acidosis
Sweet, heavy, thick odor	Draining wound	*Pseudomonas* (bacterial) infection
Musty odor	Casted body part	Infection inside cast
Fetid, sweet odor	Tracheostomy or mucous secretions	Infection of bronchial tree (*Pseudomonas* bacteria)

underlying infection. Findings from olfaction and other assessment skills allow the nurse to detect serious abnormalities.

PREPARATION FOR EXAMINATION

Proper preparation of the environment, equipment, and client ensures a smooth examination with few interruptions. A disorganized approach when preparing for a physical examination can cause errors and incomplete findings.

Environment

A physical examination requires privacy. A well-equipped examination room is preferable. Often, however, the examination occurs in the client's room, where it may be necessary to use room dividers or curtains. In the home, the nurse may perform an examination in the client's bedroom.

Adequate lighting is needed to illuminate body parts. Ideally an examination room is soundproofed so clients feel comfortable discussing their conditions. The nurse eliminates sources of noise, takes precautions to prevent interruptions from others, and makes sure the room is warm enough to maintain comfort.

Sometimes it is difficult to perform a complete examination when clients are in beds or on stretchers. Special examination tables make clients easily accessible and help them assume special positions. The tables are high and narrow. The nurse must carefully assist clients so they do not fall while getting on and off the table. A confused, combative, or uncooperative client should not be left on an examination table unsupervised.

Examination tables are often hard and uncomfortable. When the client lies supine, the head of the table can be raised about 30 degrees. The client may also use a small pillow. When examining a client in bed, the nurse can raise the bed to reach the client's body parts more easily.

Equipment

Hand washing is done before equipment preparation and the examination to reduce the transmission of microorganisms. The equipment should be readily available and arranged in an order for easy use. It should be kept as warm as appropriate. The diaphragm of the stethoscope may be briskly rubbed between the hands before it is applied to the skin. All equipment must be checked to see that it functions properly. The ophthalmoscope and otoscope require good batteries and lightbulbs. Equipment typically used is listed in Box 24-2.

Client

Physical preparation. The client's physical comfort is vital for a successful examination. Before start-

---

Box 24-2
Equipment and Supplies for Physical Assessment

Cotton applicators
Cytobrush
Disposable pad
Drapes
Eye chart (e.g., Snellen chart)
Flashlight and spotlight
Forms (e.g., physical, laboratory)
Gloves (sterile or clean)
Gown for client
Ophthalmoscope
Otoscope
Papanicolaou smear slides
Paper towels
Percussion hammer
Ruler
Safety pin
Scale with height measurement rod
Specimen containers and microscope slides
Sphygmomanometer and cuff
Stethoscope
Swabs or sponge forceps
Tape measure
Thermometer
Tissues
Tongue depressor
Tuning fork
Vaginal speculum
Water-soluble lubricant
Wristwatch with second hand or digital display

---

ing, the nurse asks if the client needs to use the toilet. An empty bladder and bowel facilitate examination of the abdomen, genitalia, and rectum. The nurse collects urine or fecal specimens at this time after explaining the proper method for collecting specimens. Each specimen is properly labeled.

Physical preparation involves being sure the client is dressed and draped properly. The client in the hospital will likely be wearing a simple gown. An outpatient will have to undress. If the examination is limited to certain body systems, it may not be necessary for the client to undress completely. The client should have privacy during undressing and plenty of time to finish. Walking into the room as the client undresses causes embarrassment. Drapes and gowns are made of linen or disposable paper. After clients have undressed and put on the gown, they should sit or lie down on the examination table with the drape over the lap or lower trunk. The examiner makes sure the client stays warm by eliminating drafts, controlling room temperature, and providing warm blankets. A seriously ill client or older adult is susceptible to chilling. The nurse should routinely ask if the client is comfortable.

Positioning. During the examination, the nurse asks clients to assume proper positions so body parts are accessible and clients stay comfortable. Table 24-3 lists the preferred positions for each part of the examination and contains figures illustrating these positions. Clients' abilities to assume positions will depend on their physical strength and degree of wellness. The nurse should be prepared to use alternative positions if the client is unable to assume the usual position for examination of a body part because of a disability or limitations. Many positions, such as the lithotomy and knee-chest position, are embarrassing and uncomfortable. Therefore clients should be kept in these positions no longer than necessary. The examiner explains the positions and assists clients in assuming them. The drapes are adjusted to be sure the area to be examined is accessible and that no body part is unnecessarily exposed. More than one position can be assumed for the same part of an examination. If clients are too weak or are physically unable to assume a position, the nurse may choose an alternative position. The nurse uses extra care to position older adults to avoid having them look into the source of light, which can cause discomfort from glare.

Psychological preparation. Because many clients find a physical examination tiring or stressful or experience anxiety about possible assessment findings, the examiner should psychologically prepare the client beforehand. A thorough explanation of the purpose and steps of each assessment lets clients know what to expect and what to do so they can cooperate. The nurse explains the examination in simple, understandable terms. Clients should feel free to ask questions and mention any discomfort. As the nurse examines each body system, a more detailed explanation is given.

The nurse's manner should be professional yet relaxed. A stiff, formal demeanor may inhibit the client's ability to communicate, but a too-casual style may fail to instill confidence (Seidel and others, 1995). When the client and nurse are of opposite gender, it may help to have a third person of the client's gender in the room. The presence of a third person assures the client the examiner will behave ethically, and the third person is a witness to the examiner's and client's conduct.

During the examination the nurse watches the client's emotional responses. The nurse observes whether the client's facial expression shows fear or concern and if body movements show anxiety. The nurse remains calm and explains each step clearly. It may be necessary to temporarily stop the examination and ask how the client feels. The client should not be forced to continue. Postponing the examination may be best, because the findings may be more accurate when the client can co-

operate and relax. If fear results from misconceptions, the nurse clarifies the purpose of the examination and how it is to be performed.

Assessment of Age-Groups

The nurse uses different interview styles and approaches to physical examination for clients of different age-groups. When assessing children, the nurse must be sensitive and anticipate the child's reaction to the examination as a strange and unfamiliar experience. Routine pediatric examinations have a focus on health promotion and illness prevention, particularly for the care of well children who receive competent parenting and have no serious health problems (Wong, 1995). The focus of an examination is on growth and development, sensory screening, dental examination, and behavioral assessment. Children who are chronically ill or disabled, foster children, or foreign-born adopted children may require additional examinations. When examining children, the following tips assist in data collection:

1. Gather all or part of the histories on infants and children from parents or guardians.
2. Perform the examination in a nonthreatening area and provide time for play to become acquainted.
3. Because parents may think they are being tested by the examiner, offer support during the examination and do not pass judgment.
4. Call children by their first name, and address the parents as "Mr. and Mrs." rather than by their first names.
5. Use open-ended questions to allow parents to share more information and describe more of the children's problems.
6. Interview older children to allow observation of parent-child interactions.
7. Interview older children, who can often provide details about their health history and severity of symptoms.
8. Treat adolescents as adults and individuals, because they tend to respond best when treated as such.
9. Remember that adolescents have the right to confidentiality. After talking with parents about historical information, speak alone with adolescents.

A comprehensive health assessment and examination of older adults should include physical data, as well as a review of growth and development, family relationships, group involvement, and religious and occupational pursuits (Ebersole and Hess, 1994). An important part of health assessment involves analysis of basic activities of daily living (ADLs) (dressing, bathing, toileting, feeding, and continence) that are fundamental to independent living. In addition, the more complex instrumental ADLs (using the telephone, preparing meals, managing money) are also assessed. Any examination of an older

TABLE 24-3
Positions for Examination

Position		Areas Assessed	Rationale	Limitations
Sitting		Head and neck, back, posterior thorax and lungs, anterior thorax and lungs, breasts, axillae, heart, vital signs, and upper extremities	Sitting upright provides full expansion of lungs and provides better visualization of symmetry of upper body parts.	Physically weakened client may be unable to sit. Examiner should use supine position with head of bed elevated instead.
Supine		Head and neck, anterior thorax and lungs, breasts, axillae, heart, abdomen, extremities, pulses	This is most normally relaxed position. It provides easy access to pulse sites.	If client becomes short of breath easily, examiner may need to raise head of bed.
Dorsal recumbent		Head and neck, anterior thorax and lungs, breasts, axillae, heart, abdomen	Position is used for abdominal assessment because it promotes relaxation of abdominal muscles.	Clients with painful disorders are more comfortable with knees flexed.
Lithotomy*		Female genitalia and genital tract	This position provides maximal exposure of genitalia and facilitates insertion of vaginal speculum.	Lithotomy position is embarrassing and uncomfortable, so examiner minimizes time that the client spends in it. Client is kept well draped.
Sims*		Rectum and vagina	Flexion of hip and knee improves exposure of rectal area.	Joint deformities may hinder client's ability to bend hip and knee.
Prone		Musculoskeletal system	This position is used only to assess extension of hip joint.	This position is poorly tolerated in clients with respiratory difficulties.
Lateral recumbent		Heart	This position aids in detecting murmurs.	This position is poorly tolerated in clients with respiratory difficulties.
Knee-chest*		Rectum	This position provides maximal exposure of rectal area.	This position is embarrassing and uncomfortable.

*Clients with arthritis or other joint deformities may be unable to assume this position.

adult should also include an evaluation of mental status.

Throughout an examination the nurse must recognize that with advancing age the body does not respond vigorously to injury or disease. Therefore older persons do not always exhibit the expected signs and symptoms (Lueckenotte, 1994). Characteristically, older adults have more blunted or atypical signs and symptoms.

Principles to use during examination of an older adult include the following:

1. Do not stereotype aging clients. Most are able to adapt to change and to learn about their health. Similarly, they are reliable historians.
2. Recognize that sensory or physical limitations can affect how quickly you are able to interview older adults and conduct examinations. Plan for more than one examination session. Sometimes it helps to give clients an initial health questionnaire before they come to a clinic or office (Ebersole and Hess, 1994).
3. Perform the examination with adequate space; this is especially important for clients with mobility aids such as a cane or walker.
4. During the examination use patience, allow for pauses, and observe for details. Recognize normalities of later life.
5. Older clients may find giving certain types of health information stressful. Illness is seen as a threat to independence and a step toward institutionalization.
6. Perform the examination near bathroom facilities if the client has an urgent need to void.
7. Be alert to signs of increasing fatigue such as sighing, grimacing, irritability, leaning against objects for support, and drooping of head and shoulders.

EXAMINATION

A physical examination, using the skills of physical assessment, is composed of individual assessments for each body system. The extent of an examination depends on its purpose and the client's condition. Clients with specific symptoms or needs require only portions of an examination. A complete health assessment follows the format of the health history (see Chapter 5). The nurse uses information from the history to focus attention on specific parts of the physical examination. For example, if the history shows that the client experiences difficulty in breathing, the nurse examines the thorax and lungs more carefully. The physical examination supplements information from the history to confirm or refute the data.

The examination should be systematic and well organized so important assessments are not omitted. A head-to-toe approach includes all body systems and helps the nurse anticipate each step. In an adult, the nurse begins by assessing the head and neck, progressing methodically down the body to include all body systems. Both sides of the body are inspected and compared for symmetry. If a client is seriously ill, the body system most at risk for being abnormal is examined first. If a client becomes fatigued, rest periods are provided. Painful procedures should be performed near the end of the examination. Assessments are recorded in specific terms on a physical assessment form or in the nurse's notes. The use of common and accepted medical abbreviations helps to keep notes brief and concise.

GENERAL SURVEY

Assessment begins when the nurse first meets the client. The nurse determines the reason for the client seeking health care. Initial data from the general survey begins with a review of the client's primary health problems. The nurse makes mental notes of the client's behavior and appearance. The examination begins with a general survey that includes observing general appearance and measuring behavior, vital signs, height, and weight. The survey provides information about characteristics of an illness, a client's hygiene and body image, emotional state, recent changes in weight, and the client's developmental status. If any abnormalities or problems are found, the affected body system is closely assessed later.

General Appearance and Behavior

Assessment of appearance and behavior can be conducted while the nurse prepares the client for the physical examination. The review of appearance and behavior includes the following:

1. *Gender and race.* A person's gender affects the type of examination performed and the manner in which assessments are made. Different physical features are related to gender and race. Certain illnesses more likely affect a specific gender or race; for example, skin cancer is 40 times higher in whites than in blacks, esophageal cancer is over three times higher among blacks than among whites, and cancer of the bladder is more common in men (American Cancer Society, 1997).
2. *Age.* Age influences normal physical characteristics. The ability to participate in some parts of the examination is also influenced by age.
3. *Signs of distress.* There may be obvious signs or symptoms indicating pain, difficulty in breathing, or anxiety. These signs help to establish priorities regarding what to examine first.
4. *Body type.* The nurse observes if a client appears trim and muscular, obese, or excessively thin. Body type can reflect level of health, age, and lifestyle.

5. *Posture.* Normal standing posture is an upright stance with parallel alignment of hips and shoulders. Normal sitting involves some degree of rounding of the shoulders. Observe whether the client has a slumped, erect, or bent posture. Posture may reflect mood or pain. Many older adults have a stooped, forward-bent posture, with hips and knees somewhat flexed and arms bent at the elbows, raising the level of the arms.

6. *Gait.* Observe the client walk into the room or along the bedside (if ambulatory). Note if movements are coordinated or uncoordinated. A person normally walks with arms swinging freely at the sides, with the head and face leading the body.

7. *Body movements.* Observe whether movements are purposeful. Note any tremors involving the extremities. Determine if any body parts are immobile.

8. *Hygiene and grooming.* Note the client's level of cleanliness by observing the appearance of the hair, skin, and fingernails. Note if the client's clothes are clean. Grooming may depend on the activities being performed just before the examination, as well as the client's occupation. Also note amount and type of cosmetics used.

9. *Dress.* Culture, lifestyle, socioeconomic level, and personal preference affect the type of clothes worn. Note if the type of clothing worn is appropriate for temperature and weather conditions.

TABLE 24-4
Clinical Indicators of Abuse

Physical Findings	Behavioral Findings
Child Sexual Abuse	
Vaginal or penile discharge	Problem in sleeping or eating
Blood on underclothing	Fear of certain people or places
Pain or itching in genital area	Play activities recreate the abuse situation
Genital injuries	Regressed behavior
Difficulty sitting or walking	Sexual acting out
Pain while urinating	Knowledge of explicit sexual matters
Foreign bodies in rectum, urethra, or vagina	Preoccupation with other's or own genitals
Venereal disease	
Domestic Abuse	
Injuries and trauma are inconsistent with reported cause	Attempted suicide
Multiple injuries involving head, face, neck, breasts, abdomen, and genitalia (black eyes, orbital fractures, broken nose, fractured skull, lip lacerations, broken teeth, strangulation marks)	Eating or sleeping disorders
	Anxiety
	Panic attacks
X-rays show old and new fractures in different stages of healing	Pattern of substance abuse (follows physical abuse)
	Low self-esteem
Burns	Depression
Human bites	Sense of helplessness
	Guilt
	Increased forgetfulness
Older Adult Abuse	
Injuries and trauma are inconsistent with reported cause (cigarette burn, scratch, bruise, or bite)	Dependent on care giver
	Physically and/or cognitively impaired
Hematomas	Combative
Bruises at various stages of resolution	Wandering
Bruises, chafing, excoriation on wrist or legs (restraints)	Verbally belligerent
Burns	Minimal social support
Fractures inconsistent with cause described	
Dried blood	
Prolonged interval between injury and medical treatment	

Data from All A: *J Gerontol Nurs* 20(7):25, 1994; Campbell J, Humphreys J: *Nursing care of survivors of family violence,* ed 2, St. Louis, 1993, Mosby; Pace H, Hoag-Apel C: *Point of View Magazine* 33(3):12, 1996.

Depressed or mentally ill persons may be unable to choose proper clothing. An older adult tends to wear extra clothing because of sensitivity to cold.

10. *Body odor.* An unpleasant body odor may result from physical exercise, poor hygiene, or certain disease pathologies. Poor oral hygiene may cause bad breath.

11. *Affect and mood.* Affect is a person's feelings as they appear to others. Mood or emotional state is expressed verbally and nonverbally. Note if verbal expressions match nonverbal behavior. Observe if mood is appropriate for the situation. Observe facial expressions while asking questions.

12. *Speech.* Normal speech is understandable and moderately paced. It shows an association with the person's thoughts. Note if the client talks rapidly or slowly. An abnormal pace may be caused by emotions or neurological impairment. Observe if the client speaks in a normal tone with clear inflection of words.

13. *Client abuse.* Abuse of children, women, and older adults is a growing health problem. It may be first suspected in clients who have suffered obvious physical injury or neglect (e.g., evidence of malnutrition or presence of bruising on the extremities or trunk). Assess for the client's fear of the spouse or partner, care giver, parent, or adult child. Note if the partner or care giver has a history of violence, alcoholism, or drug abuse. Is the person unemployed, ill, or frustrated in caring for the client? Most states mandate a report to a social service center if abuse or neglect is suspected. When abuse is suspected, interview the client in private. It is difficult to detect abuse because victims often will not complain or report that they are in an abusive situation. Clients are more likely to reveal any problems to a nurse when the suspected abuser is absent from the room. Clinical indicators for abuse are summarized in Table 24-4.

14. *Substance abuse.* Health care providers' recognition of clients who abuse alcohol, prescribed medications, or illegal drugs is typically poor. Studies have shown that only about 10% of clients who meet criteria for drug abuse are identified by primary health care providers (Caulker-Burnett, 1994). The problem affects all socioeconomic groups. A single visit to a clinic may not reveal the problem. Several visits often reveal behaviors that can be confirmed with a well-focused history and physical examination. The nurse must approach the client in a caring and nonjudgmental way, because substance abuse involves both emotional and lifestyle issues. Clients to suspect for substance abuse include those listed in Box 24-3. When abuse is suspected the nurse or examiner should ask the following questions: Have you ever felt the need to CUT DOWN on your drinking or

---

Box 24-3
Red Flags for Suspicion of Substance Abuse

Clients who frequently miss appointments

Clients who frequently request written excuses for work

Clients who have chief complaints of insomnia, "bad nerves," or pain that does not fit a particular pattern

Clients who often report lost prescriptions (e.g., tranquilizers or pain medications) or ask for frequent refills

Clients who make frequent emergency room visits

Clients who have a history of changing doctors or who bring in medication bottles prescribed by several different providers

Clients with histories of gastrointestinal bleeds, peptic ulcers, pancreatitis, cellulitis, or frequent pulmonary infections

Clients with frequent sexually transmitted diseases, complicated pregnancies, multiple abortions, or sexual dysfunction

Clients who complain of chest pains or palpitations or who have histories of admissions to rule out myocardial infarctions

Clients who give histories of activities that place them at risk for human immunodeficiency virus (HIV) infections

Clients with family history of addiction; history of childhood sexual, physical, or emotional abuse; or social and financial or marital problems

Modified from Master S, Terpstra JK: Recognition and diagnosis. In Schnoll SH and others: *Prescribing drugs with abuse liability,* Richmond, Va, 1992, DSAM, MCV-VCU.

---

drug use? Have people ANNOYED you by criticizing your drinking or drug use? Have you ever felt bad or GUILTY about your drinking or drug use? Have you ever used or had a drink first thing in the morning as an EYE-OPENER to steady your nerves or feel normal? If two or more of the CAGE questions are positive, the nurse should strongly suspect abuse and consider how to motivate the client to seek treatment (Stuart and Sundeen, 1995).

Vital Signs

Most nurses prefer measuring vital signs (see Chapter 23) before the physical examination, because positioning or moving the client can interfere with obtaining accurate values. The nurse can also measure specific vital signs during individual body system assessments.

For example, respirations may be assessed during examination of the thorax.

Height and Weight

A person's general level of health can be reflected by height and weight. Weight is a routine measure during health screenings and visits to physicians' offices or clinics. Both height and weight are routine assessments during admission to a health care setting. A nurse measures an infant's or child's height and weight to assess growth and development. In older adults, height and weight coupled with a nutritional assessment are important in determining cause and treatment for chronic disease and in assessing the older adult who has difficulty with feeding and other functional activities. The nurse should look for overall trends in height and weight changes.

A client's weight normally will vary daily because of fluid loss or retention. An assessment screens for abnormal weight changes. Before measurement, the nurse asks clients their current height and weight. The nurse also assesses if clients have had recent weight gains or losses. A weight gain of 5 lb or 2.2 kg in a day may indicate fluid-retention problems. If a change exists, the nurse assesses the amount; the period over which the change occurred; and a change in diet habits, appetite, prescription or over-the-counter drugs, or physical symptoms. It is also helpful to note if a client has a concern with weight loss or body shape (e.g., never feeling thin enough). An unusually strict caloric intake, laxative abuse, or excessive exercise could be warning signs for anorexia or bulimia.

Clients should be weighed at the same time of day, on the same scale, and in the same clothes to allow for an objective comparison of subsequent weights. Although body weight may seem routine, care should be taken to be certain of accuracy because significant medical and nursing decisions are made based on weight changes. Clients capable of bearing their own weight use a standing scale. The nurse calibrates a standard platform scale by moving the large and small weights to zero. The balance beam should be made level and steady by adjusting the calibrating knob. Electronic scales are automatically calibrated each time they are used. The client stands on the scale platform and remains still. The nurse moves the largest weight to the 50-lb or 22.5-kg increment under the client's weight. Then the smaller weight is adjusted to balance the scale at the nearest 1/4 lb or 0.1 kg (Seidel and others, 1995). Electronic scales automatically display weight within seconds.

Stretcher and chair scales are available for clients unable to bear weight. After being transferred to the scale, the client is lifted above the bed by a hydraulic device and the weight is measured on a balance beam or digital display. Caution must be used when transferring clients to and from the scales.

Infants can be weighed in baskets or on platform scales. The nurse removes an infant's clothing and weighs the infant in dry, disposable diapers to ensure accurate readings. The weight can later be adjusted for the weight of the diaper. The room should be warm to prevent chills. A light cloth or paper placed on the scale's surface prevents cross-infection from urine or feces. The nurse places infants in baskets or on platforms and holds a hand lightly above to prevent accidental falls. Weight is measured in ounces and grams.

There are different ways to measure the height of weight-bearing and non–weight-bearing clients. Clients able to stand remove their shoes. A paper towel is placed on the scale platform or floor so clients' feet remain clean. A measuring stick or tape is attached vertically to the weight scales or wall. The nurse asks the client to stand erect, exercising good posture. On a platform scale, a metal rod, attached to the back of the scale, swings out and over the crown of the client's head. A measuring stick or flat book can be placed on the client's head when a scale is unavailable. With the rod or stick placed level horizontally at a 90-degree angle to the measuring stick, the nurse measures height in inches or centimeters.

A non–weight-bearing client (such as an infant) is positioned supine on a firm surface. Portable devices are available that provide a reliable means to measure height. The nurse places the infant on the device, having the parent hold the infant's head against the headboard. With the infant's legs straight at the knees, the footboard is placed against the bottom of the infant's feet (Figure 24-4). The infant's length is recorded to the nearest 0.5 cm or ¼ inch.

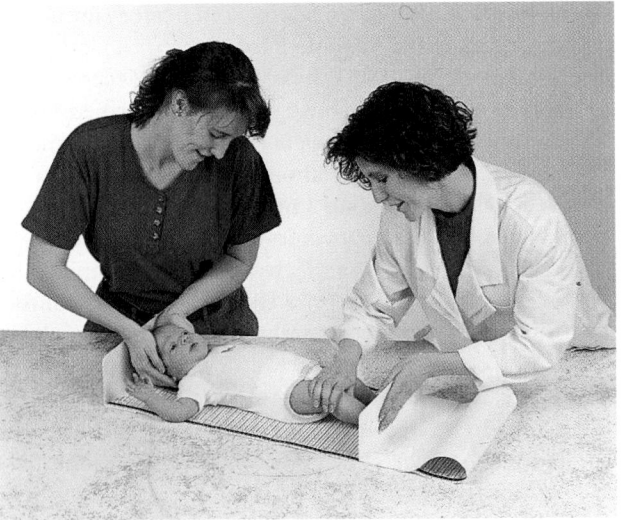

Figure 24-4. Measure of infant length. (From Seidel HM and others: *Mosby's guide to physical examination*, ed 3, St. Louis, 1995, Mosby.)

INTEGUMENT

The integument, consisting of the skin, nails, hair, and scalp, provides the body's external protection; regulates body temperature; and acts as a sensory organ for pain, temperature, and touch. The nurse may first inspect all skin surfaces or may assess the skin gradually as other body systems are examined. The physical assessment skills of inspection, palpation, and olfaction are used to assess the integument's function and integrity.

Skin

Assessment of the skin can reveal changes in oxygenation, circulation, nutrition, local tissue damage, and hydration. In a hospital setting the majority of clients are older adults, debilitated clients, or young but seriously ill. As a result there are significant risks for skin lesions resulting from trauma to the skin while administering care, from exposure to pressure during immobilization, or from reaction to medications used in treatment. Clients most at risk are the neurologically impaired; chronically ill; orthopedic clients; and clients with diminished mental status, poor tissue oxygenation, low cardiac output, and inadequate nutrition. In nursing homes and extended care facilities, clients may be at risk for many of the same problems depending on their level of mobility and presence of chronic illness. Nurses must routinely assess the skin to look for primary or initial lesions that may develop. Without proper care, primary lesions can quickly worsen to become secondary lesions that require more extensive nursing care. The development of a pressure ulcer, for example, can lengthen a hospital stay unless it is prevented or discovered early and treated properly.

The incidence of **melanoma,** an aggressive form of skin cancer, has increased about 4% every year since 1973 (American Cancer Society, 1997). In addition, the incidence of highly curable basal cell and squamous cell cancers is also increasing. Cutaneous malignancies are the most common neoplasms seen in clients (Smoller and Smoller, 1992). The nurse must incorporate a thorough skin assessment for all clients and educate them about self-examination (Box 24-4).

The condition of the client's skin reveals the need for nursing intervention. The nurse uses assessment findings to determine the type of hygiene measures required to maintain integrity of the integument (see Chapter 29). Adequate nutrition and hydration become goals of therapy if the nurse identifies alterations in the integument's status.

Adequate illumination of the skin is required for accurate observations. The recommended choice is natural or halogen lighting. For detecting skin changes in the dark-skinned client, sunlight is the best choice (Talbot and Curtis, 1996). Room temperature may also affect skin assessment. A room that is too warm may cause superficial vasodilation, resulting in an increased

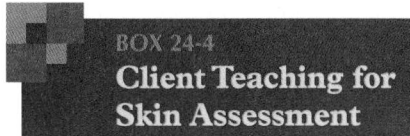

BOX 24-4

Client Teaching for Skin Assessment

- Instruct the client to conduct a monthly self-examination of the skin, noting moles, blemishes, and birthmarks.
- Tell the clients to inspect all skin surfaces. Cancerous melanomas start as small, molelike growths that increase in size, change color, become ulcerated, and bleed. A simple ABCD rule (American Cancer Society, 1997) outlines warning signals:

  A is for **asymmetry.**

  B is for **border** irregularity; edges are ragged, notched, or blurred.

  C is for **color;** pigmentation is not uniform.

  D is for **diameter,** greater than 6 millimeters.

- Tell the client to report to a physician changes in skin lesions or a sore that does not heal.
- Instruct the client to prevent skin cancer by avoiding overexposure to the sun: wear wide-brimmed hat and long sleeves; apply sunscreens with SPF greater than or equal to 15 approximately 15 minutes before going into the sun and after swimming or perspiring; avoid tanning under direct sun between 10:00 AM and 3:00 PM; and do not use indoor sunlamps, tanning parlors, or tanning pills.
- Older adults and clients with certain chronic diseases tend to have delayed wound healing.
- Instruct the client to report any lesion that bleeds or fails to heal to a physician.
- To treat excessively dry skin, tell the client to avoid hot water, use a superfatted soap (e.g., Dove), pat rather than rub the skin dry after bathing, apply mineral oil to body parts, and wear cotton clothing (Hardy, 1996).

redness of the skin. A cool environment may cause the sensitive client to develop cyanosis around the lips and nail beds (Talbot and Curtis, 1996).

Disposable gloves are required for palpation if open, moist, or draining skin lesions are present. Because the nurse inspects all skin surfaces, the client must assume several positions. The examination includes inspecting the skin's color, moisture, temperature, texture, and turgor. Vascular changes, **edema,** and lesions are also noted. Abnormalities are carefully palpated and documented. Skin odors are usually noted in skinfolds, such as the axillae or under the female client's breasts.

Health history. Before assessing the skin, the nurse asks the client about the presence of lesions, rashes, or bruises and determines whether the alterations can be linked to heat, cold, stress, exposure to toxic material or the sun, or new skin care products. The nurse also determines if there has been a recent change in skin color or trauma to the skin. If a client has been out in the sun, it is useful to know if a sunscreen has been worn. If not, the client will require education on ways to safeguard the skin. The nurse also assesses for history of allergies, use of topical medications, and a family history of serious skin disorders. The nurse uses assessment findings to determine abnormalities and the type of hygiene measures needed to maintain integrity of the integument.

Color. Skin color varies from body part to body part and from person to person. Despite individual variations, skin color is usually uniform over the body. Table 24-5 lists common variations. Normal skin pigmentation ranges from ivory or light pink to ruddy pink in white skin and from light to deep brown or black in dark skin. Sun-darkened or darker skin is common around knees and elbows.

Basal cell carcinoma is most commonly seen in sun-exposed areas and frequently occurs in a background of sun-damaged skin (Smoller and Smoller, 1992). In older adults, pigmentation increases unevenly, causing discolored skin. While inspecting the skin, the nurse must be aware that color may be masked by cosmetics or tanning agents.

The assessment of color first involves areas of the skin not exposed to the sun, such as the palms of the hands. The nurse notes if the skin is unusually pale or dark. It is more difficult to note changes such as pallor or cyanosis in clients with dark skin. Usually color hues are best seen in the palms, soles of the feet, lips, tongue, and nail beds. Areas of increased color (hyperpigmentation) and decreased color (hypopigmentation) are common. Skin creases and folds are darker than the rest of the body in the dark-skinned client.

The nurse inspects sites where abnormalities are more easily identified. For example, **pallor** is more easily seen in the face, buccal mucosa (mouth), conjunctivae, and nail beds. **Cyanosis** is best observed in the lips, nail beds, palpebral conjunctivae, and palms.

In recognizing pallor in the dark-skinned client, the nurse would observe that normal brown skin appears to be yellow-brown and normal black skin appears to be an ashen-gray. The lips, nail beds, and mucous membranes should also be assessed for generalized pallor; if pallor is present, the mucous membranes will be an ashen-gray color. Assessment of cyanosis in the dark-skinned client requires that the nurse observe areas where pigmentation occurs the least (conjunctiva, sclera, buccal mucosa, tongue, lips, nail beds, and palms and soles). In addition, the nurse should verify findings with clinical manifestations (Talbot and Curtis, 1996).

The best site to inspect for **jaundice** (yellow-orange discoloration) is the client's sclera. Normal reactive hyperemia, or redness, is most often seen in regions exposed to pressure such as the sacrum, heels, and greater trochanter.

TABLE 24-5
Skin Color Variations

Color	Condition	Causes	Assessment Locations
Bluish (cyanosis)	Increased amount of deoxygenated hemoglobin (associated with hypoxia)	Heart or lung disease, cold environment	Nail beds, lips, mouth, skin (severe cases)
Pallor (decrease in color)	Reduced amount of oxyhemoglobin	Anemia	Face, conjunctivae, nail beds, palms of hands
	Reduced visibility of oxyhemoglobin resulting from decreased blood flow	Shock	Skin, nail beds, conjunctivae, lips
Loss of pigmentation	Vitiligo	Congenital or autoimmune condition causing lack of pigment	Patchy areas on skin over face, hands, arms
Yellow-orange (jaundice)	Increased deposit of bilirubin in tissues	Liver disease, destruction of red blood cells	Sclera, mucous membranes, skin
Red (erythema)	Increased visibility of oxyhemoglobin caused by dilation or increased blood flow	Fever, direct trauma, blushing, alcohol intake	Face, area of trauma, sacrum, shoulders, other common sites for pressure ulcers
Tan-brown	Increased amount of melanin	Suntan, pregnancy	Areas exposed to sun: face, arms, areolae, nipples

The nurse inspects for any patches or areas of skin color variation. Localized skin changes, such as pallor or **erythema** (red discoloration), may indicate circulatory changes. For example, an area of erythema may be caused by localized vasodilation resulting from sunburn or fever. In the dark-skinned client, erythema is not easily observed, so the nurse must palpate the area for heat and warmth to note the presence of skin inflammation (Talbot and Curtis, 1996). An area of an extremity that appears unusually pale may result from an arterial occlusion or edema. It is important to ask if the client has noticed any changes in skin coloring. The client usually knows whether a change has occurred.

A pattern of findings that is becoming more common is that associated with clients who are chemically dependent and are intravenous (IV) drug abusers. Usually clients are in denial about their disease, and it may be difficult to recognize signs and symptoms after just one physical examination (Caulker-Burnett, 1994). A client who takes repeated IV injections may have edematous, reddened, and warm areas along the arms and legs. This pattern suggests recent injections. Evidence of old injection sites appears as hyperpigmented and shiny or scarred areas. Table 24-6 summarizes additional physical findings associated with substance abuse.

Moisture. The hydration of skin and mucous membranes helps to reveal body fluid imbalances, changes in the skin's environment, and regulation of body temperature. Moisture refers to wetness and oiliness. The skin is normally smooth and dry. Skinfolds such as the axillae are normally moist. Minimal perspiration or oiliness should be present (Seidel and others,

1995). Increased perspiration may be associated with activity, warm environments, obesity, anxiety, or excitement. The nurse uses ungloved fingertips to palpate skin surfaces and observe for dullness, dryness, crusting, and flaking. Flaking is the appearance of dandruff-like flakes when the skin surface is lightly rubbed. Scaling involves fishlike scales that are easily rubbed off the skin's surface. Both flaking and scaling are believed to indicate abnormally dry skin (Hardy, 1996). Excessively dry skin is common in older adults and persons who use excessive amounts of soap during bathing. Other factors causing dry skin include lack of humidity, exposure to sun, smoking, stress, excessive perspiration, and dehydration (Hardy, 1996). Excessive dryness can worsen existing skin conditions such as **eczema** and dermatitis.

Temperature. The temperature of the skin depends on the amount of blood circulating through the dermis. Increased or decreased skin temperature reflects an increase or decrease in blood flow. Localized erythema or redness of the skin often may be accompanied by an increase in skin temperature. A reduction in skin temperature reflects a decrease in blood flow. It is important to remember that if an examination room is cold, the client's skin temperature and color can be affected.

Temperature is more accurately assessed by palpating the skin with the dorsum or back of the hand. The nurse compares symmetrical body parts. Normally the skin is warm. Skin temperature may be the same throughout the body or may vary in one area. Assessment of skin temperature is always done for clients at risk of having impaired circulation, such as after a cast application or vascular surgery. In addition, a nurse can identify a stage I pressure ulcer early when noting warmth and erythema on an area of the skin.

Texture. The character of the skin's surface and the feel of deeper portions are its texture. The nurse determines if the client's skin is smooth or rough, thin or thick, tight or supple, and indurated (hardened) or soft by stroking it lightly with the fingertips. The texture of the skin is normally smooth, soft, and flexible in children and adults. However, the texture is usually not uniform. The palms of the hands and soles of the feet tend to be thicker. In older adults the skin becomes wrinkled and leathery because of a decrease in collagen, subcutaneous fat, and sweat glands.

Localized changes may result from trauma, surgical wounds, or lesions. When irregularities in texture such as scars or **induration** are found, the nurse asks whether the client has had a recent injury to the skin. Deeper palpation may reveal irregularities such as tenderness or localized areas of induration commonly caused by repeated intramuscular or subcutaneous injections.

TABLE 24-6
Physical Findings of the Skin Indicative of Substance Abuse

Body System	Commonly Associated Drug
Diaphoresis	Sedative hypnotic (including alcohol)
Spider angiomas	Alcohol, stimulants
Burns (especially fingers)	Alcohol
Needle marks	Opioids
Contusion, abrasions, cuts, scars	Alcohol, other sedative hypnotics
"Homemade" tatoos	Cocaine, IV opioids, (prevents detection of injection sites)
Increased vascularity of face	Alcohol

Modified from Caulker-Burnett I: Primary care screening for substance abuse, *Nurse Pract* 19(6): 42, 1994.

Turgor. **Turgor** is the skin's elasticity, which can be diminished by edema or dehydration. Normally the skin loses its elasticity with age. To assess skin turgor, a fold of skin on the back of the forearm or sternal area is grasped with the fingertips and released (Figure 24-5). Normally the skin lifts easily and snaps back immediately to its resting position. The skin stays pinched or tented when turgor is poor. The client with poor turgor does not have a resilience to the normal wear and tear on the skin. A decrease in turgor predisposes the client to skin breakdown.

Vascularity. The circulation of the skin affects color in localized areas and the appearance of superficial blood vessels. With aging, capillaries become fragile. Localized pressure areas, found after a client has lain or sat in one position, appear reddened, pink, or pale (see Chapter 38). **Petechiae** are tiny, pinpoint-sized, red or purple spots on the skin caused by small hemorrhages in the skin layers. Petechiae may indicate serious blood-clotting disorders, drug reactions, or liver disease.

Edema. Areas of the skin become swollen or edematous from fluid buildup in the tissues. Direct trauma and impairment of venous return are two common causes for edema. The nurse inspects edematous areas for location, color, and shape. The formation of edema separates the skin's surface from the pigmented and vascular layers, masking skin color. Edematous skin also appears stretched and shiny. The nurse palpates areas of edema to determine mobility, consistency, and tenderness. When pressure from the nurse's finger leaves an indentation in the edematous area, it is called *pitting edema*. To assess pitting edema, the nurse presses the edematous area firmly with the thumb for 5 seconds and releases. The depth of pitting, recorded in millime-

ters (Seidel and others, 1995), determines the degree of edema. For example, 1+ edema equals 2 mm depth.

Lesions. The skin is normally free of lesions, except common freckles or age-related changes such as skin tags or senile keratosis (thickening of skin), cherry angiomas (ruby red papules), and atrophic warts. Lesions may be primary (occurring as initial spontaneous manifestations of a pathological process), such as a wheal of an insect bite, or secondary (resulting from later formation of trauma to a primary lesion), such as a pressure ulcer. When a lesion is detected, it is inspected for color, location, texture, size, shape, type (Box 24-5), grouping (e.g., clustered or linear), and distribution (localized or generalized). Any exudate is observed for color, odor, amount, and consistency. The size is best measured by using a small, clear, flexible ruler, divided in centimeters. Lesions are measured in height, width, and depth. Palpation determines the lesion's mobility, contour (flat, raised, or depressed), and consistency (soft or hard). After a lesion is identified, it is closely inspected with good illumination. It is palpated gently, covering its entire area. If the lesion is moist or has draining fluid, gloves are worn during palpation. The nurse notes if the client complains of tenderness during palpation. Cancerous lesions frequently undergo changes in color and size. Abnormalities, especially lesions that have changed in character (e.g., color or size), are reported to a physician because further examination may be required.

Hair and Scalp

The following types of hair cover the body: terminal hair (long, coarse, thick hair easily visible on the scalp, axillae, and pubic areas) and vellus hair (small, soft, tiny hairs covering the whole body except for the palms and soles). Good lighting allows the nurse to inspect the condition and distribution of hair and integrity of the scalp. Assessment of the hair occurs during all portions of the examination. The nurse assesses the distribution, thickness, texture, and lubrication of hair. In addition, the nurse inspects for infection or infestation of the scalp.

Health history. The nurse should ask questions such as the following: Has the client noted change in growth or loss of hair? Change in texture or color? What types of hair care products are used? Has the client recently been on chemotherapy (drugs that can cause hair loss) or taken vasodilators (minoxidil) for hair growth? Has the client noted changes in diet or appetite? If a client has a hairpiece, it should be removed if inspection of the scalp is essential.

Inspection. During inspection explain that it may be necessary to separate parts of the hair to detect abnormalities. First inspect the distribution, thickness,

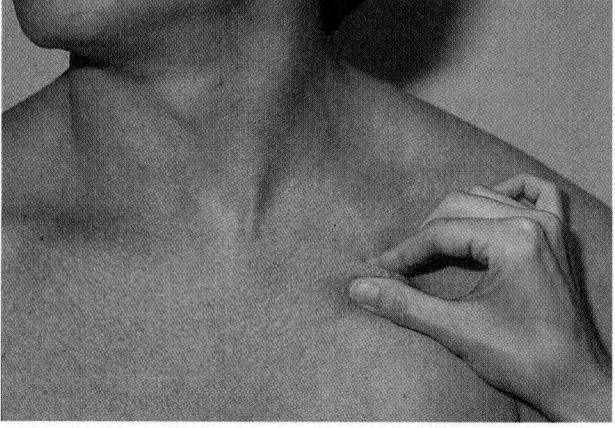

Figure 24-5. Assessment of skin turgor. (From Seidel HM and others: *Mosby's guide to physical examination,* ed 3, St. Louis, 1995, Mosby.)

Box 24-5
Types of Primary Skin Lesions

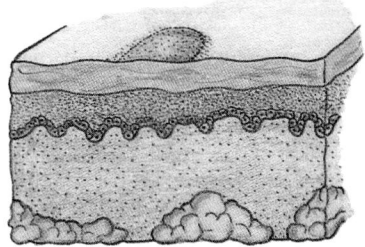

Macule: flat, nonpalpable change in skin color, smaller than 1 cm (e.g., freckle, petechia)

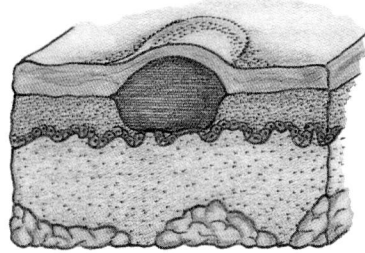

Papule: palpable, circumscribed, solid elevation in skin, smaller than 0.5 cm (e.g., elevated nevus)

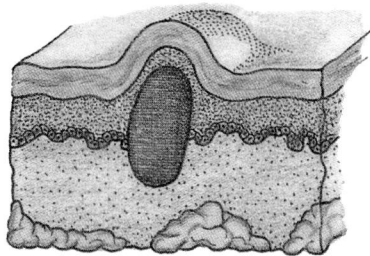

Nodule: elevated solid mass, deeper and firmer than papule, 0.2-0.5 cm (e.g., wart)

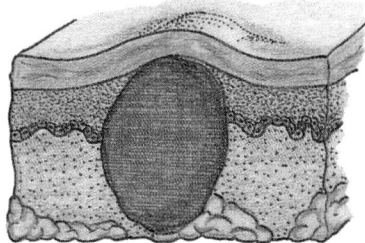

Tumor: solid mass that may extend deep through subcutaneous tissue, larger than 1-2 cm (e.g., epithelioma)

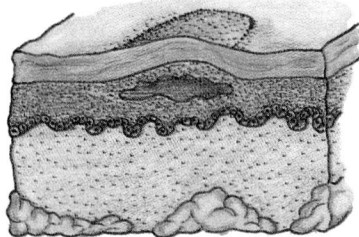

Wheal: irregularly shaped, elevated area or superficial localized edema, varies in size (e.g., hive, mosquito bite)

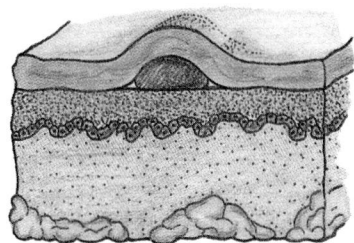

Vesicle: circumscribed elevation of skin filled with serous fluid, smaller than 0.5 cm (e.g., herpes simplex, chickenpox)

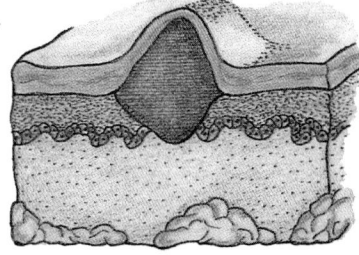

Pustule: circumscribed elevation of skin similar to vesicle but filled with pus, varies in size (e.g., acne, staphylococcal infection)

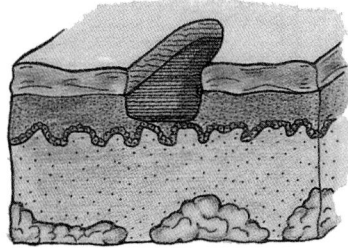

Ulcer: deep loss of skin surface that may extend to dermis and frequently bleeds and scars, varies in size (e.g., venous stasis ulcer)

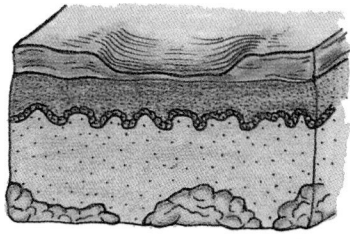

Atrophy: thinning of skin with loss of normal skin furrow with skin appearing shiny and translucent, varies in size (e.g., arterial insufficiency)

texture, and lubrication of body hair. Hair is normally distributed evenly, is neither excessively dry nor oily, and is pliant. While separating sections of scalp hair the nurse observes characteristics of color and coarseness. Normal terminal hair is black, brown, red, yellow, or variations in shades of these colors. The hair is coarse or fine and shiny. Normal variations exist in the shape of hair fibers. Clients' hair may be straight, curly, spiral, or

wavy. The hair of black persons is usually thicker and drier than the hair of whites.

In older adults, the hair becomes dull gray, white, or yellow. The hair also thins over the scalp, axillae, and pubic areas. Older men lose facial hair, whereas older women may develop hair on the chin and upper lip.

Changes may occur in the thickness, texture, and lubrication of scalp hair. Disturbances such as a febrile illness or scalp disease can result in hair loss. Conditions such as thyroid disease can alter the condition of the hair, making it fine and brittle. Baldness **(alopecia)** or thinning of the hair is usually related to genetic tendencies and endocrine disorders such as diabetes and even menopause. Poor nutrition can cause stringy, dull, dry, and thin hair. The hair is lubricated from the oil of sebaceous glands. Excessively oily hair is associated with androgen hormone stimulation. Dry, brittle hair occurs with aging and excessive use of chemical agents. The amount of hair covering the extremities may be reduced as a result of aging and arterial insufficiency and is most commonly seen over the lower extremities. In women, loss of hair should not be confused with shaven legs.

The nurse inspects the scalp for lesions, which can easily go unnoticed in thick hair. The scalp is normally smooth and inelastic, with even coloration. By carefully separating strands of hair the nurse can thoroughly examine the scalp for lesions. The nurse notes the characteristics of any scalp lesions. If lumps or bruises are found, the nurse asks if the client has experienced recent trauma to the head. Moles on the scalp are common. The nurse should warn the client that combing or brushing can cause a mole to bleed. Scaliness or dryness of the scalp is frequently caused by dandruff or psoriasis.

Careful inspection of hair follicles on the scalp and pubic areas may reveal lice or other parasites. The three types of lice are *Pediculus humanus capitis* (head lice), *Pediculus humanus corporis* (body lice), and *Pediculus pubis* (crab lice). Lice attach their eggs to hair. The head and body lice are tiny and have grayish-white bodies. Crab lice have red legs. Lice eggs look like oval particles of dandruff. The lice themselves are difficult to see. The nurse looks for bites or pustular eruptions in the follicles and in areas where skin surfaces meet, such as behind the ears and in the groin. The discovery of lice requires immediate treatment (Box 24-6).

Nails

The condition of the nails can reflect general health, state of nutrition, a person's occupation, and level of self-care. The most visible portion of the nails is the nail plate, the transparent layer of epithelial cells covering the nail bed. The vascularity of the nail bed creates the nail's underlying color. The semilunar, whitish area at the base of the nail bed from which the nail plate develops is the lunula.

Health history. Before assessing the nails the nurse asks if the client has had any recent trauma. A blow to the nail can change the shape and growth of the nail, as well as loss of all or part of the nail plate. The nurse also asks the client to describe nail-care practices. Improper care can damage nails and cuticles. It is also important to find out if clients have acrylic nails or silk wraps, because these may be areas for fungal growth. It

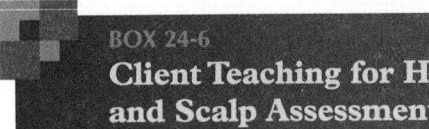

BOX 24-6
Client Teaching for Hair and Scalp Assessment

- Clients may require instruction about basic hygiene measures, including shampooing and combing of the hair (see Chapter 29).
- Instruct clients who have head lice to shampoo thoroughly with pediculicide (shampoo available at drug stores) in cold water, comb thoroughly with fine-tooth comb (following product directions), and discard comb.
- After combing remove any remaining nits or nit cases with tweezers or between the fingernails. A dilute solution of vinegar and water may help loosen nits.
- Instruct clients and parents about ways to reduce transmission of lice:
    Do not share personal care items with others.
    Vacuum all rugs, car seats, pillows, furniture, and flooring thoroughly and discard vacuum bag.
    Seal nonwashable items in plastic bags for 14 days if parents are unable to afford dry-cleaning and do not have a vacuum (Clore, 1989).
    Use thorough hand washing.
    Launder all clothing, linen, and bedding in hot soap and water and dry in a hot dryer for at least 20 minutes. Dry-clean nonwashable items (Wong, 1995).
    Do not use insecticide.
- Instruct the client that his or her partner must be notified if lice were sexually transmitted.

is helpful to know if the client has noticed changes in nail appearance or growth. Alterations may occur slowly over time. Knowing if the client has risks for nail or foot problems (e.g., diabetes, peripheral vascular disease, older adulthood) will influence the level of hygienic care recommended.

Inspection and palpation. The nurse inspects the nail bed color, the thickness and shape of the nail, the texture of the nail, and the condition of tissue around the nail. The nails are normally transparent, smooth, and convex, with surrounding cuticles smooth, intact, and without inflammation. In whites, nail beds are pink with translucent white tips. In dark-skinned clients, nail beds can be darkly pigmented with a blue or reddish hue. A brown or black pigmentation is normal with longitudinal streaks (Figure 24-6). Splinter hemorrhages can be caused by trauma, cirrhosis, diabetes mellitus, and hypertension. Vitamin, protein, and electrolyte changes can cause various lines or bands to form on nail beds.

Nails normally grow at a constant rate, but direct injury or generalized disease can slow growth. With aging, the nails of the fingers and toes become harder and thicker. Longitudinal striations develop, and the rate of nail growth slows. Nails become more brittle, dull, and opaque and may turn yellow in older adults because of insufficient calcium. Also with age the cuticle becomes less thick and wide.

Inspection of the angle between the nail and nail bed normally reveals an angle of 160 degrees (Box 24-7). A larger angle and softening of the nail bed can indicate chronic oxygenation problems. The nurse palpates the nail base to determine firmness and condition of circu-

lation. The nail base is normally firm. To palpate, the nurse gently grasps the client's finger and observes the color of the nail bed. Next, gentle, firm, quick pressure is applied with the thumb to the nail bed and released. As the pressure is applied, the nail bed appears white or blanched; however, the pink color should return immediately on release of pressure. Failure of the pinkness to return promptly indicates circulatory insufficiency. An ongoing bluish or purplish cast to the nail bed occurs with cyanosis. A white cast or pallor results from anemia.

Calluses and corns are often found on the toes or fingers. A callus is flat and painless, resulting from thickening of the epidermis. Corns are caused by friction and pressure from shoes and are usually seen over bony prominences. During the examination, the nurse instructs clients on proper nail care (Box 24-8).

Box 24-7
Abnormalities of the Nail Bed

160 degrees

Normal nail: Approximately 160-degree angle between nail plate and nail

180 degrees

180 degrees

Clubbing: Change in angle between nail and nail base (eventually larger than 180 degrees); nail bed softening, with nail flattening; often, enlargement of fingertips
Causes: Chronic lack of oxygen: heart or pulmonary disease

Beau's lines: Transverse depressions in nails indicating temporary disturbance of nail growth (nail grows out over several months)
Causes: Systemic illness such as severe infection, nail injury

Koilonychia (spoon nail): Concave curves
Causes: Iron-deficiency anemia, syphilis, use of strong detergents

Splinter hemorrhages: Red or brown linear streaks in nail bed
Causes: Minor trauma, subacute bacterial endocarditis, trichinosis

Paronychia: Inflammation of skin at base of nail
Causes: Local infection, trauma

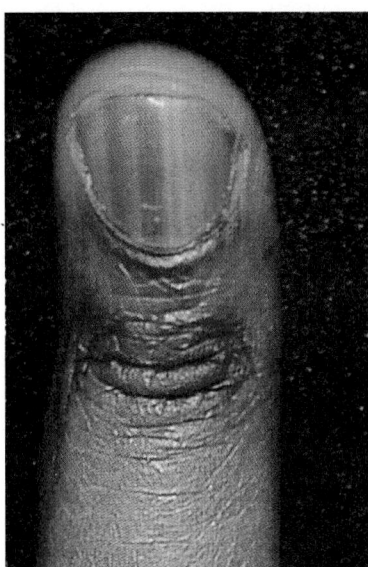

Figure 24-6. Pigmented bands in nail of client with dark skin. (From Seidel HM and others: *Mosby's guide to physical examination*, ed 3, St. Louis, 1995, Mosby.)

BOX 24-8
Client Teaching for Nail Assessment

- Instruct the client to cut nails only after soaking them about 10 minutes in warm water. (Exception: Diabetic clients are warned against soaking nails.)
- Instruct the client to avoid using over-the-counter preparations to treat corns, calluses, or ingrown toenails.
- Tell the client to cut nails straight across and even with the tops of the fingers or toes. If the client has diabetes, tell the client to file rather than cut the nails.
- Instruct the client to shape nails with a file or emery board.

HEAD AND NECK

An examination of the head and neck includes the head, eyes, ears, nose, mouth, pharynx, and neck (lymph nodes, carotid arteries, thyroid gland, and trachea). The carotid arteries can also be assessed during the assessment of peripheral arteries. The nurse needs to understand each anatomical area and its normal function. Assessment of the head and neck uses inspection, palpation, and auscultation.

Head

Health history. The history allows the nurse to screen for possible intracranial injury if necessary. The nurse asks whether the client experienced recent trauma to the head or if neurological symptoms such as headache (note onset, duration, character, pattern, and associated symptoms), dizziness, seizures, poor vision, or loss of consciousness have occurred. The history also includes a review of the client's occupation, focusing on those clients who should wear safety helmets. In addition, the nurse learns if the client participates in contact sports, cycling, roller blading, or skateboarding.

Inspection and palpation. The nurse inspects the client's head, noting the position, size, shape, and contour. The head is normally held upright and midline to the trunk. A horizontal jerking or bobbing may indicate a tremor. Holding the head tilted to one side may be an indication of unilateral hearing or visual loss. The skull is generally round with prominences in the frontal area anteriorly and the occipital area posteriorly. Local skull deformities are typically caused by trauma. In infants, a large head may result from congenital anomalies or the accumulation of cerebrospinal fluid in the ventricles (**hydrocephalus**). Adults may have enlarged jaws and facial bones resulting from **acromegaly.** The nurse palpates the skull for nodules or masses. Gentle rotation of the fingertips down the midline of the scalp and then along the sides of the head reveals abnormalities. The nurse also notes the client's facial features, looking at the eyelids, eyebrows, nasolabial folds, and mouth for shape and symmetry. It is normal for slight asymmetry to exist. If there is facial asymmetry, the nurse notes if all features on one side of the face are affected or if only a portion of the face is involved. Various neurological disorders such as a facial nerve paralysis affect different nerves that innervate muscles of the face.

Eyes

Examination of the eye includes assessment of visual acuity, visual fields, extraocular movements, and external and internal eye structures. Figure 24-7 shows a cross section of the eye. The assessment detects visual alterations and determines the level of assistance clients

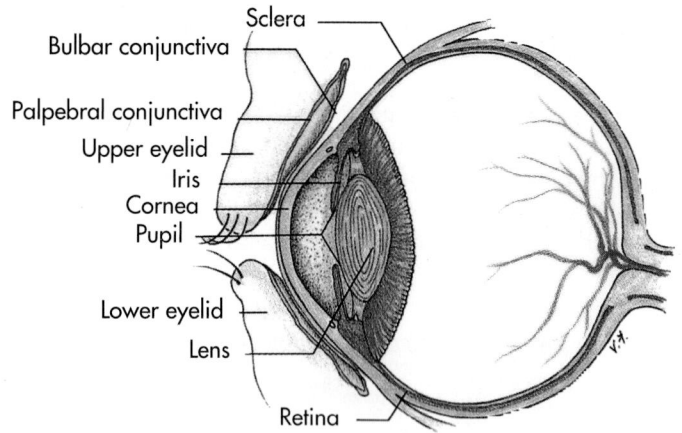

Figure 24-7. Cross section of eye.

require when ambulating or performing self-care activities. Clients with visual problems may also need special aids for reading teaching materials or instructions.

Health history. The nurse determines if the client is at risk for partial or complete visual loss by reviewing history of eye disease (e.g., glaucoma, cataracts), eye trauma, diabetes, hypertension, or eye surgery. Assessment for common symptoms of eye disease, such as eye pain, photophobia (sensitivity to light), burning, itching, excess tearing or crusting, diplopia (double vision), blurred vision, awareness of a "film" or "curtain" over the field of vision, floaters, flashing lights, or halos around lights, is critical. The nurse also reviews the client's occupational history, use of glasses or contact lenses, use of safety glasses at work and for hobbies, and regularity of visits to an ophthalmologist or optometrist (Box 24-9). The nurse also questions the client about current medications, including eye drops or ointments. The nurse should determine whether there is a family history of eye disorders or disease.

Visual acuity. The assessment of visual acuity, the ability to see small details, tests central vision. The easiest way to assess visual acuity is to ask the client to read printed material under adequate lighting. If clients use glasses or contact lenses, they should wear them. The nurse should know the language a client speaks and whether the client is literate. Asking the client to read aloud tests literacy. If the client has difficulty reading, move to the next step.

A more accurate assessment of distant vision uses a Snellen chart (paper chart or projection screen). The chart should be well lighted. Always test vision without corrective lenses first. The nurse has the client sit or stand 20 feet (6.1 m) away from the chart and try to read all of the letters beginning at any line, once with both eyes open and then with each eye separately (with opposite eye covered). The nurse notes the smallest line

- Tell clients that people under age 40 should have complete eye examinations every 3 to 5 years (or more often if family histories reveal risks such as diabetes or hypertension).
- Tell clients that people over age 40 should have eye examinations every 2 years to screen for conditions that may develop without client awareness (e.g., glaucoma).
- Tell clients that people over age 65 should have yearly eye examinations.
- Describe the typical symptoms of eye disease (see Chapter 39).
- Instruct older adults to take the following precautions because of normal visual changes: avoid driving at night, increase lighting in the home to reduce risk of falls, and paint the first and last steps of a staircase and the edge of each step in between a bright color to aid in depth perception.

in which the client can read all of the letters correctly and records the visual acuity for that line. Repeat the test with the client wearing corrective lenses. Do the test rapidly enough so that the client does not memorize the chart (Seidel and others, 1995).

If a client cannot read, the nurse uses an "E" chart or one with pictures of familiar objects. Instead of reading letters, clients tell the nurse which direction each "E" is pointing or the name of the object. The visual acuity score is recorded for each eye and both eyes. Symbol charts are frequently used to screen preschool children, and early school-age children are screened with an "E" chart; as a child advances in school, the standard Snellen chart is used.

The Snellen chart has standardized numbers at the end of each line of the chart. The numerator is the number 20, or the distance the client stands from the chart. The denominator is the distance from which the normal eye can read the chart. Normal vision is 20/20. The larger the denominator, the poorer the client's visual acuity. The nurse records acuity as *sc* (without correction) and *cc* (with correction), depending on whether the client wears glasses or contact lenses.

If clients cannot read even the largest letters or figures of a Snellen chart, the nurse tests their ability to count upraised fingers or distinguish light. The nurse holds a hand 30 cm (1 foot) from the face and instructs the client to count the upraised fingers. To check light perception, the nurse shines a penlight into the eye and then turns the light off. If the client notes when the light is turned on or off, light perception is intact.

Near vision can be assessed by asking the client to read a handheld card containing a vision-screening chart. Instruct the client to hold the card at a comfortable distance (about 14 inches, or 5 to 6 cm) from the eyes. The client reads the smallest line possible.

Visual fields. As a person looks straight ahead, all objects in the periphery can normally be seen. To assess visual fields, the nurse has the client stand or sit 2 feet (60 cm) away, facing the nurse at eye level. The client gently closes or covers one eye (e.g., the left) and looks at the nurse's eye directly opposite (client's left eye, nurse's right eye). The nurse closes the opposite eye so that the field of vision is superimposed on that of the client. The nurse moves a finger equidistant at arm's length from the nurse and client outside the field of vision, then slowly brings it back into the visual field. The client is asked to tell when the nurse's finger is seen. If the nurse sees the finger before the client does, this reveals that a portion of the client's visual field is reduced. To test temporal field vision, the object should be slightly behind the client. (NOTE: The nurse can see the finger.) The procedure is repeated for each field of vision. The examination is only approximate and presumes the nurse's visual fields are normal. Older adults commonly have loss of peripheral vision caused by changes in the lens.

Extraocular movements. Six small muscles guide the movement of each eye. Both eyes move parallel to each other in each of the six directions of gaze (Figure 24-8). The client sits or stands 2 feet away, facing the nurse. The nurse holds a finger at a comfortable distance (6 to 12 inches, or 15 to 30 cm) in front of the client's eyes. The client keeps the head in a fixed position facing the nurse and follows the movement of the finger with the eyes only. The client looks to the right, to the left, up, down, and diagonally up and down to the left and right. The nurse's finger moves smoothly and slowly within the normal field of vision. As the client gazes in each direction, the nurse observes for parallel eye movement, the position of the upper eyelid in relation to the iris, and the presence of abnormal movements such as **nystagmus.** With nystagmus a fine, rhythmical oscillation of the eyes is present. The nurse can initiate nystagmus in clients with normal eye movement by having them gaze to the far left or right. As the eyes move through each direction of gaze, the upper eyelid only covers the iris slightly. Disturbances in eye movement reflect local injury to eye muscles and supporting structures or a disorder of the cranial nerves.

The nurse can also check the alignment of the eyes by assessing the corneal light reflex. The nurse shines a penlight onto the bridge of the client's nose from 60 to 90 cm (2 to 3 feet) away in a darkened room. The client looks straight ahead. Normally light reflects on the cornea in the same spot on both eyes. If there is an abnormality, the light shines on a different spot on each eye.

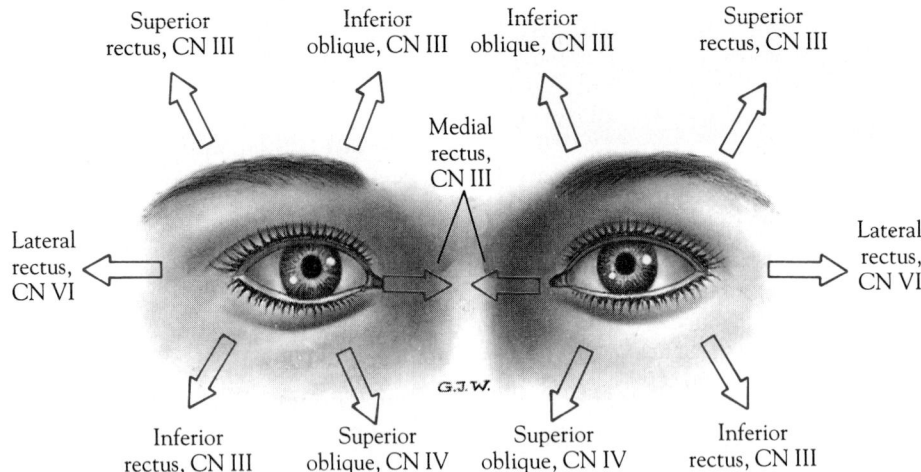

Figure 24-8. Six directions of gaze. Nurse directs client to follow finger movement through each gaze. (From Seidel HM and others: *Mosby's guide to physical examination,* ed 3, St. Louis, 1995, Mosby.)

External eye structures. To inspect external eye structures, the nurse stands directly in front of the client at eye level and asks the client to look at the nurse's face.

Position and alignment. The nurse assesses the position of the eyes in relation to one another. Normally they are parallel to each other. Bulging eyes (exophthalmos) usually indicate hyperthyroidism. The crossing of eyes (strabismus) results from neuromuscular injury or inherited abnormalities. Tumors or inflammation of the orbit can cause abnormal eye protrusion.

Eyebrows. For the remainder of the examination the client removes contact lenses. The nurse inspects the eyebrows for size, extension, texture of hair, alignment, and movement. Coarseness of hair and failure to extend beyond the temporal canthus may reveal hypothyroidism. If the brows are thinned, the client may pluck or wax the hair. Aging causes loss of the lateral third of the eyebrows. The nurse has the client raise and lower the eyebrows. The brows should raise and lower symmetrically. An inability to move the eyebrows may indicate a facial nerve paralysis.

Eyelids. The nurse inspects the eyelids for position; color; condition of surface; condition and direction of lashes; and the client's ability to open, close, and blink. When the eyes are open in a normal position, the lids do not cover the pupil, and the sclera cannot be seen above the iris. The lids are also close to the eyeball. An abnormal drooping of the lid over the pupil is called **ptosis,** caused by edema or impairment of the third cranial nerve. In the older adult, ptosis results from a loss of elasticity that accompanies aging. Defects in the position of the lid margins may be observed. An older adult frequently has lid margins that turn out (**ectropion**) or in (**entropion**). An entropion may lead to the lid's lashes irritating the conjunctiva and cornea, increasing risk of infection. The eyelashes are normally distributed evenly and curved outward away from the eye.

To inspect the surface of the upper lids, the nurse has the client close the eyes and then raises both eyebrows gently with the thumb and index finger. This stretches the skin. The lids are usually smooth and the same color as the skin. Redness indicates inflammation or infection. Lid edema may be caused by allergies or heart and kidney failure. If lesions are present, the nurse observes the size, shape, and distribution. Gloves should be worn if drainage is present.

The lids normally close symmetrically. Failure of lids to close exposes the cornea to drying. This condition is common in unconscious clients or those with facial nerve paralysis. While inspecting the lower lids, the nurse asks the client to open the eyes and observes the blink reflex. Normally a client blinks involuntarily and bilaterally as many as 20 times a minute. The blink reflex helps lubricate the cornea. The nurse reports absent or infrequent, rapid, or monocular (one-eyed) blinking.

Lacrimal apparatus. The anterior surface of the eye, composed of the sensitive cornea and conjunctiva, is moistened by tears secreted from the lacrimal gland (Figure 24-9). The gland is located in the upper, outer wall of the anterior part of the orbit. Tears flow from the gland across the eye's surface to the lacrimal duct, which is located in the nasal corner or inner canthus of the eye. The lacrimal gland can be the site of tumors or infection. The area of the gland is inspected for edema and redness and palpated gently to detect tenderness. Normally the gland cannot be felt. The nasolacrimal duct may become obstructed, blocking the flow of tears. The nurse looks for evidence of excess tearing or

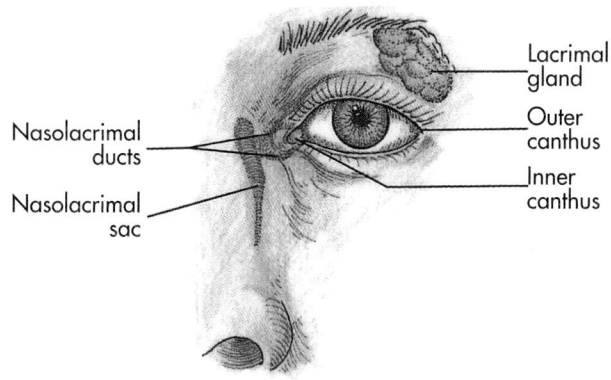

Figure 24-9. Lacrimal apparatus.

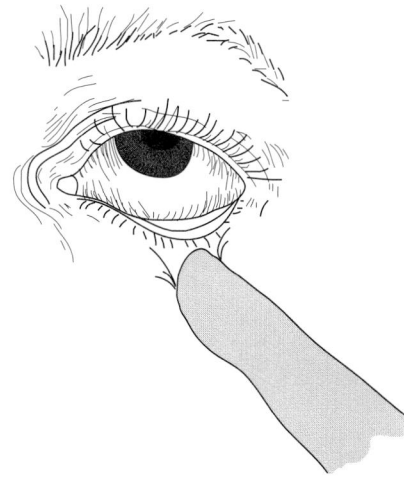

Figure 24-10. Technique for retracting the lower eyelid.

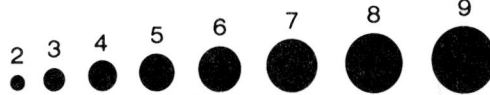

Figure 24-11. Chart depicting pupillary size in millimeters.

edema in the inner canthus. Gentle palpation of the duct at the lower eyelid just inside the orbital rim may cause a regurgitation of tears.

Conjunctiva and sclera. The bulbar conjunctiva covers the exposed surface of the eyeball up to the outer edge of the cornea. The sclera is seen under the bulbar conjunctiva and normally has the color of white porcelain in whites and light yellow in black-skinned clients. To view both structures, the nurse gently retracts both lids simultaneously with thumb and index finger pressed against the lower and upper bony orbits. If there is crusty drainage on eyelid margins, the nurse should wear gloves. A pair of new gloves should be worn to examine each eye to prevent cross-contamination. For adequate exposure the eyelids must be retracted without placing pressure directly on the eyeball. The client is asked to look up, down, and side to side. Many clients begin to blink, making the examination difficult. The nurse inspects for color, texture, and lesions.

The palpebral conjunctiva is the delicate membrane lining the eyelids. Normally the conjunctiva is transparent, enabling the nurse to view the tiny underlying blood vessels that give it a pink color. To inspect the palpebral conjunctiva, the nurse gently depresses the lower lid (Figure 24-10). Often the client can depress the eyelid to facilitate examination. The conjunctiva's color and the presence of edema or lesions are noted. A pale conjunctiva results from anemia, whereas a fiery red appearance is the result of inflammation (conjunctivitis). **Conjunctivitis** is a highly contagious infection. The crusty drainage that collects on eyelid margins can easily spread from one eye to the other. The nurse should wear gloves during the examination. Thorough hand washing is necessary before and after the examination.

Cornea. The cornea is the transparent, colorless portion of the eye covering the pupil and iris. From a side view, it looks like the crystal of a wristwatch. While the client looks straight ahead, the nurse inspects the cornea for clarity and texture while shining a penlight obliquely across the cornea's surface. The cornea is normally shiny, transparent, and smooth. In older adults,

the cornea loses its luster. Any irregularity in the surface may indicate an abrasion or tear that requires further examination by a physician. Both conditions are quite painful. The color and details of the underlying iris should be easy to see. In an older adult the iris becomes faded. A thin, white ring along the margin of the iris, called an **arcus senilis,** is common with aging but is abnormal in anyone under age 40. To test for the corneal blink reflex, see the cranial nerve test section of this chapter.

Pupils and irises. The nurse observes the pupils for size, shape, equality, accommodation, and reaction to light. The pupils are normally black, round, regular, and equal in size (3 to 7 mm in diameter) (Figure 24-11). Cloudy pupils indicate cataracts. Dilated or constricted pupils can result from neurological disorders or the effect of ophthalmic or certain systemic drugs. Pinpoint pupils are a common sign of opioid intoxication (Caulker-Burnett, 1994). When a beam of light is shined through the pupil and onto the retina, the third cranial nerve is stimulated and causes the muscles of the iris to constrict. Any abnormality along the nerve pathways from the retina to the iris alters the ability of the pupils to react to light. Changes in intracranial pressure, lesions along the nerve pathways, locally applied eye drugs, and direct trauma to the eye may alter pupillary reaction.

Pupillary reflexes (to light and accommodation) should be tested in a dimly lit room. As the client looks straight ahead, the nurse brings a penlight from the side

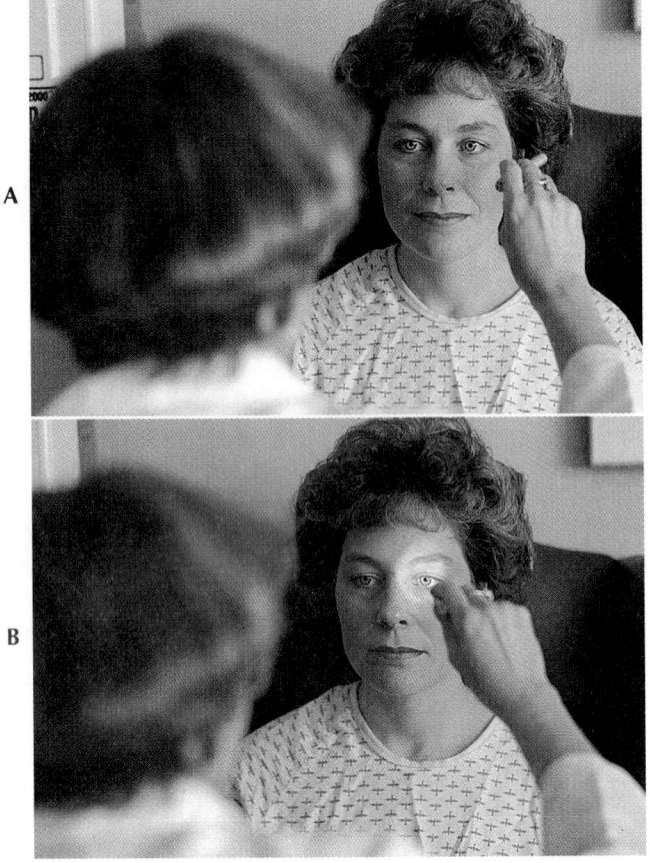

Figure 24-12. **A,** To check pupil reflexes, nurse first holds penlight to side of client's face. **B,** Illumination of pupil causes pupillary constriction.

of the client's face, directing the light onto the pupil (Figure 24-12). If the client looks at the light, there will be a false reaction to accommodation. A directly illuminated pupil constricts, and the opposite pupil constricts consensually. The nurse observes the quickness and equality of the reflex. The exam is repeated for the opposite eye.

To test accommodation, the client is asked to gaze at a distant object (the far wall) and then at a test object (finger or pencil) held by the nurse approximately 10 cm (4 inches) from the bridge of the client's nose. The pupils normally converge and accommodate by constricting when looking at close objects. The pupil responses are equal. If assessment of pupillary reaction is normal in all tests, the nurse records the abbreviation **PERRLA** (pupils equal, round, reactive to light and accommodation).

Internal eye structures. The examination of internal eye structures is beyond the scope of a new graduate nurse's practice. However, it is important to understand the purpose and the significance of findings. Clients in greatest need of the examination are those with diabetes, hypertension, and intracranial disorders. By illuminating the internal eye structures with an **ophthalmoscope,** an examiner is able to view the optic disc, the integrity of retinal vessels, the presence of retinal lesions, and the appearance of the macula and fovea centralis.

Ears

The ear assessment determines the integrity of ear structures and hearing acuity. The nurse inspects and palpates external ear structures, inspects middle ear structures with the otoscope, and tests the inner ear by

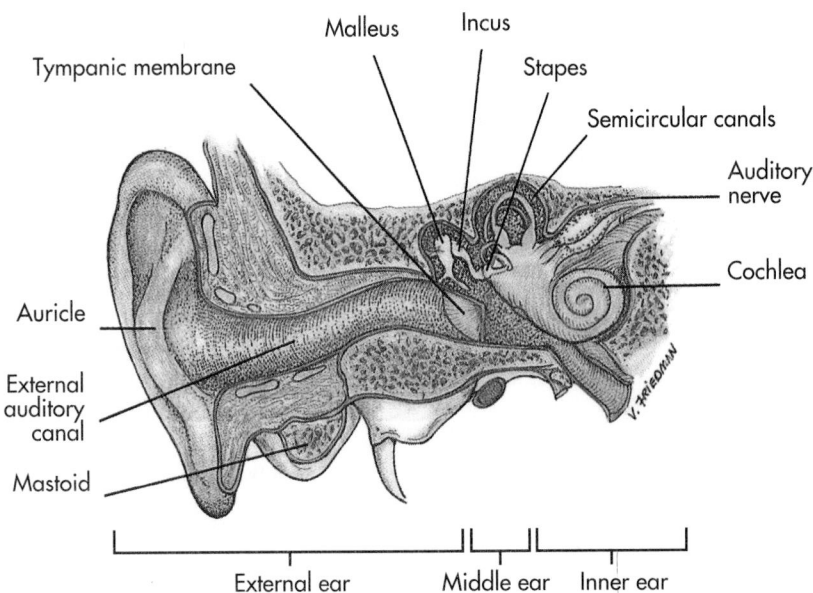

Figure 24-13. Structures of external, middle, and inner ear.

measuring the client's hearing acuity (Figure 24-13). Assessment of clients with hearing impairment provides useful data for the nurse in planning effective communication techniques.

Health history.

The client's health history includes a review of risks for hearing problems (e.g., hypoxia at birth, meningitis, intake of aspirin, aminoglycosides or other ototoxic drugs, and exposure to noise), a history of ear surgery or trauma, and the client's current exposure to high noise levels. The nurse determines if the client has ear pain, itching, discharge, tinnitus, **vertigo,** or change in hearing. The nurse notes behaviors indicative of hearing loss, such as failure to respond when spoken to, requests to repeat comments, leaning forward to hear, and child's inattentiveness or use of monotonous voice tones. If the client has had a recent hearing problem, the nurse determines the onset, contributing factors, and effect on ADLs. The nurse also assesses if the client wears a hearing aid and how the client normally cleans the ears.

Auricles.

With the client sitting, the nurse inspects the auricle's position, color, size, shape, and symmetry. It is important to examine lateral and medial surfaces and surrounding tissue. The auricles are normally of equal size and level with each other. The upper point of attachment to the head is normally in a straight line with the outer canthus or corner of the eye. Ears that are low set or at an unusual angle are a sign of chromosome abnormality (e.g., Down syndrome). The color is the same as the face without moles, cysts, deformities, or nodules. Redness is a sign of inflammation or fever. Extreme pallor can indicate frostbite. The nurse palpates the auricles for texture, tenderness, swelling, and skin lesions. The auricle is normally smooth, firm, mobile, and without lesions. If the client complains of pain, the nurse gently pulls the auricle and presses on the tragus and palpates behind the ear over the mastoid process. If palpating the external ear increases the pain, an external ear infection is likely. If palpation of the auricle and tragus does not influence the pain, the client may have a middle ear infection. Tenderness in the mastoid area can indicate mastoiditis.

The nurse inspects the opening of the ear canal for size and presence of discharge. If discharge is present, gloves should be worn during the examination. The meatus should not be swollen or occluded. A yellow, waxy substance called **cerumen** is common. Yellow or green foul-smelling discharge may indicate infection or a foreign body.

Ear canals and eardrums.

The deeper structures of the external and middle ear can be observed only with the use of an **otoscope.** A special ear speculum attaches to the battery tube of the ophthalmoscope. For best visualization the nurse selects the largest speculum that fits comfortably in the client's ear. Before inserting the speculum, the examiner checks for foreign bodies in the opening of the auditory canal.

The client must avoid moving the head during the examination to avoid damage to the canal and tympanic membrane. Infants and young children often need to be restrained. Infants should lie supine with their heads turned to one side and their arms held securely at their sides. Young children can sit on their parents' laps with their legs held between the parents' knees.

The nurse turns on the otoscope by rotating the dial at the top of the battery tube. To insert the speculum properly, the nurse asks the client to tip the head slightly to the opposite shoulder. The nurse holds the handle of the otoscope in the space between the thumb and index finger, supported on the middle finger. This leaves the ulnar side of the hand to rest against the client's head, stabilizing the otoscope as it is inserted into the canal (Seidel and others, 1995). Two grips on the otoscope may be used. In one, the examiner holds the battery tube along the client's neck with the fingers against the neck. In the other grip, the inverted otoscope is lightly braced against the side of the client's head or cheek. The nurse inserts the scope while pulling the auricle upward and backward in the adult and older child (Figure 24-14). This maneuver straightens the ear canal. In infants the nurse pulls the auricle back and down. The nurse inserts the speculum slightly down and forward, 1.0 or 1.5 cm (½ inch) into the ear canal. Care is taken not to abrade the sensitive lining of the ear canal, which can be painful. The canal normally has little cerumen and is uniformly pink with tiny hairs in the outer third of the canal. The nurse observes for color, discharge, scaling, lesions, foreign bodies, and cerumen. Normally cerumen is dry (light brown to gray and flaky) or moist (dark yellow or brown) and sticky. Dry cerumen occurs in Orientals and Native Americans about 85% of the time (Seidel and others, 1995). A

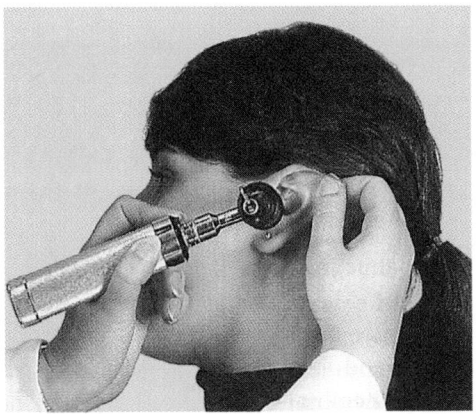

Figure 24-14. Otoscopic examination. (From Seidel HM and others: *Mosby's guide to physical examination,* ed 3, St. Louis, 1995, Mosby.)

reddened canal with discharge is a sign of inflammation or infection. In older adults, accumulated cerumen is a common problem. Buildup of cerumen can create a mild hearing loss. During the examination the nurse asks the client how the ear canal is normally cleaned (Box 24-10). The nurse should caution the client on the danger of inserting pointed objects into the canal. The use of cotton-tipped applicators to clean the ears should be avoided, because this causes impaction of cerumen deep in the ear canal.

The light from the otoscope allows visualization of the eardrum (tympanic membrane). The nurse must be familiar with the common anatomical landmarks and their appearance (Figure 24-15). The nurse moves the auricle to see the entire drum and its periphery. Because the eardrum is angled away from the ear canal, the light from the otoscope appears as a cone shape rather than a circle. The umbo is near the center of the drum, behind which is the attachment of the malleus. A knoblike structure at the top of the drum is created by the underlying short process of the malleus. The examiner should check carefully to be sure there are no tears or breaks in the eardrum's membrane. The normal eardrum is translucent, shiny, and pearly gray. It is free from tears or breaks. A pink or red bulging membrane indicates inflammation. A white color reveals pus behind it. The membrane is taut, except for the same triangular pars flaccida near the top. If the tympanic membrane is blocked by cerumen, a warm water irrigation will safely remove the wax.

Hearing acuity. The nurse can often tell if the client has a hearing loss from a response to conversation. The three types of hearing loss are conduction, sensorineural, and mixed. A conduction loss involves an interruption of sound waves as they travel from the outer ear to the cochlea of the inner ear because they are not transmitted through the outer and middle ear structures. A sensorineural loss involves the inner ear, the auditory nerve, or the hearing center of the brain.

Sound is conducted through the outer and middle ear structures, but the continued transmission of sound becomes interrupted at some point beyond the bony ossicles. A mixed loss involves a combination of conduction and sensorineural loss.

Clients working or living around loud noises are at risk for hearing loss. Older adults experience an inability to hear high-frequency sounds and consonants (e.g., s, z, t, and g). Deterioration of the cochlea and thickening of the tympanic membrane causes older adults to gradually lose hearing acuity. They are especially at risk for hearing loss caused by **ototoxicity** (injury to the auditory nerve) resulting from high-maintenance doses of antibiotics (e.g., the aminoglycosides).

To begin a hearing assessment, the nurse has the client remove any hearing aid that is worn. The nurse notes the client's response to questions. Normally the client should respond without excess requests to have the nurse repeat questions. If hearing loss is suspected, the nurse checks the client's response to the whispered voice. One ear is tested at a time while the client occludes the other ear with a finger. The nurse asks the client to gently move the finger up and down during the test. While standing 1 foot (30 cm) from the ear being tested, the nurse covers the mouth so the client is unable to read lips. After exhaling fully, the nurse whispers softly toward the unoccluded ear, reciting random numbers with equally accented syllables such as "nine-four-ten." If necessary, the nurse gradually increases voice intensity until the client correctly repeats the numbers. The other ear is then tested for comparison. Seidel and others (1995) report that clients normally hear numbers clearly when whispered. A ticking watch may be used to test hearing acuity, but the spoken word allows for more accuracy and control in testing.

If a hearing loss is present, there are tests that can be performed utilizing a tuning fork or audiometry. Both tests are best performed by either experienced practitioners or specially trained audiometry technicians.

BOX 24-10
Client Teaching for Ear and Hearing Assessment

▪ Instruct the client about the proper way to clean the outer ear (see Chapter 29), avoiding use of cotton-tipped applicators and sharp objects such as hairpins.
▪ Tell the client to avoid inserting pointed objects into the ear canal.
▪ Encourage clients over age 65 to have regular hearing checks. Explain that a reduction in hearing is a normal part of aging (see Chapter 39).
▪ Instruct family members of clients with hearing losses to avoid shouting and instead speak in low tones and to be sure the client can see the speaker's face.

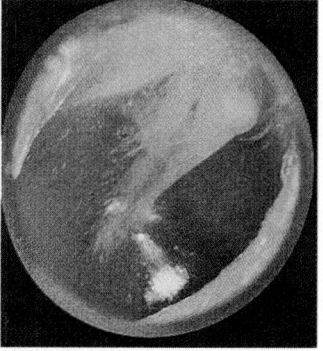

Figure 24-15. Normal tympanic membrane. (Courtesy Dr. Richard A. Buckingham, Abraham Lincoln School of Medicine, University of Illinois, Chicago.)

Nose and Sinuses

The integrity of the nose and sinuses is assessed by inspection and palpation. The client sits during the examination. A penlight allows for gross examination of each naris. A more detailed examination requires using a nasal speculum to inspect deeper nasal turbinates. A student should not use a speculum unless a qualified practitioner is present.

Health history. It is useful to know whether the client's health history indicates exposure to dust or pollutants, allergies, nasal obstruction, recent trauma, discharge, frequent infections, headaches, or postnasal drip. An assessment for a history of nosebleed (epistaxis) should include review of frequency, amount of bleeding, treatment, and difficulty stopping bleeding. The nurse also determines whether the client has a history of using nasal spray or drops, including the amount, frequency, and duration of use (Box 24-11). The nurse also asks if clients have been told that they snore or if they have difficulty breathing.

Nose. When inspecting the external nose, the nurse observes for shape, size, skin color, and presence of deformity or inflammation. The nose is normally smooth and symmetrical, with the same color as the face. Recent trauma may have caused edema and discoloration. If swelling or deformities exist, the nurse gently palpates the ridge and soft tissue of the nose by placing one finger on each side of the nasal arch and gently moving fingers from the nasal bridge to the tip. The nurse notes any tenderness, masses, and underlying deviations. Nasal structures are usually firm and stable.

Air normally passes freely through the nose as a person breathes. To assess patency of the nares, the nurse places a finger on the side of the client's nose and occludes one naris. The client is asked to breathe with the mouth closed. The nurse repeats the procedure for the other naris.

As the nurse illuminates the anterior nares, the mucosa is inspected for color, lesions, discharge, swelling, and evidence of bleeding. If discharge is present, gloves should be applied. Normal mucosa is pink and moist without lesions. Pale mucosa with clear discharge indicates allergy. A mucoid discharge indicates rhinitis. A sinus infection results in yellowish or greenish discharge. Habitual use of intranasal cocaine and opioids can cause puffiness and increased vascularity of the nasal mucosa (Master and Terpstra, 1992). For the client with a nasogastric tube, the nurse checks for local **excoriation** of the naris, characterized by redness and skin sloughing.

To view the septum and turbinates, the client tips the head back slightly to give the nurse a clearer view. Advanced clinicians may use a nasal speculum. The septum is inspected for alignment, perforation, or bleeding. Normally the septum is close to the midline and thicker anteriorly than posteriorly. The mucosa is pink and moist, with clear mucosa. A deviated septum can obstruct breathing and interfere with passage of a nasogastric tube. Perforation of the septum can occur after repeated use of intranasal cocaine. The nurse notes any polyps (tumorlike growth) or purulent drainage.

Sinuses. The examination of the sinuses is limited to palpation. In cases of allergies or infection, the interior of the sinuses becomes inflamed and swollen. The most effective way to assess for tenderness is by externally palpating the frontal and maxillary facial areas (Figure 24-16). The frontal sinus is palpated by exerting

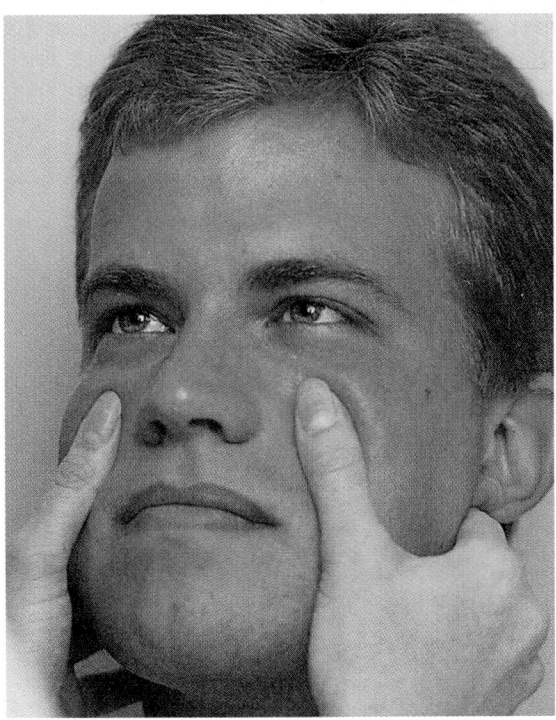

Figure 24-16. Palpation of maxillary sinuses.

pressure with the thumb up and under the client's eyebrow. Gentle upward pressure elicits tenderness easily if sinus irritation is present. Do not apply pressure to the eyes. If tenderness of sinuses is present, the nurse transilluminates the sinuses. This procedure, however, requires advanced experience.

Mouth and Pharynx

The nurse assesses the mouth and pharynx to detect signs of overall health, determine oral hygiene needs, and develop nursing therapies for clients with dehydration, restricted intake, oral trauma, or oral airway obstruction. To assess the oral cavity the nurse uses a penlight and tongue depressor or single gauze square. Gloves should be worn when contacting mucous membranes. The client may sit or lie during the examination. The nurse may assess the oral cavity while administering oral hygiene.

History. The nurse determines if the client wears dentures or retainers and if they fit comfortably. An assessment of a recent change in appetite or weight may point to a problem with chewing or swallowing. The nurse assesses the client's dental hygiene practices and when the client last visited a dentist. To rule out risks for mouth and throat cancer, the nurse asks if the client smokes or chews tobacco or smokes a pipe. The nurse also assesses for a history of pain or lesions of the mouth and pain with chewing. It helps to know if the client has a history of tonsillectomy or adenoidectomy.

Lips. The lips are inspected for color, texture, hydration, contour, and lesions. With the client's mouth closed, the nurse views the lips from end to end. Normally they are pink, moist, symmetrical, and smooth. Lip color in the dark-skinned client varies from pink to plum. Female clients should remove their lipstick before the exam. Pallor of the lips can be caused by anemia, with cyanosis caused by respiratory or cardiovascular problems. Any lesions such as nodules or ulcerations can be related to infection, irritation, or skin cancer.

Mucosa. To view the inner oral mucosa, the nurse has the client open the mouth slightly and gently pulls the lower lip away from the teeth (Figure 24-17, *A*). This process is repeated for the upper lip. The mucosa is inspected for color, hydration, texture, and lesions such as ulcers, abrasions, or cysts. Normally the mucosa is a glistening pink. Varying shades of hyperpigmentation are normal in 10% of whites after age 50 and up to 90% of blacks by the same age. Any lesions are palpated with a gloved hand for tenderness, size, and consistency.

To inspect the buccal mucosa, the nurse asks the client to open the mouth and then gently retracts the cheeks with a tongue depressor or gloved finger covered with gauze (Figure 24-17, *B*). A penlight illuminates the posterior mucosa. The surface of the mucosa must be viewed from right to left and top to bottom. Normal mucosa is glistening, pink, soft, moist, and smooth. For clients with normal pigmentation the buccal mucosa is a good site to inspect for jaundice and pallor. In older adults, the mucosa is normally dry because of reduced salivation. Thick white patches (**leukoplakia**) are often a precancerous lesion seen in heavy smokers and alcoholics. The nurse palpates for any buccal lesions by placing the index finger within the buccal cavity and the thumb on the outer surface of the cheek.

Gums and teeth. The gums or **gingivae** are examined for color, edema, retraction, bleeding, and lesions. If a client wears dentures, irregularity or lesions of the gums can create discomfort and significantly impair the ability to chew. The nurse asks the client to remove dentures for a complete assessment. Healthy gums are pink, moist, smooth, and tightly fit around

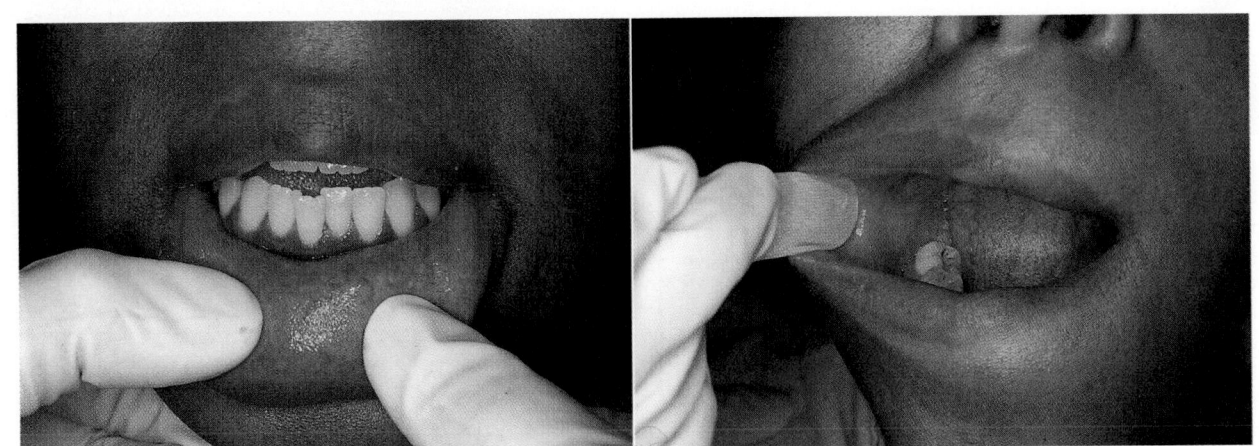

A   B

Figure 24-17. **A,** Inspection of inner oral mucosa of lower lip. **B,** Retraction allows for clear view of buccal mucosa.

each tooth. Blacks may have patchy pigmentation. In older adults the gums are usually pale. Using gloves, the nurse palpates the gums to assess for lesions, thickening, or masses. There should be no tenderness. Spongy gums that bleed easily indicate periodontal disease or vitamin C deficiency.

The nurse asks the client to clench the teeth and smile to observe teeth occlusion. The upper molars should rest directly on the lower molars, and the upper incisors slightly override the lower incisors. The position and alignment of teeth are noted. The nurse probes each tooth gently with a tongue blade when the client complains of any localized discomfort. The teeth are normally firmly set.

The quality of a client's dental hygiene is easily determined by inspecting the teeth (Box 24-12). To examine the posterior surface of the teeth, the nurse has the client open the mouth with lips relaxed. A tongue depressor may be needed to retract the lips and cheeks, especially when viewing the molars. The nurse notes the color of teeth and the presence of dental caries, tartar, and extraction sites. Normal healthy teeth are smooth, white, and shiny. A chalky white discoloration of the enamel is an early indication that caries are forming. Brown or black discolorations indicate formation of caries. A stained yellow color is from tobacco use, whereas coffee and tea cause a brown stain. In the older adult, loose or missing teeth are common because bone resorption increases. An older adult's teeth often feel rough when tooth enamel calcifies. Yellow and darkened teeth are also common in the older adult because of general wear and tear that exposes the darker underlying dentin.

Tongue and floor of mouth.

The tongue is carefully inspected on all sides, and the floor of the mouth is checked. The client first relaxes the mouth and sticks the tongue out halfway. If the client protrudes the tongue too far, the gag reflex may be elicited. Using the penlight, the nurse examines the tongue for color, size, position, texture, movement, and coating or lesions. The tongue should appear medium or dull red in color, moist, slightly rough on the top surface, and smooth along the lateral margins. The tongue remains at midline. The nurse asks the client to raise the tongue and move it from side to side. The tongue should move freely.

The undersurface of the tongue and floor of the mouth are highly vascular. Extra care is taken to inspect this area, a common site of origin for oral cancer lesions. The client lifts the tongue by placing its tip on the palate behind the upper incisors. The nurse inspects for color, swelling, and lesions such as cysts. The ventral surface of the tongue is pink and smooth with large veins between the frenulum folds. To palpate the tongue the nurse asks the client to protrude the tongue and gently grasps its tip with a gauze square. While gently pulling the tongue to one side at a time, the nurse palpates its full length and base or floor of the mouth, noting any hardening or ulceration. The tongue should have a smooth, even texture and be free of lesions.

Varicosities (swollen, tortuous veins) may be seen. Varicosities rarely cause problems but are common in the older adult.

Palate.

The client should extend the head backward, holding the mouth open so that the nurse can inspect the hard and soft palates. The hard palate or roof of the mouth is located anteriorly. The whitish hard palate should be domed shaped. The soft palate extends posteriorly toward the pharynx. It is normally light pink and smooth. The palates are observed for color, shape, texture, and extra bony prominences or defects. A bony growth, or **exostosis,** between the two palates is common.

Pharynx.

An examination of the pharyngeal structures is performed to rule out infection, inflammation, or lesions. The client tips the head back slightly, opens the mouth wide, and says "Ah." The nurse places the tip of a tongue depressor on the middle third of the tongue, taking care not to press the lower lip against the teeth (Figure 24-18). If the tongue depressor is placed too far anteriorly, the posterior part of the tongue mounds up, obstructing the view. Placing the tongue depressor on the posterior tongue elicits the gag reflex.

With a penlight, the nurse first inspects the uvula and soft palate. Both structures, which are innervated by the tenth cranial nerve (vagus), should rise centrally as the client says "Ah." The anterior and posterior tonsillar pillars are examined, and the presence or absence of tonsillar tissue is noted. The posterior pharynx is behind the pillars. Normally pharyngeal structures are smooth, pink, and well hydrated. Small irregular spots of lymphatic tissue and small blood vessels are normal.

BOX 24-12

Client Teaching for Mouth and Pharynx Assessment

- Discuss proper techniques for oral hygiene, including brushing and flossing.
- Explain the early warning signs of oral cancer, including a sore that bleeds easily and does not heal, a lump or thickening, and a red or white patch on the mucosa that persists (American Cancer Society, 1997). Difficulty chewing and swallowing are late changes.
- Encourage regular dental examinations every 6 months for children, adults, and older adults.
- Identify older clients who have difficulty in chewing and changes in the teeth. Teach clients to eat soft foods and cut food into small pieces.

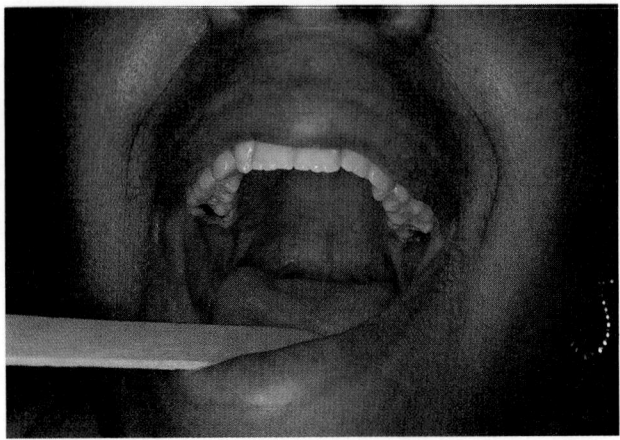

Figure 24-18. Tongue depressor allows nurse to view pharynx and posterior soft palate.

Edema, petechiae (small hemorrhages), lesions, or exudate should be noted. Clients with chronic sinus problems frequently exhibit a clear exudate that drains along the wall of the posterior pharynx. Yellow or green exudate indicates infection. A client with a typical sore throat has a reddened and edematous uvula and tonsillar pillars with possible presence of yellow exudate.

Neck

Assessment of the neck includes assessing the neck muscles, lymph nodes of the head, carotid arteries, jugular veins, thyroid gland, and trachea (Figure 24-19). An ex-amination of the carotid arteries and jugular veins can be deferred until conducting an assessment of the vascular system. The nurse inspects the neck to determine the integrity of neck structures and to examine the lymphatic system. An abnormality of superficial lymph nodes may reveal the presence of infection or malignancy. Examination of the thyroid gland and trachea also aids in ruling out malignancies. Examination is best performed with the client sitting.

Health history. The nurse determines if the client has had a recent cold or infection or feels weak or fatigued. Screening for hypothyroidism and hyperthyroidism and risk factors for human immunodeficiency virus (HIV) infection may be necessary. The nurse also assesses if the client has been exposed to radiation, toxic chemicals, or infection. The client is asked to describe any history of thyroid problems, neck or head injury, or pain of head and neck structures. Finally, the nurse asks if the client is taking thyroid medication or has a family history of thyroid disease.

Neck muscles. With the client sitting and facing the nurse, an inspection of gross neck structures is made. The nurse observes for symmetry of neck muscles, alignment of the trachea, and any subtle fullness at the neck. Any distention or prominence of jugular veins and carotid arteries is abnormal. The nurse asks the client to flex the neck with the chin to the chest, hyperextend the neck backward, and move the head laterally to each side and then sideways with the ear moving toward the shoulder. This tests the sternocleidomastoid

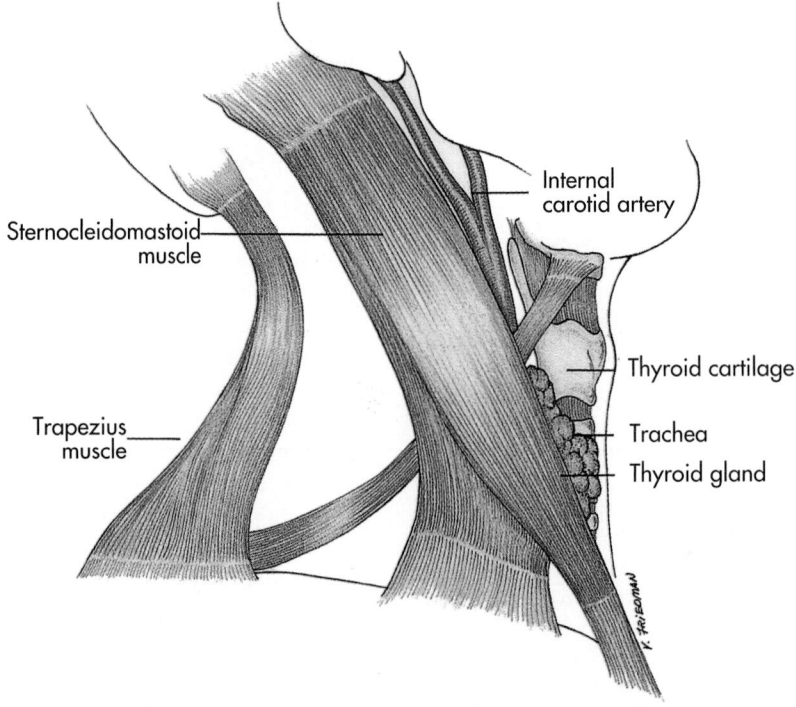

Figure 24-19. Anatomical position of major neck structures.

and trapezius muscles. The neck should move freely without discomfort.

Lymph nodes.

An extensive system of lymph nodes collects lymph from the head, ears, nose, cheeks, and lips (Figure 24-20). With the client's chin raised and head tilted slightly back, the nurse first inspects the area where lymph nodes are distributed and compares both sides. This position stretches the skin slightly over any possible enlarged nodes. Visible nodes are inspected for edema, erythema, or red streaks. Nodes are not normally visible.

A methodical approach is used to palpate the lymph nodes to avoid overlooking any single node or chain. The client relaxes muscles and tissues by keeping the neck flexed slightly forward and, if needed, toward the side of the nurse. Both sides of the neck are palpated for comparison. During palpation the nurse faces or stands to the side of the client for easy access to all nodes. Using the pads of the middle three fingers of each hand, the nurse palpates gently in a rotary motion over the nodes. Each node is checked methodically in the following sequence: occipital nodes at the base of the skull, postauricular nodes over the mastoid, preauricular nodes just in front of the ear, retropharyngeal nodes at the angle of the mandible, submaxillary nodes, and submental nodes in the midline behind the mandibular tip. The nurse tries to detect enlargement and notes the location, size, shape, surface characteristics, consistency, mobility, tenderness, and warmth of the nodes. If the skin is mobile, the nurse moves the skin over the area of the nodes (Figure 24-21) (Seidel and others, 1995). It is important to press underlying tissue in each area and not simply move the fingers over the skin. However, if excessive pressure is applied, small nodes are missed and palpable nodes are obliterated.

To palpate supraclavicular nodes the nurse asks the client to bend the head forward and relax the shoulders. The nurse may have to hook the index and third finger over the clavicle, lateral to the sternocleidomastoid muscle, to palpate these nodes. The deep cervical nodes can be palpated only with the nurse's fingers hooked around the sternocleidomastoid muscle.

Normally lymph nodes are not easily palpable. Lymph nodes that are large, fixed, inflamed, or tender indicate a problem such as local infection, systemic disease, or neoplasm (Seidel and others, 1995). Tenderness almost always indicates inflammation (Box 24-13). A problem involving a lymph node of the head and neck may mean an abnormality in the mouth, throat, abdomen, breasts, thorax, or arms. These are the areas drained by the head and neck nodes.

Thyroid gland.

The thyroid gland lies in the anterior lower neck, in front of and to both sides of the trachea. The gland is fixed to the trachea with the isthmus

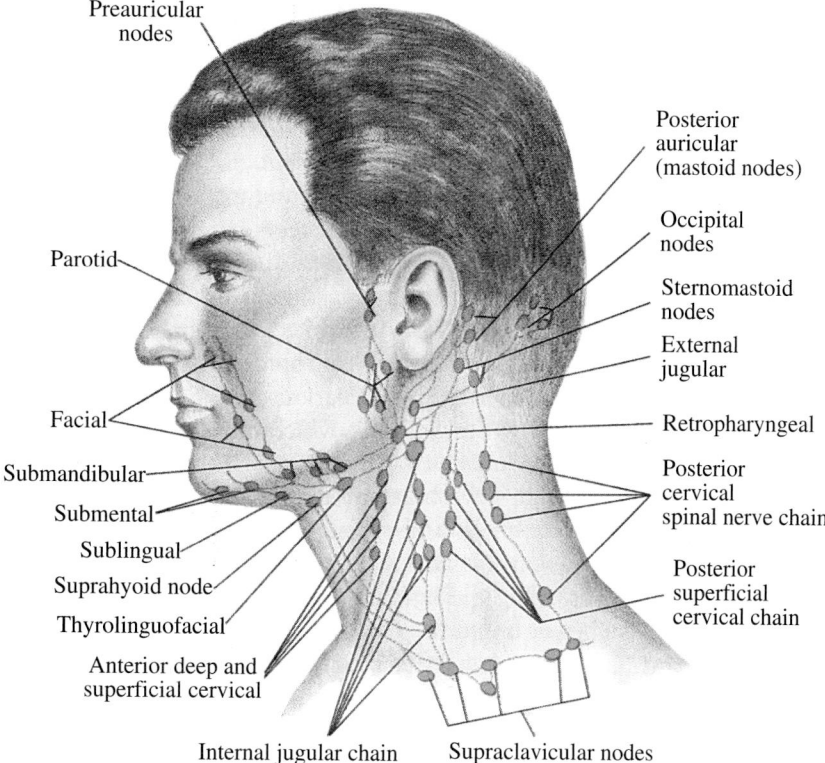

Figure 24-20. Lymphatic drainage system of the head and neck. (From Seidel HM and others: *Mosby's guide to physical examination,* ed 3, St. Louis, 1995, Mosby.)

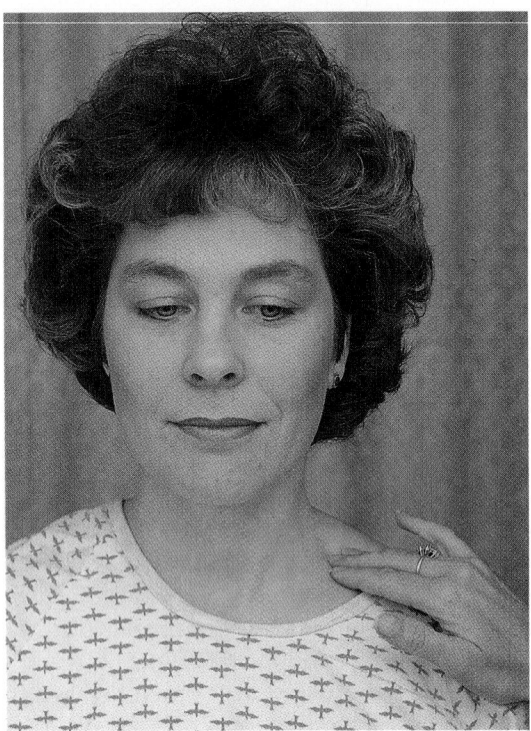

Figure 24-21. Nurse palpates lymph nodes.

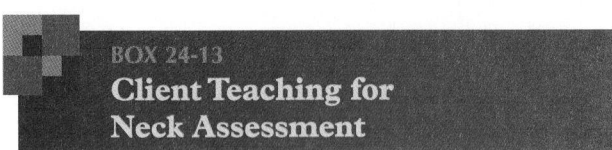

BOX 24-13
Client Teaching for Neck Assessment

▪ Stress the importance of regular compliance with medication schedule to clients with thyroid disease.
▪ Instruct clients about lymph nodes and how infection can commonly cause node tenderness.
▪ Instruct clients to call the physician when a lump or mass is noted in the neck.
▪ Teach clients risk factors for HIV infection.

overlying the trachea and connecting the two irregular, cone-shaped lobes (Figure 24-22). The nurse inspects the lower neck over the thyroid gland for obvious masses and symmetry. Offer the client a glass of water and while observing the neck, have the client swallow. This maneuver helps to visualize an abnormally enlarged thyroid gland.

More-experienced nurses can examine the thyroid by palpating for more subtle masses. Gentle palpation as the client swallows allows an examiner to feel movement of the thyroid. Displacement of the gland during swallowing allows the nurse to palpate each lobe. Thin clients often have palpable glands that should be small, smooth, and free from nodules. Enlargement of the thyroid may indicate gland dysfunction or tumor. An enlarged tender thyroid indicates thyroiditis.

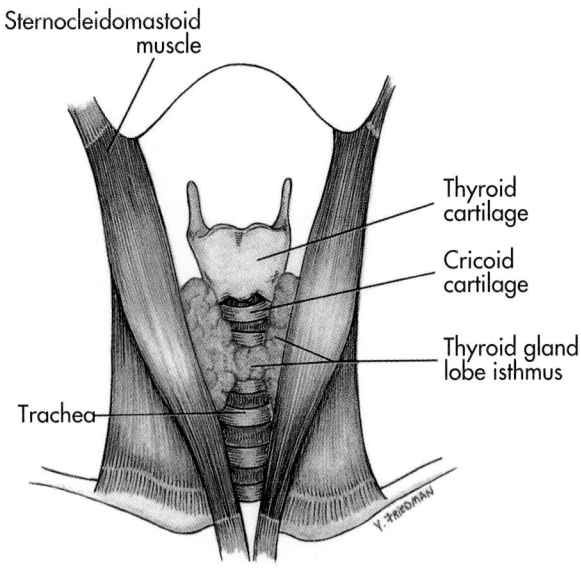

Figure 24-22. Thyroid gland.

Trachea. The trachea is a part of the upper airway that can be directly palpated. It is normally located in the midline above the suprasternal notch. Masses in the neck or mediastinum and pulmonary abnormalities can cause displacement laterally. The client may sit or lie down during palpation. The position of the trachea is determined by palpating at the suprasternal notch, slipping the thumb and index fingers to each side. The nurse notes if the finger and thumb are shifted laterally. Forceful pressure must not be applied to the trachea, because this may elicit a cough.

···THORAX AND LUNGS

Physical assessment of the thorax and lungs includes an in-depth look at ventilatory and respiratory functions of the lungs. If the lungs are affected by disease, other body systems are also affected. For example, reduced oxygenation can cause changes in mental alertness because of the brain's sensitivity to lowered oxygen levels. The nurse uses data from all body systems to determine the nature of pulmonary alterations.

Before assessing the thorax and lungs, the nurse must be familiar with the landmarks of the chest (Figure 24-23). These landmarks help the nurse locate findings and use assessment skills correctly. The client's nipples, angle of Louis, suprasternal notch, costal angle, clavicles, and vertebrae are key landmarks that provide a series of imaginary lines for sign identification. The nurse keeps a mental image of the location of the lobes of the lung and the position of each rib (Figure 24-24). The proper orientation to anatomical structures ensures a thorough assessment of the anterior, lateral, and posterior thorax.

Locating the position of each rib is critical to visual-

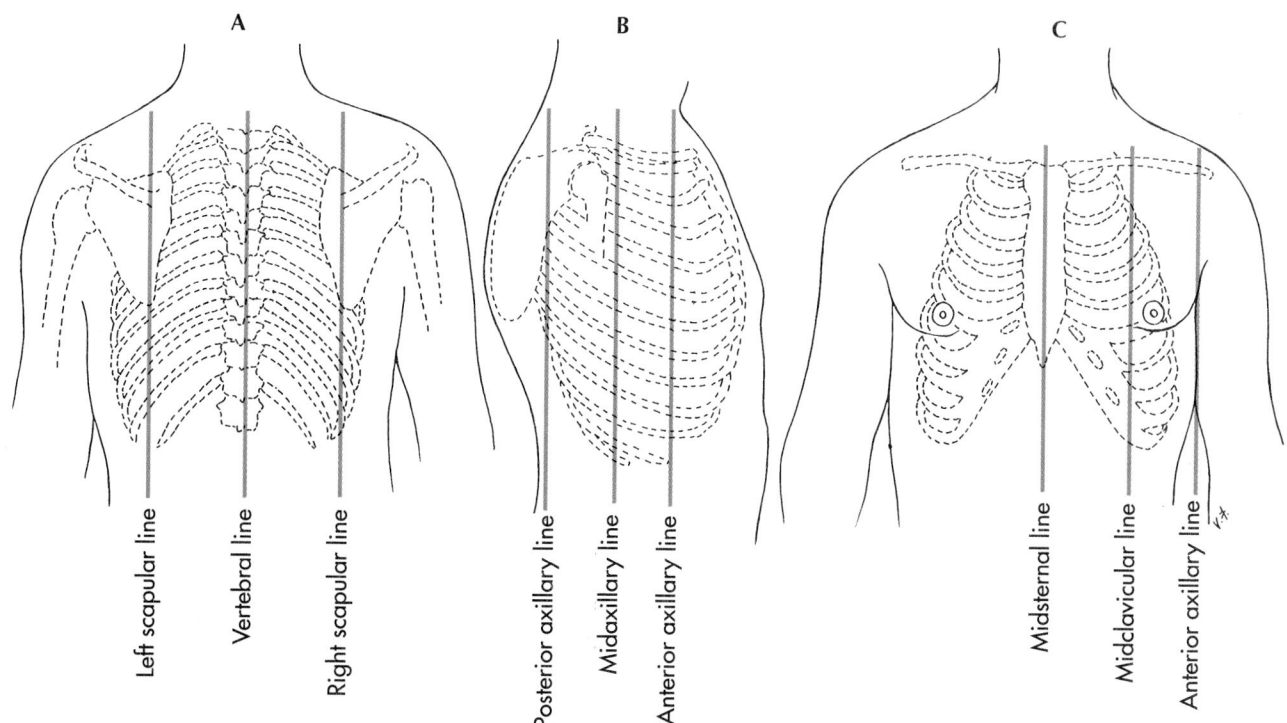

Figure 24-23. Anatomical chest wall landmarks. **A,** Posterior chest; **B,** lateral chest; **C,** anterior chest.

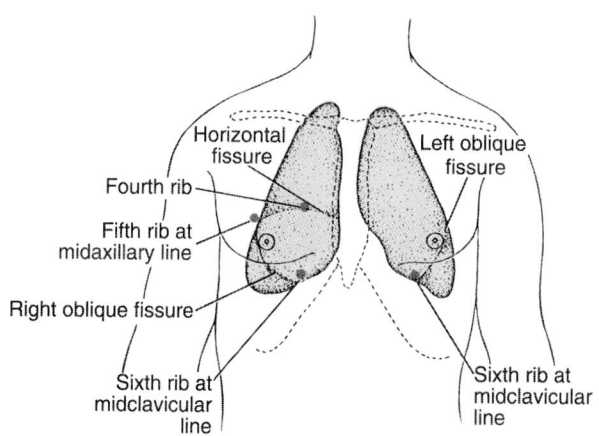

Figure 24-24. Anterior position of lung lobes in relation to anatomical landmarks.

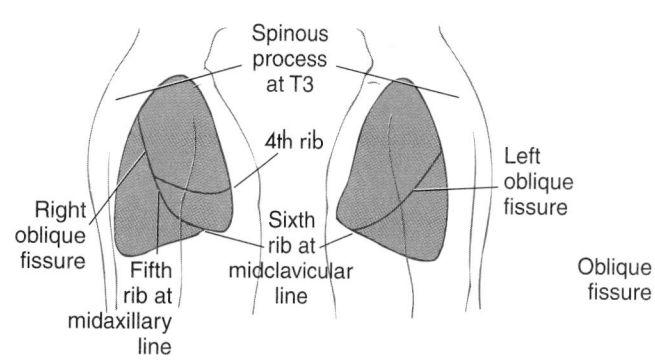

Figure 24-25. Lateral position of lung lobes in relation to anatomical landmarks.

izing the lobe of the lung being assessed. The angle of Louis, at the junction between the manubrium and the body of the sternum, is the starting point for locating the ribs anteriorly. Knowing that the second rib extends from the angle makes it easy to locate and palpate the intercostal spaces (between the ribs) in succession. The spinous process of the third thoracic vertebra and the fourth, fifth, and sixth ribs serve to locate the lung's lobes laterally (Figure 24-25). The lower lobes project laterally and anteriorly.

Posteriorly the tip or inferior margin of the scapula lies approximately at the level of the seventh rib. After the seventh rib is identified, the examiner can count upward to locate the third thoracic vertebra and align it with the inner borders of the scapula to locate the posterior lobes (Figure 24-26).

Examination requires the client to be undressed to the waist. Good lighting is needed. The examination begins with the client sitting for assessment of the posterior and lateral chest. The client may sit or lie for assessment of the anterior chest.

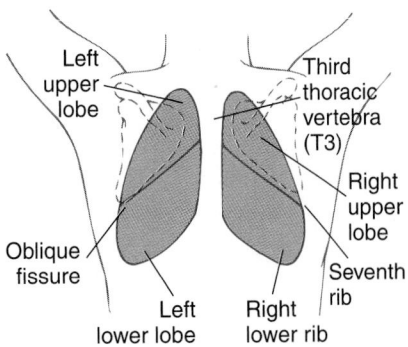

Figure 24-26. Posterior position of lung lobes in relation to anatomical landmarks.

Health History

A complete health history includes determining if the client has a history of tobacco or marijuana use, including number of years smoked, age started, number of cigarettes or cigars daily, and length of time since smoking stopped. To screen for warning signals of lung cancer, the nurse asks if the client has a persistent cough, sputum production, chest pain, or recurrent attacks of pneumonia or bronchitis. Asking the client about symptoms of **orthopnea,** shortness of breath, **dyspnea** during exertion or at rest, and poor activity tolerance can reveal other pulmonary problems. A client's risk for having lung disease is further assessed by reviewing presence of pollutants in the work environment or at home and reviewing the client's family history for cancer, tuberculosis, allergies, or chronic obstructive pulmonary disease.

Tuberculosis is on the increase in the United States. Nurses should be alert for clients at risk, including persons with HIV infection, substance abusers, residents of nursing homes, low-income individuals, and recent immigrants to the United States (American Thoracic Society, 1992; Boutotte, 1993; Hopkins and Schoener, 1996). Clients who exhibit symptoms of persistent cough, hemoptysis, unexplained weight loss, fatigue, anorexia, night sweats, and fever should be evaluated for tuberculosis and/or HIV infection.

The nursing history also includes assessment of allergies to airborne irritants, foods, drugs, or chemical substances. It is important to learn if a client has had a pneumonia or influenza vaccine and a tuberculosis test. The very young, very old, and those with chronic respiratory problems are at increased risk for disease. If the client has not been vaccinated, the nurse should educate the individual on the need for vaccination to protect against illnesses.

Posterior Thorax

The examination begins with observing for any signs or symptoms in other body systems that may indicate pulmonary problems. Reduced mental alertness, nasal flar-

ing, somnolence, and cyanosis are examples of signs assessed during other portions of the examination that can indicate oxygenation problems. The nurse begins inspecting the posterior thorax by observing the shape and symmetry of the chest from the client's back and front. The anteroposterior diameter is noted. Shape or posture can significantly impair ventilatory movement. Normally the chest contour is symmetrical, with the anteroposterior diameter one third to one half the size of the transverse or side-to-side diameter. Aging and chronic lung disease are characterized by a barrel-shaped chest (anteroposterior diameter equals transverse). Infants have an almost round shape. Abnormal contours are caused by congenital and postural alterations. A client may lean over a table or splint the side of the chest because of a breathing problem. Splinting or holding the chest wall because of pain causes a client to bend toward the affected side. Such a posture impairs ventilatory movement.

Standing at a midline position behind the client, the nurse looks for deformities, position of the spine, slope of the ribs, retraction of the intercostal spaces during inspiration, and bulging of the intercostal spaces during expiration. The spine is normally straight, and scapulae normally are symmetrical and closely attached to the chest wall. The spine normally is straight without lateral deviation. Posteriorly, the ribs tend to slope across and down. The ribs and intercostal spaces are easier to see in a thin person. Normally no bulging or active movement occurs within the intercostal spaces during breathing. Bulging indicates that the client is using great effort to breathe.

The nurse may also assess the rate and rhythm of breathing at this time (see Chapter 23). The thorax as a whole is observed. The thorax normally expands and relaxes with equality of movement bilaterally. In healthy adults the normal respiratory rates vary from 12 to 20 respirations per minute.

Palpation of the posterior thorax assesses further characteristics. The thoracic muscles and skeleton are palpated for lumps, masses, pulsations, and unusual movement. If pain or tenderness is noted, the nurse avoids deep palpation. Fractured rib fragments could be displaced against vital organs. Normally the chest wall is not tender. If a suspicious mass or swollen area is detected, it is lightly palpated for size, shape, and typical qualities of a lesion.

To measure chest excursion or depth of breathing, the nurse stands behind the client and places the thumbs along the spinal processes at the tenth rib, with the palms lightly contacting the posterolateral surfaces. The nurse's thumbs should be about 2 inches (5 cm) apart, pointing toward the spine and fingers pointing laterally (Figure 24-27, *A*). The hands are pressed toward the spine so that a small skinfold appears between the thumbs. The nurse does not slide the hands over the skin. The nurse instructs the client to take a deep breath

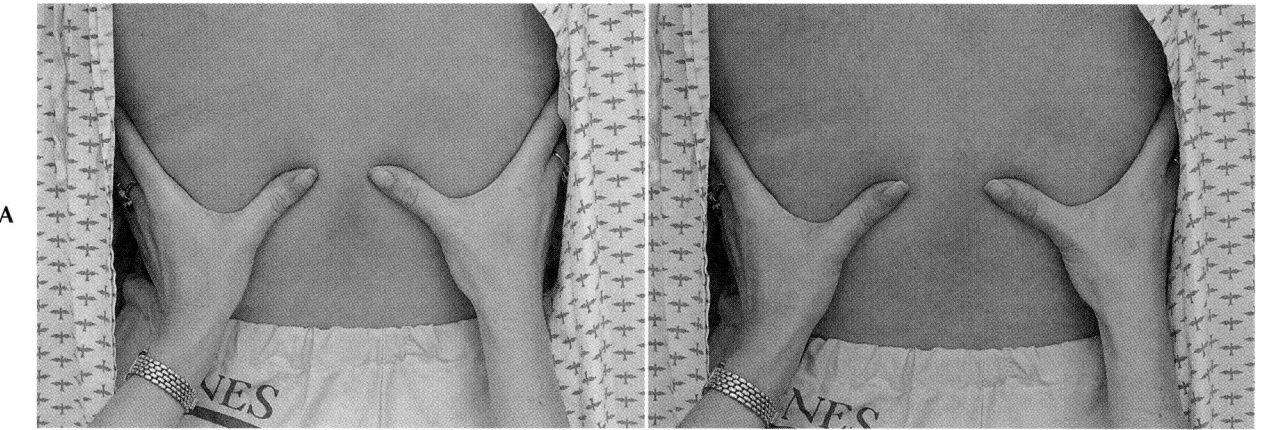

Figure 24-27. **A,** Position of nurse's hands for palpation of posterior thorax excursion. **B,** As the client inhales, the movement of chest excursion separates the nurse's thumbs.

after exhaling. The nurse notes movement of the thumbs (Figure 24-27, *B*). Chest excursion should be symmetrical, separating the thumbs 1¼ to 2 inches (3 to 5 cm). Reduced chest excursion may be caused by pain, postural deformity, or fatigue. In older adults, chest excursion normally declines because of costal cartilage calcification and respiratory muscle atrophy.

During speech the sound created by the vocal cords is transmitted through the lung to the chest wall. The sound waves create vibrations that can be palpated externally. These vibrations are called **tactile fremitus** or **vocal fremitus.** The buildup of mucous secretions, the collapse of lung tissue, or the presence of lung lesions can block the vibrations from reaching the chest wall.

To palpate for fremitus, the nurse places the ball or lower palm of the hand over symmetrical intercostal spaces, beginning at the lung apex. A firm, light touch is best. The client is asked to say "99." Normally there is a faint vibration as the client speaks. Both sides of the thorax are compared, moving from top to bottom (Figure 24-28). Only one hand is used to ensure accuracy. If the fremitus is faint, it may be necessary to ask the client to speak louder or lower the tone of voice. Tactile fremitus is symmetrical and strongest at the top near the level of the tracheal bifurcation. It is easy to assess for fremitus in a crying infant, because strong vibrations can be felt through the chest wall.

Percussion of the chest wall determines whether underlying lung tissue is air filled, fluid filled, or solid. The client folds the arms forward across the chest with the head bent forward. This position separates the scapulae further to expose more lung to assessment. Using the indirect technique, the nurse percusses in the intercostal spaces over symmetrical areas of the lung. Figure 24-28, *A,* shows how following a systematic pattern starting posteriorly allows the nurse to compare percussion notes for all lung lobes. Resonance, the sound created by air-filled lungs, is normally heard over the pos-

terior thorax. Percussion over the scapulae, ribs, or spine is dull. The chest is normally more resonant in the child than in the adult. A lung mass causes a flat sound. Conditions such as emphysema, asthma, or pneumothorax produce a hyperresonant sound because of hyperinflation of lung tissue. A dull or flat sound may suggest atelectasis, pleural effusion, pneumothorax, or asthma.

Auscultation assesses the movement of air through the tracheobronchial tree and detects mucus or obstructed airways. Normally air flows through the airways in an unobstructed pattern. Recognizing the sounds created by normal air flow allows the nurse to detect sounds caused by airway obstruction.

The nurse places the diaphragm of the stethoscope over the posterior chest wall between the ribs. The client folds the arms in front of the chest and keeps the head bent forward while taking slow, deep breaths with the mouth slightly open. The nurse listens to an entire inspiration and expiration at each position of the stethoscope (see Figure 24-28, *A*). If sounds are faint, as with an obese client, the client should be asked to breathe harder and faster temporarily. Breath sounds are much louder in children because of their thin chest walls. In children the bell works best because of a child's small chest. The same systematic pattern used in percussion should be used when comparing the right and left sides. The nurse compares the sounds in one region on one side of the body with sounds in the same region on the opposite side.

The nurse auscultates for normal breath sounds and abnormal sounds (**adventitious sounds**). Normal breath sounds differ in character, depending on the area being auscultated. Sounds normally heard over the posterior thorax include bronchovesicular and vesicular sounds. Bronchovesicular sounds are medium-pitched blowing sounds normally heard posteriorly between the scapulae. The sounds have equal inspiratory and expiratory phases. The character of bronchovesicular

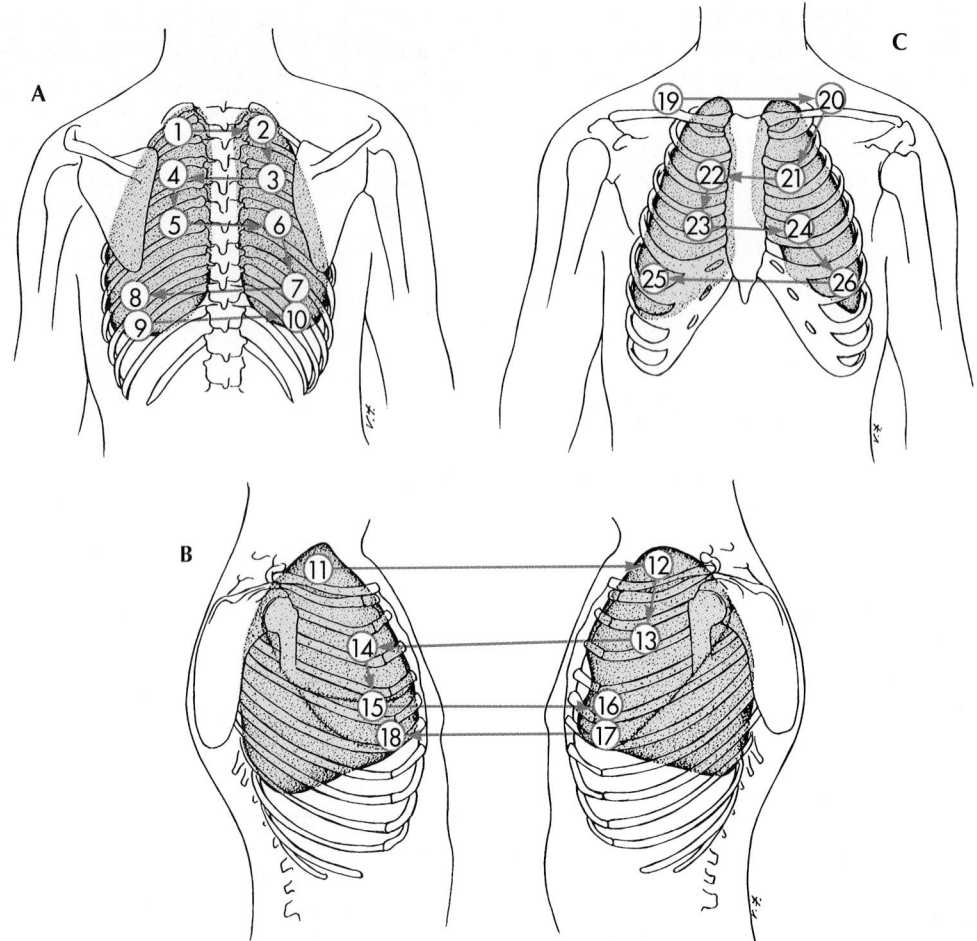

Figure 24-28. **A** to **C,** The nurse follows a systematic pattern (posterior-lateral-anterior) when comparing fremitus, percussion notes, and auscultation.

sounds is related to the larger underlying airways. Vesicular sounds are heard over the lungs' periphery. The sounds are created by air moving through the smaller airways. Vesicular sounds are soft, breezy, and low pitched, and the inspiratory phase is about three times longer than the expiratory phase.

Abnormal sounds result from air passing through moisture, mucus, or narrowed airways. They can also result from alveoli suddenly reinflating or from an inflammation between the lung's pleural linings. Adventitious sounds often occur superimposed over normal sounds. The four types of adventitious sounds include **crackles** (previously called *rales*), **rhonchi, wheezes,** and **pleural friction rub.** Each sound is caused by a specific entity and is characterized by typical auditory features (Table 24-7). The location and characteristics of the sounds should be noted, as should the absence of breath sounds (found in clients with collapsed or surgically removed lobes).

Lateral Thorax
The client sits during the lateral chest examination. Usually the nurse extends the assessment of the pos-

terior thorax to the lateral sides of the chest (Figure 24-28, *B*). The client is asked to raise the arms, which improves access to lateral thoracic structures. The nurse uses all four assessment skills. Excursion cannot be assessed laterally. Normally, percussion notes are resonant, and breath sounds are vesicular.

Anterior Thorax
The anterior thorax is inspected for the same features as the posterior thorax. The client sits or lies down with the head elevated. The nurse observes the accessory muscles of breathing: sternocleidomastoid, trapezius, and abdominal muscles. The accessory muscles move little with normal passive breathing. When a client requires effort to breathe as a result of strenuous exercise or disease (Box 24-14), the accessory muscles and abdominal muscles contract. Some clients may produce a grunting sound.

The nurse observes the width of the costal angle. It is usually larger than 90 degrees between the two costal margins. Respiratory rate and rhythm are more often assessed anteriorly (see Chapter 23). The male client's respirations are usually diaphragmatic, whereas the female's are more costal.

TABLE 24-7
Adventitious Sounds

Sound	Site Auscultated	Cause	Character
Crackles (previously called *rales*)	Are most commonly heard in dependent lobes: right and left lung bases	Random, sudden reinflation of groups of alveoli*; disruptive passage of air	Fine crackles are high-pitched fine, short, interrupted crackling sounds heard during end of inspiration, usually not cleared with coughing* Moist crackles are lower, more moist sounds heard during middle of inspiration; not cleared with coughing
Rhonchi	Are primarily heard over trachea and bronchi; if loud enough, can be heard over most lung fields	Muscular spasm, fluid, or mucus in larger airways, causing turbulence	Are loud, low-pitched, rumbling coarse sounds heard most often during inspiration or expiration; may be cleared by coughing
Wheezes	Can be heard over all lung fields	High-velocity airflow through severely narrowed bronchus	Are high-pitched, continuous musical sounds like a squeak heard continuously during inspiration or expiration; usually louder on expiration; do not clear with coughing†
Pleural friction rub	Is heard over anterior lateral lung field (if client is sitting upright)	Inflamed pleura, parietal pleura rubbing against visceral pleura	Has dry, grating quality heard best during inspiration; does not clear with coughing; heard loudest over lower lateral anterior surface

*Data from Forgacs P: The functional basis of pulmonary sounds, *Chest* 73:399, 1978.
†Data from Wilkins RL and others: *Lung sounds: a practical guide,* St. Louis, 1988, Mosby.

The nurse palpates the anterior thoracic muscles and skeleton for lumps, masses, tenderness, or unusual movement. The sternum and xiphoid are relatively inflexible. To measure chest excursion anteriorly, the nurse places the thumbs along the costal margin parallel 2½ inches (6 cm) apart with the palms touching the anterolateral chest. The thumbs are pushed toward the midline to create a skinfold. As the client inhales deeply, the thumbs should normally separate approximately 3 to 5 cm (1¼ to 2 inches), with each side expanding equally.

Tactile fremitus is assessed over the chest wall (Figure 24-28, *C*). Anterior findings differ from posterior findings because of the heart and female breast tissue. Fremitus is best felt next to the sternum at the second intercostal space, at the level of the bronchial bifurcation. It is decreased over the heart, lower thorax, and breast tissue. The nurse will not be able to sense vibrations over breast tissue and thus must retract the breasts gently during palpation. If the breasts are large, this portion of the examination may be omitted.

Percussion of the anterior thorax again follows a

- Explain the risk factors for chronic lung disease and lung cancer, including cigarette smoking, history of smoking for over 20 years, exposure to environmental pollution, and radiation exposure from occupational, medical, and environmental sources. Residential radon exposure may also increase risk, especially for cigarette smokers. Exposure to side-stream cigarette smoke increases risk for non-smokers.
- Share brochures on lung cancer from the American Cancer Society with client and family.
- Discuss the warning signs of lung cancer, such as a persistent cough, sputum streaked with blood, chest pains, and recurrent attacks of pneumonia or bronchitis.
- Counsel older adults on benefits of receiving influenza and pneumonia vaccinations because of a greater susceptibility to respiratory infection.
- Persons at risk for tuberculosis who visit clinics or health care centers should be referred for skin testing.
- Instruct clients with chronic obstructive pulmonary disease in coughing and pursed-lip–breathing exercises.

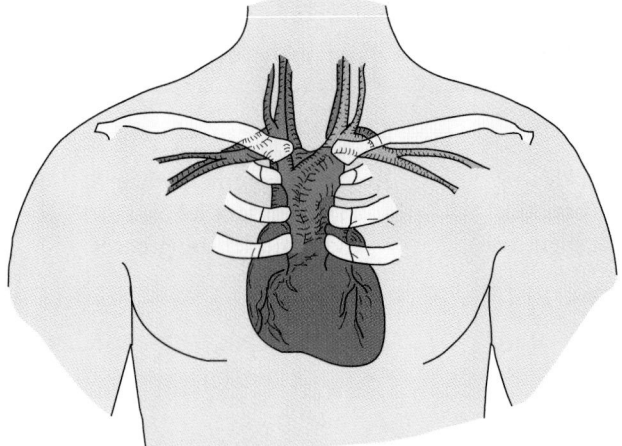

Figure 24-29. Anatomical position of the heart.

systematic pattern. The nurse should imagine the location of all internal organs anteriorly accessible to examination. The underlying liver, heart, and stomach create percussion notes different from those of the lung. Percussion may be conducted with the client in a sitting or lying position; however, the procedure is easier if the client lies down. The nurse starts above the clavicles and moves across and then down. The female's breasts are displaced as needed. The normal lung is resonant. The percussion notes over the heart and liver are dull. The gastric air bubble is tympanic.

Auscultation of the anterior thorax follows the same pattern as percussion. The client should sit, if possible, to maximize chest expansion. Special attention should be given to the lower lobes, where mucous secretions commonly gather. Bronchovesicular and vesicular sounds are heard above and below the clavicles and along the lung periphery. An additional normal breath sound, bronchial sound, can be heard over the trachea. Bronchial sounds are loud, high pitched, and hollow sounding, with expiration lasting longer than inspiration (3:2 ratio).

HEART

Assessment of heart function is closely compared with findings from the vascular examination. Alterations in either system may be manifested as changes in the other. A client with signs and symptoms of heart problems may have a life-threatening condition requiring

immediate attention. In this case, the nurse acts quickly and conducts only portions of the examination that are absolutely necessary. When a client is more stable, the nurse conducts a more thorough examination.

Assessment of cardiac function is performed through the anterior thorax. The nurse forms a mental image of the heart's exact location (Figure 24-29). In the adult the heart is located in the center of the chest (precordium) behind and to the left of the sternum, with a small section of the right atrium extending to the sternum's right. The base of the heart is the upper portion, and the apex is the bottom tip. The surface of the right ventricle comprises most of the heart's anterior surface. A section of the left ventricle shapes the left anterior side of the apex. The apex actually touches the anterior chest wall at approximately the fourth to fifth intercostal space along the midclavicular line. This is known as the apical impulse or **point of maximal impulse (PMI).**

An infant's heart is positioned more horizontally. The apex of the heart is at the third or fourth intercostal space, just to the left of the midclavicular line. By the age of 7 a child's apical impulse is in the same location as the adult's. In tall, slender persons the heart hangs more vertically and is positioned more centrally. With increased stockiness and shortness, the heart tends to lie more to the left and horizontally (Seidel and others, 1995).

To assess heart function, the nurse must understand the cardiac cycle and the physiological signs of each event (Figure 24-30). The heart normally pumps blood through its four chambers in a methodical, even sequence. Events on the left side occur just before those on the right. As the blood flows through each chamber, valves open and close, pressures within chambers rise and fall, and chambers contract. Each event creates a physiological sign. Both sides of the heart function in a coordinated fashion.

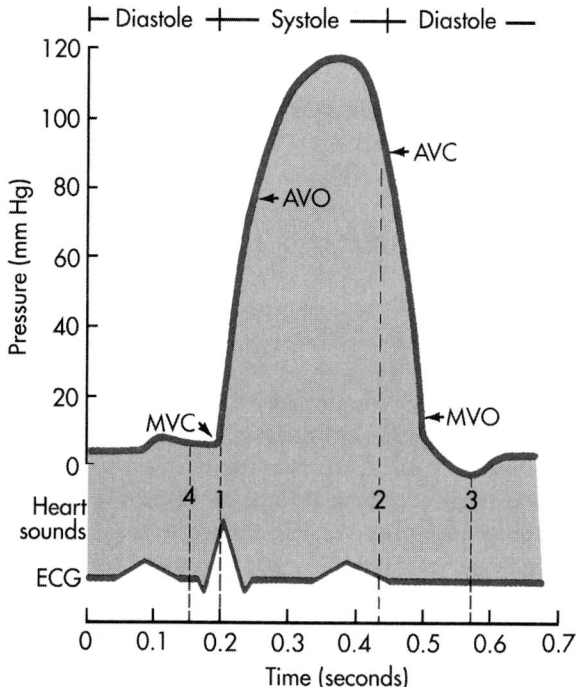

Figure 24-30. Cardiac cycle. *MVC*, Mitral valve closes; *AVO*, aortic valve opens; *AVC*, aortic valve closes; *MVO*, mitral valve opens.

There are two phases to the cardiac cycle: systole and diastole. During systole the ventricles contract and eject blood from the left ventricle into the aorta and from the right ventricle into the pulmonary artery. During diastole the ventricles relax and the atria contract to move blood into the ventricles and fill the coronary arteries.

Heart sounds occur in relation to physiological events in the cardiac cycle. As systole begins, ventricular pressure rises and closes the mitral and tricuspid valves. Valve closure causes the first heart sound (S_1), often described as "lub." The ventricles then contract and blood flows through the aorta and pulmonary circulation. After the ventricles empty, ventricular pressure falls below that in the aorta and pulmonary artery. This allows the aortic and pulmonary valves to close, causing the second heart sound (S_2), described as "dub." As ventricular pressure continues to fall, it drops below that of the atria. The mitral and tricuspid valves reopen to allow ventricular filling. Rapid ventricular filling may create a third heart sound (S_3). This is heard more often in children and young adults. An S_3 can also be heard as an abnormality in adults over 30 years of age. A fourth heart sound (S_4) may be heard when the atria contract to enhance ventricular filling. The S_4 is not normally heard in adults but may be heard in healthy older adults, children, and athletes. Because S_4 may also indicate an abnormal condition, it should be reported to a physician.

Health History

The health history should focus on risk factors for cardiovascular disease (Box 24-15). The nurse assesses the client's history of smoking, alcohol intake, caffeine intake, use of prescriptive and recreational drugs, exercise habits, and dietary patterns including fat and sodium intake. Does the client have a stressful lifestyle? If so, what are the physical demands or emotional stresses? It is important to know if the client takes medications for cardiovascular function (antidysrhythmics, antihypertensives). The nurse also assesses for signs and symptoms suggestive of heart disease, including chest pain or discomfort, **palpitations,** excess fatigue, cough, dyspnea, edema of the feet, cyanosis, fainting, or orthopnea. If the client reports chest pain, the nurse determines if it is cardiac in nature; anginal pain is usually a deep pressure or ache that is substernal and diffuse, radiating to one or both arms, the neck, or the jaw. Determine whether the client has preexisting diabetes, lung disease, obesity, or hypertension. Finally, the nurse assesses the client's personal and family history for heart disease.

Inspection and Palpation

The nurse uses inspection and palpation simultaneously. The examination begins with the client supine and the upper body elevated 45 degrees, because clients with heart disease frequently suffer shortness of breath while lying flat. The nurse stands at the client's right side. The client must not talk, especially when the nurse auscultates heart sounds. Good lighting in the room is essential.

The nurse directs attention to the anatomical sites

best suited for assessment of cardiac function. The sternal angle or angle of Louis can be felt as a ridge in the sternum approximately 2 inches below the sternal notch. The nurse slips the fingers along the angle on each side of the sternum to feel the adjacent ribs. The intercostal spaces are just below each rib. The second intercostal space allows for identification of each of the six anatomical landmarks (Figure 24-31). The second intercostal space on the right is the aortic area, and the left second intercostal space is the pulmonic area. Deeper palpation is needed to feel the spaces in obese or heavily muscled clients. After the pulmonic area is located, the nurse moves the fingers down the client's left sternal border to the third intercostal space, called the second pulmonic area. The tricuspid area is located at the fourth left intercostal space along the sternum. To find the apical area or point of maximal impulse (PMI), the nurse locates the fifth intercostal space just to the left of the sternum and moves the fingers laterally to the left midclavicular line. Some can locate the apical area with the palm of the hand, but others use the fingertips. Normally at the apical impulse the apical pulse is a light tap felt in an area 1 to 2 cm (½ inch) in diameter at the apex. Another landmark is the epigastric area at the tip of the sternum. It is typically used to palpate for aortic abnormalities.

As the nurse locates the six anatomical landmarks of the heart, each area is inspected and palpated. The nurse looks for the appearance of pulsations, viewing each area over the chest at an angle to the side. Normally, no pulsations can be seen except perhaps at the apical impulse in thin clients or at the epigastric area as a result of abdominal aorta pulsation. Palpation for pulsations is best done using the proximal halves of the four fingers together and then alternating with the ball of the hand. The nurse touches the areas gently to allow movements to lift the hand. Normally no pulsations or vibrations can be felt in the second, third, or fourth intercostal spaces. A vibration is caused by loud murmurs. If pulsations or vibrations are palpated, the nurse times their occurrence in relation to systole or diastole by auscultating heart sounds simultaneously.

The apical impulse or PMI should be felt easily. If not, the nurse has the client turn onto the left side, moving the heart closer to the chest wall. The nurse estimates the heart's size by noting the diameter of the PMI and its position relative to the midclavicular line. In cases of serious heart disease, the cardiac muscle enlarges, with the PMI found to the left of the midclavicular line. The PMI may be difficult to find in older adults because the chest deepens in its anteroposterior diameter. It may also be difficult to find in muscular or overweight clients. An infant's PMI is usually found near the third or fourth intercostal space. It is easy to palpate because of the child's thin chest wall.

Auscultation

Auscultation of the heart detects normal heart sounds, extra heart sounds, and murmurs. Concentration is needed to detect the low-intensity sounds caused by valve closure. To begin auscultation the nurse eliminates all sources of room noise and explains the procedure to relieve the client's anxiety. The nurse follows a systematic pattern beginning with the aortic area and inching the stethoscope along each of the six landmarks. The nurse must be sure to hear heart sounds clearly at each location. Then the sequence is repeated using the bell of the stethoscope. The client may be asked to assume three different positions during the examination (Figure 24-32):

Sitting up and leaning forward (good for all areas and to hear high-pitched murmurs)
Supine (good for all areas)
Left lateral recumbent (good for all areas; best position to hear low-pitched sounds in diastole)

The nurse learns to identify the first (S_1) and second (S_2) heart sounds. At normal rates, S_1 occurs after the long diastolic pause and preceding the short systolic pause. S_1 is high pitched, dull in quality, and heard best at the apex. If the nurse has difficulty hearing S_1, it can be timed in relation to the carotid pulse. It occurs just before the carotid pulsation. S_2 follows the short systolic phase and precedes the long diastolic phase. It is heard best at the aortic area.

The nurse auscultates for rate and rhythm after both sounds can be heard clearly. Each combination of S_1 and S_2 or "lub-dub" counts as one heartbeat. The nurse counts the rate for 1 minute and listens for the interval between S_1 and S_2 and then the time between S_2 and the next S_1. A regular rhythm involves regular intervals of time between each sequence of beats. There is a distinct silent pause between S_1 and S_2. Failure of the heart to beat at regular successive intervals is a **dysrhythmia.** Some dysrhythmias can be life threatening.

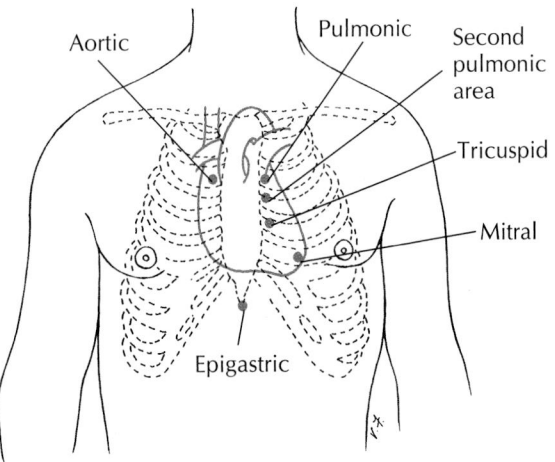

Figure 24-31. Anatomical sites for assessment of cardiac function.

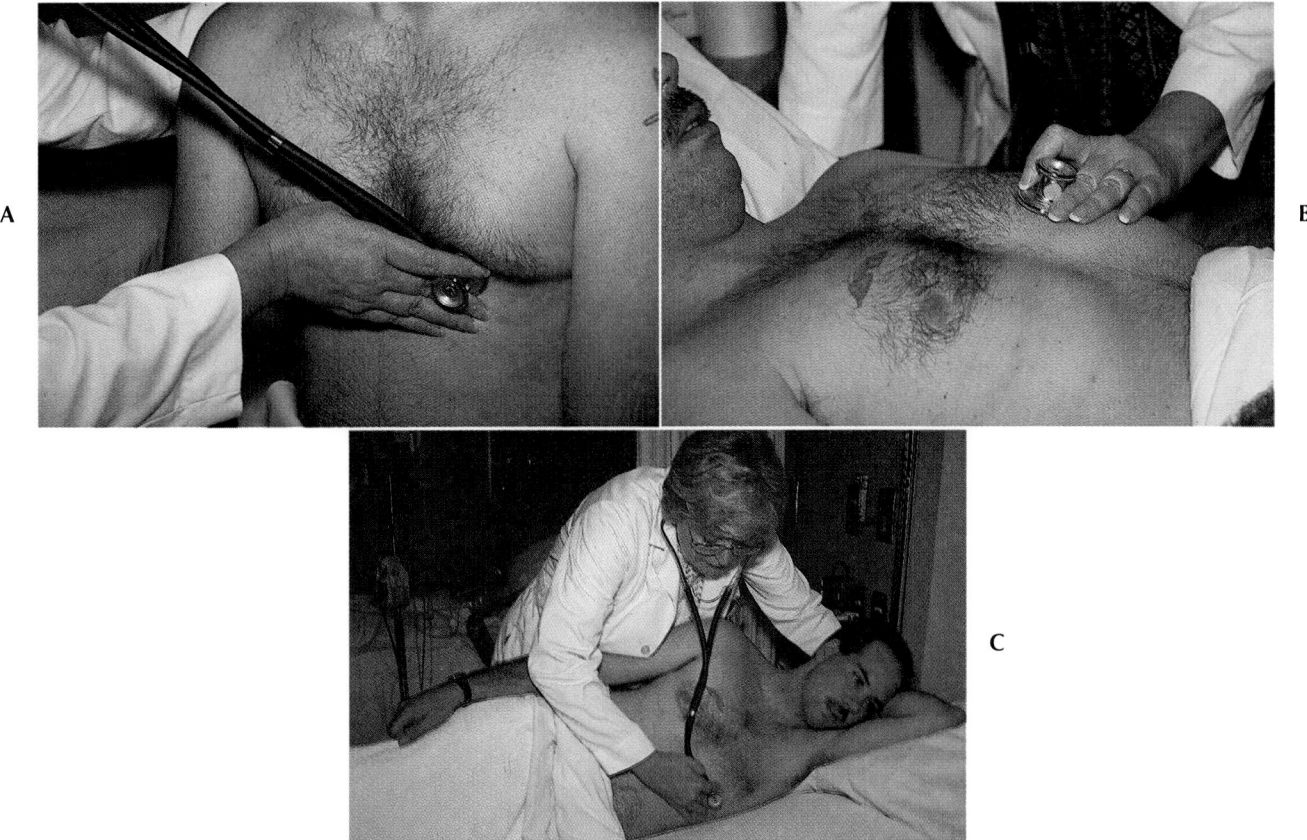

Figure 24-32. Sequences of client positions for heart auscultation. **A,** Sitting; **B,** supine; **C,** left lateral recumbent. (From Seidel HM and others: *Mosby's guide to physical examination,* ed 3, St. Louis, 1995, Mosby.)

When the heart rhythm is irregular, the nurse compares apical and radial pulse rates to determine if a pulse deficit exists. The nurse auscultates the apical pulse first and then immediately assesses the radial pulse (one examiner technique). When two examiners are available, the apical and radial rates are assessed at the same time. Compare the two rates. When a client has a pulse deficit, the radial pulse is slower than the apical because ineffective contractions fail to send pulse waves to the periphery. A difference in pulse rates is reported to the physician immediately.

The nurse also learns to assess for extra heart sounds at each auscultatory site. Using the bell of the stethoscope, the nurse listens for low-pitched sounds such as S_3 and S_4 gallops, clicks, and rubs. Auscultate over all anatomical sites. S_3 or a **ventricular gallop** occurs just after S_2 at the end of ventricular diastole. Some examiners describe the combination of S_1, S_2, and S_3 as sounding like "Ken-*tuc*-ky." It can be a sign of heart failure in adults.

S_4 or an atrial gallop occurs just before S_1 or ventricular systole. The sound of an S_4 is similar to that of "*Ten*-nessee." Physiologically it may be caused by an atrial contraction pushing against a ventricle that is not accepting blood because of heart failure or other alterations. One can often hear extra sounds more easily with the client on the left side and the stethoscope at the apical site.

Further auscultation may reveal clicks and rubs. Clicks are short, high-pitched, extra heart sounds created by mitral valve prolapse, aortic stenosis, prosthetic valves, or pulmonic disease. In contrast, rubs result from a rubbing of inflamed visceral and parietal layers of the pericardium against one another. A crackling, scratching, or grating sound (like squeaky leather or sandpaper) describes a rub (Fabius and Stunkard, 1994).

The final portion of the examination includes assessment for heart murmurs. **Murmurs** are sustained swishing or blowing sounds heard at the beginning, middle, or end of the systolic or diastolic pause. They are caused by an increased blood flow through a normal valve, forward flow through a stenotic valve or a dilated vessel or heart chamber, or backward flow through a valve that fails to close. A murmur can be asymptomatic or a sign of heart disease. Murmurs are common in children. Murmurs that occur between S_1 and S_2 are systolic, whereas murmurs that occur between S_2 and S_1 are diastolic. The nurse notes the intensity or loudness of murmurs, with grade I murmurs being barely audible and grade VI murmurs being loud enough to be heard without a stethoscope.

VASCULAR SYSTEM

Examination of the vascular system includes measuring the blood pressure (see Chapter 23) and assessing the integrity of the peripheral vascular system. The skills of inspection, palpation, and auscultation are used. The nurse notes the condition of extremities perfused by the vascular system. Disturbances in arterial perfusion or venous return cause skin and tissue changes in affected extremities. The nurse may perform portions of the vascular examination during other body system assessments.

Health History

The health history includes determining if the client has leg cramps, numbness or tingling in the extremities, or the continual sensation of cold hands or feet. These signs and symptoms may indicate vascular disease. The nurse also learns if the client has noted swelling or cyanosis of the feet, ankles, or hand or pain in the feet or legs. If the client has leg pain or cramps, the nurse asks if symptoms are aggravated by walking or standing for long periods or during sleep. This question helps to clarify if the problem is musculoskeletal or vascular in nature. For example, arterial occlusion can create muscle ischemia or claudication. This particular type of pain is a dull ache and cramping, usually appearing during sustained exercise and disappearing after a short rest. Musculoskeletal pain is not generally relieved when exercise ends. The nurse also asks if clients wear tight-fitting garters or hosiery and sit or lie in bed with their legs crossed. These activities can impair venous return. The history includes a review of the client's medical history for heart disease, hypertension, phlebitis, diabetes, or varicose veins. Finally, risk factors assessed earlier for smoking, exercise, and nutritional problems are important when assessing the vascular system.

Carotid Arteries

When the left ventricle pumps blood into the aorta, pressure waves are transmitted through the arterial system. The carotid artery reflects heart function better than peripheral arteries, because its pressure correlates with that of the aorta. The carotid artery supplies oxygenated blood to the head and neck (Figure 24-33) and is protected by the overlying sternocleidomastoid muscle.

To examine the carotid arteries, the nurse has the client sit or lie supine with the head of the bed elevated 15 to 30 degrees. One carotid artery is examined at a time. If both arteries were occluded during palpation, the client could lose consciousness as a result of inadequate circulation to the brain. The carotid arteries must

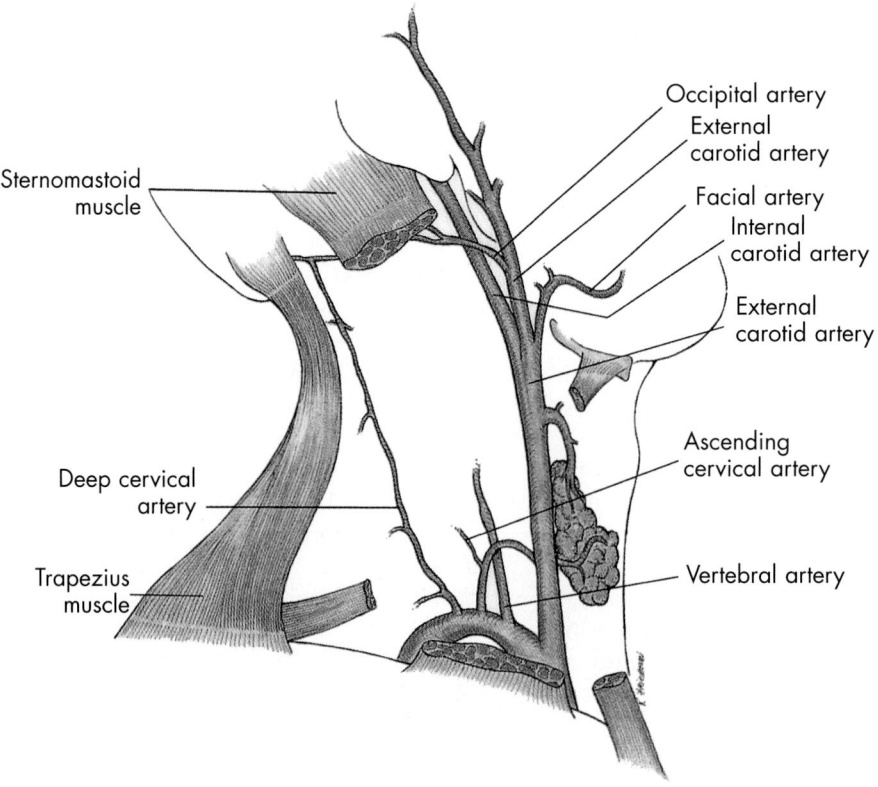

Figure 24-33. Anatomical position of the carotid artery.

not be vigorously palpated or massaged because the carotid sinus is in the upper third of the neck. The sinus sends impulses along the vagus nerve. Its stimulation can cause a reflex drop in heart rate and blood pressure, which causes **syncope** or circulatory arrest. This can be a particular problem for older adults.

The neck is first inspected for obvious pulsation of the artery. The client turns the head slightly away from the artery being examined. Sometimes the wave of the pulse can be seen. The carotid is the only site for assessing the quality of a pulse wave. Only an experienced examiner can evaluate the quality of the wave in relation to systole and diastole of the cardiac cycle. An absent pulse wave can indicate arterial occlusion (blockage) or **stenosis** (narrowing).

To palpate the pulse, ask the client to look straight ahead or turn the head slightly to the side being examined. Turning relaxes the sternocleidomastoid muscle. The nurse slides the tips of the index and middle fingers around the medial edge of the sternocleidomastoid muscle. Gently palpate to avoid occlusion of circulation (Figure 24-34).

The normal carotid pulse is localized rather than diffuse. As a strong pulse, the carotid has a thrusting quality. As the client breathes, no change occurs. Rotation of the neck or a shift from a sitting to a supine position should not change the carotid's quality. Both carotid arteries should be equal in pulse rate, rhythm, and strength and should be equally elastic. Diminished or unequal carotid pulsations may indicate **atherosclerosis** or other forms of arterial disease.

The carotid is the most commonly auscultated pulse. Auscultation is especially important for middle-age or older adults or clients suspected of having cerebrovascular disease. When the lumen of a blood vessel is narrowed, its blood flow is disturbed. As blood passes through the narrowed section, a turbulence is created, causing a blowing or swishing sound. The blowing sound is called a **bruit** (pronounced "brew-ee"). The bell of the stethoscope is placed over the carotid artery at the base of the neck and moved gradually toward the jaw. The nurse asks the client to hold the breath for a moment so that breath sounds do not obscure a bruit. Normally, no sound is heard during carotid auscultation. If a bruit is heard, the nurse gently palpates the artery lightly for a **thrill** (palpable bruit).

Jugular Veins

The most accessible veins are the internal and external jugular veins in the neck. Both veins drain bilaterally from the head and neck into the superior vena cava. The external jugular lies superficially and can be seen just above the clavicle. The internal jugular lies deeper, along the carotid artery.

Normally when a client lies in the supine position, the external jugular distends and becomes easily visible. In contrast, the jugular veins normally flatten when the client is in a sitting or standing position. A client with heart disease, however, may have distended jugular veins when sitting.

The entry-level nurse is responsible for observing for jugular venous distention. The client's jugular veins are inspected in the supine position (normally protrude), when standing (normally flat), and when sitting at a 45-degree angle (jugular veins distended only if client has right-sided heart failure) (Figure 24-35). The specific measurement of jugular venous pressure is completed by an advanced practitioner.

Peripheral Arteries

The most accurate assessment of peripheral arteries involves palpation over arteries that are close to the body surface and lie over bones. An arterial pulsation is a bounding wave of blood that diminishes in intensity with increasing distance from the heart (Seidel and others, 1995).

The nurse assesses the arterial pulses in the extremities to determine sufficiency of the entire arterial circulation. Factors such as coagulation disorders, local trauma or surgery, constricting casts or bandages, and systemic disease such as diabetes or arteriosclerosis can impair circulation to the extremities. The nurse should discuss with the client the risk for circulatory problems (Box 24-16).

The nurse examines each peripheral artery using the distal pads of the second and third fingers. The thumb may help anchor the brachial and femoral artery. The nurse applies firm pressure but avoids occluding the pulse. When it is difficult to find a pulse, it is helpful to vary pressure and feel all around the pulse site. The nurse must be sure not to palpate his or her own pulse.

Routine vital signs usually include assessment of the

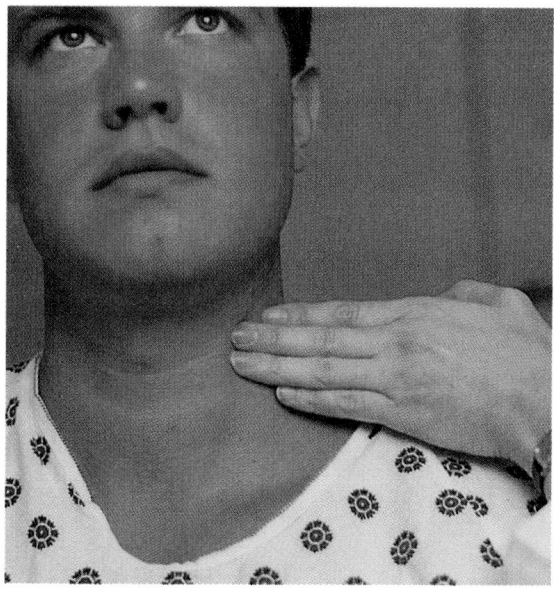

Figure 24-34. Palpation of the internal carotid artery.

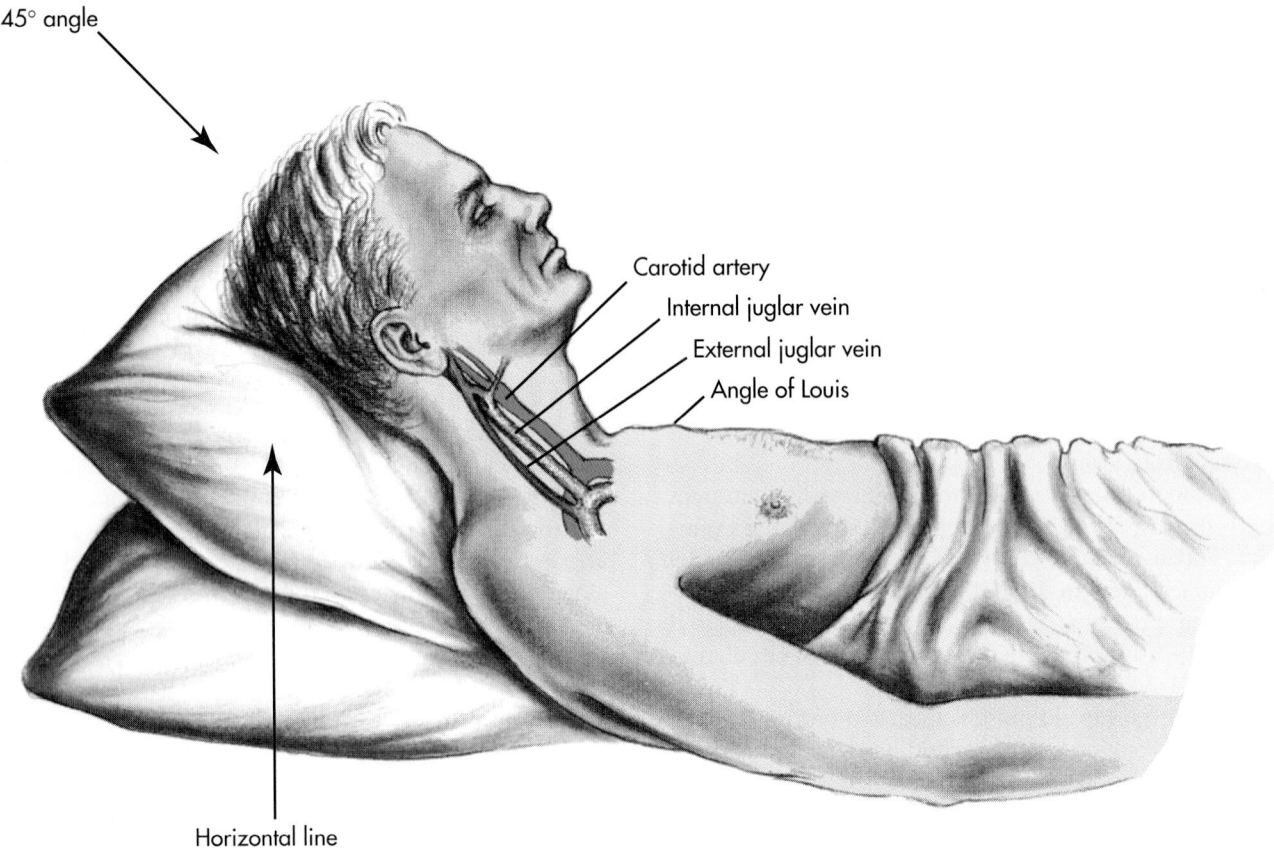

45° angle

Carotid artery

Internal jugular vein

External jugular vein

Angle of Louis

Horizontal line

Figure 24-35. Position of client to assess jugular vein distention. (From Thompson JM and others: *Mosby's manual of clinical nursing,* ed 3, St. Louis, 1993, Mosby.)

BOX 24-16
Client Teaching for Vascular Assessment

- Tell clients their blood pressure readings. Explain the normal reading for a client's age.
- Discuss implications of abnormalities.
- Instruct clients with risk or evidence of vascular insufficiency in the lower extremities to avoid tight clothing over the lower body or legs, to avoid sitting or standing for long periods, to walk regularly, and to elevate the feet when sitting.
- Advise clients to avoid cigarette smoking, because nicotine causes vasoconstriction.
- Older adults with hypertension may benefit from regular self-monitoring of blood pressure (daily, weekly, or monthly). Teach clients how to use home monitoring kits.

rate and rhythm of the radial artery, because it is easily accessible (see Chapter 23). The pulse is counted for either 30 seconds or a full minute, depending on the character of the pulse. With palpation the nurse normally feels the pulse wave at regular intervals. When an interval is interrupted by an early, late, or missed beat, the pulse rhythm is irregular. In emergencies, the carotid artery is chosen because it is accessible and closest to the heart and thus most useful in evaluating heart activity. To check local circulatory status of tissues, the nurse palpates peripheral arteries long enough to note that a pulse is present.

The nurse assesses each peripheral artery for elasticity of vessel wall, strength, and equality. The arterial wall is normally elastic, making it easily palpable. After the artery is depressed, it will spring back to shape when pressure is released. An abnormal artery may be described as hard, inelastic, or calcified.

The strength of a pulse is a measurement of the force with which blood is ejected against the arterial wall. Some examiners use a rating from 0 (zero) to 4+ (Seidel and others, 1995):

0	Absent, not palpable
1+	Pulse is diminished, barely palpable, easy to obliterate
2+	Easily palpable, normal pulse
3+	Full, increased pulse
4+	Bounding, cannot be obliterated

All peripheral pulses are measured for equality and symmetry. The left radial pulse is compared with that of the right, the left brachial pulse is compared with the left radial, and so on. Lack of symmetry may indicate impaired circulation such as a localized obstruction or an abnormally positioned artery.

In the upper extremities the brachial artery channels blood to the radial and ulnar arteries of the forearm and hand. If circulation in this artery becomes blocked, the hands will not receive adequate blood flow. If circulation in the radial or ulnar arteries becomes impaired, the hand will still receive adequate perfusion. An interconnection between the radial and ulnar arteries guards against arterial occlusion (Figure 24-36).

To locate pulses in the arm, the nurse has the client sit or lie down. The radial pulse is found along the radial side of the forearm at the wrist. In a thin individual a groove is formed lateral to the flexor tendon of the wrist. The radial pulse can be felt with light palpation in the groove (Figure 24-37). The ulnar pulse is on the opposite side of the wrist and feels less prominent (Figure 24-38). An examiner palpates the ulnar pulse only when arterial insufficiency to the hand is expected.

If a client has a weak radial or ulnar pulse, **Allen's test** can be performed to assess collateral circulation. The client makes a fist as the ulnar and radial arteries are compressed simultaneously. The client then opens the hand, and the nurse releases the ulnar artery. The hand should quickly turn pink if the ulnar artery is patent. The test may be repeated by releasing only the radial artery.

To palpate the brachial pulse, the nurse finds the groove between the biceps and triceps muscle above the elbow at the antecubital fossa (Figure 24-39). The artery runs along the medial side of the extended arm.

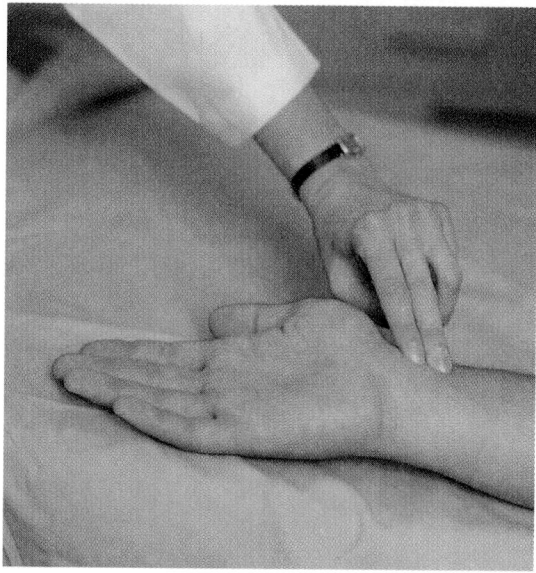

Figure 24-37. Palpation of radial pulse.

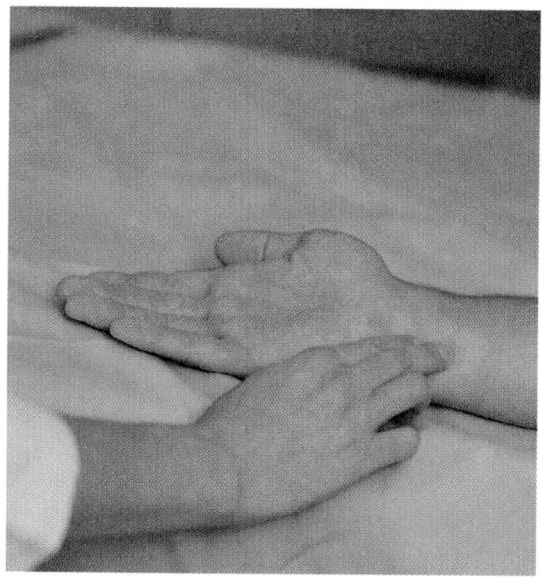

Figure 24-38. Palpation of ulnar pulse.

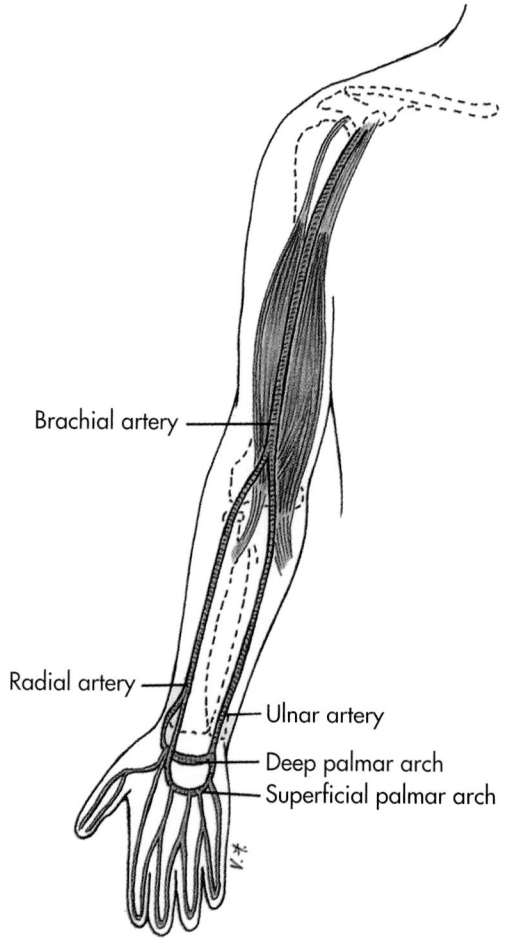

Brachial artery

Radial artery

Ulnar artery

Deep palmar arch

Superficial palmar arch

Figure 24-36. Anatomical positions of brachial, radial, and ulnar arteries.

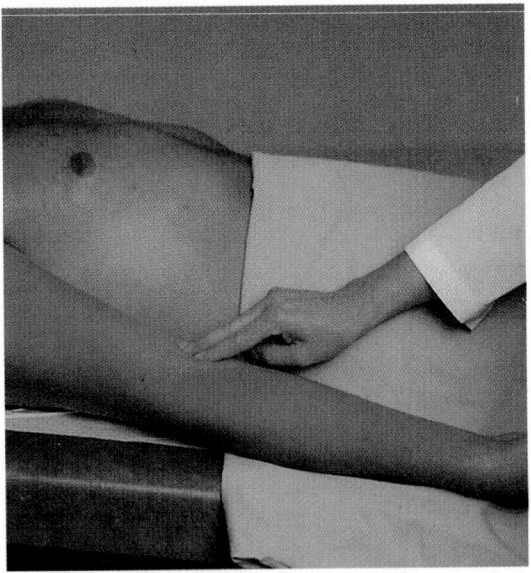

Figure 24-39. Palpation of brachial pulse.

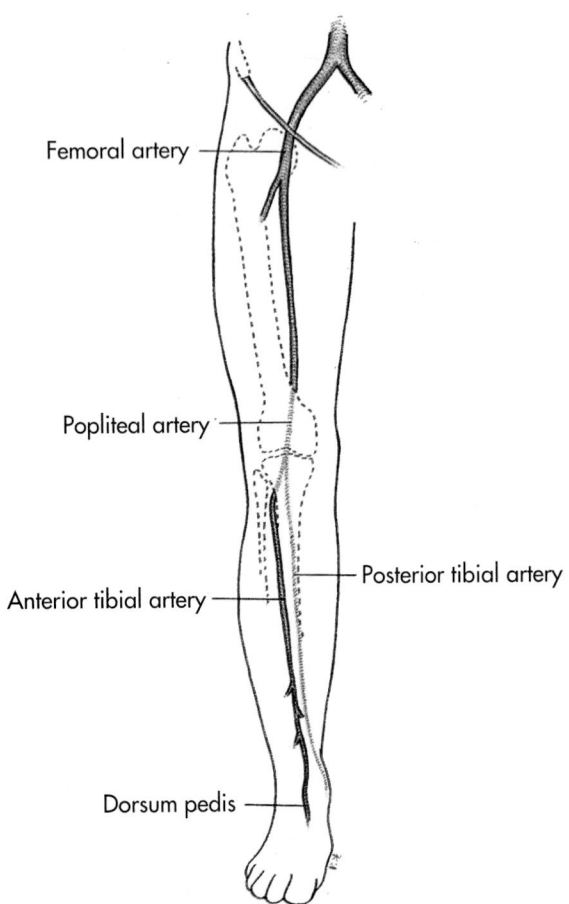

Figure 24-40. Anatomical position of femoral, popliteal, dorsalis pedis, and posterior tibial arteries.

The nurse palpates the artery with the fingertips of the first three fingers in the muscle groove.

The femoral artery is the primary artery in the leg, delivering blood to the popliteal, posterior tibial, and dorsalis pedis arteries (Figure 24-40). An interconnection between the posterior tibial and dorsalis pedis arteries guards against local arterial occlusion. The femoral pulse is found best with the client lying down with the inguinal area exposed (Figure 24-41). The femoral artery runs below the inguinal ligament, midway between the symphysis pubis and the anterosuperior iliac spine. Deep palpation may be required to feel the pulse. Bimanual palpation is effective in obese clients. The nurse places the fingertips of both hands on opposite sides of the pulse site. A pulsatile sensation can be felt as the fingertips are pushed apart by the arterial pulsation.

The popliteal pulse is found behind the knee (Figure 24-42). The client should slightly flex the knee with the foot resting on the examination table. The client may also assume a prone position with the knee slightly flexed. The client is instructed to keep leg muscles relaxed. The nurse palpates with the fingers of both hands deeply into the popliteal fossa, just lateral to the midline. The popliteal pulse is difficult to locate.

With the client's foot relaxed the nurse locates the dorsalis pedis pulse. The artery runs along the top of the foot in a line with the groove between the extensor tendons of the great toe and first toe (Figure 24-43). Often an examiner finds the pulse by placing the fingertips between the great and first toe and slowly inching up the foot. This pulse may be congenitally absent. The posterior tibial pulse is found on the inner side of each ankle (Figure 24-44). The nurse places the fingers behind and below the client's medial malleolus (ankle

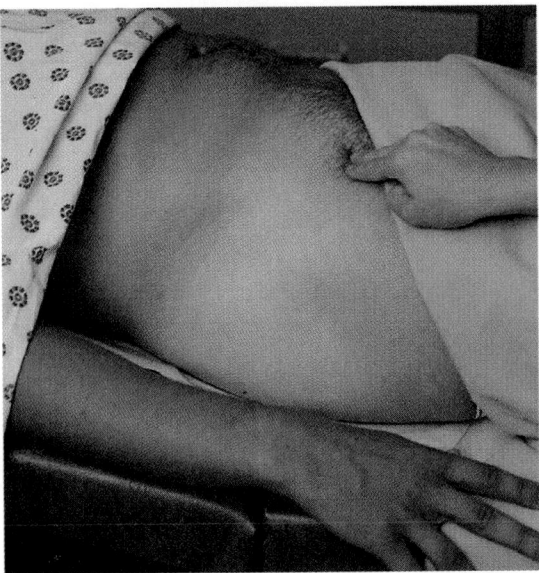

Figure 24-41. Palpation of femoral pulse.

bone). The artery is easily located with the client's foot relaxed and slightly extended.

Ultrasound Stethoscopes

If a nurse has difficulty palpating a pulse, an ultrasound stethoscope is a useful tool that can amplify sounds of a pulse wave. A thin layer of transmission gel is first applied to the client's skin at the pulse site or directly onto the transducer tip of the probe. The nurse then turns the volume control to "on" and places the tip of the probe at a 45- to 90-degree angle on the skin (Figure 24-45). The nurse moves the probe until hearing a pulsating "whooshing" sound that indicates that arterial blood flow is present.

Tissue Perfusion

The condition of the skin, mucosa, and nail beds offers useful data about the status of circulatory blood flow. The nurse first examines the face and upper extremities, looking at the color of skin, mucosa, and nail beds. The presence of cyanosis requires special attention. Central cyanosis, which indicates poor arterial oxygenation, may be caused by heart disease. It can be noted by a bluish discoloration of the lips, mouth, and conjunctivae. Peripheral cyanosis, which indicates peripheral vasoconstriction, is noted by blue lips, earlobes, and nail beds. When cyanosis is present, the nurse refers to available laboratory data on oxygen saturation to determine severity of the problem. Examination of the nails involves inspection for **clubbing,** a bulging of the tissues at the nail base. Clubbing is caused by insufficient oxygenation at the periphery

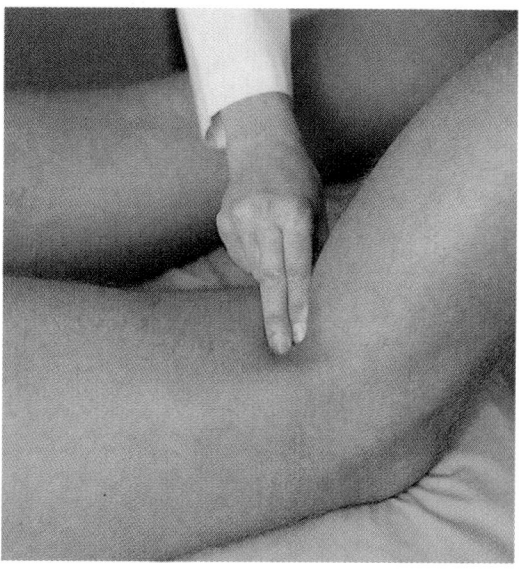

Figure 24-42. Palpation of popliteal pulse.

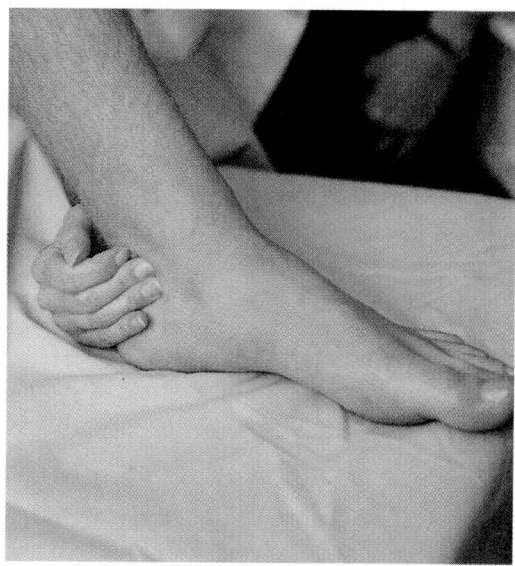

Figure 24-44. Palpation of posterior tibial pulse.

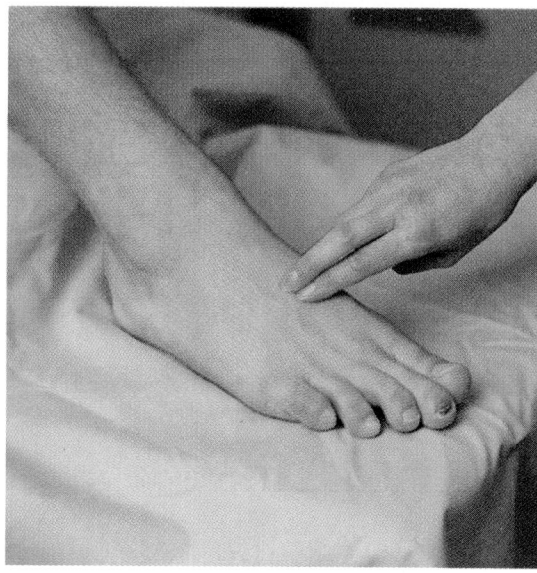

Figure 24-43. Palpation of dorsalis pedis pulse.

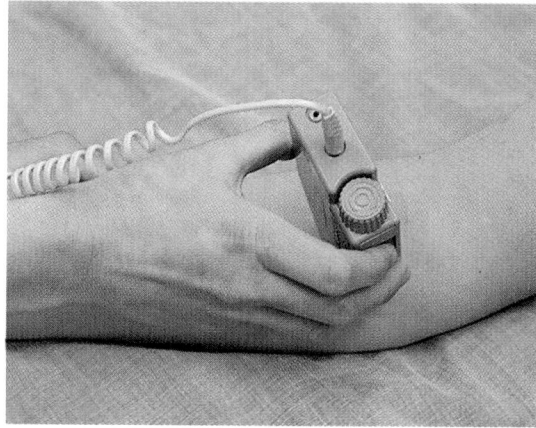

Figure 24-45. Ultrasound stethoscope in position on brachial artery.

TABLE 24-8

Signs of Venous and Arterial Insufficiency

Assessment Criterion	Venous	Arterial
Color	Normal or cyanotic	Pale; worsened by elevation of extremity; dusky red when extremity lowered
Temperature	Normal	Cool (blood flow blocked to extremity)
Pulse	Normal	Decreased or absent
Edema	Often marked	Absent or mild
Skin changes	Brown pigmentation around ankles	Thin, shiny skin; decreased hair growth; thickened nails

resulting from conditions such as congenital heart disease and chronic emphysema.

The nurse inspects the lower extremities for changes in color, temperature, and condition of the skin indicating either arterial or venous alterations (Table 24-8). This is a good time to ask the client about history of pain in the legs. If an arterial occlusion is present, the client has signs resulting from absence of blood flow. Pain will be distal to the occlusion. The three "P's" characterize an occlusion—pain, pallor, and pulselessness. Venous congestion causes tissue changes indicating inadequate circulatory flow back to the heart.

During examination of the lower extremities, the nurse also inspects skin and nail texture; hair distribution on the lower legs, feet, and toes; venous pattern; and scars, pigmentation, or ulcers. The absence of hair growth over the legs may indicate circulatory insufficiency. The nurse should not be mislead by shaven lower legs. Also, many men have less hair around the calves because of tight-fitting dress socks or jeans. Chronic recurring ulcers of the feet or lower legs are a serious sign of circulatory insufficiency and require a physician's intervention.

Peripheral Veins

The nurse assesses the status of the peripheral veins by asking the client to assume sitting and standing positions. Assessment includes inspection and palpation for varicosities, peripheral edema, and phlebitis. Varicosities are superficial veins that become dilated, especially when legs are in a dependent position. They are common in older adults because the veins normally fibrose, dilate, and stretch. They are also common in people who stand for prolonged periods. Varicosities in the anterior or medial part of the thigh and the posterolateral part of the calf are abnormal.

Dependent edema around the feet and ankles can be a sign of venous insufficiency or right-sided heart failure. Dependent edema is common in older adults and persons who spend a lot of time standing (e.g., nurses, waitresses, security guards). To assess for pitting edema the nurse uses a thumb to press firmly 1 to 2 seconds and then release over the medial malleolus or the shins. A depression left in the skin indicates edema. The severity of the edema is characterized by grading 1+ through 4+ (Figure 24-46).

Phlebitis is an inflammation of a vein that occurs commonly after trauma to the vessel wall, infection, immobilization, or prolonged insertion of IV catheters (see Chapter 31). Phlebitis promotes clot formation, a potentially dangerous situation because a clot within a deep vein of the leg can become dislodged and travel through the heart, causing a pulmonary embolus. To assess for phlebitis the nurse inspects the calves for localized redness, tenderness, and swelling over vein sites. Gentle palpation of calf muscles reveals tenderness and firmness of the muscle. The nurse may also check for Homans' sign by supporting the leg while dorsiflexing the foot. If phlebitis is present in the lower leg, forceful dorsiflexion of the foot often causes pain in the calf.

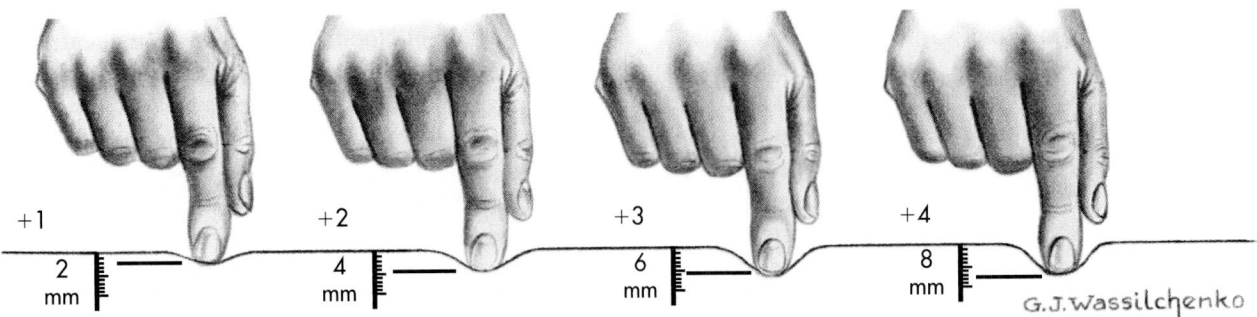

+1   2 mm   +2   4 mm   +3   6 mm   +4   8 mm

G.J.Wassilchenko

Figure 24-46. Assessing for pitting edema. (From Seidel HM and others: *Mosby's guide to physical examination*, ed 3, St. Louis, 1995, Mosby.)

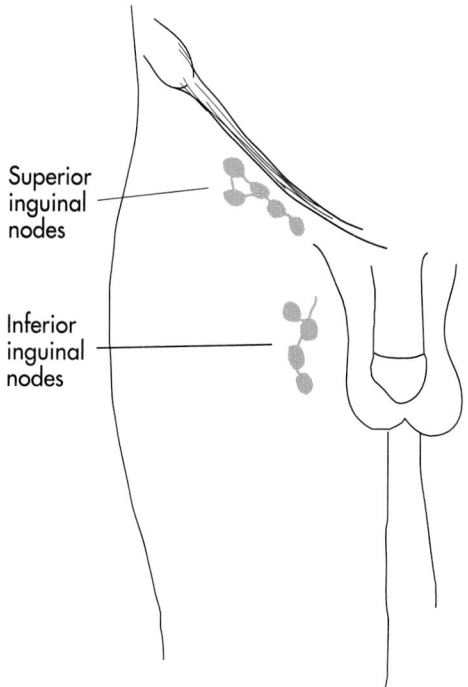

Figure 24-47. Inguinal lymph nodes.

Lymphatic System

Assessment of the lymphatic drainage of the lower extremities is performed during examination of the vascular system or during the female or male genital examination. The legs are drained by superficial and deep lymph nodes, but only two groups of superficial nodes are palpable. With the client supine, the nurse palpates the area of the superior superficial nodes in the groin area (Figure 24-47). Then the nurse moves the fingertips toward the inner thigh, feeling for any palpable inferior nodes. The nurse uses a firm but gentle pressure when palpating over each lymphatic chain. Multiple nodes are not normally palpable, although a few soft, nontender nodes are not unusual. Enlarged, hardened, tender nodes can reveal potential sites of infection or metastatic disease.

BREASTS

It is important to examine the breasts of female and male clients. A small amount of glandular tissue, a potential site for the growth of cancer cells, is located in the male breast. In contrast, the majority of the female breast is glandular tissue.

Female Breasts

New cases of breast cancer affected 180,200 (approximately one in every nine) women in the United States in 1997 (American Cancer Society, 1997). The disease is second to lung cancer as the leading cause of death in women with cancer. Early detection is the key to cure.

A major responsibility for nurses is to teach clients health behaviors such as breast self-examination (BSE) (Box 24-17). Studies suggest a minority of women actually perform BSE. Nurses should know factors that increase the likelihood of a woman performing BSE.

If the client already performs self-examinations, the nurse assesses the method she uses and the time she does the examination in relation to her menstrual cycle. The best time for a self-examination is on the last day of the menstrual period, when the breast is no longer swollen or tender from hormone elevations. If the woman is postmenopausal, she should check her breasts at the same time each month. The pregnant woman also must check her breasts on a monthly basis.

Older women may require special attention when reviewing the need for BSE. Many older women are limited by fixed incomes and thus fail to pursue regular clinical breast examination and mammography. Unfortunately, many older women ignore changes in their breasts, assuming they are a part of aging. In addition, physiological factors can affect the ease with which older women can perform BSE. Musculoskeletal limitations, diminished peripheral sensation, reduced eyesight, and changes in joint range of motion can limit palpation and inspection abilities. The nurse should find resources for older women, including free screening programs. Often family members can be taught to perform examinations.

The American Cancer Society (1997) recommends the following guidelines for the early detection of breast cancer:

1. BSE should be performed monthly by women 20 years of age and older.
2. An examination by a physician should be performed every 3 years from ages 20 to 40, and yearly for women over 40.
3. Women with a family history of breast cancer should have a yearly physician's examination.
4. Asymptomatic women should have a screening mammogram by age 40; women age 40 and over should have a mammogram annually.
5. For women age 35 or over with a history of breast cancer, a yearly examination is recommended.

The client's history should alert the nurse to any signs of breast disease and normal development changes. Because of this glandular structure, the breast undergoes changes during a woman's life. Knowledge of these changes (Box 24-18) helps the nurse complete an accurate assessment.

Health history. A health history can reveal risk factors for breast cancer, including women over age 40; women with a personal or family history of breast cancer; early-onset menarche (before age 12) or late-age menopause (after age 50); and women who have never

Box 24-17
Breast Self-Examination

Instruct client on BSE. All women 20 years and older
should perform this self-examination monthly using the
following steps:
Stand before a mirror. Look at both breasts for anything unusual, such as discharge from the nipples,
puckering, dimpling, or scaling of the skin.
To note changes in the shape of the breasts, perform
the following measures (see the illustration):
Watch in the mirror while raising the arms above the
head.
Press hands firmly on the hips and bow slightly toward the mirror while pulling the shoulders and
elbows forward.

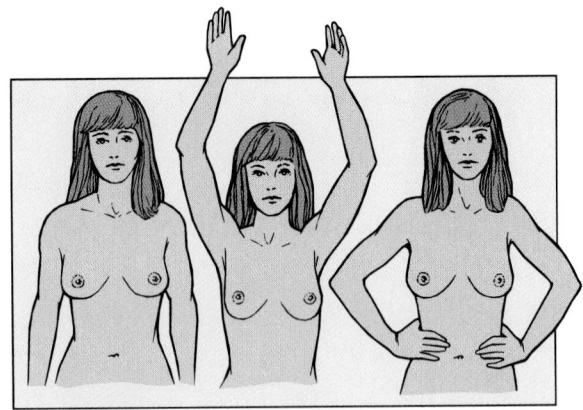

In the shower or in front of the mirror, palpate each
breast. Raise the right arm and use three or four fingers
of the left hand to explore the breast carefully (see the
illustration). Then start at the outer edge, pressing the
flat part of the fingers in small circles, moving the circles slowly around the breast, gradually working toward
the nipple (see the illustration). Pay close attention to
the area between the breast and armpit and feel for unusual lumps or masses. Repeat the process for the left
breast.
Gently palpate each nipple, looking for discharge (see the
illustration). Caution against pinching or squeezing.

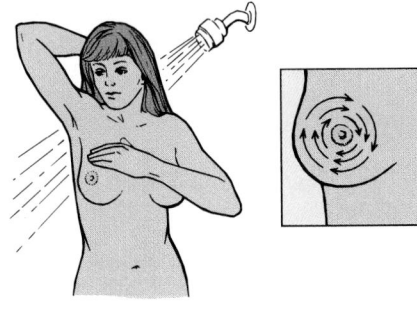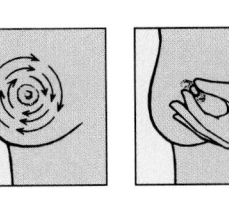

Repeat the third and fourth steps lying down. Lie flat on
the back with the right arm over the head and a small
pillow under the right shoulder. Palpate the right breast
(see the illustration). Repeat the process on the left
breast.
Call your physician if you find a lump.

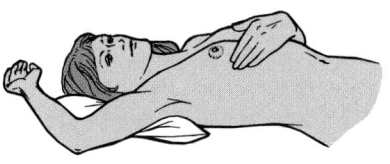

Illustrations from Payne WA, Hahn DB: *Understanding your health*, ed 2, St. Louis, 1989, Mosby.

had children, who gave birth to their first child after age
30, or who have not breast-fed their infants. A health
history should also determine whether a client (both
sexes) has a history of signs and symptoms of breast
cancer such as a lump, thickening, pain, or tenderness
of the breast; discharge, distortion, retraction, or scaling
of the nipple; or change in breast size. Determine the
client's use of medications such as oral contraceptives,
digitalis, diuretics, steroids, estrogen, or foods high in
fat. The nurse assesses the client's caffeine intake to review risk factors for fibrocystic disease. Ask if the client
performs monthly BSE. If so, determine the time of
month she performs the examination in relation to her
menstrual cycle. Have the client describe or demonstrate the method used. If the client reports a breast
mass, the nurse should perform a symptom analysis.

Inspection. The client removes the top gown
or drape to allow simultaneous visualization of both
breasts. The client may stand or sit with her arms hanging
loosely at her sides. If possible, the nurse places a mirror
in front of the client during inspection so she can see
what to look for when performing a self-examination.
To recognize abnormalities, the client must be familiar
with the normal appearance of her breasts.

The nurse describes observations or findings in relation to imaginary lines that divide the breast into four
quadrants and a tail. The lines cross at the center of the
nipple. Each tail extends outward from the upper outer
quadrant (Figure 24-48).

The breasts are inspected for size and symmetry.
Normally, the breasts extend from the third to the sixth
ribs, with the nipple at the level of the fourth intercostal

Box 24-18
Normal Changes in the Breast During a Woman's Life Span

Puberty (8 to 20 Years)*

Breasts mature in five stages. One breast may grow more rapidly than the other. The ages at which changes occur and rate of developmental progression vary.

Stage 1 (Preadolescent)

This stage involves elevation of the nipple only.

Stage 2

The breast and nipple elevate as a small mound, and the areolar diameters enlarge.

Stage 3

There is further enlargement and elevation of the breast and areola, with no separation of contour.

Stage 4

The areola and nipple project into the secondary mound above the level of the breast (may not occur in all girls).

Stage 5 (Mature Breast)

Only the nipple projects, and the areola recedes (may vary in some women).

Young Adulthood (20 to 30 Years)

Breasts reach full (nonpregnant) size. Shape is generally symmetrical. Breasts may be unequal in size.

Pregnancy

Breast size gradually enlarges to two to three times the previous size. Nipples enlarge and may become erect. Areolae darken and diameters increase. Superficial veins become prominent. A yellowish fluid (colostrum) may be expelled from the nipples.

Menopause

Breasts shrink. Tissue becomes softer, sometimes flabby.

Older Adulthood

Breasts become elongated, pendulous, and flaccid as a result of glandular tissue atrophy. The skin of the breasts tends to wrinkle, appearing loose and flabby.
Nipples become smaller, flatter, and lose erectile ability.† Nipples may invert because of shrinkage and fibrotic changes.‡

Data from:
*Wong D: *Whaley and Wong's nursing care of infants and children,* ed 5, St. Louis, 1995, Mosby.
†Seidel HM and others: *Mosby's guide to physical examination,* ed 3, St. Louis, 1995, Mosby.
‡Ebersole P, Hess P: *Toward healthy aging,* ed 4, St. Louis, 1994, Mosby.

---

space. It is common for one breast to be smaller. However, a difference in size may be caused by inflammation or a mass. As the woman becomes older, the ligaments supporting the breast tissue weaken, causing the breasts to sag and the nipples to lower.

The nurse observes the contour or shape of the breasts and notes masses, flattening, retraction, or dimpling. Breasts vary in shape from convex to pendulous or conical. Retraction or dimpling results from invasion of underlying ligaments by tumors. The ligaments fibrose and pull the overlying skin inward toward the tumor. Edema also changes the breasts' contour. To bring out the presence of retraction or changes in the shape of the breasts, the nurse asks the client to assume three positions: raise arms above the head, press hands against the hips, and extend arms straight ahead while sitting and leaning forward. Each maneuver causes a contraction of the pectoral muscles, which will accentuate the presence of any retraction.

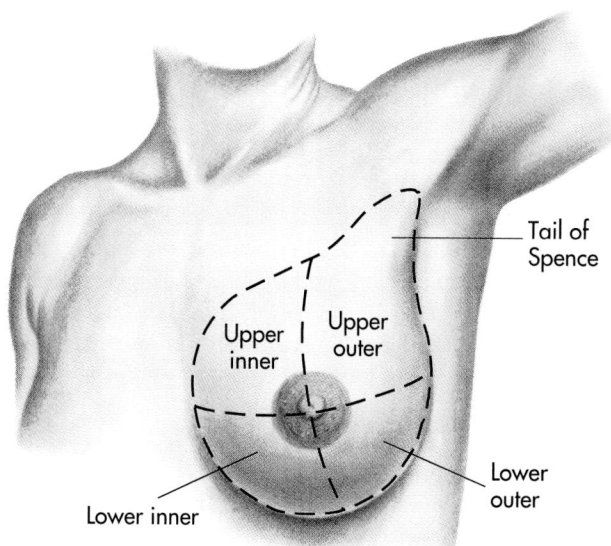

Figure 24-48. Quadrants of the left breast and axillary tail of Spence. (From Seidel HM and others: *Mosby's guide to physical examination,* ed 3, St. Louis, 1995, Mosby.)

The overlying skin is carefully inspected for color; venous pattern; and presence of edema, lesions, or inflammation. The nurse lifts each breast when necessary to observe lower and lateral aspects for color and texture changes. The breasts are the color of neighboring skin, and venous patterns are the same bilaterally. Venous patterns are more easily seen in thin clients or pregnant women. Women with large breasts often have redness and excoriation of the undersurface caused by rubbing of skin surfaces.

The nurse inspects the nipple and areola for size, color, shape, discharge, and the direction the nipples point. The normal areolae are round or oval and nearly equal bilaterally. Color ranges from pink to brown. In light-skinned women the areola turns brown during pregnancy and remains dark. In dark-skinned women the areola is brown before pregnancy (Seidel and others, 1995). Normally the nipples point in symmetrical directions, are everted, and have no drainage. If the nipples are inverted, the nurse asks if this has been a lifetime history. A recent inversion or inward turning of the nipple may indicate an underlying growth. Rashes or ulcerations are not normal on the breast or nipples. Bleeding or discharge from the nipple is noted. Clear yellow discharge 2 days after childbirth is common. While inspecting the breasts the nurse explains the characteristics seen. The client must be taught the significance of abnormal signs or symptoms.

Palpation. Palpation allows the nurse to determine the condition of underlying breast tissue and lymph nodes. Breast tissue consists of glandular tissue, fibrous supportive ligaments, and fat. Glandular tissue is organized into lobes that end in ducts opening onto the nipple's surface. The largest portion of glandular tissue is in the upper outer quadrant and tail of each breast. Suspensory ligaments connect to skin and fascia underlying the breast to support the breast and maintain its upright position. Fatty tissue is located superficially and to the sides of the breast.

A large proportion of lymph from the breasts drains into axillary lymph nodes. If cancerous lesions **metastasize** or spread, the nodes commonly become involved. The nurse learns the location of supraclavicular, infraclavicular, and axillary nodes (Figure 24-49). The axillary nodes drain lymph from the chest wall, breasts, arms, and hands. A tumor of one breast may involve nodes on the opposite side, as well as those on the same side.

To palpate lymph nodes the nurse has the client sit with arms at her sides and muscles relaxed. While facing the client and standing on the side being examined, the nurse supports the client's arm in a flexed position and abducts the arm from the chest wall. The nurse places the free hand against the client's chest wall and high in the axillary hollow (Figure 24-50). With the fingertips the nurse presses gently down over the surface

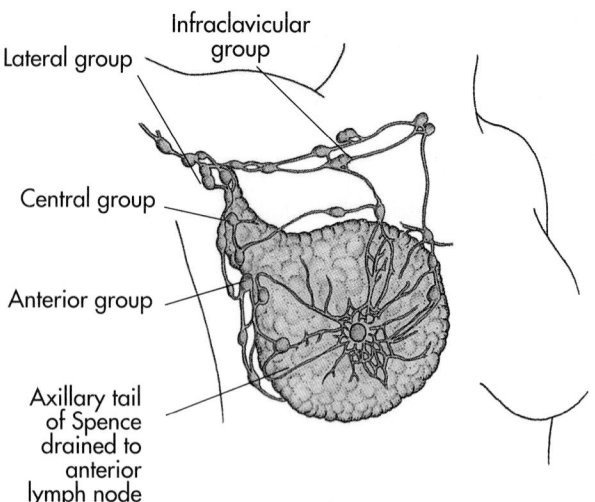

Figure 24-49. Anatomical position of axillary and clavicular lymph nodes.

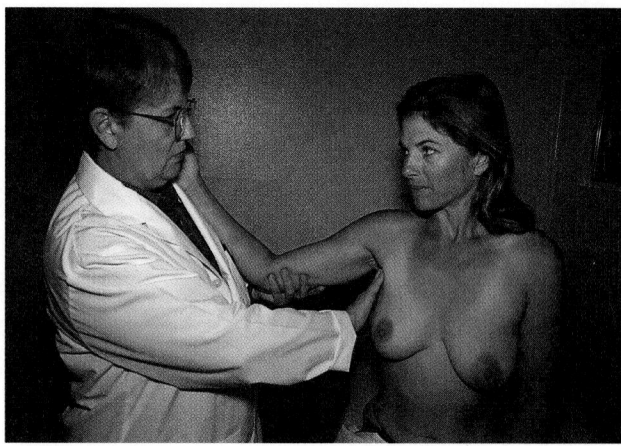

Figure 24-50. The nurse supports the client's arm and palpates axillary lymph nodes.

of the ribs and muscles. The axillary nodes are palpated with the fingertips gently rolling soft tissue. Four areas of the axilla are palpated: at the edge of the pectoralis major muscle along the anterior axillary line, the chest wall in the midaxillary area, the upper part of the humerus, and the anterior edge of the latissimus dorsi muscle along the posterior axillary line. Normally lymph nodes are not palpable. A palpable node feels like a small mass that may be hard, tender, and immobile. The nurse also palpates along the upper and lower clavicular ridges. The procedure is reversed for the client's other side.

It may be difficult for the client to learn to palpate for lymph nodes. Lying down with the arm abducted makes the area more accessible. The client is instructed to use her left hand for the right axillary and clavicular

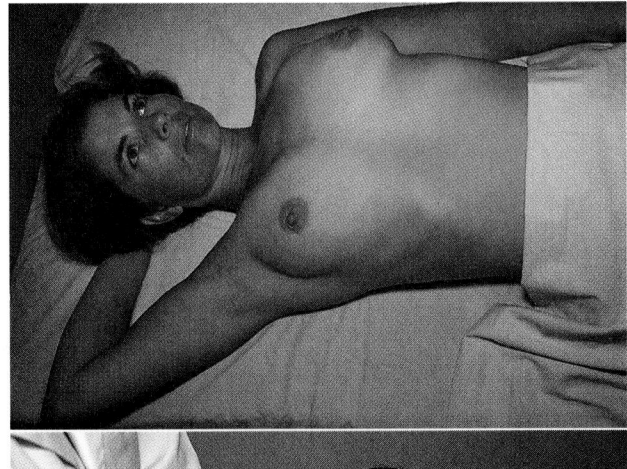

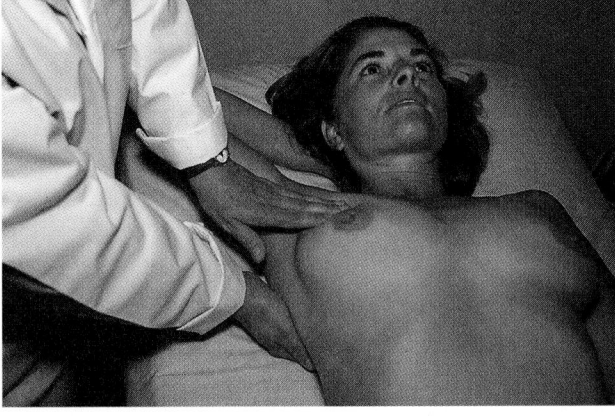

Figure 24-51. **A,** The client lies flat with arm abducted and hand under head to help flatten breast tissue evenly over the chest wall. **B,** Nurse palpates each breast in systematic fashion.

areas and vice versa. The nurse can take the client's fingertips and move them in the proper circular fashion.

Palpation of breast tissue is best performed with the client lying supine and one arm behind the head (alternating with each breast). The supine position allows the breast tissue to flatten evenly against the chest wall. The client should raise her hand and place it behind the neck to further stretch and position breast tissue evenly (Figure 24-51, *A*). The examiner often places a small pillow or towel under the client's shoulder blade to further position breast tissue.

The consistency of normal breast tissue varies widely. The breasts of a young client are firm and elastic. In an older client the tissue may feel stringy and nodular. The client's familiarity with the texture of her own breasts is most important. This familiarity is gained through monthly BSE (Box 24-19).

If the client complains of a mass, the nurse examines the opposite breast first to ensure an objective comparison of normal and abnormal tissue. The nurse uses the pads of the first three fingers to compress breast tissue gently against the chest wall, noting tissue consistency (Figure 24-51, *B*). Palpation is performed systemati-

cally in one of two ways: clockwise or counterclockwise, forming small circles with the fingers along each quadrant and the tail; or with a back-and-forth technique with the fingers moving up and down each quadrant (Figure 24-52). Whatever approach is used, the nurse must be sure to cover the entire breast and tail, directing attention to any areas of tenderness. When palpating large, pendulous breasts, the nurse uses a bimanual technique. The inferior portion of the breast is supported in one hand while the nurse uses the other hand to palpate breast tissue against the supporting hand.

During palpation the nurse notes the consistency of breast tissue. It normally feels dense, firm, and elastic. With menopause, breast tissue shrinks and becomes softer. The lobular feel of glandular tissue is normal. The lower edge of each breast may feel firm and hard. This is the normal inframammary ridge and is not a tumor. It may help to move the client's hand so she can feel normal tissue variations. Abnormal masses are palpated to determine location in relation to quadrants, diameter in centimeters, shape (e.g., round or discoid), consistency (soft, firm, or hard), tenderness, mobility, and discreteness (clear or unclear borders).

Cancerous lesions are hard, fixed, nontender, irregular in shape, and usually unilateral. A common benign condition of the breast is **fibrocystic breast disease.** This condition is characterized by bilateral lumpy, painful breasts and sometimes nipple discharge. Symptoms are more apparent during the menstrual period. When palpated, the cysts (lumps) are soft, well differentiated, and moveable. Deep cysts may feel hard.

Special attention is given to palpating the nipple and areola. The entire surface is gently palpated. The thumb and index finger compress the nipple, and the nurse notes any discharge. As the nurse examines the nipple and areola, the nipple may become erect with wrinkling of the areola. These changes are normal.

After the nurse has completed the examination, the client can demonstrate self-palpation. Observing the client's technique helps the nurse to emphasize the importance of a systematic approach. The client is urged

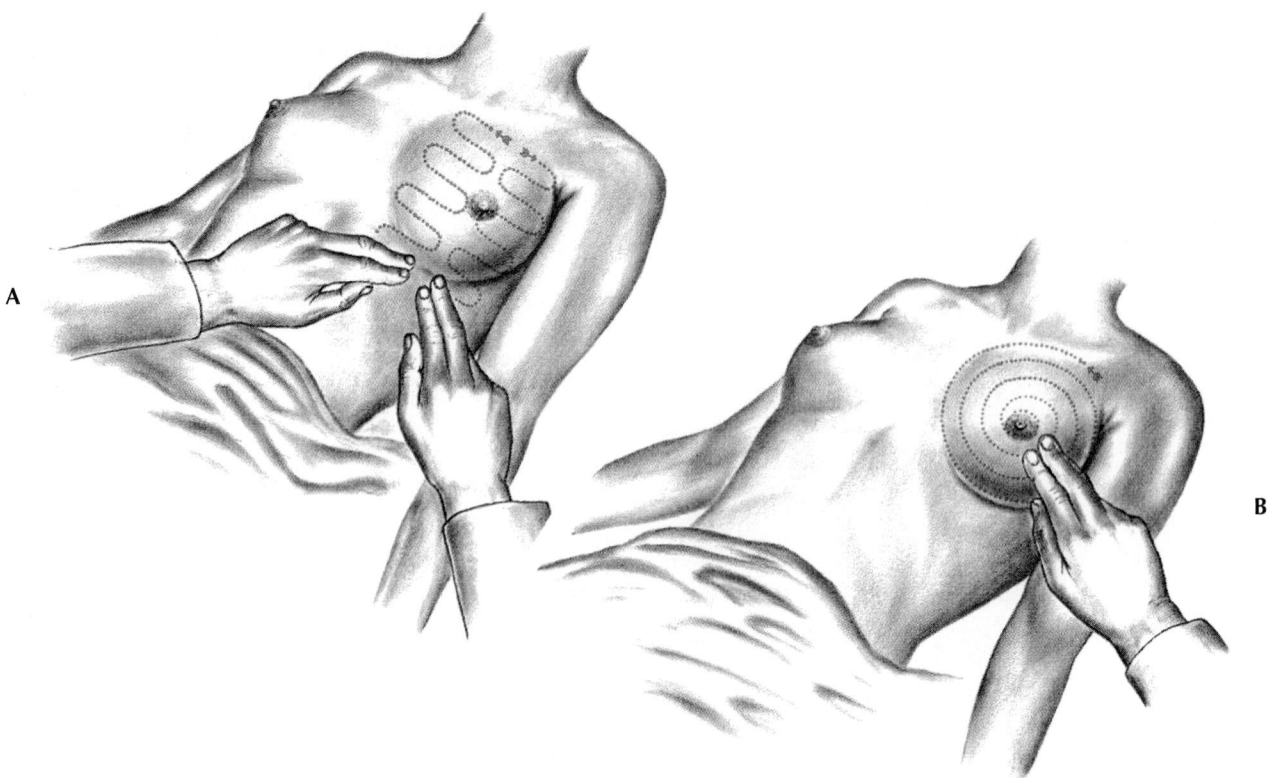

Figure 24-52. Methods for breast palpation. **A,** Back and forth; **B,** concentric circles. (From Seidel HM and others: *Mosby's guide to physical examination,* ed 3, St. Louis, 1995, Mosby.)

to see her physician if she discovers an abnormal mass during monthly self-examination. She also should know all signs and symptoms of breast cancer.

Male Breasts

Examination of the male breast is relatively easy. The nipple and areola are inspected for nodules, edema, and ulceration. An enlarged male breast may result from obesity or glandular enlargement. Breast enlargement in young males may result from steroid use. Fatty tissue feels soft, whereas glandular tissue is firm. Masses are palpated for the same characteristics as in the female breast. Because male breast cancer is relatively rare, routine self-examinations are unnecessary.

ABDOMEN

The abdominal examination can be complex because of the organs located within and near the abdominal cavity (Figure 24-53). The examiner assesses abdominal organs anteriorly and posteriorly.

A system of landmarks helps to map out the abdominal region. The xiphoid process (tip of the sternum) is the upper boundary of the anterior abdominal region. The symphysis pubis delineates the lower boundary. By dividing the abdomen into four imaginary quadrants

(Figure 24-53, *A*), the nurse can refer to assessment findings and record them in relation to each quadrant. Posteriorly the kidneys, located from the T12 to L3 vertebrae, are protected by the lower ribs and heavy back muscles. The costovertebral angle formed by the last rib and vertebral column is a landmark used during palpation of the kidney.

The examination includes an assessment of structures of the lower gastrointestinal (GI) tract in addition to the liver, stomach, kidneys, and bladder. Abdominal pain is one of the most common symptoms clients will report when seeking medical care. An accurate assessment requires matching client history data with a careful assessment of the location of physical symptoms.

During the abdominal examination, the client must be relaxed. A tightening of abdominal muscles hinders palpation. The nurse asks the client to void before beginning. The room should be warm, and the client's upper chest and legs are draped. The client lies supine or in a dorsal recumbent position with the arms at the sides and knees slightly bent. Small pillows can be placed beneath the knees. If the client places the arms under the head, the abdominal muscles may tighten. The examiner proceeds calmly and slowly, being sure there is adequate lighting. The abdomen is exposed from just above the xiphoid process down to the sym-

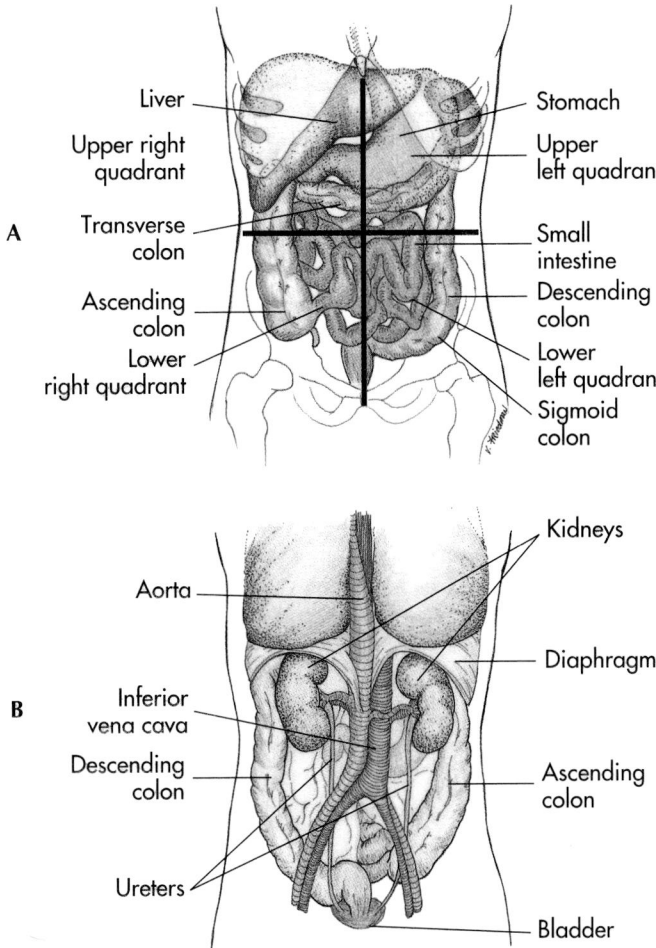

A

Liver
Upper right quadrant
Transverse colon
Ascending colon
Lower right quadrant

Stomach
Upper left quadrant
Small intestine
Descending colon
Lower left quadrant
Sigmoid colon

B

Aorta
Inferior vena cava
Descending colon
Ureters

Kidneys
Diaphragm
Ascending colon
Bladder

Figure 24-53. **A,** Anterior view of abdomen divided by quadrants. **B,** Posterior view of abdominal sections.

physis pubis. Warm hands and stethoscope further promote relaxation. The client is asked to report pain and point out areas of tenderness. Tender areas are assessed last.

The order for an abdominal examination differs slightly from previous assessments. The nurse begins with inspection and then auscultation. By using auscultation before palpation and percussion, there is less chance of altering the frequency and character of bowel sounds. During the examination the nurse needs a tape measure and marking pen.

Health History

The nurse asks whether the client has abdominal or low back pain and assesses the pain in detail (see Chapter 33). The client's normal bowel habits and stool character are also reviewed, with the nurse asking if the client uses laxatives. The nurse also determines if the client has had abdominal surgery, trauma, or diagnostic tests of the GI tract. Signs and symptoms of belching, difficulty swallowing, flatulence, bloody emesis **(hematemesis),** black tarry stools **(melena),** heartburn,

diarrhea, or constipation may reveal a pattern of a problem. The nurse also asks if the client has had a recent weight change or intolerance to diet. If the client takes antiinflammatories (e.g., aspirin, ibuprofen, steroids) and antibiotics, there may be risk for GI upset or bleeding. The nurse inquires about a family history of cancer, kidney disease, alcoholism, hypertension, or heart disease. Assess the client's usual intake of alcohol. The nurse should determine if the female client is pregnant and note her last menstrual period. The nurse also reviews a client's history for risk factors of hepatitis B virus exposure. Finally, the nurse asks the client to locate tender areas before beginning the examination.

Inspection

The nurse may be able to observe the client during routine care activities. The nurse notes the client's posture and looks for evidence of abdominal splinting, lying with the knees drawn up, or moving restlessly in bed. A client free from abdominal pain will not stoop or splint the abdomen. To inspect the abdomen for abnormal movement or shadows, the nurse stands on the client's right side and inspects from above the abdomen. By sitting down to look across the abdomen, the nurse assesses contour. The examination light is directed over the abdomen.

The nurse inspects the skin over the abdomen for color, scars, venous patterns, lesions, and **striae** (stretch marks). The skin is subject to the same color variations as the rest of the body. Venous patterns are normally faint, except in thin clients. Artificial openings may indicate drainage sites resulting from surgery or an ostomy. Scars reveal evidence of past trauma or surgery that may have created permanent changes in underlying organ anatomy. Bruising may indicate accidental injury, physical abuse, or a type of bleeding disorder. Ask if the client self-administers injections (e.g., insulin or heparin). Unexpected findings include generalized color changes such as jaundice or cyanosis. A glistening taut appearance indicates ascites.

Inspection continues with the umbilicus. The nurse notes the position; shape; color; and presence of inflammation, discharge, or protruding masses. A normal umbilicus is flat or concave with the color the same as surrounding skin.

The nurse inspects for contour, symmetry, and surface motion of the abdomen, noting any masses, bulging, or distention. A flat abdomen forms a horizontal plane from the xiphoid process to the symphysis pubis. A round abdomen protrudes in a convex sphere from a horizontal plane. A concave abdomen appears to sink into the muscular wall. Each of these findings is normal if the abdomen's shape is symmetrical. In older adults there is often an overall increased distribution of adipose tissue.

The presence of masses on only one side, or asymmetry, may indicate an underlying pathological condition.

The nurse observes the abdomen's contour while asking the client to take a deep breath and hold it. The contour should remain smooth and symmetrical. To evaluate abdominal musculature, the nurse has the client raise the head. This position causes superficial abdominal wall masses, hernias, and muscle separations to become more apparent.

Intestinal gas, tumor, or fluid in the abdominal cavity may cause distention (swelling). When distention is generalized, the entire abdomen protrudes. The skin often appears taut, as if it were stretched over. When gas causes distention, the flanks do not bulge. However, if fluid is the source of the problem, such as in ascites, the flanks bulge. The client should be asked to roll onto one side. A protuberance forms on the dependent side if fluid is the cause of the distention. The nurse asks the client if the abdomen feels unusually tight. The nurse must be careful not to confuse distention with obesity. In obesity the abdomen is large, rolls of adipose tissue are often present along the flanks, and the client does not complain of tightness in the abdomen. If abdominal distention is expected, the nurse may choose to measure the abdomen's girth by placing a tape measure around the abdomen at the level of the umbilicus. Consecutive measurements will show any increase or decrease in distention. A marking pen is used to indicate where the tape measure was applied.

The abdomen is next inspected for movement. Normally men breathe abdominally, and women breathe more costally. If the client has severe pain, respiratory movement is diminished, and the client tightens abdominal muscles to guard against the pain. The nurse also observes for peristaltic movement or aortic pulsation by looking across the abdomen from the side. These movements may be seen in thin clients; otherwise no movement is present.

Auscultation

The nurse auscultates the abdomen to listen to the bowel sounds of normal intestinal **peristalsis** and to detect vascular sounds. Clients with GI tubes connected to suction must have them temporarily turned off before beginning the examination. First the warmed diaphragm of the stethoscope is placed lightly over the lower left quadrant. The nurse asks the client not to speak. Normally, air and fluid move through the intestines, creating soft gurgling or clicking sounds that occur irregularly 5 to 35 times per minute (Seidel and others, 1995). Sounds may last ½ second to several seconds. It normally takes 5 to 20 seconds to hear a bowel sound. However, it may take 5 minutes of continuous listening before determining bowel sounds are absent. Auscultate all four quadrants to be sure no sounds are missed. The best time to auscultate is between meals. Sounds are generally described as normal, audible, absent, hyperactive, or hypoactive.

Absent sounds indicate cessation of GI motility that may result from late-stage bowel obstruction, **paralytic ileus,** or **peritonitis.** Hyperactive sounds are loud, "growling" sounds called **borborygmi,** which indicate increased GI motility. Inflammation of the bowel, anxiety, bleeding, excess ingestion of laxatives, and reaction of the intestines to certain foods cause increased motility (Box 24-20).

Bruits indicate narrowing of major blood vessels and disruption of blood flow. Presence of bruits in the abdominal area can reveal **aneurysms** or stenotic vessels. The nurse uses the stethoscope's bell to auscultate in the epigastric region and each of the four quadrants. Normally there are no vascular sounds over the aorta (midline through the abdomen) or femoral arteries (lower quadrants). Renal artery bruits can be heard by placing the stethoscope over each upper quadrant anteriorly or the costovertebral angle posteriorly (which can be done with the client sitting). A bruit should be reported immediately to a physician.

Percussion

Percussion of the abdomen maps out underlying organs and masses and reveals the presence of air in the stomach and intestines. The beginning student uses this skill in a limited fashion. Practice is needed to ensure accuracy. The nurse percusses each of the four quadrants to discriminate between the sounds of dullness and tympany. Potentially painful areas are percussed last. Tympany usually predominates because of air existing within the stomach and intestines. A dull percussion note is a medium- to high-pitched short sound heard over solid masses such as the liver, spleen, pancreas, kidneys, and a distended bladder. In addition, a dull percussion note may indicate a tumor. When dullness is

---

BOX 24-20

Client Teaching for Abdominal Assessment

- Explain factors that promote normal bowel elimination, such as diet, regular exercise, limited use of over-the-counter drugs causing constipation, establishment of a regular elimination schedule, and a good fluid intake (see Chapter 36). Stress importance for older adults.
- Caution clients about dangers of excessive use of laxatives or enemas.
- If the client has acute pain, explain activities or positions to avoid.
- If the client has chronic pain, explain measures used for pain relief (e.g., relaxation exercises, positioning) (see Chapter 33).
- Instruct the client about warning signs of colon cancer, including bleeding from the rectum, black or tarry stools, blood in the stool, and a change in bowel habits (constipation or diarrhea).

noted, it may be useful to also use palpation to complete a detailed assessment.

Percussion allows the nurse to identify borders of the liver to detect organ enlargement. The nurse starts at the client's right iliac crest and percusses upward along the midclavicular line. The percussion note changes from tympanic to dull at the liver's lower border, which is usually at the right costal margin. Extension beyond the right costal margin is an abnormality that should be reported immediately. The nurse marks the border with a marking pen. The upper border is found by percussing down from the clavicle along the intercostal spaces at the midclavicular line (Figure 24-54). This time the note changes from resonant to dull. The liver's upper border is usually found in the fifth, sixth, or seventh intercostal space. The nurse measures the distance from the upper to lower border. The distance between the points where dullness is percussed should be 6 to 12 cm (2½ to 5 inches). Diseases such as cirrhosis, cancer, and hepatitis cause liver enlargement.

The kidneys are percussed posteriorly to rule out inflammation. The client may sit or stand upright. The nurse may use direct or indirect percussion. The nurse strikes the client firmly with the ulnar surface of the partially closed fist along each costovertebral angle at the scapular lines. Normal percussion is painless. If the kidneys are inflamed, tenderness is easily elicited during percussion.

Palpation

Palpation primarily detects areas of abdominal tenderness, abnormal distention, or masses. As students become more skilled, they learn to palpate for specific organs such as the liver. Light and deep palpation are used.

The nurse performs light palpation over each abdominal quadrant. Areas previously identified as problem spots are initially avoided. The nurse lays the palm of the hand with fingers extended and approximated lightly on the abdomen. With the palmar surface of the fingers the nurse depresses ½ inch (1.3 cm) in a gentle dipping motion (Figure 24-55). The nurse avoids quick jabs and uses smooth, coordinated movements. For ticklish clients, the nurse first places the hand under the client's until palpation is tolerated. The nurse feels for muscular resistance, tenderness, and superficial organs or masses. While palpating, the nurse observes the client's face for signs of discomfort. The abdomen is normally smooth with consistent softness and nontender without masses. The older adult often lacks abdominal tone.

With experience the nurse can perform deep palpation (Figure 24-56) to delineate abdominal organs and to detect less-obvious masses. A qualified examiner must assist until the nurse becomes skilled in the technique. Short fingernails are needed. It is important for the client to be relaxed as the nurse's hands are depressed approximately 2.5 to 7.5 cm (1 to 3 inches) into the abdomen. Deep palpation is never used over a surgical incision or over extremely tender organs. It is also unwise to use deep palpation on abnormal masses. Deep pressure may cause tenderness in the healthy client over the cecum, sigmoid colon, and aorta and in the midline near the xiphoid process (Seidel and others, 1995).

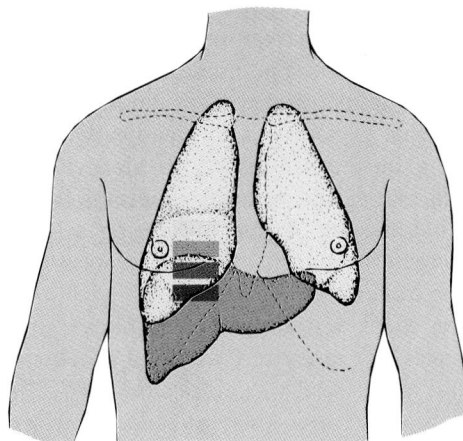

Figure 24-54. To locate the liver's upper border, the nurse percusses downward, noting the change in sound from resonance (lung) to dullness (liver).

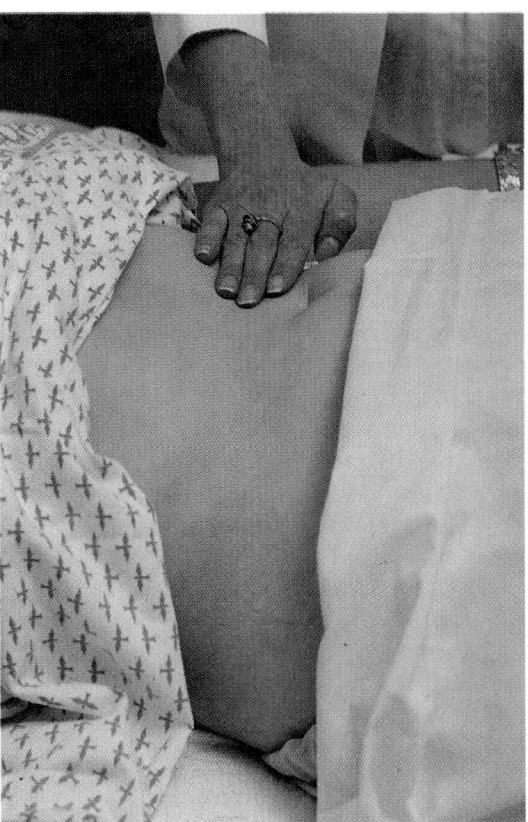

Figure 24-55. Light palpation of the abdomen.

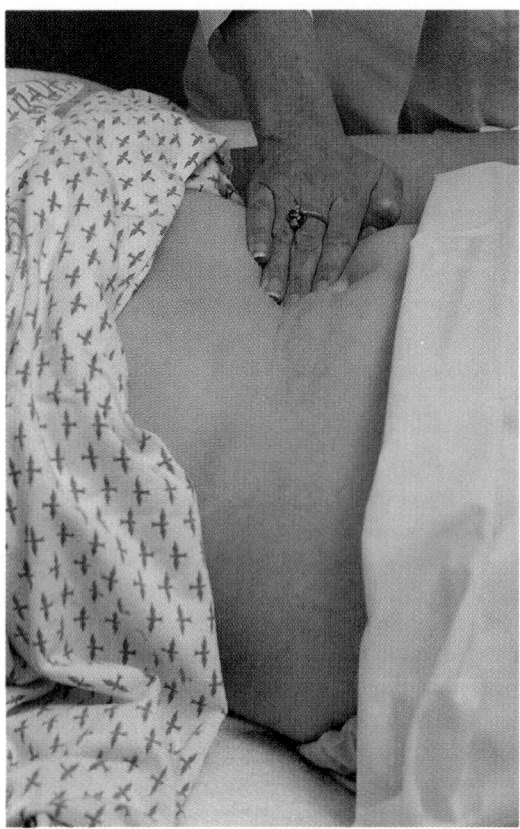

Figure 24-56. Deep palpation of the abdomen.

Each quadrant is surveyed systematically. The nurse palpates masses for size, location, shape, consistency, tenderness, pulsation, and mobility. If tenderness is found, the examiner checks for rebound tenderness. This test may be performed by having the examiner press a hand slowly and deeply into the involved area and then let go quickly. If pain is elicited with the release of the hand, the test is positive. Rebound tenderness occurs in clients with peritoneal irritation such as in appendicitis; pancreatitis; or any peritoneal injury causing bile, blood, or enzymes to enter the peritoneal cavity.

To assess aortic pulsation, the nurse palpates with the thumb and forefinger of one hand deeply into the upper abdomen just left of the midline. Normally a pulsation is transmitted forward. If there is enlargement of the aorta from an aneurysm (localized dilation of a vessel wall), the pulsation expands laterally. The nurse should not palpate a pulsating abdominal mass. In obese clients it may be necessary to palpate with both hands, one on each side of the aorta.

FEMALE GENITALIA

Examination of the female genitalia, including external and internal sex organs, can be embarrassing to the client unless the nurse uses a calm, relaxed approach.

The gynecological examination is one of the most difficult experiences for adolescents. Cultural background may further add to apprehension. For example, female Mexican Americans have a strong social value that women do not expose their bodies to men or even to other women. Similarly, Chinese Americans may believe that the examination of genitalia is offensive. The nurse must provide very thorough explanations as to the reason for the procedures used in the examination. The lithotomy position assumed during the examination is an added source of embarrassment. Comfort is achieved through correct positioning and draping. The nurse explains each portion of the examination in advance so that clients can anticipate actions. Adolescents may choose to have parents present in the examination room.

A client may require a complete examination, including assessing external genitalia and performing a vaginal examination, or the nurse may examine external genitalia while performing routine hygiene measures or preparing to insert a urinary catheter. An examination should be a part of each woman's preventive health care, because uterine and ovarian cancer cause more deaths than any other cancer of the female reproductive system (American Cancer Society, 1997).

Adolescents and young adults should be examined because of the growing incidence of sexually transmitted diseases (STDs). The average age of menarche among young girls has declined, and the majority of male and female teenagers are sexually active by age 19 (Wong, 1995). Rectal and anal assessments are easily combined with this examination, because the client can assume a lithotomy or dorsal recumbent position.

Health History

The nursing history reviews the client's previous illnesses or surgeries involving reproductive organs, including STDs. A review of the menstrual history includes age at menarche, frequency and duration of cycle, character of flow, presence of **dysmenorrhea,** pelvic pain, date of last two menstrual periods, and premenstrual symptoms. The nurse also assesses for signs of bleeding, vaginal discharge, or pain outside the normal menstrual period or after menopause. A review of the client's obstetrical history is also valuable. The nurse also asks if clients have symptoms of genitourinary problems such as burning during urination, frequency, urgency, nocturia, hematuria, incontinence, or stress incontinence.

Ask the client to describe her obstetrical history, including each pregnancy and history of abortions or miscarriages. The nurse also questions the client about current and past contraceptive practices and problems encountered. It is important to determine if the client uses safe sex practices. The nurse should discuss risks of STDs and HIV infection.

The nurse also assesses if the client has signs and

symptoms of vaginal discharge, painful or swollen peri-anal tissues, or genital lesions. A client's risks for developing cervical, endometrial, or ovarian cancer are also reviewed (Box 24-21).

Preparing the Client

This examination is best performed with the client lying on an examination table (with stirrups), or it may be performed with the client in bed with the legs supported with pillows or bath blankets. The following equipment is needed for a complete examination: examination table with stirrups; vaginal speculum of correct size; adjustable light source; sink; clean, disposable gloves; glass microscopic slides; plastic spatula and/or cytobrush; and specimen bottles with fixative spray (hairspray).

Equipment must be ready before the examination begins. The client is asked to empty her bladder so that urine is not accidentally expelled during the examination. Often it is necessary to collect a urine specimen. Assist the client to the lithotomy position, in bed or on an examination table for an external genitalia assess-

---

BOX 24-21

Client Teaching for Female Genitalia Assessment

- Instruct the client about the purpose of Papanicolaou (Pap) smears and gynecological examinations. Explain that the Pap smear is painless and should be performed annually with a pelvic examination for women who are sexually active or who are over age 18 (unless three consecutive tests are normal and physician recommends less-frequent screening).
- Counsel clients with STDs about diagnosis and treatment.
- Instruct on genital self-examination: Using a mirror, position self to examine the area covered by the pubic hair. Spread the hair apart, looking for bumps, sores, or blisters. Also, look for any warts, which may appear as small, bumpy spots and that enlarge to fleshy, cauliflower-like lesions. Next, spread the outer vaginal lips apart and look at the clitoris for bumps, blisters, sores, or warts. Also look at both sides of the inner vaginal lips. The area around the urinary and vaginal opening should be inspected for bumps, blisters, sores, or warts.
- Explain warning signs of STDs: pain or burning on urination, pain in the pelvic area, bleeding between menstruation, an itchy rash around the vagina, and vaginal discharge (different from usual).
- Teach measures to prevent STDs (e.g., male partner's use of condoms, restricting number of sexual partners, avoidance of sex with persons who have several other partners, perineal hygiene measures).
- Tell clients with STDs that they must inform their sexual partner of the need for an examination.
- Reinforce the importance of perineal hygiene (as appropriate).

---

ment. Assist the client into stirrups if a speculum examination is to be performed. Have the woman stabilize each foot in a stirrup and then have her slide the buttocks down to the edge of the examining table. The nurse places a hand at the edge of the table and instructs the client to move until touching the hand. The client's arms should be at her sides or folded across the chest to prevent tightening of abdominal muscles.

A woman suffering from pain or deformity of the joints may be unable to assume a lithotomy position. In this situation, it may be necessary to have the client abduct only one leg or to have another nurse assist in separating the client's thighs. The side-lying position may also be used with the client on the left side and the right thigh and knee drawn up to her chest.

A square drape or sheet is given to the client. She holds one corner over her sternum, the adjacent corners fall over each knee, and the fourth corner falls over the perineum. After the examination begins, the drape over the perineum is lifted. The male examiner should always have a female in attendance during the examination. A female examiner may prefer to work alone but should have a female attendant if the client is particularly anxious or emotionally unstable.

External Genitalia

The perineal area must be well illuminated. The nurse gloves both hands. The perineum is extremely sensitive and tender; the area is not touched suddenly without warning the client. It is best to touch the neighboring thigh first before advancing to the perineum.

While sitting at the end of the examination table or bed, the nurse inspects the quantity and distribution of hair growth. Preadolescents have no pubic hair. During adolescence, hair grows along the labia, becoming darker, coarser, and curlier. In an adult, hair grows in a triangle over the female perineum and along the medial surface of the thighs. Hair should be free of nits and lice.

The nurse inspects surface characteristics of the labia majora. The skin of the perineum is smooth, clean, and slightly darker than other skin. The mucous membranes appear dark pink and moist. The labia majora may be gaping or closed and appear dry or moist. They are usually symmetrical. After childbirth the labia majora are separated, causing the labia minora to become more prominent. When a woman reaches menopause, the labia majora become thinned. With advancing age they become **atrophied.** The labia majora are normally without inflammation, edema, lesions, or lacerations.

To inspect the remaining external structures, the nurse, with the nondominant hand, gently places the thumb and index finger inside the labia minora and retracts the tissues outward (Figure 24-57). The nurse should be sure to have a firm hold to avoid repeated retraction against the sensitive tissues. The nurse uses the other hand to palpate the labia minora between the thumb and second finger. On inspection the labia minora

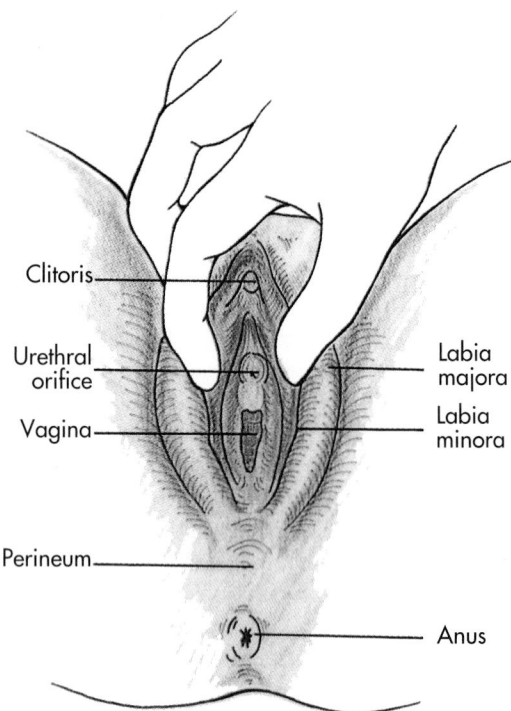

Figure 24-57. Female external genitalia.

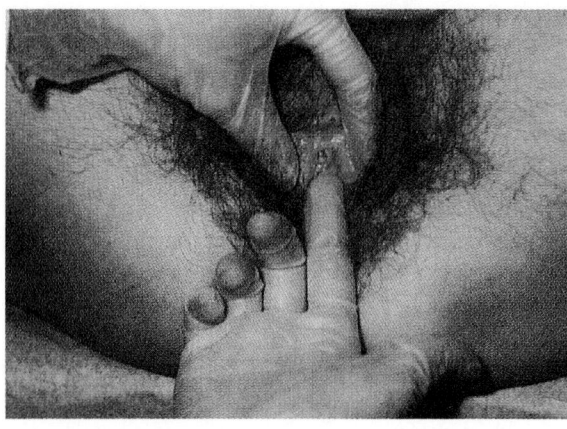

Figure 24-58. Milking the urethra and paraurethral glands. (From Seidel HM and others: *Mosby's guide to physical examination,* ed 3, St. Louis, 1995, Mosby.)

are normally thinner than the labia majora, and one side may be larger. The tissue should feel soft on palpation and without tenderness. The size of the clitoris is variable, but it normally does not exceed 2 cm in length and 0.5 cm in diameter. The nurse looks for atrophy, inflammation, or adhesions. If inflamed, the clitoris will be a bright cherry red. In young women it is a common site for syphilitic lesions or **chancres,** which appear as small open ulcers that drain serous material. Older women may have malignant changes that result in dry, scaly, nodular lesions.

The nurse inspects the urethral orifice carefully for color and position. It is normally intact and without inflammation. The urethral meatus is anterior to the vaginal orifice and is pink. It may appear as a small slit or pinhole opening just above the vaginal canal. The nurse notes any discharge, polyps, or fistulas.

The vaginal introitus is next inspected for inflammation, edema, discoloration, discharge, and lesions. Normally the introitus is a thin vertical slit or a large orifice. The tissue is moist. In women who have had several children, the opening to the vaginal canal may extend upward, blocking the view of the urethra.

With the labia retracted, the nurse examines Skene's and Bartholin's glands. Tell the client you are going to insert one finger into her vagina and that she will feel pressure. With the palm facing upward, the nurse inserts the index finger of the examining hand into the vagina as far as the second joint. Exerting upward pressure, the nurse milks Skene's glands by moving the finger outward. Discharge and tenderness are abnormal.

The examination is done on both sides of the urethra and then directly on the urethra (Figure 24-58). This technique may cause discharge to appear. If so, the nurse notes the color, odor, and consistency and obtains a culture. The nurse next changes to a clean pair of gloves.

While inspecting the vaginal orifice or introitus, the examiner notices the condition of the hymen, which is just inside the introitus. In the virgin the hymen may restrict the opening of the vagina. Only remnants of the hymen remain after sexual intercourse.

If inflammation and edema are found near the posterior end of the introitus, Bartholin's glands may be infected. The glands cannot normally be palpated. To attempt palpation the nurse places a thumb and index finger between the labia majora and introitus and palpates one side at a time.

With the gloved index and middle fingers in the vaginal orifice, the nurse asks the client to strain downward as if she were voiding. If the client lacks adequate muscular support, the vaginal walls will bulge, blocking the introitus. A portion of the vaginal wall and bladder may prolapse or fall into the orifice anteriorly; this is a **cystocele.** Bulging of the posterior wall may be caused by prolapse of the rectum **(rectocele).** Normally when a client is asked to close the vaginal orifice, the nurse palpates tension in the muscles. A woman who has undergone vaginal childbirth has less muscle tone than one who has not.

The nurse may also inspect the anus at this time, looking for lesions and hemorrhoids (see rectal examination). If the nurse performs only the external examination, the examination gloves are disposed of at this time and the client is offered perineal hygiene.

Clients who are at risk for contracting STDs should learn to perform a genital self-examination (see Box 24-21). The purpose is to detect any signs or symptoms of STDs. Many persons do not know they have an STD, and some STDs can remain undetected for years.

Speculum Examination of Internal Genitalia

An examination of internal genitalia requires much skill and practice. Usually it is performed only by advanced nurse practitioners. Beginning students will more than likely only observe the procedure or assist the examiner.

The examination involves use of a plastic or metal speculum. Consisting of two blades and an adjustable

TABLE 24-9 **Methods for Obtaining Pap Smears**	
Location	**Technique**
Outer cervix	Use plastic spatula. Place tip of longer arm in os. Rotate spatula, scraping outer surface of cervix. Apply cells to glass slide. Apply fixative solution and label slide.

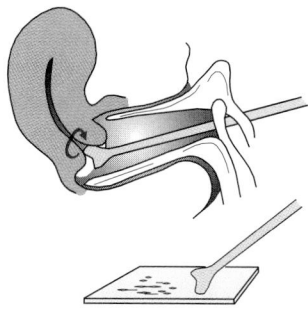

Endocervical	Use cervical brush (cytobrush). WARNING: Do *not* use on pregnant clients. Gently insert brush through os. Rotate brush 180 to 360 degrees. Apply cells by rolling and twisting brush on glass slide. Apply fixative solution and label slide.

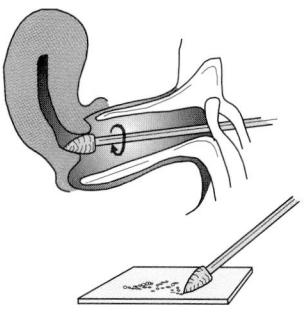

thumbscrew, the speculum is inserted into the vagina to assess the internal genitalia for cancerous lesions and other abnormalities. During the examination a **Papanicolaou (Pap) smear** is collected to test for cervical and vaginal cancer.

To assist an examiner, the nurse makes sure the client is comfortably positioned in the stirrups. A variety of speculum sizes (small, medium, large) should be available so that the examiner may select the appropriate size for the client. In addition, the nurse will have gloves, specimen slides, and a spatula and/or cytobrush close at hand. Water-soluble lubricant is only used when specimens are not being collected. Most examiners lubricate the speculum with warm water.

A Pap smear is a painless screening test for cervical cancer. Specimens are taken from the endocervix and ectocervix (Table 24-9). The examiner first collects a sample of the outer cervix or ectocervix. A plastic spatula is rotated 360 degrees against the cervical surface. Once the spatula is withdrawn, the examiner spreads the specimen lightly over a glass slide. The nurse assisting sprays the specimen with cytological fixative and labels the slide. The examiner next uses a cytobrush to collect endocervical cells. The cytobrush is inserted into the cervical os and rotated one full turn. The specimen is then spread across the slide by rolling the brush with moderate pressure. Again the specimen is sprayed and the slide is labeled. At the end of the procedure the nurse warns the client that blood spotting is normal for a few hours.

Once specimens are collected, the examiner will view the vaginal walls as the speculum is slowly withdrawn. After speculum withdrawal, the nurse assists the client to a sitting position and allows the client to redress and perform hygiene. In a hospital setting, the client may need assistance with perineal hygiene. The nurse makes sure gloves, speculum, and other disposable equipment are appropriately discarded in a receptacle. The client is informed that Pap smear results will be available in 3 to 4 days (check agency policy).

···MALE GENITALIA ....

An examination of the male genitalia assesses the integrity of the external genitalia, inguinal ring, and canal. Because the incidence of STDs in adolescents and young adults is high, an assessment of the genitalia should be a routine part of any health maintenance examination for this age-group. The nurse uses a calm and gentle approach to lessen the client's anxiety. The position and exposure obtained during the examination can be embarrassing. It often helps to minimize the client's anxiety by offering explanations of each step of the examination so the client can anticipate all actions. The genitalia are gently manipulated to avoid causing erection or discomfort. The nurse examines the genitalia carefully and completely but also briskly.

Health History

The nurse assesses the client's normal urinary pattern, including frequency of voiding, character and volume of urine, daily fluid intake, symptoms of burning, urgency and frequency, difficulty starting stream, and hematuria. The history also includes a review of previous surgery or illness involving urinary or reproductive organs, including STDs. The client's sexual history and use of safe sex habits alert the nurse to any risks for HIV or other STDs. A client's sexual performance can be influenced by a number of disorders; thus the nurse asks if the client has difficulty achieving erection or ejaculation. The nurse also reviews medications that might influence sexual performance, including diuretics, sedatives, antihypertensives, and tranquilizers. The nurse asks if the client has noted penile pain or swelling, lesions of the genitalia, or urethral discharge (signs and symptoms of STDs). The client's knowledge of testicular self-examination will guide the nurse in health teaching (Box 24-22). Ask the client if he has noticed heaviness or painless enlargement of a testis or irregular lumps (warning signs of testicular cancer). Finally, if the client reports an enlargement in the inguinal area, assess if it is intermittent or constant; associated with straining or lifting; painful; and whether pain is affected by coughing, lifting, or straining at stool (signs and symptoms indicative of inguinal hernia).

Sexual Maturity

The examination begins by having the client void. The examination room should be warm. The client lies supine with the chest, abdomen, and lower legs draped, or the client may also stand during the examination. The nurse wears disposable gloves.

First, the nurse notes the sexual maturity of the client by observing the size and shape of the penis and testes; the size, color, and texture of scrotal skin; and the character and distribution of pubic hair. The testes first increase in size in preadolescence. During this time there is no pubic hair. By the end of puberty, the testes and penis enlarge to adult size and shape and scrotal skin darkens and becomes wrinkled. With puberty, hair is coarse and abundant in the pubic area. The penis has no hair, and the scrotum has scant amounts. The nurse also inspects the skin covering the genitalia for lice, rashes, excoriations, or lesions. Normally the skin is clear, without lesions.

Penis

To inspect penile surfaces thoroughly the nurse must manipulate the genitalia or have the client assist. The nurse inspects the corona, prepuce (foreskin), glans, urethral meatus, and shaft (Figure 24-59). In uncircumcised males the foreskin is retracted to reveal the glans and urethral meatus. The nurse inspects for discharge, lesions, edema, and inflammation. The foreskin should retract easily. A bit of white cheesy smegma may be seen over the glans. If the client is circumcised, the glans is exposed and appears erythematous and is dry. The meatus is slitlike and normally positioned at the tip of the glans. The glans is smooth and pink along all surfaces. In some congenital conditions the meatus is displaced along the penile shaft. The area between the foreskin and glans is a common site for venereal lesions.

Gentle compression of the glans between the nurse's thumb and index finger opens the meatus to allow inspection for discharge, lesions, and edema. (The client may perform this maneuver.) Normally the opening is glistening and pink without discharge. Any lesion is palpated gently to note tenderness, size, consistency, and shape. When inspection of the glans is completed, the foreskin is pulled down to its original position.

The nurse continues by inspecting the entire shaft of the penis, including the undersurface, looking for any lesions, scars, or areas of edema. The shaft is palpated between the thumb and first two fingers to detect local-

---

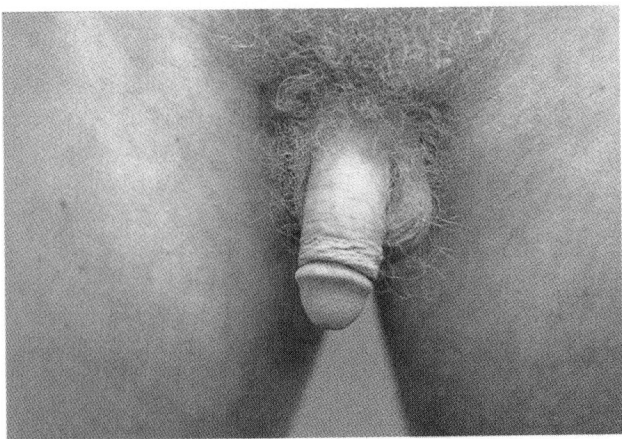

Figure 24-59. Normal male genitalia (circumcised). (From Seidel HM and others: *Mosby's guide to physical examination,* ed 3, St. Louis, 1995, Mosby.)

ized areas of hardness or tenderness. A client who has lain in bed for a prolonged time may develop dependent edema in the penile shaft. It is important for any male client to learn to perform a genital self-examination to detect signs and symptoms of STDs. Many people who have an STD do not know it. A self-examination should be a routine part of self-care (Box 24-23).

Scrotum

The nurse is especially cautious while inspecting and palpating the scrotum, because the structures that lie within the scrotal sac are very sensitive. The scrotum is a saclike structure divided internally into halves. Each half contains a testicle, epididymis, and the vas deferens, which travels upward into the inguinal ring. The left testicle is normally lower than the right. The nurse inspects the scrotum's size, color, shape, and symmetry while observing for lesions or edema.

The scrotum is gently lifted to view the posterior surface. The scrotal skin is usually loose, and the surface is coarse. The skin color is often more deeply pigmented than body skin. Tightening or loss of wrinkling may reveal edema. The scrotum's size normally changes with temperature variations as its dartos muscle contracts in

---

▪ Box 24-23
Male Genital Self-Examination

All men 15 years and older should perform this examination monthly using the following steps:

Genital Examination

Perform the examination after a warm bath or shower when the scrotal sac is relaxed.

Stand naked in front of a mirror and hold the penis in your hand and examine the head. Pull back the foreskin if uncircumcised.

Inspect and palpate the entire head of the penis in a clockwise motion, looking carefully for any bumps, sores, or blisters. Look also for any bumpy warts (see the illustration).

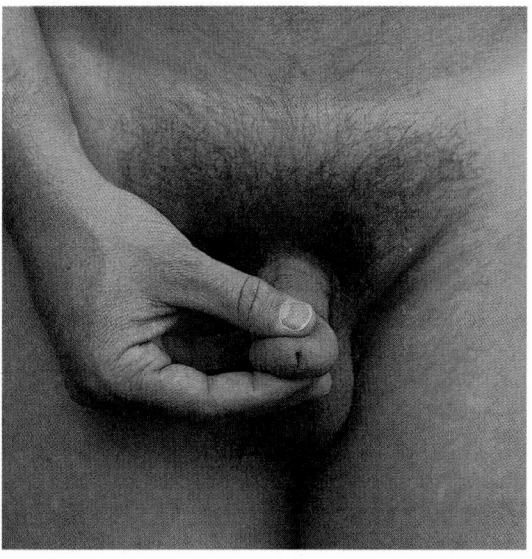

Look at the opening at the end of the penis for discharge.

Look along the entire shaft of the penis for the same signs.

Be sure to separate pubic hair at the base of the penis and carefully examine the skin underneath.

Testicular Self-Examination

Look for swelling or lumps in the skin of the scrotum while looking in the mirror.

Use both hands, placing the index and middle fingers under the testicles and the thumb on top (see the illustration).

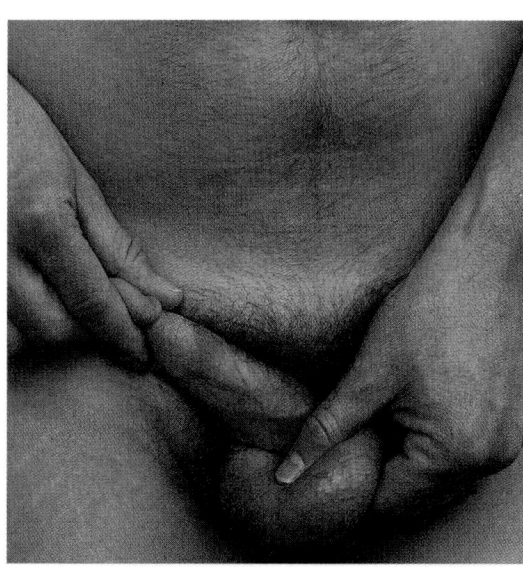

Gently roll the testicle, feeling for lumps, thickening, or a change in consistency (hardening).

Find the epididymis (a cordlike structure on the top and back of the testicle; it is not a lump).

Feel for small, pea-sized lumps on the front and side of the testicle. The lumps are usually painless and are abnormal.

Call your physician if you find a lump.

Illustrations from Seidel HM and others: *Mosby's guide to physical examination*, ed 3, St. Louis, 1995, Mosby.

cold and relaxes in warm temperature. Lumps in the scrotal skin are commonly sebaceous cysts.

Testicular cancer is a solid tumor commonly found in young men ages 18 to 34 years. Early detection is critical. Clients must learn to perform testicular self-examinations (see Box 24-23). The nurse can explain the technique while examining the client. While the client retracts the penis upward, the nurse gently palpates the testes and epididymis between the thumb and first two fingers (Figure 24-60). The nurse notes the size, shape, and consistency of tissue and asks if the client feels any tenderness. The testes should be sensitive but not tender. The underlying testicles are normally ovoid and approximately 2 by 4 cm (⅘ by 1⅗ inches) in size. The testes feel smooth and rubbery and are free from nodules. The epididymis is resilient. In the older adult the testicles decrease in size and are less firm during palpation. The most common symptoms of testicular cancer are a painless enlargement of one testis and appearance of a palpable small, hard lump about the size of a pea on the front or side of the testicle.

The nurse continues to palpate the vas deferens separately as it forms the spermatic cord toward the inguinal ring, noting nodules or swelling. It normally feels smooth and discrete.

Inguinal Ring and Canal

The external inguinal ring provides the opening for the spermatic cord to pass into the inguinal canal. The canal forms a passage through the abdominal wall, a potential site for hernia formation. A **hernia** is a pro-trusion of a portion of intestine through the inguinal wall or canal. An intestinal loop may even enter the scrotum. The client stands during this portion of the examination.

During inspection the client is asked to strain or bear down. The maneuver will help to make a hernia more visible. The nurse looks for obvious bulging. The nurse next palpates the inguinal ring and canal to be sure a hernia is not present. Standing on the right side of the client, the nurse places the index finger of the examining hand against the scrotal skin low on the right side. Gently the nurse moves the finger toward the inguinal canal with the folds of scrotal tissue covering the finger. Carrying the index finger upward along the vas deferens into the inguinal canal, the nurse follows the spermatic cord. It is important not to force the finger into the canal. When the finger reaches the farthest point along the canal, the nurse asks the client to cough and strain down. The maneuver is repeated on the left side. As the client strains, no bulging pressure will be felt. A tightening around the finger is normal.

The nurse completes the examination by palpating for inguinal lymph nodes. Small, nontender, mobile horizontal nodes may normally be found. Any abnormality may indicate local or systemic infection or malignant disease.

⋯ RECTUM AND ANUS

A good time to perform the rectal examination is after the genital examination. The procedure can be uncomfortable, so the nurse helps the client relax by explaining all steps. Usually the examination is not performed on young children or adolescents. The examination can detect colorectal cancer in its early stages. In men the rectal examination can also detect prostatic tumors.

Health History

The nursing history includes review of the client's personal history of colorectal cancer, polyps, or inflammatory bowel disease. If the client is over age 40, the nurse asks if the client has ever had a rectal examination or proctosigmoidoscopy. The client is asked about symptoms of bleeding from the rectum, black or tarry stools (melena), rectal pain, or change in bowel habits, all of which are indicative of colorectal cancer. The client's dietary habits, including intake of high-fat foods or deficient fiber content, may be linked to colon cancer. To screen male clients for possible prostate cancer the nurse asks if clients have experienced weak or interrupted urine flow; an inability to urinate; difficulty in starting or stopping the urinary stream; polyuria; nocturia; hematuria; dysuria; or continuing pain in the lower back, pelvis, or upper thighs. The nurse also reviews the client's use of laxatives, cathartics, codeine, or iron preparations, which can cause elimination problems (Box 24-24).

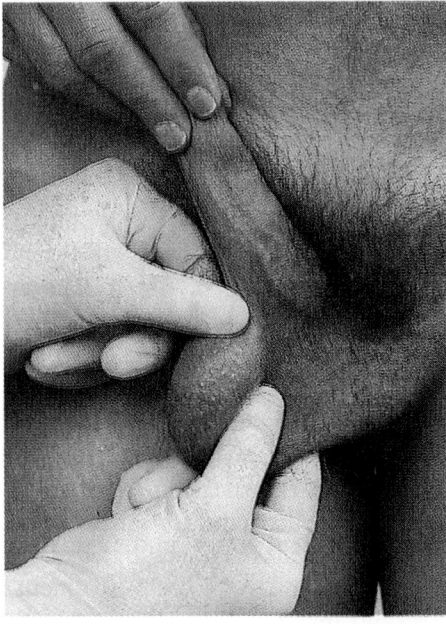

Figure 24-60. Palpating contents of scrotal sac. (From Seidel HM and others: *Mosby's guide to physical examination,* ed 3, St. Louis, 1995, Mosby.)

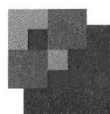

BOX 24-24

Client Teaching for Rectal and Anal Assessment

- Discuss the American Cancer Society's (1997) guidelines for early detection of colorectal cancer:

    Digital rectal examination performed yearly after age 40

    Stool blood slide test (guaiac test) performed yearly after age 50

    Proctosigmoidoscopy, involving visual inspection of the rectum and lower colon with a hollow, lighted tube, performed by a physician every 3 to 5 years after age 50, on the advice of a physician

    Know the warning signs of colorectal cancer

- Discuss dietary planning to reduce fat and increase fiber content.

- Warn clients against problems caused by overuse of laxatives, cathartic medications, codeine, or enemas.

- Discuss with male clients the American Cancer Society's (1997) guidelines for early detection of prostatic cancer:

    Digital rectal examination performed annually after age 40

    Men age 50 and over should have an annual prostate-specific antigen (PSA) blood test

    If either test is suspicious, prostate ultrasound may be performed

    Know the warning signs of prostate cancer

Inspection

Female clients may remain in the dorsal recumbent position following genitalia examination, or they may assume a side-lying (Sims') position. Men are best examined by having the client stand and bend over forward with the hips flexed and upper body resting across the examination table. A nonambulatory client can be examined in Sims' position. The nurse uses disposable gloves.

Using the nondominant hand the nurse gently retracts the buttocks to view the perianal and sacrococcygeal areas. Perianal skin is smooth and more pigmented and coarser than skin overlying the buttocks. The nurse inspects anal tissue for skin characteristics, lesions, external **hemorrhoids** (dilated veins that appear as reddened skin protrusions), ulcers, inflammation, rashes, or excoriation. Anal tissues are moist and hairless, and the anus is held closed by the voluntary sphincter. Next, the nurse asks the client to bear down as though having a bowel movement. Any internal hemorrhoids or fissures will appear at this time. Clock referents (e.g., 12 o'clock, 5 o'clock) are used to describe the location of findings. There normally is no protrusion of tissue.

Digital Palpation

Digital palpation is used to examine the anal canal and sphincters. In male clients, the prostate gland is palpated to rule out enlargement. This portion of the examination is usually reserved for advanced practitioners.

⋯MUSCULOSKELETAL SYSTEM

The musculoskeletal assessment can be done as a separate examination or integrated with other parts of the total physical examination. The nurse can also assess while performing other nursing care measures such as bathing or positioning. The assessment of musculoskeletal integrity is especially important when the client reports pain or loss of function in a joint or muscle. Frequently, muscular disorders are the result of neurological disease. For this reason a neurological assessment is often conducted simultaneously.

While examining the client's musculoskeletal function, the nurse visualizes the anatomy of bone and muscle placement and joint structure. Joints vary in their degree of mobility. Some, as in the knee, are freely moveable. The spinal vertebrae are examples of slightly moveable joints. For a complete examination the muscles and joints should be exposed and free to move. Depending on the muscle groups being assessed, the client assumes a sitting, supine, prone, or standing position.

Health History

A health history includes the client's description of any problems in bone, muscle, or joint function, including history of recent falls, trauma, lifting heavy objects, fractures, and bone or joint disease. The nurse asks the client to point out locations of any alterations. It is useful to assess the client's normal activity pattern, including the type of exercise routinely performed (Box 24-25). The nurse also assesses the nature and extent of pain or stiffness and determines if a musculoskeletal problem affects the client's ability to perform ADLs and participate in social activities. Determine if the client is involved in competitive sports (particularly involving collision and contact), fails to warm up adequately, is in poor physical condition, or had a rapid growth spurt (adolescents). The nurse should review the client's history for **osteoporosis** risk factors, including heavy alcohol use; cigarette smoking; constant dieting; calcium intake less than 500 mg daily; thin and light body frame; nulliparous; menopause before age 45; postmenopause; family history of osteoporosis; or Caucasian, Asian, or Native American ethnicity.

General Inspection

The nurse observes the client's gait and posture when entering the examination room. When a client is unaware of the nurse's observation, gait is more natural. Later a more formal test has the client walk in a straight line away from the nurse. The nurse notes how the client walks, sits, and rises from a sitting position. Normally clients walk with arms swinging freely at the sides and the head leading the body. Older adults walk with

Client Teaching for Musculoskeletal System Assessment

- Instruct the client about correct postural alignment. Consult with a physical therapist to provide the client with exercises for improving posture.
- To reduce bone demineralization, instruct older adults about a proper exercise program (e.g., walking) to be followed three or more times a week. Also encourage intake of calcium to meet the recommended daily allowance. Increased vitamin D will aid calcium absorption.
- Recommendations for calcium supplements are 1000 mg before and 1500 mg after menopause.
- Explain to clients with low back pain that they can benefit from modification of worker risk factors (e.g., lifting heavy weights, use of protective equipment), regular aerobic exercise, exercises that strengthen the back and increase trunk flexibility, and learning how to lift properly.
- Instruct the client on use of assistive devices (e.g., zippers on clothing instead of buttons, elevation of chairs to minimize bending of knees and hips) when he or she is unable to perform ADLs.
- Instruct older adults and those with osteoporosis on proper body mechanics and range of motion and moderate weight-bearing exercises (e.g., swimming and walking) to minimize trauma and subsequent bone fractures.
- Instruct older clients to pace activities to compensate for loss in muscle strength.

smaller steps and a wider base of support. Foot dragging, limping, shuffling, and the position of the trunk in relation to the legs are noted.

The nurse observes the client from the side in a standing position. The normal standing posture is an upright stance with parallel alignment of the hips and shoulders (Figure 24-61). There should be an even contour of the shoulders, level scapulae and iliac crests, alignment of the head over the gluteal folds, and symmetry of extremities. Looking sideways at the client, the nurse notes the normal cervical, thoracic, and lumbar curves. The head is held erect. As the client sits, some degree of rounding of the shoulders is normal. Older adults tend to assume a stooped, forward-bent posture, with hips and knees somewhat flexed and arms bent at the elbows, raising the level of the arms (Ebersole and Hess, 1994). Common postural abnormalities include kyphosis, lordosis, and scoliosis (Figure 24-62). **Kyphosis,** or hunchback, is an exaggeration of the posterior curvature of the thoracic spine. This postural abnormality is common in the older adult. **Lordosis,** or swayback, is an increased lumbar curvature. A lateral spinal curvature is called **scoliosis.** Loss of height is frequently the first clinical sign of osteoporosis, in which height loss occurs in the trunk as a result of vertebral fracture and collapse (Galsworthy and Wilson, 1996). Although a small amount of height loss is to be expected with aging, if the amount of loss is greater than expected, osteoporosis is likely.

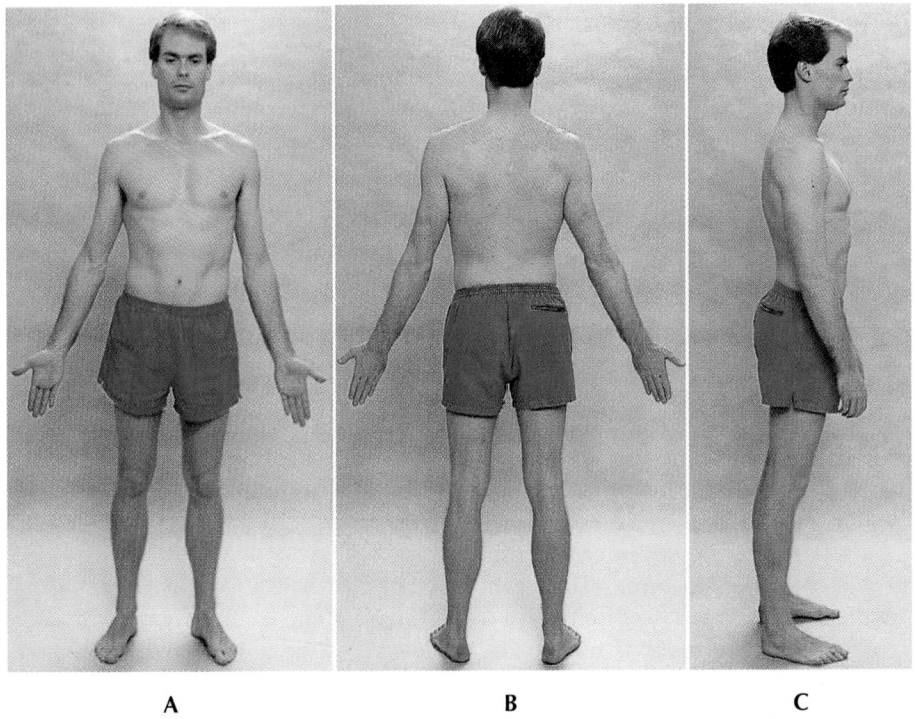

A   B   C

Figure 24-61. Inspection of overall body posture. **A,** Anterior view; **B,** posterior view; **C,** lateral view. (From Seidel HM and others: *Mosby's guide to physical examination,* ed 3, St. Louis, 1995, Mosby.)

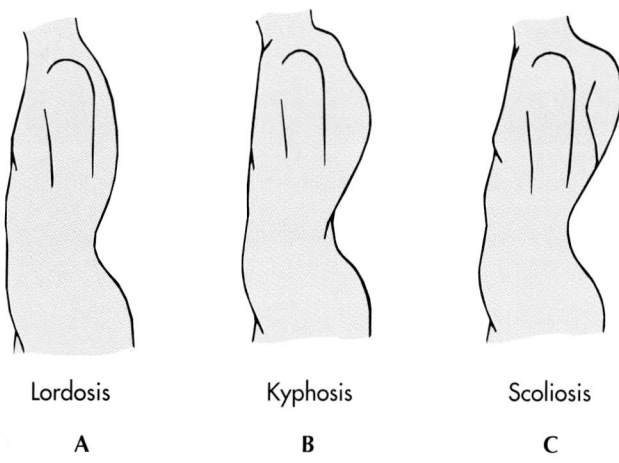

Lordosis   Kyphosis   Scoliosis

A   B   C

Figure 24-62. Common postural abnormalities. **A,** Lordosis; **B,** kyphosis; **C,** scoliosis.

During general inspection the nurse looks at the extremities for overall size, gross deformity, bony enlargement, alignment, and symmetry. There should be bilateral symmetry in length, circumference, alignment, and position and numbering of skinfolds (Seidel and others, 1995). A general review pinpoints areas requiring specialized assessment.

Palpation

The nurse applies gentle palpation to all bones, joints, and surrounding muscles in a complete examination. In the case of a focused assessment, only an involved area needs to be examined. The nurse notes any heat, tenderness, edema, or resistance to pressure. The client should feel no discomfort when palpation is applied. Muscles should be firm.

Range of Joint Motion

The nurse asks the client to put each major joint and its muscle groups through full range of motion (ROM) (Table 24-10). The examination includes comparison of both active and passive ROM. To assess ROM passively, the nurse asks the client to relax and then passively moves the joints until the end of range is felt. The same body parts are compared for equality in movement. The nurse does not force a joint into a painful position. The nurse must know each joint's normal range and the extent to which the client's joints can be moved. Ideally, the client's normal range is assessed to determine a baseline for assessing later change. Joints should be free from stiffness, instability, swelling, or inflammation. There should be no discomfort when the nurse applies pressure to bones and joints. In older adults, joints often become swollen and stiff, with reduced ROM resulting from cartilage erosion and fibrosis of synovial membranes. If a joint appears swollen and inflamed, the nurse palpates it for warmth.

Muscle Tone and Strength

The nurse assesses muscle strength and tone during ROM measurement. Tone is the slight muscular resistance felt by the examiner as the relaxed extremity is passively moved through its ROM. The client is asked to allow an extremity to relax or hang limp. This is often difficult, particularly if the client feels pain in the extremity. The extremity is supported, and each limb grasped, moving it through the normal ROM (Figure 24-63). Normal tone causes a mild, even resistance to passive movement through the entire range.

If a muscle has increased tone or **hypertonicity,** sudden passive movement of a joint is met with considerable resistance. Continued movement eventually

TABLE 24-10
Terminology for Normal Range-of-Motion Positions

Term	Range of Motion	Examples of Joints
Flexion	Movement decreasing angle between two adjoining bones; bending of limb	Elbow, fingers, knee
Extension	Movement increasing angle between two adjoining bones	Elbow, knee, fingers
Hyperextension	Movement of body part beyond its normal resting extended position	Head
Pronation	Movement of body part so that front or ventral surface faces downward	Hand, forearm
Supination	Movement of body part so that front or ventral surface faces upward	Hand, forearm
Abduction	Movement of extremity away from midline of body	Leg, arm, fingers
Adduction	Movement of extremity toward midline of body	Leg, arm, fingers
Internal rotation	Rotation of joint inward	Knee, hip
External rotation	Rotation of joint outward	Knee, hip
Eversion	Turning of body part away from midline	Foot
Inversion	Turning of body part toward midline	Foot
Dorsiflexion	Flexion of toes and foot upward	Foot
Plantar flexion	Bending of toes and foot downward	Foot

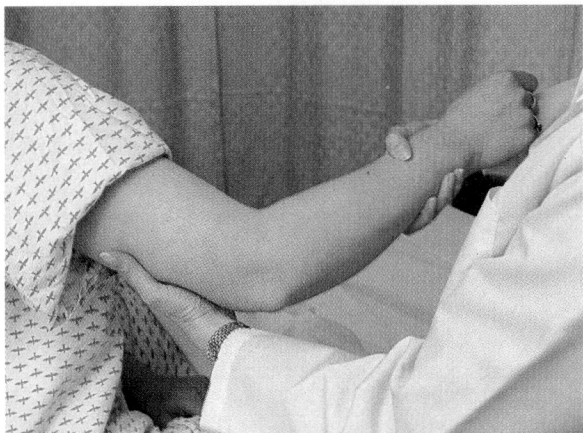

Figure 24-63. Nurse assesses muscle tone when moving the extremity passively.

causes the muscle to relax. A muscle that has little tone (**hypotonicity**) feels flabby. The involved extremity hangs loosely in a position determined by gravity.

For assessment of muscle strength the client assumes a stable position. The client performs maneuvers demonstrating strength of major muscle groups (Table 24-11). Symmetrical muscle pairs are compared for strength, based on a grading scale of 0 to 5 (Table 24-12). The arm on the dominant side is normally stronger than the arm on the nondominant side. In the older adult a loss of muscle mass causes bilateral weakness, but muscle strength remains greater in the dominant arm or leg.

Each muscle group is examined. The nurse asks the client first to flex the muscle to be examined and then to resist when the nurse applies opposing force against that flexion. It is important to not allow the client to move the joint. The nurse gradually increases pressure to a muscle group (e.g., elbow extension). The client resists the pressure applied by the nurse by attempting to move against resistance (e.g., elbow flexion). The client resists until instructed to stop. As the examiner varies the amount of pressure applied, the joint moves.

If a weakness is identified, the muscle's size is compared with its opposite counterpart by measuring the muscle body's circumference with a tape measure. A muscle that has atrophied (reduced in size) may feel soft and baggy when palpated.

NEUROLOGICAL SYSTEM

An assessment of neurological function alone can be quite time consuming. An efficient nurse integrates neurological measurements with other parts of the physical examination. Cranial nerve function can be tested during the survey of the head and neck. Mental and emotional status are observed during the nursing history.

TABLE 24-11
Maneuvers to Assess Muscle Strength

Muscle Group	Maneuver
Neck (sternocleido-mastoid)	Place hand firmly against client's upper jaw. Ask client to turn head laterally against resistance.
Shoulder (trapezius)	Place hand over midline of client's shoulder, exerting firm pressure. Have client raise shoulders against resistance.
Elbow	
Biceps	Pull down on forearm as client attempts to flex arm.
Triceps	As client's arm is flexed, apply pressure against forearm. Ask client to straighten arm.
Hip	
Quadriceps	When client is sitting, apply downward pressure to thigh. Ask client to raise leg up from table.
Gastrocnemius	Client sits, holding shin of flexed leg. Ask client to straighten leg against resistance.

Many variables must be considered when deciding the extent of the examination. A client's level of consciousness influences the ability to follow directions. General physical status influences tolerance to assessment. The client's chief complaint also helps to determine the need for a thorough neurological assessment. If the client complains of headache or a recent loss of function in an extremity, a complete neurological review is needed. The nurse will require use of special equipment including reading material, vials of aromatic substances (e.g., vanilla extract, coffee), opposite tip of cotton swab or tongue blade broken in half, Snellen eye chart, penlight, vials of sugar or salt, tongue blade, two test tubes (one containing hot water, the other containing cold), cotton balls or cotton-tipped applicators, tuning fork, and reflex hammer.

Health History

The nurse gathers a health history that includes a screening for symptoms of headache, seizures, tremors, dizziness, vertigo, numbness or tingling of body parts, visual changes, weakness, pain, or changes in speech. The presence of any symptom then requires a more de-

TABLE 24-12
Muscle Strength

Muscle Function Level	Scales		
	Grade	% Normal	Lovett Scale
No evidence of contractility	0	0	0 (zero)
Slight contractility, no movement	1	10	T (trace)
Full range of motion, gravity eliminated*	2	25	P (poor)
Full range of motion with gravity	3	50	F (fair)
Full range of motion against gravity, some resistance	4	75	G (good)
Full range of motion against gravity, full resistance	5	100	N (normal)

From Barkauskas VH and others: *Health and physical assessment,* St. Louis, 1994, Mosby.
*Passive movement.

tailed review (e.g., onset, severity, precipitating factors or sequence of events). The client's use of analgesics, alcohol, sedatives, hypnotics, antipsychotics, antidepressants, nervous system stimulants, or recreational drugs is reviewed. The nurse also assesses if the client's family has noticed any recent changes in the client's behavior (e.g., increased irritability, mood swings, memory loss, or change in energy level). The nurse asks about any noticeable changes in vision, hearing, smell, taste, and touch. A history of head or spinal cord trauma, meningitis, congenital anomalies, neurological disease, or psychiatric counseling will focus the nurse's assessment of select findings. If an older adult client displays sudden acute confusion (delirium), review history for drug toxicity, serious infections, metabolic disturbances, heart failure, and severe anemia.

Mental and Emotional Status

A great deal can be learned about mental capacities and emotional state by interacting with the client. A nurse can ask questions during an examination to gather data and observe the appropriateness of emotions and thoughts. There are special assessment tools designed to assess a client's mental status. Kahn and other's (1960) Mental Status Questionnaire (MSQ) is a 10-item instrument and a widely used tool. Folstein and others (1975) developed the Mini–Mental State (MMS) to measure orientation and cognitive function (Box 24-26). A maximum score on the MMS is 30. Clients with scores of 21 or less generally reveal cognitive impairment requiring further evaluation.

To ensure an objective assessment the nurse considers the client's cultural and educational background, values, beliefs, previous experiences, and current level of coping. Such factors influence response to questions. An alteration in mental or emotional status may reflect a disturbance in cerebral functioning. The cerebral cortex controls and integrates intellectual and emotional functioning. Primary brain disorders, medications, and metabolic changes are examples of factors that may change cerebral function.

Level of Consciousness

The level of consciousness exists along a continuum from full awakeness, alertness, and cooperation to unresponsiveness to any form of external stimuli. The nurse converses with a client, asking questions about events involving the client or concerns about any health problem. A fully conscious client responds to questions quickly, and ideas are expressed logically. With a lowering of the client's consciousness, the nurse uses the Glasgow Coma Scale (GCS) for an objective measurement of consciousness on a numerical scale (Table 24-13). The client must be as alert as possible before testing. Caution is needed in using the scale if a client has sensory losses (e.g., vision or hearing).

The GSC allows the nurse to evaluate a client's neurological status over time. The higher the score, the better the client's neurological function. The nurse asks short, simple questions, such as "What is your name?" or "Where are you?" The nurse also asks the client to follow simple commands, such as "Move your toes."

If the client's consciousness is lowered to the point of being unable to follow commands, the nurse tries to elicit a response by applying firm pressure with a thumb over the root of the client's fingernail. The normal response to painful stimuli is withdrawal of the body part from the stimulus.

Behavior and Appearance

Behaviors, moods, hygiene, grooming, and choice of dress reveal pertinent information about mental status. The nurse remains perceptive of the client's mannerisms and actions during the entire physical assessment. The nurse notes both nonverbal and verbal behaviors. Does the client respond appropriately to directions? Does the client's mood vary with no apparent cause? Does the client show concern about appearance?

Box 24-26
Folstein's Mini–Mental State

"Mini–Mental State"

Maximum
Score

Orientation

5 ( ) What is the (year) (season) (date) (day) (month)?

5 ( ) Where are we (state) (county) (town) (hospital) (floor)?

Registration

3 ( ) Name 3 objects; 1 second to say each. Then ask the patient to repeat all 3 after you have said them. Give 1 point for each correct answer. Then repeat them until he learns all 3. Count trials and record.

Attention and Calculation

5 ( ) Serial 7's. 1 point for each correct. Stop after 5 answers. Alternatively, spell "world" backwards.

Recall

3 ( ) Ask for the 3 objects repeated above. Give 1 point for each correct.

Language

9 ( ) Name a pencil and a watch (2 points)
Repeat the following: "No ifs, ands, or buts" (1 point)
Follow a 3-stage command:
"Take a paper in your right hand, fold it in half, and put it on the floor" (3 points)
Read and obey the following:
"Close your eyes" (1 point)
Write a sentence (1 point)
Copy design (1 point)

Total Score

Assess level of consciousness along a continuum

Alert	Drowsy	Stupor	Coma

Instructions for Administration of Mini–Mental State Examination

Orientation

Ask for the date. Then ask specifically for parts omitted, e.g., "Can you also tell me what season it is?" One point for each correct.

Ask in turn "Can you tell me the name of this hospital?" (town, county, etc.). One point for each correct.

Registration

Ask the patient if you may test his memory. Then say the names of 3 unrelated objects, clearly and slowly, about 1 second for each. After you have said all 3, ask him to repeat them. This first repetition determines his score (0-3), but keep saying them until he can repeat all 3, up to 6 trials. If he does not eventually learn all 3, recall cannot be meaningfully tested.

Attention and Calculation

Ask the patient to begin with 100 and count backwards by 7. Stop after 5 subtractions (93, 86, 79, 72, 65). Score the total number of correct answers.

If the patient cannot or will not perform this task, ask him to spell the word "world" backwards. The score is the number of letters in correct order, e.g., dlrow = 5, dlorw = 3.

Recall

Ask the patient if he can recall the 3 words you previously asked him to remember. Score 0-3.

Language

Naming: Show the patient a wristwatch and ask him what it is. Repeat for pencil. Score 0-2.

Repetition: Ask the patient to repeat the sentence after you. Allow only one trial. Score 0 or 1.

3-Stage command: Give the patient a piece of plain blank paper and repeat the command. Score 1 point for each part correctly executed.

Reading: On a blank piece of paper print the sentence "Close your eyes" in letters large enough for the patient to see clearly. Ask him to read it and do what it says. Score 1 point only if he actually closes his eyes.

Writing: Give the patient a blank piece of paper and ask him to write a sentence for you. Do not dictate a sentence; it is to be written spontaneously. It must contain a subject and verb and be sensible. Correct grammar and punctuation are not necessary.

Copying: On a clean sheet of paper, draw intersecting pentagons, each side about 1 inch, and ask him to copy it exactly as it is. All 10 angles must be present and 2 must intersect to score 1 point. Tremor and rotation are ignored.

Estimate the patient's level of sensorium along a continuum, from alert on the left to coma on the right.

From Folstein MF and others: Mini–mental state: a practical method for grading the cognitive state of patients for the clinician, *J Psychiatr Res* 12:189, 1975.

TABLE 24-13
Glasgow Coma Scale

Action	Response	Score
Eyes open	Spontaneously	④
	To speech	3
	To pain	2
	None	1
Best verbal response	Oriented	⑤
	Confused	4
	Inappropriate words	3
	Incomprehensible sounds	2
	None	1
Best motor response	Obeys commands	⑥
	Localized pain	5
	Flexion withdrawal	4
	Abnormal flexion	3
	Abnormal extension	2
	Flaccid	1
	TOTAL SCORE	⑮

Is the client's hair clean and neatly groomed, and are the nails trim and clean? The client should behave in a manner expressing concern and interest in the examination. The client should make eye contact with the nurse and express appropriate feelings that correspond to the situation. Normally the client will show some degree of personal hygiene.

Choice and fit of clothing may reflect socioeconomic background or personal taste rather than deficiency in self-concept or self-care. The nurse avoids being judgmental and focuses assessment on the appropriateness of clothing for the weather. Older adults may neglect their appearance because of a lack of energy, finances, or reduced vision.

Language. Normal cerebral function allows a person to understand spoken or written words and to express the self through written words or gestures. The nurse observes the client's voice inflection, tone, and manner of speech. The client's voice should have inflections, be clear and strong, and increase in volume appropriately. Speech should be fluent. When communication is clearly ineffective (e.g., omission or addition of letters and words, misuse of words, hesitations), the nurse assesses for **aphasia.** Injury to the cerebral cortex may result in aphasia.

The two types of aphasia are sensory (or receptive) and motor (or expressive). With receptive aphasia a person cannot understand written or verbal speech. With expressive aphasia a person understands written and verbal speech but cannot write or speak appropriately when attempting to communicate. A client may suffer a combination of receptive and expressive aphasia. Assessment requires the nurse to ask the client to name familiar objects when the nurse points at them. The client may also be asked to respond to simple verbal commands, such as "Stand up." Finally, the nurse may ask the client to read a simple sentence out loud. Normally a client names objects correctly, follows commands, and reads sentences correctly.

Intellectual Function
Intellectual function includes memory, knowledge, abstract thinking, association, and judgment. Each aspect of function is tested with a specific technique. However, because cultural and educational background influences the ability to respond to test questions, the nurse does not ask questions related to concepts or ideas with which the client is unfamiliar.

Memory. The nurse assesses immediate recall and recent and remote memory. Immediate recall is reflected in the ability of the client to repeat a series of numbers in the order they are presented or in reverse order. Clients can normally recall five to eight digits forward or four to six digits backward.

The nurse asks if the client's memory can be tested. Then the nurse says clearly and slowly the name of three unrelated objects. After the nurse says all three, the client is asked to repeat each. This is continued until the client is successful. Then, later in the assessment, the nurse asks the client to repeat the three words again. The client should be able to identify the three words. Another test for recent memory involves asking the client to recall events occurring during the same day (e.g., what was eaten for breakfast). Information may need to be validated with a family member.

To assess past memory, the nurse can ask the client to recall the mother's maiden name, a birthday, or a special date in history. It is best to ask open-ended questions rather than simple yes/no questions. A client should have immediate recall of such information. With older adults, a nurse should not interpret a hearing loss as confusion. Good communication techniques are necessary throughout the examination to ensure the client clearly understands all the directions and testing.

Knowledge. The nurse can assess the client's knowledge by asking how much is known about the illness or the reason for hospitalization. By assessing a client's knowledge, the nurse determines the client's ability to learn or understand. If there is an opportunity to teach information, the nurse can test the client's mental status by asking for feedback during a follow-up visit.

Abstract thinking. Interpreting abstract ideas or concepts reflects the capacity for abstract thinking. A higher level of intellectual functioning is required for an individual to explain common sayings such as "A stitch in time saves nine" or "Don't count your chickens before they're hatched." The nurse notes whether the client's explanations are relevant and concrete. The client with altered mentation will probably interpret the phrase literally or will merely rephrase the words.

Association. Another higher level of intellectual function involves finding similarities or associations between concepts (e.g., a dog is to a beagle as a cat is to a Siamese). The nurse names related concepts and asks the client to identify their associations. Questions should be appropriate to the client's level of intelligence.

Judgment. Judgment requires a comparison and evaluation of facts and ideas to understand their relationships and to form appropriate conclusions. The nurse attempts to measure the client's ability to make logical decisions with questions such as "Why did you decide to seek health care?" or "What would you do if you suddenly became ill at home?" Normally a client can make logical decisions.

Cranial Nerve Function

The nurse may assess all 12 cranial nerves or test a single nerve or related group of nerves. A dysfunction in one nerve reflects an alteration at some point along the cranial nerve's distribution. Measurements used to assess the integrity of organs within the head and neck also assess cranial nerve function. A complete assessment involves testing the 12 cranial nerves in order of their number. To remember the order of the nerves, this simple phrase can be used: "On old Olympus' towering tops a Finn and German viewed some hops." The first letter of each word in the phrase is the same as the first letter of the names of the cranial nerves listed in order (Table 24-14).

Sensory Function

The sensory pathways of the central nervous system conduct the sensations of pain, temperature, position, vibration, and crude and finely localized touch. Different nerve pathways relay the various types of sensations. Most clients require only a quick screening of sensory function, unless there are symptoms of reduced sensation, motor impairment, or paralysis.

Normally a client has sensory responses to all stimuli tested. Sensations are felt equally on both sides of the body in all areas. All sensory testing is performed with the client's eyes closed so that the client is unable to see when or where a stimulus strikes the skin (see Table 24-15 on p. 552). Stimuli are then applied in a random, unpredictable order to maintain the client's attention and to prevent detection of a predictable pattern. The client tells the nurse when, what, and where each stimulus is felt. The nurse compares symmetrical areas of the body while applying stimuli to the arms, trunk, and legs.

Motor Function

An assessment of motor function includes measurements made during the musculoskeletal examination. In addition, cerebellar function is determined. The cerebellum coordinates muscular activity, maintains balance and equilibrium, and helps to control posture. Clients with any degree of motor dysfunction are at risk for injury (Box 24-27).

Balance. The nurse assesses balance by asking the client to stand with the feet together and arms at the sides, with eyes open and closed. Standing close to the client prevents an accidental fall. Slight swaying of the body is expected in Romberg's test. A loss of balance (positive Romberg) causes a client to fall to the side.

A second test for balance involves asking the client to stand on one foot while the eyes are closed, with the arms held straight at the sides. The test is repeated on the opposite foot. Normally balance is maintained for 5 seconds with slight swaying. Another possible test to assess balance and gross motor function is to ask the client to walk a straight line by placing the heel of one foot directly in front of the toes of the other foot (heel-to-toe walking).

Coordination. To avoid confusion, the nurse demonstrates each assessment maneuver and then has the client repeat them while observing for smoothness and balance in the client's movement. In older adults normally slow reaction time may cause movements to be less rhythmical.

To assess fine motor function, the nurse has the client extend the arms out to the sides and touch each forefinger alternately to the nose (first with eyes open, then with eyes closed). Normally the client alternately touches the nose smoothly. Performing rapid, rhythmical, alternating movements demonstrates coordination in the upper extremities. While sitting, the client begins by patting the knees with both hands. Then the client alternately turns up the palm and back of the hands while continuously patting. The maneuver should be done smoothly and regularly with increasing speed.

BOX 24-27
Client Teaching for Neurological System Assessment

- Explain to family or friends the implications of any behavioral or mental impairment shown by the client.
- If the client has sensory or motor impairments, explain measures to ensure safety (e.g., use of ambulation aids, use of safety bars in bathrooms or on stairways).
- Teach older adults to plan enough time to complete tasks, because reaction time is slowed.
- Teach older adults to observe skin surface for areas of trauma, because their perception of pain is reduced.

TABLE 24-14
Cranial Nerve Function and Assessment

Number	Name	Type	Function	Method
I	Olfactory	Sensory	Sense of smell	Ask client to identify different nonirritating aromas such as coffee and vanilla.
II	Optic	Sensory	Visual acuity	Use Snellen chart or ask client to read printed material while wearing glasses.
III	Oculomotor	Motor	Extraocular eye movement	Assess directions of gaze.
			Pupil constriction and dilation	Measure pupil reaction to light reflex and accommodation.
IV	Trochlear	Motor	Upward and downward movement of eyeball	Assess directions of gaze.
V	Trigeminal	Sensory and motor	Sensory nerve to skin of face	Lightly touch cornea with wisp of cotton. Assess corneal reflex. Measure sensation of light pain and touch across skin of face.
			Motor nerve to muscles of jaw	Palpate temples as client clenches teeth.
VI	Abducens	Motor	Lateral movement of eyeballs	Assess directions of gaze.
VII	Facial	Sensory and motor	Facial expression	As client smiles, frowns, puffs out cheeks, and raises and lowers eyebrows, look for asymmetry.
			Taste	Have client identify salty or sweet taste on front of tongue.
VIII	Auditory	Sensory	Hearing	Assess ability to hear spoken word.
IX	Glossopharyngeal	Sensory and motor	Taste	Ask client to identify sour or sweet taste on back of tongue.
			Ability to swallow	Use tongue blade to elicit gag reflex.
X	Vagus	Sensory and motor	Sensation of pharynx	Ask client to say "Ah." Observe palate and pharynx movement.
			Movement of vocal cords	Assess speech for hoarseness.
XI	Spinal accessory	Motor	Movement of head and shoulders	Ask client to shrug shoulders and turn head against passive resistance.
XII	Hypoglossal	Motor	Position of tongue	Ask client to stick out tongue to midline and move it from side to side.

An additional maneuver for upper extremity coordination involves touching each finger with the thumb of the same hand in rapid sequence. The client moves from the index finger to the little finger and back with one hand tested at a time. The client's dominant hand is slightly less awkward when performing this movement. Movement should be smooth and in succession.

Lower extremity coordination is tested with the client lying supine, legs extended. The nurse places a hand at the ball of the client's foot. The client taps the nurse's hand with the foot as quickly as possible. Each foot is tested for speed and smoothness. The feet do not normally move as rapidly or evenly as the hands.

Reflexes

Reflex testing assesses the integrity of sensory and motor pathways of the reflex arc and specific spinal cord segments. When a muscle and tendon are stretched, nerve impulses travel along afferent nerve pathways to the dorsal horn of the spinal cord segment. Impulses synapse and travel to the efferent motor neuron in the spinal cord. A motor nerve then sends the impulses back to the muscle, causing the reflex response. Experience is needed to test reflexes accurately.

The two categories of normal reflexes are deep tendon reflexes, elicited by mildly stretching a muscle and tapping a tendon, and cutaneous reflexes, elicited by

TABLE 24-15
Assessment of Sensory Nerve Function

Function	Equipment	Method	Precautions
Pain	Broken tongue blade or wooden end of cotton applicator	Ask client to voice when dull or sharp sensation is felt. Alternately apply sharp and blunt ends of tongue blade to skin's surface. Note areas of numbness or increased sensitivity.	Remember that areas where skin is thickened, such as heel or sole of foot, may be less sensitive to pain.
Temperature	Two test tubes, one filled with hot water and the other with cold	Touch skin with tube. Ask client to identify hot or cold sensation.	Omit test if pain sensation is normal.
Light touch	Cotton ball or cotton-tipped applicator	Apply light wisp of cotton to different points along skin's surface. Ask client to voice when sensation is felt.	Apply at areas where skin is thin or more sensitive (e.g., face, neck, inner aspect of arms, top of feet and hands).
Vibration	Tuning fork	Apply stem of vibrating fork to distal interphalangeal joint of fingers and interphalangeal joint of great toe, elbow, and wrist. Have client voice when and where the vibration is felt.	Be sure client feels vibration and not merely pressure.
Position		Grasp finger or toe, holding it by its sides with thumb and index finger. Alternate moving finger or toe up and down. Ask client to state when finger is up or down. Repeat with toes.	Avoid rubbing adjacent appendages as finger or toe is moved. Do not move joint laterally; return to neutral position before moving again.
Two-point discrimination	Two broken tongue blades	Lightly apply one or both tongue blade tips simultaneously to skin's surface. Ask client if one or two pricks are felt. Find the distance at which client can no longer distinguish two points.	Apply blade tips to same anatomical site (e.g., fingertips, palm of hand, or upper arms). Minimum distance at which client can discriminate two points varies (2 to 8 mm on fingertips).

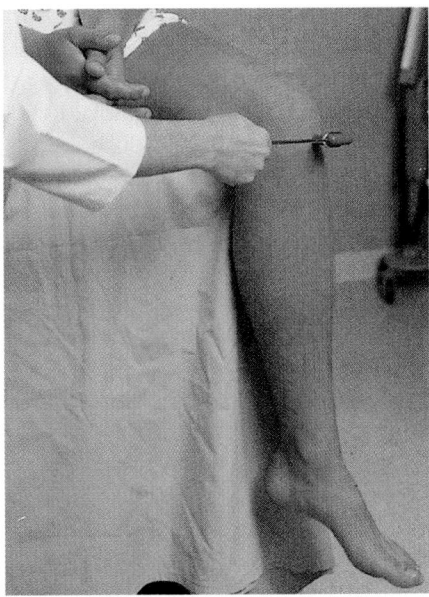

Figure 24-64. Position for testing patellar tendon reflex. Lower leg will normally extend.

stimulating the skin superficially. Reflexes are graded as follows:

0   No response
1+ Low normal with slight muscle contraction
2+ Normal with visible muscle twitch and movement of the arm or leg
3+ Brisker than normal; may not indicate disease
4+ Hyperactive and very brisk; often associated with spinal cord disorders

When reflexes are being assessed, the client relaxes as much as possible to avoid voluntary movement or muscle tensing. The nurse positions the limbs to slightly stretch the muscle being tested. The reflex hammer is held loosely between the nurse's thumb and fingers so it can swing freely and tap the tendon briskly (Figure 24-64). The nurse compares the symmetry of the reflex from one side of the body to the other. Reflexes are graded based on the degree of response. In older adults, reflexes are normally slowed. Reflexes can be hyperactive in clients with alcohol, cocaine, or opioid

TABLE 24-16
Assessment of Common Reflexes

Type	Procedure	Normal Reflex
Deep Tendon Reflexes		
Biceps	Flex client's arm up to 45 degrees at elbow with palms down. Place your thumb in antecubital fossa at base of biceps tendon and your fingers over the biceps muscle. Strike triceps tendon with reflex hammer.	Flexion of arm at elbow
Triceps	Flex client's arm at the elbow, holding arm across chest, or hold upper arm horizontally and allow lower arm to go limp. Strike triceps tendon just above elbow.	Extension at elbow
Patellar	Have client sit with legs hanging freely over side of table or chair, or have client lie supine and support knee in a flexed 90-degree position. Briskly tap patellar tendon just below patella.	Extension of lower leg
Achilles	Have client assume same position as for patellar reflex. Slightly dorsiflex client's ankle by grasping toes in palm of your hand. Strike Archilles tendon just above heel at the ankle malleolus.	Plantar flexion of foot
Cutaneous Reflexes		
Plantar	Have client lie supine with legs straight and feet relaxed. Take handle end of reflex hammer and stroke lateral aspect of sole from heel to ball of foot, curving across ball of foot toward big toe.	Plantar flexion of all toes
Gluteal	Have client assume side-lying position. Spread buttocks apart and lightly stimulate perineal area with cotton applicator.	Contraction of anal sphincter
Abdominal	Have client stand or lie supine. Stroke abdominal skin with base of cotton applicator over lateral borders of rectus abdominus muscle toward midline. Repeat test in each abdominal quadrant.	Contraction of rectus abdominus muscle with pulling of umbilicus toward stimulated side

intoxication (Caulker-Burnett, 1994). Practitioners often use stick figures to record reflexes. Table 24-16 summarizes common deep tendon and cutaneous reflexes.

AFTER THE EXAMINATION

The nurse may record findings from the physical assessment during the examination or at the end. Special forms are available to record data. The nurse reviews all findings before assisting the client with dressing in case of a need to recheck any information or gather additional data. Physical assessment findings are integrated into the plan of care.

After completing the assessment, the nurse gives the client time to dress. The hospitalized client may need help with hygiene and returning to bed. When the client is comfortable, it helps to share a summary of the assessment findings. If the findings have revealed serious abnormalities such as a highly irregular heart rate, the client's physician should be consulted before any findings are revealed. It is the physician's responsibility to make definitive medical diagnoses. The nurse can explain the type of abnormality found and the need for the physician to conduct an additional examination.

The nurse may delegate support staff to clean the examination area. Infection-control practices are used in removing materials or instruments soiled with potentially infectious wastes. If the client's bedside was the site for the examination, the nurse clears away soiled items from the bedside table and makes sure the bed linen is dry and clean. The client may appreciate a clean gown and the opportunity to wash the face and hands. Afterward, the nurse washes hands.

The nurse checks to be sure the recording of the assessment is complete. If entry of items into the assessment form was delayed, the nurse enters them at this time to avoid forgetting important information. If entries were made periodically during the examination, they are reviewed for accuracy and thoroughness. Significant findings are communicated to appropriate medical and nursing personnel, either verbally or in the client's written care plan.

The client often needs a number of ancillary examinations such as x-ray film examinations, laboratory tests, or ultrasonography after a physical examination. The tests provide additional screening information to rule out and to help diagnose specific abnormalities found during the examination. The nurse explains the purpose of these tests and the sensations that the client can expect.

Key Terms

acromegaly	kyphosis
adventitious sounds	leukoplakia
Allen's test	lordosis
alopecia	melanoma
aneurysms	melena
aphasia	metastasize
arcus senilis	murmurs
atherosclerosis	nystagmus
atrophied	ophthalmoscope
auscultation	orthopnea
basal cell carcinoma	osteoporosis
borborygmi	otoscope
bruit	ototoxicity
cerumen	pallor
chancres	palpation
clubbing	palpitations
conjunctivitis	Papanicolaou (Pap)
crackles	smear
cyanosis	paralytic ileus
cystocele	percussion
dysmenorrhea	peristalsis
dyspnea	peritonitis
dysrhythmia	PERRLA
ectropion	petechiae
eczema	phlebitis
edema	pleural friction rub
entropion	point of maximal im-
erythema	pulse (PMI)
excoriation	ptosis
exostosis	rectocele
fibrocystic breast	rhonchi
disease	scoliosis
gingivae	stenosis
hematemesis	striae
hemorrhoids	syncope
hernia	tactile fremitus
hydrocephalus	thrill
hypertonicity	turgor
hypotonicity	ventricular gallop
induration	vertigo
inspection	vocal fremitus
jaundice	wheezes

■ Key Concepts

Baseline assessment findings reflect the client's functional abilities when the nurse first assesses the client and serve as the basis for comparison with subsequent assessment findings.

Assessment data are used to make nursing diagnoses, select appropriate nursing interventions, and evaluate the outcomes of nursing care.

Physical assessment of a child or infant requires the nurse to apply principles of physical growth and development.

The nurse recognizes that the normal process of aging affects physical findings collected from an older adult.

Client teaching should be integrated throughout the examination to help clients learn about health promotion and disease prevention.

The nurse can use time more efficiently by integrating physical assessment with routine nursing care.

Inspection requires good lighting, full exposure of the body part, and a careful comparison of the part with its counterpart on the opposite side of the body.

Palpation involves the use of parts of the hand to detect different types of physical characteristics.

Percussion is the detection of differences in density of underlying tissues by listening to sounds produced while striking the body's surface.

A good stethoscope should have earpieces that fit snugly, flexible thick-walled tubing of the proper length, and a chestpiece with a bell and diaphragm.

Through auscultation the nurse assesses the character of sounds created in various body organs.

A physical examination should be performed only after proper preparation of the environment and equipment and after preparing the client physically and psychologically.

Throughout the examination the nurse should keep the client warm, comfortable, and informed of each step of the assessment process.

The client assumes various positions during the physical examination to provide greater accessibility of body parts and increase accuracy in assessment.

The nurse should use a systematic approach when conducting a physical assessment.

A competent examiner learns to combine assessments of different body systems simultaneously.

Information from the nursing history helps the nurse to focus on body systems likely to be affected.

When assessing a seriously ill client, the nurse concentrates on the body systems most likely to be affected.

Accuracy in assessing the thorax, heart, and abdomen is enhanced by creating a mental image of internal organs in relation to external anatomical landmarks.

When assessing heart sounds, the nurse imagines events occurring during the cardiac cycle.

The carotid arteries should never be palpated simultaneously.

When examining a woman's breasts, the nurse explains the techniques for breast self-examination.

The abdominal assessment differs from other portions of the examination in that auscultation follows inspection.

During assessment of the genitalia, the nurse explains the technique for genital self-examination.

Assessment of musculoskeletal function can be easily conducted when observing the client ambulate or participate in other active movements.

The nurse assesses mental and emotional status by interacting with the client throughout the examination.

At the end of the examination the nurse provides for the client's comfort and then completes a detailed review of physical assessment findings.

Critical Thinking Activities

1. A 32-year-old client entering a neighborhood clinic exhibits the following symptoms: frequent productive cough, fatigue, decreased appetite, and persistent fever. What focused assessment should the nurse conduct?

2. The nurse is performing an abdominal assessment and observes a pulsating midline abdominal mass. What is the nurse's next line of action?

3. What physical examination techniques does the nurse use during the following situations: evaluating a client's oral hygiene, a client with a cast on the lower leg, a client found on the floor, and a client reporting abdominal pain?

4. An elderly woman with reduced visual acuity would have difficulty performing what aspect of breast self-examination?

5. A 75-year-old black male is being visited 1 week postoperatively by the home health nurse to assess peripheral vascular status following a femoral-popliteal bypass graft for arterial insufficiency. What assessment data need to be obtained by the nurse?

6. Explain the different findings the nurse might gather when assessing coordination in a 40-year-old versus an 80-year-old.

References

All A: A literature review: assessment and intervention in elder abuse, *J Gerontol Nurs* 20(7):25, 1994.

American Cancer Society: *1997 Cancer facts and figures,* New York, 1997, The Society.

American Thoracic Society: Control of tuberculosis in the United States, *Am Rev Resp Dis* 146(6):1623, 1992.

Barkauskas VH and others: *Health and physical assessment,* St. Louis, 1994, Mosby.

Boutotte J: TB the second time around . . . and how you can help to control it, *Nurs 93* 23(5):42, 1993.

Campbell J, Humphreys J: *Nursing care of survivors of family violence,* ed 2, St. Louis, 1993, Mosby.

Caulker-Burnett I: Primary care screening for substance abuse, *Nurse Pract* 19(6):42, 1994.

Clore E: Dispelling the common myths about pediculosis, *J Pediatr Health Care* 3:28, 1989.

Ebersole P, Hess P: *Toward healthy aging,* ed 4, St. Louis, 1994, Mosby.

Fabius D, Stunkard J: Uncovering the secrets of snaps, rubs, and clicks, *Nurs 94* 24(7):45, 1994.

Folstein MF and others: Mini–Mental State: a practical method for grading the cognitive state of patients for the clinician, *J Psychiatr Res* 12:189, 1975.

Forgacs P: The functional basis of pulmonary sounds, *Chest* 73:399, 1978.

Galsworthy T, Wilson P: Osteoporosis: it steals more than bone, *Am J Nurs* 96(6):27, 1996.

Hardy M: What can you do about your patient's dry skin? *J Gerontol Nurs* 22(5):10, 1996.

Hopkins ML, Schoener L: Tuberculosis and the elderly living in long-term care facilities, *Geriatr Nurs* 17(1):27, 1996.

Kahn RL and others: Brief objective measures for the determination of mental status in the aged. *Am J Psychiatry* 117:326-328, 1960.

Lueckenotte A: *Pocket guide to gerontologic assessment,* ed 2, St. Louis, 1994, Mosby.

Master S, Terpstra J: Recognition and diagnosis. In Schnoll S and others: *Prescribing drugs with abuse liability,* Richmond, Va, 1992, DSAM, MCV-VCU.

Pace H, Hoag-Apel C: Stemming the tide of domestic violence, *Point of View Magazine* 33(3):12, 1996.

Payne WA, Hahn DB: *Understanding your health,* ed 2, St. Louis, 1989, Mosby.

Seidel HM and others: *Mosby's guide to physical examination,* ed 3, St. Louis, 1995, Mosby.

Smoller J, Smoller BR: Skin malignancies in the elderly: diagnosable, treatable, and potentially curable, *J Gerontol Nurs* 18(5):19, 1992.

Stuart G, Sundeen S: *Principles and practice of psychiatric nursing,* ed 5, St. Louis, 1995, Mosby.

Talbot L, Curtis L: The challenges of assessing skin indicators in people of color, *Home Healthcare Nurs* 14(3):167, 1996.

Thompson JM and others: *Mosby's manual of clinical nursing,* ed 3, St. Louis, 1993, Mosby.

Wilkins RL and others: *Lung sounds: a practical guide,* St. Louis, 1988, Mosby.

Wong D: *Whaley and Wong's nursing care of infants and children,* ed 5, St. Louis, 1995, Mosby.

Infection Control

OBJECTIVES

Mastery of content in this chapter will enable the student to:

- Define the key terms listed.
- Identify the body's normal defenses against infection.
- Discuss the events in the inflammatory response.
- Describe the signs and symptoms of a localized or systemic infection.
- Describe characteristics of each link of the infection chain.
- Assess clients at risk for acquiring an infection.
- Explain conditions that could precipitate the onset of nosocomial infections.
- Describe strategies for Standard Precautions.
- Identify principles of surgical asepsis.
- Describe nursing interventions designed to break each link in the infection chain.
- Correctly perform isolation barrier techniques.
- Perform proper procedures for hand washing.
- Properly apply a surgical mask and gloves.
- Describe infection control interventions unique to health promotion versus acute care versus restorative care settings.

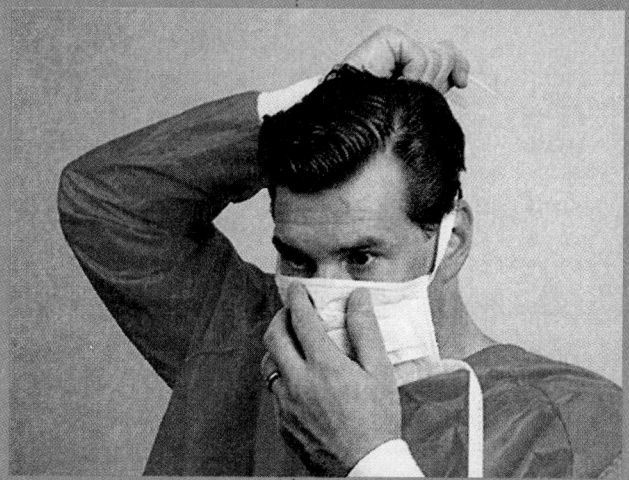

Current trends in health care delivery have increased interest in infection control and prevention practices. Many clients previously seen in traditional settings are now receiving health care in the home or outpatient facilities. Increases in drug-resistant microorganisms and concern about occupational exposure to tuberculosis, human immunodeficiency virus (HIV), or hepatitis have stimulated a concern about transmission of infections. Regulatory and accrediting agencies have established an increased focus on infection control and prevention. The cost of infections is being carefully watched by health care insurers, government providers, and clients. Today's nurse has an opportunity to participate in cost-effective quality health care by focusing on strategies that prevent and control infections.

Infection control and prevention are some of the most important functions a nurse can perform. Although advocacy for the client is an obvious priority, the nurse can be at risk for contact with infectious material or exposure to a communicable disease. Knowledge of the infectious process and the critical thinking skills involved in aseptic technique and barrier protection cannot be overemphasized. This chapter will emphasize techniques for control and prevention of infections and the critical thinking skills necessary to achieve these goals.

···SCIENTIFIC KNOWLEDGE BASE

Nature of Infection

An **infection** is the invasion of a susceptible host by pathogens or **microorganisms,** resulting in disease. The principal infecting agents are bacteria, viruses, fungi, and protozoa (Table 25-1). It is important to know the difference between an infection and a colonization. If a microorganism is present or invades a host, grows, and/or multiplies but does not cause disease or infection, this is referred to as a **colonization.**

TABLE 25-1
Common Pathogens and Some Infections or Diseases They Produce

Organism	Major Reservoir(s)	Major Diseases/Infections
Bacteria		
Staphylococcus aureus	Skin, hair, upper respiratory	Wound infection, abscess, cellulitis, osteomyelitis, pneumonia, food poisoning
Staphylococcus epidermidis	Skin	IV line infection, bacteremia, endocarditis
Streptococcus pyogenes	Skin, upper respiratory, perianal	Wound infection, impetigo, strep throat, puerperal sepsis (postpartum sepsis)
Escherichia coli	Colon	Gastroenteritis, urinary tract infection
Pseudomonas aeruginosa	Water, soil	Wound or burn infections, urinary tract infection, pneumonia
Neisseria gonorrhoeae	Genitourinary tract, rectum, mouth	Sexually transmitted disease (gonorrhea), pelvic inflammatory disease, septic arthritis
Chlamydia trachomatis	Genitourinary tract, rectum	Sexually transmitted disease (chlamydia), pelvic inflammatory disease, neonatal eye and lung infections
Mycobacterium tuberculosis	Droplet nuclei from lungs	Tuberculosis
Viruses		
Hepatitis A virus	Feces	Hepatitis A
Hepatitis B virus	Blood and some body fluids	Hepatitis B
Hepatitis C virus	Blood	Hepatitis C
Herpes simplex virus (Types I and II)	Lesions of mouth, skin, genitals	Cold sores, herpetic whitlow, sexually transmitted disease
Varicella-zoster virus	Vesicle fluid, respiratory tract infection	Varicella (chickenpox) primary infection, herpes zoster (shingles) reactivation
Fungi		
Candida albicans	Skin, mouth, genital tract	Bacteremia, pneumonia, wound infection
Protozoa		
Plasmodium falciparum	Blood, infected female *Anopheles* mosquito	Malaria

From Keroack M, Rosen-Kotlainen H: Microbiology/laboratory diagnostics. In Olmsted R, editor: *APIC infection control and applied epidemiology,* St. Louis, 1996, Mosby.

Disease or infections result only if the **pathogens** multiply and alter normal tissue function. If the infectious disease can be transmitted directly from one person to another, it is considered a contagious or **communicable disease** (Bobo, 1995).

Chain of Infection

The presence of a pathogen does not mean that an infection will begin. Development of an infection occurs in a cyclical process that depends on the following elements: the infectious agent or pathogen, reservoir for pathogen growth, portal of exit from the reservoir, means of transmission or vehicle, portal of entry, and a susceptible host (Figure 25-1). Infection develops if this chain stays intact. The nurse's efforts to control and prevent infections are directed at breaking this chain.

Infectious agent. Microorganisms on the skin are categorized as **resident flora** (normally present and stable in number) or **transient flora** (picked up when a person contacts another object). Resident pathogens are mostly found in superficial skin layers, but about 10% to 20% inhabit deep epidermal layers (Larson, 1995). They are not easily removed by hand washing unless considerable friction is used. Transient organisms attach loosely to the skin in dirt and grease or under fingernails and can be removed easily with thorough hand washing. The development of an infectious disease depends on the number of organisms, their **virulence** or ability to produce disease, their ability to enter and survive in the host, and the susceptibility of the host.

Reservoir. Places where microorganisms can survive, multiply, and await transfer to a susceptible host are called *reservoirs*. Common reservoirs are humans and animals (hosts), insects, food, water, and organic matter on inanimate surfaces (fomites). Frequent reservoirs for nosocomial infections include health care workers, clients, equipment, and the environment. Human reservoirs are divided into two types: those with acute or symptomatic disease and those who show no signs of disease but are **carriers** of the disease. Microorganisms or disease can be transmitted in either case.

Portal of exit. After microorganisms find a site in which to grow and multiply, they must find a portal of exit if they are to enter another host and cause disease. Microorganisms can exit through a variety of sites such as skin and mucous membranes, respiratory tract, gastrointestinal tract, reproductive tract, and blood.

Mode of transmission. The mode of transmission is the most fragile of the links of the chain and the most important for the nurse to understand. Many times there is little that a nurse can do about the infectious agent or the susceptible host, but by practicing infection control and prevention techniques, such as hand washing, the mode of transmission can be interrupted (Box 25-1). Certain infectious diseases tend to be transmitted more commonly by specific modes. However, the same microorganism may be transmitted by more than one route. For example, the virus that causes chickenpox may be spread by airborne route in droplet nuclei and also by direct contact with vesicle fluid.

Portal of entry. Organisms can enter the body through the same routes they use for exiting. Common portals of entry include nonintact skin, mucous membranes, genitourinary (GU) tract, gastrointestinal (GI) tract, or respiratory tract. For example, obstruction to the flow of urine from a urinary catheter allows organisms to ascend up the urethra. Factors that reduce the body's defenses enhance the chances that pathogens will enter.

Susceptible host. Susceptibility to an infectious agent depends on the individual's degree of resistance to pathogens. Although everyone is constantly in contact with large numbers of organisms, an infection does not develop until an individual becomes susceptible to the strength and numbers of those microorganisms. A person's natural defenses against infection and certain risk factors (see Assessment section) affect susceptibility.

A host is no longer considered susceptible if it has acquired **immunity** from either a natural or artificially induced event. Natural active immunity results from having a certain disease, such as measles, and mounting an immune response that usually lasts a lifetime. Natural passive immunity is the acquisition of an **antibody** by one person from another, such as the baby that is born with its mother's antibodies. These antibodies are acquired through the placenta during the last months of pregnancy. This type of immunity is of short duration, usually lasting only a few weeks to months.

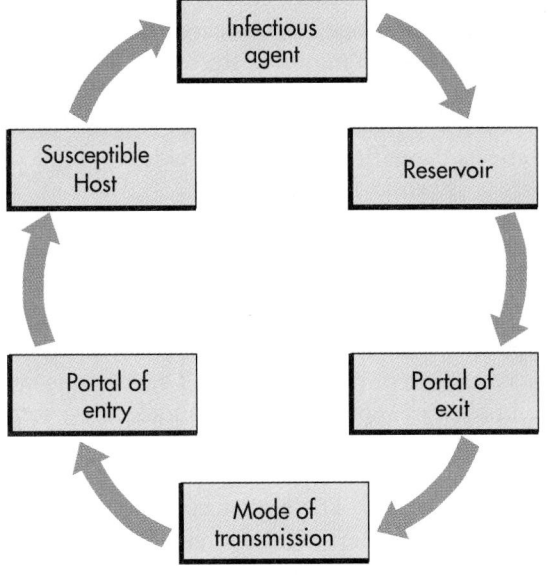

Figure 25-1. Chain of infection.

Box 25-1
Modes of Transmission

Routes and Means
Contact
Direct
Person-to-person (fecal-oral) or physical contact
  between source and susceptible host (e.g.,
  touching client)
Indirect
Personal contact of susceptible host with contami-
  nated inanimate object (e.g., needles or sharps,
  or dressings)
Droplet
Large particles that travel up to 3 feet and come in
  contact with susceptible host (e.g., coughing,
  sneezing, or talking)

Air
Droplet nuclei suspended in air (e.g., coughing,
  sneezing, or talking)

Vehicles
Contaminated items
Water
Drugs, solutions
Blood
Food (improperly handled, stored, or cooked)

Vector
External mechanical transfer (flies)
Internal transmission such as parasitic conditions
  between vector and host such as:
  Mosquito
  Tick
  Flea

Modified from Jackson M: General principles of epidemiology. In
Olmsted R, editor: *APIC infection control and applied epidemiology,*
St. Louis, 1996, Mosby.

Box 25-2
Course of Infection

Incubation Period
There is an interval between entrance of pathogen
into the body and appearance of first symptoms
(e.g., chickenpox 2 to 3 weeks, common cold 1 to
2 days, influenza 1 to 3 days, and mumps 18 days).

Prodromal Stage of Illness
There is an interval from the onset of nonspecific
signs and symptoms (malaise, low-grade fever, and
fatigue) to more specific symptoms; during this time,
microorganisms grow and multiply, and a client is
more capable of spreading disease to others.

Full Stage of Illness
Client manifests signs and symptoms specific to type
of infection (e.g., common cold manifested by sore
throat, sinus congestion, rhinitis; mumps manifested
by earache, high fever, parotid and salivary gland
swelling).

Convalescence
Acute symptoms of infection disappear; length of recovery depends on severity of infection and client's
general state of health; recovery may take several
days to months.

From Benenson A: *Control of communicable disease manual,* Washington, DC, 1995, APHA.

An antitoxin or immune globulin (e.g., tetanus antitoxin or hepatitis B immune globulin) may be given
when a person requires a short-term immunity to a certain disease. This type of immunity is called *artificial
passive immunity.* Artificial active immunity is when an
individual receives a vaccine, (e.g., polio vaccine) and
the person's immune system is stimulated to produce
an antibody. The duration of artificial active immunity
is variable and depends on the vaccine. Sometimes a
booster is needed to maintain protection (e.g., diphthe-
ria, measles).

Course of Infection

By understanding the infection chain, the nurse can assist in the control and prevention of infection. The
nurse assesses the risk for infection and takes appropri-

ate actions to prevent its spread. Infections follow a progressive course (Box 25-2). The severity depends on the
extent of the infection, the **pathogenicity** and virulence of the causative microorganisms, and the host's
susceptibility.

If infection is localized, such as in a wound, antibiotic therapy and proper wound care may control the infection's spread and minimize the illness. The client will
experience only localized symptoms such as pain, tenderness, and swelling at the wound site. An infection
that affects the entire body instead of just a single organ
or part is systemic and can be fatal.

Defenses Against Infection

The body has normal defenses against infection. Normal flora, body system defenses, and inflammation are
nonspecific defenses that protect against microorganisms, regardless of prior exposure. The immune system
is composed of separate cells and molecules, some of
which fight specific pathogens.

Normal flora. The body usually contains normal
flora or large numbers of microorganisms that reside on
the surface and deep layers of the skin, in the saliva and

oral mucosa, and in the intestinal walls. Normal flora do not cause disease but instead help to maintain health. For example, the skin's flora inhibit multiplication of organisms landing on the skin. The number of flora maintains a sensitive balance with other microorganisms to prevent infection. Any factor that disrupts this balance places a person at serious risk for infection. For example, the use of broad-spectrum antibiotics for the treatment of infection can eliminate or change normal bacterial

flora, leading to **supra infection.** Microorganisms resistant to antibiotics can then cause serious infection (Cooper, 1995).

Body system defenses. The skin, respiratory tract, and gastrointestinal tract are easily accessible to microorganisms, but they also have unique defenses against infection, physiologically suited to their structure and function (Table 25-2). Any condition that

---

TABLE 25-2
Normal Body System Defense Mechanisms Against Infection

Defense Mechanisms	Action	Factors That May Alter Defense
Skin		
Intact multilayered surface, body's first line of defense against infection	Provides mechanical barrier to microorganisms	Cuts, abrasions, puncture wounds, areas of maceration
Shedding of outer layer of skin cells	Removes organisms that adhere to skin's outer layers	Failure to bathe regularly
Sebum	Contains fatty acid that kills some bacteria	Excessive bathing
Mouth		
Intact multilayered mucosa	Provides mechanical barrier to microorganisms	Lacerations, trauma, extracted teeth
Saliva	Washes away particles containing microorganisms	Poor oral hygiene, dehydration
	Contains microbial inhibitors (e.g., lysozyme)	
Respiratory Tract		
Cilia lining upper airways, coated by sticky mucous blanket	Trap inhaled microbes and sweep them outward in mucus to be expectorated or swallowed	Smoking, high concentration of oxygen and carbon dioxide, decreased humidity, cold air
Macrophages	Engulf and destroy microorganisms that reach lung's alveoli	Smoking
Urinary Tract		
Flushing action of urine flow	Washes away microorganisms on lining of bladder and urethra	Obstruction to normal flow by urinary catheter placement, obstruction from growth or tumor, or delayed micturition
Intact multilayered epithelium	Provides barrier to microorganisms	Introduction of urinary catheter, continual movement of catheter in urethra
Gastrointestinal Tract		
Acidity of gastric secretions	Chemically destroys microorganisms incapable of surviving low pH	Administration of antacids
Rapid peristalsis in small intestine	Prevents retention of bacterial contents	Delayed motility from impaction of fecal contents in large bowel or mechanical obstruction by masses
Vagina		
At puberty, normal flora cause vaginal secretions to achieve low pH	Acidic secretions inhibit growth of many microorganisms	Antibiotics and birth control pills that disrupt normal flora

impairs an organ's specialized defenses increases susceptibility to infection.

Inflammation. The body's cellular response to injury or infection is **inflammation.** Inflammation is a protective vascular reaction that delivers fluid, blood products, and nutrients to interstitial tissues in an area of injury. This process neutralizes and eliminates pathogens or **necrotic** tissues and establishes a means of repairing body cells and tissues. Signs of inflammation include swelling, redness, heat, pain or tenderness, and loss of function in the affected body part. When inflammation becomes systemic, other signs and symptoms may develop; these include fever, leukocytosis (increased number of white blood cells), malaise, anorexia, nausea, vomiting, and lymph node enlargement.

The inflammatory response may be triggered by many physical agents (e.g., temperature extremes and radiation), chemical agents (e.g., gastric acid or poisons), and microorganisms. Inflammation involves a series of well-coordinated events, including vascular and cellular responses, formation of inflammatory **exudate,** and tissue repair (Table 25-3).

Immune response. When a foreign material **(antigen)** enters the body, a series of responses changes the body's biological makeup so that reactions to future antigens are different from the first. In an immune response, the antigen is neutralized, destroyed, or eliminated. There are two types of immunity: cell mediated and humoral. In cell-mediated immunity, T-cells, a form of **lymphocyte,** or white blood cell, bind with antigens. The T-cell becomes sensitized and releases lymphocytes, which attract macrophages and cause them to destroy antigens. In humoral immunity, B-lymphocytes cause synthesis of the antibodies that destroy antigens. After a B-cell binds with an antigen, it causes formation of plasma cells and memory B-cells. Plasma cells synthesize and secrete antibodies for greater immunity. Memory B-cells prepare the body against future invasion.

Nosocomial Infection

Clients in health care settings, especially acute care hospitals and long-term care facilities, may be at a higher risk for infection than those clients seen in the home setting. Clients often have multiple illnesses and are elderly and poorly nourished, thus more susceptible to infections. In addition, many clients have a lowered resistance to microorganisms because of underlying medical conditions (e.g., HIV, diabetes mellitus, malignancies) that impair the body's immune response. Many invasive devices such as intravenous catheters or urinary catheters impair the body's natural defenses against microorganisms. Several invasive diagnostic exams such as bronchoscopy or gastroscopy and treatment with broad-spectrum antibiotics have also been demonstrated to increase the risk for certain infections (Schaffer and others, 1996).

TABLE 25-3
Inflammation

Physiological Response	Signs and Symptoms
Vascular and Cellular Response	
Arterioles supplying infected or injured area dilate, delivering blood and leukocytes.	Redness Warmth
Tissue necrosis causes release of histamine, bradykinin, prostaglandin, and serotonin, which increase blood vessel permeability.	Edema
Fluid, protein, and cells enter interstitial spaces to cause swelling.	Pain
White blood cells (WBCs) enter tissues and phagocytose microorganisms. More WBCs are released into bloodstream.	WBC count normally 5000 to 10,000/mm³; 15,000 to 20,000/mm³ common with inflammation
Phagocytic release of pyrogens from bacteria occurs.	Fever
Inflammatory Exudate	
Fluid, dead cells, and WBCs form exudate at inflammatory site that later clears with lymphatic drainage.	Serous or sanguineous exudate
Tissue Repair	
Damaged cells are replaced with healthy new cells. Cells mature to take on structural characteristics and appearance of injured cells.	Tissue defects heal and close

A client who develops an infection that was not present or incubating at the time of admission is said to have a **nosocomial infection.** A community-acquired infection is one that was present in a client when admitted to a health care facility. An **iatrogenic infection** is a type of nosocomial infection resulting from a diagnostic or therapeutic procedure; an example could be a urinary tract infection that develops after catheter insertion. The incidence of nosocomial infections may be lowered if nurses conscientiously practice hand washing and aseptic techniques.

Nosocomial infections may be exogenous or endogenous. An **exogenous infection** arises from microorganisms outside the individual, such as *Salmonella, Clostridium tetani,* and *Aspergillus,* which do not exist as normal flora. **Endogenous infections** can occur when part of the client's flora becomes altered and an overgrowth results (e.g., infections caused by enterococci, yeasts, and streptococci). This often happens when the client receives broad-spectrum antibiotics that can alter normal flora. When sufficient numbers of microorganisms normally found in one body cavity or lining are transferred to another body site, an endogenous infection develops. The number of microorganisms needed to cause a nosocomial infection depends on the virulence of the organism, the host's susceptibility, and the body site affected (Box 25-3).

Asepsis.

The nurse's efforts to minimize the onset and spread of infection are based on the principles of aseptic technique. **Aseptic technique** is an effort to keep the client as free from exposure to infection-causing pathogens as possible. The term **asepsis** means the absence of disease-producing microorganisms. The two types of aseptic technique that the nurse practices are medical asepsis and surgical asepsis.

Medical asepsis (clean techniques) includes procedures used to reduce the number of microorganisms and prevent their spread. Hand washing, barrier techniques, and routine environmental cleaning are examples of medical asepsis. Principles of medical asepsis are commonly followed in the home, such as in the case of washing hands before preparing food or disinfecting a surface after a blood spill.

Surgical asepsis (sterile techniques) are methods used during client care, including surgery, to prevent microbial contamination of an open wound or a sterile item. These techniques can be practiced by nurses in the operating room or at the bedside. Surgical asepsis demands the highest level of aseptic technique and requires that all areas be kept as free as possible of infectious microorganisms. In medical asepsis, an area or object is considered contaminated only if it is suspected of containing pathogens (e.g., a used bedpan, wet piece of gauze). In surgical asepsis, an area or object may be considered contaminated if touched by an object that is not sterile (e.g., a tear in a surgical glove during a procedure, a sterile instrument placed on an unsterile surface).

The nurse is responsible for providing the client with

Box 25-3
Examples of Sites and Potential Causes for Nosocomial Infections*

Surgical or Traumatic Wound Infections

Improper surgical technique
Improper skin preparation before surgery (shaving or incorrect antiseptic scrub)
Improper aseptic technique during dressing change

Primary Bloodstream Infection/Sepsis

Improper skin prep before insertion of intravascular access device
Failure to change intravenous site when inflammation first appears
Contamination of intravenous fluids, needles, or catheters
Improper technique during the insertion of drug additive into intravenous fluids
Improper care of peritoneal or hemodialysis shunts
Improper technique when adding stopcocks or connecting tubes to intravenous fluids
Use of multiple lumen central venous catheters

Pneumonia

Improper aseptic technique during suctioning
Displacement of NG tube
Use of H_2 blocker/antacids
Client risk factors such as immobility or decreased gag reflex

Urinary Tract Infection

Improper insertion of urinary catheter
Open or disconnected drainage system
Improper specimen collection technique
Obstruction of drainage
Reflux of urine into bladder
Contaminated catheter or equipment

Bone and Joint Infection

Improper aseptic technique during pin care or dressing care

Cardiovascular System Infection

Improper hand washing technique
Improper aseptic technique during dressing change or following cardiac surgery

Central Nervous System Infection

Improper aseptic techniques during dressing changes or during monitoring of intracranial monitoring device

Gastrointestinal System Infection

Contaminated food or water
Overuse of antibiotics

Skin and Soft Tissue

Improper skin care
Client risk factors such as poor nutrition and hydration

*All forms of nosocomial infection can result from improper hand washing and use of contaminated equipment.

a safe environment. The effectiveness of aseptic practices depends on the nurse's critical thinking skills and consistency in practicing effective aseptic techniques. It is easy to forget key procedural steps or to take shortcuts that break aseptic procedures when hurried. In addition, clients often present challenges in clinical practice where problem solving is needed to adapt approaches so that infection control principles are maintained. The nurse's failure to use good technique places clients at risk for an infection that can seriously impair their recovery.

The nurse should also assume responsibility for monitoring other health care team members who care for the client. The nurse is the primary person at the client's bedside and is in a prime position to remind or educate others regarding possible isolation procedures for the client and to reinforce proper technique when procedures are performed.

NURSING KNOWLEDGE BASE

The experience of having a serious infection can invoke feelings of apprehension, anxiety, frustration, and hostility in clients or their families. These feelings can worsen when clients are placed in isolation. The solitude of protective isolation limits normal social interactions. Emotional reactions are likely to occur. For example, clients may display hostile behaviors or show signs of depression. The seemingly unreasonable demands made by some clients may be extremely distressing to health care workers. Family members may fear the possibility of developing the infection themselves and may avoid contact with the client. Even the simple procedures of proper hand washing, gloving, or masking may communicate feelings of rejection. The nurse can help clients and families reduce some of these feelings by discussing the disease process, explaining isolation procedures, and maintaining a friendly, understanding manner.

Cultural, religious, or social beliefs can not only influence how a client reacts to an infectious disease but can also influence infection prevention. For example, although diversity exists within the group, Latino or Hispanic clients may be less likely to seek medical treatment for infectious diseases such as acquired immunodeficiency syndrome (AIDS) or hepatitis. The reason for this could be linked to the perceived cultural stigma associated with high-risk behaviors such as homosexual or bisexual activities, or the fact that many Hispanics have limited access to health care or health prevention programs (COSSMHO, 1991).

In another example, social support may promote adherence to treatment for infectious diseases. Rubel and Garro (1992) report that during an outbreak of pulmonary tuberculosis (TB) on a Navajo Indian reservation, traditional healers received specific education about TB control practices. These healers then incorporated recommended interventions into the traditional health beliefs of the community.

Why a client may react to an infection or infectious disease is important for a nurse to know in establishing a plan of care. The challenge for the nurse is to identify and support those behaviors that maintain human health or prevent infections.

NURSING PROCESS

Assessment

The nurse assesses the client's susceptibility to and defenses against infection (Box 25-4). A review of the medical history with the client and family may reveal a recent exposure to a communicable disease. By evaluating signs and symptoms, the nurse can determine whether a client's clinical condition may indicate the onset or extension of an infection. The assessment should also include risk factors for infections. During the interview process, the nurse also has an opportunity to assess the client's and family's knowledge of a known infection or disease.

Because a client's nutritional health can directly influence susceptibility to infection, a thorough diet history is necessary. The nurse should determine a client's normal daily nutrient intake and whether preexisting problems such as impaired swallowing or oral pain alter food intake.

Laboratory data should be assessed as soon as available (Table 25-4). Laboratory values such as increased white blood cells (WBCs) and/or a positive blood culture may indicate infection. When assessing laboratory data, the age of the client should be considered. For example, in the older adult, smaller amounts of bacteria such as *Salmonella* can cause gastrointestinal (GI) infections because of decreased bactericidal gastric acids and deterioration of the mucosal layer of the stomach (Rusnak, 1996).

Sometimes positive laboratory results may indicate the client's risk for infection and the need for the use of barrier precautions or isolation. The nurse can consult with the infection control professional or refer to the facility's policy for assistance. The early recognition of infection assists the nurse in making the correct nursing diagnosis and establishing a treatment plan. In addition, the nurse can alert other members of the health care team to the need for further investigation of the client's condition, facilitating initiation of prompt therapy and barrier protection.

The nurse must also assess ways in which an infection affects client and family needs. Clients with chronic or serious infection such as tuberculosis or AIDS may experience psychological and social problems from self-imposed isolation or rejection by friends and family. Clients or their families may not be able to afford the cost of medical care. In home care settings, clients and families may not have the opportunity for the physical or emotional support necessary to facilitate adjustment to disease. As soon as possible after entry

Box 25-4
Factors Affecting Susceptibility to Infection

Age

Infants have immature immune systems.

Children acquire more immunity but are susceptible to infectious diseases such as mumps and measles.

Young and middle-age adults have refined body system defenses and immunity.

Older adults' immune responses decline, and the structure and function of major organs change.

Heredity

Certain congenital and genetic chromosomal disorders can have an effect on humoral or cellular immunity.

Clients with diabetes, some types of which are hereditary, can be more at risk for infections and delayed wound healing.

Cultural Practices

Various cultural or religious beliefs or practices can influence clients' decisions to seek treatment for an infection or to use methods to prevent infections (e.g., a Native American or Latino client may seek treatment from a "healer" rather than a physician, or the decision of whether to use a condom may be determined by the client's religious belief).

Nutritional Status

A reduction in protein, carbohydrates, and fats as a result of illness, inadequate diet, or debility, increases a client's susceptibility to infection and delays wound repair.

Stress

Increased stress elevates cortisone levels, causing decreased resistance to infection.

Continuous stress exhausts energy stores.

Rest and Exercise

Inadequate rest and exercise can increase stress and decrease body functions such as elimination and circulation.

Inadequate Defenses

Primary and secondary defenses may be altered (e.g., broken skin or mucosa, traumatized tissue, suppressed immune response).

Personal Habits

Smoking inhibits respiratory ciliary action and decreases resistance to respiratory infections.

Alcohol ingestion can impair the effect of antibiotics.

Risky sexual behavior, such as multiple sex partners, increases the chance for exposure to HIV.

Environmental Factors

Crowded living conditions, and adequacy and safety of water supply can influence the client's susceptibility to infections.

Inadequate refrigeration and cooking facilities can increase a client's exposure to food-borne illness such as *Shigella* or *E. coli.*

Immunization/Disease History

Clients who have not received recommended immunizations are at risk for vaccine-preventable diseases such as measles, mumps, and rubella.

Older adults with underlying medical conditions can decrease their susceptibility to influenza and pneumococcal pneumonia through immunizations.

Recent exposure to a communicable disease may increase the client's susceptibility.

Medical Therapies

Certain drugs, such as cortisone, and certain invasive therapies, such as intravenous catheters or surgeries, can increase the risk for infection.

Clinical Appearance/Data

Localized infections usually present with redness, swelling, and pain or tenderness. There may be a purulent drainage from wounds or lesions.

Systemic infections may present with fever, chills, nausea and vomiting, loss of appetite, or lymph node enlargement.

Clinical data may show an increase in WBCs, positive culture, or a positive x-ray.

into the health care system, the nurse should assess the client's and family's ability to adjust to the disease and the need for resources to manage health problems.

Client expectations. The nurse assesses the clients' expectations concerning their care and involves them in all aspects of care planning. Some clients and their families may wish to know more about the disease process, whereas others may only want to know the interventions necessary to treat the infection. Clients may be concerned about the level of discomfort from an infection and the potential for available relief. Clients

TABLE 25-4

Laboratory Tests to Screen for Infection

Laboratory Value	Normal (Adult) Values	Indication of Infection
WBC count	5000-10,000/mm³	Increased in acute infection, decreased in certain viral or overwhelming infections
Erythrocyte sedimentation rate	Up to 15 mm/hr for men and 20 mm/hr for women	Elevated in presence of inflammatory process
Iron level	60-90 μg/dl	Decreased in chronic infection
Cultures of urine and blood	Normally sterile, without microorganism growth	Presence of infectious microorganism growth
Cultures of wound, sputum, and throat	Possible normal flora	Presence of infectious microorganism growth
Differential Count (Percentage of Each Type of WBC)		
Neutrophils	55%-70%	Increased in acute suppurative infection, decreased in overwhelming bacterial infection (older adult)
Lymphocytes	20%-40%	Increased in chronic bacterial and viral infection, decreased in sepsis
Monocytes	2%-8%	Increased in protozoal, rickettsial, and tuberculosis infections
Eosinophils	1%-4%	Increased in parasitic infection
Basophils	0.5%-1%	Normal during infection

should be encouraged to verbalize their expectations so that interventions can be established to meet clients' priorities.

▪ Nursing Diagnosis

Following assessment, the nurse reviews all findings and analyzes data to identify relevant nursing diagnoses. For the nursing diagnosis *risk for infection,* defining characteristics include risk factors such as inadequate primary defenses (e.g., broken skin or stasis of body fluids), inadequate secondary defenses (e.g., decreased hemoglobin and white blood cells), or chronic disease.

Clusters of defining characteristics lead to the selection of a nursing diagnosis. The related factors, revealed in the assessment, ensure individualization of the diagnosis. For example, the nurse may diagnose *risk for infection related to intravenous catheter placement* in a client with a decreased WBC count, multiple intravenous catheters, and inflammation around a single catheter site. The related factor, *intravenous catheter placement,* will direct the nurse to change the catheter regularly and take measures to minimize microorganism transfer through the intravenous system. If the nursing diagnosis happened to be *risk for infection related to malnutrition,* the nurse's choice of interventions would include use of nutritional support. An accurate related factor ensures a more appropriate care plan.

Infection or its associated treatment may be the related factor for a number of nursing diagnoses (see nursing diagnoses box). In the case of the diagnosis *social isolation,* the related factor may be the isolation precautions used for the client. Nursing interventions would then be directed at minimizing the effect isolation has on the client's ability to socialize.

The presence of an actual infection poses a collaborative problem in which the nurse intervenes. An actual infection might be indicated by objective data such as an elevated temperature, open draining wound, inflammation of a wound site, and laboratory values revealing an increased WBC count. Subjective findings might include client complaint of chills, malaise, or tenderness at the wound site. The nurse works with physicians, dietitians, and other team members in monitoring the infection, providing therapies such as antibiotic administration and wound care, and implementing appropriate infection control measures.

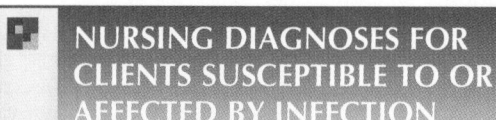

NURSING DIAGNOSES FOR CLIENTS SUSCEPTIBLE TO OR AFFECTED BY INFECTION

Body image disturbance
Infection, risk for
Nutrition, altered: less than body requirements
Skin integrity, impaired
Social isolation
Tissue integrity, impaired

Planning

The client's care plan is based on each nursing diagnosis and related factor. Specific goals and outcomes are identified, priorities are set, and appropriate interventions are proposed. Nursing interventions are selected in collaboration with the client, family, and other health care team members. For example, in an acute care setting, the goal for the diagnosis might be "to control or decrease the progression of infection" and the outcome might be "client's wound drainage decreases in 3 days." In this plan, other members of the health care team such as the infection control nurse or the enterostomy therapist might be involved.

In home care, a formal plan of care is needed to ensure that quality, comprehensive, and cost-effective care is provided to the client. The client's self-care abilities and resources, such as the ability to ambulate or follow instruction, should be incorporated into the plan. For example, if the goal is "increase resistance to infection," an outcome could be "client achieves 2600-calorie balanced diet." In the home care setting, it is particularly important to determine if the client has facilities to ensure appropriate hygiene measures can be followed.

Implementation

The nurse's role includes those activities designed to control and prevent infection. These techniques include helping clients and families gain knowledge of the disease process, in addition to measures needed to prevent an infection from occurring.

Health promotion. Good infection control begins with prevention. The nurse has the opportunity to review with clients and their families approaches designed to prevent or reduce infections. These include preventive measures to strengthen the host's defenses such as nutrition, recommended immunizations, stress reduction, and regular rest and exercise. In addition, the nurse can explain infection control principles such as food safety designed to prevent infections from occurring in the home care setting.

Nutrition. Nutrition is a major determinant of a person's resistance to infection. Some increased risks for infection usually associated with aging may in fact be related to nutrition. Throughout the world, malnutrition is a major cause of immunosuppression. Deficiencies in calorie-protein intake have dramatic effects on cell-mediated immunity and can affect all aspects of the immune response (Chandra, 1993).

Low serum albumin levels and weight loss can be associated with the risk of development of nosocomial infections and immune system deficiencies (Gorse and others, 1989). A proper diet is one that promotes optimal immune functioning and consists of a variety of foods from the seven food groups. Two or three servings each of food from the protein and dairy groups are recommended each day (see Chapter 34).

Nurses, either alone or in collaboration with dietitians, should design education programs specific to clients' needs. After assessment and input from the client, the nurse can teach the client the importance a proper diet plays in maintaining immunity and preventing infection.

Stress reduction. Stress reduction is another way clients can improve their immune system and prevent infections. Stress is often associated with an individual's ability to prevent a disease (Ickovic and Rodin, 1992). The nurse can recommend stress reduction programs that are suitable for the client's age, physical condition, and expressed interest. Stress reduction as a health promotion activity can enhance both physical and mental health (see Chapter 22).

Immunization. Immunization programs for infants and children have decreased the occurrence of many childhood, vaccine-preventable diseases. New vaccines such as hepatitis A and varicella have provided immunity to both adults and children for highly communicable diseases. In addition, specific vaccines such as influenza and pneumococcal pneumonia have decreased the mortality and morbidity previously seen in older adults or clients with underlying medical problems such as chronic obstructive pulmonary disease (COPD). Table 25-5 lists some of the recommended childhood and adult immunizations. Nurses should advise clients about the advantages of immunizations but should be aware of the contraindications for particular vaccines, especially for pregnant or lactating women.

Adequate rest and regular exercise. Adequate rest and regular exercise contribute to the prevention of infection. The Centers for Disease Control and Prevention (1993) stress that physical exercise increases lung capacity, circulation, energy, and endurance. It also decreases stress and improves appetite, sleeping, and elimination. Balancing the need for regular exercise is the need for rest and sleep. Some clients may need education stressing the importance of sleep and rest for infection prevention.

Infection control in the home. The nurse can instruct clients and their families on how to prevent and control infections in the home, especially those relating to the kitchen. Items that should be discussed include the following:

1. Clean frequently around sinks using household disinfectants or diluted bleach.
2. Discard sponges and dish mops frequently, or disinfect in a dishwasher at least once a week or after use for cleaning up blood from meat or poultry.
3. If dishes are hand washed, air dry rather than using a dish towel.
4. Keep a supply of paper cups and paper towels close to the sink rather than sharing glasses or hand towels.
5. Discard any food in the refrigerator that does

TABLE 25-5
Recommended Vaccines, Indications, and Administration Guidelines*

Vaccine	Type	Indications	Frequency	Route†
Diphtheria-tetanus-pertussis (DTP)	Toxoid/inactivated whole bacteria	Infants and children up to the age of 6 months	3 doses 6 months	IM
DPT-*Haemophilus influenzae* type b conjugate (DPT-Hib)	Toxoid/inactivated whole bacteria and bacterial polysaccharide conjugated to protein	Infants and children up to the age of 6 months	3 doses 2, 4, 6 months	IM
Diphtheria-tetanus-acellular pertussis (DtaP)	Toxoid/inactivated bacterial components	Infants, children, and adults	5 doses at ages 2, 4, 6, 15-18 months, and 4-6 years; booster every 10 years	IM
Haemophilus influenzae type b conjugate (Hib)	Bacterial polysaccharide conjugated to protein	Infants at least 2 months old; children and adults who may be at risk for *H. influenzae* infections	1-3 doses depending on age; booster need depends on age and number of doses in primary series	IM
Hepatitis A	Inactivated virus	Children and adults who are at increased risk for HAV or are traveling to developing countries	2-3 doses; differs according to age and manufacturer's formulation; need for booster unknown	IM
Hepatitis B	Inactivated virus	Infants, children, and adults, including health care workers, who are at increased risk for HBV	3-4 doses depending on manufacturer's formulation and receiver's response rate	IM (deltoid)
Influenza	Inactivated virus or viral components	Persons <6 months of age who because of age or underlying medical conditions are at increased risk for complications of flu; additionally, all health care workers and persons over 65 should be immunized	Annually, fall and winter during flu season	IM

Vaccine	Type	Recommendations	Route
Measles-mumps-rubella	Active virus	Children over the age of 12 months and nonimmune adults born before 1957	SQ
Meningococcal	Bacterial polysaccharide of serotypes A, C, Y, W-135	Military recruits, travelers to countries where *N. meningitides* is prevalent, control measure for serogroup C outbreak	SQ
Pneumococcal	Bacterial polysaccharide of 23 pneumococcal types	Single dose, booster need depends on age and risk for serious pneumococcal infections	IM or SQ
Poliovirus vaccine, inactivated (IPV)	Inactivated virus	All persons over the age of 65, persons over the age of 2 who are at increased risk for complications from *Streptococcus pneumoniae*	
		All infants, children, and nonimmune adults	SQ
		Two schedule options depending on whether child/adult can take live virus: 2 doses IVP, 2 and 4 months, followed by 2 doses of OPV Or 4 doses IPV at 2, 4, 12-18 months, and 4-6 years Adults, the first 3 doses should be at least 4 weeks apart	
Poliovirus vaccine oral (OPV)	Activated virus	Vaccination option for children and adults See schedule above If given alone, 3 doses OPV at ages 2, 4, 6-18 months	PO
Tetanus-diphtheria (Td or DT)	Inactivated toxin	Adults and children over the age of 1 year 3 doses for those not previously immunized, booster every 10 years	IM
Varicella	Active virus	All children over the age of 12 months, all nonimmune health care workers Single dose	IM

Data from Advisory Committee on Immunization Practices, Centers for Disease Control and Prevention: *MMWR* 4/4/97, 3/28/97, 7/12/96, 2/14/97, 1/3/97, 12/27/96, 11/22/96.
*This does not include all recommendations for childhood or adult immunizations. Check with physician about schedule and any contraindications for vaccines.
†*IM*, intramuscular; *SQ*, subcutaneous; *PO*, by mouth.

not look or smell good even if it is not past its expiration date.

6. Wash all raw fruits and vegetables before consumption.

7. If possible, thaw all foods, especially meat, in the refrigerator and avoid thawing and refreezing food products. Wash hands immediately after touching raw or thawing meat.

8. Chill cooked perishable leftover food at an internal temperature of less than 45° F within 2 to 4 hours after preparation.

9. Use only pasteurized milks and processed juices and ciders.

10. Cutting boards should be cleaned with hot, soapy water and a disinfectant after use. Use separate cutting boards for meats and raw vegetables.

Acute care. A client with an infection may have many needs. By monitoring the infection's course carefully, the nurse can choose the most appropriate measures to maintain or restore the client's health. To prevent an infection from developing or spreading, the nurse minimizes the numbers and kinds of organisms transmitted to potential infection sites. Eliminating reservoirs of infection, controlling portals of exit and entry, and avoiding actions that transmit microorganisms prevent bacteria from finding a site to grow. Disinfection and sterilization of supplies and good hand washing are examples of aseptic methods used to control the spread of microorganisms.

When a client develops an infection, the nurse continues preventive care so that health care personnel and other clients do not acquire the infection. Good hand washing and use of barrier precautions, such as gloves or masks, minimize exposure of staff and clients to infection. Clients with communicable diseases and infections that are easily transmissible to others require special precautions. Isolation precautions involve control of a client's environment by forming barriers against bacterial spread. Interventions for the older adult require recognition of risk factors that are caused by the aging process (Box 25-5).

Treatment of an infection includes identification and elimination of the organism and support of the client's defenses. The nurse collects specimens of body fluids or drainage from infected body sites for cultures. When the disease process or causative organism has been identified, the physician prescribes the antibiotic drug most effective for the situation. The nurse administers antibiotics carefully, watching for allergic reactions, assessing the progress of the client's infection, and administering the drugs by the proper methods.

Systemic infections, those that affect the body as a whole, require measures to prevent the complications of fever (see Chapter 23). Maintaining intake of fluids prevents dehydration resulting from diaphoresis. Increased

BOX 25-5
Gerontological Nursing Practice

The older adult experiences a number of age-associated physiological changes that influence susceptibility to infection. These changes include the following:

▪ There are decreased tears to flush and remove debris from the eye and a decrease in lysozymes that affect certain microorganisms. A decreased blink reflex can lead to corneal dryness. Caution clients and families to observe for eye infections and use artificial tears when necessary.

▪ Drying of the oral mucosa and recession and weakening of gingival tissues require frequent oral hygiene and regular dental care.

▪ An increased chest diameter and rigidity, weakened cough, decreased ability to swallow, and decreased elastic tissue surrounding alveoli predispose older adults to ventilatory problems. Aspiration and postoperative pneumonia are common complications. When caring for older adult clients, elevate the head of the bed and encourage the client to ambulate as soon as possible (unless contraindicated). Instruct and assist client in deep breathing and coughing techniques.

▪ A decrease in production of digestive juices and a reduction in intestinal motility affect removal of potential pathogens in the bowel. Clients and families should learn about safe food preparation and eat foods that are nutritionally good and easy to digest.

▪ A thinning of the dermal and epidermal skin layers, along with a decrease in skin elasticity predisposes older adults to skin tearing. Rigorous nursing care is necessary to prevent pressure ulcers in bedridden clients (see Chapter 38).

▪ With aging there is a decreased production of T-lymphocytes and B-lymphocytes. With reduced immunity it is important for older adults to receive regular immunizations and medical checkups.

Modified from Rusnak P: Long-term care. In Olmstead R, editor: *APIC infection control and applied epidemiology,* St. Louis, 1996, Mosby.

metabolism requires an adequate nutritional intake. Rest preserves energy for the healing process.

Localized infections often require measures to facilitate removal of infectious organisms. Wet-to-dry dressings (see Chapter 38) are used to remove infected drainage from wound sites. Application of heat compresses promotes blood flow to an infected site and thus the delivery of blood components needed to fight an infection. Drainage tubes may be inserted to remove infected drainage from body cavities. The nurse uses medical and surgical aseptic techniques to manage wounds and ensures the correct handling of infected drainage or body fluids.

During any infection, the nurse supports the client's body defense mechanisms. For example, if a client is known to have diarrhea, the nurse must maintain skin integrity to prevent breakdown and entrance of microorganisms. Routine hygiene measures such as cleansing the oral cavity, bathing, and skin lubrication further protect the skin and mucous membranes from organism spread.

Medical asepsis. The nurse follows certain principles and procedures to prevent infection and control its spread. Basic medical aseptic techniques break the infection chain. The nurse uses precautions for all clients, even when an infection has not been diagnosed. Aggressive preventive measures can be highly effective in reducing nosocomial infections.

Control or elimination of infectious agents. With the increased use of disposable equipment, nurses may be less aware of disinfection and sterilization procedures. The proper cleaning, disinfection, and sterilization of contaminated objects significantly reduce and often eliminate microorganisms. In large health care centers, a central supply department does most of the disinfection and sterilization of reusable supplies, which in most cases involve surgical aseptic techniques. However, nurses also use medical aseptic techniques in preparing items. Many of these principles also apply in the home.

Cleaning. Cleaning is the process of removing foreign materials (e.g., organic material such as blood or inorganic material such as soil) from objects. Generally, this is accomplished by the use of water, a detergent, and proper mechanical scrubbing action. Cleaning must occur before disinfection and sterilization procedures (Rutala, 1996). The nurse should check the health care facility's policy before cleaning. In most institutions, technicians will clean equipment. When cleaning objects soiled by blood or body fluids, the nurse applies personal protection equipment (PPE) such as gloves, goggles, and mask to protect from splashing fluids.

Disinfection and sterilization. Physical and chemical processes are used for disinfection and sterilization. Both processes disrupt the internal functioning of microorganisms by destroying cell proteins. **Disinfection** is a process that eliminates almost all pathogenic organisms on objects, with the exception of bacterial spores. **Sterilization** is a process that eliminates or destroys all forms of microbial life (Rutala, 1996). Examples of sterilization are processing items using moist heat, dry heat, or ethylene oxide (ETO). The level of disinfection and sterilization required depends on the type and use of the contaminated item (Box 25-6). The nurse has the responsibility of checking for package integrity and/or outdates before using an object designated as sterile. Items not meeting the criteria for being sterile should be disposed of or sent to the sterilization processing department (check agency policy).

Control or elimination of reservoirs. To control or eliminate infection in reservoir sites, the nurse eliminates sources of body fluids, drainage, or solutions that might harbor microorganisms. The nurse also carefully

---

Box 25-6

Categories for Sterilization, Disinfection, and Cleaning

Critical Items—Sterilization
Items that enter sterile tissue or the vascular system present a high risk of infection if the items are contaminated with any microorganisms and spores. Items must be sterile. These items include surgical instruments, cardiac and urinary catheters, needles, and implants.

Semicritical Items—Disinfection
Items that come in contact with skin that is not intact or with mucous membranes also present risks. These objects must be free of all microorganisms (except bacterial spores). These items include respiratory therapy equipment, endotracheal tubes, gastrointestinal endoscopes, and reusable mercury thermometers.

Noncritical Items—Cleaning
Items that come in contact with intact skin but not with mucous membranes must be clean. These items include bedpans, blood pressure cuffs, crutches, linens, and food utensils.

---

discards disposable articles that become contaminated with infectious material (Box 25-7).

Control of portals of exit. To control organisms exiting through the respiratory tract, the nurse avoids talking, sneezing, or coughing directly over a surgical wound or sterile dressing field. The nurse also teaches clients to protect others when they sneeze or cough and gives clients disposable wipes or tissues to control spread of microorganisms. A nurse who has a mild cold and continues to work with clients should wear a mask, especially when changing a dressing or performing a sterile procedure. The nurse should refrain from working with clients who are highly susceptible to infection.

Another way of controlling the exit of microorganisms is the careful handling of body fluids such as urine, feces, and wound drainage. Nurses should at least wear disposable gloves and wash their hands if there is a chance of contact with any blood or body fluids. Contaminated items should be bagged appropriately.

Control of transmission. Effective strategies require nurses to know the modes of transmission of microorganisms and the ways of control. In any health care setting, a client should have a personal set of care items. Sharing thermometers, bedpans, urinals, bath basins, and eating utensils can easily lead to transmission of infection. Glass thermometers, even when individually used, require special care. Because the client's mucus can become a source for microorganism growth,

Control and Prevention to Reduce Reservoirs of Infection

Hand washing. Use appropriate soap and warm water to wash hands before and after client care.

Bathing. Use soap and water to remove drainage, dried secretions, excess perspiration, or sediment from antiseptics.

Dressing changes. Change dressings that become wet and soiled (see Chapter 38).

Contaminated articles. Place tissues, soiled dressings, or soiled linen in moisture-resistant bags for proper disposal.

Contaminated needles. Place syringes, hypodermic needles, and intravenous needles in puncture-proof containers. (Do not recap needles or attempt to break them.)

Bedside unit. Keep table surfaces clean and dry.

Bottled solutions. Do not leave bottles open for long periods. Keep solutions tightly capped. Date solutions once opened.

Surgical wounds. Keep drainage tubes and collection bags patent to prevent accumulation of serous fluid under the skin's surface.

Drainage bottles and bags. Empty and rinse suction bottles according to agency policy. Empty all drainage systems on each shift unless otherwise ordered by a physician.

the thermometer should be washed in soap and water and dried after each use.

Because certain microorganisms travel easily through the air, linens or bedclothes should not be shaken. Dusting done with a treated or dampened cloth will prevent dust particles from entering the air.

To prevent transmission of microorganisms through indirect contact, soiled items and equipment must not touch the nurse's clothing. A common error is to carry dirty linen in the arms against the uniform. Special linen bags should be used, or soiled linen should be carried with the hands held out from the body. Clean or soiled linen should never be put on the floor.

Hand washing. The most important and most basic technique in preventing and controlling transmission of pathogens is hand washing. Hand washing is a vigorous, brief rubbing together of all surfaces of lathered hands, followed by rinsing under a stream of water (Larson, 1996). The need for hand washing depends on the following: the intensity of contact with the client or contaminated object, the degree or amount of contamination that could occur with that contact, the susceptibility of the client or health care worker to infection, and the procedure or activity to be performed (Larson, 1996). For example, if a nurse simply touches an object

that is not visibly soiled, hand washing is not required. In contrast, contact with any client, especially one with wound drainage, requires thorough hand washing. Larson (1995) recommends that hands be washed in the following situations:

1. When visibly soiled
2. Before and after client contact
3. Before performing invasive procedures such as urinary catheterization or placement of an intravascular catheter (antimicrobial soap is recommended)
4. After contact with a source of microorganisms (blood or body fluid, mucous membranes, nonintact skin, or inanimate objects that might be contaminated)
5. After removing gloves (wearing gloves does not remove the need to wash hands)

The Centers for Disease Control and Prevention (CDC) note that washing hands for at least 10 to 15 seconds is necessary to remove transient microorganisms from the skin. Hands that are more heavily soiled may require a longer time for washing (Garner, 1996b). The frequency of washing also affects the type and number of microorganisms on the hands. Larson (1996) states that health care workers who wash their hands eight times a day are less likely to carry gram-negative bacteria on their hands. Hands may be routinely washed with soap in any convenient form (liquid, powder, bar, or leaflet). Skill 25-1 lists the correct steps for hand washing.

Use of antimicrobial soap (antiseptic) is encouraged when nurses work in special care units, perform invasive procedures, or care for clients who are **immunocompromised,** have damage to their integumentary system (wounds), or are infected or colonized with epidemiologically significant organisms (e.g., methicillin-resistant *S. aureus* [MRSA], vancomycin-resistant enterococcus [VRE]). There are several effective antimicrobials, including chlorhexidine gluconate, alcohols, and iodophor. Certain antimicrobial soaps can irritate the skin, and the need for antimicrobial soap must be evaluated against potential skin irritations.

Isolation and barrier protection. Regardless of the health care setting, there is always a risk of transmission of microorganisms or disease to clients or health care workers. When a client has a known infection, nurses follow specific infection control practices, but not all sources of infection are obvious. The majority of microorganisms that cause infections or disease are found in colonized body substances of clients, regardless of whether a culture has confirmed an infection and a diagnosis has been made. Because of increased attention to the prevention of blood-borne pathogens and tuberculosis, the CDC and the Occupational Safety and Health Administration (OSHA) have stressed the importance of barrier protection (CDC, 1994; OSHA, 1991).

Hand Washing

Delegation Considerations

Hand washing can be delegated to unlicensed assistive personnel.

- Instruct, assist, and monitor care provider in proper method of hand washing.
- Instruct care provider to inform nurse if any skin irritation from soaps or antimicrobials is encountered.

Equipment

- Easy-to-reach sink with warm running water
- Antimicrobial or regular soap
- Paper towels or air dryer
- Clean orangewood stick (optional)

STEPS	RATIONALE
1. Inspect surface of hands for breaks or cuts in skin or cuticles. Report and cover lesions before providing client care.	Open cuts or wounds can harbor high concentrations of microorganisms. Agency policy may prevent nurses from caring for high-risk clients. If dermatitis occurs, additional interventions may be needed.
2. Inspect hands for heavy soiling.	Requires lengthier hand washing.
3. Inspect nails for length.	Nails should be short and filed because most microbes on hands come from beneath the fingernails.
4. Assess client's risk for or extent of infection (e.g., white blood cell count, extent of open wounds, known medical diagnosis).	Use of antimicrobial soaps is encouraged for clients who are immunosuppressed (Larson, 1995).
5. Push wristwatch and long uniform sleeves above wrists. Avoid wearing rings. If worn, remove during washing.	Provides complete access to fingers, hands, wrists. Wearing of rings increases number of microorganisms on hands (Garner, 1996a).
6. Stand in front of sink, keeping hands and uniform away from sink surface. (If hands touch sink during hand washing, repeat.)	Inside of sink is a contaminated area. Reaching over sink increases risk of touching edge, which is contaminated.
7. Turn on water. Turn faucet on or push knee pedals laterally or press pedals with foot to regulate flow and temperature (see illustration).	

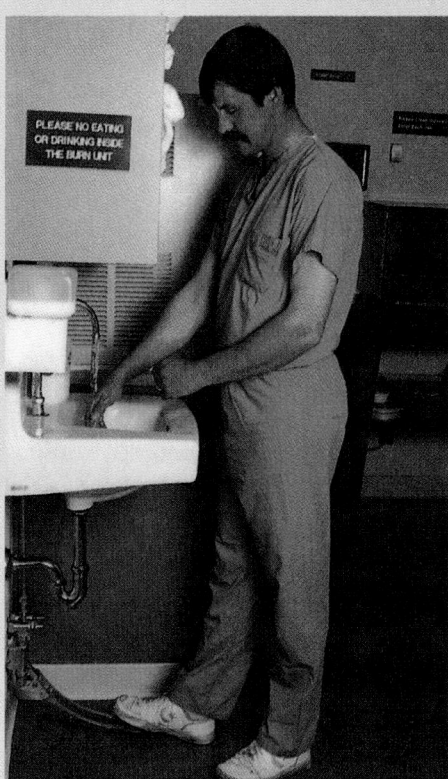

Step 7

Continued

STEPS	RATIONALE
8. Avoid splashing water against uniform.	Microorganisms travel and grow in moisture.
9. Regulate flow of water so that temperature is warm.	Warm water removes less of the protective oils than hot water.
10. Wet hands and wrists thoroughly under running water. Keep hands and forearms lower than elbows during washing.	Hands are the most contaminated parts to be washed. Water flows from least to most contaminated area, rinsing microorganisms into sink.
11. Apply a small amount of soap or antiseptic, lathering thoroughly (see illustration). Soap granules and leaflet preparations may be used.	The use of antiseptic exclusively can be drying to the hands and can cause skin irritations. The decision whether to use an antiseptic should depend on the procedure to be performed and the client's immune status.
12. Wash hands using plenty of lather and friction for at least 10 to 15 seconds. Interlace fingers and rub palms and back of hands with circular motion at least 5 times each. Keep fingertips down to facilitate removal of microorganisms.	Soap cleanses by emulsifying fat and oil and lowering surface tension. Friction and rubbing mechanically loosen and remove dirt and transient bacteria. Interlacing fingers and thumbs ensures that all surfaces are cleansed.
13. Areas underlying fingernails are often soiled. Clean them with fingernails of other hand and additional soap or clean orangewood stick.	Area under nails can be highly contaminated, which will increase the risk of infections for the nurse or the client.

CRITICAL DECISION POINT

Do not tear or cut skin under or around nail.

14. Rinse hands and wrists thoroughly, keeping hands down and elbows up (see illustration).	Rinsing mechanically washes away dirt and microorganisms.

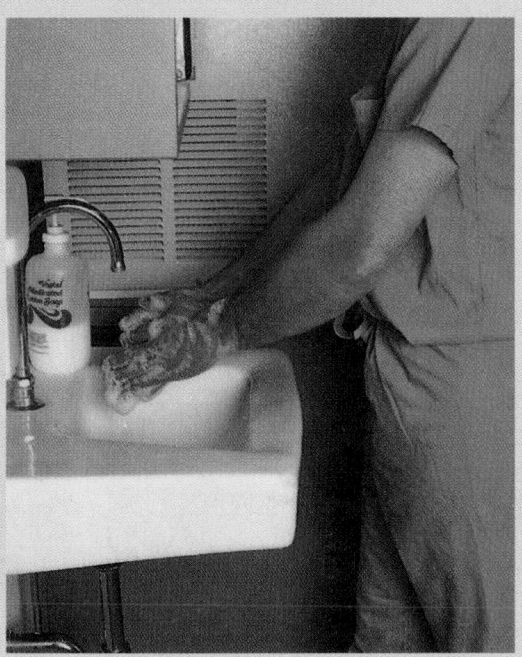

Step 11

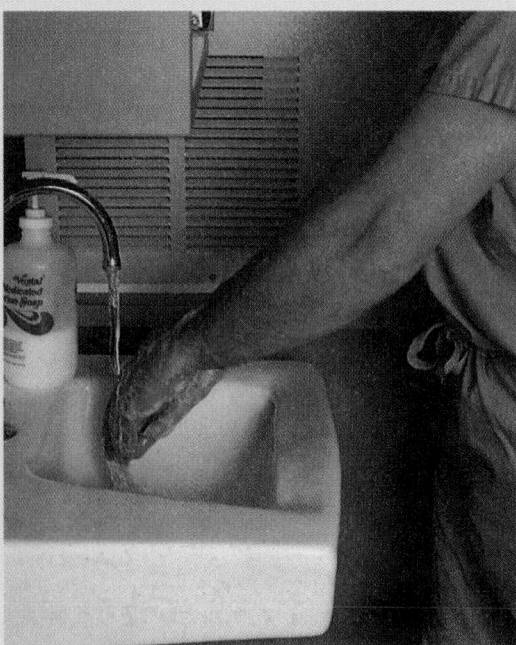

Step 14

STEPS	RATIONALE
15. Optional: repeat steps 5 through 13 and extend period of washing if hands are heavily soiled.	
16. Dry hands thoroughly from fingers to wrists and forearms with paper towel, single-use cloth, or warm air dryer.	Drying from cleanest (fingertips) to least clean (forearms) area avoids contamination. Drying hands prevents chapping and roughened skin.
17. If used, discard paper towel in proper receptacle.	Prevents transfer of microorganisms.
18. Turn off water with foot or knee pedals. To turn off hand faucet, use clean, dry paper towel; avoid touching handles with hands.	Wet towel and hands allow transfer of pathogens by capillary action.
19. If hands are dry or chapped, a small amount of lotion or barrier cream can be applied.	Use small individual-use container of lotion because large, refillable containers have been associated with nosocomial infections.
20. Inspect surfaces of hands for obvious signs of soil or other contaminants.	Determines if hand washing is adequate.
21. Inspect hands for dermatitis or cracked skin.	Indicates complications from excess hand washing.

Recording and Reporting

- It is not necessary to record or report this procedure.
- Report any dermatitis to employee health and/or infection control per agency policy.

Home Care Considerations

- Evaluate the hand washing facilities in the home to determine possibility of contamination, the proximity of the facilities to the client, and available supplies in the area.
- Evaluate the availability of warm running water and soap when conducting home visits and anticipate the need for alternative hand washing products such as alcohol-based hand rubs and detergent-containing towels.
- Instruct the client and primary care giver in proper techniques and situations for hand washing.

Isolation or barrier protection includes the appropriate use of gloves, masks or respirators, eyewear, and gowns. Nurses should assess the need for barrier precautions based on potential transmission of infection for all clients, regardless of their diagnosis. Unfortunately, as the emphasis on barrier protection has increased, so also has the price of these devices. The nurse should be aware of the cost of these items and use only those that are needed to prevent transmission of an organism or disease. For example, since tuberculosis (TB) is transmitted by droplet nuclei, only a mask or respirator is needed as a barrier protection. When the nurse also uses gloves or gowns, this does nothing to prevent the transmission of TB but does increase the cost of care for the client.

In 1996 the CDC published revised guidelines for isolation precautions. Although primarily intended for care of clients in acute care, these recommendations could be applied to clients in all health care settings. These guidelines can be modified in facilities, according to need and as dictated by state or local regulations (HICPAC, 1996; Garner, 1996b).

The new recommendations contain two tiers of precautions (Table 25-6). The first and most important tier is called Standard Precautions and is designed to be used for care of all clients, in all settings, regardless of diagnosis. **Standard Precautions** are the primary strategies for prevention of infection transmission.

Standard Precautions apply to contact with blood, body fluid, nonintact skin, and mucous membranes. These precautions combine the major features of the previous categories—Universal Precautions and Body Substance Isolation—and provide protection for the health care worker as directed by OSHA.

The second tier is transmission categories designed for care of clients with specific types of infection. The precautions are used for clients known or suspected to be infected or colonized with microorganisms transmitted by droplets or by airborne route, or by contact with contaminated surfaces or dry skin.

TABLE 25-6
CDC Isolation Guidelines

Standard Precautions (Tier One)

Standard precautions apply to blood, all body fluids, secretions, excretions (except sweat), nonintact skin, and mucous membranes.

Hands are washed between client contacts; after contact with blood, body fluids, secretions, and excretions and after contact with equipment or articles contaminated by them; and immediately after gloves are removed.

Gloves are worn when touching blood, body fluids, secretions, excretions, nonintact skin, mucous membranes, or contaminated items. Gloves should be removed and hands washed between client care.

Masks, eye protection, or face shields are worn if client care activities may generate splashes or sprays of blood or body fluid.

Gowns are worn if soiling of clothing is likely from blood or body fluid. Wash hands after removing gown.

Client care equipment is properly cleaned and reprocessed and single-use items are discarded.

Contaminated linen is placed in a leak-proof bag and handled to prevent skin and mucous membrane exposure.

All sharp instruments and needles are discarded in a puncture-resistant container. CDC recommends that needles be disposed of uncapped or that a mechanical device be used for recapping.

A private room is unnecessary unless the client's hygiene is unacceptable. Check with an Infection Control Professional.

Transmission Categories (Tier Two)

Category	Disease	Barrier Protection
Airborne precautions	Droplet nuclei smaller than 5 microns; measles; chickenpox (varicella); disseminated varicella zoster; pulmonary or laryngeal TB	Private room, negative airflow of at least six exchanges per hour, mask or respiratory protection device (see CDC TB Guidelines)
Droplet precautions	Droplets larger than 5 microns, diphtheria (pharyngeal); rubella; streptococcal pharyngitis, pneumonia, or scarlet fever in infants and young children; pertussis; mumps; mycoplasma pneumonia; meningococcal pneumonia or sepsis; pneumonic plague	Private room or cohort clients; mask
Contact precautions	Direct client or environmental contact; colonization or infection with multidrug-resistant organism; respiratory syncytial virus; shigella and other enteric pathogens; major wound infections; herpes simplex; scabies, varicella zoster (disseminated)	Private room or cohort clients; gloves, gowns

Modified from Garner JS: Guidelines for isolation precautions for hospitals, *Infect Control Hosp Epidemiol* 17(1):54, 1996b.

There are three types of transmission-based precautions: **airborne, droplet,** and **contact.** They may be used singly or in combination for diseases (e.g., chickenpox) that have multiple routes of transmission. When used either singly or in combination, they are to be used in addition to Standard Precautions.

Because of the resurgence of TB, the CDC (1994) has produced guidelines for the prevention of transmission of TB in the health care worker and stresses the importance of isolation for the known or suspected TB client in a special negative-pressure room. The CDC has made further recommendations for the venting and exchange of air in these rooms. The doors should be closed to control direction of air flow. A special high filtration particulate respirator is worn when entering a respiratory isolation room or when caring for a cough-producing client.

Respirators must be able to fit health care workers with different facial sizes and characteristics. When worn correctly, particulate respirators and masks (Figures 25-2 and 25-3) have a tighter face seal and filter at a higher level than routine surgical masks (OSHA, 1995).

Additional guidelines for prevention of transmission of certain drug-resistant organisms have been published by the CDC (HICPAC, 1996). These guidelines, primarily for microorganisms such as vancomycin-resistant enterococcus (VRE), are more stringent than other published recommendations.

With the development of Standard Precautions, all

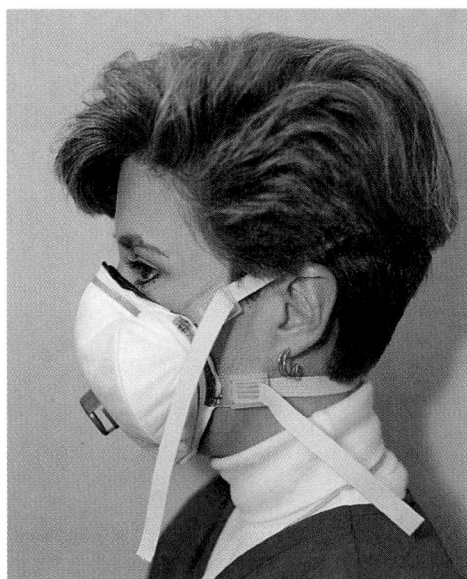

Figure 25-2. Disposable HEPA air-purifying respirator

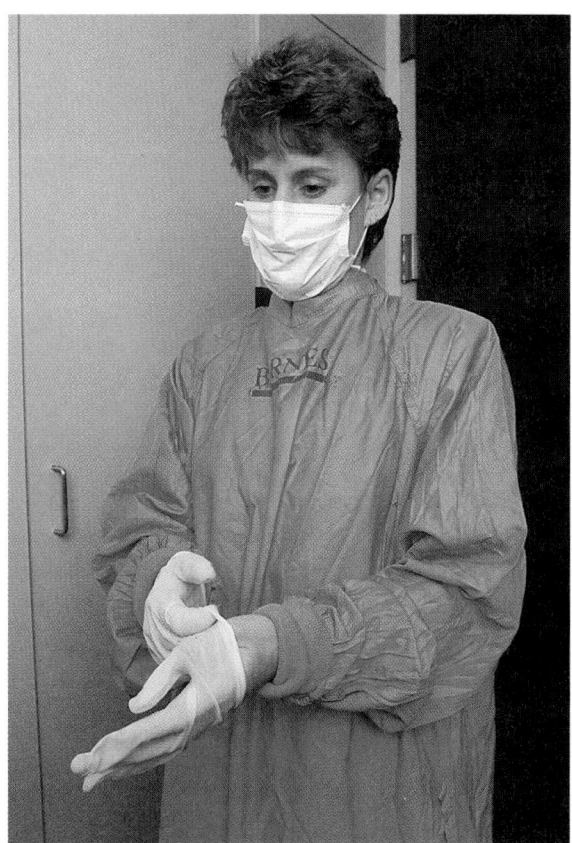

Figure 25-3. Nurse wearing an N-95 respirator.

clients are potentially in some type of isolation room. Regardless of the type of isolation or barrier protection used, the nurse must follow certain basic principles when delivering care in a client's room (Box 25-8). The nurse should understand how certain diseases are transmitted and what barriers are needed to prevent transmission. For example, a nurse would not routinely need to wear a gown or gloves when giving oral medications but may need these barriers when changing a dressing from a draining wound. However, gloves are appropriate when assisting a client with an oral medication if the client has a visible draining oral herpes simplex lesion. The nurse should assess cost of items used for barriers before use and use only those items that are needed.

Care should be taken to avoid exposing an article brought into a client's room to an infectious material. Any contaminated article (e.g., blood pressure cuff) should be bagged according to agency policy and sent for decontamination. A contaminated article should not be used or brought into the room of another client.

Before isolation measures are instituted, the client and family must understand the nature of the client's condition, the purposes of the barriers, and ways to carry out specific precautions. If the client and family can participate in maintaining isolation precautions, there is a greater chance of reducing the spread of infection and lowering the client's risk of complications. The client and family are taught the proper way to wash hands and apply gloves, masks, or gowns. Each procedure should be demonstrated, and the client and family should be given an opportunity to practice. The nurse also explains methods of transmission of infectious organisms so that the client understands the difference between contaminated and clean objects.

The nurse also provides for the client's sensory stimulation during isolation. Reading materials, a radio or television set, a clock, and hobby materials should be available. The room environment should be clean and pleasant looking. The room drapes or shades should be opened and excess supplies or equipment removed. The nurse must take the opportunity to listen to the client's concerns or interests; if the nurse rushes through care or shows a lack of interest in the client's needs, the client will feel rejected and even more isolated.

The nurse explains the client's potential risk of depression or loneliness to family members. Visitors should be encouraged to avoid negative expressions or actions concerning isolation. The nurse advises family members on ways to provide meaningful stimulation.

Protective environment. When Standard Precautions are in place, all clients are treated as though they are potentially infected. In addition, if a client has a disease that could be transmitted by an airborne route, a private room is recommended for reducing the possibility of transmission of infection, separating susceptible clients from those who might have an infection. In addition, this room may be required to have negative-pressure airflow to prevent infectious particles from floating out of the room. There also may be special rooms for highly susceptible clients such as transplant recipients. When a private room is recommended, the

Box 25-8

Procedural Guidelines for Caring for a Client on Isolation Precautions

1. Assess isolation indications (i.e., current laboratory tests or client's history of exposure).
2. Review precautions necessary for the specific isolation system and consider care measures to be performed while in client's room.
3. Review nurses' notes or confer with colleagues regarding client's emotional state and adjustment to isolation.
4. Wash hands and prepare all equipment to be taken into client's room.
5. Apply gown, mask, gloves, and goggles as appropriate:
   a. Apply gown, being sure it covers all outer garments. Pull sleeves down to wrist. Tie securely at neck and waist.
   b. Apply disposable gloves. (NOTE: Unpowdered, latex-free gloves should be worn if the client or the health care worker has a latex allergy). If worn with gown, bring glove cuffs over edge of gown sleeves.
   c. Apply either surgical mask or respirator around mouth and nose. (Type of mask or respirator will depend on type of isolation and facility policy.)
   d. Apply goggles snugly around face and eyes.
6. Enter client's room. Arrange supplies and equipment. (If equipment will be removed from room for reuse, place on clean paper towel.)
7. Explain purpose of isolation and necessary precautions to client and family. Offer opportunity to ask questions. Assess for evidence of emotional problems that may be caused by being in isolation.
8. Assess vital signs.
   a. If client is infected or colonized with a resistant organism (e.g., vancomycin-resistant enterococcus [VRE], methicillin-resistant *S. aureus* [MRSA], etc.), equipment remains in room. Proceed to assess vital signs by routine procedures. Avoid contact of stethoscope or blood pressure cuff with infective material.
   b. If stethoscope is to be reused, clean diaphragm or bell with alcohol. Set aside on clean surface.
   c. Individual or disposable thermometers should be used.
9. Administer medications (see Chapter 26):
   a. Give oral medication in wrapper or cup.
   b. Dispose of wrapper or cup in plastic-lined receptacle.
   c. Administer injection, being sure gloves are worn.
   d. Discard syringe and uncapped needle or sheathed needle into special container.
   e. If gloves are not worn and hands contact contaminated article or body fluids, wash hands immediately.
10. Administer hygiene, encouraging the client to discuss questions or concerns about isolation. Informal teaching can be used at this time.
    a. Avoid allowing gown to become wet.
    b. Remove linen from bed; if excessively soiled, avoid contact with gown. Place in impervious linen bag.
    c. Change gloves and wash hands if they become excessively soiled and further care is necessary.
11. Collect specimens:
    a. Place specimen containers on clean paper towel in client's bathroom.
    b. Follow procedure for collecting specimen of body fluids.
    c. Transfer specimen to container without soiling outside of container. Place container in a plastic bag and place label on the outside of bag or as per facility policy.
12. Dispose of linen and trash bags as they become full:
    a. Use sturdy, moisture-resistant single bags to contain soiled articles.
    b. Tie bags securely at top in knot.
13. Resupply room as needed.
14. Leave isolation room.
    a. Remove eyewear or goggles.
    b. Untie gown at waist. Remove one glove by grasping cuff and pulling glove inside out over hand. Discard glove. With ungloved hand, tuck finger inside cuff of remaining glove and pull it off, inside out.
    c. Untie mask strings; drop mask into trash receptacle. (Do not touch outer surface of mask.)
    d. Untie neck strings of gown. Allow gown to fall from shoulders. Remove hands from sleeves without touching outside of gown. Hold gown inside at shoulder seams and fold inside out; discard in laundry bag.
    e. Wash hands minimum of 10 seconds.
    f. Explain to client when you plan to return to room. Ask whether client requires any personal care items, books, or magazines.
    g. Leave room and close door, if necessary. (Door should be closed if client is on airborne precautions.)
    h. All contaminated supplies and equipment should be disposed of in a manner that prevents spread of microorganisms to other persons (see agency policy).

nurse posts a card on the client's room door, listing the precautions for the isolation category (check agency policy). The card is a handy reference for health care workers and visitors and alerts all who enter the room of any special precautions.

The isolation room or an adjoining anteroom should contain hand washing, bathing, and toilet facilities. Soap and antiseptic solutions should also be available. Personnel and visitors wash their hands before coming to the client's bedside and again before leaving the room. If toilet facilities are unavailable, there are special procedures for handling portable commodes, bedpans, or urinals (check agency policy). Personal protective equipment (PPE) should be stored in an anteroom between the room and hallway or in a convenient location close to the point of use. The nurse resupplies PPE as needed.

Each client care room, including those used for isolation, contains a special impervious bag for soiled or contaminated linen, as well as a trash container with plastic liners. These receptacles prevent transmission of microorganisms by preventing seepage to and soiling of the outside surface. A disposable, rigid container should be available in the room to discard used needles, sharps, and syringes.

Depending on the microorganism and mode of transmission, the nurse critically evaluates what articles or equipment can be taken into an isolation room. For example, the Hospital Infection Control Practices Advisory Committee (HICPAC) of CDC recommends dedicated articles be taken into an isolation room of a client infected or colonized with vancomycin-resistant enterococci (HICPAC, 1995).

Personal protective equipment. Gowns prevent the soiling of clothing during contact with the client. Gowns or coverups protect health care workers from coming in contact with infected blood and body fluids or materials. Gowns used for barrier protection are made of a fluid-resistant material and should be changed immediately if damaged or heavily contaminated. Depending on agency policy, isolation gowns or coverups can be disposable or reusable.

Isolation gowns usually open at the back and have ties or snaps at the neck and waist to keep the gown closed and secure. A gown should be long enough to cover all outer garments. Long sleeves with tight-fitting cuffs provide added protection. No special technique is required for applying a gown as long as it is fastened securely. Occasionally, a nurse reuses an isolation gown but only for the same client. The nurse must evaluate the cost of the gown and coverup and can reuse the isolation gown for the same client if the gown is not visibly soiled.

Masks or respirators should be worn when splashing or spraying of blood or a body fluid is anticipated. Additionally, the mask protects the health care worker from inhaling microorganisms from a client's respiratory tract and prevents the transmission of pathogens from the nurse's respiratory tract. Occasionally, a client who is susceptible to infection may wear a mask to prevent inhalation of pathogens. Clients requiring respiratory precautions should wear masks when ambulating or being transported outside of their room to protect other clients and personnel.

Masks may prevent the transmission of infections caused by direct contact with mucous membranes. A mask discourages the wearer from touching the nose or mouth. A properly applied mask fits snugly over the mouth and nose so that pathogens and body fluids cannot enter or escape through the sides (Box 25-9). If a person wears glasses, the top edge of the mask fits below the glasses so they will not cloud over as the person exhales. Talking should be kept to a minimum while wearing a mask. A mask that has become moist is ineffective and should be discarded. Clients and family members should be warned that a mask can cause a sensation of smothering. If family members become uncomfortable, they should leave the room and discard the mask.

Nurses apply gloves when there is a risk of exposure to blood, body fluids, or potentially infectious material. In addition, gloves are recommended when the nurse has scratches or breaks in the skin; when performing venipuncture, finger, or heel sticks; and when the nurse is inexperienced (CDC, 1988). In most cases disposable, single-use gloves are worn. Gloves may be worn alone or in combination with other PPE. When other PPE is necessary, the nurse first dons a mask and eyewear (if required), washes and dries the hands, applies a gown (if required), and then applies gloves. Disposable gloves are easily applied and designed to fit either hand. However, the glove's thin rubber can tear easily. The glove cuffs should be pulled up over the wrists or cuffs of a gown.

After contacting infectious material, the nurse changes gloves and washes hands if care is not completed. If the nurse's actions do not involve more client contact, reapplying gloves is unnecessary. Clients and their families can be taught the reasons for wearing gloves and the correct method for applying gloves.

Many gloves used for barrier protection or surgical asepsis are made of latex. Before applying latex gloves, nurses should assess the potential for latex allergies. The symptoms range from mild dermatitis to severe anaphylactic shock. Clients and health care workers can become sensitized to latex by repeated contact or by inhaling aerosolized latex allergens.

The ANA (1996) provides the following suggestions for nurses to avoid becoming latex allergic:

1. Whenever possible, wear powder-free gloves (they are lower in protein allergens).
2. Wear gloves that are appropriate for the task (e.g., avoid use for cleaning).

Box 25-9

Procedural Guidelines for Donning a Surgical-Type Mask

1. Find top edge of mask (usually has thin metal strip along edge). Pliable metal fits snugly against bridge of nose
2. Hold mask by top two strings or loops. Tie two top ties at top of back of head (see illustration), with ties above ears. (Alternative: slip loops over each ear.)

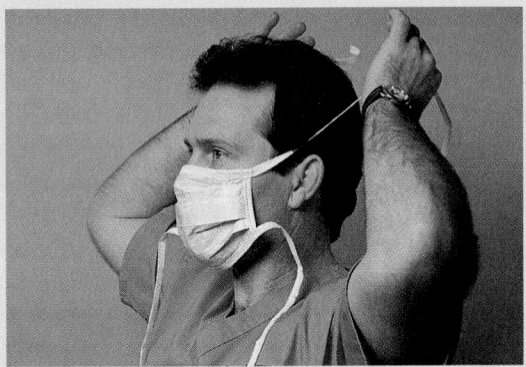

Step 2

3. Tie two lower ties snugly around neck with mask well under chin (see illustration).

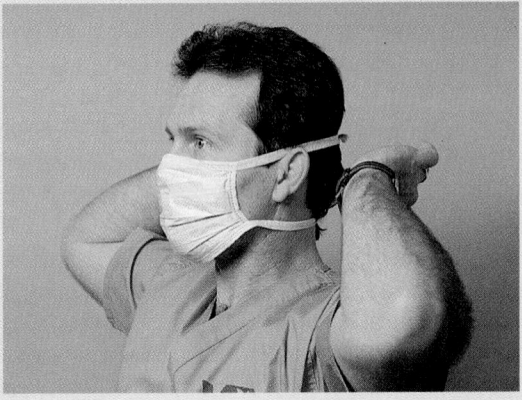

Step 3

4. Gently pinch upper metal band around bridge of nose.
NOTE: Mask should be changed if wet, moist, or contaminated.

---

3. Wash with a pH-balanced soap immediately after removing gloves.
4. Apply only non–oil-based hand care products (oil-based products break down latex allergens).
5. If a reaction or dermatitis occurs, report to employee health and/or seek medical treatment immediately.

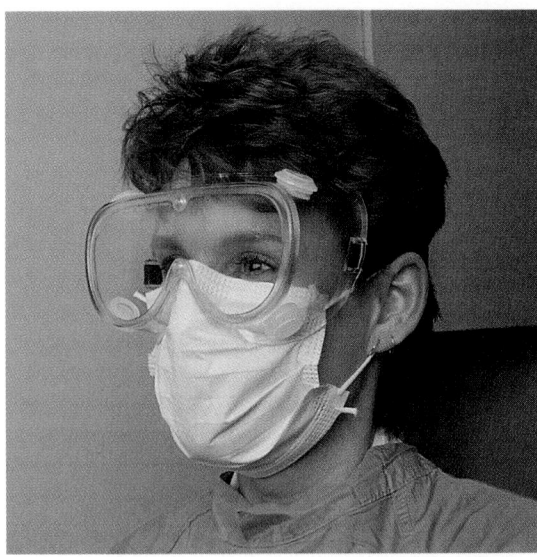

Figure 25-4. Nurse wearing protective goggles and mask.

Eyewear and face shields, properly fitted, should be worn to protect the nurse during procedures in which the eyes or face could be splattered by blood or other infectious material (Figure 25-4). OSHA (1991) requires health care organizations to enforce policy requiring employees to protect their eyes, nose, or mouth during procedures in which splattering could occur. In many instances, care givers purchase their own eyewear with prescription lenses. Regular glasses are insufficient. Glasses must have side shields to prevent material from entering the eye between the glasses and face. Nurses working in high-risk areas such as operating rooms, emergency, labor and delivery, or trauma units should be especially careful to protect themselves from exposure.

Specimen collection. A client with a suspected or actual infectious disease may undergo many laboratory studies. Body fluids and materials suspected of containing infectious organisms are collected for culture and sensitivity tests. The specimen is placed in a special medium that promotes the growth of organisms. A laboratory technologist then identifies the type of microorganisms growing in the culture. Additional sensitivity test results indicate the antibiotics to which the organisms are resistant or sensitive so that the proper medications will be used in the client's treatment.

The nurse obtains all culture specimens with sterile equipment. Collecting fresh material from the site of infection, as in the case of wound drainage, ensures that the specimen will not be contaminated by resident flora. All specimen containers should be sealed tightly to prevent spillage and contamination of the outside of the container (Box 25-10). In each case, a clean container remains outside the client's room or on a clean paper towel in the client's bathroom. After the specimens are transferred to containers, the nurse labels each specimen properly with the client's name, client identifier, date and time, and type of specimen. Nurses place the specimen containers in labeled impervious bags before transporting them to the laboratory.

Bagging. Bagging articles generally is the same for all clients' rooms regardless of whether the room is an isolation room. If an item is contaminated, the nurse uses special bagging procedures for removing it from the client's environment. Bagging articles prevents accidental exposure of personnel to contaminated articles and prevents contamination of the surrounding environment. Garner (1996a) recommends that a single bag is adequate for discarding or wrapping items if the bag is impervious and sturdy and if the article can be placed in the bag without contaminating the outside of the bag. The nurse typically places reusable equipment such as stethoscopes, forceps, or suction bottles in single bags according to agency policy.

All soiled linen should be placed in a designated waterproof impervious bag in the client's room, not overfilling the bag. Linen that is visibly soiled with blood or body fluids should be handled, transported, and processed in a manner that will prevent exposure of skin or mucous membrane and/or contamination of the health care worker's clothing. Double bagging still may be required in some hospitals. However, Garner (1996a) recommends that instead of rigid rules and regulations, hygienic and common-sense handling, storage, and processing of clean and soiled linen should be followed. A standard-sized linen bag, not overfilled, tied securely and intact is adequate to prevent infection transmission. The nurse should consult agency policy and any applicable regulations for the proper procedure.

Biohazardous waste includes both infectious and medical waste that must be disposed of in special red bags. Red-bagged or infectious trash must be disposed of by incineration and special handling. These special procedures are a high expense for health care facilities. The following waste materials should be considered infectious or medical waste (Schmidt, 1996):

1. Cultures, including discarded cultures of infectious organisms
2. Pathological waste, such as discarded human tissue, organs, and body parts
3. Blood and blood products, including discarded serum or plasma and materials containing free-flowing blood
4. Sharps, including discarded needles, syringes, scalpels, blood vials, broken or unbroken glass, and pipettes
5. Selected isolation material, discarded waste material from clients with highly communicable diseases

Removal of protective equipment. The method of removing protective clothing, gloves, mask, eyewear,

---

Box 25-10
Specimen Collection Techniques*

Wound Specimen

Clean site with sterile water or saline prior to wound specimen collection. Wear gloves and use cotton-tipped swab or syringe to collect as much drainage as possible. Have clean test tube or culture tube on clean paper towel. After swabbing center of wound site, grasp collection tube by holding it with paper towel. Carefully insert swab without touching outside of tube. After securing tube's top, transfer tube into bag for transport and then wash hands.

Blood Specimen

Wearing gloves, use syringe and culture media bottles to collect up to 10 ml of blood per culture bottle (check agency policy). After prepping, perform venipuncture at two different sites to decrease likelihood of both specimens being contaminated with skin flora. Place blood culture bottles on bedside table or other surface; swab off bottle tops with alcohol. Inject appropriate amount of blood into each bottle. Remove gloves and transfer specimen into clean, labeled bag for transport. Wash hands.

Stool Specimen

Wearing gloves, use clean cup with seal top (need not be sterile) and tongue blade to collect small amount of stool, approximately the size of a walnut. Place cup on clean paper towel in client's bathroom. Using tongue blade, collect needed amount of feces from client's bedpan. Transfer feces to cup without touching cup's outside surface. Dispose of tongue blade, and place seal on cup. Transfer specimen into clean bag for transport. Remove gloves and wash hands.

Urine Specimen

Wearing gloves, use syringe and sterile cup to collect 1 to 5 ml of urine. Place cup or tube on clean towel in client's bathroom. If client has a urinary catheter, use syringe to collect specimen. Have client follow procedure to obtain a clean-voided specimen (see Chapter 35) if not catheterized. Transfer urine into sterile container by injecting urine from syringe or pouring it from used collection cup. Secure top of container and transfer specimen into clean, labeled bag for transport. Remove gloves and wash hands.

*Agency policies may differ on type of containers and amount of specimen material required.
From Pagana KD, Pagana TJ: *Diagnostic testing and nursing implications,* ed 4, St. Louis, 1994, Mosby.

and gown before leaving an isolation room depends on the protective equipment worn by the nurse at the time. In the example in which all four protective items are worn, the nurse first removes the gloves because they are most likely to be contaminated. If the nurse unties a gown with gloves still on, there is a chance of contaminating hair or a portion of the uniform. When gloves are pulled off, the cuff should be grasped with the other gloved hand and pulled off, turning the glove inside out. The nurse tucks the fingers of the ungloved hand inside the cuff of the remaining glove and pulls it off, turning the glove inside out (Figure 25-5). The gloves are discarded in a plastic-lined receptacle.

Isolation masks are disposable and made of a specially prepared paper or natural fiber. The nurse unties the top string first, then the bottom, and pulls the mask away from the face while holding the strings. The outside surface of the mask should not be touched. The nurse simply discards the mask in a plastic-lined receptacle. Check agency policy for frequency of disposal of HEPA and other types of respirators.

To remove a gown, the nurse first unties the waist and neck ties. The nurse allows the gown to fall gently from the shoulders. Care should be taken to remove the hands from the sleeves without touching the outside of the gown (Figure 25-6). The sleeves should not be allowed to turn inside out. The gown is held at the shoulder seams and folded in half with the outside surfaces touching to reduce contact with the soiled gown. The gown is then discarded in an appropriate receptacle.

The last step is to remove eyewear. Some goggles and glasses are reusable. The nurse refers to agency policy for cleaning procedures. Once eyewear is removed, the nurse completes a thorough hand washing.

Transporting clients. Clients infected with highly communicable organisms, such as TB, should leave their rooms only for essential purposes such as diagnostic procedures or surgery. Before transferring the client to a wheelchair or stretcher, the nurse gives the client the appropriate barrier protection. For example, a client who is infected by an organism transmitted by the respiratory tract must wear a mask. Personnel transporting the client should practice the appropriate precautions while in the client's room. Personnel in diagnostic areas or the operating room should be notified that the client is on isolation. The nurse records the type of isolation on the client's chart and explains ways to avoid transmitting infection during transport.

Control of portals of entry. Many measures that control the exit of microorganisms also control the entrance of pathogens. The nurse evaluates the client and

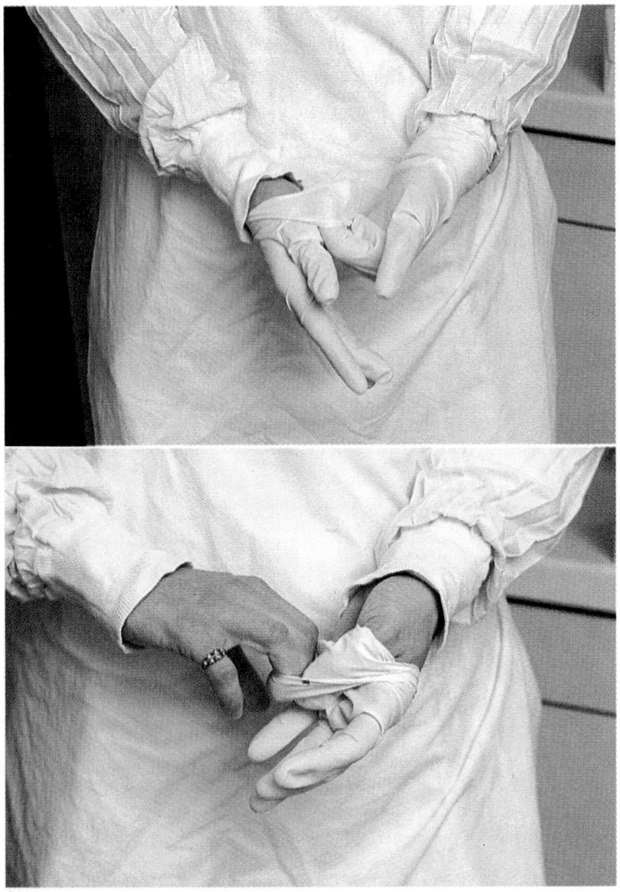

Figure 25-5. Removing disposable gloves. **A,** Nurse places gloved finger inside cuff to pull first glove off hand. **B,** Second glove is removed as nurse slides finger inside glove cuff and pulls.

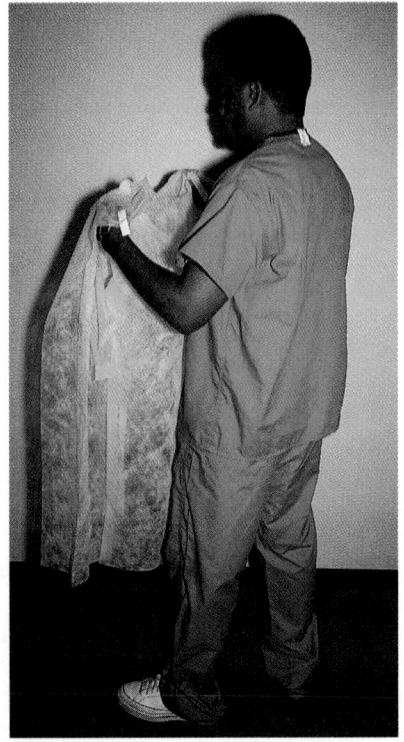

Figure 25-6. Nurse removing isolation gown.

provides interventions to control and prevent organisms from gaining a portal of entry (Box 25-11).

Protection of the susceptible host. A client's resistance to infection improves by the nurse's initiating measures that protect normal body defense mechanisms. In the acute care setting, many of the interventions are designed to either promote existing body defense mechanisms or control exposure to microorganisms. Regular bathing removes transient microorganisms from the skin. Lubrication helps to keep the skin hydrated and intact. Regular oral hygiene removes proteins in the saliva that attract microorganisms. Flossing removes tartar and plaque that can cause infection. An adequate fluid intake promotes normal urine formation and a resultant outflow of urine to flush the bladder and urethra of microorganisms. For immobilized or dependent clients, regular coughing and deep breathing exercises remove mucus from lower airways.

Role of the infection control and prevention department. Most health care facilities employ health professionals who are specially trained in the area of infection control. Their roles and responsibilities include providing consultations, educational offerings, and program development in infection control and prevention.

Health promotion in health care workers and clients. A health care worker who becomes ill can expose susceptible clients to any of a number of infectious diseases. An institution's employee health service provides the following programs to assist in infection control:

1. *Placement evaluation.* A health assessment evaluates an employee's risk for acquiring or transmitting an infectious disease in the workplace.
2. *Employee health and safety education.* Departments coordinate educational programs to orient personnel at all levels to the policies and procedures for infection control.
3. *Immunization programs.* An immunization program safeguards personnel and protects clients from becoming infected by personnel.
4. *Work restrictions and control of job-related illnesses.* When an employee is exposed to an infectious disease, the employee health service must determine whether the employee can continue working. The hospital has the responsibility of preventing the spread of infection to clients and employees.
5. *Protocols for management of job-related exposures to infectious diseases.* Hospitals have the responsibility of providing prompt follow-up for job-related exposures to such diseases as AIDS, hepatitis, and TB.
6. *Health counseling.* Hospital personnel should know about infection risks. Personnel with certain clinical conditions require health counseling.

Surgical asepsis. Surgical asepsis or aseptic technique is designed to eliminate all microorganisms, including spores and pathogens, from an object and to protect an area from these microorganisms. Surgical asepsis requires more precautions than medical asepsis. Breaks in technique could result in contamination, thus increasing the client's risk for infection (Crow and others, 1995).

Although surgical asepsis is commonly practiced in the operating room, labor and delivery area, and major diagnostic areas, the nurse may also use surgical aseptic techniques at the client's bedside (e.g., when inserting intravenous catheters). Surgical asepsis is indicated during procedures that require intentional perforation of the client's skin (e.g., surgical incision), when the skin's integrity is broken related to trauma or burns, and during procedures that involve insertion of a catheter or surgical instruments into sterile body cavities (Decastro and others, 1996).

A nurse in an operating room follows a series of steps toward sterile techniques, such as applying a mask, protective eyewear, and a cap; performing a surgical scrub; and applying a sterile gown and gloves. In contrast, a nurse performing a sterile dressing change at a client's

---

Box 25-11
Infection Control of Portals of Entry

Intact Skin and Mucosa

Keep skin clean and well lubricated.

Avoid positioning clients on tubes or objects that might cause breaks in skin.

Use dry, wrinkle-free linen.

Offer frequent oral hygiene (see Chapter 29).

Provide frequent position changes for clients with impaired mobility.

Urinary Tract

Teach women to clean rectum and perineum by wiping from area of least contamination (urinary meatus) toward area of most contamination (rectum).

Do not allow urine in drainage bags and tubes to flow back into the bladder. Never raise a drainage system above the level of the bladder.

Keep points of connection between catheter or drain and tubing closed.

Invasive Tubes and Lines

When obtaining specimens from drainage tubes or inserting needles into intravenous lines, disinfect tubes and ports by wiping them liberally with a disinfectant solution before entering the system.

Wound Care

Keep draining wounds covered so that drainage is contained.

Clean outward from a wound site using a clean swab for each application.

bedside may only wash his or her hands and apply sterile gloves. Regardless of the procedures followed in different settings, the use of surgical asepsis depends on the nurse developing an aseptic conscience. The nurse must always recognize the importance of strict adherence to aseptic principles. The nurse can also be an excellent role model and client advocate, reinforcing proper practice for other care givers.

Preparation for sterile procedures. In the operating room, control of aseptic technique is more easily enforced. In treatment rooms and at the bedside it is important to have a client's full cooperation. Therefore the nurse must assess the client's understanding of sterile procedure and the reasons for not moving or interfering with the procedure. Special precautions, such as masking the client or changing the clients's position, may be necessary to prevent contamination during procedures. The nurse determines whether a client has undergone a sterile procedure in the past. The nurse explains how the procedure will be performed and what the client can do to avoid contaminating sterile objects:

1. Avoid sudden movements of body parts covered by sterile drapes.
2. Refrain from touching sterile supplies, drapes, or the nurse's sterile gloves and gown.
3. Avoid coughing, sneezing, or talking over a sterile area.

Certain sterile procedures may last for an extended time. The nurse assesses the client's needs (e.g., pain control, elimination) and anticipates factors that may disrupt a procedure. If a client is in pain, the nurse tries to administer analgesics no more than 30 minutes before a sterile procedure begins. Clients often assume relatively uncomfortable positions during sterile procedures. The nurse helps the client to assume the most comfortable position possible. Finally, the client's condition may result in events that contaminate a sterile field (e.g., the client with a respiratory infection who transmits organisms by coughing or breathing). The nurse anticipates such a problem (e.g., offering a mask to the client before the procedure begins).

Principles of surgical asepsis. When beginning a surgically aseptic procedure, the nurse follows certain principles to ensure maintenance of asepsis. Failure to follow each principle conscientiously endangers clients, placing them at risk for an infection. Principles of surgical asepsis include the following:

1. *A sterile object remains sterile only when touched by another sterile object.* The following principles guide the nurse in placement and handling of sterile objects:
   - Sterile touching sterile remains sterile; for example, sterile gloves are worn to handle objects on a sterile field.
   - Sterile touching clean becomes contaminated; for example, if the tip of a syringe touches the surface of a clean disposable glove, the syringe is contaminated.
   - Sterile touching contaminated becomes contaminated; for example, when the nurse touches a sterile object with an ungloved hand, the object is contaminated.
   - Sterile touching questionable is contaminated; for example, when a tear or break in the covering of a sterile object is found, it is discarded or reprocessed regardless of whether the object appears untouched.
2. *Only sterile objects may be placed on a sterile field.* All items are properly sterilized before use. The package or container holding a sterile object must be intact and dry. A package that is torn, punctured, wet, or open is unsterile.
3. *A sterile object or field out of the range of vision or an object held below a person's waist is contaminated.* Nurses never turn their backs on a sterile tray or leave it unattended. Any object held below waist level is considered contaminated because it cannot be viewed at all times. Sterile objects should be kept either on or out over the sterile field.
4. *A sterile object or field becomes contaminated by prolonged exposure to the air.* The nurse avoids activities that may create air currents, such as excessive movements or rearranging linen after a sterile object or field becomes exposed. When sterile packages are opened, the nurse minimizes the number of people walking into the area. Microorganisms also travel by droplet through the air. No one should talk, laugh, sneeze, or cough over a sterile field or when gathering and using sterile equipment. When opening a tray and adding sterile equipment, the nurse should wear a mask. Microorganisms traveling through the air can fall on sterile items or fields if the nurse reaches over the work area.
5. *A sterile object or field becomes contaminated by capillary action when a sterile surface comes in contact with a wet contaminated surface.* Moisture seeps through a sterile package's protective covering, allowing microorganisms to travel to the sterile object. When stored sterile packages become wet, the nurse discards the objects immediately or sends the equipment for resterilization. Spilling solution over a sterile drape contaminates the field unless the drape cannot be penetrated by moisture.
6. *Because fluid flows in the direction of gravity, a sterile object becomes contaminated if gravity causes a contaminated liquid to flow over the object's surface.* To avoid contamination during a surgical hand scrub, the surgical nurse holds the hands above the elbows. This allows water to flow downward without contaminating the nurse's hands and fingers. The principle of water flow by gravity is also the reason

for drying from fingers to elbows with the hands held up, after the scrub.

7. *The edges of a sterile field or container are contaminated.* A 2.5-cm (1-inch) border around a sterile towel or drape is considered contaminated. The edges of sterile containers become exposed to air after they are open and are thus contaminated. After a sterile needle is removed from its protective cap or after forceps are removed from a container, the objects must not touch the container's edge. The lip of an opened bottle of solution also becomes contaminated after it is exposed to air. When pouring a sterile liquid, the nurse first pours a small amount of solution and discards it. The solution washes away any microorganisms on the bottle lip. The nurse then pours a second time to fill a container with the desired amount of solution.

Performing sterile procedures. All of the equipment needed during a procedure should be assembled beforehand. The nurse should anticipate requirements so that equipment is not left unattended. A few extra supplies should be available, in case objects accidentally become contaminated. Before the sterile procedure, each step should be explained so that the client can cooperate fully. If an object becomes contaminated during the procedure, the nurse should not hesitate to discard it or send it back for reprocessing.

Donning and removing caps and masks. For sterile procedures on a general nursing division, the nurse may wear a surgical mask without a cap. For sterile surgical procedures, the nurse first applies a clean cap that covers all the hair and then the surgical mask. A mask must fit snugly around the face and nose to prevent contamination by droplet nuclei. After a mask is worn for several hours, the area over the mouth and nose often becomes moist, which promotes the spread of microorganisms. When operating room nurses' masks become wet, nurses must change them with the aid of the circulating room nurse or by stepping out of the room at an appropriate time. Before permanently removing a mask and cap, the nurse removes sterile gloves to prevent contamination of the hair, neck, and facial area. After untying the mask, the nurse holds it by the ties and discards it with the cap then washes hands thoroughly.

Opening sterile packages. Sterile items such as syringes, gauze dressings, or irrigation trays are packaged in paper or plastic containers impervious to microorganisms as long as they are dry and intact. Plastics are pliable and resistant to tearing. Some agencies wrap reusable sterile items in a double thickness of linen. Sterile items are kept in clean, enclosed storage cabinets and are separated from dirty equipment. If the integrity of the sterile package is questionable (e.g., wet, torn, discolored), the item should not be used. If moisture is found after opening a sterile tray, these items should be discarded or resterilized according to agency policy.

Before opening a sterile item, the nurse washes the hands thoroughly. The nurse assembles the supplies in the work area such as at a bedside table or counter top. Sterile supplies should not be opened in a confined space where a dirty object might fall on or strike them.

Opening a sterile item on a flat surface. Sterile packaged items can be opened without contaminating the contents. Commercially packaged items are usually designed so that the nurse only has to tear away or separate the paper or plastic cover. The item is held in one hand while the wrapper is pulled away with the other (Figure 25-7). Care is then taken to keep the inner contents sterile before use. See Box 25-12 for guidelines in opening items wrapped in linen or paper.

To close a package, the nurse reverses the order of the steps used to unwrap an item. The nurse does not touch the inside contents or reach over the field. This practice may be used in an operating room or at the client's bedside.

Preparing a sterile field. To perform sterile procedures, the nurse needs a sterile work area for handling and placing sterile items. A sterile field is an area free of microorganisms and prepared to receive sterile items. A field may be created by using the inner surface of a sterile wrapper laid flat or by preparing a sterile drape. Drapes are available in cloth, paper, and plastic. The ideal drape is waterproof.

When preparing a sterile field, the nurse may use gloved or ungloved hands. Gloved hands make the procedure easier because the nurse can touch the entire drape. If gloves are not worn, the nurse may touch only a 1-inch border along the drape's edge. The most important principle to follow in preparing a field is to avoid contamination by not reaching over a drape, not allowing the drape to touch the uniform, and not allowing the drape's sterile surface to touch the client. See Box 25-13 for preparation of a sterile field.

Adding sterile supplies to a sterile field. Occasionally the nurse will add sterile supplies to a sterile field. For example, after opening a gauze pack wrapped in linen, the nurse may add sterile instruments to the

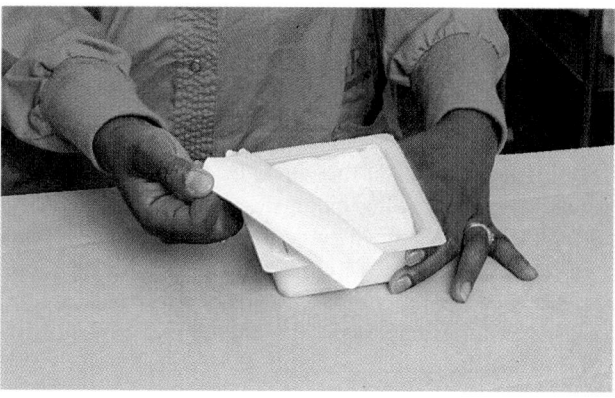

Figure 25-7. Opening a commercially packaged sterile item.

Box 25-12

Procedural Guidelines for Opening Wrapped Sterile Items

1. Place item flat in center of work surface.
2. Remove any tape or seal indicating sterilization date.
3. Grasp the outer surface of the tip of the outermost flap.
4. Open the outer flap away from the body, keeping the arm outstretched and away from the sterile field (see illustration).

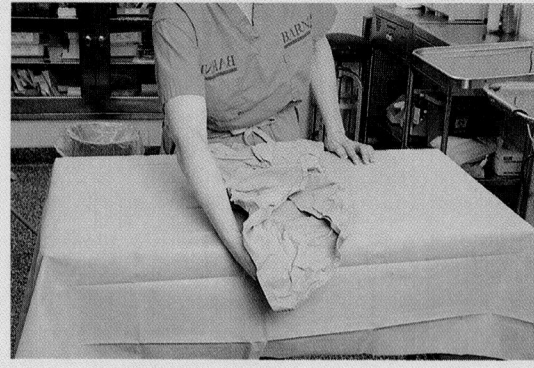

Step 4

5. Grasp the outside surface of the first side flap.
6. Open the side flap, allowing it to lie flat on the work surface. Keep the arm to the side and not over the sterile surface. Do not allow flaps to spring back over the sterile contents (see illustration).

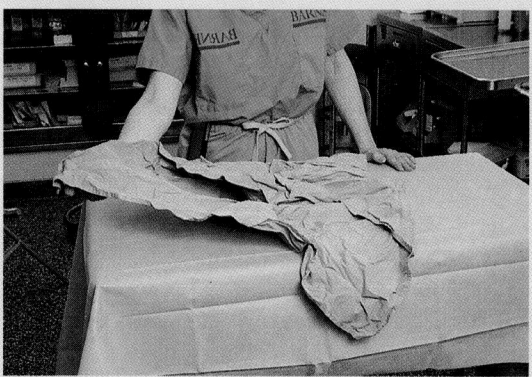

Step 6

7. Grasp the outside surface of the second flap (again keeping the arm to the side) and allow it to lie flat on table surface.
8. Grasp the outside surface of the last innermost flap.
9. Stand away from the sterile package and pull the flap back, allowing it to fall flat on the surface (see illustration).
10. Use the inner surface of the package (except for the 1-inch border around the edges) as a field to add additional items because it is sterile. Grasp the 1-inch border to move the field over the work surface.

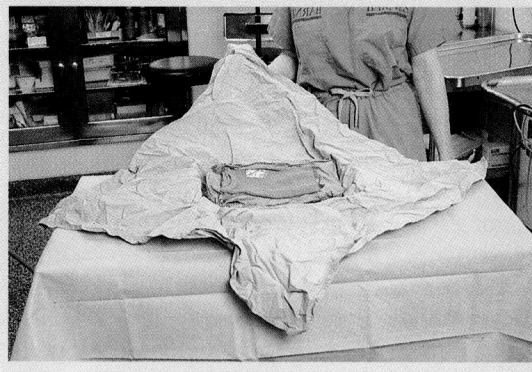

Step 9

field. To add supplies, the nurse opens the item to be transferred by grasping its outside wrapper in the nondominant hand. After the wrapper is peeled over on the nondominant hand, the item is still sterile and the nurse can safely drop the item onto the sterile field. If the wrapper is long and could fall on the sterile field, the nurse takes the dominant hand and carefully holds the wrapper around the wrist of the nondominant hand (Figure 25-8). When transferring sterile items, the nurse must carefully place objects onto the sterile field. An object that comes in contact with the edge of the sterile field must be discarded.

Pouring sterile solutions. A bottle containing a sterile solution is sterile on the inside and contaminated on the outside, including the bottle's neck. The inside of the bottle cap is also sterile. After a cap or lid is opened, it is held in the hand or placed sterile side (inside) up on a clean surface. This means that the inside of the lid

Box 25-13

Procedural Guidelines for Preparation of a Sterile Field

1. Wash hands.
2. Place pack containing sterile drape on work surface and open as described under "Opening a sterile item on a flat surface."
3. With fingertips of one hand, pick up the folded top edge of the sterile drape.
4. Gently lift the drape up from its outer cover and let it unfold by itself without touching any object. Discard the outer cover with the other hand.

5. With the other hand, grasp an adjacent corner of the drape and hold it straight up and away from the body (see illustration).
6. Holding the drape, first position and lay the bottom half over the intended work surface (see illustration).
7. Allow the top half of the drape to be placed over the work surface last (see illustration).
8. Grasp the 1-inch border around the edge to position as needed.

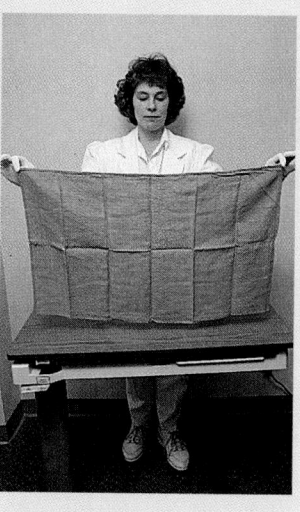
Step 5

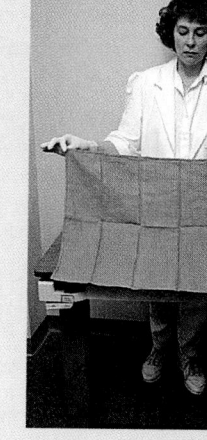
Step 6

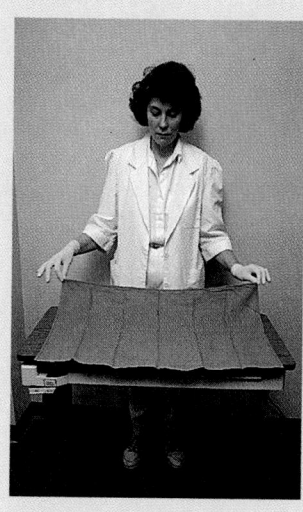
Step 7

can be seen as it rests on the table surface. A bottle cap or lid should never rest sterile side down on a sterile surface because the outer edge of the cap is unsterile and would contaminate the surface. Likewise, placing a sterile cap sterile side down on an unsterile surface may increase the chances of the inside of the cap becoming contaminated.

The bottle should be held with its label in the palm of the hand to prevent the solution from wetting and fading the label. Before pouring the solution into the container, the nurse pours a small amount (1 to 2 ml) into a disposable cup or plastic-lined waste receptacle. The discarded solution cleans the lip of the bottle. The edge of the bottle is kept away from the edge or inside of the receiving container. The nurse pours the solution slowly to avoid splashing the drape or field. The bottle should also be kept low to reduce splashing during pouring. The bottle should be held outside the edge of the sterile field.

Surgical hand washing. Surgical hand washing or scrubs are performed to reduce resident flora and tran-

sient flora from the hands and forearms (Skill 25-2) before assisting with a surgical procedure. Regular hand washing may be satisfactory before routine sterile procedures on a general nursing division. The optimum duration of the surgical hand wash is unclear and may

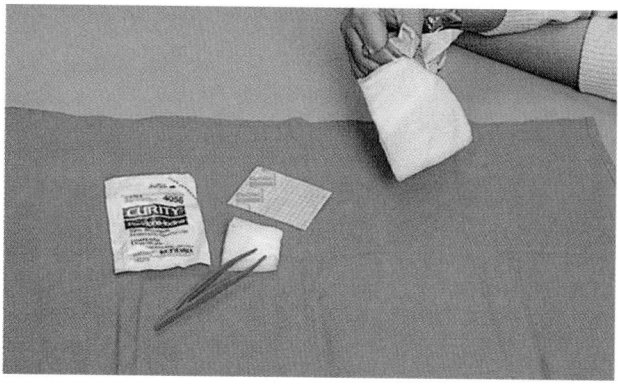

Figure 25-8. Adding item to a sterile field, being sure NOT to hold arm over sterile field.

.... Skill 25-2
Surgical Hand Washing

Delegation Considerations

The circulating nurse must always be a registered nurse. The role of the scrub nurse can be delegated to a surgical technologist or licensed practical nurse. Nonlicensed personnel can assist the registered nurse in the circulating role by opening sterile supplies, setting up sterile fields, and running errands under the direction of the registered nurse.

Equipment

- Deep sink with foot or knee controls for dispensing water and soap (faucets should be high enough for hands and forearms to fit comfortably)
- Antiseptic detergent (nonirritating, broad-spectrum, fast-acting, effective in reducing skin microorganisms, and having a residual effect) (Association of Operating Room Nurses, 1995)
- Surgical scrub brush with plastic nail pick
- Paper mask and cap or hood
- Sterile towel
- Proper scrub attire
- Protective eyewear (glasses or goggles)

STEPS	RATIONALE
1. Consult institutional policy regarding required length of time for hand wash.	Guidelines vary regarding ideal time needed for surgical scrub.
2. Be sure fingernails are short, clean, and healthy. Artificial nails should be removed.	Long nails and chipped or old polish increase number of bacteria residing on nails. Long fingernails can puncture gloves, causing contamination. Artificial nails are known to harbor gram-negative microorganisms and fungus.

CRITICAL DECISION POINT

Remove nail polish if chipped or worn longer than 4 days because it may harbor microorganisms (Association of Operating Room Nurses, 1995).

3. Inspect hands for presence of abrasions, cuts, or open lesions.	These conditions increase likelihood of more microorganisms residing on skin surfaces.
4. Apply surgical shoe covers, cap or hood, face mask, and protective eyewear.	Mask prevents escape into air of microorganisms that can contaminate hands. Other protective wear prevents exposure to blood and body fluid splashes during the procedure.
5. Turn on water using knee or foot controls and adjust to comfortable temperature.	
6. Wet hands and arms under running lukewarm water and lather with detergent to 5 cm (2 inches) above elbows. (Hands need to be above elbows at all times.)	Water runs by gravity from fingertips to elbows. Hands become cleanest part of upper extremity. Keeping hands elevated allows water to flow from least to most contaminated areas. Washing a wide area reduces risk of contaminating overlying gown that the nurse later applies.
7. Rinse hands and arms thoroughly under running water. **Remember to keep hands above elbows.**	Rinsing removes transient bacteria from fingers, hands, and forearms.
8. Under running water, clean under nails of both hands with nail pick. Discard after use (see illustration).	Removes dirt and organic material that harbor large numbers of microorganisms.

STEPS	RATIONALE
9. Wet clean brush and apply antimicrobial detergent. Scrub the nails of one hand with 15 strokes. Holding brush perpendicular, scrub the palm, each side of the thumb and fingers, and the posterior side of the hand with 10 strokes each. The arm is mentally divided into thirds and each third is scrubbed 10 times (see illustration). Entire scrub should last 5 to 10 minutes. Rinse brush and repeat the sequence for the other arm. A two-brush method may be substituted. Check agency policy.	Scrubbing loosens resident bacteria that adhere to skin surfaces. Ensures coverage of all surfaces. Scrubbing is performed from cleanest area (hands) to marginal area (upper arms).
10. Discard brush and rinse hands and arms thoroughly (see illustration). Turn off water with foot or knee control and back into room entrance with hands elevated in front of and away from the body.	After touching skin, brush is considered contaminated. Rinsing removes resident bacteria. Prevents accidental contamination.

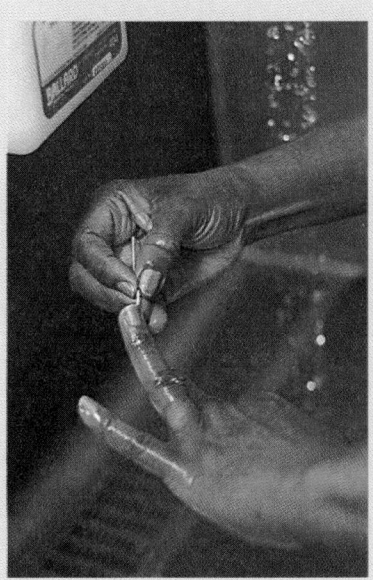

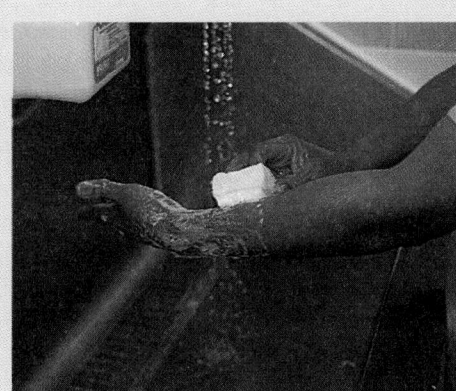

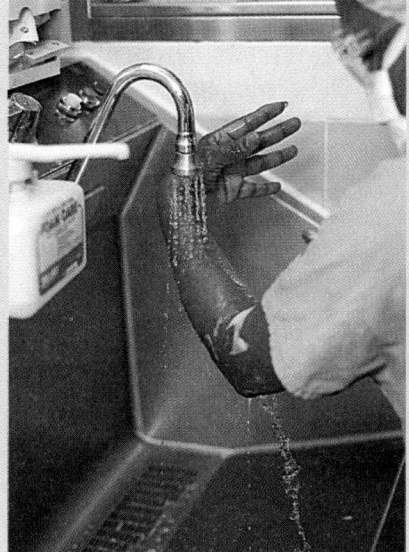

| Step 8 | Step 9 | Step 10 |

11. Bending slightly forward at the waist, use a sterile towel to dry one hand thoroughly, moving from fingers to elbow. Dry in a rotating motion. Dry from cleanest to least clean area.	Drying prevents chapping and facilitates donning of gloves. Leaning forward prevents accidental contact of arms with scrub attire.
12. Repeat drying method for other hand, using a different area of the towel or a new sterile towel.	Prevents accidental contamination.
13. Inspect hands for dermatitis or cracked skin.	Indicates complications from excessive hand washing.
14. Observe the client for signs of localized wound infection.	Signs of infection include redness, heat, swelling, pain, and drainage.

Recording and Reporting

- It is not necessary to record or report this procedure.

- Report any dermatitis to employee health or infection control per agency policy.

depend on the antimicrobial used. Larson (1996) recommends applying antimicrobial soap to wet hands and forearms and applying friction for at least 2 minutes. The nurse should check agency policy before the procedure. For maximum elimination of bacteria, the nurse removes all jewelry and keeps fingernails short, clean, and free of polish.

Donning sterile gloves. After the nurse scrubs the hands, sterile gloves act as an additional barrier to bacterial transfer. However, bacteria multiply rapidly under gloves and can contaminate a wound or sterile object through a puncture. Use of antiseptic detergents retards bacterial growth under gloves.

There are two gloving methods: open and closed. Nurses commonly use the open method in the clinical area before changing dressings, inserting catheters, or suctioning a client's airway. Both methods are acceptable in operating rooms, but closed gloving is more frequently used for initial gloving and the open method for changing a contaminated glove during an operative procedure. Box 25-14 reviews steps for open gloving. Gloves are made in whole and half sizes, and it is important to choose the right size glove. The glove should not stretch so tightly that it can easily tear; yet it should be tight enough that objects can be picked up.

Sebazco (1996) stresses that before donning latex gloves, the client and the health care worker should be aware of potential latex allergies. Studies have shown that for those individuals who are highly sensitive to latex, local and even systemic reaction can occur when someone removes a pair of latex gloves in close proximity to that individual. It is believed that latex particles can become suspended in the air on glove powder particles (Beezhold and others, 1994).

After a sterile procedure the nurse disposes of gloves in the following manner to minimize hand contamination:

1. The outside of one cuff is grasped with the other gloved hand (taking care not to touch the wrist).
2. The glove is peeled off, turned inside out, and discarded in the proper receptacle.
3. The fingers of the bare hand tuck inside the remaining glove's cuff. (The outside of the glove is not touched.)
4. The glove is peeled off, turned inside out, and discarded in the proper receptacle.

Sterile gowning. The nurse wears a sterile gown in the operating and delivery rooms so that sterile objects can be easily handled with less risk of contamination. The sterile gown acts as a barrier to microorganisms. The nurse dons a gown after applying a mask, goggles, and cap and after surgical hand washing. The nurse can pick up only the inside surface of the gown at the collar. The gown is held straight up at arm's length away from the body. The nurse holds the gown by the inside open shoulder seams while placing each hand through the armholes.

The hands are kept inside the cuffs so that gloves can later be applied (closed method). Only a certain portion of the gown—the area from the anterior waist to but not including the collar and the anterior surface of the sleeves—is considered sterile. A circulating nurse in the operating room ties the back of the nurse's gown to prevent contamination.

Restorative care.
The need for infection control is also present when clients are in the restorative phase of their care. Nurses in long-term care or home health settings can contribute to quality health care by practicing skills and techniques necessary to prevent infections.

Long-term care. Some of the same risks for infections that are present in acute care can apply in a long-term care facility, such as skilled nursing homes (Rusnak, 1996). These facilities are required to have an active infection control program designed to monitor and prevent infections of their residents.

Certain risks of nosocomial infections are increased because of the usual age of clients seen in long-term care facilities. For example, in older adults there are several age-associated physical changes that can alter the natural barriers to infections (see Box 25-5).

Some of the major infections common to clients in long-term care are urinary tract infections, pressure ulcer infections, and pneumonia. The nurse can play an important role in the control of these infections by using critical thinking skills and knowledge of how these infections can be prevented.

Urinary tract infections. The leading cause of nosocomial infections in long-term care and the most common cause of bacteremia in older adults are urinary tract infections (UTIs) (Rusnak, 1996). Most UTIs are caused by endogenous intestinal organisms, such as *E. coli*, which contaminate the periurethral area. Contamination is enhanced by clients whose hygiene may be compromised because of immobility or confusion. Microorganisms may also enter the bladder of catheterized clients through the lumen of a urinary catheter. Additionally, personnel can transfer organisms from one client to another because of inadequate hand washing after handling catheter bags and tubing or cleaning incontinent clients. Chapter 35 summarizes guidelines for preventing UTIs.

Pressure ulcer infections. The second leading cause of infections in long-term care facilities are pressure ulcer infections (Rusnak, 1996). Pressure ulcers are soft-tissue lesions in which cell death has occurred because of decreased blood supply (see Chapter 38). Ulcers may vary in severity from a redness of the skin to ulceration extending through the muscle into the bone. Regardless of the depth of the pressure ulcer, it may or may not be infected. Signs and symptoms of an infected ulcer may include purulent drainage, pain, induration, swelling, or heat surrounding the lesion. See Chapter 38 for a review of nursing interventions in the treatment and prevention of pressure ulcers.

Box 25-14

Procedural Guidelines for Open Gloving

1. Consider the procedure to be performed and consult agency policy on use of gloves.
2. Inspect hands for cuts, open lesions, or abrasions.
3. Assess if the client or health care worker has a known allergy to latex.
4. Examine glove package to ensure package is not wet, torn, or discolored.
5. Perform thorough hand washing and determine correct glove size and type of glove material to be used.
6. Remove outer glove package wrapper by carefully separating and peeling apart sides.
7. Grasp inner package and lay it on clean, flat surface just above waist level. Open package, keeping gloves on wrapper's inside surface.
8. Identify right and left glove. Each glove has cuff approximately 5 cm (2 inches) wide. Glove dominant hand first.
9. With thumb and first two fingers of nondominant hand, grasp edge of cuff of the glove for the dominant hand. Touch only glove's inside surface.
10. Carefully pull glove over dominant hand (see illustration) leaving a cuff and being sure the cuff does not roll up wrist. Be sure thumb and fingers are in proper spaces (see illustration).
11. With gloved dominant hand, slip fingers underneath second glove's cuff (see illustration).
12. Carefully pull second glove over nondominant hand (see illustration). Do not allow fingers and thumb of gloved dominant hand to touch any part of exposed nondominant hand. Keep thumb of dominant hand abducted.
13. After second glove is on, interlock hands (see illustration). Cuffs usually fall down after application. Be sure to touch only sterile sides.

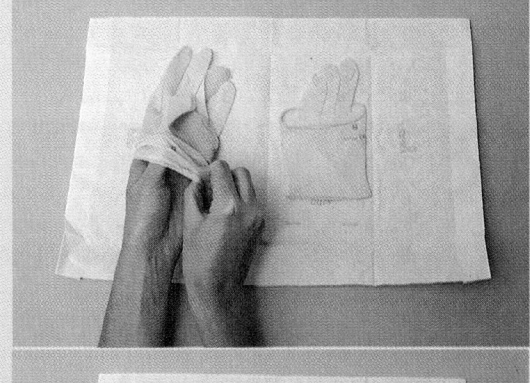

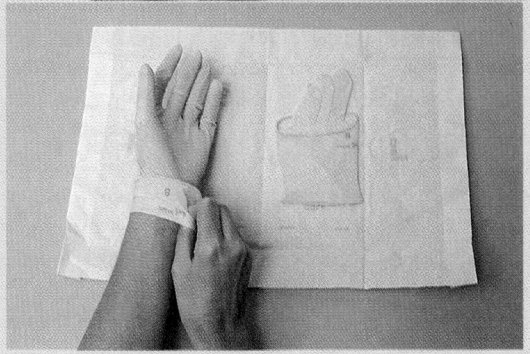

Step 10

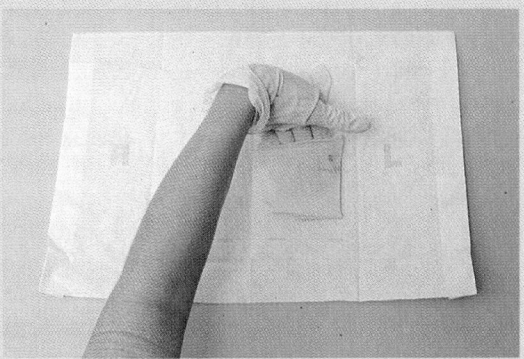

Step 11

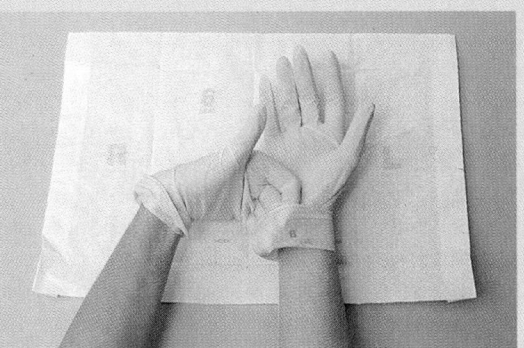

Step 12

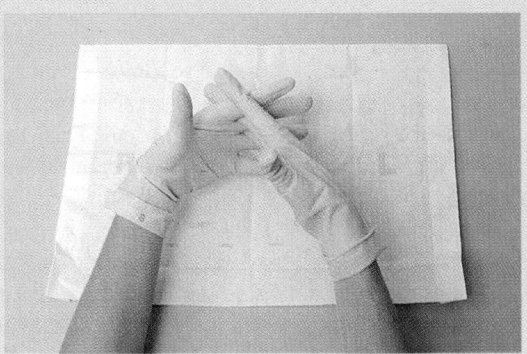

Step 13

Pneumonia. The third most common infection seen in long-term care clients is pneumonia. Mortality (death) in older adults is significantly higher than in younger persons. In 80% of older adults, pneumonia onset is sudden, with shaking chills, high fever, and a productive cough. In about 15% to 20% of clients, onset may be gradual and signs and symptoms may be atypical: no temperature elevation, confusion, fatigue, and increased respirations (Rusnak, 1996). Common causes of pneumonia in clients in long-term care facilities include aspiration of endogenous organisms (e.g., *S. aureus* and *Streptococcus pneumoniae*) that colonize the oropharyngeal area, direct contact with respiratory droplets from an infected individual, and direct contact with contaminated equipment or hands of direct care givers. Chapter 30 summarizes nursing interventions for preventing pneumonia in long-term care clients.

If a client has a respiratory infection that can be contagious to other clients, a private room is indicated and clients with similar infections can be cohorted (housed in same room).

Home health. The provision of nursing services in the home setting is increasing every year. Nurses practicing in the home care setting have several infection control and prevention challenges. For example, environmental factors such as inadequate sanitation, poor hygiene, contaminated supplies, insect or rodent infestation, exposure to heat or cold, and family members with infectious diseases can increase the client's susceptibility to an infection. In the home situation, principles of infection control should be taught to the client and all the care givers in the family.

Client education. Client education must include information regarding infection control practices at home. Aseptic technique becomes almost second nature to the nurse practicing it daily. However, the client is less aware of the factors that promote the spread of infection or of the ways to prevent its transmission. The home does not always lend itself to the practice of aseptic technique. A nurse must often help a client to improvise with the resources available to maintain hygienic techniques. For example, a client may use a laundered washcloth instead of expensive sterile gauze to wash around his or her open wound.

After clients are at home, they determine their own adherence to infection control practices. The nurse educates clients about infection and techniques to prevent onset of infection or to control its spread (Box 25-15). Family members must also become involved in the teaching plan. Teaching efforts involve a common-sense approach to controlling and preventing infection (Goldbrick and Turner, 1995).

Hand washing. There may be occasions, as in some home care situations, in which soap and running water are not available. In those instances, the nurse should anticipate the need for cleansing the hands with an alcohol-based handrub or detergent-containing

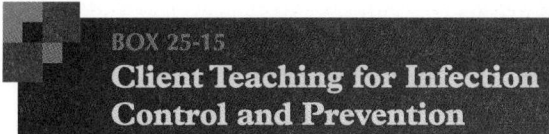

BOX 25-15
Client Teaching for Infection Control and Prevention

- Teach client basic hand washing practices (when and how).
- Instruct client about hygiene practices that reduce organism growth and spread.
- Provide a simple explanation of clean versus contaminated items.
- Discuss the client's susceptibility to infection.
- Explain that family members are at risk for acquiring infections.
- Teach the application of aseptic principles to self-care activities such as wound care and medication administration.
- Instruct client about proper methods for food handling and storage.
- Discuss preventive health care (e.g., diet, immunizations).

towel until hands can be thoroughly washed using soap and warm water.

Clients and their families in the home care setting should be instructed to wash their hands in the following situations: before and after dressing changes, after going to the bathroom, before eating or handling medication, and after handling or caring for pets. The nurse should explain and demonstrate the correct procedure for hand washing.

Equipment cleaning and disinfecting. The same principles for cleaning and disinfecting apply regardless of the health care setting (Rutala, 1996). All items must be thoroughly cleaned before any disinfection process. Modification to routine disinfection can be made in the home care setting (Garofalo, 1996). Products and processes suitable for disinfection in the home include boiling water for 10 minutes; bleach, usually in a 1:10 solution; acetic acid (vinegar); isopropyl alcohol (70%); and commercial disinfectants that contain phenolic solutions.

Disposal of infectious or hazardous waste. Infectious or hazardous waste, including needles and sharps, must be disposed of as outlined by local and state regulations (Garofalo, 1996). When home care nurses are giving injections, an agency may choose to provide a rigid sharps container for the home. When full, the closed container may be removed by the home care nurse (check state laws regarding transportation of sharps). Clients and their families can be taught to dispose of needles in capped glass or plastic bottles or containers containing a 1:10 bleach solution. Contaminated dressings and items soiled with blood or body fluid should be wrapped or placed in plastic bags before disposal.

Wound care. Although a large variety of wound care practices exist in home care, many wounds are treated using clean, rather than sterile technique. Sterile technique is required if ordered by a physician and for fresh wounds. Wound care protocol depends on the following: type of wound, economics, skill of client and family, and preference of home care team. Clients and their families should be able to successfully demonstrate techniques before performing the procedure.

◼ Evaluation

Client care. As the nurse delivers care to the client, it is important to evaluate the result of interventions so that the nurse can either continue, revise nursing care therapies, or determine that a problem has been resolved. Evaluation of nursing care is based on the goals and outcomes established during the planning phase of the nursing process. Because a client's condition can change at any time, evaluation is ongoing. The nurse must use assessment skills to determine the client's progress over time.

The nurse will use evaluative measures for each of the established expected outcomes. The information gathered determines the status of each client goal. For example, if the goal is "wound heals within 2 weeks" and the outcome is "client's wound drainage decreases in 3 days," the evaluative measure involves the nurse inspecting the amount of drainage on a dressing or measuring the amount of drainage collected in a drainage device.

The nurse's evaluation will determine if interventions should continue, if revisions are needed in therapies, if new therapies are required, or if the client has developed new nursing diagnoses.

Client expectations. The nurse should always remember to ask the client if expectations of care have been met. Has the client gained the information he or she desires to understand therapies and to manage treatment of an infection at home? Does the client believe that the nurse performed knowledgeably and competently? Was the client on isolation treated with respect and dignity? The nurse must not assume to know the client's expectations. The nurse's evaluation reviews expectations gathered during assessment and then reassesses the client's perceptions and opinions about care.

Key Terms

airborne precautions	infection
antibody	inflammation
antigen	isolation
asepsis	lymphocyte
aseptic technique	medical asepsis
carriers	microorganisms
colonization	necrotic
communicable disease	nosocomial infection
contact precautions	pathogenicity
disinfection	pathogens
droplet precautions	resident flora
endogenous infection	Standard Precautions
exogenous infection	sterilization
exudate	supra infection
flora	surgical asepsis
iatrogenic infection	transient flora
immunity	virulence
immunocompromised	

◼ Key Concepts

Normal body flora resist infection by releasing antibacterial substances and inhibiting multiplication of pathogenic microorganisms.

Immunity to infection is measured by the capacity to produce antibodies in response to exposure to an antigen.

An infection can develop as long as the six elements comprising the infection chain are uninterrupted.

A microorganism's virulence depends on its ability to resist attack by the body's normal defenses.

Microorganisms are transmitted by direct and indirect contact, by airborne spread, and by vectors and contaminated vehicles.

Increasing age, poor nutrition, stress, inherited conditions, chronic disease, and treatments or conditions that compromise the immune response increase susceptibility to infection.

Gloves, gowns, and masks in combination with eye protection devices such as goggles or glasses with solid side shields should be worn when in contact with blood or potentially infectious material or whenever splashes or spray of blood or potentially infectious material may be generated.

Invasive procedures, medical therapies, long hospitalization, and contact with health care personnel increase a hospitalized client's risk for acquiring a nosocomial infection.

Surgical asepsis requires more stringent techniques than medical asepsis and is directed toward eliminating microorganisms.

Continued

Key Concepts—cont'd

The CDC recommends that all clients be considered as potentially infected with HIV and other blood-borne pathogens; therefore health care workers should reduce the risk of exposure to blood and body fluids.

Standard Precautions involve using barrier protection with all clients regardless of presence of infection.

Following aseptic principles is the key to a nurse's success in preventing clients from acquiring infections.

A client receiving isolation precautions is subject to sensory deprivation because of the restricted environment.

Lack of hand washing is the main cause of nosocomial infections.

An infection control health professional provides educational and consultative services to maintain aseptic practices.

If the skin is broken or if the nurse performs an invasive procedure into a body cavity normally free of microorganisms, surgical aseptic practices are enforced.

A sterile object becomes contaminated by direct contact with a clean or contaminated object, by exposure to airborne microorganisms, or by contact with a wet surface containing microorganisms.

Critical Thinking Activities

1. During a home care visit, it is reported that several members of a family have had diarrhea and vomiting after eating a dinner of turkey and stuffing. After further investigation, it is determined that the turkey was thawed at room temperature instead of following the recommendation to thaw in the refrigerator and that the stuffing was placed in the turkey's cavity before the turkey was completely thawed. The nurse reports this immediately to the physician, and stool cultures are ordered. Three members of the family are diagnosed as having *Salmonella* food-borne illness. Describe in this case (using the chain of infection) how the infection occurred and how the nurse can assist the clients in preventing further food-borne illness.

2. In the following client care situations, select the appropriate personal protective equipment (PPE) and give the rationale: (a) starting an IV catheter,

   (b) blood pressure checks on a client with hepatitis B, (c) changing the bed linen for an incontinent client, (d) entering the room of a client with meningococcal meningitis, (e) entering the room of a client with *Mycobacterium avium,* (f) emptying a suction bottle containing bloody fluid, and (g) changing an infected wound dressing on a client in a home situation.

3. Mrs. Smith is admitted for a major surgical procedure. During the admission procedure, the nurse notices that Mrs. Smith has a productive cough that she says she has had for about 6 weeks. She further states that she has occasionally seen blood in her sputum and has lost weight over the past 4 weeks. Mrs. Smith also tells the nurse that one of the members of her immediate household has been recently diagnosed with tuberculosis. With this additional history, what should the nurse do?

References

Advisory Committee on Immunization Practices, CDC: *MMWR*: 4/4/97, 3/28/97, 2/14/97, 1/3/97, 12/27/96, 11/22/96, 7/12/96.

American Nurses Association (ANA): *Latex allergy, WP-70M, 1996*, Washington, DC, 1996, The Association.

Association of Operating Room Nurses: Recommended practices for surgical hand scrubs, *AORN standards and recommended practices for perioperative nursing*, Denver, 1995, The Association.

Beezhold D and others: The transfer of protein allergens from latex gloves, *AORN J* 59(30):605, 1994.

Benenson A: *Control of communicable disease manual*, Washington, DC, 1995, APHA.

Bobo L: The microbiologic environment. In Soule B and others, editors: *Infections and nursing practice*, St. Louis, 1995, Mosby.

Centers for Disease Control and Prevention (CDC): Update: universal precautions for prevention of transmission of human immunodeficiency virus, hepatitis B, and other bloodborne pathogens in health care setting, *MMWR* 37(24):377, 1988.

Centers for Disease Control and Prevention (CDC): Physical activity and the prevention of coronary heart disease, *MMWR* 42(35):669, 1993.

Centers for Disease Control and Prevention (CDC): Guidelines for preventing the transmission of tuberculosis in health care facilities, *MMWR* 43(RR-13):1, 1994.

Chandra R: Symposium on nutrition and immunity in serious illness, *Proc Nutr Soc* 52:77, 1993.

Cooper B: Antimicrobial chemotherapeutics. In Soule B and others, editors: *Infections and nursing practice*, St. Louis, 1995, Mosby.

COSSMHO (National Coalition of Hispanic and Human Service Organizations): *HIV/AIDS: the impact on Hispanics in selected states*, Washington, DC, 1991, The Coalition.

Crow S and others: Antisepsis, disinfection, sterilization. In Soule B and others, editors: *Infections and nursing practice*, St. Louis, 1995, Mosby.

DeCastro M and others: Aseptic technique. In Olmsted R, editor: *APIC infection control and applied epidemiology*, St. Louis, 1996, Mosby.

Garner J: Isolation systems. In Olmsted R, editor: *APIC infection control and applied epidemiology*, St. Louis, 1996a, Mosby.

Garner JS: Guidelines for isolation precautions for hospitals, *Infect Control Hosp Epidemiol* 17(1):54, 1996b.

Garofalo K: Home care. In Olmsted R, editor: *APIC infection control and applied epidemiology*, St. Louis, 1996, Mosby.

Goldbrick B, Turner J: Education and behavior changes in prevention and control of infection. In Soule B and others, editors: *Infections and nursing practice*, St. Louis, 1995, Mosby.

Gorse GJ and others: Association of malnutrition with nosocomial infection, *Infect Control Hosp Epidemiol* 10:194, 1989.

Hospital Infection Control Practices Advisory Committee (HICPAC): Recommendations for preventing the spread of vancomycin-resistant organisms, *Am J Infect Control* 23:87, 1995.

Hospital Infection Control Practices Advisory Committee (HICPAC): Guidelines for isolation precautions in hospitals, *Am J Infect Control* 24:24, 1996.

Ickovic J, Rodin J: Women and AIDS in the USA: epidemiology, natural history, and mediating mechanisms, *Health Psychol* 11(1):1, 1992.

Jackson M: General principles of epidemiology. In Olmsted R, editor: *APIC infection control and applied epidemiology*, St. Louis, 1996, Mosby.

Keroack M, Rosen-Kotlainen H: Microbiology/laboratory diagnostics. In Olmsted R, editor: *APIC infection control and applied epidemiology*, St. Louis, 1996, Mosby.

Larson E: APIC guidelines for hand washing and hand antisepsis in health care settings, *Am J Infect Control* 23(4):251, 1995.

Larson E: Antiseptic. In Olmsted R, editor: *APIC infection control and applied epidemiology*, St. Louis, 1996, Mosby.

Occupational Safety and Health Administration (OSHA): Occupational exposure to blood borne pathogens: final rule, 29CRF 1919:1030, *Federal Register* 56:64175, 1991.

Occupational Safety and Health Administration (OSHA): Respiratory protective devices: final rules and notice, *Federal Register* 60:30336, 1995.

Pagana KD, Pagana TJ: *Diagnostic testing and nursing implications*, ed 4, St. Louis, 1994, Mosby.

Rubel A, Garro I: Social and cultural factors in successful control of tuberculosis, *Public Health Report* 107(6):626, 1992.

Rusnak P: Long term care. In Olmsted R, editor: *APIC infection control and applied epidemiology*, St. Louis, 1996, Mosby.

Rutala W: Disinfection and sterilization of patient-care items, *Infect Control Hosp Epidemiol* 17(6):377, 1996.

Schaffer S and others: *Infection prevention and safe practice*, St. Louis, 1996, Mosby.

Schmidt E: Medical waste management. In Olmsted R, editor: *APIC infection control and applied epidemiology*, St. Louis, 1996, Mosby.

Sebazco S: Latex allergy. In Olmsted R, editor: *APIC infection control and applied epidemiology*, St. Louis, 1996, Mosby.

CHAPTER

26

Administering Medications

OBJECTIVES

Mastery of content in this chapter will enable the student to:

- Define the key terms listed.
- Discuss the nurse's legal responsibilities in medication prescription and administration.
- Describe the physiological mechanisms of medication action, including absorption, distribution, metabolism, and excretion of medications.
- Differentiate toxic, idiosyncratic, allergic, and side effects of medications.
- Discuss developmental factors that influence pharmacokinetics.
- Discuss factors that influence medication actions.
- Discuss methods of educating a client about prescribed medications.
- Describe the roles of the pharmacist, physician, and nurse in medication administration.
- Describe factors to consider when choosing routes of medication administration.
- Correctly calculate a prescribed medication dosage.
- Discuss factors to include in assessing a client's needs for and response to medication therapy.
- List the "five rights" of medication administration.
- Correctly prepare and administer subcutaneous, intramuscular, and intradermal injections; intravenous medications; oral and topical skin preparations; eye, ear, and nose drops; vaginal instillations; rectal suppositories; and inhalants.

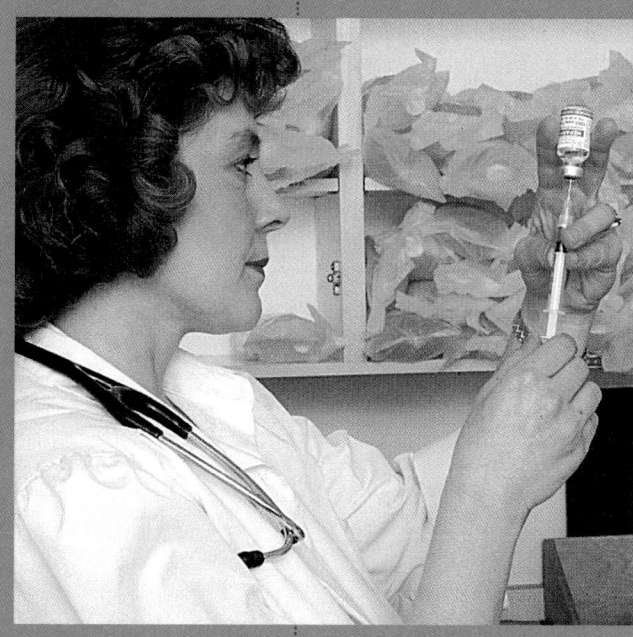

Clients with acute or chronic alterations in their health use many modalities to help restore or maintain their health. A medication is a substance used in the diagnosis, treatment, cure, relief, or prevention of health alterations. In fact, medications are the primary modality clients associate with restoration of health. No matter where clients receive their health care—hospitals, clinics, or home—the nurse plays an essential role in medication administration, medication teaching, and evaluating clients and the role medications play in restoration or maintenance of their health. The role of the nurse in medication activities is modified based on the setting of the client-nurse interaction.

In the primary care setting, the client often self-administers medications. The nurse is responsible for evaluating the effects of the medications on the client's health status and for teaching clients about their medications and their side effects, ensuring client compliance with medication regimens, and evaluating client technique when the client administers medication by routes that are not given by mouth. In the acute care setting, nurses spend a great deal of time in administering medication to clients. The nurse also ensures that clients are adequately prepared to administer their medications when they return to the community. In the home care setting clients usually administer their own medications. When clients cannot administer their own medications, family members or home health aides may be responsible for doing so. The nurse provides assessment of the effect the medications have in restoring or maintaining health, as well as providing continued education to the client, family, or home health care personnel in medication purpose and side effects.

SCIENTIFIC KNOWLEDGE BASE

Medications administered to clients are used, almost exclusively, to prevent, diagnose, or treat disease. Because medication administration and evaluation are essential to nursing practice, nurses need to have knowledge about the actions and effects of the medications they deliver to clients. This could not be done if the nurse did not have an understanding of the life sciences. Moreover, to safely and accurately administer medications to clients, nurses must have an understanding of pharmacokinetics (the movement of drugs in the human body), growth and development, nutrition, and mathematics. The nursing process organizes the nurse's thoughts and actions and forms the foundation for medication administration.

Application of Pharmacology in Nursing Practice

Names. A medication may have as many as three different names. A medication's chemical name pro-

vides an exact description of the medication's composition and molecular structure. Chemical names are rarely used in clinical practice. An example of a chemical name is N-acetyl-para-aminophenol, which is commonly known as Tylenol. The generic or nonproprietary name is given, with United States Adopted Name Council (USANC) approval, by the manufacturer who first develops the medication. Acetaminophen is an example of a generic name. It is the generic name for Tylenol. The generic name becomes the official name that is listed in official publications such as the *United States Pharmacopeia* (USP). The trade name, brand name, or proprietary name is the name under which a manufacturer markets a medication. The trade name has the symbol ®, at the upper right of the name, indicating that the manufacturer has copyrighted the medication's name

The nurse finds medications under a variety of different nomenclatures or names and must be careful to obtain the exact name and spelling for a particular medication.

Classification. Nurses learn to categorize medications with similar characteristics by their class. Medication classification indicates the effect of the medication on a body system, the symptoms the medication relieves, or the medication's desired effect. For example, clients who have non–insulin-dependent diabetes often take medications to lower their blood sugar level. This class of medication is called *oral hypoglycemic agent*. Usually each class contains more than one medication that can be prescribed for a type of health problem. For example, there are more than eight different types of oral hypoglycemic agents. The physical and chemical composition of medications within a class may be slightly different. A health care provider chooses a particular oral hypoglycemic medication based on client characteristics, cost, efficacy, dosing frequency, or prescriber experience with the medication.

A medication may also be part of more than one class. For example, aspirin is an analgesic, an antipyretic, and an antiinflammatory medication.

Medication forms. Medications are available in a variety of forms or preparations. The form of the medication determines its route of administration. The composition of a medication is designed to enhance its absorption and metabolism. Many medications are made in several forms such as tablets, capsules, elixirs, and suppositories. When administering a medication, the nurse must be certain to use the proper form (Table 26-1).

Medication Legislation and Standards

Federal regulations. The role of the U.S. government in regulation of the pharmaceutical industry is

TABLE 26-1
Forms of Medication

Form	Description
Caplet	Solid dosage for oral use; shaped like a capsule and coated for ease of swallowing.
Capsule	Solid dosage form for oral use; medication in a powder, liquid, or oil form and encased by a gelatin shell; capsule colored to aid in product identification.
Elixir	Clear fluid containing water and/or alcohol; designed for oral use; usually has a sweetener added.
Enteric-coated	Tablet for oral use is coated with materials that do not dissolve in the stomach; coatings dissolve in the intestine, where medication is absorbed.
Extract	Concentrated drug form made by removing the active portion of a drug from its other components (e.g., a fluid extract is a drug made into a solution from a vegetable source).
Glycerite	Solution of drug combined with glycerin for external use; contains at least 50% glycerin.
Intraocular disk	A small, flexible oval consisting of two soft, outer layers and a middle layer containing medication. When moistened by ocular fluid, it releases medication for up to 1 week.
Liniment	Preparation usually containing alcohol, oil, or soapy emollient that is applied to skin.
Lotion	Drug in liquid suspension applied to protect skin.
Ointment (salve)	Semisolid preparation, thicker and stiffer than ointment; absorbed through skin more slowly than ointment.
Paste	Semisolid preparation, thicker and stiffer than ointment; absorbed through skin more slowly than ointment.
Pill	Solid dosage form containing one or more drugs, shaped into globules, ovoids, or oblong shapes; true pills are rarely used; they have been replaced by tablets.
Solution	Liquid preparation that may be used orally, parenterally, externally, or inhaled; can also be instilled into a body organ or cavity (e.g., bladder irrigations); contains water with one or more dissolved compounds; must be sterile for parenteral use.
Suppository	Solid dosage form mixed with gelatin and shaped in form of pellet for insertion into body cavity (rectum or vagina); melts when it reaches body temperature, releasing drug for absorption.
Suspension	Finely divided drug particles dispersed in a liquid medium; when suspension is left standing, particles settle to the bottom of the container; commonly an oral medication and is not to be given intravenously.
Sustained-release	Solid dosage form that contains small particles of the drug coated with material that requires a varying amount of time to dissolve.
Syrup	Medication dissolved in a concentrated sugar solution; may contain flavoring to make drug more palatable.
Tablet	Powdered dosage form compressed into hard disks or cylinders; in addition to primary drug, contains binders (adhesive to allow powder to stick together), disintegrators (to promote tablet dissolution), lubricants (for ease of manufacturing), and fillers (for convenient tablet size).
Transdermal disk or patch	Medication contained within semipermeable membrane disk or patch, which allows medications to be absorbed through skin slowly over long periods.
Tincture	Alcohol or water-alcohol drug solution.
Troche (lozenge)	Flat, round dosage form containing drug, flavoring, sugar, and mucilage; dissolves in mouth to release drug.

to protect the health of the people by ensuring that medications are safe and effective. The first U.S. law to regulate medications was the Pure Food and Drug Act. This law simply requires all medications to be free of impure products. Subsequent legislation has set standards related to safety, potency, and efficacy. Enforcement of medication laws rests with the Food and Drug Administration (FDA) by ensuring that all medications on the market undergo vigorous review before they are allowed to be dispensed to the public.

In 1993 the FDA instituted the MedWatch program. This voluntary program encourages nurses and other health care professionals to report when a medication, product, or medical event causes serious harm to a client. The MedWatch form is available to report such events (Figure 26-1).

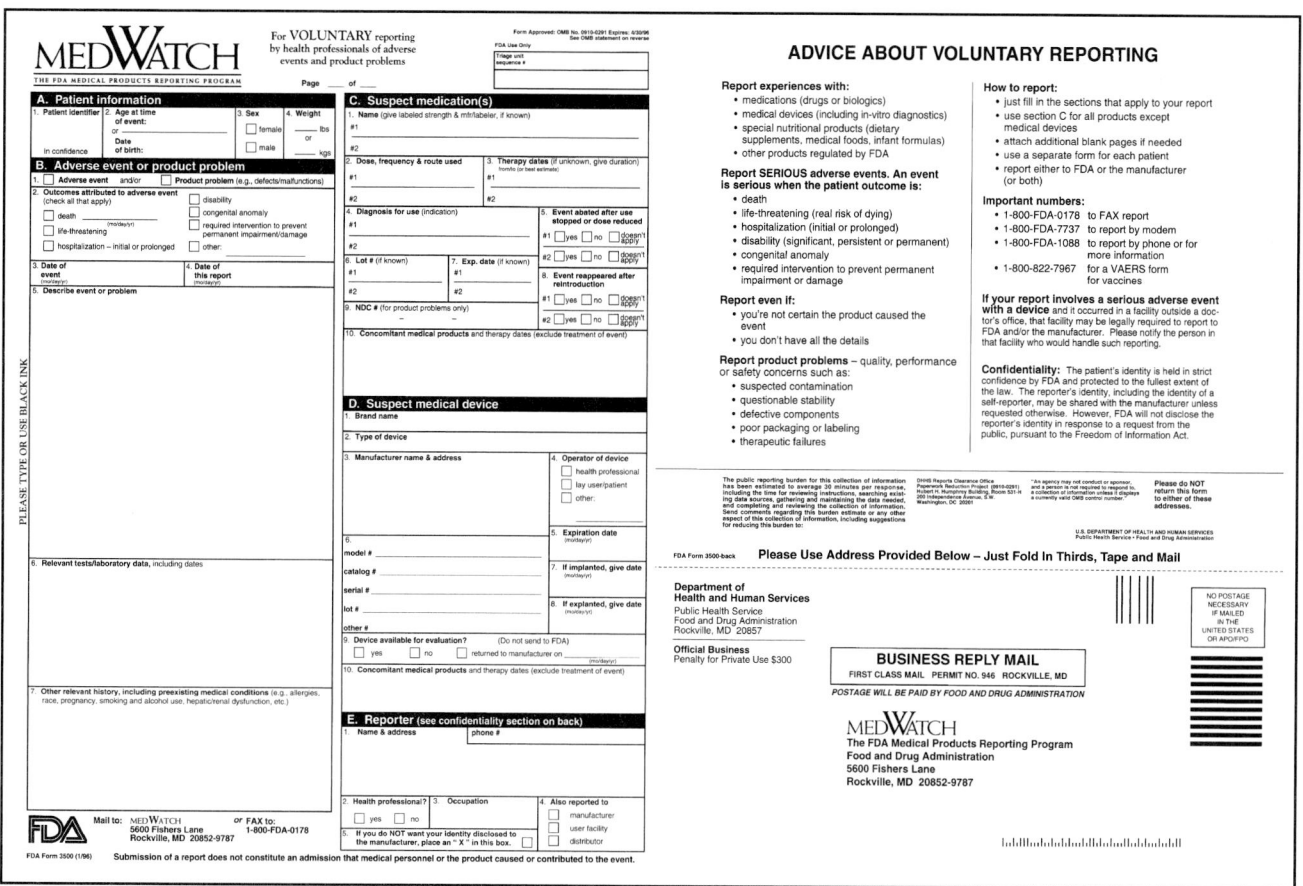

Figure 26-1. MedWatch form. FDA form 3500 (1/96). (Courtesy FDA, MedWatch, Rockville, Md.)

State and local regulation of medication.

State and locality medication laws must conform with federal legislation. States can also have additional controls, including control of substances not regulated by the federal government. Local governmental bodies also regulate the use of alcohol and tobacco.

Health care institutions and medication laws.

Health care institutions establish individual policies that must meet federal, state, and local regulations. The size of an institution, the types of services it provides, and the types of professional personnel it employs influence these policies. Institutional policies are often more restrictive than governmental controls. An institution is concerned primarily with preventing health problems resulting from medication use. For example, a common institutional policy is the automatic discontinuation of antibiotic therapy after a set number of days. Although a physician may reorder the antibiotic, this policy helps to control unnecessarily prolonged medication therapy.

Medication regulations and nursing practice.

State **nurse practice acts** have the most influence over nursing practice by defining the scope of a nurse's professional functions and responsibilities. In general, most nurse state practice acts are purposefully broad so as not to limit the professional responsibilities of the nurse. For example, most nurse practice acts state that nurses can "execute medical regime prescribed by a licensed physician" (New Jersey Department of Law and Public Safety, 1995). Institutions and agencies may interpret specific actions allowed under the acts, but they cannot modify, expand, or restrict the act's intent. The primary intent of the state nurse practice acts is to protect the public from unskilled, undereducated, and unlicensed nurses.

The nurse is responsible for following legal provisions when administering controlled substances or narcotics (medications that affect the mind and behavior), which are carefully controlled through federal and state guidelines. Violations of the Controlled Substances Act are punishable by fines, imprisonment, and loss of nurse licensure. Hospitals and other health care institutions have policies for the proper storage and distribution of narcotics (Box 26-1).

Nontherapeutic medication use.

Some people use medications for purposes other than their proper one. In the past the misuse or abuse of medications was

Box 26-1
Guidelines for Safe Narcotic Administration and Control

Store all narcotics in a locked, secure cabinet or container. (Computerized, locked cabinets are now available.)

Nurses in charge carry a set of keys (or a special computer entry code) for the narcotics cabinet.

During an institution's change of shift, the nurse going off duty counts all narcotics with the nurse coming on duty. Both nurses sign the narcotic record to indicate that the count is correct.

Discrepancies in narcotic counts are reported immediately.

A special inventory record is used each time a narcotic is dispensed.

The record is used to document the client's name, date, time of drug administration, name of drug, dosage, and signature of nurse dispensing the drug.

The form provides an accurate ongoing count of narcotics used and remaining.

If only one part of a premeasured dosage of a controlled substance is given, a second nurse witnesses disposal of the unused portion and documents such on the record form.

---

related to use for therapeutic qualities, such as the relief of pain or reduction in anxiety. At present, factors such as peer pressure, curiosity, and the pursuit of pleasure are motivators for nontherapeutic medication use. Problems with medication use are not limited to heroin, cocaine, and other "hard" medications. Millions of people in the United States and Canada consume alcohol daily. Our society is medication conscious, as shown by the frequent advertisements for pain relievers, decongestants, and antacids on television.

Nurses have ethical and legal responsibilities to understand the problems of persons using medications improperly. When caring for clients with suspected **medication abuse** or **medication dependence,** nurses must be aware of their own values and attitudes about the willful use of potentially harmful substances. Nurses cannot develop therapeutic relationships with clients if personal values interfere with acceptance or understanding of their needs. Knowing the physical, psychological, and social changes resulting from medication abuse allows nurses to identify clients with medication problems.

A problem involving the misuse of medications by health professionals also exists. Stress in the workplace, personal problems, and the strong desire to perform well are some of the factors that may cause nurses to

rely on medications. Nurses must recognize and understand the problems of colleagues who suffer from medication abuse. At present, many programs are available to assist these nurses toward recovery. These programs may be offered through the institution's Employee's Assistance Program, the state board of nursing, or community agencies.

Pharmacokinetics as the Basis of Medication Actions

For medications to be therapeutically useful they must be taken into a client's body; absorbed and distributed to cells, tissues, or a specific organ; and alter its physiological functions. **Pharmacokinetics** is the study of how medications enter the body, reach their site of action, are metabolized, and exit the body. The nurse uses knowledge of pharmacokinetics when timing medication administration, selecting the route of administration, judging the client's risk for alterations in medication action, and observing the client's response.

Absorption. **Absorption** refers to passage of medication molecules into the blood from its site of administration. Factors that influence medication absorption are the route of administration, ability of the medication to dissolve, blood flow to the site of administration, body surface area, and lipid solubility of medication.

Route of administration. Medications can be administered by various routes. Each route has a different rate of absorption. When medications are placed on the skin, absorption is slow because of the physical makeup of the skin. Medications placed on the mucous membranes and respiratory airways are quickly absorbed, because these tissues contain many blood vessels. Because orally administered medications must pass through the gastrointestinal (GI) tract to be absorbed, the overall rate of absorption may be slowed. Intravenous injection produces the most rapid absorption, because this route provides immediate access to the systemic circulation.

Ability of the medication to dissolve. The ability of an oral medication to dissolve depends largely on its form or preparation. Solutions and suspensions already in a liquid state are absorbed more readily than tablets or capsules. Acidic medications pass through the gastric mucosa rapidly. Medications that are basic are not absorbed before reaching the small intestine.

Blood flow to the area of absorption. When tissue contains many blood vessels, medications are absorbed more rapidly. This occurs because blood is constantly moving in a vessel, allowing for more medication-free blood. This facilitates the passage of blood into the medication.

Body surface area. When a medication is in contact with a large surface area, the medication will be absorbed at a faster rate. This explains why the majority of medications are absorbed in the small intestine rather than the stomach.

Lipid solubility of a medication. Medications that are highly lipid soluble are absorbed easier because they readily cross the cell membrane, which is made of a lipid layer.

Another factor that may affect absorption of a medication is whether food is in the stomach. Some oral medications are absorbed more easily when administered between meals, because food can change the structure of a medication and impair its absorption. Some medications when administered together may interfere with each other and impair the absorption of one or both.

Nurses often have knowledge of factors that may alter or impair absorption of the medications that have been prescribed for their client. The nurse uses this knowledge to ensure that all prescribed medications are administered correctly. It may be appropriate for the nurse to administer medications given half an hour before, half an hour after, and with meals or withhold medications if absorption is not likely to occur.

Distribution.

After a medication is absorbed, it is distributed within the body to tissues and organs and ultimately to its specific site of action. The rate and extent of distribution depend on the physical and chemical properties of medications and the physiology of the person taking the medication.

Circulation. Once a medication enters the bloodstream it is carried throughout the tissue and organs of the body. How fast it gets there depends on the vascularity of the various tissues and organs. When conditions exist that limit blood flow, or intended sites of action are poorly perfused, the distribution of a medication is inhibited. Consider the client who has a tumor. Solid tumors have poor blood supply and may not respond to therapy intended to destroy them.

Membrane permeability. To be distributed to an organ a medication must pass all of the biological membranes an organ or tissue has. Some membranes may serve as barriers to the passage of medications. The blood-brain barrier allows only fat-soluble medications to pass into the brain and cerebral spinal fluid. Central nervous system (CNS) infections require treatment with antibiotics injected directly into the subarachnoid space in the spinal cord. Older clients may experience adverse effects (e.g., confusion) as a result of the change in the permeability of the blood-brain barrier, with easier passage of fat-soluble medications. The placental membrane is a nonselective barrier to medications. Fat-soluble and non–fat-soluble agents may cross the placenta and produce fetal deformities, respiratory depression, and, with narcotic abuse, withdrawal symptoms.

Protein binding. The degree to which medications bind to serum proteins such as albumin affects medication distribution. Most medications bind to this protein to some extent. When medications bind to albumin, they cannot exert any pharmacological activity. The unbound or "free" medication is the active form of the medication. Older adults have a decrease in albumin in the bloodstream, probably caused by change in liver function. The same is true for clients with liver disease or malnutrition. Because of the potential for more medication being unbound, the older adult may be at risk for an increase in medication activity, toxicity, or both.

Metabolism.

After a medication reaches its site of action, it becomes metabolized into a less active or inactive form that is more easily excreted. **Biotransformation** occurs under the influence of enzymes that **detoxify,** degrade (break down), and remove biologically active chemicals. Most biotransformation occurs within the liver, although the lungs, kidneys, blood, and intestines also metabolize medications. The liver is especially important because its specialized structure oxidizes and transforms many toxic substances. The liver degrades many harmful chemicals before they become distributed to the tissues. If a decrease in liver function occurs, such as with aging or liver disease, a medication may be eliminated more slowly, resulting in an accumulation of the medication. If the organs that metabolize medications are altered, clients are at risk for medication toxicity. For example, a small sedative dose of a barbiturate may cause a client with liver disease to lapse into a hepatic coma.

Excretion.

After medications are metabolized, they exit the body through the kidneys, liver, bowel, lungs, and exocrine glands. The chemical makeup of a medication determines the organ of excretion. Gaseous and volatile compounds such as nitrous oxide and alcohol exit through the lungs. Deep breathing and coughing (see Chapter 40) help the postoperative client to eliminate anesthetic gases more rapidly. The exocrine glands excrete lipid-soluble medications. When medications exit through sweat glands, the skin may become irritated. The nurse assists the client in good hygiene practices (see Chapter 29) to promote cleanliness and skin integrity.

If a medication is excreted through the mammary glands, there is a risk that a nursing infant will ingest the chemicals. Mothers should check on the safety of any medication used while breast-feeding.

The GI tract is another route for medication excretion. Many medications enter the hepatic circulation to be broken down by the liver and excreted into the bile. After chemicals enter the intestines through the biliary tract, they may be reabsorbed by the intestines. Factors that increase peristalsis (e.g., laxatives, enemas) accelerate medication excretion through the feces, whereas factors that slow peristalsis (e.g., inactivity, improper diet) may prolong a medication's effects.

The kidneys are the main organs for medication

excretion. Some medications escape extensive metabolism and exit unchanged in the urine. Other medications must undergo biotransformation in the liver before being excreted by the kidney. If renal function declines, a client is at risk for medication toxicity. If the kidney cannot adequately excrete a medication, it may be necessary to reduce the dose. Maintenance of an adequate fluid intake (50 ml/kg/day) promotes proper elimination of medications for the average adult.

Types of Medication Action

Medications vary considerably in the way they act and their types of action. Factors other than characteristics of the medication also influence medication actions. A client may not respond in the same way to each successive dose of a medication. Likewise, the same medication dosage may cause very different responses in different clients. Box 26-2 lists important variables that influence medication action. It is important for the nurse to understand all the effects that medications have when taken by clients.

Therapeutic effects. The **therapeutic effect** is the expected or predictable physiological response a medication causes. Each medication has a desired therapeutic effect for which it is prescribed. For example, nitroglycerin is used to reduce the cardiac workload and increase myocardial oxygen supply. A single medication may have many therapeutic effects. For example, aspirin is an analgesic, antipyretic, antiinflammatory, and

reduces platelet aggregation (clumping). It is important for the nurse to know for which therapeutic effect a medication is prescribed. This will allow the nurse to properly teach the client about the medication's intended effect.

Side effects. A **side effect** is when a medication predictably will cause unintended, secondary effects. Side effects may be harmless or injurious. If the side effects are serious enough to negate the beneficial effects of a medication's therapeutic action, the prescriber may discontinue the medication. Clients often stop taking medications because of side effects.

Adverse effects. **Adverse effects** are generally considered severe responses to medication. For example, a client may become comatose when a drug is ingested. When adverse responses to medications occur, the prescriber must discontinue the medication. Some adverse effects are unexpected effects that were not discovered during drug testing. When this situation occurs, health care providers are obligated to report the adverse effect to the FDA (see Figure 26-1, p. 599).

Toxic effects. **Toxic effects** may develop after prolonged intake of a medication or when a medication accumulates in the blood because of impaired metabolism or excretion. Excess amounts of a medication within the body may have lethal effects, depending on the medication's action. For example, toxic levels of

---

◼ Box 26-2
Factors Influencing Drug Actions

Genetic Differences

A person's genetic makeup can influence drug metabolism. Members of a family may share a sensitivity to a medication.

Physiological Variables

Sex, age, body weight, nutritional status, and disease states all affect drug actions.

Hormonal differences between men and women affect drug metabolism.

Children require lower drug doses than adults. The changes accompanying aging alter the influence of drugs.

There is a direct relationship between the amount of medication administered and the amount of body tissue in which it is distributed. Proper drug metabolism relies on good nutrition.

Diseases that impair the function of organs responsible for normal pharmacokinetics also impair drug action.

Environmental Conditions

Stress and the exposure to heat and cold affect drug actions. Clients receiving vasodilators, for example, require lower drug dosages in warm weather.

The setting in which a drug is administered can influence a client's reaction. If a person is alone or isolated, more pain medication may be needed than if he or she is in a room with other clients.

Psychological Factors

A client's attitude, reaction to the meaning of a drug, and the nurse's behavior affect drug actions. If a client understands and accepts the need for a drug and if it is administered with a supportive behavior, the drug's effect is enhanced.

Diet

Drug and nutrient interactions can alter a drug's action or the effect of a nutrient. For example, mineral oil decreases the absorption of fat-soluble vitamins.

morphine may cause severe respiratory depression and death. Antidotes are available to treat specific types of medication toxicity. For example, Narcan is used to reverse the effects of opioid toxicity.

Idiosyncratic reactions.
Medications may cause unpredictable effects such as an **idiosyncratic reaction** in which a client overreacts or underreacts to a medication or has a reaction different from normal. For example, a child receiving an antihistamine (e.g., Benadryl) may become extremely agitated or excited instead of drowsy. It is impossible to assess clients for idiosyncratic responses.

Allergic reactions.
Allergic reactions are another unpredictable response to a medication; they make up 5% to 10% of all medication reactions. A client can become sensitized immunologically to the initial dose of a medication. With repeated administration the client develops an allergic response to the medication, its chemical preservatives, or a metabolite. The medication or chemical acts as an antigen, triggering the release of the body's antibodies. A client's **medication allergy** may be mild or severe. Allergic symptoms vary, depending on the individual and the medication. Among the different classes of medications, antibiotics cause a high incidence of allergic reactions. Common, mild allergy symptoms are summarized in Table 26-2. Severe or **anaphylactic reactions** are characterized by sudden constriction of bronchiolar muscles, edema of the pharynx and larynx, and severe wheezing and shortness of breath. Antihistamines, epinephrine, and bronchodilators may be used to treat anaphylactic reactions.

The client may also become severely hypotensive, necessitating emergency resuscitation measures. A client with a known history of an allergy to a medication should avoid reexposure and wear an identification bracelet or medal (Figure 26-2), which alerts nurses and physicians to the allergy if the client is unconscious when receiving medical care.

Medication interactions.
When one medication modifies the action of another medication, a **medication interaction** occurs. Medication interactions are common in individuals taking several medications. A medication may potentiate or diminish the action of other medications and may alter the way in which another medication is absorbed, metabolized, or eliminated from the body. When two medications have a **synergistic effect,** or act synergistically, the effect of the two medications combined is greater than the effect of the medications when given separately. For example, alcohol is a CNS depressant that has a synergistic effect on antihistamines, antidepressants, barbiturates, and narcotic analgesics.

A medication interaction is not always undesirable. Often a physician orders combination medication therapy to create a medication interaction for the client's therapeutic benefit. For example, a client with moderate hypertension typically receives several medications such as diuretics and vasodilators that act together to control blood pressure.

Medication dose responses.
After a nurse administers a medication, it undergoes absorption, distribution, metabolism, and excretion. Except when administered intravenously, medications take time to enter the bloodstream. The quantity and distribution of a medication in different body compartments change constantly. When a medication is prescribed, the goal is a constant blood level within a safe therapeutic range. Repeated doses are required to achieve a constant therapeutic **concentration** of a medication, because a portion of a medication is always being excreted. The highest serum concentration (peak concentration) of the

TABLE 26-2	
Mild Allergic Reactions	

Symptom	Description
Urticaria (hives)	Raised, irregularly shaped skin eruptions with varying sizes and shapes; have reddened margins and pale centers
Eczema (rash)	Small, raised vesicles that are usually reddened; often distributed over entire body
Pruritus	Itching of skin; accompanies most rashes
Rhinitis	Inflammation of mucous membranes lining nose; causes swelling and clear, watery discharge

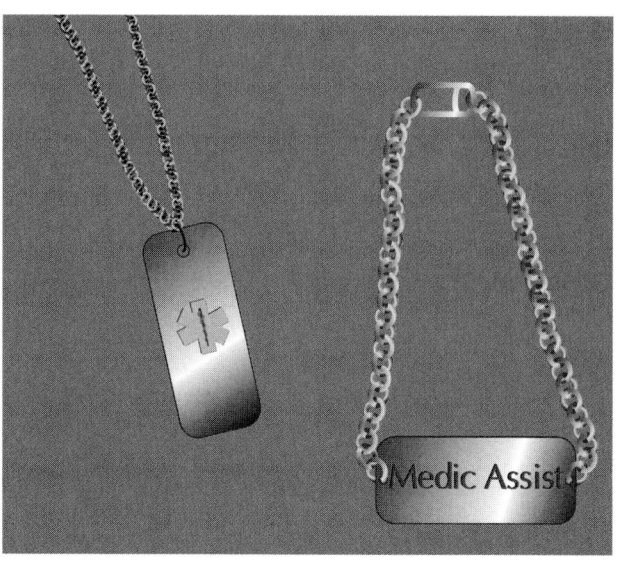

Figure 26-2. Identification bracelet and medal.

medication usually occurs just before the last of the medication is absorbed (Clark and others, 1996). After peaking, the serum medication concentration falls progressively. With intravenous **infusions,** the peak concentration occurs quickly, but the serum level also begins to fall immediately (Figure 26-3).

All medications have a **serum half-life,** which is the time it takes for excretion processes to lower the serum medication concentration by half. To maintain a therapeutic plateau, the client must receive regular fixed doses. For example, it has been shown that pain medications are most effective when they are given "around the clock" rather than when the client intermittently complains of pain. In this way an almost constant level of pain medication is maintained. After an initial medication dose the client receives each successive dose when the previous dose reaches its half-life.

The client and nurse must follow regular dosage schedules and adhere to prescribed doses and dosage intervals. Dosage schedules are set by the agency in which the nurse is employed. Table 26-3 lists common dosage schedules used in acute care settings. When teaching clients about dosage schedules the nurse uses language that is familiar to the client. For example, when teaching a client about b.i.d. medication dosing the nurse instructs the client to take a medication in the morning and again in the evening. Knowledge of the time intervals of medication action also helps the nurse to anticipate a medication's effect. With this knowledge the nurse can instruct the client when to expect a re-

sponse. Table 26-4 lists common terms associated with medication actions.

Routes of Administration

The route prescribed for administering a medication depends on the medication's properties and desired effect and on the client's physical and mental condition

TABLE 26-3
Common Dosage Administration Schedule

Abbreviation	Meaning
AC, ac	Before meals
ad lib	As desired
BID, bid	Twice a day
h	Hour
HS, hs	Hour of sleep
PC, pc	After meals
p.r.n.	Whenever there is a need
qAM	Every morning, every AM
qd, od	Every day
qh	Every hour
q2h	Every 2 hours
q4h	Every 4 hours
q6h	Every 6 hours
q8h	Every 8 hours
QID, qid	4 times a day
QOD, qod	Every other day
STAT	Give immediately
TID, tid	3 times a day

TABLE 26-4
Terms Associated With Medication Actions

Term	Meaning
Onset	Time it takes after a drug is administered for it to produce a response
Peak	Time it takes for a drug to reach its highest effective concentration
Trough	Minimum blood serum concentration of a drug reached just before the next scheduled dose
Duration	Time during which the drug is present in a concentration great enough to produce a response
Plateau	Blood serum concentration of a drug reached and maintained after repeated fixed doses

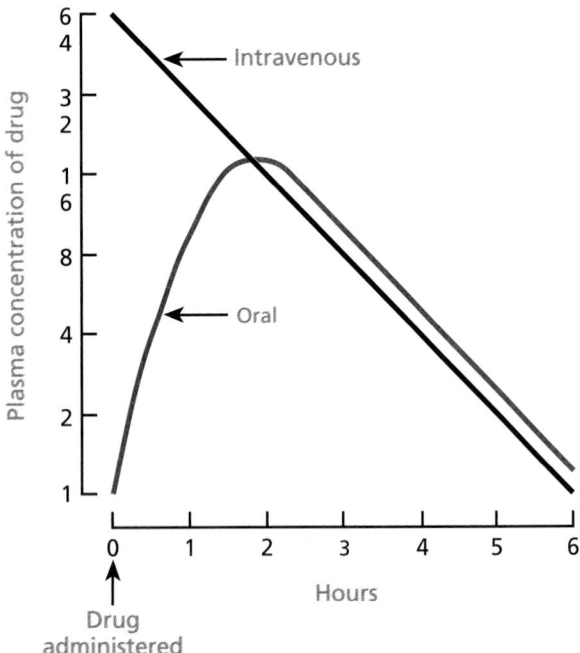

Figure 26-3. Curve showing therapeutic blood levels. (From Clark JB and others: *Pharmacologic basis of nursing practice,* ed 5, St. Louis, 1996, Mosby.)

(Table 26-5). A nurse collaborates with the physician in determining the best route for a client's medication, as in the following hypothetical situation:

The client, Mr. Huels, has progressively worsened physically. His temperature is 39.28° C. He complains of nausea and is unable to tolerate oral fluids. The nurse checks Mr. Huels' order, which reads,

"Aspirin 600 mg orally for temperature above 38.5° C." On the basis of the assessment, the nurse believes that because Mr. Huels is nauseated, he will not be able to tolerate an oral dose of aspirin. By consulting the physician, the nurse acquires an order for a rectal suppository instead. A rectal suppository enables the nurse to administer aspirin to decrease the fever without increasing the client's symptoms of nausea.

TABLE 26-5

Factors Influencing Choice of Administration Routes

Advantages	Disadvantages
Oral, Buccal, Sublingual Routes	
Routes are convenient and comfortable for client. Routes are economical. Medications may produce local or systemic effects. Routes rarely cause anxiety for client.	These routes are avoided when client has alterations in GI function (e.g., nausea, vomiting), reduced motility (after general anesthesia or bowel inflammation), gastric suction, surgical resection of portion of GI tract, and reduced ability to swallow. Oral medications may irritate lining of GI tract, discolor teeth, or have unpleasant taste.
SQ, IM, IV, ID Routes	
Routes provide means of administration when oral drugs are contraindicated. More rapid absorption occurs than with topical or oral routes. IV infusion provides drug delivery when client is critically ill. If peripheral perfusion is poor, IV route is preferred over injections.	There is risk of introducing infection, drugs are expensive, and these routes are avoided in clients with bleeding tendencies. There is risk of tissue damage with SQ injections. IM and IV routes are dangerous because of rapid absorption. These routes cause considerable anxiety in many clients, especially children.
Skin	
Topical	
Topical skin applications primarily provide local effect. Route is painless. Limited side effects occur.	Extensive applications may be bulky and cause difficulty in maneuvering. Clients with skin abrasions are at risk for rapid drug absorption and systemic effects.
Transdermal	
Transdermal applications provide prolonged systemic effects, with limited side effects.	Application leaves oily or pasty substance on skin and may soil clothing.
Mucous Membranes*	
Therapeutic effects are provided by local application to involved sites. Aqueous solutions are readily absorbed and capable of causing systemic effects. Mucous membranes provide route of administration when oral drugs are contraindicated.	Mucous membranes are highly sensitive to some drug concentrations. Insertion of rectal and vaginal medication often causes embarrassment. Client with ruptured eardrum cannot receive irrigations. Rectal suppositories are contraindicated if client has had rectal surgery or if active rectal bleeding is present.
Inhalation	
Inhalation provides rapid relief for local respiratory problems. Route provides easy access for introduction of general anesthetic gases.	Some local agents can cause serious systemic effects.

*Includes eyes, ears, nose, vagina, rectum, buccal, sublingual routes.

Oral routes

Oral administration. The oral route is the easiest and the most commonly used. Medications are given by mouth and swallowed with fluid. Oral medications have a slower onset of action and a more prolonged effect than parenteral medications. Clients generally prefer the oral route.

Sublingual administration. Some medications are designed to be readily absorbed after being placed under the tongue to dissolve (Figure 26-4). A medication given by **sublingual** route should not be swallowed, or the desired effect will not be achieved. Nitroglycerin is commonly given by sublingual route. A drink should not be taken by the client until the medication is completely dissolved.

Buccal administration. Administration of a medication by the **buccal** route involves placing the solid medication in the mouth and against the mucous membranes of the cheek until the medication dissolves (Figure 26-5). Clients should be taught to alternate cheeks with each subsequent dose to avoid mucosal irritation. Clients are also warned not to chew or swallow the medication or to take any liquids with it. A buccal medication acts locally on the mucosa or systemically as it is swallowed in a person's saliva.

Parenteral routes.
Parenteral administration involves injecting a medication into body tissues. The four major sites of injection include the following:

1. **Subcutaneous (SQ):** Injection into tissues just below the dermis of the skin
2. **Intramuscular (IM):** Injection into a muscle
3. **Intravenous (IV):** Injection into a vein
4. **Intradermal (ID):** Injection into the dermis just under the epidermis

Some medications may be administered into body cavities through other routes, including epidural, intraperitoneal, intrathecal or intraspinal, intracardiac, intrapleural, intraarterial, intraosseous, and intraarticular routes. Nurses with advanced training or in advanced practice may administer medications by these routes. Medication routes such as intracardiac or intraarticular are usually limited to physician administration. Regardless of whether the nurse actually administers the medication by these routes, the nurse often remains responsible for monitoring the integrity of the system of medication delivery, understanding the therapeutic value of the medication, and evaluating the client's response to the therapy.

Topical administration. Medications applied to the skin and mucous membranes generally have local effects. The topical medication is applied to the skin by painting or spreading it over an area, applying moist dressings, soaking body parts in a solution, or giving medicated baths. Systemic effects can occur if a client's skin is thin, if the medication concentration is high, or if contact with the skin is prolonged.

Some medications (e.g., nitroglycerin, scopolamine, estrogens) have systemic effects because they are applied topically by a **transdermal disk** or patch. The disk secures the medicated ointment to the skin. These topical applications may be applied for as little as 24 hours or as long as 7 days.

Medications can be applied to mucous membranes in a variety of ways, including the following:

1. By directly applying a liquid or ointment (e.g., eye drops, gargling, swabbing the throat)
2. By inserting a medication into a body cavity (e.g., placing a suppository in rectum or vagina, inserting medicated packing into vagina)
3. By instilling fluid into body cavity (e.g., ear drops, nose drops, bladder or rectal **instillation** [fluid is retained])
4. By irrigating a body cavity (e.g., flushing eye, ear, vagina, bladder, or rectum with medicated fluid [fluid is not retained])
5. Spraying (e.g., instillation into nose and throat)

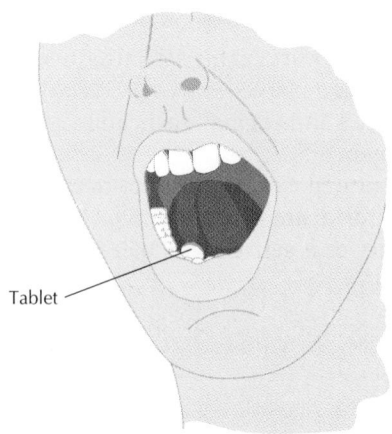

Tablet

Figure 26-4. Sublingual administration of a tablet.

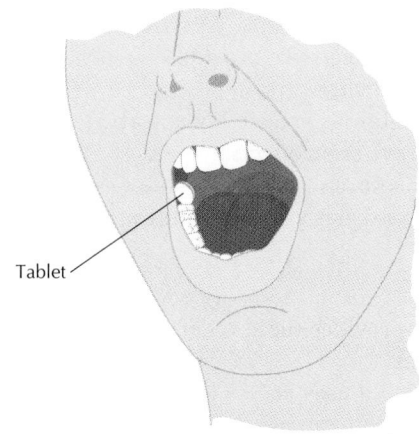

Tablet

Figure 26-5. Buccal administration of a tablet.

Inhalation route.

The deeper passages of the respiratory tract provide a large surface area for medication absorption. Medications can be administered through the nasal passages, oral passage, or tubes that have been placed into the client's mouth to the trachea (Figure 26-6). Medications that are administered by the **inhalation** route are readily absorbed and work rapidly because of the rich vascular alveolar-capillary network present in the pulmonary tissue. Inhaled medications may have local or systemic effects.

Intraocular route.

Intraocular medication delivery involves inserting a medication similar to a contact lens into the client's eye. The eye medication disk has two soft outer layers that have medication enclosed in them. The disk is inserted into the client's eye, much like a contact lens. The disk can remain in the client's eye for up to 1 week. Pilocarpine, a medication used to treat glaucoma, is the most common medication disk seen.

Systems of Medication Measurement

The proper administration of a medication depends on the nurse's ability to compute medication doses accurately and measure medications correctly. A careless mistake in placing a decimal point or adding a zero to a dose can lead to a fatal error. The nurse is responsible for checking the dose before giving a medication.

The metric, apothecary, and household systems of measurement are used in medication therapy. Most nations, including Canada, use the metric system as their standard of measurement. Although the U.S. Congress has not officially adopted the metric system, most health professionals in the United States use it. **Prescriptions** to be self-administered are often written in household measures for clients. The **apothecary system** is rarely used.

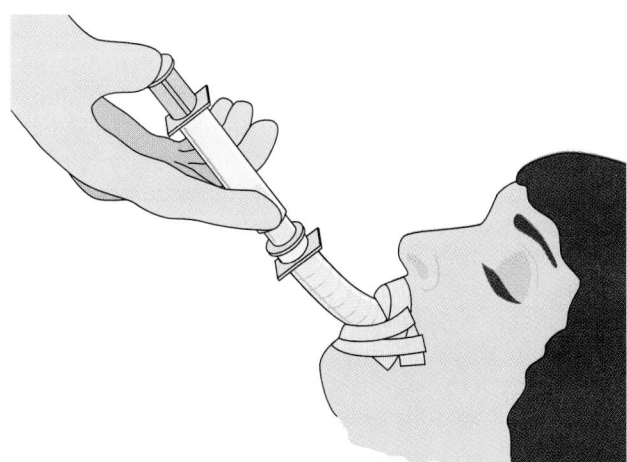

Figure 26-6. Medication being instilled through endotracheal tube using the syringe method.

Metric system.

As a decimal system the **metric system** is the most logically organized. Metric units can easily be converted and computed through simple multiplication and division. Each basic unit of measurement is organized into units of 10. Multiplying or dividing by 10 forms secondary units. In multiplication, the decimal point moves to the right; in division, the decimal moves to the left. For example:

$$10.0 \text{ mg} \times 10 = 100.0 \text{ mg}$$
$$10.0 \text{ mg} \div 10 = 1.0 \text{ mg}$$

The basic units of measurement in the metric system are the meter (length), liter (volume), and gram (weight). For medication calculations the nurse uses only the volume and weight units. In the metric system, small or large letters are used to designate basic units:

$$\text{Gram} = \text{g or Gm}$$
$$\text{Liter} = \text{l or L}$$

Small letters are abbreviations for other units:

$$\text{Milligram} = \text{mg}$$
$$\text{Milliliter} = \text{ml}$$

A system of Latin prefixes designates subdivision of the basic units: deci- ($\frac{1}{10}$ or 0.1), centi- ($\frac{1}{100}$ or 0.01), and milli- ($\frac{1}{1000}$ or 0.001). Greek prefixes designate multiples of the basic units: deka- (10), hecto- (100), and kilo- (1000). When writing medication doses in metric units, physicians and nurses use fractions or multiples of a unit. Fractions are always in decimal form:

$$500 \text{ mg or } 0.5 \text{ g, not } \frac{1}{2} \text{ g}$$
$$10 \text{ ml or } 0.01 \text{ L, not } \frac{1}{100} \text{ L}$$

When fractions are used, a zero is always placed in front of the decimal to prevent error.

Household measurements.

Household units of measure are familiar to most people. The disadvantage with household measures is their inaccuracy. Household utensils such as teaspoons and cups often vary in size. Scales to measure pints or quarts are often not well calibrated. Household measures include drops, teaspoons, tablespoons, and cups for volume and pints and quarts for weight. Although pints and quarts are considered household measures, they are also used in the apothecary system.

The advantage of household measurements is their convenience and familiarity. When the accuracy of a medication dose is not critical, it is safe to use household measures. For example, many over-the-counter (OTC) medications can safely be measured by this method. Table 26-6 gives common equivalents from each measurement unit.

Solutions.

The nurse uses solutions of various concentrations for **injections, irrigations,** and infusions.

TABLE 26-6

Equivalents of Measurement

Metric	Apothecary	Household
1 ml	15-16 minims (℥)	15 drops (gtt)
4-5 ml	1 fluidram (f℥)	1 teaspoon (tsp)
16 ml	4 fluidrams (f℥)	1 tablespoon (tbsp)
30 ml	1 fluid ounce (f℥)	2 tablespoons (tbsp)
240 ml	8 fluid ounces (f℥)	1 cup (c)
480 ml (approximately 500 ml)	1 pint (pt)	1 pint (pt)
960 ml (approximately 1 L)	1 quart (qt)	1 quart (qt)
3840 ml (approximately 5 L)	1 gallon (gal)	1 gallon (gal)

A **solution** is a given mass of solid substance dissolved in a known volume of fluid or a given volume of liquid dissolved in a known volume of another fluid. When a solid is dissolved in a fluid, the concentration is in units of mass per units of volume (e.g., g/ml, g/L, mg/ml). A concentration of a solution may also be expressed as a percentage. A 10% solution, for example, is 10 g of solid dissolved in 100 ml of solution. A proportion also expresses concentrations. A $\frac{1}{1000}$ solution represents a solution containing 1 g of solid in 1000 ml of liquid or 1 ml of liquid mixed with 1000 ml of another liquid.

Clinical Calculations

To administer medications it is often necessary for the nurse to have a understanding of basic arithmetic to calculate medication dosages, mix solutions, and perform a variety of other activities. This skill is important because medications are not always dispensed in the unit of measure in which they are ordered. This occurs because medication companies package and bottle certain standard equivalents. For example, the physician may order 250 mg of a medication that is available only in grams. The nurse is responsible for converting available units of volume and weight to the desired doses. Therefore the nurse should be aware of approximate equivalents in all major measurement systems.

Conversions Within One System

Converting measurements within one system is relatively easy. In the metric system the nurse simply divides or multiplies. To change milligrams to grams, the nurse divides by 1000, moving the decimal 3 points to the left.

$$1000 \text{ mg} = 1 \text{ g}$$
$$350 \text{ mg} = 0.35 \text{ g}$$

To convert liters to milliliters, the nurse multiplies by 1000 or moves the decimal 3 points to the right.

$$1 \text{ L} = 1000 \text{ ml}$$
$$0.25 \text{ L} = 250 \text{ ml}$$

To convert units of measurement within the apothecary or household system, the nurse must consult an equivalent table. For example, when converting fluid ounces to quarts the nurse must first know that 32 ounces is the equivalent of 1 quart. To convert 8 ounces to a quart measurement, for example, the nurse divides 8 by 32 to get the equivalent, $\frac{1}{4}$ or 0.25 quart.

Conversion between systems. The nurse must frequently determine the proper dose of a medication by converting weights or volumes from one system of measurement to another. Often, metric units must be converted to equivalent household measures for use at home. To make actual medication calculations, it is necessary to work with units in the same measurement system. Tables of equivalent measurements are available in all health care institutions. The pharmacist is also a good resource.

Before making a conversion, the nurse compares the measurement system available with that ordered. For example, the prescriber orders Robitussin 30 ml. To provide proper instruction to the client, the nurse must convert "ml" to common household measurement. To convert "ml" to tablespoon, the nurse must know the equivalent, 30 ml = 2 tablespoons or refer to a table such as the one in Table 26-7.

Dosage calculations. There are many formulas that can be used to calculate medication dosages. The following basic formula can be applied when preparing solid or liquid forms:

$$\frac{\text{Dose ordered}}{\text{Dose on hand}} \times \frac{\text{Amount on}}{\text{hand}} = \frac{\text{Amount to}}{\text{administer}}$$

The dose ordered is the amount of pure medication prescribed. The dose on hand is the weight or volume of medication available in units supplied by the pharmacy; it may be expressed on the medication label as the contents of a tablet or capsule or as the amount of medication dissolved per unit volume of liquid. The amount on hand is the basic unit or quantity of the medication that contains the dose on hand. For solid medications the amount on hand may be one capsule; the amount of liquid on hand may be a milliliter or liter depending on the container. The amount to administer is the actual amount of available medication the nurse will administer. The amount to administer is always expressed in the same unit as the amount on hand.

The following example illustrates how to apply the formula. The prescriber orders the client to receive

TABLE 26-7
Ways to Prevent Drug Administration Errors

Precaution	Rationale
Read drug labels carefully.	Many products come in similar containers, colors, and shapes.
Question administration of multiple tablets or vials for single dose.	Most doses are one or two tablets or capsules or one single-dose vial. Incorrect interpretation of order may result in excessively high dose.
Be aware of drugs with similar names.	Many drug names sound alike (e.g., digoxin and digitoxin, Keflex and Keflin, Orinase and Ornade).
Check decimal point.	Some drugs come in quantities that are multiples of one another (e.g., Coumadin in 2.5- and 25-mg tablets, Thorazine in 30- and 300-mg spansules).
Question abrupt and excessive increases in dosages.	Most dosages are increased gradually so that physician can monitor therapeutic effect and response.
When new or unfamiliar drug is ordered, consult resource.	If prescriber is also unfamiliar with drug, there is greater risk of inaccurate dosages being ordered.
Do not administer drug ordered by nickname or unofficial abbreviation.	Many prescribers refer to commonly ordered medications by nicknames or unofficial abbreviations. If nurse or pharmacist is unfamiliar with name, wrong drug may be dispensed and administered.
Do not attempt to decipher illegible writing.	When in doubt, ask prescriber. Unless nurse questions order that is difficult to read, chance of misinterpretation is great.
Know clients with same last names. Also have clients state their full names. Check name bands carefully.	It is common to have two or more clients with same or similar last names. Special labels on Kardex or medication book can warn of potential problem.
Do not confuse equivalents.	When in hurry, it may be easy to misread equivalents (e.g., milligram instead of milliliter).

Demerol 50 mg IM (dose ordered). The medication is available only in ampules containing 100 mg (dose on hand) in 1 millimeter (amount on hand). The formula is applied as follows:

$$\frac{50 \text{ mg}}{100 \text{ mg}} \times 1 \text{ ml} = \text{Volume in milliliter to administer}$$

To simplify the $^{50}/_{100}$ fraction, divide numerator and denominator by 50:

$$\frac{1}{2} \times 1 \text{ ml} = \frac{1}{2} \text{ ml to administer}$$

Syringes are calibrated only in decimals. After converting the fraction $\frac{1}{2}$ to 0.5, the nurse can more accurately draw up the correct dose.

Another example demonstrates how the formula applies with solid dose forms. The physician orders 0.125 mg PO of digoxin. The medication is available in tablets containing 0.25 mg.

$$\frac{0.125 \text{ mg}}{0.250 \text{ mg}} \times 1 \text{ Tablet} = \text{Tablets to administer}$$

The fraction $^{0.125}/_{0.250}$ equals $\frac{1}{2}$ or 0.5. Therefore,

$$0.5 \times 1 \text{ Tablet} = 0.5 \text{ or } \frac{1}{2} \text{ tablet to be administered}$$

Many tablets come with scores or indentations across the center of the tablet. A scored tablet is easy to break in half for divided doses. In some institutions pharmacists are responsible for scoring tablets. The potential for giving an incorrect dosage is high when the nurse estimates amounts by breaking unscored tablets.

Often, liquid medications come prepared in volumes greater than 1 ml. The formula still applies. For example, the order states, "Erythromycin suspension 250 mg PO." The pharmacy delivers 100-ml bottles with the labels stating, "5 ml contains 125 mg of erythromycin."

$$\frac{250 \text{ mg}}{125 \text{ mg}} \times 5 \text{ ml} = \text{Volume to administer}$$

The fraction $^{250}/_{125}$ equals 2. Therefore,

$$2 \times 5 \text{ ml} = 10 \text{ ml to administer}$$

Here the nurse ignores the total volume available and instead uses the values noted on the label. If the nurse calculated the dose on the basis of 100 ml available, the following error would occur:

$$\frac{250 \text{ mg}}{125 \text{ mg}} \times 100 \text{ ml} = 200 \text{ ml to administer}$$

On the basis of this calculation the client would receive 20 times the desired dose. The nurse should always double-check calculations or confer with another professional if an answer seems unreasonable.

Pediatric Dosages

Calculating children's medication dosages requires caution. Children are unable to metabolize many medications as readily as adults. The child's body size also requires smaller dosages. In most cases the prescriber will calculate the dose for a child before ordering the medication. However, nurses should be aware of the formulas used to calculate pediatric dosages and recheck all dosages before administration. Most medication references list the normal ranges for pediatric dosages.

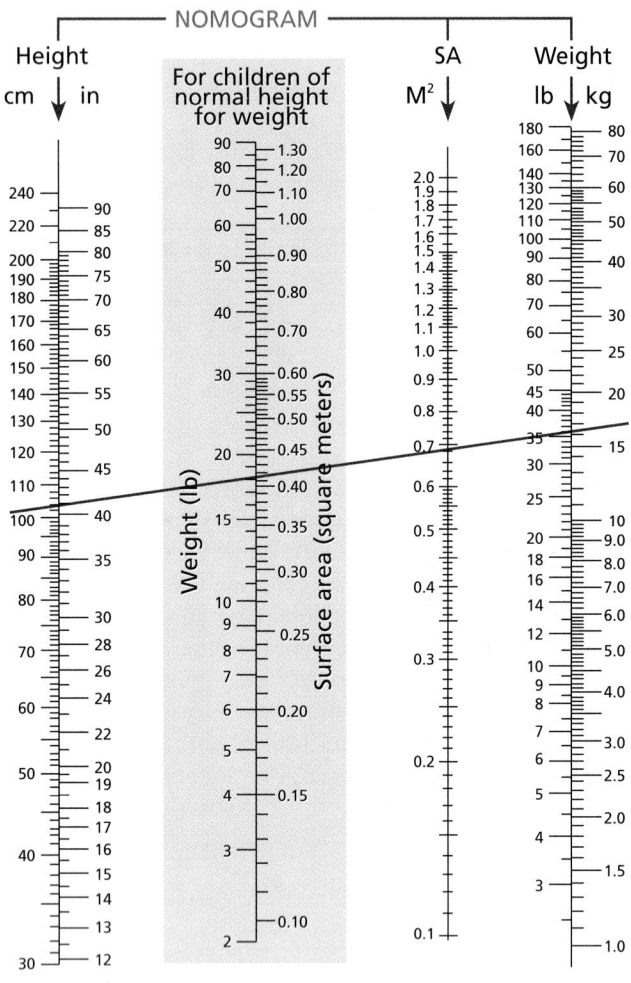

Figure 26-7. West nomogram for estimation of surface areas in children. A straight line is drawn between height and weight. The point where the line crosses the surface area column is the estimated body surface area. (From Behrman RE, Vaughan VC, editors: *Nelson textbook of pediatrics*, ed 13, Philadelphia, 1987, WB Saunders; modified from data of Boyd E, by West CD.)

The most accurate method of calculating pediatric dosages is based on a child's body surface area. Body surface area is estimated on the basis of the child's height and weight. A standard nomogram (e.g., the West nomogram) can be used for estimation of a child's body surface area (Figure 26-7).

To calculate a pediatric dose the nurse uses the following formula. The formula is a ratio of the child's body surface area compared with the body surface area of an average adult (1.7 square meters, or 1.7 m²).

$$\text{Child's dose} = \frac{\text{Surface area of child}}{1.7 \text{ m}^2} \times \text{Normal adult dose}$$

For example, a prescriber orders ampicillin for a child weighing 12 kg. The normal adult dose for ampicillin is 250 mg. The West nomogram shows that a child weighing 12 kg has a surface area of 0.54 m². Using this information the nurse then can calculate the appropriate child's dose.

$$\text{Child's dose} = \frac{0.54 \text{ m}^2}{1.7 \text{ m}^2} \times 250 \text{ mg}$$

The m² units are canceled out.

$$\text{Child's dose} = \frac{0.54}{1.7} \times 250 \text{ mg}$$

$$\frac{0.54}{1.7} = 0.3$$

$$\text{Child's dose} = 0.3 \times 250 \text{ mg} = 75 \text{ mg}$$

Administering Medications

The nurse does not have sole responsibility for medication administration. The prescriber* and pharmacist also help to ensure the right medication gets to the right client. However, the nurse administering medications is accountable for knowing what medications are prescribed, their therapeutic and nontherapeutic effects, and the client's needs and abilities.

Prescriber's role. The physician or nurse practitioner prescribes the client's medications. The prescriber writes an order on a form in the client's medical record, in an order book, on a legal prescription pad, or through a computer terminal. Where allowed, a prescriber may also order a medication by telephone or by giving the nurse a verbal order.

The nurse enters and signs all telephone and verbal orders, writes the name of the prescriber ordering the medication, and later has the prescriber countersign the order. Most institutions require a prescriber's signature within 24 hours after the order is made.

---

*Refers to physician, advanced practice nurses (e.g., nurse practitioner, clinical nurse specialist), or physician's assistant.

Institutional policies vary regarding the personnel who can take verbal or telephone orders. Generally, nursing students cannot take medication orders. No medication is to be given without an order. If the technology is available, a physician may fax orders to the unit.

Common abbreviations are used when writing orders. The abbreviations indicate dosage frequencies or times, routes of administration, and special information for giving the medication (see Table 26-4).

Types of orders in acute care agencies. Four common types of medication orders are based on the frequency and/or urgency of medication administration.

Standing orders. A standing order is carried out until the physician cancels it by another order or until a prescribed number of days elapse. A standing order may indicate a final date or number of treatments or dosages. Many institutions have policies for automatically discontinuing standing orders. The following are examples of standing orders:

Tetracycline 500 mg PO q6h and Decadron 10 mg qd × 5 days

P.R.N. orders. The physician may order a medication when a client requires it. This is a p.r.n. order. The nurse uses objective assessment, subjective assessment, and discretion in determining whether the client needs the medication. Often the physician sets minimum intervals for the time of administration. This means the medication cannot be given any more often than what is prescribed. Examples of p.r.n. orders are:

Morphine sulfate 2 mg SQ q3-4h p.r.n. for incisional pain and Maalox 30 ml p.r.n. for gastric discomfort.

When medications are administered, the nurse documents the assessment made and the time of medication administration. The nurse should make frequent evaluation of the effectiveness of the medication and record findings in the appropriate record.

Single (one-time) orders. A physician will often order a medication to be given only once at a specified time. This is common for preoperative medications or medications given before diagnostic examinations. For example:

Versed 25 mg IM on call to OR and Valium 10 mg PO at 0900.

STAT orders. A STAT order signifies that a single dose of a medication is to be given immediately and only once. STAT orders are often written for emergencies when the client's condition changes suddenly. For example:

Give Apresoline 10 mg IM STAT.

Some conditions change the status of a client's medication orders. For example, surgery automatically cancels all of a client's preoperative medications (see Chapter 40). Because the client's condition changes after surgery, the physician must write new orders. When a client is transferred to another health care agency or a different service within a hospital or is discharged, the physician should review the medications and write new orders as indicated.

Prescriptions. The physician writes prescriptions for clients who are to take medications outside the hospital. The prescription includes more detailed information than a regular order, because the client must understand how to take the medication and when to refill the prescription if necessary. The parts of a prescription are included in Figure 26-8.

Pharmacist's role. The pharmacist prepares and distributes prescribed medications. Pharmacists may also assess the medication plan and evaluate the client's medication-related needs (American Pharmaceutical Association, 1994). The pharmacist is responsible for filling prescriptions accurately and for being sure that prescriptions are valid.

Distribution systems. Systems for storing and distributing medications vary. Pharmacists provide the medications, but nurses distribute medications to clients. Institutions providing nursing care have a special area for stocking and dispensing medications. Special medication rooms, portable locked carts, computerized medication cabinets, and individual storage units next to clients' rooms are some of the facilities used. Nurses must make sure that storage areas are locked when unattended.

Stock supply. With a stock system, medications are available in larger, multidose containers. This system is not only time consuming but also costly, because a nurse must dispense each medication separately for a client. This type of system of medication delivery has been associated with a high rate of medication errors and is not commonly used at present (Perini and Vermeulen, 1994).

Unit dose. The unit-dose system uses portable carts containing a drawer with a 24-hour supply of medications for each client. The unit dose is the ordered dose of medication the client receives at one time. Each tablet or capsule is wrapped in a foil or paper container. At a designated time each day the pharmacist refills the drawers in the cart with a fresh supply. The cart also contains limited amounts of p.r.n. and stock medications for special situations. The unit-dose system is designed to reduce the number of medication errors and saves steps in dispensing medications.

Computer-controlled dispensing systems. Computer-controlled dispensing systems are used successfully throughout the country (Figure 26-9). They are especially useful for the delivery and control of **narcotics.** Each nurse has a security code allowing access

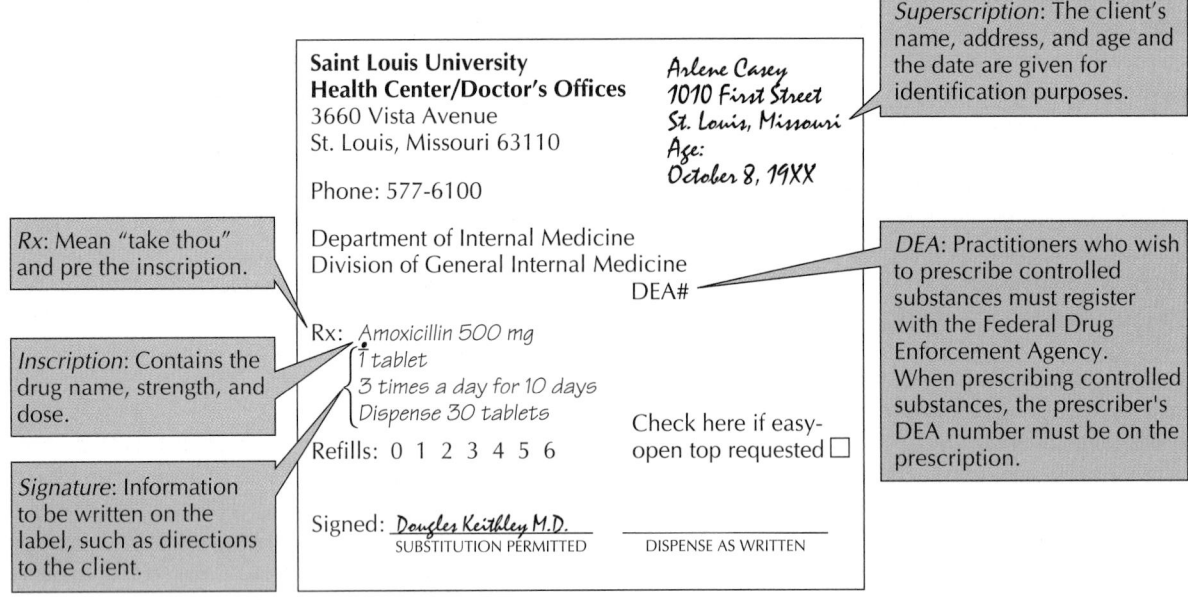

Superscription: The client's name, address, and age and the date are given for identification purposes.

Saint Louis University Health Center/Doctor's Offices
3660 Vista Avenue
St. Louis, Missouri 63110

Phone: 577-6100

Arlene Casey
1010 First Street
St. Louis, Missouri
Age:
October 8, 19XX

Rx: Mean "take thou" and pre the inscription.

Department of Internal Medicine
Division of General Internal Medicine
                              DEA#

DEA: Practitioners who wish to prescribe controlled substances must register with the Federal Drug Enforcement Agency. When prescribing controlled substances, the prescriber's DEA number must be on the prescription.

Inscription: Contains the drug name, strength, and dose.

Rx: *Amoxicillin 500 mg*
      1 tablet
      3 times a day for 10 days
      Dispense 30 tablets

Refills: 0 1 2 3 4 5 6

Check here if easy-open top requested ☐

Signature: Information to be written on the label, such as directions to the client.

Signed: *Douglas Keithley M.D.*
              SUBSTITUTION PERMITTED   DISPENSE AS WRITTEN

Figure 26-8. Example of a medication prescription. (Courtesy Saint Louis University Medical Center, St. Louis.)

to the system. The client's identification number is entered next. In these systems the nurse is then allowed to select the desired medication, dosage, and route. The system delivers the medication to the nurse, records it, and charges it to the client.

Nurses may also scan bar codes to identify the client, medication (name, dosage, route), and nurse administering the medication (Abdoo, 1992). This information is then automatically recorded on a computerized database.

Nurse's role. Since the nurse spends the most time with clients, the nurse is the most appropriate health care worker to administer medications. The administration of medications to clients requires knowledge and a set of skills that are unique to a nurse. The nurse assesses the client's ability to self-administer medications, determines whether a client should receive a medication at a given time, administers medications correctly, and monitors the effects of prescribed medications. Client and family education about proper medication administration and monitoring is an integral part of the nurse's role. The nurse uses the nursing process to integrate medication therapy into care.

CRITICAL THINKING IN MEDICATION ADMINISTRATION

Knowledge

The nurse uses the knowledge learned from many disciplines when administering medications. It is this knowledge that helps the nurse to understand why a particular medication has been prescribed for a client and how this medication will alter the client's physiology so as to exert its therapeutic effect. For example, in physiology you may have learned that potassium is a major intracellular ion. When a client does not have enough potassium in the body, the client may experi-

Figure 26-9. Computer-controlled dispensing system.

ence signs and symptoms that are associated with hypokalemia, such as muscle fatigue or weakness. Medications may be prescribed that may restore the client's potassium level to normal.

Knowledge about child development may show that children often perceive medication administration as a negative experience. The nurse uses principles from child development to ensure that the child cooperates with medication administration.

Experience

The nursing student often has limited experience with medication administration as it applies to professional practice. The clinical experience provides the student with the opportunity to use the nursing process as it applies to medication administration. As the student nurse gains experiences in medication administration, psychomotor skills (the "how-to") become more refined. However, psychomotor skills represent a small part of medication administration. Client attitudes, knowledge, physical and mental status, and client responses can make medication administration a complex experience.

Attitudes

To administer medications safely to clients, certain cognitive skills are essential.

Accountability and responsibility. The nurse accepts full responsibility for all actions that are delivered, including the administration of medications. When a nurse administers a medication to a client, the nurse accepts the responsibility that the medication or the nursing actions in administering it will not harm the client in any way. The nurse does not assume that the medication that is ordered for the client is the correct medication or the correct dose. The nurse could be held accountable for administering an ordered medication that is obviously inappropriate for the client. Because of this, the nurse should be familiar with the therapeutic effect, usual dosage, anticipated changes in laboratory data, and side effects of all medications that are administered. The nurse is also responsible for ensuring that clients have been properly informed about all aspects of self-administration.

Demonstrating accountability and acting responsibly in professional practice would mean that the nurse acknowledges when errors in professional practice occur. Most of the errors made by nurses are medication errors. A **medication error** is any event that could cause or lead to a client receiving inappropriate medication therapy or failing to receive appropriate medication therapy (Edgar and others, 1994). Most medication errors occur when a nurse fails to follow routine procedures such as checking dosage calculations, deciphering illegible handwriting, or administering medications with which the nurse is unfamiliar (see Table 26-7). Unfortunately, many medication errors are never identified.

When an error occurs, it should be acknowledged immediately and reported to the appropriate hospital personnel (e.g., nurse manager and physician). Measures to counteract the effects of the error may be necessary. The nurse is also responsible for completing an incident report describing the nature of the incident. Incident reports assist administrative personnel in identifying hospital system problems that contribute to medication errors.

Institutional policy may place limitations on the nurse's ability to administer certain types of medications, by certain routes, or in certain units of the acute care setting. Most settings have nursing procedure manuals that outline policies to define the classes of medications nurses employed by the agency may and may not administer.

Standards

Standards are those actions that ensure safe nursing practice. To ensure safe medication administration the nurse should be aware of a nursing standard called the "five rights" of medication administration:

1. The right medication
2. The right dose
3. The right client
4. The right route
5. The right time

Right medication. When medications are first ordered, the nurse compares the medication recording form or computer orders with the physician's written orders. When administering medications, the nurse compares the label of the medication container with the medication form. The nurse does this three times: (1) before removing the container from the drawer or shelf, (2) as the amount of medication ordered is removed from the container, and (3) before returning the container to storage. With unit-dose prepackaged medications, the nurse checks the label with the medicine form a third time even though there is no permanent container. Unit-dose medications may be checked before opening at the client's bedside.

Nurses administer only the medications they prepare. If an error occurs, the nurse who administers the medication is responsible for its effects. If a client questions the medication a nurse prepares, it is important not to ignore these concerns. An alert client will know whether a medication is different from those received before. In most cases the client's medication order has been changed; however, the client's questions might reveal an error. The nurse should withhold the medication until the preparation can be rechecked against the prescriber's orders.

Clients who self-administer medications should keep them in their original labeled containers, separate from other medications, to avoid confusion.

The nurse should never prepare medications from unmarked containers or containers with illegible labels. If a client refuses a medication, the nurse should discard it rather than return it to the original container. Unit-dose packaged medications can be saved if they are unopened.

Right dose. The unit-dose system is designed to minimize errors. When a medication must be prepared from a larger volume or strength than needed or when the prescriber orders a system of measurement different from what the pharmacist supplies, the chance of error increases. When performing medication calculations or conversions, the nurse should have another qualified nurse check the calculated doses.

After calculating dosages, the nurse should prepare the medication using standard measurement devices. Graduated cups, syringes, and scaled droppers can be used to measure medications accurately. At home, clients should use kitchen measuring spoons rather than teaspoons and tablespoons, which vary in volume.

When it is necessary to break a scored tablet, the break should be even. A tablet may be cut in half by using a knife edge or by using a cutting device. Tablets that do not break evenly are discarded. The two halves are given in successive doses if the second half was repackaged and labeled.

Often a nurse prepares a tablet by crushing it so that it can be mixed in food. The crushing device should always be cleaned completely before the tablet is crushed. Remnants of previously crushed medications may increase a medication's concentration or result in the client receiving a portion of an unprescribed medication. Crushed medications should be mixed with very small amounts of food or liquid. The client's favorite foods or liquids should not be used, because a medication may alter their taste and decrease the client's desire for them.

Right client. An important step in administering medications safely is being sure the medication is given to the right client. It is difficult to remember every client's name and face. To identify a client correctly, the nurse should check the medication administration form against the client's identification bracelet (Figure 26-10) and ask the client to state his or her name.

If an identification bracelet becomes smudged or illegible, or is missing, the nurse must acquire a new one for the client. When asking the client's name, the nurse should not merely speak the name and assume that the client's response indicates that he or she is the right person. Instead, the nurse should ask the client to state his or her full name.

Right route. If a prescriber's order does not designate a route of administration, the nurse should consult the prescriber. Likewise, if the specified route is not the

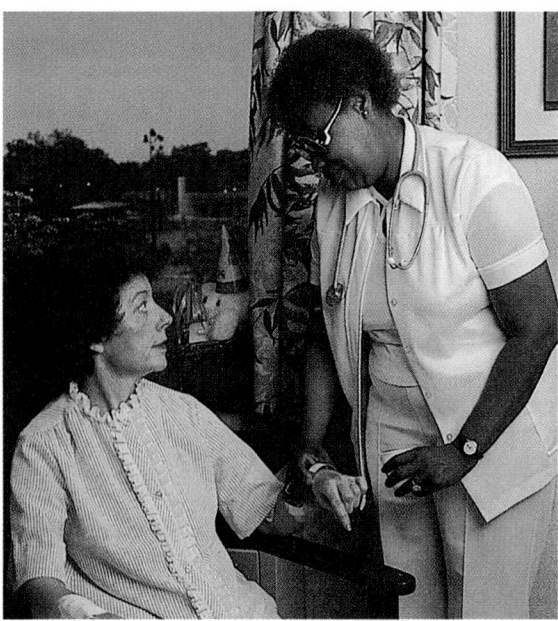

Figure 26-10. Before administering any medications, the nurse checks the client's identification and allergy bracelet.

recommended route, the nurse should alert the prescriber immediately.

When the nurse administers injections, precautions are necessary to ensure that the medications are given correctly. It is also important to prepare injections only from preparations designed for parenteral use. The injection of a liquid designed for oral use can produce local complications, such as a sterile abscess, or fatal systemic effects. Medication companies label parenteral medications "for injectable use only."

Right time. The nurse must know why a medication is ordered for certain times of the day and whether the time schedule can be altered. For example, two medications are ordered, one q8h (every 8 hours) and the other t.i.d. (3 times a day). Both medications are to be given 3 times within a 24-hour period. The prescriber intends the q8h medication to be given around the clock to maintain therapeutic blood levels of the medication. In contrast, the t.i.d. medication is given during the waking hours. Each institution has a recommended time schedule for medications ordered at frequent intervals.

The prescriber often gives specific instructions about when to administer a medication. A preoperative medication to be given on call means that the nurse is to administer the medication when the operating room notifies the nursing division. A medication ordered PC (after meals) is to be given within half an hour after a meal when the client has a full stomach. A STAT medication is to be given immediately.

Medications that must act at certain times are given

priority. For example, insulin should be given at a precise interval before a meal. All routinely ordered medications should be given within 30 minutes of the times ordered (30 minutes before or after the prescribed time).

Some medications require the nurse's clinical judgment in determining the proper time for administration. A p.r.n. sleeping medication should be administered when the client is prepared for bed or at a time appropriate for maximum benefit. A nurse also uses judgment when administering p.r.n. analgesics. For example, the nurse may need to obtain a STAT order from the prescriber if the client requires a medication before the p.r.n. interval has elapsed.

At home a client may have to take several medications throughout the day. The nurse helps to plan schedules based on preferred medication intervals and the client's daily schedule. For clients who have difficulty remembering when to take medications, the nurse can make a chart that lists the times when each medication is to be taken or prepare a special container to hold each timed dose.

Professional standards influence the activities of medication administration. The American Nurses Association's (ANA's) *Standard of Nursing Practice* (see Chapter 10), based on the nursing process, also applies to the activity of medication administration. Other professional nursing standards may also apply.

Maintaining Clients' Rights

In accordance with the *Patient's Bill of Rights* (see Chapter 12) and because of the potential risks related to medication administration, a client has the right to:

1. Be informed of medication name, purpose, action, and potential undesired effects
2. Refuse a medication regardless of the consequences
3. Have qualified nurses or physicians assess a medication history, including allergies
4. Be properly advised of the experimental nature of medication therapy and to give written consent for its use
5. Receive labeled medications safely without discomfort in accordance with the "five rights" of medication administration (see section on medication delivery)
6. Receive appropriate supportive therapy in relation to medication therapy
7. Not receive unnecessary medications

NURSING PROCESS

◼ Assessment

To determine the need for and potential response to medication therapy, the nurse assesses many factors.

History. Before administering medications the nurse obtains or reviews the client's medical history. A client's medical history may provide indications or contraindications for medication therapy. Disease or illness may place clients at risk for adverse medication effects. For example, if a client has a gastric ulcer, compounds containing aspirin will increase the likelihood of bleeding. Long-term health problems such as diabetes or arthritis, which require medications, suggest to the nurse the type of medications a client is taking. A client's surgical history may indicate use of medications. For example, after a thyroidectomy a client may require hormone replacement.

History of allergies. If the client has a history of allergies to medication, the nurse informs other members of the health care team. Food allergies should also be carefully documented, because many medications have ingredients also found in food sources. One example is shellfish. If clients are allergic to shellfish, the client may be sensitive to any product containing iodine such as Betadine or dyes used in radiological testing. Another example is dye used in food products (e.g., candy, soda). In a hospital, clients wear identification bands listing medications to which they are allergic. All allergies should be noted on the nurse's admission notes, medication records, and physician's history. The nurses should also inquire about the client's knowledge and use of medical alert bracelet.

Medication history. The nurse assesses information about each medication the client takes, including length of time drug has been taken, current dosage schedule, and whether the client has experienced ill effects. In addition, the nurse reviews drug data, including action, purpose, normal dosages, routes, side effects, and nursing implications for administration and monitoring. Common questions to ask are: Is the smallest possible dose ordered (a question pertinent to older adults)? Can a certain medication interact with other medications being used? Are there special instructions for administering the medication? Often, several resources must be consulted to gather needed information. Pharmacology textbooks, nursing journals, the *Physicians' Desk Reference* (PDR), medication package inserts, and the pharmacist are valuable resources. The nurse is responsible for knowing as much as possible about each medication given. Many nursing students prepare or purchase cards containing medication data to use as a quick resource.

Diet history. A diet history reveals normal eating patterns and food preferences. The nurse can then plan the dosage schedule more effectively and advise the client in avoiding foods that may interact with medications.

Client's perceptual or coordination problems. For a client with perceptual or coordination limitations, self-administration may be difficult. The nurse must assess the client's ability to prepare doses and take medications correctly. If the client is unable to self-administer medications, the nurse may need to assess whether family or friends will be available to assist.

Client's current condition. The ongoing physical or mental status of a client may affect whether a medication is given or how it is administered. The nurse should assess a client carefully before giving any medication. For example, the nurse checks blood pressure before giving an antihypertensive. A client who is nauseated may be unable to swallow a tablet. Assessment findings also serve as a baseline in evaluating the effects of medication therapy.

Client's attitude about medication use. The client's attitude about medications may reveal a level of medication dependence or drug avoidance. Clients may not express their feelings about taking a particular medication, particularly if dependence is a problem. The nurse should observe the client's behavior for evidence of medication dependence or avoidance (see Box 26-2). The nurse should also be aware that the client's cultural beliefs about Western medicine can interfere with medication compliance (see Chapter 18).

Client's knowledge and understanding of medication therapy. The client's knowledge and understanding of medication therapy influence the willingness or ability to follow a medication regimen. Unless a client understands a medication's purpose, the importance of regular dosage schedules and proper administration methods, and the possible side effects, compliance is unlikely. When assessing knowledge of a medication, the nurse asks: What is it for? How is it taken? When is it taken? What side effects have there been? Has the client ever stopped taking doses? Is there anything else the client does not understand and would like to know about the medication? When the client does not take medication properly, the nurse should also review resources available for purchase of medications.

Client's learning needs. By assessing the client's level of knowledge about a medication and the resources available to take medications regularly, the nurse determines the need for instruction. It may be necessary for the nurse to explain the action and purpose of the medication, expected side effects, correct administration techniques, and ways to help the client to remember the medication regimen. In addition, clients might require instruction on ways to adjust a medication schedule to their lifestyle. If a client has been placed on a newly prescribed medication, instruction may need to be more involved.

▪ Nursing Diagnosis

Assessment provides data about the client's condition, ability to self-administer medications, and medication use patterns, which can be used to determine actual or potential problems with medication therapy. Certain data are defining characteristics, which when clustered together reveal nursing diagnoses (see nursing diagnoses box). For example, a client's admission of missing a dose, evidence that a medication has not reversed symptoms, or evidence that the client has not progressed indicates noncompliance regarding a medication regimen. Once the diagnosis is selected, the nurse identifies the related factor. The related factors of inadequate resources versus lack of knowledge require different interventions. If the client's noncompliance is related to inadequate finances, the nurse will collaborate with family members, social workers, or community agencies to help a client receive necessary medications. If the related factor is lack of knowledge, the nurse will implement an extensive teaching plan and follow-up.

▪ Planning

The nurse organizes care activities to ensure the safe administration of medications. Hurrying to give clients medications can lead to errors. The nurse reviews the client's plan of care to determine when hygiene activities, treatments, and diagnostic tests are needed. The nurse can also plan to use time during medication administration to teach clients about their medications. It is important to collaborate with the client's family or friends when instruction is given. Family members will often reinforce the importance of medication regimens in the home setting. When clients are hospitalized, it is important for the nurse to not postpone instruction until the day of discharge. For the client to understand medications and self-administration guidelines, there must be time for questions and discussion. Early planning is critical.

In the community the nurse ensures that the client knows where and how to obtain medications. The nurse also ensures that clients know how to read medication labels. Whether a client attempts self-administration or the nurse assumes responsibility for administering med-

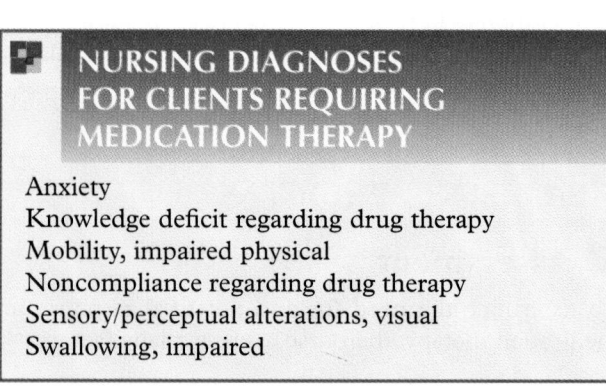

▪ **NURSING DIAGNOSES FOR CLIENTS REQUIRING MEDICATION THERAPY**

Anxiety
Knowledge deficit regarding drug therapy
Mobility, impaired physical
Noncompliance regarding drug therapy
Sensory/perceptual alterations, visual
Swallowing, impaired

ications, the following goals and expected outcomes must be met:

1. Client and family understand medication therapy.
2. Client gains therapeutic effect of the prescribed medications without discomfort or complications.
3. Client has no complications related to the route of administration.
4. Client safely self-administers medications.

Implementation

Health promotion activities. The nurse, in promoting or maintaining the client's health, identifies factors that may improve or diminish well-being. Health beliefs, personal motivations, socioeconomic factors, and habits (e.g., smoking) can influence the client's compliance with the medication regimen.

Teaching the client and family about the benefit of a medication and the knowledge needed to take it correctly can promote adherence to the regimen and foster independence. Integrating the client's health beliefs and cultural practices into the treatment plan can assist the nurse in establishing a schedule or routine with the client. The nurse may make referrals to community resources if the client is unable to afford, or cannot get out to obtain, necessary medications.

Client and family teaching. Unless a client is properly informed about medications, he or she may take the medications incorrectly or not at all. The nurse provides information about the purpose of medications and their actions and effects. Many health care institutions offer easy-to-read leaflets on specific types of medications. A client must know how to take a medication properly and the effects if he or she fails to do so. For example, after receiving a prescription for an antibiotic, a client must understand the importance of taking the full prescription. Failure to do this can lead to a worsening of the condition, as well as the development of bacteria resistant to the medication.

Nurses teach proper self-administration of medications to clients who depend on daily injections. The client learns to prepare and administer an injection correctly using aseptic technique. Family members or friends should be taught to give injections in case the client becomes ill or physically unable to handle a syringe. Nurses can provide specially designed equipment such as syringes with enlarged calibrated scales for easier reading or braille-labeled medication vials for clients with visual alterations.

Clients must be aware of the symptoms of medication side effects or toxicity. For example, clients taking anticoagulants learn to notify the physician immediately when signs of bleeding or bruising develop. Family members should be informed of medication side effects such as changes in behavior, because they are often the first persons to recognize such effects. Clients are better able to cope with problems caused by medications if they understand how and when to act. All clients should learn the basic guidelines for medication safety. These guidelines ensure the proper use and storage of medications in the home (Box 26-3).

Acute care activities. One rationale for hospitalization may be to have expert nursing observation and documentation of responses to medications (Benner, 1984). When a nurse receives a medication order, several nursing interventions are essential for safe and effective medication administration.

Receiving medication orders. A medication order is required for any medication to be administered by a nurse. Before any other interventions, the nurse ensures that the medication order contains all of the elements in Box 26-4. If the medication order is incomplete the nurse should inform the prescriber and ensure completeness before carrying out any medication order. Some medication orders can be given verbally or by telephone by the prescriber to the nurse. A verbal order is a medication or treatment order received by the nurse in the presence of the prescriber. Verbal orders are entered into the client's medical record by the registered nurse and transcribed the same way as if the prescriber wrote the order himself or herself. Telephone orders are medication or treatment orders given to the nurse by the prescriber, generally after the nurse updates the prescriber about a change in the client's condition. The nurse follows institutional policy regarding the receiving, recording, and transcription of verbal and telephone orders. Generally, verbal and telephone orders must be signed by the provider within 24 hours. When the prescriber is present, a verbal order is discouraged and the order should be written. Student nurses are prohibited from receiving verbal and telephone orders.

Correct transcription and communication of orders. The nurse or a designated unit secretary

---

BOX 26-3
Client Teaching for Safe Medication Administration

- Keep each drug in its original labeled container.
- Protect drugs from exposure to heat and light, as required.
- Check that labels are legible.
- Discard outdated medications.
- Always finish a prescribed drug unless otherwise instructed, and never save a drug for future illnesses.
- Dispose of drugs in a sink or toilet, and never place drugs in the trash within reach of children.
- Never give a family member a drug prescribed for another.
- Refrigerate drugs that require it.
- Read labels carefully and follow all instructions.
- Notify physician or practitioner of side effects.

Box 26-4
Components of Drug Orders

A medication order is incomplete unless it has the following parts:

Client's full name. The client's full name distinguishes the client from other persons with the same last name.

Date that the order is written. The day, month, year, and time must be included. Designating the time that an order is written helps clarify when certain orders are to stop automatically. If an incident occurs involving a medication error, it is easier to document what happened when this information is available.

Drug name. The physician will order a generic or trade-name drug. Correct spelling is essential in preventing confusion with drugs with similar spelling.

Dosage. The amount or strength of the medication is included.

Route of administration. The physician uses common abbreviations for drug routes. Accuracy is important because some drugs are administered by more than one route.

Time and frequency of administration. The nurse needs to know when to initiate drug therapy. Orders for multiple doses establish a routine schedule for drug administration.

Signature of physician or advanced practice nurse. The signature makes the order a legal request.

writes the physician's complete order on the appropriate medication form, called a medication administration record (MAR) (Figure 26-11). The transcribed order includes the client's name, room, and bed number and the medication name, dosage, frequency, and route of administration. Each time a medication dosage is prepared, the nurse refers to the medication form. With the unit-dose system, only one transcription is necessary, limiting the opportunity for errors. When transcribing orders, the nurse should be sure that names, dosages, and symbols are legible. The nurse rewrites any smudged or illegible transcriptions.

In some institutions a computer printout lists all currently ordered medications with dosage information. Orders are entered directly into the computer, preventing the need for transcription of orders. The same printout may be used to record medications given.

A registered nurse checks all transcribed orders against the original order for accuracy and thoroughness. If an order seems incorrect or inappropriate, the nurse consults the prescriber. The nurse who gives the wrong medication or an incorrect dose is legally responsible for the error.

Accurate dosage calculation and measurement. When measuring liquid medications, the nurse uses standard measuring containers. The procedure for medication measurement is systematic to lessen the chance of error. The nurse calculates each dose when preparing the medication, pays close attention to the process of calculation, and avoids interference from other nursing activities.

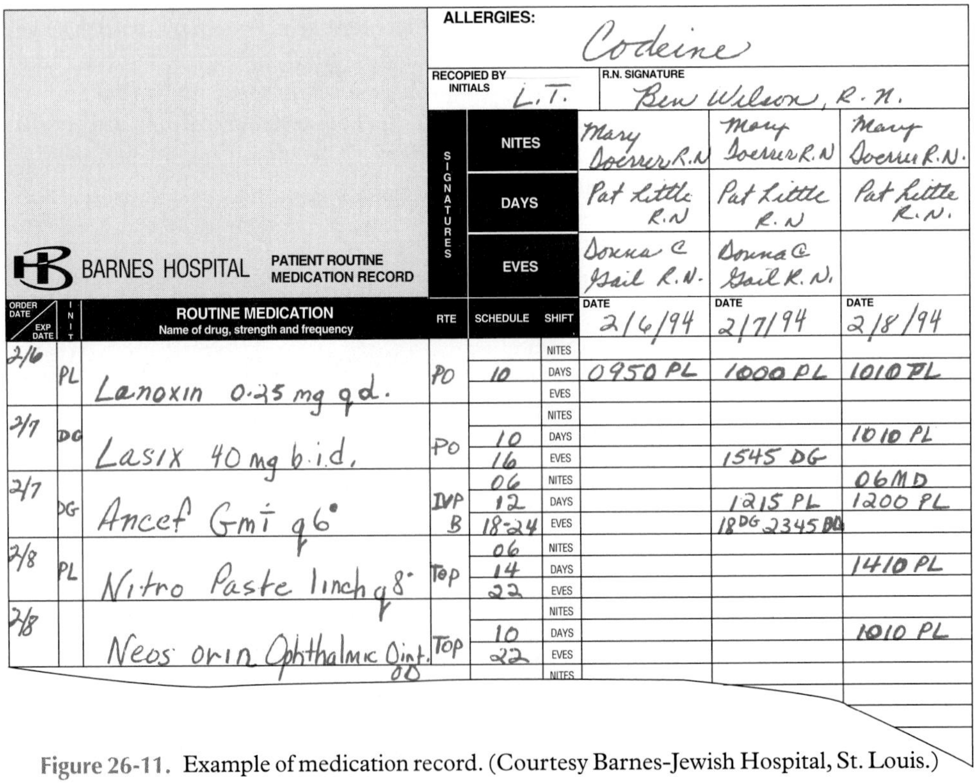
BARNES HOSPITAL PATIENT ROUTINE MEDICATION RECORD

ALLERGIES: Codeine

RECOPIED BY INITIALS: L.T. | R.N. SIGNATURE: Ben Wilson, R.N.

SIGNATURES			
NITES	Mary Doerrer R.N	Mary Doerrer R.N	Mary Doerrer R.N.
DAYS	Pat Little R.N	Pat Little R.N	Pat Little R.N.
EVES	Donna C Gail R.N.	Donna C Gail R.N.	

ORDER DATE / EXP DATE	INIT	ROUTINE MEDICATION Name of drug, strength and frequency	RTE	SCHEDULE	SHIFT	DATE 2/6/94	DATE 2/7/94	DATE 2/8/94
2/6	PL	Lanoxin 0.25 mg q.d.	PO		NITES			
				10	DAYS	0950 PL	1000 PL	1010 PL
					EVES			
2/7	DG	Lasix 40 mg b.i.d.	PO		NITES			
				10	DAYS			1010 PL
				16	EVES		1545 DG	
2/7	DG	Ancef Gm i q6°	IVPB	06	NITES			06 MD
				12	DAYS		1215 PL	1200 PL
				18-24	EVES		18 DG 2345 BD	
2/8	PL	Nitro Paste 1 inch q8°	Top	06	NITES			
				14	DAYS			1410 PL
				22	EVES			
2/8		Neosporin Ophthalmic Oint. OU	Top		NITES			
				10	DAYS			1010 PL
				22	EVES			

Figure 26-11. Example of medication record. (Courtesy Barnes-Jewish Hospital, St. Louis.)

Correct administration. For safe administration, the nurse uses aseptic technique and proper procedures when handling and giving medications. For example, certain medications require the nurse to perform assessments (e.g., assessing heart rate before giving antidysrhythmic medications).

Recording medication administration. After administering a medication, the nurse records it immediately on the appropriate record form (see Figure 26-11). **The nurse never charts a medication before administering it.** Recording immediately after administration prevents errors.

The recording of a medication includes the name of the medication, dosage, route, and exact time of administration. Often the medication forms are prepared and the nurse need only record the time. Agency policies may also require that the nurse record the location of an injection.

If a client refuses a medication or is undergoing tests or procedures that result in a missed dose, the nurse explains the reason the medication was not given in the nurse's notes. Some agencies require the nurse to circle the prescribed administration time on the medication record when a dose is missed.

Restorative care activities.
Because of the numerous types of restorative care settings, medication administration activities vary. Clients with functional limitations may require the nurse to fully administer all medications. In the home health and rehabilitation settings the client usually administers his or her own medications. Regardless of the type of medication activity, the nurse remains responsible for medication instruction. The nurse is also responsible for monitoring compliance with medications and determining the effectiveness of medications that have been prescribed.

Special considerations for administering medications to specific age-groups.
A client's developmental level is a factor in the way nurses administer medications. Knowledge of a client's developmental needs helps the nurse to anticipate responses to medication therapy.

Infants and children. Children vary in age; weight; surface area; and the ability to absorb, metabolize, and excrete medications. Children's medication dosages are lower than those of adults, so special caution is needed when preparing medications for them. Medications are usually not prepared and packaged in standardized dose ranges for children. Preparing an ordered dosage from an available amount requires careful calculation.

A child's parents are valuable resources for learning the best way to give a child medications. Sometimes it is less traumatic for the child if a parent gives the medication and the nurse supervises. Depending on the route of administration, tips exist for effective medication administration for children (Box 26-5).

Box 26-5
Tips for Administering Drugs to Children

Oral Medications

Liquids are safer to swallow to avoid aspiration.

Offer juice, a soft drink, or a frozen juice bar after a drug is swallowed.

Carbonated beverages poured over finely crushed ice reduce nausea.

When mixing drugs with palatable flavorings such as syrup or honey, use only a small amount. (The child may refuse to take all of a larger mixture. Avoid mixing the drug with food or liquids the child enjoys because the child may then refuse them.)

A plastic disposable syringe is the most accurate device for preparing liquid dosages. (Cups, teaspoons, and droppers are inaccurate.)

When administering liquid drugs, a spoon, plastic cup, or syringe (without needle) are useful.

Injections

Be very careful when selecting intramuscular injection sites. Infants and small children have underdeveloped muscles.

Children can be unpredictable and uncooperative. Have someone available to hold a child if needed.

Always awaken a sleeping child before giving an injection.

Distracting the child with conversation or a toy may reduce pain perception.

Give the injection quickly and do not fight with the child.

Older adults. Older adults also require special consideration during medication administration. In addition to physiological changes of aging (Figure 26-12), behavioral and economic factors influence an older person's use of medications. Ebersole and Hess (1994) describe five behavioral patterns of medication use characteristic of the older client.

Polypharmacy. **Polypharmacy** means that the client is taking many medications, prescribed or not, in an attempt to treat several disorders simultaneously. When this occurs, there is a high risk of medication interactions with other medications and with foods that the client may eat. There is also an increased risk of the client having an adverse reaction to the medications.

Self-prescribing of medications. A variety of symptoms can be experienced by older clients (e.g., pain, constipation, insomnia, indigestion). All of these symptoms are amenable to OTC medications. Older adults often attempt to seek relief from problems by using OTC preparations, folk medicines, and herbs.

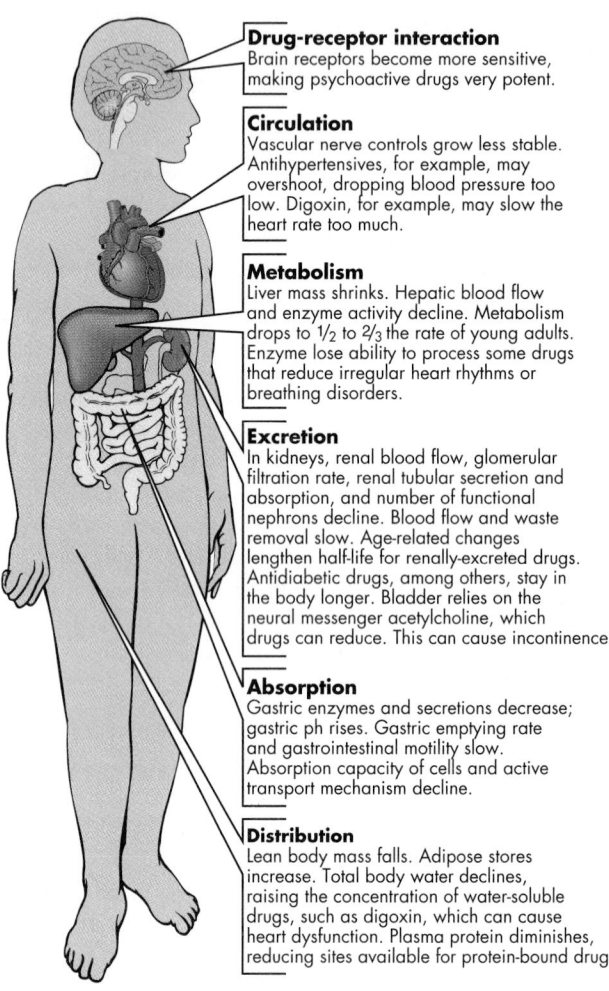

Drug-receptor interaction
Brain receptors become more sensitive, making psychoactive drugs very potent.

Circulation
Vascular nerve controls grow less stable. Antihypertensives, for example, may overshoot, dropping blood pressure too low. Digoxin, for example, may slow the heart rate too much.

Metabolism
Liver mass shrinks. Hepatic blood flow and enzyme activity decline. Metabolism drops to 1/2 to 2/3 the rate of young adults. Enzyme lose ability to process some drugs that reduce irregular heart rhythms or breathing disorders.

Excretion
In kidneys, renal blood flow, glomerular filtration rate, renal tubular secretion and absorption, and number of functional nephrons decline. Blood flow and waste removal slow. Age-related changes lengthen half-life for renally-excreted drugs. Antidiabetic drugs, among others, stay in the body longer. Bladder relies on the neural messenger acetylcholine, which drugs can reduce. This can cause incontinence.

Absorption
Gastric enzymes and secretions decrease; gastric ph rises. Gastric emptying rate and gastrointestinal motility slow. Absorption capacity of cells and active transport mechanism decline.

Distribution
Lean body mass falls. Adipose stores increase. Total body water declines, raising the concentration of water-soluble drugs, such as digoxin, which can cause heart dysfunction. Plasma protein diminishes, reducing sites available for protein-bound drugs.

Figure 26-12. Aging body and drug use. (From Lewis SM and others: *Medical-Surgical nursing,* ed 4, St. Louis, 1996, Mosby.)

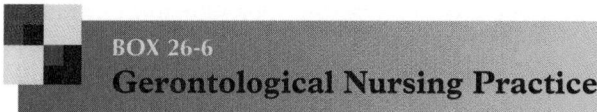

BOX 26-6
Gerontological Nursing Practice

- Space oral medications so that not more than one or two are taken at one time.
- Have client drink a little fluid *before* taking oral medications (to ease swallowing).
- Encourage the client to drink at least 5 to 6 ounces of fluid after taking medications (to ensure that the medications have left the esophagus and are in the stomach and to speed absorption of the medication).
- Do not routinely give analgesics for pain every 4 hours. Because of delayed absorption and distribution and the half-life of the medication, there may be an adverse cumulative effect.
- If the client has difficulty swallowing a large capsule or tablet, ask the physician to substitute a liquid medication if possible (cutting the tablet in half or crushing it and placing it in applesauce or fruit juice may distort the action of some medications, reduce the dose, or cause choking or aspiration of particles of medication or applesauce).
- Teach alternatives to medications, such as the following:
  Proper diet instead of vitamins
  Exercise instead of laxatives
  Bedtime snacks instead of hypnotics
  Decrease in weight, salt, fats, stress, and smoking and increased exercise instead of hypertensive agents (if approved by the physician)

Modified from Ebersole P, Hess P: *Toward health aging: human needs and nursing response,* ed 5, St. Louis, 1998, Mosby.

Over-the-counter medications. It is known that OTC medications are used by 75% of older adults to relieve symptoms. Many of these OTC preparations have ingredients that, when used inappropriately, may cause undesirable side effects or adverse reactions or may be contraindicated in the client's condition.

Misuse of medications. Forms of misuse by older adults include overuse, underuse, erratic use, and contraindicated use.

Noncompliance. Noncompliance is defined as a deliberate misuse of medication. Of older adults, 75% intentionally do not adhere to their medication regimen by altering the dose either because of ineffectiveness or uncomfortable side effects. Box 26-6 outlines tips for administering medications to the older adult client.

▪ Evaluation

The nurse monitors a client's response to medications on an ongoing basis. This requires that the nurse know the therapeutic action and common side effects of each medication. A change in a client's condition can be physiologically related to health status or may result from medications or both. The nurse must be alert for reactions in a client taking several medications. The goal of safe and effective medication administration involves a careful evaluation of technique and the client's response to therapy and ability to assume responsibility for self-care.

To evaluate the effectiveness of nursing interventions when meeting established goals of care, the nurse uses evaluative measures to identify if client outcomes were met. Many different evaluation measures can be used to evaluate client response to medications: direct observation of behavior or response, rating scales (e.g., pain scale) and checklists, and oral questioning. The type of measurement used varies with the action being evaluated, the reading skill and knowledge level of the client, and cognitive and psychomotor ability. The most common type of measurement that the nurse uses is a physiological measure. Examples of physiological measure are blood pressure, heart rate, and visual acuity. Client statements can also be used as evaluative measures. Table 26-8 contains examples of goals, expected outcomes, and corresponding evaluative measures.

TABLE 26-8
Example Evaluations for Client Goals

Goal	Expected Outcomes	Evaluative Measure With Example
Client and family understand drug therapy.	Client and family describe information about drug, dosage, schedule, purpose, and adverse effects.	Written measurement: Have client write out medication schedule for a 24-hour period. Oral questioning: Ask client to describe purpose, dosage, and adverse effects of each prescribed medication.
	Client and family identify situations that require medical intervention.	Oral questioning: Have family describe what to do when a client has adverse effects from a medication.
	Client and family demonstrate appropriate administration technique.	Direct observation: Have client demonstrate filling of an insulin syringe and self-injection.
Client safely self-administers medications.	Client follows prescribed treatment regimen.	Anecdotal notes: Have family keep log of client's compliance with therapy for 1 week.
	Client performs techniques correctly.	Direct observation: Observe client instill eye drops.
	Client identifies available resources for obtaining necessary medication.	Oral questioning: Ask family to identify how to contact local pharmacy, community clinic, or American Cancer Society for necessary medications.

ORAL ADMINISTRATION

The easiest and most desirable way to administer medications is by mouth (Skill 26-1). Clients usually are able to ingest or self-administer oral medications with a minimum of problems. Most tablets and capsules should be swallowed and administered with approximately 60 to 100 ml of fluid (as allowed). However, there may be situations that contraindicate the client's receiving medications by mouth. The primary contraindications to giving oral medications include the presence of GI alterations, the inability of a client to swallow food or fluids, and the use of gastric suction. An important precaution to take when administering any oral preparation is to protect clients from aspiration. Aspiration occurs when food, fluid, or medication intended for GI administration is inadvertently administered into the respiratory tract. The nurse protects the client from aspiration by evaluating the client's ability to manage oral medications. Box 26-7 includes techniques the nurse can use to protect the client from aspirating. Properly positioning the client is also essential in preventing aspiration. The nurse positions the client in a seated position when administering oral medications, if not contraindicated by the client's condition. The lateral position can also be used when the client's swallow, gag, and cough reflexes are intact. A client who has difficulty swallowing should be evaluated by appropriate personnel (e.g., speech therapist) before receiving oral preparations.

Box 26-7
Assessments to Protect the Client From Aspiration

Determine the client's ability to swallow:
   Ask the client to repeat certain sounds that require the same muscle movements as swallowing: "me-me-me" (for the lips); "la-la-la" (for the tongue); "ga-ga-ga" (for the soft palate and pharynx).
   Assess the swallowing reflex by having the client slide the tongue backward along the palate.
   Position your thumb and index finger on the client's larynx, and ask the client to swallow. Normally the larynx will elevate.
Assess the client's cough:
   See Chapter 30 on proper techniques of coughing.
Determine the presence of a gag reflex:
   Assess the gag reflex by stroking the posterior pharyngeal wall with a tongue blade. *Never check the gag reflex in a client who doesn't exhibit an intact cough or swallow reflex.* To protect the airway the client must have all three: a positive cough, gag, and swallow reflex.

Modified from Gauwitz DG: How to protect the dysphagic stroke patient, *Am J Nurs* 95:34, 1995.

Administering Oral Medications

Delegation Considerations
Administering medications by the oral route requires problem solving and knowledge application unique to professional nursing. For this procedure delegation to unlicensed personnel is not appropriate.

Equipment
- Medication cart or tray
- Disposable medication cups
- Glass of water, juice, or preferred liquid
- Drinking straw
- Pill-crushing or pillating device (optional)
- Paper towels
- MAR or computer printout

STEPS	RATIONALE
1. Assess for any contraindications to client receiving oral medication: Is client able to swallow? Is client suffering from nausea/vomiting? Is client diagnosed as having bowel inflammation or reduced peristalsis? Has client had recent GI surgery? Does client have gastric suction?	Alterations in GI function interfere with drug distribution, absorption, and excretion. Clients with GI suction might not receive benefit from the medication because it may be suctioned from the GI tract before it can be absorbed.
a. Check the client's swallow, cough, and gag reflexes (see Box 26-7) if in doubt about client's ability to manage oral medications. Withhold medication if swallow, cough, or gag is impaired and notify physician.	
2. Assess client's medical history, history of allergies, medication history, and diet history.	These factors can influence how certain drugs act. Information also reflects client's need for medications.

CRITICAL DECISION POINT
Drug allergies should be listed on *each* page of the MAR and prominently displayed on the client's medical record.

3. Gather and review assessment and laboratory data that may influence drug administration.	Physical examination or laboratory data may contraindicate drug administration.

CRITICAL DECISION POINT
If contraindications exist, withhold medication and inform prescriber.

4. Assess client's knowledge regarding health and medication usage.	Determines client's need for drug education. Also assists in identifying client's adherence to drug therapy at home. Assessment may reveal drug use problems such as drug tolerance. This occurs when a client desires more and more medication to achieve the desired effect. Other drug use problems are noncompliance, abuse, addiction, or dependence.
5. Assess client's preferences for fluids.	Offering fluids during drug administration increases client's fluid intake. Fluids ease swallowing and facilitate absorption from the GI tract. Fluid restrictions must be maintained.

STEPS	RATIONALE
6. Check accuracy and completeness of each MAR or computer printout with prescriber's written medication order. Check client's name, drug name and dosage, route of administration, and time for administration.	The order sheet is the most reliable source and only legal record of drugs client is to receive.
7. Prepare medications:	
a. Wash hands.	Reduces transfer of microorganisms.
b. Arrange medication tray and cups in medication preparation area or move medication cart to position outside client's room.	Organization of equipment saves time and reduces error.
c. Unlock medicine drawer or cart.	Medications are safeguarded when locked in cabinet or cart.
d. Prepare medications for one client at a time. Keep all pages of MARs or computer printouts for one client together.	Prevents preparation errors.
e. Select correct drug from stock supply or unit-dose drawer. Compare label of medication with MAR or computer printout (see illustration).	Reading label and comparing it with transcribed order reduces errors.
f. Calculate drug dose as necessary. Double-check calculation.	Double-checking reduces risk of error.
g. To prepare tablets or capsules from a floor stock bottle, pour required number into bottle cap and transfer medication to medication cup. Do not touch medication with fingers. Extra tablets or capsules may be returned to bottle. Medications that need to be broken to administer half the dosage can be broken, using a gloved hand, or cut with a pillating device (see illustration). Tablets that are to be broken in half must be prescored. Prescored tablets are identified by a manufactured line that transverses the center of the tablet.	Drugs are very expensive; avoid waste.

Continued

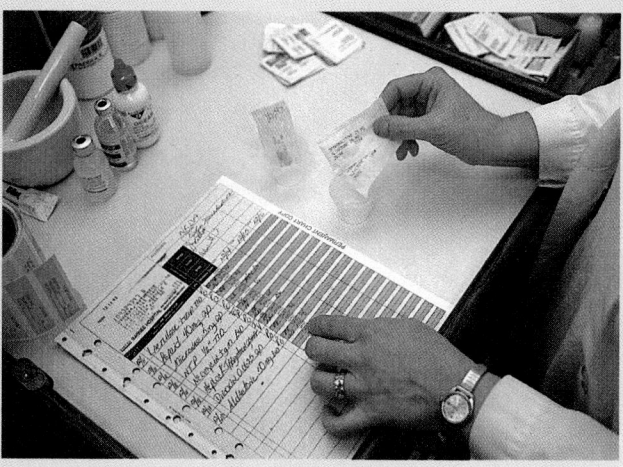

Step 7e

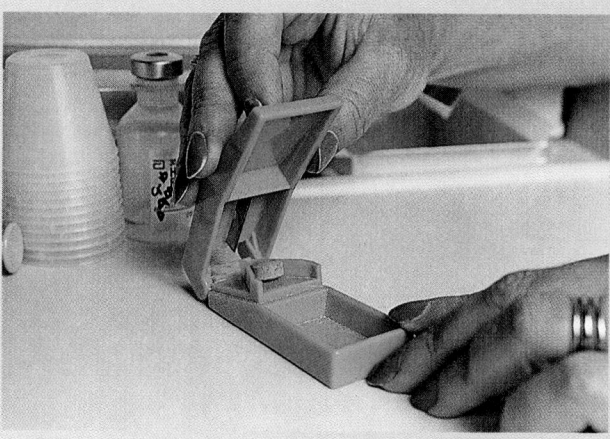

Step 7g

Administering Oral Medications

STEPS	RATIONALE
h. To prepare unit-dose tablets or capsules, place packaged tablet or capsule directly into medicine cup. (Do not remove wrapper; see illustration.)	Wrapper maintains cleanliness of medications and identifies drug name and dosage.
i. All tablets or capsules to be given to client at same time may be placed in one medicine cup except for those requiring preadministration assessments (e.g., pulse rate or blood pressure).	Keeping medications that require preadministration assessments separate from others makes it easier for the nurse to withhold drugs as necessary.
j. If client has difficulty swallowing or liquid medications are not an option, use pill-crushing device such as a mortar and pestle to grind pills. If a pill-crushing device is not available, place tablet between two medication cups and grind with a blunt instrument. Mix ground tablet in small amount of soft food (custard or applesauce.)	Large tablets can be difficult to swallow. Ground tablet mixed with palatable soft food is usually easier to swallow.

CRITICAL DECISION POINT

Not all drugs can be crushed (e.g., capsules, enteric-coated drugs). Consult with pharmacist when in doubt.

k. Prepare liquids:	
(1) Remove bottle cap from container and place cap upside down.	Prevents contamination of inside of cap.
(2) Hold bottle with label against palm of hand while pouring.	Spilled liquid will not soil or fade label.
(3) Hold medication cup at eye level and fill to desired level on scale (see illustration). Scale should be even with fluid level at its surface or base of meniscus, not edges.	Ensures accuracy of measurement.
(4) Discard any excess liquid into sink. Wipe lip and neck of bottle with paper towel.	Prevents contamination of bottle's contents and prevents bottle cap from sticking.

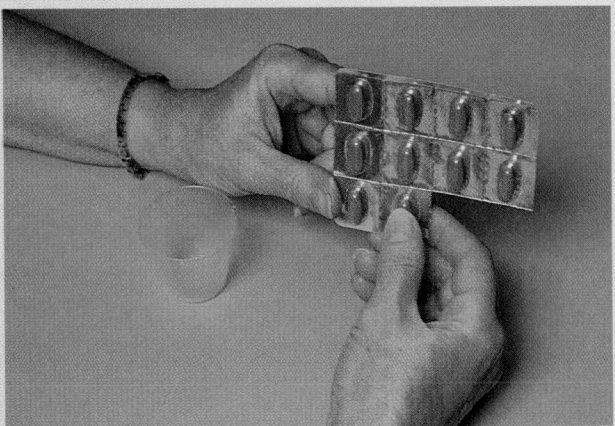

Step 7h

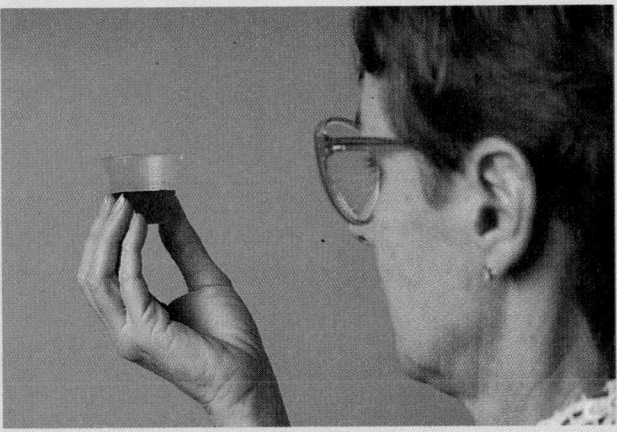

Step 7k(3)

STEPS	RATIONALE

(5) Some liquid medications are in unit-dose containers. Draw up volumes of less than 10 ml in syringe without needle (see illustration).

Step 7k(5)

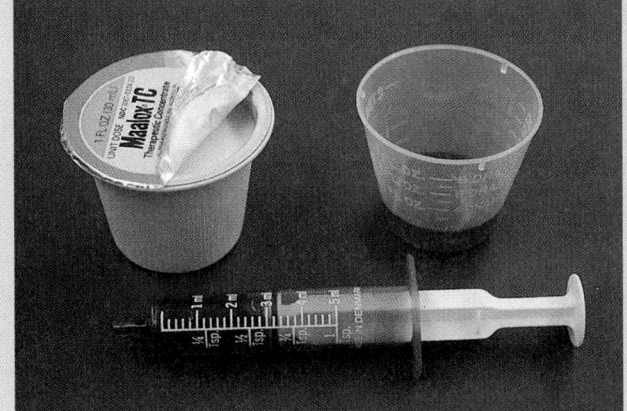

l. When preparing narcotics, check narcotic record for previous drug count and compare with supply available.

Controlled substance laws require careful monitoring of dispensed narcotics.

m. Check expiration date on all medications.

Medications used past expiration date may be inactive or harmful to client.

n. Compare MAR or computer printout with prepared drug and container.

Reading label second time reduces error.

o. Return stock containers or unused unit-dose medications to shelf or drawer and read label again.

Third check of label reduces administration errors.

p. Do not leave drugs unattended.

Nurse is responsible for safekeeping of drugs.

8. Administering medications:

a. Take medications to client at correct time.

Medications are administered within 30 minutes before or after prescribed time to ensure intended therapeutic effect. STAT or single-order medications should be given at time ordered.

b. Identify client by comparing name on MAR or computer printout with name on client's identification bracelet (see Figure 26-10). Ask client to state name.

Identification bracelets are made at time of client's admission and are most reliable source of identification. Replace any missing or faded identification bracelets.

c. Explain purpose of each medication and its action to client. Allow client to ask any questions about drugs.

Client has right to be informed, and client's understanding of purpose of each medication improves compliance with drug therapy.

d. Assist client to sitting or side-lying position if sitting is contraindicated.

Sitting position prevents aspiration during swallowing.

e. Administer drugs properly:

(1) Client may wish to hold solid medications in hand or cup before placing in mouth.

Client can become familiar with medications by seeing each drug.

(2) Offer water or juice to help client swallow medications. Give cold carbonated water if available and not contraindicated.

Choice of fluid promotes client's comfort and can improve fluid intake. Carbonated water helps passage of tablet through esophagus.

(3) For sublingual-administered drugs, have client place medication under tongue and allow it to dissolve completely. Caution client against swallowing tablet.

Drug is absorbed through blood vessels of undersurface of tongue. If swallowed, drug is destroyed by gastric juices or so rapidly detoxified by liver that therapeutic blood levels are not attained.

Continued

Administering Oral Medications

STEPS	RATIONALE
(4) For buccal-administered drugs, have client place medication in mouth against mucous membranes of the cheek until it dissolves (see Figure 26-5). Avoid administering liquids until buccal medication has dissolved.	Buccal medications act locally on mucosa or systemically as they are swallowed in saliva.
(5) Mix powdered medications with liquids at bedside and give to client to drink.	When prepared in advance, powdered drugs may thicken and even harden, making swallowing difficult.
(6) Caution client against chewing or swallowing lozenges.	Drug acts through slow absorption through oral mucosa, not gastric mucosa.
(7) Give effervescent powders and tablets immediately after dissolving.	Effervescence improves unpleasant taste of drug and often relieves GI problems.
f. If client is unable to hold medications, place medication cup to the lips and gently introduce each drug into the mouth, one at a time. Do not rush.	Administering single tablet or capsule eases swallowing and decreases risk of aspiration.
g. If tablet or capsule falls to the floor, discard it and repeat preparation.	Drug is contaminated when it touches floor.
h. Stay until client has completely swallowed each medication. Ask client to open mouth if uncertain whether medication has been swallowed.	Nurse is responsible for ensuring that client receives ordered dosage. If left unattended, client may not take dose or may save drugs, causing risk to health.
i. For highly acidic medications (e.g., aspirin), offer client nonfat snack (e.g., crackers) if not contraindicated by client's condition.	Reduces gastric irritation.
j. Assist client in returning to comfortable position.	Maintains client's comfort.
k. Dispose of soiled supplies and wash hands.	Reduces transmission of microorganisms.
9. Return within 30 minutes to evaluate client's response to medications.	Evaluates drug's therapeutic benefit and can detect onset of side effects or allergic reactions.
10. Ask client or family member to identify drug name and explain purpose, action, dosage schedule, and potential side effects of drug.	Determines level of knowledge gained by client and family.
11. Always notify prescriber when the client exhibits a toxic effect or allergic reaction, or with the onset of side effects. Withhold further doses.	Notification alerts prescriber to modify or discontinue medication.

Recording and Reporting
- Record administration of oral medications on MAR, placing nurse's initials or signature.
- Record the reason any drug is withheld and follow agency's policy for proper recording.

Home Care Considerations
- All clients should learn the basic guidelines for drug safety:
    - Keep each drug in its original, labeled container.
    - Be sure labels are legible.

Discard any outdated medications.
Always finish a prescribed drug unless otherwise instructed. Never save a drug for future illnesses.
Dispose of drugs by taking them to the pharmacy. Do not place drugs in the trash within reach of children.
Do not give a family member a drug prescribed for another.
Refrigerate medications that require it.
Read labels carefully and follow all instructions.

Box 26-8

Procedural Guidelines for Giving Drugs Through a Nasogastric Tube, J-Tube, G-Tube, or Small-Bore Feeding Tube

1. Administer medications in a liquid form (suspension, elixir, or solution) when possible to prevent tube obstruction.
2. Read medication labels carefully before crushing a tablet or opening a capsule.
3. Do *not* crush buccal or sublingual tablets.
4. Do *not* crush enteric-coated or sustained-action medications.
5. Dissolve crushed tablets and powders in warm water.
6. Dissolve soft, gelatin capsules in warm water.
7. Irrigate the tube before and after all medication is given with 50 to 150 ml of water.
8. Avoid giving syrups or medications with a pH of less than 4.
9. Do not attempt to give whole or undissolved medications.

Data from Petrosin BM and others: *Crit Care Nurs Q* 12:1, 1989.

For clients with nasogastric feeding tubes, liquid medications are preferred but some tablets can be crushed and capsules opened to mix in a solution for administration (Box 26-8).

TOPICAL MEDICATION APPLICATIONS

Topical medications are medications applied locally, most often to intact skin. They can be in the form of lotions, pastes, or ointments (see Table 26-1). They can also be applied to mucous membranes.

Skin Applications

Because many locally applied medications such as lotions, pastes, and ointments can create systemic and local effects, the nurse should apply these medications using gloves and applicators. Sterile technique is used if the client has an open wound.

Skin encrustation and dead tissues harbor microorganisms and block contact of medications with the tissues to be treated. Simply applying new medications over previously applied medications does little to prevent infection or offer therapeutic benefit. Before applying medications, the nurse cleans the skin thoroughly by washing the area gently with soap and water, soaking an involved site, or locally debriding tissue.

When applying ointments or pastes, the nurse spreads the medication evenly over the involved surface and covers the area well without applying an overly thick layer. Opaque ointments prevent visualization of underlying skin. Prescribers may order a gauze dressing to be applied over the medication to prevent soiling of clothes and wiping away of the medication. Each type of medication, whether an ointment, lotion, powder, or other type, should be applied a specific way to ensure proper penetration and absorption. The nurse applies lotions and creams by smearing them lightly onto the skin's surface; rubbing may cause irritation. A liniment is applied by rubbing it gently but firmly into the skin. A powder is dusted lightly to cover the affected area with a thin layer. During any application the nurse should assess the skin thoroughly. To record administration, the area applied, name of medication, and condition of skin should be noted.

Nasal Instillation

Clients with nasal sinus alterations may receive medications by spray, drops, or tampons (Skill 26-2). The most commonly administered form of nasal instillation is decongestant spray or drops, used to relieve symptoms of sinus congestion and colds. Clients must be cautioned to avoid abuse of medications, because overuse can lead to a rebound effect in which the nasal congestion worsens. When excess decongestant solution is swallowed, serious systemic effects may also develop, especially in children. Saline drops are safer as a decongestant for children than nasal preparations that contain sympathomimetics (e.g., Afrin, Neo-Synephrine).

It is easier to have the client self-administer sprays, because the client can control the spray and inhale as it enters the nasal passages. For clients who use nasal sprays repeatedly, the nurse checks the nares for irritation. Nasal drops are effective in treating sinus infections. The nurse learns the proper way of positioning clients to permit the medication to reach the affected sinus. Severe nosebleeds are usually treated with packing or nasal tampons, which are treated with epinephrine, to reduce blood flow. Usually a physician places nasal tampons.

Eye Instillation

Common medications used by clients are eye drops and ointments, including OTC preparations such as artificial tears and vasoconstrictors (e.g., Visine, Murine). However, many clients receive prescribed **ophthalmic** medications for eye conditions such as glaucoma or after cataract extraction. A large percentage of clients receiving eye medications are older adults. Age-related problems including poor vision, hand tremors, and difficulty grasping or manipulating containers affect the ease with which the older adult can self-administer eye medications. The nurse instructs clients and family members about the proper techniques for administering eye medications (Skill 26-3). The nurse may deter-

Text continued on p. 633

.... **Skill 26-2**
Administering Nasal Instillations

Delegation Considerations
Administration of nasal drops and ointments requires problem solving and knowledge application unique to professional nursing. For this procedure delegation to unlicensed personnel is not appropriate.

Equipment
- Prepared medication with clean dropper or spray container
- Facial tissue
- Small pillow (optional)
- Washcloth (optional)
- Gloves (optional, only if client has extensive nasal drainage)
- MAR or computer printout

STEPS	RATIONALE
1. For nasal drops, determine which sinus is affected by referring to medical record.	Affects client's position during drug instillation.
2. Assess client's history of hypertension, heart disease, diabetes mellitus and hyperthyroidism.	These conditions can contraindicate use of decongestants that stimulate CNS. Side effects of transient hypertension, tachycardia, palpitations, and headache may occur.
3. Inspect condition of nose and sinuses. Palpate sinuses for tenderness.	Provides baseline to monitor effects of medication. Presence of discharge interferes with drug absorption.
4. Assess client's knowledge regarding use of nasal instillations and technique for instillation and willingness to learn self-administration.	May necessitate health teaching regarding use of drugs. Motivation influences teaching approach.
5. Explain procedure to client regarding positioning and sensations to expect, such as burning or stinging of mucosa, or choking sensation as medication trickles into throat.	Helps client anticipate experience of procedure to reduce anxiety.
6. Wash hands. Arrange supplies and medications at bedside.	Reduces transmission of microorganisms; ensures smooth, orderly procedure.
7. Instruct client to clear or blow nose gently unless contraindicated (e.g., risk of increased intracranial pressure or nosebleeds).	Removes mucus and secretions that can block distribution of medication.
8. Administer nasal drops:	
a. Assist client to supine position.	Position provides access to nasal passages.
b. Position head properly:	
(1) For access to posterior pharynx, tilt client's head backward.	
(2) For access to ethmoid or sphenoid sinus, tilt head back over edge of bed or place small pillow under client's shoulder and tilt head back (see illustration).	
(3) For access to frontal and maxillary sinus, tilt head back over edge of bed or pillow with head turned toward side to be treated (see illustration).	Position allows medication to drain into affected sinus.
c. Support client's head with nondominant hand.	Prevents straining of neck muscles.
d. Instruct client to breathe through mouth.	Mouth breathing reduces chance of aspirating nasal drops into trachea and lungs.
e. Hold dropper 1 cm (½ inch) above nares and instill prescribed number of drops toward midline of ethmoid bone.	Avoids contamination of dropper. Instilling toward ethmoid bone facilitates distribution of medication over nasal mucosa.

STEPS	RATIONALE

f. Have client remain in supine position 5 minutes.
g. Offer facial tissue to blot runny nose, but caution client against blowing nose for several minutes.

Prevents premature loss of medication through nares.
Allows maximal amount of medication to be absorbed.

9. Assist client to a comfortable position after drug is absorbed.

Restores comfort.

10. Dispose of soiled supplies in proper container and wash hands.

Maintains neat, orderly environment. Reduces spread of microorganisms.

11. Observe client for onset of side effects 15 to 30 minutes after administration.

Drugs absorbed through mucosa can cause systemic reaction.

12. Ask if client is able to breathe through nose after decongestant administration. May be necessary to have client occlude one nostril at a time and breathe deeply.

Determines effectiveness of decongestant medication.

13. Reinspect condition of nasal passages between instillations.

Condition of mucosa reveals response to medication.

14. Ask client to review risks of overuse of decongestants and methods for administration.

Feedback ensures that client can self-administer drugs properly.

15. Have client demonstrate self-medication.

Feedback demonstrates learning.

Recording and Reporting
- Record medication administration, including drug name, concentration, number of drops, nostril into which drug was instilled, and time of administration.
- Record client's response in nurse's notes.
- Report any unusual systemic effects to nurse in charge or physician.

Home Care Considerations
- Instruct client to expect timely resolution of problems. Instruct client on signs to observe of persistent

or worsening problem. Clear nasal discharge indicates sinus problem. Yellow or greenish discharge indicates infection.
- Use OTC nasal sprays or nose drops for only one illness; bottles become easily contaminated with bacteria.
- Instruct clients that each family member should have a different dropper or spray applicator. Applicators should be washed or rinsed after each use.

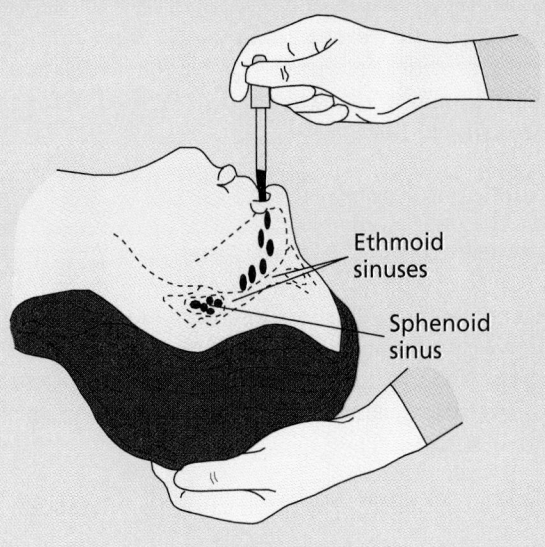

Ethmoid sinuses
Sphenoid sinus

Step 8b(2)

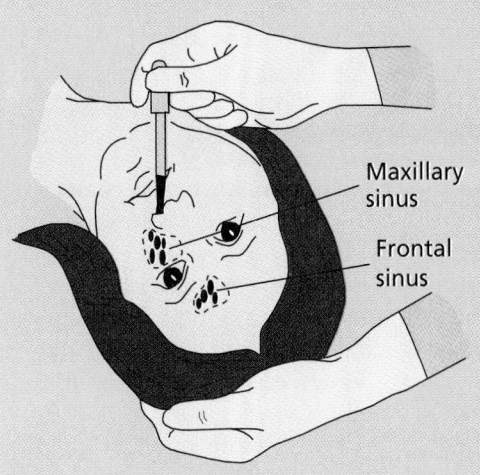

Maxillary sinus
Frontal sinus

Step 8b(3)

Skill 26-3

Administering Ophthalmic Medications

Delegation Considerations
Administration of eye drops and ointments requires problem solving and knowledge application unique to professional nursing. For this procedure delegation to unlicensed personnel is not appropriate.

Equipment
- Medication bottle with sterile eye dropper or ointment tube
- Medicated intraocular disk
- Cotton ball or tissue
- Washbasin filled with warm water and washcloth
- Eye patch and tape (optional)
- Clean gloves
- MAR or computer printout

STEPS	RATIONALE
1. Review prescriber's medication order for number of drops (if a liquid), and eye (right = O.D.; left = O.S.; both = O.U.) to receive medication.	Ensures correct administration of medication.
2. Assess condition of external eye structures. (May also be done just before drug instillation.)	Provides baseline to later determine if local response to medications occurs. Also indicates need to clean eye before drug application.
3. Determine whether client has any known allergies to eye medications. Also ask if client has allergy to latex.	Protects client from risk of allergic drug response. Will require use of nonlatex gloves.
4. Determine whether client has any symptoms of visual alterations.	Certain eye medications act to either lessen or increase these symptoms. Nurse must be able to recognize change in client's condition.
5. Assess client's level of consciousness and ability to follow directions.	If client becomes restless or combative during procedure, a greater risk of accidental eye injury exists.
6. Assess client's knowledge regarding drug therapy and desire to self-administer medication.	Client's level of understanding may indicate need for health teaching. Motivation influences teaching approach.
7. Assess client's ability to manipulate and hold dropper.	Reflects client's ability to learn to self-administer drug.
8. Explain procedure to client.	Relieves anxiety about medication being instilled into eye.
9. Wash hands and arrange supplies at bedside; apply clean gloves.	Reduces transmission of microorganisms; ensures a smooth, orderly procedure.
10. Ask client to lie supine or sit back in chair with head slightly hyperextended.	Position provides easy access to eye for medication instillation and minimizes drainage of medication through tear duct.

CRITICAL DECISION POINT

Do not hyperextend the neck of a client with cervical spine injury.

11. If crusts or drainage are present along eyelid margins or inner canthus, gently wash away. Soak any crusts that are dried and difficult to remove by applying damp washcloth or cotton ball over eye for a few minutes. Always wipe clean from inner to outer canthus.	Crusts or drainage harbors microorganisms. Soaking allows easy removal and prevents pressure from being applied directly over eye. Cleansing from inner to outer canthus avoids entrance of microorganisms into lacrimal duct.
12. Hold cotton ball or clean tissue in nondominant hand on client's cheekbone just below lower eyelid.	Cotton or tissue absorbs medication that escapes eye.

STEPS	RATIONALE
13. With tissue or cotton resting below lower lid, gently press downward with thumb or forefinger against bony orbit.	Technique exposes lower conjunctival sac. Retraction against bony orbit prevents pressure and trauma to eyeball and prevents fingers from touching eye.
14. Ask client to look at ceiling.	Action retracts sensitive cornea up and away from conjunctival sac and reduces stimulation of blink reflex.
15. Instill eye drops while explaining steps to client:	
a. With dominant hand resting on client's forehead, hold filled medication eye dropper or ophthalamic solution approximately 1 to 2 cm (½ to ¾ inch) above conjunctival sac (see illustration).	Helps prevent accidental contact of eyedropper with eye structures, thus reducing risk of injury to eye and transfer of infection to dropper. Ophthalmic medications are sterile.
b. Drop prescribed number of medication drops into conjunctival sac.	Conjunctival sac normally holds 1 or 2 drops. Provides even distribution of medication across eye.
c. If client blinks or closes eye or if drops land on outer lid margins, repeat procedure.	Therapeutic effect of drug is obtained only when drops enter conjunctival sac.
d. After instilling drops, ask client to close eye gently.	Helps to distribute medication. Squinting or squeezing of eyelids forces medication from conjunctival sac.
e. When administering drugs that cause systemic effects, apply gentle pressure with your finger and clean tissue on the client's nasolacrimal duct for 30 to 60 seconds.	Prevents overflow of medication into nasal and pharyngeal passages. Prevents absorption into systemic circulation.
16. Instill eye ointment:	
a. Ask client to look at ceiling.	Action retracts sensitive cornea up and away from conjunctival sac and reduces stimulation of blink reflex.
b. Holding ointment applicator above lower lid margin, apply thin stream of ointment evenly along inner edge of lower eyelid on conjunctiva (see illustration) from the inner canthus to outer canthus.	Distributes medication evenly across eye and lid margin.
c. Have client close eye and rub lid lightly in circular motion with cotton ball, if rubbing is not contraindicated.	Further distributes medication without traumatizing eye.

Continued

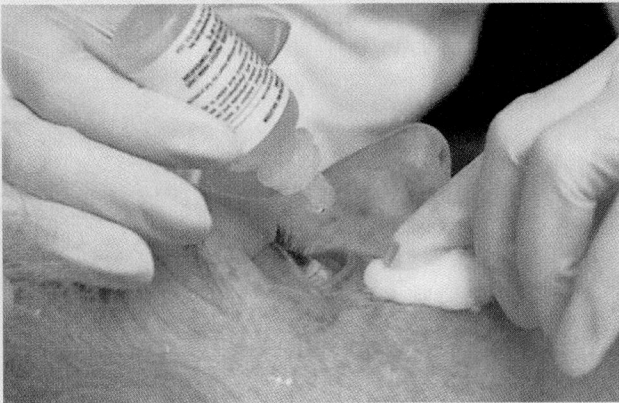

Step 15a

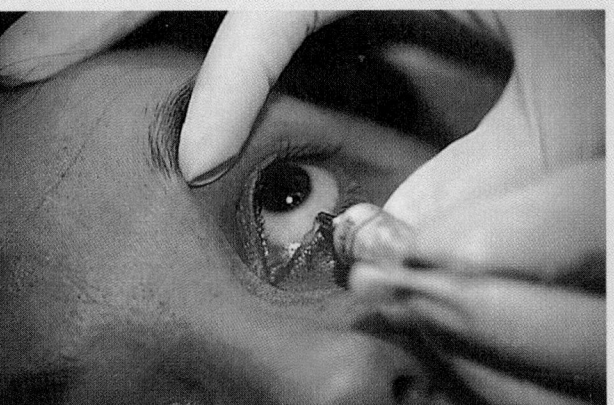

Step 16b

Skill 26-3—cont'd
Administering Ophthalmic Medications

STEPS	RATIONALE
17. Intraocular disk 　a. Application:	
(1) Open package containing the disk. Gently press your fingertip against the disk so that it adheres to your finger. Position the convex side of the disk on your fingertip (see illustration).	Allows nurse to inspect disk for damage or deformity.
(2) With your other hand, gently pull the client's lower eyelid away from the eye. Ask client to look up.	Prepares conjunctival sac for receiving medicated disk.
(3) Place the disk in the conjunctival sac, so that it floats on the sclera between the iris and lower eyelid (see illustration).	Ensures delivery of medication.
(4) Pull the client's lower eyelid out and over the disk (see illustration).	Ensures accurate medication delivery.

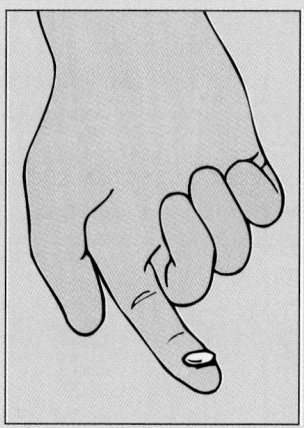

Step 17a(1)

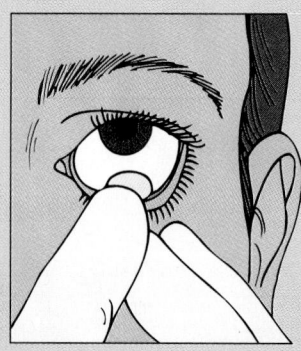

Step 17a(3)

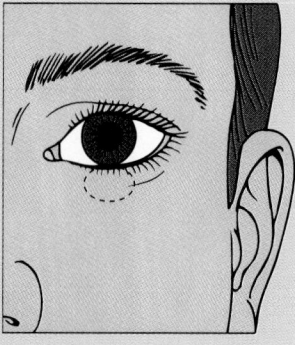

Step 17a(4)

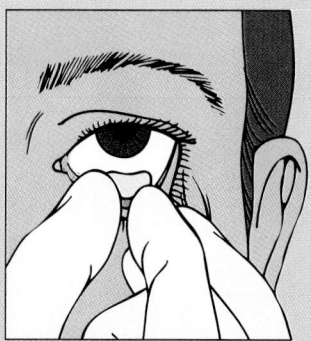

Step 17b(4)

STEPS	RATIONALE

CRITICAL DECISION POINT

You should not be able to see the disk at this time. Repeat Step 4 if you can see the disk.

   b. Removal:
     (1) Wash hands and put on gloves.
     (2) Explain procedure to client.
     (3) Gently pull on the client's lower eyelid to expose the disk.
     (4) Using your forefinger and thumb of your opposite hand, pinch the disk and lift it out of the client's eye (see illustration).

STEPS	RATIONALE
18. If excess medication is on eyelid, gently wipe it from inner to outer canthus.	Promotes comfort and prevents trauma to eye.
19. If client had eye patch, apply clean one by placing it over affected eye so entire eye is covered. Tape securely without applying pressure to eye.	Clean eye patch reduces chance of infection.
20. Remove gloves, dispose of soiled supplies in proper receptacle, and wash hands.	Maintains neat environment at bedside and reduces transmission of microorganisms.
21. Note client's response to instillation; ask if any discomfort was felt.	Determines if procedure was performed correctly and safely.
22. Observe response to medication by assessing visual changes and noting any side effects.	Evaluates effects of medication.
23. Ask client to discuss drug's purpose, action, side effects, and technique of administration.	Determines client's level of understanding.
24. Have client demonstrate self-administration of next dose.	Provides feedback regarding competency with skill.

Recording and Reporting
- Record drug, concentration, number of drops, time of administration, and eye (left, right, or both) that received medication on MAR.
- Record appearance of eye in nurse's notes.

Home Care Considerations
- If eye drops are stored in refrigerator, rewarm to room temperature before administering.
- Many clients lack confidence in their ability to instill drops without supervision. The nurse teaches others, such as a family member, to instill drops into the client's eye.

mine the client and family's ability to self-administer through a return demonstration of the procedure. Showing clients each step of the procedure for instilling eye drops can improve their compliance. The following principles can be applied when administering eye medications:

1. The cornea of the eye is richly supplied with pain fibers and thus very sensitive to anything applied to it. Avoid instilling any form of eye medication directly onto the cornea.

2. The risk of transmitting infection from one eye to the other is high. Avoid touching the eyelids or other eye structures with eye droppers or ointment tubes.

3. Use eye medication only for the client's affected eye.

4. Never allow a client to use another client's eye medications.

Some medications are administered intraocularly. Medications delivered this way resemble a contact lens.

Box 26-9

Procedural Guidelines for Administering Ear Medications

Ear Drops

1. Have client assume side-lying position (if not contraindicated by client's condition) with ear to be treated facing up, or client may sit in chair or at the bedside.
2. Straighten ear canal by pulling auricle down and back (children) or upward and outward (adult).
3. Instill prescribed drops holding dropper 1 cm (½ inch) above ear canal (see illustration).

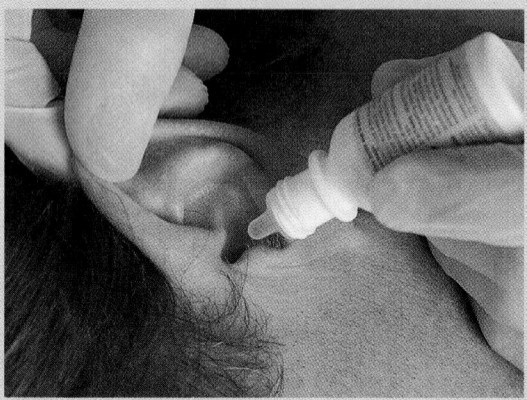

Step 3

4. Ask client to remain in side-lying position 2 to 3 minutes. Apply gentle massage or pressure to tragus of ear with finger.
5. At times the prescriber orders insertion of portion of cotton ball into outermost part of canal. Do not press cotton into canal. Remove cotton after 15 minutes.

Ear Irrigations

1. Assess the tympanic membrane or review medical record for history of eardrum perforation, which would contraindicate ear irrigation.
2. Assist client to assume sitting or lying position with head tilted or turned toward affected ear. Place towel under client's head and shoulder and have client hold basin under affected ear.
3. Fill irrigating syringe with solution (approximately 50 ml).
4. Gently grasp auricle and straighten ear canal by pulling it down and back (children) or upward and outward (adult).
5. Slowly instill irrigating solution by holding tip of syringe 1 cm (½ inch) above opening of ear canal. Allow fluid to drain out during instillation. Continue until canal is cleansed or all solution is used.

The nurse places the medication onto the conjunctival sac where it remains in place for up to 1 week. Currently, medications such as pilocarpine are administered this way. The client receiving medications in this way requires teaching about monitoring for adverse reactions to the disk as well as methods of insertion and removal. Skill 26-3 reviews the steps the nurse uses for administering an intraocular disk.

Ear Instillation

Internal ear structures are very sensitive to temperature extremes. Failure to instill ear drops or irrigating fluid at room temperature may cause vertigo (severe dizziness) or nausea. Although the structures of the outer ear are not sterile, it is wise to use sterile drops and solutions in case the eardrum is ruptured. The entrance of nonsterile solutions into middle ear structures could result in infection. With ear drainage, the nurse should check with the physician to be sure the client does not have a ruptured eardrum. A nurse should never occlude the ear canal with the dropper or irrigating syringe. Forcing medication into an occluded ear canal creates pressure that may injure the eardrum. Box 26-9 reviews guidelines for administering ear drops and ear irrigations.

External ear structures of children differ from those of adults. When instilling drops or irrigating solutions, the nurse must straighten the ear canal. In infants and young children the nurse straightens the cartilaginous canal by grasping the auricle of the ear and pulling it gently down and backward. In adults the ear canal is longer and composed of underlying bone and is straightened by pulling the auricle upward and backward. Failure to straighten the canal properly may prevent medicinal solutions from reaching the deeper external ear structures.

Vaginal Instillation

Vaginal medications are available as suppositories, foam, jellies, or creams. Suppositories come individually packaged in foil wrappers. Storage in a refrigerator prevents the solid, oval-shaped suppositories from melting. After a suppository is inserted into the vaginal cavity, body temperature causes it to melt and be distributed and absorbed. Foam, jellies, and creams are administered with an applicator or inserter (Figure 26-13). A suppository is given with a gloved hand in accordance with Standard Precautions (Figure 26-14). Clients often prefer administering their own vaginal medications and should be given privacy. After instillation of the medication, a client may wish to wear a perineal pad to collect drainage. Because vaginal medications are often given to treat infection, discharge may be foul smelling. Aseptic technique should be followed, and the client should be offered frequent opportunities to maintain perineal hygiene (see Chapter 29).

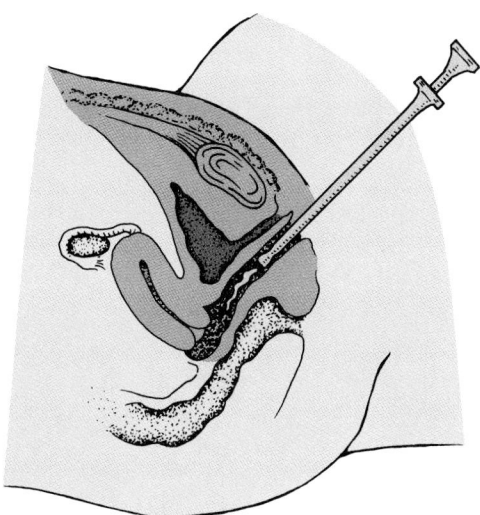

Figure 26-13. Instillation of medication in vaginal canal.

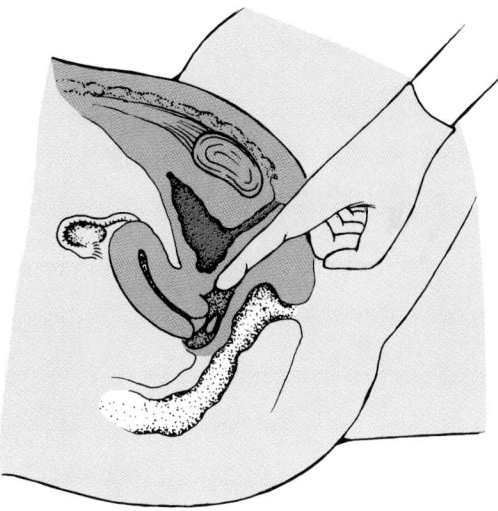

Figure 26-14. Insertion of a suppository into the vaginal canal.

Rectal Instillation

Rectal suppositories are thinner and more bullet shaped than vaginal suppositories. The rounded end prevents anal trauma during insertion. Rectal suppositories contain medications that exert local effects such as promoting defecation or systemic effects such as reducing nausea. Rectal suppositories are stored in the refrigerator until administered.

During administration, the nurse must place the suppository past the internal anal sphincter and against the rectal mucosa. Otherwise the suppository may be expelled before it can dissolve and be absorbed into the mucosa. With practice a nurse learns to recognize the sensation of the sphincter relaxing around the finger. The suppository should not be forced into a mass of fecal material. It may be necessary to clear the rectum with a small cleansing enema before a suppository can be inserted.

⋯ADMINISTERING MEDICATIONS BY INHALATION

Medications administered with hand-held inhalers are dispersed through an aerosol spray, mist, or powder that penetrates lung airways. The alveolar-capillary network absorbs medications rapidly. **Metered-dose inhalers (MDIs)** are usually designed to produce local effects such as bronchodilation. However, some medications can create serious systemic side effects.

Clients who receive medications by inhalation frequently suffer chronic respiratory disease such as chronic asthma, emphysema, or bronchitis. Medications given by inhalation provide these clients with control of airway obstruction, and because these clients depend on medications for disease control, they must learn about them and ways to administer them safely (Skill 26-4).

An MDI delivers a measured dose of medication with each push of a canister. Approximately 5 to 10 pounds of pressure must be used to activate the aerosol. This is important for the nurse to know, because hand strength diminishes with age and from the effects of chronic respiratory disease. The nurse evaluates whether clients have enough hand strength to use the MDI appropriately (see Skill 26-4).

⋯ADMINISTERING MEDICATIONS BY IRRIGATION

Medications may be used to irrigate or wash out a body cavity and are delivered through a stream of solution. Irrigations most commonly use sterile water, saline, or antiseptic solutions on the eye, ear, throat, vagina, and urinary tract. If there is a break in the skin or mucosa, the nurse uses aseptic technique. When the cavity to be irrigated is not sterile, as in the case with the ear canal (see Box 26-9) or vagina, clean technique is acceptable. In health care settings, however, use sterile solutions. Irrigations can cleanse an area, instill a medication, or apply hot or cold to injured tissue.

⋯PARENTERAL ADMINISTRATION OF MEDICATIONS

Parenteral administration of medications is the administration of medications by injection. When medications are administered this way, it is an invasive procedure

Using Metered Dose Inhalers

Delegation Considerations
Administering MDI and supervising clients who self-administer MDIs require problem solving and knowledge application unique to professional nursing. Delegation to unlicensed personnel is not appropriate.

Equipment
- MDI with medication canister
- Aerochamber (optional)
- Facial tissues (optional)
- Wash basin or sink with warm water
- Paper towel
- MAR or computer printout

STEPS	RATIONALE
1. Assess client's ability to hold, manipulate, and depress canister and inhaler.	Any impairment of grasp or presence of hand tremors interferes with client's ability to depress canister within inhaler.
2. Assess client's readiness to learn: client asks questions about medication, disease, or complications; requests education in use of inhaler; is mentally alert; participates in own care.	Affects client's ability to understand explanations and actively participate in teaching process.
3. Assess client's ability to learn: client should not be fatigued, in pain, or in respiratory distress; assess level of understanding of technical vocabulary terms.	Mental or physical limitations affect client's ability to learn and methods nurse uses for instruction.
4. Assess client's knowledge and understanding of disease and purpose and action of prescribed medications.	Knowledge of disease is essential for client to realistically understand use of inhaler.
5. Assess drug schedule and number of inhalations prescribed for each dose.	Influences explanations nurse provides for use of inhaler.
6. If previously instructed in self-administration of inhaled medicine, assess client's technique in using an inhaler.	Nurse's instruction may require only simple reinforcement, depending on client's level of dexterity.
7. Instruct client in comfortable environment by sitting in chair in hospital room or sitting at kitchen table in home.	Client will be more likely to remain receptive of nurse's explanation.
8. Provide adequate time for teaching session.	Prevents interruptions. Instruction should occur when client is receptive.
9. Wash hands and arrange equipment needed.	Reduces transfer of microorganisms and saves time.
10. Allow client opportunity to manipulate inhaler, canister, and spacer device. Explain and demonstrate how canister fits into inhaler.	Client must be familiar with how to use equipment.
11. Explain what metered dose is, and warn client about overuse of inhaler, including drug side effects.	Client must not arbitrarily administer excessive inhalations because of risk of serious side effects. If drug is given in recommended doses, side effects are uncommon.
12. Explain steps for administering inhaled dose of medication (demonstrate steps when possible):	Use of simple, step-by-step explanations allows client to ask questions at any point during procedure.
a. Remove mouthpiece cover from inhaler.	
b. Shake inhaler well.	Ensures fine particles are aerosolized.
c. Have client take a deep breath and exhale.	Prepares the client's airway to receive the medication.

STEPS	RATIONALE
d. Instruct the client to position the inhaler in one of two ways. (1) Open lips and place inhaler in mouth with opening toward back of throat (see illustration). (2) Position the device 1 to 2 inches from the mouth (see illustration).	Directs aerosol spray toward airway. Positioning the mouthpiece 1 to 2 inches from the mouth is considered the best way to deliver the medication.
e. With the inhaler properly positioned, have client hold inhaler with thumb at the mouthpiece and the index finger and middle finger at the top. This is called a three-point or lateral hand position.	MDIs work best when clients use a three-point or lateral hand position to activate canisters (Statz, 1984).
f. Instruct client to tilt head back slightly, inhale slowly and deeply through mouth, and depress medication canister fully.	Medication is distributed to airways during inhalation. Inhalation through mouth rather than nose draws medication more effectively into airways.
g. Hold breath for approximately 10 seconds.	Allows tiny drops of aerosol spray to reach deeper branches of airways.
h. Exhale through pursed lips.	Keeps small airways open during exhalation.
13. Explain steps to administer inhaled dose of medication using a spacer such as an ae__ __mber (demonstrate when possible):	
a. Remove mouthpiece cover fro__ __nd mouthpiece of aerochamber.	Inhaler fits into end of aerochamber.
b. Insert MDI into end of aer__	Aerochamber is a spacer that traps medication released from the MDI; the client then inhales the drug from the device. These devices deposit up to 80% more medication in the lungs rather than in the oropharynx (Weixler, 1994).
c. Shake inhaler well.	Ensures fine particles are aerosolized.
d. Place aerochamber mou hpiece in mouth and close lips. Do not insert beyond raised lip on mouthpiece. Avoid covering small exhalation slots with the lips (see illustration).	Medication should not escape through mouth.

Continued

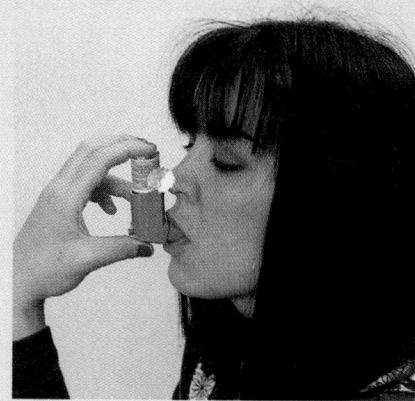

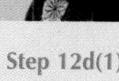

Step 12d(1)

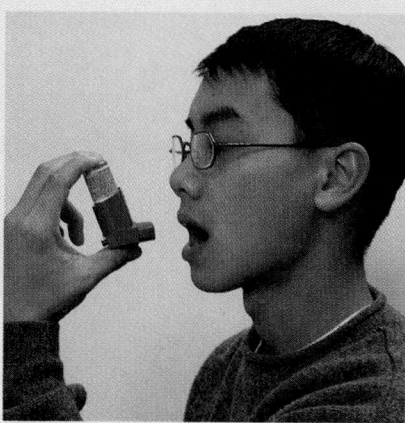

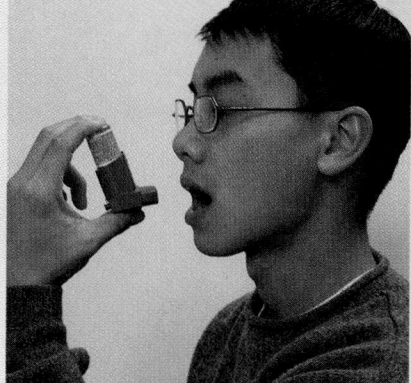

Step 12d(2)

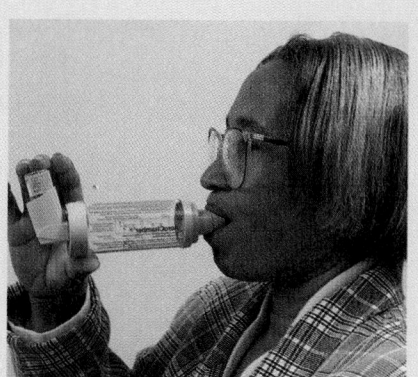

Step 13b

Skill 26-4—cont'd
Using Metered Dose Inhalers

STEPS	RATIONALE
e. Breathe normally through aerochamber mouthpiece.	Allows client to relax before delivering medication.
f. Depress medication canister, spraying one puff into aerochamber.	Emits spray that allows finer particles to be inhaled. Large droplets are retained in aerochamber.
g. Breathe in slowly and fully (for 5 seconds).	Ensures particles of medication are distributed to deeper airways.
h. Hold full breath for 5 to 10 seconds.	Ensures full drug distribution.
14. Instruct client to wait 2 to 5 minutes between inhalations or as ordered by prescriber.	Drugs must be inhaled sequentially. First inhalation opens airways and reduces inflammation. Second or third inhalation penetrates deeper airways.
15. Instruct client against repeating inhalations before next scheduled dose.	Drugs are prescribed at intervals during day to provide constant drug levels and minimize side effects. Beta-adrenergic MDIs are used either on an "as needed" basis or regularly every 4 to 6 hours.
16. Explain that client may feel gagging sensation in throat caused by droplets of medication on pharynx or tongue.	Results when inhalant is sprayed and inhaled incorrectly.
17. Instruct client in removing medication canister and cleaning inhaler in warm water.	Accumulation of spray around mouthpiece can interfere with proper distribution during use.
18. Ask if client has any questions.	Clarifies misconceptions or misunderstanding.
19. Have client explain and demonstrate steps in use of inhaler.	Return demonstration provides feedback for measuring client's learning.
20. Ask client to explain drug schedule.	Improves likelihood of compliance with therapy.
21. Ask client to describe side effects of medication and criteria for calling physician.	Will allow client to recognize signs of overuse and need to seek medical support when drugs are ineffective.
22. After medication instillation, assess client's respirations and auscultate lungs.	Determines status of breathing pattern and adequacy of ventilation.

Recording and Reporting
▪ Document in nurse's notes what skills were taught and client's ability to perform skills.
▪ Record time when client used MDI (amount of puffs).

▪ Report any undesirable effects from medication.

Home Care Considerations
▪ Teach clients how to determine fullness of canisters, using displacement in water (see illustration).

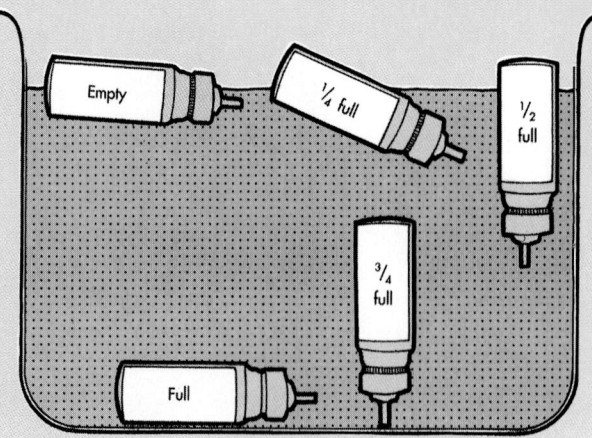

that must be performed using aseptic techniques (Box 26-10). After a needle pierces the skin, there is risk of infection. Each type of injection requires certain skills to ensure that the medication reaches the proper location. The effects of a parenterally administered medication can develop rapidly, depending on the rate of medication absorption. The nurse closely observes the client's response.

Equipment

A variety of syringes and needles are available, each designed to deliver a certain volume of a medication to a specific type of tissue. The nurse uses judgment when determining the syringe or needle that will be most effective.

Syringes. Syringes consist of a cylindrical barrel with a tip designed to fit the hub of a hypodermic needle and a close-fitting plunger. Syringes, in general, are classified as being Luer-lok or non–Luer-lok. This name is based on the design on the syringe's tip. Luer-lok syringes (Figure 26-15, *A*) require special needles, which are twisted onto the tip and lock themselves in place. This design prevents the inadvertent removal of the needle. Non–Luer-lok syringes (Figure 26-15, *B-D*) require needles that slip onto the tip. Most health care institutions use disposable, single-use plastic syringes, which are inexpensive and easy to manipulate.

The nurse fills a syringe by aspiration, pulling the plunger outward while the needle tip remains immersed in the prepared solution. The nurse may handle the outside of the syringe barrel and the handle of the plunger. To maintain sterility, the nurse avoids letting any unsterile object touch the tip or inside of the barrel, the hub, the shaft of the plunger, or the needle (Figure 26-16).

Syringes come in a number of sizes, from 0.5 to 60 ml. It is unusual to use a syringe larger than 5 ml for an SQ or IM injection. A 2- to 3-ml syringe is usually adequate. A larger volume creates discomfort. The nurse uses large syringes to administer certain IV medications, add medications to IV solutions, and irrigate wounds or drainage tubes. A 2.5- or 3-ml hypodermic syringe often comes prepackaged with a needle attached. However, the nurse may change needle sizes. The hypodermic has two scales along the barrel; one is divided into minims and the other into tenths of a milliliter.

Insulin syringes (see Figure 26-15, *C* and *D*) hold 0.5 to 1 ml and are calibrated in units. Insulin syringes that hold 0.5 ml are known as low-dose

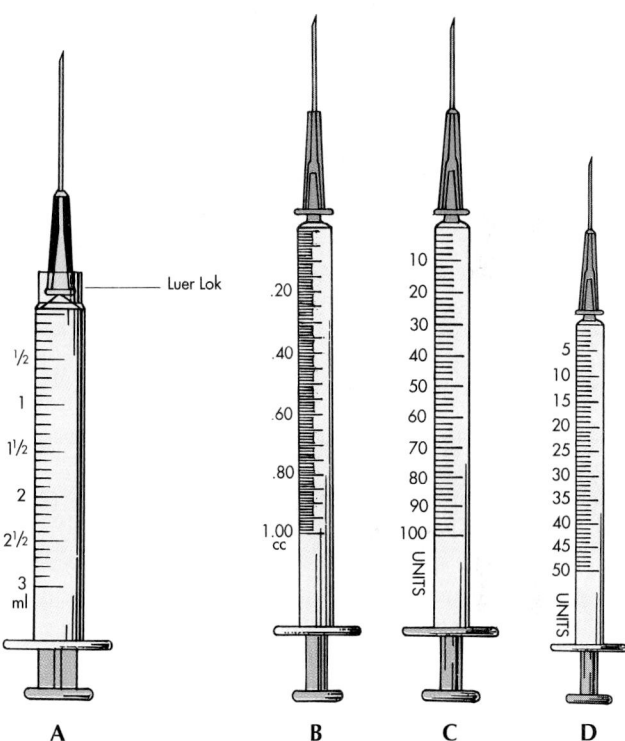

Figure 26-15. Types of syringes. **A,** Luer-lok syringe marked in 0.1 (tenths). **B,** Tuberculin syringe marked in 0.01 (hundredths) for doses of less than 1 ml. **C,** Insulin syringe marked in units (100). **D,** Insulin syringe marked in units (50).

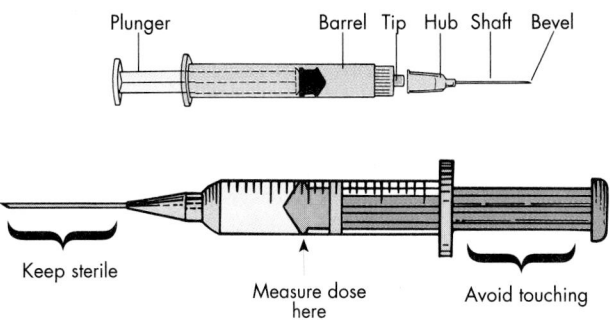

Figure 26-16. Parts of a syringe.

> ### Box 26-10
> ## Preventing Infection During an Injection
>
> To prevent contamination of solution, draw medication from ampule quickly. Do not allow it to stand open.
>
> To prevent needle contamination, avoid letting needle touch contaminated surface (e.g., outer edges of ampule or vial, outer surface of needle cap, nurse's hands, counter top, table surface).
>
> To prevent syringe contamination, avoid touching length of plunger or inner part of barrel. Keep tip of syringe covered with cap or needle.
>
> To prepare skin, wash skin soiled with dirt, drainage, or feces with soap and water and dry. Use friction and a circular motion while cleaning with an antiseptic swab. Swab from center of site, and move outward in a 2-inch radius.

syringes (50 micrograms per 0.5 ml). Most insulin syringes are U-100s, designed for use with U-100 strength insulin. Each milliliter of solution contains 100 units of insulin.

The tuberculin syringe (see Figure 26-15, *B*) has a long, thin barrel with a preattached thin needle. The syringe is calibrated in sixteenths of a minim and hundredths of a milliliter and has a capacity of 1 ml. The nurse uses a tuberculin syringe to prepare small amounts of potent medications. A tuberculin syringe is also useful when preparing small precise doses for infants or young children.

Needles. Needles come packaged in individual sheaths to allow flexibility in choosing the right needle for a client. Some needles are preattached to standard-size syringes. Most needles are made of stainless steel and are disposable.

The needle has three parts: the hub, which fits onto the tip of a syringe; the shaft, which connects to the hub; and the bevel or slanted tip (see Figure 26-16). The tip of a needle, or the bevel, is always slanted. The bevel creates a narrow slit when injected into tissue and quickly closes when the needle is removed to prevent leakage of medication, blood, or serum. A short beveled tip is best for IV injections, because it is not easily occluded against the inside of a blood vessel wall. Long beveled tips are sharper and narrower, which minimizes discomfort when entering tissue used for SQ or IM injections.

Needles vary in length from $\frac{1}{4}$ to 3 inches (Figure 26-17). The nurse chooses the needle length according to the client's size and weight and the type of tissue into which the medication is to be injected. A child or slender adult generally requires a shorter needle. The nurse uses longer needles (1 to $1\frac{1}{2}$ inches) for IM injections and a shorter needle ($\frac{3}{8}$ to $\frac{5}{8}$ inch) for SQ injections.

The smaller the needle gauge, the larger the needle diameter (see Figure 26-17). The selection of a gauge depends on the viscosity of fluid to be injected or infused. An IM injection usually requires a 19- to 23-gauge needle, depending on the viscosity of the medication. SQ injections require smaller-diameter needles such as a 25-gauge needle. A 26-gauge needle is used for an ID injection.

Disposable injection units. Disposable, single-dose, prefilled syringes are available for some medications. The nurse must be careful to check the medication and concentration, because all prefilled syringes appear very similar. With these syringes the nurse does not have to prepare medication dosages, except perhaps to expel portions of unneeded medications.

The Tubex and Carpoject injection systems include a reusable plastic mechanism that holds prefilled, disposable, sterile cartridge-needle units (Figure 26-18).

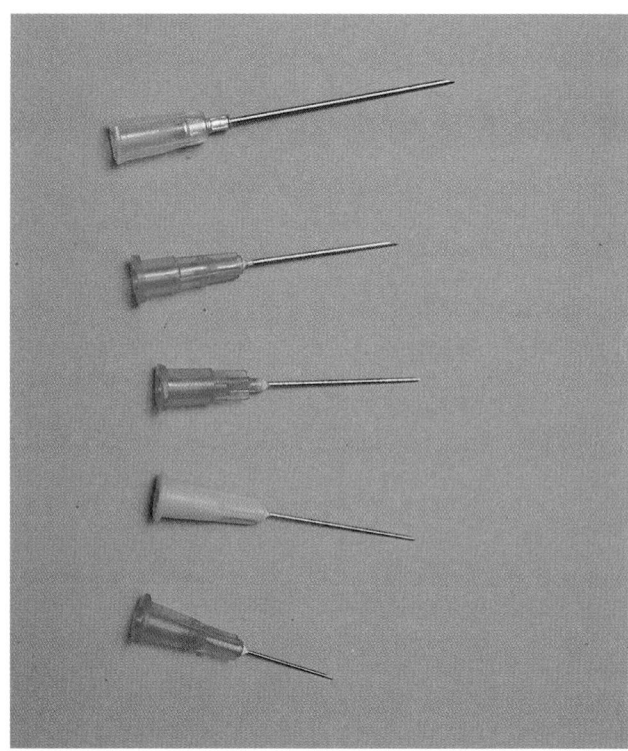

Figure 26-17. Hypodermic needles (*top to bottom*): 19 gauge, $1\frac{1}{2}$-inch length; 20 gauge, 1-inch length; 21 gauge, 1-inch length; 23 gauge, 1-inch length; and 25 gauge, $\frac{5}{8}$-inch length.

The nurse slips the cartridge into the syringe, secures it (following package directions), and checks for air bubbles in the syringe. The nurse advances the plunger to expel excess medication as in a regular syringe. A new type of injection system involves screwing a plungerlike device into the end of a prefilled vial containing a needle. After the medication is given, the entire unit is disposed of in a receptacle. This design reduces the risk of needle-stick injuries.

Preparing an Injection From an Ampule

Ampules contain single doses of medication in a liquid. Ampules are available in several sizes, from 1 ml to 10 ml or more (Figure 26-19, *A*). An ampule is made of glass with a constricted neck that must be snapped off to allow access to the medication. A colored ring around the neck indicates where the ampule is prescored to be broken easily. Aspiration of the medication into a syringe occurs easily and may be completed with a filter needle (if required by institutional policy).

Preparing an Injection From a Vial

A vial is a single-dose or multidose container with a rubber seal at the top (Figure 26-19, *B*). A metal cap

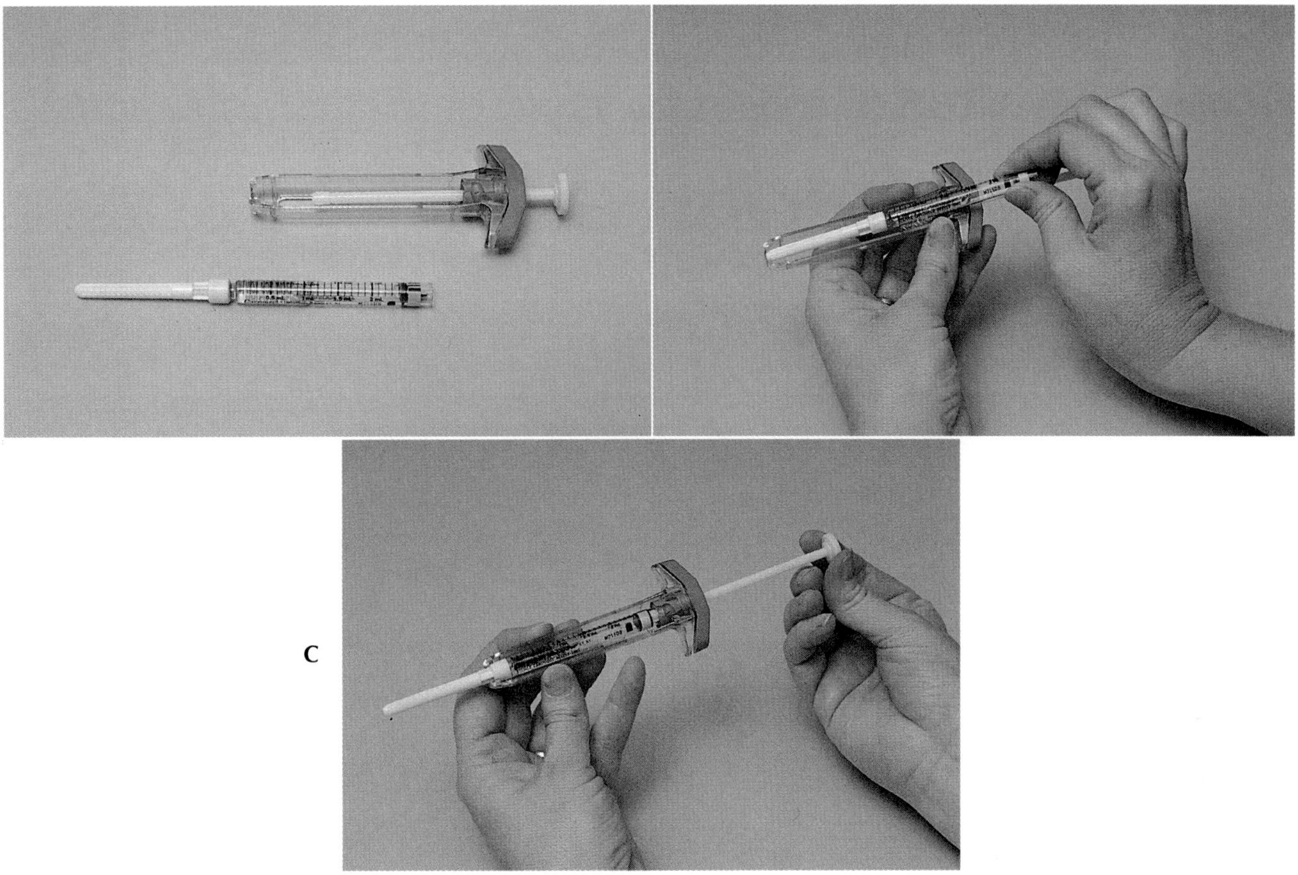

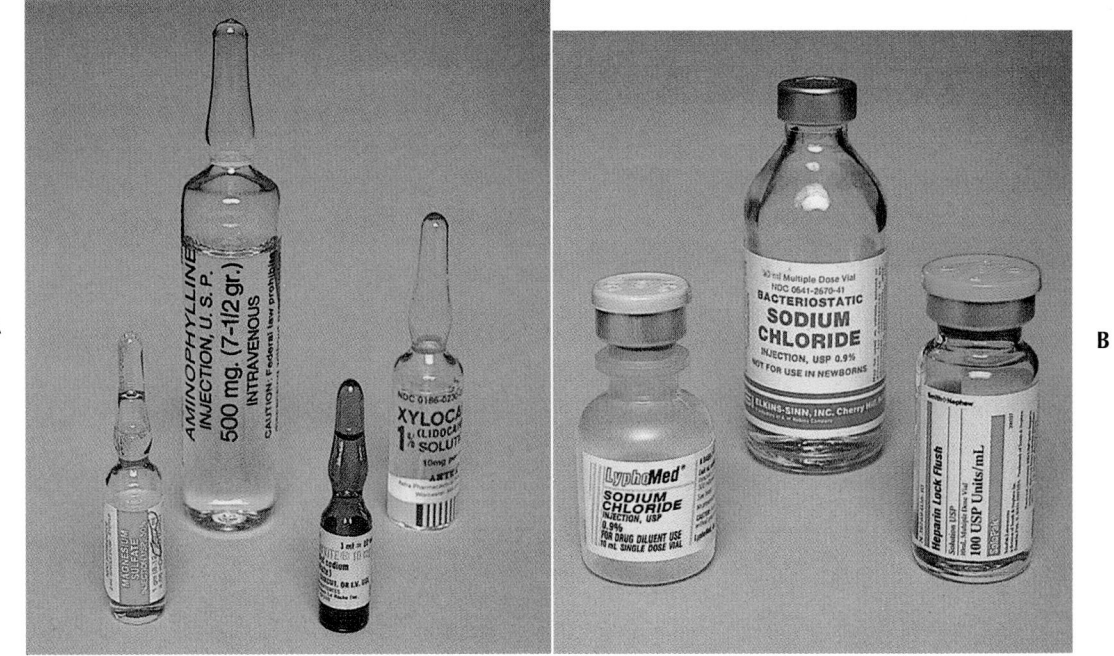

Figure 26-18. **A,** Carpoject syringe and prefilled sterile cartridge with needle. **B,** Assembling the Carpoject. **C,** Cartridge locks at needle end; plunger screws into opposite end.

Figure 26-19. **A,** Medication in ampules. **B,** Medication in vials. Rubber top must be cleansed with alcohol when vial is reused.

Skill 26-5
Preparing Injections

Delegation Considerations

Preparing injections from ampules and vials requires problem solving and knowledge application unique to professional nursing. For this procedure delegation to unlicensed personnel is not appropriate.

Equipment
Medication in an Ampule
- Syringe and two needles (filter needle optional)
- Small gauze pad or alcohol swab

Medication in a Vial
- Syringe and two needles (filter needle optional)
- Small gauze pad or alcohol swab
- Diluent (e.g., normal saline or sterile water) (optional)

Both
- MAR or computer printout

STEPS	RATIONALE
1. Check client's name and drug name, dosage, route of administration, and time of administration.	Ensures correct administration of medication.
2. Review pertinent information related to medication, including action, purpose, side effects, and nursing implications.	Allows nurse to administer drug properly and to monitor client's response.
3. Assess client's body build, muscle size, and weight.	Determines type and size of syringe and needles for injection.
4. Prepare medication.	
A. Ampule preparation:	
(1) Tap top of ampule lightly and quickly with finger until fluid moves from neck of ampule (see illustration).	Dislodges any fluid that collects above neck of ampule. All solution moves into lower chamber.
(2) Place small gauze pad around neck of ampule.	Placing pad around neck of ampule protects nurse's fingers from trauma as glass tip is broken off.
(3) Snap neck of ampule quickly and firmly away from hands (see illustration).	Protects nurse's fingers and face from shattering glass.
(4) Draw up medication quickly.	System is open to airborne contaminants.

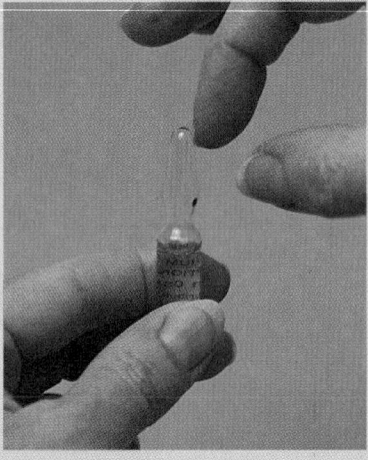

Step 4A(1)

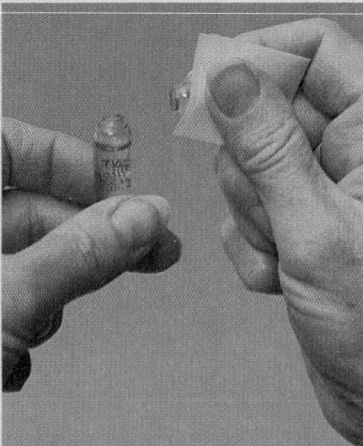

Step 4A(3)

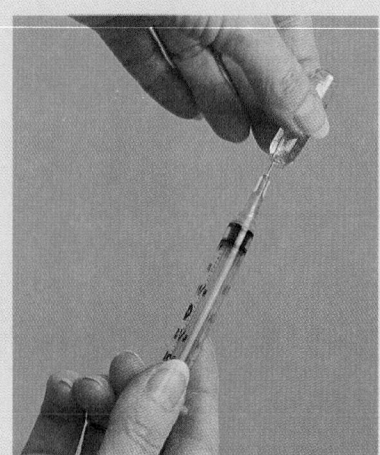

Step 4A(6)

STEPS	RATIONALE
(5) Hold ampule upside down, or set it on a flat surface. Insert syringe or filter needle (see agency policy) into center of ampule opening. Do not allow needle tip or shaft to touch rim of ampule.	Broken rim of ampule is considered contaminated. When ampule is inverted, solution does dribble out if needle tip or shaft touches rim of ampule.
(6) Aspirate medication into syringe by gently pulling back on plunger (see illustration).	Withdrawal of plunger creates negative pressure within syringe barrel, which pulls fluid into syringe.
(7) Keep needle tip under surface of liquid. Tip ampule to bring all fluid within reach of the needle.	Prevents aspiration of air bubbles.
(8) If air bubbles are aspirated, do not expel air into ampule.	Air pressure may force fluid out of ampule and medication will be lost.
(9) To expel excess air bubbles, remove needle from ampule. Hold syringe with needle pointing up. Tap side of syringe to cause bubbles to rise toward needle. Draw back slightly on plunger, and then push plunger upward to eject air. Do not eject fluid.	Withdrawing plunger too far will remove it from barrel. Holding syringe vertically allows fluid to settle in bottom of barrel. Pulling back on plunger allows fluid within needle to enter barrel so fluid is not expelled. Air at top of barrel and within needle is then expelled.
(10) If syringe contains excess fluid, use sink for disposal. Hold syringe vertically with needle tip up and slanted slightly toward sink. Slowly eject excess fluid into sink. Recheck fluid level in syringe by holding it vertically.	Medication is safely dispersed into sink. Position of needle allows medication to be expelled without flowing down needle shaft. Rechecking fluid level ensures proper dose.
(11) Cover needle with its safety sheath or cap. Change needle on syringe or use filter needle if you suspect medication is on needle shaft.	Prevents contamination of needle. New needle prevents tracking medication through skin and SQ tissues.

B. Vial containing a solution:

STEPS	RATIONALE
(1) Remove cap covering top of unused vial to expose sterile rubber seal, keeping rubber seal sterile. If a multidose vial that has been used before is being used again, firmly and briskly wipe surface of rubber seal with alcohol swab and allow it to dry.	Vial comes packaged with cap to prevent contamination of rubber seal. Cap cannot be replaced after seal removal. Allowing alcohol to dry prevents needle from being coated with alcohol and mixing with medication.
(2) Pick up syringe and remove needle cap. Pull back on plunger to draw amount of air into syringe equivalent to volume of medication to be aspirated from vial.	Air must first be injected into vial to prevent buildup of negative pressure in vial when aspirating medication.
(3) With vial on flat surface, insert tip of needle with beveled tip entering first through center of rubber seal (see illustration on p. 644). Apply pressure to tip of needle during insertion.	Center of seal is thinner and easier to penetrate. Injecting beveled tip first and using firm pressure prevent coring of rubber seal, which could enter vial or needle.
(4) Inject air into the vial's airspace, holding on to plunger. Hold plunger with firm pressure; plunger may be forced backward by air pressure within the vial.	Air must be injected before aspirating fluid. Injecting into vial's airspace prevents formation of bubbles and inaccuracy in dosage.

Continued

Skill 26-5—cont'd
Preparing Injections

STEPS	RATIONALE
(5) Invert vial while keeping firm hold on syringe and plunger (see illustration). Hold vial between thumb and middle fingers of nondominant hand. Grasp end of syringe barrel and plunger with thumb and forefinger of dominant hand to counteract pressure in vial.	Inverting vial allows fluid to settle in lower half of container. Position of hands prevents forceful movement of plunger and permits easy manipulation of syringe.
(6) Keep tip of needle below fluid level.	Prevents aspiration of air.
(7) Allow air pressure from the vial to fill syringe gradually with medication. If necessary, pull back slightly on plunger to obtain correct amount of solution.	Positive pressure within vial forces fluid into syringe.
(8) When desired volume has been obtained, position needle into vial's airspace; tap side of syringe barrel carefully to dislodge any air bubbles. Eject any air remaining at top of syringe into vial.	Forcefully striking barrel while needle is inserted in vial may bend needle. Accumulation of air displaces medication and causes dosage errors.
(9) Remove needle from vial by pulling back on barrel of syringe.	Pulling plunger rather than barrel causes plunger to separate from barrel, resulting in loss of medication.
(10) Hold syringe at eye level, at 90-degree angle, to ensure correct volume and absence of air bubbles. Remove any remaining air by tapping barrel to dislodge any air bubbles (see illustration). Draw back slightly on plunger; then push plunger upward to eject air. Do not eject fluid.	Holding syringe vertically allows fluid to settle in bottom of barrel. Pulling back on plunger allows fluid within needle to enter barrel so fluid is not expelled. Air at top of barrel and within needle is then expelled.

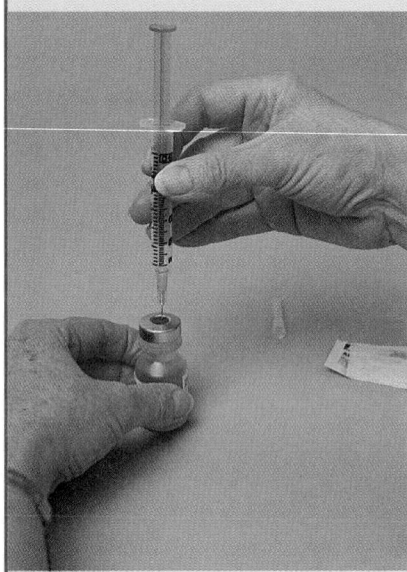

Step 4B(3)

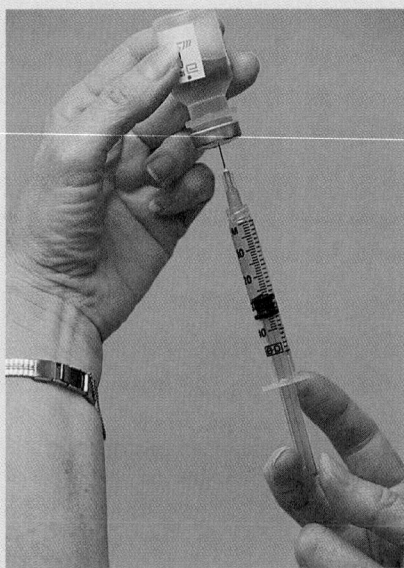

Step 4B(5)

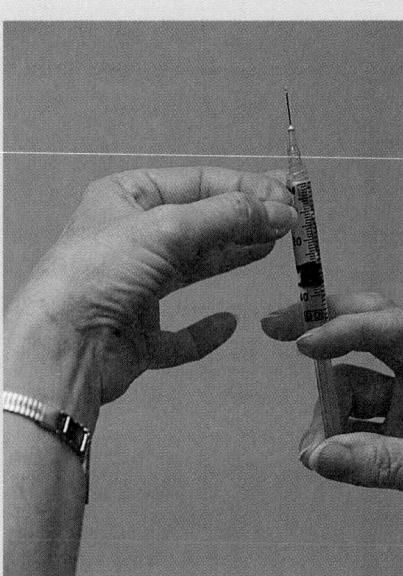

Step 4B(10)

STEPS	RATIONALE
(11) If medication is to be injected into client's tissue, change needle to appropriate gauge and length according to route of medication.	Inserting needle through a rubber stopper may dull beveled tip. New needle is sharper. Because no fluid is along shaft, needle will not track medication through tissues.
(12) For multidose vial, make label that includes date of mixing, concentration of drug per milliliter, and nurse's initials.	Ensures that future doses will be prepared correctly. Some drugs must be discarded after certain number of days after mixing of vial.
C. Vial containing a powder (reconstituting medications):	
(1) Remove cap covering vial of powdered medication and cap covering vial of proper diluent.	Cap prevents contamination of rubber seal.
(2) Draw up diluent into syringe following Steps 4B(2) through 4B(10).	Prepares diluent for injection into vial containing powdered medication.
(3) Insert tip of needle through center of rubber seal of vial of powdered medication. Inject diluent into vial. Remove needle.	Diluent begins to dissolve and reconstitute medication.
(4) Mix medication thoroughly. Roll in palms. Do not shake.	Ensures proper dispersal of medication throughout solution.
(5) Reconstituted medication in vial is ready to be drawn into new syringe. Read label carefully to determine dose after reconstitution.	Once diluent has been added, concentration of medication (mg/ml) determines dose to be given.
5. Dispose of soiled supplies. Place broken ampule and/or used vials and used needle in puncture-proof and leak-proof container. Clean work area and wash hands.	Proper disposal of glass and needle prevents accidental injury to staff. Controls transmission of infection.

protects the seal until it is ready for use. Vials contain liquid or dry forms of medications. Medications that are unstable in solution are packaged dry. The vial label specifies the solvent or diluent used to dissolve the medication and the amount of diluent needed to prepare a desired medication concentration. Normal saline and sterile distilled water are solutions commonly used to dissolve medications.

Unlike the ampule, the vial is a closed system, and air must be injected into it to permit easy withdrawal of the solution. Failure to inject air when withdrawing creates a vacuum within the vial that makes withdrawal difficult (Skill 26-5).

To prepare a powdered medication, the nurse draws up the amount of diluent or solvent recommended on the vial's label. The nurse injects the diluent into the vial in the same manner as injecting air into the vial. Most powdered medications dissolve easily, but it may be necessary to withdraw the needle to mix the contents thoroughly. Gently shaking or rolling the vial between the hands will dissolve the powdered medication. The needle is reinserted to draw up the dissolved medication. After mixing multidose vials the nurse makes a label that includes the date and time of mixing and the concentration of medication per milliliter. Multidose vials may require refrigeration after the contents are reconstituted.

Mixing Medications

If two medications are compatible, it is possible to mix them in one injection. Most nursing units have charts that list common compatible medications. If there is any uncertainty about medication compatibilities, consult a pharmacist.

Mixing medications from two vials. The nurse applies the following principles when mixing medications from two vials:

1. Do not contaminate one medication with another.
2. Ensure the final dosage is accurate.
3. Maintain aseptic technique.

Only one syringe is needed to mix medications from two vials (Figure 26-20). The nurse takes a syringe and aspirates the volume of air equivalent to the first medication's dose (vial A). The nurse injects the air into vial A, making sure the needle does not touch the solution. The nurse withdraws the needle, aspirates air equivalent to the second medication's dose (vial B), and then injects the volume of air into vial B. The nurse immediately withdraws the medication from vial B into the syringe. At this point the medication from vial A has not contaminated vial B. The nurse applies a new sterile needle to the syringe and inserts it into vial A, being careful not to push the plunger and expel the medication within the syringe into the vial. The nurse then withdraws the desired amount of medication from vial A into the syringe. If a vial has excess positive pressure, the plunger may move before the nurse is ready, causing an accidental withdrawal of too much of the med-

ication. After withdrawing the necessary amount, the nurse withdraws the needle, applies a new needle, and sheathes the syringe.

Mixing medications from one vial and one ampule.
Mixing medications from a vial and an ampule is simple because it is not necessary to add air to withdraw medication from an ampule. The nurse prepares medication from the vial first and then, using the same syringe and needle, withdraws medication from the ampule. This technique prevents contamination of the solution in the vial and the needle.

Insulin preparation.
Insulin is the hormone used to treat diabetes mellitus. It must be administered by injection, because it is broken down and destroyed in the GI tract. In the United States and Canada, the medication is available in 100 units per milliliter of solution. When preparing insulin, the correct syringe must be used; a 100-unit scaled syringe is used to prepare 100-unit insulin.

Insulin is classified by rate of action, including rapid, intermediate, and long-acting. A client with diabetes

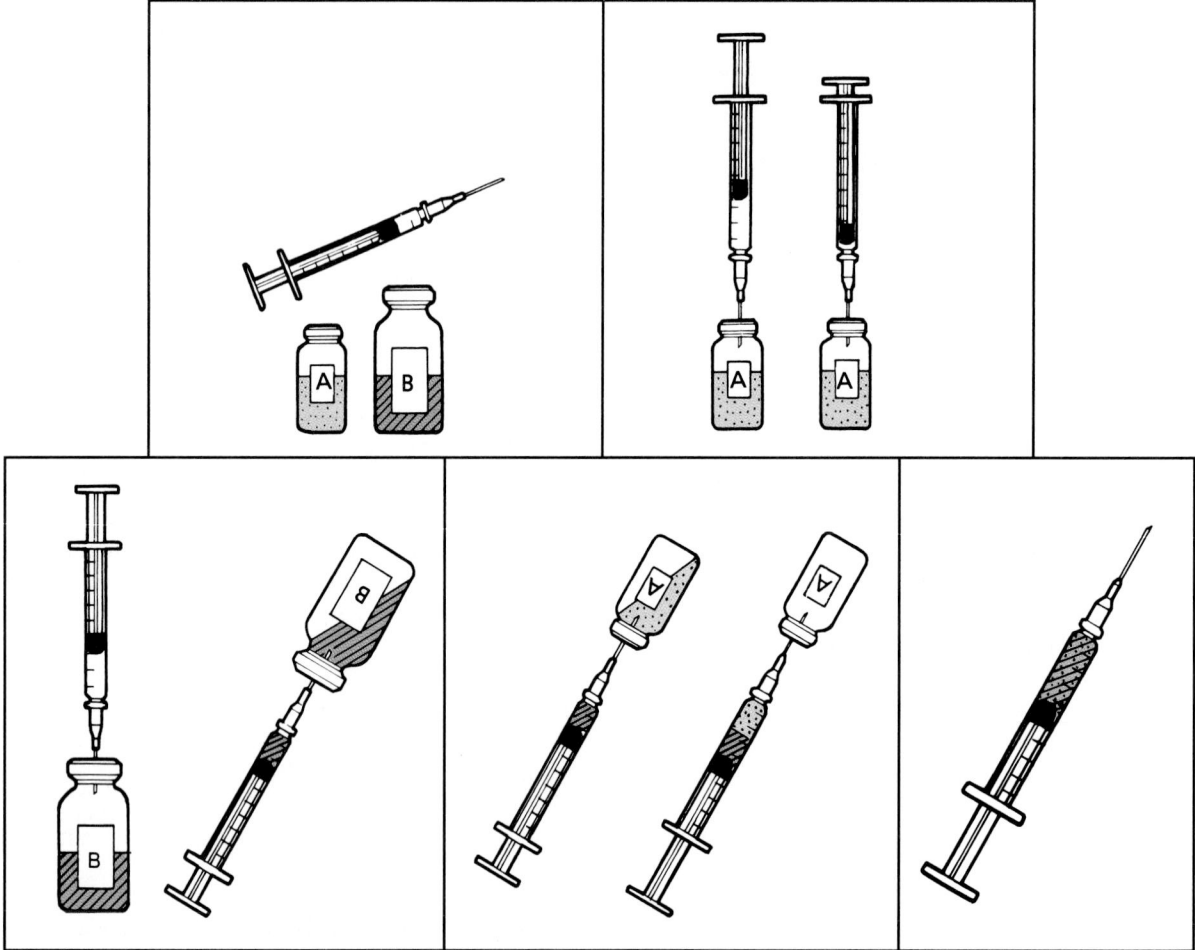

Figure 26-20. Steps in mixing medications from two vials.

may require more than one type of insulin. For example, by receiving a rapid-acting (regular) and an intermediate-acting (NPH) insulin, a client receives more sustained control of blood sugar over 24 hours.

Regular unmodified insulin is a clear solution that acts rapidly and can be given either subcutaneously or intravenously. Other types of insulin are cloudy because of the addition of a protein, which slows absorption. These slower-acting insulin preparations can be given only subcutaneously.

Insulin is ordered by specific dosage at select times or by a sliding scale. A sliding scale dictates a certain dosage based on the client's blood sugar level. Only regular insulin is used for sliding scales. Before mixing different types of insulin, each vial should be rotated at least 1 minute between both hands. This resuspends the modified insulin preparations and helps to warm the medication. The nurse should not shake insulin vials. Shaking causes bubbles to form, which take up space in a syringe and alter the dosage. Box 26-11 describes the guidelines used for mixing two kinds of insulin in the same syringe.

Administering Injections

Each injection route is unique in regard to the type of tissues into which the medication is injected. The characteristics of the tissues influence the rate of medication absorption and thus the onset of medication action. Before injecting a medication the nurse should know the volume of the medication to administer, the medication's characteristics and viscosity, and the location of anatomical structures underlying injection sites (Skill 26-6).

A nurse's inability to administer injections correctly can have negative consequences. Failure to select an injection site in relation to anatomical landmarks can result in nerve or bone damage during needle insertion. If the nurse fails to aspirate the syringe before injecting a medication, the medication may accidentally be injected directly into an artery or vein. Injecting too large a volume of medication for the site selected causes extreme pain and may result in local tissue damage.

Many clients, particularly children, fear injections. Clients with serious or chronic illness often are given several injections daily. The nurse may be able to minimize the client's discomfort in the following ways:

1. Using a sharp-beveled needle in the smallest suitable length and gauge
2. Positioning the client as comfortably as possible to reduce muscular tension
3. Selecting the proper injection site, using anatomical landmarks
4. Diverting the client's attention from the injection through conversation
5. Inserting the needle quickly and smoothly to minimize tissue pulling

---

Box 26-11

Procedural Guidelines for Mixing Two Kinds of Insulin in One Syringe

1. Lente insulins (Semilente, Lente, Ultralente) may be mixed with each other, in any ratio.
2. Regular insulin may be mixed with any ratio.
3. Mixing of regular and Lente insulin is not recommended except for clients already adequately controlled on such a mixture. This is caused by the binding of Lente insulin with regular insulin, delaying onset of action.

To prepare insulin from two vials, the nurse or client follows these steps:

1. With an insulin syringe and needle, inject air, equal to the dose of insulin to be withdrawn, into the vial of modified insulin (cloudy vial). Do not touch the tip of the needle to the solution.
2. Remove the syringe from the vial of modified insulin.
3. With the same syringe, inject air, equal to the dose of insulin to be withdrawn, into the vial of unmodified (regular) insulin (clear vial). Then withdraw the correct dose.
4. Remove the syringe from the unmodified (regular) insulin. Carefully remove air bubbles in the syringe to ensure correct dosage.
5. Return to the vial of modified insulin and withdraw the correct dose.
6. Administer mixture of insulins within 5 minutes of preparing it. Regular insulin binds with modified (NPH) insulin, thus reducing the action of the regular insulin.

Always prepare the unmodified (regular) insulin first. This prevents adding modified insulin to the unmodified (regular) vial. If two modified forms are mixed, it makes no difference which vial is prepared first.

Modified from White JR, Campbell RK. In Haire-Joshu D, editor: *Management of diabetes mellitus: perspectives of care across the life span*, ed 2, St. Louis, 1996, Mosby.

---

6. Holding the syringe steady while the needle remains in tissues
7. Injecting the medication slowly and steadily
8. Massaging the injected area gently for several seconds unless contraindicated

Subcutaneous injections. SQ injections involve placing medications into the loose connective tissue under the dermis (see Skill 26-6). Because SQ tissue is not

Administering Injections

Delegation Considerations
Administering injections requires problem solving and knowledge application unique to professional nursing. For this procedure delegation to unlicensed personnel is not appropriate.

Equipment
- Proper size syringe and needle:
    SQ: Syringe (1 to 3 ml) and needle (27 to 25 gauge, $\frac{3}{8}$ to $\frac{5}{8}$ inch)

IM: Syringe 2 to 3 ml for adult, 0.5 to 1 ml for infants and small children. Two needles: 21 to 23 gauge, 1 to $1\frac{1}{2}$ inches for adults; 1 inch for children

ID: 1-ml tuberculin syringe with preattached 26- or 27-gauge needle
- Small gauze pad and/or alcohol swab
- Vial or ampule of medication or skin test solution
- Disposable gloves
- MAR or computer printout

STEPS	RATIONALE
For all injections:	
1. Review physician's medication order for client's name, drug name, dose, time, and route of administration.	Ensures safe and correct administration of medication.
2. Assess client's history of allergies and know substances client is allergic to and normal allergic reaction.	Certain substances have similar compositions; nurse should not administer any substance to which client is known to be allergic.
3. Check date of expiration for medication vial or ampule.	Drug potency may increase or decrease when outdated.
4. Observe verbal and nonverbal responses toward receiving injection.	Injections can be painful. Clients may have anxiety, which can increase pain.
5. Assess for contraindications.	
A. For subcutaneous injections: Assess for factors such as circulatory shock or reduced local tissue perfusion. Assess adequacy of client's adipose tissue.	Reduced tissue perfusion interferes with drug absorption and distribution. Physiological changes of aging or client illness may influence the amount of SQ tissue a client possesses. This influences methods for administering injections.
B. For intramuscular injections: Assess for factors such as muscle atrophy, reduced blood flow, or circulatory shock.	Atrophied muscle absorbs medication poorly. Factors interfering with blood flow to muscles impair drug absorption.
6. Prepare correct medication dose from ampule or vial (see Skill 26-5). Check carefully. Be sure all air is expelled.	Ensures that medication is sterile. Preparation techniques differ for ampule and vial.
7. Identify client by checking identification armband and asking client's name. Compare with MAR.	Ensures correct client receives ordered drug.
8. Explain steps of procedure and tell client injection will cause a slight burning or sting.	Helps minimize client's anxiety.
9. Close room curtain or door.	Provides privacy.
10. Wash hands thoroughly.	Reduces transfer of microorganisms.
11. Keep sheet or gown draped over body parts not requiring exposure.	Proper selection of injection site may require exposure of body parts.

STEPS	RATIONALE

12. Select appropriate injection site. Inspect skin surface over sites for bruises, inflammation, or edema.

   a. SQ: Palpate sites for masses or tenderness. Avoid these areas. For daily insulin, rotate site daily. Be sure needle is correct size by grasping skinfold at site, with thumb and forefinger. Measure fold from top to bottom. Needle should be one-half length.

   b. IM: Note integrity and size of muscle and palpate for tenderness or hardness. Avoid these areas. If injections are given frequently, rotate sites.

   c. ID: Note lesions or discolorations of forearm. Select site three to four fingerwidths below antecubital space and a handwidth above wrist.

CRITICAL DECISION POINT

Injection sites should be free of abnormalities that may interfere with drug absorption. Site used repeatedly can become hardened from lipohypertrophy (increased growth in fatty tissue). An ID site should be clear so that results of skin test can be seen and interpreted correctly. Do not use an area that is bruised or has signs associated with infection.

13. Assist client to comfortable position:

   a. SQ: Have client relax arm, leg, or abdomen, depending on site chosen for injection. — Relaxation of site minimizes discomfort.

   b. IM: Have client lie flat, on side, or prone, depending on site chosen. — Reduces strain on muscle and minimizes discomfort of injections.

   c. ID: Have client extend elbow and support it and forearm on flat surface. — Stabilizes injection site for easiest accessibility.

   d. Talk with client about subject of interest. — Distraction reduces anxiety.

CRITICAL DECISION POINT

Ensure that client's position is not contraindicated by medical condition.

14. Relocate site using anatomical landmarks. — Injection into correct anatomical site prevents injury to nerves, bones, and blood vessels.

15. Cleanse site with an antiseptic swab. Apply swab at center of the site and rotate outward in a circular direction for about 5 cm (2 inches) (see illustration, p. 650). — Mechanical action of swab removes secretions containing microorganisms.

16. Hold swab or gauze between third and fourth fingers of nondominant hand. — Gauze or swab remains readily accessible when needle is withdrawn.

17. Remove needle cap or sheath from needle by pulling it straight off. — Preventing needle from touching sides of cap prevents contamination.

Continued

Skill 26-6—cont'd
Administering Injections

STEPS	RATIONALE
18. Hold syringe between thumb and forefinger of dominant hand	
a. SQ: Hold as dart, palm down (see illustration) or hold syringe across tops of fingertips.	Quick, smooth injection requires proper manipulation of syringe parts.
b. IM: Hold as dart, palm down.	
c. ID: Hold bevel of needle pointing up.	With bevel up, medication is less likely to be deposited into tissues below dermis.
19. Administer injection:	
A. Subcutaneous:	
(1) For average-size client, spread skin tightly across injection site or pinch skin with nondominant hand.	Needle penetrates tight skin easier than loose skin. Pinching skin elevates SQ tissue and may desensitize area.
(2) Inject needle quickly and firmly at 45- to 90-degree angle. Then release skin, if pinched.	Quick, firm insertion minimizes discomfort. (Injecting medication into compressed tissue irritates nerve fibers.)
(3) For obese client, pinch skin at site and inject needle at 90-degree angle below tissue fold.	Obese clients have fatty layer of tissue above SQ layer.
(4) After needle enters site, grasp lower end of syringe barrel with nondominant hand. Move dominant hand to end of plunger. Avoid moving syringe while slowly pulling back on plunger to aspirate drug (see illustration). If blood appears in syringe, remove needle, discard medication and syringe, and repeat procedure. *Exception: Do not aspirate when giving heparin.*	Properly performed injection requires smooth manipulation of syringe parts. Movement of syringe may displace needle and cause discomfort. Aspiration of blood into syringe indicates IV placement of needle. SQ and IM injections are not for IV use (dermis is relatively vascular). Aspiration of heparin injection may cause the needle to move, creating tissue damage and bleeding.
(5) Inject medication slowly.	

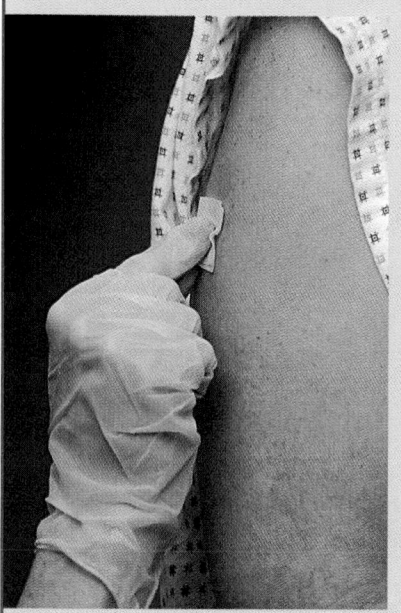

Step 15

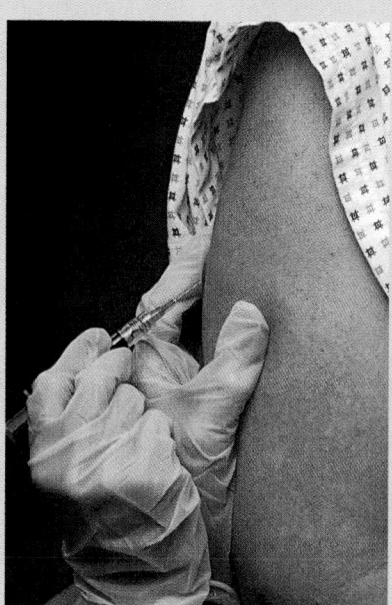

Step 18a

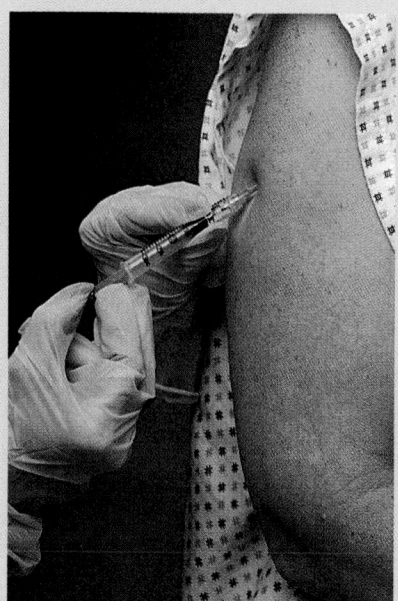

Step 19A(4)

STEPS	RATIONALE
B. Intramuscular:	
(1) Position nondominant hand at proper anatomical landmarks and pull skin down to administer in a Z-track. Inject needle quickly at 90-degree angle into muscle.	Speeds insertion and reduces discomfort. Creates zigzag path through tissues that seals needle track to avoid tracking of medication.
(2) If client's muscle mass is small, grasp body of muscle between thumb and fingers.	Ensures that medication reaches muscle mass.
(3) Aspirate as in Step 19A(4).	
(4) Inject medication slowly.	
(5) Wait 10 seconds. Then smoothly and steadily withdraw needle while placing antiseptic swab or dry gauze gently above or over injection.	Support of tissues around infection site minimizes discomfort during needle withdrawal. Some advocate use of dry gauze to minimize client discomfort associated with alcohol on non-intact skin.
C. Intradermal:	
(1) With nondominant hand, stretch skin over site with forefinger or thumb.	Needle pierces tight skin more easily.
(2) With needle almost against client's skin, insert it slowly at a 5- to 15-degree angle until resistance is felt. Then advance needle through epidermis to approximately 3 mm (⅛ inch) below skin surface. Needle tip can be seen through skin.	Ensures needle tip is in dermis.
(3) Inject medication slowly. Normally, resistance is felt. If not, needle is too deep; remove and begin again.	Slow injection minimizes discomfort at site. Dermal layer is tight and does not expand easily when solution is injected.
(4) While injecting medication, notice that small bleb approximately 6 mm (½ inch) resembling mosquito bite appears on skin's surface (see illustration).	Bleb indicates medication is deposited in dermis.
20. Withdraw needle while applying alcohol swab or gauze gently over site. Support of tissue around injection site minimizes discomfort during needle withdrawal.	Some advocate the use of dry gauze to minimize client discomfort associated with alcohol on nonintact skin.

Continued

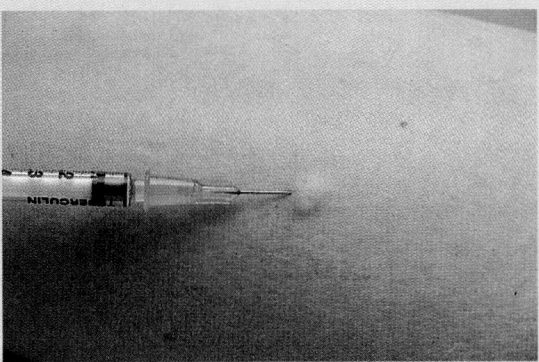

Step 19C(4)

Administering Injections

STEPS	RATIONALE
21. Do not massage site after SQ injection of heparin or insulin or after IM or ID injection. Apply bandage over ID site.	Massage of site after heparin injection may cause bleeding; massage after insulin injection may increase absorption of insulin. Massage of IM site may cause underlying tissue damage. Massage of ID site may disperse medication into underlying tissue layers and alter test results.
22. Assist client to comfortable position.	Gives client sense of well-being.
23. Discard uncapped needle or needle enclosed in safety shield and attached syringe into puncture- and leak-proof receptacle. When nurse is unable to leave client's bedside, a one-handed technique can be used to recap a needle.	Needles should not be recapped before disposal. Safety shields prevent needle-stick injuries.
24. Remove disposable gloves and wash hands.	Reduces transmission of microorganisms.
25. Stay with client and observe for any allergic reactions.	Severe anaphylactic reaction is characterized by dyspnea, wheezing, and circulatory collapse.
26. Return to room and ask if client feels any acute pain, burning, numbness, or tingling at injection site.	Continued discomfort may indicate injury to underlying bones or nerves.
27. Inspect site, noting any bruising or induration.	Bruising or induration indicates complication associated with injection. Notify nurse in charge or health care provider. Provide warm compress to site.
28. Return to evaluate client's response to medication in 10 to 30 minutes. IM medications absorb quickly; undesired effects may also develop rapidly.	Nurse's observations determine efficacy of drug action.
29. Ask client to explain purpose and effects of medication.	Evaluates client's understanding of information taught.
30. *For ID injections,* Use skin pencil and draw circle around perimeter of injection site. Read site within 48 to 72 hours of injection.	Site must be read at various intervals to determine test results. Pencil mark makes site easy to find.

Recording and Reporting
- Chart medication dose, route, site, time, and date given in medication record.
- Report any undesirable effects from medication to nurse in charge or physician.
- Record client's response to medications in nurse's notes.

Home Care Considerations
- Clients with hypertrophy of the skin from repeated insulin injections (common with beef or pork formulations) should be taught not to use the site for 6 months.

as richly supplied with blood as the muscles, medication absorption is somewhat slower than with IM injections. However, medications are absorbed completely if the client's circulatory status is normal. Because SQ tissue contains pain receptors, the client may experience some discomfort.

The best SQ injection sites include the outer posterior aspect of the upper arms, the abdomen from below the costal margins to the iliac crests, and the anterior aspects of the thighs (Figure 26-21). The site most frequently recommended for heparin injections is the abdomen (Figure 26-22). Other sites include the scapular areas of the upper back and the upper ventral or dorsal gluteal areas. The injection site chosen should be free of skin lesions, bony prominences, and large underlying muscles or nerves.

Use of the same part of the body for a sequence of injections provides more consistency in the absorption of the insulin. For example, if the morning insulin is injected into the client's arm, then a subsequent injection should also be given in the arm. The injections are to be given at least an inch away from the previous site. No injection site should be used again for at least 1 month.

Only small doses (0.5 to 1 ml) of water-soluble medications should be given subcutaneously, because the tissue is sensitive to irritating solutions and large volumes of medications. Collection of medications within the tissues can cause sterile abscesses, which appear as hardened, painful lumps under the skin.

A client's body weight indicates the depth of the SQ layer. Therefore the nurse must choose the needle length and angle of insertion based on weight. Generally a 25-gauge ⅝-inch needle inserted at a 45-degree angle (Figure 26-23) or a ½-inch needle inserted at a 90-degree angle deposits medications into the SQ tissue of a normal-size client. A child may require only a ½-inch needle. If the client is obese, the nurse often pinches the tissue and uses a needle long enough to insert through fatty tissue at the base of the skinfold. The preferred needle length is one half the width of the skinfold. With this method the angle of insertion may be between 45 and 90 degrees. Thin clients may have insufficient tissue for SQ injections. The upper abdomen is the best site for injection with this type of client.

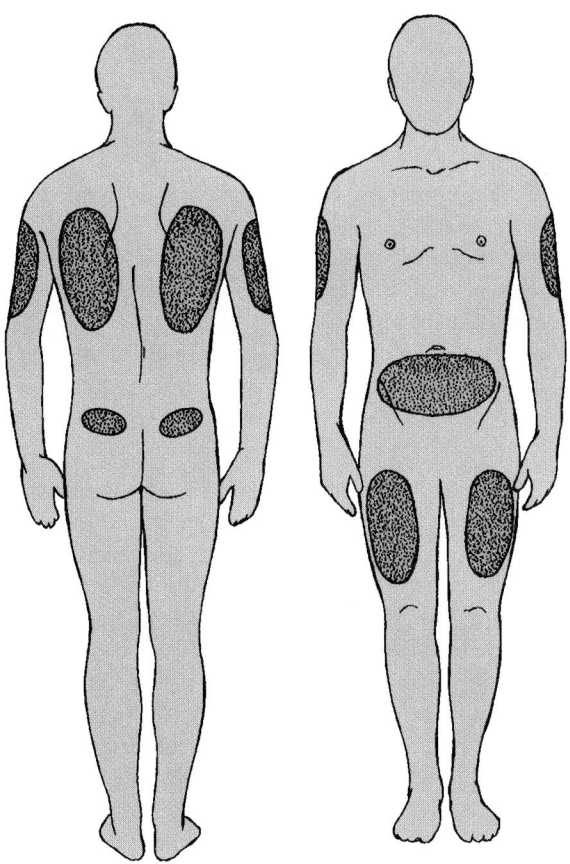

Figure 26-21. Sites recommended for SQ injections.

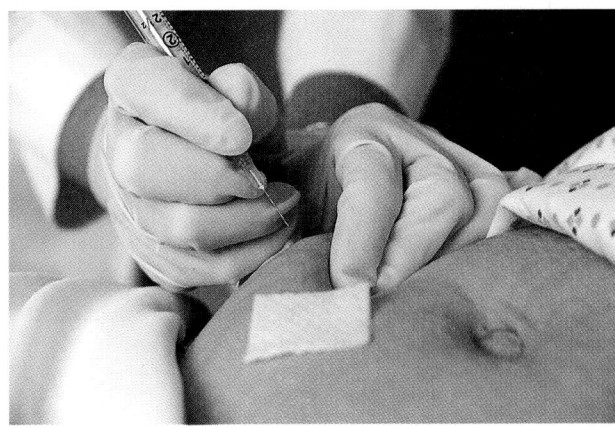

Figure 26-22. Giving SQ heparin in the abdomen.

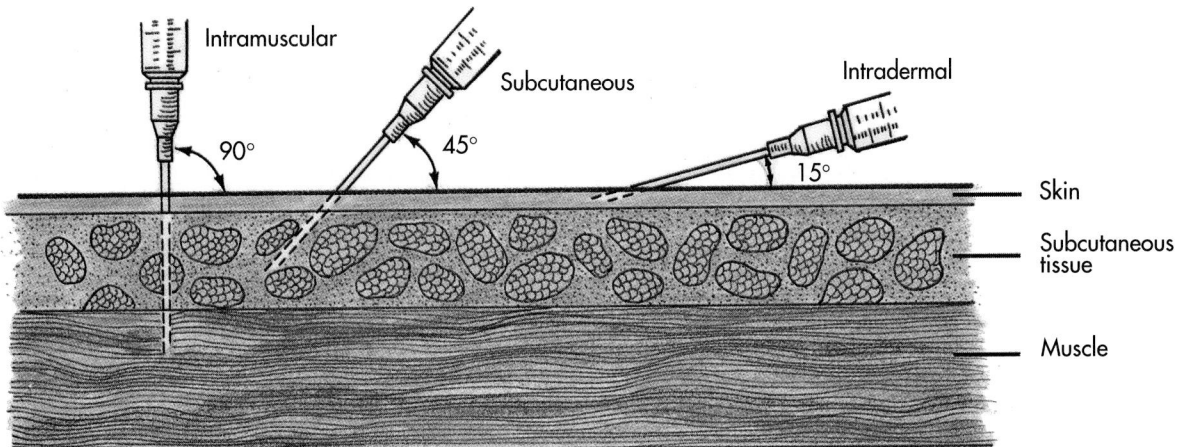

Figure 26-23. Comparison of angles of insertion for IM (90 degrees), SQ (45 degrees), and ID (15 degrees) injections.

Insulin syringes generally come with 26- to 29-gauge needles. To ensure the insulin reaches the SQ tissue, the nurse follows this rule: if 2 inches of tissue can be grasped, the needle should be inserted at a 90-degree angle; if 1 inch of tissue can be grasped, the needle should be inserted at a 45-degree angle.

Intramuscular injections. The IM route provides faster medication absorption than the SQ route because of muscle's greater vascularity. There is less danger of causing tissue damage when medications enter deep muscle, but the risk of inadvertently injecting medications directly into blood vessels exists. The nurse uses a longer and heavier-gauge needle to pass through SQ tissue and penetrate deep muscle tissue (see Skill 26-6). Weight and the amount of adipose tissue can influence needle size selection. For example, an obese client may require a needle 3 inches long, and a thin client may only require a $\frac{1}{2}$- to 1-inch needle.

The angle of insertion for an IM injection is 90 degrees (see Figure 26-23). Muscle is less sensitive to irritating and viscous medications. A normal, well-developed client can tolerate 3 ml of medication into a larger muscle without severe muscle discomfort. A larger volume of medication is unlikely to be absorbed properly. Children, older adults, and thin clients can tolerate only 2 ml of an IM injection. Wong (1995) recommends giving no more than 1 ml to small children and older infants.

The nurse assesses the integrity of a muscle before giving an injection. The muscle should be free of tenderness. Repeated injections in the same muscle can cause severe discomfort. With the client relaxed, the nurse can palpate the muscle to rule out any hardened lesions. The nurse can minimize discomfort during an injection by helping the client assume a position that will help reduce muscle strain.

Sites. When selecting an IM site, the nurse considers the following: Is the area free of infection or necrosis? Are there local areas of bruising or abrasions? What is the location of underlying bones, nerves, and major blood vessels? What volume of medication is to be administered? Each site has certain advantages and disadvantages (Box 26-12).

Ventrogluteal. The ventrogluteal muscle involves the gluteus medius and minimus, is situated deep and away from major nerves and blood vessels, and is a safe site for all clients. Research has shown that injuries such as fibrosis, nerve damage, abscess, tissue necrosis, muscle contraction, gangrene, and pain have been associated with all the common IM sites except the ventrogluteal site (Beyea and Nicoll, 1995). The ventrogluteal site is the preferred injection site for adults and anyone over 7 months old (Beyea and Nicoll, 1996).

The nurse locates the muscle by placing the heel of the hand over the greater trochanter of the client's hip with the wrist perpendicular to the femur. The right

---

> **Box 26-12**
> ## Characteristics of Intramuscular Sites
>
> **Vastus Lateralis**
> Lacks major nerves and blood vessels
> Rapid drug absorption
>
> **Ventrogluteal**
> A deep site, situated away from major nerves and blood vessels
> Less chance of contamination in incontinent clients or infants
> Easily identified by any prominent bony landmark
>
> **Deltoid**
> Easily accessible but muscle not well developed in most clients
> Used for small amounts of drugs
> Not used in infants or children with underdeveloped muscles
> Potential for injury to radial and ulnar nerves or brachial artery

hand is used for the left hip, and the left hand is used for the right hip. The nurse points the thumb toward the client's groin and fingers toward the client's head, points the index finger to the anterosuperior iliac spine, and extends the middle finger back along the iliac crest toward the buttock. The index finger, the middle finger, and the iliac crest form a V-shaped triangle, and the injection site is the center of the triangle (Figure 26-24). The client may lie on the side or back. Flexing of the knee and hip helps the client relax this muscle.

Vastus lateralis. The vastus lateralis muscle is another injection site used in the adult client and children. The muscle is thick and well developed, is located on the anterior lateral aspect of the thigh, and extends in an adult from a handbreadth above the knee to a handbreadth below the greater trochanter of the femur (Figure 26-25). The middle third of the muscle is the suggested site for injection. The width of the muscle usually extends from the midline of the thigh and the midline of the thigh's outer side. With young children or cachectic clients, it helps to grasp the body of the muscle during injection to be sure that the medication is deposited in muscle tissue. To help relax the muscle, the nurse asks the client to lie flat with the knee slightly flexed or to assume a sitting position.

Dorsogluteal. The dorsogluteal muscle has been a traditional site for IM injections; however, a risk exists of striking the underlying sciatic nerve or major blood vessels. Insertion of a needle into the sciatic nerve can cause permanent or partial paralysis of the involved leg. In clients with flabby, sagging tissues the site is difficult to locate. This site is not being recommended for use in this text.

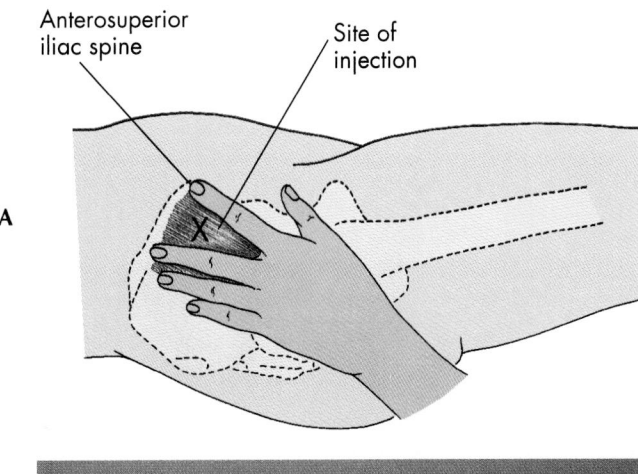

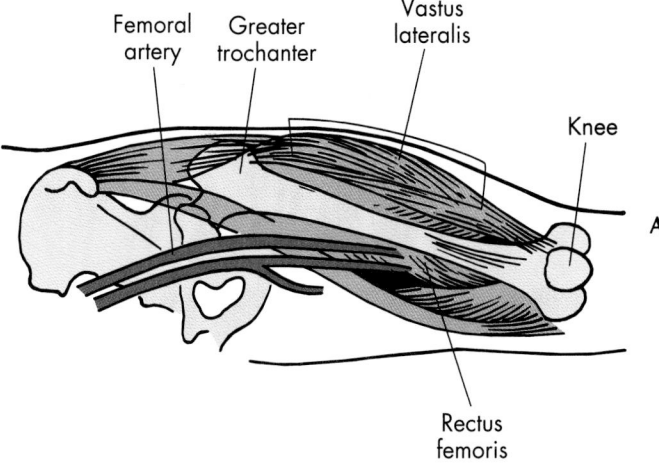

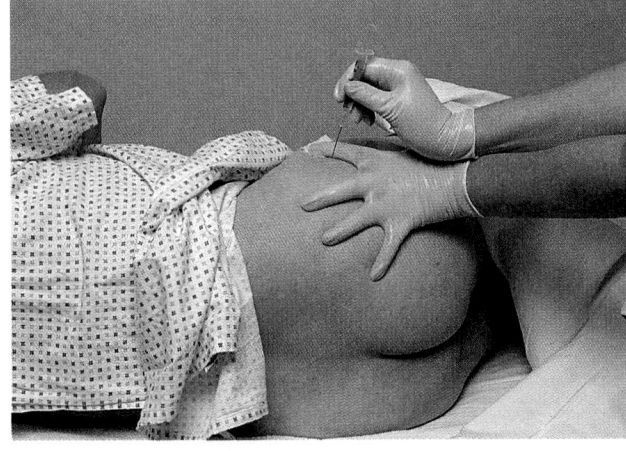

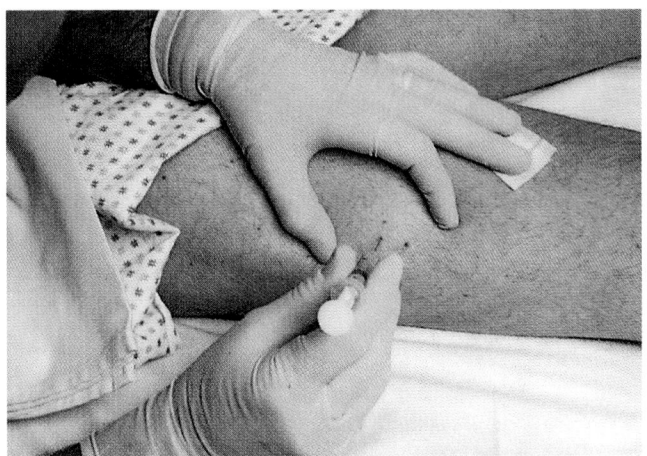

Figure 26-24. **A,** Landmarks for ventrogluteal site. **B,** Locating IM injection for ventrogluteal site.

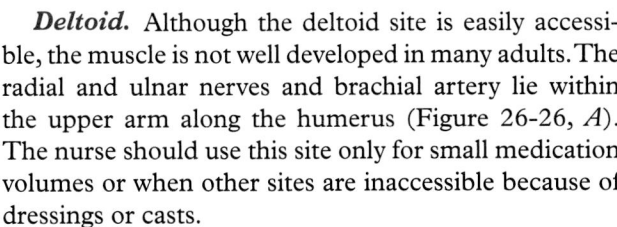

Figure 26-25. **A,** Landmarks for vastus lateralis site. **B,** Giving IM injection in vastus lateralis muscle.

Deltoid. Although the deltoid site is easily accessible, the muscle is not well developed in many adults. The radial and ulnar nerves and brachial artery lie within the upper arm along the humerus (Figure 26-26, *A*). The nurse should use this site only for small medication volumes or when other sites are inaccessible because of dressings or casts.

To locate the deltoid muscle, the nurse fully exposes the client's upper arm and shoulder. A tight-fitting sleeve should not be rolled up. The nurse has the client relax the arm at the side and flex the elbow. The client may sit, stand, or lie down (Figure 26-26, *B*). The nurse palpates the lower edge of the acromion process, which forms the base of a triangle in line with the midpoint of the lateral aspect of the upper arm. The injection site is in the center of the triangle, about 2.5 to 5 cm (1 to 2 inches) below the acromion process (see Figure 26-26, *A*). The nurse may also locate the site by placing four fingers across the deltoid muscle, with the top finger along the acromion process. The injection site is then three fingerwidths below the acromion process.

Technique in intramuscular injections

Z-track method. It is recommended that when giving IM injections, the **Z-track injection** method be used to minimize irritation by sealing the medication in muscle tissue. The nurse selects an IM site, preferably in larger, deeper muscles such as the ventrogluteal muscle. A new needle must be applied to the syringe after preparing the medication so that no solution remains on the outside needle shaft. After preparing the site with an antiseptic swab, the nurse pulls the overlying skin and SQ tissues approximately 2.5 to 3.5 cm (1 to 1½ inches) laterally to the side. Holding the skin taut with the nondominant hand, the nurse injects the needle deep into the muscle. With practice the nurse learns to hold the syringe and aspirate with one hand. The nurse injects the medication and air slowly if there is no blood return on aspiration. The needle remains inserted for 10 seconds to allow the medication to disperse evenly. The nurse then releases the skin after withdrawing the needle. This leaves a zigzag path that seals the needle track where tissue planes slide across each other (Figure 26-27). The medication cannot escape from the muscle tissue.

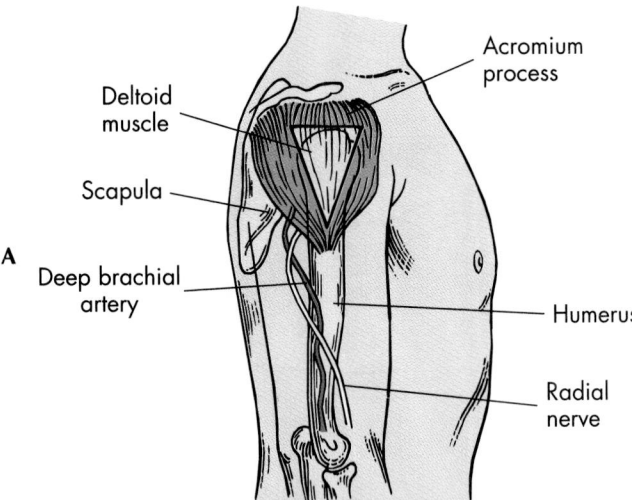

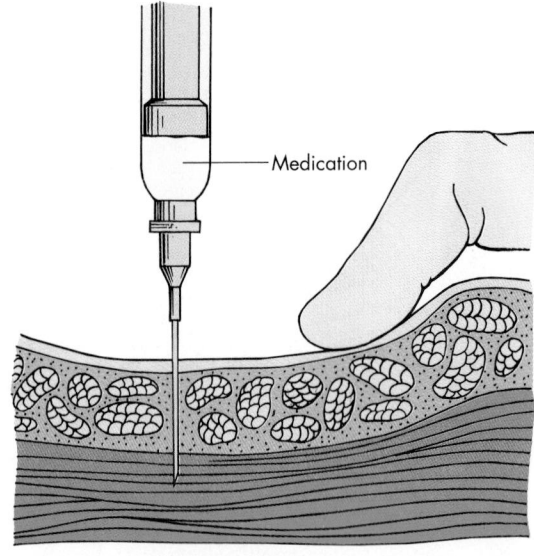

During Injection

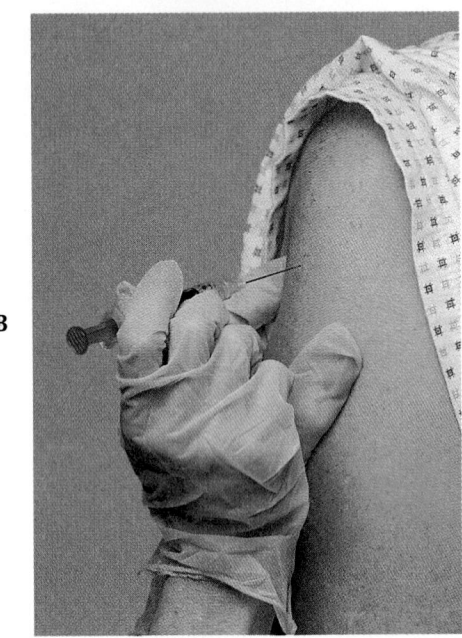

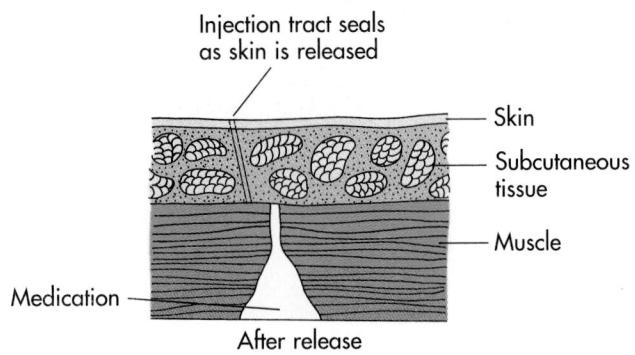

Figure 26-27. Z-track method of injection prevents deposit of medication into sensitive tissues.

Figure 26-26. **A,** Landmarks for deltoid site. **B,** Giving IM infection in deltoid muscle.

sembling a mosquito bite should appear on the skin's surface (see Skill 26-6). If a bleb does not appear or if the site bleeds after needle withdrawal, there is a good chance the medication entered SQ tissues. In this case, test results will not be valid.

Safety in administering medications by injection

Intradermal injections. The nurse typically gives ID injections for skin testing (e.g., tuberculin screening, allergy tests). Because these medications are potent, they are injected into the dermis, where blood supply is reduced and medication absorption occurs slowly. A client may have a severe anaphylactic reaction if the medications enter the circulation too rapidly.

Skin testing requires that the nurse be able to clearly see the injection sites for changes in color and tissue integrity. ID sites should be lightly pigmented, free of lesions, and relatively hairless. The inner forearm and upper back are ideal locations.

The nurse uses a tuberculin or small hypodermic syringe for skin testing. The angle of insertion for an ID injection is 5 to 15 degrees (see Figure 26-23, p. 653). As the nurse injects the medication, a small bleb re-

Needleless devices. Approximately one million accidental needle-stick and sharps injuries occur annually in health care settings (Jagger, 1992). These injuries commonly occur when nurses forget and recap needles, mishandle IV lines and needles, or contact stray needles left at a client's bedside. The risk of exposure of health care workers to blood-borne pathogens has led to the development of "needleless devices" or special needle-safety devices.

Special syringes are designed with a sheath or guard that covers the needle after it is withdrawn from the skin (Figure 26-28). The needle is immediately covered, eliminating the chance for a needle-stick injury. The syringe and sheath are disposed of together in a recepta-

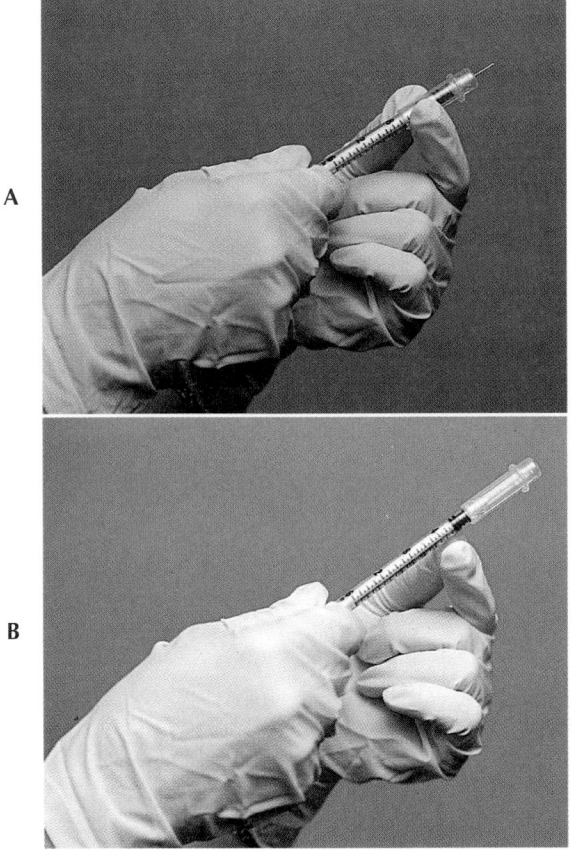

A

B

Figure 26-28. Needle with plastic guard to prevent needle-sticks. **A,** Position of guard before injection. **B,** After injection the guard locks in place, covering the needle.

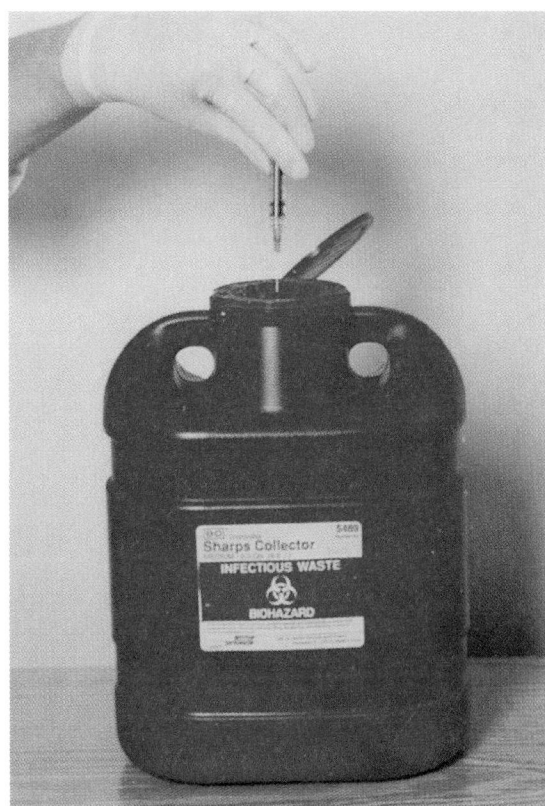

Figure 26-29. Sharps disposal using only one hand.

cle. The CDC and OSHA have recommended use of "needleless" devices to reduce the risk to health care workers of needle-sticks and sharps injuries (Owens-Schwab and Fraser, 1993).

Needles and other instruments considered "sharps" are always disposed of into clearly marked, appropriate containers (Figure 26-29). Containers should be puncture proof and leak proof. A needle should never be forced by anyone into a full needle-disposal receptacle. Used needles and syringes are never placed in any wastebasket, in the nurse's pocket, on a client's meal tray, or at the client's bedside.

One-handed needle recapping technique. In administering injections it may be necessary, for client safety reasons, to recap a contaminated needle. For example, the nurse may be assisting with emergency measures at the bedside and cannot reach a disposal container. If a commercially made recapping device is not available, then the following procedure is recommended to reduce the risk of accidental needle-sticks (Craft, 1990):

1. Position the needle cap on its side at the edge of a table or counter.

2. Hold the syringe with the dominant hand and scoop up the cap with the tip of the needle, being careful not to contaminate a sterile needle (Figure 26-30).
3. Press the syringe, needle, and cover against a flat, vertical surface (e.g., a wall or cabinet door) to get the cap firmly in place.

To reduce the temptation of using two hands, it is suggested that the nondominant hand be held behind the back during the recapping procedure. Craft (1990) also recommends that needle-sticks may be prevented by the nurse carefully assessing the client and the environment and properly disposing of materials in puncture-proof containers as soon as possible.

Intravenous Administration

The nurse administers medications intravenously by the following methods:

1. As mixtures within large volumes of IV fluids
2. By injection of a bolus, or small volume, of medication through an existing IV infusion line or intermittent venous access (heparin or saline lock)
3. By "piggyback" infusion of a solution containing the prescribed medication and a small volume of IV fluid through an existing IV line

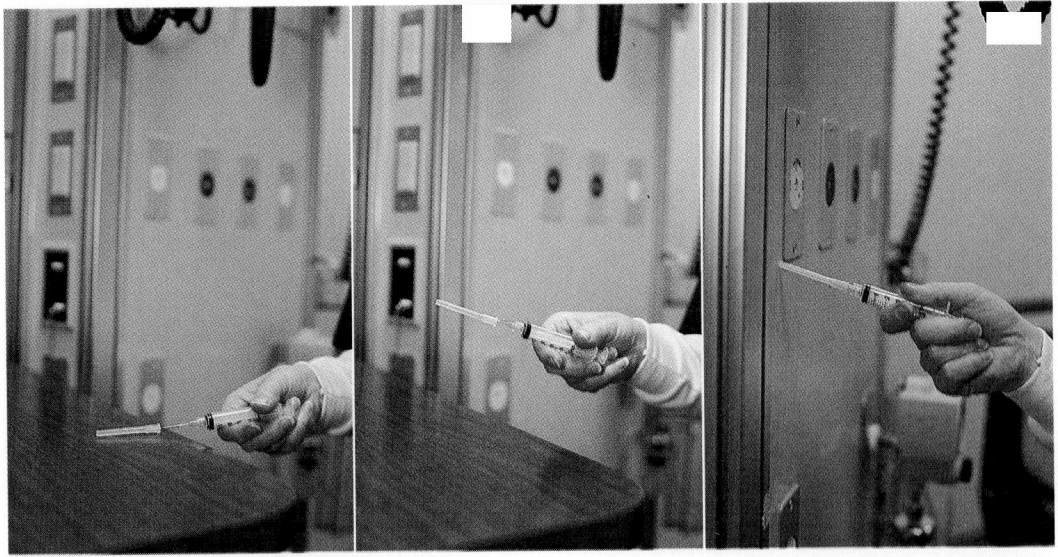

Figure 26-30. The scoop technique to prevent needle-stick injuries.

In all three methods the client has either an existing IV infusion line or an IV access site such as an intermittent infusion (heparin or saline lock). In most institutions, policies and procedures list persons who may give IV medications and the situations in which they may be given. These policies are based on the medication, capability and availability of staff, and type of monitoring equipment available.

Chapter 31 describes the technique for performing venipuncture and establishing continuous IV fluid infusions. Medication administration is only one reason for supplying IV fluids. IV fluid therapy is used primarily for fluid replacement in clients unable to take oral fluids and as a means of supplying electrolytes and nutrients.

When using any method of IV medication administration, the nurse must observe clients closely for symptoms of adverse reactions. After a medication enters the bloodstream, it begins to act immediately, and there is no way to stop its action. Thus the nurse takes special care to avoid errors in dose calculation and preparation. The nurse should double-check the "five rights" of safe medication administration and know the desired action and side effects. If the medication has an antidote, it must be available during administration. When administering potent medications, the nurse assesses vital signs before, during, and after infusion.

Administering medications by the IV route has advantages. Often the nurse uses the IV route in emergencies when a fast-acting medication must be delivered quickly. The IV route is also best when it is necessary to establish constant therapeutic blood levels. Some medications are highly alkaline and irritating to muscle and SQ tissue. These medications cause less discomfort when given intravenously.

Large-volume infusions. Of the three methods of administering IV medications, mixing medications in large volumes of fluids is the safest and easiest. Medications are diluted in large volumes (500 ml or 1000 ml) of compatible IV fluids such as normal saline or lactated Ringer's solution (Skill 26-7). In most institutions the pharmacist adds medications to the primary container of IV solution to ensure asepsis. Because the medication is not in a concentrated form, the risk of side effects or fatal reactions is minimal when infused over the prescribed time frame. Vitamins and potassium chloride are two types of medications commonly added to IV fluids. However, there is a danger with continuous infusion; if the IV fluid is infused too rapidly, the client may suffer circulatory fluid overload.

Intravenous bolus. An IV bolus involves introducing a concentrated dose of a medication directly into the systemic circulation (Box 26-13). Because a bolus requires only a small amount of fluid to deliver the medication, it is an advantage when the amount of fluid the client can take is restricted. The IV bolus is the most dangerous method for administering medications, because there is no time to correct errors. In addition, a bolus may cause direct irritation to the lining of blood vessels. Before administering a bolus the nurse confirms placement of the IV line. This involves obtaining a blood return through the IV catheter or needle. A blood return occurs by slowly pulling back on the syringe plunger and blood appears in the syringe. The inability to obtain a blood return suggests that the needle or catheter is in the client's tissues or resting against the vein wall. A medication should never be given intravenously if the insertion site appears puffy or edematous or the IV fluid cannot flow at the proper rate.

Adding Medications to Intravenous Fluid Containers

. . . . .

Delegation Considerations

Adding medications to IV fluid containers requires problem solving and knowledge application unique to professional nursing. For this procedure delegation to unlicensed personnel is not appropriate. (In some institutions the pharmacist may add drugs to primary containers of IV solutions to ensure asepsis.)

Equipment
- Vial or ampule of prescribed medication

- Syringe of appropriate size (5 to 20 ml)
- Sterile needle (1 to 1½ inch, 19 to 21 gauge) with special filters (optional)
- Correct diluent (e.g., sterile water, normal saline)
- Sterile IV fluid container (bag or bottle, 50 to 1000 ml in volume)
- Alcohol or antiseptic swab
- Label to attach to IV bag or bottle
- MAR or computer printout

STEPS	RATIONALE
1. Check physician's order to determine type of IV solution to use and type of medication and dosage.	Client's overall physical condition dictates type of IV solution used. Ensures safe and accurate drug administration.
2. Collect information necessary to administer drug safely, including action, purpose, side effects, normal dose, time of peak onset, and nursing implications.	Allows nurse to give drug safely and to monitor client's response to therapy.
3. When more than one medication is to be added to IV solution, assess for compatibility of medications.	Drugs often are incompatible when mixed together. Chemical reactions that occur result in clouding or crystallization of IV fluids. Check hospital policy for approved drug compatibility list.
4. Assess client's systemic fluid balance, as reflected by skin hydration and turgor, body weight, pulse, and blood pressure.	Danger of continuous IV infusions is that fluids may infuse too rapidly, causing circulatory overload.
5. Assess client's history of drug allergies.	IV administration of drugs causes rapid effects. Allergic response can be immediate.
6. Assess IV insertion site for signs of infiltration or phlebitis (see Chapter 31).	An intact, properly functioning site ensures medication is given safely.
7. Assess client's understanding of purpose of drug therapy.	May reveal need for education.
8. Wash hands thoroughly.	Reduces transfer of microorganisms.
9. Assemble supplies in medication room.	Ensures procedure will be orderly, with less likelihood of contaminating supplies.
10. Identify client by reading identification band and asking name. Compare with medication ticket.	
11. Prepare prescribed medication from vial or ampule (see Skill 26-5).	Ensures accurate delivery of medication.
12. Add medication to new container (usually done in medication room or at medication cart):	
a. *Solutions in a bag:* Locate medication injection port on plastic IV solution bag. Port has small rubber stopper at end. Do not select port for the IV tubing insertion or air vent.	Medication injection port is self-sealing to prevent introduction of microorganisms after repeated use.
b. *Solutions in bottles:* Locate injection site on IV solution bottle, which is often covered by a metal or plastic cap.	Accidental injection of medication through main tubing port or air vent can alter pressure within bottle and cause fluid leaks through air vent. Cap seals bottle to maintain its sterility.

Continued

.... Skill 26-7—cont'd
Adding Medications to Intravenous
Fluid Containers

STEPS	RATIONALE
c. Wipe off port or injection site with alcohol or antiseptic swab (see illustration).	Reduces risk of introducing microorganisms into bag during needle insertion.
d. Remove needle cap or sheath from syringe and insert needle of syringe through center of injection port or site; inject medication (see illustration).	Injection of needle into sides of port may produce leak and lead to fluid contamination.
e. Withdraw syringe from bag or bottle.	Open tubing port in bottle provides direct route for microorganisms to enter solution. Bags have self-sealing port.
f. Mix medication and IV solution by holding bag or bottle and turning it gently end to end.	Allows even distribution of medication.
g. Complete medication label with name and dose of medication, date, time, and nurse's initials. Stick it on bottle or bag. *Optional (check agency policy): Apply a flow strip that identifies the time the solution was hung and intervals indicating fluid levels (see illustration).* Spike bag or bottle with IV tubing.	Label can be easily read during infusion of solution. Informs nurses and physicians of contents of bag or bottle.

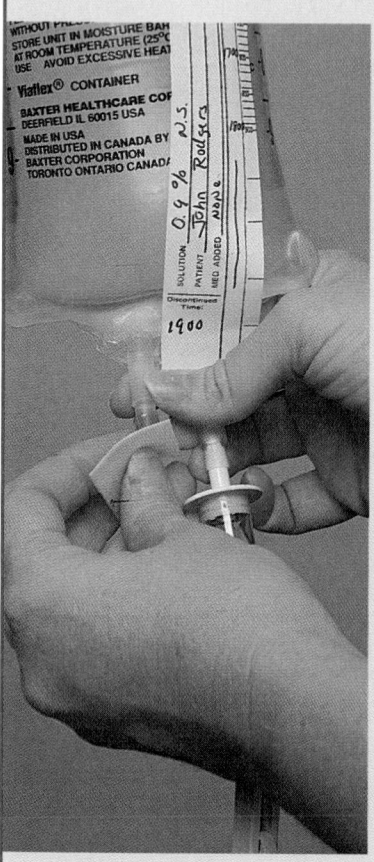

Step 12c

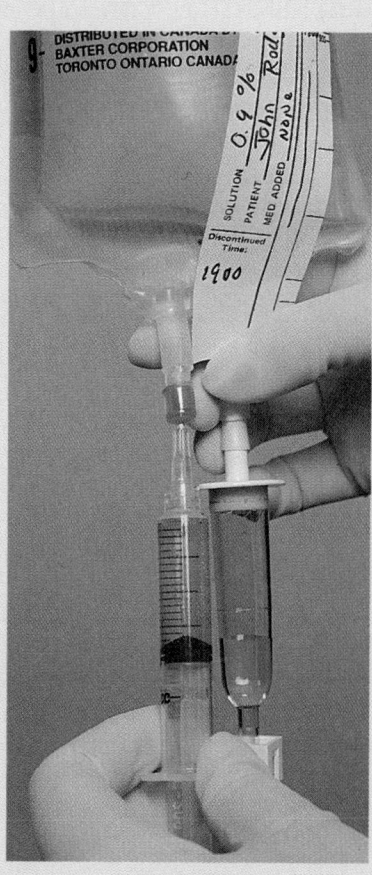

Step 12d

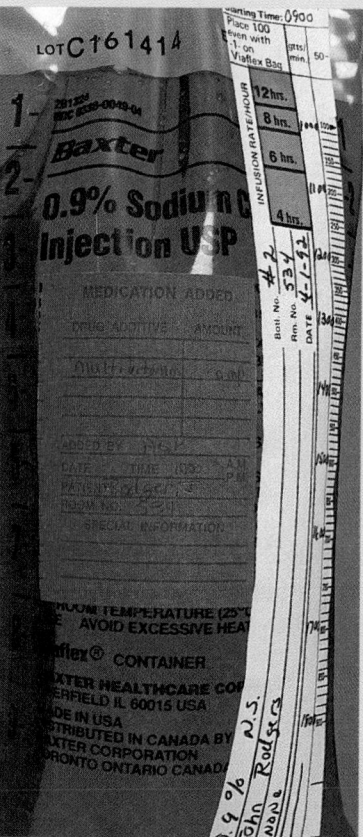

Step 12g

STEPS	RATIONALE
13. Bring assembled items to client's bedside.	Ensures correct client receives ordered medication.
14. Prepare client by explaining that medication is to be given through existing IV line or one to be started. Explain that no discomfort should be felt during drug infusion. Encourage client to report symptoms of discomfort.	Most IV medications do not cause discomfort when diluted. However, potassium chloride can be irritating. Pain at insertion site may be early indication of infiltration.
15. Regulate infusion at ordered rate.	Prevents rapid infusion of fluid.
16. Add medication to existing container:	
a. Prepare vented IV bottle or plastic bag:	
(1) Check volume of solution remaining in bottle or bag.	Proper minimal volume is needed to dilute medication adequately.
(2) Close off IV infusion clamp.	Prevents medication from directly entering circulation as it is injected into bag or bottle.
(3) Wipe off medication port with an alcohol or antiseptic swab.	Mechanically removes microorganisms that could enter container during needle insertion.
(4) Insert syringe needle through injection port and inject medication.	Injection port is self-sealing and prevents fluid leaks.
(5) Lower bag or bottle from IV pole and gently mix. Rehang bag.	Ensures medication is evenly distributed.
b. Complete medication label and stick it to bag or bottle.	Informs nurses and physicians of contents of bag or bottle.
c. Regulate infusion to desired rate.	Prevents rapid infusion of fluid.
17. Properly dispose of equipment and supplies. Do not cap needle of syringe. Specially sheathed needles are discarded as a unit with needle covered.	Proper disposal of needle prevents injury to nurse and client. Capping of needles increases risk of needlestick injuries.
18. Wash hands.	Reduces transmission of microorganisms.
19. Observe client for signs or symptoms of drug reaction.	IV medications can cause rapid effects.
20. Observe for signs and symptoms of fluid volume excess.	Rapid uncontrolled infusion can cause circulatory overload.
21. Periodically return to client's room to assess IV insertion site and rate of infusion.	Over time IV site may become infiltrated or needle malpositioned. Flow rate may change according to client's position or volume left in container.
22. Observe for signs or symptoms of IV infiltration.	Infiltrated drugs can injure tissue.

Recording and Reporting

- Record solution and medication added to parenteral fluid on appropriate form.
- Report any side effects to nurse in charge or physician.

Box 26-13

Procedural Guidelines for Giving Medications by Intravenous Bolus

1. Check physician's order for type of medication to be administered, dosage, and route.
2. Wash hands and apply gloves.
3. Prepare a syringe with ordered medication and 2 syringes with saline. Carefully read package directions for proper dilution of medication.
4. Carefully check client's identification by looking at armband and asking name.
5. Assess IV insertion site for signs of infiltration or phlebitis. If present, do not give medication; restart IV line or intermittent venous access in another site.
6. Attach small-gauge needles (21 or 25 gauge) to syringes to insert through IV tubing ports if needleless values are not available.
7. Administer IV push through IV lock:
    Clean off injection port with antiseptic swab.
    Connect syringe to needleless port or insert needle through tubing port.
    Aspirate for blood return.
    Clear lock with 1 ml saline. (A central venous port may require 5 to 10 ml saline.)
    Attach medication syringe and administer medication over recommended time.
    Clear lock with another 1 ml saline.
    Option: Inject 1 ml heparin, 10 units/ml (may be omitted depending on institution's policy).
8. Start IV push through existing line:
    Select injection port closest to client.
    Clean off injection port with antiseptic swab.
    Occlude IV line by pinching tubing just above injection port.
    Administer medication over specified time recommended. (Check manufacturer's directions.) Use a watch to time administration.
    Insert spring into port and gently aspirate for blood return, then inject medication slowly.
9. Dispose of gloves and wash hands.
10. Observe client closely for adverse reactions as the drug is administered and for several minutes thereafter.
11. Dispose of uncapped needles or needle enclosed in safety shield and attached syringes in proper container.
12. Record drug, dosage, route, time administered, and length of time medication is given on medication form. Note adverse reactions.

Accidental injection of a medication into the tissues around a vein can cause pain, sloughing of tissues, and abscesses, depending on the medication's composition.

The rate of administration of an IV bolus medication is usually determined by the amount of medication that can be given each minute. The nurse should look up each medication to determine the recommended concentration and rate of administration. The purpose for which a medication is prescribed and any potential adverse effects related to the rate or route of administration must be considered when a nurse gives a medication by IV push.

Volume-controlled infusions. Another way of administering IV medications is through small amounts (50 to 100 ml) of compatible IV fluids. The fluid is within a secondary fluid container separate from the primary fluid bag. The container connects directly to the primary IV line or to a separate tubing that inserts into the primary line. Three types of containers are volume-control administration sets (e.g., Volutrol, Pediatrol), piggy-back and/or tandem sets, and mini-infusors. Using volume-controlled infusions has the following advantages:

1. Reduces risk of rapid-dose infusion by IV push; medications are diluted and infused over longer time intervals (e.g., 30 to 60 minutes)
2. Allows for administration of medications (e.g., antibiotics) that are stable for a limited time in solution
3. Allows for control of IV fluid intake

Piggyback. A piggyback is a small (25 to 100 ml) IV bag or bottle connected to a short tubing line that connects to the *upper* Y-port of a primary infusion line or to an intermittent venous access (Figure 26-31). The piggyback tubing is a microdrip or macrodrip system (see Chapter 31). The set is called a "piggyback" because the small bag or bottle is set higher than the primary infusion bag or bottle. In the piggyback setup the main line does not infuse when the piggybacked medication is infusing. The port of the primary IV line contains a back-check valve that automatically stops flow of the primary infusion once the piggyback infusion flows. After the piggyback solution infuses and the solution within the tubing falls below the level of the primary infusion drip chamber, the back-check valve opens and the primary infusion again flows.

Tandem. A tandem setup is a small (25 to 100 ml) IV bag or bottle connected to a short tubing line to the *lower* Y-port of a primary infusion line or to an intermittent venous access. The tandem set is placed at the same height as the primary infusion bag or bottle. In the tandem setup the tandem and the main line infuse simultaneously. The nurse must monitor the tandem setup closely. If the tandem setup is not immediately clamped when the medication is infused, the IV solution from the primary line will back up into the tandem line.

Administering Intravenous Medications by Piggyback, Intermittent Intravenous Infusion Sets, and Miniinfusion Pumps

Delegation Considerations

Administering medications by IV fluid by piggyback, intermittent intravenous infusion sets, and miniinfusion pumps requires problems solving and knowledge application unique to professional nursing. For this procedure delegation is not appropriate.

Equipment

Piggyback, Tandem, or Miniinfusion Pump

- Gloves (for connecting IV tubing)
- Medication prepared in 5- to 150-ml labeled infusion bag or syringe
- Short microdrip or macrodrip tubing set for piggyback (may have needleless system attachment)
- Needleless device
- Needles (21 or 23 gauge, only if stopcocks or other needleless methods are not available)

- Stopcocks
- Miniinfusion pump
- Adhesive tape (optional)
- Antiseptic swab
- IV pole or rack
- MAR or computer printout

Volume-Control Administration Set

- Gloves (for connecting IV tubing)
- Volutrol or Burette
- Infusion tubing (may have needleless system attachment)
- Syringe (5 to 20 ml)
- Vial or ampule of ordered medication
- Medication label
- MAR or computer printout

STEPS	RATIONALE
1. Check physician's order to determine type of IV solution to be used, type of medication, dose, route, and time of administration.	Client's overall physical condition dictates type of IV solution used. Ensures safe and accurate drug administration.
2. Collect information necessary to administer drug safely, including action, purpose, side effects, normal dose, time of peak onset, and nursing implications.	Allows nurse to give drug safely and to monitor client's response to therapy.
3. Assess patency of client's existing IV infusion line by noting infusion rate of main IV line.	IV line must be patent and fluids must infuse easily for medication to reach venous circulation effectively.
4. Assess IV insertion site for signs of infiltration or phlebitis: redness, pallor, swelling, tenderness on palpation.	Confirmation of placement of IV needle or catheter and integrity of surrounding tissues ensures medication is administered safely.
5. Assess client's history of drug allergies.	Effects of medications can develop rapidly after IV infusion. Nurse should be aware of clients at risk.
6. Assess client's understanding of purpose of drug therapy.	May reveal need for education.
7. Assemble supplies at bedside. Prepare client by informing client that medication will be given through IV equipment	Drug preparation usually is not required. Nurse may assemble infusion tubing and bag of medication in medication room or client's room. Allows client to understand procedure and minimizes anxiety.
8. Wash hands and apply gloves.	Reduces transmission of infection. During handling of IV tubing there is some risk of blood exposure.
9. Check client's identification by looking at armband and asking client's name.	Ensures drug is administered to correct client.
10. Explain purpose of medication and side effects to client and explain that medication is to be given through existing IV line. Encourage client to report symptoms of discomfort at site.	Keeps client informed of planned therapies.

Continued

Administering Intravenous Medications by Piggyback, Intermittent Intravenous Infusion Sets, and Miniinfusion Pumps

STEPS	RATIONALE
11. Administer Infusion:	
A. Piggyback or tandem infusion:	
(1) Connect infusion tubing to medication bag (see Chapter 31). Allow solution to fill tubing by opening regulator flow clamp.	Infusion tubing should be filled with solution and free of air bubbles to prevent air embolus.
(2) Hang piggyback medication bag above level of primary fluid bag. (Hook may be used to lower main bag.) Hang tandem infusion at same level as primary fluid bag (see illustration).	Height of fluid bag affects rate of flow to client.
(3) Connect tubing of piggyback or tandem infusion to appropriate connector on primary infusion line:	
(a) *Stopcock:* Wipe off stopcock port with alcohol swab and connect tubing. Turn stopcock to open position.	Stopcock eliminates need for needle.
(b) *Needleless system:* Wipe off needleless port, and insert tip of piggyback or tandem infusion tubing (see illustration).	The CDC strongly recommends needleless connections to prevent accidental needle-stick injuries. Establishes route for IV medication to enter main IV line.

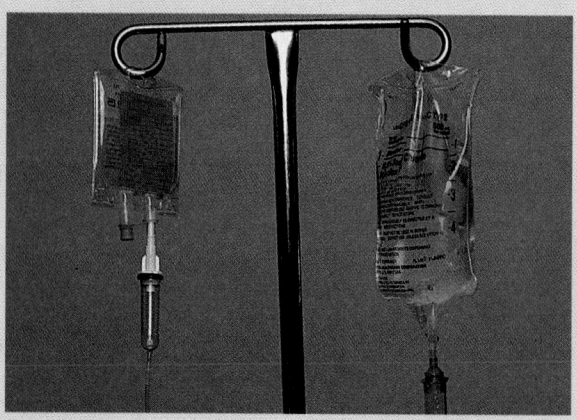

Step 11A(2)

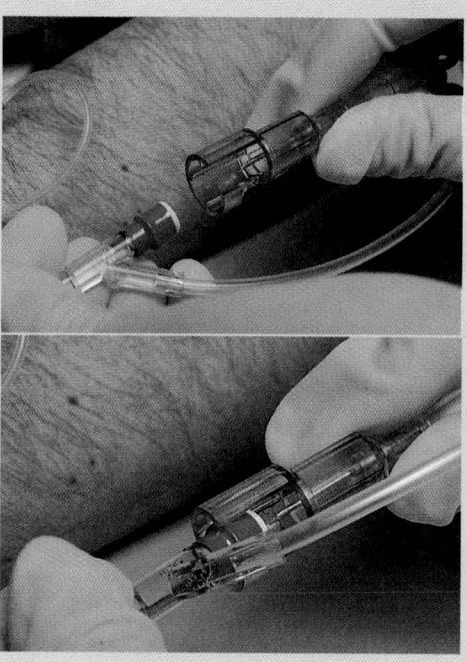

Step 11A(3)(b)

STEPS	RATIONALE
(c) *Tubing port:* Connect sterile needle to end of piggyback or tandem infusion tubing, remove cap, cleanse injection port on main IV line, and insert needle through center of port.	Prevents introduction of microorganisms during needle insertion.
(4) Regulate flow rate of medication solution by adjusting regulator clamp. (Usually medication should infuse within 20 to 90 minutes.)	Provides slow, intermittent infusion of medication in 20 to 90 minutes; maintains therapeutic blood levels.
(5) After medication has infused, check flow regulator on primary infusion. Back-check valve on piggyback stops flow of the primary infusion until second medication infuses. The tandem and primary infusions flow together until the tandem set empties. The primary infusion should automatically begin to flow after the piggyback or tandem solution is empty.	Valve prevents backup of medication into main infusion line. Checking flow rate ensures proper administration of IV fluids.
(6) Regulate main infusion line to desired rate, if necessary.	Infusion of piggyback may interfere with the main line infusion rate.
(7) Leave secondary bag and tubing in place for future drug administration or discard in appropriate containers.	Establishment of secondary line produces route for microorganisms to enter main line. Repeated changes in tubing increase risk of infection transmission (check agency policy).

B. Volume-control administration set (e.g., Volutrol):

STEPS	RATIONALE
(1) Assemble supplies in medication room.	Controls risk of contaminating IV solution.
(2) Prepare medication from vial or ampule (see Skill 26-5).	Ensures medication is sterile.
(3) Explain procedure to client. Encourage client to report symptoms of discomfort at site.	Keeps client informed of planned therapies.
(4) Fill Volutrol with desired amount of fluid (50 to 100 ml) by opening clamp between Volutrol and main IV bag (see illustration, p. 649).	Small volume of fluid dilutes IV medication and reduces risk of too-rapid infusion.
(5) Close clamp and check to be sure clamp on air vent of Volutrol chamber is open.	Prevents additional leakage of fluid into Volutrol. Air vent allows fluid in Volutrol to exit at regulated rate.
(6) Clean injection port on top of Volutrol with antiseptic swab.	Prevents introduction of microorganisms during needle insertion.
(7) Remove needle cap or sheath and insert syringe needle through port, then inject medication (see illustration, p. 649). Gently rotate Volutrol between hands.	Rotating mixes medication with solution in Volutrol to ensure equal distribution.
(8) Regulate IV infusion rate to allow medication to infuse in 30 to 90 minutes.	For optimal therapeutic effect, drug should infuse in prescribed time interval.

Continued

Skill 26-8—cont'd
Administering Intravenous Medications by Piggyback, Intermittent Intravenous Infusion Sets, and Miniinfusion Pumps

STEPS	RATIONALE
(9) Label Volutrol with name of drug, dosage, total volume including diluent, and time of administration.	Alerts nurses to drug being infused. Prevents other medications from being added to Volutrol.
(10) Dispose of uncapped needle or needle enclosed in safety shield and syringe in proper container.	Prevents accidental needle-sticks.
C. Miniinfusor administration:	
(1) Connect prefilled syringe to miniinfusion tubing.	Special tubing designed to fit syringe delivers medication to main IV line.
(2) Carefully apply pressure to syringe plunger, allowing tubing to fill with medication.	Ensures tubing is free of air bubbles to prevent air embolus.
(3) Place syringe into miniinfusor pump (follow product directions). Be sure syringe is secure (see illustration).	
(4) Connect miniinfusion tubing to main IV line.	
(a) *Stopcock:* Wipe off stopcock port with alcohol swab and connect tubing. Turn stopcock to open position.	Stopcock reduces risk of needle-stick injuries.
(b) *Needleless system:* Wipe off needleless port and insert tip of miniinfusor tubing.	Needleless system reduces risk of needle-stick injuries.
(c) *Tubing port:* Connect sterile needle to miniinfusion tubing, remove cap, cleanse injection port on main IV line, and insert needle through center of port.	Cleansing reduces transmission of microorganisms.

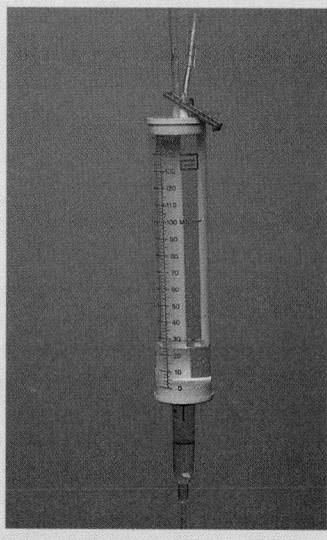

Step 11B(4)

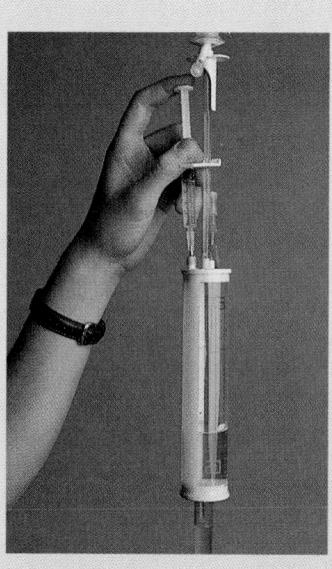

Step 11B(7)

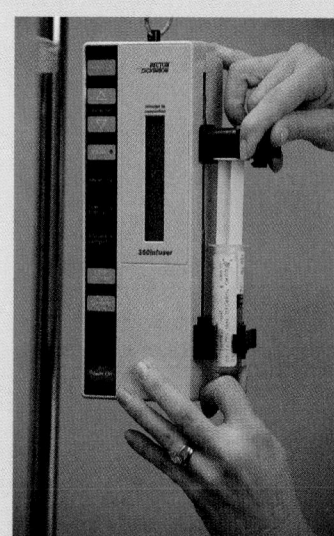

Step 11C(3)

STEPS	RATIONALE
(5) Explain purpose of medication and side effects to client and explain that medication is to be given through existing IV line. Ask client to report symptoms of discomfort at site.	Informs client of planned therapies.
(6) Hang infusion pump with syringe on IV pole alongside main IV bag. Press button on pump to begin infusion. *Optional: Set alarm.*	Pump automatically delivers medication at safe, constant rate based on volume in syringe. (Alarm is used if medication is delivered into heparin/saline lock.)
(7) After medication has infused, check flow regulator on primary infusion. The infusion should automatically begin to flow once the pump stops. Regulate main infusion line to desired rate as needed. (NOTE: If stopcock is used, turn off mini-infusion line.)	Maintains patency of primary IV line.
(8) Remove disposable gloves. Wash hands.	Reduces transmission of infection.
12. Observe client for signs of adverse reactions.	IV medications act rapidly.
13. During 20 to 90 minutes of infusion, periodically check infusion rate and condition of IV site.	IV must remain patent for proper drug administration. Development of infiltration necessitates discontinuing infusion.
14. Ask client to explain purpose and side effects of medication.	Evaluates client's understanding of instruction.

Recording and Reporting

- Record drug, dose, route, and time administered on MAR or computer printout.
- Record volume of fluid in medication bag or Volutrol on intake and output form.
- Report any adverse reactions to nurse in charge or physician.

Home Care Considerations

- Ensure that all needles contaminated by blood are disposed of in puncture-resistant containers (e.g., coffee can).
- Piggyback tubing and intravenous container should be disposed of in non-puncture container or according to agency policy.

Volume-control administration. Volume-control administration (e.g., Volutrol, Buretrol, Pediatrol) sets are small (50 to 150 ml) containers that attach just below the primary infusion bag or bottle. The set is attached and filled in a manner similar to that used with a regular IV infusion. However, the priming filling of the set is different, depending on the type of filter (floating valve or membrane) within the set. Follow package directions for priming sets (see Skill 26-8).

Miniinfusor pump. The miniinfusor pump is battery operated and delivers medications to be given in very small amounts of fluid (5 to 60 ml) within controlled infusion times using standard syringes (see Skill 26-8).

Intermittent venous access. An intermittent venous access (commonly called a heparin lock or saline lock) is an IV catheter with a small "well" or chamber covered by a rubber diaphragm (Figure 26-32). Special rubber-seal injection caps serve as wells and can be inserted into most IV catheters (see Chapter 31). Advantages to intermittent venous access include the following:

1. Cost savings resulting from the omission of continuous IV therapy
2. Convenience to the nurse by eliminating constant monitoring of flow rates

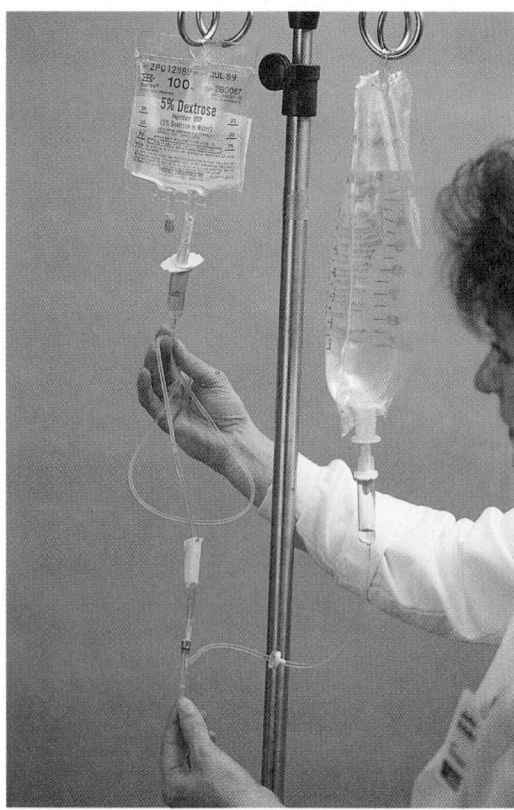

Figure 26-31. Tandem/piggyback setup.

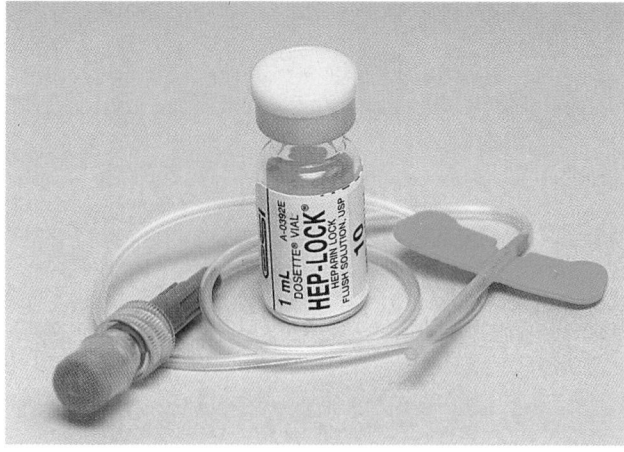

Figure 26-32. Intermittent lock covered with a rubber diaphragm. Requires a needle to flush.

3. Increased mobility, safety, and comfort for client by eliminating the need for a continuous IV

After an IV bolus or piggyback medication has been administered through an intermittent venous access, the access must be flushed with a solution to keep it patent. Traditionally, heparin has been used. It is now widely accepted that normal saline is as effective as heparin as a flush solution for peripheral catheters (Shoaf and Oliver, 1992).

Normally, checking for a blood return in an IV lock before bolus administration is unnecessary. However, if the needle site becomes puffy or the client complains of discomfort, the well must be aspirated for a blood return.

Key Terms

absorption	medication interaction
adverse effects	metered-dose inhalers
anaphylactic reactions	(MDIs)
apothecary system	metric system
biotransformation	narcotics
buccal	nurse practice acts
concentration	ophthalmic
detoxify	parenteral admin-
idiosyncratic reaction	istration
infusions	pharmacokinetics
inhalation	polypharmacy
injections	prescriptions
instillation	serum half-life
intradermal (ID)	side effect
intramuscular (IM)	solution
intraocular	subcutaneous (SQ)
intravenous (IV)	sublingual
irrigations	synergistic effect
medication abuse	therapeutic effect
medication allergy	toxic effects
medication dependence	transdermal disk
medication error	Z-track injection

■ Key Concepts

Learning medication classifications improves understanding of nursing implications for administering medications with similar characteristics.

All controlled substances are handled according to strict procedures that account for each medication.

The nurse applies understanding of the physiology of medication action when timing administration, selecting routes, initiating actions to promote medication efficacy, and observing responses to medications.

The older adult's body undergoes structural and functional changes that alter medication actions and influence the manner in which nurses provide medication therapy.

Children's medication doses are computed on the basis of body surface area or weight.

Medications given parenterally are absorbed more quickly than medications administered by other routes.

Each medication order should include the client's name; the order date; the medication name, dosage, route, and time of administration; and the physician's signature.

A medication history reveals allergies, medications a client is taking, and the client's compliance with therapy.

The "five rights" of medication administration ensure accurate preparation and administration of medication doses.

Nurses administer only medications they prepare, and prepared medications are never left unattended.

Medications should be charted immediately after administration.

A nurse uses clinical judgment in determining the best time to administer p.r.n. medications.

The nurse reports a medication error immediately.

When preparing medications, the nurse checks the medication container label against the MAR or computer printout three times.

The Z-track method for IM injections protects SQ tissues from irritating parenteral fluids.

Failure to select injection sites by anatomical landmarks may lead to tissue, bone, or nerve damage.

■ Critical Thinking Activities

1. You are working with a critical care nurse who has been floated to your unit. You observe this nurse drawing up 0.25 mg of digoxin into a 3-ml syringe. The nurse does not dilute the medication and is preparing to give this medication by IV bolus. You tell her that neither you nor any other nurse has given digoxin by IV bolus. She tells you that she does almost every day. Would you intervene in this situation? What rationale would you use to justify your position?

2. Fifteen minutes after you have hung an IV antibiotic, the client is itching and clawing at the skin and hair. You determine that the client may be having an allergic reaction to the antibiotic. What steps would you take immediately? Why?

3. You have prepared an IM injection for your client. You did not assess the client before preparing the medication. You draw the medication up in a syringe with a 1½-inch, 21-gauge needle. When you arrive to give the injection, you find that the client is cachectic and has very little muscle mass anywhere. How would you proceed with your assessment and intervention? Give your rationale.

4. Your client is receiving insulin at home and has run out of syringes. You have some 1-ml tuberculin syringes on hand. The client needs to receive 18 units of NPH and 4 units of regular insulin. How would you draw this up? How many tenths of a milliliter of each insulin would you draw up?

References

Abdoo YM: Designing a patient care medication and recording system that uses bar code technology, *Comp Nurs* 10(3):116, 1992.

American Pharmaceutical Association: Summary of the final report of the scope of pharmacy practice project, *Am J Hosp Pharm* 51:2179, 1994.

Behrman RE, Vaughan VC, editors: *Nelson textbook of pediatrics*, ed 13, Philadelphia, 1987, WB Saunders.

Benner P: *From novice to expert: excellence in clinical nursing practice*, Redwood City, Calif, 1984, Addison-Wesley.

Beyea SC, Nicoll LH: Administration of medication via the intramuscular route: an integrative review of the literature and research-based protocol for the procedure, *Appl Nurs Res* 8(1):23, 1995.

Beyea SC, Nicoll LH: Back to basics: administering IM injections the right way, *Am J Nurs* 96(1):34, 1996.

Clark JB and others: *Pharmacologic basis of nursing practice*, ed 5, St. Louis, 1996, Mosby.

Craft K: Do you really know how to handle sharps? *RN* 53(8):33, 1990.

Ebersole P, Hess P: *Toward healthy aging: human needs and nursing response*, ed 4, St. Louis, 1994, Mosby.

Edgar TA and others: Experience with a national medication error reporting program, *Am J Hosp Pharm* 51:1335, 1994.

Gauwitz DG: How to protect the dysphagic stroke patient, *Am J Nurs* 95:34, 1995.

Jagger J: *Preventable needlesticks, preventable HIV infection, preventable deaths among health care workers.* Testimony before Rep. Ron Wyden, Hearings in Washington, DC, 1992.

Lewis SM and others: *Medical-surgical nursing*, ed 4, St. Louis, 1996, Mosby.

New Jersey Department of Law and Public Safety, Division of Consumer Affairs: *Statues (N.J.S.A. 45:11-23 et seq.) and regulations (N.J.A.C. 13:37)*, Board of Nursing, 1995.

Owens-Schwab E, Fraser VJ: Needles and needle protection devices: a second look at efficacy and selection, *Infect Control Hosp Epidemiol* 14(11):657, 1993.

Perini V, Vermeulen LC: Comparison of automated medication-management systems, *Am J Hosp Pharm* 51:1883, 1994.

Petrosin BM and others: *Crit Care Nurs Q* 12:1, 1989.

Shoaf J, Oliver S: Efficacy of normal saline injection with and without heparin for maintaining intermittent intravenous site, *Appl Nurs Res* 5(1):9, 1992.

Statz E: Hand strength and metered dose inhalers, *Am J Nurs* 84:8000, 1984.

Weilitz PB, Dettenmeier PA: Test your knowledge of tracheostomy takes, *Am J Nurs* 94(2):46, 1994.

Weixler D: Correcting metered-dose inhaler misuse, *Nursing 94* 24:7, 1994.

White JR, Campbell RK. In Haire-Joshu D, editor: *Management of diabetes mellitus: perspectives of care across the life span*, ed 2, St. Louis, 1996, Mosby.

Wong DL: *Whaley and Wong's nursing care of infants and children*, ed 5, St. Louis, 1995, Mosby.

Body Mechanics

OBJECTIVES

Mastery of content in this chapter will enable
the student to:

- Define the key terms listed.
- Describe the role of the skeleton, skeletal
  muscles, and nervous system in the regulation
  of movement.
- Discuss physiological and pathological
  influences on body alignment and joint
  mobility.
- Assess clients for impaired body alignment and
  mobility.
- Formulate nursing diagnoses for clients
  experiencing problems with impaired body
  alignment and mobility.
- Write a nursing care plan for a client with
  impaired body alignment and mobility.
- Describe the interventions for maintaining
  proper alignment, assisting a client to move up
  in bed, repositioning a client needing
  assistance, and transferring a client from a bed
  to a chair.
- Evaluate the nursing care plan for maintaining
  body alignment and mobility.

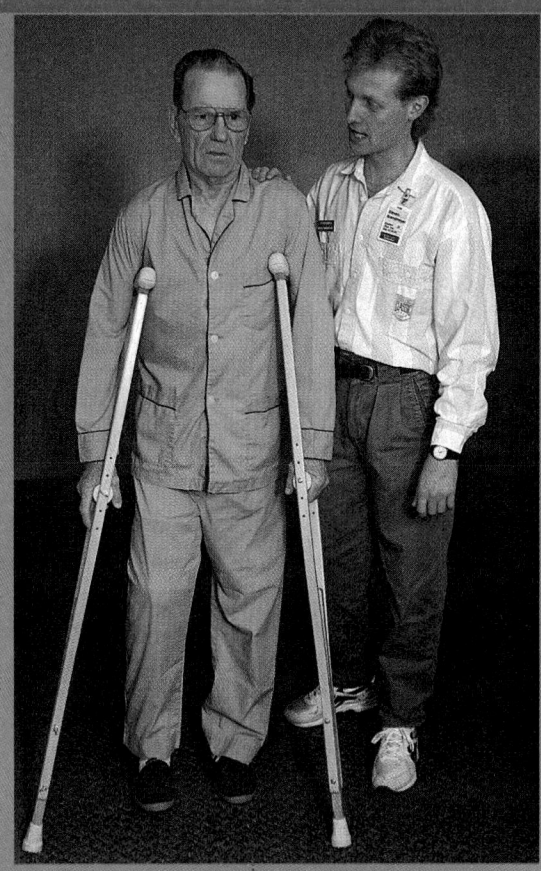

The actions of walking, turning, lifting, or carrying are essential components in the provision of nursing care. Such activities require muscle exertion by the nurse. To reduce the risk of injury to the client or nurse, the nurse must know and practice proper **body mechanics**. This includes knowledge of the actions of various muscle groups, understanding of the factors involved in the coordination of body movement, and familiarity with the integrated functioning of the skeletal, muscular, and nervous systems.

OVERVIEW OF BODY MECHANICS

The coordinated efforts of the musculoskeletal and nervous systems to maintain balance, posture, and body alignment during lifting, bending, moving, and performing activities of daily living provide the foundation for body mechanics. The proper implementation of these activities reduces the risk of injury to the musculoskeletal system and facilitates body movements, allowing physical mobility without muscle strain and excessive use of muscle energy.

Body Alignment

Body alignment refers to the relationship of one body part to another body part along a horizontal or vertical line. Correct alignment reduces strain on musculoskeletal structures, maintains adequate **muscle tone**, and contributes to balance.

Body Balance

Body balance is achieved when a relatively low **center of gravity** is balanced over a wide, stable base of support, and a vertical line falls from the center of gravity through the base of support. The base of support is the foundation. When the vertical line from the center of gravity does not fall through the base of support, the body loses balance.

Body balance is also enhanced by posture. The term **posture** means maintaining optimal body position. It means a position that most favors function, requires the least muscular work to maintain, and places the least strain on muscles, ligaments, and bones (Thibodeau and Patton, 1996).

The nurse maintains proper body alignment and posture by using two simple techniques. First, the base of support can easily be widened by separating the feet to a comfortable distance. Second, balance is increased by bringing the center of gravity closer to the base of support. This is achieved by bending the knees and flexing the hips until the person is squatting and still maintaining proper back alignment by keeping the trunk erect. The nervous system is responsible for muscle tone and regulates and coordinates the amount of pull exerted by the individual muscles (Thibodeau and Patton, 1996).

Coordinated Body Movement

Weight is the force exerted on a body by gravity. When an object is lifted, the lifter must overcome the object's weight and be aware of its center of gravity. In symmetrical objects, the center of gravity is located at the exact center of the object. The force of weight is always directed downward. An object that is unbalanced has its center of gravity away from the midline and falls without support. Because people are not geometrically perfect, their centers of gravity are usually at 55% to 57% of standing height and are located in the midline. Like unbalanced objects, clients who fail to maintain a balance with their center of gravity are unsteady, placing them at risk for falling. Nurses must be able to identify such clients and intervene with them in such a way that safety is maintained.

Friction

Friction is a force that occurs in a direction to oppose movement. As the nurse turns, transfers, or moves a client up in bed, friction must be overcome. A nurse can reduce friction by following some basic principles. The greater the surface area of the object to be moved, the greater the friction. If a client is unable to assist in moving up in bed, the client's arms should be placed across the chest. This decreases surface area and reduces friction.

A passive or immobilized client produces greater friction to movement. Thus when possible, the nurse should use some of the client's strength and mobility when lifting, transferring, or moving the client up in bed. This can be done by explaining the procedure and telling the client when to move. For instance, friction is decreased if the client can bend his or her knees as the nurse assists him or her to move up in the bed.

Friction can also be reduced by lifting rather than pushing a client. Lifting has an upward component and decreases the pressure between the client and the bed or the chair. The use of a lift sheet reduces friction because the client is more easily moved along the bed's surface.

REGULATION OF MOVEMENT

Coordinated body movement involves the integrated functioning of the skeletal, muscular, and nervous systems. Because these three systems cooperate so closely in mechanical support of the body, they are often considered as a single functional unit.

Skeletal System

Bones perform five functions in the body: support, protection, movement, mineral storage, and hematopoiesis (blood cell formation). In the discussion of body mechanics two of these functions, support and movement, are most important. In support, bones serve as the framework and contribute to the shape, alignment, and positioning of the body parts. In movement, bones with their **joints** constitute levers for muscle attachment. As muscles contract and shorten, they pull on bones, producing joint movement (Thibodeau and Patton, 1996).

Joints. An articulation or joint is the connection between bones. Each joint is classified according to its structure and degree of mobility. On the basis of connective structures, joints are classified as fibrous, cartilaginous, and synovial (Huether and McCance, 1996). Fibrous joints fit closely together and are fixed, permitting little, if any, movement. The cartilaginous joint has little movement but is elastic and uses cartilage to unite separate body surfaces. Cartilaginous joints are found where bones are exposed to a constant pressure, such as the costosternal joints between the sternum and the ribs or the symphysis pubis.

The synovial or true joint is a freely movable joint and the body's most mobile, numerous, and anatomically complex joint. There are seven structural characteristics of synovial joints: joint capsule, synovial membrane, articular cartilage, joint cavity, menisci, ligaments, and bursae (Thibodeau and Patton, 1996).

Ligaments. Ligaments are white, shiny, flexible bands of fibrous tissue that bind joints and connect bones and cartilages. Ligaments are elastic and aid joint flexibility and support. In some areas of the body, ligaments also have a protective function. For example, ligaments between vertebral bodies prevent damage to the spinal cord during back movement.

Tendons. Tendons are white, glistening, fibrous bands of tissue that connect muscle to bone. Tendons are strong, flexible, and inelastic, and occur in various lengths and thicknesses. The Achilles tendon is the thickest and strongest tendon in the body.

Cartilage. Cartilage is nonvascular, supporting connective tissue with the flexibility of a firm, plastic material. The gristlelike nature of cartilage permits it to sustain weight and serve as a shock-absorber pad between articulating bones. It is located chiefly in the joints and in the thorax, trachea, larynx, nose, and ear (Thibodeau and Patton, 1996).

Skeletal Muscle

When we walk, talk, run, breathe, or participate in physical activity, we do so by the contraction of skeletal muscle. There are over 600 skeletal muscles in the body. In addition to facilitating movement, these muscles determine the form and contour of our bodies. Most of our muscles span at least one joint and attach to both articulating bones. When contraction occurs, one bone is fixed while the other moves. The origin is the point of attachment that remains still; the insertion is the point that moves when the muscle contracts (Thibodeau and Patton, 1996).

Muscles concerned with movement. The muscles of movement are located near the skeletal region, where movement is caused by a lever system (Thibodeau and Patton, 1996). The lever system makes the work of moving a weight or load easier. It occurs when specific bones, such as the humerus, ulna, and radius, and the associated joints, such as the elbow, act as a lever. Thus the force applied to one end of the bone to lift a weight at another point tends to rotate the bone in the direction opposite that of the applied force. Muscles that attach to bones of leverage provide the necessary strength to move the object.

Muscles concerned with posture. Gravity pulls on parts of the body all the time; the only way the body can be held in position is for muscles to exert pull on bones in the opposite direction. Muscles accomplish this counterforce by maintaining a low level of sustained contraction. Poor posture places more work on muscles to counteract the force of gravity. This leads to fatigue and can eventually interfere with bodily functions and cause deformities.

Muscle groups. The antagonistic, synergistic, and antigravity muscle groups are coordinated by the nervous system and maintain posture and initiate movement. Antagonistic muscles bring about movement at the joint. During movement, the active mover muscle contracts while its antagonist relaxes. For example, when flexing the arm the active mover, the biceps brachii, contracts and its antagonist, the triceps brachii, relaxes. During **extension** of the arm, the active mover, now the triceps brachii, contracts and the new antagonist, the biceps brachii, relaxes.

Synergistic muscles contract to accomplish the same movement. When the arm is flexed, the strength of the contraction of the biceps brachii is increased by contraction of the synergistic muscle, the brachialis. Thus with synergistic muscle activity there are now two active movers, the biceps brachii and the brachialis, which contract while the antagonistic muscle, the triceps brachii, relaxes.

Antigravity muscles are involved with joint stabilization. These muscles continuously oppose the effect of gravity on the body and permit a person to maintain an upright or sitting posture. In an adult the antigravity muscles are the extensors of the leg, the gluteus maximus, the quadriceps femoris, the soleus muscles, and the muscles of the back.

Skeletal muscles support posture and carry out voluntary movement. The muscles are attached to the skeleton by tendons, which provide strength and permit motion. The movement of the extremities is voluntary and requires coordination from the nervous system.

Nervous System

Movement and posture are regulated by the nervous system. The major voluntary motor area, located in the cerebral cortex, is the precentral gyrus or motor strip. A majority of motor fibers descend from the motor strip and cross at the level of the medulla. Thus the motor fibers from the right motor strip initiate voluntary movement for the left side of the body, and motor fibers from the left motor strip initiate voluntary movement for the right side of the body.

Transmission of the impulse from the nervous system to the musculoskeletal system is an electrochemical event and requires a neurotransmitter. Basically, neurotransmitters are chemicals such as acetylcholine that transfer the electric impulse from the nerve across the myoneural junction to stimulate the muscle, causing movement.

Movement can be impaired by disorders that alter neurotransmitter production, transfer from the neurotransmitter to the muscle, or activation of muscle activity. Parkinsonism is an example of such a disorder.

Proprioception. Posture is also regulated by the nervous system and requires coordination of proprioception and balance. Proprioception is the awareness of the position of the body and its parts (Huether and McCance, 1996). Proprioception is monitored by proprioceptors located on nerve endings in muscles, tendons, and joints. As a person carries out activities of daily living, proprioceptors monitor muscle activity and body position. For example, the proprioceptors on the soles of the foot contribute to correct posture while standing or walking. In standing, pressure is continuous on the bottom of the feet. The proprioceptors monitor the pressure, communicating this information through the nervous system to the antigravity muscles. The standing person remains upright until deciding to change position. As a person walks, the proprioceptors on the bottom of the feet monitor pressure changes. Thus when the bottom of the moving foot comes in contact with the walking surface, the individual automatically moves the stationary foot forward. The proprioceptors allow people to walk without having to watch their feet.

Balance. When standing, running, lifting, or performing activities of daily living, a person must have adequate balance. **Balance** is assisted through control by the nervous system, specifically by the cerebellum and the inner ear. The major function of the cerebellum is to coordinate all voluntary movement, particularly highly skilled movements, such as those required in skiing.

Within the inner ear are the semicircular canals, three fluid-filled structures that assist in maintaining balance. Fluid within the canals has a certain inertia, and when the head is suddenly rotated in one direction, the fluid remains stationary for a moment, whereas the canal turns with the head. This allows a person to change position suddenly without losing balance.

Principles of body mechanics. Using principles of body mechanics during routine activities also prevents injury. The nurse teaches colleagues and clients' families to lift, transfer, or position clients properly. A nurse teaching a client's family to transfer the client from bed to chair can increase and reinforce the family's knowledge by consistently demonstrating proper body mechanics.

Whether the nurse is moving an immobilized client, assisting a client from the bed to the chair, or teaching a client to carry out activities of daily living efficiently, knowledge of basic principles of body mechanics is crucial. The nurse also incorporates knowledge of physiological and pathological influences on body alignment and mobility (Box 27-1).

PATHOLOGICAL INFLUENCES ON BODY MECHANICS

Many pathological conditions affect body alignment and mobility. These conditions include congenital defects; disorders of bones, joints, and muscle; central nervous system damage, and musculoskeletal trauma.

Congenital Defects
Congenital abnormalities affect the efficiency of the musculoskeletal system in regard to alignment, balance,

---

| **Box 27-1** |
| **Principles of Body Mechanics** |

The wider the base of support, the greater the stability of the nurse.

The lower the center of gravity, the greater the stability of the nurse.

The equilibrium of an object is maintained as long as the line of gravity passes through its base of support.

Facing the direction of movement prevents abnormal twisting of the spine.

Dividing balanced activity between arms and legs reduces the risk of back injury.

Leverage, rolling, turning, or pivoting requires less work than lifting.

When friction is reduced between the object to be moved and the surface on which it is moved, less force is required to move it.

Reducing the force of work reduces the risk of injury.

Maintaining good body mechanics reduces fatigue of the muscle groups.

Alternating periods of rest and activity helps to reduce fatigue.

and appearance. Osteogenesis imperfecta is an inherited disorder that affects bone. Bones are porous, short, bowed, and deformed; as a result, children experience curvature of the spine and shortness of stature. Scoliosis is a structural curvature of the spine associated with vertebral rotation. Muscles, ligaments, and other soft tissues become shortened. Balance and mobility are affected in proportion to the severity of abnormal spinal curvatures (Huether and McCance, 1996).

Disorders of Bones, Joints, and Muscles

Osteoporosis is a well-known and well-publicized disorder of aging in which the density or mass of bone is reduced. The bone remains biochemically normal but has difficulty maintaining integrity and support. The cause is uncertain and theories vary from hormonal imbalances to insufficient intake of nutrients (Huether and McCance, 1996).

Osteomalacia is a metabolic disease characterized by inadequate and delayed mineralization resulting in compact and spongy bone. Mineral calcification and deposition do not occur. Replaced bone consists of soft material rather than rigid bone.

Joint mobility can be altered by inflammatory and noninflammatory joint diseases and by articular disruption. Inflammatory joint disease (e.g., arthritis) is characterized by inflammation or destruction of the synovial membrane and articular cartilage, and systemic signs of inflammation. Noninflammatory diseases have none of these characteristics, and the synovial fluid is normal (Huether and McCance, 1996). Joint degeneration, which can occur with inflammatory and noninflammatory disease, is marked by changes in articular cartilage combined with overgrowth of bone at the articular ends. Degenerative changes commonly affect weight-bearing joints.

Articular disruption may be as mild as a sprain or as severe as dislocation. Articular disruption involves trauma to the articular capsules, such as a tear in a sprain or a separation in a dislocation. Articular disruption usually results from trauma but can also be congenital, as with congenital hip dysplasia.

Central Nervous System Damage

Damage to any component of the central nervous system that regulates voluntary movement results in impaired body alignment and mobility. For example, the motor strip in the cerebrum can be damaged by trauma from a head injury. The amount of voluntary motor impairment is directly related to the amount of destruction of the motor strip. A client with a right-sided cerebral hemorrhage and damage to the right motor strip may have left-sided hemiplegia. However, a client with a right-sided head injury may only have cerebral edema (but not destruction) of the motor strip. With extensive physical therapy, voluntary movement gradually returns to the left side.

Musculoskeletal Trauma

Musculoskeletal trauma can result in bruises, contusions, sprains, and fractures. A fracture is a disruption of bone tissue continuity. Fractures most commonly result from direct external trauma. They can also occur because of some deformity of the bone, as with pathological fractures of osteoporosis.

CRITICAL THINKING AND APPLICATION OF BODY MECHANICS

Each of us at some time in our lives has experienced a sense of disequilibrium while performing activities. Many times clients are cautious or hesitant to ask for assistance in performing simple tasks of daily living. Such feelings are often felt but unexpressed by clients of different ethnic groups. It may be difficult for them to be dependent upon others for self-care. For some female clients modesty is of utmost importance and the client may resent being unnecessarily exposed. As a result, tasks may remain undone. The nurse must be careful in regarding such responses as indifference or noncompliance. Clients already at risk from existing health interruptions need protection from further injury because of a disruption in body mechanics.

As the nurse begins the process of problem solving for client care, a variety of concepts must be considered and woven together to provide the best outcome for the client. Knowledge of the musculoskeletal system and health interruptions that create problems for the client in the area of body mechanics lay the foundation for planning and decision making. Standards of care provide guidelines for the provider. The nurse's experiences and attitude affect the problem-solving approach with clients and must be reevaluated with each new client.

Any acquired or congenital condition that affects the structure of the musculoskeletal or nervous system impairs to some degree body alignment or joint mobility. The impairment can be temporary, such as casting of an extremity, or permanent, as in contractures. For clients with limited range of motion or mobility, the nursing care plan should include interventions that maintain the present level of alignment and joint mobility and increase the level of motor function.

The nurse must remember clients have the capacity for recovery in spite of the loss of some physical function. Restoration of functioning begins early in the care of clients experiencing disruption in their ability to perform self-care. Encouragement, support, commitment, and perseverence are important attitudes in critical thinking for these clients.

When intervening with clients experiencing problems with body mechanics who may be dependent upon the nurse for assistance with positioning, turning, or ambulation, perseverance is one attitude the nurse must possess. Hourly responsibility for turning often becomes repetitive and the nurse may lose sight of its importance. Perseverance is especially important in the delegation of these activities to unlicensed health care providers or family members. To make certain the task is performed and is performed correctly is an essential nursing function.

Another attitude for the nurse to demonstrate is one of creativity. Since problems with mobility are often prolonged, the more creative the nurse's approach on improving mobility skills, the greater the chance of success. This is especially important for the child client. Strides toward greater mobility can become a game with stickers and pretty colors to visualize successes.

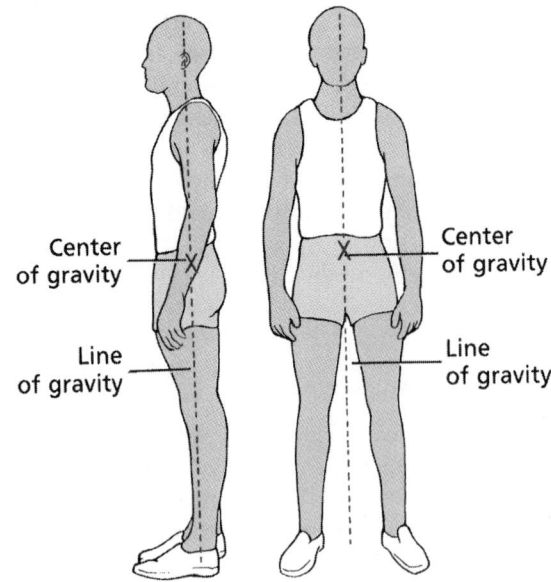

Figure 27-1. Correct body alignment when standing.

NURSING PROCESS

▪ Assessment

Assessment of body alignment and posture can be carried out with the client standing, sitting, or lying down. Through the assessment, the nurse will be able to determine normal physiological changes in growth and development; deviations related to poor posture, trauma, muscle damage, or nerve dysfunction; and any learning needs of clients. In addition, during assessment the nurse can provide opportunities for clients to observe their posture and obtain important information about other factors that contribute to poor alignment, such as fatigue, malnutrition, and psychological problems.

The first step in assessing body alignment is to put the client at ease so unnatural or rigid positions are not assumed. When assessing body alignment of an immobilized or unconscious client, pillows and positioning supports should be removed from the bed if not contraindicated and the client placed in the **supine** position.

Standing. Assessment for the standing client includes the following: the head is erect and midline; body parts are symmetrical; the spine should be straight with normal curvatures (cervical concave, thoracic convex, lumbar concave); the abdomen is comfortably tucked; the knees should be in a straight line between the hips and ankles and slightly flexed; the feet should be flat on the floor and pointed directly forward and slightly apart to maintain a wide base of support; the arms should hang comfortably at the sides (Figure 27-1). The client's center of gravity is in the midline, and the line of gravity is from the middle of the forehead to a midpoint between the feet. Laterally, the line of gravity runs vertically from the middle of the skull to the posterior third of the foot (Thompson and Wilson, 1996).

Sitting. Assessment of the client in the sitting position includes the following: the head is erect, and the neck and vertebral column are in straight alignment; the body weight is distributed on the buttocks and thighs; the thighs are parallel and in a horizontal plane (be careful to avoid pressure on the popliteal nerve and blood supply); the feet are supported on the floor; the forearms are supported on the armrest, in the lap, or on a table in front of the chair.

Assessment of alignment in the sitting position is particularly important for the client with muscle weakness, muscle paralysis, or nerve damage. A client with these alterations has diminished sensation in affected areas and is unable to perceive pressure or decreased circulation. Proper sitting alignment reduces the risk of musculoskeletal system damage in such a client.

Recumbent. Assessment of the client in the recumbent position requires that the client be placed in the lateral position with all but one pillow and all positioning supports removed from the bed. The vertebrae should be in straight alignment without observable curves. This assessment provides baseline data concerning the client's body alignment.

Conditions that create a risk of damage to the musculoskeletal system when lying down include impaired mobility (e.g., traction), decreased sensation (e.g., hemiparesis from a stroke), impaired circulation (e.g., diabetes), and lack of voluntary muscle control (e.g., spinal cord injuries).

When a client is unable to change position voluntarily, the nurse assesses the position of body parts while the client is lying down. The vertebrae should be in straight alignment without any observable curves. The extremities should be in alignment and not crossed over one another. The head and neck should be aligned without excessive flexion or extension.

Mobility. Assessment of mobility enables the nurse to determine the client's coordination and balance while walking, the ability to carry out activities of daily living, and the ability to participate in an exercise program. The assessment of mobility has three components: range of joint motion, **gait**, and exercise.

Range of motion. Assessing range of motion (ROM) is one of the first assessment techniques used to determine the degree of damage or injury to a joint. The nurse assesses ROM to collect data to answer questions about joint stiffness, swelling, pain, limited movement, and unequal movement (see Chapter 24).

Limited range of motion may indicate inflammation such as arthritis, fluid in the joint, altered nerve supply, or contractures. Increased mobility (beyond normal) of a joint may indicate connective tissue disorders, ligament tears, or possible joint fractures.

Gait. Gait is the manner or style of walking, including rhythm, cadence, and speed. Assessing gait allows the nurse to draw conclusions about balance, posture, and the ability to walk without assistance (see Chapter 24). The nurse should note conformity, a regular smooth rhythm, symmetry in the length of leg swing, smooth swaying related to the gait phase, and a smooth, symmetrical arm swing (Johnson and Wilson, 1996).

Exercise. Exercise is physical activity for conditioning the body, improving health, maintaining fitness, or providing therapy for correcting a deformity or restoring the overall body to a maximal state of health. When a person exercises, physiological changes occur in body systems (Box 27-2).

During exercise, muscle tone, size, and strength increase. As a result the person is able to exercise longer with each strengthening of the muscles. Joint mobility is also enhanced because the exercise itself requires movement of body parts.

Activity tolerance. **Activity tolerance** is the kind and amount of exercise or work a person is able to perform. Assessment of activity tolerance is necessary when planning physical activity for clients with acute or chronic illness. This assessment provides the nurse with baseline data about the client's activity patterns and assists in determining which factors (physical, psychological, or motivational) are affecting activity tolerance (Ackley and Ladwig, 1997). Box 27-3 lists factors affecting activity tolerance.

Client expectations. In assessing the client's expectations concerning body alignment and joint mobil-

---

Box 27-2
Effects of Exercise

Cardiovascular System
Increased cardiac output
Improved myocardial contraction, thereby strengthening cardiac muscle
Decreased resting heart rate
Improved venous return

Pulmonary System
Increased respiratory rate and depth followed by a quicker return to resting state
Improved alveolar ventilation
Decreased work of breathing
Improved diaphragmatic excursion

Metabolic System
Increased basal metabolic rate
Increased use of glucose and fatty acids
Increased triglyceride breakdown
Increased gastric motility
Increased production of body heat

Musculoskeletal System
Improved muscle tone
Increased joint mobility
Improved muscle tolerance to physical exercise
Possible increase in muscle mass
Reduced bone loss

Activity Tolerance
Improved tolerance
Decreased fatigue

Psychosocial Factors
Improved tolerance to stress
Reports of "feeling better"
Reports of decrease in illness (e.g., colds, influenza)

Data from Huether SE, McCance KL: *Understanding pathophysiology*, St. Louis, 1996, Mosby; Hoeman SP: *Rehabilitation nursing: process and application*, St. Louis, 1996, Mosby.

---

ity, the nurse will first need insight into the client's perception of what is normal or acceptable to the client in regard to mobility. For example, one of the factors affecting posture, alignment, and mobility is freedom from pain. If exercising is painful or tiresome to the client, compliance and commitment to desired interventions may be lacking. Clients may be content with their present range of motion or mobility and may not perceive a need for improvement. Unless there is a real threat to health maintenance, forcing the client to accept the nurse's perspective is a breach of standards of care.

Box 27-3
Factors Influencing Activity Tolerance

Physiological Factors
Skeletal abnormalities
Muscular impairments
Endocrine or metabolic illnesses (e.g., diabetes mellitus or thyroid disease)
Hypoxemia
Decreased cardiac function
Decreased endurance
Impaired physical stability
Pain
Sleep pattern disturbance
Prior exercise patterns
Infectious processes and fever

Emotional Factors
Anxiety
Depression
Chemical addictions
Motivation

Developmental Factors
Age
Sex

Pregnancy
Physical growth and development of muscle and skeletal support

Modified from Phipps WJ and others: *Medical surgical nursing,* St. Louis, 1996, Mosby.

NURSING DIAGNOSES FOR CLIENTS WITH IMPROPER BODY MECHANICS AND IMPAIRED JOINT MOBILITY

Activity intolerance
Body image disturbance
Injury, risk for
Mobility, impaired physical
Pain
Skin integrity, impaired

Nursing Diagnosis

Assessment of the client's body alignment and joint mobility provides related clusters of data or defining characteristics that lead the nurse into the identification of nursing diagnoses (see nursing diagnoses box).

Alterations in body alignment and joint mobility can result from developmental changes, postural abnormalities, abnormalities in bone formation, impaired muscle development, damage to the central nervous system, or direct trauma to the musculoskeletal system. In some instances alterations in joint mobility or alignment may be one of the defining characteristics of a separate nursing diagnosis and not the actual nursing diagnosis. Nursing diagnoses often focus on the individual's ability to move. The diagnostic label should direct nursing interventions. For example, in the nursing care plan the diagnostic label *impaired physical mobility* is supported by the characteristics: difficulty in extending shoulder during activities of daily living and reduced range of joint motion. The related-to factor is supported by the assessment of pain on movement. Another diagnostic label, *risk for injury,* is supported by improper use of body mechanics, impaired balance, or dizziness.

Planning

Once the nursing diagnoses have been defined, the nurse and client set goals and expected outcomes to direct interventions. The plan should include consideration of any risks for injury to the client. It should also take into consideration preexisting health concerns. It is especially important to have knowledge of the client's home environment when planning therapies to maintain or improve body alignment and mobility. The client's family should be included in the care plan. For some clients with alterations in joint mobility, family members may be the providers of care.

Planning also involves an understanding of the client's need to maintain motor function and independence. Collaboration with others members of the health care team, for example, physical or occupational therapists, will be especially important for these clients. Long-term rehabilitation may be necessary. The nurse individualizes a plan of care directed at meeting the actual or potential needs of the client (see care plan).

Implementation

Health promotion activities. In recent years, the rate of injuries in occupational settings has increased dramatically. Half of all back pain is associated with manual lifting tasks (Gassett and others, 1996). The most common back injury is strain on the lumbar muscle group, which includes the muscles around the lumbar vertebrae. Injury to these areas affects the ability to bend forward, backward, and side to side. The ability to rotate the hips and lower back is also decreased. To protect the client and the nurse, proper body mechanics must be learned and mastered (Box 27-4).

Lifting techniques. Before lifting, the nurse should assess the weight to be lifted and what assistance, if any, is needed. If help is needed, the nurse should assess if a second person is adequate or if mechanical assistance is needed. Once the amount of needed assistance is determined, these steps are followed:

SAMPLE NURSING CARE PLAN

Assessment

Joseph Indelicato is a 72-year-old man hospitalized for surgery on his right knee. Over the past 5 years, he has continued to experience pain and decreased mobility. He is now 2 days postoperative following right total knee replacement. His incision is healing and there is no edema or erythema. He rates his **pain as 6 to 7 on a 10-point scale,** and is using a **patient-controlled analgesia pump.** He uses a **continuous passive motion (CPM) machine four times a day.** His degree of **knee flexion is now 60 degrees.** He is able to **ambulate to the bathroom with the aid of a walker.**

Nursing Diagnosis

Impaired physical mobility related to pain and limited joint motion.

Planning

Goal

Client will gain optimal range of joint motion (ROJM) of right knee.

Client will maintain optimum level of comfort.

Expected Outcomes

Client will gain a minimum of 90 degrees flexion in right knee.

Client will ambulate full length of hall by discharge.

Client's pain will be 3 to 4 on a 10-point scale by discharge.

Client's pain will be controlled by oral analgesics.

Implementation

Steps

1. Provide analgesics 30 minutes before ROJM exercises or use of CPM machine.
2. Teach client and family muscle strengthening exercises.
3. Teach client and family proper positioning and joint alignment.

Rationale

Peak actions of analgesic will occur as client begins exercise.

Exercise improves circulation to the area and strengthens extremity for ambulation.

Prevents deformity and loss of function.

Evaluation

Measure degree of knee flexion.
Observe client's ROJM or use of CPM machine.
Observe client ambulate.
Ask client to rate level of pain on a 10-point scale.

Defining characteristics are shown in bold type.

---

1. Tighten stomach muscles and tuck pelvis; this provides balance and protects the back.
2. Bend at the knees; this helps to maintain the nurse's center of gravity and lets the strong muscles of the legs do the lifting (Figure 27-2).
3. Keep the weight to be lifted as close to the body as possible; this action places the weight in the same plane as the lifter and close to the center of gravity for balance.
4. Maintain the trunk erect and the knees bent so that multiple muscle groups work together in a synchronized manner (Gassett and others, 1996).
5. Avoid twisting. Twisting can overload your spine and lead to serious injury.

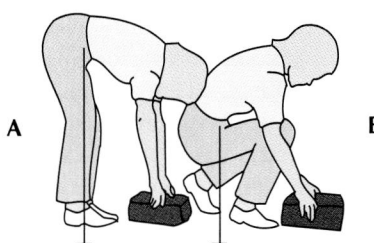

Figure 27-2. Incorrect **(A)** and correct **(B)** body position for lifting.

Client Teaching for Body Mechanics

- People are more likely to do something if they believe they will be able to perform successfully. They also have to believe that a skill or action will make a positive difference.
- Clients should exercise joints only as ordered by the physician. Increases in discomfort should be reported immediately and not attributed to the exercise activity.
- Family members should be taught the safe use of adaptive aids (e.g., transfer belts, lifts) to assist with transfers and activities in the home.
- Mobility aids are valuable in promoting energy conservation and decreasing fatigue, further promoting compliance with activity.
- Clients and care providers should assess and stabilize their centers of gravity to promote safety in lifting and positioning.

6. The best height for lifting vertically is approximately 2 feet off the ground and close to the lifter's center of gravity (Gassett and others, 1996).

To reach an object overhead the nurse should do the following:

1. Use a safe, stable step stool or ladder for elevation. Avoid standing on tiptoe with the feet together. This decreases the base of support, elevates the center of gravity, and decreases balance.
2. Stand as close to the shelf as possible. This decreases the amount of time the nurse must support the weight of the object with the arms.
3. Transfer the weight of the object from the shelf to the arms and over the base of support. This maintains the nurse's base of support and aligns the weight of the object close to the nurse's center of gravity.

Acute care

Positioning techniques. Clients with impaired nervous or musculoskeletal system functioning, clients with increased weakness, or those restricted to bed rest benefit from therapeutic positioning by the nurse (Hoeman, 1996). During client positioning, the nurse must determine areas of bony prominences where pressure, friction, and shear cause the most wear and tear. Through the use of proper positioning and pressure-relief methods, these areas can be protected.

In general, clients should be repositioned every 2 hours if they are in bed and every 20 to 30 minutes if they are sitting in a chair. Those clients with contractures

or who are at greater risk for skin breakdown over bony prominences need repositioning more frequently. Additional variables influencing frequency of position changes include level of comfort, amount of spontaneous movement, presence of edema, loss of sensation, and overall physical and mental status (Hoeman, 1996).

Several devices are available for the nurse to use in maintaining good body alignment for clients while clients are being positioned (Table 27-1). Various positions are described in the following paragraphs. The methods of positioning clients are described in Skill 27-1.

Fowler's position. The head of the client's bed is elevated 45 to 60 degrees and the client's knees are slightly elevated, avoiding pressure on the popliteal vessels. The head rests against the mattress or a small pillow for support. Pillows can be used to maintain natural alignment of the hands, wrists, and forearms. Supports must permit flexion of the hips and proper alignment of the normal curves in the cervical, thoracic, and lumbar vertebrae (Metzler, 1996).

Supine position. The supine position is when the client rests on the back. A small, flat pillow supports the head, neck, and upper shoulders (Hoeman, 1996). Pillows, trochanter rolls (see Table 27-1), and hand rolls or arm splints are used to increase comfort and reduce injury to the skin or musculoskeletal system. (Metzler, 1996). The risk of aspiration is greater with this position; thus the supine position should be avoided.

The mattress should be firm enough to support the cervical, thoracic, and lumbar vertebrae. Pressure on the back of the legs should be avoided. A foot support is used to prevent **footdrop,** maintain proper alignment, and provide freedom of movement for the feet.

Prone position. Before placing a client in the **prone** position, the nurse should assess the client record for any possible complications such as increasing intracranial pressure or cardiopulmonary disease (Hoeman, 1996). The client is assisted to lie on the abdomen. The head is turned to the side. This facilitates respiration and drainage of oral secretions. A pillow is placed under the head for comfort and relief from pressure. As an alternative, a wedge can be placed under the client's chest, or arms flexed over the head, if it is more comfortable. Place a pillow under the lower leg; this promotes relaxation. If a pillow is unavailable, the client's ankles should be in **dorsiflexion** over the end of the mattress. Body alignment is poor when the ankles are continuously in **plantar flexion** and the lumbar spine remains in **hyperextension.** Lung expansion may be compromised in this position, especially in the obese.

Lateral position. In the lateral (or side-lying) position, the client is supported on the right or left side with the opposite arm, thigh, and knee flexed and resting on the bed. A pillow is placed under the head to keep the head, neck, and spine in alignment. The upper arm is flexed and supported with a pillow (Metzler, 1996). The upper leg is flexed at the hip and knee and positioned on

Text continued on p. 689

TABLE 27-1
Devices Used for Proper Positioning

Devices	Uses and Descriptions
Pillows	Pillows are readily available in most health care facilities, including the home. They should be of appropriate size for the body part to be positioned. Pillows provide support, elevate body parts, and can splint incisional areas, reducing postoperative pain during activity or coughing and deep breathing.
Foot boots	**Foot boots** maintain feet in dorsiflexion. Boots are made of rigid plastic or heavy foam and keep the foot flexed at the proper angle. The nurse should remove the foot boots 2 or 3 times a day to assess skin integrity and joint mobility.
Trochanter rolls	**Trochanter rolls** prevent external rotation of legs when clients are in the supine position. To form a trochanter roll, a cotton bath blanket or a sheet is folded lengthwise to a width extending from the greater trochanter of the femur to the lower border of the popliteal space (Figure 27-3). The blanket is placed under the buttocks and then rolled away from the client until the thigh is in the neutral position or an inward position with the patella facing upward.
Sandbags	**Sandbags** provide support and shape to body contours; they immobilize extremities and maintain specific body alignment. Sandbags are filled plastic tubes that can be shaped to body contours. They can be used in place of, or in addition to, trochanter rolls.
Hand rolls	**Hand rolls** maintain the thumb slightly adducted and in opposition to the fingers; they maintain fingers in a slightly flexed position (Figure 27-4). Hand rolls can be made by folding a washcloth in half, rolling it lengthwise, and securing the roll with tape. The roll is placed against the palmar surface of the hand. The nurse evaluates the position of the hand roll to make certain the hand is indeed in a functional position.
Hand-wrist splints	**Hand-wrist splints** are individually molded for the client to maintain proper alignment of the thumb in slight **adduction** and the wrist in slight dorsiflexion. These splints should be used only for the client for whom the splint was made.
Trapeze bar	The **trapeze bar** descends from a securely fastened overhead bar attached to the bed frame (Figure 27-5). The trapeze allows the client to use upper extremities to raise the trunk off the bed, to assist in transfer from bed to wheelchair, or to perform upper arm strengthening exercises.
Side rails	**Side rails** are bars positioned along the sides of the length of the bed. They ensure client safety and are useful for increasing mobility. In addition, they provide assistance in rolling from side to side or sitting up in bed.
Bed boards	**Bed boards** are plywood boards placed under the entire surface area of the mattress. They are useful for increasing back support and alignment, especially with a soft mattress.
Wedge pillow	A wedge or abductor pillow is a triangular-shaped pillow made of heavy foam. It is used to maintain the legs in **abduction** following total hip replacement surgery.

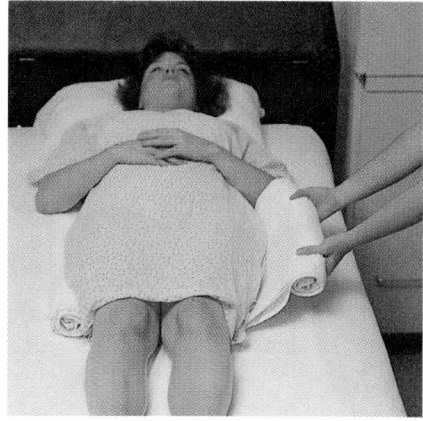

Figure 27-3. Trochanter roll.

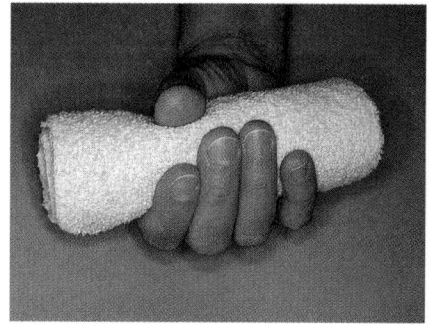

Figure 27-4. Hand roll.

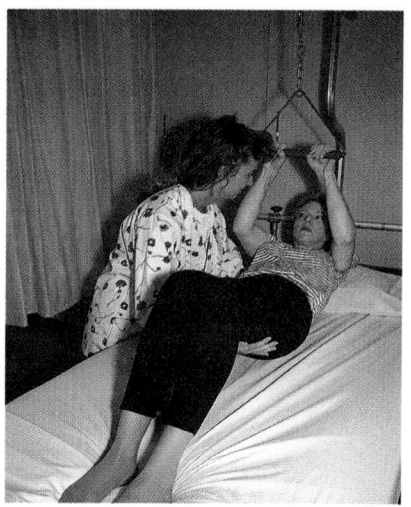

Figure 27-5. Client using a trapeze bar.

Positioning Clients in Bed

Delegation Considerations

The skills of moving and positioning clients in bed can be delegated to unlicensed assistive personnel. Clients who have spinal cord trauma usually require transfer and moving by professional nurses.

- Caution care giver about level of the bed for selected skills.
- Caution care giver to maintain proper body mechanics.
- Instruct care giver on moving and positioning in bed.

Equipment

- Pillows
- Footboard (optional)
- High-top sneakers
- Trochanter roll
- Sandbag
- Hand rolls
- Side rails
- Drawsheet

STEPS	RATIONALE
1. Assess client's body alignment and comfort level while client is lying down.	Provides baseline data for later comparisons. Determines ways to improve position and alignment.
2. Assess for risk factors that may contribute to complications of immobility:	Increased risk factors require client to be repositioned more frequently.
a. Paralysis: hemiparesis resulting from cerebrovascular accident (CVA); decreased sensation	Paralysis impairs movement, muscle tone changes; sensation is affected. Because of difficulty in moving and poor awareness of involved body part, client is unable to protect and position body part for self.
b. Impaired mobility: traction or arthritis or other contributing disease processes	Traction or arthritic changes of affected extremity result in decreased ROJM.
c. Impaired circulation	Decreased circulation predisposes client to pressure sores.
d. Age: very young, aged	Premature and young infants require frequent turning because their skin is fragile. Normal physiological changes associated with aging predispose older adults to greater risks for developing complications of immobility.
e. Client's level of consciousness	Determines needs for special aids or devices. Clients with altered levels of consciousness may not understand instructions and may be unable to help.
3. Assess client's physical ability to help with moving and positioning.	Enables nurse to use client's mobility and strength. Determines need for additional help. Ensures client and nurse safety.
4. Raise level of bed to comfortable working height.	Raises level of work toward nurse's center of gravity.
5. Remove all pillows and devices used in previous position.	Reduces interferences from bedding during positioning procedure.
6. Get extra help as needed.	Provides for client and nurse safety.
7. Explain procedure to client.	Helps to decrease anxiety and increase cooperation.
8. Position client in bed.	
A. Move immobile client up in bed (one nurse):	
(1) Place client on back with head of bed flat. Stand on one side of bed.	Enables nurse to assess body alignment. Reduces gravity's pull on client's upper body.
(2) Remove pillow from under head and shoulders and place pillow at head of bed.	Prevents striking client's head against head of bed.

STEPS	RATIONALE
(3) Begin at client's feet. Face foot of bed at 45-degree angle. Place feet apart with foot nearest head of bed behind other foot (forward-backward stance). Flex knees and hips as needed to bring arms level with client's legs. Shift weight from front to back leg, and slide client's legs diagonally toward head of bed.	Positioning is begun at client's legs because they are lighter and easier to move. Facing direction of movement ensures proper balance. Shifting nurse's weight reduces force needed to move load. Diagonal motion permits pull in direction of force. Flexing knees lowers nurse's center of gravity and uses thigh muscles rather than back muscles.
(4) Move parallel to client's hips. Flex knees and hips as needed to bring arms level with client's hips.	Maintains nurse's correct body alignment. Brings nurse closer to object to be moved and lowers center of gravity. Uses thigh muscles rather than back muscles.
(5) Slide client's hips diagonally toward head of bed.	Aligns client's hips and feet.
(6) Move parallel to client's head and shoulders. Flex knees and hips as needed to bring arms level with client's body.	Maintains nurse's proper body alignment. Brings nurse closer to object to be moved. Lowers nurse's center of gravity. Uses thigh muscles rather than back muscles.
(7) Slide arm closest to head of bed under client's neck, with hand reaching under and supporting client's shoulder.	Supports client's head and neck, maintaining alignment and preventing injury during movement.
(8) Place other arm under client's upper back.	Supports client's body weight and reduces friction during movement.
(9) Slide client's trunk, shoulders, head, and neck diagonally toward head of bed.	Realigns client's body on one side of bed.
(10) Elevate side rail. Move to other side of bed and lower side rail.	Protects client from falling out of bed.
(11) Repeat procedure, switching sides until client reaches desired position in bed.	
(12) Center client in middle of bed, moving body in same three sections.	Maintains proper body alignment. Provides ample room for turning, positioning, and other nursing activities.
B. Assist client to move up in bed (one or two nurses):	
(1) Place client on back with head of bed flat.	Enables nurse to assess body alignment. Reduces gravity's pull on client's upper body.
(2) Remove pillow from under head and shoulders and place pillow at head of bed.	Prevents striking client's head against head of bed.
(3) Face head of bed.	Facing direction of movement prevents twisting of nurse's body while moving client.
(a) Each nurse should have one arm under client's shoulders and one arm under client's thighs.	
(b) Alternative position: position one nurse at client's upper body. Nurse's arm nearest head of bed should be under client's head and opposite shoulder; other arm should be under client's closest arm and shoulder. Position other nurse at client's lower torso. The nurse's arms should be under client's lower back and torso.	Prevents trauma to client's musculoskeletal system by supporting shoulder and hip joints and evenly distributing weight.

Continued

········· Skill 27-1—cont'd
Positioning Clients in Bed
· · · · · ·

STEPS	RATIONALE
(4) Place feet apart, with foot nearest head of bed behind other foot (forward-backward stance).	Wide base of support increases nurse's balance. Stance enables nurse to shift body weight as client is moved up in bed, thereby reducing force needed to move load.
(5) Flex knees and hips. Shift weight from front to back leg, and move client and drawsheet or pullsheet to desired position in bed.	Facing direction of movement ensures proper balance. Shifting weight reduces force needed to move load. Flexing knees lowers nurses' center of gravity and uses thighs instead of back muscles.
C. Position client in supported Fowler's position (see illustration):	
(1) Elevate head of bed 45 to 60 degrees.	Increases comfort, improves ventilation, and increases client's opportunity to socialize or relax.
(2) Rest head against mattress or on small pillow.	Prevents flexion contractures of cervical vertebrae.
(3) Use pillows to support arms and hand if client does not have voluntary control or use of hands and arms.	Prevents shoulder dislocation from effect of downward pull of unsupported arms, promotes circulation by preventing venous pooling, and prevents flexion contractures of arms and wrists.
(4) Position pillow at lower back.	Supports lumbar vertebrae and decreases flexion of vertebrae.
(5) Place small pillow or roll under thigh.	Prevents hyperextension of knee and occlusion of popliteal artery from pressure from body weight.
(6) Place small pillow or roll under ankles.	Prevents prolonged pressure of mattress on heels.

CRITICAL DECISION POINT

To keep feet in proper alignment, place footboard at bottom of client's feet or apply high-top sneakers on client's feet.

D. Position hemiplegic client in supported Fowler's position:	
(1) Elevate head of bed 45 to 60 degrees.	Increases comfort, improves ventilation, and increases client's opportunity to relax.
(2) Position client in sitting position as straight as possible.	Counteracts tendency to slump toward affected side. Improves ventilation and cardiac output; decreases intracranial pressure. Improves client's ability to swallow and helps to prevent aspiration of food, liquids, and gastric secretions.
(3) Position head on small pillow with chin slightly forward. If client is totally unable to control head movement, hyperextension of the neck must be avoided.	Prevents hyperextension of neck. Too many pillows under head may cause or worsen neck flexion contracture.

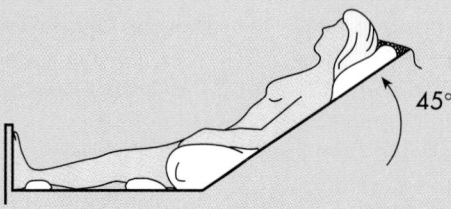

45°

Step 8C

STEPS	RATIONALE
(4) Provide support for involved arm and hand on overbed table in front of client. Place arm away from client's side and support elbow with pillow.	Paralyzed muscles do not automatically resist pull of gravity as they do normally. As a result, shoulder subluxation, pain, and edema may occur.
(a) Position *flaccid* hand in normal resting position with wrist slightly extended, arches of hand maintained, and fingers partially flexed; may use section of rubber ball cut in half; clasp client's hands together.	Maintains hand in functional position. Prevents contractures.
(b) Position *spastic* hand with wrist in neutral position or slightly extended; fingers should be extended with palm down or may be left in relaxed position with palm up.	Maintains hand in functional position. Inhibits flexor spasticity.
(5) Flex knees and hips by using pillow or folded blanket under knees.	Ensures proper alignment. Flexion prevents prolonged hyperextension, which could impair joint mobility.
(6) Support feet in dorsiflexion with firm pillow, footboard, or high-top sneakers.	Prevents footdrop. Stimulation of ball of foot by hard surface has tendency to increase muscle tone in client with extensor spasticity of lower extremity.

E. Position client in supine position:

STEPS	RATIONALE
(1) Place client on back with head of bed flat.	Necessary for placing client in supine position.
(2) Place small rolled towel under lumbar area of back.	Provides support for lumbar spine.
(3) Place pillow under upper shoulders, neck, or head.	Maintains correct alignment and prevents flexion contractures of cervical lumbar spine.
(4) Place trochanter rolls or sandbags parallel to lateral surface of client's thighs.	Reduces external rotation of hip.
(5) Place small pillow or roll under ankle to elevate heels.	Reduces pressure on heels, helping to prevent pressure sores.
(6) Support feet in dorsiflexion with firm pillow, footboard, or high top sneakers.	Prevents footdrop.
(7) Place pillows under pronated forearms, keeping upper arms parallel to client's body (see illustrations).	Reduces internal rotation of shoulder and prevents extension of elbows. Maintains correct body alignment.

Continued

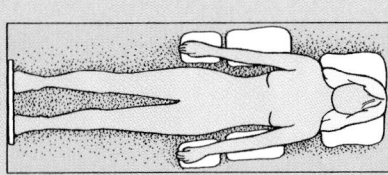

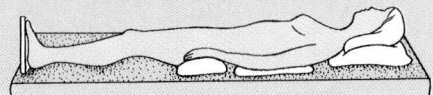

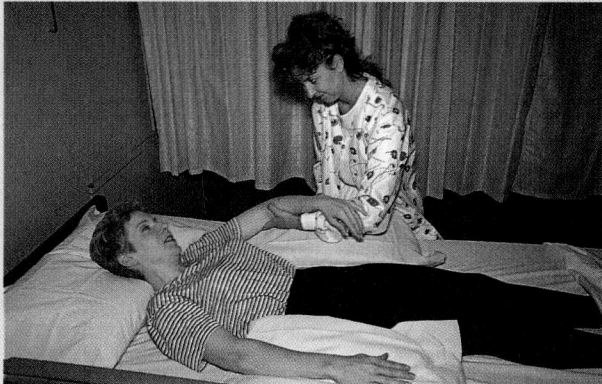

Step 8E(7)

Positioning Clients in Bed

STEPS	RATIONALE
(8) Place hand rolls in client's hands. Consider physical therapy referral for use of hand splints.	Reduces extension of fingers and abduction of thumb. Maintains thumb slightly adducted and in opposition to fingers.
F. Position hemiplegic client in supine position:	
(1) Place head of bed flat.	Necessary for positioning in supine position.
(2) Place folded towel or small pillow under shoulder or affected side.	Decreases possibility of pain, joint contracture, and subluxation. Maintains mobility in muscles around shoulder to permit normal movement patterns.
(3) Keep affected arm away from body with elbow extended and palm up. (Alternative is to place arm out to side, with elbow bent and hand toward head of bed.)	Maintains mobility in arm, joints, and shoulder to permit normal movement patterns. (Alternative position counteracts limitation of ability of arm to rotate outward at shoulder [external rotation]. External rotation must be present to raise arm overhead without pain.)
(4) Place folded towel under hip of involved side.	Diminishes effect of spasticity in entire leg by controlling hip position.
(5) Flex affected knee 30 degrees by supporting it on pillow or folded blanket.	Slight flexion breaks up abnormal extension pattern of leg. Extensor spasticity is most severe when client is supine.
(6) Support feet with soft pillows at right angle to leg.	Maintains foot in dorsiflexion and prevents footdrop. Pillows prevent stimulation to ball of foot by hard surface, which has tendency to increase muscle tone in client with extensor spasticity extremity.
G. Position client in prone position:	
(1) Roll client over arm positioned close to body, with elbow straight and hand under hip. Position on abdomen in center of bed.	Positions client correctly so alignment can be maintained.
(2) Turn client's head to one side and support head with small pillow (see illustration).	Reduces flexion or hyperextension of cervical vertebrae.
(3) Place small pillow under client's abdomen below level of diaphragm (see illustration).	Reduces pressure on breasts of some female clients and decreases hyperextension of lumbar vertebrae and strain on lower back. Improves breathing by reducing mattress pressure on diaphragm.
(4) Support arms in flexed position level at shoulders.	Maintains proper body alignment. Support reduces risk of joint dislocation.

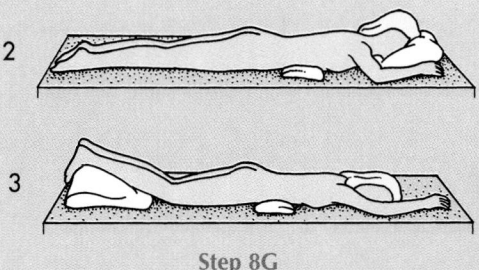

Step 8G

STEPS	RATIONALE
(5) Support lower legs with pillow to elevate toes (see illustration).	Reduces external rotation of legs and mattress pressure on toes.
H. Position hemiplegic client in prone position:	
(1) Move client toward unaffected side.	Ensures proper client alignment in center of bed when client is rolled onto abdomen.
(2) Roll client onto side.	
(3) Place pillow on client's abdomen.	Prevents sagging of abdomen when client is rolled over; decreases hyperextension of lumbar vertebrae and strain on lower back.
(4) Roll client onto abdomen by positioning involved arm close to client's body, with elbow straight and hand under hip. Roll client carefully over arm.	Prevents injury to affected side.
(5) Turn head toward involved side.	Promotes development of neck and trunk extension, which is necessary for standing and walking.
(6) Position involved arm out to side, with elbow bent, hand toward head of bed, and fingers extended (if possible).	Counteracts limitation of arms ability to rotate outward at shoulder (external rotation). External rotation must be present to raise arm over head without pain.
(7) Flex knees slightly by placing pillow under legs from knees to ankles.	Flexion prevents prolonged hyperextension, which could impair joint mobility.
(8) Keep feet at right angle to legs by using pillow high enough to keep toes off mattress and use high-top sneakers.	Maintains feet in dorsiflexion.
I. Position client in lateral (side-lying) position:	
(1) Lower head of bed completely or as low as client can tolerate.	Provides position of comfort for client and removes pressure from bony prominence on back.
(2) Position client to side of bed.	Provides room for client to turn to side.
(3) Turn client onto side.	

Continued

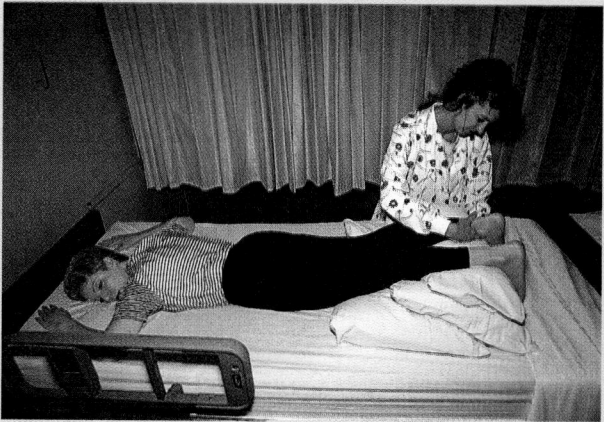

Step 8G(5)

.... **Skill 27-1—cont'd**

Positioning Clients in Bed

STEPS	RATIONALE

CRITICAL DECISION POINT

Clients at risk for pressure ulcer development require the 30-degree lateral position (see Chapter 38).

(4) Roll client onto side toward nurse by flexing client's knees and placing one hand on client's hip and one hand on client's shoulder.	Client is positioned so leverage on hip makes turning easy. Rolling client toward nurse lessens trauma to tissues.
(5) Place pillow under client's head and neck.	Maintains alignment. Reduces lateral neck flexion. Decreases strain on sternocleidomastoid muscle.
(6) Bring shoulder blade forward.	Prevents client's weight from resting directly on shoulder joint.
(7) Position both arms in slightly flexed position. Upper arm is supported by pillow level with shoulder; other arm, by mattress.	Decreases internal rotation and adduction of shoulder. Supporting both arms in slightly flexed position protects joint. Ventilation is improved because chest is able to expand more easily.
(8) Place tuck-back pillow behind client's back. (Make by folding pillow lengthwise. Smooth area is slightly tucked under client's back.).	Provides support to maintain client on side.
(9) Place pillow under semiflexed upper leg level at hip from groin to foot (see illustrations).	Flexion prevents hyperextension of leg. Maintains leg in correct alignment. Prevents pressure on bony prominence.
(10) Place sandbag parallel to plantar surface of dependent foot. Place high-top sneakers on client's feet.	Maintains dorsiflexion of foot. Prevents footdrop.
J. Position client in Sims' (semiprone) position:	
(1) Lower head of bed completely.	Provides for proper body alignment while client is lying down.
(2) Place client in supine position.	Prepares client for position.
(3) Position client in lateral position, lying partially on abdomen.	Client is rolled only partially on abdomen.

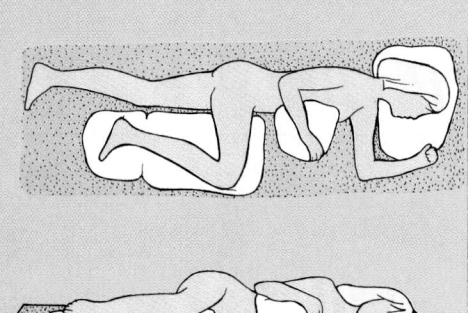

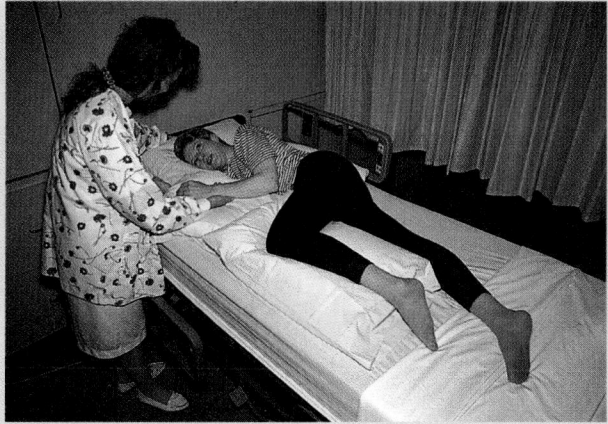

Step 8I(9)

STEPS	RATIONALE
(4) Place small pillow under client's head.	Maintains proper alignment and prevents lateral neck flexion.
(5) Place pillow under flexed upper arm, supporting arm level with shoulder.	Prevents internal rotation of shoulder. Maintains alignment.
(6) Place pillow under flexed upper legs, supporting leg level with hip.	Prevents internal rotation of hip and adduction of leg. Flexion prevents hyperextension of leg. Reduces mattress pressure on knees and ankles.
(7) Place sandbags parallel to plantar surface of foot (see illustration).	
(8) Place high-top sneakers on client's feet.	Maintains foot in dorsiflexion. Prevents footdrop.
(9) Wash hands.	Reduces transmission of infection.
(10) Lower bed and raise side rails.	Provides for client safety.
(11) Observe client's body alignment, position, and level of comfort.	Determines effectiveness of positioning. Additional supports (e.g., pillows, bath blankets), may be added or removed to promote comfort and correct body alignment.
(12) Assess for areas of erythema or breakdown involving skin.	Provides ongoing observation regarding client's skin and musculoskeletal systems. Indicates complications of immobility or improper positioning of body part.

Recording and Reporting

- Record each position change, including amount of assistance needed and client's response and tolerance.
- Record and report any signs of redness in areas such as over bony prominences.

Home Care Considerations

- For clients who need positioning at home, teach family the importance of body mechanics for themselves and the client.
- Teach family about the signs of skin breakdown and the importance of safety during positioning for clients with decreased sensation.

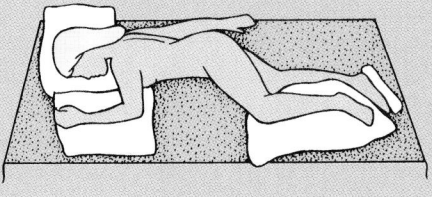

Step 8J(7)

a small pillow (Hoeman, 1996). Clients who are obese or older may not be able to tolerate this position for any length of time.

Sims' position. In the Sims' position the client is semiprone on the right or left side with the opposite arm, thigh, and knee flexed and resting on the bed. The Sims' position differs from the side-lying position in the distribution of the client's weight. In this position the client's weight is placed on the anterior ilium, humerus, and clavicle.

Improper positioning can cause unnecessary harm to clients, especially if they have certain preexisting conditions such as peripheral vascular disease or diabetes. Positions that compromise peripheral blood flow may damage nerves as well (Metzler, 1996). Every time a client is repositioned, make certain to check total body alignment and placement of extremities.

Transfer techniques. Nurses often provide care for immobilized clients whose position must be changed, who must be moved up in bed, or who must be transferred from a bed to a chair or a bed to a stretcher. Proper use of body mechanics enables the nurse to move, lift, or transfer clients safely and also protects the nurse from injury to the musculoskeletal system.

Nurses use many transfer techniques. The following general guidelines should be followed in any transfer procedure:

1. Mentally review the transfer steps before beginning to ensure the safety of both the client and the nurse.
2. Assess the client's mobility and strength to determine the assistance he or she can offer during transfer.
3. Determine the amount and type of assistance required of the nurse.
4. Explain the procedure and describe what is expected of the client.
5. Raise the side rail on the side of the bed opposite the nurse to prevent the client from falling out of bed on that side.
6. Position the level of the bed to a comfortable and safe height.
7. Assess client for correct body alignment and pressure areas after the transfer.

Clients require various levels of assistance to move up in bed or to the side-lying position, or to sit up at the side of the bed. To determine what the client is able to do alone and how many people are needed to help move the client, the nurse assesses how the client tolerates exertion. Next, the nurse determines whether the client comprehends what is expected of him or her. Then the nurse determines the comfort level of the client. The nurse also evaluates personal strengths and knowledge of the procedure. Finally, the nurse determines whether the client is too heavy or too immobile for the nurse to complete the procedure alone. In doubtful cases the nurse should always request some assistance from another person. Skill 27-2 describes the methods nurses most commonly use when moving clients in bed.

Some clients require the use of mechanical devices to assist with lift or transfer procedures. The most commonly used device is the pneumatic lift (Hoyer lift). A client is positioned on a one- or two-piece sling connected by chains to a crossbar on the lift. The hydraulic mechanism carries the client in a seated position for transfer (Hoeman, 1996). Newer lifts allow the client to stand.

Transferring a client from a bed to a chair. Transfer of a client from bed to chair by one nurse requires assistance from the client and should not be attempted with clients unable to assist or comprehend instructions (see Skill 27-2). The nurse explains the procedure to the client before attempting transfer. The environment is also prepared by moving obstacles out of the way. The chair is placed next to the bed with the chair back parallel to the head of the bed. This placement allows the nurse to pivot with the client and to transfer the client's weight quickly to the chair.

A safe transfer is the first priority. The nurse who is doubtful about personal strength or the client's ability to help should request assistance. The client should sit and dangle his or her feet at the side of the bed for a minute before standing. Then the client should stand at the side of the bed for another minute so that he or she can quickly be lowered back into it in case of dizziness or fainting.

Transferring a client from a bed to a stretcher. An immobilized client who must be transferred from bed to stretcher or bed to bed requires a three-person carry (see Skill 27-2). This technique is best implemented when personnel are of a similar height. If their centers of gravity are within the same plane, they can lift as a team.

Caution is used when the client has spinal cord trauma. If the client must be moved, the three-person carry is used and spinal alignment is maintained during the transfer.

The client should be prepared for the transfer and asked to help (e.g., by folding the arms over the chest). The environment should be free from obstacles, and unnecessary equipment should be removed from the bed. The stretcher should be placed at a right angle to the bed so the lifters can pivot toward the stretcher and transfer the client easily. Use of a smooth board or glide can also assist with transferring.

As with all procedures, safety is the priority. Safety is increased in the three-person carry if all the lifters work together. Therefore one person should assume the leadership role and direct the other two.

Restorative care

Joint mobility. The easiest intervention to maintain or improve joint mobility for clients and one that can be coordinated with other activities is the use of range-of-motion exercises. In **active range-of-motion exercises,** the client is able to move his or her joints. The nurse moves each joint in **passive range-of-motion exercises.** The use of these exercises enables the nurse to systematically assess and improve the client's joint mobility.

Joints that are not moved periodically can develop contractures, a permanent shortening of a muscle followed by the eventual shortening of associated ligaments and tendons. Over time, the joint may become fixed in one position and the client loses normal use of the joint. For the client who does not have voluntary motor control, passive range-of-motion exercises are the exercises of choice.

The older adult has a decline in physical activity and changes in joints that may predispose the client to problems with mobility, and joint flexibility may be limited.

Text continued on p. 697

Transfer Techniques

Delegation Considerations

The skills of safe and effective transfer techniques can be delegated to unlicensed assistive personnel. Clients who have spinal cord trauma usually require transfer and moving by professional nurses.

▪ Caution care giver about level of the bed for selected skills.
▪ Caution care giver to maintain proper body mechanics.
▪ Instruct care giver on safe transfer techniques.

Equipment

▪ Transfer belt (if needed), sling or lap board (as needed), nonskid shoes, bath blankets, pillows
▪ Wheelchair: position chair at 45-degree angle to bed, lock brakes, remove footrests, lock bed brakes
▪ Stretcher: position at right angle (90 degrees) to bed, lock brakes on stretcher, lock brakes on bed
▪ Mechanical/hydraulic lift: use frame, canvas strips or chains, and hammock or canvas strips

STEPS	RATIONALE
1. Assess the client for the following: a. Muscle strength b. Joint mobility c. Presence of paralysis or paresis d. Orthostatic hypotension e. Activity tolerance f. Level of consciousness g. Level of comfort h. Ability to follow instructions	Provides information to the nurse relative to the client's abilities, physical status, ability to comprehend, and the number of individuals needed to provide safe transferring.
2. Identify clients at greatest risk for problems with transfering.	Provides information to the nurse relative to clients who may require intervention beyond the unlicensed care provider, for example, physical therapy department.
3. Explain procedure to client.	Promotes cooperation, encourages assistance, and enhances understanding of procedure.
4. Close door or curtain.	Maintains privacy.
5. Wash hands.	Reduces transfer of microorganisms.
6. Transfer client. A. **Assist client to sitting position (bed at waist level):**	
(1) Place client in supine position.	Enables nurse to assess client's body alignment continually and to administer additional care, such as suctioning or hygiene needs.
(2) Face head of bed and remove pillows.	Proper positioning reduces twisting of the nurse's body when moving the client. Pillows may cause interference when the client is sitting up in bed.
(3) Place feet apart with foot nearer bed behind other foot.	Improves nurse's balance and allows transfer of body weight as client is moved to sitting position.
(4) Place hand farther from client under shoulders, supporting client's head and cervical vertebrae.	Maintains alignment of head and cervical vertebrae and allows for even lifting of client's upper trunk.
(5) Place other hand on bed surface.	Provides support and balance.
(6) Raise client to sitting position by shifting weight from front to back leg.	Improves nurse's balance, overcomes inertia, and transfers weight in direction in which client is moved.
(7) Push against bed using arm that is placed on bed surface.	Divides activity between nurse's arms and legs and protects back from strain. By bracing one hand against mattress and pushing against it as client is lifted, part of weight that would be lifted by nurse's back muscles is transferred through nurse's arms onto mattress.

Continued

.... **Skill 27-2—cont'd**
Transfer Techniques

STEPS	RATIONALE
B. Assist client to sitting position on side of bed with bed in low position:	
(1) With client in supine position, raise head of bed 30 degrees.	Decreases amount of work needed by client and nurse to raise client to sitting position.
(2) Turn client to side, facing nurse on side of bed on which client will be sitting (see illustration).	Prepares client to move to side of bed and protects from falling.
(3) Stand opposite client's hips. Turn diagonally so nurse faces client and far corner of foot of bed.	Places nurse's center of gravity nearer client. Reduces twisting of nurse's body because nurse is facing direction of movement.
(4) Place feet apart with foot closer to head of bed in front of other foot.	Increases balance and allows nurse to transfer weight as client is brought to sitting position on side of bed.
(5) Place arm nearer head of bed under client's shoulder, supporting head and neck.	Maintains alignment of head and neck as nurse brings client to sitting position.
(6) Place other arm nearer head and neck (see illustration).	Supports hip and prevents client from falling backward during procedure.
(7) Move client's lower legs and feet over side of bed. Pivot toward rear leg, allowing client's upper legs to swing downward.	Decreases friction and resistance. Weight of client's legs when off bed allows gravity to lower legs, and weight of legs assists in pulling upper body into sitting position.
(8) At same time, shift weight to rear leg and elevate client (see illustration).	Allows nurse to transfer weight in direction of motion.
(9) Remain in front of client until client regains balance.	Reduces risk of falling.
C. Transfer client from bed to chair with bed in low position:	
(1) Assist client to sitting position on side of bed. Have chair in position at 45-degree angle to bed.	Positions chair within easy access for transfer.
(2) Apply transfer belt or other transfer aids, if needed.	Transfer belt allows nurse to maintain stability of client during transfer and reduces risk of falling. Client's arm should be in sling if flaccid paralysis is present.

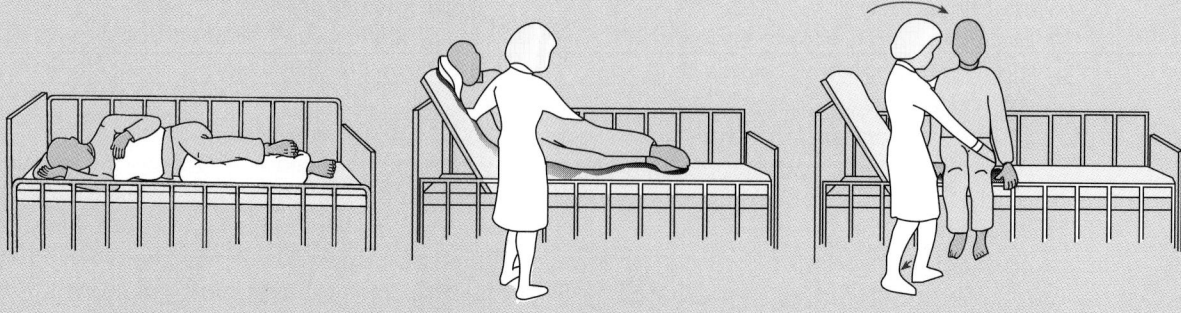

Step 6B(2)   Step 6B(6)   Step 6B(8)

STEPS	RATIONALE
(3) Ensure that client has stable nonskid shoes. Weight-bearing or strong leg is placed forward, with weak foot back.	Nonskid soles decrease risk of slipping during transfer. Always have clients wear shoes during transfer; bare feet increase risk of falls. Client will stand on stronger, or weight-bearing, leg.
(4) Spread feet apart.	Ensure balance with wide base of support.
(5) Flex hips and knees, aligning knees with client's knees (see illustration).	Flexion of knees and hips lowers nurse's center of gravity to object to be raised; aligning knees with client's allows for stabilization of knees when client stands.
(6) Grasp transfer belt from underneath, if used, or reach through client's axillae and place hands on client's scapulas.	Lifting client with hands on scapulas reduces pressure on axillae and maintains client stability. Clients with upper extremity paralysis or paresis should never be lifted by or under arms. Transfer belt is grasped at each side to provide movement of client at center of gravity.
(7) Rock client up to standing position on count of three while straightening hips and legs and keeping knees slightly flexed (see illustration). Client may be instructed to use hands to push up if applicable.	Rocking motion gives client's body momentum and requires less muscular effort to lift client.
(8) Maintain stability of client's weak or paralyzed leg with knee.	Ability to stand can often be maintained in paralyzed or weak limb with support of knee to stabilize.
(9) Pivot on foot farther from chair.	Maintains support of client while allowing adequate space for client to move.
(10) Instruct client to use armrests on chair for support and ease into chair (see illustration).	Increases client stability.
(11) Flex hips and knees while lowering client into chair (see illustration).	Prevents injury to nurse from poor body mechanics.

Continued

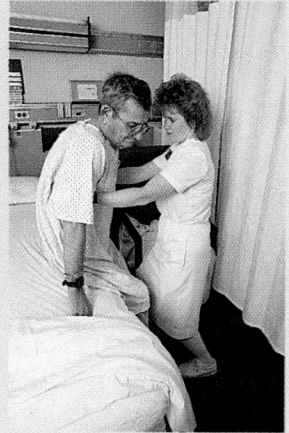
Step 6C(5)

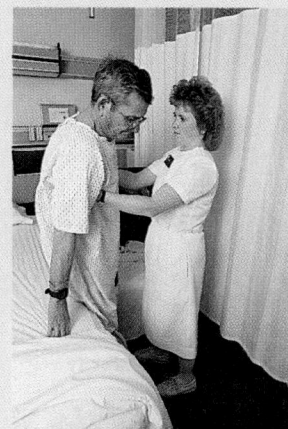
Step 6C(7)

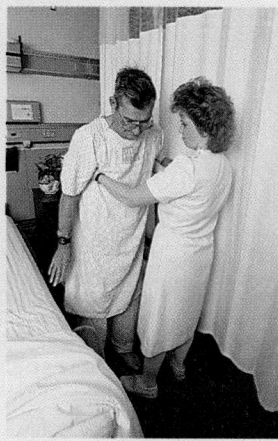
Step 6C(10)

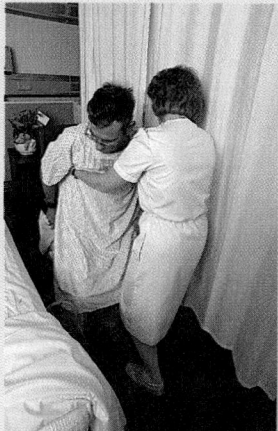
Step 6C(11)

Skill 27-2—cont'd
Transfer Techniques

STEPS	RATIONALE
(12) Assess client for proper alignment for sitting position. Provide support for paralyzed extremities. Lap board or sling will support flaccid arm. Stabilize leg with bath blanket or pillow.	Prevents injury to client from poor body alignment.
(13) Praise client's progress, effort, performance.	Continued support and encouragement provide incentive for client perseverance.
D. Perform three-person carry from bed to stretcher (bed at stretcher level):	
(1) Three nurses stand side by side facing side of client's bed. Individuals performing the procedure should be of equal height.	Prevents twisting of nurses' bodies. Client's alignment is maintained.
(2) Each person assumes responsibility for one of three areas: head and shoulders, hips, and thighs and ankles.	Distributes client's body weight evenly.
(3) Each person assumes wide base of support with foot closer to stretcher in front and knees slightly flexed.	Increases balance and lowers center of gravity of person lifting.
(4) Arms of lifters are placed under client's head and shoulders, hips, and thighs and ankles, with fingers securely around other side of client's body (see illustration).	Distributes client's weight over forearms of lifters.

CRITICAL DECISION POINT

Spinal cord injuries must be stabilized before transfer.

(5) Lifters roll client toward their chests. On count of three, client is lifted and held against nurses' chests.	Moves workload over lifters' base of support. Enables lifters to work together and safely lift client.
(6) On second count of three, nurses step back and pivot toward stretcher, moving forward if needed.	Transfers weight toward stretcher.

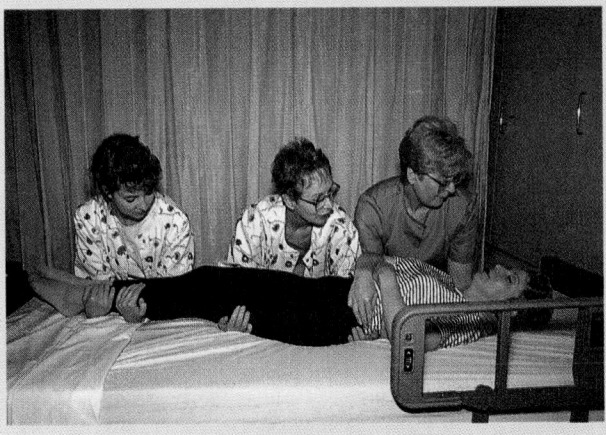

Step 6D(4)

STEPS	RATIONALE
(7) Nurses gently lower client onto center of stretcher by flexing knees and hips until elbows are level with edge of stretcher.	Maintains nurses' alignment during transfer.
(8) Nurses assess client's body alignment, place safety straps across body, and raise side rails.	Reduces risk of injury from poor alignment or falling.
E. Use mechanical/hydraulic lift to transfer client from bed to chair:	
(1) Bring lift to bedside.	Ensures safe elevation of client off bed. (Before using lift, be thoroughly familiar with its operation.)
(2) Position chair near bed, and allow adequate space to maneuver lift.	Prepares environment for safe use of lift and subsequent transfer.
(3) Raise bed to high position with mattress flat. Lower side rail.	Allows nurse to use proper body mechanics.
(4) Keep bed side rail up on side opposite nurse.	Maintains client safety.
(5) Roll client away from nurse.	Positions client for use of lift sling.
(6) Place hammock or canvas strips under client to form sling (see illustration). With two canvas pieces, lower edge fits under client's knees (wide piece), and upper edge fits under client's shoulders (narrow piece).	Two types of seats are supplied with mechanical/hydraulic lift: hammock style is better for clients who are flaccid, weak, and need support; canvas strips can be used for clients with normal muscle tone. Hooks should face away from client's skin. Place sling under client's center of gravity and greatest portion of body weight.
(7) Raise bed rail.	Maintains client safety.
(8) Go to opposite side of bed and lower side rail.	
(9) Roll client to opposite side and pull hammock (strips) through.	Completes positioning of client on mechanical/hydraulic sling.
(10) Roll client supine onto canvas seat.	Sling should extend from shoulders to knees (hammock) to support client's body weight equally.
(11) Remove client's glasses, if appropriate.	Swivel bar is close to client's head and could break eyeglasses.

Continued

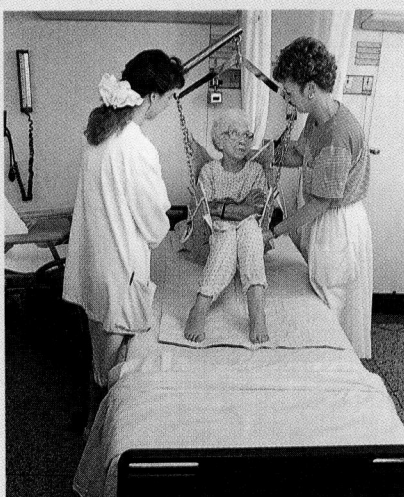

Step 6E(6)

STEPS	RATIONALE
(12) Place lift's horseshoe bar under side of bed (on side with chair).	Positions lift efficiently and promotes smooth transfer.
(13) Lower horizontal bar to sling level by releasing hydraulic valve. Lock valve.	Positions hydraulic lift close to client. Locking valve prevents injury to client.
(14) Attach hooks on strap (chain) to holes in sling. Short chains or straps hook to top holes of sling; longer chains hook to bottom of sling.	Secures hydraulic lift to sling.
(15) Elevate head of bed.	Positions client in sitting position.
(16) Fold client's arms over chest.	Prevents injury to paralyzed arms.
(17) Pump hydraulic handle using long, slow, even strokes until client is raised off bed.	Ensures safe support of client during elevation (see illustration).
(18) Use steering handle to pull lift from bed and maneuver to chair.	Moves client from bed to chair.
(19) Roll base around chair.	Positions lift in front of the chair in which client is to be transferred.
(20) Release check valve slowly (turn to left) and lower client into chair (see illustration).	Safely guides client into back of chair as seat descends.
(21) Close check valve as soon as client is down and straps can be released.	If valve is left open, boom may continue to lower and injure client.
(22) Remove straps and mechanical/hydraulic lift.	Prevents damage to skin and underlying tissues from canvas or hooks.
(23) Check client's sitting alignment.	Prevents injury from poor posture.
7. Wash hands.	Reduces transmission of microorganisms.
8. With each transfer, assess client's tolerance and level of tiredness.	Increased activity may elevate heart rate and blood pressure.
9. With each transfer, evaluate client's alignment.	

Recording and Reporting
▪ Record each transfer and position change, including amount of assistance needed and client's response.
▪ Record and report any signs of redness over bony prominences, etc.

Home Care Considerations
▪ For clients who need head of bed elevated at home, teach family about use of pillows or bed blocks.
▪ Teach family the importance of body mechanics for themselves and the client.

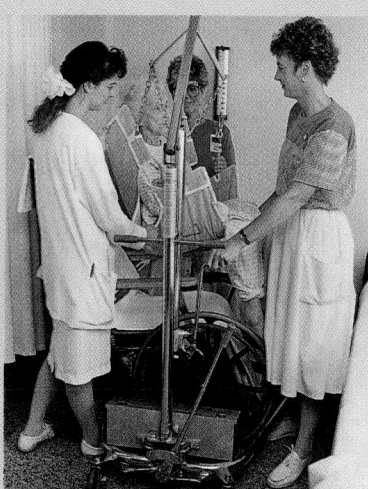

Step 6E(20)

The nurse can recommend approaches that help older adults to use proper body mechanics and prevent injury (Box 27-5).

Mechanical devices are available for specific joints, which place these joints through continuous passive range of motion (CPM). These CPM machines are used postoperatively to place joints through a selective repetitive range of motion. The machine can be set to certain degrees of joint mobility with increasing joint mobility or flexion as the goal. The most common clients who use the CPM machine are those who have undergone some form of total joint replacement surgery.

Unless contraindicated, the nursing care plan should include exercising each joint through as nearly a full range of motion as possible. Passive range-of-motion exercises should be initiated as soon as the client loses the ability to move the extremity or joint. The following guidelines apply to the use of range of motion exercises:

1. Provide explanation to the client; this elicits co-operation and assistance.
2. Start slowly; movements should be smooth and easy.
3. Flexion of the joint can continue until slight resistance is felt; do not move a joint to the point of pain; avoid hyperextending the joint.
4. Work from distal joints to proximal joints on one extremity at a time.
5. Provide support for joints distal to the joint being manipulated.
6. Assess client closely for signs of generalized fatigue.
7. When exercises are completed, make certain to leave joints in correct alignment position.

Table 27-2 details range-of-motion exercises for each area and illustrates the motion of each joint.

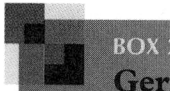

BOX 27-5
Gerontological Nursing Practice

- Encourage the older adult client to avoid prolonged sitting, to get up and stretch. Frequent stretching decreases joint contractures.
- Be sure client maintains proper body alignment when sitting. Proper alignment minimizes joint and muscle stress.
- Teach clients how to use stronger joints or larger muscle groups to manipulate spray cans, container lids, etc. Efficient distribution of workload decreases joint stress and pain.
- Some studies have demonstrated that nonstrenuous exercise (such as ROM) may improve memory or the ability to recall for up to 30 minutes or more (Dawe and Moore-Orr, 1995).
- Provide resources for planned exercise programs. Proper exercise activities slow further bone loss and prevent fractures in the older adult with osteoporosis.

Walking. Joint mobility is also increased by walking. In the normal walking posture the head is erect, the cervical, thoracic, and lumbar vertebrae are aligned, the hips and knees have appropriate flexion, and the arms swing freely in alternation with the legs. Illness or trauma can reduce activity tolerance, necessitating a need for assistance with walking or the use of mechanical devices such as crutches, canes, or walkers.

Assisting a client to walk. Assisting the client to walk requires preparation. The nurse assesses the client's activity tolerance, strength, coordination, and balance to determine the type of assistance needed. The nurse should also assess the client's orientation and determine if there are any signs of distress. This would preclude attempts at ambulation.

The nurse evaluates the environment for safety prior to ambulation; this includes the removal of obstacles, a clean and dry floor, and the establishment of rest points should the client's activity tolerance become less than expected. The client should also wear supportive, non-slipping shoes. Resting points should be established in the event the client's activity tolerance is less than was estimated or the client becomes dizzy.

When preparing a client for ambulation, dangling is an important technique. The client should be assisted to a position of sitting at the side of the bed and should rest for 1 to 2 minutes before standing. The longer the period of immobility, the greater the physiological changes. This is especially true regarding changes in circulation. When the client has been flat for extended periods, blood pressure may drop when the client stands (see Chapter 23). Dangling helps to prevent this. After standing, the client should remain stationary for a minute or two before moving. If the client becomes dizzy, the bed is still nearby and the nurse can quickly ease him or her back to bed.

Several methods are used for assisting a client with ambulation. The nurse should provide support at the waist so the client's center of gravity remains midline. This can be achieved when the nurse places both hands at the client's waist or uses a gait belt. A gait belt is a leather belt that encircles the client's waist and has handles attached for the nurse to hold while the client ambulates. Clients should not lean to one side because then their center of gravity is no longer midline, which distorts their balance, and their risk of falling is increased.

The client who appears unsteady or complains of dizziness should be returned to the closest bed or a chair. If the client has a syncopal episode or begins to fall, the nurse should assume a wide base of support with one foot in front of the other, thus supporting the client's body weight. The nurse gently lowers the client to the floor, protecting the client's head. Although lowering a client to the floor is not difficult, the student should practice this technique with a friend or classmate before attempting it in a clinical setting (see Figure 27-6, p. 702).

Text continued on p. 702

TABLE 27-2
Range-of-Motion Exercises

Body Part	Type of Joint	Type of Movement	Range (degrees)	Primary Muscles
Neck, cervical spine	Pivotal	Flexion: bring chin to rest on chest	45	Sternocleidomastoid
		Extension: return head to erect position	45	Trapezius
		Hyperextension: bend head back as far as possible	10	Trapezius
		Lateral flexion: tilt head as far as possible toward each shoulder	40-45	Sternocleidomastoid
		Rotation: turn head as far as possible in circular movement	180	Sternocleidomastoid, trapezius
Shoulder	Ball and socket	Flexion: raise arm from side position forward to position above head	180	Coracobrachialis, biceps brachii, deltoid, pectoralis major
		Extension: return arm to position at side of body	180	Latissimus dorsi, teres major, triceps brachii
		Hyperextension: move arm behind body, keeping elbow straight	45-60	Latissimus dorsi, teres major, deltoid
		Abduction: raise arm to side to position above head with palm away from head	180	Deltoid, supraspinatus
		Adduction: lower arm sideways and across body as far as possible	320	Pectoralis major

TABLE 27-2

Range-of-Motion Exercises—cont'd

Body Part	Type of Joint	Type of Movement	Range (degrees)	Primary Muscles
		Internal rotation: with elbow flexed, rotate shoulder by moving arm until thumb is turned inward and toward back	90	Pectoralis major, latissimus dorsi, teres major, subscapularis
		External rotation: with elbow flexed, move arm until thumb is upward and lateral to head	90	Infraspinatus, teres major, deltoid
		Circumduction: move arm in full circle (**Circumduction** is combination of all movements of ball-and-socket joint.)	360	Deltoid, coracobrachialis, latissimus dorsi, teres major
Elbow	Hinge	Flexion: bend elbow so that lower arm moves toward its shoulder joint and hand is level with shoulder	150	Biceps brachii, brachialis, brachioradialis
		Extension: straighten elbow by lowering hand	150	Triceps brachii
Forearm	Pivotal	Supination: turn lower arm and hand so that palm is up	70-90	Supinator, biceps brachii
		Pronation: turn lower arm so that palm is down	70-90	Pronator teres, pronator quadratus
Wrist	Condyloid	Flexion: move palm toward inner aspect of forearm	80-90	Flexor carpi ulnaris, flexor carpi radialis
		Extension: move fingers so that fingers, hands, and forearm are in same plane	80-90	Extensor carpi ulnaris, extensor carpi radialis brevis, extensor carpi radialis longus
		Hyperextension: bring dorsal surface of hand back as far as possible	89-90	Extensor carpi radialis brevis, extensor carpi radialis longus, extensor carpi ulnaris
		Abduction (radial flexion): bend wrist medially toward thumb	Up to 30	Flexor carpi radialis, extensor carpi radialis brevis, extensor carpi radialis longus
		Adduction (ulnar flexion): bend wrist laterally toward fifth finger	30-50	Flexor carpi ulnaris, extensor carpi ulnaris

Continued

TABLE 27-2
Range-of-Motion Exercises—cont'd

Body Part	Type of Joint	Type of Movement	Range (degrees)	Primary Muscles
Fingers	Condyloid hinge	Flexion: make fist	90	Lumbricales, interosseus volaris, interosseus dorsalis
		Extension: straighten fingers	90	Extensor digiti quinti proprius, extensor digitorum communis, extensor indicis proprius
		Hyperextension: bend fingers back as far as possible	30-60	
		Abduction: spread fingers apart	30	Interosseus dorsalis
		Adduction: bring fingers together	30	Interosseus volaris
Thumb	Saddle	Flexion: move thumb across palmar surface of hand	90	Flexor pollicis brevis
		Extension: move thumb straight away from hand	90	Extensor pollicis longus, extensor pollicis brevis
		Abduction: extend thumb laterally (usually done when placing fingers in abduction and adduction)	30	Abductor pollicis brevis
		Adduction: move thumb back toward hand	30	Adductor pollicis obliquus, adductor pollicis transversus
		Opposition: touch thumb to each finger of same hand		Opponeus pollicis, opponeus digiti minimi
Hip	Ball and socket	Flexion: move leg forward and up	90-120	Psoas major, iliacus, iliopsoas, sartorius
		Extension: move back beside other leg	90-120	Gluteus maximus, semitendinosus, semimembranosus
		Hyperextension: move leg behind body	30-50	Gluteus maximus, semitendinosus, semimembranosus

TABLE 27-2
Range-of-Motion Exercises—cont'd

Body Part	Type of Joint	Type of Movement	Range (degrees)	Primary Muscles
		Abduction: move leg laterally away from body	30-50	Gluteus medius, gluteus minimus
		Adduction: move leg back toward medial position and beyond if possible	30-50	Adductor longus, adductor brevis, adductor magnus
		Internal rotation: turn foot and leg toward other leg	90	Gluteus medius, gluteus minimus, tensor fasciae latae
		External rotation: turn foot and leg away from other leg	90	Obturatorius internus, obturatorius externus
		Circumduction: move leg in circle		Psoas major, gluteus maximus, gluteus medius, adductor magnus
Knee	Hinge	Flexion: bring heel back toward back of thigh	120-130	Biceps femoris, semitendinosus, semimembranosus, sartorius
		Extension: return leg to the floor	120-130	Rectus femoris, vastus lateralis, vastus medialis, vastus intermedius
Ankle	Hinge	Dorsal flexion: move foot so that toes are pointed upward	20-30	Tibialis anterior
		Plantar flexion: move foot so that toes are pointed downward	45-50	Gastrocnemius, soleus
Foot	Gliding	Inversion: turn sole of foot medially	10 or less	Tibialis anterior, tibialis posterior
		Eversion: turn sole of foot laterally	10 or less	Peroneus longus, peroneus brevis
Toes	Condyloid	Flexion: curl toes downward	30-60	Flexor digitorum, lumbricalis pedis, flexor hallucis brevis
		Extension: straighten toes	30-60	Extensor digitorum longus, extensor digitorum brevis, extensor hallucis longus
		Abduction: spread toes apart	15 or less	Abductor hallucis, interosseus dorsalis
		Adduction: bring toes together	15 or less	Adductor hallucis, interosseus plantaris

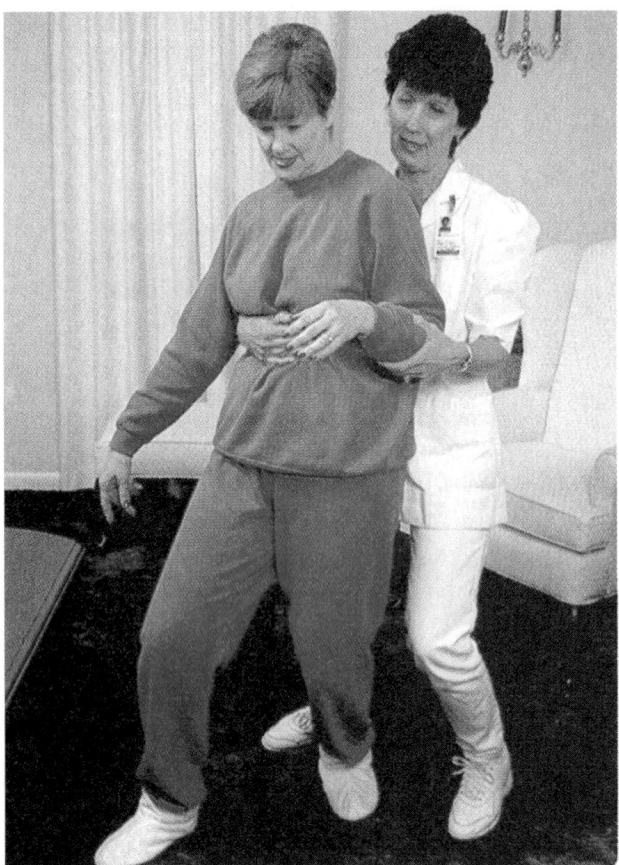

Figure 27-6. Ease the client down to the floor by bending your knees, keeping your back straight. (From Birchenall JM, Streight ME: *Mosby's textbook for the home care aide,* St. Louis, 1997, Mosby.)

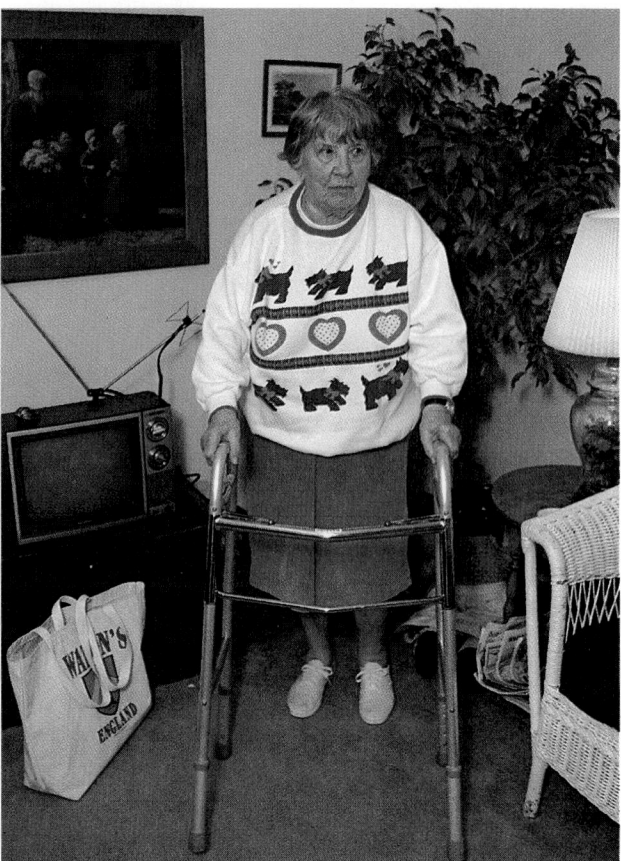

Figure 27-7. Client using a walker.

Clients with hemiplegia (one-sided paralysis) or hemiparesis (one-sided weakness) need assistance in ambulating. The nurse stands by the client's affected side and supports the client by holding one arm around the client's waist and the other arm around the inferior aspect of the client's upper arm so that the nurse's hand is supporting the client's axilla. The client's unaffected arm is left free to enable the client to assist. Providing support by holding the client's arm is incorrect because, if the client should experience syncope or fall, the nurse cannot easily support the weight and lower the client to the floor. In addition, if the client falls with the nurse holding the arm, the shoulder joint may be dislocated.

A nurse who has even the slightest doubt about his or her strength and ability to ambulate a client alone should request help. The two-nurse method helps to distribute the client's weight evenly. The two nurses stand on either side of the client. Each nurse's near arm is around the client's waist, and the other arm is around the inferior aspect of the client's arm so that the hands of both nurses are supporting the client's axillae.

Assistive devices for walking. Walkers are extremely light, movable devices, about waist high and

made of metal tubing (Figure 27-7). They have four widely placed, sturdy legs. The client holds the handgrips on the upper bars, takes a step, moves the walker forward, and takes another step.

Canes are lightweight, easily movable devices about waist high, made of wood or metal. Two common types of canes are the single straight-legged cane and the quad cane. The single straight-legged cane is more common and is used to support and balance a client with decreased leg strength. This cane should be kept on the stronger side of the body. For maximum support when walking, the client places the cane forward 15 to 25 cm (6 to 10 inches), keeping body weight on both legs. The weaker leg is moved forward to the cane so that body weight is divided between the cane and the stronger leg. The stronger leg is then advanced past the cane so the weaker leg and the body weight are supported by the cane and weaker leg. During walking, the client continually repeats these three steps. The client must be taught that two points of support, such as both feet or one foot and the cane, are present at all times.

The quad cane provides the most support and is used when there is partial or complete leg paralysis or some hemiplegia (Figure 27-8). The same three steps used with the straight-legged cane are taught to the client.

Crutches are often needed to increase mobility. The use of crutches may be temporary, such as after ligament damage to the knee. However, crutches may be needed permanently by a client with paralysis of the lower extremities. A crutch is a wooden or metal staff. The two types of crutches are the double adjustable Lofstrand or forearm crutch (Figure 27-9) and the axillary wooden or metal crutch. The forearm crutch has a handgrip and a metal band that fits around the client's forearm. The metal band and the handgrip are adjusted to fit the client's height. The axillary crutch has a padded curved surface at the top, which fits under the axilla. A handgrip in the form of a crossbar is held at the level of the palms to support the body. It is important that crutches be measured for the appropriate length and that clients be taught to use their crutches safely, to achieve a stable gait, to ascend and descend stairs, and to rise from a sitting position.

Measuring for crutches. The axillary crutch is the more common crutch used. Measurements include the client's height, the angle of elbow flexion, and the distance between the crutch pad and the axilla. When crutches are fitted, the length of the crutch should be from three to four finger-widths from the axilla to a point 15 cm (6 inches) lateral to the client's heel (Hoeman, 1996) (Figure 27-10).

The handgrips should be positioned so the client's body weight is not supported by the axillae. Pressure on the axillae increases risk to underlying nerves, which could result in partial paralysis of the arm. Correct position of the handgrips is determined with the client upright, supporting weight by the handgrips with the elbows slightly flexed (20 to 25 degrees). Elbow flexion may be verified with a goniometer (Figure 27-11). When the height and placement of the handgrips have been determined, the nurse should again verify that the distance between the crutch pad and the client's axilla is three to four finger-widths (Figure 27-12).

Crutch safety. Before being allowed to walk independently with crutches, the client should be taught the following safety guidelines:

1. Clients with axillary crutches must be aware of the dangers of pressure on the axilla. Therefore they must not use crutches that fit improperly or lean on their crutches to support body weight.

2. Crutch-dependent clients should be taught to inspect the crutch tips routinely. The rubber tips should be securely attached to the crutches. When the tips are worn, they should be replaced immediately. Rubber crutch tips increase surface friction and prevent the crutches from slipping.

3. Crutch tips should remain dry. If the tips become wet, the client should dry them. Water decreases surface friction and increases the risk that the crutches will slip.

4. The structure of the crutches should also be

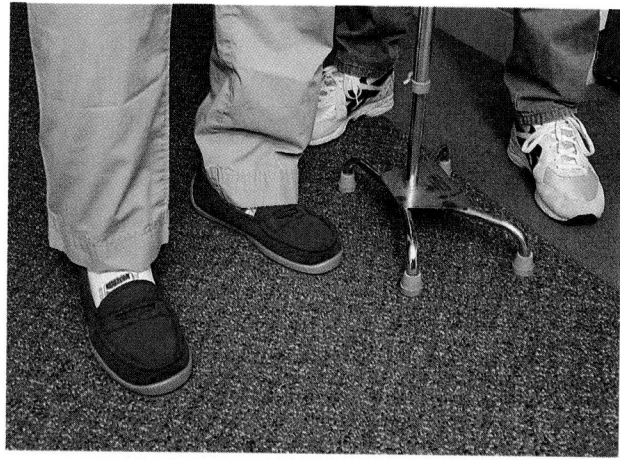

Figure 27-8. Quad cane.

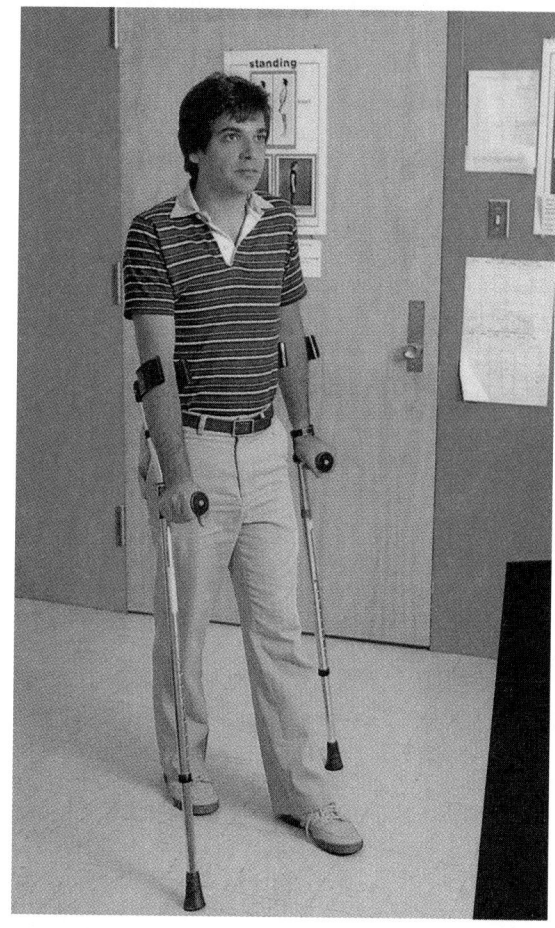

Figure 27-9. Double adjustable Lofstrand or forearm crutch.

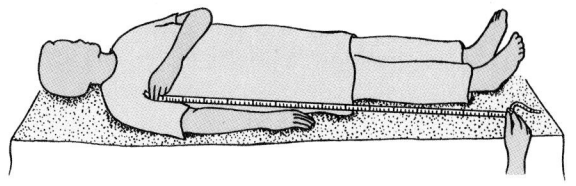

Figure 27-10. Measuring crutch length.

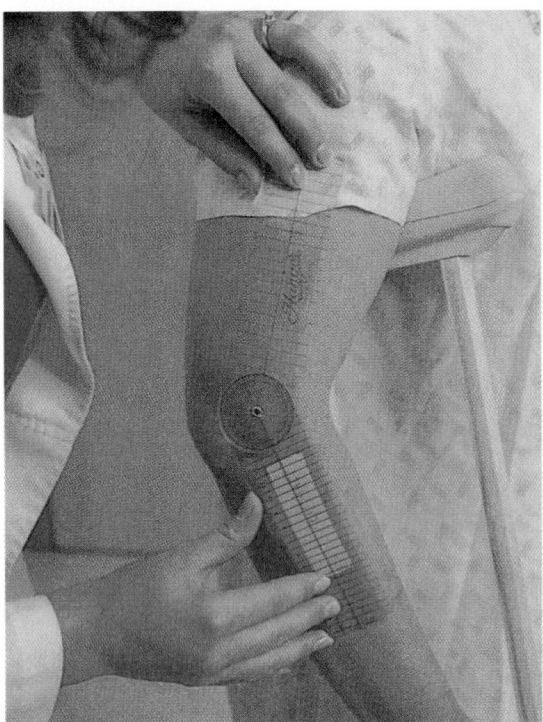

Figure 27-11. Using the goniometer to verify correct degree of elbow flexion for crutch use.

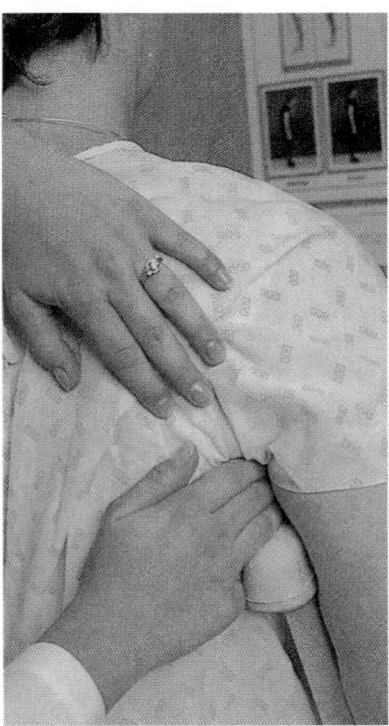

Figure 27-12. Verifying correct distance between crutch pads and axilla.

routinely inspected. Cracks in a wooden crutch decrease the crutch's ability to support weight. Bends in aluminum crutches can alter body alignment, increasing the risk of further damage to the musculoskeletal system.

5. Clients should be given a list of medical suppliers in their community. This allows the clients to obtain repairs, new rubber tips, handgrips, and crutch pads.

6. Crutch-dependent clients should always have spare crutches and tips on hand.

Crutch gait. The **crutch gait** is assumed by alternately bearing weight on one or both legs and on the crutches. The gait selected by the physician is determined by assessing the client's physical and functional abilities and the disease or injury that resulted in the need for crutches. This section summarizes the basic crutch stance and the four standard gaits: four-point alternating gait, three-point alternating gait, two-point gait, and swing-through gait.

The basic crutch stance is the tripod position, formed when the crutches are placed 15 cm (6 inches) in front of and 15 cm to the side of each foot (Figure 27-13). This position improves the client's balance by providing a wider base of support. The body alignment of the client in the tripod position includes erect head and neck, straight vertebrae, and extended hips and knees. No weight should be borne by the axillae. The tripod position is used before crutch walking.

Four-point alternating or four-point gait gives stability to the client but requires weight bearing on both legs. Each leg is moved alternately with each opposing crutch so that three points of support are on the floor at all times (Figure 27-14).

Three-point alternating or three-point gait requires the client to bear all of the weight on one foot. In a three-point gait, weight is borne on both crutches and then on the uninvolved leg, and the sequence is repeated (Figure 27-15). The affected leg does not touch the ground during the early phase of the three-point gait. Gradually the client progresses to touchdown and full weight bearing on the affected leg.

The two-point gait requires at least partial weight bearing on each foot (Figure 27-16). The client moves a crutch at the same time as the opposing leg, so the crutch movements are similar to arm motion during normal walking.

The swing-through or swing-through gait is frequently used by paraplegics who wear weight-supporting braces on their legs. With weight placed on the supported legs, the client places the crutches one stride in front and then swings to or through the crutches while they support the client's weight.

Crutch walking on stairs. When ascending stairs on crutches, the client usually uses a modified three-point gait (Figure 27-17). The client stands at the bottom of the stairs and transfers body weight to the crutches. The unaffected leg is advanced between the crutches to the stairs. The client then shifts weight from

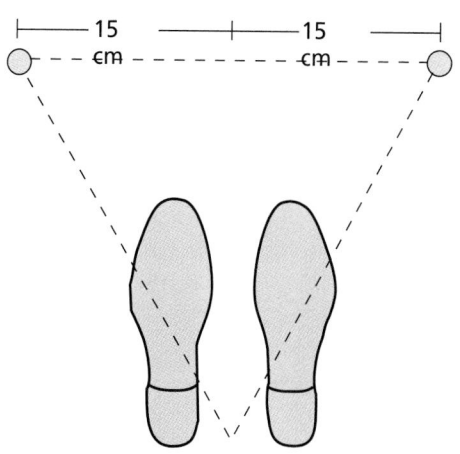

Figure 27-13. Tripod position, basic crutch stance.

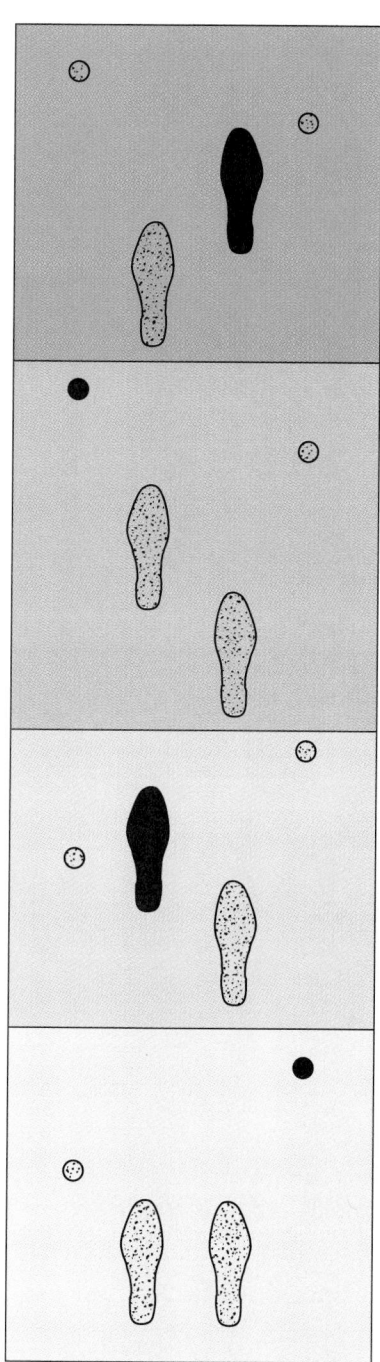

Figure 27-14. Four-point alternating gait. Solid feet and crutch tips show foot and crutch tip moved in each of the four phases.

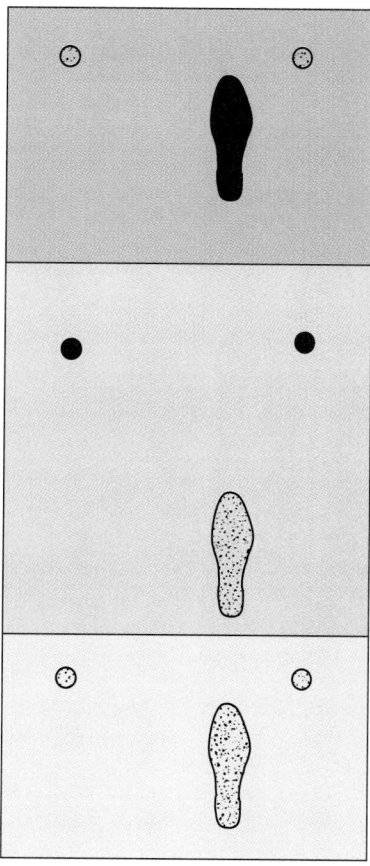

Figure 27-15. Three-point gait with weight borne on unaffected leg. Solid foot and crutch tips show weight-bearing in each phase.

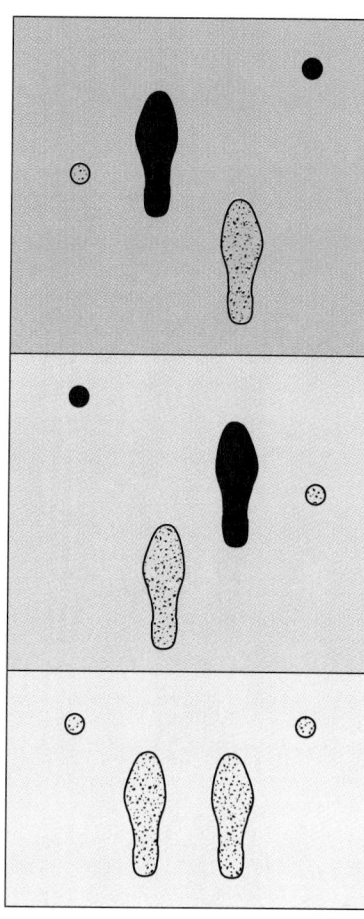

Figure 27-16. Two-point gait with weight borne partially on each foot and each crutch advancing with opposing leg. Solid areas indicate leg and crutch tips bearing weight.

the crutches to the unaffected leg. Finally, the client aligns both crutches on the stairs. This sequence is repeated until the client reaches the top of the stairs.

To descend the stairs (Figure 27-18), a three-phase sequence is also used. The client transfers body weight to the unaffected leg. The crutches are placed on the stair, and the client begins to transfer body weight to the crutches, moving the affected leg forward. Finally, the unaffected leg is moved to the stairs with the crutches. Again, the client repeats the sequence until reaching the bottom of the stairs.

Because in most cases clients will need to use

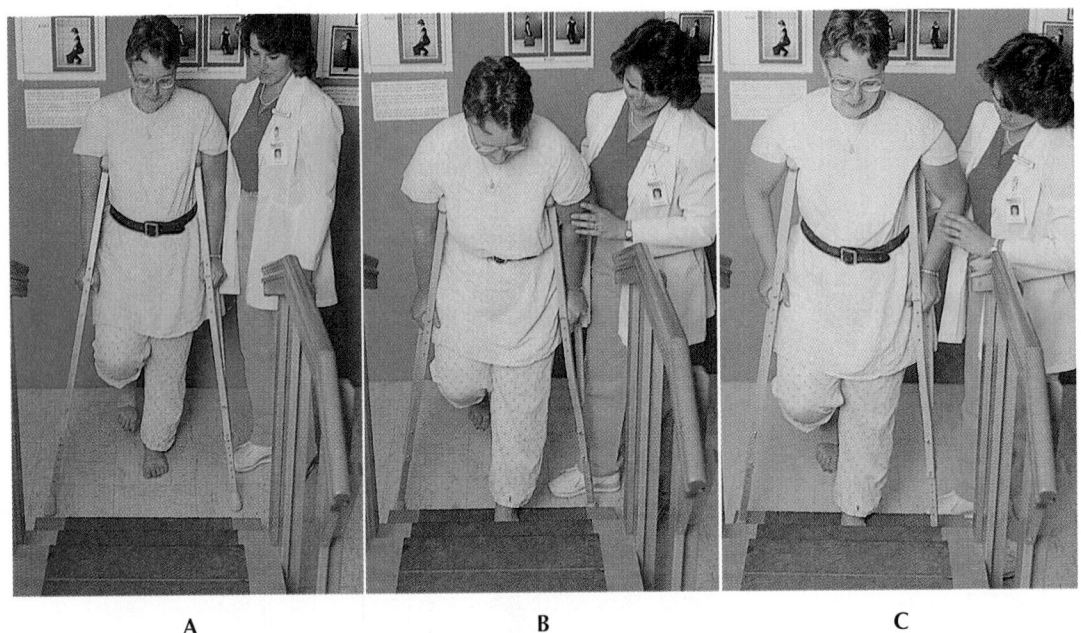

| A | B | C |

Figure 27-17. Ascending stairs. **A,** Weight is placed on crutches. **B,** Weight is transferred from crutches to unaffected leg on stairs. **C,** Crutches are aligned with unaffected leg on stairs.

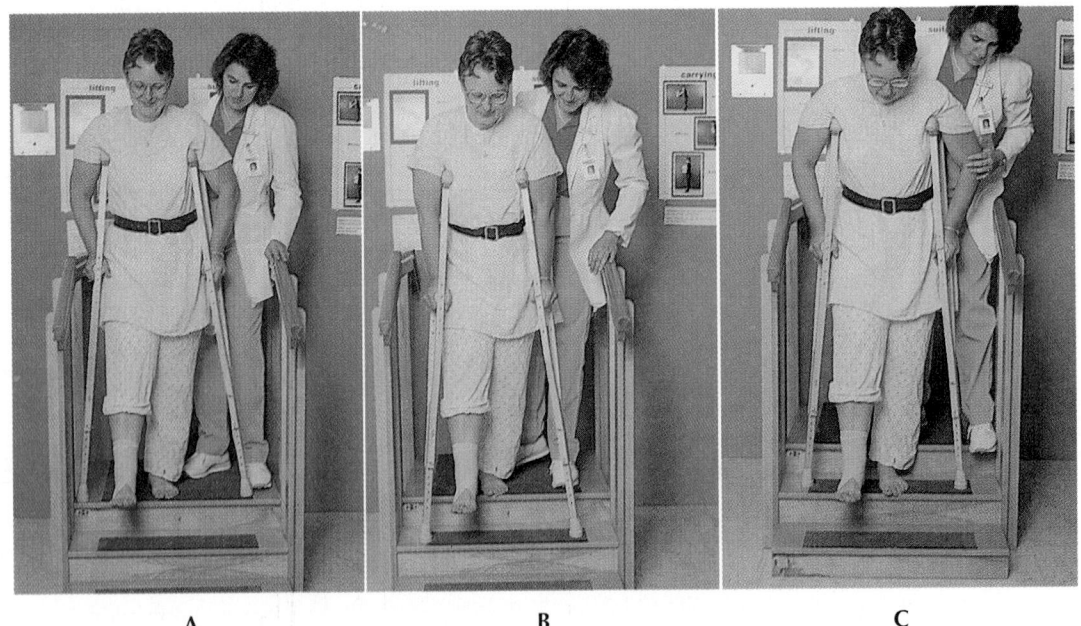

| A | B | C |

Figure 27-18. Descending stairs. **A,** Body weight on unaffected leg. **B,** Body weight transferred to crutches. **C,** Unaffected leg aligned on stairs with crutches.

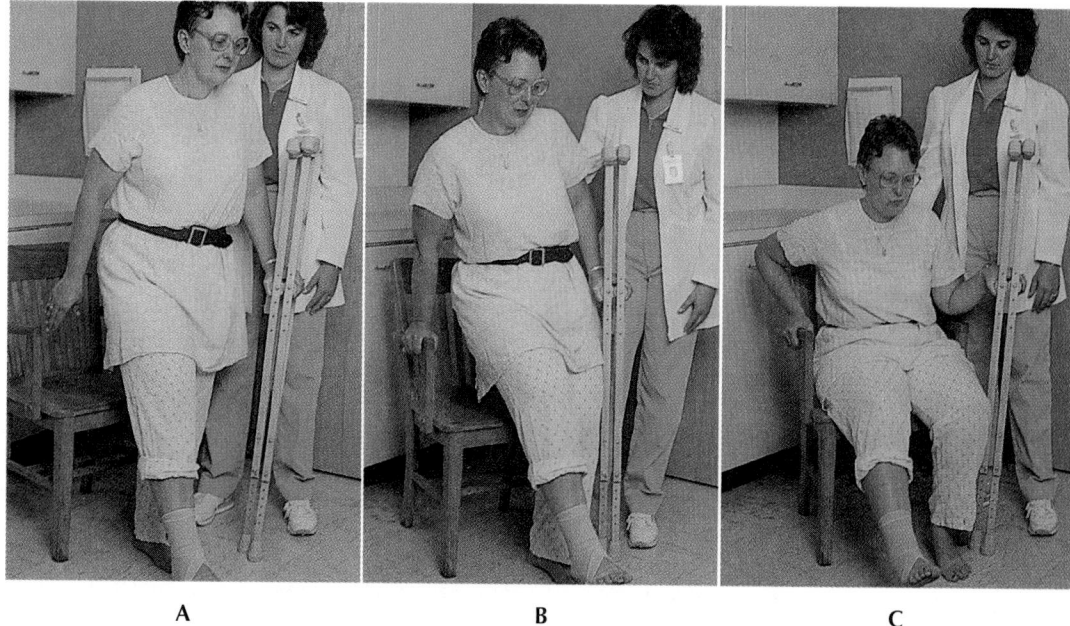

Figure 27-19. Sitting in a chair. **A,** Both crutches are held by one hand. Client transfers weight to crutches and unaffected leg. **B,** Client grasps arm of chair with free hand and begins to lower herself into chair. **C,** Client completely lowers herself into chair.

crutches for some time, they should be adequately taught to use crutches on stairs before discharge. This instruction applies to all crutch-dependent clients, not only those who have stairs in their homes.

Sitting in a chair with crutches. As with crutch walking and crutch walking up and down stairs, the procedure for sitting in a chair involves phases and requires the client to transfer weight (Figure 27-19). First, the client gets positioned at the center front of the chair with the posterior aspect of the legs touching the chair. Then the client holds both crutches in the hand opposite the affected leg. If both legs are affected, as with a paraplegic who wears weight-supporting braces, the crutches are held in the hand on the client's stronger side. With both crutches in one hand, the client supports body weight on the unaffected leg and crutches. While still holding the crutches, the client grasps the arm of the chair with the remaining hand and lowers the body into the chair. To stand, the procedure is reversed, and the client, when fully erect, should assume the tripod position before beginning to walk.

▪ Evaluation

For the client with alterations in body mechanics or joint mobility, the effectiveness of nursing interventions is measured by the success of meeting the client's expected outcomes and goals of care. For some clients, maintenance of joint mobility will be easily accomplished and will not be a priority goal. For others, return of joint mobility and maintenance of body align-

ment will be the most important outcome and all interventions will be directed toward its accomplishment.

For the nurse to evaluate the client's perception of the interventions, the nurse must first have knowledge of the client's expectations concerning joint mobility, posture, or body alignment. What is acceptable or anticipated on the part of the nurse may be vastly different from what the client and family members anticipate or can accept.

Key Terms

abduction	hand rolls
active range of motion	hand-wrist splints
activity tolerance	hyperextension
adduction	joints
balance	muscle tone
bed board	passive range of motion
body mechanics	plantar flexion
center of gravity	posture
circumduction	prone
crutch gait	range of motion
dorsiflexion	sandbags
extension	side rails
foot boot	supine
footdrop	trapeze bar
friction	trochanter roll
gait	

▪ Key Concepts

The term *body mechanics* describes the coordinated efforts of the musculoskeletal and nervous systems as a person moves, lifts, bends, assumes a standing, sitting, or lying position, and completes activities of daily living.

Muscles primarily associated with movement are located near the skeletal region, where movement results from leverage, which is characteristic of the movement of the upper extremities.

Muscles primarily associated with posture are located in the lower extremities, trunk, neck, and back.

Balance is assisted through nervous system control by the cerebellum and inner ear.

Body alignment is the positioning of joints, tendons, ligaments, and muscles in various body positions.

Body balance is achieved when there is a wide base of support, the center of gravity falls within the base of support, and a vertical line falls from the center through the base of support.

Developmental stages influence body alignment and mobility.

Pathological conditions that affect body alignment and mobility include postural abnormalities, altered bone formation, altered joint mobility, impaired muscle development, damage to the central nervous system, and direct trauma to the musculoskeletal system.

Assessment of a client's mobility enables the nurse to determine the client's coordination, balance, and ability to complete activities of daily living and makes it possible to evaluate or plan an exercise program.

Range of joint motion is the maximal movement possible at a joint in one of the three planes of the body: sagittal, frontal, and transverse.

Assessing gait allows the nurse to draw some conclusions about the client's balance, posture, and ability to walk without assistance.

Clients with impaired body alignment require nursing interventions to maintain them in the supported Fowler's, supine, prone, side-lying, and Sims' positions.

Transfer techniques require the nurse to use correct body mechanics to move the client in bed, from bed to chair, and from bed to stretcher.

Mechanical devices, such as canes and walkers, require specific nursing interventions to promote walking.

▪ Critical Thinking Activities

1. Jon, who is 82 years old, is being released from the hospital today. He is going home with his daughter, who will be caring for him. He is unable to transfer to a chair without assistance. List and discuss the guidelines to be given to Jon's daughter concerning body mechanics safety for herself and for her father. What transfer techniques would you encourage her to use?

2. You are assisting a client to ambulate to the bathroom. The client is 2 days postoperative from major abdominal surgery. Halfway to the bathroom the client complains of dizziness and begins to fall to the floor. What is your initial response? What would you chart regarding this incident?

3. You are assigned to a client who has a trapeze bar across the bed, trochanter rolls, a footboard, and side rails. Explain the rationale for each of these devices in maintaining proper body alignment.

4. Before your client with a full-leg cast can go home, he or she must be taught to ambulate with crutches and a three-point gait. Develop a teaching plan for your client.

References

Ackley BJ, Ladwig GB: *Nursing diagnosis handbook: a guide to planning care,* ed 3, St. Louis, 1997, Mosby.

Birchenall JM, Streight ME: *Mosby's textbook for the home care aide,* St. Louis, 1997, Mosby.

Dawe D, Moore-Orr R: Low-intensity, range of motion exercise: invaluable nursing care for elderly patients, *J Adv Nurs* 21(4):675, 1995.

Gassett RS and others: Ergonomics and body mechanics in the work place, *Nurs Clin North Am* 27-4(10):861, 1996.

Hoeman SP: *Rehabilitation nursing; process and application,* St. Louis, 1996, Mosby.

Huether SE, McCance KL: *Understanding pathophysiology,* St. Louis, 1996, Mosby.

Johnson JM, Wilson SF: *Health assessment for nursing practice,* St. Louis, 1996, Mosby.

Metzler DJ: Positioning your patient properly, *Am J Nurs* 96(3):33, 1996.

Phipps WJ and others: *Medical surgical nursing,* St. Louis, 1996, Mosby.

Thibodeau GA, Patton KT: *Anatomy and physiology,* ed 3, St. Louis, 1996, Mosby.

Thompson JM, Wilson SF: *Health assessment for nursing practice,* St. Louis, 1996, Mosby.

Basic Human Needs

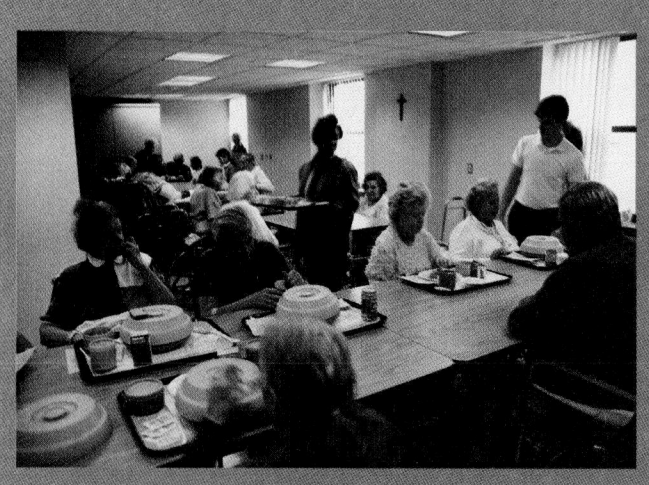

UNIT

6

28

Safety

OBJECTIVES

Mastery of content in this chapter will enable the student to:

- Define the key terms listed.
- Describe how unmet basic physiological needs of oxygen, fluids, nutrition, and temperature can threaten safety.
- Discuss methods to reduce physical hazards and the transmission of pathogens.
- Discuss present methods of pollution control.
- Discuss the specific risks to safety as they pertain to developmental age.
- Identify factors to assess when a client should be placed in restraints.
- Describe four categories of safety risks in a health care agency.
- Describe assessment activities designed to identify a client's physical, psychological, and cognitive status as it relates to safety status.
- State nursing diagnoses associated with risks to safety.
- Develop a nursing care plan for clients whose safety is threatened.
- Describe nursing interventions specific to the client's age for reducing risk of falls, fires, poisonings, and electrical hazards.
- Describe methods to evaluate interventions designed to maintain or promote safety.

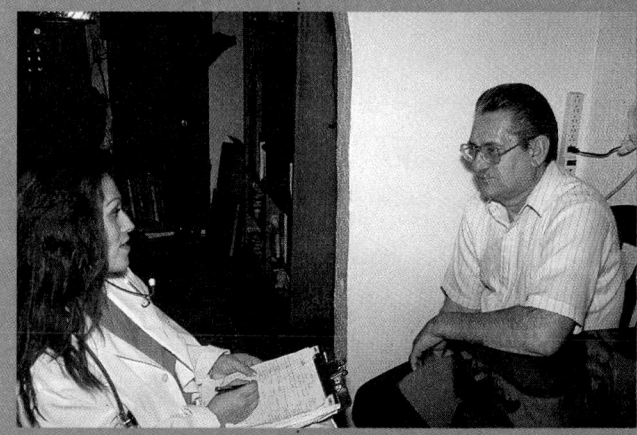

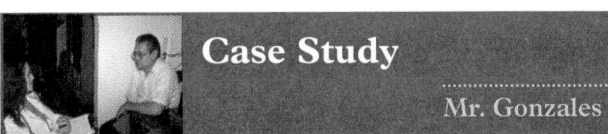

Case Study

Mr. Gonzales is a 68-year-old man who lives alone in a senior apartment building since his wife died 6 months ago. He and his wife had been born in Mexico but came to live in the United States shortly after they were married. He is retired from a produce warehouse where he worked for 37 years. He and his wife raised three sons, who have all married and have families of their own. The closest son is 45 minutes away by car. Mr. Gonzales is generally healthy but has some hearing loss from the noisy warehouse job and some "arthritis." He expects to live at least as long as his father, who lived to be 92 years old. Since his wife's death, Mr. Gonzales attends Catholic mass every day at his parish church where his wife had attended daily. Hearing the mass in Spanish is comforting to him.

Joani Green, a 25-year-old married mother of two, is currently a senior nursing student at the local college. As part of the clinical requirements for the home care course, she and her partner are conducting health screenings and providing health promotion education for the residents of the apartment building where Mr. Gonzales lives.

Safety is a basic human need that is often described as freedom from psychological and physical injury. The nurse can increase a client's safety by including interventions for a safe environment in the plan of care and as part of all nursing activities.

SCIENTIFIC KNOWLEDGE BASE

Vulnerable groups that often require the nurse's help in achieving a safe environment include infants, children, the ill, the disabled, the illiterate, the poor, and the older adult. To be effective the nurse needs to understand factors contributing to a safe environment in the home or health care agency and then thoroughly assess the environment for threats to safety. Also of importance is the nurse's understanding of sensory function and how alterations in that function can affect safety (see Chapter 39). A safe environment includes meeting basic human needs, reducing physical hazards, reducing transmission of pathogens, and controlling pollution.

Basic Human Needs

Basic human needs that may be at risk from a variety of hazards include the physiological needs of oxygen, nutrition, optimal temperature, and appropriate humidity.

An environmental hazard that may threaten available oxygen is **carbon monoxide,** a colorless, odorless, poisonous gas produced by the combustion of carbon or organic fuels. This gas binds strongly with hemoglobin, preventing the formation of oxyhemoglobin and thus reducing the supply of oxygen delivered to the tissues (see Chapter 30). Carbon monoxide is most commonly introduced into the client's environment by an improperly functioning furnace or by automobile exhaust fumes.

Other environmental threats to safety arise in connection with nutritional needs. Unrefrigerated perishable foods or food products with expired dates for use may contain harmful organisms. Improper home handling of raw meat or poultry may increase the threat of disease. Unwashed fresh vegetables and fruits can harbor insecticides, dirt, and pathogens.

Temperature extremes, which frequently occur during the winter and summer, affect comfort, productivity, and safety. Exposure to severe cold for prolonged periods causes frostbite and **hypothermia** (see Chapter 23). The risk of hypothermia is increased by advanced age, acute or chronic illness, and alcohol consumption. Exposure to extreme heat can change the body's electrolyte balance and raise the core body temperature, resulting in heatstroke or **heat exhaustion.**

Another environmental variable that may affect the client's health and safety is **relative humidity,** the amount of water vapor in the air compared with the maximum amount of water vapor the air could contain at the same temperature. The skin's moisture evaporates more quickly as the relative humidity decreases. People at risk from high environmental temperatures, such as older adults or the very young, should avoid extremely hot, humid environments or heat exhaustion may result.

Reduction of Physical Hazards

Physical hazards in an environment may threaten a client's safety and result in physical or psychological injury. Possible hazards to be assessed include inadequate lighting, clutter, and lack of security measures.

Inadequate lighting can cause eyestrain as the client carries out daily activities and can increase the risk of injury from falls. The risk of crime is also higher in poorly lit areas. The nurse should evaluate the adequacy of illumination in areas where the client moves and works, particularly outside walkways, steps, garages, doorways, and interior halls and staircases.

The client's home should be assessed for clutter, because injuries frequently result from inadvertent contact with objects on stairs, floors, bedside tables, closet shelves, refrigerator tops, and bookshelves. The risk of injury from clutter is greatest for older adults; clients with impaired vision; and clients who require adaptive aids for ambulation. Clients with impaired mobility are at great risk for falls. The nurse should assess the condition of stairways, bathrooms, and limited-access areas to be sure safety devices are in place. For example, handrails around toilets and grab bars in showers can help.

Pathogens. Pathogens and parasites pose a threat to client safety. A **pathogen** is any microorganism capable of producing an illness (see Chapter 25). Pathogens can be found in water, food, people, insects, and animals. Factors to be assessed include food sanitation, insect and rodent control, and human waste disposal.

Improperly processed or contaminated food can cause illness and death by transmitting pathogens and parasites. **Food poisoning** is the toxic process resulting from ingesting a food contaminated by toxic substances or by bacteria containing toxins.

Insects and rodents are carriers of pathogens. For example, the Anopheles mosquito is a carrier of malaria, and the rat or mouse can transmit rat-bite fever. Uncontrolled mosquito and rodent populations increase the risk of these diseases.

Sanitation. The transmission of pathogens and parasites is also controlled by adequate disposal of human waste through proper construction and repair of sewers and drains. Without a satisfactory sewer and waste system, the population is at risk for illnesses such as typhoid fever and hepatitis.

Health care agencies are also faced with problems concerning the processing of biohazardous wastes. Needles, surgical dressings, and syringes must be disposed of in such a manner that neither the general population nor employees are at risk for exposure. Bed linens and client gowns contaminated by body fluids must be properly cleansed or disposed of to reduce threats to safety.

Pollution. A healthy environment is free of air, water, or noise pollution. A **pollutant** is a harmful, chemical, or waste material discharged into the water or atmosphere. **Air pollution** is the contamination of the environmental atmosphere with pollutants. In urban regions, industrial wastes and vehicle exhausts commonly contribute to air pollution. Cigarette smoke is the primary indoor air pollutant. Prolonged exposure to air pollution increases the risk for pulmonary disease.

Water pollution. **Water pollution** is the contamination of lakes, rivers, and streams, usually by industrial pollutants. Properly functioning water-treatment facilities filter harmful contaminants from the water, but flooding may damage a treatment station, requiring boiling of drinking water.

Noise pollution. **Noise pollution** occurs when the noise level in an environment becomes uncomfortable to its inhabitants. Noise levels are measured in units of sound intensity called *decibels.* Noise level tolerances vary among individuals and are influenced by health status.

Land pollution. **Land pollution** is the depositing of trash and other hazardous wastes on and in the soil, causing contamination of the soil and groundwater.

⋯NURSING KNOWLEDGE BASE⋯⋯⋯⋯⋯

Threats to safety are influenced by developmental stage, lifestyle habits, mobility status, sensory impairments, and safety awareness. In the United States, accidents are the leading cause of death in people between 1 and 34 years of age and the fifth leading cause overall (U.S. Bureau of the Census, 1996). It is important for the nurse to be aware of the threats to safety and to teach parents and other care givers to take appropriate action to lessen the dangers.

Development Level

Infant, toddler, and preschooler. Home accidents kill, disfigure, and permanently disable thousands of children each year, with children between 1 and 5 years of age being at greatest risk for death. Accidents involving children are largely preventable, but parents frequently need to be shown the specific dangers by nurses and other health care professionals. As the infant grows, accident potential increases. The newborn's accident potential is influenced by people or external agents, but growth and the acquisition of new motor skills place the active toddler and preschooler at risk for injuries. Accident prevention thus requires health education for parents and removal of dangers where possible.

School-age child. When children enter school, their environment expands to include the school and the means of transportation to and from school. Children should be taught to cross the street safely and to refrain from talking to or accepting rides or gifts from strangers. School-age children involved in team and contact sports should be taught to play safely and to use protective safety equipment. Bicycle-related injuries, especially head injuries, account for a large number of primarily preventable causes of long-term disability and death (Logedon, 1995).

Adolescent. As children enter adolescence, they begin to develop a sense of identity and personal values, which may conflict with parental values. In addition, the adolescent begins to separate emotionally from the family, and the peer group begins to have a stronger influence.

Adolescent behavior is characterized by wide variations that swing from childlike to mature behavior (Wong, 1997). Moodiness and confusion are typical adolescent behavior patterns. When assessing for possible substance abuse, the nurse must look for environmental and psychological clues. Environmental clues include drug-oriented magazines, beer and liquor bottles, drug paraphernalia, blood spots on clothing, and the continual wearing of long-sleeved shirts in hot weather and dark glasses indoors. Psychosocial clues include failing grades, change in dress, increased absenteeism from school, increased aggressiveness, changes in interpersonal relationships, isolation, erratic behavior, avoidance of eye contact, bragging about drug abuse, and increased time spent in the bathroom.

Adult. The threats to an adult client's safety are frequently related to lifestyle habits. The client who excessively uses alcohol or drugs, for example, is at greater risk for motor vehicle accidents. The adult experiencing a high level of stress is at greater risk for accidents, as well as certain stress-related illnesses such as headaches, gastrointestinal disorders, and infections (see Chapter 22).

Older adult. Accidental injury from falls, driving accidents, and thermal injuries account for many hospitalizations of older adults, most of whom are unable to return to their previous level of independence (Ebersole and Hess, 1994). Falls are the second leading cause of accidental death among the older adult population (Brady and others, 1993). Fifty percent of accidents are caused by environmental factors such as broken stairs, icy sidewalks, inadequate lighting, throw rugs, and exposed electrical cords (Edelman and Mandle, 1994). Older adults are more likely to fall because of physiological changes or acute or chronic diseases that result in weakness. In addition, changes in mental status related to multiple medications or emotional responses that can accompany a loss can increase the risk of falls (Ebersole and Hess, 1994; Edelman and Mandle, 1994).

Other Risk Factors

Lifestyle. Lifestyle can increase safety risks. At greater risk of injury are people who drive or operate machinery while under the influence of chemical substances, who work at jobs that are inherently more dangerous, and who are risk takers or daredevils. In addition, people experiencing great stress or anxiety are more accident prone because they often are too preoccupied with stressors to notice the source of potential accidents, such as a cluttered stair or a stop sign.

Mobility. A client with impaired mobility has many kinds of safety risks. Immobilization can predispose a client to other physiological and emotional hazards, which in turn can further restrict mobility and independence (see Chapter 37). A client with impaired mobility is at risk for injury when entering motor vehicles and buildings not equipped for the handicapped.

Physically challenged clients are also at greater risk for automobile and other kinds of accidents.

Sensory impairments. Clients with visual, hearing, or communication impairments are at greater risk for injury. Such clients may not be able to perceive a potential danger or express needs for assistance (see Chapter 39).

Safety awareness. Some clients are unaware of safety precautions, such as keeping medicine, poisonous plants, or other poisons away from children or reading the expiration date on food products. A complete nursing assessment should help the nurse to identify the client's level of knowledge regarding home safety so that deficiencies can be corrected with an individualized care plan.

Allergic reactions. The majority of insect bites and stings are not serious, but the danger of death resulting from insect allergy always exists. Immediate emergency medical treatment is required for an allergic reaction (Wong, 1997). When doing any health assessment, the nurse must also include information about allergies to foods, latex, medications, and insect venom (see Chapter 24). A complete assessment should include allergies to foods, medications, and insect venom.

Risks in the Health Care Agency

Clients in health care settings are at risk for falls, client-inherent accidents, procedure-related accidents, and equipment-related accidents. The nurse learns to recognize factors associated with these risks and to take steps to prevent or minimize accidents.

Falls. Falls account for 29% to 89% of all incidents reported in hospitals (Brady and others, 1993). Brians and others (1991) have developed a risk assessment tool for early recognition of potential falls (Box 28-1). Such tools might enable the nurse to assess potential risks before accidents and injuries result.

Client-inherent accidents. Client-inherent accidents are accidents other than falls in which the client is the primary factor. Examples are self-inflicted cuts, injuries, and burns; ingestion or injection of foreign substances; self-mutilation or setting fires; and pinching fingers in drawers or doors.

Procedure-related accidents. Procedure-related accidents occur during therapy. They include medication and fluid administration errors, improper application of external devices, and improper performance of procedures such as dressing changes. The nurse can prevent many procedure-related accidents by using good judgment and following agency guidelines.

Box 28-1
Risk for Falls Assessment Tool

Tool 1: Risk Assessment Tool for Falls

Directions: Place a check mark in front of elements that apply to your client. The decision of whether a client is at risk for falls is based on your nursing judgment. *Guideline:* A client who has a check mark in front of an element with an asterisk (*) or four or more of the other elements would be identified as at risk for falls.

General Data

_____ Age over 60
_____ History of falls before admission*
_____ Postoperative/admitted for operation
_____ Smoker

Physical Condition

_____ Dizziness/imbalance
_____ Unsteady gait
_____ Diseases/other problems affecting weight-bearing joints
_____ Weakness
_____ Paresis
_____ Seizure disorder
_____ Impairment of vision
_____ Impairment of hearing
_____ Diarrhea
_____ Urinary frequency

Mental Status

_____ Confusion/disorientation*
_____ Impaired memory or judgment
_____ Inability to understand or follow directions

Medications

_____ Diuretics or diuretic effects
_____ Hypotensive or CNS suppressants (e.g., narcotic, sedative, psychotropic, hypnotic, tranquilizer, antihypertensive, antidepressant)
_____ Medication that increases GI motility (e.g., laxative)

Ambulatory Devices Used

_____ Cane
_____ Crutches
_____ Walker
_____ Wheelchair
_____ Geriatric (geri) chair
_____ Braces

Tool 2: Reassessment Is Safe "Kare" (Risk) Tool

Directions: Place a check mark in front of any element that applies to your client. A client who has a check mark in front of any of the first four elements would be identified as at risk for falls. In addition, when a high-risk client has a check mark in front of the element "Use of a wheelchair," the client is considered to be at greater risk for falls.

_____ Unsteady gait/dizziness/imbalance
_____ Impaired memory or judgment
_____ Weakness
_____ History of falls
_____ Use of a wheelchair

Data from Brians LK and others: The development of the RISK tool for fall prevention, *Rehabil Nurs* 16(2):67, 1991.

Equipment-related accidents. Equipment-related accidents result from the malfunction, disrepair, or misuse of equipment or from an electrical hazard. To avoid injury, personnel should not operate monitoring or therapy equipment without instruction.

CRITICAL THINKING IN CLIENT CARE

Synthesis

Synthesis is "the putting together of elements and parts so as to form a whole" (Bloom, 1954/1981). The synthesis of knowledge, experience, and other elements of critical thinking helps the nurse to make clinical decisions. Data are collected, analyzed, and synthesized, to make clinical decisions in providing for client safety.

Knowledge. There must be a complete picture of the client, including physical, psychological, and environmental information to guide the nurse in providing care and protecting the client from injury. The nurse must consider a wide variety of factors before choosing those that will be included in the plan of care. Because every client is different, with various strengths and weaknesses, the nurse must prioritize among the possible factors that are threats to safety and concentrate on those that are probable threats.

Experience. The nurse uses experience to recall incidents that occurred with another client or family member and the specific circumstances that led to the situation. Experience alerts the nurse to recognize risks and to take appropriate corrective measures. A nurse's grandmother may have fallen because her slipper became entangled in a throw rug at the top of the stairs. The nurse would then use the experience of the grandmother's fall and apply the knowledge gained when assessing a client's home for safety hazards during a home visit.

Attitudes. The nurse must view all situations as opportunities to protect the client. Once they occur, injuries may cause pain, immobility, loss of income, or even death. After considering a client's specific strengths and weaknesses, the client's environment, and the developmental stage, the nurse needs to work with the client and family to determine creative solutions that will protect the client's safety.

Standards. The American Nurses Association (ANA) *Standards of Nursing Practice* (see Chapter 10) include the concept of safety, stating that interventions are implemented in a safe and appropriate manner. The ethical standards that would impact safety issues are included in the ANA *Code of Ethics* (see Chapter 11) in the statement of the nurse's responsibility to safeguard the client and the public when health care and safety are affected by the incompetent, unethical, or illegal practice of any person. The nurse is also responsible for maintaining competence in nursing to minimize potential hazards related to lack of knowledge and skill.

NURSING PROCESS

Assessment

The nurse, in considering threats to client safety, must review all client factors and environmental factors to decrease the risk of injury. A nursing history that includes data about the past and present level of wellness, family history, changes in life patterns, sociocultural history, spiritual health, and mental and emotional reactions will be completed. This information will highlight possible areas of concern. Other basic information such as age and developmental level will aid the nurse in determining client factors that affect safety (Box 28-2). An assessment of the environment will be important to detect potential hazards in the health care agency or in the home.

Client expectations. Safety is a basic human need; however, expectations for one's safety may differ. In some cases a client's expectations of what is safe may not be appropriate. In such instances the nurse must intervene and educate both the client and family regarding safe practices as they concern everyday decisions, use of medications and medical equipment, and the client's environment. People usually do not purposefully put themselves in jeopardy. However, when clients are uninformed or inexperienced, threats to their safety can occur.

Box 28-2

Physical Assessment Findings in the Older Adult That Increase the Risk of Accidents

Musculoskeletal Changes
Muscle strength decreases
Joints become less mobile
Posture changes; some kyphosis is common
ROM is limited

Nervous System Changes
All voluntary or autonomic reflexes are slower
Decreased ability to respond to multiple stimuli
Decreased sensitivity of touch

Sensory Changes
Peripheral vision and lens accommodation decrease
Lens may develop opacity
Stimuli threshold for light touch and pain increases
Hearing is impaired as high-frequency tones are
    less perceptible

Genitourinary Changes
Increased nocturia
Increased occurrence of incontinence

Modified from Ebersole P, Hess P: *Toward healthy aging: human needs and nursing responses,* ed 4, St. Louis, 1994, Mosby.

Successful critcal thinking requires a synthesis of knowledge, experience, information gathered from clients, and critical thinking and standards. Clinical judgments require the nurse to anticipate what information is needed, to analyze data, and to then make decisions regarding client care. The client expects competent and informed care. In the following case study, Joani incorporates previous knowledge and experiences in providing care for Mr. Gonzales.

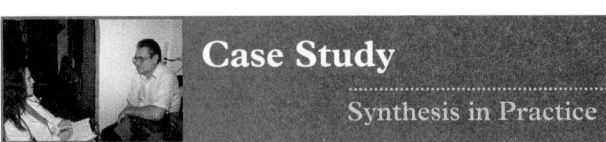

Case Study

Synthesis in Practice

Joani Green has completed the health screening on Mr. Gonzales. She knows she needs to incorporate knowledge about environmental risks as they relate to her client's age, level of independence, health status, and expectations. In addition, Mr. Gonzales is the third client Joani has cared for in the home, and she also has an experiential basis for practice. As Joani integrates knowledge with previous experience, she remembers that the client values his independence. As a result Joani is able to develop a plan

Continued

of care to meet Mr. Gonzales's safety needs while assisting him in maintaining his independence. At his apartment, Joani makes an inspection of the environmental hazards. She discovers that the lighting is poor and that several throw rugs are placed near the chairs and the bedside. The health screening has revealed that Mr. Gonzales has decreased visual acuity and has not had a new pair of glasses for 3 years.

◼ Nursing Diagnosis

The nursing diagnosis should include specific causative or contributing factors so that nursing care measures can be individualized. For example, the nursing diagnosis *risk for injury* could be related to altered mobility, or it could be related to sensory alteration (e.g., visual). Correct identification of the causative factor (such as altered mobility) would lead to selecting such nursing interventions as teaching and performing range-of-motion (ROM) exercises or proper use of safety devices such as side rails, canes, or crutches. Visual impairment as the related factor would lead to selecting different interventions such as keeping the area well lighted; orienting the client to the surroundings; or keeping eyeglasses clean, handy, and well protected. Not identifying the correct causative factor increases the risk of injury. For example, the nurse who does not have the home environment evaluated for hazards may be sending the client back home only to return with an additional injury (see nursing diagnoses box).

◼ Planning

Clients with actual or potential risks to safety require a nursing care plan with interventions to prevent threats to safety and meet safety needs. Planning and goal setting need to be done in collaboration with the client, family, and other members of the health care team. The total plan should address all aspects of client needs and utilize resources of the health care team and the community when appropriate. The client who is an active participant in reducing the threats to safety will be more

◼ NURSING DIAGNOSES FOR CLIENTS WITH SAFETY RISKS

Body temperature, altered, risk for
Home maintenance management, impaired
Injury, risk for
Knowledge deficit
Poisoning, risk for
Sensory/perceptual alteration
Suffocation, risk for
Thought processes, altered
Trauma, risk for

alert to potential hazards. Clients need to learn how to identify and select resources within their community that will enhance safety. For example, in a senior center other members are alerted to a spill on the floor. Another example is the neighbor who makes it a part of his or her day to check on an older neighbor during times of extreme weather.

The nurse must consider the role of the environment and the family when planning care. For example, the nurse may see that one way to assist the client is to have the client sleep in a bedroom closest to the bathroom. However, this may not be possible. In collaboration with the family, the alternative of a bedside commode may be used.

To develop the care plan, priority goals for the client that are most important in terms of risk to safety and health promotion should be identified. An example of a client-centered goal is *Client's potential for injury will be reduced* (see care plan, p. 719).

◼ Implementation

Nursing interventions are directed toward maintaining the client's safety in all types of settings. Nursing measures for providing a safe environment include health promotion, developmental interventions, and environmental protection. Each of these areas of implementation is appropriate for health promotion and acute and restorative care settings.

Health promotion. The emphasis in health care today is on health promotion. Wellness (which is synonymous with health promotion) depends on safety. Edelman and Mandle (1994) describe passive and active strategies aimed at health promotion. Passive strategies are implemented through government legislation (e.g., sanitation and clean water laws). Active strategies are those in which the individual is actively involved through changes in lifestyle and participating in wellness programs.

The nurse participates by supporting legislation and acting as a positive role model. Because environmental and community values have the greatest impact on health promotion, community and home health nurses can assess and recommend safety measures in the home, school, neighborhood, and workplace.

Developmental interventions

Infant, toddler, and preschooler. Growing, curious children depend on adults to protect them from injury. Nurses can frequently educate young parents or guardians about reducing risks of injuries for children. Nurses working in prenatal clinics and in community health programs can teach parents to promote safety in their homes. The pediatric nurse can also teach the child about safety. Nursing interventions that should be incorporated into the care plan for safety of a child are illustrated in Figures 28-1 and 28-2.

CASE STUDY NURSING CARE PLAN

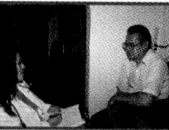

Risk for Injury

Assessment

Mr. Gonzales is a 68-year-old man **with diminished visual acuity** who lives in an apartment with **throw rugs on the floors and poor lighting.** He states that he cannot read the labels on his medication bottles very well and sometimes takes his medication from memory. When observed walking, he **does not pick his feet very high up off the floor, and his movements appear stiff.**

Nursing Diagnosis

Risk for injury related to altered mobility and decreased visual acuity.

Goal

Client's environment will be adapted to motor, sensory, and cognitive developmental needs (within 2 months).

Expected Outcomes

Client will list hazards within 1 week.
Modifiable hazards will be reduced 100% within 1 month.

Implementation

Steps

1. Review with client the potential risks for accidents in the home.
   a. Remove throw rugs.
   b. Increase lighting to a minimum of 75 watts per light.
2. Stress importance of safeproofing the home and give specific instructions for prevention of burns, falls, and poisoning.

Rationale

Accurate home assessment more readily identifies threats to safety than teaching alone (Wong, 1997).

Advance guidance is important in preventing potential injuries (Edelman and Mandle, 1994).

Evaluation

Observe environment for elimination of threats to safety.
Reassess motor, sensory, and cognitive status for appropriate environmental modifications.

Defining characteristics are shown in bold type.

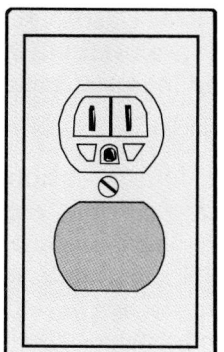

Figure 28-1. Safety covers for electrical outlets.

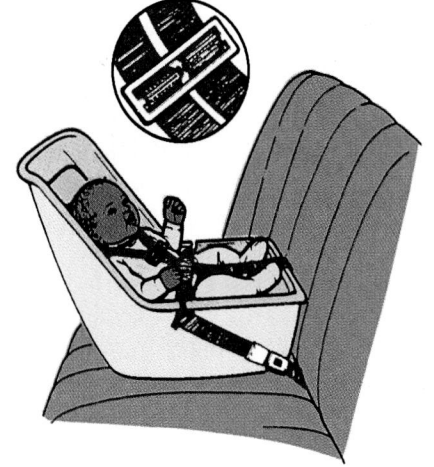

Figure 28-2. Infant car seat.

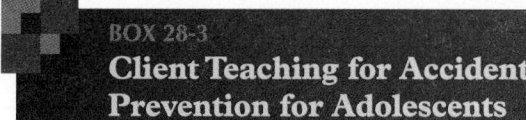

BOX 28-3
Client Teaching for Accident Prevention for Adolescents

- Enroll teenagers in a driver's education course and make practice drives with them in good and bad weather. Teach them to handle a motor vehicle in a skid.
- Teach them to wear seat belts while driving or as passengers.
- Instruct them not to drive after using a psychoactive substance or enter an automobile when the driver has been using such substances.
- Form a contract with teenagers: if they drink at a party, they will call home for a ride with no questions asked.
- Help them to develop safe eating, sleeping, and relaxation habits.
- Inform them of the dangers of psychoactive substances.
- Recognize changes in adolescents' behavior and mood.
- Listen to them.
- Do not try to be a buddy; remain a parent.

BOX 28-4
Gerontological Nursing Practice

- Older adult clients frequently have visual impairments that increase their risk for accidents. The nurse will teach clients to keep living areas well lighted and free of clutter, to keep eyeglasses in good condition, and to avoid night driving.
- Older adults have musculoskeletal changes that make movement difficult and increase the risk of falling. The nurse will teach clients to use assistive devices in proper working order (canes, rails in tub and bathroom, and elevated seats).
- Older adults have sensory impairments that increase their risks for burns. The nurse will advise clients to avoid smoking in bed, to lower thermostats on water heaters, to avoid overloading electrical outlets, and to install and maintain smoke detectors in the house.
- Older adults may have slowed reaction time. The nurse will teach clients safety tips for avoiding automobile accidents.
- Older adults frequently have some impairment of memory that increases their risk for accidental poisoning. The nurse will teach clients about the proper handling and storage of food and safe methods of scheduling and taking medications.
- Older adults have physiological changes that result in slower metabolism of drugs. The nurse teaches clients about drug interactions and signs and symptoms of drug toxicity to report to their health care provider.

School-age child. School-age children increasingly explore their environment. They have friends outside their immediate neighborhood; they may walk to school; and they become more active in school, church, and community activities.

Adolescent. When children approach adolescence, much of their time is spent away from home and with their peer group. During adolescence young persons learn to drive. Risks to the adolescent's safety therefore involve many factors outside the home. Box 28-3 lists measures by which nurses and parents can help the adolescent to prevent accidents.

Adult. Risks to young and middle-age adults frequently result from lifestyle factors such as child rearing, high stress states, inadequate nutrition, and abuse of drugs or alcohol. Adults need to be taught that their safety is in fact threatened, and as a result their lifestyle needs to be modified.

Older adult. Most injuries to older adults involve falls, auto accidents, and burns (Ebersole and Hess, 1994). Advancing age and the concurrent physiological changes in vision, hearing, mobility, reflexes, circulation, and the ability to make quick judgments all predispose older adults to falls (Box 28-4) (see Chapter 20). Steinmetz and Hobson (1994) reported mental status change and mobility deficit as the most frequent risk factor for falls. Certain disease states common to older adults, such as arthritis or cerebrovascular accidents, increase chances of injury. In addition, the effects of many medications such as sedatives, diuretics, and laxatives given to older adults make falls more likely. Nursing interventions designed to prevent falls and compensate for the physiological changes of aging are listed in Table 28-1.

The nurse should also provide information regarding neighborhood resources for the older adult (Ebersole and Hess, 1994). Older adults frequently relocate to new neighborhoods and must get acquainted with new resources such as modes of transportation and church schedules. In addition, the food resources of some older adults (e.g., Meals on Wheels) make the difference in their ability to maintain an independent lifestyle. Although retired from their jobs, older adults have a wealth of past experiences to aid volunteer organizations. In addition, some retirees may enjoy reentering the work force in a new capacity. Information about assistance resources, such as daily "hello" programs, emergency services, and elder abuse hot lines are often helpful. Nurses able to provide this information to older adults assist them in maintaining an independent lifestyle.

Environmental interventions. Nursing interventions directed at eliminating environmental threats include general preventive measures such as meeting basic needs, reducing physical hazards, reducing pathogen and parasite transmission, and controlling pollution effects. They also include specific measures to reduce the risk of accidental injuries from falls, fires, poisoning, and electrical hazards.

TABLE 28-1
Measures to Prevent Falls by Older Adults

Measure	Rationale
Stairs	
Install treads with uniform depth of 9 inches (22.5 cm) and 9-inch risers (vertical face of steps).	If stairs are of uniform size, older adult does not have to continually adjust vision.
Install uniform-textured or plain-colored surfaces on each tread, and mark edge of tread with contrasting color.	Uniform textures or color help to decrease vertigo. Marking edge of tread provides obvious visual clue to end of stair.
Ensure proper lighting of each tread. Block sun or light-bulb glare with translucent shades or screen, or use lower-wattage bulbs.	Older adults' vision is unable to adjust quickly to changes in lighting.
Ensure adequate head room so that users do not have to duck to negotiate stairs.	Sudden changes in head position may result in dizziness.
Remove protruding objects from staircase walls.	Decreased peripheral vision may prevent client from seeing object.
Maintain outdoor walkways and stairs in good condition and free of holes, cracks, and splinters.	Decreased visual acuity can prevent client from seeing any structural defect.
Handrails	
Install smooth but slip-resistant handrail at least 2 inches (5 cm) from wall.	Two-inch distance allows client to grasp handrail firmly for support.
Secure handrail firmly so that user's weight is supported, especially at bottom and top of stairway.	Older adult has greatest risk of falling at top and bottom of stairs, because center of gravity is being shifted and balance is unstable.
Install grab rails in bathroom near toilet and tub.	This enables client to have support while rising from sitting to standing position.
Floor Coverings	
Ensure clients wear properly fitting shoes or slippers with nonskid surface.	Reduces chances of slipping.
Secure all carpeting, mats and tile; place nonskid backing under small rugs.	Sudden slip may cause dizziness and inability to regain balance.
Orientation	
Place disoriented clients in room near nurses' station.	Provides for more frequent observation on the part of nursing staff.
Maintain close supervision of confused clients.	Confused client often attempts to wander out of bed or room.

General preventive measures. Nursing interventions can contribute to a safer environment by helping the client to meet the basic physiological needs of oxygen, humidity, nutrition, and temperature. To ensure that oxygen availability is not threatened, the client's furnace should be periodically inspected for proper functioning. To achieve a comfortable level of humidity in the home, the client might attach a humidifier to the furnace or, in the case of upper respiratory tract infection, use a room humidifier while the client sleeps. The nurse can teach basic techniques for food handling and preparation so that nutritional needs are met safely. Education regarding frostbite, hypothermia, heatstroke, and heat exhaustion can help clients to avoid conditions caused by temperature extremes.

Adequate lighting and security measures in and around the home, including the use of night-lights, exterior lighting, and locks on doors and windows, enable the client to reduce the risk of injury from falls or crime. The nurse should also encourage removing clutter from halls, stairs, traffic areas, and furniture such as bedside tables to further reduce the risk of falls.

Nurses use effective and efficient methods to control pathogen transmission. These include techniques of medical asepsis, removing or destroying disease-causing organisms or infected material, and surgical asepsis, protection against infection by the use of sterile techniques.

The nurse should provide information about any potential threat from air, water, and noise pollution in the client's environment so the client can eliminate the pollutant where possible and otherwise limit exposure.

Specific safety concerns. The nurse should take measures to help the client to avoid falls, fires, poisons, and electrical hazards.

Falls. Modifications in the client's home or health care environment can easily reduce the risk of falls. A heavy or debilitated client in a bed or wheelchair or on a toilet should be properly secured or supported. Excess furniture and equipment should be removed, and a weakened client should wear rubber-soled shoes or slippers for walking or transferring. Clients should be instructed to inspect canes, walkers, and crutches to be sure the rubber tip is intact.

With clients in the home or hospital, certain safeguards can be implemented or taught to the family to minimize the risk of falls (Box 28-5). In addition, confused and disoriented clients or clients who repeatedly try to remove medical devices (e.g., oxygen equipment, IV lines, dressings) may require the use of restraints and side rails to keep them from falling out of bed.

Restraints. A physical **restraint** is a device used to immobilize a client or extremity and restrain the level of activity. Because of the risks of restraints, current legislation is moving toward reducing the use of restraints in nursing homes and extended care facilities (National Citizens' Coalition for Nursing Home Reform, 1993). In addition, regulatory agencies such as the Joint Commission on Accreditation of Healthcare Organizations (JCAHO) are enforcing standards for the safe use of restraints in inpatient settings. The impetus is for health care organizations to move to a more "restraint free" environment. Nurses should use alternatives such as more frequent observation, involvement of family during visitation, frequent reorientation, and introducing familiar stimuli within the environment to reduce behaviors, such as confusion, that often lead to restraint use. The use of restraints involves a psychological adjustment for the client and family, and the nurse should assist them in adapting to this change when it is necessary. Nursing homes must now obtain informed consents from family members before using restraints. As with other procedures, the nurse must follow specific guidelines when using physical restraints (Skill 28-1). The overall objectives for restraint use include the following:

1. Reduce the risk of client injury from falls
2. Prevent interruption of therapy such as traction, IV infusions, nasogastric tube feeding, or Foley catheter
3. Prevent the confused or combative client from removing life support equipment
4. Reduce the risk of injury to others by the client

In keeping with current trends toward health promotion, improved assessment techniques and modifications of the environment are being offered as alternatives to restraints (Box 28-6, p. 727). A device known as the **AMBULARM** may be used for the client who climbs out of bed unassisted and is in danger of falling. This device is worn on the leg and signals when the leg is in a dependent position such as over the side rail or on the floor. This device may allow the family to avoid physical restraints and the client to avoid a fall.

For legal purposes the nurse must be familiar with agency policy and procedures for appropriate use and monitoring of restraints. Institutions require a physician's order that is time limited and designates the patient behavior for which restraints are to be used. When making an independent judgment to apply restraints, the nurse should document the assessment of the client's activity and behavior, the conclusions about the client's status, the nursing action, and the fact that the action was explained to the client and family. In addition, the nurse should note the type of restraint selected and where it was applied.

Side rails. Chapter 27 discusses side rails as a device for increasing the client's mobility and stability in bed or when moving from bed to chair. Side rails also help to prevent the unconscious client from falling out of bed. However, the use of side rails alone for a disoriented client may cause only more confusion and further injury. Frequently a confused client or one determined to get out of bed because of pain, toileting needs, or anxiety attempts to climb over the side rail or climbs out at the foot of the bed. Either attempt usually results in a fall. Nursing interventions to reduce a client's confusion should first focus on the cause of the confusion.

BOX 28-5
Client Teaching for Reducing Risk of Falls

- Instruct family to place bedside tables and overbed tables close to the client.
- Encourage the client to rise from the bed or chair slowly to prevent dizziness resulting from postural hypotension.
- Tell the family to remove clutter from bedside tables, hallways, bathrooms, and grooming areas.
- Encourage the family to mount grab bars around the toilets and showers; instruct the client on how to use them.
- Advise that rugs and carpets be securely attached to floors and stairs.
- Advise that bath mats and nonskid strips be attached to bathtubs and the floors of shower stalls.
- Advise that electrical cords be secured against the baseboards so that the client cannot easily trip over them.
- Ensure that the call bell is within easy reach of the hospitalized client, who should be shown the location of emergency call bells in bathrooms. Nurses must respond to call lights quickly, especially for clients needing assistance to the bathroom.
- Ensure that wheelchairs remain locked when transporting a client from bed to wheelchair or back to bed.
- Instruct care givers to check that side rails are up and safety straps are secured around the client who is on a stretcher.

Delegation Considerations

Use of restraints is an intervention with elements that *can* be delegated and elements that *cannot* be delegated. Elements that *cannot* be delegated because they require problem solving and knowledge application unique to professional nursing include the following:

- Assessment of safety needs
- Selection of appropriate interventions
- Evaluation of effectiveness of restraint
- Ongoing assessment to prevent complications of restraint use

Elements that *can* be delegated to unlicensed personnel include the following:

- Instruct care provider to inform nurse if any skin excoriation is present under or around restraint location.
- Instruct care provider in proper way to remove and reapply restraint to provide skin care and allow supervised movement.

Equipment
- Proper restraint
- Padding

STEPS	RATIONALE
1. Assess if a client needs a restraint.	Restraints are used when other measures have failed to prevent interruption of therapy such as traction, IV infusions, or nasogastric tube feedings; to prevent confused or combative client from self-injury by falling out of bed or wheelchair; to prevent client from removing Foley catheters, surgical drains, or life support equipment; and to reduce risk of injury to others by client.
2. Review agency policies regarding restraints. Check the physician's order for purpose of restraint and the type and duration of restraint.	A physician's order is necessary to apply restraints. The least restrictive type of restraint should be ordered. Because restraints limit the client's ability to move freely, the nurse must make clinical judgments appropriate to the client's condition and agency policy. If the nurse restrains a client in an emergency situation, a physician's order should be obtained as soon as possible.
3. Review the manufacturer's instructions before entering the client's room.	The nurse should be familiar with all devices used for client care and protection. Incorrect application of a restraining device may result in client injury or death.
4. Inspect the area where the restraint is to be placed. Assess condition of skin underlying area on which restraint is to be applied.	Restraints may compress and interfere with functioning of devices or tubes. Provides baseline assessment data regarding skin integrity. Enables nursing personnel an objective measure against subsequent skin assessment.
5. Explain to the client and family the need for the restraint. Attempt to obtain consent.	Helps minimize client anxiety during application of device and minimize family concern during maintenance of restraint.
6. Place client in proper body alignment.	Proper body alignment should be maintained to prevent contractures and neurovascular injury.

Continued

STEPS	RATIONALE
7. Pad bony prominences before applying restraints.	Padding protects skin from irritation.
8. Apply restraint, making sure it is not over an IV line or other device (e.g., dialysis shunt).	IV lines and other therapeutic devices may be occluded.
a. **Jacket (Vest or Posey) restraint:** vestlike garment. The front and back of the garment should be labeled as such (see illustration). Apply over clothing or hospital gown.	Restrains client while lying or reclining in bed and while sitting in chair or wheelchair. Proper application prevents suffocation or choking. Clothing or gown prevents friction against the skin.
b. **Belt restraint:** device that secures client to bed or stretcher. Avoid placing belt too tightly across client's chest or abdomen (see illustration).	Restrains center of gravity and prevents client from rolling off stretcher or sitting up while on stretcher or from falling out of bed. Tight application may interfere with ventilation.
c. **Extremity (ankle or wrist) restraint:** restraint designed to immobilize one or all extremities. Commercially available limb restraints are composed of sheepskin with foam padding (see illustration).	Maintains immobilization of extremity to protect client from injury from fall or accidental removal of therapeutic device (e.g., IV tube or Foley catheter).
d. In an emergency, if a commercial extremity restraint is not immediately available, a clove-hitch restraint can be constructed by making a figure eight with gauze and picking up loops. Place padding around extremity, then place loops of clove hitch directly over padded surface (see illustration).	

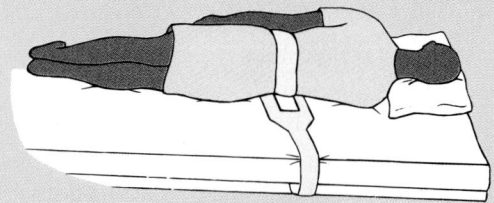

Step 8b

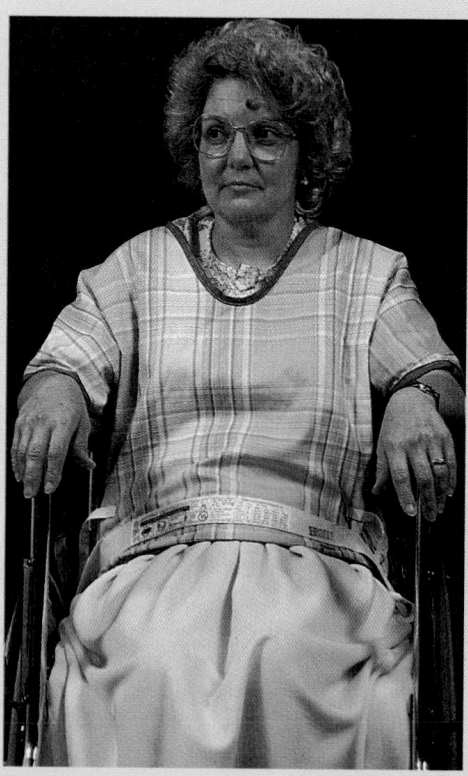

Step 8a

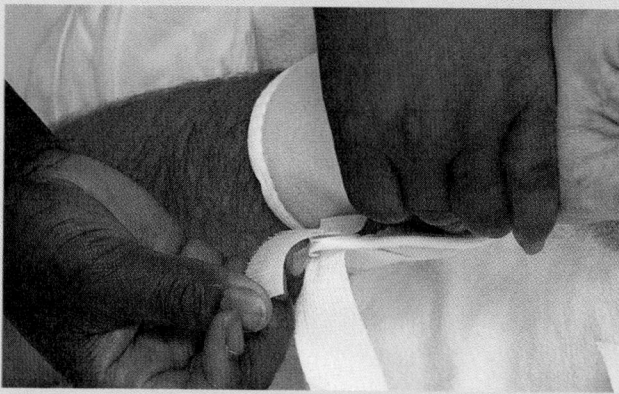

Step 8c

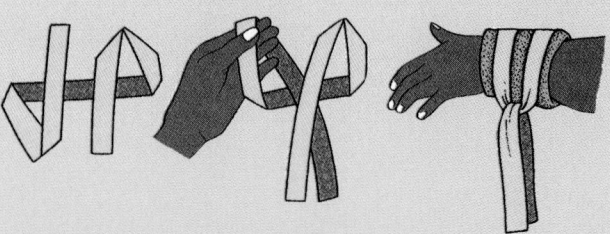

Step 8d

STEPS	RATIONALE

CRITICAL DECISION POINT

A clove-hitch configuration should not tighten as the client moves.
If tightening occurs, the device is not constructed properly.

e. **Mitten restraint:** thumbless mitten device to restrain client's hands (see illustration)

Prevents clients from dislodging invasive equipment, removing dressings, or scratching, yet allows greater movement than a wrist restraint.

9. Attach restraints to bed frame, which moves when the head of the bed is raised or lowered (see illustration). **Do not attach to side rails.**

The client may be injured if the restraint is secured to the side rail and it is lowered.

10. When the client is in a chair, the jacket restraint should be secured by placing the ties under the armrests and securing at the back of the chair (see illustration).

Prevents client from sliding; restraint ties up the back of the chair.

CRITICAL DECISION POINT

If the ties are not under the armrests, clients may be able to slide the ties
up the back of the chair and free themselves.

11. Secure the restraints with a quick-release tie (see illustration, p. 726).

Allows for quick release in an emergency.

12. Insert two fingers under the secured restraint (see illustration, p. 726).

Checking for constriction prevents neurovascular injury.
A tight restraint may cause contriction and impede circulation.

Continued

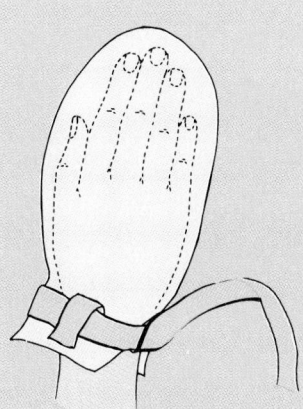

Step 8e

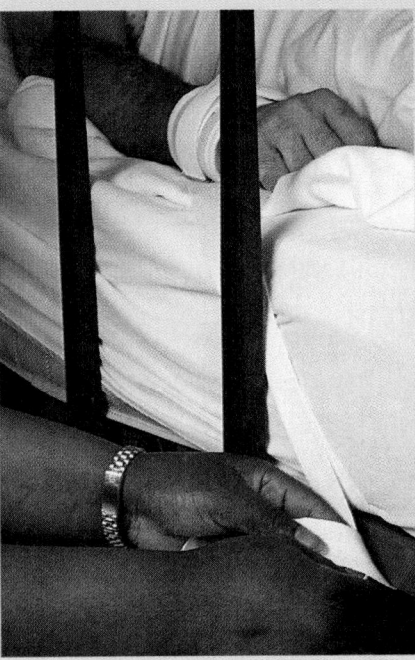

Step 9

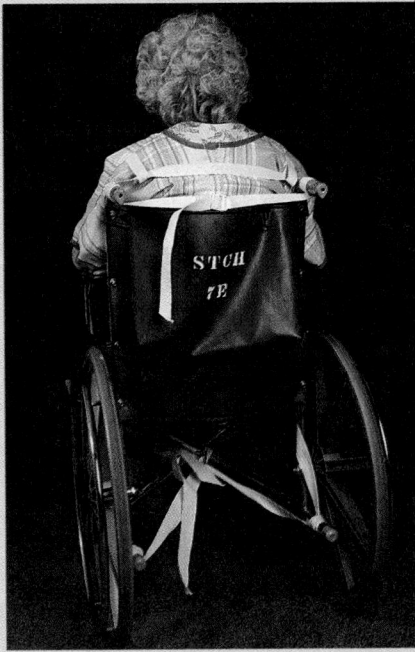

Step 10

Skill 28-1—cont'd
Use of Restraints

STEPS	RATIONALE
13. Every 30 minutes, proper placement of the restraint and skin integrity, pulses, temperature, color, and sensation of the restrained body part should be assessed.	Frequent assessment prevent complications, such as suffocation, skin breakdown, and impaired circulation.
14. Restraints should be removed for 30 minutes every 2 hours. If the client is violent and noncompliant, remove one restraint at a time and/or have staff assistance while removing restraints. Client should not be left unattended at this time.	Provides opportunity to change client's position and perform full ROM.
15. Secure call bell or intercom system within reach.	Allows client, family, or care giver to obtain assistance quickly.
16. Leave bed or chair with wheels locked. Bed should be in the lowest position.	Locked wheels prevent bed or chair from moving if client attempts to get out. If client falls when bed is in the lower position, the chances of injury are reduced.
17. Wash hands.	Reduces the transmission of microorganisms.
18. Inspect client for any injury, including all hazards of immobility, while restraints are in use.	Client should be free of injury and not exhibit any signs of immobility complications. Use of restraints should be seen as a temporary measure and use discontinued as soon as possible (Stolley, 1995).
19. Observe IV catheters and urinary catheters to determine that they are positioned correctly and that therapy remains uninterrupted.	

Recording and Reporting
▪ Record client behaviors that place client at risk for injury.
▪ Document client's response and expected or unexpected outcomes after restraint is applied.

Home Care Considerations
▪ Plan care with family. If possible, the use of an AMBULARM may free the client from physical restraints.

▪ Instruct family (or other care provider) in use of alternatives to restraints (Box 28-6).
▪ If physical restraints are necessary, instruct the family (or other care provider) in proper application and observation of possible complications related to restraint use. Also inform care provider whom to contact if any abnormal findings occur.

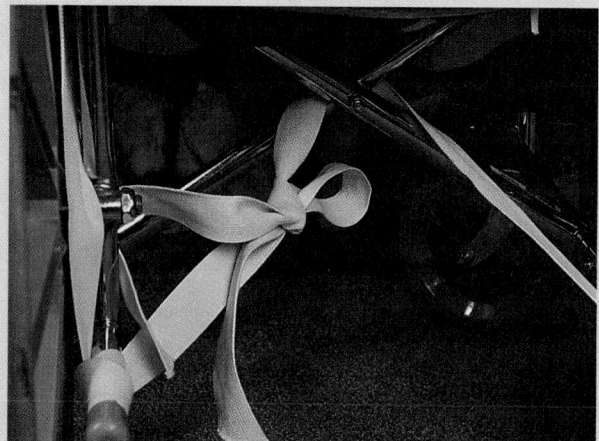

Step 11

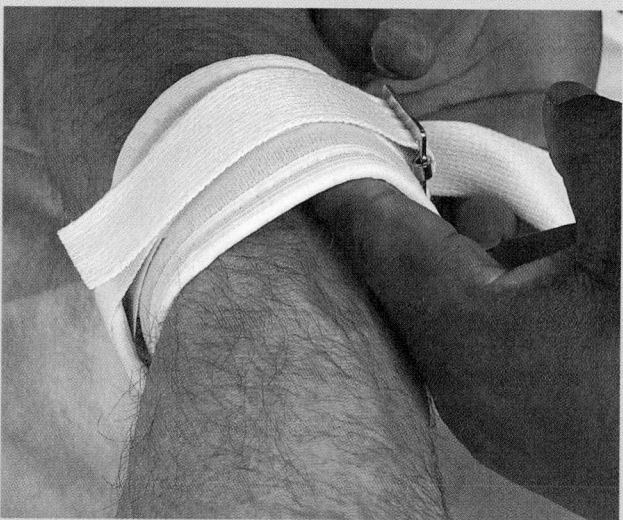

Step 12

Box 28-6
Alternatives to Restraints

Orient clients and families to surroundings; explain all procedures and treatments to them.

Encourage family and friends to stay, or utilize sitters for clients who need supervision.

Assign confused or disorientated clients to rooms near the nurses' station. Observe these clients frequently.

Provide appropriate visual and auditory stimuli (e.g., family pictures, clock, radio).

Eliminate bothersome treatments as soon as possible. For example, discontinue tube feedings and begin oral feedings as quickly as the client's condition allows.

Use relaxation techniques (e.g., massage).

Institute exercise and ambulation schedules as the client's condition allows.

Maintain toileting routines.

Consult with physical and occupational therapists to enhance clients' abilities to carry out activities of daily living.

Evaluate all medications clients are receiving to determine if the medication is having the desired therapeutic effect.

Conduct ongoing assessment and evaluation of clients' care and their ongoing response to care.

Modified from Stolley J: Freeing your patients from restraints, *Am J Nurs* 95(2):27, 1995.

Frequently, nurses mistake confusion for a client's attempt to explore his or her environment or to self-toilet. If all efforts to reduce confusion or restlessness fail, restraints may become necessary.

Fires. A fire is always possible in the home or hospital. Accidental home fires typically result from smoking in bed, careless extinguishing of cigarette butts in trash cans, grease fires, or electrical fires resulting from faulty wiring or appliances. Institutional fires typically result from a client smoking in bed or from an electrical or anesthetic-related fire.

If a fire occurs in a health care agency, the nurse first protects clients from injury. When detecting a fire, the nurse should report its exact location after rescuing any client in immediate danger.

The interventions described are directed toward fires occurring in health care agencies, but the same principles apply for fires in the home. It is important to have a plan of action in the event of fire.

When hospital or institutional fires occur, all personnel are mobilized to evacuate clients. Clients who are close to the fire, regardless of its size, are at risk of injury and should be moved to another area. If a client requires oxygen but not life support, the nurse discontinues the oxygen, which is combustible and can fuel an existing fire. If the client is on life support, the nurse may need to maintain the client's respiratory status manually with an Ambu bag (see Chapter 30) until the client is moved away from the fire. Ambulatory clients can be directed to walk by themselves to a safe area and in some cases may be able to assist in moving clients in wheelchairs. Bedridden clients are generally moved from the scene by a stretcher, their bed, or a wheelchair. If none of these methods is appropriate, the clients must be carried from the area. If a client must be carried, the nurse should be careful not to overextend physical limits for lifting because injury to the nurse can result in further injury to the client. If fire department personnel are on the scene, they can help to evacuate the clients.

After a fire has been reported and clients are out of danger, nurses and other personnel must take measures to contain or put out the fire, such as closing doors and windows, turning off oxygen and electrical equipment, and using a fire extinguisher. The three basic types of fires for which extinguishers are used are paper and rubbish (type A), grease and anesthetic gas (type B), and electrical (type C). The appropriate extinguisher must be used for each type.

The best intervention is to prevent fires. Nursing measures aimed at primary prevention include complying with the agency's smoking policies and keeping combustible materials away from heat sources. Some agencies have fire doors that are held open by magnets and close automatically when a fire alarm sounds. It is important to keep equipment away from these doors.

Poisoning. A **poison** is any substance that impairs health or destroys life when ingested, inhaled, or absorbed by the body. Specific antidotes or treatments are available for only some types of poisons. The capacity of body tissue to recover from poison determines the reversibility of the effect. Poisons can impair the respiratory, circulatory, central nervous, hepatic, gastrointestinal, and renal systems of the body. Accidental poisonings are a greater risk for the toddler, preschooler, and young school-age child. The nurse can help parents to reduce the risk of accidental poisoning by teaching them to keep hazardous substances out of the reach of children. With adolescents and young or middle-age adults, poisonings are often caused by insect or snake bites. Drug and other substance poisonings in these age groups are commonly related to suicide attempts or drug experimentation. Older adults are also at risk for poisoning, because diminished eyesight may cause an accidental ingestion of a toxic substance. The impaired memory of some older adult clients may result in an accidental overdose of prescribed medications.

The nurse should teach parents that calling a **poison control center** for information before attempting home remedies can save their child's life. There are guidelines

Box 28-7

Procedural Guidelines for Intervening in Accidental Poisoning

1. Assess for signs or symptoms of accidental ingestion of harmful substances.
2. Identify the type and amount of substance ingested to help determine the correct type and amount of antidote needed.
3. Call the poison control center before attempting any intervention. Poison control centers have information needed to treat poisoned clients or to offer referral to treatment centers.
4. If instructed to induce vomiting:
   a. Infants up to 12 months: ipecac administered only under direction of a physician
   b. Children (1 to 12 years): 1 tablespoon (15 ml) of ipecac
   c. Adults: 2 tablespoons (30 ml) of ipecac
5. Give oral fluids to assist vomiting (if directed):
   a. Children (1 to 12 years): 5 to 15 ml/kg; up to 8 oz of water
   b. Adults: 16 oz of water
6. If requested to do so, save vomitus and deliver to poison control center. Laboratory analysis can determine further treatment.
7. Position victim with head turned to side to reduce risk of aspiration.
8. Vomiting is never induced with the following substances: lye, household cleaners, grease or petroleum products, or furniture polish.
9. Vomiting is never induced in an unconscious victim, because vomiting increases risk of aspiration.
10. If instructed by poison control center to take person to emergency room, call ambulance. Ambulance personnel will be able to provide emergency measures if needed. In addition, parent or guardian may be too upset to drive safely.

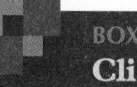

BOX 28-8
Client Teaching for Prevention of Electrical Hazards

- Discuss the methods of grounding appliances and other equipment.
- Provide examples of common hazards, such as frayed cords, visibly damaged equipment, and overloaded outlets.
- Discuss guidelines to prevent electrical shocks:
   Use extension cords only when absolutely necessary, and tape to ground with electrical tape.
   Never run electrical wiring under carpets.
   Never pull a plug using the cord; always grasp the plug itself.
   Never use electrical appliances near sinks, bathtubs, or other water supplies.
   Never operate unfamiliar equipment or appliances.
   Always disconnect before cleaning equipment or appliances.

▪ Evaluation

Client care. Nursing interventions for reducing threats to safety are evaluated by comparing the client's response to the expected outcomes for each goal of care. When expected outcomes are not met, interventions must be revised. The nurse applies evaluative measures to determine a client's progress toward outcomes and goals. Examples of goals, outcomes, and corresponding evaluative measures include the goal *Client's environment is adapted to motor, sensory, and cognitive developmental needs.* An outcome for this goal could be *Modifiable hazards in the home are reduced by 100% within 2 weeks.* Evaluative measures could include *Observe environment for elimination of threats to safety;* and *Reassess motor, sensory, and cognitive status for appropriate environmental modifications.*

Although the nurse evaluates the client's outcome by comparing what was planned with what resulted, the nurse also evaluates how well he or she was able to implement the plan. The nurse will examine the planned interventions for appropriateness and effectiveness in each situation. The accomplishment of goals and outcomes are validation of effective care for the nurse.

Client expectations. The client has come to expect the highest-quality care from the nurse and the health care system. Expectations as a result of care may include restoration of health, reduction in risks for falling, safer home environment, and improved recognition of safety risks. Clients are often unaware of the dangers to be found in their homes and workplaces, and many will make the necessary adjustments to keep themselves and loved ones safe and injury free once the dangers have been identified.

for accepted interventions for accidental poisonings the nurse may teach to a parent or guardian (Box 28-7). In addition, the parent may be instructed to give milk to neutralize an acid substance or lemon juice or vinegar to neutralize an alkaline substance.

Electrical hazards. Much of the equipment used in health care settings is electrical and must be well maintained in a safe condition to prevent electrical hazards. Properly **grounded** and functional electrical equipment decreases the risk of electrical injury and fire. Client teaching will decrease incidence of electrical injury in the home (Box 28-8).

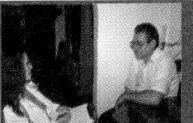

Case Study

It has been 2 weeks since the plan of care was implemented for Mr. Gonzales. The hazards have been identified and modifications made. With regular exercise, Mr. Gonzales has found that his walking has improved and now he feels safer about leaving the apartment. The new medication labels have made it easier for Mr. Gonzales to tell his several medications apart. His new glasses will arrive within a few days. The client is currently injury free and now feels better about living to a "ripe old age" like his father. He understands that he can make changes in his environment that will keep him safe. Joani Green, student nurse, has a sense of accomplishment in a job well done.

Documentation Note

Mr. Gonzales' home has improved lighting and the throw rugs are removed. During good weather and during daylight hours he exercises in his neighborhood. He is able to list all medications by name, dose, when taken, and significant side effects. No reports of injury.

Key Terms

air pollution	noise pollution
AMBULARM	pathogen
carbon monoxide	poison
food poisoning	poison control center
grounded	pollutant
heat exhaustion	relative humidity
hypothermia	restraint
land pollution	water pollution

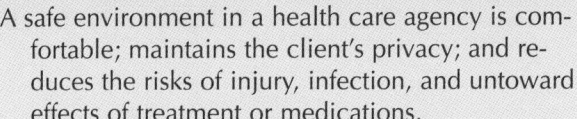

Key Concepts

A safe environment in a health care agency is comfortable; maintains the client's privacy; and reduces the risks of injury, infection, and untoward effects of treatment or medications.

A safe health care environment reduces the length of treatment or hospitalization, the frequency of treatment-related accidents, the potential for lawsuits, the number of work-related injuries to personnel, and the overall cost of health service.

Safety in the home reduces the risk of accidents, illnesses, and the need for health care services.

In the community, a safe environment is one in which basic needs are achievable, physical hazards are reduced, transmission of pathogens and parasites is reduced, pollution is controlled, and sanitation is maintained.

The transmission of pathogens and parasites is reduced through medical and surgical asepsis, immunization, food sanitation, insect and rodent control, and disposal of human wastes.

Every developmental stage involves specific safety risks the nurse should assess.

Children under 5 years of age are at greatest risk for home accidents that may result in severe injury and death.

The school-age child is at risk for injury at home, at school, and traveling to and from school.

Adolescents are at risk from injury from the effects of drug and alcohol abuse.

Threats to an adult's safety are frequently associated with lifestyle habits.

Risks of injury for older adults are directly related to the physiological changes of the aging process.

Risks to client safety within a health care agency include falls and client-inherent, procedure-related, and equipment-related accidents.

Nursing interventions for promoting safety are individualized for developmental stage, lifestyle, and the environment.

Nursing interventions are developed to modify environment for protection from falls, fires, poisonings, and electrical hazards.

The nursing care plan to promote safety is continually evaluated to identify new or continued risks to the client.

Physical restraints should be used only as a last resort, when clients' behavior places them at risk for injury.

Critical Thinking Activities

1. The newest admission to the nursing unit is an older adult woman with arthritis and limited mobility. She is legally blind but is mentally alert. What are some nursing interventions that will help protect her safety while in the nursing unit?
2. During your clinical experience in maternal-child health you have the opportunity to teach new parents about safety and the newborn. Your time is limited, because your clients will be discharged before you return tomorrow. What will you teach today, and what will you teach in 3 days when you make a follow-up home visit?
3. You enter a client's room to answer the call bell and see the client frantically pointing to the trash can next to the bed. You smell smoke and see small flames. What do you do next?

References

Bloom BS, editor: *Taxonomy of educational objectives: book 1: cognitive domain,* New York, 1954/1981, Longman.

Brady R and others: Geriatric falls: prevention strategies for the staff, *J Gerontol Nurs* 19(9):26,1993.

Brians L and others: The development of the RISK tool for fall prevention, *Rehabil Nurs* 16(2):67, 1991.

Ebersole P, Hess P: *Toward healthy aging: human needs and nursing response,* ed 4, St. Louis, 1994, Mosby.

Edelman CL, Mandle CL: *Health promotion throughout the life span,* ed 3, St. Louis, 1994, Mosby.

Logedon M: Use of bicycle helmets, *Kentucky Nurs* 43(2):23, 1995.

National Citizens' Coalition for Nursing Home Reform: *Avoiding physical restraint use: new standards in care and alternative care approaches to reduce use of restraints,* Washington, DC, 1993, U.S. Government Printing Office.

Steinmetz H, Hobson S: Prevention of falls among the community dwelling elderly: an overview, *Phys Occup Ther Geriatrics* 12(4):13,1994.

Stolley J: Freeing your patients from restraints, *Am J Nurs* 95(2):27, 1995.

U.S. Bureau of the Census: *Statistical abstract of the U.S. 1993,* ed 116, Washington, DC, 1996, U.S. Department of Commerce.

Wong D: *Whaley and Wong's essentials of pediatric nursing,* ed 5, St. Louis, 1997, Mosby.

Hygiene

OBJECTIVES

Mastery of content in this chapter will
enable the student to:

- Define the key terms listed.
- Identify common skin problems and related interventions.
- Describe factors that influence personal hygiene practices.
- Discuss conditions that may put a client at risk for impaired skin integrity.
- Describe the types of bathing techniques used for various physical conditions and for clients of various age-groups.
- Perform a complete bed bath and back rub.
- Discuss factors that influence the condition of the nails and feet.
- Explain the importance of foot care for the diabetic client.
- Describe the methods used for cleaning and cutting the nails.
- Discuss conditions that may put a client at risk for impaired oral mucous membranes.
- Discuss measures used to provide special oral hygiene.
- Assist with or provide oral hygiene.
- List common hair and scalp problems and their related interventions.
- Offer hygiene to meet the needs of clients requiring eye, ear, and nose care.
- Describe how hygiene care for the older adult client may differ from that for the younger client.
- Make an occupied and unoccupied hospital bed.

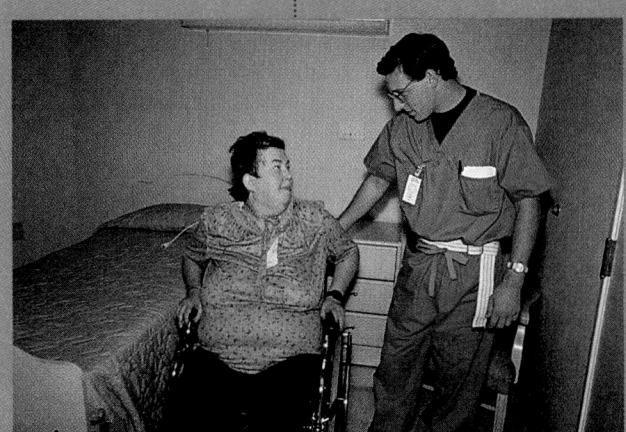

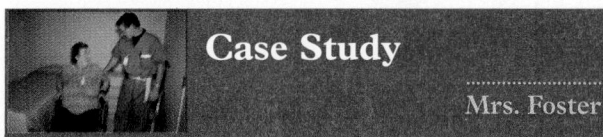

Case Study

Mrs. Foster

Mrs. Foster is a 49-year-old woman who has been a resident in a skilled nursing facility for the past 3 years. She has a medical history of multiple sclerosis. Recently she had increased dental problems and had three root canal procedures. Mrs. Foster is married and has three daughters. Her family lives approximately 2 hours from the facility. Today she related the "need to feel better about herself."

James Joseph is a freshman nursing student assigned to the skilled nursing facility. James is 20 years old and single. James has had some experience working with clients who have been in a skilled nursing facility. James has a part-time job in a facility near his home. He knows how important it is for clients to feel comfortable and have their basic needs met.

To provide basic hygiene, James needs to learn about what is important to Mrs. Foster's comfort. When hygiene needs are not fulfilled, clients will experience low self-esteem and have difficulties dealing with individuals in their environment. Clients should be given opportunities to maintain self-care needs. At an optimal level of functioning with assistance, this client is at risk for potential self-care deficits, impaired skin integrity, and altered health maintenance. During hygiene the nurse is able to interact with the client to assess the client's readiness to learn and to teach health promotion practices. The nurse preserves as much of the client's independence as possible, ensures privacy, and fosters physical well-being.

SCIENTIFIC KNOWLEDGE BASE

Good physical hygiene is necessary for comfort, safety, and well-being. Whereas well people are usually capable of meeting their own hygiene needs, ill people may require assistance. Several factors influence hygiene practice. The nurse determines a client's ability to perform self-care and provides hygiene care according to the client's needs and preferred practices.

The skin and mucosa cells exchange oxygen, nutrients, and fluids with underlying blood vessels. The cells require adequate nutrition, hydration, and circulation to resist injury and disease. The skin often reflects a change in physical condition by alterations in color, thickness, texture, turgor, temperature, and hydration.

Care of the Skin
The skin is an active organ. The skin protects, secretes, excretes, regulates temperature, and is a sense organ (Table 29-1). The three primary layers of the skin are the epidermis, dermis, and subcutaneous tissue.

The epidermis shields underlying tissue against water loss and injury and prevents entry of microorganisms. The dermis contains nerve fibers, blood vessels, sebaceous and sweat glands, and hair follicles. Subcutaneous tissue insulates and cushions the skin.

Care of the Feet and Nails
The feet and nails often require special attention to prevent infection, odor, and injury. Problems result from abuse or poor care.

The feet are important to physical and emotional health. Foot pain can often change a walking gait, causing strain on different muscle groups. Discomfort while standing or walking can lead to physical and emotional stress.

The nails are epithelial tissues that grow from the root of the nail bed, located in the skin at the nail groove. A normal healthy nail is transparent, smooth, and convex, with a pink nail bed and translucent white tip. Disease can cause changes in the shape, thickness, and curvature of the nail (see Chapter 24).

Care of the Oral Cavity and Teeth
The oral cavity is lined with mucous membranes continuous with the skin. The oral or **buccal cavity** consists of the lips surrounding the opening of the mouth, the cheeks running along the side walls of the cavity, the tongue and its muscles, and the hard and soft palate. The oral mucosa is normally light pink and moist.

Care of the Hair
Hair growth, distribution, and pattern can indicate general health status (Chapter 24). Hormonal changes, emotional and physical stress, aging, infection, and certain illnesses can affect hair characteristics. The hair shaft is an inert structure. Changes in its color or condition are caused by hormonal and nutrient deficiencies to the hair follicle. Table 29-5 on p. 766 describes common hair and scalp problems and nursing interventions.

NURSING KNOWLEDGE BASE

Personal preferences for hygiene can be influenced by a number of factors. No two individuals perform hygiene in the same way, and the nurse can provide individualized care only after knowing the client's unique practices.

Hygiene care is never routine. During the bath the nurse assesses physical conditions such as skin turgor and condition, areas of potential skin breakdown, and tissue perfusion. Because hygiene care often requires intimate contact with the client, the nurse uses communication skills to promote the therapeutic relationship and to learn about a client's emotional needs.

TABLE 29-1
Functions of the Skin and Implications for Care

Function/Description	Implications for Care
Protection Epidermis is relatively impermeable layer that prevents entrance of micro-organisms. Although microorganisms reside on skin surface and in hair follicles, relative dryness of surface inhibits bacterial growth. *Sebum* removes bacteria from hair follicles. Acidic pH of skin further slows bacterial growth.	Weakening of epidermis occurs by scraping or stripping its surface as by use of dry razors, tape removal, or improper turning or positioning techniques. Excessive dryness causes cracks and breaks in skin and mucosa that allow bacteria to enter. Emollients soften and prevent moisture loss, soaking improves moisture retention, and hydration of mucosa prevents dryness. However, constant exposure to moisture causes maceration or softening, which interrupts dermal integrity and promotes ulcers and bacterial growth. Bed linen and clothing should be kept dry. Misuse of soap, detergents, cosmetics, deodorant, and depilatories can cause chemical irritation. Alkaline soaps neutralize protective acid condition of skin. Cleansing removes excess oil, sweat, dead skin cells, and dirt that can promote bacterial growth.
Sensation Skin contains sensory organs for touch, pain, heat, cold, and pressure.	Friction should be minimized to avoid loss of stratum corneum, which can increase risk of pressure ulcers. Smoothing linen removes sources of mechanical irritation. The nurse should remove rings to prevent injuring client's skin. Bath water should not be too hot or cold.
Temperature Regulation Body temperature is controlled by radiation, evaporation, conduction, and convection.	Factors that interfere with heat loss can alter temperature control. Wet bed linen or gowns interfere with convection and conduction. Excess blankets or bed coverings can interfere with heat loss through radiation and conduction. Coverings can conserve heat.
Excretion and Secretion Sweat promotes heat loss by evaporation. Sebum lubricates skin and hair.	Perspiration and oil can harbor microorganism growth. Bathing removes excess body secretions, although excessive bathing can cause dry skin.

During hygiene care the nurse can also assess readiness to learn about health promotion practices. The nurse must also consider clients' specific physical limitations, beliefs, values, and habits. Individual hygiene preferences do not significantly affect health and can usually be included in the plan of care. The nurse preserves as much of the client's independence as possible, ensures privacy, and fosters physical well-being.

Body Image

A client's general appearance may reflect the importance hygiene holds for that person. Body image is persons' subjective concept of their physical appearance. These images can change frequently and can affect the way in which personal hygiene is maintained. The client's body image may change as the result of surgery, illness, or a change in functional status. Because of these factors the nurse must make an extra effort to promote hygiene.

Social Practices

Social groups also influence hygiene preferences and practices. During childhood, hygiene is influenced by family customs. As children enter the adolescent years, hygienic practices are influenced by dating and peer groups. Later in life, friends and work groups shape the expectations people have about their personal appearance. Older adults' hygiene practices may change because of living arrangements.

Socioeconomic Status

A person's economic resources influence the type and extent of hygiene practices used. The nurse should determine whether the client can afford supplies such as deodorant, shampoo, toothpaste, and so on. In the home environment there may be a need to modify the home with safety devices, such as safety bars, nonskid surfaces in the bath, or the addition of a tub chair.

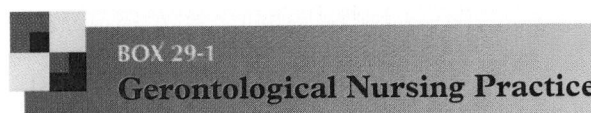

- The turnover rate for the stratum corneum declines by 50% as the client ages. This decline results in slower healing, reduced barrier protection, and delayed absorption of medications or chemicals placed on the skin (Lueckenotte, 1997).
- Older clients produce less sebum and perspire less and thus generally need to bathe less frequently. However, personal preference must always be considered.
- Older clients' skin is often more fragile; avoid hot water, and use only a mild cleansing agent. Some authorities suggest the use of bath oils; use with caution because this increases the danger of falling in a slippery tub.
- The majority of older clients have some degree of itching and skin sensitivity; hydrocortisone cream, superfatted soaps, and petrolatum can offer relief.
- Dryness and redness are a common problem as skin ages, which worsens in cold, dry air; humidity should be kept above 40% (PPPUA, 1993).
- Elder abuse affects between 1 and 2 million persons a year (Anetzberger and others, 1993); unexplained bruises and skin trauma should not be ignored.

Cultural Variables

A client's cultural beliefs and personal values influence hygiene care. People from diverse cultural backgrounds follow different self-care practices (see Chapter 18). In North America it is common to bathe or shower daily, whereas in some other cultures it is customary to completely bathe only once a week.

Personal Preferences

Each client has individual desires and preferences about when to bathe, shave, and perform hair care. Clients select different products according to personal preferences and needs. These desires should assist the nurse in delivering individualized care for the client. In addition, the nurse should also assist the client in developing new hygiene practices when indicated by an illness or condition.

Knowledge

Knowledge about the importance of hygiene and its implications for well-being influences hygiene practices. However, knowledge alone is not enough. The client also must be motivated to maintain self-care. Often learning about an illness or condition and its influence on the individual encourages the client to improve hygiene. For example, the client with diabetes is aware of the effect of the illness on circulation and the long-term potential of injury. As a result the client is motivated to learn about proper foot hygiene and nail care.

Physical Condition

People with certain illnesses or those who have undergone surgery may lack the physical energy and dexterity to perform hygienic care. A client whose arm is in a cast or traction requires assistance with hygiene. Chronic illnesses, such as cardiac disease, cancer, or neurological disorders, may exhaust or incapacitate the client and require the nurse to perform total hygiene.

⋯CRITICAL THINKING IN CLIENT CARE

Synthesis

The nurse must synthesize knowledge, draw from experience, use critical thinking attitudes, and be knowledgeable of standards of practice. The nurse uses practical experience and knowledge from scientific and nursing domains to provide individualized nursing care for clients requiring assistance with hygiene. The hygiene needs and practices of the clients may be different than those of the nurse; therefore the nurse accepts and respects these differences.

Knowledge. It is imperative that the nurse understand the implications of proper hygiene on the client's total health status. Proper hygiene promotes skin integrity, a sense of well-being, and improved body image. Knowledge about hygiene practices, which may include cultural, developmental, and pathophysiologic factors, can provide a scientific basis for identifying and meeting clients' hygiene needs.

The nurse uses knowledge from basic sciences to determine how changes in mobility, aging, exposure to the environment, and disease affect the skin. To effectively identify the hygiene needs of individualized clients, the nurse also uses specific knowledge and techniques of communication theory and knowledge of cultural influence with regard to hygiene. The principles in establishing a trusting relationship will enhance client care, and basic understanding of the principles of self-concept is important in identifying and meeting the client's hygiene needs. The nurse must also consider the client's values in setting hygiene priority needs in regard to skin integrity and mobility.

The diabetic client has specialized needs for nail and foot care. The pathophysiology of diabetes and the impact of the illness on the client's circulation provide the nurse with the scientific knowledge base needed to implement proper foot care practices.

Experience. Nursing students have experienced their own specific hygiene needs. In addition, they may have assisted family members with their hygiene. Usually an early clinical experience involves providing hygiene to a client. As the student increases the experiential knowledge base, the ability to provide individualized hygiene increases.

Attitudes. There are multiple critical thinking attitudes that apply to hygiene care. For example, the nurse uses creativity to collaborate with the client to determine the best way to meet hygiene needs. The nurse is nonjudgmental and confident when providing care. Because clients' individual physical strength and hygiene practices may differ, it is important that the nurse establish flexibility in the client's schedule to identify needs for periods of rest to lessen the chance of exhaustion during hygiene.

Standards. The nurse is a client advocate in maintaining standards of care. During hygiene care the nurse promotes client independence while maintaining safety. The nurse must be mindful of the client's limitations. These concerns for the client establish and maintain self-concept, independence, and mutual respect through advocacy.

NURSING PROCESS AND SKIN CARE

▣ Assessment

Nursing assessment is an ongoing process. The nurse does not assess all body regions before a bath or hair shampooing; however, the nurse does routinely observe the condition of the skin whenever care to the client is given. The nurse must also determine whether the client can tolerate hygiene procedures, which can often be exhausting.

Most assessment occurs while the nurse cares for the client's hygiene needs. For example, during oral care the condition of the teeth and mucosa can be observed. Hygiene care allows the nurse to assess for a variety of health care problems and thus helps to set health care priorities.

Physical assessment of skin. While assisting a client with personal hygiene, the nurse assesses all external body surfaces. Using inspection and palpation (see Chapter 24), the nurse looks for alterations, determines the need for hygiene, and notes skin changes in response to therapies.

The nurse observes the skin's color, texture, thickness, turgor, temperature, and hydration. The nurse gives special attention to the characteristics most influenced by hygiene measures. Is the skin dry from too much bathing? Are there calluses of the feet that may benefit from soaking?

Certain conditions place clients at risk for impaired skin integrity (see Chapter 38). Nurses must be partic-

ularly alert when assessing clients with reduced sensation, vascular insufficiency, and immobility. The development of pressure ulcers is a common complication that extends hospital stays.

While inspecting the skin, the nurse notes the presence and condition of lesions (see Chapter 24). Certain common skin problems affect how hygiene is administered (Table 29-2). Special care is also given to assess less obvious surfaces, such as under the female client's breasts or around perineal tissues (see Chapter 38). The nurse who observes skin problems should explain proper skin care to the client. The nurse may also educate the client about avoiding irritants, which can worsen the skin condition.

Developmental changes. Age influences the normal condition of the skin and the type of hygiene required. The neonate's skin is relatively immature and thin. The epidermis and dermis are loosely bound together. The nurse must handle the neonate carefully during bathing to avoid friction, which can result in bruising. A break in the skin can easily cause infection.

The toddler's skin layers are more tightly bound together and thus have a greater resistance to infection and skin irritation. However, because the child is more active and does not have regular hygiene habits, care givers must be attentive.

During adolescence, growth and maturation of the skin are increased. Sebaceous glands become more active, resulting in **acne.** Eccrine and apocrine sweat glands become fully functional during puberty. More frequent bathing and use of antiperspirants become necessary to reduce body odors.

The condition of an adult's skin depends on hygiene practices and exposure to environmental irritants. Normally the skin is elastic, well hydrated, firm, and smooth. With age the skin loses its resiliency and moisture, and sebaceous and sweat glands become less active. This encourages dry, cracked skin. Daily bathing, inadequate fluid and nutrition, and the use of some soap products may cause the skin of an older adult client to become too dry (Box 29-1). The epithelium thins and elastic collagen fibers shrink, making the skin fragile and subject to bruising and breaking. The nurse uses caution when turning and repositioning an older adult client.

Cultural considerations. A client's cultural heritage influences hygiene practices. For example, clients may desire certain oils or lotions during their bath. When caring for clients from difference cultures, nurses need to be sensitive to the client's normal practices, such as when and how often bathing is performed, the extent of bathing, and the use of personal care practices. Most of these preferences can be incorporated into the client's hygiene.

TABLE 29-2
Common Skin Problems

Problem	Characteristics	Implications	Interventions
Dry skin	Flaky, rough texture on exposed areas such as hands, arms, legs, or face.	Skin may become infected if epidermal layer is allowed to crack.	Bathe less frequently. Use superfatted soap (e.g., Dove) for cleansing. Rinse body of all soap well because residue left can cause irritation and breakdown. Add moisture to air through use of humidifier. Increase fluid intake when skin is dry. Use moisturizing lotion to aid healing process; lotion forms protective barrier and helps maintain fluid within skin. Use creams to clean skin that is dry or irritated by soaps and detergents.
Acne	Inflammatory, papulo-pustular skin eruption, usually involving bacterial breakdown of sebum; appears on face, neck, shoulders, and back.	Infected material within pustule can spread if area is squeezed or picked. Permanent scarring can result.	Wash hair and skin each day with hot water and soap to remove oil. Use cosmetics sparingly because oily cosmetics or creams accumulate in pores and tend to make conditions worse. Dietary restrictions may need to be implemented. Foods found to aggravate condition should be eliminated from diet. Use prescribed topical antibiotics for severe acne.
Hirsutism	Excessive growth of body and facial hair, especially in women.	Hirsutism may cause negative body image by giving female a male appearance.	The following may be used to remove unwanted hair: depilatories (can cause infection, rashes, or dermatitis), shaving (safest method), electrolysis (permanently removes hair by destroying hair follicles), tweezing (lasts temporarily), and bleaching (lasts temporarily).
Skin rashes	Skin eruption that may result from overexposure to sun or moisture or from allergic reaction; may be flat or raised, localized or systemic, pruritic or nonpruritic.	If skin is continually scratched, inflammation and infection may occur. Rashes can also cause discomfort.	Wash area thoroughly, and apply antiseptic spray or lotion to prevent further itching and aid healing process. Warm soaks may relieve inflammation.
Contact dermatitis	Inflammation of skin characterized by abrupt onset with erythema, pruritus, pain, and appearance of scaly oozing lesions; seen on face, neck, hands, forearms, and genitalia.	Dermatitis is often difficult to eliminate because person is usually in continual contact with substance causing skin reaction. Substance may be hard to identify.	Condition usually disappears when exposure to causative agents (e.g., cleansers, soaps) is avoided.
Abrasion	Scraping or rubbing away of epidermis; may result in localized bleeding and later weeping of serous fluid.	Infection occurs easily as result of loss of protective skin layer.	Nurses should always be careful not to scratch clients with their jewelry or fingernails. Wash abrasions with mild soap and water. Dressing or bandage could increase risk of infection because of retained moisture.

When caring for clients with dark skin pigmentation, the nurse must be aware of unique assessment characteristics and techniques. It is important to provide meticulous skin assessment in clients who are at risk for pressure ulcers (see Chapters 37 and 38). Understanding of normal skin assessment characteristics in clients with dark skin pigmentation can assist in early identification of impaired skin integrity (Box 29-2).

Assessment of self-care ability. When a client becomes unable to bathe or perform personal skin care, the nurse provides assistance. To determine whether a client requires a bed bath instead of a tub bath or shower, the nurse should assess balance, activity tolerance, and muscle strength and coordination. The degree of assistance needed by a client during bathing may also depend on vision, the ability to sit without support, hand grasp, and range of motion (ROM) of extremities. If cognitive function is impaired, the nurse's help will probably be needed.

Client expectations. With all nursing care, it is important to know the client's expectations. Hygiene is a very personal aspect of care, and clients may indeed have varying expectations. When providing skin care, determine the client's preferences for soaps, lotions,

showers, or tub bath. How much privacy does the client wish? Is it important to have hygiene completed before family members visit, or does the client wish the family to assist with hygiene practices? The client has certain expectations in all aspects of hygiene, including bathing, nail care, oral hygiene, and hair care. Whenever possible, try to incorporate the client's routine practices into hygiene care. Sometimes extra time is needed to offer the client a daily shampoo. However, hygiene may be one aspect of care where flexibility is easier to achieve.

··························

Successful critical thinking requires a synthesis of knowledge, experience, information gathered from clients, and critical thinking attitudes and standards. Clinical judgments require the nurse to anticipate what information is needed, to analyze the data, and then to make decisions regarding client care. The client expects competent and informed care. James incorporates previous knowledge and experience in providing care for Mrs. Foster.

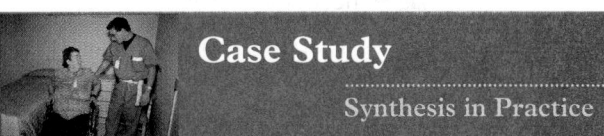

Case Study

Synthesis in Practice

Before entering Mrs. Foster's room, James reviews and synthesizes knowledge about the impact of chronic illness on body image and independence, reviews principles of communication, and reviews the pathophysiology for pressure ulcers.

When James arrives in Mrs. Foster's room, he finds her in bed facing the wall. Mrs. Foster does not want to talk; in fact, she is having a difficult time trying not to cry. Initially James begins to straighten up the environment, giving Mrs. Foster some private time.

Previous clinical experience has taught James that clients need to have an opportunity to determine how nursing care is implemented. James engages Mrs. Foster into some discussion regarding how she would like her morning care. James learns that Mrs. Foster was incontinent of stool during the night, and although the nurses did provide perineal care, Mrs. Foster still feels "dirty" and would like a shower. The night nurses told her she would have to wait until her routine shower day, which is 2 days away. At this point in time James feels that assisting Mrs. Foster with a shower is his first priority.

James continues to synthesize knowledge and use previous clinical experience to appropriately analyze assessment data and make his nursing diagnoses. He maintains accurate information and incorporates good communication skills, which will ensure meeting standards for quality care.

Box 29-2

Cultural Considerations: Skin Assessment for the Client With Intact Darkly Pigmented Skin

Assess localized skin color changes:
    Skin color changes
    Color darker than surrounding skin, purplish,
       bluish, eggplant
    Taut
    Shiny
    Induration
Assess for edema (nonpitting swelling)
Importance of lighting for skin assessment:
    Use natural or halogen light
    Avoid fluorescent lamps, which can give the skin
       a bluish tone
Assess skin temperature:
    Initially may feel warmer than surrounding skin
    Subsequently may feel cooler than surrounding
       skin
    Use the back of your hand and fingers and, if
       client's condition permits, no gloves when do-
       ing this assessment

Data from Bennett MA: Report of the task force on the implications for darkly pigmented intact skin in the prediction and prevention of pressure ulcers, *Adv Wound Care* 8(6):34, 1995.

Nursing Diagnosis

An assessment reveals the condition of the skin and the client's need for and ability to maintain personal hygiene. The nurse reviews all data gathered (e.g., the client's risk for physical immobilization, presence of secretions, or altered circulation and sensation). Clustering defining characteristics reveals the diagnosis of *impaired skin integrity*. Accurate selection of a diagnosis ensures the client's needs are met (see nursing diagnoses box).

NURSING DIAGNOSES FOR SKIN INTEGRITY AND THE NEED FOR THOROUGH SKIN CARE

Self-care deficit, bathing/hygiene
Skin integrity, impaired
Skin integrity, impaired, risk for
Tissue integrity, impaired
Tissue perfusion, altered, peripheral

A nursing diagnosis is accurate only if the appropriate related factors are selected. The diagnosis influences the nursing therapies chosen. For the diagnosis *bathing/hygiene self-care deficit related to decreased mobility*, the nurse must incorporate principles that will increase mobility to enhance self-care and independence. Frequent turning or repositioning, using a proper support surface, and removing underlying tubing are good measures. In contrast, the diagnosis *impaired skin integrity related to exposure to body excretions* requires a nurse to choose different therapies. Frequent skin cleansing, controlling sources of wound drainage or incontinence, and timely bed linen changes would be good measures to control the irritation of excretions. Selecting an incorrect related factor for a diagnosis can result in inappropriate and ineffective nursing care.

Planning

After the nursing diagnoses are identified and individualized, the nurse and the client set goals and expected outcomes to direct nursing interventions. The plan for providing skin care should focus on the types or methods of care and on the many care measures the nurse can perform while a client bathes. The nurse can teach, provide emotional support, and assist with ROM exercises.

Considering a client's hygiene preferences before planning is important. The type of hygiene the client desires or requires will determine the supplies and equipment the nurse must prepare. The normal lifestyle before admission and preferences by the client will be incorporated into the care plan.

The client's condition influences the plan for delivering hygiene (see care plan). A seriously ill client usually needs a daily bath because body secretions accumulate, and the client is unable to maintain cleanliness. An older adult client at home may require a visit from the nurse to assist with a tub bath. The nurse must also provide for necessary assistance for clients who are weakened or have poor muscle strength.

Implementation

Health promotion and restorative care. Nurses can instruct clients to follow a few general rules to promote skin health and restore optimal function. Clients should bathe daily unless contraindicated, preferably in the morning. They should use lotions to moisturize dry skin and bathe in a warm environment, avoiding cold drafts. Drinking at least eight glasses of water daily helps to maintain hydration. Clients should always inspect their skin for any changes in skin color and texture, and report abnormalities to their primary care provider. The client should handle the skin gently, avoiding excessive rubbing. Finally, clients should be encouraged to eat nutritious foods rich in vitamins and minerals.

Bathing a client. Bathing may be done for cleanliness or for a specific therapy, depending on the type of bath. The extent of the bath and the methods used for bathing depend on the client's physical abilities, health problems, and the degree of hygiene required. A **complete bed bath** is for clients who are dependent and require total hygiene care (Skill 29-1).

A **partial bed bath** involves bathing only body parts that would cause discomfort or odor if left unbathed. Aging or dependent clients in need of only partial hygiene or self-sufficient bedridden clients unable to reach all body parts receive partial bed baths.

The tub bath or shower can be used to give a more thorough bath than a bed bath. Washing and rinsing all body parts are easier. Safety is of primary concern because the surface of a tub or shower stall is slippery. Clients vary in how much help they will need. Regardless of the type of bath the client receives, the nurse should use the following guidelines:

1. Provide privacy. Close the door, or pull room curtains around the bathing area. While bathing the client, expose only the areas being bathed.
2. Maintain safety. Keep side rails up while away from the client's bedside. (This is particularly important for dependent or unconscious clients.) Place the call light in the client's reach if leaving the room temporarily.
3. Maintain warmth. The room should be kept warm because the client is partially uncovered and may easily be chilled. Control drafts, and keep windows closed. Keep client covered, only exposing the body part being washed during the bath.

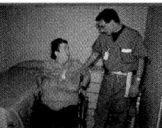

CASE STUDY NURSING CARE PLAN

Skin Care

Assessment

Mrs. Foster is very concerned about her physical appearance. She wants to "look her best." She is **in a wheelchair** and **does not have the coordination or muscle strength to independently transfer or stand.** Her skin is intact, but there is **prolonged erythema over ischial pressure areas bilaterally.** Her **skin is dry, fingernails and toenails are very brittle,** and **she is frequently incontinent of stool and urine.**

Nursing Diagnosis

Risk for impaired skin integrity related to impaired mobility and incontinence.

Planning

Goal

Client's skin remains intact.

Expected Outcomes

Client's skin is without increased erythema.
Client's skin remains dry.
Client's skin is odor free.
Client feels clean and dry.

Implementation

Steps	Rationale
1. Provide perineal care after each diarrheal episode.	Minimizing skin exposure to moisture decreases irritation and susceptibility to injury (PPPUA, 1993).
2. Change linen after diaphoresis or diarrheal episode.	Changing linen keeps skin free of moisture, which promotes bacterial growth (NPUAP, 1989).
3. Apply lotion to areas that can easily become dried and chapped.	Lotion reduces drying and chapping of skin. Dry, chapped skin impairs skin integrity and is port of entry for bacteria.
4. Monitor length of time any area of redness persists. Determine turning and positioning interval. Turning interval − hypoxia time = suggest interval (e.g., 2 hours − 30 min = 1½ hr).	Repositioning reduces pressure and allows for normal hyperemic response (Maklebust, 1991).
5. Do **not** massage reddened area.	Massage increases breaks in capillaries in underlying tissues (Maklebust, 1991; USDHHS, 1992).

Evaluation

Observe skin for pressure and moisture after each position change, according to turning interval, every 1½ hours.
Inspect skin for breakdown.
Ask client how her skin feels after skin care.

Defining characteristics are shown in bold type.

---

4. Promote the client's independence as much as possible during bathing activities. Offer assistance as needed.
5. Anticipate needs. Bring a new set of clothing and hygiene products to the bedside or bathroom.

Perineal care. **Perineal care** is usually part of the complete bed bath (Skill 29-2). Clients most in need of perineal care are at greatest risk for acquiring an infection (e.g., clients who have indwelling urinary catheters or who are recovering from rectal or genital surgery or childbirth). A client able to perform self-care should be allowed to do so. Many nurses are embarrassed about providing perineal care, particularly to clients of the opposite sex. This should not cause the nurse to overlook the client's hygiene needs. A professional, dignified attitude can reduce embarrassment and put the client and the nurse at ease.

If a client performs self-care, various problems such as vaginal or urethral discharge, skin irritation, and unpleasant odors may go unnoticed. The nurse must be

Text continued on p. 747

Bathing a Client

Delegation Considerations

Skills of bathing may be delegated to unlicensed assistive personnel.

- Inform care provider about early signs of impaired skin integrity, and tell provider to have nurse reassess the skin when changes are noted.
- Review procedure for application of moisturizing lotions.
- Warn against massaging reddened areas.
- Review type of bath and client's ability to participate.

Equipment

- Two washcloths
- Two bath towels
- Bath blanket
- Soap and soap dish
- Toiletry items (deodorant, powder, lotion, cologne)
- Clean hospital gown or client's own pajamas or gown
- Laundry bag
- Disposable gloves (when risk for contacting body fluids)

STEPS	RATIONALE
1. Assess client's tolerance for activity, discomfort level, cognitive ability, and musculoskeletal function.	Determines client's ability to perform self-care and level of assistance required from nurse. Also determines type of bath to administer (e.g., tub bath or partial bed bath).
2. Review orders for specific precautions concerning client's movement or positioning.	Prevents accidental injury to client during bathing activities. Determine level of assistance required by client.
3. Explain procedure, and ask client for suggestions on how to prepare supplies. If partial bath, ask how much of bath client wishes to complete.	Promotes client's cooperation and participation.
4. Adjust room temperature and ventilation, close room doors and windows, and draw room divider curtain.	Warm room that is free of drafts prevents rapid loss of body heat during bathing. Privacy ensures client's mental and physical comfort.
5. Prepare equipment and supplies.	Avoids interrupting procedure or leaving client unattended to retrieve missing equipment.
6. Bathe client.	
A. Complete or partial bed bath:	
(1) Offer client bedpan or urinal. Provide towel and washcloth.	Client will feel more comfortable after voiding. Prevents interruption of bath.
(2) Wash hands.	Reduces transmission of microorganisms.

CRITICAL DECISION POINT

Apply gloves if drainage or secretions appear on client's skin.

(3) Lower side rail closest to you, and assist client in assuming comfortable position, maintaining body alignment. Bring client toward side closest to nurse. Place hospital bed in high position.	Aids nurse's access to client. Maintains client's comfort throughout procedure. Nurse does not have to reach across bed, thus minimizing strain on back muscles.
(4) Loosen top covers at foot of bed. Place bath blanket over top sheet. Fold and remove top sheet from under blanket. If possible, have client hold bath blanket while withdrawing sheet.	Removal of top linens prevents their becoming soiled or moist during bath. Blanket provides warmth and privacy.

STEPS	RATIONALE
(5) If top sheet is to be reused, fold it for replacement later. If not, dispose in laundry bag, taking care not to allow linen to contact uniform.	Proper disposal prevents transmission of micro-organisms.
(6) Remove client's gown or pajamas. If an extremity is injured or has reduced mobility, begin removal from *unaffected* side. If client has IV tube, remove gown from arm *without* IV first; then lower IV container and slide gown covering affected arm over tubing and container. Rehang IV container and check flow rate (see illustrations).	Provides full exposure of body parts during bathing. Undressing unaffected side first allows easier manipulation of gown over body part with reduced ROM.
(7) Pull side rail up. Fill washbasin two thirds full, with warm water. Have client place fingers in water to test temperature tolerance. Place plastic container of bath lotion in bath water to warm, if desired.	Raising side rail maintains client's safety as nurse leaves bedside. Warm water promotes comfort, relaxes muscles, and prevents unnecessary chilling. Testing temperature prevents accidental burns. Bath water warms lotion for application to client's skin.

Continued

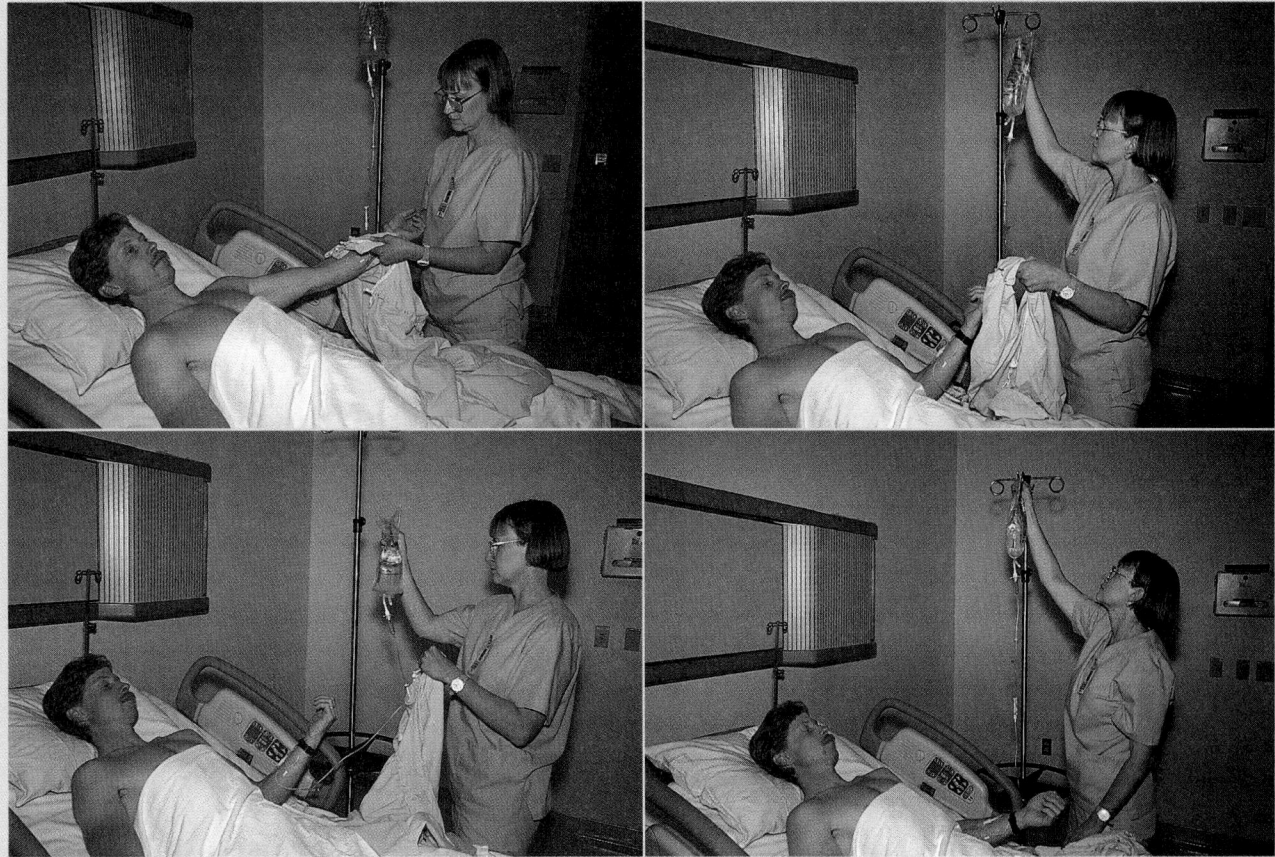

Step 6A(6)

STEPS	RATIONALE
(8) Remove pillow if allowed, and raise head of bed 30 to 45 degrees. Place bath towel under client's head. Place second bath towel over client's chest.	Removal of pillow makes it easier to wash client's ears and neck. Placement of towels prevents soiling of bed linen and bath blanket.
(9) Fold washcloth around fingers of nurse's hand to form mitt (see illustration). Immerse mitt in water and wring thoroughly.	Mitt retains water and heat better than loosely held washcloth; keeps cold edges from brushing against client and prevents splashing.
(10) Wash client's eyes with plain warm water. Inquire if client is wearing contact lenses. If so, perform eye care as described in Skill 29-6. Use different section of mitt for each eye. Move mitt from inner to outer canthus (see illustration). Soak any crusts on eyelid for 2 to 3 minutes with damp cloth before attempting removal. Dry eye thoroughly but gently.	Soap irritates eyes. Use of separate sections of mitt reduces infection transmission. Bathing eye from inner to outer canthus prevents secretions from entering nasolacrimal duct. Pressure can cause internal injury.
(11) Ask if client prefers to use soap on face. Wash, rinse, and dry well forehead, cheeks, nose, neck, and ears. (Men may wish to shave at this point or after bath.)	Soap tends to dry face, which is exposed to air more than other body parts.
(12) Remove bath blanket from client's arm that is closest to nurse. Place bath towel lengthwise under arm.	Prevents soiling of bed.
(13) Bathe arm with soap and water using long, firm strokes from distal to proximal areas (fingers to axilla). Raise and support arm above head (if possible) while thoroughly washing axilla.	Soap lowers surface tension and facilitates removal of debris and bacteria when friction is applied during washing. Long, firm strokes stimulate circulation. Movement of arm exposes axilla and exercises joint's normal ROM.

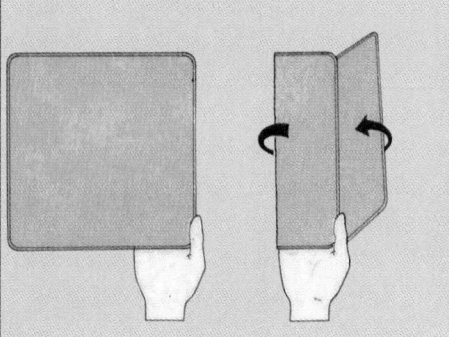

Step 6A(9)

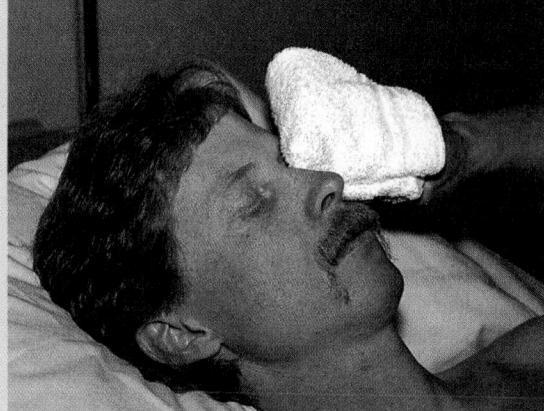

Step 6A(10)

STEPS	RATIONALE
(14) Rinse and dry arm and axilla thoroughly. If client uses deodorant or talcum powder, apply it.	Alkaline residue from soap discourages growth of normal skin bacteria (Barnes, 1987). Excess moisture causes skin maceration or softening. Deodorant controls body odor.
(15) Fold bath towel in half, and lay it on bed beside client. Place basin on towel. Immerse client's hand in water. Allow hand to soak for 3 to 5 minutes before washing hand and fingernails (see Skill 29-3). Remove basin and dry hand well.	Soaking softens cuticles and calluses of hand, loosens debris beneath nails, and enhances feeling of cleanliness. Thorough drying removes moisture from between fingers.
(16) Raise side rail, and move to other side of bed. Lower side rail, and repeat steps 12 through 15 for other arm.	
(17) Check temperature of bath water, and change water if necessary.	Warm water maintains client's comfort.
(18) Cover client's chest with bath towel, and fold bath blanket down to umbilicus. With one hand, lift edge of towel away from chest. With mitted hand, bathe chest using long, firm strokes. Take special care to wash skinfolds under female client's breasts. It may be necessary to lift breast upward while bathing underneath it. Keep client's chest covered between wash and rinse periods. Dry well.	Draping prevents unnecessary exposure of body parts. Towel maintains warmth and privacy. Secretions and dirt collect easily in areas of tight skinfolds. Skinfolds are susceptible to excoriation if breasts are pendulous.
(19) Place bath towel lengthwise over chest and abdomen. (Two towels may be needed.) Fold blanket down to just above pubic region.	Prevents chilling and exposure of body parts.
(20) With one hand, lift bath towel. With mitted hand, bathe abdomen, giving special attention to bathing umbilicus and abdominal folds. Stroke from side to side. Keep abdomen covered between washing and rinsing. Dry well.	Moisture and sediment that collect in skinfolds predispose skin to maceration and irritation.
(21) Apply clean gown or pajama top.	Maintains client's warmth and comfort. Dressing affected side first allows easier manipulation of gown over body part with reduced ROM.

CRITICAL DECISION POINT

If one extremity is injured or immobilized, always dress affected side first. This step may be omitted until completion of bath; gown should not become soiled during remainder of bath.

| (22) Cover chest and abdomen with top of bath blanket. Expose near leg by folding blanket toward midline. Be sure perineum is draped. | Prevents unnecessary exposure. |

Continued

Skill 29-1—cont'd
Bathing a Client

STEPS	RATIONALE
(23) Bend client's leg at knee by positioning nurse's arm under leg. While grasping client's heel, elevate leg from mattress slightly, and slide bath towel lengthwise under leg. Ask client to hold foot still. Place bath basin on towel on bed, and secure its position next to foot to be washed.	Towel prevents soiling of bed linen. Support of joint and extremity during lifting prevents strain on musculoskeletal structures. Sudden movement by client could spill bath water. (Omit this step if client is unable to hold leg in basin.)
(24) With one hand supporting lower leg, raise it and slide basin under lifted foot. Make sure foot is firmly placed on bottom of basin. Allow foot to soak while washing leg. If client is unable to hold leg, do not immerse; simply wash with washcloth (see illustration).	Proper positioning of foot prevents pressure being applied from edge of basin against calf. Soaking softens calluses and rough skin.
(25) Unless contraindicated, use long, firm strokes in washing from ankle to knee and from knee to thigh. Dry well.	Promotes venous return.

CRITICAL DECISION POINT

Clients with history of deep vein thromboses or hypercoagulation disorders should not have their lower extremities washed with long firm strokes.

(26) Cleanse foot, making sure to bathe between toes. Clean and clip nails as needed (see Skill 29-3). Dry well. If skin is dry, apply lotion. Do not massage any reddened area on client's skin.	Secretions and moisture may be present between toes. Lotion helps retain moisture and soften skin.
(27) Raise side rail, and move to other side of the bed. Lower side rail, and repeat steps 22 through 26 for other leg and foot.	
(28) Cover client with bath blanket, raise side rail for client's safety, and change bath water.	Decreased bath water temperature can cause chilling. Clean water reduces microorganism transmission.

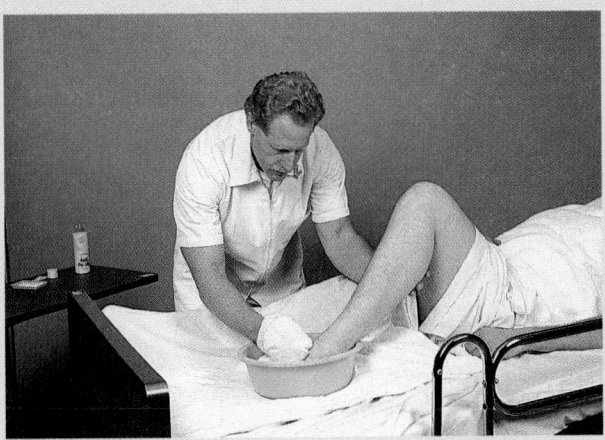

Step 6A(24)

STEPS	RATIONALE
(29) Lower side rail. Assist client in assuming prone or side-lying position (as applicable). Place towel lengthwise along client's side.	Exposes back and buttocks for bathing.
(30) Keep client draped by sliding bath blanket over shoulders and thighs. Wash, rinse, and dry back from neck to buttocks using long, firm strokes. Pay special attention to folds of buttocks and anus. Give a back rub.	Maintains warmth, and prevents unnecessary exposure. Skinfolds near buttocks and anus may contain fecal secretions that harbor microorganisms.
(31) Apply disposable gloves if not done previously.	Prevents contact with microorganisms in body secretions.
(32) Assist client in assuming side-lying or supine position. Cover chest and upper extremities with towel and lower extremities with bath blanket. Expose only genitalia. (If client can wash, covering entire body with bath blanket may be preferable.) Wash, rinse, and dry perineum (see Skill 29-2). Pay special attention to skinfolds. Apply water-repellent ointment to area exposed to moisture.	Maintains client's privacy. Clients capable of performing partial bath usually prefer to wash their own genitalia. Water-repellent ointments (e.g., A & D, Pericare) protect skin from moisture.
(33) Dispose of gloves in receptacle.	Prevents transmission of infection.
(34) Apply additional body lotion or oil as desired.	Moisturizing lotion prevents dry, chapped skin.
(35) Assist client in dressing. Comb client's hair. Women may want to apply makeup.	Promotes client's body image.
(36) Make client's bed (see Skills 29-7 and 29-8).	Provides clean environment.
(37) Remove soiled linen, and place in dirty-linen bag. Clean and replace bathing equipment. Replace call light and personal possessions. Leave room as clean and comfortable as possible.	Prevents transmission of infection. Clean environment promotes client's comfort. Keeping call light and articles of care within reach promotes client's safety.
(38) Wash hands.	Reduces transmission of microorganisms.
B. Tub bath or shower:	
(1) Consider client's condition, and review orders for precautions concerning client's movement or positioning.	Prevents accidental injury to client during bathing.
(2) Check tub or shower for cleanliness. Use cleaning techniques outlined in agency policy. Place rubber mat on tub or shower bottom. Place disposable bath mat or towel on floor in front of tub or shower.	Cleaning prevents transmission of microorganisms. Mats prevent slipping and falling.
(3) Collect all hygienic aids, toiletry items, and linens requested by client. Place within easy reach of tub or shower.	Placing items close at hand prevents possible falls when client reaches for equipment.
(4) Assist client to bathroom if necessary. Have client wear robe and slippers to bathroom.	Assistance prevents accidental falls. Wearing robe and slippers prevents chilling.

Continued

Skill 29-1—cont'd
Bathing a Client

STEPS	RATIONALE
(5) Demonstrate how to use call signal for assistance.	Bathrooms are equipped with signaling devices in case client feels faint or weak or needs immediate assistance. Clients prefer privacy during bath if safety is not jeopardized.
(6) Place "occupied" sign on bathroom door.	Maintains client's privacy.
(7) Provide shower seat or tub chair if needed (see illustration). Fill bathtub halfway with warm water. Ask client to test water, and adjust temperature if water is too warm. Explain which faucet controls hot water. If client is taking shower, turn shower on, and adjust water temperature before client enters shower stall.	Adjusting water temperature prevents accidental burns. Older adults and clients with neurological alterations (e.g., spinal cord injury) are at high risk for burns as a result of reduced sensation. Use of assistive devices facilitates bathing and minimizes physical exertion.
(8) Instruct client to use safety bars when getting in and out of tub or shower. Caution client against use of bath oil in tub water.	Prevents slipping and falling. Oil causes tub surfaces to become slippery.
(9) Instruct client not to remain in tub longer than 20 minutes. Check on client every 5 minutes.	Prolonged exposure to warm water may cause vasodilation and pooling of blood, leading to lightheadedness or dizziness.
(10) Return to bathroom when client signals, and knock before entering.	Provides privacy.
(11) For client who is unsteady, drain tub of water before client attempts to get out of it. Place bath towel over client's shoulders. Assist client in getting out of tub as needed, and assist with drying.	Prevents accidental falls. Client may become chilled as water drains.

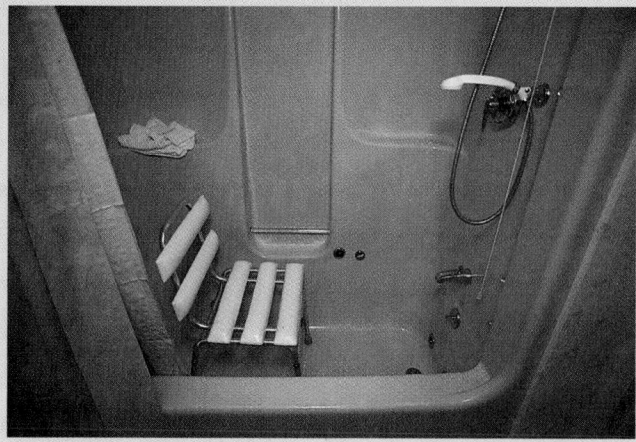

Step 6B(7)

STEPS	RATIONALE

CRITICAL DECISION POINT

Weak or unstable clients need extra assistance in getting out of a tub. Planning for additional personnel is essential before attempting to assist the client from the tub.

STEPS	RATIONALE
(12) Assist client as needed in donning clean gown or pajamas, slippers, and robe. (In home setting, client may don regular clothing.)	Maintains warmth to prevent chilling.
(13) Assist client to room and comfortable position in bed or chair.	Maintains relaxation gained from bathing.
(14) Clean tub or shower according to agency policy. Remove soiled linen and place in dirty-linen bag. Discard disposable equipment in proper receptacle. Place "unoccupied" sign on bathroom door. Return supplies to storage area.	Prevents transmission of infection through soiled linen and moisture.
(15) Wash hands.	Reduces transfer of microorganisms.
7. Observe skin, paying particular attention to areas that were previously soiled, reddened, or showed early signs of breakdown.	Techniques used during bathing should leave skin clean and clear.
8. Observe ROM during bath.	Measures joint mobility.
9. Ask client to rate level of comfort.	

Recording and Reporting
- Record bath on flow sheet. Note level of assistance required.
- Record condition of skin and any significant findings (e.g., reddened areas, bruises, nevi, or joint or muscle pain).

- Report evidence of alterations in skin integrity to nurse in charge or physician.

Home Care Considerations
- Assess client's tub and shower area for need for adaptive devices, such as grab bars, shower chair, or handheld shower.

---

alert for complaints of burning during urination, localized soreness or excoriation, or perineal pain. The nurse also inspects vaginal and perineal areas and bed linen for signs of discharge.

Back rub. A back rub usually follows the bath (see Chapter 33). It promotes relaxation, relieves muscular tension, stimulates skin circulation, and is generally well tolerated by even critically ill clients (Tyler and others, 1990). During the back rub the nurse can assess skin condition.

An effective back rub takes 3 to 5 minutes. The nurse should first ask whether the client would like a back rub because some clients dislike physical contact.

The nurse should also consult the client's record for contraindications.

Bathing an infant. An infant can be bathed in much the same way as an adult, either by a sponge bath or in a small tub. However, there are special precautions. Because an infant's temperature control mechanisms are still immature, prolonged exposure of body parts may cause rapid cooling. When giving a bath, the nurse keeps the infant covered as much as possible, and the nurse should work quickly. Bathing a newborn by immersion causes less heat loss and less crying. The infant's thin, sensitive skin requires gentle handling and avoiding substances that might irritate the skin. Care of

Skill 29-2
Providing Perineal Care

Delegation Considerations

Skills of perineal care can be delegated to unlicensed assistive personnel.
- Inform and assist care provider in proper way to position male and female clients.
- Inform care provider about proper positioning of indwelling catheter during perineal care.
- Instruct care provider to inform nurse if any perineal drainage, excoriation, or rash is observed.

Equipment
- Washbasin
- Soap dish with soap
- Two or three washcloths
- Bath towel
- Bath blanket
- Waterproof pad or bedpan
- Toilet tissue or diaper wipes
- Disposable gloves

Additional supplies are needed when pericare is given other than during a bath:
- Cotton balls or swabs
- A solution bottle or container filled with warm water or prescribed rinsing solution
- Waterproof bag

STEPS	RATIONALE
1. Identify clients at risk for developing infection of genitalia, urinary tract, or reproductive tract (e.g., presence of indwelling catheter, fecal incontinence).	Secretions that accumulate on surface of skin surrounding female and male genitalia act as reservoir for infection. Tissues traumatized by surgery or by presence of foreign object provide route for introduction of infectious organisms.
2. Assess client's cognitive and musculoskeletal function.	Determines client's ability to perform self-care and determines level of assistance required from nurse.
3. Assess genitalia for signs of inflammation, skin breakdown, or infection (see Chapter 24).	Determines extent of perineal care required by client.
4. Assess client's knowledge of importance of perineal hygiene.	Clients at risk for infection in perineal area may be unaware of importance of cleanliness. Reflects client's need for education.
5. Explain procedure and its purpose to client.	Helps minimize anxiety during procedure that is often embarrassing to nurse and client.
6. Prepare necessary equipment and supplies.	Used when administering a bed bath.
7. Pull curtain around client's bed, or close room door. Assemble supplies at bedside.	Maintains client's privacy and ensures orderly procedure.
8. Raise bed to comfortable working position. Lower side rail, and assist client in assuming side-lying position, placing towel lengthwise along client's side and keeping client covered with bath blanket.	Facilitates good body mechanics. Provides easy access to genitalia.
9. Apply disposable gloves.	Eliminates transmission of microorganisms.
10. If fecal material is present, enclose in a fold of underpad or toilet tissue, and remove with disposable wipes. Cleanse buttocks and anus, washing front to back (see illustration). Cleanse, rinse, and dry area thoroughly. If needed, place an absorbent pad under client's buttocks. Remove and discard underpad, and replace with clean one.	Cleansing reduces transmission of microorganisms from anus to urethra or genitalia.
11. Change gloves when they are soiled.	

STEPS	RATIONALE
12. Fold top bed linen down toward foot of bed, and raise client's gown above genital area.	Exposes perineal area for easy accessibility.
a. "Diamond" drape client by placing bath blanket with one corner between client's legs, one corner pointing toward each side of bed, and one corner over client's chest. Tuck side corners around client's legs and under hips.	Prevents unnecessary exposure of body parts and maintains client's warmth and comfort during procedure.
b. Raise side rail. Fill washbasin with warm water.	Prevents client from falling. Proper water temperature prevents burns to perineum.
c. Place washbasin and toilet tissue on overbed table. Place washcloths in basin.	Equipment placed within nurse's reach prevents accidental spills.
13. Provide perineal care.	
A. Female perineal care:	
(1) Assist client to dorsal recumbent position.	Provides easy access to genitalia.
(2) Lower side rail, and help client flex knees and spread legs. Note restrictions or limitations in client's positioning.	Provides full exposure of female genitalia. Minimize degree of abduction in female if position causes pain because of arthritis or reduced joint mobility.
(3) Fold lower corner of bath blanket up between client's legs onto abdomen. Wash and dry client's upper thighs.	Minimizes transmission of microorganisms. Keeping client draped until procedure begins minimizes anxiety. Buildup of perineal secretions can soil surrounding skin surfaces.
(4) Wash labia majora. Use nondominant hand to gently retract labia from thigh; with dominant hand, wash carefully in skinfolds. Wipe in direction from perineum to rectum (front to back). Repeat on opposite side using separate section of washcloth. Rinse and dry area thoroughly.	Skinfolds may contain body secretions that harbor microorganisms. Wiping from perineum to rectum (front to back) reduces chance of transmitting fecal organisms to urinary meatus.
(5) Separate labia with nondominant hand to expose urethral meatus and vaginal orifice. With dominant hand, wash downward from pubic area toward rectum in one smooth stroke (see illustration). Use separate section of cloth for each stroke. Cleanse thoroughly around labia minora, clitoris, and vaginal orifice.	Cleansing method reduces transfer of microorganisms to urinary meatus. (For menstruating women or clients with indwelling urinary catheters, cleanse with cotton balls.)

Continued

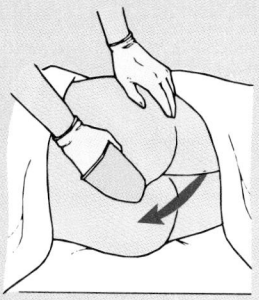

Step 10

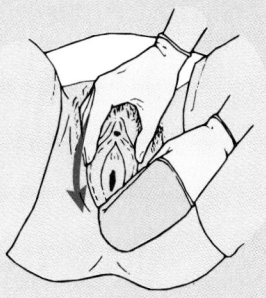

Step 13A(5)

.... **Skill 29-2—cont'd**
Providing Perineal Care

STEPS	RATIONALE
(6) If client uses bedpan, pour warm water over perineal area. Dry perineal area thoroughly, using front-to-back method.	Rinsing removes soap and microorganisms more effectively than wiping. Retained moisture harbors microorganisms.
(7) Fold lower corner of bath blanket back between client's legs and over perineum. Ask client to lower legs and assume comfortable position.	
B. Male perineal care:	
(1) Lower side rails, and assist client to supine position. Note restriction in mobility.	Provides full exposure of male genitalia.
(2) Fold lower corner of bath blanket up between client's legs and onto abdomen. Wash and dry client's upper thighs.	Minimizes transmission of microorganisms. Keeping client draped until procedure begins minimizes anxiety. Buildup of perineal secretions can soil surrounding skin surfaces.
(3) Gently raise penis, and place bath towel underneath. Gently grasp shaft of penis. If client is uncircumcised, retract foreskin. If client has an erection, defer procedure until later.	Towel prevents moisture from collecting in inguinal area. Gentle but firm handling reduces chance of client having an erection. Secretions capable of harboring microorganisms collect underneath foreskin.
(4) Wash tip of penis at urethral meatus first. Using circular motion, cleanse from meatus outward (see illustration). Discard washcloth, and repeat with clean cloth until penis is clean. Rinse and dry gently.	Direction of cleansing moves from area of least contamination to area of most contamination, preventing microorganisms from entering urethra.
(5) Return foreskin to its natural position.	Tightening of foreskin around shaft of penis can cause local edema and discomfort.

CRITICAL DECISION POINT

After administering perineal care, the nurse needs to make sure the foreskin is in its natural position. This is extremely important in those clients with decreased sensation in their lower extremities.

(6) Wash shaft of penis with gentle but firm downward strokes. Pay special attention to underlying surface of penis. Rinse and dry penis thoroughly. Instruct client to spread legs apart slightly.	Vigorous massage of penis can lead to erection, which can embarrass client and nurse. Underlying surface of penis may have greater accumulation of secretions. Abduction of legs provides easier access to scrotal tissues.

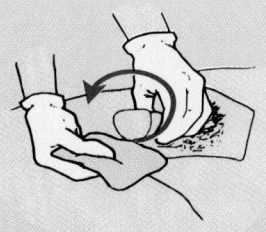

Step 13B(4)

STEPS	RATIONALE
(7) Gently cleanse scrotum. Lift it carefully, and wash underlying skinfolds. Rinse and dry.	Pressure on scrotal tissues can be painful to client. Secretions collect between skinfolds.
(8) Fold bath blanket back over client's perineum, and assist client in turning to side-lying position.	Draping promotes comfort and minimizes client's anxiety. Side-lying position provides access to anal area.
14. If client has had urinary or bowel incontinence, apply thin layer of skin barrier containing petrolatum or zinc oxide over anal and perineal skin.	Protects skin from excess moisture and toxins from urine or stool (Maklebust, 1991).
15. Remove disposable gloves, and dispose in proper receptacle.	Moisture and body secretions on gloves can harbor microorganisms.
16. Assist client in assuming a comfortable position, and cover with sheet.	Client's comfort helps to minimize stress of procedure.
17. Remove bath blanket, and dispose of all soiled bed linen. Return unused equipment to storage area.	Reduces transmission of microorganisms.
18. Inspect surface of external genitalia and surrounding skin after cleansing.	Thick secretions may cover underlying skin lesions or areas of breakdown. Evaluation determines need for additional hygiene.
19. Ask if client feels sense of cleanliness.	Evaluates client's comfort level.
20. Observe for abnormal drainage or discharge from genitalia.	Evaluates presence of infection.

Recording and Reporting

■ Record procedure and presence of any abnormal findings (e.g., character and amount of discharge or condition of genitalia).
■ Record appearance of suture line, if present.
■ Report any break in suture line or presence of abnormalities to nurse in charge or physician.

Home Care Considerations

■ For clients who require bathing, assess perineum at every visit because of the risk for infection and skin breakdown. When appropriate, teach care giver how to make this assessment, and instruct care giver to do this assessment daily.

---

the umbilical cord is a special consideration for the newborn. The neonate must have sponge baths until the cord falls off and the skin heals. Immersing the umbilicus in a tub of water before the skin heals can cause a serious infection. The nurse gives special care to infants who have been circumcised. A small amount of bleeding normally occurs from the penis. The physician applies a sterile gauze dressing with petrolatum jelly around the circumcised area. The nurse instructs the parents to periodically clean the penis with moistened cotton balls until the dressing can be removed permanently (Wong, 1997).

■ Evaluation

The evaluation component for all hygiene activities includes not only actual client care but also how the cli-

ent's expectations were met. Combining both of these aspects of evaluation is important in determining the success or revision of the plan of care.

Client care. During and after bathing and skin care, the nurse evaluates the success of interventions. The process is dynamic because the client's condition may change. The nurse must always be prepared to revise the care plan based on the evaluation. For example, if a client's skin continues to be reddened over the sacrum, more frequent turning may be necessary. Systematic evaluation requires the nurse to determine if expected outcomes have been met.

Client expectations. During assessment the nurse collects data on the client's expectations of care. After hygiene care the nurse needs to determine if the client's expectations were met. For example, this evaluation can be done by asking the client if hygiene preferences were met or if family members were able to assist as desired. In addition, the nurse should ask the client about the care provided, thus determining if the client's expectations were met or whether the client had additional needs.

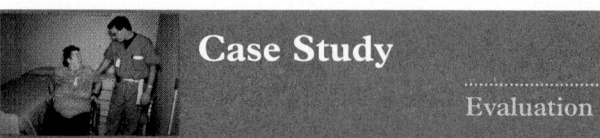

Case Study

Evaluation

James is able to provide Mrs. Foster with a shower and modifies her plan of care to include a shower every other day. Mrs. Foster tells James that she really appreciates having more frequent showers and that they really help her feel and do her best. Although Mrs. Foster is very tired and needs a rest period after the shower, she feels it is worth it. Mrs. Foster knows that James provides the extra effort to her care and the subsequent modification of the care plan, and she is happy and feels somewhat in control of her care.

Documentation Note

Assisted Mrs. Foster in a shower. Nursing care plan was modified to include shower every other day followed by a 30-minute rest period. Physical and occupational therapy times were moved to accommodate shower and rest periods. Mrs. Foster went to the dining room for lunch.

⋯NURSING PROCESS FOR CARE OF THE FEET AND NAILS

Foot care can be incorporated into the client's daily hygiene routine. Often people are unaware of foot or nail problems until pain or discomfort occurs. Problems can result from abuse or poor care of the feet and hands, such as biting nails or trimming them improperly, exposure to harsh chemicals, and wearing poorly fitting shoes.

■ Assessment

The nurse assesses clients for nail and foot problems by reviewing developmental factors contributing to alterations, determining the client's type of footwear, and assessing hygiene care practices. The nurse inspects the condition of the nails and looks for lesions, dryness, inflammation, or cracking (Table 29-3).

■ Nursing Diagnosis

After a thorough assessment, the nurse gathers and clusters all defining characteristics of specific foot and nail problems. These may include the presence or absence of discomfort or pain, swelling, lesion formation, changes in mobility, or altered circulation. The nurse selects the appropriate nursing diagnosis based on these factors (see nursing diagnoses box).

The related factors help the nurse to plan care for the client. For the diagnosis *impaired skin integrity related to improper nail-cutting practices,* the nurse designs interventions to evaluate the client's nail-cutting technique and foot care practices. In contrast, *impaired skin integrity related to friction of shoes* requires the nurse to

TABLE 29-3
Common Foot and Nail Problems

Condition	Characteristics	Implications	Interventions
Callus	Thickened portion of epidermis, consisting of mass of horny, keratotic cells; usually flat, painless, and found on undersurface of foot or on palm of hand; caused by local friction or pressure.	Foot calluses may cause discomfort when wearing tight-fitting shoes.	Wear gloves when using tools or objects that may create friction on palms. Wear comfortable shoes. Soak callus in warm water and Epsom salts to soften cell layers (soaking of feet is contraindicated with diabetic clients). Use pumice stone to remove callus after it softens. Applications of creams or lotions can reduce re-formation. Use of orthotic devices (e.g., foam insoles, metatarsal pads, various cushioning devices) redistributes weight and pressure away from callus area.

TABLE 29-3

Common Foot and Nail Problems—cont'd

Condition	Characteristics	Implications	Interventions
Corns	Keratosis caused by friction and pressure from shoes; mainly on toes, over bony prominence; usually cone shaped, round, and raised. Calluses with painful core.	Conical shape compresses underlying dermis, making it thin and tender. Pain is aggravated by tight-fitting shoes. Tissue can become attached to bone if allowed to grow. Client may suffer alteration in gait because of pain.	Surgical removal may be necessary, depending on severity of pain and size of corn. Use oval corn pads carefully, since they increase pressure on toes and reduce circulation.
Plantar warts	Fungating lesion that appears on sole of foot; caused by papillomavirus.	Warts may be contagious, are painful, and make walking difficult.	Treatment ordered by physician may include topical applications to acids, electrodesiccation (burning with electric spark), cryotherapy (freezing) with carbon dioxide or liquid nitrogen, or laser therapy (Osterman and Stuck, 1990).
Athlete's foot (tinea pedis)	Fungal infection of foot; scaliness and cracking of skin between toes and on soles of feet; small blisters containing fluid may appear, apparently induced by constricting footwear (e.g., sneakers).	Athlete's foot can spread to other body parts, especially hands. It is contagious and frequently recurs.	Feet should be well ventilated. Drying feet well after bathing and applying powder help prevent infection. Wearing clean socks or stockings reduces incidence. Physician may order application of griseofulvin, miconazole nitrate, or tolnaftate.
Ingrown nails	Toenail or fingernail growing inward into soft tissue around nail; results from improper nail trimming, poor shoe fit, or heredity.	Ingrown nails can cause localized pain when pressure is applied.	Treatment is frequent hot soaks in antiseptic solution and removal of portion of nail that has grown into skin. Instruct client on proper nail trimming techniques. Professional podiatry may be needed.
Ram's horn nails	Unusually long curved nails.	Attempt by nurse to cut nails may damage nail bed and/or cause infection.	Refer client to podiatrist.
Paronychia	Inflammation of tissue surrounding nail after hangnail or other injury; occurs in people who frequently have their hands in water; common in diabetic clients.	Area can become infected.	Treatment is hot compresses or soaks and local application of antibiotic ointments. Paronychia can be prevented by careful manicuring.
Foot odors	Result of excess perspiration promoting microorganism growth. Faulty foot hygiene or improper footwear may also contribute.		Frequent washing, use of foot deodorants and powders, and clean footwear will prevent or reduce this problem.

NURSING DIAGNOSES FOR FOOT AND NAIL PROBLEMS

Infection, risk for
Knowledge deficit regarding foot/nail care
Mobility, impaired physical
Pain
Self-care deficit, bathing/hygiene
Skin integrity, impaired
Skin integrity, impaired, risk for

take a different approach. The nurse should assess the type, size, and quality of shoes worn, observe the client while walking, and make recommendations to reduce any source of friction. Effective nursing care and appropriate nursing interventions result from selecting the correct related factors for a nursing diagnosis.

Planning

The nurse may provide foot and nail care during the bed bath or at another time according to the client's preference. Many home health nurses visit clients at home to provide foot and nail care. Some foot and nail care problems are too complex for nursing intervention and require consultation with a podiatrist.

Implementation

Health promotion and restorative care. For proper foot and nail care, clients should be instructed to protect the feet from injury, keep the feet clean and dry, and wear footwear that fits properly. The nurse can also help the client learn the proper way to inspect the feet for lesions, dryness, or signs of infection. Any of these conditions should be reported to the nurse. Finally, to maintain and promote foot and nail health, clients should visit a podiatrist when necessary.

Foot and nail care involves soaking to soften cuticles and layers of horny cells, thorough cleansing, drying, and proper nail trimming. The nurse may provide the care in bed for an immobilized client or have the client sit in a chair (Skill 29-3). The nurse must take time during the procedure to teach the client proper techniques for cleaning and nail trimming. Measures to prevent infection and promote good circulation should be stressed.

A client with diabetes or peripheral vascular disease is at risk for foot and nail problems because of impaired circulation (Christensen and others, 1991). Although ongoing good foot care can help prevent toe amputation, studies have shown that many clients have not learned proper care. The nurse instructs clients on the following precautions during foot and nail care:

1. Wash the feet daily using lukewarm water; **do not soak.** Thoroughly pat the feet dry, and dry well between the toes.
2. Do not cut corns or calluses or use commercial removers. Consult a physician or podiatrist.
3. If the feet perspire, apply a bland foot powder.
4. If dryness is noted along the feet or between the toes, apply lanolin, baby oil, or even corn oil, and rub gently into the skin.
5. File the toenails straight across and square; do not use scissors or clippers. Consult a podiatrist as needed.
6. Do not use over-the-counter preparations to treat athlete's foot or ingrown toenails. Consult a physician or podiatrist.
7. Avoid wearing elastic stockings, knee-high hose, or constricting garters. Do not cross the legs. Both impair circulation to the lower extremities.
8. Inspect the feet daily, including tops and soles of the feet, heels, and the area between the toes. Use a mirror to inspect all surfaces.
9. Wear clean socks or stockings daily. Socks should be dry and free of holes or darns that might cause pressure.
10. Do not walk barefoot.
11. Wear shoes that fit properly. Soles of shoes should be flexible and should not slip. Lamb's wool can be used between toes that rub or overlap. Shoes should be sturdy, closed in, and not restrictive.
12. Exercise regularly to improve circulation to the lower extremities. Walk slowly, elevate, rotate, flex, and extend the feet at the ankle. Dangle the feet over the side of the bed 1 minute, then extend both legs and hold them parallel to the bed while lying supine for 1 minute, and finally rest 1 minute.
13. Avoid applying hot-water bottles or heating pads to the feet; use extra coverings instead.
14. Minor cuts should be washed immediately and dried thoroughly. Only mild antiseptics (e.g., Neosporin ointment) should be applied to the skin. Avoid iodine or Mercurochrome. Contact a physician to treat cuts or lacerations.

Evaluation

A client's response to nail and foot care is best evaluated over several days. Existing medical problems may take time to improve. Evaluation based on expected outcomes requires the nurse to determine the success of the interventions. Based on evaluative findings, the nurse must be prepared to revise the care plan. For example, if the client continues to have discomfort while walking, a different style of footwear may be needed. The nurse also instructs the client about ways to evaluate nail and foot care practices to prevent further problems.

Performing Nail and Foot Care

Delegation Considerations

The skill of nail and foot care of the nondiabetic client can be delegated to unlicensed assistive personnel. If the client is diabetic, this skill should not be delegated to unlicensed personnel.

- Inform and assist care provider in proper way to use nail clippers.
- Instruct care provider to report immediately any cuts in skin.

Equipment

- Washbasin
- Emesis basin
- Washcloth
- Bath or face towel
- Nail clippers
- Orange stick
- Emery board or nail file
- Body lotion
- Disposable bath mat
- Paper towels
- Disposable gloves

STEPS	RATIONALE
1. Inspect all surfaces of fingers, toes, feet, and nails. Pay particular attention to areas of dryness, inflammation, or cracking. Also inspect areas between toes, heels, and soles of feet.	Integrity of feet and nails determines frequency and level of hygiene required. Heels, soles, and sides of feet are prone to irritation from ill-fitting shoes.
2. Assess color and temperature of toes, feet, and fingers. Assess capillary refill of nails. Palpate radial and ulnar pulse of each hand and dorsalis pedis pulse of foot; note character of pulses.	Assesses adequacy of blood flow to extremities. Circulatory alterations may change integrity of nails and increase client's chance of localized infection when break in skin integrity occurs.
3. Observe client's walking gait. Have client walk down hall or walk straight line (if able).	Painful disorders of feet can cause limping or unnatural gait.
4. Ask female clients about whether they use nail polish and polish remover frequently.	Chemicals in these products can cause excessive dryness.
5. Assess type of footwear worn by clients: Are socks worn? Are shoes tight or ill fitting? Are garters or knee-high nylons worn? Is footwear clean?	Types of shoes and footwear may predispose client to foot and nail problems (e.g., infection, areas of friction, ulcerations).
6. Identify client's risk for foot or nail problems:	Certain conditions increase likelihood of foot or nail problems.
a. Older adult	Poor vision, lack of coordination, or inability to bend over contributes to difficulty in performing foot and nail care. Normal physiological changes of aging also result in nail and foot problems.
b. Diabetes	Vascular changes associated with diabetes reduce blood flow to peripheral tissues. Break in skin integrity places diabetic at high risk for skin infection.
c. Heart failure, renal disease	Both conditions can increase tissue edema, particularly in dependent areas (e.g., feet). Edema reduces blood flow to neighboring tissues.
d. Cerebrovascular accident, stroke	Presence of residual foot or leg weakness or paralysis results in altered walking patterns. Altered gait pattern causes increased friction and pressure on feet.
7. Assess type of home remedies client uses for existing foot problems:	Certain preparations or applications may cause more injury to soft tissue than initial foot problem.
a. Over-the-counter liquid preparations to remove corns	Liquid preparations can cause burns and ulcerations.
b. Cutting of corns or calluses with razor blade or scissors	Cutting of corns or calluses may result in infection caused by break in skin integrity.

Continued

Performing Nail and Foot Care

STEPS	RATIONALE
c. Use of oval corn pads	Oval pads may exert pressure on toes, thereby decreasing circulation to surrounding tissues.
d. Application of adhesive tape	Skin of older adult is thin and delicate and prone to tearing when adhesive tape is removed.
8. Assess client's ability to care for nails or feet: visual alterations, fatigue, musculoskeletal weakness.	Determines client's ability to perform self-care and degree of assistance required from nurse.
9. Assess client's knowledge of foot and nail care practices.	Determines client's need for health teaching.

CRITICAL DECISION POINT

Diabetic clients should not soak hands and feet.

STEPS	RATIONALE
10. Explain procedure to client, including fact that proper soaking requires several minutes.	Client must be willing to place fingers and feet in basins for 10 to 20 minutes. Client may become anxious or fatigued.
11. Obtain physician's order for cutting nails if agency policy requires it.	Client's skin may be accidentally cut. Certain clients are more at risk for infection, depending on their medical condition.
12. Wash hands. Arrange equipment on overbed table.	Easy access to equipment prevents delays.
13. Pull curtain around bed or close room door (if desired).	Maintaining client's privacy reduces anxiety.
14. Assist ambulatory client to sit in bedside chair. Help bed-bound client to supine position with head of bed elevated. Place disposable bath mat on floor under client's feet or place towel on mattress.	Sitting in chair facilitates immersing feet in basin. Bath mat protects feet from exposure to soil or debris.
15. Fill washbasin with warm water. Test water temperature.	Warm water softens nails and thickened epidermal cells, reduces inflammation of skin, and promotes local circulation. Proper water temperature prevents burns.
16. Place basin on bath mat or towel, and help client place feet in basin. Place call light within client's reach.	Clients with muscular weakness or tremors may have difficulty positioning feet. Client's safety is maintained.
17. Adjust overbed table to low position, and place it over client's lap. (Client may sit in chair or lie in bed.)	Easy access prevents accidental spills.
18. Fill emesis basin with warm water, and place basin on paper towels on overbed table.	Warm water softens nails and thickened epidermal cells.
19. Instruct client to place fingers in emesis basin and place arms in comfortable position.	Prolonged positioning can cause discomfort unless normal anatomical alignment is maintained.
20. Allow client's feet and fingernails to soak for 10 to 20 minutes. Rewarm after 10 minutes.	Softening of corns, calluses, and cuticles ensures easy removal of dead cells and easy manipulation of cuticle.
21. Clean gently under fingernails with orange stick while fingers are immersed (see illustration). Remove emesis basin, and dry fingers thoroughly.	Orange stick removes debris under nails that harbors microorganisms. Thorough drying impedes fungal growth and prevents maceration of tissues.
22. With nail clippers, clip fingernails straight across and even with tops of fingers (see illustration). Shape nails with emery board or file. If client has circulatory problems, do not cut nail; file the nail only.	Cutting straight across prevents splitting of nail margins and formation of sharp nail spikes that can irritate lateral nail margins. Filing prevents cutting nail too close to nail bed.

STEPS	RATIONALE
23. Push cuticle back gently with orange stick.	Reduces incidence of inflamed cuticles.
24. Move overbed table away from client.	Provides easier access to feet.
25. Put on disposable gloves, and scrub callused areas of feet with washcloth.	Gloves prevent transmission of fungal infection. Friction removes dead skin layers.
26. Clean gently under nails with orange stick. Remove feet from basin, and dry thoroughly.	Removal of debris and excess moisture reduces chances of infection.
27. Clean and trim toenails using procedures in steps 21 and 22. Do not file corners of toenails.	Shaping corners of toenails may damage tissues.
28. Apply lotion to feet and hands, and assist client back to bed and into comfortable position.	Lotion lubricates dry skin by helping to retain moisture.
29. Remove disposable gloves, and place in receptacle. Clean and return equipment and supplies to proper place. Dispose of soiled linen in hamper. Wash hands.	Reduces transmission of infection.
30. Inspect nails and surrounding skin surfaces after soaking and nail trimming.	Evaluates condition of skin and nails. Allows nurse to note any remaining rough nail edges.
31. Ask client to explain or demonstrate nail care.	Evaluates client's level of learning techniques.
32. Observe client's walk after toenail care.	Evaluates level of comfort and mobility achieved.
33. Record procedure and observations (e.g., breaks in skin, inflammation, ulcerations).	Documents procedure, client's response, and presence of abnormalities requiring additional therapy.
34. Report any breaks in skin or ulcerations to nurse in charge or physician.	These abnormalities can seriously increase client's risk of infection and must be carefully observed.

Recording and Reporting

- Record procedure and observations (e.g., breaks in skin, inflammation, ulcerations).
- Report any breaks in skin or ulcerations to nurse in charge or physician. These are serious in client with peripheral vascular illnesses and illnesses in which client's circulation is impaired. Special foot care treatments may be needed.

Home Care Considerations

- Alternative therapies: moleskin applied to areas of feet that are under friction is less likely to cause pressure than corn pads; spot adhesive bandages can guard against friction, but they do not have padding to protect against pressure; wrapping small pieces of lamb's wool around toes reduces irritation of soft corns between toes.
- If client is ambulatory, instruct to soak feet in bathtub. When client's mobility is limited, a large basin or pan can be used.

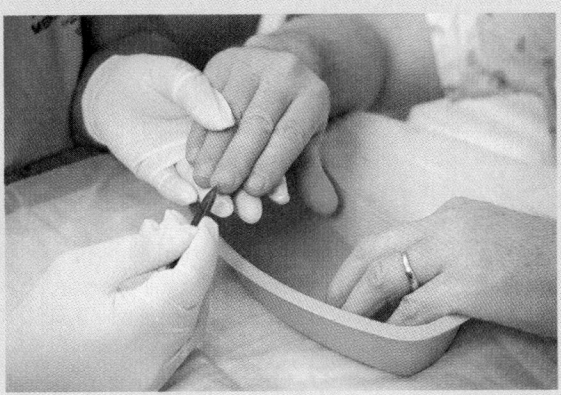

Step 21

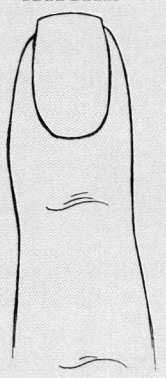

Step 22

NURSING PROCESS FOR ORAL HYGIENE

Oral hygiene helps to maintain the healthy state of the mouth, teeth, gums, and lips. Brushing cleans the teeth of food particles, plaque, and bacteria. It also massages the gums and relieves discomfort resulting from unpleasant odors and tastes. Complete oral hygiene enhances well-being and stimulates the appetite. The nurse's responsibilities in oral hygiene are maintenance and prevention. The nurse can help clients to maintain good oral hygiene by teaching correct techniques or by performing hygiene for weakened or disabled clients.

Assessment

A thorough assessment for problems related to oral hygiene should be included in every client's care (Table 29-4). During the assessment the nurse can inform the client about good oral hygiene habits. The nurse may also refer the client to a specialist if common oral problems are found (see Box 29-3). Early identification of poor oral hygiene practices and common oral problems can reduce the risk of gum disease and **dental caries** or cavities.

Nursing Diagnosis

The nurse's assessment can reveal if the client is at risk for or has an actual alteration in oral integrity. These findings may also indicate the client's need for assistance with oral hygiene care. The nurse clusters all defining characteristics to select appropriate nursing diagnoses for the client's problems (see nursing diagnoses box).

The nurse should carefully select a nursing diagnosis appropriate for the related factors displayed by the

---

Box 29-3
Common Oral Problems

Dental Caries (Cavities)
Caries are most common among young people.
Buildup of plaque causes acid destruction of tooth enamel. Initially appears as chalky, white discoloration of the tooth.

Periodontal Disease (Pyorrhea)
Periodontal disease is most common after age 35.
It involves destruction of gingiva (gums) and other supporting structures with bleeding gums, inflammation, and receding gum lines.

Other Problems
Stomatitis (inflammation of the mouth)
Glossitis (inflammation of the tongue)
Gingivitis (inflammation of the gums)
Halitosis (bad breath)
Cheilosis (cracked lips)
Oral malignancy (mouth lumps or ulcers)

TABLE 29-4
Risk Factors for Oral Problems

Type of Client	Risk Factors
Clients who are paralyzed, seriously ill, or have physical restrictions to upper extremities (e.g., cast or dressing)	Client lacks upper extremity strength or dexterity needed to perform oral hygiene (Phipps, 1995).
Unconscious, confused, combative, or depressed clients	Client is unable or unwilling to attend to personal hygiene needs.
Diabetic clients	Client is prone to dryness of mouth, gingivitis, periodontal disease, and loss of teeeth (Phipps, 1995).
Clients who cannot take anything by mouth or are on fluid restrictions, have nasogastric tubes, receive continuous nasal oxygen, or are mouth-breathers	Client is prone to dehydration and drying of mucous membranes. Thick secretions develop on tongue and gums. Lips become cracked and reddened.
Clients undergoing radiation therapy	Radiation therapy causes soreness, mild erythema, swollen mucosa, dysphagia, dryness, taste changes, and possible oral infection.
Clients receiving chemotherapeutic drugs	Chemotherapeutic drugs cause ulcerations and inflammation of mucosa and possible oral infection.
Clients experiencing oral surgery, trauma to mouth, placement of oral endotracheal tubes or airways	Tissues in oral cavity become traumatized with swelling, ulcerations, inflammation, and possible bleeding.
Clients with immunosuppression (e.g., HIV, organ transplantation)	Immunosuppression and immunosuppressant drugs may increase risk for oral infection.

> ### NURSING DIAGNOSES FOR ORAL HYGIENE PROBLEMS
>
> Body image distrubance
> Infection, risk for
> Knowledge deficit regarding oral hygiene
> Nutrition, altered: less than body requirements
> Oral mucous membrane, altered
> Pain
> Self-care deficit, bathing/hygiene

client. Selection influences the choice of nursing interventions. For example, for the diagnosis *altered oral mucous membrane related to trauma,* the nurse must design therapies to prevent further mucosal injury. Special rinses, suctioning, and nutritional support may be ordered. In contrast, *altered mucous membrane related to ineffective oral hygiene* requires the nurse to take a different approach. Observing the client brushing and flossing, teaching good oral care practices, and helping the client to select the proper oral care equipment can assist the client to improve oral hygiene.

Planning

Developing a care plan for maintaining oral hygiene involves considering the client's personal preferences and physical and emotional status. The nurse must establish a good relationship with the client to assist with oral hygiene. Some clients are sensitive about the condition of their mouth and are reluctant to let someone else administer oral hygiene care. In many cases clients are also unaware they are at risk for serious dental and periodontal disease and thus need instruction.

Implementation

Good oral hygiene involves cleanliness, comfort, and the moisturizing of mouth structures. Proper care will prevent oral disease. Unfortunately, clients in hospitals or long-term care facilities often do not receive the aggressive care they need. Oral care must be provided on a regular basis.

Health promotion and restorative care.
To encourage health promotion and restoration, the nurse should instruct clients to brush their teeth after each meal and before bedtime and to floss once daily. Clients should also reduce their intake of carbohydrates, especially sweet snacks. Acidic fruits in the client's diet can reduce plaque formation. All clients should visit a dentist regularly every 6 months for checkups.

Diet. To prevent tooth decay, clients may have to change eating habits (e.g., reducing intake of carbohydrates, especially sweet snacks between meals). A well-balanced diet ensures the integrity of oral tissues.

Brushing. Thorough toothbrushing at least 4 times a day (after meals and at bedtime) is basic to an effective oral hygiene program. A toothbrush should have a straight handle and brush small enough to reach all areas of the mouth. Older adult clients with reduced dexterity and grip may require an enlarged handle with an easier grip.

Clients who receive cancer chemotherapy, radiation, or immunosuppression agents may develop stomatitis and may require certain modifications to oral care. These modifications reduce the discomfort of stomatitis (Skill 29-4).

All tooth surfaces should be brushed thoroughly. Commercially made foam rubber toothbrushes are useful for clients with sensitive gums. Electric toothbrushes can be used, but the nurse must check for electrical hazards. Lemon-glycerin sponges should be avoided because they dry mucous membranes and erode tooth enamel. Moi-Stin is a salivary supplement that improves moisture and texture of the tongue and mucosa.

When teaching clients about mouth care, the nurse should recommend they do not share toothbrushes with family members or drink directly from a bottle of mouthwash. Cross-contamination occurs easily. The amount of assistance needed by the client when brushing the teeth may vary (see Skill 29-4).

Unconscious clients need special attention. While providing hygiene to an unconscious client, the nurse must protect the client from choking and aspirating. The safest technique is to have two nurses provide the care. One does the actual cleaning, and the other removes secretions with suction equipment. While cleansing the oral cavity, the nurse should never use fingers to hold the mouth open. A human bite is highly contaminated. It may be necessary to perform mouth care at least every 2 hours. The nurse explains the steps of mouth care and the sensations the client will feel. The nurse also tells the client when the procedure is completed (Skill 29-5).

Flossing. Dental flossing is necessary to remove plaque and tartar between teeth. Flossing involves inserting waxed or unwaxed dental floss between all tooth surfaces, one at a time. The seesaw motion used to pull floss between teeth removes plaque and tartar from tooth enamel. If toothpaste is applied to the teeth before flossing, fluoride can come in direct contact with tooth surfaces, aiding in cavity prevention. Flossing once a day is sufficient. Because it is important to clean all teeth surfaces thoroughly, the nurse should not rush to complete flossing. Placing a mirror in front of the client will help the nurse to demonstrate the proper methods for holding the floss and cleaning between the teeth.

Denture care.
Clients should be encouraged to clean their dentures on a regular basis to avoid gingival infection and irritation. When clients become disabled,

Providing Oral Hygiene

Delegation Considerations
Skills of brushing teeth can be delegated to unlicensed assistive personnel.
- Inform and assist care provider in proper way to provide toothbrushing.
- Instruct care provider on how to recognize impaired integrity of oral mucosa.

Equipment
- Soft-bristled toothbrush
- Nonabrasive fluoride toothpaste or dentifrice
- Dental floss
- Water glass with cool water
- Normal saline or fluoride mouthwash (optional; follow client's preference)
- Emesis basin
- Face towel
- Paper towels
- Disposable gloves

STEPS	RATIONALE
1. Wash hands and apply disposable gloves.	Reduces transmission of microorganisms. Gloves prevent contact with microorganisms in blood or saliva.
2. Inspect integrity of lips, teeth, buccal mucosa, gums, palate, and tongue (see Chapter 24).	Determines status of client's oral cavity and extent of need for oral hygiene.
3. Identify presence of common oral problems: a. Dental caries—chalky white discoloration of tooth or presence of brown or black discoloration b. Gingivitis—inflammation of gums c. Periodontitis—receding gum lines, inflammation, gaps between teeth d. Halitosis—bad breath e. Cheilosis—cracking of lips f. Stomatitis—inflammation of the mouth	Helps determine type of hygiene client requires and information client requires for self-care.
4. Remove gloves and wash hands.	Prevents spread of microorganisms.
5. Assess risk for oral hygiene problems:	Certain conditions increase likelihood of impaired oral cavity integrity and need for preventive care.
a. Dehydration, inability to take fluids or food by mouth (NPO)	Causes excess drying and fragility of mucous membranes; increases accumulation of secretions on tongue and gums.
b. Presence of nasogastric or oxygen tubes; mouth breathers	Causes drying of mucosa (Harrell and Damon, 1989).
c. Chemotherapeutic drugs	These drugs kill rapidly multiplying cells, including cancerous tumors and cells lining oral cavity and gastrointestinal tract. Drug effects can lead to stomatitis (Dudjak, 1987).
d. Calcium channel blockers, dilantin, some amphetamines used to treat hyperactivity in children, and cyclosporine used by organ transplant recipients.	Produces gum overgrowth.
e. Over-the-counter lozenges, cough drops, antacids, and chewable vitamins.	Medications contain large amounts of sugar. Repeated daily use increases sugar or acid content in mouth.
f. Radiation therapy to head and neck	Reduces salivary flow and lowers pH of saliva; can lead to stomatitis and tooth decay (Danielson, 1988).
g. Presence of artificial airway	Increases irritation to gums and mucosa. Excess secretions accumulate on teeth and tongue.
h. Blood-clotting disorders (e.g., leukemia, aplastic anemia)	Predisposes to inflammation and bleeding of gums.
i. Oral surgery, trauma to mouth	Break in mucosa increases risk of infection. Vigorous brushing can disrupt suture lines.

STEPS	RATIONALE

    j. Aging

    k. Diabetes mellitus

    Prone to dryness of mouth, gingivitis, periodontal disease, and loss of teeth.

6. Determine client's oral hygiene practices:

    a. Frequency of toothbrushing and flossing

    b. Type of toothpaste or dentifrice used

    c. Last dental visit

    d. Frequency of dental visits

    e. Type of mouthwash or moistening preparation

    Allows nurse to identify errors in technique, deficiencies in preventive oral hygiene, and client's level of knowledge regarding dental care.

    Lemon-glycerin preparations can be detrimental. Glycerin is an astringent that dries and shrinks mucous membranes and gums. Lemon exhausts salivary reflex and can erode tooth enamel (Poland, 1987). Mouthwash provides pleasant aftertaste but can dry mucosa after extended use if it has an alcohol base (Blaney, 1986).

7. Asseses client's ability to grasp and manipulate toothbrush. Assessment determines level of assistance required from nurse.

    Older adult clients or persons with musculoskeletal or nervous system alterations may be unable to hold toothbrush with firm grip or manipulate brush.

8. Prepare equipment at bedside.

9. Explain procedure to client and discuss preferences regarding use of hygiene aids.

    Some clients feel uncomfortable about having the nurse care for their basic needs. Client involvement with procedure minimizes anxiety.

10. Place paper towels on overbed table, and arrange other equipment within easy reach.

11. Raise bed to comfortable working position. Raise head of bed (if allowed) and lower side rail. Move client, or help client move closer. Side-lying position can be used.

    Raising bed and positioning client prevent nurse from straining muscles. Semi-Fowler's position helps prevent client from choking or aspirating.

12. Place towel over client's chest.

13. Apply gloves.

    Prevents contact with microorganisms or blood in saliva.

14. Apply toothpaste to brush, holding brush over emesis basin. Pour small amount of water over toothpaste.

    Moisture aids in distribution of toothpaste over tooth surfaces.

15. Client may assist by brushing. Hold toothbrush bristles at 45-degree angle to gum line (see illustration). Be sure tips of bristles rest against and penetrate under gum line. Brush inner and outer surfaces of upper and lower teeth by brushing from gum to crown of each tooth. Clean biting surfaces of teeth by holding top of bristles parallel with teeth and brushing gently back and forth (see illustration). Brush sides of teeth by moving bristles back and forth (see illustration).

    Angle allows brush to reach all tooth surfaces and to clean under gum line where plaque and tartar accumulate. Back-and-forth motion dislodges food particles caught between teeth and along chewing surfaces.

Continued

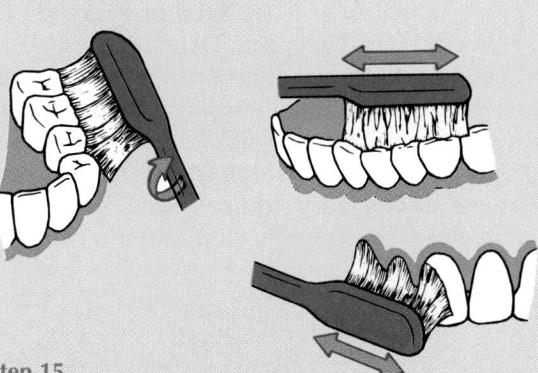

Step 15

.... **Skill 29-4—cont'd**

Providing Oral Hygiene

STEPS	RATIONALE
16. Have client hold brush at 45-degree angle and lightly brush over surface and sides of tongue. Avoid initiating gag reflex.	Microorganisms collect and grow on tongue's surface and contribute to bad breath. Gagging may cause aspiration of toothpaste.
17. Allow client to rinse mouth thoroughly by taking several sips of water, swishing water across all tooth surfaces, and spitting into emesis basin.	Irrigation removes food particles.
18. Allow client to gargle to rinse mouth with mouthwash as desired.	Mouthwash leaves pleasant taste in mouth.
19. Assist in wiping client's mouth.	Promotes sense of comfort.
20. Allow client to floss.	Reduces tartar on tooth surfaces.
21. Allow client to rinse mouth thoroughly with cool water and spit into emesis basin. Assist in wiping client's mouth.	Irrigation removes plaque and tartar from oral cavity.
22. Assist client to comfortable position, remove emesis basin and bedside table, raise side rail, and lower bed to original position.	Provides for client comfort and safety.
23. Wipe off overbed table, discard soiled linen and paper towels in appropriate containers, remove soiled gloves, and return equipment to proper place.	Proper disposal of soiled equipment prevents spread of infection.
24. Wash hands.	Reduces transmission of microorganisms.
25. Ask client if any area of oral cavity feels uncomfortable or irritated.	Pain indicates more chronic problem.
26. Apply gloves and inspect condition of oral cavity.	Determines effectiveness of hygiene and rinsing.
27. Ask client to describe proper hygiene techniques.	Evaluates client's learning.
28. Observe client brushing.	Evaluates client's ability to use correct technique.

Recording and Reporting

▪ Record procedure on flow sheet. Note condition of oral cavity in nurses' notes.
▪ Report bleeding or presence of lesions to nurse in charge or physician.

Home Care Considerations

▪ Assess oral cavity at each visit to determine the effects of medications on the structures of the oral cavity.

the nurse or care giver must assume responsibility for denture care (Box 29-4). Dentures are the client's personal property and need to be handled with care because they can be easily broken. Dentures must be removed at night to give the gums a rest and prevent bacterial buildup. To prevent warping, dentures should be kept covered in water when they are not worn, and they should always be stored in an enclosed, labeled cup with the cup placed in the client's bedside stand. Discourage clients from removing their dentures and placing them on a napkin or tissue because they could be easily thrown away.

■ Evaluation

The expected outcomes of oral hygiene may not be seen for several days. Repeated cleansing is often needed to remove thick encrustations on the tongue and to restore the mucosa's normal hydration. The nurse evaluates the success of interventions to maintain mucosa integrity or to prevent further injury to the oral mucosa. The care plan is designed to be changed when the client's condition changes. If interventions are not successful, the nurse may have to initiate more aggressive actions. For instance, it will take weeks of rigorous hygiene to reduce the incidence of dental caries.

Performing Mouth Care for an Unconscious or Debilitated Client

Delegation Considerations

Skills of brushing teeth of an unconscious or debilitated client can be delegated to unlicensed assistive personnel.

- After checking for gag reflex, inform care provider in proper way to position clients for mouth care.
- Instruct care provider on how to use the oral suction catheter for clearing oral secretions.
- Instruct care provider on how to recognize impaired integrity of oral mucosa.

Equipment

- Antiinfective solution (e.g., diluted hydrogen peroxide) that loosens crusts
- Small soft-bristled toothbrush
- Sponge toothette or tongue blade wrapped in single layer of gauze
- Padded tongue blade
- Face towel
- Paper towels
- Emesis basin
- Water glass with cool water
- Water-soluble lip lubricant
- Small-bulb syringe (optional)
- Suction machine equipment (optional)
- Disposable gloves

STEPS	RATIONALE
1. Wash hands. Apply disposable gloves.	Reduces transmission of microorganisms. Gloves prevent contact with microorganisms in blood or saliva.
2. Test for presence of gag reflex by placing blade on back half of tongue.	Reveals whether client is at risk for aspiration.

CRITICAL DECISION POINT

Clients with impaired gag reflex require oral care as well. The nurse must determine the type of suction apparatus needed at the bedside to protect the client's airway against aspiration.

STEPS	RATIONALE
3. Inspect condition of oral cavity (see Chapter 24).	Determines condition of oral cavity and need for hygiene.
4. Remove gloves. Wash hands.	Prevents spread of infection.
5. Assess client's risk for oral hygiene problems (see Skill 29-4).	Certain conditions increase likelihood of alterations in integrity of oral cavity structures and may require more frequent care.
6. Position client on side (Sims' position) with head turned well toward dependent side and head of bed lowered. Raise side rail.	Allows secretions to drain from mouth instead of collecting in back of pharynx. Prevents aspiration.
7. Explain procedure to client.	Allows debilitated client to anticipate procedure without anxiety. Unconscious client may retain ability to hear.
8. Wash hands, and apply disposable gloves.	Reduces transfer of microorganisms.
9. Place paper towels on overbed table and arrange equipment. If needed, turn on suction machine, and connect tubing to suction catheter.	Prevents soiling of table top. Equipment prepared in advance ensures smooth, safe procedure.
10. Pull curtain around bed, or close room door.	Provides privacy.
11. Raise bed to its highest horizontal level; lower side rail.	Use of good body mechanics with bed in high position prevents injury.
12. Position client close to side of bed; turn client's head toward mattress.	Proper positioning of head prevents aspiration.

Continued

· · · · · · · · Skill 29-5—cont'd
Performing Mouth Care for an Unconscious or Debilitated Client

STEPS	RATIONALE
13. Place towel under client's head and emesis basin under chin.	Prevents soiling of bed linen.
14. Carefully separate upper and lower teeth with padded tongue blade by inserting blade, quickly but gently, between back molars. Insert when client is relaxed, if possible. Do not use force (see illustration).	Prevents client from biting down on nurse's fingers and provides access to oral cavity.

CRITICAL DECISION POINT

Never use fingers to separate client's teeth.

STEPS	RATIONALE
15. Clean mouth using brush or sponge toothettes moistened with peroxide and water. Clean chewing and inner tooth surfaces first. Clean outer tooth surfaces. Swab roof of mouth, gums, and inside cheeks. Gently swab or brush tongue but avoid stimulating gag reflex (if present). Moisten clean swab or toothette with water to rinse. (Bulb syringe may also be used to rinse.) Repeat rinse several times.	Brushing action removes food particles between teeth and along chewing surfaces. Swabbing helps remove secretions and crusts from mucosa and moistens mucosa. Repeated rinsing removes peroxide that can be irritating to mucosa.
16. Suction secretions as they accumulate, if necessary.	Suction removes secretions and fluid that can collect in posterior pharynx.
17. Apply thin layer of water-soluble jelly to lips (see illustration).	Lubricates lips to prevent drying and cracking.
18. Inform client that procedure is completed.	Provides meaningful stimulation to unconscious or less responsive client.
19. Remove gloves, and dispose in proper receptacle.	Prevents transmission of microorganisms.
20. Reposition client comfortably, raise side rail, and return bed to original position.	Maintains client's comfort and safety.

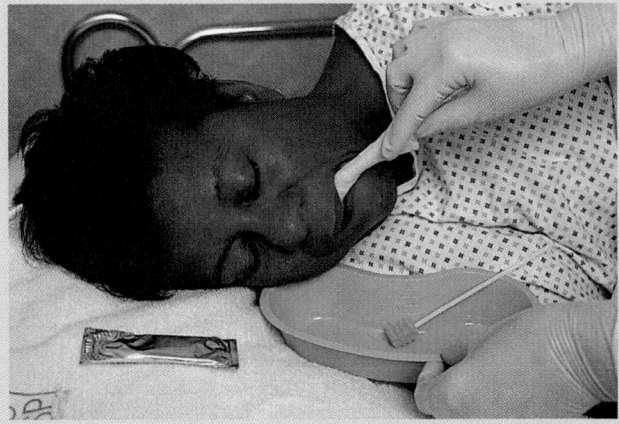

Step 14

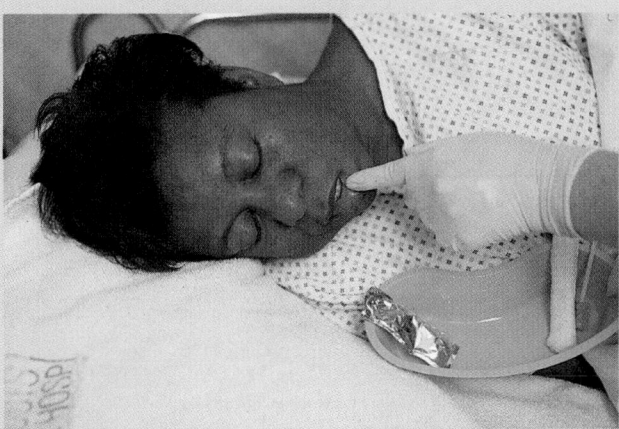

Step 17

21. Clean equipment and return to its proper place. Place soiled linen in proper receptacle.	Proper disposal of soiled equipment prevents spread of infection.
22. Wash hands.	Reduces transmission of microorganisms.
23. Apply gloves, and inspect oral cavity.	Determines efficacy of cleansing. Once thick secretions are removed, underlying inflammation or lesions may be revealed.
24. Ask debilitated client if mouth feels clean.	Evaluates level of comfort.
25. Assess client's respirations on an ongoing basis.	Ensures early recognition of aspiration.

Recording and Reporting

▪ Record procedure, including pertinent observations (e.g., presence of bleeding gums, dry mucosa, ulcerations, crusts on tongue).

▪ Report any unusual findings to nurse in charge or physician.

Home Care Considerations

▪ Irrigate cavity with bulb syringe; a gravy baster may be substituted.

▪ Mouth care should be given at least twice a day. Care givers can get nonprescription oral care solutions (e.g., carbamide peroxide solutions) at most pharmacies.

Box 29-4

Procedural Guidelines for Cleaning Dentures

Equipment: Soft-bristled toothbrush, denture toothbrush, emesis basin or sink, denture dentifrice or toothpaste, water glass, 4 × 4 inch gauze, washcloth, denture cup, disposable gloves

1. Clean dentures for client during routine mouth care. Dentures need to be cleansed as often as natural teeth.

2. Fill emesis basin with tepid water. (If using sink, place washcloth in bottom of sink, and fill sink with approximately 1 inch of water.)

3. Remove dentures: If client is unable to do this independently, don gloves, grasp upper plate at front with thumb and index finger wrapped in gauze, and pull downward. Gently lift lower denture from jaw, and rotate one side downward to remove from client's mouth. Place dentures in emesis basin or sink.

4. Apply dentifrice or toothpaste to denture, and brush surfaces of dentures (see illustration). Hold dentures close to water. Hold brush horizontally, and use back-and-forth motion to cleanse biting surfaces. Use short strokes from top of denture to biting surfaces of teeth to clean outer tooth surface. Hold brush verti-

cally, and use short strokes to clean inner tooth surfaces. Hold brush horizontally, and use back-and-forth motion to clean undersurface of dentures.

5. Rinse dentures thoroughly in tepid water.

6. Return dentures to client, or store in tepid water in denture cup.

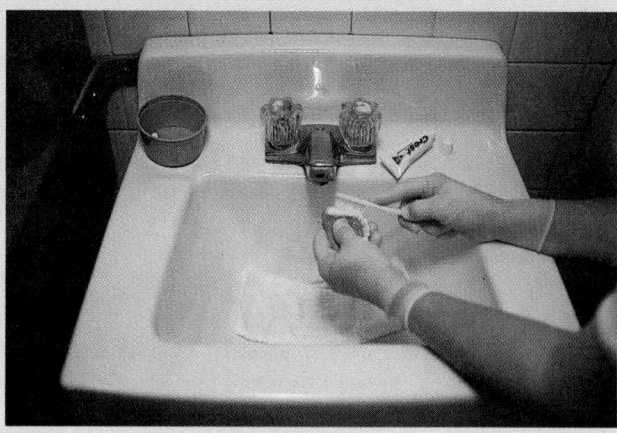

Step 4

NURSING PROCESS AND HAIR CARE

A person's appearance and feeling of well-being often depend on the way the hair looks and feels. Illness or disability may prevent a client from maintaining daily hair care. An immobilized client's hair soon becomes tangled. Dressings may leave sticky blood or antiseptic solutions on the hair. Proper hair care is important to the client's body image. Brushing, combing, and shampooing are basic hygiene measures for all clients.

■ Assessment

Before performing hair care, the nurse must assess the condition of the hair and scalp (Table 29-5). Findings will reveal the frequency and extent of care needed. A client's self-care ability can be altered by conditions such as arthritis, fatigue, and the presence of physical encumbrances (e.g., cast or IV). The nurse assesses the client's physical ability to perform hair care. It is also essential to consider a client's personal hair care practices so every effort can be made to maintain the client's preferred appearance (Box 29-5).

Cultural practices. When caring for clients from different cultures, it is important to learn as much as possible about and be sensitive to the client's customs, beliefs, and practices. Ask the client about preferred hair care methods or any cultural restrictions. For example, African Americans usually have dry hair. Special lanolin conditioners may be used to maintain conditioning.

TABLE 29-5
Hair and Scalp Problems

Problem	Characteristics	Implications	Interventions
Dandruff	Scaling of the scalp accompanied by itching; in severe cases, dandruff on eyebrows.	Dandruff causes embarassment; if dandruff enters eyes, conjunctivitis may develop.	Shampoo regularly with medicated shampoo; in severe cases seek physician's advice.
Ticks	Small gray-brown parasites that burrow into skin and suck blood.	Ticks transmit Rocky Mountain spotted fever, Lyme disease, and tularemia.	Do not pull ticks from skin; sucking apparatus remains and may become infected; place drop of oil or ether on tick, or cover it with petrolatum to ease removal.
Pediculosis capitis (head lice)	Tiny grayish white parasitic insects that attach to hair strands; eggs look like oval particles, resemble dandruff; bites or pustules may be observed behind ears and at hairline.	Head lice are difficult to remove and if not treated may spread to furniture and other people.	Use medicated shampoo for eliminating lice; repeat 12 to 24 hours later; change bed linens, using isolation precautions required by agency.
Pediculosis corporis (body lice)	Tend to cling to clothing so may not be easily seen; body lice suck blood and lay eggs on clothing and furniture.	Client itches constantly; scratches on skin may become infected; hemorrhagic spots may appear on skin where lice are sucking blood.	Client should bathe or shower thoroughly; after skin is dried, apply lotion for eliminating lice; after 12 to 24 hours another bath or shower should be taken; bag infested clothing or linen until laundered.
Pediculosis pubis (crab lice)	Found in pubic hair; crab lice are grayish white with red legs.	Lice may spread through bed linen, clothing, or furniture or sexual contact.	Shave hair off affected area; cleanse as for body lice; if lice were sexually transmitted, partner must be notified.
Alopecia	Balding patches in periphery of hair line; hair becomes brittle and broken; caused by improper use of hair curlers and picks, tight braiding, hot styling tools, certain diseases.	Patches of uneven hair growth and loss alter client's appearance.	Stop hair care practices that damage hair.

NURSING DIAGNOSES FOR HAIR AND SCALP CARE

Body image disturbance
Infection, risk for
Pain
Self-care deficit, dressing/grooming
Skin integrity, impaired

Nursing Diagnosis

Assessment of the hair and scalp indicates the client's need for and ability to maintain personal grooming. Conditions of the hair and scalp may reveal findings such as coarse or silky hair or the presence or absence of secretions, lacerations, or infestations. The nurse reviews and clusters all defining characteristics to select appropriate nursing diagnoses (see nursing diagnoses box). The diagnoses may focus primarily on grooming and comfort. However, when abnormalities of the scalp are identified, nursing diagnoses focus on scalp integrity.

Selecting appropriate related factors influences the nurse's care plan. For the diagnosis *impaired skin integrity related to parasite infestation,* the nurse must design actions to remove the infestation. Shampooing and showering with special products, isolating all linens, and client teaching are good measures. The diagnosis *impaired skin integrity related to scalp laceration* will require measures to promote healing. Maintaining an intact suture line, preventing infection, and removing secretions may be necessary. Nursing interventions are designed to meet actual alterations or alterations a client may be at risk of developing.

Planning

Good hair care practices must be performed routinely to meet the client's hygiene needs. The nurse should remember the client is aware of appearance at all times.

Therefore an effective plan allows the client to initiate and participate in hygiene measures.

Implementation

Health promotion and restorative care

Brushing and combing. Frequent brushing helps to keep hair clean and distributes oil evenly along hair shafts. Combing prevents hair from tangling. The client should be encouraged to maintain routine hair care. However, clients with limited mobility and poor coordination and those who are confused or seriously weakened by illness require help. Clients in a hospital or extended care facility appreciate the opportunity to have their hair brushed and combed before being seen by others.

Long hair can easily become matted after a client is confined to bed, even for a short period. When lacerations or incisions involve the scalp, blood and topical medications can also cause tangling. Frequent brushing and combing keep long hair neatly groomed. Braiding can help to avoid repeated tangles. The nurse asks permission before braiding a client's hair.

To brush hair the nurse parts the hair into two sections and separates each into two more sections. It is easier to brush smaller sections of hair. Brushing from the scalp toward the hair ends minimizes pulling. Moistening the hair with water or alcohol frees tangles for easier combing. The nurse never cuts a client's hair without written consent.

Shampooing. Frequency of shampooing depends on a client's daily routines. The nurse should remind hospitalized clients that staying in bed, excess perspiration, or treatments that leave blood or solutions in the hair may require more frequent shampooing. For clients at home, the nurse's greatest challenge may be to find ways the client can shampoo the hair without injury.

If the client is able to take a shower or bath, the hair can usually be shampooed without difficulty. A shower chair may be used for the ambulatory client who becomes tired or faint. Handheld shower nozzles allow clients to wash the hair during a tub bath or shower. Clients allowed to sit in a chair can usually be shampooed in front of a sink. If the client is forced to sit at

Box 29-6

Procedural Guidelines for Shampooing Hair of Bed-Bound Client

Equipment: Bath towels, washcloths, shampoo and hair conditioner (optional), water pitcher, plastic shampoo trough, washbasin, bath blanket, waterproof pad, clean comb and brush, hair dryer (optional)

1. Before washing client's hair, determine that there are no contraindications to this procedure. Certain medical conditions, such as head and neck injuries, spinal cord injuries, and arthritis, could place the client at risk for injury during shampooing because of positioning and manipulation of client's head and neck.
2. Inspect the hair and scalp prior to initiating the procedure. This determines the presence of any conditions that may require the use of special shampoos or treatments (e.g, for the removal of dried blood, dandruff).
3. Place waterproof pad under client's shoulders, neck, and head (see illustration). Position client supine, with head and shoulders at top edge of bed. Place plastic trough under client's head and washbasin at end of trough. Be sure trough spout extends beyond edge of mattress.

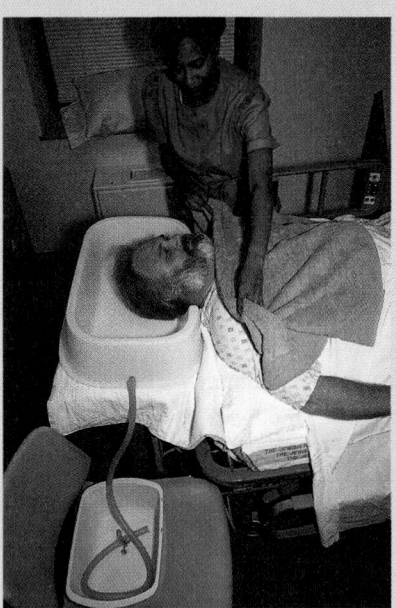

Step 3

4. Place rolled towel under client's neck and bath towel over client's shoulders.
5. Brush and comb client's hair.
6. Obtain warm water.

7. Ask client to hold face towel or washcloth over eyes.
8. Slowly pour water from water pitcher over hair until it is completely wet (see illustration). If hair contains matted blood, don gloves, apply peroxide to dissolve clots, and then rinse hair with saline. Apply small amount of shampoo.

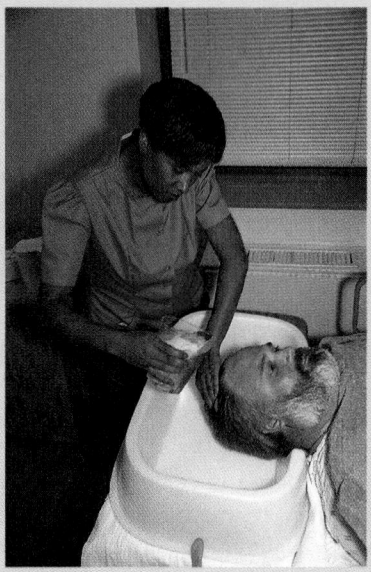

Step 8

9. Work up lather with both hands. Start at hairline, and work toward back of neck. Lift head slightly with one hand to wash back of head. Shampoo sides of head. Massage scalp by applying pressure with fingertips.
10. Rinse hair with water. Make sure water drains into basin. Repeat rinsing until hair is free of soap.
11. Apply conditioner or cream rinse if requested, and rinse hair thoroughly.
12. Wrap client's head in bath towel. Dry client's face with cloth used to protect eyes. Dry off any moisture along neck or shoulders.
13. Dry client's hair and scalp. Use second towel if first becomes saturated.
14. Comb hair to remove tangles, and dry with dryer if desired.
15. Apply oil preparation or conditioning product to hair, if desired by client.
16. Assist client to comfortable position, and complete styling of hair.

the bedside, the hair can be shampooed as the client leans forward over a washbasin.

If a client is unable to sit but can be moved, the nurse may transfer the client to a stretcher for transportation to a sink or shower equipped with a handheld nozzle. The nurse places a towel or small pillow under the client's head and neck, allowing the head to hang slightly over the stretcher's edge. Caution is needed with clients with neck injuries because hyperextension of the neck could cause further injury.

If the client is unable to sit in a chair or be transferred to a stretcher, shampooing must be done with the client in bed. Many institutions require a physician's order for the procedure (Box 29-6).

Shaving. Shaving facial hair can be done after the bath or shampoo. Women may prefer to shave their legs or axillae while bathing. When assisting a client, the nurse should take care to avoid cutting the client with razor blades. Clients prone to bleeding (e.g., those receiving anticoagulants or high doses of aspirin) should use an electric razor. Before using an electric razor, the nurse should check for electrical hazards. Electric razors should be used on only one client because of infection control considerations.

When a razor blade is used for shaving, the skin must be softened to prevent pulling, scraping, or cuts. For example, placing a warm washcloth over the male client's face for a few seconds, followed by application of shaving cream or a lathering of mild soap, softens the skin. If the client is unable to shave, the nurse may perform the shave. To avoid causing discomfort or razor cuts, the nurse gently pulls the skin taut and uses short, firm razor strokes in the direction the hair grows. Short downward strokes work best to remove hair over the upper lip. A client usually can explain to the nurse the best way to move the razor across the skin.

Mustache and beard care. Clients with mustaches or beards require daily grooming. Keeping these areas clean is important because food particles and mucus can easily collect in the hair. If the client is unable to carry out self-care, the nurse should do so at the client's request. The nurse never shaves off a mustache or beard without the client's consent.

Hair and scalp care. To best promote and restore hair and scalp health, clients should be instructed to keep hair clean, combed, and brushed regularly. Clients may also need to know how to check for and remove parasites (see Table 29-5). The nurse should tell clients they need to notify the primary health care provider of changes in the texture and distribution of hair.

Evaluation

Evaluative measures for care of a client's hair are dynamic and change as the client's condition changes. As the care plan is being developed, the nurse must always be prepared to make necessary changes. For example, if the client becomes unable to provide care because of immobility, the nurse initiates and maintains good hair grooming techniques until the client or family is able to do so.

NURSING PROCESS AND CARE OF THE EYES, EARS, AND NOSE

Special attention is given to cleansing the eyes, ears, and nose during the client's bath. Care focuses on preventing infection and maintaining normal organ function.

Assessment

The nurse carefully inspects all external eye structures. Normally the conjunctivae are clear and not inflamed. The eyelid margins are in close approximation with the eyeball, and the lashes are turned outward. The lid margins are normally without inflammation, drainage, or lesions. Flaking skin around the eyebrows may indicate dandruff.

Assessment of the external ear structures includes inspecting the auricle, external ear canal, and tympanic membrane. When performing hygiene, the nurse is most concerned with presence of accumulated cerumen or drainage in the ear canal, local inflammation, or pain.

The nurse inspects the nares for signs of inflammation, discharge, lesions, edema, and deformity. The nasal mucosa is normally pink, clear, and without discharge. For clients with any form of tubing exiting the nose, the nurse should observe for tissue sloughing, localized tenderness, inflammation, and even bleeding.

Use of sensory aids. For clients who wear eyeglasses, contact lenses, artificial eyes, or hearing aids, the nurse assesses the client's knowledge and methods used to care for the aids, as well as any problems caused by them. The nurse's findings may indicate a need for client education.

Self-care ability. The nurse assesses a client's physical ability to perform eye, ear, and nose care, as well as care of any sensory aids. Clients who are unable to grasp small objects, have limited upper extremity mobility, have reduced vision, or are seriously fatigued require assistance.

Nursing Diagnosis

The nurse's assessment may reveal an actual alteration in the function of sensory organs, a problem in the client's ability to perform personal hygiene, or a deficit in the client's understanding of how to perform hygiene. Clustering defining characteristics such as physical limitation, visual impairment, or irritation of the eyes, ears, or nares helps the nurse to form accurate nursing diagnoses (see nursing diagnoses box on p. 770).

NURSING DIAGNOSES FOR EYE, EAR, OR NOSE PROBLEMS

Infection, risk for
Knowledge deficit regarding personal hygiene
Pain
Self-care deficit, bathing/hygiene
Sensory/perceptual alterations (visual, auditory, or olfactory)

BOX 29-7
Gerontological Nursing Practice

- Maintaining and improving eyesight are important aspects of an independent and satisfying life for older adults.
  Encourage regular eye examinations.
  Discuss vision changes that occur naturally with aging.
  Describe signs and symptoms of major eye diseases associated with aging.
- Twenty-five percent to 40% of people 65 years of age and older are hearing impaired (Ney, 1993); speak slowly and articulate carefully. However, do not shout, and do not assume that *all* older clients have difficulty hearing.
- Ear wax tends to be drier in older people, impacts more easily, and takes longer to soften. Complaints of feeling of fullness, itching or ringing, and "blocked hearing" warrant regular assessment (Mahoney, 1993).

Planning

The client's personal preference and habits are considered when the nurse plans hygiene care. When bathing a client, the nurse uses extra care to avoid injury to the eyes, ears, or nose. These areas are sensitive to irritating or painful stimuli. Children and older adult clients are especially susceptible. In the home environment family members or friends should be familiar with a client's hygiene routines. Sensory aids must be clean and functional for the client to interact within the environment.

Implementation

Health promotion and restorative care. To maintain optimal health, clients should be instructed in the proper methods of caring for the eyes, ears, and nose. Clients with specific health concerns involving these structures should see the appropriate specialist regularly for checkups and ongoing care. When active, clients should know the best ways of protecting these sensitive organs (e.g., eye protective devices). Older adults experience a variety of changes in sensory function (see Chapter 39). The nurse adapts practice approaches to consider their special needs (Box 29-7).

Basic eye care. Cleansing the eyes simply involves washing with a clean washcloth moistened in water. Soap may cause burning and irritation (see Skill 29-1). Direct pressure should never be applied over the eyeball because it may cause serious injury.

The unconscious client may require more frequent eye care. Secretions may collect along the lid margins and inner canthus when the blink reflex is absent or when the eye does not totally close. It may be necessary to place an eye patch over the involved eye to prevent corneal drying and irritation. Lubricating eyedrops may be given according to the physician's orders.

Eyeglasses. Glasses are made of hardened glass or plastic that is impact resistant to prevent shattering. Nevertheless, because of the cost, the nurse should be careful when cleaning glasses and should protect them from breakage or other damage when they are not worn. Glasses should be put in a case and in a drawer of the bedside table when not in use.

Warm water is sufficient for cleaning glass lenses. A soft cloth is best for drying to prevent scratching the lens. Plastic lenses in particular are scratched easily, and special cleansing solutions and drying tissues are available.

Contact lenses. A contact lens is a small, round, sometimes colored disk that fits over the cornea of the eye. Clients who cannot remove their own lenses require assistance. Care includes cleaning, proper application and removal, and storage (Skill 29-6).

Nose care. The client can usually remove secretions from the nose by gently blowing into a soft tissue. The nurse cautions the client against harsh blowing that creates pressure capable of injuring the eardrum, nasal mucosa, and even sensitive eye structures. Bleeding from the nares is a key sign of harsh blowing.

If the client is unable to remove nasal secretions, the nurse assists by using a wet washcloth or a cotton-tipped applicator moistened in water or saline. The applicator should never be inserted beyond the length of the cotton tip. Excessive nasal secretions can also be removed by gentle suctioning.

When clients have tubes inserted through the nose, the nurse should change the tape anchoring the tube at least once a day. When tape becomes moist from nasal secretions, the skin and mucosa can easily become macerated. Friction causes tissue sloughing. The nurse should know how to tape tubing correctly to minimize tension or friction on the nares (see Chapter 34). When sloughing occurs, it may be necessary for the nurse to remove the tube and insert one through the other naris.

Evaluation

Evaluation of eye, ear, and nose care must be based on the client's existing sensory function and the expected outcomes for the care plan's goals. Hygiene care alone will not improve sensory function beyond a client's baseline level. The evaluation process is ongoing. The nurse revises the care plan when the client's needs

. . . .
Caring for the Client With Contact Lenses

Delegation Considerations

The skills of caring for eye and ear prostheses can be delegated to unlicensed assistive personnel.

- Inform and assist care provider in proper way to care for eye and ear prostheses.
- Stress to care provider that careful handling of these devices is of utmost importance to prevent physical injury to the client and damage to the devices.
- Inform care provider of types of findings to report (e.g., eye pain, eye socket drainage).

Equipment

- Clean lens storage container

- Bath towel
- Suction cup (optional)
- Sterile saline solution
- Sterile lens cleaning solution
- Sterile lens rinsing solution
- Sterile lens disinfectant
- Sterile enzyme solution (depends on care regimen)
- Sterile wetting solution (depends on care regimen)
- Cotton ball or cotton-tipped applicator
- Emesis basin
- Disposable gloves

STEPS	RATIONALE
1. Place towel just below client's face.	Catches lens if one should accidentally fall from eye.
2. Stand at client's side. Inspect eye, or ask client if contact lens is in place.	Lenses are generally comfortable to wear, and client may forget they are in place. Prolonged wear may cause injury to eye.

CRITICAL DECISION POINT

Unconscious or confused clients entering the health care setting should be carefully assessed; lenses are often difficult to assess if clear (untinted).

3. Ask if client feels any eye discomfort, and assess length of time client normally wears lenses.	Scratched lens can cause corneal irritation and abrasion. Accumulation of dust or debris between lens and cornea causes irritation. Continuous wearing of certain types of lenses can irritate cornea.
4. Ask if client is able to manipulate and hold contact lens.	Determines level of assistance required in care.
5. Assess client for any unusual visual signs/symptoms (reduced visual acuity, blurred vision, halos, photophobia).	May indicate underlying visual alteration or need to change lens prescription. A reduction in visual acuity calls for referral.
6. Assess types of medications prescribed for client: sedatives, hypnotics, muscle relaxants, antihistamines, anticholinergics, and antidepressants.	Sedatives, hypnotics, and muscle relaxants reduce blink reflex and thus reduce lubrication of cornea. Antihistamines, anticholinergics, and antidepressants can reduce tear production.
7. After lenses are removed (see Step 11), inspect eye for signs of corneal irritation (e.g., redness, pain, swelling of eyelids and conjunctivae, discharge, and excess tearing).	Signs/symptoms indicate corneal irritation or abrasion.

CRITICAL DECISION POINT

If pain persists or worsens after removal of lenses, an immediate referral to the ophthalmologist should be made. Severe pain may indicate corneal epithelium disruption or infection (Cohen and Krachmer, 1992).

Continued

Caring for the Client With Contact Lenses

STEPS	RATIONALE
8. Discuss procedure with client.	Client can assist in planning by explaining technique that may aid removal and insertion. Client may be anxious as nurse retracts eyelids and manipulates lenses.
9. Have client assume supine or sitting position in bed or chair.	Provides easy access for nurse while retracting eyelids and manipulating lenses.
10. Assemble supplies at bedside.	Provides easy access to supplies.
11. Remove lenses.	
A. Soft lenses:	
(1) Wash hands. Apply disposable gloves if there are cuts, scratches, or dermatological lesions on nurse's hands.	Reduces transmission of microorganisms.
(2) Add a few drops of sterile saline solution to client's eye.	Lubricates eye to facilitate lens removal.
(3) Tell client to look straight ahead.	Eases tipping of lens during removal.
(4) Using middle finger, retract lower eyelid.	Exposes lower edge of lens.
(5) With pad of index finger of same hand, slide lens off cornea onto white of eye.	Positions lens for easy grasping. Use of finger pad (rather than fingernail) prevents injury to cornea and damage to lens.
(6) Pull upper eyelid down gently with thumb of other hand, and compress lens slightly between thumb and index finger.	Causes soft lens to double up. Air enters underneath lens to release suction.
(7) Gently pinch lens, and lift out.	Protects lens from damage. Avoid allowing lens edges to stick together. Soft lenses can be easily torn.
(8) Clean and rinse lens. Place lens in proper storage case compartment: *R* for right lens and *L* for left lens (see illustration).	Ensures proper lens will be reinserted into correct eye. Proper storage prevents cracking or tearing.
a. After removing one lens from case, apply one or two drops of cleaning solution to lens in palm of hand (use cleanser recommended by lens manufacturer or eye care practitioner).	Removes tear components, including mucus, lipids, and proteins that collect on lens.
b. Rub lens gently but thoroughly on both sides for 20 to 30 seconds. Use index finger (soft lenses) or little finger or cotton-tipped applicator soaked with cleaning solution (rigid lenses) to clean inside lens. Be careful not to touch or scratch lens with fingernail.	It is easier to manipulate and clean lens using fingertips. Cleans microorganisms from all surfaces.
c. Holding lens over emesis basin, rinse thoroughly with manufacturer-recommended rinsing solution (soft lenses) or cold tap water (rigid lenses).	Removes debris and cleaning solution from lens surface. Rinsing methods and solutions differ for each type of lens.
d. Place lens in proper storage case compartment and fill with storage solution recommended by manufacturer or eye care practitioner.	Disinfects lens, removes residue, enhances wetability of lens, and prevents scratches to lens that can be caused by a dry case.
(9) Repeat Steps (2) through (8) for other lens. Secure cover over storage case. Label with client's name and room number.	Proper storage prevents damage to or loss of lenses.

STEPS	RATIONALE

    (10) Assess appearance and condition of eyes after lenses are removed.

    (11) Dispose of towel, remove gloves, and wash hands. — Reduces transmission of infection.

B. Rigid lenses:

    (1) Wash hands, and apply gloves if needed. — Reduces transmission of microorganisms.

    (2) Be sure lens is positioned directly over cornea. — Correct position of lens allows easy removal from eye.

CRITICAL DECISION POINT

If lens is not positioned directly over cornea, have client close eyelids, place index and middle fingers of one hand on eyelid just beside the lens and beneath it, and gently but firmly massage lens back into place.

    (3) Place index finger on outer corner of client's eye, and draw skin gently back toward ear (see illustration). — Tightens eyelid against eyeball.

    (4) Tell client to blink. Do not release pressure on eyelid until blink is completed. — Maneuver should cause lens to dislodge and pop out. Lid margins must clear top and bottom of lens until the blink.

    (5) If lens fails to pop out, gently retract eyelid beyond edges of lens. Press lower eyelid gently against lower edge of lens. — Pressure causes upper edge of lens to tip forward.

    (6) Allow both eyelids to close slightly, and grasp lens as it rises from eye. Cup lens in hand. — Maneuver causes lens to slide off easily. Protects lens from breakage.

CRITICAL DECISION POINT

A lens suction cup can be used to remove lenses from the eyes of confused or unconscious clients. Gently apply suction cup to lens surface, and lift out.

Continued

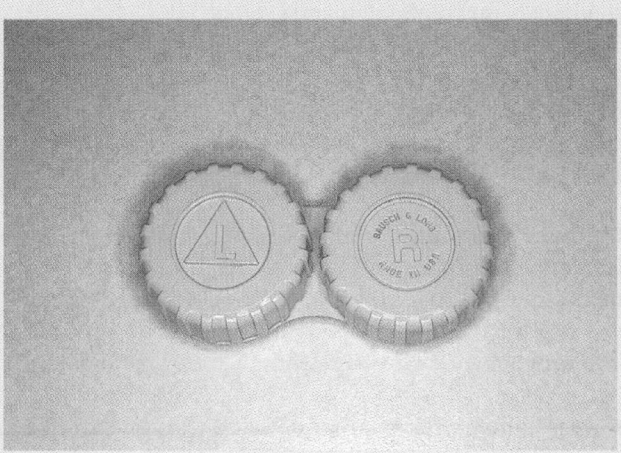

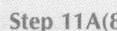

Step 11A(8)

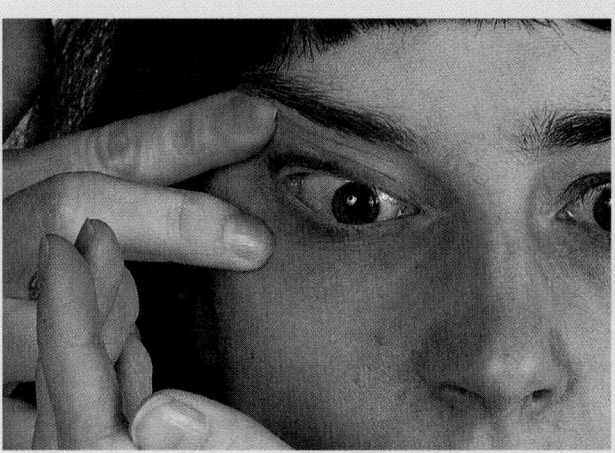

Step 11B(3)

Caring for the Client With Contact Lenses

STEPS	RATIONALE
(7) Clean and rinse lens (see Step 11A[8]). Place lens in proper storage case compartment: *R* for right lens and *L* for left lens. Center lens in storage case, convex side down.	Both lenses may not have the same prescription. Proper storage prevents breaking, scratching, chipping, and discoloration.
(8) Repeat Steps (2) through (7) for other lens. Secure cover over storage case. Label with client's name and room number.	Proper storage prevents damage to or loss of lenses.
(9) Dispose of towel, remove gloves, and wash hands.	Reduces spread of infection and keeps client's environment neat.
12. Ask client if lens feels comfortable after removal and reinsertion of lenses.	Determines if any debris is caught between lens and cornea. Lens should be removed if client experiences discomfort.
13. Inspect eye (over time) for signs of ocular infection.	
14. Assess client's visual acuity (see Chapter 24).	Determines improvement in visual perception.
15. Observe client for signs of eye injury.	

Recording and Reporting
- Record or report any signs/symptoms of visual alterations noted during procedure.
- Record on nursing care plan or Kardex times of lens insertion and removal if client is going to surgery or special procedure.

Home Care Considerations
- Clients must be taught not to wear lenses in presence of noxious or irritating vapors or fumes because these irritants can cause damage to lens surface.

change. For example, if the client's hearing is altered because of a faulty hearing aid, the nurse may need to seek advice from other health care providers to correct the problem.

········ ## CLIENT'S ROOM ENVIRONMENT

Attempting to make a client's room as comfortable as the home is one of the nurse's priorities. The client's room should be comfortable, safe, and large enough to allow the client and visitors to move about freely. The nurse can control room temperature, ventilation, noise, and odors to create a more comfortable environment. Keeping the room neat and orderly also contributes to the client's sense of well-being.

Maintaining Comfort
The nature of what constitutes a comfortable environment depends on the client's age, severity of illness, and level of normal daily activity. Depending on the client's age and physical condition, the room temperature should be maintained between 20° and 23° C (68° and 74° F). Infants, older adults, and the acutely ill may need a warmer room. However, certain critically ill clients benefit from cooler room temperatures to lower the body's metabolic demands.

A good ventilation system keeps stale air and odors from lingering in the room. The nurse must protect the acutely ill, infants, and older adults from drafts by ensuring they are adequately dressed and covered with a lightweight blanket.

Good ventilation also reduces lingering odors caused by draining wounds, vomitus, bowel movements, and unemptied bedpans and urinals. Room deodorizers can help remove many unpleasant odors. Nurses should always empty and rinse bedpans or urinals promptly. Thorough hygiene measures are the best way to control body or breath odors. Most health care institutions now prohibit smoking. Before using room deodorizers the nurse should determine that the client is not allergic to or sensitive to the deodorizer itself.

Ill clients seem to be more sensitive to common

hospital noises. Until the client is familiar with hospital noises, the nurse should try to control the noise level. The nurse also explains the source of any unfamiliar noises.

Proper lighting is necessary for everyone's safety and comfort. A brightly lit room is usually stimulating, but a darkened room is best for rest and sleep. Room lighting can be adjusted by closing or opening drapes, regulating overbed and floor lights, and closing or opening room doors.

Room Equipment

A typical hospital room contains certain basic pieces of furniture: overbed table, bedside stand, chairs, lamp, and bed. The overbed table rolls on wheels and can be adjusted to various heights over the bed or a chair. Usually two storage areas are under the tabletop. The table provides ideal working space for the nurse performing procedures. It also provides a surface on which to place meal trays, toiletry items, and objects frequently used by the client. The bedpan and urinal should not be placed on the overbed table. The bedside stand is used to store the client's personal possessions and hygiene equipment. The telephone, water pitcher, and drinking cup are commonly found on a bedside stand.

Most hospital rooms contain an armless straight-backed chair and an upholstered lounge chair with arms. The lounge chair is used by the client and visitors and is usually placed at the foot of the bed or beside it. Straight-backed chairs are convenient when temporarily transferring the client from the bed, such as during bed making.

Each room usually has an overbed light and a floor or table lamp. Movable lights that extend over the bed from the wall should be positioned for easy reach but moved aside when not in use. Gooseneck or special examination lights are portable standing lights used to provide extra light during bedside procedures.

Other equipment usually found in a client's room includes a call light, a television set or radio, a blood pressure gauge, oxygen and vacuum wall outlets, and personal care items. Special equipment designed for comfort or positioning clients includes footboards and foot boots (Figure 29-1), special mattresses, and bed boards.

Beds. Seriously ill clients may remain in bed for a long time. Because a bed is the piece of equipment used most by a client, it should be designed for comfort, safety, and adaptability for changing positions.

The typical hospital bed has a firm mattress on a metal frame that can be raised and lowered horizontally. Different bed positions are used to promote lung expansion, postural drainage, and other interventions (Table 29-6).

The position of a bed is usually changed by electrical controls on the side or foot of the bed or on a bedside table. Clients can thus raise or lower sections of

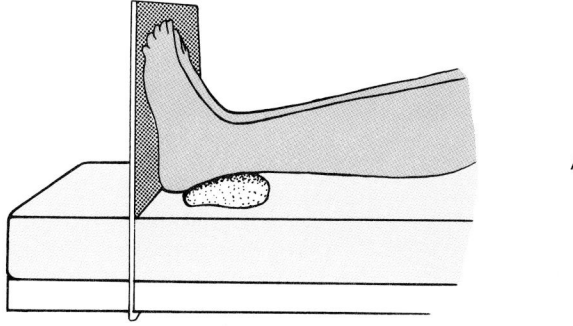

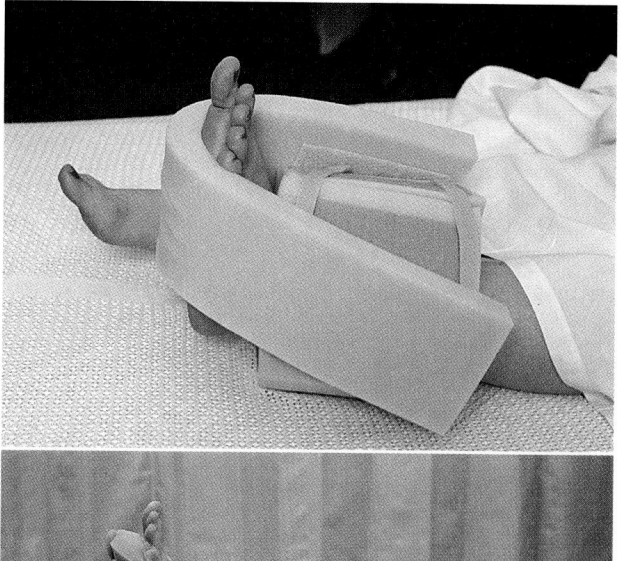

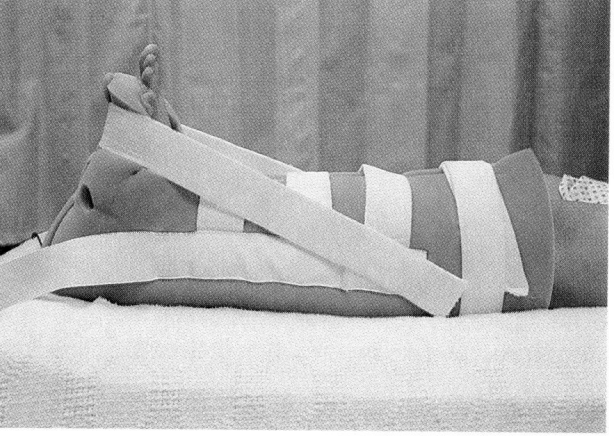

Figure 29-1. **A,** Footboard. **B,** Foot boots. **C,** Foot boot with lower leg extension.

the bed without expending much energy. Nurses should instruct clients on the proper use of controls and caution them against raising the bed to a position that might cause harm. The greater height of a hospital bed prevents undue musculoskeletal strain on the nurse and client.

Beds contain safety features such as locks on the wheels or casters. Wheels should be locked when the bed is stationary to prevent accidental movement. Side rails protect clients from accidental falls. The headboard can be removed from most beds. This is important when the medical team must have easy access to the head such as during cardiopulmonary resuscitation.

TABLE 29-6
Common Bed Positions

Position	Description	Uses
Fowler's	Head of bed raised to angle of 45 degrees or more; semisitting position.	Preferred while client eats; used during nasogastric tube insertion and nasotracheal suction; promotes lung expansion.
Semi-Fowler's	Head of bed raised approximately 30 degrees; incline less than Fowler's position.	Promotes lung expansion.
Trendelenburg's	Entire bed tilted downward with head of bed down.	For postural drainage; facilitates venous return in clients with poor peripheral perfusion.
Reverse Trendelenburg's	Entire bed frame tilted downward with foot of bed down.	Used infrequently; promotes gastric emptying and prevents esophageal reflux.
Flat	Entire bed frame parallel with floor.	For clients with vertebral injuries and in cervical traction; used by hypotensive clients; generally preferred by clients for sleeping.

Bed making. A client's bed should be kept as clean and comfortable as possible. This requires frequent inspections to be sure linen is clean, dry, and free of wrinkles.

The nurse usually makes a bed in the morning after the client's bath or while the client is bathing, in a shower, sitting in a chair eating, or out of the room for procedures or tests. Throughout the day the nurse straightens linen that becomes loose or wrinkled. The bed linen should also be checked for food particles after meals and for wetness or soiling. Linen that becomes soiled or wet should be changed.

When changing the bed linen, the nurse follows basic principles of asepsis by keeping soiled linen away from the uniform. Soiled linen is placed in special linen containers before discarding it in the linen hamper. To avoid air currents, which can spread microorganisms, the nurse never fans linen. To avoid transmitting infection, the nurse should not place soiled linen on the floor. If clean linen touches the floor, it is immediately discarded.

During bed making, the nurse must use proper body mechanics. The bed should always be raised to its high-est position before changing linen so the nurse does not have to bend or stretch over the mattress. When making an occupied bed the nurse should also use principles of body mechanics (see Chapter 27).

The client's privacy, comfort, and safety are important when making a bed. Using side rails, keeping call lights within the client's reach, and maintaining the proper bed position help promote comfort and safety. After making a bed the nurse always returns it to the lowest horizontal position to prevent accidental falls.

When possible the nurse should make the bed while it is unoccupied (Skill 29-7). If the client is confined to bed, the nurse organizes bed-making activities to conserve time and energy (Skill 29-8). When making an unoccupied bed the nurse follows the same basic principles as for bed making. The surgical, recovery, or postoperative bed is a modified version of the unoccupied bed. The top covers are folded to one side or fanfolded to the bottom third of the bed. After a client is discharged, all bed linen is sent to the laundry, the mattress and bed are cleaned by housekeeping personnel, and new bed linen is applied.

Text continued on p. 786

Making an Unoccupied Bed

Delegation Considerations
The skill of bed making can be delegated to unlicensed assistive personnel.
- Instruct care provider on how to transfer client from bed to chair. Review any precautions or activity restrictions for client.
- Tell care provider what to do if wound drainage, dressing material, drainage tubes, or intravenous (IV) tubing becomes dislodged or is found in the linens.
- Instruct care provider on what to do if client becomes fatigued.

Equipment
- Linen bag(s)
- Mattress pad (needs to be changed only when soiled)
- Bottom sheet (flat or fitted)
- Drawsheet (optional)
- Top sheet
- Blanket
- Bedspread
- Waterproof pads or bath blankets (optional)
- Pillowcases
- Bedside chair or table
- Disposable gloves (optional, if linens are soiled)

STEPS	RATIONALE
1. Assess if client is incontinent or has excess drainage on bed linen.	Determines need for protective waterproof pads or bath blankets on bed.
2. Assess activity orders and physical mobility.	Determines level of activity allowed, including whether client should be out of bed.
3. If client is in bed, explain that you wish to change bed while client is sitting up. Ask if client feels able to sit in chair and assist as necessary.	Client should not feel inconvenienced by procedure. Client may feel anxious if uncomfortable or fatigued.
4. Prepare needed equipment and supplies.	
5. Wash hands.	Reduces transmission of microorganisms.
6. Assemble and arrange equipment on bedside chair or table. Remove unnecessary equipment, such as overbed table.	Provides for smooth procedure and ensures comfort. Placing linen on clean surface minimizes spread of infection.
7. Lower side rail on near side of bed, and remove call light.	Provides easy access to bed.
8. Adjust bed height to comfortable working position.	Minimizes strain on nurse's back and muscles.
9. On near side, loosen linen, starting at top of bed. Move along sides and then down toward foot. Move to other side of bed, lower side rail, and loosen linen.	Makes linen easier to remove.
10. Remove breadspread and blanket separately by folding each into ball or folded square and discarding into linen bag if they are not to be reused. Do not allow uniform to come in contact with soiled linen. Avoid fanning or shaking linen.	Reduces transmission of microorganisms.
11. If spread or blanket is to be reused, fold neatly. Place folded spread or blanket over back of chair.	Facilitates replacement and prevents wrinkling.
12. Remove soiled pillowcases by grasping closed end with one hand and slipping pillow out with other. Discard pillowcases in linen bag and place pillows on table.	Minimizes contact with soiled linen.
13. Fold each piece of remaining bed linen separately into ball or folded square, and discard into linen bag.	Attempting to fold all soiled linen at once creates bulky bundle that is difficult to discard and may easily come in contact with uniform.
14. Slide mattress toward head of bed.	If mattress slides toward foot of bed when head of bed is raised, it is difficult to tuck in linen.

Continued

Making an Unoccupied Bed

STEPS	RATIONALE
15. Wipe off moisture on mattress with washcloth moistened in antiseptic solution; dry thoroughly.	Reduces transmission of microorganisms.
16. Stand at side of bed where linen is placed. Spread mattress pad over mattress.	Time is saved by making half of bed first and then moving to opposite side.
17. Smooth out all wrinkles in pad.	Wrinkles or folds of linen are source of chronic irritation against client's skin.
18. Unfold bottom sheet lengthwise and place vertical center crease lengthwise along center of bed. Fold sheet's top layer toward opposite side of bed. Smooth bottom layer of sheet across mattress on near side; bring edge over side of mattress. Allow it to hang 25 cm (10 inches) over mattress edge. Lower hem of bottom sheet should lie seam down, even with bottom edge of mattress (see illustration). Pull remaining top portion of sheet over top edge of mattress.	Method of unfolding linen saves nurse's time and energy. Making one side of bed at a time avoids excess movement. Proper placement of linen ensures adequate length will be available to cover opposite side of bed. Keeping seam edge down eliminates source of irritation to client's skin. If bottom edge of sheet is not tucked in, it can later be changed without removing top linen.
19. While standing at head of bed, miter top corner of bottom sheet:	Mitered corner is not loosened easily.
a. Face head of bed diagonally. Place hand away from head of bed under top corner of mattress near mattress edge and lift.	
b. With other hand, tuck top edge of bottom sheet smoothly under mattress so side edges of sheet above and below mattress would meet if brought together.	
c. Face side of bed, and pick up top edge of sheet approximately 45 cm (18 inches) down from top of mattress (see illustration).	
d. Lift sheet, and lay it on top of mattress to form neat, triangular fold, with lower base of triangle even with mattress side edge (see illustration).	
e. Tuck lower edge of sheet, hanging free below mattress, under mattress. Tuck with palms down without pulling triangular fold (see illustration).	
f. Hold portion of sheet covering side edge of mattress in place with one hand. With other hand, pick up top of triangular linen fold, and bring it down over side of mattress. Tuck this portion under mattress (see illustration).	

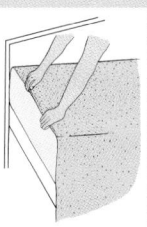

Step 18

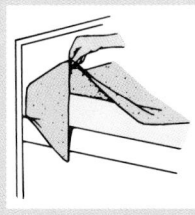
Step 19c

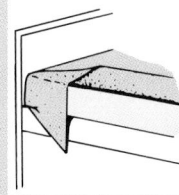
Step 19d

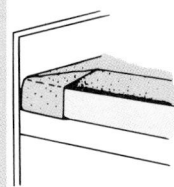
Step 19e

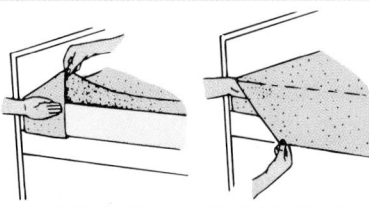
Step 19f

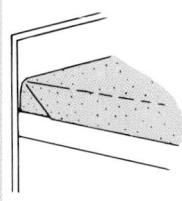
Step 20

STEPS	RATIONALE
20. Tuck remaining portion of sheet under mattress. Keep linen smooth (see illustration).	Folds can irritate client's skin.
21. Open drawsheet so it unfolds in half. Lay center fold along middle of bed lengthwise. Fanfold top layer at center of bed. Smooth bottom layer of drawsheet over mattress.	Drawsheet is used to lift and reposition client. Placement under client's torso distributes most of body weight over sheet.
22. Tuck excess edge under mattress, keeping palms down.	Anchors sheet in place to prevent sliding and wrinkling.
23. Move to opposite side of bed.	
24. Spread fanfolded bottom sheet smoothly over edge of mattress from head to foot of bed.	Wrinkles can cause irritation.
25. Miter top corner of bottom sheet (see Step 19). When tucking corner, be sure sheet is taut.	Taut sheet eliminates wrinkles and folds that can rub client's skin.
26. Facing side of bed, grasp remaining edge of bottom sheet, lean back, keeping back straight, and pull when tucking excess linen tightly under mattress. Proceed from head to foot of bed. (Avoid lifting mattress during tucking to ensure tight fit.)	Prevents injury to nurse.
27. Smooth folded drawsheet over bottom sheet. Grasp edge of drawsheet with palms down, lean back, and tuck sheet under mattress. Tuck first at middle, then at top, and then at bottom.	Tucking first at top or bottom may pull sheet sideways, causing poor fit. Loose bed sheets reduce friction and help to prevent pressure ulcers.
28. If needed, apply waterproof pad or bath blanket over drawsheet.	Pad collects body secretions and drainage, protecting linen from becoming soiled.
29. Move to side of bed when linen is located. Place top sheet over bed with vertical center fold lengthwise down middle of bed. Open sheet out from head to foot, being sure top edge of sheet is seam up and even with top edge of mattress. Spread excess sheet over bottom edge of mattress. (Do not fan top sheet over the bed.)	Placement ensures equal distribution of sheet over bed. Positioning sheet with seam up prevents irritation of client's skin. Fanning creates air currents that can spread microorganisms throughout room.
30. Make horizontal toe pleat: Stand at foot of bed and fan fold in sheet 5 to 10 cm (2 to 4 inches) across bed. Pull sheet up from bottom to make fold. Fold should be approximately 15 cm (6 inches) from bottom edge of mattress.	Allows for free movement of client's feet and prevents friction against surface of toes.
31. Tuck in remaining portion of sheet on one side of foot of mattress (optional).	Anchors top sheet so that client can move freely.
32. Place blanket on bed, unfolding it so that crease runs lengthwise along middle of bed. Top edge should be parallel with edge of top sheet and 15 to 20 cm (6 to 8 inches) down from top mattress edge. Spread blanket evenly over bed.	Blanket provides adequate warmth. Cuff will be formed with sheet folded over top edge of blanket and spread.
33. Place spread over bed according to Step 32. Be sure top edge of spread extends about 2.5 cm (1 inch) above blanket's edge. Then tuck top edge of spread over and under top edge of blanket.	Spread gives bed a neat appearance and provides extra warmth.
34. Make cuff by turning edge of top sheet down over top edge of blanket and spread.	Smooth cuff protects client's face from irritation.

Continued

Skill 29-7—cont'd
Making an Unoccupied Bed

STEPS	RATIONALE
35. Standing on one side at foot of bed, lift mattress corner slightly with one hand, and with other hand tuck top sheet, blanket, and spread together under mattress. Be sure toe pleats of sheet are not pulled out so that linens are loose enough for client to move.	Pressure sores can develop on client's toes and heels if feet rub between tight-fitting bed sheets. Lifting mattress too high can loosen bottom linen.
36. Make modified mitered corner with top sheet, blanket, and spread: Pick up side edge of top sheet, blanket, and spread approximately 45 cm (18 inches) up from foot of mattress. Lift linens to form triangular fold, and lay it on bed. Tuck loose edge hanging down under side of mattress. Pick up triangular fold, and bring it down over mattress, holding linen in place along side of mattress. Do not tuck tip of triangle (see illustration).	Modified mitered corner secures top linen but keeps even edge of top sheet, blanket, and spread draped over mattress. 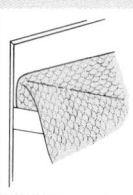 Step 36
37. Go to other side of bed. Spread sheet, blanket, and spread out evenly. Fold top edge of spread over blanket, and make cuff with top sheet (as in Step 34). Make modified mitered corner at foot of bed (as in Step 36).	Nurse saves time and energy by completing one side of bed at time.
38. Apply clean pillowcase. With one hand, grasp pillowcase at center of closed end. Gather case, turning it inside out over hand holding it. With same hand, pick up middle of one end of pillow. Pull pillowcase down over pillow with other hand. Be sure corners of case fit evenly over pillow.	This method makes it easy to slide case smoothly over pillow.
39. Position pillows at center of head of bed.	Maintains neat appearance.
40. Place call light within client's reach, and return bed to comfortable height.	Provides for client's safety.
41. If client is to return to bed, fold back top covers to one side, or fanfold them down to bottom third of bed.	Folding back covers makes it easy for client to return to bed.
42. Rearrange furniture, and place any personal items within easy reach.	Neat environment promotes sense of well-being.
43. Discard dirty linen in linen hamper or chute. Wash hands.	Prevents transmission of microorganisms.
44. Evaluate client's tolerance to sitting up in chair. Compare heart rate to previous resting rate; ask if client feels weak, dizzy, or fatigued; assess blood pressure if client complains of dizziness or weakness.	Client's inability to tolerate exertion, even low levels of exercise, may be reflected in changes in vital signs or subjective report of symptoms.
45. Assist client in returning to bed.	

Recording and Reporting
- Bed making need not be documented. Record client's vital signs and symptoms only if there are changes.

Home Care Considerations
- Review with care giver the available linen and laundry facilities within the client's home.
- Review with care giver an approximate schedule for linen change and indications for linen change.

Making an Occupied Bed

Delegation Considerations
The skills of bed making and making an occupied bed can be delegated to unlicensed assistive personnel.
- Inform care provider how to properly position clients during occupied bed-making procedure.
- Tell care provider what to do if wound drainage, dressing material, drainage tubes, or intravenous (IV) tubing becomes dislodged or is found in the linens.
- Instruct care provider on what to do if client becomes fatigued.
- Stress safety procedures, for example, use of side rails in making an occupied bed, location of call system for easy access in the event that staff assistance is needed.
- Instruct care provider to report any changes in client's level of consciousness, breathing patterns, level of pain, or dizziness.

Equipment
- Linen bag(s)
- Mattress pad (needs to be changed only when soiled)
- Bottom sheet (flat or fitted)
- Drawsheet
- Top sheet
- Blanket
- Bedspread
- Waterproof pads and/or bath blankets (optional)
- Pillowcases
- Bedside chair or table
- Disposable gloves (optional)

STEPS	RATIONALE
1. Determine if client is incontinent or has excess drainage on bed linen.	Determines need for protective waterproof pads or extra bath blankets on bed.
2. Check chart for orders or specific precautions for movement and positioning.	Ensures safety and use of proper body mechanics for nurse and client.
3. Explain procedure to client, noting that client will be asked to turn on side to roll over linen.	Minimizes anxiety and promotes cooperation.
4. Prepare needed equipment and supplies.	
5. Wash hands.	Minimizes spread of infection.
6. Assemble and arrange equipment on bedside chair or table. Remove unnecessary equipment.	Provides for smooth procedure and ensures comfort.
7. Draw room curtain around bed or close door.	Maintains privacy, thus promoting emotional and physical comfort.
8. Lower side rail on near side of bed. Remove call light.	Provides easy access to bed and linen.
9. Adjust bed height to comfortable working position.	Minimizes strain on nurse's back. It is easier to remove and apply linen evenly to bed in flat position.
10. Loosen top linen sheet at foot of bed.	Makes linen easier to remove.
11. Remove bedspread and blanket separately by folding them into squares and placing them in linen bag (if not to be reused). Do not allow linen to contact uniform. Do not fan or shake linen.	Reduces transmission of microorganisms.
12. If blanket and spread are to be reused, fold by bringing top and bottom edges together. Fold into neat squares and place folded linen over back of chair.	Facilitates replacement and prevents wrinkling.
13. Cover client with bath blanket in following manner. Unfold bath blanket over top sheet. Ask client to hold top edge of bath blanket. If client is unable to help, tuck top of bath blanket under shoulder. Grasp top sheet under bath blanket at client's shoulders, and bring sheet down to foot of bed. Remove sheet, and discard it in linen bag.	Bath blanket provides warmth and keeps body parts covered during linen removal.

Continued

Making an Occupied Bed

STEPS	RATIONALE
14. With assistance from another nurse, slide mattress toward head of bed.	If mattress slides toward foot of bed when head of bed is raised, it is difficult to tuck linen and is uncomfortable for client.
15. Position client on the side on far side of bed, facing away. Adjust pillow under head. Be sure farthest side rail is up.	Provides space for placement of clean linen. Side rail ensures safety.
16. Loosen bottom linens, moving from head to foot of bed.	
17. Fanfold first drawsheet and then bottom sheet toward client. Tuck edges of linen just under buttocks, back, and shoulders. Do not fanfold mattress pad if it is to be reused.	Provides maximum work space for placing clean linen. Later, when client turns to other side, soiled linen can be easily removed.
18. Wipe off moisture on mattress with towel and appropriate disinfectant.	Reduces transmission of microorganisms.
19. Apply clean linen to exposed half of bed:	
a. Place clean mattress pad on bed by folding it lengthwise with center crease in middle of bed. Fanfold top layer over mattress. (If pad is reused, simply smooth out wrinkles.)	Applying linen over bed in successive layers minimizes energy and time nurse uses in bed making.
b. Unfold bottom sheet lengthwise so center crease is situated lengthwise along center of bed. Fanfold sheet's top layer toward center of bed alongside client. Smooth bottom layer of sheet over mattress, and bring edge over near side (see illustration). Allow sheet's edge to hang about 25 cm (10 inches) over mattress edge. Lower hem of bottom sheet should lie seam down and even with bottom edge of mattress.	Proper positioning of linen on one side ensures that adequate linen will be available to cover opposite side of bed. Keeping seam edges down eliminates irritation to client's skin.

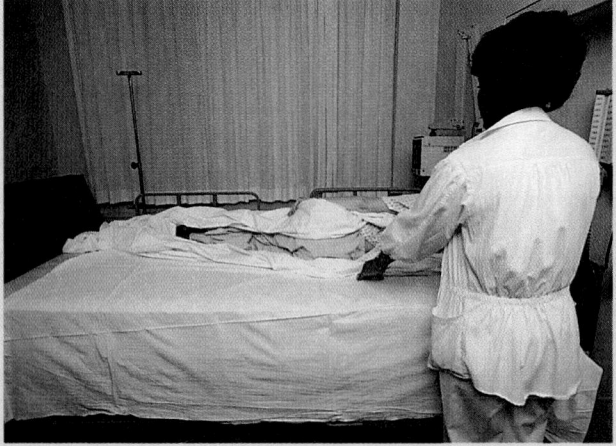

Step 19b

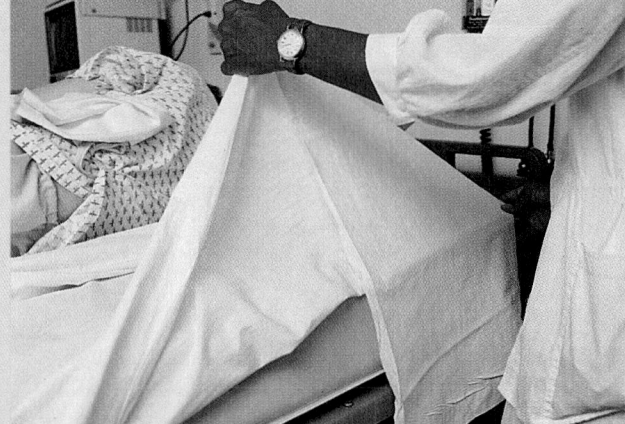

Step 20d

STEPS	RATIONALE
20. Miter bottom sheet at head of bed:	Mitered corner cannot be loosened easily, even if client moves about frequently in bed.
a. Face head of bed diagonally. Place hand away from head of bed under top corner of mattress, near mattress edge, and lift.	
b. With other hand, tuck top edge of bottom sheet smoothly under mattress so side edges of sheet above and below mattress would meet if brought together.	
c. Face side of bed, and pick up top edge of sheet at approximately 45 cm (18 inches) down from top of mattress.	
d. Lift sheet, and lay it on top of mattress to form neat triangular fold, with lower base of triangle even with mattress side edge (see illustration, p. 782).	
e. Tuck lower edge of sheet, which is hanging free below mattress, under mattress. Tuck with palms down without pulling triangular fold.	
f. Hold portion of sheet covering side edge of mattress in place with one hand. With other hand, pick up top of triangular linen fold, and bring it down over side of mattress. Tuck this portion of sheet under mattress.	

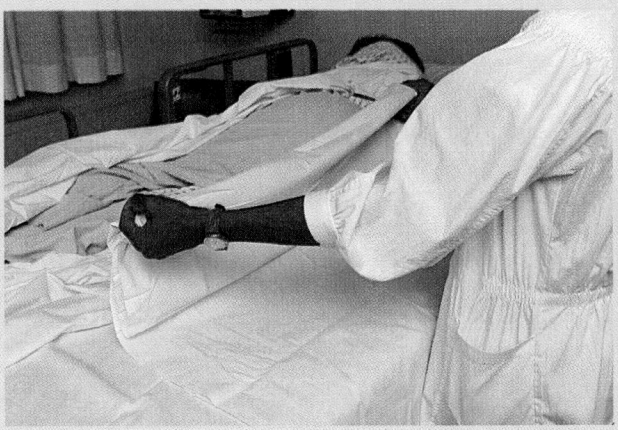

Step 22

STEPS	RATIONALE
21. Tuck remaining portion of sheet under mattress, moving toward foot of bed. Keep linen smooth.	Folds of linen are source of irritation.
22. Open drawsheet so it unfolds in half. Lay center fold along middle of bed lengthwise, and position sheet so it will be under buttocks and torso (see illustration). Fanfold top layer toward client with edge alongside back. Smooth bottom layer out over mattress and tuck excess edge under mattress (keep palms down).	Drawsheet is used to lift and reposition client. Placement distributes most of body weight over sheet.
23. Place waterproof pad over drawsheet with center fold against client's side. Fanfold far half toward client.	Used to protect bed linen from soiling.
24. Raise side rail on working side, and go to other side.	Maintains safety.
25. Lower side rail. Assist client to roll slowly onto other side, over folds of linen.	Exposes opposite side of bed for removal of soiled linen and placement of clean linen.
26. Loosen edges of soiled linen from underneath mattress.	Makes linen easier to remove.
27. Without allowing dirty linen to touch uniform, remove soiled linen by folding it into a bundle or square, with soiled side turned in. Discard it in linen bag.	Reduces transmission of microorganisms.
28. Spread clean, fanfolded linen smoothly over edge of mattress from head to foot of bed.	Smooth linen will not irritate client's skin.
29. Assist client in rolling back into supine position. Reposition pillow.	Client's comfort is maintained.

Continued

.... Skill 29-8—cont'd
Making an Occupied Bed

STEPS	RATIONALE
30. Miter top corner of bottom sheet (see Step 20). When tucking corner, be sure sheet is smooth and free of wrinkles.	Wrinkles and folds can cause mechanical irritation to skin.
31. Facing side of bed, grasp remaining edge of bottom sheet, keep back straight, and pull as excess linen is tucked under mattress (see illustration). Proceed from head to foot of bed. (Avoid lifting mattress during tucking to ensure fit.)	Proper use of body mechanics while tucking linen prevents injury to nurse.
32. Smooth fanfolded drawsheet over bottom sheet. Grasp edge of sheet with palms down, lean back, and tuck sheet under mattress. Tuck from middle to top and to bottom.	Tucking first at top or bottom may pull sheet sideways, causing poor fit.
33. Place top sheet over client with center fold lengthwise down middle of bed. Open sheet from head to foot, and unfold it over client.	Sheet should be equally distributed over bed by correctly positioning center fold.
34. Without allowing dirty linen to touch uniform, ask client to hold clean top sheet, or tuck sheet around shoulders. Remove bath blanket, and discard it into linen bag (see illustration).	Sheet prevents exposure of body parts. Having client hold sheet encourages participation in care.
35. Place blanket on bed, unfolding it so that crease runs lengthwise along middle of bed. Unfold blanket to cover client. Top edge should be parallel with edge of top sheet and 15 to 20 cm (6 to 8 inches) down from top sheet's edge.	Blanket should be placed to cover client completely and provide adequate warmth.
36. Place spread over bed according to Step 31. Be sure top edge of spread extends about 2.5 cm (1 inch) above blanket's edge. Tuck top edge of spread over and under top edge of blanket.	Spread gives bed neat appearance and provides extra warmth.
37. Make cuff by turning edge of top sheet down over top edge of blanket and spread.	Smooth cuff protects client's face from rubbing against blanket or spread.

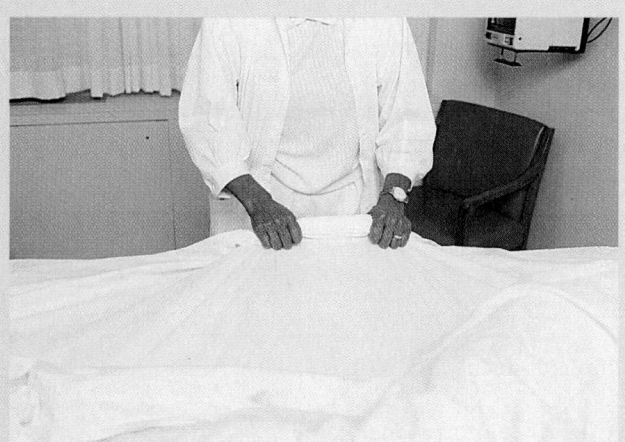

Step 31

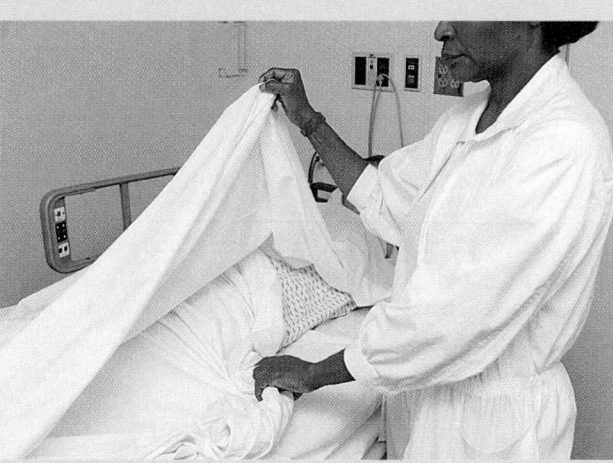

Step 34

STEPS	RATIONALE
38. Standing on one side at foot of bed, lift mattress corner slightly with one hand, and tuck top linens under mattress. Top sheet and blanket are tucked under together. Be sure linens are loose enough to allow for movement of client's feet. (Horizontal toe pleat may be made [see Skill 29-7, Step 30].)	Tucking all top linens together makes neat-appearing bed. Pressure sores can develop on client's toes and heels from feet rubbing between tight-fitting bed sheets.
39. Make modified mitered corner with top sheet, blanket, and spread:	
a. Pick up side edge of top sheet, blanket, and spread approximately 45 cm (18 inches) up from foot of mattress. Lift linens to form triangular fold, and lay it on bed.	Modified mitered corner secures top linen but keeps an even edge of blanket and top sheet draped over mattress.
b. Tuck lower edge of sheet, which is hanging free below mattress, under mattress. Do not pull triangular fold.	
c. Pick up triangular fold, and bring it down over mattress while holding linen in place along side of mattress. Do not tuck tip of triangle.	
40. Raise side rail. Make other side of bed; spread sheet, blanket, and bedspread out evenly; fold top edge of spread over blanket, and make cuff with top sheet (see Step 37); make modified corner at foot of bed (see Step 39).	Side rail protects client from accidental falls.
41. Change pillowcase:	
a. Have client raise head. While supporting neck with one hand, remove pillow.	Prevents injury during flexion and extension of neck.
b. Remove soiled case and discard in linen bag.	
c. Grasp clean pillowcase at center of closed end. Gather case, turning it inside out over hand holding it. With same hand pick up middle of one end of pillow. Pull pillowcase down over pillow with other hand and be sure pillow corners fit evenly in corners of pillowcase.	Method makes it easy to slide pillowcase over pillow. Poorly fitting case constricts fluffing and expansion of pillow.
42. Support client's head under neck, and place pillow under head.	Prevents hyperextension of neck muscles.
43. Place call light within client's reach; return bed to comfortable position.	Ensures safety and comfort.
44. Open room curtains. Rearrange furniture. Place personal items within easy reach on overbed table or bedside stand. Return bed to comfortable height.	Promotes sense of well-being.
45. Discard dirty linen in linen hamper or chute; wash hands.	Prevents transmission of microorganisms.

Recording and Reporting

- Bed making need not be documented. Record the client's vital signs and symptoms only if there are changes.

Home Care Considerations

- Assess the primary care giver's ability to safely make an occupied bed.
- Assess the home laundry facilities to plan for the frequency with which the linen can be laundered.
- Assess the amount of linen in the home for the anticipated amount of linen changes needed.

Linens. Before bed making, it is important to collect not only bed linens but also the client's personal linens. Linens are pressed and folded to prevent the spread of microorganisms and to make bed making easier. Bed linens have a center crease that the nurse places in the center of the bed from the head to the foot. The linens unfold easily to the sides, with creases often fitting over the mattress edge. New linens are applied whenever there is soiling.

Key Terms

acne	oral hygiene
buccal cavity	partial bed bath
complete bed bath	perineal care
dental caries	subcutaneous layer

■ Key Concepts ■

The nurse provides clients' daily hygiene needs if they are unable to care for themselves adequately.

Providing hygiene care gives the nurse the chance to assess external body surfaces and the client's emotional state.

While providing daily hygiene needs, the nurse uses teaching and communication skills to develop a relationship with the client.

The client's personal preferences must always be considered when the nurse plans daily hygiene care.

The nurse must maintain privacy and comfort when providing the client's daily care.

During assessment of the skin and oral mucosa, the nurse observes characteristics influenced by hygiene.

Clients who are immobilized and poorly nourished and who have reduced sensation or peripheral circulation are at risk for altered skin integrity.

Gloves should be worn by nurses during hygiene care when the risk of contacting body fluids is high and should always be worn during perineal care.

Clients with diabetes need special nail and foot care.

When administering oral care to unconscious clients, the nurse takes measures to prevent aspiration.

Clients who wear contact lenses must learn proper self-care techniques to avoid corneal injury.

Evaluation of hygiene care is based on the client's sense of comfort, relaxation, well-being, and understanding of hygiene techniques.

■ Critical Thinking Activities ■

1. Mr. Roberts, an 80-year-old widower who lives alone, is admitted to the intensive care unit. He is obese and has poor hygiene. His skin is rough and dry with some areas of excoriation. What are the most important assessments to be made in the situation? What appropriate interventions may be used?

2. Mrs. John, a 30-year-old woman, is admitted to the neurological unit following a spinal cord injury. She is now a quadriplegic. In terms of hygiene needs, what are the priorities in taking care of Mrs. John?

3. Mr. Green, a 52-year-old man, has been on long-term therapy for peripheral vascular disease. He has been on coumarin therapy. What home care instructions are essential in his discharge planning in regard to hygiene?

References

Anetzberger GJ and others: Elder mistreatment: a call for help, *Patient Care* 27(11):93, 1993.

Barnes SH: Patient and family education for the patient with a pressure necrosis, *Nurs Clin North Am* 22:163, 1987.

Bennett MA: Report of the task force on the implication for darkly pigmented intact skin in the prediction and preventions of pressure ulcers, *Adv Wound Care* 8(6):34, 1995.

Blaney GM: Mouthcare—basic and essential, *Geriatric Nurs* 7:242, 1986.

Christensen MH and others: How to care for the diabetic foot, *Am J Nurs* 91(3):50, 1991.

Cohen E, Krachmer J: Red eyes and contact lenses, *Patient Care* 26(9):143, 1992.

Danielson LH: Oral care and older adults, *J Gerontol Nurs* 7:242, 1988.

Dudjak LA: Mouthcare for mucositis due to radiation therapy, *Cancer Nurs* 10:131, 1987.

Harrell JS, Damon JF: Prediction of patients' need for mouth care, *West J Nurs Res* 11:748, 1989.

Lueckenotte AG: *Gerontologic nursing*, St. Louis, 1997, Mosby.

Mahoney DF: Cerumen impaction: prevalence and detection in nursing homes, *J Gerontol Nurs* 54(12):56, 1993.

Maklebust J: Pressure ulcer update, *RN* 41(12):56, 1991.

National Pressure Ulcer Advisory Panel (NPUAP): Pressure ulcer incidence, economics, risk assessment: consensus development conference statement, *Decubitus* 2(2):24, 1989.

Ney DF: Cerumen impaction, ear hygiene practices, and hearing acuity, *Geriatric Nurs* 14(2):70, 1993.

Osterman HM, Stuck RM: The aging foot, *Orthop Nurs* 9:43, 1990.

Panel for the Prediction and Prevention for Pressure Ulcers in Adults (PPPUA): Assessing risk and preventing pressure ulcers, *Patient Care* 27(7):36, 1993.

Phipps W and others: *Medical-surgical nursing concepts and clinical practice*, ed 5, St. Louis, 1995, Mosby.

Poland JM: Comparing Moi-Stir to lemon glycerin swabs, *Am J Nurs* 87:422, 1987.

Tyler D and others: Effects of a one minute backrub on mixed venous oxygen saturation and heart rate, *Heart Lung* 19(5):562, 1990.

U.S. Department of Health and Human Services: *Prediction and prevention*, Pub No. 92-0047, 92-0050, Rockville, Md, 1992, PHS, Agency for Health Care Policy and Research.

Wong DL: *Whaley and Wong's essentials of pediatric nursing*, ed 6, St. Louis, 1997, Mosby.

30

Oxygenation

OBJECTIVES

Mastery of content in this chapter will enable the student to:

- Define the key terms listed.
- Identify physiological processes in maintaining cardiac output, myocardial blood flow, and coronary artery circulation.
- Describe the electrical conduction system of the heart.
- Identify physiological processes involved in ventilation, perfusion, and exchange of respiratory gases.
- Explain the ways a client's level of health, age, lifestyle, and environment can affect tissue oxygenation.
- Identify causes and effects of disturbances in conduction, altered cardiac output, impaired valvular function, myocardial ischemia, and impaired tissue perfusion.
- Identify causes and effects of hyperventilation, hypoventilation, and hypoxemia.
- Perform a nursing assessment of the cardiopulmonary system.
- Develop nursing diagnoses for altered oxygenation.
- Describe nursing interventions to maintain or restore cardiopulmonary function.
- Develop evaluation criteria for a care plan for the client with altered oxygenation.

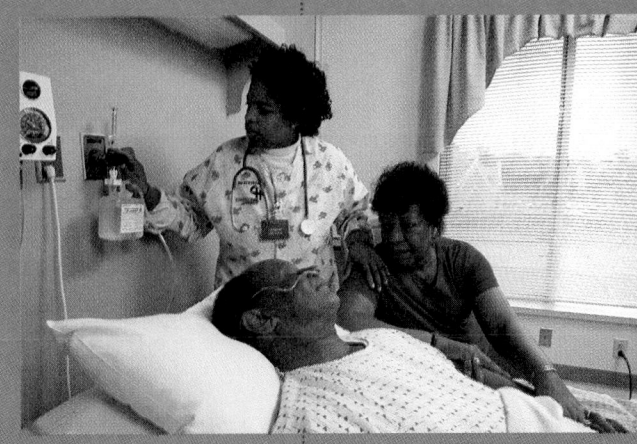

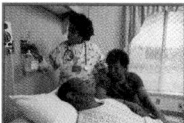

Case Study

....
Mr. King

Mr. King, age 74, came to the hospital 2 days ago with complaints of chest pain, weakness, and a high temperature. Mr. King is a retired bookbinder, who resides in a mobile home with his wife. Both have preexisting health conditions that put them at risk for pneumonia. Mrs. King is diabetic and takes insulin twice a day. Mr. King has a history of alcohol abuse but at present is not drinking. Both individuals are heavy smokers and have been for greater than 50 years. Currently they are not utilizing any external support systems outside the home. Mrs. King performs most of the household duties and grocery shops once a week with the help of her daughter. Mr. King used to help out with the housework, and he loves to tinker in the garden; however, lately he has been unable to do either. His wife states, "All he seems to be able to do is sit in his chair and watch TV."

Mary Brown is a junior nursing student assigned to her first hospital-based clinical experience. Mary has had some experience in health assessment and client teaching related to health promotion activities from her recent clinical rotation in a clinic. In the previous clinical experience, clients were motivated to adjust their at-risk health behaviors, such as smoking or poor diet. Mary feels confident when she arrives in the clinical area this morning because Mr. King has similar health needs to the clinical experiences she has had. However, when Mary goes to meet Mr. King and performs her morning assessment, she is overwhelmed. This client is in a great deal of respiratory distress. It seems that every breath is a struggle for this client. Everything that Mary has planned to do seems of less importance. The client is extremely anxious. His wife is at his side anticipating Mary's every move and demanding some action.

SCIENTIFIC KNOWLEDGE BASE

Oxygen is a basic human need and is required for life. The nurse often encounters clients who are unable to meet oxygen needs. To help clients meet their oxygen needs, the nurse must understand cardiac and respiratory physiology.

Cardiovascular Physiology

The function of the cardiac system is to deliver oxygen, nutrients, and other substances to the tissues and remove the waste products of cellular metabolism through the cardiac pump, the circulatory vascular system, and the integration of other systems (e.g., respiratory, digestive, and renal systems) (McCance and Huether, 1994).

Structure and function. The right ventricle pumps blood to the pulmonary circulation while the left ventricle pumps blood to the systemic circulation, supplying oxygen and nutrients to the tissues and removing wastes from the body (Figure 30-1). The circulatory system exchanges respiratory gases, nutrients, and waste products between the blood and the tissues.

Myocardial pump. The pumping action of the heart is essential to maintain oxygen delivery. Decreased pump effectiveness, such as in coronary artery disease and cardiomyopathic conditions, results in a diminished stroke volume, the volume of the blood ejected from the ventricles. Hemorrhage and dehydration decrease pump effectiveness by reducing the amount of blood ejected from the ventricles.

Myocardial blood flow. To maintain adequate blood flow to the pulmonary and systemic circulations, myocardial blood flow must supply sufficient oxygen

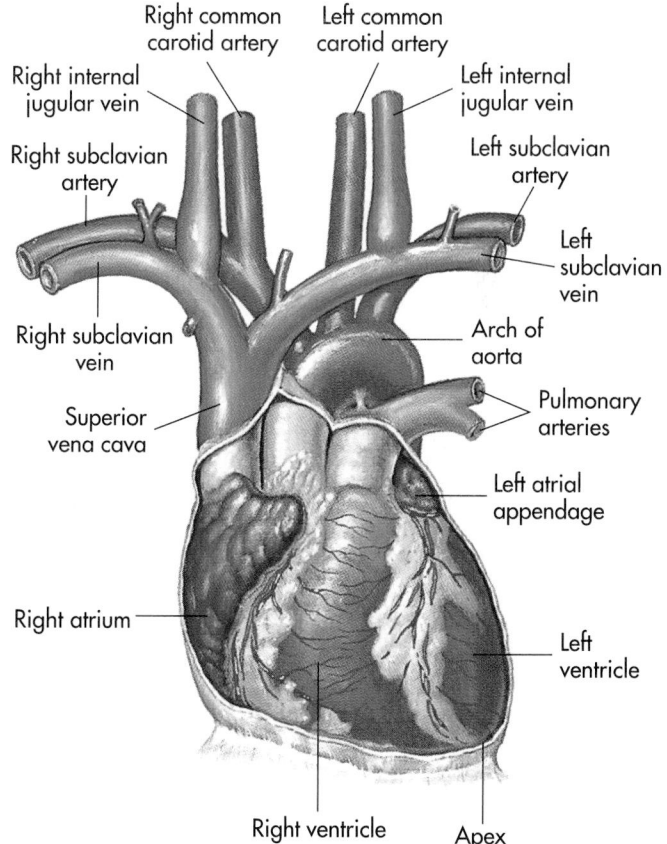

Figure 30-1. Diagram showing serially connected pulmonary and systemic circulations. Right heart chambers propel unoxygenated blood through the pulmonary circulation; left heart chambers propel oxygenated blood through the systemic circulation. (From Canobbio MM: *Cardiovascular disorders,* St. Louis, 1990, Mosby.)

and nutrients to the myocardium itself. The one-way flow of blood through the heart is ensured by the four heart valves.

Coronary artery circulation. Blood flow through the atria and ventricles does not supply oxygen and nutrients to the myocardium itself. The coronary circulation is the branch of the systemic circulation that supplies oxygen and nutrients to and removes waste from the myocardium.

Systemic circulation. The arteries and veins of the systemic circulation deliver nutrients and oxygen to and remove waste from the tissues. Oxygenated blood flows from the left ventricle by way of the aorta and into the large systemic arteries. These arteries branch into smaller arteries, arterioles, and finally the smallest vessels, the capillaries. At the capillary level the exchange of respiratory gases, nutrients, and waste occurs, and the tissues are oxygenated. The waste products exit the capillary network by way of the venules that join to form veins. These veins form the larger veins, which carry deoxygenated blood to the right side of the heart, where it is returned to pulmonary circulation.

Regulation of blood flow. The amount of blood ejected from the left ventricle each minute is the **cardiac output.** The normal cardiac output is 4 to 6 L/min in the healthy 150-lb (70-kg) adult at rest. The circulating volume of blood changes according to the oxygen and metabolic needs of the body.

Cardiac index is the adequacy of the cardiac output for an individual. The cardiac index equals cardiac output divided by a person's body surface area. The normal range of the cardiac index is 2.5 to 4.0 L/min/m³ (Urban and others, 1995).

Stroke volume is the amount of blood ejected from the ventricle with each contraction. It can be affected by the amount of blood in the left ventricle at the end of diastole (preload), the resistance to left ventricular ejection (afterload), and myocardial contractility.

Preload is essentially the end-diastolic volume. As the ventricles fill, they stretch. The greater the stretch on the ventricle, the greater the contraction and the greater the stroke volume (Starling's law). In clinical situations the preload and subsequent stroke volume can be manipulated by changing the amount of circulating blood volume.

Afterload is the resistance to left ventricular ejection, the work the heart must overcome to fully eject blood from the left ventricle. The diastolic aortic pressure is a good clinical measure of afterload. In a client with an acute hypertensive crisis, the afterload is increased, increasing the cardiac workload. Afterload in this situation can be reduced by decreasing systemic blood pressure.

Myocardial contractility also affects stroke volume and cardiac output. Poor contraction decreases the amount of blood ejected by the ventricles during each contraction. Myocardial contractility can be increased

by drugs that increase the force of contraction. Myocardial contractility can be decreased by injury to the myocardial muscle, such as an acute myocardial infarction. The myocardium of the older adult is more rigid and slower in recovering its contractility (Lueckenotte, 1994).

Heart rate affects blood flow because of the interaction between rate and diastolic filling time. With a sustained heart rate greater than 160 beats/min, diastolic filling time decreases, decreasing stroke volume and cardiac output. The heart rate of the older adult is slow to increase under stress. To compensate for this, the stroke volume may increase to increase the cardiac output and blood pressure (Lueckenotte, 1996).

Conduction system. The rhythmic relaxation and contraction of the atria and ventricles depend on continuous, organized transmission of electrical impulses. These impulses are generated and transmitted by the conduction system.

The heart's conduction system generates the necessary action potentials that conduct the impulses required to initiate the electrical mechanical chain of events. The autonomic nervous system influences the rate of impulse generation, the transmission speed through the conductive pathway, and the strength of contractions. Sympathetic nerve fibers, which increase the impulse generation rate and the impulse transmission speed, supply the atria and ventricles. Parasympathetic fibers from the vagus nerve, which decrease this rate, also supply these parts along with the sinoatrial and atrioventricular nodes (McCance and Huether, 1994).

The conduction system originates with the **sinoatrial (SA) node,** the "pacemaker" of the heart. The SA node is in the right atrium next to the entrance of

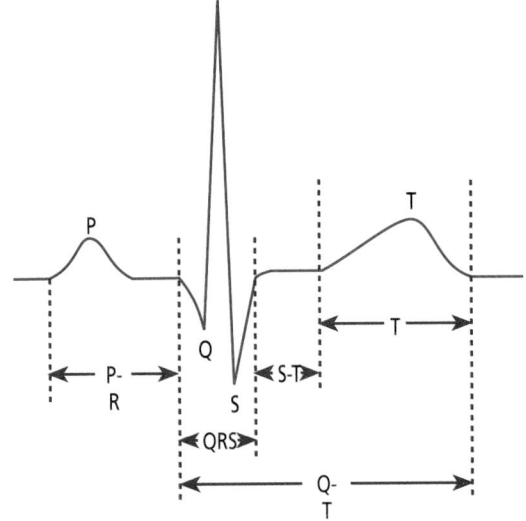

Figure 30-2. Normal ECG waveform. (From Canobbio MM: *Cardiovascular disorders,* St. Louis, 1990, Mosby.)

the superior vena cava (McCance and Huether, 1994). Impulses are initiated at the SA node at an intrinsic rate of 60 to 100 beats/min. The resting adult rate is approximately 75 beats/min.

The electrical impulses are then transmitted through the atria along intraarterial pathways to the **atrioventricular (AV) node.** The AV node mediates impulses between the atria and the ventricles. It assists atrial emptying by delaying the impulse before transmitting it through the **bundle of His** and the ventricular **Purkinje network.**

The electrical activity of the conduction system is recorded on an **electrocardiogram (ECG).** An ECG monitors the regularity and path of the electrical impulse through the conduction system; however, it does not reflect muscular work of the heart. The normal sequence on the ECG is called **normal sinus rhythm (NSR)** (Figure 30-2).

Respiratory Physiology

Most cells in the body obtain much of their energy from chemical reactions involving oxygen and the elimination of carbon dioxide. The exchange of respiratory gases occurs between environmental air and the blood. There are three steps in the process of oxygenation: ventilation, perfusion, and diffusion (McCance and Huether, 1994). For the exchange of respiratory gases

to occur, the organs, nerves, and muscles of respiration must be intact and the central nervous system must be able to regulate the respiratory cycle (Figure 30-3).

Structure and function. Respiration can be altered by conditions or diseases that change the structure and function of the lung. The respiratory muscles, pleural space, lungs, and alveoli (Figure 30-4) are essential for ventilation, perfusion, and exchange of respiratory gases (Box 30-1).

Ventilation. Ventilation is the process of moving gases into and out of the lungs. **Ventilation** requires coordination of the muscular and elastic properties of the lung and thorax and intact innervation. The major inspiratory muscle of respiration is the diaphragm. It is innervated by the phrenic nerve, which exits the spinal cord at the fourth cervical vertebra.

Work of breathing. Breathing is the effort required to expand and contract the lungs. The work of breathing is determined by the degree of compliance of the lungs, airway resistance, presence of active expiration, and use of accessory muscles of respiration.

Compliance. The degree of elasticity or expandability of the lungs and thorax is called **compliance.** Compliance is decreased in diseases such as pulmonary edema, interstitial and pleural fibrosis, and congenital

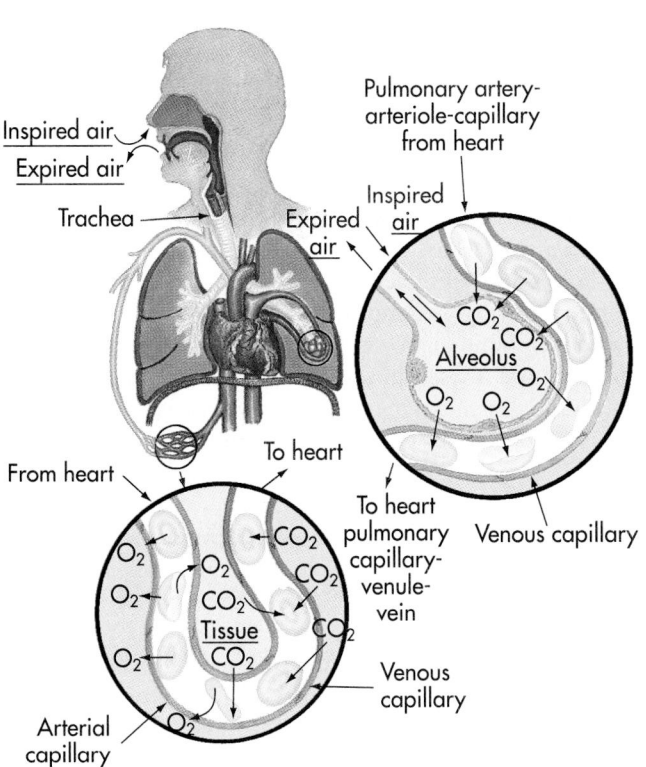

Figure 30-3. Structures of the pulmonary system. The circle denotes the alveoli. (Modified from Wilson SF, Thompson JM: *Mosby's clinical nursing series: respiratory disorders,* St. Louis, 1990, Mosby.)

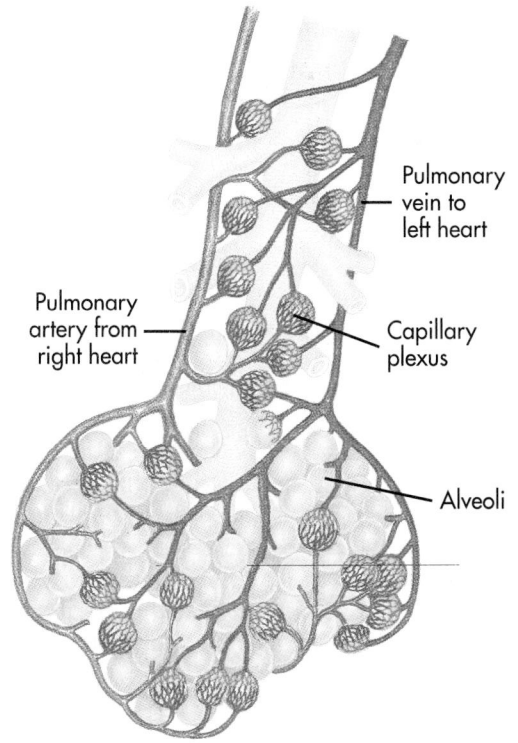

Figure 30-4. Alveoli at the terminal end of the lower airway. (From Thompson J and others: *Mosby's manual of clinical nursing,* ed 3, St. Louis, 1993, Mosby.)

Box 30-1
Major Anatomical Structures of the Thorax and Their Functions

Inspiratory Muscles
Diaphragm

Contraction causes the diaphragm to descend, creating a negative pleural pressure and increasing the vertical dimension of the lungs, which contributes to lung inflation. The increase in vertical dimension and the decrease in intrapulmonary pressure (negative with respect to atmospheric pressure) cause air to enter the lungs.

External Intercostal

Contraction elevates the anterior ends of the ribs, causing them to move upward and outward. This increases the anteroposterior dimension of the thorax.

Accessory Muscles

Accessory muscles include the scalene, sternocleidomastoid, and trapezius muscles. Contraction elevates the first two ribs and the sternum.

Expiratory Muscles
Internal Intercostal

Contraction pulls ribs down and in, thereby decreasing the anteroposterior diameter of the thorax.

Abdominal Respiratory

Abdominal respiratory muscles contract to depress lower ribs, force the diaphragm up, and decrease the vertical dimension of the thoracic cavity.

Pleural Space

The pleural space is a potential space that is only a thin film of liquid lying between the outer layer of the lung (visceral pleura) and the inner layer of the chest cavity (parietal pleura). It permits a smooth, gliding movement of the lungs along the chest wall. Normally, air is not present in the pleural space.

Lungs
Left (Two Lobes) and Right (Three Lobes)

The lungs transfer oxygen from the atmosphere into the alveoli and carbon dioxide from the alveoli to the lungs to be excreted as a waste product. They also filter toxic material from circulation and metabolize compounds such as angiotensin I, bradykinin, and prostaglandins.

Alveoli

Alveoli transfer oxygen and carbon dioxide to and from the blood through the alveolar membrane. These tiny air sacs expand during inspiration, greatly increasing the surface area over which exchange of gases occurs.

---

or traumatic structural abnormalities, such as kyphosis or fractured ribs.

Surfactant is the chemical produced in the lung by alveolar type II cells that maintains the surface tension of the alveoli, keeps them dry, and keeps them from collapsing. When surfactant is decreased, alveoli can become fluid filled, non–easily distensible, or can collapse.

Airway resistance. The pressure difference between the mouth and the alveoli in relation to the rate of flow of inspired gas is called **airway compliance.** Airway resistance can be increased by an airway obstruction, small airway disease (e.g., asthma), and tracheal edema. When resistance is increased, the amount of air traveling through the anatomical airways is decreased.

Expiration is normally a passive process that depends on elastic recoil properties and requires little or no muscle work. Elastic recoil is produced by elastic fibers in lung tissue and by surface tension in the fluid film lining the alveoli (Dettenmeier, 1992). Clients with advanced chronic obstructive pulmonary disease lose the elastic recoil of the lung and the thorax. As a result the client's work of breathing is increased.

Accessory muscles of respiration can increase lung volume during inspiration. Clients with chronic obstructive pulmonary disease, especially emphysema, frequently use these muscles to increase lung volume. During assessment the nurse may observe the client's clavicles being elevated during inspiration; as the clavicles elevate, the apices of the lungs distend and inspiratory lung volume is increased.

Decreased compliance, increased airway resistance, active expiration, or use of accessory muscles increases the work of breathing, resulting in an increased energy expenditure. To meet this expenditure the body increases its metabolic rate and the need for oxygen as well as the elimination of carbon dioxide. This sequence is a vicious cycle for a client with impaired ventilation, causing further deterioration of respiratory status and ability to oxygenate adequately.

Lung volumes. Normal lung volumes are measured through pulmonary function testing. Spirometry measures the volume of air entering or leaving the lungs. Variations in lung volumes may be associated with pregnancy, exercise, obesity, and obstructive or restrictive conditions of the lung. The amount of surfactant, degree of compliance, and strength of respiratory muscles can affect lung pressures and volumes within the lungs.

Pressures. Gases move into and out of the lung through pressure changes. Intrapleural pressure is less than atmospheric pressure, which is 760 mm Hg at sea level and is referred to as negative pressure. For air to flow into the lungs, intrapleural pressure must become more negative, setting up a pressure gradient between the atmosphere and alveoli. Inspiratory airflow is increased because air from the atmosphere, which is at a greater pressure, enters the alveoli during inspiration.

Perfusion. The primary function of pulmonary circulation is to move blood to and from the alveolar-capillary membrane so gas exchange can occur. Pulmonary circulation is a reservoir for blood so the lung can increase its blood volume without large increases in pulmonary artery or venous pressures. The pulmonary circulation also acts as a filter, removing small thrombi before they reach vital organs.

Pulmonary circulation. Pulmonary circulation begins at the pulmonary artery, which receives poorly oxygenated mixed venous blood from the right ventricle. Blood flow through this system depends on the pumping ability of the right ventricle, which has an output of approximately 4 to 6 L/min. The flow continues from the pulmonary artery through the pulmonary arterioles to the pulmonary capillaries, where blood comes in contact with the alveolocapillary membrane and the exchange of respiratory gases occurs. The oxygen-rich blood then circulates through the pulmonary venules and pulmonary veins, returning to the left atrium.

Distribution. Pressures within the pulmonary circulation system are low in comparison to those in the systemic circulatory system. The normal pulmonary systolic arterial pressure is between 20 and 30 mm Hg, the diastolic pressure is less than 12 mm Hg, and the mean pressure is less than 20 mm Hg (Daily and Schroeder, 1994). The walls of the pulmonary vessels are thinner than those in the systemic circulation and contain less smooth muscle because of the low pressure and resistance. The lung accepts the total cardiac output from the right ventricle and, except in cases of alveolar hypoxia, does not direct blood flow from one region to another.

Exchange of respiratory gases. Respiratory gases are exchanged in the alveoli of the lungs and the capillaries of the body tissues. Oxygen is transferred from the lungs to the blood, and carbon dioxide is transferred from the blood to the alveoli to be exhaled as waste product. At the tissue level, oxygen is transferred from the blood to tissues, and carbon dioxide is transferred from tissues to the blood to return to the alveoli and be exhaled. This transfer is dependent on the process of diffusion.

Diffusion. **Diffusion** is the movement of molecules from an area of high concentration to an area of low concentration. Diffusion of respiratory gases occurs at the alveolocapillary membrane, and the rate of diffusion can be affected by thickness of the membrane.

Increased thickness of the membrane impedes diffusion because gases take longer to transfer across. Clients with pulmonary edema, pulmonary infiltrates, or a pulmonary effusion have an increased thickness of the alveolocapillary membrane, resulting in slowed diffusion, slowed exchange of respiratory gases, and impaired delivery of oxygen to tissues.

The surface area of the membrane can be altered as a result of a chronic disease (e.g., emphysema), an acute disease (e.g., pneumothorax), or a surgical process (e.g., lobectomy). When fewer alveoli are functioning, the surface area is decreased.

Oxygen transport. The oxygen transport system consists of the lungs and cardiovascular system. Delivery depends on the amount of oxygen entering the lungs (ventilation), blood flow to the lungs and tissues (perfusion), rate of diffusion, and oxygen-carrying capacity. The capacity of the blood to carry oxygen is influenced by the amount of dissolved oxygen in the plasma, amount of hemoglobin, and tendency of hemoglobin to bind with oxygen (Ahrens, 1990).

Only a relatively small amount of required oxygen, about 3%, is dissolved in the plasma. Most oxygen is transported by hemoglobin, which serves as a carrier for oxygen and carbon dioxide. The hemoglobin molecule combines with oxygen to form oxyhemoglobin. The formation of oxyhemoglobin is easily reversible, allowing hemoglobin and oxygen to dissociate, which frees oxygen to enter tissues.

Carbon dioxide transport. Carbon dioxide diffuses into red blood cells and is rapidly hydrated into carbonic acid (H_2CO_3) because of carbonic anhydrase. The carbonic acid then dissociates into hydrogen (H^+) and bicarbonate (HCO_3^-) ions. The hydrogen ion is buffered by hemoglobin, and the HCO_3^- diffuses into the plasma (see Chapter 31). In addition, some of the carbon dioxide in red blood cells reacts with amino acid groups, forming carbamino compounds. This reaction can occur rapidly without the presence of an enzyme. Reduced hemoglobin (deoxyhemoglobin) can combine with carbon dioxide more easily than can oxyhemoglobin, and therefore venous blood transports most of the carbon dioxide.

Regulation of respiration. The main purpose of respiratory regulation is to supply sufficient oxygen to meet the body's demands, such as during exercise, infection, or pregnancy. Respiratory regulation promotes exhalation of metabolically produced carbon dioxide, which is a determinant of acid-base status (see Chapter 31).

Respiration is controlled by neural and chemical regulators. Neural regulation includes the central nervous system control of respiratory rate, depth, and rhythm. Chemical regulation involves the influence of chemicals such as carbon dioxide and hydrogen ions on the rate and depth of respiration (Box 30-2).

Factors Affecting Oxygenation
Adequacy of circulation, ventilation, perfusion, and transport of respiratory gases to the tissues are influenced by multiple factors.

Pathophysiological and physiological factors.
Any condition that affects cardiopulmonary functioning directly affects the body's ability to meet oxygen demands. The general classifications of cardiac disorders include disturbances in conduction, impaired valvular function, myocardial hypoxia, cardiomyopathic conditions, and peripheral tissue hypoxia. Respiratory disorders include hyperventilation, hypoventilation, and hypoxia.

▪ Box 30-2
Neural and Chemical Regulation of Respiration

Neural Regulation
Neural regulation maintains rhythm and depth of respiration, as well as the balance between inspiration and expiration.

Cerebral Cortex
Voluntary control of respiration delivers impulses to the respiratory motor neurons by way of the spinal cord. Voluntary control of respiration accommodates speaking, eating, and swimming.

Medulla Oblongata
Automatic control of respiration occurs continuously.

Chemical Regulation
Chemical regulation maintains appropriate rate and depth of respirations based on changes in the blood's carbon dioxide (CO_2), oxygen (O_2), and hydrogen ion (H^+) concentration.

Chemoreceptors
Chemoreceptors are located in the medulla, aortic body, and carotid body. Changes in chemical content of O_2, CO_2, and H^+ stimulate chemoreceptors, which in turn stimulate neural regulators to adjust the rate and depth of ventilation to maintain normal arterial blood gas levels. Chemical regulation can occur during physical exercise and in some illnesses. It is a short-term adaptive mechanism.

Other pathophysiological processes affecting a client's oxygenation include alterations that affect the oxygen-carrying capacity of blood (e.g., anemia), increases in the body's metabolic demands (e.g., fever, infection), and alterations that affect the client's chest wall movement or the central nervous system.

Decreased oxygen-carrying capacity. Hemoglobin carries 97% of oxygen to tissues. Any process that decreases or alters hemoglobin, such as anemia or inhalation of toxic substances, decreases the oxygen-carrying capacity of blood.

Carbon monoxide is the most common toxic inhalant decreasing the oxygen-carrying capacity of blood. Hemoglobin tends to bind with carbon monoxide 210 times more than with oxygen, creating a functional anemia (Ahrens and Rutherford, 1993). Because of the bond's strength, carbon monoxide is not easily dissociated from hemoglobin, making the hemoglobin unavailable for oxygen transport.

Decreased inspired oxygen concentration. When the concentration of inspired oxygen declines, the oxygen-carrying capacity of the blood is decreased. Decreases in the fraction of inspired oxygen concentration (F_IO_2) can be caused by an upper or lower airway obstruction limiting delivery of inspired oxygen to alveoli, decreased environmental oxygen (as occurs at high altitudes), or decreased inspiration as the result of an incorrect oxygen concentration setting on respiratory therapy equipment.

Hypovolemia. Hypovolemia is a reduced circulating blood volume resulting from extracellular fluid losses that occurs in conditions such as shock and severe dehydration. If the fluid loss is significant, the body tries to adapt by increasing the heart rate and peripheral vasoconstriction to increase the volume of blood returned to the heart and increase the cardiac output.

Increased metabolic rate. Increases in metabolic activity of the body result in an increased oxygen demand. When the body systems are unable to meet this increased demand, the level of oxygenation declines. An increased metabolic rate is a normal response of the body to pregnancy, wound healing, and exercise because the body is building tissue. Most people can meet the increased oxygen demand and do not display signs of oxygen deprivation.

Fever increases the tissues' need for oxygen, and as a result carbon dioxide production also increases. If the febrile state persists, the metabolic rate remains high and the body begins to break down protein stores, resulting in muscle wasting and decreased muscle mass. Respiratory muscles such as the diaphragm and intercostals are also wasted. The body attempts to adapt to the increased carbon dioxide levels by increasing the rate and depth of respiration to eliminate the excess carbon dioxide. The client's work of breathing increases, and the client will eventually display signs and symptoms of hypoxemia. Those clients with pulmonary diseases are at greater risk for hypoxemia and hypercapnia. Assessment reveals increased rate and depth of respiration, use of the accessory muscles of respiration, use of pursed-lip breathing, and decreased activity tolerance.

Conditions affecting chest wall movement. Any condition that reduces chest wall movement can result in decreased ventilation. If the diaphragm cannot fully descend with breathing, the volume of inspired air decreases and less oxygen is delivered to the alveoli and subsequently to tissues.

Pregnancy. As the fetus grows during pregnancy, the greater size of the uterus pushes abdominal contents up against the diaphragm. In the last trimester of pregnancy the inspiratory capacity declines, resulting in dyspnea on exertion and increased fatigue.

Obesity. Obese clients often have reduced lung volumes from the heavy lower thorax and abdomen, particularly when in recumbent and supine positions. Obese clients have a reduction in compliance as a result of encroachment of the abdomen into the chest, increased work of breathing, and decreased lung volumes and may have fatigue and carbon dioxide retention (Burns and others, 1994).

Musculoskeletal abnormalities. Musculoskeletal impairments in the thoracic region reduce oxygenation. Such impairments may result from abnormal structural configurations, trauma, muscle diseases, and diseases of the nervous system.

Abnormal structural configurations. Abnormal structural configurations impairing oxygenation include those that affect the rib cage, such as pectus excavatum, and those that affect the spinal column, such as kyphosis. The angle of curvature in kyphosis can progress with time, resulting in severe hypoventilation and hypoxemia.

Trauma. Trauma to the chest wall can also impede inspiration. The person with multiple rib fractures can develop a flail chest, a condition in which fractures cause instability in part of the chest wall and paradoxical breathing. In paradoxical breathing, the lung underlying the injured area contracts on inspiration and bulges on expiration, resulting in hypoxia.

Chest wall or upper abdomen incisions may also decrease chest wall movement. The client may use shallow respirations to minimize chest wall movement to avoid pain. Excessive or high doses of narcotic analgesics may depress the respiratory center, thus decreasing respiratory rate and chest wall expansion.

Muscle diseases. Muscle diseases such as muscular dystrophy affect tissue oxygenation of tissues by decreasing the client's ability to expand and contract the chest. Ventilation is impaired, and atelectasis, hypercapnia, and hypoxemia can occur.

Nervous system diseases. Myasthenia gravis, Guillain-Barré syndrome, and poliomyelitis are examples of nervous system diseases that can affect respiratory functioning and result in hypoventilation. These diseases impair nervous and muscular control. When the nerves and muscles of the respiratory system are affected, impaired ventilation (hypoventilation) occurs.

Disease or trauma involving the medulla oblongata and spinal cord may result in impaired respiration. When the medulla oblongata is affected, neural regulation of respiration is damaged and abnormal breathing patterns may develop. Damage to the spinal cord can affect respiration in two ways. If the phrenic nerve is damaged, the diaphragm may not descend, thus reducing inspiratory lung volumes and causing hypoxemia. Cervical trauma at C3 to C5 can result in paralysis of the phrenic nerve. Spinal cord trauma below the fifth cervical vertebra usually leaves the phrenic nerve intact but damages nerves that innervate the intercostal muscles, preventing anteroposterior chest expansion.

Influences of chronic disease. Oxygenation can be decreased as a direct consequence of chronic disease. It can also be decreased as a secondary effect, as with anemia. The physiological response to chronic hypoxemia is the development of a secondary polycythemia or an increase in red blood cells. This adaptive response is the body's attempt to increase the amount of circulating hemoglobin to increase the available oxygen-binding sites.

⋯NURSING KNOWLEDGE BASE

Total health is affected by many factors, including health beliefs and individual behaviors, physical and psychological stressors, and environmental factors. To provide the most effective care, the nurse needs to understand the relationship of different needs and the factors that determine the priorities for the client. The nurse also identifies actual and potential risk factors that predispose a person or group to illness.

The nurse who understands how clients react to illness can minimize the effects of illness and assist the client and family to maintain or return to the highest level of functioning.

Developmental Factors

The developmental stage of the client and the normal aging process can affect tissue oxygenation.

Premature infants. Premature infants are at risk for hyaline membrane disease, which is thought to be caused by a surfactant deficiency. The surfactant-synthesizing ability of the lungs develops late in pregnancy, about the seventh month, and may therefore be lacking in preterm infants.

Infants and toddlers. Infants and toddlers are at risk for upper respiratory tract infections as a result of frequent exposure to other children and exposure to secondhand smoke (Huebner, 1994; Whatling, 1994). In addition, during the teething process some infants develop nasal congestion, which can encourage bacterial growth and increase the potential for respiratory tract infection. Upper respiratory tract infections are usually not dangerous, and infants and toddlers recover with little difficulty.

School-age children and adolescents.
School-age children and adolescents are exposed to respiratory infections and respiratory risk factors such as second-hand smoke and the increased risk to begin cigarette smoking. A healthy child usually does not have adverse pulmonary effects from respiratory infections. A person who starts smoking in adolescence and continues to smoke into middle age, however, has an increased risk for cardiopulmonary disease and lung cancer.

Young and middle-age adults.
Young and middle-age adults are exposed to cardiopulmonary risk factors: an unhealthy diet, lack of exercise, stress, and smoking. Reducing these modifiable factors may decrease the client's risk for cardiac or pulmonary diseases.

Older adults.
The cardiac and respiratory systems change throughout the aging process. In the arterial system atherosclerotic plaques develop and the systemic blood pressure may rise.

Chest wall compliance is decreased in the older client as a result of osteoporosis and the calcification of the costal cartilages. The respiratory muscles weaken, and the pulmonary vascular circulation becomes less distensible. The trachea and large bronchi become enlarged from the calcification of the airways, and alveoli enlarge, decreasing the surface area available for gas exchange. In addition, the number of functional cilia is reduced. Decreased ciliary action and effectiveness of cough mechanisms put the older adult at increased risk for respiratory infections (Lueckenotte, 1996).

Ventilation and transfer of respiratory gases decline with age. Osteoporotic changes of the thoracic cage and kyphosis of the vertebrae occur normally with aging. With these changes the lungs are unable to expand fully, leading to lower oxygenation levels (Table 30-1).

TABLE 30-1
Changes in the Aging Lung

Function	Pathophysiological Change	Key Clinical Findings
Breathing mechanics	Decreased chest wall compliance Loss of elastic recoil Decreased respiratory muscle mass and strength	Decreased vital capacity Increased reserve volume Decreased expiratory flow rates
Oxygenation	Increased ventilation/perfusion mismatch Decreased cardiac output Decreased mixed venous oxygen Increased physiological dead space Decreased alveolar surface area Decreased carbon dioxide diffusion capacity	Decreased PaO_2 Increased alveolar-arterial oxygen gradient Decreased cardiac output
Ventilation control and breathing pattern	Decreased responsiveness of central and peripheral chemoreceptors to hypoxemia and hypercapnia	Deceased tidal volume Increased respiratory rate Increased minute ventilation
Lung defense mechanisms	Decreased number of cilia and effectiveness of the mucociliary clearance Diminished cough reflex Decreased humoral and cellular immunity Decreased IgA production	Decreased airway clearance Increased risk for infection Increased risk of aspiration
Sleep and breathing	Decreased ventilatory drive Decreased tone of upper airway muscles Decreased arousal	Increased risk of apnea, hypopnea, and arterial oxygen desaturation during sleep Increased risk of aspiration Snoring Obstructive sleep apnea
Exercise capacity	Muscle deconditioning and efficiency Decreased muscle mass Decreased reserves	Decreased maximum oxygen consumption Breathlessness at low exercise levels

Data from Pierson DJ: Effects of aging on the respiratory system. In Pierson DJ, Kacmarek RM, editors: *Foundations of respiratory care,* New York, 1992, Churchill Livingstone.

Behavioral Factors

Lifestyle behaviors may directly or indirectly affect the body's ability to meet oxygen requirements. Lifestyle factors that influence respiratory function include nutrition, exercise, cigarette smoking, substance abuse, and stress.

Nutrition. Nutrition affects cardiopulmonary function in several ways. Severe obesity decreases lung expansion, and the increased body weight increases oxygen demands to meet metabolic needs. The malnourished client may experience respiratory muscle wasting, resulting in decreased muscle strength and respiratory excursion. Cough efficiency is reduced secondary to respiratory muscle weakness, putting the client at risk for retention of pulmonary secretions. Diets high in fat increase cholesterol and atherogenesis in the coronary arteries. Clients who are obese and malnourished clients are also at risk for anemia. Diets high in carbohydrates may play a role in increasing the carbon dioxide load for clients with carbon dioxide retention. As carbohydrates are metabolized, an increased load of carbon dioxide is created and excreted via the lungs (Weilitz, 1993).

Exercise. Exercise increases the body's metabolic activity and oxygen demand. The rate and depth of respiration increase, enabling the person to inhale more oxygen and expire excess carbon dioxide.

A physical exercise program has many benefits (see Chapter 37). People who exercise 3 to 4 times per week for 20 to 40 minutes have a lower pulse rate, lower blood pressure, decreased cholesterol, increased blood flow, and greater oxygen extraction by working muscles. Fully conditioned people can increase oxygen consumption by 10% to 20% because of increased cardiac output and increased efficiency of the myocardial muscle.

Cigarette smoking. Cigarette smoking is associated with a number of diseases, including heart disease, chronic obstructive lung disease, and lung cancer. Cigarette smoking can worsen peripheral vascular and coronary artery diseases. The risk of lung cancer is 10 times greater for a person who smokes than for a nonsmoker (Dettenmeier, 1992). Exposure to sidestream smoke increases the risk of lung cancer in the nonsmoker.

Substance abuse. Excessive use of alcohol and other drugs can impair tissue oxygenation in two ways. First, the person who has chronic substance abuse often has a poor nutritional intake. With the resultant decrease in intake of iron-rich foods, hemoglobin production declines. Second, excessive use of alcohol and certain other drugs can depress the respiratory center, reducing the rate and depth of respiration and the amount of inhaled oxygen. Substance abuse by either smoking or inhaling causes direct injury to lung tissue that can lead to permanent lung damage and impaired oxygenation.

Anxiety. A continuous state of severe anxiety increases the body's metabolic rate and the oxygen demand. The body responds to anxiety and other stresses by an increased rate and depth of respiration. Most people can adapt, but some, particularly those with chronic illnesses or acute life-threatening illnesses such as a **myocardial infarction,** cannot tolerate the oxygen demands associated with anxiety.

Environmental Factors

The environment can also influence oxygenation. The incidence of pulmonary disease is higher in smoggy, urban areas than in rural areas. In addition, the client's workplace may increase the risk for pulmonary disease.

Alterations in Cardiac Functioning

Alterations in cardiac functioning are caused by illnesses and conditions that affect cardiac rhythm, strength of contraction, blood flow through the chambers, myocardial blood flow, and peripheral circulation.

Disturbances in conduction. Some disturbances in conduction are the result of electrical impulses that do not originate from the SA node. These rhythm disturbances are called **dysrhythmias,** meaning a deviation from the normal sinus heart rhythm (Table 30-2). Dysrhythmias may occur as a primary conduction disturbance; as a response to ischemia, valvular abnormality, anxiety, and drug toxicity; as a result of caffeine, alcohol, or tobacco use; or as a complication of acid-base or electrolyte imbalance (see Chapter 31).

Dysrhythmias are classified by cardiac response and site of impulse origin. Cardiac response can be either tachycardia (greater than 100 beats/min), bradycardia (less than 60 beats/min), premature (early beat), or blocked (delayed or absent beat).

Altered cardiac output. Failure of the myocardium to eject sufficient volume to the systemic and pulmonary circulations can result in heart failure. Failure of the myocardial pump results from primary coronary artery disease, cardiomyopathic conditions, valvular disorders, and pulmonary disease.

Left-sided heart failure. Left-sided heart failure is an abnormal condition characterized by impaired functioning of the left ventricle caused by elevated pressures and pulmonary congestion. If left ventricle failure is significant, the amount of blood ejected from the left ventricle drops greatly, resulting in decreased cardiac output.

TABLE 30-2
Common Basic Cardiac Dysrhythmias

Rhythm Characteristics	Etiology	Clinical Significance	Management
Sinus Tachycardia Regular rhythm, rate 100-180 beats/min (higher in infants), normal P wave, normal QRS complex	Rate increase may be normal response to exercise, emotion, or stressors such as pain, fever, pump failure, hyperthyroidism, and certain drugs (e.g., caffeine, nitrates, atropine, epinephrine, isoproterenol, nicotine)	May have hemodynamic consequence in client with damaged heart that is unable to sustain increased workloads (increased myocardial oxygen consumption) brought on by persistent increases in heart rate	Correct underlying factors; remove offending drugs

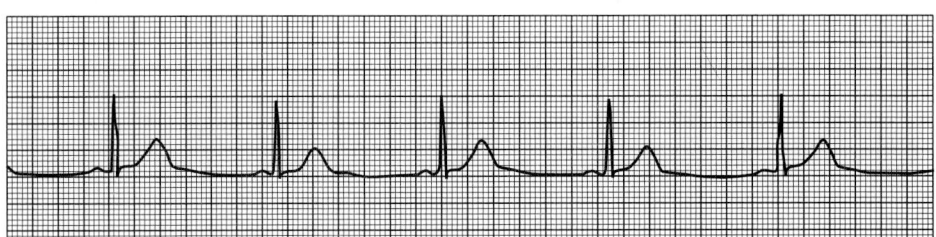

Sinus Bradycardia Regular rhythm, rate less than 60 beats/min, normal P wave, normal PR interval, normal QRS complex	Rate decrease may be normal response to sleep or in well-conditioned athlete; abnormal drops in rate may be caused by diminished blood flow to SA node, vagal stimulation, hypothyroidism, increased intracranial pressure, or pharmacological agents (e.g., digoxin, propranolol, quinidine, procainamide)	No clinical significance unless associated with signs of impaired cardiac output and symptoms of dizziness, syncope, chest pain	Correct underlying causes; administer atropine, 0.5-1.0 mg IV; may need to implant transvenous pacemaker

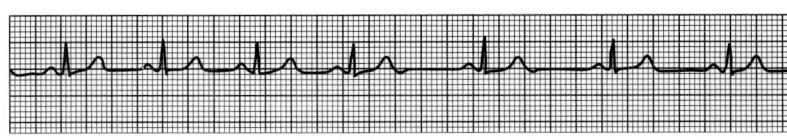

Sinus Dysrhythmia Irregular rhythm; possibly phasic with respiration, slowing during inspiration and increasing with expiration; rate of 60-100 beats/min; normal P wave; normal PR interval; normal QRS complex	Sinus rhythm with cyclic variation caused by vagal impulses that influence rhythm during respiration; occurs commonly in children, young adults, and older adults; usually disappears as heart rate increases	No clinical significance unless heart rate decreases and symptoms of dizziness occur with decreased rate	None is indicated unless heart rate decreases and symptoms occur

Modified from Canobbio MM: *Cardiovascular disorders,* St. Louis, 1990, Mosby.

TABLE 30-2

Common Basic Cardiac Dysrhythmias—cont'd

Rhythm Characteristics	Etiology	Clinical Significance	Management

Supraventricular Tachycardia (SVT)

Sudden, rapid onset of tachycardia with stimulus originating above AV node; regular rhythm; rate 150-250 beats/min; P wave uniform, possibly buried in preceding T wave; PR interval variable, often difficult to measure; normal QRS complex	May begin and end spontaneously or be precipitated by excitement, fatigue, or caffeine, smoking, or alcohol use	Usually no significant impairment; client complains of palpitations and shortness of breath; if persistent or occurring in client with preexisting organic heart disease, may cause decrease in cardiac output and/or blood pressure, resulting in pump failure or shock	Perform vagal stimulation with carotid sinus massage. Physician may order drugs to decrease ventricular response with medication to block AV conduction: verapamil, 5-10 mg IV push; propranolol slowly IV in 1-mg increments up to 4 mg (contraindicated in clients with heart failure); edrophonium, test dose 1 mg followed by 10 mg IV. Perform cardioversion if resistant to preceding measures

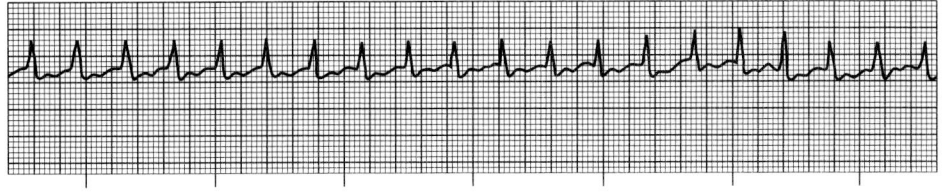

Premature Ventricular Contractions (PVCs)

Irregular rhythm with ectopic beats followed by full compensatory pause; rate normal or increased depending on number of ectopic beats; P wave absent in ectopic beat; PR interval absent; QRS complex widened and distorted; T wave in opposition to R wave	Caused by irritable focus within ventricle, commonly associated with myocardial infarction; other causes include hypoxia, hypocalcemia, acidosis	PVCs occurring frequently (more than 6/min) or in pairs, indicating increased ventricular irritability	Try to suppress PVCs; if PVCs frequent, administer IV bolus of lidocaine (50-100 mg) followed by continuous IV infusion; administer additional antiarrhythmic agents as needed

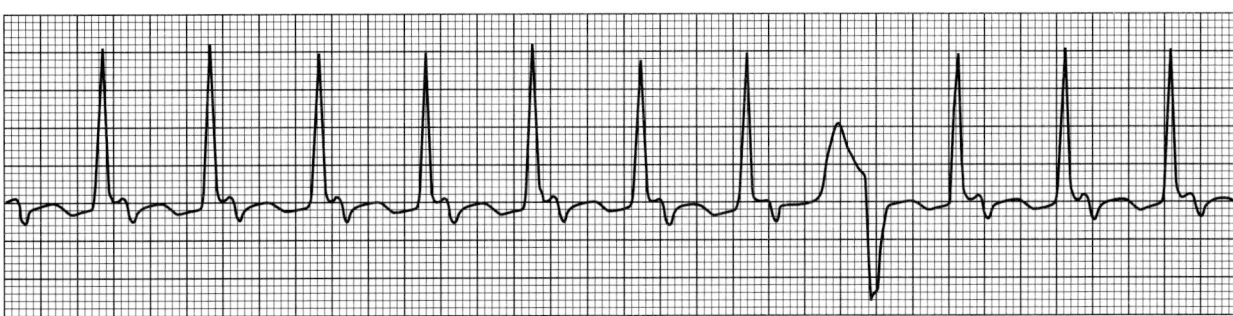

Ventricular Tachycardia

Rhythm slightly irregular, rate 100-200 beats/min, P wave absent, PR interval absent, QRS complex wide and bizarre, >0.12 second	Caused by irritable ventricular foci firing repetitively, commonly caused by myocardial infarction	Often a forerunner of ventricular fibrillation; if condition persistent and rapid, causes decreased cardiac output because of decreased ventricular filling time	Most episodes terminate abruptly without treatment; administer IV bolus of lidocaine (75-100 mg) followed by continuous IV drip; perform cardioversion

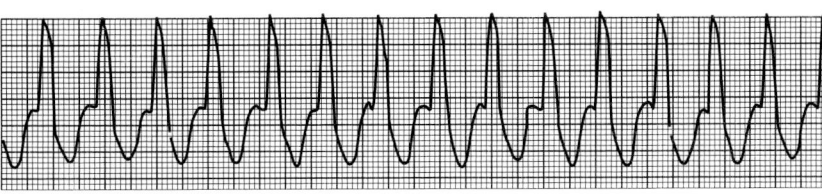

Right-sided heart failure. Right-sided heart failure results from impaired functioning of the right ventricle characterized by venous congestion in the systemic circulation. Right-sided heart failure more commonly results from pulmonary disease or as an outcome of left-sided failure.

Impaired valvular function. Valvular heart disease is an acquired or congenital disorder of a cardiac valve characterized by stenosis and obstructed blood flow or valvular degeneration and regurgitation of blood (Canobbio, 1990). When stenosis occurs in the semilunar valves (aortic and pulmonic valves), the adjacent ventricles must work harder to move the ventricular volume beyond the stenotic valve. When regurgitation occurs, there is a backflow of blood into an adjacent chamber.

Myocardial ischemia. Myocardial ischemia results when the supply of blood to the myocardium from the coronary arteries is insufficient to meet the oxygen demands of the organ. Two common manifestations of this ischemia are angina pectoris and myocardial infarction.

Alterations in Respiratory Functioning

Alterations in respiratory functioning are caused by illnesses and conditions that affect ventilation or oxygen transport. The three primary alterations are hyperventilation, hypoventilation, and hypoxia.

Hyperventilation. The goal of ventilation is to produce a normal arterial carbon dioxide tension ($PaCO_2$) and maintain a normal arterial oxygen tension (PaO_2) (Dettenmeier, 1992). Hyperventilation and hypoventilation refer to alveolar ventilation.

Hyperventilation is a state of ventilation in excess of that required to eliminate the normal venous carbon dioxide produced by cellular metabolism. Hyperventilation can be induced by anxiety, infections, drugs, an acid-base imbalance, and hypoxia associated with pulmonary embolus or shock. Acute anxiety can lead to hyperventilation and may cause loss of consciousness from excess carbon dioxide exhalation. Fever can cause hyperventilation. For each increase of 1° F, there is a 7% increase in the metabolic rate, thereby increasing carbon dioxide production. The clinical response is increased rate and depth of respiration.

Hyperventilation can also be chemically induced. Salicylate (aspirin) poisoning causes excessive stimulation of the respiratory center as the body attempts to compensate for excessive carbon dioxide. Amphetamines also increase ventilation by raising carbon dioxide production.

Hyperventilation can also occur as the body tries to compensate for metabolic acidosis by producing a respiratory alkalosis. Ventilation increases to reduce the amount of carbon dioxide available to form carbonic acid (see Chapter 31).

Alveolar hyperventilation produces many signs and symptoms (Box 30-3). Hemoglobin does not release oxygen to tissues as readily, and tissue hypoxia results. As symptoms worsen, the client may become more agitated, which further increases the respiratory rate and can result in respiratory alkalosis.

Hypoventilation. Hypoventilation occurs when alveolar ventilation is inadequate to meet the body's oxygen demand or to eliminate sufficient carbon dioxide. As alveolar ventilation decreases, $PaCO_2$ is elevated. Severe atelectasis can produce hypoventilation. **Atelectasis** is a collapse of the alveoli that prevents more respiratory exchange of oxygen and carbon dioxide. As alveoli collapse, less of the lung can be ventilated and hypoventilation occurs.

In clients with chronic obstructive pulmonary disease, the inappropriate administration of excessive oxygen can result in hypoventilation. These clients have adapted to a high carbon dioxide level, and their carbon dioxide–sensitive chemoreceptors are essentially not functioning. Their stimulus to breathe is a decreased PaO_2. If excessive oxygen is administered, the oxygen requirement is satisfied and the stimulus to breathe is negated. High concentrations of oxygen (e.g., greater than 24% to 28% [1 to 3 L/min]) prevent the PaO_2 from falling and obliterate the stimulus to breathe, resulting in hypoventilation. The excessive retention of carbon dioxide may lead to a respiratory arrest.

Signs and symptoms of hypoventilation are listed in Box 30-4. If untreated, the client's status can rapidly decline. Convulsions, unconsciousness, and death can result.

Treatment for hyperventilation and hypoventilation begins by treating the underlying cause, then improving

---

Box 30-3

Signs and Symptoms of Alveolar Hyperventilation

Tachycardia
Shortness of breath
Chest pain
Dizziness
Light-headedness
Decreased concentration
Paresthesia
Numbness (extremities, circumoral)
Tinnitus
Blurred vision
Disorientation
Tetany (carpopedal spasm)

Box 30-4
Signs and Symptoms of Alveolar Hypoventilation

Dizziness   Cardiac dysrhythmias
Headache (may be occip-   Electrolyte imbalances
    ital only on awakening)   Convulsions
Lethargy   Coma
Disorientation   Cardiac arrest
Decreased ability to fol-
    low instructions

Box 30-5
Signs and Symptoms of Hypoxia

Restlessness   Increased pulse rate
Apprehension, anxiety   Increased rate and
Decreased ability to   depth of respiration
    concentrate   Elevated blood pressure
Decreased level of con-   Cardiac dysrhythmias
    sciousness   Pallor
Increased fatigue   Cyanosis
Dizziness   Clubbing
Behavioral changes   Dyspnea

tissue oxygenation, restoring ventilatory function, and achieving acid-base balance.

Hypoxia. **Hypoxia** is inadequate tissue oxygenation at the cellular level. This can result from a deficiency in oxygen delivery or oxygen utilization at the cellular level. Hypoxia can be caused by (1) a decreased hemoglobin level and lowered oxygen-carrying capacity of the blood; (2) a diminished concentration of inspired oxygen, which may occur at high altitudes; (3) the inability of the tissues to extract oxygen from the blood, as with cyanide poisoning; (4) decreased diffusion of oxygen from the alveoli to the blood, as in pneumonia; (5) poor tissue perfusion with oxygenated blood, as with shock; or (6) impaired ventilation, as with multiple rib fractures or chest trauma.

The clinical signs and symptoms of hypoxia include apprehension, restlessness, inability to concentrate, declining level of consciousness, dizziness, and behavioral changes (Box 30-5). The client with hypoxia is unable to lie down and appears fatigued and agitated. Vital sign changes include an increased pulse rate and increased rate and depth of respiration. During early stages of hypoxia the blood pressure is elevated unless the condition is caused by shock. As the hypoxia worsens, the respiratory rate may decline as a result of respiratory muscle fatigue.

Cyanosis, a blue discoloration of the skin and mucous membranes caused by the presence of desaturated hemoglobin in capillaries, is a late sign of hypoxia. The presence or absence of cyanosis is not a reliable measure of oxygenation status. Central cyanosis, observed in the tongue, soft palate, and conjunctiva of the eye, where blood flow is high, indicates hypoxemia. Peripheral cyanosis, seen in the extremities, nail beds, and earlobes, is often the result of vasoconstriction and stagnant blood flow.

Hypoxia is a life-threatening condition. Untreated, it can produce cardiac dysrhythmias that result in death. Hypoxia is managed by administration of oxygen and treatment of the underlying cause, such as airway obstruction.

CRITICAL THINKING IN CLIENT CARE

Synthesis

The care of clients with impaired oxygenation requires the nurse to synthesize knowledge from the basic and other sciences, integrate previous learning experiences, apply critical thinking attitudes when caring for clients who may have unhealthy lifestyles, and provide care according to standards of practice.

Knowledge. When caring for clients with cardiopulmonary problems, the nurse incorporates and applies knowledge from physiology and pathophysiology; nutrition; and fluid, electrolyte, and acid-base balance. In addition, the nurse uses knowledge about health promotion to prevent or reduce at-risk behaviors in clients with cardiopulmonary problems. Last, the nurse must also investigate and use knowledge about restorative care to assist clients in attaining and maintaining optimal cardiopulmonary function.

Experience. Most students have been exposed to individuals who have had problems with breathing. There is a high percentage of individuals who have respiratory diseases such as asthma or chronic obstructive pulmonary disease due to environmental triggers or cigarette smoking. Clients who require nursing management in the community setting are usually stable, whereas the acute care setting requires the nurse and client to deal with an exacerbation of the disease.

Attitudes. The critical thinking attitudes of accountability, creativity, perseverance, and integrity may be used when providing nursing care. The nurse is accountable for the health care information given to clients about cardiopulmonary risk factors. For example, when providing care to a client who smokes and has pulmonary disease, the nurse is accountable for the approach taken to help the client decrease smoking, as well as the smoking cessation information provided.

The nurse uses creativity in providing care to promote and maintain an optimal level of oxygenation. As a client advocate the nurse may encounter difficult client problems. The attitude of perseverance is important to find effective client-centered solutions. For example, when a client has severe cardiac or pulmonary disease and has a limited income, solutions for promoting health and maintaining client independence are complex. The nurse's own personal integrity and professional values can identify realistic creative solutions.

Standards. The American Lung Association has specific guidelines for pulmonary rehabilitation so that the client can control and alleviate symptoms and pathophysiological complications and to achieve optimal ability to carry out activities of daily living. Methods used are exercise reconditioning, inspiratory muscle training, breathing retraining, nutrition counseling, smoking cessation, and psychosocial management.

NURSING PROCESS AND OXYGENATION

▣ Assessment

The nursing assessment of a client's cardiopulmonary functioning should include data collected from the following areas:

- Nursing history of the client's normal and present cardiopulmonary function, past impairments in circulatory or respiratory functioning, and measures the client may use to optimize oxygenation
- Physical examination of the client's cardiopulmonary status (see Chaper 24)
- Review of laboratory and diagnostic test results, such as complete blood count, ECG, pulmonary function test, sputum, and oxygenation such as arterial blood gases or pulse oximetry

Nursing history. The nursing history should focus on the client's ability to meet oxygen needs. The nursing history for cardiac or respiratory problems is detailed in the following sections. At the end of each section are examples of questions to ask during the nursing history.

Pain. Cardiac pain does not occur with respiratory variations. It is most often on the left side of the chest and radiates. Pericardial pain resulting from an inflammation of the pericardial sac is usually nonradiating and may occur with inspiration.

Pleuritic chest pain is peripheral and may radiate to the scapular regions. It is worsened by inspiratory maneuvers, such as coughing, yawning, and sighing. Pleuritic pain is often caused from an inflammation or infection in the pleural space and is described as knifelike,

lasting from a minute to hours, and always associated with inspiration.

Musculoskeletal pain may be present following exercise, rib trauma, and prolonged coughing episodes. The pain is also aggravated by inspiratory movements and may easily be confused with pleuritic chest pain.

- Have you ever had pain in your chest? Explain.
- Where and when do you feel the pain? Does it radiate? Describe the pain.

Refer to history of cardiac function for additional questions to rule out cardiac origin.

Breathing patterns. Dyspnea is a clinical sign of hypoxia and manifests as breathlessness. Dyspnea can be associated with clinical signs such as exaggerated respiratory effort, use of the accessory muscles of respiration, nasal flaring, and marked increases in the rate and depth of respirations. The use of a visual analog scale can help clients to make an objective assessment of their dyspnea. The visual analog scale is a 100-mm vertical line with 0 equated with no dyspnea and the 100-mm marker equated with the worst breathlessness the client has experienced. Measurement of dyspnea on the analog scale helps to show changes in the clients' status.

Orthopnea is an abnormal condition in which the person must use multiple pillows when lying down or must sit to breathe. The presence of orthopnea is usually quantified by the number of pillows required to sleep, such as two- or three-pillow orthopnea.

Wheezing is characterized by a high-pitched musical sound caused by high-velocity movement of air through a narrowed airway. Wheezing may be associated with asthma, acute bronchitis, or pneumonia. Wheezing can occur on inspiration, expiration, or both. The nurse should determine any precipitating factors such as respiratory infection, allergens, exercise, or stress.

- What types of activities bring on the shortness of breath? Is it gradual or sudden? Is it constant or intermittent?
- Does the shortness of breath interfere with your daily activities?
- Have you ever noticed shortness of breath or times when it is hard to breathe? Does anything seem to trigger these episodes?
- Does the shortness of breath interfere with your activities? Is it harder to inhale or exhale, or is it equally affected?
- How many pillows do you require when you lie down to sleep?

Fatigue. Fatigue is a subjective sensation in which the client reports a loss of endurance. Fatigue in the client with cardiopulmonary alterations is often an early sign of worsening of the chronic underlying process. To provide an objective measure of fatigue, the client may be asked to rate the fatigue on a scale of 1 to 10, with 10 being the worst level of fatigue and 1 representing no fatigue.

- When did you first notice the fatigue?
- Was the onset sudden or gradual?
- Have you noticed any recent changes in your activity level?

Risk factors. The nurse needs to investigate familial and environmental risk factors such as a family history of cardiovascular or lung disease. Document which blood relatives have had the disease and their present level of health or age at time of death. Other family risk factors include the presence of infectious diseases, particularly tuberculosis. The nurse should determine who in the client's household has been infected and the status of the treatment.

- Do you exercise? How often and what kind?
- Do you smoke? How much? How long?
- Describe your usual eating habits.
- How would you describe your personality? How do you relax?
- Have you ever had high blood pressure?
- In your family, is there a history of diabetes, heart disease, hyperlipidemia, or hypertension?

Environmental exposure to many inhaled substances is closely linked with respiratory disease. The nurse should investigate exposures in the client's home and workplace.

An employment history assesses exposure to substances such as asbestos, coal, cotton fibers, chemical fumes, or chemical inhalants. It is particularly important with middle-age and older adults, who may have worked in places without regulations to protect workers from carcinogens.

- Do you smoke? How long?
- Are you exposed to the smoke from others in your home?
- Are there environmental conditions that may affect your breathing where you work?
- Have you recently traveled to countries or areas of the United States where you may have been exposed to uncommon respiratory diseases?

Cough. **Cough** is a sudden, audible expulsion of air from the lungs. The person breathes in, the glottis is partially closed, and the accessory muscles of expiration contract to expel the air forcibly. Coughing is a protective reflex to clear the trachea, bronchi, and lungs of irritants and secretions. The carina, the point of bifurcation of the right and left mainstem bronchus, is the most sensitive area for cough production.

Cough is classified according to the time when the client most frequently coughs. Clients with chronic sinusitis may cough only in the early morning or immediately after rising from sleep. This clears the airway of mucus resulting from sinus drainage. Clients with chronic bronchitis generally produce sputum all day, although greater amounts are produced after rising from a semirecumbent or flat position. This is the result of the dependent accumulation of sputum in the airways and is associated with reduced mobility (see Chapter 37).

A **productive cough** results in sputum production, material coughed up from the lungs that may be swallowed or expectorated. Sputum contains mucus, cellular debris, and microorganisms and may contain pus or blood. The nurse must collect data about the type and quantity of sputum (Box 30-6).

If **hemoptysis** (bloody sputum) is reported, the nurse determines if it is associated with coughing and bleeding from the upper respiratory tract, from sinus drainage, or from the gastrointestinal tract **(hematemesis).** In addition, the hemoptysis should be described according to amount, color, and duration and whether it is mixed with sputum.

- Do you have a cough? How would you describe the cough? Do you cough up anything? What color is this material?
- Is your cough associated with position, with anxiety, or with talking or activity?

Respiratory infections. Determine if the client has had a Pneumovax or flu vaccine in the past. The nurse also asks about any known exposure to tuberculosis and the results of the tuberculin skin test.

Determine the client's risk for human immunodeficiency virus (HIV) infection. Clients with a history of intravenous drug use, multiple unprotected sexual partners, or a homosexual lifestyle are at risk of developing HIV infection. Clients may not display any symptoms of HIV infection until they present with *Pneumocystis carinii* or *Mycobacterium* pneumonia.

Box 30-6
Sputum Characteristics

Color		Quantity
Clear	Green	Same as usual
White	Brown	Increased
Yellow	Red	Decreased
Streaked with blood		
		Consistency
Changes in Color		Frothy
Same color throughout		Watery
the day		Tenacious, thick
Clearing with coughing		
Progressively darker		**Presence of Blood**
		Occasional
Odor		Early morning
None		Bright or dark red
Foul		Blood-tinged

TABLE 30-3
Inspection of Cardiopulmonary Status

Abnormality	Cause
Eyes	
Xanthelasma (yellow lipid lesions on eyelids)	Associated with hyperlipidemia
Corneal arcus (whitish opaque ring around junction of cornea and sclera)	Abnormal finding in young to middle-age adults associated with hyperlipidemia (normal finding in older adults with arcus senilis)
Pale conjunctivae	Associated with anemia
Cyanotic conjunctivae	Associated with hypoxemia
Petechiae on conjunctivae	Associated with fat embolus or bacterial endocarditis
Skin	
Peripheral cyanosis	Vasoconstriction and diminished blood flow
Central cyanosis	Hypoxemia
Decreased skin turgor	Dehydration (normal finding in older adults as a result of decreased skin elasticity)
Dependent edema	Associated with right- and left-sided heart failure
Periorbital edema	Associated with kidney disease
Fingertips and Nail Beds	
Cyanosis	Decreased cardiac output or hypoxia
Splinter hemorrhages	Bacterial endocarditis
Clubbing	Chronic hypoxemia
Mouth and Lips	
Cyanotic mucous membranes	Decreased oxygenation (hypoxia)
Pursed-lip breathing	Associated with chronic lung disease
Neck Veins	
Distention	Associated with right-sided heart failure
Nose	
Flaring nares	Air hunger, dyspnea
Chest	
Retractions	Increased work of breathing, dyspnea
Asymmetry	Chest wall injury

Medication use. The nurse assesses clients' knowledge and ability to correctly take medication (see Chapter 26). Of particular importance is the nurse's assessment of clients' understanding of potential side effects of the medications.

Common drugs that can be monitored by measuring blood levels include theophylline preparations, digitalis preparations, and phenobarbital. Illicit drugs, particularly parenterally administered narcotics, which are often diluted with talcum powder, can cause pulmonary disorders resulting from the irritant effect of talcum powder on lung tissues.

Client expectations. The perception the client has regarding his or her health and its maintenance will determine the teaching strategy required. It makes a difference whether one is threatened by the symptoms or incidence rates or utilizes a denial mechanism.

The client's unwillingness to adhere to a treatment schedule must be assessed. In addition, what does the client expect from the care giver? Does the client expect health to improve or expect supportive care? Does the client want to be an active participant in care or want family members to make decisions and provide care?

Physical examination. The physical examination performed to assess level of tissue oxygenation includes evaluation of the entire cardiopulmonary system (see Chapter 24) (Tables 30-3 to 30-6).

Diagnostic tests. Tests are conducted to determine adequacy of the cardiac conduction system, myocardial contraction, and blood flow; to measure the adequacy of ventilation and oxygenation; and to visualize structures of the respiratory system.

TABLE 30-4

Assessment of Breathing Patterns

Patterns	Causes
Eupnea—normal respiratory rate; adult range of 12-20 breaths/min; normal tidal volume of 5-7 ml/kg body weight*	
Tachypnea—increased respiratory rate above client's normal rate; shallow respirations	Exercise, pregnancy, fever, pulmonary diseases, anxiety, neurological conditions, bronchoconstriction
Bradypnea—decreased respiratory rate below client's normal rate	Drug overdose, central nervous system dysfunction, airway obstruction
Kussmaul's respiration—abnormally deep, very rapid sighing type of respiration; increased tidal volume and rate	Diabetic ketoacidosis
Ataxic respirations—uncoordinated respiratory patterns; no coordinated rate or depth of respiration	Central nervous system disorders
Cheyne-Stokes respiration—breathing pattern characterized by alternating periods of apnea and deep rapid breathing; cycle beginning with slow, shallow breaths that gradually increase to abnormal depth and rate; respiration gradually subsiding as breathing slows and becomes shallow	Congestive heart failure, bronchopneumonia, drug overdose, sleep, central nervous system damage

*From Luce JM and others: *Intensive respiratory care*, ed 2, Philadelphia, 1993, WB Saunders.

TABLE 30-5

Assessment of Abnormal Chest Wall Movement

Abnormality	Cause
Retraction—visible sinking in soft tissues of chest between and around firmer tissue and cartilaginous and bony ribs; retractions having specific beginning point and worsening with need for increased inspiratory effort; possibly found at intercostal space, intraclavicular space, trachea, and substernally*	Any condition that causes increased inspiratory effort (e.g., airway obstruction, asthma, tracheobronchitis)
Paradoxical breathing—asynchronous breathing; chest contraction during inspiration and expansion during expiration	Flail chest
Increased anteroposterior diameter	Senile emphysema or chronic obstructive pulmonary disease

*Infants can experience sternal and substernal retractions with only slight inspiratory effort because of chest pliability.

TABLE 30-6
Respiratory Pattern

Type/ Pattern	Rate (Breaths per Minute)	Clinical Significance
Eupnea	16-20	Normal
Tachypnea	>35	Respiratory failure Response to fever Anxiety Shortness of breath Respiratory infection
Bradypnea	<10	Sleep Respiratory depression Drug overdose Central nervous system (CNS) lesion
Apnea	Periods of no respiration lasting >15 seconds	May be intermittent such as in sleep apnea Respiratory arrest
Hypernea	16-20	Can result from anxiety or response to pain Can cause marked respiratory alkalosis, paresthesia, tetany, confusion
Kussmaul's	Usually >35, may be slow or normal	Tachypnea pattern associated with diabetic ketoacidosis, metabolic acidosis, or renal failure
Cheyne-Stokes	Variable	Increasing and decreasing pattern caused by alterations in acid-base status. Underlying metabolic problem or neurocerebral insult
Biot's	Variable	Periods of apnea and shallow breathing caused by CNS disorder; found in some healthy clients
Apneustic	Increased	Increased inspiratory time with short grunting expiratory time; seen in CNS lesions of the respiratory center

From Weilitz PB: *Pocket guide to respiratory care*, St. Louis, 1991, Mosby.

Successful critical thinking requires a synthesis of knowledge, experience, information gathered from clients, and critical thinking attitudes and standards. Clinical judgments require the nurse to anticipate what information is needed, to analyze the data, and to then make decisions regarding client care. The client expects competent and informed care. Mary incorporates previous knowledge and experience in providing care for Mr. King.

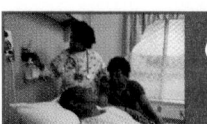

Case Study
Synthesis in Practice

Mr. King's history reveals risk factors of a 40-year history of smoking two packs a day, and he currently continues this habit. He has had multiple respiratory infections in the past 5 years, and he complains of chronic cough, especially in the early mornings.

Mary's knowledge of physiology and pathophysiology enables her to realize that the shortness of breath is because the infection is obstructing his alveolocapillary membrane, preventing oxygenation of blood in some parts of his lung. She also is aware of his preexisting chronic obstructive pulmonary disease and the effects of his smoking. Mary realizes how bad smoking is for this individual, and knowledge from the area of health promotion and restoration can assist her in promoting smoking cessation for Mr. King.

From clinical experiences Mary knows the impact of support systems in assisting clients to cope with chronic illnesses. Mary can use creativity and independent thinking to incorporate community and family resources into the plan of care for Mr. King. Mary will need to inquire about his social supports and the availability of smoking cessation programs in his community.

▪ Nursing Diagnosis

Clients with an altered level of oxygenation may have nursing diagnoses that are primarily from a cardiovascular or pulmonary origin (see nursing diagnoses box). Each nursing diagnosis is based on specific defining characteristics and includes the related etiology. The diagnostic label is validated by the defining characteristics or signs and symptoms.

During the assessment process, the nurse must collect data to accurately reflect the client's needs. For example, the diagnosis of *ineffective airway clearance related to the presence of tracheobronchial secretions secondary to infection* is supported by objective findings of productive cough, dyspnea, crackles, tachypnea, changes in depth of respiration, and pleuritic pain. The ability of the client to bring

<table>
<tr><td>

NURSING DIAGNOSES FOR CARDIOPULMONARY DYSFUNCTION

Activity intolerance
Airway clearance, ineffective
Breathing pattern, ineffective
Cardiac ouput, decreased
Gas exchange, impaired
Infection, risk for

</td></tr>
</table>

up sputum is a crucial part of treatment for pneumonia. Pleuritic pain can interfere with the client's ability to rest and can impair the ability to cough and clear the airway, resulting in worsening infection.

Another example of a related nursing diagnosis is *activity intolerance related to imbalance between oxygen supply and demand.* The objective findings include an inability to move secretions, restlessness, tachycardia, dyspnea, use of accessory muscles, and hypoxia (PaO_2 less than 60 mm Hg). Clients will avoid physical effort because dyspnea may be precipitated by exercise. Consequently their level of fitness decreases, they become weak, and they have difficulty with normal activities of daily living. As the level of exercise tolerance is increased, the degree of dyspnea and shortness of breath may actually diminish. Identifying the appropriate related factor can enable the nurse to design nursing interventions to maximize the balance between the client's oxygen supply and demand.

Planning

Clients with impaired oxygenation require a nursing care plan directed toward meeting the actual or potential oxygenation needs of the client. Individual goals are derived from client-centered needs. The goals are related to improving a client's airway, level of independence, tolerance to activity, and tissue oxygenation, to name a few (see care plan, p. 808).

Impaired levels of oxygenation affect all aspects of the client's life, not just the physical component. Designing collaborative nursing interventions with physical and occupational therapy can improve the client's level of functioning. Respiratory therapy can assist in designing measures to improve breathing and cough control. When planning care for clients with impaired oxygenation, the nurse needs to be sensitive to the needs of the client as well as the family. Many times social service can be of assistance in identifying resources within the community.

Implementation

Nursing interventions for promoting and maintaining adequate oxygenation are included in the domain of nursing: administering and monitoring therapeutic interventions and regimens (Benner, 1984). These include independent nursing actions such as health promotion and prevention behaviors, positioning, coughing techniques, and interdependent or dependent interventions such as oxygen therapy, lung inflation techniques, hydration, medications, and chest physiotherapy.

Health promotion in a primary care setting. Maintaining the client's optimal level of health is important in reducing the number and severity of respiratory symptoms. Prevention of respiratory infections is foremost in maintaining optimal health. The nurse provides client education to help clients make choices for improving health practices (Box 30-7).

Influenza and pneumococcal vaccine. Annual influenza vaccines are recommended for older clients and those with chronic illnesses; however, the value of vaccination of immunocompromised clients is not completely understood. HIV-positive clients may receive the flu vaccine; however, they may require a second vaccine to gain protection (Centers for Disease Control and Prevention, 1993). HIV-positive clients can also receive

---

BOX 30-7
Client Teaching for Cardiopulmonary Health Promotion

- Educate the client about the importance of regular blood pressure checkups and taking blood pressure medications as prescribed.
- Educate the client about the importance of monitoring the serum cholesterol and triglyceride levels.
- Educate the client about the basic food groups and recommended servings of each.
- Educate client about low-fat, low-salt, proper caloric diet, and provide sample menus.
- Educate client about need for regular aerobic exercise 3 to 4 times per week for 30 to 40 minutes.
- Discuss strategies for minimizing and reducing stress in the client's life, such as setting realistic goals, relaxation and meditation techniques, and getting adequate amounts of rest, relaxation, and sleep.
- Discuss the importance and benefits of pneumococcal vaccine and annual influenza vaccine.
- Discuss the importance of monitoring pollution indexes and limiting exposure on days when the index is high.
- Discuss the need to avoid smoking and secondhand smoke exposure.
- If clients smoke, enroll them in a structured smoking cessation program.
- Discuss strategies to avoid or control secondary infection exposure, such as avoiding prolonged exposure to crowds during the flu season.
- Educate the client about the need to cover the mouth and nose with a scarf when going out into cold air.

CASE STUDY NURSING CARE PLAN

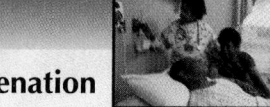

Oxygenation

Assessment
Mr. King is in respiratory distress as evidenced by **dyspnea, cough, prolonged expiration, audible expiratory wheezing, diminished breath sounds** over right lower lobe, **anxiety, sputum-producing cough, hyperresonance, cyanosis** of nail beds and mucous membranes, and **use of accesory muscles during breathing.** His vital signs are pulse rate 120, temperature 102° F, **respiratory rate 36,** and blood pressure 110/45.

Nursing Diagnosis
Impaired gas exchange related to increased pumonary secretions.

Planning

Goal

Client's excessive pulmonary secretions will return to baseline levels within 3 days.

Expected Outcomes

Client's sputum will be clear, white within 48 hours.

Client's adventitious lung sounds will disappear within 48 hours.

Client's respiratory rate will be between 20 and 28 within 24 hours.

Client will be able to clear airway by coughing in 24 hours.

Implementation

Steps

1. Instruct client to turn and cough every 2 hours.

2. Perform percussion with routine position changes.

3. Increase fluid intake to 1500 ml within 24 hours.

Rationale

Major complication of reduced mobility is retained pulmonary secretions, which predisposes client to atelectasis and pneumonia (Dettenmeier, 1992).

Percussion provides mechanical force to loosen secretions adhered to walls of airways and aids secretion removal (Dettenmeier, 1992).

Fluids and humidification help liquefy secretions for easy removal (Luce and others, 1993).

Evaluation
Auscultate client's lungs.
Observe client's cough.
Observe color of client's sputum.
Observe client's respirations.

Defining characteristics are shown in bold type.

---

the pneumococcal vaccination. Persons who should not be vaccinated include those with a known hypersensitivity to eggs or other components of the vaccine and adults with an acute febrile illness (Centers for Disease Control and Prevention, 1993).

Both the influenza vaccine and pneumococcal vaccine can be used in pregnant women. There are no contraindications to the pneumococcal vaccine (Centers for Disease Control and Prevention, 1991), and influenza vaccine can be given after the first trimester (Centers for Disease Control and Prevention, 1993). However, in all cases it is important to consult the client's obstetrician before administering either vaccine.

Environmental pollutants. Avoiding exposure to secondhand smoke is essential to maintaining optimal cardiopulmonary function. Most businesses and restaurants now ban smoking or have separate areas designated as smoking areas. If clients are exposed to secondhand smoke in their home environments, counseling and support may be necessary to assist the smoker in successful smoking cessation or alterations in behavior patterns such as smoking outside.

Exposure to chemicals and pollutants in the work environment must be considered. Nurses educate clients on the benefits of wearing protective devices, such as particulate filter masks to reduce inhalation of particles.

Acute care. Clients with acute pulmonary illnesses require nursing interventions directed toward halting the pathological process, such as a respiratory tract infection; shortening the duration and severity of the illness, such as hospitalization with pneumonia; and preventing complications from illness or treatments, such as nosocomial infection resulting from invasive procedures.

Dyspnea management. Dyspnea is difficult to measure and treat. Treatment modalities need to be individualized for each client, and more than one therapy is usually implemented. The underlying process that causes or worsens dyspnea must be treated and stabilized initially, then four additional therapies should be administered:

1. Pharmacological measures (e.g., bronchodilators, steroids, mucolytics, antianxiety drugs)
2. Oxygen therapy for dyspnea associated with exercise
3. Physical techniques (e.g., cardiopulmonary reconditioning, breathing techniques, cough control)
4. Psychosocial techniques (e.g., relaxation techniques, biofeedback, meditation) to lessen the sensation of dyspnea

Maintenance of a patent airway. The airway is patent when the trachea, bronchi, and large airways are free from obstructions. Three types of interventions are used to maintain a patent airway: coughing techniques, suctioning, and insertion of an artificial airway.

Coughing techniques. Coughing maintains a patent airway by permitting the client to remove secretions from both the upper and lower airways. The normal series of events in the cough mechanisms are deep inhalation, closure of the glottis, active contraction of the expiratory muscles, and glottis opening. Deep inhalation increases lung volume and airway diameter, allowing the air to pass partially obstructing mucus plugs or other foreign matter. Contraction of the expiratory muscles against the closed glottis causes a high intrathoracic pressure to develop. When the glottis opens, a large flow of air is expelled at a high speed, providing momentum for mucus to move to the upper airways, where it can be expectorated or swallowed.

The effectiveness of coughing is evaluated by sputum expectoration, the client's report of swallowed sputum, or clearing of adventitious sounds by auscultation. Clients with chronic pulmonary diseases, upper respiratory tract infections, and lower respiratory tract infections should be encouraged to deep breathe and cough at least every 2 hours while awake. Clients with a large amount of sputum should be encouraged to cough every hour while awake and every 2 to 3 hours while asleep until the acute phase of mucus production has ended.

Cascade cough. With the cascade cough, the client takes a slow, deep breath and holds it for 2 seconds while contracting expiratory muscles. Then the client opens the mouth and performs a series of coughs throughout exhalation, thereby coughing at progressively lowered lung volumes. This technique promotes airway clearance and a patent airway in clients with large volumes of sputum.

Huff cough. The huff cough stimulates a natural cough reflex and is generally effective only for clearing central airways. While exhaling, the client opens the glottis by saying the word *huff*. With practice the client inhales more air and may be able to progress to the cascade cough.

Quad cough. The quad cough technique is used for clients without abdominal muscle control, such as those with spinal cord injuries. While the client breathes out with a maximal expiratory effort, the client or nurse pushes inward and upward on the abdominal muscles toward the diaphragm, causing the cough.

Suctioning techniques. When a client is unable to clear respiratory tract secretions with coughing, the nurse must use suctioning to clear the airways. The three primary suctioning techniques are oropharyngeal and nasopharyngeal suctioning, orotracheal and nasotracheal suctioning, and suctioning of an artificial airway (Skill 30-1).

These techniques are based on common principles. Because the oropharynx and trachea are considered sterile, sterile technique is required for suctioning. The mouth is considered clean, and therefore the suctioning of oral secretions should be performed after suctioning of the oropharynx and trachea. Each type of suctioning requires the use of a round-tipped catheter with a number of holes along the side of the catheter at the distal end. Frequency of suctioning is determined by client assessment. If secretions are identified by inspection or auscultation techniques, suctioning is required. Sputum is not produced continuously or every 1 or 2 hours but occurs as a response to a pathological condition. Therefore there is no rationale for routine suctioning of all clients every 1 to 2 hours.

Oropharyngeal and nasopharngeal suctioning. The oropharynx extends behind the mouth from the soft palate above the level of the hyoid bone and contains the tonsils. The nasopharynx is located behind the nose and extends to the level of the soft palate. Oropharyngeal or nasopharyngeal suctioning is used when the client is able to cough effectively but is unable to clear secretions by expectorating or swallowing.

Orotracheal and nasotracheal suctioning. Orotracheal or nasotracheal suctioning is necessary when the client with pulmonary secretions is unable to cough and does not have an artificial airway (Skill 30-1). A catheter is passed through the mouth or nose into the trachea. The nose is the preferred route because stimulation of the gag reflex is minimal. The procedure is

Text continued on p. 816

Suctioning

Delegation Considerations
This skill requires problem solving and knowledge application unique to a professional nurse. For this skill, delegation is inappropriate.

Equipment
- Appropriate-size suction catheter (smallest diameter that will remove secretions effectively) or Yankauer catheter (oral suction)
- Small Y-adapter (if catheter does not have a suction control port)
- Water-soluble lubricant
- Two sterile gloves or one sterile and one nonsterile glove
- Sterile basin
- Sterile normal saline solution or water (about 100 ml)
- Clean towel or paper drape
- Portable or wall suction
- Connecting tube (6 feet)
- Nasal or oral airway (if indicated)
- Mask or face shield

STEPS	RATIONALE
1. Assess signs and symptoms of upper and lower airway obstruction requiring nasotracheal or orotracheal suctioning, including respiratory rate or adventitious sounds, nasal secretions, drooling, gastric secretions or vomitus in mouth.	Physical signs and symptoms result from decreased oxygen to tissues as well as pooling of secretions in upper and lower airways.
Assess signs and symptoms associated with hypoxia and hypercapnia: apprehension, anxiety, decreased ability to concentrate, lethargy, decreased level of consciousness (especially acute), increased fatigue, dizziness, behavioral changes (especially irritability), increased pulse rate or rate of breathing, decreased depth of breathing, elevated blood pressure, cardiac dysrhythmias, pallor, cyanosis, and dyspnea.	
2. Determine factors that normally influence upper or lower airway functioning.	
a. Fluid status	Fluid overload may increase amount of secretions. Dehydration promotes thicker secretions.
b. Lack of humidity	The environment influences secretion formation and gas exchange, necessitating airway suctioning when the client cannot clear secretions effectively.
c. Infection	Clients with respiratory infections are prone to increased secretions that are thicker and sometimes more difficult to expectorate.
d. Anatomy	Abnormal anatomy can impair normal drainage of secretions. For example, nasal swelling, deviated septum, or facial fractures may impair nasal drainage. Tumors in or around the lower airway may impair secretion removal by occluding or externally compressing the lumen of the airway.
3. Assess client's understanding of procedure.	Reveals need for client instruction and encourages cooperation.
4. Obtain physician's order if indicated by agency policy.	Some institutions require a physician's order for tracheal suctioning.
5. Explain to client how procedure will help clear airway and relieve breathing problems and that temporary coughing, sneezing, gagging, or shortness of breath is normal. Encourage client to cough out secretions. Practice coughing, if able. Splint surgical incisions, if necessary.	Encourages cooperation and minimizes risks, anxiety, and pain.

STEPS	RATIONALE
6. Assist client to assume position comfortable for nurse and client (usually semi-Fowler's or sitting upright with head hyperextended, unless contraindicated).	Reduces stimulation of gag reflex, promotes client comfort and secretion drainage, prevents aspiration and nurse strain. Hyperextension facilitates insertion of catheter into trachea.
7. Place towel across client's chest.	Reduces transmission of microorganisms by protecting gown from secretions.
8. Wash hands, and apply face shield if splashing is likely.	Reduces transmission of microorganisms.
9. Connect one end of connecting tubing to suction machine, and place other end in convenient location near client. Turn suction device on, and set vacuum regulator to appropriate negative pressure.	Excessive negative pressure damages nasopharyngeal and tracheal mucosa and can induce greater hypoxia.
10. If indicated, increase supplemental oxygen therapy to 100% or as ordered by physician. Encourage client's deep breathing.	These measures reduce suction-induced hypoxemia.
11. Prepare suction catheter:	
a. Open suction kit or catheter with use of aseptic technique. If sterile drape is available, place it across client's chest or on the overbed table. Do not allow the suction catheter to touch any nonsterile surfaces.	Maintains asepsis and reduces transmission of microorganisms.
b. Unwrap or open sterile basin and place on bedside table. Be careful not to touch inside of basin. Fill with about 100 ml of sterile normal saline solution or water.	Saline or water is used to clean tubing after each suction pass.
c. Open lubricant. Squeeze small amount onto open sterile catheter package without touching package.	Prepares lubricant while maintaining sterility. Water-soluble lubricant is used to avoid lipoid aspiration pneumonia.
12. Apply sterile glove to each hand, or apply nonsterile glove to nondominant hand and sterile glove to dominant hand.	Reduces transmission of microorganisms and allows nurse to maintain sterility of suction catheter.
13. Pick Yankauer or suction catheter with dominant hand without touching nonsterile surfaces. Pick up connecting tubing with nondominant hand. Secure catheter to tubing (see illustration).	Maintains catheter sterility. Connects catheter to suction.

Continued

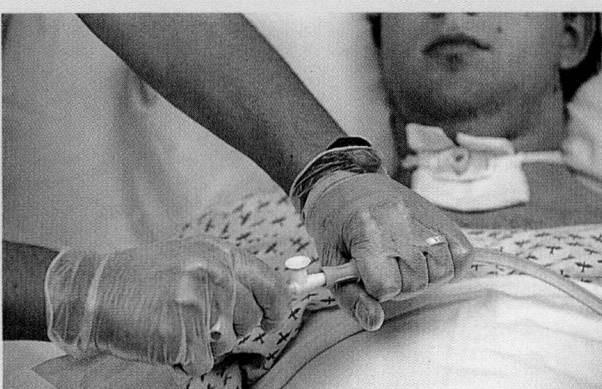

Step 13

.... **Skill 30-1—cont'd**
Suctioning

STEPS	RATIONALE
14. Suction small amount of normal saline solution from basin.	Ensures equipment function. Lubricates internal catheter and tubing.
15. Coat distal 6 to 8 cm (2 to 3 inches) of catheter with water-soluble lubricant. Do not lubricate Yankauer catheter.	Lubricates catheter for easier insertion.
16. Suction airway.	
A. Oropharyngeal:	
(1) Insert catheter into mouth along gum line to pharynx. Move catheter around mouth until secretions are cleared (see illustration). Encourage client to cough. Replace oxygen mask.	Catheter provides continuous suction. Take care not to allow suction tip to invaginate oral mucosal surfaces. Coughing moves secretions from lower airway into mouth and upper airway.

CRITICAL DECISION POINT

Be careful not to dislodge any oral tubing or tubing in posterior pharynx, such as nasogastric tubes.

(2) Rinse catheter with water in cup or basin until connecting tubing is cleared of secretions. Turn off suction. May need to wash face if secretions are present on client's skin.	Rinses catheter and reduces probability of transmission of microorganisms. Clean suction tubing enhances delivery of set suction pressure. Prevents skin breakdown.
B. Nasopharyngeal and nasotracheal:	
(1) Remove oxygen delivery device, if applicable, with nondominant hand. Without applying suction and using dominant thumb and forefinger, gently but quickly insert catheter into naris during inhalation with slight downward slant or through mouth. Do not force through naris (see illustration).	

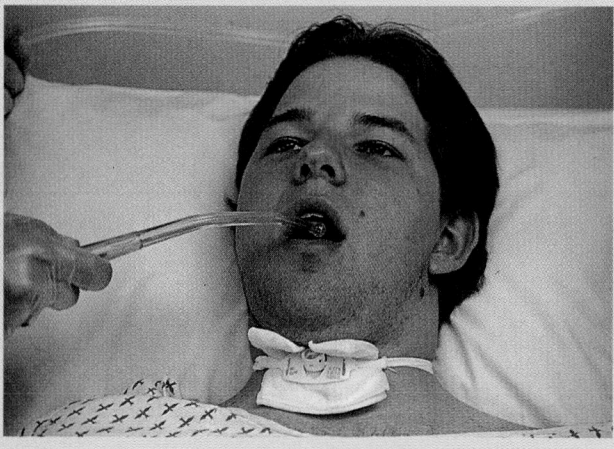

Step 16A(1)

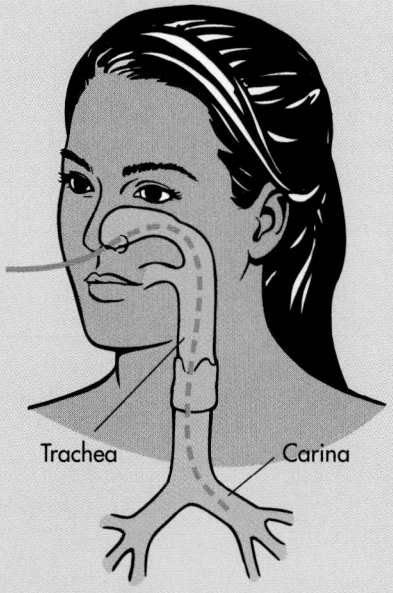

Trachea   Carina

Step 16B(1)

STEPS	RATIONALE

CRITICAL DECISION POINT

Be sure to insert catheter during client inhalation, especially if inserting catheter into trachea, because epiglottis is open. Do not insert during swallowing, or catheter will most likely enter esophagus. *NEVER* APPLY SUCTION DURING INSERTION.

(a) Nasopharyngeal suctioning: in adults, insert catheter about 16 cm; in older children, 8 to 12 cm (3 to 5 inches); in infants and young children, 4 to 8 cm (2 to 3 inches). Rule of thumb is to insert catheter distance from tip of nose (or mouth) to base of ear lobe.

(b) Nasotracheal suctioning: in adults, insert catheter about 20 cm; in older children, 14 to 20 cm (5.5 to 8 inches); in young children and infants, 8 to 14 cm (3 to 5.5 inches).

(c) Positioning: in some instances turning client's head to right helps nurse suction left mainstem bronchus; turning head to left helps nurse suction right mainstem bronchus.

    If resistance is felt after insertion of catheter for maximum recommended distance, catheter has probably hit carina. Pull catheter back 1 cm before applying suction.

(Rationale for (c):) Application of suction pressure while introducing catheter into trachea increases risk of damage to mucosa and increases risk of hypoxia because of removal of entrained oxygen present in airways. Epiglottis is open on inspiration and facilitates insertion into trachea. Client should cough. If client gags or becomes nauseated, catheter is most likely in esophagus and must be removed.

CRITICAL DECISION POINT

Use the nasal approach and perform tracheal suctioning before pharyngeal suctioning whenever possible. The mouth and pharynx contain more bacteria than the trachea does. If copious oral secretions are present before beginning the procedure, suction mouth with Yankauer suction device.

(2) Apply intermittent suction for up to 10 to 15 seconds by placing and releasing nondominant thumb over vent of catheter and slowly withdrawing catheter while rotating it back and forth between dominant thumb and forefinger. Encourage client to cough. Replace oxygen device, if applicable.

(Rationale:) Intermittent suction and rotation of catheter prevent injury to mucosa. If catheter "grabs" mucosa, remove thumb to release suction. Suctioning longer than 10 seconds can cause cardiopulmonary compromise, usually from hypoxemia or vagal overload.

(3) Rinse catheter and connecting tubing with normal saline or water until cleared.

(Rationale:) Removes secretions from catheter. Secretions that remain in suction catheter or connecting tubing decrease suctioning efficiency.

Continued

Suctioning

STEPS	RATIONALE
(4) Assess for need to repeat suctioning procedure. Allow adequate time between suction passes for ventilation and oxygenation. Ask client to deep breathe and cough.	Observe for alterations in cardiopulmonary status. Suctioning can induce hypoxemia, dysrhythmias, laryngospasm, and bronchospasm. Deep breathing reventilates and reoxygenates alveoli. Repeated passes clear the airway of excessive secretions but can also remove oxygen and may induce laryngospasm.
(5) When pharynx and trachea are sufficiently cleared of secretions, perform oropharyngeal suctioning to clear mouth of secretions. Do not suction nose again after suctioning mouth.	Removes upper airway secretions. More microorganisms are generally present in mouth.
C. Endotracheal or tracheal tube:	
(1) Hyperinflate and/or hyperoxygenate client before suctioning, using manual resuscitation Ambu-bag connected to oxygen source or sigh mechanism on mechanical ventilator. Some mechanical ventilators have a button that when pushed delivers 100% oxygen for a few minutes and then resets to the previous value.	Hyerinflation decreases atelectasis caused by negative pressure of suctioning. Preoxygenation converts large proportion of resident lung gas to 100% oxygen to offset amount used in metabolic consumption while ventilator or oxygenation is interrupted, as well as to offset volume lost during suction procedure.
(2) Open swivel adapter or if necessary remove oxygen or humidity delivery device with nondominant hand.	Exposes artificial airway.
(3) Without applying suction, gently but quickly insert catheter using dominant thumb and forefinger into artificial airway (best to time catheter insertion with inspiration) until resistance is met or client coughs; then pull back 1 cm (½ in).	Application of suction pressure while introducing catheter into trachea increases risk of damage to tracheal mucosa, as well as increased hypoxia related to removal of entrained oxygen present in airways. Pulling back stimulates cough and removes catheter from mucosal wall.
(4) Apply intermittent suction by placing and releasing nondominant thumb over vent of catheter; slowly withdraw catheter while rotating it back and forth between dominant thumb and forefinger. Encourage client to cough. Watch for respiratory distress.	Intermittent suction and rotation of catheter prevent injury to tracheal mucosal lining. If catheter "grabs" mucosa, remove thumb to release suction.

CRITICAL DECISION POINT

If the client develops respiratory distress during the suction procedure, immediately withdraw the catheter and supply additional oxygen and breaths as needed. Oxygen can be administered directly through the catheter in an emergency. Disconnect suction and attach oxygen at prescribed flow rate through the catheter.

(5) Close swivel adapter, or replace oxygen delivery device. Encourage client to deep breathe, if able. Some clients respond well to several manual breaths from the mechanical ventilator or Ambu-bag.	Reoxygenates and reexpands alveoli. Suctioning can cause hypoxemia and atelectasis.

STEPS	RATIONALE
(6) Rinse catheter and connecting tubing with normal saline until clear. Use continuous suction.	Removes catheter secretions. Secretions left in tubing decrease suction and provide environment for microorganism growth. Secretions left in connecting tube decrease suctioning efficiency.
(7) Assess client's cardiopulmonary status for secretion clearance and complications. Repeat Steps (1) through (7) once or twice more to clear secretions. Allow adequate time (at least 1 full minute) between suction passes for ventilation and reoxygenation.	Suctioning can induce dysrhythmias, hypoxia, and bronchospasm and impair cerebral circulation or adversely affect hemodynamics. Repeated passes with suction catheter clear airway of excessive secretions and promote improved oxygenation.
(8) Perform nasopharyngeal and oropharyngeal suctioning. After nasopharyngeal and oropharyngeal suctioning are performed, catheter is contaminated; do not reinsert into endotracheal or tracheostomy tube.	Removes upper airway secretions.
17. When suctioning is completed, roll catheter around fingers of dominant hand. Pull glove off inside out so that catheter remains coiled in glove. Pull off other glove over first glove in same way to seal in contaminants. Discard in appropriate receptacle. Turn off suction device.	Reduces transmission of microorganisms.
18. Remove towel, place in laundry or appropriate receptacle, and reposition client. (Nurse may need to wear clean gloves for personal care.)	Reduces transmission of microorganisms. Promotes comfort.
19. If indicated, readjust oxygen to original level because client's blood oxygen level should have returned to baseline.	Prevents absorption atelectasis and oxygen toxicity while allowing client time to reoxygenate blood.
20. Reposition client as indicated by condition. Nurse may need to reapply clean gloves for client's personal care.	Promotes comfort. Sims' position encourages drainage and reduces risk of aspiration.
21. Discard remainder of normal saline into appropriate receptacle. If basin is disposable, discard into appropriate receptacle. If basin is reusable, rinse and place in soiled utility room.	
22. Remove and discard face shield, and wash hands.	Reduces transmission of microorganisms.
23. Place unopened suction kit on suction machine or at head of bed according to institution preference.	Provides immediate access to suction catheter.
24. Compare client's respiratory assessments before and after suctioning.	Identifies physiological effects of suction procedure to restore airway patency.
25. Ask client if breathing is easier and if congestion is decreased.	Provides subjective confirmation that airway obstruction is relieved with suctioning procedure.
26. Observe airway secretions.	Provides data to document presence or absence of respiratory tract infection.

Recording and Reporting

▪ Record the amount, consistency, color, and odor of secretions and client's response to procedure; document client's presuctioning and postsuctioning respiratory status.

Home Care Considerations

▪ Normal saline may be made at home by adding 2 tsp of table salt to 1 qt of boiled water. Store in jar that has been sterilized (i.e., boiled). Several quart or pint jars can be processed at one time if prepared with home canning equipment.

similar to nasopharyngeal suctioning, but the catheter tip is moved farther into the client to suction the trachea.

Tracheal suctioning. Tracheal suctioning is accomplished through an artificial airway such as a tracheostomy tube. Two methods of suctioning are currently used. Open suctioning involves using a freshly opened sterile suction catheter that is handled with a sterile glove. Closed suctioning involves a multiple-use catheter that is encased in a plastic sheath and used for 24 hours. Closed suctioning is most often used on clients who require mechanical ventilation to support their respiratory efforts because it permits continuous delivery of oxygen while suctioning is performed (Figure 30-5).

Artificial airways. An artificial airway is indicated for clients with decreased level of consciousness, airway obstruction, mechanical ventilation, and removal of tracheal bronchial secretions (Skill 30-1).

Oral airway. The oral airway, the simplest type of artificial airway, prevents obstruction of the trachea by displacement of the tongue into the oropharynx (Figure 30-6). The oral airway extends from the teeth to the oropharynx, maintaining the tongue in the normal position. The correct size airway must be used. Proper oral airway size is determined by measuring the distance from the corner of the mouth to the angle of the jaw just below the ear. The length is equal to the distance from the flange of the airway to the tip (Weilitz, 1991). If the airway is too small, the tongue is not held in the anterior portion of the mouth; if too large, it may force the tongue toward the epiglottis and obstruct the airway.

The airway is inserted by turning the curve of the airway toward the cheek and placing it over the tongue. When the airway is in the oropharynx, the nurse turns it so the opening points downward. Correctly placed, the airway moves the tongue forward, away from the oropharynx, and the flange, the flat portion of the airway, rests against the client's teeth. Incorrect insertion merely forces the tongue back into the oropharynx.

Tracheal airway. Tracheal airways include endotracheal, nasotracheal, and tracheal tubes. These allow easy access to the client's trachea for deep tracheal suctioning. Because of the artificial airway, the client no longer has normal humidification of the tracheal mucosa. The nurse should ensure that humidity is being supplied to the airway through nebulization or with the oxygen delivery system. This humidification is protective and helps reduce the risk of airway plugging.

Mobilization of pulmonary secretions. The ability of a client to mobilize pulmonary secretions may make the difference between a short-term illness and a long recovery involving complications.

Hydration. Maintenance of adequate systemic hydration keeps mucociliary clearance, the body's natural mechanism for removing mucus and cellular debris from the respiratory tract, normal. In clients with adequate hydration, pulmonary secretions are thin, white, watery, and easily removable with minimal coughing. Excessive coughing to clear thick, tenacious secretions is fatiguing and energy depleting. The best way to maintain thin secretions is to provide a fluid intake of 1500 to 2000 ml/day, unless contraindicated by cardiac status. Adequacy of hydration can be determined by the color, consistency, and ease of secretion expectoration.

Humidification. **Humidification** is the process of adding water to gas. Temperature is the most important factor affecting the amount of water vapor a gas can hold. The percentage of water in the gas in relation to its capacity for water is the relative humidity. Air or oxygen with a high relative humidity keeps the airways moist and helps loosen and mobilize pulmonary secretions.

Humidification is necessary for clients receiving oxygen therapy. Oxygen delivered to the upper airways, such as with a nasal catheter, nasal cannula, or face mask, can be humidified by bubbling it through water. Generally humidification is added when oxygen flow rates exceed 4 L/min.

When humidity is used, the nurse needs to ensure that sterile saline for inhalation is used for humidifica-

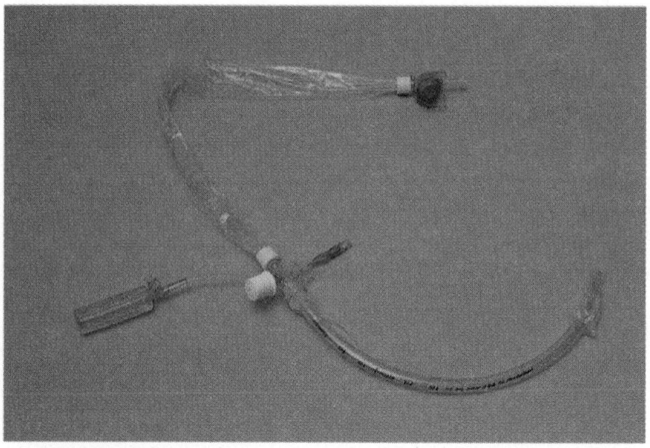

Figure 30-5. Ballard tracheal care closed suction.

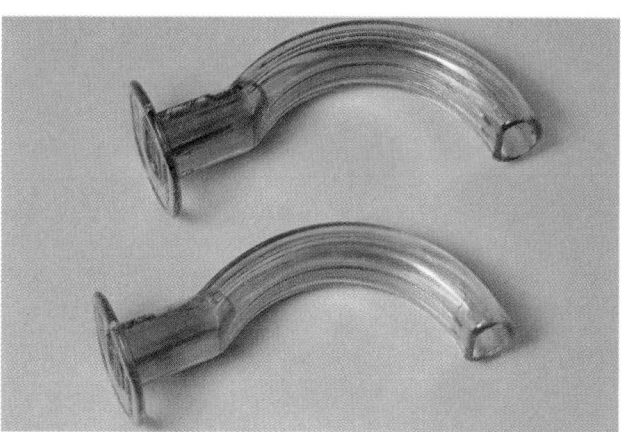

Figure 30-6. Artificial oral airways.

tion and the solution is changed according to agency procedures. Humidification can be a source for nosocomial infections in clients because the moist environment supports the growth of pathogens.

Nebulization. **Nebulization** is a process of adding moisture or medications to inspired air by mixing particles of varying sizes with the air. A nebulizer uses the aerosol principle to suspend a maximum number of water drops or particles of the desired size in inspired air. The moisture added to the respiratory system through nebulization improves clearance of pulmonary secretions. Nebulization is often used for administration of bronchodilators and mucolytic agents.

When the thin layer of fluid that supports the mucus layer over the cilia is allowed to dry, the cilia are damaged and cannot adequately clear the airway. Humidification through nebulization enhances mucociliary clearance.

Maintenance or promotion of lung expansion. Nursing interventions to maintain or promote lung expansion include positioning and chest physiotherapy, procedures using equipment such as incentive spirometry, and invasive procedures such as management of a chest tube.

Positioning. In the healthy, completely mobile person, adequate ventilation and oxygenation are maintained by frequent position changes during daily activities. However, when a person's illness or injury restricts mobility, there is an increased risk for respiratory impairment. Frequent changes of position are simple and cost-effective methods for reducing the risks of stasis of pulmonary secretions and decreased chest wall expansion.

The most effective position for clients with cardiopulmonary diseases is the 45-degree semi-Fowler's position (Burns and others, 1994), using gravity to assist in lung expansion and reduce pressure from the abdomen on the diaphragm. When the client uses this position, the nurse needs to ensure that the client does not slide down in bed, which could reduce lung expansion. Clients with unilateral lung disease, such as pneumothorax or atelectasis affecting one lung should be positioned with the "good lung down." This promotes better perfusion of the healthy lung, improving oxygenation. In the presence of pulmonary abscess or hemorrhage, place the affected lung down to prevent drainage toward the healthy lung (Yeaw, 1992).

Incentive spirometry. **Incentive spirometry** is a method of encouraging voluntary deep breathing by providing visual feedback to clients about inspiratory volume. Incentive spirometry promotes deep breathing to prevent or treat atelectasis in the postoperative client; however, studies have shown no respiratory benefit to postoperative incentive spirometry when compared to deep breathing and early ambulation (Bell, 1993).

Flow-oriented incentive spirometers consist of one or more plastic chambers that contain freely moving colored balls. The client inhales slowly and with an even flow to elevate the balls and to keep them floating as long as possible to ensure a maximally sustained inhalation.

Volume-oriented incentive spirometry devices have a bellows that is raised to a predetermined volume by an inhaled breath. An achievement light or counter is used to provide feedback. Some devices are constructed so the light will not turn on unless the bellows is held at a minimum desired volume for a specified period to enhance lung expansion.

Incentive spirometry encourages clients to breathe to their normal inspiratory capacities. A postoperative inspiratory capacity one half to three fourths of the preoperative volume is acceptable because of postoperative pain. Administration of pain medications prior to incentive spirometry will help the client achieve deep breathing by reducing pain and splinting.

Chest physiotherapy. **Chest physiotherapy (CPT)** is a group of therapies used in combination to mobilize pulmonary secretions (Box 30-8). These therapies include postural drainage, chest percussion, and vibration. CPT should be followed by productive coughing or suctioning the client who has a decreased ability to cough. CPT is recommended for clients who produce greater than 30 ml of sputum per day or have evidence of atelectasis by chest x-ray film.

Chest percussion. **Chest percussion** involves striking the chest wall over the area being drained. The hand is positioned so that the fingers and thumb touch and the hand is cupped (Figure 30-7). Percussion on the surface of the chest wall sends waves of varying amplitude and frequency through the chest, changing the consistency and location of the sputum. Chest percussion is performed by alternating hand motion against the chest wall (Figure 30-8). Percussion is performed over a single layer of clothing, not over buttons, snaps, or zippers. The single layer of clothing prevents slapping

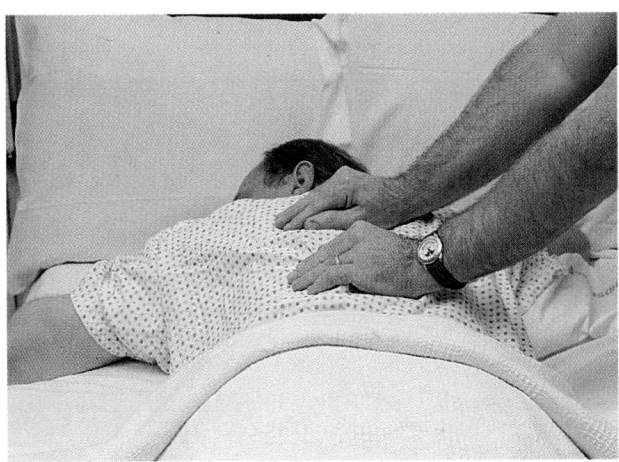

Figure 30-7. Hand position for chest wall percussion during physiotherapy.

Assessment Criteria for Chest Physiotherapy

Nursing care and selection of CPT skills are based on specific assessment findings. The following guidelines help the nurse in physical assessment and subsequent decision making:

1. *Know the client's normal range of vital signs.* Conditions such as atelectasis and pneumonia requiring CPT can affect vital signs. The degree of change is related to the level of hypoxia, overall cardiopulmonary status, and tolerance to activity.

2. *Know the client's medications.* Certain medications, particularly diuretics and antihypertensives, cause fluid and hemodynamic changes. These may decrease the client's tolerance to the positional changes and postural drainage. Chronic steroid use increases the client's risk of pathological rib fractures and often contraindicates rib shaking.

3. *Know the client's medical history.* Certain conditions such as increased intracranial pressure, spinal cord injuries, and abdominal aneurysm resection contraindicate the positional changes of postural drainage. Thoracic trauma or surgery may also contraindicate percussion, vibration, and rib shaking.

4. *Know the client's level of cognitive function.* Participation in controlled cough techniques requires the client to follow instructions. Congenital or acquired cognitive limitations may alter the client's ability to learn and participate in these techniques.

5. *Be aware of the client's exercise tolerance.* CPT maneuvers are fatiguing. When the client is not used to physical activity, initial tolerance to the maneuvers may be decreased. However, with gradual increases in activity and planned CPT, client tolerance to the procedure improves.

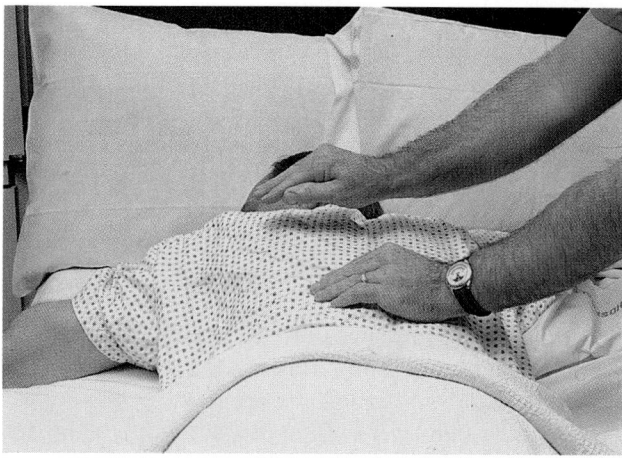

Figure 30-8.   Chest wall percussion, alternating motion against the client's chest wall.

the client's skin. Thicker or multiple layers of material dampen the vibrations.

Caution should be taken to percuss the lung fields and not the scapular regions, or trauma may occur to the skin and underlying musculoskeletal structures. Percussion is contraindicated in clients with bleeding disorders, osteoporosis, or fractured ribs.

Vibration. **Vibration** is a fine, shaking pressure applied to the chest wall only during exhalation. This technique is thought to increase the velocity and turbulence of exhaled air, facilitating secretion removal (Dettenmeier, 1992). Vibration increases the exhalation

of trapped air and may shake mucus loose and induce a cough. Vibration is not recommended in infants and young children.

Postural drainage. **Postural drainage** is the use of positioning techniques that draw secretions from specific segments of the lungs and bronchi into the trachea. Coughing or suctioning normally removes secretions from the trachea. The procedure for postural drainage can include most lung segments (Table 30-7). Because clients may not require postural drainage of all lung segments, the procedure is based on clinical assessment findings. For example, clients with left lower lobe atelectasis may require postural drainage of only the affected region, whereas a child with cystic fibrosis may require postural drainage of all segments.

Chest tubes. A **chest tube** is a catheter inserted through the thorax to remove air and fluids from the pleural space and to reestablish normal intrapleural and intrapulmonic pressures. Chest tubes are used after chest surgery and chest trauma and for pneumothorax or hemothorax to promote lung expansion (Skill 30-2).

A **pneumothorax** is a collection of air or other gas in the pleural space. The gas causes the lung to collapse because it obliterates the negative intrapleural pressure and a counterpressure is exerted against the lung, which is then unable to expand. There are a variety of mechanisms for a pneumothorax. It may occur spontaneously or from chest trauma.

A client with a pneumothorax usually feels pain as atmospheric air irritates the parietal pleura. The pain may be sharp and pleuritic. Dyspnea is common and worsens as the size of the pneumothorax increases.

Hemothorax is an accumulation of blood and fluid in the pleural cavity between the parietal and visceral pleurae, usually as the result of trauma. It produces a counterpressure and prevents the lung from full expansion. In addition to pain and dyspnea, signs and symptoms of shock can develop if blood loss is severe.

Care of Clients With Chest Tubes

Delegation Considerations
This skill requires problem solving and knowledge application unique to a professional nurse and should not be delegated. For this skill, the nurse must be sure the care provider knows the following:
- Inform and assist care provider in the proper positioning of a client with chest tubes to facilitate drainage.
- Instruct care provider in the appropriate setup of drainage equipment for the type of system to be used.
- Instruct care provider to inform nurse of any changes in the vital signs, chest tube drainage, or excessive bubbling in water-seal chamber.

Equipment
- Chest drainage system (bottles or disposable system)
- Suction source and setup (wall canister or portable)
- Nonsterile gloves
- Sterile irrigation saline or sterile water (500-ml bottle)
- 2-inch tape
- Sterile gauze sponges
- 2 shodded hemostats

STEPS	RATIONALE
1. Assess client for respiratory distress and chest pain, breath sounds over affected lung area, and stable vital signs (see Chapter 24).	Signs and symptoms reflect improvement in respiratory distress and chest pain after insertion of chest tube.
2. Observe for increased respiratory distress.	Signs and symptoms of increased respiratory distress and/or chest pain, decrease in breath sounds over the affected and nonaffected lungs, marked cyanosis, asymmetric chest movements, presence of subcutaneous emphysema around tube insertion site or neck, hypotension, and tachycardia. Notify physician immediately.
3. Observe:	
a. Chest tube dressing.	Ensures that tubing is patent.
b. Tubing for kinks, dependent loops, or clots.	Maintains a patent, freely draining system, preventing fluid accumulation in chest cavity.
c. Chest drainage system, which should be upright and below level of tube insertion.	System must be in this position to function properly.
4. Provide two shodded hemostats for each chest tube, attached to top of client's bed with adhesive tape. Chest tubes are only clamped under specific circumstances:	Shodded hemostats have a covering to prevent hemostat from penetrating chest tube.
a. To assess air leak.	
b. To quickly empty or change collection bottle or chamber; performed by nurse who has received training in procedure.	
c. To change disposable systems; have new system ready to be connected before clamping tube so that transfer can be rapid and drainage system reestablished.	
d. To change a broken water-seal bottle in the event that no sterile solution container is available.	
e. To assess if client is ready to have chest tube removed (which is done by physician's order); the nurse must monitor client for recreation of pneumothorax.	

Continued

Skill 30-2—cont'd
Care of Clients With Chest Tubes

STEPS	RATIONALE
5. Position the client.	Permits optimal drainage of fluid and/or air.
a. Semi-Fowler's position to evacuate air (pneumothorax).	Air rises to highest point in chest. Pneumothorax tubes are usually placed on the anterior aspect at midclavicular line, second or third intercostal space.
b. High Fowler's position to drain fluid (hemothorax).	Permits optimal drainage of fluid. Posterior tubes are placed on midaxillary line, eighth or ninth intercostal space.
6. Maintain tube connection between chest and drainage tubes intact and taped.	Secures chest tube to drainage system and reduces risk of air leak causing breaks in airtight system.
a. Water-seal vent must be without occlusion.	Permits displaced air to pass into atmosphere.
b. Suction-control chamber vent must be without occlusion when suction is used.	Provides safety factor of releasing excess negative pressure into atmosphere.
7. Coil excess tubing on mattress next to client. Secure with rubber band and safety pin or system's clamp.	Prevents excess tubing from hanging over edge of mattress in dependent loop. Drainage could collect in loop and occlude drainage system.
8. Adjust tubing to hang in straight line from top of mattress to drainage chamber. If chest tube is draining fluid, indicate time (e.g., 0900) that drainage was begun on drainage bottle's adhesive tape or on write-on surface of disposable commercial system.	Provides a baseline for continuous assessment of type and quality of drainage.
9. Strip or milk chest tube only if indicated:	Stripping is controversial and should be peformed only if the hospital policy permits it and there is a physician's order. Stripping creates a high degree of negative pressure and has potential of pulling lung tissue or pleura into drainage holes of chest tube.
a. Postoperative mediastinal chest tubes are manipulated if nursing assessment indicates obstruction of drainage secondary to clots or debris in tubing.	
b. Postoperative assessment is done every 15 minutes for the first 2 hours. This assessment interval then changes based on client's status.	

CRITICAL DECISION POINT

Review agency policy before milking or stripping chest tubes.

10. Wash hands.	Reduces transmission of infection.
11. Observe:	
a. Chest tube dressing, tubing, and chest tube drainage system, which should be upright and below level of tube insertion.	Ensures that the tube is patent, and notes any drainage. Maintains tubing free of kinks and dependent loops. Note presence of clots or debris in tubing.
b. Water seal for fluctuations with client's inspiration and expiration.	Fluid should rise in water seal with inspiration and fall with expiration, indicating that system is functioning properly.
c. Bubbling in water-seal bottle or chamber (Table 30-8).	When system is initially connected to client, bubbles are expected in chamber from air that was present in system and in client's intrapleural space. After a short period, bubbling will stop. Fluid will continue to fluctuate in water seal on inspiration and expiration until lung is reexpanded or system becomes occluded.

STEPS	RATIONALE
d. Type and amount of fluid drainage. Nurse should note color and amount of drainage, client's vital signs, and skin color.	Sudden gush of drainage may be retained blood and not active bleeding. Increase in drainage can be result of client position.
(1) Less than 50 to 300 ml/hr immediately postoperative in mediastinal chest tube; approximately 500 ml in first 24 hours; dark red drainage is expected early in postoperative period, turning serous with time.	Reexpansion of lungs forces drainage into tube. Coughing can also cause large gushes of drainage.
(2) Between 100 and 300 ml of fluid may drain in posterior chest tube during first 2 hours after insertion; rate will decrease after 2 hours; 500 to 1000 ml can be expected in first 24 hours; drainage will be grossly bloody during first several hours after surgery and then change to serous.	Excessive amounts and/or continued presence of frank, bloody drainage after first several hours of surgery should be reported to physician, along with client's vital signs and respiratory status.
e. Bubbling in the suction-control chamber (when suction is being used) (Table 30-8).	Suction-control chamber has constant, gentle bubbling. Tubing to suction source should be free of obstruction, and suction source should be turned on to appropriate setting.

Recording and Reporting
- Record in nurse's notes patency of chest tubes, presence of drainage, presence of fluctuations, client's vital signs, chest dressing status, type of suction, and level of comfort.

Home Care Considerations
- If client goes home with chest tube (i.e., empyema), teach client and family to care for chest tube and drainage bottle.

The one-bottle system is the simplest closed drainage system because the single bottle serves as a collector and a water seal (Figure 30-9, *A*). During normal respiration the fluid should ascend with inspiration and descend with expiration. The one-bottle system is used for smaller amounts of drainage, such as empyema.

A two-bottle system permits the liquid to flow into the collection bottle, and air flows into the water-seal bottle (Figure 30-9, *B*). Fluctuations in the water-seal tube are still anticipated. The two-bottle system allows more accurate measurement of chest drainage and is used when larger amounts of drainage are expected.

A three-bottle system is used to evaluate any volume of air or fluid with controlled suction (Figure 30-9, *C*). The suction-control bottle contains a long tube, submerged under water, and vented to the atmosphere. There are two short tubes; one tube connects bottles two and three, and the second tube is connected to an external suction source. The suction pressure causes

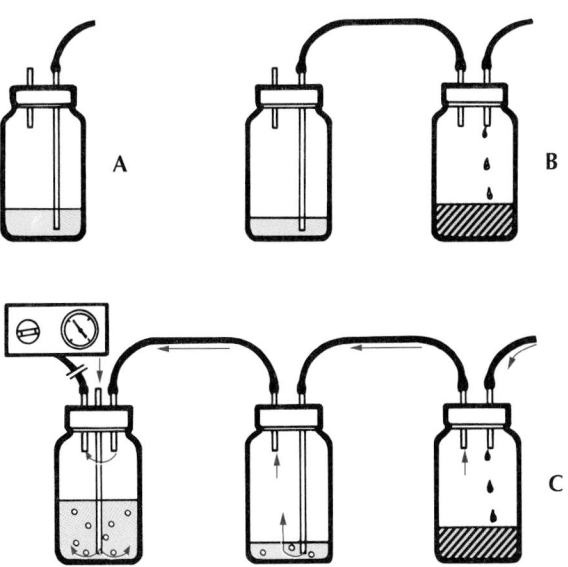

Figure 30-9.   Chest tube drainage. **A,** One-bottle system. **B,** Two-bottle system. **C,** Three-bottle system with suction.

TABLE 30-7
Positions for Postural Drainage

Lung Segment	Position of Client	Lung Segment	Position of Client
Adult			

Lung Segment	Position of Client	Lung Segment	Position of Client
Bilateral	High Fowler's	Right middle lobe—posterior segment	Prone with thorax and abdomen elevated

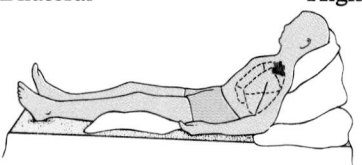
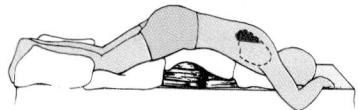

Apical segments Right upper lobe—anterior segment	Sitting on side of bed Supine with head elevated	Both lower lobes—anterior segments	Supine in Trendelenburg's

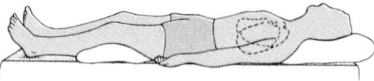
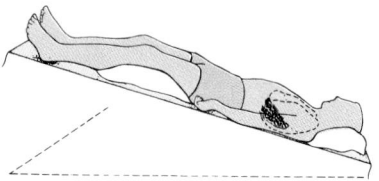

Left upper lobe—anterior segment	Supine with head elevated	Left lower lobe—lateral segment	Right side lying in Trendelenburg's position

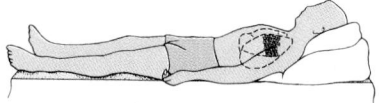
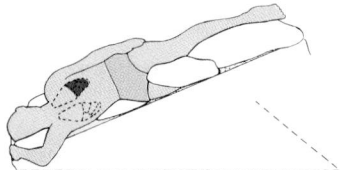

Right upper lobe—posterior segment	Side lying with right side of chest elevated on pillows	Right lower lobe—lateral segment	Left side lying in Trendelenburg's position

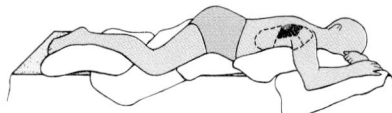
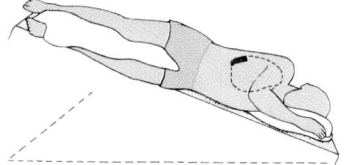

Left upper lobe—posterior segment	Side lying with left side of chest elevated on pillows	Right lower lobe—posterior segment	Prone with right side of chest elevated in Trendelenburg's position

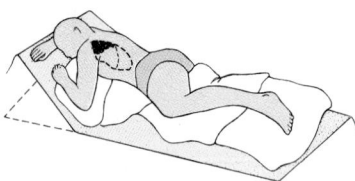
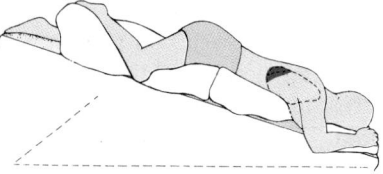

Right middle lobe—anterior segment	Three-fourths supine position with dependent lung in Trendelenburg's position	Both lower lobes—posterior segment	Prone in Trendelenburg's position

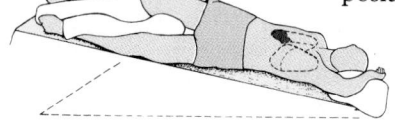
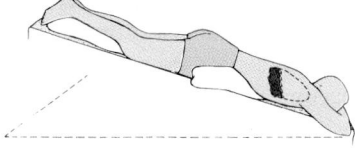

TABLE 30-7
Positions for Postural Drainage—cont'd

Lung Segment	Position of Client	Lung Segment	Position of Client
Child		Bilateral lobes— anterior segments	Lying supine on nurse's lap, back supported with pillow
Bilateral—apical segments	Sitting on nurse's lap, leaning slightly forward flexed over pillow		
Bilateral—middle anterior segments	Sitting on nurse's lap, leaning against nurse		

gentle, continuous bubbling in bottle three. Suction pressure is measured in centimeters of water and is equated with length of the long tube submerged in water. Usually -15 to -20 cm H_2O is used for adults. This means the long tube is submerged in 15 to 20 cm H_2O. Children require lesser amounts of pressure.

The disposable systems, such as a Thora-Sene III or Pleur-Evac chest drainage system (DeKental), are a one-piece molded plastic unit that duplicates the three-bottle system (Figure 30-10). The disposable units appear to be the system of choice because they are cost-effective and some facilitate autotransfusion, a common practice in open heart surgeries. Knowledge of the basics of chest tube management and troubleshooting maneuvers reduces the client's risk of complications (Table 30-8).

Special considerations. Clamping chest tubes is contraindicated when the client is ambulating or being transported. The nurse should handle the chest drainage unit or bottles carefully and maintain the drainage device below the client's chest. If the tubing disconnects from the bottles, the nurse should instruct the client to exhale as much as possible and to cough. This maneuver rids the pleural space of as much air as possible. The nurse needs to cleanse the tips of the tubing and reconnect them to the bottles quickly. If the chest tube breaks, quickly submerge the end of the tubing in a container of water to reestablish the seal. Clamping the chest tube may result in a tension pneumothorax, which is a life-threatening event.

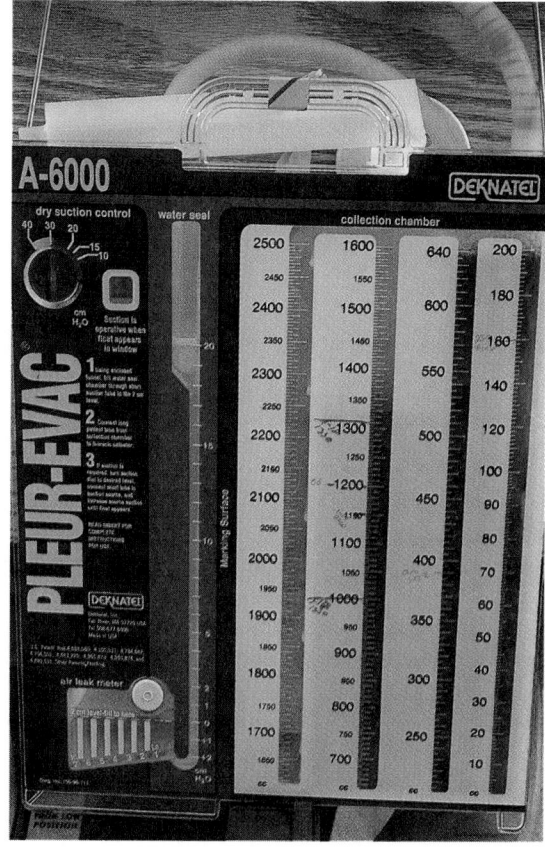

Figure 30-10. Disposable, commercial chest drainage system.

TABLE 30-8
Problem Solving With Chest Tubes

Problem	Solution
Air leak is present.	Locate leak.
Continuous bubbling is seen in water-seal bottle/chamber, indicating that leak is between client and water seal.	Tighten loose connections between client and water seal. Loose connections cause air to enter system. Leaks are corrected when constant bubbling stops.
Bubbling continues, indicating that air leak has not been corrected.	Cross-clamp chest tube close to client's chest. If bubbling stops, air leak is inside client's thorax or at chest tube insertion site. *Unclamp tube and notify physician immediately.* Reinforce chest dressing. Leaving chest tube clamped causes a tension pneumothorax and mediastinal shift.
Bubbling continues, indicating that leak is not in the client's chest or at the insertion site.	Gradually move clamps down drainage tubing away from client and toward suction-control chamber, moving one clamp at a time. When bubbling stops, leak is in section of tubing or connection distal to the clamp. Replace tubing or secure connection and release clamp.
Bubbling continues, indicating that leak is not in tubing.	Leak is in drainage system. Change drainage system.
Tension pneumothorax is present. Severe respiratory distress Chest pain Absence of breath sounds on affected side Hyperresonance on affected side Mediastinal shift to unaffected side Tracheal shift to unaffected side Hypotension Tachycardia	Determine that chest tubes are not clamped, kinked, or occluded. Obstructed chest tubes trap air in intrapleural space when air leak originates within client. Notify physician immediately. Prepare immediately for another chest tube insertion; obtain a flutter (Heimlich) valve or large-gauge needle for short-term emergency release of air in intrapleural space; have emergency equipment (e.g., oxygen and code cart) near client.
Dependent loops of drainage tubing have trapped fluid.	Drain tubing contents into drainage bottle. Coil excess tubing on mattress, and secure in place.
Water seal is disconnected.	Connect water seal, and tape connection.
Water-seal bottle is broken.	Insert distal end of water-seal tube into sterile solution so that tip is 2 cm below surface, and set up new water-seal bottle. If no sterile solution is available, double clamp chest tube while preparing new bottle.
Water-seal tube is no longer submerged in sterile fluid.	Add sterile solution to water-seal bottle until distal tip is 2 cm under surface, or set water-seal bottle upright so that tip is submerged.

Removal of chest tubes requires client preparation. A recent study investigated clients who reported sensations during chest tube removal. The most frequent sensations reported include burning, pain, and a pulling sensation (Gift and others, 1991).

Maintenance and promotion of oxygenation. Promotion of lung expansion, mobilization of secretions, and maintenance of a patent airway assist the client in meeting oxygenation needs. Some clients, however, also require oxygen therapy to keep a healthy level of tissue oxygenation.

Goals of oxygen therapy. The goal of oxygen therapy is to prevent or relieve hypoxia. Any client with impaired tissue oxygenation can benefit from controlled oxygen administration. Oxygen is not a substitute for other treatments, however, and should be used only when indicated. Oxygen should be treated as a drug. It is expensive and has dangerous side effects. As with any drug, the dosage or concentration of oxygen should be continuously monitored. The nurse should routinely check the physician's orders to verify that the client is receiving the prescribed oxygen concentration. The five rights of medication administration also pertain to oxygen administration (see Chapter 26).

Safety precautions with oxygen therapy. Oxygen is a highly combustible gas. Although it will not spontaneously burn or cause an explosion, it can easily cause a fire to ignite in a client's room if it contacts a spark from a cigarette or electrical equipment. Oxygen in high concentrations has a great combustion potential and fuels fire readily.

With increasing use of home oxygen therapy, clients and health care professionals must be aware of these dangers of combustion. The nurse should promote safety by using the following measures:

1. "No smoking" signs should be placed on the client's room door and over the bed. The client, visitors, roommates, and all personnel should be informed that smoking is not permitted in areas where oxygen is in use.
2. The nurse determines that all electrical equipment in the room is functioning correctly and is properly grounded (see Chapter 28).
3. The nurse should know the fire procedures and the location of the closest fire extinguisher.
4. The nurse should always check the oxygen level of portable tanks before transporting to ensure there is enough remaining in the tank.

Supply of oxygen. Oxygen is supplied to the client's bedside either by oxygen tanks or through a permanent wall-piped system. Oxygen tanks are transported on wide-based carriers that allow the tank to be placed upright at the client's bedside. Regulators are used to control the amount of oxygen delivered. One common type is an upright flow meter with a flow-adjustment valve at the top. A second type is a cylinder indicator with a flow-adjustment handle.

Methods of oxygen delivery. Oxygen can be delivered to the client by nasal cannula, nasal catheter, face mask, or mechanical ventilator (Table 30-9).

Home oxygen. Indications for home oxygen therapy include an arterial partial pressure (PaO_2) of 55 mm Hg or less or an arterial oxygen saturation (SaO_2) of 88% or less on room air at rest, on exertion, or with exercise (Dettenmeier, 1992).

When home oxygen is required, it is usually delivered by nasal cannula. When a client has a permanent tracheostomy, however, a T tube or tracheostomy collar is necessary. Three types of oxygen systems are used: compressed oxygen, liquid oxygen, and oxygen concentrators. The advantages and disadvantages of each type are assessed, along with the client's needs and community resources, before placing a certain delivery system in the home. In the home the major consideration is the oxygen delivery source.

Clients requiring home oxygen need extensive teaching to be able to continue oxygen therapy at home efficiently and safely. This includes oxygen safety, regulation of the amount of oxygen, and how to use the prescribed home oxygen delivery system. The nurse coordinates the efforts of the client and the family, home care nurse, home respiratory therapist, and home oxygen equipment vendor. The social worker usually assists with arranging the home care nurse and oxygen vendor.

Restoration of cardiopulmonary functioning. If a client's hypoxia is severe and prolonged, cardiac arrest may result. A cardiac arrest is a sudden cessation of cardiac output and circulation. When this occurs, oxygen is not delivered to the tissues, carbon dioxide is not transported from tissues, tissue metabolism becomes anaerobic, and metabolic and respiratory acidosis occur. Permanent heart, brain, and other tissue damage occurs within 4 to 6 minutes.

Cardiac resuscitation. Cardiac arrest is characterized by an absence of pulse and respiration. If the nurse determines that the client has cardiac arrest, **cardiopulmonary resuscitation (CPR)** must be initiated. CPR is a basic emergency procedure of artificial respiration and manual external cardiac massage (Skill 30-3). The "ABCs" of CPR are establish an airway, initiate breathing, and maintain circulation. When an airway cannot be established, the nurse must reassess proper head position and assess for airway obstruction. There is no clinical benefit to cardiac compressions if an airway cannot be established.

Restorative care.
Restorative care may emphasize cardiopulmonary reconditioning as a structured rehabilitation program. **Cardiopulmonary rehabilitation** is actively assisting the client to achieve and maintain an optimal level of health through controlled physical exercise, nutrition counseling, relaxation and stress management techniques, prescribed medications, and oxygen administration. As physical reconditioning occurs, the client's physical symptoms, anxiety, depression, or somatic concerns should decrease. Goals of rehabilitation are defined by the client and the rehabilitation team.

Respiratory muscle training. Respiratory muscle training improves strength and endurance, resulting in improved activity tolerance. Respiratory muscle training may prevent respiratory failure in clients with chronic obstructive pulmonary disease.

One method for respiratory muscle training is the **incentive spirometer resistive breathing device (ISRBD).** Resistive breathing is achieved by placing a restrictive breathing device into a volume-dependent incentive spirometer. Muscle training is achieved when the client uses the ISRBD on a scheduled routine, for example, twice a day for 15 minutes or 4 times a day for 15 minutes (Celli, 1994).

Breathing exercises. Breathing exercises include techniques to improve ventilation and oxygenation. The three basic techniques are deep breathing and coughing exercises, pursed-lip breathing, and diaphragmatic

Text continued on p. 832

TABLE 30-9

Oxygen Delivery Systems

Delivery System	Indications	O₂ Concentration (Flow Rate)	Considerations
Nasal cannula	Simple, comfortable device to deliver low-concentration O₂ (less than 6 L/min)	24% (1 L/min) 28% (2 L/min) 32% (3 L/min) 36% (4 L/min) 40% (5 L/min) 44% (6 L/min)	Flow rates greater than 4 L/min often cause drying effect on mucosa; humidify oxygen; be alert for skin breakdown over ears and in nares; questionable efficiency in mouth breathers.
Nasal catheter	Continuous uninterrupted O₂ therapy; insertion of a catheter into the nose to the nasopharynx	Approximately 30% (6 L/min)	Rarely used; causes pain on insertion and trauma to nasal mucosa; catheter needs to be changed every 8 hours, alternating nostrils.
Transtracheal O₂ (TTO)	For chronic lung diseases; small, IV-size catheter inserted directly into trachea	Flow requirements may be reduced to 60% to 80%, which greatly increases amount of time available from portable source of O₂.	No O₂ lost to atmosphere; clients achieve adequate oxygenation at lower rates (more efficient, less expensive, and produces fewer side effects); clients more likely to use O₂ because of mobility, comfort, and cosmetic improvement.
Oxygen masks	Administer O₂, humidity, or heated humidity		
Simple face mask	Short-term O₂ therapy	30% to 60% (6-8 L/min)	Contraindicated for clients with carbon dioxide retention; effective for mouth breathers (Figure 30-11).
Plastic face mask with a reservoir bag	Delivers high concentrations of O₂	80% to 90% (10 L/min)	Frequently inspect the bag to make sure it is inflated (Figure 30-12).
Venturi mask	Can deliver precise, high-flow rates of O₂; adapters can be applied to increase humidification.	24% (2 L/min) 28% (3 L/min) 30% (4 L/min) 35% (6 L/min) 40% (8 L/min) 45% (10 L/min) 55% (14 L/min)	Mask must be removed when client eats (Figure 30-13).

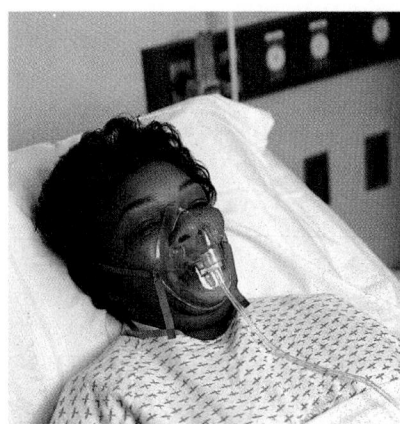

Figure 30-11.   Simple face mask.

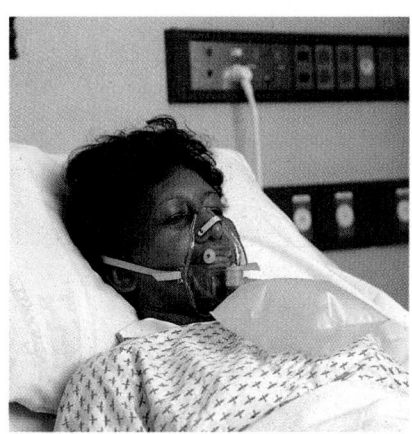

Figure 30-12.   Plastic face mask with inflated reservoir bag.

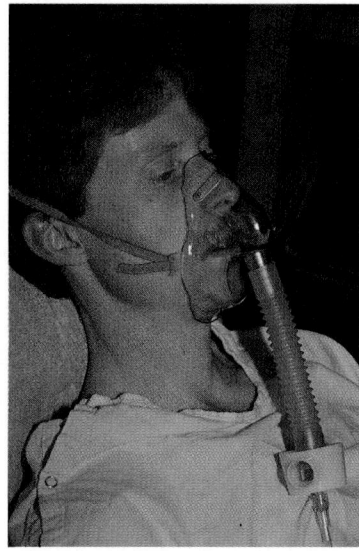

Figure 30-13.   Venturi mask.

Cardiopulmonary Resuscitation

Delegation Considerations
This skill of cardiopulmonary resuscitation can be performed by assistive personnel.
- Caution the care provider to make certain the client is indeed pulseless before initiating chest compressions.
- Review the procedures for opening the airway if the client has any risk for cervical neck trauma.
- Caution the provider regarding the differences between infants, children, and adults.

Equipment
- Ambu-bag, if available
- CPR pocket mask or barrier device, if available
- Chest compression board, if available
- Gloves, if available
- Resuscitation cart, if available
- Face shield, if available

STEPS	RATIONALE
1. Determine if client is unconscious by shaking client and shouting, "Are you OK?"	Confirms that client is unconscious as opposed to intoxicated, sleeping, or hearing impaired.
2. Activate emergency medical services.	The majority of adult victims are in ventricular fibrillation and need defibrillation and antiarrhythmic drugs as soon as possible.
3. Determine breathlessness and carotid or brachial (use with infants) pulse.	Presence of pulse and respirations contraindicates initiation of CPR.
4. Place victim on hard surface such as floor, ground, or backboard. Victim must be flat. If necessary, logroll victim to flat, supine position using spine precautions.	External compression of heart is facilitated. Heart is compressed between sternum and spinal vertebrae, which must be on a hard and firm surface.
5. Assume correct and comfortable position.	Nurse may be administering CPR for extended period, particularly in community setting. Correct, comfortable position decreases skeletal muscle fatigue and promotes more effective compressions.
A. **One-person rescue**	
(1) Position to face victim, on knees, parallel to victim's sternum.	Allows rescuer to quickly move back and forth from victim's mouth to sternum.
B. **Two-person rescue**	
(1) One person faces victim, kneeling parallel to victim's head. Second person moves to opposite side and faces victim, kneeling parallel to victim's sternum.	Allows one rescuer to maintain breathing while other maintains circulation, without getting in each other's way.
6. If available, apply gloves and face shield.	Reduces transmission of microorganisms.
7. Open airway:	
a. If no head or neck trauma, use head tilt–chin lift method (AHA, 1994) (see illustration).	The tongue is the most common cause of airway obstruction in the unconscious client. Airway obstruction from tongue is relieved. If necessary, remove foreign body.

Continued

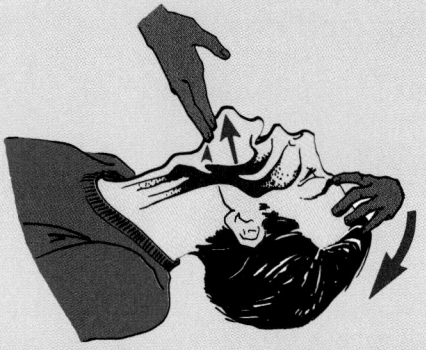

Step 7a

Cardiopulmonary Resuscitation

STEPS	RATIONALE
b. Jaw thrust maneuver (see illustration) can be used by health professionals but is not taught to general public. Grasp angles of victim's lower jaw and lift with both hands, displacing the mandible forward while tilting the head backward.	When head and/or neck trauma is suspected, this maneuver opens the airway while maintaining proper head and neck alignment, thus reducing the risk of further damage to the neck.
8. If readily available, insert oral airway.	Maintains tongue on anterior floor of mouth and prevents obstruction of posterior airway by tongue.
9. If the victim does not resume breathing, administer artificial respiration.	Airtight seal is formed, and air is prevented from escaping through nose.

A. Mouth-to-mouth

Adult

(1) Pinch victim's nose with the thumb and index fingers, and occlude mouth with nurse's mouth or use CPR pocket mask. Maintain head tilt–chin lift while administering breaths so air enters lungs and not stomach. Blow two slow full breaths into victim's mouth (each breath should take 0.5 to 2 seconds); allow victim to exhale between breaths. Continue giving 12 breaths per minute (AHA, 1994).

Hyperventilation is promoted and assists in maintaining adequate blood oxygen levels. In most adults this volume is 800 to 1200 ml and is sufficient to make the chest rise.

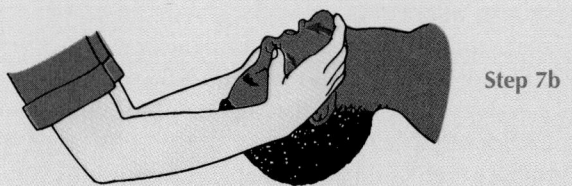

Step 7b

Child

(2) Place nurse's mouth over child's mouth (see illustration), or use CPR pocket mask. For mouth-to-mouth resuscitation of child, administer two slow breaths lasting 1 to 1½ seconds with a pause between. Continue giving 20 breaths per minute (AHA, 1994).

Airtight seal is formed, and air is prevented from escaping from nose.

Infant

(3) Because an infant's air passages are smaller and resistance to flow is quite high, making recommendations about the force or volume of the rescue breaths is difficult. Place nurse's mouth over infant's nose and mouth. However, three factors should be remembered: (1) rescue breaths are the single most important maneuver in assisting a nonbreathing child, (2) an appropriate volume is one that makes the chest rise and fall, and (3) slow breaths provide an adequate volume at the lowest possible pressure, thereby reducing the risk of gastric distention.

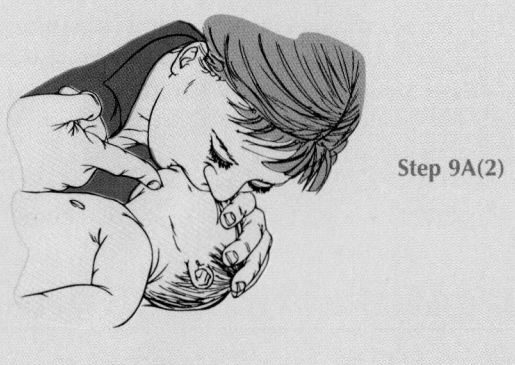

Step 9A(2)

B. Mouth-to-nose

(1) Keep the victim's head tilted with one hand on the forehead. Use the other hand to lift the jaw and close the mouth. Seal nurse's lips around the victim's nose and blow. Allow passive exhalation.

In some victims (those whose mouth cannot be opened or whose jaws or mouth is seriously injured) mouth-to-nose can be a more effective method of ventilation.

STEPS	RATIONALE

CRITICAL DECISION POINT

It may be necessary to open the victim's mouth on occasion to allow trapped exhaled air to escape.

C. Ambu-bag
   Adult and child
   (1) For Ambu-bag resuscitation use proper size face mask and apply it under chin, up and over victim's mouth and nose.

Airtight seal is formed; as bag is compressed, oxygen enters client.

   (2) Observe for rise and fall of chest wall with each respiration (see illustration). Listen for air escaping during exhalation, and feel for flow of air. If lungs do not inflate, reposition head and neck and check for visible airway obstruction, such as vomitus.

Repositioning ensures airway is properly opened and that artificial respirations are entering lungs.

10. Suction secretions if necessary, or turn victim's head to one side, unless contraindicated.

Suctioning prevents airway obstruction. Turning client's head to one side allows gravity to drain secretions.

11. Check for presence of carotid (adults) or brachial (infants) pulse after restoring breathing.

Carotid artery pulse is the most easily accessible and persists when other peripheral pulses are no longer palpable.

12. If pulse is absent, initiate chest compressions:
   a. Assume correct hand position:

Places hands and fingers over heart in proper position. Prevents xiphoid process and rib fracture, which can further compromise cardiopulmonary status.

   Adult
   (1) Place hands 1 to 2 cm above xiphoid process on sternum (see illustration). Keep hands parallel to chest and fingers above chest. Interlocking fingers is helpful. Keep fingers off of the chest wall. Extend arms and lock elbows. Maintain arms straight and shoulders directly over victim's sternum.

Continued

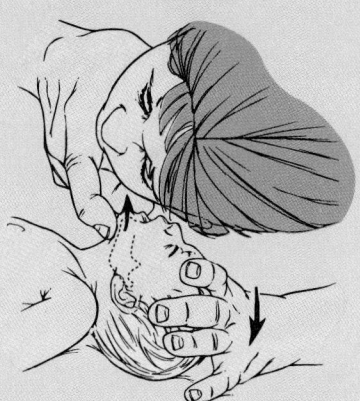

Step 9C(2)

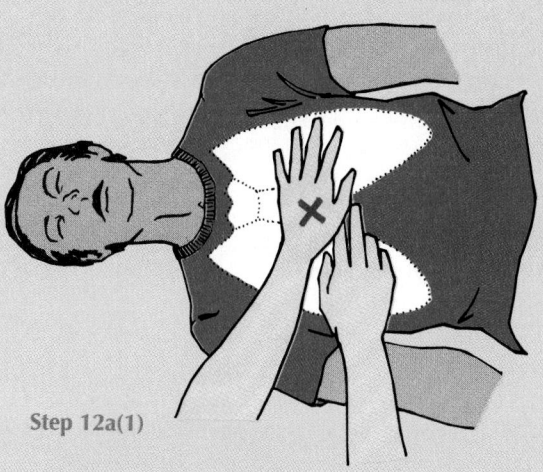

Step 12a(1)

STEPS	RATIONALE

CRITICAL DECISION POINT

It is critical to keep the hands off of the xiphoid process by marking that area with two fingers of one hand and then placing the heel of the other hand next to them. The hand marking the xiphoid process can then be moved and placed on top of the other hand.

Child

(2) Place heel of one hand 1 to 2 cm above xiphoid process (see illustration). Maintain head tilt with other hand, if possible, to maintain patent airway.

Infant

(3) Place index and middle fingers of one hand on sternum above xiphoid process. Fingers should be 1 cm below nipple line and perpendicular to sternum and not slanted (see illustration).

b. Compress sternum to proper depth from shoulders and then release pressure, maintaining contact with skin to ensure ongoing proper placement of hands. Do not rock, but transmit weight vertically down.
 (1) Adult and adolescent: 4 to 5 cm (1½ to 2 inches) (see illustration).
 (2) Older child: 3 to 4 cm (1 to 1½ inches).
 (3) Toddler and preschooler: 2 to 4 cm (¾ to 1½ inches).
 (4) Infant: 1 to 2 cm (½ to 1 inch).

c. Maintain proper rate of compression:
 (1) Adult and adolescent: 80 to 100 per minute (count "one 1000; two 1000").
 (2) Older child: 100 per minute.
 (3) Child: 100 per minute.
 (4) Infant: at least 100 per minute.

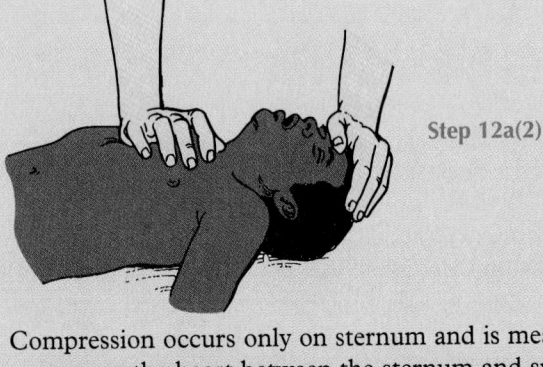

Step 12a(2)

Compression occurs only on sternum and is meant to squeeze the heart between the sternum and spine. Pressure necessary for external compression is created by nurse's upper arm muscle strength and upper body. When the compression is released, the heart fills.

Proper number of compressions per minute should be delivered to ensure adequate cardiac output.

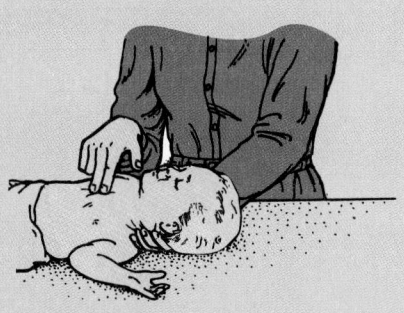

Step 12a(3)

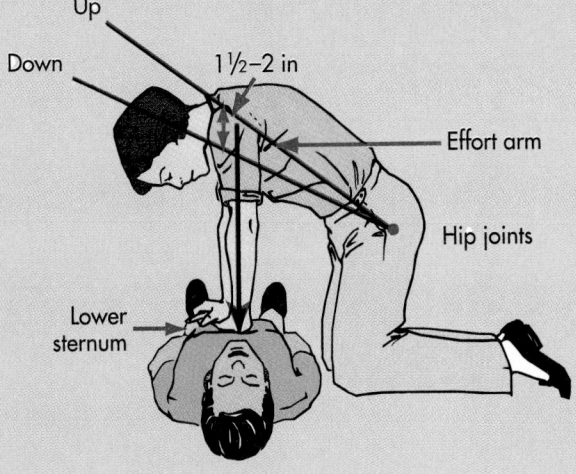

Step 12b(1)

STEPS	RATIONALE

CRITICAL DECISION POINT

Ratio of compressions to breaths for two rescuers is 5 to 1; for one rescuer, the ratio is 15 to 2.

STEPS	RATIONALE

d. Continue mouth-to-mouth or Ambu-bag ventilations.
  (1) Adult and adolescent: every 5 seconds (12 per minute).
  (2) Older child: every 4 seconds (15 per minute).
  (3) Child: every 3 seconds (20 per minute).
  (4) Infant and toddler: every 3 seconds (20 per minute).
	Promotes adequate ventilations to excrete waste gas and supply oxygen.

13. Palpate for carotid or brachial pulse with each external chest compression for first full minute (two-person rescue). If carotid pulse is not palpable, compressions are not strong enough or hand position is incorrect.	Assessment of pulse validates that adequate stroke volume is achieved with each compression.
14. Continue CPR until relieved, until victim regains spontaneous pulse and respirations, until the rescuer is exhausted and unable to perform CPR effectively, or until physician discontinues CPR.	Artificial cardiopulmonary function is maintained.
15. Remove and discard into appropriate receptacle: gloves, face shield, and pocket mask.	Reduces transmission of microorganisms.
16. Assess carotid pulse at 5-minute intervals following first minute of CPR.	Documents adequacy of external cardiac compressions.
17. CPR is not interrupted for more than 5 seconds.	Maintain adequacy of oxygenation and circulation.

Recording and Reporting

- Immediately report arrest indicating exact location of victim.
  In hospital setting, follow hospital policy.
  In community setting, dial 911 or other emergency number.
- Record in nurse's notes and appropriate code sheet onset of arrest, medication and other treatments given, procedures performed, and victim's response.

Home Care Considerations

- Assess the home environment to determine the presence of a suitable backboard and the client's room to determine if there is sufficient room to pull the client to the floor, if necessary, to perform CPR.
- A mouthpiece for CPR should be kept handy during all home health visits, and family should be advised to obtain mouthpieces when appropriate.
- If a client is at high risk for cardiopulmonary arrest, the family or care givers should be instructed and certified in CPR.
- The client and family should keep emergency numbers taped to the phone. These numbers may include fire department, ambulance, hospital, and physician. Instruct client and family on whom to call.

breathing (Celli, 1994). Deep breathing and coughing exercises are routine for postoperative clients (see Chapter 40).

Pursed-lip breathing involves deep inspiration and prolonged expiration through pursed lips to prevent alveolar collapse. While sitting up, the client is instructed to take a deep breath and to exhale slowly through pursed lips. Clients need to gain control of the exhalation phase so that exhalation is longer than inhalation (Dettenmeier, 1992). The client is usually able to perfect this technique by counting inhalation time and gradually increasing the count during exhalation.

Diaphragmatic breathing is more difficult and requires the client to relax intercostal and accessory respiratory muscles while taking deep inspirations. The client concentrates on expanding the diaphragm during controlled inspiration. The client is taught to place one hand flat below the breast bone above the waist and the other hand 2 to 3 cm below the first hand. The client is asked to inhale while the lower hand moves outward during inspiration. The client observes for inward movement as the diaphragm ascends. These exercises are initially taught with the client in the supine position and then practiced while the client sits and stands. The exercise is often used with the pursed-lip breathing technique.

◼ Evaluation

Client care. Nursing interventions and therapies are evaluated by comparing the client's progress to the goals and desired outcomes of the nursing care plan. When nursing measures directed to improve oxygenation are unsuccessful, the nurse must immediately modify the nursing care plan. New interventions are then developed. The nurse should not hesitate to notify the physician about a client's deteriorating oxygenation status. Prompt notification can avoid an emergency situation or even the need for CPR.

For the client with alterations in oxygenation the successful management of a client with chronic obstructive pulmonary disease depends on achieving three major goals: reduction of airflow obstruction, prevention or management of complications, and improvement in the client's quality of life.

The nurse must realize that the client with chronic cardiopulmonary disease presents one of nursing's greatest challenges. To begin with, these clients need a lot of nursing care when they are acutely ill. But because of the chronic nature of the disease, nurses cannot think in terms of recovery. Nurses have to recognize that they are dealing with a debilitating disease that gets progressively worse. Nurses who care for these clients will not see the dramatic cure but will be part of clients' improving the quality of their life in small but significant ways.

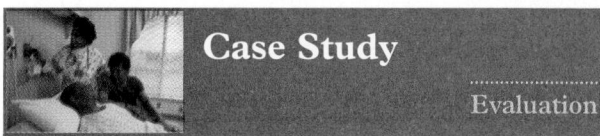

Case Study
Evaluation

Mary cares for Mr. King throughout his hospital stay. He is able to go home with improved activities of daily living. He does not require supplemental oxygen use at home. Because he participated in breathing exercises, he practices purse-lipped breathing, his breathing is more controlled, and his subsequent anxiety is relieved.

Mr. King is afebrile, white blood cells are within normal limits, and sputum cultures are negative at discharge. He is able to describe ways to prevent respiratory infections, since they aggravate airways and may precipitate an episode of acute respiratory failure.

While Mary observes Mr. King prepare for discharge, it is quite evident that Mr. King is using the various breathing techniques that they have worked on together. His wife even appears less anxious and states she feels as though for the first time they have taken a step (even though small) to improve the quality of their lives.

Documentation Note
Mr. King discharged to home. Able to state the purpose of breathing exercise and each medication, able to list causes and symptoms of respiratory tract infection. Has an appointment in 1 week with a community-based rehabilitation program. Scheduled to see his physician in 2 weeks. Prescriptions explained and given to client. Accompanied to the exit. Left with wife and son.

Client expectations. The goals that are set for clients must be individualized and realistic. Clients need to know how to cope with this chronic disease. Before any teaching program can be effective, clients must want to learn. The nurse needs to ask these clients if they would like to know more about chronic obstructive pulmonary disease and how to control it. Inform these clients that it is possible to gain greater independence, improve mobility, decrease dyspnea, and decrease the frequency of acute respiratory infections. Does the client need to view the knowledge offered by the nurse as being helpful and useful? Presenting an individualized education program, based on assessment data, helps to ensure that clients will comprehend, learn, use, and ultimately benefit from the education.

Key Terms

accessory muscles	chest tube	hypovolemia	pneumothorax
afterload	compliance	hypoxia	postural drainage
airway compliance	cough	humidification	preload
atelectasis	cyanosis	incentive spirometer	productive cough
atrioventricular (AV)	diaphragmatic	resistive breathing	pulmonary function
node	breathing	device (ISRBD)	tests
bundle of His	diffusion	incentive spirometry	Purkinje network
cardiac index	dyspnea	left-sided heart failure	pursed-lip breathing
cardiac output	dysrhythmias	myocardial	right-sided heart failure
cardiopulmonary	electrocardiogram	contractility	sinoatrial (SA) node
rehabilitation	(ECG)	myocardial infarction	stroke volume
cardiopulmonary	hematemesis	myocardial ischemia	surfactant
resuscitation (CPR)	hemoptysis	nebulization	valvular heart disease
chest percussion	hemothorax	normal sinus rhythm	ventilation
chest physiotherapy	hyperventilation	(NSR)	vibration
(CPT)	hypoventilation	orthopnea	wheezing

Key Concepts

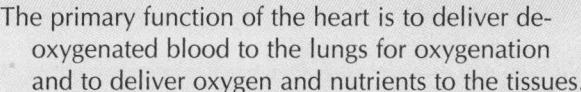

The primary function of the heart is to deliver deoxygenated blood to the lungs for oxygenation and to deliver oxygen and nutrients to the tissues.

Cardiac output is altered by preload, afterload, contractility, and heart rate.

Cardiac dysrhythmias are classified by cardiac activity and site of impulse origin.

The primary function of the lungs is to transfer oxygen from the atmosphere into the alveoli and carbon dioxide out of the body as a waste product.

Ventilation is the process of providing adequate oxygenation from the alveoli to the blood.

Compliance, or the ability of the lungs to expand and contract, depends on the function of musculoskeletal and neurological systems and on the other physiological factors.

The process of inspiration (active process) and expiration (passive process) is achieved with lung changes in pressures and volumes.

Respiration is controlled by the central nervous system and by chemicals within the blood.

Decreased hemoglobin levels alter the client's ability to transport oxygen.

Impaired chest wall movement reduces the level of tissue oxygenation.

Hyperventilation is a respiratory rate greater than that required to maintain normal levels of carbon dioxide.

Hypoventilation causes carbon dioxide retention.

Hypoxia occurs if the amount of oxygen delivered to tissues is too low.

The nursing assessment includes information about the client's cough, dyspnea, fatigue, wheezing, chest pain, environmental exposures, respiratory infection, cardiopulmonary risk factors, use of medications, and physical functioning.

Pursed-lip breathing is an effective intervention to control breathing and increase oxygenation.

Breathing exercises improve ventilation, oxygenation, and sensations of dyspnea.

Relaxation techniques and imagery are valuable interventions in controlling dyspnea and anxiety in clients with chronic obstructive pulmonary disease.

Nebulization delivers small drops of water or particles of medication to the airways.

Chest physiotherapy includes postural drainage, percussion, and vibration to mobilize pulmonary secretions.

Coughing and suctioning techniques are used to maintain a patent airway.

Oxygen therapy is used to improve levels of tissue oxygenation and is delivered by nasal cannula, nasal catheter, or oxygen mask.

Cardiac arrest requires the use of CPR.

Critical Thinking Activities

1. Referring to the advantages and disadvantages of various oxygen delivery devices outlined in Table 30-9, make a recommendation for each of the following clients requiring supplemental oxygen:
   a. A 42-year-old client requiring short-term, low-flow oxygen therapy after abdominal surgery.
   b. A 20-year-old client with a fractured nose and multiple chest contusions. The physician has prescribed F_IO_2 of 50% to 60%.
2. How can you determine whether Yankauer or endotracheal suctioning would be most beneficial for a client without an artificial airway?
3. After entering a client's tracheostomy with a suction catheter, the client begins to cough and his face turns red. What would you do?
4. While caring for a client with a chest tube to water-seal drainage and 20 cm of wall suction, you note excessive bubbling in the water-seal bottle. The client has had the chest tube for 24 hours, after undergoing lung surgery.
   a. What should you do, and why?
   b. During ambulation you note that the drainage is serous and the volume for the last 8 hours is approximately 500 ml. What should your response be?

References

Ahrens TS: SvO$_2$ monitoring: is it being used appropriately? *Crit Care Nurse* 10(7):70, 1990.

Ahrens TS, Rutherford K: *Essentials of Oxygenation*, Boston, 1993, Jones & Bartlett.

American Heart Association: *Basic life support for health care providers*, Dallas, 1994, The Association.

Bell DA: Do incentive spirometers reduce the rate of postoperative pulmonary complications? *Perspect Respir Nurs* 4(3):1, 1993.

Benner P: *From novice to expert*, Philadelphia, 1984, Addison-Wesley.

Burns SM and others: Effect of body position on spontaneous respiratory rate and tidal volume in patients with obesity, abdominal distention and ascites, *Am J Crit Care* 3(2):102, 1994.

Canobbio MM: *Cardiovascular disorders*, St. Louis, 1990, Mosby.

Celli BR: Physical reconditioning of patients with respiratory diseases: legs, arms, and breathing retraining, *Respir Care* 39(5):481, 1994.

Centers for Disease Control and Prevention: Update on adult immunization, *MMWR* 40(RR-12), 1991.

Centers for Disease Control and Prevention: Prevention and control of influenza: part I, vaccines, *MMWR* 42(RR-6):1, 1993.

Daily EK, Schroeder JS: *Techniques in bedside hemodynamic monitoring*, ed 6, St. Louis, 1994, Mosby.

Dettenmeier PA: *Pulmonary nursing care*, St. Louis, 1992, Mosby.

Gift A and others: Sensations during chest tube removal, *Heart Lung* 20(2):131, 1991.

Huebner A: Where there's smoke . . . tobacco smoke in the air is a hazard to children. *Am Baby Expectant New Parents* 56(7):28, 1994.

Luce JM and others: Intensive respiratory care, ed 2, Philadelphia, 1993, WB Saunders.

Lueckenotte AG: *Textbook of gerontologic nursing*, St. Louis, 1996, Mosby.

McCance KL, Huether SE: *Pathophysiology: the biologic basis for disease in adults and children*, ed 2, St. Louis, 1994, Mosby.

Pierson DJ: Effects of aging on the respiratory system. In Pierson DJ, Kacmarek RM, editors: *Foundations of respiratory care*, New York, 1992, Churchill Livingstone.

Thompson J and others: *Mosby's manual of clinical nursing*, ed 3, St. Louis, 1993, Mosby.

Urban NA and others: *Guidelines for critical care nursing*, St. Louis, 1995, Mosby.

Weilitz PB: *Pocket guide to respiratory care*, St. Louis, 1991, Mosby.

Weilitz PB: Pulmonary embolism and chest trauma. In Ahrens, Prentice D: *Critical care certification preparation and review*, ed 3, Norwalk, Conn, 1993, Appleton & Lange.

Whatling J: Childhood asthma and passive smoking, *Nurs Standard* 8(46):25, 1994.

Wilson SF, Thompson JM: *Mosby's clinical nursing series: respiratory disorders*, St. Louis, 1990, Mosby.

Yeaw EMJ: How position affects oxygenation: good lung down? *Am J Nurs* 92(3):27, 1992.

CHAPTER

31

Fluid, Electrolyte, and Acid-Base Balances

OBJECTIVES

Mastery of content in this chapter will
enable the student to:

- Define the key terms listed.
- Describe the mechanisms by which fluids and
  electrolytes are moved and regulated.
- Describe the processes involved in acid-base
  balance.
- Discuss common disturbances in fluid,
  electrolyte, and acid-base balances.
- Discuss variables that affect fluid, electrolyte,
  and acid-base balances.
- Discuss clinical assessments for fluid,
  electrolyte, and acid-base imbalances.
- List and discuss nursing interventions for
  clients with fluid, electrolyte, and acid-base
  imbalances.
- Measure and record fluid intake and output.
- Describe procedures for initiating and
  maintaining intravenous therapy.
- Discuss complications of intravenous therapy.
- Describe the procedure for initiating a blood
  transfusion and the complications of blood
  therapy.

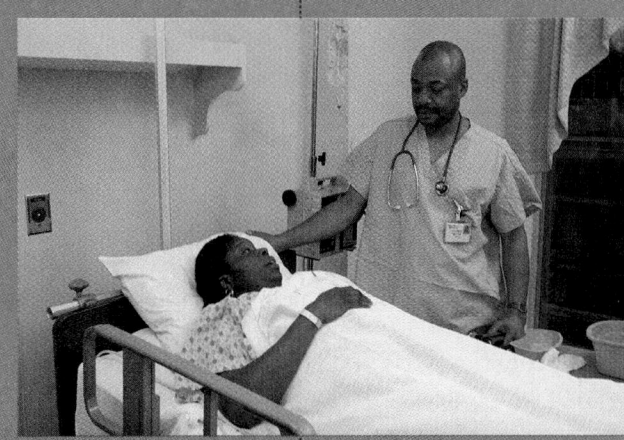

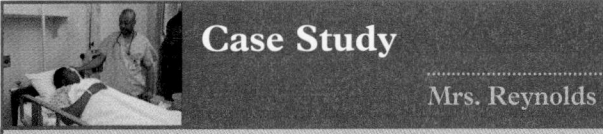

Case Study

Mrs. Reynolds

Susan Reynolds, a 42-year-old black married accountant, has just been admitted to the medical-surgical unit with a history of nausea, loss of appetite for 3 days, and vomiting and diarrhea for 2 days. She feels her symptoms are related to "bad food" she must have had on her recent business trip. Past surgical history includes a cesarean section 9 years ago without complications. Past medical history includes hypertension controlled by Lasix 40 mg once a day and a no-salt-added diet. After obtaining a blood sample for electrolytes, complete blood count, and electocardiogram (ECG), the doctor has admitted the client for observation and has ordered that she remain NPO and have an intravenous (IV) infusion of 0.45% normal saline at 125 ml/hour and be placed on intake and output (I&O) recordings and vital signs every 4 hours, with daily weights done at 7 AM.

Robert is a junior nursing student assigned to Mrs. Reynolds. He is 35 years old, married with three young children, and a former paramedic. Although this is somewhat of a career change for him, after two semesters of medical-surgical nursing he has enjoyed each rotation and he is sure a career in nursing is for him.

Fluid, electrolyte, and acid-base balances within the body are necessary to maintain health and function in all body systems. These are maintained by the intake and output of water and electrolytes, their distribution in the body, and the regulation of renal and pulmonary functions. Imbalances may result from many factors, including illnesses, altered fluid intake, or prolonged episodes of vomiting or diarrhea. Acid-base balance is necessary for many physiological processes, and imbalances can alter respiration, metabolism, and the function of the central nervous system.

SCIENTIFIC KNOWLEDGE BASE

Water is the largest single component of the body; 60% of the average adult weight is fluid. A healthy, mobile, well-oriented adult is usually capable of maintaining normal fluid, electrolyte, and acid-base balances because of the body's adaptive physiological mechanisms.

Distribution of Body Fluids

Body fluids are distributed in two distinct compartments, one containing **intracellular fluids** and the other **extracellular fluids.** Intracellular fluid (ICF) comprises all fluid within body cells. This fluid contains dissolved solutes essential to fluid and electrolyte balance and metabolism. It makes up about 40% of body weight (McCance and Huether, 1994).

Extracellular fluid (ECF) is all fluid outside a cell, which is divided into two smaller compartments: interstitial and intravascular fluids. **Interstitial fluid** is the fluid between cells and outside the blood vessels, whereas **intravascular fluid** is blood plasma. Other extravascular fluids are the lymph, transcellular, and organ fluids (McCance and Huether, 1994). ECF makes up about 20% of the total body weight.

Composition of Body Fluids

As water moves through the compartments of the body, it contains substances that are sometimes called minerals or salts but are technically known as electrolytes (Christensen and Kockrow, 1995). An **electrolyte** is an element or compound that, when melted or dissolved in water or another solvent, separates into **ions** and is able to carry an electric current. Positively charged electrolytes are **cations.** Negatively charged electrolytes are **anions.** Although the accumulation of electrolytes differs in ECF and ICF, the total number of anions and cations in each fluid compartment should be the same

Electrolytes are commonly measured in **milliequivalents per liter (mEq/L).** This value represents the number of grams of the specific electrolyte **(solute)** dissolved in a liter of plasma **(solution).** The solution in which a solute is dissolved is called the **solvent** (Weldy, 1996).

Movement of Body Fluids

Fluids and electrolytes constantly shift from compartment to compartment to meet a variety of metabolic needs. The movement of fluids depends on cell membrane permeability.

Diffusion is a process in which a solute (gas or substance) in a solution moves from an area of higher concentration to an area of lower concentration, evenly distributing the solute in the solution. For example, when you pour a small amount of cream into a cup of black coffee, the cream mixes or diffuses through the whole cup of coffee (Weldy, 1996). The difference in the two concentrations is known as a **concentration gradient.** Fluids and electrolytes diffuse across cellular membranes. For a substance to cross the membrane, the membrane must be permeable to it.

Osmosis is the movement of water across a semipermeable membrane from an area of lower concentration to one that has a higher concentration. Osmosis equalizes the concentration of molecules (ions) on each side of the membrane. Boiling a hot dog is an example of osmosis. The concentration of molecules inside the hot dog is greater than in water. The water passes through the hot dog skin, which is a semipermeable membrane, in an attempt to equalize the number of molecules on both sides of the membrane. Finally, when the hot dog can hold no more water, the skin, or semipermeable membrane, ruptures (Christensen and Kockrow, 1995).

When you have a more concentrated solution on one side of a selectively permeable membrane and a less concentrated solution on the other side, there is a pull called **osmotic pressure** that draws the water through the membrane to the more concentrated side. When the solutions on both sides of the semipermeable membrane have established equilibrium, or are equal in concentration, they are **isotonic.** The measure of a solution's ability to create osmotic pressure and thus affect the movement of water is termed **osmolality. Osmolarity,** another term used to describe the concentration of solutions, reflects the number of molecules in a liter of solution and is measured in milliosmoles per liter (mOsm/L). Osmolality is the measure used to evaluate serum and urine in clinical practice. Changes in extracellular osmolality may result in changes in both ECF and ICF volume.

Solutions are classified as hypertonic, isotonic, or hypotonic. **Hypertonic** (a solution of higher osmotic pressure) solutions pull fluid from cells; isotonic (a solution of same osmotic pressure) solutions expand the body's fluid volume without causing a fluid shift from one compartment to another; and **hypotonic** (a solution of lower osmotic pressure) solutions move into the cells, causing them to enlarge. Each of these actions occurs through osmosis.

Diffusion and osmosis are passive processes that do not require energy from the body's cells. **Active transport** is the movement of molecules or ions "uphill" against osmotic pressures to areas of higher concentration. An example of active transport found in the body is the sodium-potassium-ATPase pump, which moves sodium to the outside of the cell and then returns potassium to the inside of the cell.

Hydrostatic pressure is the force of the fluid pressing outward against a surface. When there is a difference in the hydrostatic pressure on two sides of a membrane, water and diffusible solutes move out of the solution that has the higher hydrostatic pressure. This process is called **filtration.** At the arterial end of the capillary, the hydrostatic pressure is greater than the **colloid osmotic pressure (oncotic pressure),** causing fluid and diffusible solutes to move out of the capillary into the interstitial space. At the venous end, the colloid osmotic pressure (oncotic pressure), or pull, is greater than the hydrostatic pressure, and fluids and some solutes move into the capillary from the interstitial space. The excess fluid and solutes remaining in the interstitial space are returned to the intravascular compartment by the lymph channels (Weldy, 1996). The

pressure at the capillary bed is called *colloid osmotic pressure,* because blood plasma proteins are not allowed to pass freely since the capillary membrane is impermeable to proteins (colloids). This activity enhances the osmotic pressure by forcing the blood proteins to stay within the capillary.

Regulation of Body Fluids

Body fluids are regulated by fluid intake, hormonal controls, and fluid output. This physiological balance is termed **homeostasis** (Horne and others, 1997). In health, the body is able to respond to disturbances in fluids and electrolytes to prevent or repair damage.

Fluid intake. Fluid intake is regulated primarily through the thirst mechanism. Thirst is the conscious desire for water and is one of the major factors that determines fluid intake (Weldy, 1996). The **osmoreceptors** continually monitor the serum osmotic pressure, and when osmolality increases, the hypothalamus is stimulated. Increased plasma osmolality can occur with any condition that interferes with the oral ingestion of fluids, or it can occur with the intake of hypertonic fluids. The hypothalamus will also be stimulated when excess fluid is lost, and **hypovolemia** occurs as in excessive vomiting and hemorrhage. In addition, the stimulation of the renin-angiotensin-aldosterone mechanism, potassium depletion, psychological factors, and oropharyngeal dryness initiate the sensation of thirst (Figure 31-1).

The average adult's fluid intake is about 2200 to 2700 ml per day; oral intake accounts for 1100 to 1400 ml, solid foods about 800 to 1000 ml, and oxidative metabolism 300 ml daily (Horne and others, 1997). Water oxidation (oxidative metabolism) is the by-product of cellular metabolism of ingested solid foods. Fluid intake requires an alert state. Infants, clients with neurological or psychological problems,

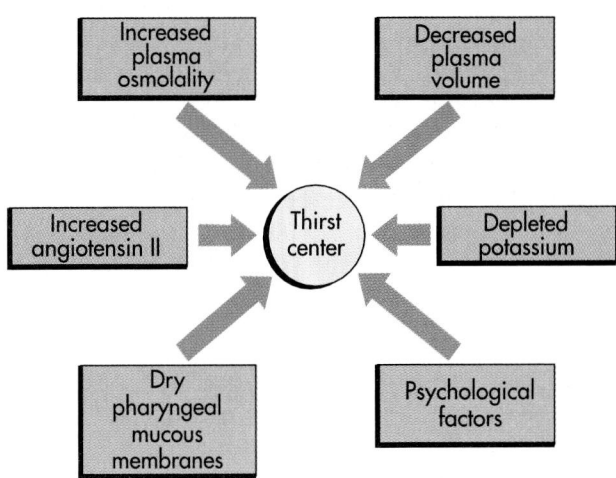

Figure 31-1. Stimuli affecting the thirst mechanism.

and some older adults are unable to perceive or respond to the thirst mechanism; they are at risk for **dehydration.**

Hormonal regulation. **Antidiuretic hormone (ADH)** stored in the posterior pituitary gland is released in response to changes in the blood osmolarity. The osmoreceptors in the hypothalamus are stimulated when there is an increase in the osmolarity to release the hormone ADH. The ADH works directly on the renal tubules and collecting ducts to make them more permeable to water. This in turn causes water to return to the systemic circulation, diluting the blood and decreasing its osmolarity. The client will experience a decrease in urinary output as the body tries to compensate. When the blood has been sufficiently diluted, the osmoreceptors stop the release of ADH.

Aldosterone is released by the adrenal cortex in response to increased plasma potassium levels or as a part of the renin-angiotensin-aldosterone mechanism to counteract hypovolemia. It acts on the distal portion of the renal tubule to increase the reabsorption (saving) of sodium and the secretion and excretion of potassium and hydrogen. Because sodium retention leads to water retention, the release of aldosterone acts as a volume regulator (Horne and others, 1997).

Renin, a proteolytic enzyme, responds to decreased renal perfusion secondary to a decrease in extracellular volume. Renin acts to produce **angiotensin** I, which causes some vasoconstriction. However, angiotensin I almost immediately becomes reduced by an enzyme that converts angiotension I into angiotensin II. Angiotensin II then causes massive selective vasoconstriction of many blood vessels and relocates and increases the blood flow to the kidney, improving renal perfusion. In addition, angiotensin II also stimulates the release of aldosterone.

Fluid output regulation. Fluid output occurs through four organs of water loss: kidneys, skin, lungs, and gastrointestinal (GI) tract. The kidneys are the major regulatory organs of fluid balance. They receive approximately 180 L of plasma to filter each day and produce 1200 to 1500 ml of urine.

Water loss from the skin is regulated by the sympathetic nervous system, which activates sweat glands. Water loss from the skin can be a sensible or insensible loss. An average of 500 to 600 ml of sensible and insensible fluid is lost via the skin each day (Horne and others, 1997). **Insensible water loss** is continuous and is not perceived by the person but can increase significantly with fever or burns (Horne and others, 1997). **Sensible water loss** occurs through excess perspiration and can be perceived by the client or by the nurse through inspection. The amount of sensible perspiration is directly related to the stimulation of the sweat glands.

The lungs expire about 400 ml of water daily. This insensible water loss may increase in response to changes in respiratory rate and depth. In addition, devices for giving oxygen can increase insensible water loss from the lungs.

Under normal conditions, the GI tract accounts for only 100 to 200 ml of fluid loss each day, yet it plays a vital role in fluid regulation because it is the site of nearly all fluid gain. In disease, however, the GI tract may become a site of major fluid loss because approximately 3 to 6 L of isotonic fluid is secreted into and reabsorbed out of the GI tract daily.

Regulation of Electrolytes

Cations. Major cations within the body fluids include sodium (Na^+), potassium (K^+), calcium (Ca^{++}), and magnesium (Mg^{++}). Cations interchange when one cation leaves the cell and is replaced by another. This occurs because cells tend to maintain electrical neutrality.

Sodium regulation. Sodium is the most abundant cation (90%) in ECF. Sodium ions are the major contributors to maintaining water balance through their effect on serum osmolality, nerve impulse transmission, regulation of acid-base balance, and participation in cellular chemical reactions (McCance and Huether, 1994). Sodium is regulated by dietary intake and aldosterone secretion. The normal extracellular sodium concentration is 135 to 145 mEq/L.

Potassium regulation. Potassium is the predominant intracellular cation. It regulates many metabolic activities and is necessary for glycogen deposits in the liver and skeletal muscle, transmission and conduction of nerve impulses, normal cardiac rhythms, and skeletal and smooth muscle contraction (McCance and Huether, 1994). A relatively small amount (approximately 2%) of potassium is located within the ECF (Horne and others, 1997). The normal range for serum potassium concentrations is 3.5 to 5 mEq/L. Potassium is regulated by dietary intake and renal excretion. The body does not conserve potassium well, so any condition that increases urine output will result in a decreased serum potassium.

Calcium regulation. Calcium is stored in bone, plasma, and body cells. Ninety-nine percent of calcium is located in bone, and only 1% is located in ECF. Approximately 50% of calcium in the plasma is bound to protein, primarily albumin, and 40% is free ionized calcium. The remaining small percentage is combined with nonprotein anions such as phosphate, citrate, and carbonate (Horne and others, 1997). Normal serum ionized calcium is 4 to 5 mEq/L. Normal total calcium is 8.5 to 10.5 mg/dl. Calcium is necessary for bone and teeth formation, blood clotting, hormone secretion, cell membrane integrity, cardiac conduction, transmission of nerve impulses, and muscle contraction.

Magnesium regulation. Magnesium is essential for enzyme activities, neurochemical activities, and cardiac and skeletal muscle excitability. Plasma concentrations of magnesium range from 1.5 to 2.5 mEq/L. Serum magnesium is regulated by dietary intake, renal mechanisms, and actions of PTH.

Anions. The three major anions of body fluids are chloride (Cl^-), bicarbonate (HCO_3^-), and phosphate (PO_4^{3-}), ions.

Chloride regulation. Chloride is the major anion in ECF. The transport of chloride follows sodium. Normal concentrations of chloride range from 95 to 108 mEq/L. Serum chloride is regulated by dietary intake and the kidneys. A person with normal renal function who has a high chloride intake will excrete a higher amount of urine chloride.

Bicarbonate regulation. Bicarbonate is the major chemical base buffer within the body. The bicarbonate ion is found in ECF and ICF. The bicarbonate ion is an essential component of the carbonic acid–bicarbonate buffering system essential to acid-base balance. The kidneys regulate bicarbonate. Normal arterial bicarbonate levels range between 22 and 26 mEq/L; venous bicarbonate is measured as carbon dioxide content, and the normal value is 24 to 30 mEq/L.

Phosphorus-phosphate regulation. Nearly all the phosphorus in the body exists in the form of phosphate (PO_4^{3-}), and the terms *phosphorus* and *phosphate* often are used interchangeably (Horne and others, 1997). Phosphate is a buffer anion found primarily in ICF, with a small amount found in ECF. It assists in acid-base regulation. Phosphate and calcium help to develop and maintain bones and teeth. Calcium and phosphate are inversely proportional; if one rises, the other falls. Phosphate also promotes normal neuromuscular action and participates in carbohydrate metabolism. Phosphate is normally absorbed through the GI tract. It is regulated by dietary intake, renal excretion, intestinal absorption, and PTH. The normal serum level is 2.5 to 4.5 mg/dl.

Regulation of Acid-Base Balance

For optimal functioning of the cells, metabolic processes maintain a steady balance between acids and bases. Arterial pH is an indirect measurement of hydrogen ion (H^+) concentration (i.e., the greater the concentration, the more acidic the solution and the lower the pH; the lower the concentration, the more alkaline the solution and the higher the pH). pH is also a reflection of the balance between carbon dioxide (CO_2), which is regulated by the lungs, and bicarbonate (HCO_3^-), a base regulated by the kidneys (Horne and others, 1997). Acid-base balance exists when the net rate at which the body produces acids or bases equals the rate at which acids or bases are excreted. This balance results in a stable concentration of hydrogen ions (H^+) in body fluids that is expressed as the pH value. Normal hydrogen ion level is necessary to maintain cell

membrane integrity and the speed of cellular enzymatic reactions. A pH is a scale for measuring the acidity or alkalinity of a fluid. A pH value of 7 is neutral; below 7 is acid, and above 7 is alkaline. Normal values in arterial blood range from 7.35 to 7.45.

The three general types of acid-base regulators within the body are chemical, biological, and physiological buffering systems. A **buffer** is a substance or a group of substances that can absorb or release H^+ to correct an acid-base imbalance.

Chemical regulation. The largest chemical buffer in ECF is the carbonic acid and bicarbonate buffer system (Figure 31-2). This system can be expressed as the following:

$$CO_2 + H_2O \rightleftarrows H_2CO_3 \rightleftarrows H^+ + HCO_3^-$$
$$\text{Carbon} + \text{Water} \rightleftarrows \text{Carbonic} \rightleftarrows \text{Hydrogen} + \text{Bicarbonate}$$
$$\text{dioxide} \qquad\qquad \text{acid} \qquad\qquad \text{ion}$$

The carbonic acid–bicarbonate buffer system is the first buffering system to react to change in the pH of ECF, and it reacts within seconds. The excretion of carbon dioxide that results from metabolism is controlled primarily by the lungs. The excretion of hydrogen and bicarbonate ions is controlled by the kidneys.

Biological regulation. Biological buffering occurs when hydrogen ions are absorbed or released by cells. Biological buffering occurs after chemical buffering and takes 2 to 4 hours. The hydrogen ion has a positive charge and must be exchanged with another positively charged ion, frequently potassium (K^+). In conditions with excess acid, a hydrogen ion enters the cell and a potassium ion leaves the cell and enters the ECF, thus causing an elevated serum potassium. The release of fatty acids that occurs with diabetic ketoacidosis and starvation is an example.

A second biological buffer is the hemoglobin-oxyhemoglobin system. Carbon dioxide diffuses into the red blood cell (RBC) and forms carbonic acid. The carbonic acid dissociates into hydrogen and bicarbonate ions. The hydrogen ions attach to hemoglobin, and the bicarbonate ion becomes available for

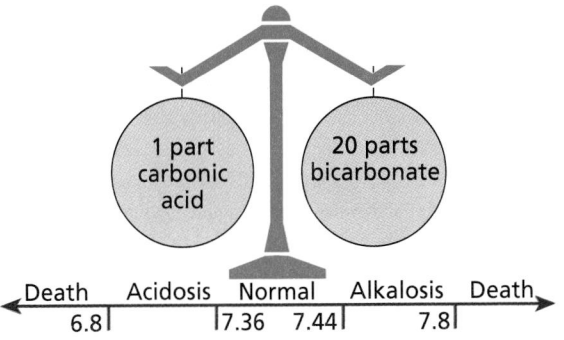

Figure 31-2. Carbonic acid-bicarbonate ratio and pH.

buffering by exchanging with extracellular chloride (Kokko and Tannen, 1990).

Another biological buffer is the chloride shift within RBCs. When blood is oxygenated in the lungs, bicarbonate diffuses into the cells and chloride travels from the hemoglobin to the plasma to maintain electrical neutrality. The reverse occurs when carbon dioxide moves into the red cell in tissue capillary beds. This process is referred to as the *chloride shift* and is a reciprocal exchange between these anions (Gröer and Shekleton, 1989).

Physiological regulation.

The two physiological buffers in the body are the lungs and the kidneys. The lungs adapt rapidly to an acid-base imbalance; they act to return the pH to normal before the action of the biological buffers. Ordinarily, increased levels of hydrogen ions and carbon dioxide provide the stimulus for respiration. When the concentration of hydrogen ions is altered, the lungs react to correct the imbalance by altering the rate and depth of respiration. For example, in alkalosis, the body compensates by reducing the respiratory rate, and thus carbon dioxide is retained. Carbon dioxide combines with water in the blood to form carbonic acid, which helps to correct the alkaline excess.

The kidneys take from a few hours to several days to regulate acid-base imbalance. They reabsorb bicarbonate in cases of acid excess and excrete it in cases of acid deficit. In addition, the kidneys use a phosphate ion (PO_4^{3-}) to excrete hydrogen ions by forming phosphoric acid (H_3PO_4); sulfuric acid (H_2SO_4) may also be excreted. Finally, the kidneys convert ammonia (NH_3^-) to ammonium (NH_4) by attaching a hydrogen ion to ammonia (Price and Wilson, 1992).

Disturbances in Electrolyte, Fluid, and Acid-Base Balances

Disturbances in electrolyte, fluid, or acid-base balances seldom occur alone and can disrupt normal body processes. When there is a loss of body fluids because of burns, illnesses, or trauma, the client is also at risk for electrolyte imbalances. In addition, some untreated electrolyte imbalances (e.g., potassium loss) result in acid-base disturbances.

Electrolyte imbalances

Sodium imbalances. Hyponatremia is a lower-than-normal concentration of sodium in the blood (serum), which can occur with a net sodium loss or net water excess (Table 31-1). It occurs frequently in seriously ill clients. Clinical indicators and treatment depend on the cause of hyponatremia and whether it is associated with a normal, decreased, or increased ECF volume (Horne and others, 1997). The usual situation is a loss of sodium without a loss of fluid, and this results in a decrease in the osmolality of ECF. The body

initially adapts by reducing water excretion and thus sodium excretion to maintain serum osmolality at near-normal levels. As the sodium loss continues, the body continues to preserve the blood and interstitial (tissue) volume. As a result, the sodium in ECF becomes diluted.

Hypernatremia is a greater-than-normal concentration of sodium in ECF that can be caused by excess water loss or an overall sodium excess (see Table 31-1). When the cause of hypernatremia is increased aldosterone secretion, sodium is retained and potassium is excreted. When hypernatremia occurs, the body attempts to conserve as much water as possible through renal reabsorption.

Potassium imbalances. Hypokalemia is one of the most common electrolyte imbalances in which an inadequate amount of potassium circulates in ECF (see Table 31-1). When severe, hypokalemia can affect cardiac conduction and function. Because the normal amount of serum potassium is so small, there is little tolerance for fluctuations. The most common cause is the use of potassium-wasting diuretics such as thiazide and loop diuretics.

Hyperkalemia is a greater-than-normal amount of potassium in the blood. Severe hyperkalemia produces marked cardiac conduction abnormalities (see Table 31-1). The primary cause of hyperkalemia is renal failure, because any decrease in renal function diminishes the amount of potassium the kidney can excrete.

Calcium imbalances. Hypocalcemia represents a drop in serum and/or ionized calcium. It can result from several illnesses, some of which directly affect the thyroid and parathyroid glands (see Table 31-1). Another cause is renal insufficiency (in which the kidneys' inability to excrete phosphorus causes the phosphorus level to rise and the calcium level to decline). Signs and symptoms can be related to the physiological role of serum calcium in neuromuscular function.

Hypercalcemia is an increase in the total serum concentration of calcium and/or ionized calcium. Hypercalcemia is frequently a symptom of an underlying disease resulting in excess bone resorption with release of calcium (see Table 31-1).

Magnesium imbalances. Disturbances in magnesium levels are summarized in Table 31-1. Symptoms are the result of changes in neuromuscular excitability.

Chloride imbalances. Hypochloremia occurs when the serum chloride level falls below normal. Vomiting or prolonged and excessive nasogastric or fistula drainage can result in hypochloremia because of the loss of hydrochloric acid. The use of loop and thiazide diuretics also results in increased chloride excretion as sodium is excreted. When serum chloride levels fall, metabolic alkalosis results as the body adapts by increasing reabsorption of the bicarbonate ion to maintain electrical neutrality.

TABLE 31-1
Electrolyte Imbalances

Causes	Signs and Symptoms
Hyponatremia Kidney disease resulting in salt-wasting Adrenal insufficiency GI losses Increased sweating Use of diuretics, especially when combined with low-sodium diet Psychogenic polydipsia Syndrome of inappropriate ADH (SIADH)	*Physical examination:* apprehension, personality change, postural hypotension, postural dizziness, abdominal cramping, nausea and vomiting, diarrhea, tachycardia, convulsions and coma, and fingerprints remaining on sternum after palpation *Laboratory findings:* serum sodium level < 135 mEq/L, serum osmolality < 280 mOsm/kg, and urine specific gravity < 1.010 (if not caused by SIADH)
Hypernatremia Ingestion of large amounts of concentrated salt solutions Iatrogenic administration of hypertonic saline solution parenterally Excess aldosterone secretion Diabetes insipidus Increased sensible and insensible water loss Water deprivation	*Physical examination:* thirst, dry and flushed skin, dry and sticky tongue and mucous membranes, fever, agitation, convulsions, restlessness, and irritability *Laboratory findings:* serum sodium levels > 145 mEq/L, serum osmolality > 295 mOsm/kg, and urine specific gravity > 1.030 (if not caused by diabetes insipidus)
Hypokalemia Use of potassium-wasting diuretics Diarrhea, vomiting, or other GI losses Alkalosis Excess aldosterone secretion Polyuria Extreme sweating Excessive use of potassium-free IV solutions Treatment of diabetic ketoacidosis with insulin	*Physical examination:* weakness and fatigue, decreased muscle tone, intestinal distention, decreased bowel sounds, ventricular dysrhythmias, paresthesias and weak, irregular pulse *Laboratory findings:* serum potassium level < 3.5 mEq/L and ECG abnormalities (e.g., ventricular dysrhythmias)*
Hyperkalemia Renal failure Fluid volume deficit Massive cellular damage such as from burns and trauma Iatrogenic administration of large amounts of potassium intravenously Adrenal insufficiency Acidosis, especially diabetic ketoacidosis Rapid infusion of stored blood Use of potassium-sparing diuretics	*Physical examination:* anxiety, dysrhythmias, paresthesia, weakness, abdominal cramps, and diarrhea *Laboratory findings:* serum potassium level > 5.3 mEq/L and ECG abnormalities (bradycardia, heart block, dysrhythmias); eventually QRS pattern widens and cardiac arrest occurs*
Hypocalcemia Rapid administration of blood transfusions containing citrate Hypoalbuminemia Hypoparathyroidism Vitamin D deficiency Pancreatitis Alkalosis	*Physical examination:* numbness and tingling of fingers and circumoral region, hyperactive reflexes, positive Trousseau's sign (carpopedal spasm with hypoxia), positive Chvostek's sign (contraction of facial muscles when facial nerve is tapped), tetany, muscle cramps, and pathological fractures (chronic hypocalcemia) *Laboratory findings:* serum calcium level < 4.0 mEq/L or 8.5 mg/100 ml and ECG abnormalities

*Data from Horne MM and others: *Mosby's pocket guide series: fluid, electrolyte, and acid-base balance,* ed 3, St. Louis, 1997, Mosby.

Continued

TABLE 31-1
Electrolyte Imbalances—cont'd

Causes	Signs and Symptoms
Hypercalcemia Hyperparathyroidism Malignant neoplastic disease Paget's disease Osteoporosis Prolonged immobilization Acidosis	*Physical examination:* anorexia, nausea and vomiting, weakness, lethargy, low back pain (from kidney stones), decreased level of consciousness, personality changes, and cardiac arrest *Laboratory findings:* serum calcium level > 5 mEq/L or 10.5 mg/100 ml; x-ray examination showing generalized osteoporosis, widespread bone cavitation, radiopaque urinary stones; and elevated blood urea nitrogen (BUN) level > 25 mg/100 ml and elevated creatinine level > 1.5 mg/100 ml caused by fluid volume deficit (FVD) or renal damage caused by urolithiasis; ECG abnormalities
Hypomagnesemia Inadequate intake: malnutrition and alcoholism Inadequate absorption: diarrhea, vomiting, nasogastric drainage, fistulas; diseases of small intestine Excessive loss resulting from thiazide diuretics Aldosterone excess Polyuria	*Physical examination:* muscular tremors, hyperactive deep tendon reflexes, confusion and disorientation, dysrhythmias, and positive Chvostek's and Trousseau's sign *Laboratory findings:* serum magnesium level < 1.5 mEq/L
Hypermagnesemia Renal failure Excess oral or parenteral intake of magnesium	*Physical examination:* physical findings that are more frequent in acute elevations in magnesium levels: hypoactive deep tendon reflexes, decreased depth and rate of respirations, hypotension, and flushing *Laboratory findings:* serum magnesium level > 2.5 mEq/L

Hyperchloremia occurs when the serum chloride level rises above normal, which usually occurs when the serum bicarbonate value falls or sodium level rises. Hypochloremia and hyperchloremia rarely occur as single disease processes but are commonly associated with acid-base imbalance. There is no single set of symptoms associated with these two alterations.

Fluid disturbances. The basic types of fluid imbalances are isotonic and osmolar. Isotonic deficit and excess exist when water and electrolytes are gained or lost in equal proportions. In contrast, osmolar imbalances are losses or excesses of only water so that the concentration (osmolality) of the serum is affected. Table 31-2 lists the causes and symptoms of common disturbances.

Acid-Base Imbalances
Arterial blood gas (ABG) analysis is the best way of evaluating acid-base balance. When we measure ABGs, we look at six components. Deviation from a normal value will indicate that the client is experiencing an acid-base imbalance. These six components are pH, $PaCO_2$, PaO_2, oxygen saturation, base excess, and HCO_3^-.

pH. pH measures H^+ concentration in the body fluids. Even a slight change can be potentially life threatening. An increase in concentration of hydrogen ions (H^+) makes a solution more acidic; a decrease makes the solution more alkaline. Normal pH value is 7.35 to 7.45 (acidic is <7.35, and alkalotic is >7.45).

$PaCO_2$. $PaCO_2$ is the partial pressure of carbon dioxide in arterial blood and is a reflection of the depth of pulmonary ventilation. Normal range is 35 to 45 mm Hg. When the $PaCO_2$ is less than 35, it is an indicator that hyperventilation has occurred. As rate and depth of respiration increase, more carbon dioxide is exhaled and the carbon dioxide concentration decreases. When the $PaCO_2$ is more than 45, hypoventilation has occurred. As rate and depth of respiration decrease, less carbon dioxide is exhaled and more is retained, increasing the concentration of carbon dioxide.

TABLE 31-2
Fluid Disturbances

Causes	Signs and Symptoms
Isotonic Imbalances	
Fluid Volume Deficit (FVD)—Water and Electrolytes Lost in Equal or Isotonic Proportions	
Losses from the GI system, such as from diarrhea, vomiting, or drainage from fistulas or tubes Loss of plasma or whole blood, such as with burns or hemorrhage Excessive perspiration Fever Decreased oral intake of fluids Use of diuretics	*Physical examination:* postural hypotension, tachycardia, dry mucous membranes, poor skin turgor, thirst, confusion, rapid weight loss, slow vein filling, lethargy, oliguria, weak pulse *Laboratory findings:* urine specific gravity > 1.025, increased hematocrit level $> 50\%$, and increased BUN level > 25 mg/100 ml (hemoconcentration)
Fluid Volume Excess (FVE)—Water and Sodium Retained in Isotonic Proportions	
Congestive heart failure Renal failure Cirrhosis of the liver Increased serum aldosterone and steroid levels Excessive sodium intake or administration	*Physical examination:* rapid weight gain, edema (especially in dependent areas), hypertension, polyuria (if renal mechanisms are normal), neck vein distention, increased venous pressure, crackles in lungs *Laboratory findings:* decreased hematocrit level $< 38\%$ and decreased BUN level < 10 mg/100 ml (hemodilution)
Osmolar Imbalances	
Hyperosmolar Imbalance—Dehydration	
Diabetes insipidus Interruption of neurologically driven thirst drive Diabetic ketoacidosis Osmotic diuresis Administration of hypertonic parenteral fluids or tube feeding formulas	*Physical examination:* dry and sticky mucous membranes, flushed and dry skin, thirst, elevated body temperature, irritability, convulsions, coma *Laboratory findings:* increased serum sodium level > 145 mEq/L and increased serum osmolality > 295 mOsm/kg
Hypoosmolar Imbalance—Water Excess	
SIADH Excess water intake	*Physical examination:* decreased level of consciousness, convulsions, coma *Laboratory findings:* decreased serum sodium level < 135 mEq/L and decreased serum osmolality < 280 mOsm/kg

PaO₂. PaO_2 is the partial pressure of oxygen in arterial blood. It has no primary role in acid-base regulation if it is within normal limits. A PaO_2 less than 60 can lead to anaerobic metabolism, resulting in lactic acid production and metabolic acidosis. There is a normal decline in PaO_2 in older adults. Hypoxemia also may cause hyperventilation, resulting in respiratory alkalosis (Horne and others, 1997). Normal range is 80 to 95 mm Hg.

Oxygen saturation. Saturation is the point at which hemoglobin is saturated by oxygen (O_2). It can be affected by changes in temperature, pH, and $PaCO_2$. When the PaO_2 falls below 60 mm Hg, there is a large drop in saturation (Horne and others, 1997). Normal range is 95% to 99%.

Base excess. Base excess is the amount of blood buffer (hemoglobin and bicarbonate) that exists. A high value indicates alkalosis, and a low value indicates acidosis. Normal range is ± 2.

Bicarbonate. Serum bicarbonate (HCO_3^-) is the major renal component of acid-base balance and is excreted and reproduced by the kidneys to maintain a normal acid-base environment. Normal range is 22 to 26 mEq/L. Less than 24 mEq/L usually indicates metabolic acidosis, and more than 28 mEq/L indicates metabolic alkalosis.

Types of acid-base imbalances. The four primary types of acid-base imbalance are respiratory acidosis, respiratory alkalosis, metabolic acidosis, and

TABLE 31-3
Acid-Base Imbalances

Causes	Signs and Symptoms
Respiratory Acidosis ***Hypoventilation Resulting From Primary Respiratory Problems*** Atelectasis (obstruction of small airways often caused by retained mucus) Pneumonia Cystic fibrosis Respiratory failure Airway obstruction Chest wall injury ***Hypoventilation Resulting From Factors Outside of the Respiratory System*** Drug overdose with a respiratory depressant Paralysis of respiratory muscles caused by various neurological alterations Head injury Obesity	*Physical examination:* confusion, dizziness, lethargy, headache, ventricular dysrhythmias, warm and flushed skin, muscular twitching, convulsions, and coma *Laboratory findings:* arterial blood gas alterations: pH < 7.35, partial pressure of carbon dioxide in arterial blood ($PaCO_2$) > 45 mm Hg, arterial partial pressure of oxygen (PaO_2) < 80 mm Hg, and bicarbonate level normal (if uncompensated) or > 26 mEq/L (if compensated)
Respiratory Alkalosis ***Hyperventilation Resulting From Primary Respiratory Problems*** Asthma Pneumonia Inappropriate mechanical ventilator settings ***Hyperventilation Resulting From Factors Outside of the Respiratory System*** Anxiety Hypermetabolic states Disorders of the central nervous system (head injuries, infections) Salicylate overdose	*Physical examination:* dizziness, confusion, dysrhythmias, tachypnea, numbness and tingling of extremities, convulsions, and coma *Laboratory findings:* arterial blood gas alterations: pH > 7.45, $PaCO_2$ < 35 mm Hg, PaO_2 normal, and bicarbonate level normal (if short lived or uncompensated) or < 22 mEq/L (if compensated)
Metabolic Acidosis ***High Anion Gap*** Starvation Diabetic ketoacidosis Renal failure Lactic acidosis from heavy exercise Use of drugs (methanol, ethanol, formic acid, paraldehyde, aspirin) ***Normal Anion Gap*** Renal tubular acidosis Diarrhea	*Physical examination:* headache, lethargy, confusion, dysrhythmias, tachypnea with deep respirations, abdominal cramps, and flushed skin *Laboratory findings:* arterial blood gas alterations: pH < 7.35, $PaCO_2$ normal (if uncompensated) or < 35 mm Hg (if compensated), PaO_2 normal or increased (with rapid, deep respirations), bicarbonate level < 22 mEq/L, and oxygen saturation normal
Metabolic Alkalosis Excessive vomiting Prolonged gastric suctioning Hypokalemia or hypercalcemia Excess aldosterone Use of drugs (steroids, sodium bicarbonate, diuretics)	*Physical examination:* dizziness; dysrhythmias; numbness and tingling of fingers, toes, and circumoral region; muscle cramps; tetany *Laboratory findings:* arterial blood gas alterations: pH > 7.45, $PaCO_2$ normal (if uncompensated) or > 45 mm Hg (if compensated), PaO_2 normal, and bicarbonate level > 26 mEq/L

metabolic alkalosis (Table 31-3). **Respiratory acidosis** is marked by an increased arterial carbon dioxide concentration ($PaCO_2$), excess carbonic acid (H_2CO_3), and an increased hydrogen ion concentration (decreased pH). With respiratory acidosis, the cerebrospinal fluid and brain cells become acidic, causing neurological changes. Hypoxemia occurs because of respiratory depression, resulting in further neurological impairments. Electrolyte changes such as hyperkalemia and hypercalcemia may accompany the acidosis.

Respiratory alkalosis is marked by decreased $PaCO_2$ and increased pH. Like respiratory acidosis, respiratory alkalosis can begin outside the respiratory system (e.g., anxiety with hyperventilation) or within the respiratory system (e.g., initial phase of an asthma attack).

Metabolic acidosis results because of the high acid content of the blood, which also causes a loss of sodium bicarbonate, the alkaline half of the carbonate buffer system (Weldy, 1996). In an attempt to identify the cause of the metabolic acidosis, an analysis of serum electrolytes to detect an anion gap may be helpful. **Anion gap** reflects unmeasurable anions present in plasma and is calculated by subtracting the sum of chloride and bicarbonate from the amount of plasma sodium concentration (Table 31-4) (Horne and others, 1997).

Metabolic alkalosis is marked by the heavy loss of acid from the body or by increased levels of bicarbonate. The most common cause is vomiting.

NURSING KNOWLEDGE BASE

Fluid and electrolyte imbalances may affect anyone regardless of age, sex, color, or religion. Infants, severely ill adults, disoriented or immobile clients, and older adults are frequently at greater risk because of their inability to respond independently to the early warnings of an impending problem. Over time, the body's adaptive compensatory mechanisms can no longer maintain fluid and electrolyte or acid-base balance adequately, and the client's health becomes compromised. The severity and long-term effects on the client's health that have been compromised will influence a client's ability to return to a state of optimal functioning. Prolonged or severe compromises may lead to irreversible chronic health problems that may not only change the lifestyle of the client but may also have an impact on the care giver(s), guardians, parents, families, and/or friends.

CRITICAL THINKING IN CLIENT CARE

Synthesis

A client's condition can change very quickly with a fluid and electrolyte imbalance. Multiple factors can be involved; therefore the nurse needs to recognize that clinical decision making using the nursing process will need to include a synthesis of knowledge, experience, attitudes, and intellectual and professional standards to provide safe, quality care.

Knowledge. Providing care for the client with a fluid and electrolyte imbalance or acid-base imbalance requires the nurse to synthesize previously learned knowledge from chemistry, physiology, and pharmacology when considering the factors that might have contributed to the health problem. For example, a client who has experienced a few days of diarrhea and vomiting may have had a loss of appetite and nausea a couple of days earlier that restricted an adequate amount of fluid intake. The client might also have been taking a potassium-wasting diuretic, which has as a side effect serum potassium loss. The nurse's knowledge that potassium cannot be stored or well regulated by the body, GI secretions are very high in potassium, and potassium's role is vital in the functioning of the body's major organs leads the nurse to understand that untreated vomiting and diarrhea for some clients can be life threatening.

Experience. Professional experience assists the nurse when caring for clients with fluid and electrolyte or acid-base imbalances. Clients' clinical signs and symptoms help the nurse to more quickly make clinical decisions when the same signs and symptoms are again

TABLE 31-4 **Anion Gap**		
Anion Gap Type	**Values**	**Causes**
Normal anion gap	12 (±2) mEq/L	Diarrhea, renal tubular acidosis, or pancreatic fistula causing a direct loss of HCO_3^-; addition of chloride-containing acids
Increased anion gap	>14 mEq/L	Lactic acidosis, uremia, diabetic ketoacidosis (DKA), or salicylate and methanol toxicity, resulting in accumulation of nonvolatile acids with decrease in HCO_3^-

From Horne MM and others: *Mosby's pocket guide series: fluid, electrolyte, and acid-base balance*, ed 3, St. Louis, 1997, Mosby.

seen with new clients. Reflecting back on the way in which a client presented with a clinical problem makes the nurse more adept at problem solving in the future.

Attitudes. The two attitudes best used when caring for clients with fluid and electrolyte and acid-base imbalance are accountability and integrity. Accountability is important when performing vital signs, documenting I&O, or calculating IV flow rates accurately. Integrity is necessary when supporting clients' need for privacy during voiding or defecation or attempting to minimize a client's embarrassment because of the malodorous vomitus and diarrhea.

Standards. The use of IV therapy for a client experiencing an alteration in fluid and electrolyte or acid-base balance is standard practice. The nurse must be familiar with the standards of care involved in appropriately establishing, maintaining, and monitoring IV lines and fluid therapy. The Centers for Disease Control and Prevention (Pearson, 1996) have written guidelines for the prevention of intravascular device–related infection. Such guidelines, integrated into the nurse's practice, ensure safe and appropriate care for clients.

NURSING PROCESS

▣ Assessment

The nurse understands the importance of fluid, electrolyte, and acid-base balance to homeostasis. By gathering assessment data the nurse will identify clients at risk and clarify all appropriate nursing diagnoses.

Nursing history. The nursing assessment begins with a client history, which is designed to reveal any risk factors or preexisting conditions that may cause or contribute to a disturbance of fluid and electrolytes and acid-base balance. The nurse will explore with the client any factors that may cause a disturbance and integrate the information with knowledge of fluid volume regulation, electrolyte concentration, and acid-base regulation.

The nurse first considers the client's age. An infant's proportion of total body water is greater that that of children or adults, but they are not protected from fluid loss because they ingest and excrete a relatively greater daily water volume than adults (Horne and others, 1997). They are thus at greater risk for FVD and hyperosmolar imbalance, because body water loss is proportionately greater per kilogram of weight. Children ages 2 through 12 have less stable regulatory responses to imbalance. In the event of high fevers or diarrhea, children have a narrow range of tolerance for severe fluid or electrolyte alterations. Adolescents have increased metabolic processes and increased water production. Girls have greater fluid changes because of hormonal changes.

Older adults experience a number of age-related changes that can affect fluid and electrolyte and acid-base balance. The kidneys have a decrease in glomerular filtration rate and in the number of filtering nephrons (Lueckenotte, 1996). These changes can mean that in the presence of sodium depletion or overload the older adult may be unable to maintain homeostasis and the imbalance is instead worsened. In addition, older adults are at risk for decreased excretion of medications, which can lead to imbalances causing metabolic or respiratory acidosis, FVD and hyperosmolar imbalance, and hyponatremia and hypernatremia (Horne and others, 1997). The changes in lung function that accompany aging can lead to respiratory acidosis and the inability to compensate for metabolic acidosis.

Chronic disease (e.g., cancer, CHF, renal disease) becomes a focus of the nursing history, because a variety of conditions can create fluid and electrolyte and acid-base imbalances. In the presence of chronic disease the nurse must review the normal pathology of such conditions to understand how fluid and electrolyte and acid-base status may be affected. The nurse determines how long the client has suffered the disease and the type of treatment currently being administered. In addition to chronic health problems, the nurse determines if the client has a history of GI alterations (e.g., diarrhea, vomiting, colostomy), nasogastric suctioning, or intestinal drainage. Any condition that results in the loss of GI fluids predisposes the client to dehydration and a variety of electrolyte disturbances.

Recent surgery, head and chest trauma, and second- or third-degree burns are conditions that place clients at high risk for fluid and electrolyte alterations. The stress response of surgery causes fluid balance changes in the second to fifth postoperative day. Aldosterone, glucocorticoids, and ADH are increasingly secreted, causing sodium and chloride retention, potassium excretion, and decreased urinary output.

The nurse should also include certain environmental factors in the nursing history. Clients who have participated in vigorous exercise or who have become exposed to temperature extremes may have clinical signs of fluid and electrolyte alterations. Exposure to environmental temperatures exceeding 28° to 30° C (82.4° to 86° F) results in excessive sweating with weight loss. A body weight loss over 7% decreases the ability of the cooling mechanism to conserve water.

A client's current dietary history is an important component of nursing assessment. Recent changes in appetite or the ability to chew and swallow can affect nutritional status and fluid hydration. Dieting can lead to acidosis, because rapid water loss can lead to hyperosmolar fluid imbalance.

Lifestyle factors should also be inclined in the nurse's history. If a client already has preexisting medical risks, a history of smoking or alcohol consumption can further impair the client's ability to adapt to acid-base alterations. Alcohol and tobacco use can ultimately cause respiratory depression, which can result in respiratory acidosis.

A final category to include in the assessment is a history of medication use (Box 31-1). If the assessment reveals a medication that is likely to cause an electrolyte or acid-base disorder, the nurse will also closely examine laboratory values. In addition, the nurse will assess the client's knowledge of side effects and adherance to medication schedules.

Physical examination. A thorough examination is necessary, because fluid and electrolyte or acid-base disturbances can affect all body systems (see Chapter 24). While examining each system, the nurse carefully considers the signs and symptoms to expect as a result of any imbalance. For example, an examination of the oral cavity will likely reveal signs of dehydration if the nurse suspects the client is experiencing a fluid loss. Table 31-5 summarizes possible physical findings for clients with fluid and electrolyte and acid-base imbalance.

Measuring fluid intake and output. Measuring and recording all liquid I&O during a 24-hour period is an important part of the client's assessment database for fluid and electrolyte balance. It is important to note trends in the I&O (e.g., a gradually decreasing urine output can indicate that the body is trying to adapt to an FVD or hyperosmolar fluid imbalance). Accurate I&O measurements identify both

clients at risk for and clients who are experiencing fluid, electrolyte, and acid-base disturbances.

For clients in health care settings, the nurse neither needs to nor should wait for a physician's order to begin I&O measurements. Generally, I&O is routinely measured for clients after surgery, clients whose conditions are unstable, clients who have a temperature elevation, clients whose fluids are restricted, or clients who are receiving diuretic or IV therapy. The nurse also measures I&O for clients with chronic cardiopulmonary or renal illnesses and clients whose health status has deteriorated.

Oral intake includes all liquids taken by mouth, such as gelatin, ice cream, soup, juice, and water. Liquid intake also includes fluids given through nasogastric or jejunostomy feeding tubes (see Chapter 34), liquids given as IV fluids (including both continuous infusions and intermittent IV piggybacks), and blood or its components. Liquid output includes urine, diarrhea, vomitus, gastric suction, and drainage from postsurgical wounds or other tubes (see Chapter 38).

Ambulatory clients' urinary output is recorded after each trip to the bathroom. These clients are instructed to save their urine in a container so that the nurse can record the amount, or clients may be instructed to measure and record their own output. When a client has an indwelling Foley catheter, drainage tube, or suction, that output is recorded at the end of each nursing shift or more frequently (e.g., every hour) as the client's condition requires. The nurse should measure, not estimate, I&O.

In the hospital, forms for recording I&O are attached to the bedside chart or room door (Figure 31-3). The 24-hour total is calculated at midnight or 6 AM depending on agency policy.

Taking I&O measurements is a procedure requiring help from the client and family. The nurse explains the reasons that measurements are needed and instructs the client and family to not empty any container with voided fluid but to ask the nurse to do so. A client using a toilet should be instructed to use a calibrated insert, which attaches to the rim of the toilet bowl. After each urination the client notifies the nurse, who measures, records, and empties the urine and rinses the insert. Occasionally, clients may also be instructed to measure and record their own output. It is important for the client to have good vision and motor skills to ensure accuracy.

Occasionally clients receive a specific amount of a liquid medication every 1 to 2 hours. A client receiving tube feedings may receive numerous liquid medications, and water may be used to flush the tube with the medications. Over a 24-hour period, these liquids can amount to a significant intake and should always be recorded on the I&O record.

Recording I&O is essential for obtaining an accurate database. This information helps to maintain an

---

Box 31-1

Medications That Cause Fluid and Electrolyte and Acid-Base Disturbances

Diuretics—metabolic alkalosis and hyperkalemia

Steroids—metabolic alkalosis

Potassium supplements—GI disturbances, including intestinal and gastric ulcers and diarrhea

Respiratory center depressants such as narcotic analgesics—decreased rate and depth of respirations, resulting in respiratory acidosis

Antibiotics—nephrotoxicity (e.g., vancomycin, methicillin, aminoglycosides); hyperkalemia and/or hypernatremia (e.g., azlocillin, carbenicillin, piperacillin, ticarcillin, Unasyn)*

Calcium carbonate (Tums)—mild metabolic alkalosis with nausea and vomiting*

Magnesium hydroxide (Milk of Magnesia)—hypokalemia*

*Data from McKenry LM, Salerno E: *Mosby's pharmacology in nursing*, ed 19, St. Louis, 1995, Mosby.

TABLE 31-5
Physical and Behavioral Nursing Assessment for Fluid, Electrolyte, and Acid-Base Imbalances

Assessment	Imbalance
Weight Changes	
2%-5% loss	Mild FVD★
5%-10% loss	Moderate FVD★
10%-15% loss	Severe FVD★
15%-20% loss	Death★
2% gain	Mild FVE
5% gain	Moderate FVE
8% gain	Severe FVE
Head	
History:	
Headache	FVD,★ metabolic or respiratory acidosis, metabolic alkalosis
Dizziness	FVD,★ respiratory acidosis or alkalosis, hyponatremia
Observation:	
Irritability	Metabolic or respiratory alkalosis, hyperosmolar imbalance, hypernatremia, hypokalemia
Lethargy	FVD,★ metabolic acidosis or alkalosis, respiratory acidosis, hypercalcemia
Confusion, disorientation	FVD,★ hypomagnesemia, metabolic acidosis, hypokalemia
Eyes	
Inspection:	
Sunken, dry conjunctivae, decreased or absent tearing	FVD
Periorbital edema, papilledema	FVE
History:	
Blurred vision	FVE
Throat and Mouth	
Inspection:	
Sticky, dry mucous membranes, dry cracked lips, decreased salivation	FVD, hypernatremia
Longitudinal tongue furrows	
Cardiovascular System	
Inspection:	
Flat neck veins	FVD
Distended neck veins	FVE
Dependent body parts: legs, sacrum, back	
Slow venous filling	FVD★
Palpation:	
Edema (dependent body parts: back, sacrum, legs)	FVE★
Dysrhythmias (also noted as ECG changes)	Metabolic acidosis, respiratory alkalosis and acidosis, potassium imbalance, hypomagnesemia
Increased pulse rate	Metabolic alkalosis, respiratory acidosis, hyponatremia, FVD, FVE, hypomagnesemia
Decreased pulse rate	Metabolic alkalosis, hypokalemia
Weak pulse	
Decreased capillary filling	FVD, hypokalemia
Bounding pulse	FVD
	FVE

★Data from Horne M and others: *Mosby's pocket guide series: fluid, electrolyte, and acid-base balance,* ed 3, St. Louis, 1997, Mosby.

TABLE 31-5

Physical and Behavioral Nursing Assessment for Fluid, Electrolyte, and Acid-Base Imbalances—cont'd

Assessment	Imbalance
Cardiovascular System—cont'd	
Auscultation:	
Blood pressure low or without orthostatic changes	FVD, hyponatremia, hyperkalemia, hypermagnesemia
Third heart sound	FVE
Hypertension	FVE
Respiratory System	
Inspection:	
Increased rate	FVE, respiratory alkalosis, metabolic acidosis
Dyspnea	FVE
Auscultation:	
Crackles	FVE
Gastrointestinal System	
History:	
Anorexia	Metabolic acidosis
Abdominal cramps	Metabolic acidosis
Inspection:	
Sunken abdomen	FVD
Distended abdomen	Third-space syndrome
Vomiting	FVD, hypercalcemia, hyponatremia
Diarrhea	Hyponatremia
Auscultation:	
Hyperperistalsis with diarrhea, or hypoperistalsis	FVD, hypokalemia
Renal System	
Inspection:	
Oliguria or anuria	FVD, FVE
Diuresis (if kidneys are normal)	FVE
Increased urine specific gravity	FVD
Neuromuscular System	
Inspection:	
Numbness, tingling	Metabolic alkalosis, hypocalcemia, potassium imbalances
Muscle cramps, tetany	Hypocalcemia, metabolic or respiratory alkalosis
Coma	Hyperosmolar or hypoosmolar imbalances, hyponatremia
Tremors	Respiratory acidosis, hypomagnesemia
Palpation:	
Hypotonicity	Hypokalemia, hypercalcemia★
Hypertonicity	Hypocalcemia, hypomagnesemia, metabolic alkalosis
Percussion:	
Decreased or absent deep tendon reflexes	Hypercalcemia, hypermagnesemia
Increased or hyperactive deep tendon reflexes	Hypocalcemia, hypomagnesemia
Skin	
Body temperature:	
Increased	Hypernatremia, hyperosmolar imbalance, metabolic acidosis
Decreased	FVD
Inspection:	
Dry, flushed	FVD, hypernatremia, metabolic acidosis
Palpation:	
Inelastic skin turgor, cold, clammy skin	FVD

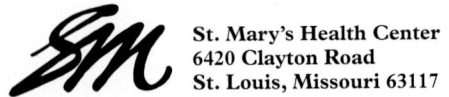

PATIENT LABEL

INTAKE AND OUTPUT SUMMARY

	DATE 6-10-XX	2200 – 0600	0600 – 1400	1400 – 2200	24 Hr.	
INTAKE	P.O. Intake	120	800	650	1570	**TOTAL INTAKE**
	Tube Feedings					
	Hyperalimentation					
	I.V. Primary					
	I.V.P.B.	50		50	100	**1670**
	Blood/Blood Products					
OUTPUT	Urine	325	700	500	1525	**TOTAL OUTPUT**
	Emesis					
	G.I. Suction					
	Drainage	50	75	30	155	**1855**
	Chest tube	75	50	50	175	

	DATE	2200 – 0600	0600 – 1400	1400 – 2200	24 Hr.	
INTAKE	P.O. Intake					**TOTAL INTAKE**
	Tube Feedings					
	Hyperalimentation					
	I.V. Primary					
	I.V.P.B.					
	Blood/Blood Products					
OUTPUT	Urine					**TOTAL OUTPUT**
	Emesis					
	G.I. Suction					
	Drainage					

	DATE	2200 – 0600	0600 – 1400	1400 – 2200	24 Hr.	
INTAKE	P.O. Intake					**TOTAL INTAKE**
	Tube Feedings					
	Hyperalimentation					
	I.V. Primary					
	I.V.P.B.					
	Blood/Blood Products					
OUTPUT	Urine					**TOTAL OUTPUT**
	Emesis					
	G.I. Suction					
	Drainage					

	DATE	2200 – 0600	0600 – 1400	1400 – 2200	24 Hr.	
INTAKE	P.O. Intake					**TOTAL INTAKE**
	Tube Feedings					
	Hyperalimentation					
	I.V. Primary					
	I.V.P.B.					
	Blood/Blood Products					
OUTPUT	Urine					**TOTAL OUTPUT**
	Emesis					
	G.I. Suction					
	Drainage					

Figure 31-3. Twenty-four-hour I&O record. (Courtesy St. Mary's Health Center, St. Louis.)

ongoing evaluation of the client's hydration status to prevent severe imbalances. I&O recording can be delegated to unlicensed personnel. The nurse is responsible to make sure staff members can correctly measure and calculate I&O and are aware of the need to be accurate and timely.

Laboratory studies. The nurse reviews laboratory tests to obtain further objective data about fluid, electrolyte, and acid-base balances (Box 31-2). These tests include serum and urinary electrolyte levels, hematocrit, blood creatinine level, BUN levels, urine specific gravity, and ABG readings. Serum electrolytes are measured to determine the hydration status, the electrolyte concentration of the blood plasma, and acid-base balance. The frequency with which these electrolytes are measured depends on the severity of the client's illness. Serum electrolyte tests are routinely performed on any client entering a hospital to screen for alterations and to serve as a baseline for future comparisons.

The complete blood count (CBC) is a determination of the number and type of red and white blood cells per cubic millimeter of blood. When the client does not have anemia, the hematocrit can be an indication of the hydration status of the client. The hematocrit will increase (become more concentrated) in situations where fluid is lost, whereas it will decrease in situations in which fluid is excessively retained in the vascular space.

Blood creatinine levels are useful in measuring kidney function. Creatinine is a normal by-product of muscle metabolism and is excreted by the kidneys at fairly constant levels, regardless of factors such as fluid intake, diet, or exercise. Therefore it provides a measure of renal function that is relatively independent of the hydration status of the client or the client's dietary intake.

BUN is the amount of nitrogenous substance present in the blood as urea. It is a rough indicator of kidney function.

Serum osmolality measures the concentration of the plasma. The osmolality will decrease when the client is experiencing hypoosmolar fluid imbalance (water excess) or hyponatremia. Decreased serum osmolality results in the movement of fluid into body cells (cellular edema) by osmosis. The osmolality will increase with a hyperosmolar fluid imbalance (water deficit) or hypernatremia or other gains of solutes such as glucose. This will result in the movement of fluid out of body cells into the interstitial space (cellular shrinkage). Both cellular edema and shrinkage will disrupt normal cell processes.

The urine specific gravity test measures the urine's degree of concentration and evaluates the kidneys' ability to conserve or excrete water. The specific gravity, measured at the bedside using a urinometer, normally ranges between 1.010 and 1.025.

Box 31-2
Laboratory Data for Fluid, Electrolyte, and Acid-Base Imbalances

Fluid and Electrolytes

Altered concentrations of sodium, potassium, magnesium, calcium, phosphates, chloride, and bicarbonate (venous CO_2 contentions)

Increase in hematocrit, BUN, sodium, and osmolality in serum (related to loss of ECF fluid or gain of solutes)

Decrease in hematocrit, BUN, sodium, and osmolality in serum (related to gain of ECF fluid or loss of solutes)

Concentrated urine demonstrated by urine specific gravity > 1.030

Dilute urine demonstrated by a specific gravity < 1.012

Metabolic Alkalosis

pH > 7.45

$PaCO_2$ normal or > 45 mm Hg if lungs are compensating

PaO_2 normal

O_2 saturation (SaO_2) normal

HCO_3^- > 26 mEq/L

K^+ < 3.5 mEq/L

Metabolic Acidosis

pH < 7.35

$PaCO_2$ normal or < 35 mm Hg if lungs are compensating

PaO_2 normal

SaO_2 normal

HCO_3^- < 22 mEq/L

K^+ > 5.3 mEq/L

K^+ < 3.5 mEq/L

Respiratory Alkalosis

pH > 7.45

$PaCO_2$ < 35 mm Hg

PaO_2 normal

SaO_2 normal

HCO_3^- normal

K^+ < 3.5 mEq/L

Respiratory Acidosis

pH < 7.35

$PaCO_2$ > 45 mm Hg

PaO_2 normal or < 80 mm Hg, depending on cause of acidosis

SaO_2 normal or < 95%, depending on cause of acidosis

HCO_3^- normal if early respiratory acidosis or > 26 mEq/L if kidneys are compensating

K^+ > 5.3 mEq/L

ABG analysis provides information on the status of acid-base balance and the effectiveness of ventilatory function in providing normal oxygen–carbon dioxide exchange. The nurse should understand that an ABG result gets evaluated in a systematic approach. First, the pH is examined; less than 7.35 is considered acidic, and greater than 7.45 is considered alkalosis. Next the $PaCO_2$ is checked; the pH and $PaCO_2$ should move in opposite directions (e.g., as pH increases, the $PaCO_2$ should decrease). The HCO_3^- (bicarbonate) is evaluated. The pH and HCO_3^- should move in the same direction. If the $PaCO_2$ and the HCO_3^- are both abnormal, then the value that corresponds more closely to the pH is examined. The value that more closely corresponds to the pH and deviates more from the norm usually points to the primary disturbance responsible for altering the pH.

Client expectations. Often a fluid and electrolyte or acid-base disturbance is so serious or acute that the client's condition prevents a review of his or her expectations. However, if a client is alert enough to discuss care with the nurse, a review of expectations may reveal short-term needs (e.g., provision of comfort from nausea) or long-term needs (e.g., understanding how to prevent alterations from occurring in the future). The client must be able to understand the implications of fluid and electrolyte or acid-base changes to be able to express expectations of care. The client's trust in the nurse is strengthened through the nurse's competent response to sudden changes in the client's condition.

....

Successful critical thinking requires a synthesis of knowledge, experience, information gathered from clients, and critical thinking attitudes and standards. Clinical judgments require the nurse to anticipate what information is needed, analyze the data, and then make decisions regarding client care. The client expects competent and informed care. Robert incorporates previous knowledge and experience in providing care for Mrs. Reynolds.

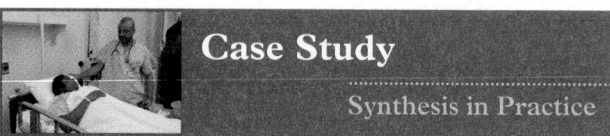

Case Study

Synthesis in Practice

Robert spends time the evening before his clinical assignment to review Mrs. Reynolds' clinical condition. The nursing history found in the medical record reveals that Mrs. Reynolds' loss of appetite, episodes of diarrhea, and continued use of Lasix (a non–potassium-sparing diuretic) for hypertension have placed her at risk for a fluid and electrolyte imbalance. The cause of her GI symptoms is unclear, although the physician plans further diagnostic tests. Robert reviews the physiology of potassium as an

electrolyte and studies the pathology of potassium excess and deficiency. He also reads recommendations in his pharmacology text on how to minimize the risk of hypokalemia when diuretics are taken. Robert anticipates the need to be able to perform a concise physical assessment of this client tomorrow and to be prepared to manage and monitor her IV therapy. He knows the client education will eventually be important for this client, because her therapy for hypertension will likely continue.

Just 4 weeks ago, Robert cared for a client with ulcerative colitis. Although Mrs. Reynolds' condition is different, both clients had diarrhea. Robert knows that Mrs. Reynolds will require careful monitoring of I&O, as well as stabilization of GI function. The lessons learned from his previous client will help Robert to be more alert should Mrs. Reynolds' clinical condition change under his care.

Robert knows the importance of being accountable in completing an examination, assessing and documenting I&O, assessing vital signs, and administering medications in a timely manner. A well-organized approach to Mrs. Reynolds' care will minimize the chance of errors being made.

As a last step in preparation, Robert checks the procedure for IV therapy. His instructor has reviewed new standards for dressing changes, and Robert wants to be sure he is familiar with the new technique.

▪ Nursing Diagnosis

When caring for clients with suspected fluid, electrolyte, and acid-base imbalances, it is particularly important that the nurse be skilled in using critical thinking to formulate nursing diagnoses (see nursing diagnoses box). The assessment data that establish the risk for or the actual presence of a nursing diagnosis in these areas may be subtle, and patterns and trends emerge only when the nurse consciously looks for them because many body systems will be involved. For example, relevant assessment data for the nursing diagnosis *fluid volume deficit* could include the presence of insufficient oral intake, weight loss, dry skin and mucous membranes, inelastic skin turgor, decreased blood pressure, and increased heart rate. The serum sodium and osmolality could be elevated. The urine could be dark, with an elevated specific gravity. The volume of the urine could be decreasing over a period of days.

In addition to the accurate clustering of assessment data, the nurse must precisely identify the related factor for the nursing diagnosis to plan appropriate nursing care. For example, for the nursing diagnosis *fluid volume deficit*, the related factor could be *diarrhea* or *vomiting*. If the related factor were diarrhea, nursing interven-

NURSING DIAGNOSES FOR CLIENTS WITH FLUID, ELECTROLYTE, AND ACID-BASE ALTERATIONS

Breathing pattern, ineffective
Cardiac output, decreased
Fluid volume deficit
Fluid volume deficit, risk for
Fluid volume excess
Gas exchange, impaired
Management of therapeutic regimen, individuals: ineffective
Oral mucous membrane, altered
Skin integrity, impaired
Skin integrity, impaired, risk for
Tissue integrity, impaired
Tissue perfusion, altered, peripheral

tions would include administering ordered antidiarrheal medications, providing oral fluids containing electrolytes and glucose, and teaching the client to use careful hand washing and to avoid dairy products. In contrast, if the related factor were vomiting, the nurse would administer antiemetics, remove sights and odors that could induce nausea, and provide a small amount of fluids containing electrolytes. When choosing which nursing diagnosis is appropriate, the nurse needs to prioritize the client's needs based on the assessment performed.

Planning

During the planning process the nurse works with the client in establishing goals and expected outcomes for each nursing diagnosis. The client's clinical condition will determine which of the diagnoses takes the greatest priority. Many nursing diagnoses in the area of fluid and electrolyte and acid-base balance are of highest priority, because the consequences for the client can be serious or even life threatening. Each goal should be measurable and achievable. Consultation with the client's physician may assist in setting realistic time frames for the goals of care, particularly when the client's physiological status is unstable.

During planning the nurse collaborates as much as possible with the client and family. The family can be particularly helpful in identifying subtle changes in a client's behavior associated with any imbalances (e.g., anxiety, confusion, irritability). The nurse also incorporates client preferences and resources into the plan of care (see care plan on p. 854).

For those clients with acute disturbances, discharge planning must begin early. In the hospital the nurse anticipates the needs of the client and family so that care can continue in the home or long-term care setting with few disruptions. For example, a client might be discharged home with IV therapy. In such a situation the nurse must determine the knowledge and skills of the family member or friend who is to assume care-giving responsibilities and make a referral to home IV therapy as soon as possible.

The nurse also collaborates closely with other members of the health care team, such as the physician, dietitian, and pharmacist. The dietitian can be a valuable resource in recommending food sources to either increase or reduce intake of certain electrolytes. Chapter 34 describes various therapeutic diets (e.g., low sodium). The pharmacist can assist the nurse and physician in identifying medications or combinations of medications likely to cause electrolyte or acid-base disturbances. Furthermore, the pharmacist can offer information regarding client education on side effects to anticipate for those drugs prescribed to the client. The physician will direct the treatment of any fluid and electrolyte or acid-base alteration.

Implementation

Health promotion. Health promotion activities in the area of fluid, electrolyte, and acid-base imbalances focus primarily on client teaching. Clients and care givers need to recognize risk factors for these imbalances and implement appropriate preventive measures. For example, parents of infants need to understand that GI losses can quickly lead to serious imbalances; therefore when vomiting or diarrhea occur in the infant, the parent needs to recognize the risk and promptly seek health care to restore normal balance. Even the healthy adult is at risk for developing imbalances when subjected to elevated environmental temperatures. Nurses need to advise them to supplement the fluid loss from perspiration by increasing oral fluids such as water, maintaining adequate environmental ventilation, and refraining from excessive activity during this period of time.

Clients with chronic health alterations are at particularly high risk for developing changes in their fluid, electrolyte, and acid-base balance. They need to understand their own risk factors and measures to take to avoid imbalances. For example, the client with renal failure must avoid excess intake of fluid, sodium, potassium, and phosphorus. Through diet education these clients learn the types of foods to avoid and the volume of fluid they are permitted daily. Clients with chronic health diseases need to be made aware of early signs and symptoms of fluid, electrolyte, and acid-base imbalances. For example, a client with heart disease should be instructed to obtain an accurate body weight each day at the approximate same time and to inform the physician of significant changes of weight from one day to another. Increase in weight, shortness of breath, orthopnea, and dependent edema are all associated with fluid retention.

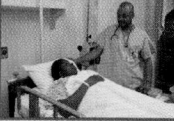

Fluid and Electrolyte Imbalance

Assessment

Mrs. Reynolds' vital signs are temperature 99.6° F, **pulse 100** and regular, **blood pressure 110/60** with no changes when the client stands. The client's skin is intact, without discoloration, but **turgor is decreased.** Inspection of **mucous membranes** shows them to be **dry,** with thick mucus. Respirations were 18 and nonlabored with bilateral breath sounds clear to auscultation. Bowel sounds were present in all four quadrants but hyperactive before one loose bowel movement this morning. The perianal area is slightly reddened. Mrs. Reynolds has had no nausea or vomiting since yesterday and only two loose stools since midnight. Twenty-four-hour intake equaled 2450 ml, with output of 2200 ml **(urine output was only 1000 ml).** Mrs. Reynolds voids without difficulty, with **dark yellow urine.** Robert also reviewed laboratory results: **hematocrit 44%** (suggesting hypovolemia); potassium 3.6 mEq/L and sodium 138 mEq/L (both low normal because of prolonged vomiting and diarrhea). Mrs. Reynolds' ECG showed a normal sinus rhythm, and her admission **weight** of 143 lb was **down** only **1 lb** this morning. The client's Lasix is on hold this morning pending the next potassium level.

Nursing Diagnosis

Fluid volume deficit related to excessive diarrhea, vomiting, and use of potassium-wasting diuretic.

Planning

Goal

Client's fluid and electrolyte levels will return to normal limits by discharge.

Expected Outcomes

Mucous membranes will be moist, and skin turgor will recoil normally within 48 hours.

Blood pressure will remain within 10% of baseline during position changes within 24 hours.

Urine output will equal intake within 48 hours.

Hematocrit, potassium, and sodium levels will return to normal ranges within 48 hours.

Implementation

Steps

1. Monitor and maintain IV fluids (0.45% normal saline) at 125 ml/hour.

2. Administer antidiarrheal medication (Lomotil) after each liquid stool as ordered.

3. Provide comfort measures: oral hygiene every 2 hours while awake or as client desires, lip balm to lips, A&D ointment to perianal area.
4. Monitor I&O and vital signs every 8 hours.
5. Begin client teaching regarding types of foods that offer source of potassium.

Rationale

Replacement of body fluid restores blood volume and normal serum electrolyte levels; use of hypotonic fluid allows fluid to move into body cells, relieving cellular dehydration.

Lomotil inhibits intestinal propulsive motility by acting on smooth muscle and decreases transit time (McKenry and Salerno, 1995).

Local hydration lubrication keep mucous membranes moist and intact.

Documents progress of treatment regimen.

Lasix is a potassium-wasting diuretic. Body cannot store potassium, thus requiring diet supplements rich in potassium (Christensen and Kockrow, 1995).

Evaluation

Inspect oral mucous membranes.

Palpate skin turgor.

Auscultate blood pressure with client lying, sitting, and standing.

Measure urine output, and note color of urine with each void.

Monitor daily laboratory test results.

Defining characteristics are shown in bold type.

Acute care. Although fluid, electrolyte, and/or acid-base imbalance can occur in all settings, changes in the acute care health delivery system place more demanding expectations on the nurse. Today the nurse must manage the client's complex medical care in a shorter span of time while being expected to perform more difficult technological skills.

Daily weight and intake and output measurement. When implementing specific measures to increase or reduce fluid, two nursing interventions are necessary: daily weight and I&O measurements. Clients with fluid and electrolyte alterations should be weighed daily. Daily weights are the single most important indicator of fluid status (Horne and others, 1997). Weight should be determined at the same time each day with the same scale after the client voids. The scale should be calibrated each day or routinely. The client should wear the same clothes or clothes that weigh the same; if a bed scale is used, the same number of sheets should be used on the scale with each weighing.

I&O records provide additional information about fluid balance. I&O measurements, when examined for trends, can indicate whether excess fluid volume is excreted in the form of urine or whether excretion of fluids through the kidneys has diminished. The I&O is not as accurate as daily weights in assessing daily fluid balance.

Enteral replacement of fluids. Oral replacement of fluids and electrolytes is appropriate as long as the client is not so physiologically unstable that oral fluids cannot be replaced rapidly. Oral replacement of fluids is contraindicated when the client is vomiting, has a mechanical obstruction of the GI tract, is at risk for aspiration, or has impaired swallowing. Clients unable to tolerate solid foods may still be able to ingest fluids.

When replacing fluids by mouth in a client with a fluid deficit, it is wise to choose fluids with adequate calories and electrolyte content (e.g., fruit juices, gelatin, and replacements like Pedialyte and Gastrolyte). However, it is important to remember that liquids containing lactose, caffeine, or low-sodium content may not be appropriate when the client has diarrhea.

A feeding tube may be appropriate when the client's GI tract is healthy but the client cannot ingest fluids (e.g., after oral surgery or with impaired swallowing). Fluids can also be replaced through a gastrostomy or jejunostomy feeding tube, or they can be administered via a small-bore nasogastric feeding tube.

Restriction of fluids. Clients who retain fluids and have FVE require restricted fluid intake. Fluid restriction is often difficult for clients, particularly if they take drugs that dry the oral mucous membranes or if they breathe through the mouth. The nurse should explain the reasons fluids are restricted. In addition, the client needs to know the amount of fluid permitted orally and should understand that ice chips, gelatin, and ice cream are considered fluid. The client should help to decide the amount of fluid with each meal, between meals, before bed, and with medications. Frequently clients on fluid restriction can swallow a number of pills with as little as 1 oz (30 ml) of liquid.

A good rule of thumb for fluid restrictions is to allow half of the allotted total oral fluids between 7 AM and 3 PM, the period when clients usually are more active, receive two meals, and take most of their oral medications. An additional two fifths of the allotted total fluid is permitted between 3 PM and 11 PM. This permits fluids with meals and evening visitors. Between 11 PM and 7 AM, the remainder is permitted. The nurse should also make sure that clients receive the type of fluids they like best (unless contraindicated). Clients on fluid restriction require mouth care frequently to moisten mucous membranes, decrease the chance of mucosal drying and cracking, and achieve comfort.

Parenteral replacement of fluids and electrolytes. Fluid and electrolytes may be replaced through infusion directly into the blood rather than via the digestive system. Parenteral replacement includes TPN, IV fluid and electrolyte therapy, and blood and blood component administration.

With increasing risk to health care workers for transmission of the human immunodeficiency virus (HIV), the cause of acquired immunodeficiency syndrome (AIDS); hepatitis B virus (HBV); and other infectious diseases, standard precautions must be practiced when administering parenteral fluids (see Chapter 25).

Vascular access devices. **Vascular access devices** are catheters, cannulas, or infusion ports designed for long-term repeated access to the vascular system. These devices are more effective than peripherally placed catheters for administering medications and solutions that are irritating to veins and for the delivery of long-term IV therapy. Increased use of central venous catheters and implanted infusion ports (Figure 31-4) requires nurses to be educated in the care of these devices.

Total parenteral nutrition. TPN is a nutritionally adequate hypertonic solution consisting of glucose and other nutrients and electrolytes given through an indwelling peripheral or central IV catheter. TPN is used

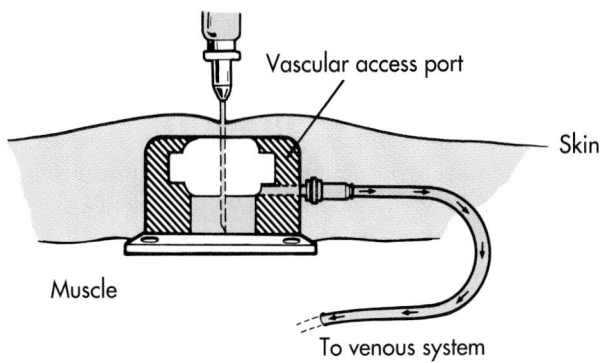

Figure 31-4. Example of implantable vascular access device.

as an intervention in severe cases of malnutrition. Chapter 34 fully describes its administration.

Intravenous therapy. The goal of IV fluid administration is to correct or prevent fluid and electrolyte disturbances. It allows for direct access to the vascular system, permitting the infusion of continuous fluids over a period of time. IV fluid therapy must be continuously regulated because of continual changes in the client's fluid and electrolyte balance.

When IV fluid administration is required, the nurse must know the correct ordered solution, equipment needed, and procedures required to initiate an infusion, regulate the infusion rate, maintain the system, identify and correct problems, and discontinue the infusion.

Administration of Intravenous Therapy

Types of solutions. Many prepared IV solutions are available for use (Table 31-6). IV solutions fall into the following categories: isotonic, hypotonic, and hypertonic. Isotonic solutions are those that have the same effective osmolality as body fluids. Hypotonic solutions are those that have an effective osmolality less than body fluids. Hypertonic solutions are those that have an effective osmolality greater than body fluids (Horne and others, 1997).

In general, isotonic fluids are used most commonly for extracellular volume replacement (e.g., FVD after prolonged vomiting). The decision to use a hypotonic or hypertonic solution is based on the specific fluid and electrolyte imbalance. For example, the client with a hypertonic fluid imbalance will generally receive a hypotonic IV to dilute the ECF and rehydrate the cells. All IV fluids should be given carefully, especially hypertonic solutions, because these pull fluid into the vascular space by osmosis, resulting in an increased vascular volume that can lead to pulmonary edema, particularly in clients with heart or renal failure.

Certain additives, most commonly vitamins and potassium chloride (KCl), are frequently added to IV solutions. A physician's order includes required additives. For example:

Bottle #1: 1000 ml D_5 ½ NS with 20 mEq KCl and 1 ampule of multivitamins at 125 ml/hour

Clients with normal renal function who are receiving nothing by mouth should have potassium added to IV solutions. The body cannot conserve potassium, and even when the serum level falls, the kidneys continue to excrete potassium. If there is no potassium intake orally or parenterally, hypokalemia can develop quickly. Conversely, the nurse should verify that the client has adequate urine output before administering an IV solution containing potassium, because hyperkalemia can quickly develop.

Equipment. Correct selection and preparation of IV equipment assists in safe and quick placement of an IV line. Because fluids are instilled into the blood-

TABLE 31-6
Intravenous Solutions

Solution	Concentration	Other Names
Dextrose in Water Solutions		
Dextrose 5% in water*	Isotonic	D_5W
Dextrose 10% in water	Hypertonic	$D_{10}W$
Saline Solutions		
0.45% sodium chloride (half normal saline)	Hypotonic	½ NS 0.45% NS
0.9% sodium chloride† (normal saline)	Isotonic	NS 0.9% NS 0.9% NaCl
3%-5% sodium chloride	Hypertonic	3%-5% NS 3%-5% NaCl
Dextrose in Saline Solutions		
Dextrose 5% in 0.9% sodium chloride	Hypertonic	$D_5$0.9% NaCl $D_5$0.9% NS D_5NS
Dextrose 5% in 0.45% NaCl sodium chloride	Hypertonic	$D_5$0.45% NaCl $D_5$0.45% NS D_5½NS
Multiple Electrolyte Solutions		
Lactated Ringer's‡	Isotonic	LR
Dextrose 5% in Lactated Ringer's	Hypertonic	D_5LR

*Dextrose is quickly metabolized, leaving free water to be distributed evenly in all fluid compartments (Horne and others, 1997).
†Although it is isotonic because the total concentration of electrolytes equals plasma concentration, it contains 154 mEq of both sodium and chloride, which is a higher concentration of these electrolytes than is found in the plasma, which can cause FVE (Metheny, 1992).
‡Contains sodium, potassium, calcium, chloride, and lactate.

stream, sterile technique is necessary; the nurse must therefore have all equipment organized and at the bedside. The nurse who must leave the bedside to obtain another piece of equipment must start the procedure again.

IV equipment includes needles or catheters, tourniquet, gloves, dressings, solution containers, various types of tubing, and IV pumps or volume control devices. Injectable medications such as the antibiotic ampicillin may be added to a small IV solution bag and "piggybacked" into the main line to be administered over a 30- to 60-minute period (see Chapter 26). The type and amount of solution depend on the medication added and the client's physiological status.

Different types of tubing are used to administer medications or IV fluids. A solution given rapidly needs to be infused with macrodrip tubing, which delivers large drops (standard drop size is 10 or 15 gtt/ml depending on the manufacturer) so that a rapid rate can be maintained. In contrast, microdrip tubing provides a standard drop size of 60 gtt/ml. Microdrip tubing is used to allow precise regulation of IV fluids even at slow rates. In addition, clients may require IV extension tubing to increase mobility or to facilitate changes in position. IV pumps or volume control devices are used with children, with clients with renal or cardiac failure, or with critically ill clients to prevent sudden uncontrolled rapid infusion of large volumes of fluid. (Additional information on IV pumps and volume control devices is presented in the section on regulating the infusion flow rate.)

Initiating the intravenous line. After the equipment is collected at the bedside, the nurse prepares to place the IV line by assessing the client for a venipuncture site (Skill 31-1). Common IV puncture sites include the hand and the arm (Figure 31-5, *A* and *B*). The use of the foot (Figure 31-5, *C*) for an IV site is common with pediatric clients but is avoided in the adult because of the danger of thrombophlebitis (Pearson, 1996). The nurse assessing the client for potential venipuncture sites for IV infusion should consider conditions, cautions, and contraindications that exclude certain sites. Because very young children and older adults have fragile veins, the nurse should avoid sites that are easily moved or bumped such as the dorsal surface of the hand (Box 31-3). Venipuncture is contraindicated in a site that has signs of infection, infiltration, or thrombosis. An infected site is red, tender, swollen, and pos-

BOX 31-3
Gerontological Nursing Practice

- In older clients, use the smallest gauge catheter or needle possible (e.g., 24 to 26 gauge). This is less traumatizing to the vein and allows better blood flow to provide increased hemodilution of the IV fluids or medications. This gauge can be used for hourly flow rates of 75 to 100 ml/hour.
- Avoid the back of the older adult's hand or the dominant arm for venipuncture, because these sites greatly interfere with the older adult's independence.
- If the older adult has fragile skin and veins, use minimal tourniquet pressure.
- When the older adult has lost subcutaneous tissue, the veins lose stability and will roll away from the needle. To stabilize the vein, apply traction to the skin below the projected insertion site.
- Using an angle of 5 to 15 degrees on insertion is helpful, because the older adult's veins are more superficial.
- In the older person with fragile skin, prevent skin tears by minimizing the amount of tape used.

Modified from Coulter K: Intravenous therapy for the elder patient: implications for the intravenous nurse, *J Intraven Nurs* 15(suppl): S18, 1992.

sibly warm to the touch. Exudate may be present. An infected site is not used because of the danger of introducing bacteria from the skin surface into the bloodstream. Avoid using an extremity with a vascular (dialysis) graft/fistula or on the side of a mastectomy. IVs should be placed at the most distal point when possible. Using a distal site first allows for the use of proximal sites later if the client would need a venipuncture site change.

Text continued on p. 867

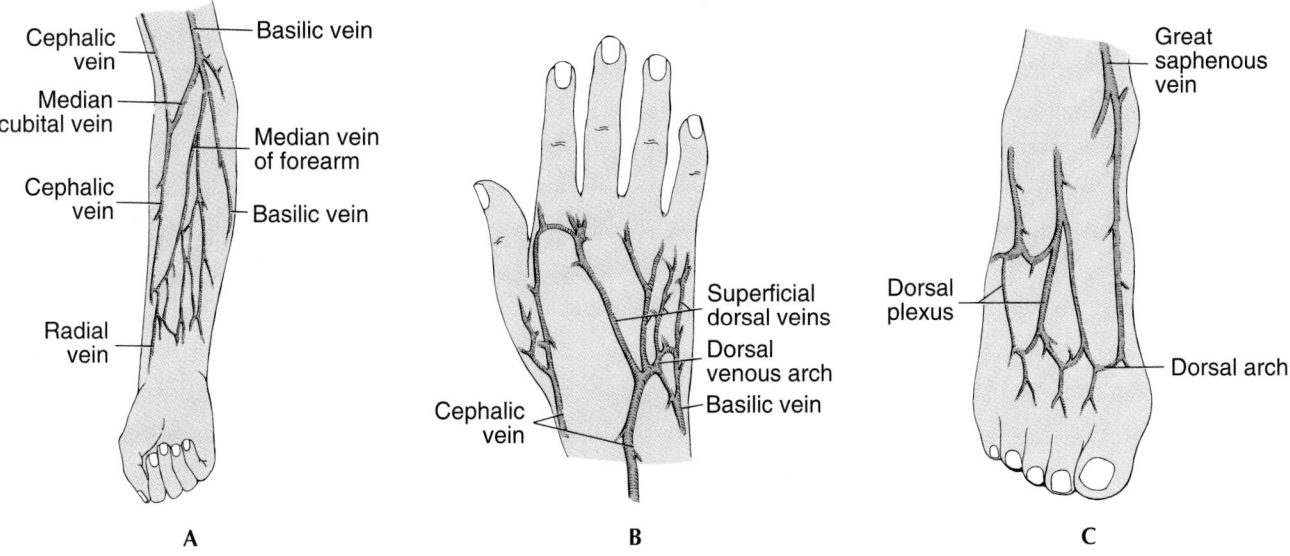

Figure 31-5. Common IV sites. **A,** Inner arm. **B,** Dorsal surface of hand. **C,** Dorsal surface of foot (used only for pediatric clients).

Initiating a Peripheral Intravenous Infusion

Delegation Considerations

The skills of initiating IV therapy requires problem solving and knowledge application unique to professional nursing. For this procedure delegation is not appropriate.

Equipment
- Correct IV solution (with time tape attached)
- Proper catheter for venipuncture (will vary with client's body size and reason for IV fluid administration)

For IV fluid infusion
- Administration set (choice depends on type of solution and rate of administration; infants and children require microdrip tubing, which provides 60 gtt/ml)
- 0.22 μm filter (if required by agency policy or if particulate matter is likely)
- Extension tubing (used when a longer IV line is necessary)
- Alcohol and povidone-iodine cleaning swabs or sticks
- Disposable gloves
- Tourniquet (can be a source of contamination; use a single-use product)
- Arm board, if needed (used to maintain wrist or elbow joint position when ONC is placed close to or over a joint; will help prevent infiltration of IV)

- Nonallergenic tape
- Towel (to place under client's hand or arm)
- IV pole, rolling or ceiling mounted
- Special client gown with snaps at shoulder seams (makes removal with IV tubing easier), if available
- Needle disposal container (also called sharps container)

Gauze dressing only
- 2 × 2 or 4 × 4 sterile gauze sponge

Transparent dressing
- Transparent dressing

For heparin or normal saline lock
- Injection cap (also called IV plug)
- IV loop or short piece of extension tubing, if necessary
- 1 to 3 ml of normal saline or heparin flush (10 to 100 U/ml as ordered)
- Syringes and 25-gauge needles
- Optional: IV kit
    Some agencies use an IV start kit, which contains a sterile drape to place under the client's arm, cleansing and antiseptic preparations, dressings, and a small roll of sterile, precut tape

STEPS	RATIONALE
1. Review client's medical record for physician's order stating type and amount of IV fluid and rate of fluid administration. In addition, nurse follows "five rights" for administration of medications (see Chapter 26).	An order requesting the initiation of a peripheral IV access and administration of an IV solution must be made by a physician before the implementation of this procedure.
2. Identify the client whose potential for fluid and electrolyte imbalance may require IV fluid therapy. Observe for signs and symptoms indicating fluid or electrolyte imbalances.	
a. Greater than 2% decrease in body weight	Daily weights document fluid loss or retention. Change in body weight of 1 kg corresponds to 1 L of fluid loss or retention (Horne and Swearingen, 1997).
b. Dry skin and mucous membranes	May signal FVD.
c. Flattened neck veins	Suggests FVD.
d. Blood pressure changes; tachycardia	Elevated blood pressure may indicate FVE because of increase in stroke volume. Decreased blood pressure may indicate FVD because of a decrease in stroke volume. Tachycardia may indicate FVD.
e. Irregular pulse rhythm	May occur with potassium, calcium, and/or magnesium abnormalities.
f. Inelastic skin turgor (after pinching, fails to return to normal position within 3 seconds)	With FVD, the pinched skin stays elevated for several seconds.

STEPS	RATIONALE

CRITICAL DECISION POINT

This is a less reliable indicator for older adults because their skin is less elastic naturally due to aging.

g. Anorexia, nausea, and vomiting	May occur with acute FVD or FVE.
h. Thirst	Symptomatic of FVD.
i. Decreased urine output	Monitoring urinary output is one method of assessing fluid balance. During dehydration, kidneys attempt to restore fluid balance by reducing urine production. Average daily adult urine output is 1500 ml; urine output of less than 400 ml/24 hours (oliguria) signals the retention of metabolic wastes (Horne and Swearingen, 1997).
j. Behavior changes	Restlessness and confusion may occur with FVD or acid-base imbalance.
3. Obtain information about composition of IV fluids, purposes for administration, potential incompatibilities, and side effects to monitor for.	This allows detection of an inadvisable IV fluid order and helps to determine priority assessments.
4. Determine client's understanding of the reason for IV fluids, what to expect during the venipuncture, and the client's psychological readiness for venipuncture and IV therapy.	Determines teaching needs and need for special psychological support.
5. Assess for the following risk factors: child or older adult, presence of heart failure or renal failure, or low platelet count.	Persons at extremes in age develop fluid imbalances more rapidly, because they have proportionately larger ECF volume; persons with heart failure may require fluid restriction and cannot adapt to sudden increases in vascular volume, and persons with renal failure cannot eliminate excess ECF. A low platelet count predisposes clients to bleeding at IV site.
6. Prepare client and family by explaining the procedure, its purpose, and what is expected of client.	Decreases anxiety and promotes cooperation.
7. Identify accessible vein for placement of IV needle or catheter by inspection; this will most likely require application of a tourniquet. The most appropriate veins to utilize are cephalic, basilic, and median cubital for adults. For infants, the most appropriate veins include scalp and foot veins.	Pearson (1996) reports that the site at which a catheter is placed influences subsequent risk of catheter-related infection.

CRITICAL DECISION POINT

Never use foot veins in adults unless ordered by a physician.

a. Avoid bony prominences.	Selection of appropriate vein promotes ease of placement of IV needle or catheter.
b. Use most distal portion of vein first.	If damage to the vein occurs, the proximal site of the same vein is still usable.
c. Avoid placing IV catheter near client's wrist or antecubital fossa, if possible.	Frequent bending of the wrist or arm increases the likelihood of infiltration and phlebitis and has a high potential to affect the IV flow rate.

Continued

Initiating a Peripheral Intravenous Infusion

STEPS	RATIONALE
d. For peripheral catheters, upper extremity insertions pose less of a risk of phlebitis than lower extremity insertions. In adults, hand veins have a lower risk of phlebitis than upper arm or wrist veins (Pearson, 1996).	
e. Avoid placing IV in client's dominant arm, if possible.	Allows greater freedom of movement.
f. Avoid using an extremity where sensation is decreased, such as one affected by hemiparesis experienced after a stroke.	Ability to perceive pain helps in early detection of complications.
g. Avoid inserting IV through an infection, rash, or any break in the skin.	Increases the risk for IV-related bacteremia.
h. Avoid previously accessed veins, injured veins, or sclerotic veins. Insert proximal to injured areas.	
8. Assist client to comfortable sitting or lying position.	
9. Wash hands.	Reduces transmission of microorganisms.
10. Organize equipment on clean clutter-free bedside stand or overbed table.	Reduces risk of contamination and accidents.
11. Change client's gown to the more easily removed gown with snaps at the shoulder, if available.	Use of a special IV gown facilitates safe removal of the gown.
12. Open sterile packages using sterile aseptic technique.	Maintains sterility of equipment and reduces spread of microorganisms.
13. Check IV solution, using "five rights" of drug administration (see Chapter 26). Make sure prescribed additives, such as potassium and vitamins, have been added. Check solution for color, clarity, and expiration date. Check bag for leaks, which is best if done before reaching the bedside.	IV solutions are medications and should be carefully checked to reduce risk of error. Solutions that are discolored, contain particles, or are expired are not to be used. Leaky bags present an opportunity for infection and must not be used.
14. Open infusion set, maintaining sterility of both ends of tubing. Many sets allow for priming of tubing without removal of end cap.	Prevent bacteria from entering infusion equipment and bloodstream.
15. Place roller clamp (see illustration) about 2 to 4 cm (1 to 2 inches) below drip chamber and move roller clamp to "off" position (see illustrations).	Close proximity of roller clamp to drip chamber allows more accurate regulation of flow rate. Moving clamp to "off" prevents accidental spillage of fluid.
16. Remove protective sheath over IV tubing port on plastic IV solution bag (see illustration). For bottled IV solution, remove metal cap and metal and rubber disks beneath cap.	Provides access for insertion of infusion tubing into solution.
17. Insert infusion set into fluid bag or bottle. Remove protector cap from tubing insertion spike (keeping spike sterile), and insert spike into opening of IV bag (see illustration). Cleanse rubber stopper on bottled solution with antiseptic, and insert spike into black rubber stopper of IV bottle.	Prevents contamination of solution from contaminated insertion spike.
18. Prime infusion tubing by filling with IV solution. Compress drip chamber and release, allowing it to fill one-third to one-half full (see illustration).	Creates suction effect; fluid enters drip chamber to prevent air from entering tubing.

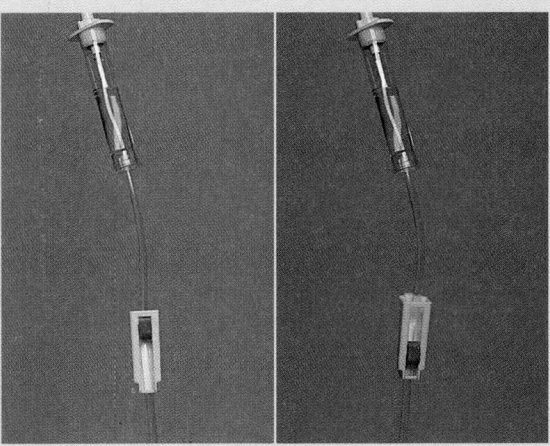

Step 15

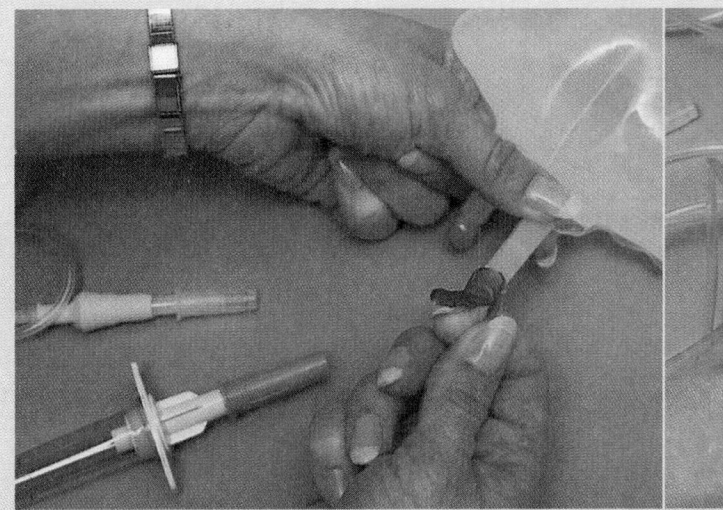

Step 16

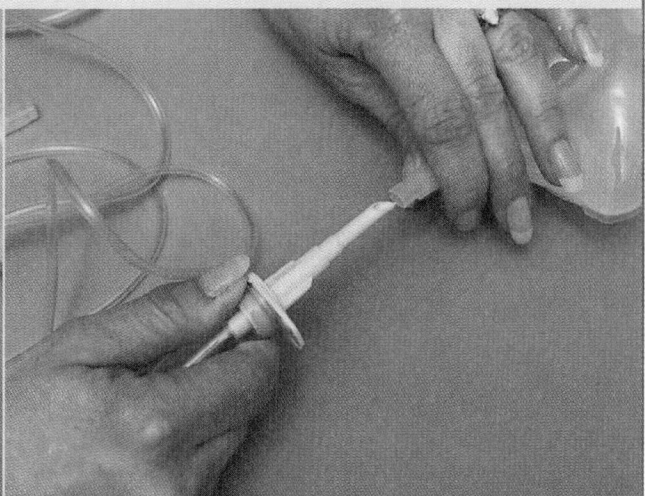

Step 17

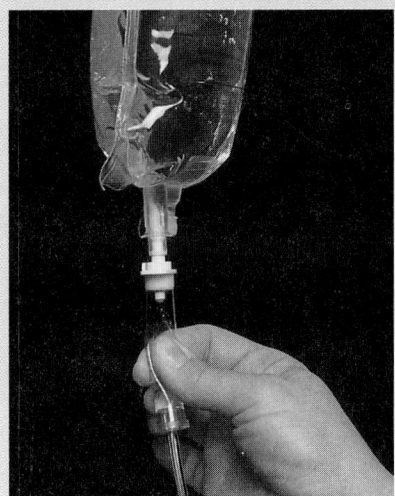

Step 18

Continued

Initiating a Peripheral Intravenous Infusion

STEPS	RATIONALE
19. Remove tubing protector cap (some tubing can be primed without removal) and slowly release roller clamp to allow fluid to travel from drip chamber through tubing to needle adapter. Return roller clamp to "off" position after tubing is primed (filled with IV fluid).	Slow fill of tubing decreases turbulence and chance of bubble formation. Removes air from tubing and permits tubing to fill with solution. Closing the clamp prevents accidental loss of fluid.
20. Be certain tubing is clear of air and air bubbles. To remove small air bubbles, firmly tap IV tubing where air bubbles are located. Check entire length of tubing to ensure that all air bubbles are removed.	Large air bubbles can act as emboli.
21. Replace tubing cap protector on end of tubing.	Maintains system sterility.
22. Optional: prepare heparin or normal saline lock for infusion. If a loop or short extension tubing is needed because of an awkward IV site placement, use sterile technique to connect the IV plug to the loop or short extension tubing. Inject 1 to 3 ml normal saline through the plug and through the loop or short extension tubing.	Removes air to prevent introduction into the vein. Do the same with the saline plug.
23. Select most distal site of vein to be used.	If sclerosing or damage to vein occurs, a more proximal site of same vein is still usable.
24. If large amount of body hair is present at needle insertion site, clip it.	Reduces risk of contamination from bacteria on hair. Also assists in maintaining an intact dressing and makes removal of tape less painful.

CRITICAL DECISION POINT

Do not shave area. Shaving may cause microabrasions, predisposing to infection.

STEPS	RATIONALE
25. If possible, place extremity in dependent position.	Permits venous dilation and visibility.
26. Place tourniquet 10 to 12 cm (4 to 5 inches) above insertion site. Tourniquet should obstruct venous, not arterial, flow. Check presence of distal pulse.	Diminished arterial flow prevents venous filling. The pressure of the tourniquet should cause the vein to dilate. Further methods for vein dilation are listed in Step 29.
27. Apply disposable gloves. Eye protection and mask may be worn (see agency policy).	Decreases exposure to HIV, hepatitis, and other blood-borne organisms (CDC, 1987) and prevents spraying of blood on nurse's mucous membranes.
28. Place needle adapter end of infusion set nearby on sterile gauze or sterile towel.	Permits smooth, quick connection of infusion to IV needle once vein is punctured.
29. Select well-dilated vein. Methods to foster vein dilation include:	
a. Stroking the extremity from distal to proximal below the proposed venipuncture site.	Increases the volume of blood in the vein at the venipuncture site.
b. Opening and closing fist.	Muscle contraction increases the amount of blood in the extremity.
c. Light tapping over the vein.	Fosters venous dilation.
d. Applying warmth to the extremity for several minutes (e.g., with a warm washcloth).	Increases blood supply and fosters venous dilation.

STEPS	RATIONALE
30. (If area of insertion appears to need cleansing, use soap and water first.) Then cleanse insertion site using firm, circular motion (middle to outward) with povidone-iodine solution; refrain from touching the cleansed site; allow the site to dry for at least 2 minutes. If the client is allergic to iodine, use 70% alcohol and allow to dry for 60 seconds (see illustration).	Povidone-iodine is a topical antiinfective that reduces skin surface bacteria; touching the cleansed area would introduce organisms from the nurse's hand to the site. Povidone-iodine must dry to be effective in reducing microbial counts (Baranowski, 1993).
31. Perform venipuncture. Anchor vein by placing thumb over vein and by stretching the skin against the direction of insertion 2 to 3 inches distal to the site.	Places needle parallel to vein. When vein is punctured, risk of puncturing posterior vein wall is reduced.

    Butterfly needle: Hold needle at 20- to 30-degree angle with bevel up slightly distal to actual site of venipuncture.

    ONC: Insert ONC (see illustrations) with bevel up at 20- to 30-degree angle slightly distal to actual site of venipuncture in the direction of the vein.

    Needleless IV catheter safety device: Insert using same position as for ONC.

CRITICAL DECISION POINT

No more than three attempts at inserting an IV should be made by a single nurse (check agency policy).

Continued

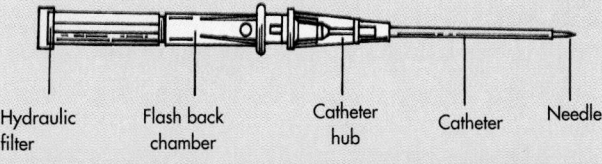

Hydraulic filter   Flash back chamber   Catheter hub   Catheter   Needle

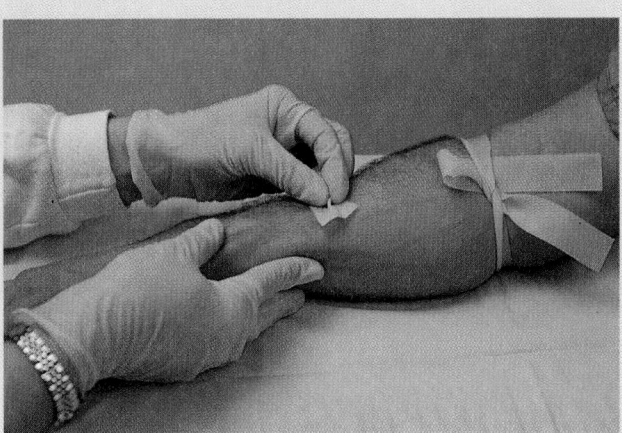

Step 30

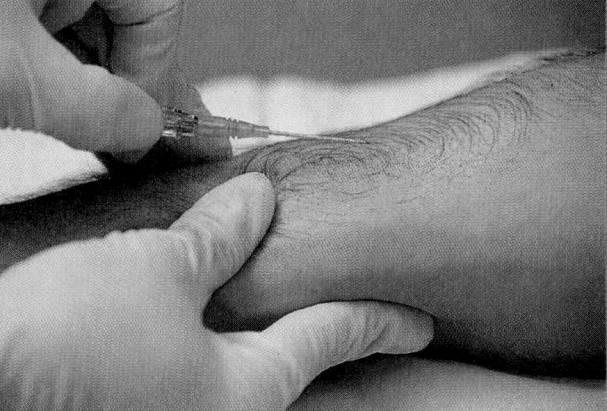

Step 31

.... Skill 31-1—cont'd
Initiating a Peripheral Intravenous Infusion

STEPS	RATIONALE
32. Look for blood return through tubing of butterfly needle or flashback chamber of ONC, indicating that needle has entered vein (see illustration). Lower needle until almost flush with skin. Advance butterfly needle until hub rests at venipuncture site. Advance ONC catheter $1/4$ inch into vein and then loosen stylet. Advance catheter into vein until hub rests at venipuncture site (see illustration). Do not reinsert the stylet once it is loosened. (If available, advance the safety device by using push-off tab to thread the catheter.)	Increased venous pressure from tourniquet increases backflow of blood into catheter or tubing. Reinsertion of the stylet can cause catheter breakage in the vein.
33. Stabilize the catheter with one hand by placing pressure on the hub or on the vein above the insertion site. Release tourniquet and remove stylet from ONC. Do not recap the stylet. For a safety device, slide the catheter off the stylet while gliding the protective guard over the stylet. A click indicates the device is locked over the stylet.	Permits venous flow, reduces backflow of blood, and allows connection with administration set.
34. Quickly connect needle adapter of administration set or heparin lock to hub of ONC or butterfly tubing. Do not touch point of entry of needle adapter.	Prompt connection of infusion set maintains patency of vein. Maintains sterility.
35. Bloodless method: Hold pressure over tip of inserted catheter with your thumb; with your index finger and thumb remove cap and attach tubing to catheter hub (see illustration).	Prevents risk of exposure to blood.
36. Release roller clamp slowly to begin infusion at a rate to maintain patency of IV line (not necessary with a heparin lock).	Permits venous flow and prevents clotting of vein and obstruction of flow of IV solution.

CRITICAL DECISION POINT

Be sure to calculate rate so as not to infuse IV solution too rapidly or too slowly.

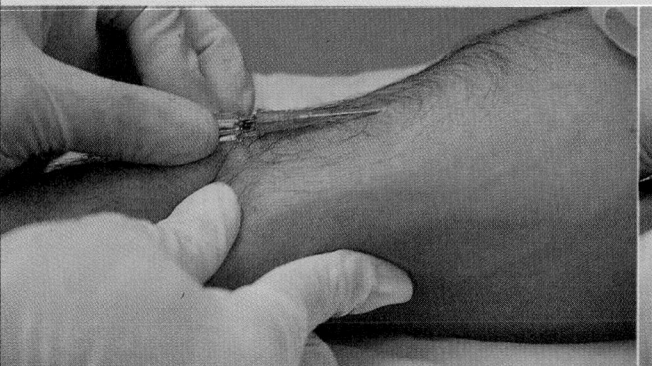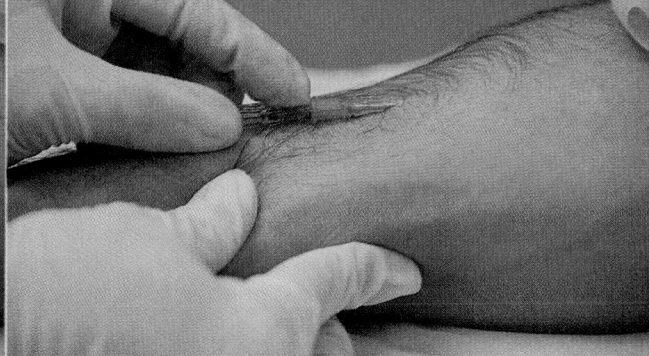

Step 32

STEPS	RATIONALE

37. Secure IV catheter or needle (procedures can differ; follow agency policy):

A. Gauze dressing:

(1) Place narrow piece (½ inch) of tape under catheter hub with sticky side up and cross tape over catheter (see illustration).

Prevents accidental removal of catheter from vein. Prevents back-and-forth motion, which can irritate the vein and introduce bacteria on the skin into the vein.

(2) Place second piece of narrow tape directly across hub of catheter.

Further prevents displacement of catheter.

(3) Place 2 × 2 or 4 × 4 gauze sponge over insertion site and catheter hub and secure completely with 1-inch piece of tape. Do not cover connection between IV tubing and catheter hub.

Occlusive dressing protects site from bacterial contamination. Connection between administration set and hub needs to be uncovered to facilitate changing the tubing if necessary. Pearson (1996) no longer recommends application of antimicrobial ointment to catheter site.

Continued

B. Transparent dressing:

(1) Apply dressing to site first (no tape) (see illustration). Dressing is molded around catheter hub to secure catheter from movement.

(2) Apply one piece of tape across edge of dressing closest to the hub. Proceed to use two ½-inch pieces of tape around connection and catheter. Apply 1-inch piece of tape over hub for security.

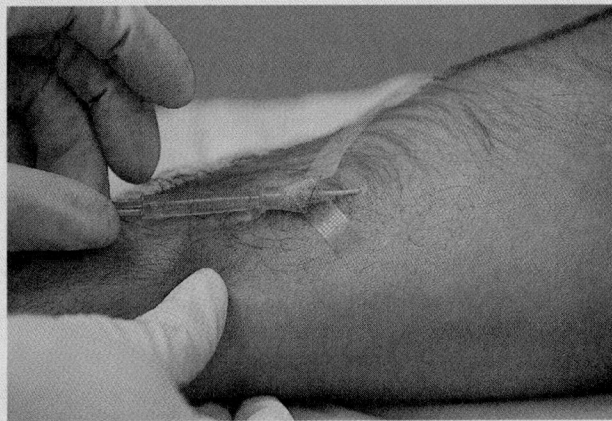

Step 37A(1)

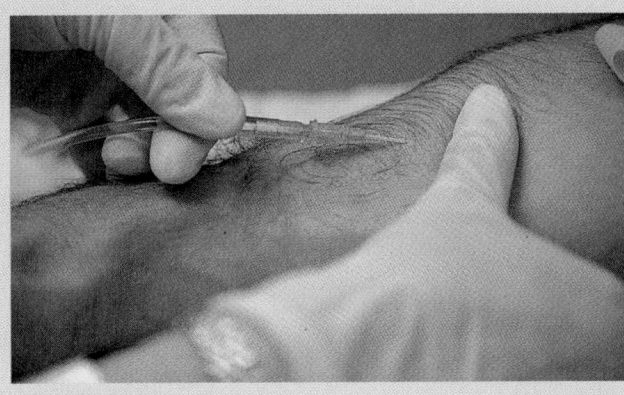

Step 35

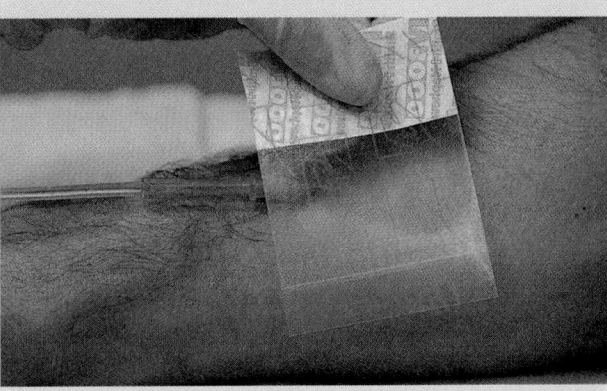

Step 37B(1)

Skill 31-1—cont'd
Initiating a Peripheral Intravenous Infusion

STEPS	RATIONALE
38. Secure loop: secure a loop of infusion tubing to dressing with piece of 1-inch tape. Place tape on tape, not on dressing (reduces the action of the transparent film if placed on top of it).	Stabilizes connection of administration set to catheter. Prevents weight of tubing from pulling catheter or needle out of venipuncture site.
39. For *IV fluid administration* adjust flow rate to correct drops per minute (Skill 31-2).	Maintains correct rate of flow for IV solution. Flow can fluctuate, so it must be checked at intervals.
a. For *heparin lock* flush with 1 to 3 ml of heparin (10 to 100 U/ml).	
b. For *saline lock* flush with 1 to 3 ml of sterile normal saline.	Maintains patency of IV catheter.
40. Write date and time, gauge size and size of catheter, and placement of IV line and dressing.	Documents when IV was inserted and when subsequent dressing changes are needed.
41. Dispose of used needles in appropriate sharps container. Discard supplies. Remove gloves and wash hands.	Reduces transmission of microorganisms and protects staff from injury.
42. Observe client every hour to determine if fluid is infusing correctly.	
a. Check if correct amount of solution is infused as prescribed by looking at time tape.	
b. Count flow rate.	
c. Check patency of IV catheter or needle: briefly compress cannulated vein proximal to site. Observe for slowing or cessation of IV rate.	Compression results in mechanical obstruction of vein. When IV catheter is patent, compression results in slowing or cessation of flow rate. No change in flow rate may indicate infiltration.
d. Also observe client during compression of vessel for signs of discomfort.	
e. Inspect insertion site for absence of infiltration, phlebitis, or inflammation.	Provides continuous evaluation of type and amount of fluid delivered to client. Hourly inspection prevents accidental fluid overload or inadequate infusion rate and identifies early incidence of vein inflammation or tissue damage.
43. Observe client every hour to determine response to therapy (i.e., measure vital signs, conduct post-procedure assessments).	IV fluids and additives are given to maintain or restore fluid and electrolyte balance. They can also cause unexpected effects, which can be serious.

Recording and Reporting

- Record in nurse's notes number of attempts for insertion, type of fluid, insertion site by vessel, flow rate, size and type of catheter or needle, and when infusion was begun. A special parenteral therapy flow sheet may be used (Figure 31-6).
- Record client's response to IV fluid, amount infused, and integrity and patency of system every 4 hours or according to agency policy.
- Report to oncoming nursing staff: type of fluid, flow rate, status of venipuncture site, amount of fluid remaining in present solution, expected time to hang next IV bag or bottle, and any side effects.

Home Care Considerations

- See Box 31-4.
- Teach care giver to apply pressure with sterile gauze if catheter falls out and, if client is on anticoagulant therapy, to tape several pieces of sterile gauze in place for at least 20 minutes or until bleeding stops.
- Teach client and care giver to perform tub bath without getting IV tubing wet and to unplug pump first if one is used. For showering, the client must insert hand and forearm into a plastic bag. Tape bag in place to ensure that IV site is completely covered.
- Teach client and family to monitor I&O using household measuring devices.

A venipuncture is a technique in which a vein is punctured through the skin by a sharp rigid stylet (e.g., butterfly needle, metal needle), a partially covered plastic catheter (over-the-needle catheter [ONC]), or a needle attached to a syringe. Large catheters placed into a central vein such as the subclavian vein are used to deliver large volumes of fluids and TPN or to administer irritating medications. Although these catheters are inserted by physicians, nurses are responsible for maintaining them. When veins are fragile or collapse, venipuncture becomes extremely difficult, but it is also a life-saving measure. For these difficult clients, venipuncture should be performed by an experienced practitioner. The general purposes of venipuncture are to

ST. JOHN'S HOSPITAL
Springfield, Illinois

I.V. MAINTENANCE RECORD

I.V. FLUID & I.V. MEDICATION

Site Code	R.J. or L.J. – Right or Left Jugular R.S.V. or L.S.V. – Right or Left Subclavian Vein R.L.L. or L.L.L. – Right or Left Lower Leg R.H. or L.H. – Right or Left Hand R.F.A. or L.F.A. – Right or Left Forearm R.U.A. or L.U.A. – Right or Left Upperarm R.F. or L.F. – Right or Left Foot R.S., L.S. or M.S. – Right, Left or Mid Scalp R.F.V. or L.F.V. – Right or Left Femoral Vein R.A.C. or L.A.C. – Right or Left Antecubital R.W. or L.W. – Right or Left Wrist K.V.O. – Keep Vein Open H.L. – Heparin Lock P.B. – Piggyback P. – Push
Triple Lumen Catheter	Proximal - 18 gauge (White): Draw blood, Blood Adm, Medications Middle - 18 gauge (Blue): TPN, Medications Distal - 16 gauge (Brown): Blood Adm., Colloids, Viscous Fluids, CVP Monitoring, Medications

Signature:

Allergy:

No. of last I.V. __________ Letter of last expander __________

No. of last Blood/Component __________

DATE		
Night Nurse		
Day Nurse		
Evening Nurse		

Order Date		Amount, Solution, Infusing Time or Rate, Medication, Dose, Time	Site(s)			Pump	Time	Time
		One Time I.V. Meds.						
	No.	I.V. Fluids						
		I.V. TUBING CHANGE. (Indicate I.V. No. & Time)						
	Stop Date	Intermittent & PRN I.V. Meds.						
		I.V.P.B. TUBING CHANGE (Indicate Drug & Time)						

Continued

Figure 31-6. IV maintenance record. (Courtesy St. John's Hospital, Springfield, Ill.)

collect a blood specimen, to instill a medication, to start an IV infusion, or to inject a radiopaque or radioactive tracer for special examinations. Skill 31-1 describes **venipuncture** for IV fluid infusion.

Regulating the infusion flow rate. After the IV infusion is secured and the line is patent, the nurse must regulate the rate of infusion according to the physician's orders (Skill 31-2). An infusion rate that is too slow can lead to further cardiovascular and circulatory collapse in a critically ill client who has FVD or hyperosmolar imbalance or who is in shock. An IV that is running too slowly can also become clotted off more easily. An infusion rate that is too rapid can result in

FVE. The nurse calculates the infusion rate to prevent too-slow or too-rapid administration of IV fluids. The minimal rate used to keep a vein open and patent is about 10 to 15 ml/hour using a microdrip infusion set.

Infusion devices assist the nurse to maintain correct flow rate of IV fluids, prevent runaway and obstructed IV infusions, and alert the nurse when an IV bag or bottle is empty (Millam, 1990). Many electronic infusion devices record the volume of the fluid infused. An **infusion pump** is designed to deliver a measured amount of fluid over a period of time (i.e., ml/hr). The pump has a drop sensor and an alarm that will sound if drops are not detected at the appropriate rate. There are also

I.V. SITE ASSESSMENT		
SITE CODE		**TYPE CODE**

SITE CODE			TYPE CODE	
R.J. or L.J. – Right or Left Jugular			M.C. – Medicut	H.C. – Hickman Catheter
R.S.V. or L.S.V. – Right or Left Subclavian Vein	K.V.O. – Keep Vein Open		A.C. – Angiocath	B.C. – Broviac Catheter
R.L.L. or L.L.L. – Right or Left Lower Leg	H.L. – Heparin Lock		S.V. – Scalpvein	M.L.C. – Multi-lumen Catheter
R.H. or L.H. – Right or Left Hand	P.B. – Piggyback		A.S. – Angio-set	M.L.P. – Multi-lumen Proximal
R.F.A. or L.F.A. – Right or Left Forearm	P. – Push			
R.U.A. or L.U.A. – Right or Left Upperarm	Cath – Catheter		C.D. – Cutdown	M.L.M. – Multi-lumen Middle
R.F. or L.F. – Right or Left Foot				
R.S., L.S. or M.S. – Right, Left or Mid Scalp			I.C. – Intracath	M.L.D. – Multi-lumen Distal
R.F.V. or L.F.V. – Right or Left Femoral Vein				
R.A.C. or L.A.C. – Right or Left Antecubital			I.P. – Infuse A Port	I. – Introducer
R.W. or L.W. – Right or Left Wrist	NA – Not Applicable			

Document on each site once each shift & P.R.N.   No space is to be left blank.   Place "NA" in spaces which do not apply.

Date	Time	I.V. Site Start / d/c	Site Code	Cath Size	Type Code	Site Day	Cap Change	Dressing Change	I.V. Site: s̄ tenderness redness, edema, drainage	Signature

Figure 31-6, cont'd IV maintenance record.

Regulating Intravenous Flow Rate

Delegation Considerations
The skill of regulating IV therapy requires problem solving and knowledge application unique to professional nursing. For this procedure delegation is not appropriate.

Equipment
▪ Watch with second hand
▪ Paper and pencil
▪ IV infusion pump (optional)
▪ Volume control device (optional)

STEPS	RATIONALE
1. Observe for patency of IV line and needle or catheter:	For fluid to infuse at proper rate, IV line and needle must be free of kinks, knots, and clots.
a. Open drip regulator and observe for rapid flow of fluid from solution into drip chamber, then close drip regulator to prescribed rate.	Rapid flow of fluid into drip chamber indicates patency of IV line. Closing drip chamber to prescribed rate prevents fluid overload.
b. Compress cannulated vein slightly proximal to the end of the catheter and observe the drip chamber.	Cessation of drops from drip chamber indicates catheter or needle is in vein. If fluid continues to drip, infiltration may be present and further assessment is needed.
2. Check client's medical record for correct solution, additives, and time of infusion. Usual order includes solution for 24 hours, usually divided into 2 or 3 L. Occasionally, IV order contains only 1 L to keep vein open (KVO). Record also shows time over which each liter is to infuse.	"Five rights" for drug administration ensure correct fluids are given to correct client.
3. Check client's knowledge of how positioning of the IV site affects flow rate.	Fosters client participation in maintaining most effective position of arm with IV equipment.
4. Verify with client how venipuncture site feels (e.g., determine if there is pain or burning).	Pain or burning may be early indication of phlebitis. Includes client in decision making.
5. Have paper and pencil to calculate flow rate.	The beginning student is unfamiliar with IV fluid rates and should use mathematical calculations to obtain correct rate.

6. Know calibration (drop factor) in drops per milliliter (gtt/ml) of infusion set:
Microdrip: 60 gtt/ml
Macrodrip: (Metheny, 1992):
  Abbott: 15 gtt/ml
  Travenol: 10 gtt/ml
  McGaw: 15 gtt/ml
	Microdrip tubing, also called pediatric tubing, universally delivers 60 gtt/ml and is used when small or very precise volumes are to infused. However, there are different commercial parenteral administration sets for macrodrip tubing. Macrodrip tubing should be used when large quantities or fast rates are necessary.

CRITICAL DECISION POINT

Know which company's infusion set your agency uses.

7. Select one of the following formulas to calculate flow rate after determining ml/hr:
ml/hr = total infusion (ml)/hour of infusion
  (a) ml/hr/60 minutes = ml/minute
  (b) Drop factor × ml/minute = drops/minute
          OR
ml/hr × drop factor/60 minutes = drops/minute
	Once hourly rate has been determined, these formulas give correct flow rate.

Continued

Skill 31-2—cont'd
Regulating Intravenous Flow Rate

STEPS	RATIONALE

8. Read physician's orders and follow "five rights" for correct solution and proper additives.
IV fluids are usually ordered for 24-hour period, indicating how long each liter of fluid should run; for example, IV order for client is:
  Bottle 1: 1000 ml D_5W with 20 mEq KCl to run 8 hours
  Bottle 2: 1000 ml D_5W with 20 mEq KCl to run 8 hours
  Bottle 3: 1000 ml D_5W with 20 mEq KCl to run 8 hours
  Total 24-hour IV intake: 3000 ml
	IV fluids are medications; following "five rights" decreases chance of medication error.
	Determines volume of fluid that should infuse hourly.

9. Determine hourly rate by dividing volume by hours; for example:
  1000 ml/8 = 125 ml/hr
  or if 3 L is ordered for 24 hours
  3000/24 = 125 ml = 125 ml/hour
	Provides even infusion of fluid over prescribed hourly rate.

10. Place adhesive or fluid indicator tape on IV bottle or bag next to volume markings (see illustration).	Time taping IV bag gives nurse visual cue as to whether fluids are being administered over correct period of time. Time tapes should be used for all IV infusions, including those on therapies infused via electronic infusion devices.

CRITICAL DECISION POINT

Do not use felt-tip pens or permanent markers on IV bags, because ink could contaminate the solution (Millam, 1992).

11. After hourly rate has been determined, calculate minute rate based on drop factor of infusion set. Microdrip infusion set has a drop factor of 60 gtt/ml. Regular drip or macrodrip infusion set used in this example has drop factor of 15 gtt/ml.	Allows nurse to calculate minute flow rate based on this formula: Total volume × Drop factor/infusion time in minutes

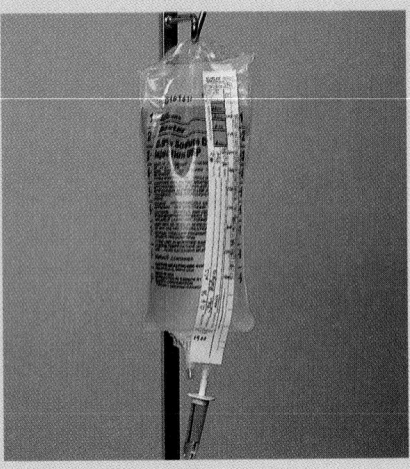

Step 10

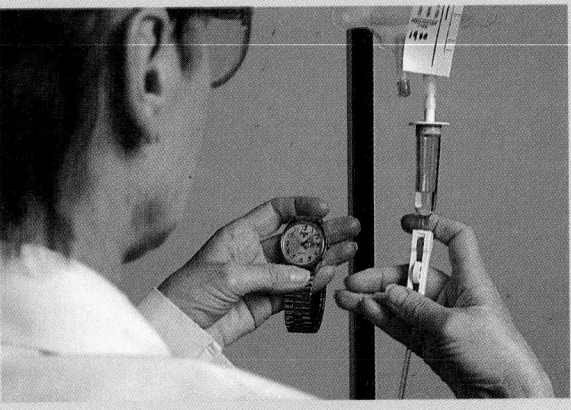

Step 12

STEPS	RATIONALE

Using formula, calculate minute flow rates: Bottle 1:1000 ml with 20 mEq KCl

Microdrip:

125 ml × 60 gtt/ml/60 minutes =

7500 gtt/60 minutes = 125 gtt/minute

When using microdrip, ml/hour always equals gtt/minute.

Macrodrip:

125 ml × 15 gtt/ml/60 minutes =

31 to 32 gtt/minute

Volume is multiplied by drop factor and the product is divided by time (in minutes).

12. Time flow rate by counting drops in drip chamber for 1 minute by watch, then adjust roller clamp to increase or decrease rate of infusion (see illustration).

Determines if fluids are administered too slowly or too fast.

13. Follow this procedure for infusion controller or pump:

    a. Place electonic eye on drip chamber below origin of drop and above fluid level in chamber, or consult manufacturer's directions for setup of the infusion (see illustration). If a controller is used, ensure that IV bag is 36 inches above the IV site.

The electronic eye counts the number of drops flowing from administration set to ensure that proper rate infuses. IV controller works by gravity.

    b. IV infusion tubing is placed within ridges of control box in direction of flow (i.e., portion of tubing nearest IV bag at top and portion of tubing nearest client at bottom) or consult manufacturer's directions for use of pump (see illustration). Required drops per minute or volume per hour are selected, door to control chamber is closed, power button is turned on, and start button is pressed.

Infusion pumps move fluid by compressing and milking IV tubing, thus propelling fluid through tubing.

Continued

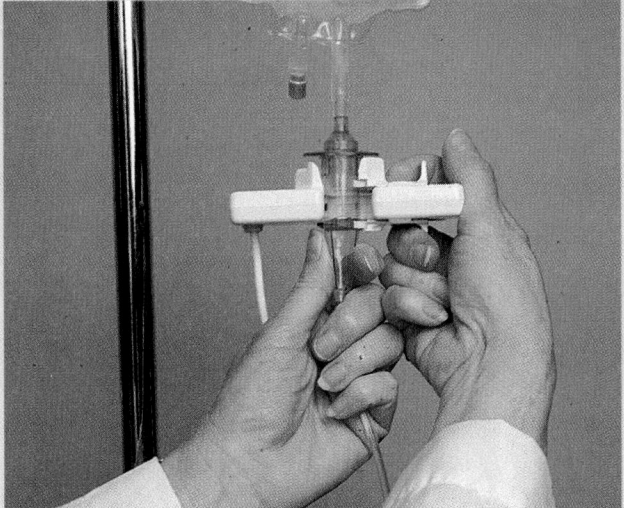

Step 13a

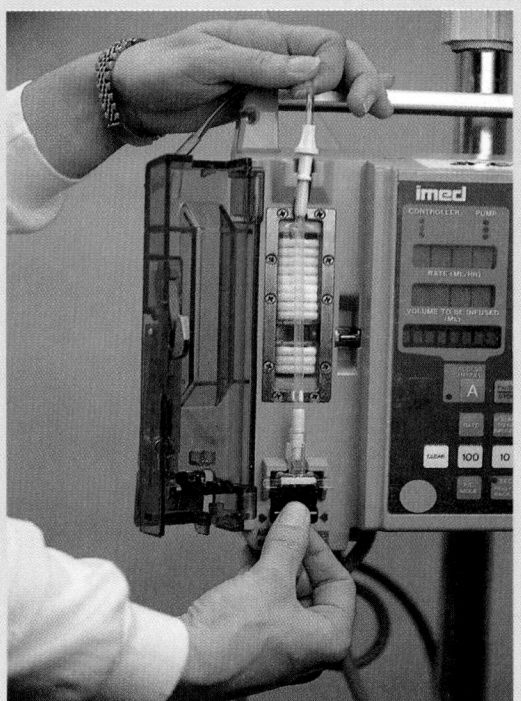

Step 13b

.... Skill 31-2—cont'd
Regulating Intravenous Flow Rate

STEPS	RATIONALE

CRITICAL DECISION POINT

Special infusion tubing is required for some pumps (check agency policy).

c. Drip regulator must be open while infusion controller or pump is in use.

d. Monitor infusion rates and IV site for infiltration according to agency policy.

Infusion controllers or pumps are not infallible and do not replace frequent, accurate nursing assessments. Infusion pumps may continue to infuse IV fluids after an infiltration has begun.

e. Assess patency and integrity of system when alarm sounds.

Alarm indicates that electronic eye has not noted precise number of drops from drip chamber, or there is an empty solution bag or bottle, kink in tubing, closed drip regulator, infiltrated or clotted needle, and/or air in the tubing.

14. Follow this procedure for volume control device:

a. Place volume control device between IV bag and insertion spike of infusion set (see illustration).

Reduces risk of sudden increase in fluid volume.

b. Place 2 hours' allotment of fluid into device.

Prevents IV line from running dry if nurse does not return in exactly 60 minutes. In addition, if there is accidental increase in flow rate, client receives at most only a 2-hour allotment of fluid.

c. Assess system at least hourly; add fluid to volume control device. Regulate flow rate.

Maintains patency of system.

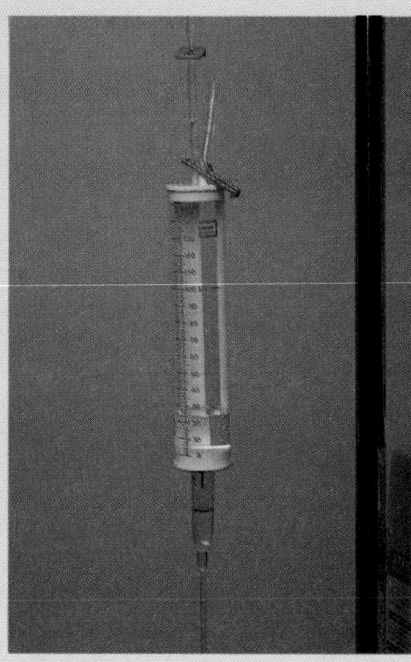

Step 14a

STEPS	RATIONALE
15. Observe client for signs of overhydration or dehydration to determine response to therapy and restoration of fluid and electrolyte balance.	Signs and symptoms of dehydration or overhydration warrant changing rate of fluid infused.
16. Evaluate for signs of infiltration: inflammation at site, clot in catheter, kink or knot in infusion tubing.	Prevents decrease or cessation of flow rate.

Recording and Reporting

- Record name of solution, rate of infusion, drops/minute, and ml/hour in nurse's notes every 4 hours or according to agency policy.
- Immediately record in nurse's notes any new IV fluid rates.
- Document use of any EID or controlling device and number on that device.
- At change of shift or when leaving on break, report rate of infusion to nurse in charge or next nurse assigned to care for client.

Home Care Considerations

- Ensure that client is able and willing to operate the EID (if applicable) and administer IV therapy or that there is a reliable care giver or nursing support personnel at home to provide this IV therapy care.
- Teach client and primary care giver to time drops per minute using watch with second hand.

alarms to alert the nurse to increased system pressure that can occur with an infiltration (IV fluid seeping into the tissue instead of the vascular space).

A second type of infusion device is an IV controller (i.e., dial-a-flow) that delivers fluid with the aid of gravity. IV controllers deliver fluids based on a determination of ml/hr. The rate of infusion with an IV controller depends on the height of the IV fluid container, IV tubing size, and fluid viscosity. The IV controller is less precise than the IV pump in delivering IV fluids with precision. With either device, the client requires close monitoring to verify the correct infusion of the IV solution and to detect the occurrence of any complication.

Patency of the IV needle or catheter means that there are no clots at the tip of the needle or catheter and that the catheter or needle tip is not against the vein wall. A blocked catheter or needle can affect the rate of infusion of the IV fluids. IV flow rates can also be affected by the patency of the IV needle or catheter, infiltration, a knot or kink in the tubing, the height of the solution, and the position of the client's extremity. The nurse can assess patency by lowering the IV bag below the level of the IV insertion site and observing for a blood return. If no blood return occurs and fluid does not flow easily from the drip chamber when the roller clamp is opened, several problems may exist: a too-tight IV

dressing may be impeding the flow, a clot may be occluding the cannula of the IV catheter, or the catheter tip may be occluded against the wall of the vein. The tubing and area around the insertion site should be inspected for anything that could obstruct the flow of IV fluids. A knot or kink in the tubing can decrease the flow rate. Occasionally the tubing is kinked under a dressing, which requires the nurse to remove the dressing to locate the problem. The flow rate frequently resumes after the tubing is straightened. The client may also occlude the tubing by lying or sitting on it. The height of the IV bag can also affect flow rates. Raising the bag usually increases the rate because of increased hydrostatic pressure.

The position of the extremity, particularly at the wrist or elbow, can decrease flow rates. Occasionally the use of an arm board helps to keep the joint extended. Sometimes it is more comfortable for the client to have an infusion started in a new location rather than dealing with a site that causes problems. However, before discontinuing the infusion hampered by an extremity position, the nurse should start the infusion in another site to verify that the client has other accessible veins.

An infiltration may be present when the insertion site is cool, clammy, swollen, and in some cases painful. An infiltration occurs when the needle or catheter has dislodged from the vein and is in the subcutaneous space. When an infiltration occurs, the IV line must be discontinued and a new line inserted. Factors that alter IV flow rates can occur with any client at any time. When caring for a client with an infusion, the nurse should assess the site and the infusion rate at least every hour.

Children, older adults, clients with severe head trauma, and clients susceptible to volume overload must be protected from sudden increases in infusion volumes. The nurse needs to understand that when certain IV controller devices are opened, the IV fluid will infuse rapidly. If this is not controlled, an excessive amount of solution can infuse. Sudden increases can occur accidentally. For example, a restless client may loosen the roller clamp with a sudden movement and increase the flow rate, or the flow rate may be accidentally increased if the client ambulates. A sudden increase in IV infusion rate causes a rapid increase in vascular volume, which can make the client critically ill or even cause death. Volume control devices, such as a Volutrolor buret, can prevent sudden excessive increases in the volume of IV solution infused.

Maintaining the system. After the IV line is in place and the flow rate is regulated, the nurse must maintain the system. This is achieved by (1) keeping the system sterile; (2) changing solutions, tubing, and site dressings; and (3) assisting the client with self-care activities so as to not disrupt the system.

The nurse plays an important role in maintaining the integrity of an IV to prevent infection from developing. Figure 31-7 demonstrates the potential sites for contamination of an intravascular device. The client's microflora and contamination by insertion are initially controlled for in the procedure for IV insertion. However, the other factors are controlled through conscientious use of infection-control principles. This begins

with the use of thorough hand washing before and after the nurse handles any component of the IV system.

The integrity of the IV system must always be maintained. The nurse never disconnects a tubing because it becomes tangled or because it might be more convenient in positioning or moving a client. If a client needs more room to maneuver, extension tubings can be added to an IV line. Stopcocks are available for connecting more than one IV solution to a single IV access site. An IV tubing should be inserted into each port on a stopcock; otherwise the port should be plugged with a sterile cap. Do not allow a port to remain exposed to air.

IV tubing also contains injection ports through which needles can be inserted for medication injection. An injection port must be cleaned thoroughly with 70% alcohol or povidone-iodine solution before accessing the system (Pearson, 1996).

Clients receiving IV therapy over several days will require frequent changing of solutions. It is important for the nurse to organize tasks so that this can be done in plenty of time before the solution runs out and possibly becomes clotted. The CDC (Pearson, 1996) has no recommendation for the hang time of IV fluids; however, the nurse should refer to agency policy. Skill 31-3 reviews steps for changing IV solutions.

IV tubing administration sets can remain sterile for 72 hours (Pearson, 1996). The exception is tubing containing blood, blood products, and lipid emulsions, which are more likely to promote bacterial growth. Agency policy may require more frequent tubing changes. It is easier to change tubing when a new IV bag or bottle is being hung (Skill 31-3). To prevent entry of bacteria into the bloodstream, sterility must be maintained during tubing and solution changes.

The dressings over IV sites are applied to reduce the

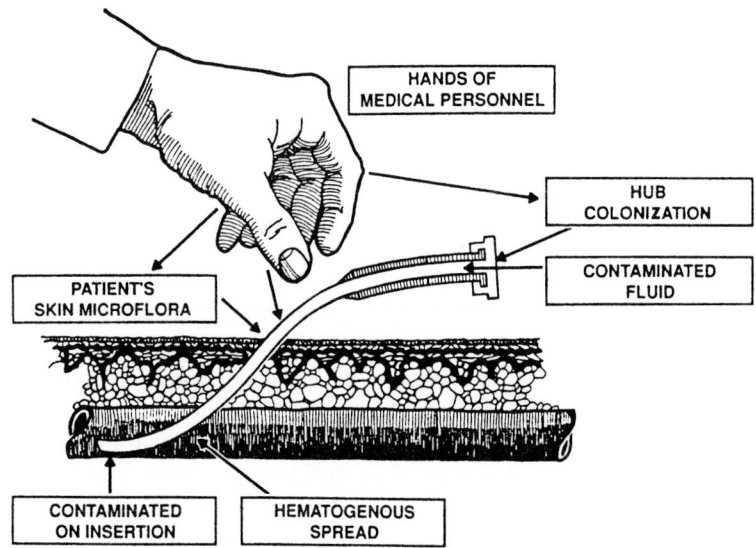

Figure 31-7. Potential sites for contamination of an intravascular device.

Changing Intravenous Solution and Infusion Tubing

Delegation Considerations
The skill of changing IV solutions and tubing requires problem solving and knowledge application unique to professional nursing. For this procedure delegation is not appropriate.

Equipment
IV infusion
- Bottle/bag of IV solution as ordered by physician
- Time tape

- Infusion tubing
- 0.22 μm filter and extension tubing (if necessary)

Heparin flush
- Injection cap, loop, or short extension tubing (if necessary)

Normal saline flush
- Syringes
- 2 sterile 2 × 2 gauze pads
- Tape
- Disposable nonsterile gloves

STEPS	RATIONALE
Changing IV Solution	
1. Check physician's orders.	Ensures that correct solution will be used.
2. If order is written for KVO or to keep open (TKO), note date and time when solution was last changed.	A hang time is no longer recommended by the CDC (Pearson, 1996) to ensure sterility of solutions in bag or bottle. Refer to agency policy.
3. Determine the compatibility of all IV fluids and additives by consulting appropriate literature or the pharmacy.	Incompatibilities can cause physical, chemical, and therapeutic client changes.
4. Determine client's understanding of need for continued IV therapy.	Reveals need for client instruction.
5. Assess patency of current IV access site.	If patency is not verified, a new IV access site may be needed. Notify physician.
6. Have next solution prepared at least 1 hour before needed. If prepared in pharmacy, be sure it has been delivered to the client's hospital unit. Check that solution is correct and properly labeled. Check solution expiration date.	Adequate planning reduces risk of clot formation in vein caused by empty IV bag. Checking prevents medication error.
7. Prepare to change solution when less than 50 ml of fluid remains in bottle or bag.	Prevents air from entering tubing and vein from clotting from lack of flow.
8. Prepare client and family by explaining the procedure, its purpose, and what is expected of client.	Decreases anxiety and promotes cooperation.
9. Be sure drip chamber is at least half full.	Provides fluid to vein while bag is changed.
10. Wash hands.	Reduces transmission of microorganisms.
11. Prepare new solution for changing. If using plastic bag, remove protective cover from IV tubing port. If using glass bottle, remove metal cap and metal and rubber disks.	Permits quick, smooth, and organized change from old to new solution.
12. Move roller clamp to stop flow rate.	Prevents solution remaining in drip chamber from emptying while changing solutions.
13. Remove old IV fluid container from IV pole.	Brings work to nurse's eye level.
14. Quickly remove spike from old solution bag or bottle and, without touching tip, insert spike into new bag or bottle.	Reduces risk of solution in drip chamber running dry and maintains sterility.

CRITICAL DECISION POINT

If spike is contaminated, a new IV tubing set is required.

Continued

.... **Skill 31-3—cont'd**
Changing Intravenous Solution and Infusion Tubing

STEPS	RATIONALE
15. Hang new bag or bottle of solution.	Gravity assists with delivery of fluid into drip chamber.
16. Check for air in tubing. If bubbles form, they can be removed by closing the roller clamp, stretching the tubing downward, and tapping the tubing with the finger (the bubbles rise in the fluid to the drip chamber) (see illustration). For a larger amount of air, insert a needle and syringe into a port below the air and aspirate the air into the syringe. Swab port with alcohol and allow to dry before inserting needle into port. Reduce air in tubing by priming slowly instead of allowing a wide-open flow.	Reduces risk of air embolus. Use of an air-eliminating filter also reduces this risk.
17. Make sure drip chamber is one-third to one-half full. If the drip chamber is too full, pinch off tubing below the drip chamber, invert the container, squeeze the drip chamber (see illustration), hang up the bottle, and release the tubing.	Reduces risk of air entering tubing.
18. Regulate flow to prescribed rate.	Maintains measures to restore fluid balance and deliver IV fluid as ordered.
19. Observe client for signs of overhydration or dehydration to determine response to IV fluid therapy.	Provides ongoing evaluation of client's fluid and electrolyte status.
20. Observe IV system for patency and development of complications (e.g., infiltration or phlebitis).	Provides ongoing evaluation of IV system.

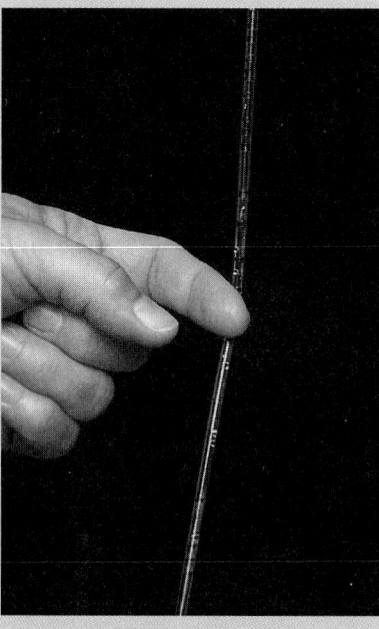

Step 16

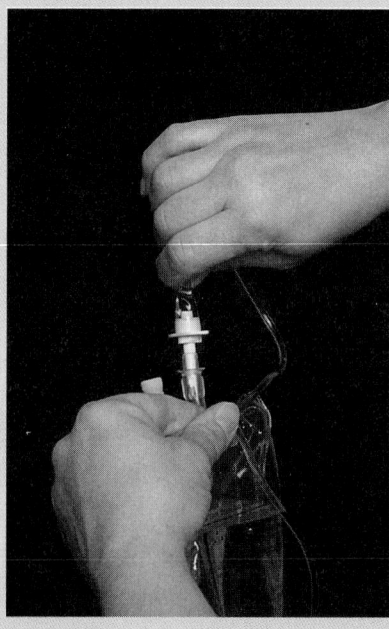

Step 17

STEPS	RATIONALE
Changing IV Tubing	
21. Determine when new infusion set is needed:	The CDC (Pearson, 1996) recommends tubing change no more often than 72-hour intervals.
a. Agency policy will indicate frequency of routine change for IV administration sets and heparin flushes.	
b. Puncture of infusion tubing.	Punctured tubing results in fluid leakage and bacterial contamination.
c. Contamination of tubing.	Contamination of tubing allows entry of bacteria into client's bloodstream.
22. Observe for occlusions in tubing. Such occlusions can occur after infusion of packed red cells, whole blood, albumin, or other blood components.	Whole blood or blood component product can occlude or partially occlude tubing, because viscous solutions adhere to walls of tubing and decrease the size of the lumen.
23. Prepare client and family by explaining the procedure, its purpose, and what is expected of client.	Decreases anxiety, promotes cooperation, and prevents sudden movement of extremity, which could dislodge IV needle or catheter.
24. Wash hands.	Reduces transmission of microorganisms.
25. Open new infusion set, keeping protective coverings over infusion spike and connector and connector site for butterfly needle or IV catheter.	Provides nurse with ready access to new infusion set and maintains sterility of infusion set.
26. Apply nonsterile, disposable gloves.	Reduces risk of exposure to HIV, hepatitis, and other blood-borne bacteria (CDC, 1987; Garner, 1996).
27. If needle or catheter hub is not visible, remove IV dressing. Do not remove tape securing needle or catheter to skin.	Needle hub must be accessible to provide smooth transition when removing old and inserting new tubing.
28. For IV infusion:	
a. Move roller clamp on new IV tubing to "off" position.	Prevents spillage of solution after bag or bottle is spiked.
b. Slow rate of infusion by regulating drip rate on old tubing. Be sure rate is at KVO rate.	Prevents complete infusion of solution that remains in tubing, which can increase risk of occlusion of IV catheter or needle.
c. With old tubing in place, compress drip chamber and fill chamber.	Provides surplus of fluid in drip chamber so there is enough fluid to maintain IV patency while changing tubing.
d. Remove old tubing from solution and hang or tape drip chamber on IV pole 36 inches above IV site.	Allows fluid to continue to flow through IV catheter while nurse is preparing new tubing.
e. Place insertion spike of new tubing into old solution bag opening and hang solution bag on IV pole.	Permits flow of fluid from solution into new infusion tubing.
f. Compress and release drip chamber on new tubing; slowly fill drip chamber one-third to one-half full.	Allows drip chamber to fill and promotes rapid, smooth flow of solution through new tubing.
g. Slowly open roller clamp, remove protective cap from needle adapter (if necessary), and flush tubing with solution. Replace cap.	Removes air from tubing and replaces it with fluid.
h. Turn roller clamp on old tubing to "off" position.	Prevents spillage of fluid as tubing is removed from needle hub.

Continued

Changing Intravenous Solution and Infusion Tubing

STEPS	RATIONALE
29. For heparin lock: a. If a loop or short extension tubing is needed because of an awkward IV site placement, use sterile technique to connect the new injection cap to the loop or tubing. b. Swab injection cap with alcohol. Insert syringe with 1 to 3 ml saline and inject through the injection cap into the loop or short extension tubing.	Removes air to prevent introduction into the vein.
30. Stabilize hub of catheter or needle and apply pressure over vein just above insertion site. Gently pull out old tubing (see illustration). Maintain stability of hub and quickly insert needle adapter of new tubing or heparin lock into hub (see illustration).	Prevents accidental displacement of catheter or needle. Prevents clot formation in catheter or needle and back flow of blood.
31. Open roller clamp on new tubing. Allow solution to run rapidly for 30 to 60 seconds.	Permits IV solution to enter catheter to prevent catheter occlusion.
32. Regulate IV drip according to physician's orders and monitor rate hourly.	Maintains infusion flow at prescribed rate.
33. If necessary, apply new dressing.	Reduces risk of bacterial infection from skin.
34. Discard old tubing in proper container.	Reduces accidental transmission of microorganisms.
35. Remove and dispose of gloves. Wash hands.	Reduces transmission of microorganisms.
36. Evaluate flow rate and observe connection site for leakage.	Maintains prescribed rate of flow of IV fluid and determines if fit is secure.

Recording and Reporting

▪ Record changing of tubing and solution on client's record. A special parenteral therapy flow sheet may be used.

▪ Place a piece of tape or preprinted label with the date and time of tubing change and attach to tubing below the level of drip chamber.

Home Care Considerations

▪ Emphasize to client and family the importance of changing solutions when IV tubing still contains fluid.

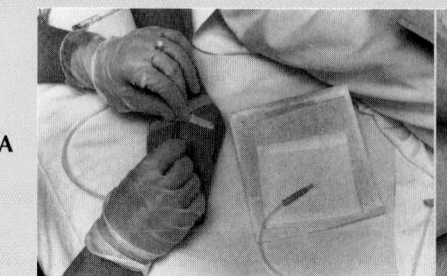 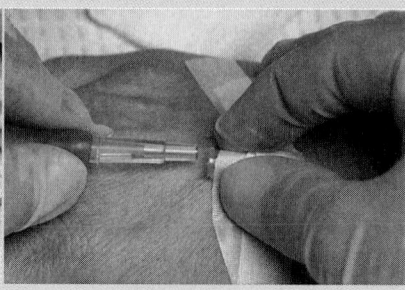

Step 30

entrance of bacteria into the insertion site. The two forms of dressings are gauze and transparent. Transparent dressings reliably secure the IV device, allow continuous visual inspection of the IV site, become less easily soiled or moistened, and require less frequent changes than standard gauze (Pearson, 1996). Either form of dressing must be changed when the IV device is removed or replaced or when the dressing becomes damp, loosened, or soiled (Pearson, 1996). Agency policy may require IV dressings to be routinely changed within a certain time frame (e.g., 48 to 72 hours) (Skill 31-4).

To prevent the accidental disruption of an IV system, the nurse may need to assist the client with hygiene, comfort measures, meals, and ambulation. Because a client with an infusion in the arm finds it difficult to meet hygiene needs, the nurse should help with bathing and changing gowns. It helps to use a gown specifically made with snaps along the top sleeve seam to facilitate changing the gown without disturbing the venipuncture site. Regular gowns are changed by following these six steps for maximum arm mobility and speed:

1. Remove the sleeve of the gown from the arm without the IV.
2. Remove the sleeve of the gown from the arm with the IV.
3. Remove the IV bottle or bag from its stand and pass it and the tubing through the sleeve. (If this involves removing the tubing from an IV pump, use the roller clamp to slow the infusion to prevent the accidental infusion of a large volume of solution or medication).
4. Place the IV bottle or bag and tubing through the sleeve of the clean gown and hang it on its stand. (If the IV is connected to a pump, reassemble and open the roller clamp. Turn the pump on.)
5. Place the arm with the IV through the gown sleeve.
6. Place the arm without the IV through the gown sleeve. (Breaking the integrity of an IV line to change a gown leads to contamination.)

The client with an arm or a hand infusion is able to walk, unless contraindicated. A walking IV pole (a standard IV pole with wheels) is needed. The nurse helps the client get out of bed and places the pole next to the involved arm. The client is instructed to hold on to the pole with the involved hand and to push it while walking. The nurse should assess the equipment to make sure that the IV bag is at the proper height, that there is no tension on the tubing, and that the flow rate is correct. The nurse should instruct the client to report any blood in the tubing, a stoppage in the flow, or increased discomfort. IV catheters and drugs, especially antibiotics and potassium, can cause discomfort and burning sensations at the IV site. Clients must be reassured that

occasional discomfort is normal. Sometimes discomfort is relieved by repositioning the extremity, but occasionally it is necessary to start a new IV line in a larger vein.

Complications of intravenous therapy. An **infiltration** occurs when IV fluids enter the subcutaneous space around the venipuncture site. This is manifested as swelling (from increased tissue fluid) and pallor (caused by decreased circulation) around the venipuncture site. Fluid may be flowing through the IV line at a decreased rate or may have stopped flowing. Pain may also be present and usually results from edema and increases proportionately as the infiltration continues.

When infiltration occurs, the infusion must be discontinued and, if IV therapy is still necessary, the catheter or needle is reinserted into another extremity. To reduce discomfort, the nurse raises the extremity, which promotes venous drainage. To help decrease the edema, the nurse wraps the extremity in a warm towel for 20 minutes, which increases circulation and reduces pain and edema.

Phlebitis is an inflammation of the vein. Selected risk factors for phlebitis include the type of catheter material, chemical irritation of additives and drugs given intravenously (e.g., antibiotics), and the anatomical position of the catheter. Placement of the IV at the wrist creates the highest risk (Maki and Ringer, 1991). Signs and symptoms include pain, increased skin temperature over the vein, and, in some instances, redness traveling along the path of the vein. When phlebitis develops, the IV line must be discontinued and a new line inserted in another vein. Warm, moist heat on the site of phlebitis can offer some relief to the client (see Chapter 38). Phlebitis can be dangerous, because blood clots (thrombophlebitis) can occur and in some cases may result in emboli. Phlebitis is prevented by the routine removal and rotation of IV sites. The CDC (Pearson, 1996) recommends replacing peripheral venous catheters and rotating sites every 48 to 72 hours.

FVE occurs when the client has received a too-rapid administration of IV solutions. The assessment findings include shortness of breath, crackles in the lungs, and tachycardia. The nurse should slow the rate of infusion, notify the physician, raise the head of the bed, and monitor vital signs.

Bleeding can occur around the venipuncture site during the infusion or through the catheter, needle, or tubing if these become inadvertently disconnected. Bleeding is common in clients who have received heparin or who have a bleeding disorder. If bleeding occurs around the venipuncture site and the catheter is within the vein, a pressure dressing may be applied over the site to control the bleeding. Bleeding from a vein is usually a slow, continuous seepage and is not serious.

Discontinuing intravenous infusions. Discontinuing an infusion is necessary after the prescribed amount of fluid has been infused, when an infiltration occurs, if phlebitis is present, or if the infusion catheter

Changing a Peripheral Intravenous Dressing

Delegation Considerations
The skill of changing a peripheral IV dressing requires problem solving and knowledge application unique to professional nursing. For this procedure delegation is not appropriate.

Equipment
- Povidone-iodine swab stick
- Alcohol swab stick
- Adhesive remover (if needed)
- Strips of nonallergenic tape
- Disposable gloves

For gauze dressing
- Sterile 2 × 2 gauze pad
  OR
- Sterile 4 × 4 gauze pad

For transparent dressing
- Sterile transparent dressing

STEPS	RATIONALE
1. Determine when dressing was last changed. Many institutions require nurse to write date and time on dressing and date the device was first placed.	Provides information regarding length of time present dressing has been in place. In addition, nurse is able to plan for dressing change.
2. Observe present dressing for moisture and intactness.	Moisture is a medium for bacterial growth and renders dressing contaminated.
3. Observe IV system for proper functioning or complications: kinks in infusion tubing or IV catheter. Palpate the catheter site through the intact dressing for inflammation or subjective complaints of pain or burning.	Unexplained decrease in flow rate requires the nurse to investigate placement and patency of the IV catheter. Pain can be associated with both phlebitis and infiltration.
4. Inspect exposed catheter site for swelling or infiltration.	Indicates fluid infusing into surrounding tissues. Will require removal of IV catheter.
5. Assess client's understanding of need for continued IV infusion.	Determines need for client instruction.
6. Explain procedure and purpose to client and family. Explain that affected extremity must be held still and how long procedure will take.	Decreases anxiety, promotes cooperation, and gives client time frame around which personal activities can be planned.
7. Wash hands. Apply disposable gloves.	Reduces transmission of microorganisms.
8. Remove tape, gauze, and/or transparent dressing from old dressing one layer at a time, leaving tape that secures IV needle or catheter in place. Be cautious if catheter tubing becomes tangled between two layers of dressing.	Prevents accidental displacement of catheter or needle.
9. Observe insertion site for signs and/or symptoms of infection, namely redness, swelling, and exudate.	

STEPS	RATIONALE
10. If infiltration, phlebitis, or clot occurs or if ordered by physician, discontinue infusion.	
11. If IV is infusing properly, gently remove tape securing needle or catheter. Stabilize needle or catheter with one finger. Use adhesive remover to cleanse skin and remove adhesive residue, if needed.	Exposes venipuncture site. Stabilization prevents accidental displacement of catheter or needle. Adhesive residue decreases ability of new tape to adhere tightly to skin.
12. Keep one finger over catheter at all times until tape is replaced.	Prevents decannulation from vein.
13. Using circular motion, cleanse peripheral IV insertion site with alcohol, then povidone-iodine solution starting at insertion site and working outward creating concentric circles. Allow each solution to dry for 2 minutes.	Circular motion prevents cross-contamination from skin bacteria near venipuncture site. Povidone-iodine is a topical antiinfective that reduces skin surface bacteria; the solution must be dry to be effective in reducing microbial counts (Baranowski, 1993).

CRITICAL DECISION POINT

Do not tape over connection of access tubing or port to IV catheter.

14. Gauze dressing:	
a. Place single strip of ½-inch nonallergenic tape under peripheral IV catheter with sticky side up to anchor IV catheter or needle.	Prevents accidental displacement of catheter or needle.
b. Place a second piece of sterile tape directly across catheter at hub.	Further prevents accidental displacement of catheter.
c. Place 2 × 2 or 4 × 4 gauze over venipuncture site.	Provides barrier against bacteria.
15. Transparent dressing:	
a. Place a piece of sterile tape directly across catheter hub.	Further prevents accidental displacement of catheter.
b. Place transparent dressing over venipuncture site. Apply in the direction of hair growth.	Provides barrier against bacteria. Reduces discomfort when dressing is removed.
16. Remove and discard gloves.	
17. Anchor IV tubing with additional pieces of tape. When using polyurethane dressing, minimize the tape placed over dressing.	Prevents accidental displacement of IV needle or catheter or separation of IV tubing from needle adapter.
18. Place date and time of dressing change and size and gauge of catheter directly on dressing.	Documents dressing change.
19. Discard equipment and wash hands.	Reduces transmission of microorganisms.
20. Observe functioning and patency of IV system in response to changing dressing.	Validates that IV is patent and functioning correctly.
21. Monitor client's body temperature.	Elevated temperature indicates an infection that may be associated with bacterial contamination of the venipuncture site.

or needle develops a clot at its tip. The nurse discontinuing an infusion first applies disposable gloves and then removes the tape and dressing in the same manner as for the daily infusion dressing changes. The nurse then moves the roller clamp to the "off"/closed position to prevent spillage of IV fluid. The nurse places a sterile 2×2 gauze pad over the venipuncture site and, using the other hand, withdraws the catheter needle by pulling straight back away from the puncture site. If necessary, alcohol or soap and water can be used to remove dried blood or other drainage from around the site. Alcohol is not used on the IV site, because it can cause stinging and prolongs bleeding (Phillips, 1993). The nurse elevates the extremity and applies pressure to the site for 1 to 2 minutes to control bleeding and prevent hematoma formation. Clients who have received heparin require longer pressure because of the action of heparin on blood-clotting mechanisms. If needed, the nurse applies a bandage over a sterile cotton ball or applies a larger sterile dressing over the venipuncture site. The nurse records the amount of fluid infused and the time of the discontinuation.

Blood replacement. Blood replacement or transfusion is the IV administration of whole blood or a component such as plasma, packed RBCs, or platelets. The objectives for blood transfusions include (1) to increase circulating blood volume after surgery, trauma, or hemorrhage; (2) to increase the number of RBCs and to maintain hemoglobin levels in clients with severe anemia; and (3) to provide selected cellular components as replacement therapy (e.g., clotting factors, platelets, albumin).

Blood groups and types. The most important grouping for transfusion purposes is the ABO system, which includes A, B, O, and AB blood types. The determination of blood groups is based on the presence or absence of A and B red cell antigens. Individuals with A antigens, B antigens, or no antigens belong to groups A, B, and O respectively. The person with A and B antigens has AB blood.

Individuals with type A blood naturally produce anti-B antibodies in their plasma. Similarly, type B individuals naturally produce anti-A antibodies. A type O individual has neither type A nor type B antigen and thus is considered a universal blood donor. An AB type individual produces neither antibody, which is why type AB individuals can be universal recipients and receive any type of blood. If blood that is mismatched with the client's blood is transfused, a **transfusion reaction** occurs. The transfusion reaction is an antigen-antibody reaction and can range from a mild response to severe anaphylactic shock.

Another consideration when matching for blood transfusions is the Rh factor, an antigenic substance in the erythrocytes of most people. A person with the factor is Rh positive, whereas a person without it is Rh negative.

Autologous transfusion. **Autologous transfusion** (autotransfusion) is the collection and reinfusion of a client's own blood. The blood for an autologous transfusion can be obtained by preoperative donation up to 5 weeks before the planned surgery (e.g., open heart, orthopedic, plastic, gynecological). The client donates 1 to 5 units of his or her own blood depending on the type of surgery and the ability of the client to maintain an acceptable hematocrit. The blood will be tested for HIV and HBV. An autologous transfusion can also be obtained during perioperative blood salvage (e.g., during vascular and orthopedic surgery, organ transplant surgery, and traumatic injuries) and reinfused during the surgery. Blood can also be salvaged postoperatively from mediastinal and chest-tube drains and after joint and spinal surgery.

Autologous transfusions are safer for the client because they decrease the risk of complications such as mismatched blood and exposure to blood-borne infectious agents.

Blood transfusions. Transfusing blood or blood components is a nursing procedure. The nurse is responsible for assessment before, during, and after the transfusion and for regulation of the transfusion.

If the client has an IV line in place, the nurse should assess the venipuncture site for signs of infection or infiltration. The nurse should also determine whether the venipuncture was performed with an 18- or 19-gauge catheter. The large catheter is needed because blood is thicker and stickier than IV fluids. The nurse should determine that the IV catheter is patent and functioning properly. The tubing for blood administration has an in-line filter (Figure 31-8). The tubing should be filled with 0.9% normal saline to prevent **hemolysis** of RBCs.

Pretransfusion assessment also includes obtaining information from the client. The nurse asks whether the client knows the reason for the blood transfusion and whether the client has ever had a previous transfusion or transfusion reaction. A client who has had a transfusion reaction is usually at no greater risk for a reaction with a subsequent transfusion. However, the client may be anxious about the transfusion, requiring nursing intervention. Before giving a transfusion, the nurse explains the procedure and instructs the client to report any side effects (e.g., chills, dizziness, fever) once the transfusion begins. The nurse also checks to be sure the client has signed an informed consent.

Because of the danger of transfusion reactions, it is very important to use specific precautions in administering blood or blood products. The nurse must obtain the client's baseline vital signs before the transfusion begins. This data will allow the nurse to determine when changes in vital signs occur, which can indicate that a transfusion reaction is developing. To ensure that the right client receives the correct type of blood or blood product, a thorough procedure is used to check the identity of the blood products, the client, and the

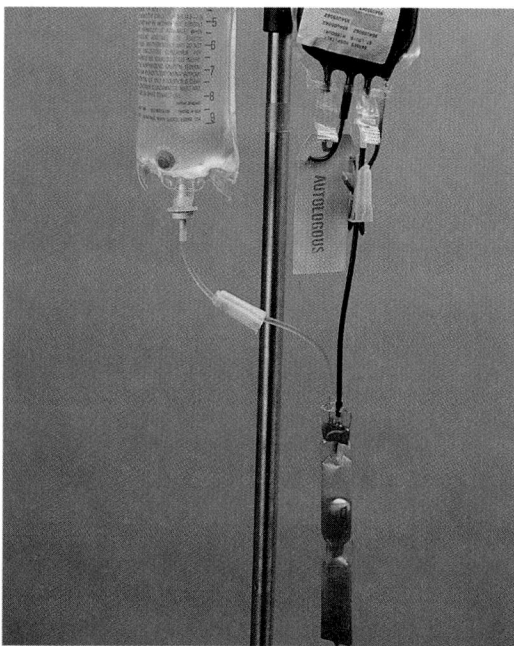

Figure 31-8. Tubing for blood administration has an in-line filter.

compatibility of the blood and the client. The nurse, although not involved in the blood labeling process, is responsible for determining that the blood delivered to the client corresponds to the client's blood type listed in the medical record. Two registered nurses or one registered nurse and a licensed practical nurse (see agency policy) must together check the label on the blood product against the client's identification number, blood group, and complete name. If even a minor discrepancy exists, the blood should not be given and the blood bank is immediately notified.

Initiation of a transfusion begins slowly to allow for the early detection of a transfusion reaction. The nurse maintains the infusion rate, monitors for side effects, assesses vital signs, and promptly records all findings. The nurse usually stays with the client during the first 15 minutes, the time when a reaction is most likely to occur. The nurse will continue to monitor the client and obtain vital signs periodically during the transfusion as directed by agency policy. If a transfusion reaction is anticipated or suspected, the nurse will obtain vital signs more frequently (Table 31-7).

The rate of transfusion is usually specified in the physician's orders. Ideally a unit of whole blood or packed RBCs is tranfused in 2 hours. This time can be lengthened to 4 hours if the client is at risk for FVE. Beyond 4 hours there is a risk of the blood becoming contaminated.

When clients have a severe blood loss such as with hemorrhage, they may receive rapid transfusions through a central venous pressure catheter. A blood-warming device is often necessary, because the tip of the central ve-

nous pressure catheter lies in the superior vena cava, above the right atrium. Rapid administration of cold blood can result in cardiac dysrhythmia (LaRocca and Otto, 1989).

Transfusion reactions. A transfusion reaction is a systemic response by the body to incompatible blood. Causes include red cell incompatibility or allergic sensitivity to the components of the transfused blood or to the potassium or citrate preservative in the blood. Blood transfusion can also result in the transmission of infectious disease. Several types of reactions can result from blood transfusions (see Table 31-7).

A second category of reactions includes diseases transmitted by infected blood donors who are asymptomatic. Diseases transmitted through transfusions are malaria, hepatitis, and AIDS. Because all units of blood collected must undergo serological testing and screening for HIV and HBV, the risk of acquiring blood-borne infections from blood transfusions is reduced.

Circulatory overload is a risk when a client receives massive whole blood or packed RBC transfusions for massive hemorrhagic shock or when a client with normal blood volume receives blood. Clients particularly at risk for circulatory overload are older adults and those with cardiopulmonary diseases.

Blood transfusion reactions are life threatening, but prompt nursing intervention can maintain the client's physiological stability (see Table 31-7):

1. If a blood reaction is suspected, the nurse **stops the transfusion immediately.**
2. The nurse keeps the IV line open by "piggy-backing" 0.9% normal saline directly into the IV line.
3. The nurse **should not** turn off the blood and simply turn on the 0.9% normal saline that is connected to the Y-tubing infusion set. This would cause blood remaining in the Y-tubing to infuse into the client. Even a small amount of mismatched blood can cause a major reaction.
4. The nurse has the physician notified immediately.
5. The nurse remains with the client, observing signs and symptoms and monitoring vital signs as often as every 5 minutes.
6. The nurse prepares to administer emergency drugs such as antihistamines, vasopressors, fluids, and steroids per physician order.
7. The nurse prepares to perform cardiopulmonary resuscitation.
8. The nurse obtains a urine specimen and sends it to the laboratory.
9. The blood container, tubing, attached labels, and transfusion record are saved and returned to the laboratory.
10. The nurse must document the transfusion reaction, how it was treated, and the outcome.

TABLE 31-7
Acute Transfusion Reactions

Reaction	Cause	Clinical Manifestations	Management	Prevention
Acute hemolytic	Infusion of ABO-incompatible whole blood, RBCs, or components containing 10 ml or more of RBCs. Antibodies in the recipient's plasma attach to antigens on transfused RBCs causing RBC destruction.	Chills, fever, low back pain, flushing, tachycardia, tachypnea, hypotension, vascular collapse, hemoglobinuria, hemoglobinemia, bleeding, acute renal failure, shock, cardiac arrest, death.	Treat shock, if present. Draw blood samples for serologic testing slowly to avoid hemolysis from the procedure. Send urine specimen to the laboratory. Maintain BP with IV colloid solutions. Give diuretics as prescribed to maintain urine flow. Insert indwelling catheter or measure voided amounts to monitor hourly urine output. Dialysis may be required if renal failure occurs. Do not transfuse additional RBC-containing components until transfusion service has provided newly crossmatched units.	Meticulously verify and document patient identification from sample collection to component infusion.
Febrile, non-hemolytic (most common)	Sensitization to donor white blood cells, platelets or plasma proteins.	Sudden chills and fever (rise in temperature of greater than 1° C), headache, flushing, anxiety, muscle pain.	Give antipyretics as prescribed—avoid aspirin in thrombocytopenic patients. **Do not restart transfusion.**	Consider leukocyte-poor blood products (filtered, washed, or frozen).
Mild allergic	Sensitivity to foreign plasma proteins.	Flushing, itching, urticaria (hives).	Give antihistamine as directed. If symptoms are mild and transient, transfusion may be restarted slowly. Do not restart transfusion if fever or pulmonary symptoms develop.	Treat prophylactically with antihistamines.
Anaphylactic	Infusion of IgA proteins to IgA-deficient recipient who has developed IgA antibody.	Anxiety, urticaria, wheezing, progressing to cyanosis, shock, possible cardiac arrest.	Initiate CPR, if indicated. Have epinephrine ready for injection (0.4 ml of a 1:1000 solution subcutaneously or 0.1 ml of 1:1000 solution diluted to 10 ml with saline for IV use). **Do not restart transfusion.**	Transfuse extensively washed RBC products, from which all plasma has been removed. Alternatively, use blood from IgA-deficient donor.

From National Blood Resource Education Programs: *Transfusion therapy guidelines for nurses,* NIH Pub. No. 90-2668a, September 1990.
ABO, Blood group consisting of groups A, AB, B, and O; *RBCs,* red blood cells; *BP,* blood pressure; *IV,* intravenous; *IgA,* immunoglobulin A; *CPR,* cardiopulmonary resuscitation.

TABLE 31-7
Acute Transfusion Reactions—cont'd

Reaction	Cause	Clinical Manifestations	Management	Prevention
Circulatory overload	Fluid administered faster than the circulation can accommodate.	Cough, dyspnea, pulmonary congestion (rales), headache, hypertension, tachycardia, distended neck veins.	Place patient upright with feet in dependent position. Administer prescribed diuretics, oxygen, morphine. Phlebotomy may be indicated.	Adjust transfusion volume and flow rate based on patient size and clinical status. Have tranfusion service divide unit into smaller aliquots for better spacing of fluid input.
Sepsis	Transfusion of contaminated blood components.	Rapid onset of chills, high fever, vomiting, diarrhea, and marked hypotension and shock.	Obtain culture of patient's blood and send bag with remaining blood to transfusion service for further study. Treat septicemia as directed—antibiotics, IV fluids, vasopressors, steroids.	Collect, process, store, and transfuse blood products according to blood banking standards and infuse within 4 hr of starting time.

Interventions for acid-base imbalances. Nursing interventions to promote acid-base balance support prescribed medical therapies and are aimed at reversing the acid-base imbalance that exists. Such imbalances can be life threatening and require rapid correction. The nurse must maintain a functional IV line and frequently check the physician's orders for new medications or fluids. Prescribed drugs, such as insulin or sodium bicarbonate, and fluid and electrolyte replacement should be given promptly. Chapter 30 reviews appropriate therapies for clients with respiratory acidosis.

The nurse also monitors clients closely for changes in acid-base balance. Clients with acid-base disturbances usually require repeated ABG analysis. This procedure provides arterial blood samples for analysis of hydrogen ion concentration.

Arterial blood gases. ABG determination requires the removal of a sample of blood from an artery to assess the client's acid-base status and the adequacy of ventilation and oxygenation. Arterial blood is drawn from a peripheral artery (usually the radial) or from an arterial line inserted by a physician. In some agencies, nurses are responsible for radial artery punctures. Beginning nursing students do not draw arterial samples but frequently assist in the sampling process and care for the client after the procedure. After the specimen is obtained, care is taken to prevent air from entering the syringe because this will affect the blood gas analysis. To reduce metabolism of cells, the syringe is submerged in crushed ice and transported immediately to the laboratory. The nurse applies pressure to the puncture site for at least 5 minutes to reduce the risk of hematoma formation. The nurse might also reassess the radial pulse after pressure has been removed.

Restorative care. After experiencing acute alterations in fluid and electrolyte or acid-base balance, clients often require ongoing maintenance to prevent a recurrence of health alterations. Older adults and the chronically ill require special considerations to prevent complications from developing.

Home intravenous therapy. IV therapy is often continued in the home setting for clients requiring long-term hydration, parenteral nutrition (see Chapter 34), or long-term medication administration. A home IV therapy nurse will work closely with the client to ensure that a sterile IV system is maintained and that complications can be avoided or recognized promptly. Box 31-4 summarizes client education guidelines for home IV therapy.

Nutritional support. Most clients who have had electrolyte disorders or metabolic acid-base disturbances require ongoing nutritional support. Depending on the type of disorder, fluid or food intake may be encouraged or restricted (see Chapter 34). The client needs a nutritionally well-balanced diet. If clients are still responsible for preparing their own meals, they should learn to look at the lists of the nutrient content of foods and to read the lables of commercially prepared foods.

BOX 31-4
Client Teaching for Home Intravenous Therapy

- Explain to client and care giver the importance of IV therapy in maintaining hydration and access for the delivery of medications.
- Emphasize the risks involved when the IV system is not kept sterile.
- Be sure the client and/or care giver is able to manipulate the required equipment.
- Instruct client or care giver on how to change IV solutions, tubing, and dressing when they become soiled or dislodged (NOTE: The home health nurse may be able to visit frequently enough to perform scheduled tubing and dressing changes.)
- Instruct client and care giver about signs and symptoms of infiltration, phlebitis, and infection and to notify the home health nurse immediately.
- Instruct client and care giver to notify the home health nurse if the infusion slows or stops or if blood is seen in the tubing.
- Teach client with care giver's assistance how to ambulate, perform hygiene, and participate in other activities of daily living without dislodging or disconnecting catheter and tubing.

Medication safety. Numerous drugs contain constituents or create potential side effects that can alter fluid and electrolyte balance. Clients with chronic disease who are receiving multiple medications and those with renal or liver disorders are at significant risk for alterations to develop. Once clients return to a restorative care setting, whether in the home, long-term care, or a nursing home, drug safety becomes very important. Client and family education is essential to provide information on knowing what is contained in a drug and what side effects to observe for. The nurse should review all medications with clients and encourage them to consult with their local pharmacist, especially if they try a new over-the-counter medication.

▪ Evaluation

Client care. The evaluation of a client's clinical status is especially important if an acute alteration in fluid and electrolyte or acid-base disturbance exists. The client's condition can change very quickly, and the nurse must be able to recognize the signs and symptoms of impending problems. To do this well, the nurse integrates knowledge of known alterations, the effects of medications and fluids, and the client's presenting clinical status. The nurse will perform evaluative measures to determine if changes have occurred from the last client assessment. For example, assessment of heart rate and rhythm, muscle tone, bowel sounds, and peripheral sensation can detect if a client with hypokalemia is showing signs of improvement. The physical signs and symptoms of hypokalemia should begin to disappear or lessen in intensity if the hypokalemia is being managed.

For clients with less acute alterations, evaluation likely occurs over a longer period of time. In this situation the nurse's evaluation may be focused more on behavioral changes (e.g., the client's ability to follow dietary restrictions and medication schedules). The family's ability to anticipate alterations and prevent problems from recurring is also an important element to evaluation.

The client's level of progress determines whether the nurse needs to continue or revise the plan of care. If goals are not met as a result of the failure to meet expected outcomes, the nurse may increase the frequency of an intervention (e.g., provide more fluids to a dehydrated client), introduce a new therapy (e.g., initiate insertion of an IV), or discontinue a therapy (e.g., consult with physician in discontinuing a diuretic). Once outcomes have been met, the nurse can resolve the nursing diagnosis and focus on other priorities.

Client expectations. The nurse routinely reviews with the client his or her success in meeting the client's expectations of care. "Tell me if I have helped you feel more comfortable," is a question that the nurse might raise if the client's expectations revolve around comfort and symptom management. If the client's concerns involve having a better understanding of a chronic problem, the nurse's evaluation might focus on the client's satisfaction with educational offerings. Often the client's level of satisfaction with care also depends on the nurse's success in involving family and friends. If the client has concerns about returning home or to a different care setting, it will be important to evaluate if the client feels prepared for the transition from acute care.

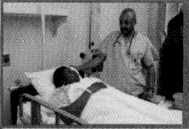

Case Study

Evaluation

Robert returns to the clinical area the next day and evaluates Mrs. Reynolds' progress. She remarks, "I feel much better. I have had no nausea since I saw you last and no diarrhea since yesterday morning." The IV of 0.45% normal saline is still in place, infusing at 125 ml/hour. However, the physician has just visited and ordered the rate to be reduced to 40 ml/hour. Mrs. Reynolds' 24-hour intake since yesterday is 2800 ml, and her output is 2200 ml. During examination Robert notices the oral mucosa is still slightly dry; skin turgor has returned to normal. The perianal area no longer shows redness. Mrs. Reynolds' vital signs are blood pressure 126/78, pulse 88, and respirations 18. She is afebrile. The serum potassium drawn at 6 AM was 4.0.

Robert tells Mrs. Reynolds he is pleased with her progress. He prepares her for breakfast, during which she receives her first soft foods since entering the hospital. Robert plans time to discuss with Mrs. Reynolds the information she has learned from their discussion about food sources for potassium. Robert asks, "After discussing the importance of potassium in your diet, tell me what food you would select that might include potassium." Mrs. Reynolds is again able to identify six different sources of potassium that she would be able to routinely include in her diet.

Documentation Note

Client denies nausea and reports feeling better. No diarrheal stool since yesterday morning. On inspection, oral mucosa remains dry, without lesions or inflammation. Skin turgor is normal. Bowel sounds are normal in all four quadrants, and abdomen is soft to palpation. Perianal area is intact, with no redness. IV of 0.45% normal saline is infusing in left forearm at 125 ml/hour, without tenderness or inflammation at site. Client is able to identify six food sources for potassium to include in her diet.

Key Terms

active transport
aldosterone
angiotensin
anion gap
anions
antidiuretic hormone (ADH)
autologous transfusion
buffer
cations
colloid osmotic pressure
concentration gradient
dehydration
diffusion
electrolyte
extracellular fluids
filtration
fluid volume deficit (FVD)
fluid volume excess (FVE)
hemolysis
homeostasis
hydrostatic pressure
hypertonic
hypotonic
hypovolemia
infiltration

infusion pump
insensible water loss
interstitial fluid
intracellular fluids
intravascular fluid
ions
isotonic
metabolic acidosis
metabolic alkalosis
milliequivalents per liter (mEq/L)
oncotic pressure
osmolality
osmolarity
osmoreceptors
osmosis
osmotic pressure
phlebitis
renin
respiratory acidosis
respiratory alkalosis
sensible water loss
solute
solution
solvent
transfusion reaction
vascular access devices
venipuncture

■ Key Concepts

Body fluids are distributed in ECF and ICF compartments.

Body fluids are composed of electrolytes, minerals, cells, and water.

Body fluids are regulated through fluid intake, output, and hormonal regulation.

Volume disturbances include isotonic and osmolar deficits and excesses.

Electrolytes are regulated by dietary intake and hormonal controls.

Chronic and serious illnesses increase the risk of fluid, electrolyte, and acid-base imbalances.

Clients who are very young or very old are at greater risk for fluid, electrolyte, and acid-base imbalances.

Assessment for fluid, electrolyte, and acid-base alterations includes the nursing history; physical and behavioral assessment; measurements of I&O; daily weights; and specific laboratory data such as measurement of serum osmolality, serum electrolytes, BUN, urine specific gravity, and ABGs.

FVD and osmolar imbalances can be corrected by enteral or parenteral administration of fluid.

Common complications of IV therapy include infiltration, phlebitis, infection, FVE, and bleeding at the infusion site.

Blood transfusions are given to replace fluid volume loss from hemorrhage, treat anemia, or replace coagulation factors.

Administration of blood or blood products requires the nurse to follow a specific procedure to identify transfusion reactions quickly.

In addition to transfusion reactions, the risks of transfusion include hyperkalemia, hypocalcemia, FVE, and infection.

Treatment for electrolyte disturbances includes dietary and pharmacological interventions.

Acid-base balance depends on the hydrogen ion concentration in the blood.

Acid-base imbalances are buffered by chemical, biological, and physiological buffering systems, especially the lungs and kidneys.

The body's chemical buffering system responds first to acid-base abnormalities.

Respiratory acidosis is characterized by increased carbon dioxide and hydrogen ion concentrations.

Respiratory alkalosis is characterized by decreased carbon dioxide and hydrogen ion concentrations.

Metabolic acidosis is characterized by a decrease in bicarbonate level and increase in hydrogen ion concentration.

Metabolic alkalosis is characterized by an increase in bicarbonate level and decrease in hydrogen ion concentration.

The goals of therapy for acid-base imbalances are to treat the underlying illness and to restore the arterial pH to normal.

■ Critical Thinking Activities

1. MaryBeth is a 24-year-old healthy adult. While at work she received a phone call that her husband had been involved in a serious accident. When she got to the hospital, Caroline, the ER nurse, noticed that she was pale, breathing rapidly, and complaining of dizziness. What is the cause of her symptoms? Which intervention would you expect the physician to initiate? How will this correct her problem?

2. Mr. St. John is admitted to the hospital after his wife found him confused, with an increase in his breathing and a fever. She states, "He has had a terrible cold for 2 weeks now." His temperature is 102° F, heart rate 110, respirations 30, and blood pressure 128/64. His serum electrolytes are within normal limits, and his ABG reveals: pH 7.25, PO_2 88, PCO_2 55, HCO_3 24. What does

Mr. St. John's ABG indicate? Why would the physician order a chest x-ray for Mr. St. John? If left untreated, could Mr. St. John's problem be life threatening?

3. Justin is receiving IV fluids because he is NPO after surgery earlier today. His IV fluid order is 1000 ml lactated Ringer's with 20 mEq KCl to run over 8 hours. What IV tubing should be used to administer these fluids in terms of drop size? The nurse hangs a new bag of IV fluids at 5 PM. At 8 PM, the nurse notes that 375 ml has infused from the bag. Are these fluids on time?

4. While starting an IV, Alexandra begins to advance the ONC and notes that the area immediately around the insertion site is swelling. What should she do?

References

Baranowski L: Central venous access device: current technologies, users, and management strategies, *J Intraven Nurs* 16(3):167, 1993.

Centers for Disease Control: Recommendations for prevention of HIV transmission in health care settings, *MMWR* 36 (suppl 25):35, 1987.

Christensen B, Kockrow E: *Foundations of nursing,* ed 2, St. Louis, 1995, Mosby.

Coulter K: Intravenous therapy for the elder patient: implications for the intravenous nurse, *J Intraven Nurs* 15(suppl): S18, 1992.

Garner J: Guideline for isolation precautions in hosptials, *Infect Control Hosp Epidemiol* 17(1):53, 1996.

Gröer MW, Shekleton ME: *Basic pathophysiology: a holistic approach,* St. Louis, 1989, Mosby.

Horne MM and others: *Mosby's pocket guide series: fluid, electrolyte, and acid-base balance,* ed. 3, St. Louis, 1997, Mosby.

Kokko JP, Tannen RL: *Fluids and electrolytes,* Philadelphia, 1990, WB Saunders.

LaRocca JC, Otto SE: *Pocket guide to intravenous therapy,* St. Louis, 1989, Mosby.

Lueckenotte A: *Gerontologic nursing,* St. Louis, 1996, Mosby.

Maki DG, Ringer M: Risk factors for infusion-related phlebitis with small peripheral venous catheters: a randomized controlled trial, *Ann Intern Med* 114(10):845, 1991.

McCance KL, Huether SE: *Pathophysiology: the biologic basis for disease in adults and children,* ed 2, St. Louis, 1994, Mosby.

McKenry LM, Salerno E: *Mosby's pharmacology in nursing,* ed 19, St. Louis, 1995, Mosby.

Metheny NM: *Fluid and electrolyte balance: nursing considerations,* ed 3, Philadelphia, 1992, JB Lippincott.

Millam DA: Controlling the flow: electronic infusion devices, *Nursing 90* 20(8):65, 1990.

Millam DA: Starting IVs: how to develop your venipuncture experience, *Nurs 92* 22(9):33, 1992.

Pearson ML: Hospital infection control practices, Advisory Committee, Guideline for Prevention of Intravascular-Device—Related Infections, *Infect Control Hosp Epidemiol* 17(7):438, 1996.

Phillips LD: *Manual of IV therapeutics,* Philadelphia, 1993, FA Davis.

Price SA, Wilson LM: *Pathophysiology: clinical concepts of disease processes,* ed 3, St. Louis, 1992, Mosby.

Weldy NJ: *Body fluids and electrolytes: a programmed presentation,* ed 7, St. Louis, 1996, Mosby.

Sleep

OBJECTIVES

Mastery of content in this chapter will enable the student to:

- Define the key terms listed.
- Compare the characteristics of rest and sleep.
- Explain the effect the 24-hour sleep-wake cycle has on biological function.
- Discuss mechanisms that regulate sleep.
- Describe the normal stages of sleep.
- Explain the functions of sleep.
- Compare and contrast the characteristics of sleep for different age-groups.
- Identify factors that normally promote and disrupt sleep.
- Discuss characteristics of common sleep disorders.
- Gather a sleep history for a client.
- Describe interventions appropriate in promoting sleep for clients with various sleep disorders.
- Discuss differences in nursing interventions used for clients of different age-groups.
- Develop a teaching plan to improve a client's sleep hygiene.
- Describe ways to evaluate sleep therapies.

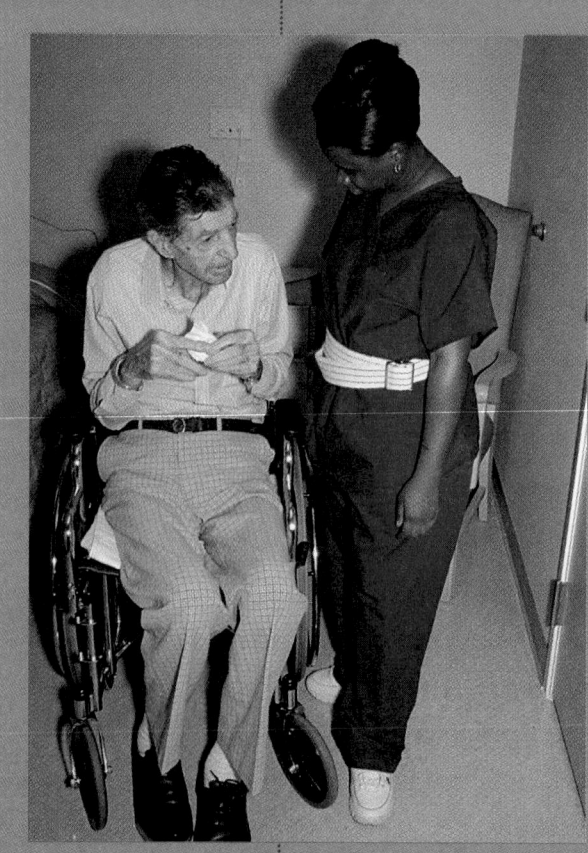

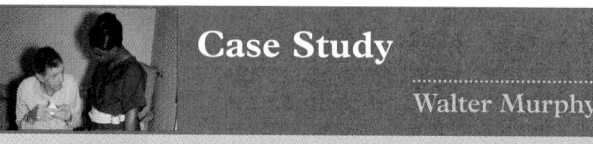

Case Study

Walter Murphy

Walter Murphy is an 82-year-old client who has resided in the local nursing home for the last 3 months. His wife, Mary, still lives at home but visits Walter on a daily basis. Walter is confined to a wheelchair as a result of osteoarthritis and a mild stroke, experienced just 1 year ago. Even though he has physical limitations, he is alert and oriented. Over the last several weeks, Mary has found her husband to be very sleepy when she visits him just before lunchtime. Walter tells Mary that he has trouble falling asleep at night, and once he does fall asleep, he reawakens frequently during the night. Mary is concerned because her husband does not seem as alert or interested during her visit.

Anna is a 23-year-old junior student assigned to the nursing home for her second semester in nursing school. She has had experience in nursing homes, having worked in one center as a nurse assistant during the last two summers. Anna is assigned to care for Mr. Murphy over the next 4 weeks.

Physical and emotional health depends on adequate sleep and rest. Without proper amounts of rest and sleep, the ability to concentrate, make judgments, and participate in daily activities decreases. To help a client gain needed rest and sleep, a nurse must understand the nature of sleep, the factors influencing it, and the client's sleep habits. Nurses care for clients who often have preexisting sleep disturbances and for clients who develop sleep problems as a result of illness or exposure to the environment of a health care agency (e.g., hospital or long-term care). The nurse must use an individualized approach based on clients' personal sleep habits and pattern of sleep to provide effective sleep therapies.

SCIENTIFIC KNOWLEDGE BASE

Sleep and Rest

When people are at rest, they usually feel mentally relaxed, free from anxiety, and physically calm. Rest does not imply inactivity, although everyone often thinks of it as settling down in a comfortable chair or taking a brief nap. When people are at rest, they are in a state of mental and physical activity that leaves them feeling refreshed, rejuvenated, and ready to resume the activities of the day. All persons have their own habits for obtaining rest, for example, reading a book, practicing medi-

tation or relaxation exercise (see Chapter 33), or taking a long walk.

Sleep is a recurrent, altered state of consciousness that occurs for sustained periods. When persons obtain proper sleep, they feel that their energy has been restored. Some experts believe that these feelings of energy restoration imply that sleep provides time for the repair and recovery of body systems for the next period of wakefulness.

Physiology of Sleep

Sleep is a cyclical physiological process that alternates with longer periods of wakefulness. The sleep-wake cycle influences and regulates body functions and behavioral responses.

Circadian rhythms. People experience cyclical rhythms as part of their everyday life. The most familiar rhythm is the 24-hour, day-night cycle known as the diurnal or **circadian rhythm.** Circadian rhythms influence the pattern of major biological and behavioral functions including fluctuation and predictability of body temperature, heart rate, blood pressure, hormone secretion, sensory acuity, and mood.

All circadian rhythms, including the sleep-wake cycle, are affected by light and temperature as well as external factors such as social activities and environmental stressors. All persons have **biological clocks** that synchronize their sleep cycles. Some people can fall asleep at 8 PM, whereas others go to bed at midnight or early in the morning. Different people also function best at different times of the day.

Health care agencies (e.g., hospitals, nursing homes) usually do not adapt care to an individual's sleep-wake cycle preferences. Typical care routines interrupt sleep or prevent clients from falling asleep at their usual times. The unfamiliar environment also creates numerous noises that disrupt or prevent sleep. If a person's sleep-wake cycle is altered significantly, a poor quality of sleep can result. Nonplanned reversals in the sleep-wake cycle such as sleeping during the day can indicate serious illness.

The biological rhythm of sleep frequently becomes synchronized with other body functions. Changes in body temperature, for example, correlate with sleep patterns. Normally, body temperature peaks in the afternoon, decreases gradually, and then drops sharply after a person falls asleep. When the sleep-wake cycle becomes disrupted (e.g., by working rotating shifts), other physiological functions may change as well. For example, the person may experience a decreased appetite and lose weight. Failure to maintain the individual's usual sleep-wake cycle can adversely affect the client's overall health.

Sleep regulation. Sleep involves a sequence of physiological states maintained by highly integrated central nervous system (CNS) activity that is associated with changes in the peripheral nervous, endocrine, cardiovascular, respiratory, and muscular systems (Robinson, 1993). Each sequence can be identified by specific physiological responses and patterns of brain activity. The control and regulation of sleep may depend on the interrelationship between two cerebral mechanisms that intermittently activate and suppress the brain's higher centers to control sleep and wakefulness (Figure 32-1). One mechanism, the **reticular activating system (RAS),** causes wakefulness, whereas the other, the **bulbar synchronizing region (BSR),** causes sleep.

While persons try to fall asleep, they close their eyes and assume relaxed positions. Stimuli to the RAS in the upper brainstem decline. If the room is dark, quiet, and at a comfortable temperature, activation of the RAS further declines. At some point the BSR takes over, causing sleep. Persons will generally not reawaken until their usual sleep cycle is finished or stimuli in the environment (e.g., traffic outside, chirping of birds) stimulate the RAS to awaken the individual.

Stages of sleep. Different levels of brain, muscle, and eye activity are associated with different stages of sleep (Sleep Research Society, 1993). Normal sleep involves two phases: nonrapid eye movement **(NREM sleep)** and rapid eye movement **(REM sleep)** (Box 32-1). During NREM a sleeper progresses through four stages during a typical 90-minute sleep cycle. The quality of sleep from stage 1 through stage 4 becomes increasingly deep. Lighter sleep is characteristic of stages 1 and 2, when a person is more easily arousable. Stages 3 and 4 involve a deeper sleep called slow-wave sleep from which a person is more difficult to arouse. REM sleep is the phase at the end of each

90-minute sleep cycle. Memory consolidation (Karni and others, 1994) and psychological restoration may occur at this time.

Sleep cycle. Normally an adult's routine sleep pattern begins with a presleep period during which the person is aware only of a gradually developing sleepiness. This period normally lasts 10 to 30 minutes, but if a person has difficulty falling asleep, it may last an hour or more.

Once asleep, the person usually passes through four to six complete sleep cycles, each consisting of four stages of NREM sleep and a period of REM sleep. The cyclical pattern usually progresses from stage 1 through stage 4 of NREM, followed by a reversal from stage 4 to 3 to 2, ending with a period of REM sleep (Figure 32-2).

With each successive cycle, stages 3 and 4 shorten, and the period of REM lengthens. REM sleep may last up to 60 minutes during the last sleep cycle. Not all people progress consistently through the usual stages of sleep. For example, a sleeper may fluctuate back and forth for short intervals between NREM stages 2, 3, and 4 before entering REM sleep. The amount of time spent in each stage varies. Shifts from stage to stage tend to accompany body movements, and shifts to light sleep tend to occur suddenly, whereas shifts to deep sleep tend to be gradual (Closs, 1988). The number of sleep cycles depends on the total amount of time that the person spends sleeping.

Functions of Sleep

The purpose of sleep is still unclear. One theory suggests that sleep is a time of restoration and preparation for the next period of wakefulness (Anch and others, 1988). During NREM sleep, biological functions slow. A healthy adult's normal heart rate throughout the day averages 70 to 80 beats/min. However, during sleep the heart rate falls to 60 beats/min, thus preserving cardiac function.

Sleep may also restore biological processes. During deep slow-wave (NREM stage 4) sleep, the body releases human growth hormone for the repair and renewal of epithelial and specialized cells such as brain cells (Mendleson, 1987; Born and others, 1988). Protein synthesis and cell division for the renewal of tissues may also occur during rest and sleep.

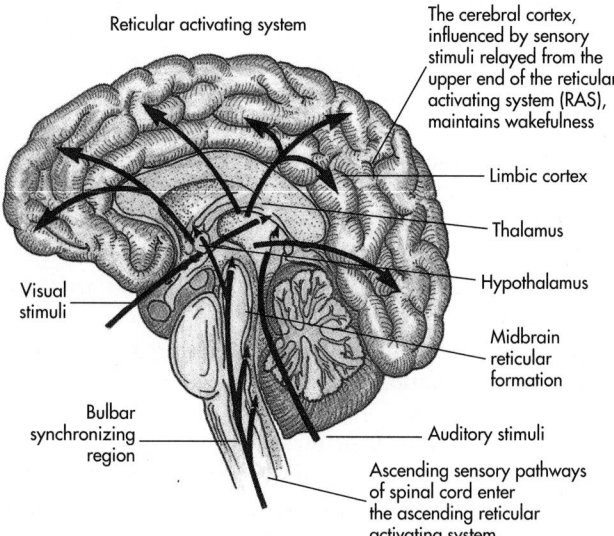

Figure 32-1. The RAS and BSR control sensory input, intermittently activating and suppressing the brain's higher centers to control sleep and wakefulness.

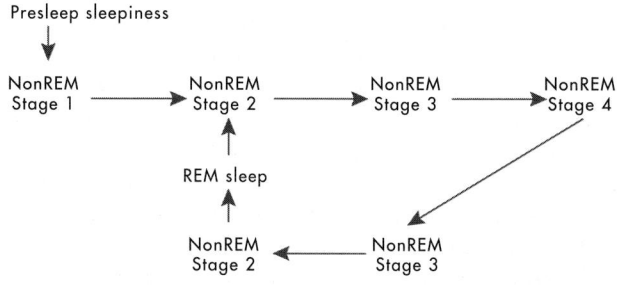

Figure 32-2. The stages of the adult sleep cycle.

Box 32-1
Stages of the Sleep Cycle

Stage 1: NREM

Stage includes lightest level of sleep.

Stage lasts a few minutes.

Decreased physiological activity begins with gradual fall in vital signs and metabolism.

Person is easily aroused by sensory stimuli such as noise.

Awakened, person feels as though daydreaming has occurred.

Stage 2: NREM

Stage 2 is period of sound sleep.

Relaxation progresses.

Arousal is still relatively easy.

Stage lasts 10 to 20 minutes.

Body functions continue to slow.

Stage 3: NREM

Stage 3 involves initial stages of deep sleep.

Sleeper is difficult to arouse and rarely moves.

Muscles are completely relaxed.

Vital signs decline but remain regular.

Stage lasts 15 to 30 minutes.

Stage 4: NREM

Stage 4 is deepest stage of sleep.

It is very difficult to arouse sleeper.

If sleep loss has occurred, sleeper will spend considerable portion of night in this stage.

Vital signs are significantly lower than during waking hours.

Stage lasts approximately 15 to 30 minutes.

Sleepwalking and enuresis may occur.

REM Sleep

Vivid, full-color dreaming may occur in REM. Less vivid dreaming may occur in other stages.

Stage usually begins about 90 minutes after sleep has begun.

It is typified by autonomic response of rapidly moving eyes, fluctuating heart and respiratory rates, and increased or fluctuating blood pressure.

Loss of skeletal muscle tone occurs.

Gastric secretions increase.

It is very difficult to arouse sleeper.

Duration of REM sleep increases with each cycle and averages 20 minutes.

REM sleep appears to be important for cognitive restoration. REM sleep is associated with changes in cerebral blood flow, increased cortical activity, increased oxygen consumption, and epinephrine release. This association may assist with memory storage and learning. During sleep, the brain filters stored information about the day's activities.

The benefits of sleep often go unnoticed until a person develops a problem resulting from sleep deprivation. A loss of REM sleep can lead to feelings of confusion. Various body functions (e.g., motor performance, memory, equilibrium) appear to be altered when prolonged sleep loss occurs. Traffic, home, and work-related accidents due to falling asleep have been estimated to cost billions of dollars a year in the United States alone (Leger, 1994; Webb, 1995).

Dreams. While dreams occur during both NREM and REM sleep, the dreams of REM sleep are more vivid and elaborate and are believed to be functionally important to the consolidation of long-term memory. REM dreams may progress in content throughout the night from dreams about current events to emotional dreams of childhood or the past. Personality can influence the quality of dreams; for example, a creative person may have creative dreams, and a depressed person may dream of helplessness.

Dreams may help people sort out immediate concerns (e.g., dreams about work problems) or erase certain fantasies or nonsensical memories (e.g., living in a make-believe world). Since most dreams are forgotten, many people have little dream recall and don't believe they dream at all. To remember a dream, a person must consciously think about it on awakening. People who recall dreams vividly usually awaken just after a period of REM sleep.

⋯NURSING KNOWLEDGE BASE

Normal Sleep Requirements and Patterns

Sleep duration and quality vary among persons of all age-groups. Figure 32-3 shows the change in the distribution of sleep stages during life.

Neonates. The neonate up to the age of 3 months averages about 16 hours of sleep a day. Approximately 50% of this sleep is REM sleep, which stimulates the higher brain centers.

Infants. Infants usually develop a nighttime pattern of sleep by 3 months of age. The infant may take several naps during the day but usually sleeps an average of 8 to 10 hours during the night. About 30% of sleep time is spend in the REM cycle. Awakening commonly occurs early in the morning, although the infant may waken during the night.

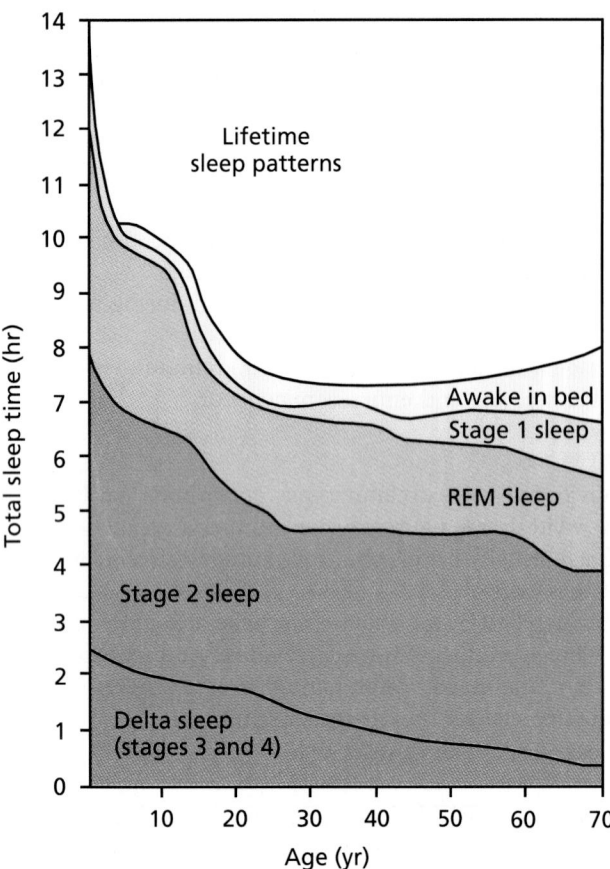

Figure 32-3. Distribution of sleep stages over the life span. (Adapted with permission from Berman TM and others: Sleep disorders: take them seriously, *Patient Care* 24:85, © 1990, Medical Economics.)

Toddlers. By the age of 2 years, children usually sleep through the night and take daily naps. Total sleep averages 12 hours a day. Naps may be eliminated at 3 years. It is common for toddlers to awaken during the night. The percentage of REM sleep continues to fall. Toddlers may be unwilling to go to bed at night.

Preschoolers. A preschooler sleeps an average 12 hours a night (about 20% is REM). By the age of 5, the preschooler rarely takes daytime naps (Wong, 1995) except in cultures where a siesta is the custom. The preschooler usually has difficulty relaxing or quieting down after long, active days. A preschooler also has problems with bedtime fears, waking during the night, and nightmares.

School-age children. The school-age child usually does not require a nap. A 6-year-old averages 11 to 12 hours of sleep nightly, whereas an 11-year-old sleeps about 9 to 10 hours (Wong, 1995). The 6- or 7-year-old can usually be persuaded to go to bed by encouraging quiet activities. The older child often resists sleeping because of an unawareness of fatigue or a need to be independent.

Adolescents. Typically teenagers get about $7\frac{1}{2}$ hours of sleep per night (Carskadon, 1990a). At a time when sleep needs actually increase, the typical adolescent is subject to a number of changes that often reduce the time spent sleeping (Carskadon, 1990b). Usually parents no longer set a specific bedtime. School demands, after-school social activities, and part-time jobs may lessen time available for sleep. Teens go to bed later and rise earlier during the high school years. Because of lifestyle demands that shorten the time available for sleep and probably physiological need, teens often experience excessive daytime sleepiness (EDS). School performance, vulnerability to accidents, and behavioral problems can be the result of EDS due to insufficient sleep.

Young adults. Most young adults average 6 to $8\frac{1}{2}$ hours of sleep a night, but this can vary. Young adults rarely take regular naps. Approximately 20% of sleep time is spent in REM sleep, which remains consistent throughout the remainder of life. Healthy young adults require adequate sleep to participate in the day's busy activities. However, lifestyle demands often interrupt usual sleep patterns, causing insomnia.

Middle-age adults. During mid-adulthood the total time spent sleeping at night begins to decline. The amount of stage 4 sleep begins to fall, a decline that continues with advancing age. Sleep disturbances are often initially diagnosed among people in this age range even when the symptoms of a disorder have been present for several years. Members of this age-group may rely on sleeping medications.

Older adults. Complaints of sleeping difficulties increase with age. More than 50% of persons age 65 and older report regular problems with sleep (Ancoli-Israel, 1997). Older adults have less stage 3 and stage 4 NREM sleep; some older adults have almost no stage 4, or deep sleep. Episodes of REM sleep tend to shorten. Older adults awaken more often during the night, and it may take more time for them to fall asleep. Their sleep efficiency (the amount of time asleep given the amount of time in bed) is reduced, and the number of naps taken during the day is increased (Ancoli-Israel, 1997). Tests show that older adults do not have an increased need for sleep, but the ability to sleep is reduced.

As people age, their circadian clock advances, causing **advanced sleep phase syndrome.** The syndrome is common in older adults and is a common reason behind the complaint of waking early in the morning and being unable to get back to sleep (Campbell and Dawson, 1992). People with advanced sleep phase syndrome get sleepy early in the evening (e.g., 8 or 9 PM). If they were to go to bed at that time, they would sleep for about 8 hours and wake up around 4 or 5 AM. However, when people with advanced sleep phase syndrome stay up until their customary 10 or 11 PM, their bodies still awaken at 4 or 5 AM. They thus receive only 5 to 6 hours of sleep, the amount of time they are in bed before their advanced sleep-wake cycle wakes them up (Ancoli-Israel, 1997).

Factors Affecting Sleep

A number of factors (physical, psychological, and environmental) affect the quantity and quality of sleep. Often more than one factor combine to cause a sleep problem.

Physical illness. Any illness or condition that causes pain, difficulty breathing, nausea, or mood problems such as anxiety or depression can result in sleep problems. Persons with such alterations may have trouble falling or staying asleep. Illnesses also may force clients to sleep in positions to which they are unaccustomed. Table 32-1 summarizes illnesses and conditions that have the potential for causing sleep alterations.

Drugs and substances. A considerable number of drugs cause either sleepiness, insomnia, or fatigue as a side effect (Box 32-2). Medications prescribed for sleep often cause more problems than benefits. L-Tryptophan, a natural protein found in foods such as milk, cheese, and meats, may help a person sleep.

Lifestyle. A person's daily routine may influence sleep patterns. An individual who alternately works day and night shifts, for example, often has difficulty adjusting to the altered sleep schedule. Other alterations in routine that can disrupt sleep patterns include performing unaccustomed heavy work, engaging in late-night social activities, and changing evening mealtime.

Usual sleep patterns and excessive daytime sleepiness. In the last 100 years the amount of sleep obtained nightly by U.S. citizens has decreased over 20% (National Commission on Sleep Disorders Research, 1993). Many Americans are sleep deprived and experience excessive sleepiness during the day. EDS often results in impairment of waking function, poor work or school performance, accidents while driving or using equipment, and behavioral or emotional problems. Feelings of sleepiness are usually most intense upon awakening from or right before going to sleep and about 12 hours after the midsleep period.

Sleepiness becomes pathological when it occurs at times when persons need or want to be awake. Persons who temporarily experience sleep deprivation as a result of an active social evening or lengthened work schedule usually feel sleepy the next day. However, they may be able to overcome these feelings even though they have difficulty performing tasks and remaining attentive. Chronic lack of sleep is much more serious than temporary sleep deprivation and can cause serious alterations in the ability to perform daily activities. EDS is most difficult to overcome during sedentary tasks (e.g., driving).

Emotional stress. Worry over personal problems or situations can disrupt sleep. Emotional stress causes tension and often leads to frustration when sleep does not come. Stress may also cause a person to try too hard to fall asleep, to awaken frequently during the sleep cycle, or to oversleep. Continued stress may cause poor sleep habits.

Environment. The physical environment in which a person sleeps has a significant influence on the ability

TABLE 32-1	
Illnesses and Conditions That Can Alter Sleep	
Illness/Condition	**Nature of Sleep Alteration**
Respiratory disease (e.g., emphysema, asthma, bronchitis, allergic rhinitis, common cold)	Shortness of breath requires use of 2 to 3 pillows to raise head. Rhythm of breathing may be altered. Nasal congestion and sore throat impair breathing and ability to relax.
Coronary heart disease with episodes of chest pain and irregular heart rates	Frequent awakenings and sleep stage changes during sleep as well as significant alterations in all stages of sleep (Landis, 1988).
Hypertension	Early morning awakening and fatigue.
Hypothyroidism	Decreases stage 4 sleep.
Hyperthyroidism	Takes more time to fall asleep.
Nocturia (reduced bladder tone, diabetes, urethritis, prostate disease)	Awakenings at night to urinate; difficulty returning to sleep.
Gastric reflux	Burning pain in lower esophagus; increases when lying flat in bed.
Depression	Awakenings in early morning with inability to return to sleep; worsened by anxiety or agitation.

Box 32-2
Drugs and Their Effects on Sleep

Hypnotics
Interfere with reaching deeper sleep stages
Provide only temporary (1-week) increase in quantity of sleep
Eventually cause "hangover" during day; excess drowsiness, confusion, decreased energy
May worsen sleep apnea in older adults

Diuretics
Cause nocturia

Antidepressants and Stimulants
Suppress REM sleep
Decrease total sleep time

Alcohol
Speeds onset of sleep
Disrupts REM sleep
Awakens person during night and causes difficulty returning to sleep

Caffeine
Prevents person from falling asleep
May cause person to awaken during night

Beta-Blockers
Cause nightmares
Cause insomnia
Cause awakening from sleep

Benzodiazepines
Increase sleep time
Increase daytime sleepiness

Narcotics (Morphine/Demerol)
Suppress REM sleep
Cause increased daytime drowsiness

Antihistamines
Cause drowsiness
Excess amounts can cause insomnia

Nasal Decongestants
Cause daytime sleepiness

to fall and remain asleep. Good ventilation, a comfortable temperature, and a darkened or softly lit room are essential for restful sleep. The size, firmness, and position of a bed can also affect sleep quality. Hospital beds are often harder than those at home. If a person usually sleeps with another individual, sleeping alone during times of illness or a stay in a health care agency can cause wakefulness. However, sleeping with a restless or snoring bed partner can also disrupt sleep.

Sound influences sleep. The level of noise needed to awaken a person depends on the stage of sleep (Webster and Thompson, 1986). Low noises are more likely to arouse a person from stage 1 sleep, whereas louder noises awaken a person in stage 3 or 4 sleep. Some persons require silence to fall asleep, whereas others prefer background noise such as soft music or television.

In hospitals and other health care facilities, noise creates a problem for clients. In 1974 the U.S. Environmental Protection Agency recommended that hospital noise be maintained at 40 to 45 decibels during the day and at less than 35 decibels at night (Pope, 1995). Griffin (1992) reported that average hospital noise, measured over 24 hours, ranged from 57.2 decibels in a postanesthesia care unit to 58 to 72 decibels in an intensive care unit. Conversation between health care staff measures about 50 decibels. Schnelle and others (1993) studied a nursing home environment and found that an average of 32 noises per night per resident were recorded at the level of loud speech or above (60 decibels).

Noise in health care settings is usually new or strange to the client. This problem is greatest the first night a client stays in a hospital or other facility, when clients often experience increased total wake time, increased awakening, and decreased REM sleep and total sleep time. Nursing activities are a source of increased sound levels. The intensive care setting is perhaps one of the loudest, where close proximity of clients, noise from confused and ill clients, and ringing of alarm systems and telephones make the environment very unpleasant.

Exercise and fatigue. A person who is moderately fatigued usually achieves restful sleep, especially if the fatigue results from enjoyable work or exercise. Exercising 2 hours or more before bedtime allows the body to cool down and maintains a state of fatigue that promotes relaxation. However, excess fatigue resulting from exhausting or stressful work can make falling asleep difficult. This can be a common problem for grade-school and adolescent children.

Food and caloric intake. Following good eating habits is important for proper health, including sleep. Eating a large, heavy, and/or spicy meal at night may result in indigestion that interferes with sleep. Caffeine and alcohol consumed in the evening have insomnia-producing effects. Coffee, tea, cola, and chocolate contain caffeine and xanthines, substances that cause sleeplessness as a result of CNS stimulation. Food allergies may cause insomnia. In infants, nighttime waking and crying may be caused by a milk allergy, requiring that breast milk of a nonmilk formula be used. Other foods that often result in an insomnia-producing allergy in children and adults include corn, wheat, nuts, chocolate, eggs, seafood, red and yellow food dyes, and yeast (Hauri and Linde, 1990). It may take up to 2 weeks to restore normal sleep when a food causing allergy is eliminated.

Weight loss or gain influences sleep patterns. When a person gains weight, sleep periods become longer with fewer interruptions. Weight loss can cause short and fragmented sleep. Certain sleep disorders may be the result of the semistarvation diets popular in a weight-conscious society.

Sleep Disorders

Sleep disorders are conditions that, if untreated, cause disturbed nighttime sleep that results in one of three problems: insomnia; abnormal movements or sensation during sleep or when awakening at night; or excessive daytime sleepiness (Naylor and Aldrich, 1994). The occurrence of sleep disorders is becoming a significant health problem especially for persons living in stressful environments. Sleep disorders have been classified into four major categories (American Sleep Disorders Association, 1990) (Box 32-3). The dyssomnias are primary disorders that have their origin in different body systems and are subdivided into three groups. The intrinsic sleep disorders include disorders of initiating and maintaining sleep. Extrinsic sleep disorders develop from external factors, which if removed, lead to resolution of the sleep disorder. The circadian rhythm sleep disorders arise from a misalignment between the timing of sleep and what is desired by the individual or is a societal norm. The parainsomnias are undesirable behaviors that occur usually during sleep. Many medical and psychiatric sleep disorders are associated with sleep and wake disturbances. These sleep disturbances are divided into those associated with psychiatric, neurological, or other medical disorders. The proposed sleep disorders are newly described disturbances still under study.

Insomnia. **Insomnia** is a symptom experienced by clients who have chronic difficulty falling asleep, frequent awakenings from sleep, and/or a short sleep or nonrestorative sleep (Zorick, 1994). The person with insomnia complains of EDS, as well as insufficient quantity and quality of sleep. Frequently, however, the client gets more sleep than is realized. Insomnia may signal an underlying physical or psychological disorder.

People may experience transient or temporary insomnia as a result of situational stresses such as work or

---

Box 32-3
Classification of Sleep Disorders

Dyssomnias
Intrinsic Sleep Disorders

Psychophysiological insomnia
Narcolepsy
Obstructive sleep apnea syndrome
Periodic limb movement disorder

Extrinsic Sleep Disorders

Inadequate sleep hygiene
Insufficient sleep syndrome
Hypnotic-dependent sleep disorders
Alcohol-dependent sleep disorders

Circadian Rhythm Sleep Disorders

Time-zone change (jet lag) syndrome
Shift-work sleep disorder
Delayed sleep phase syndrome

Parasomnias
Arousal Disorders

Sleepwalking
Sleep terrors

Sleep-Wake Transition Disorders

Sleeptalking
Nocturnal leg cramps

Parasomnias Usually Associated With REM Sleep

Nightmares
REM sleep behavior disorder

Other Parasomnias

Sleep bruxism (teeth grinding)
Sleep enuresis (bed-wetting)
Sudden infant death syndrome

Sleep Disorders Associated With Medical/Psychiatric Disorders
Associated With Psychiatric Disorders

Mood disorders
Anxiety disorders

Associated With Neurological Disorders

Dementia
Parkinsonism

Associated With Other Medical Disorders

Nocturnal cardiac ischemia
Chronic obstructive pulmonary disease

Proposed Sleep Disorders

Menstruation-associated sleep disorders
Sleep choking syndrome

Data from American Sleep Disorders Association: *The international classification of sleep disorders: diagnostic and coding manual,* Rochester, NY, 1990, Allen Press.

family problems. Insomnia may recur, but between episodes the client is able to sleep well. A temporary case of insomnia caused by a stressful event can, however, lead to chronic difficulty in obtaining sufficient sleep.

Insomnia is often associated with poor sleep habits. If the condition continues, the fear of not being able to sleep can be enough to cause wakefulness. During the day a person with chronic insomnia may feel sleepy, fatigued, depressed, and anxious.

There are several treatment approaches for insomnia. It is important to treat underlying emotional or medical problems that may be causing the insomnia. Treatment can also be directed at the symptoms, including improved sleep hygiene measures, biofeedback, and relaxation techniques. When insomnia develops secondary to inappropriate health behaviors (e.g., drug dependence), treatment is directed at changing the behavior (e.g., withdrawal of the drug).

Sleep apnea. **Sleep apnea** is a disorder in which the individual cannot breathe and sleep at the same time (Ancoli-Israel, 1997). There is a lack of airflow through the nose and mouth for periods from 10 seconds to 1 to 2 minutes in length. There can be 10 or 15 to more than 100 respiratory events per hour of sleep (Ancoli-Israel, 1997). There are three types of sleep apnea: central, obstructive, and mixed.

The most common form, obstructive sleep apnea, is characterized by cessation of airflow despite the effort to breathe. It occurs when muscles or structures of the oral cavity or throat relax during sleep. The upper airway becomes partially or completely blocked, and nasal airflow is diminished (hypopnea) or stopped (apnea). The person tries to breathe because chest and abdominal movement continues, which often results in loud snoring sounds. When breathing is partially or completely diminished, each successive diaphragmatic movement becomes stronger until the obstruction is relieved. Structural abnormalities such as a deviated septum, nasal polyps, or enlarged tonsils may predispose a client to obstructive apnea. EDS is the most common complaint of people with obstructive sleep apnea.

Obstructive apnea causes a serious decline in the arterial oxygen level (see Chapter 30). Clients are at risk for cardiac dysrhythmias, right heart failure, pulmonary hypertension, angina attacks, stroke, and hypertension.

Central sleep apnea is caused by cessation of diaphragmatic and intercostal respiratory effort as a result of dysfunction of the brain's respiratory control center. The impulse to breathe temporarily fails. Nasal airflow and chest wall movement cease, with oxygen saturation of the blood also falling. Central sleep apnea is seen in clients with brainstem injury, muscular dystrophy, and encephalitis, as well as in people who breathe normally during the day. It is the least common sleep apnea. People with central sleep apnea tend to awaken during

sleep and complain of insomnia and EDS. Mild and intermittent snoring is also present.

The client with sleep apnea is often deprived of deep sleep. In addition to complaints of EDS, sleep attacks, fatigue, morning headaches, and decreased sex drive are common. Treatment includes therapy for underlying cardiac or respiratory complications and emotional problems. Sleep hygiene and a weight loss program may help. The treatment of choice is use of a nasal continuous positive airway pressure (CPAP) device at night.

Narcolepsy. **Narcolepsy** is a CNS dysfunction of mechanisms that regulate the sleep and wake states. EDS is the most common complaint associated with narcolepsy. During the day a person may suddenly feel an overwhelming wave of sleepiness and fall asleep. REM sleep can occur within 15 minutes of falling asleep. **Cataplexy,** or sudden muscle weakness during intense emotions such as anger or laughter, is a symptom of narcolepsy that may occur at any time during the day. If the cateplectic attack is severe, the client may lose voluntary muscle control and fall to the floor.

A person with narcolepsy often falls asleep uncontrollably at inappropriate times. Unless this disorder is understood, a sleep attack can easily be mistaken for laziness, lack of interest in activities, or drunkenness. Typically symptoms first occur in adolescence and may be confused with the EDS that is thought to be common in teens. Narcoleptics are treated with stimulants that may only partially increase wakefulness and reduce sleep attacks and with medications that suppress cataplexy and the other REM-related symptoms.

Sleep deprivation. **Sleep deprivation** is a problem many clients have as a result of the dyssomnias. Causes may include illness (e.g., fever, difficulty breathing, pain), emotional stress, medications, environmental disturbances (e.g., frequent nursing care), and variability in the timing of sleep as a result of shift work. Physicians and nurses may be particularly prone to sleep deprivation because of long work schedules and rotating shifts.

Hospitalization, especially in intensive care units, makes clients vulnerable to the extrinsic and circadian sleep disorders (Wood, 1992). Sleep deprivation involves decreases in the quantity and quality of sleep as well as inconsistency in the timing of sleep. When sleep becomes interrupted or fragmented, changes in the normal sequencing of the sleep cycles occur. A cumulative sleep deprivation develops.

Individuals respond to sleep deprivation differently. Clients may experience a variety of physiological and psychological symptoms (Box 32-4). The severity of symptoms is often related to the duration of sleep deprivation. The most effective treatment for sleep deprivation is elimination or correction of factors that disrupt the sleep pattern. Nurses play an important role in identifying treatable sleep deprivation problems.

Parasomnias. The parasomnias are sleep problems that are more common in children compared with adults. One common exception is sleep **bruxism** (tooth grinding), frequently seen in adults experiencing continuous stress. Sudden infant death syndrome (SIDS) is believed to be related to apnea, hypoxia, and cardiac arrhythmias caused by abnormalities in the autonomic nervous system that occur during sleep (Gillis and Flemons, 1994).

Parainsomnias that occur among older children include somnambulism (sleepwalking), night terrors, nightmares, nocturnal enuresis (bed-wetting), and tooth grinding (bruxism). Specific treatment for these disorders varies. However, in all cases it is important to support clients and maintain their safety.

CRITICAL THINKING IN CLIENT CARE

Synthesis

It is not uncommon for almost any client to have experienced some type of sleep disorder. However, it is important not to overlook such a problem or consider it as normal. The nurse must apply knowledge, experience, and appropriate critical thinking attitudes and standards to make the correct clinical judgments for clients.

Knowledge. To make decisions about a client's sleep problems, it is important to synthesize knowledge regarding the physiology and functions of sleep, as well as factors that affect sleep. Knowledge of the pathophysiology of select disease processes further helps in understanding the mechanisms for certain sleep problems. In addition, the nurse should have a good knowledge of pharmacological information because many of the medications clients receive can contribute to sleeping difficulties.

Another important area of knowledge to synthesize is that of a client's cultural orientation. Infant care practices such as co-sleeping and the practice of regular siestas or naps are examples of cultural variations influencing sleep. The nurse should anticipate how such cultural factors will ultimately influence an individual client's ability to sleep.

Experience. Each of us knows of factors that have either disrupted or promoted our ability to sleep. This personal experience can be valuable when assessing clients' sleep problems or in selecting therapies for sleep promotion. Previous clinical experience with clients helps the nurse to appreciate that environmental and lifestyle variations significantly affect the quality and quantity of sleep a client receives. For example, having cared for a client in pain or who is anxious because of impending surgery might provide lessons the nurse can apply when caring for future clients.

Attitudes. When dealing with sleep problems, it may take a long period of time to find effective therapies. Chronic insomnia, for example, is not easily eliminated in a short period. Perseverance is an important critical thinking attitude to use if the nurse is to help find effective solutions for the client. The problems posed by sleep disturbances also often require creative approaches. An original idea may be necessary, for example, to minimize or control environmental stressors in the client's sleep environment.

Standards. When learning about a client's sleep problem, the nurse must utilize numerous intellectual standards in conducting the nursing assessment. It is important for the nurse to conduct a detailed sleep assessment to understand the nature of the sleep problem as well as potential causes and solutions. A clear, precise, specific, and accurate assessment will also be very important so that an appropriate plan of care can be established.

NURSING PROCESS

▮ Assessment

The nurse assesses a client's sleep pattern using the nursing history to gather information about factors that usually influence sleep. Sleep is a subjective experience. Only the client can report whether it is sufficient and restful. If the client is satisfied with the amount and quality of sleep received, it may be considered normal (Closs, 1988). If a client admits to or the nurse suspects a sleep problem, a more detailed history is needed.

Assessment is aimed at understanding the characteristics of any sleep problem and the client's usual sleep habits so that ways for promoting sleep can be incorporated into nursing care.

Sources for sleep assessment.
Clients are the best resources for describing a sleep problem and any change from their usual sleep and waking patterns. Bed partners can offer information on clients' sleep patterns that may reveal the nature of certain disorders. The nurse should ask bed partners whether clients have restful sleep or problems such as going to the bathroom frequently or having pauses in breathing during sleep.

A child's sleep history is usually gathered from parents. Some parents may not know that there is a wide variability in the sleeping patterns of infants and may need reassurance if their infant seems to sleep less than others but is otherwise healthy and thriving (Parkinson, 1994). Older children often are able to relate their fears or worries that prevent them from falling asleep. If children frequently awaken in the middle of bad dreams, parents can identify the problem without necessarily knowing the meanings of the dreams. Parents can also describe typical behavior patterns that foster or impair sleep. With chronic sleep problems, parents can relate the duration of the problem, its progression, and children's responses. Parents of infants may need to keep a 24-hour log of their infant's waking and sleeping behavior over a period of several days.

Sleep history.
Clients may report that they enjoy adequate sleep. In this situation the sleep history can be brief. A determination of usual bedtime, normal bedtime rituals, preferred environment for sleeping, and what time the client usually rises give the nurse information for planning care conducive to sleep. When a sleep problem is suspected, the nurse assesses the quality and characteristics of sleep in greater depth.

Sleep pattern.
A sleep history begins with clients' self-report of their sleep pattern. Most persons can give a reasonably accurate estimate of their sleep patterns, particularly if any changes have occurred. An effective, subjective method for assessing sleep quality is the use of a visual analog scale (Closs, 1988). The nurse draws a straight horizontal line about 100 mm (4 inches) long. Opposing statements such as "best night's sleep" and "worst night's sleep" are at each end of the line. Clients are asked to place a mark along the horizontal line at the point that best matches their perception of the previous night's sleep. The distance of the mark along the line in millimeters offers a numerical value for satisfaction with sleep. The scale can be repeatedly used to show change in sleep over time.

It is important to have clients describe their usual sleep pattern should there be significant changes cre-

ated by a sleep disorder. To assess the client's sleep pattern, the nurse asks the following questions:

1. What time do you usually get in bed?
2. What time do you usually fall asleep? Do you do anything special to help you fall asleep?
3. How many times do you awaken during sleep? Why do you think you awaken? What do you do about awakening?
4. What time do you typically wake up?
5. What time do you get out of bed and stay up once you have awakened?
6. What is the average number of hours you sleep?
7. During the last week what time did you usually go to bed, fall asleep, and awaken?
8. During the last week, how much difficulty did you have going to sleep?

The nurse compares assessment data with the pattern usually found for other clients of the same age and looks for patterns that might suggest problems. Clients with sleep problems may show patterns very different from their usual one, or the change may be relatively minor. Hospitalized clients usually need or want more sleep as a result of illness. However, some may require less sleep because they are less active. Clients who are ill may think that it is important to try to sleep more than what is usual for them, eventually making sleeping difficult.

Description of sleeping problems.
When a client admits to or the nurse suspects a sleep problem, the nursing history must be detailed. Open-ended questions help a client to describe a problem more fully. A general description of the problem followed by more focused questions usually reveals specific sleep characteristics.

To begin, the nurse needs to understand the nature of the sleep problem, its signs and symptoms, its onset and duration, its severity, predisposing factors or causes, and the overall effect on the client. Assessment questions might include the following:

1. *Nature of the problem:* Tell me what type of problem you have with your sleep. Tell me why you think you are not getting enough sleep. Describe for me a recent typical night's sleep. How is this sleep different from what you are used to?
2. *Signs and symptoms:* Do you have difficulty falling asleep, staying asleep, or waking up? Have you been told that you snore loudly? Do you have headaches when awakening? Does your child awaken from nightmares?
3. *Onset and duration:* When did you notice the problem? How long has this problem lasted?
4. *Severity:* How long does it take you to fall asleep? How often during the week do you have trouble falling asleep?
5. *Predisposing factors:* Tell me what you do just before going to bed. Have you recently had any changes at work, school, or home? How would you describe

your current mood, and have you noticed any recent changes? What medications or recreational drugs do you take regularly? Do you eat foods (e.g., spicy or greasy foods) or drink liquids (e.g., alcohol, caffeinated beverages) that might disrupt your sleep? If so, how much do you eat/drink daily?

6. *Effect on client:* How has the loss of sleep affected you? (Ask a spouse or friend: Have you noticed any changes in the client's behavior since the sleep problem started?) Do you feel excessively sleepy or irritable or have trouble concentrating? Do you have trouble staying awake, or have you fallen asleep at inappropriate times?

Sleep log. In addition to the sleep history, a client and bed partner may be asked to keep a sleep-wake log for 1 to 2 weeks (Douglas and others, 1990). The log is completed daily to provide information on day-to-day variations in sleep-wake patterns over extended periods. Entries in the log often include 24-hour information about various waking and sleeping health behaviors such as physical activities, mealtimes, type and amount of intake (alcohol and caffeine), time and length of daytime naps, evening and bed routines, the time the client tries to fall asleep, time and number of awakenings, and the time of morning awakening. A partner can help to complete the sleep-wake log. The log is most helpful if the client is motivated to complete it thoroughly. Use of a tape recorder is a helpful option for clients with visual impairment or who have difficulty writing. The log is not used with acutely ill clients who have short hospital stays.

Physical illness. The nurse assesses for any physical or psychological problems that may be affecting a client's sleep. A review of known medical conditions can reveal if there are symptoms (e.g., pain, shortness of breath, incontinence, fear) that are interfering with the client's normal sleep pattern. The nurse also assesses the client's medication history, including a description of over-the-counter and prescribed drugs. If a client takes medications to aid sleep, the nurse gathers information about the type and amount of medication that is being used.

If the client has recently undergone surgery, the nurse can expect the client to experience some disturbance in sleep. The effect on sleep depends on the severity of pain experienced after surgery (Closs, 1992).

Current life events. Changes in lifestyle can disrupt a client's sleep. A person's family situation or occupation may offer a clue to the nature of a sleep problem. Changes in job responsibilities, rotating shifts, or the recent birth of a child or loss of a family member can contribute to a sleep disturbance. Questions about social activities, recent travel, or mealtime schedules also help clarify the sleep assessment.

Emotional and mental status. If a client is anxious, fearful, excitable, or angry, mental preoccupations can seriously disrupt sleep. The client may be experiencing emotional stress related to illness or situational crises such as loss of a job or loved one. The nurse asks clients to explore feelings with regard to family relationships, job, or other meaningful situations. When a sleep disturbance is related to an emotional problem, the key is to treat the primary problem, and its resolution should improve sleep (Ancoli-Israel, 1997).

Bedtime routines. The nurse asks about what the client does to prepare for sleep. The nurse assesses habits that are beneficial compared with those that have been found to disturb sleep. Watching television may promote sleep for one person but keep another individual wide awake. Sometimes pointing out that a particular habit may be interfering with sleep can help clients to find ways to change or eliminate habits that disrupt sleep.

A client's activity or exercise pattern before bedtime offers additional information about sleep quality. Does the client perform strenuous exercise within 2 hours of going to sleep? Does the client usually spend 1 to 2 hours cooling down or relaxing before sleep?

Bedtime environment. The nurse asks the client to describe preferred bedroom conditions, for example, keeping the bedroom dark or softly lit and closing the door. The client may listen to a radio or watch TV or may prefer a quiet environment if noise prevents the client from falling asleep. The nurse also asks about room temperature and ventilation.

The nurse also assesses the type of bed in which the person sleeps. Does the client sleep in the same bed every night? Is the mattress comfortable? Does the client need several pillows or cushions in bed to sit up during sleep? Does the client use a lounge chair to sleep? Information about the sleeping environment helps the nurse design better sleeping conditions.

In the health care setting, the nurse determines whether environmental stimuli are disrupting the client's sleep. A roommate who stays up late or has multiple visitors, the presence of electrical equipment at a client's bedside, and the likelihood of noise coming from an outside hallway are examples of factors to consider that can be reduced or controlled.

Behaviors of sleep deprivation. Some clients may be unaware of how their sleep problems are affecting their behavior. The nurse observes for behaviors such as irritability, disorientation (similar to a drunken state), and slurred speech. If sleep deprivation has lasted a long time, psychotic behavior such as delusions and paranoia may develop. For example, a client may report seeing strange objects or colors in the room. The client may act afraid when the nurse enters the room.

Client expectations. After assessing the client's sleep history, the nurse should also learn the client's expectations regarding nursing care. For example, the nurse might ask, "Now that I understand more about your sleep habits and the recent problems you have had, what is it that you expect from us regarding your care?" or "In order to improve your sleep, what do you feel is most important that we do for you?" The client may have a different view on the relationship of sleep and health from that of the nurse. Examining client expectations helps to clarify any misconceptions the nurse might have. In the hospital setting, clients might be more concerned about being sure the nurses are checking their condition routinely than about whether the nurses awaken them from sleep. The nurse will plan nursing care, being sure the client's expectations are fully addressed.

....

Successful critical thinking requires a synthesis of knowledge, experience, information gathered from clients, and critical thinking attitudes and standards. Clinical judgments require the nurse to anticipate what information is needed, to analyze the data, and then to make decisions regarding client care. The client expects competent and informed care. Anna incorporates previous knowledge and experience in providing care for Mr. Murphy.

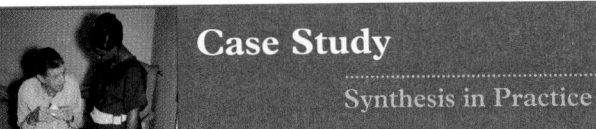

Case Study

Synthesis in Practice

As Anna prepares to conduct an assessment of Mr. Murphy, she knows it is important to consider how sleep is altered in older adults. Since they typically have less deep sleep and more awakenings to begin with, it will be important to consider what factors in the nursing home environment may be disrupting sleep. In addition, she has learned that the pain of Mr. Murphy's osteoarthritis can be a contributing factor to any possible sleep disturbance. His immobility resulting from the stroke may add to any discomfort. Anna also plans to assess Mr. Murphy's medications carefully to determine if any drugs might be adding to a sleep alteration.

From Anna's experience in a nursing home, she knows that a resident's sleep is often fragmented. Furthermore, she has read in a journal article that multiple factors affect sleep in the nursing home client, including physical illness, dementia, depression, high prevalence of sleep-disordered breathing, chronic bed rest, circadian rhythm disturbances, and the noise and lighting of the nursing home environment (Ancoli-Israel, 1997). She wants to be sure that her assessment considers all potential factors influencing Mr. Murphy's sleep pattern. Anna plans to include Mr. Murphy's wife in the assessment to learn more about Mrs. Murphy's perceptions of changes in Mr. Murphy's behavior. A complete assessment must be clear and precise; thus Anna plans to talk with Mr. Murphy more than one time to gather the necessary information and to keep her client from becoming fatigued. ▪

Nursing Diagnosis

Assessment will reveal clusters of data that include defining characteristics for a sleep problem or other nursing diagnoses that result from disturbed sleep. If a sleep pattern disturbance is identified, it is helpful for the nurse to specify the exact condition (see nursing diagnoses box). By specifying the nature of a sleep disturbance, the nurse can design more effective interventions.

Assessment should also identify the probable cause or related factor for the sleep disturbance, such as a noisy environment, a high intake of caffeine, or stress involving work. These causes become the focus of interventions for minimizing or eliminating the problem. For example, a hospitalized client who experiences insomnia as a result of a noisy sleeping environment might benefit from interventions such as controlling hospital equipment noise or reducing interruptions. If the insomnia is related to worry over a threatened marital separation, the nurse's interventions might involve introducing coping strategies. If the probable cause or related factors are incorrectly defined, the client may not benefit from care.

Planning

After identifying all relevant nursing diagnoses for a client, the nurse develops a plan of care (see care plan). An individualized care plan can be developed only after the nurse understands the client's normal and current sleep pattern, the client's perception of that sleep pattern, and the factors disrupting sleep. Together the nurse and client develop realistic goals and outcomes for care and select interventions most likely to promote rest and sleep in the home or health care setting. For example, the goal of "client establishes a healthy sleep pattern" will include outcomes such as "client will fall asleep within $1/2$ hour of planned time" and "client will have less than two awakenings during the night." The outcomes will serve as measurable guidelines to determine goal achievement.

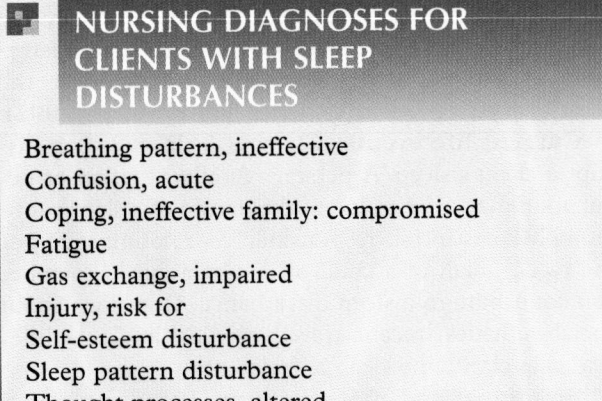

NURSING DIAGNOSES FOR CLIENTS WITH SLEEP DISTURBANCES

Breathing pattern, ineffective
Confusion, acute
Coping, ineffective family: compromised
Fatigue
Gas exchange, impaired
Injury, risk for
Self-esteem disturbance
Sleep pattern disturbance
Thought processes, altered

CASE STUDY NURSING CARE PLAN

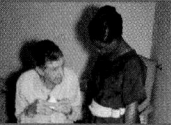

Insomnia

Assessment

Anna learns that Mr. Murphy usually slept from 10:30 PM to 6:00 AM when he was at home, usually awakening once or twice during the night to urinate. He rarely had difficulty falling asleep, but according to this wife, listening to music helped him relax. Since being in the nursing home he now reports, **"I have so much trouble falling asleep. It probably takes over an hour."** When asked if he awakens during the night, Mr. Murphy responds, "Are you kidding? No one can sleep here; something is always going on." Mr. Murphy admits to **awakening as many as 3 or 4 times during the night.** The client estimates he received maybe **4 hours of sleep the previous night.** He denies that he is having discomfort from the osteoarthritis but is **having difficulty** changing positions and **getting comfortable.** While Mr. Murphy describes his situation, he **yawns frequently** and states, **"I really feel tired."** Anna asks him to rate the quality of the previous night's sleep, and he places a **mark on the analog scale, near "worst night's sleep."** Anna notices during the assessment that Mr. Murphy's roommate is frequently calling out to anyone who passes the room door. The roommate's television is also on.

Nursing Diagnosis

Sleep pattern disturbance (insomnia) related to excessive environmental stimuli.

Plan

Goal

Client will obtain a sense of restfulness following sleep within 1 month.

Expected Outcomes

Client will have fewer than two self-reported awakenings during the night within 2 weeks.

Client will report being able to fall asleep within $\frac{1}{2}$ hour of going to sleep within 2 weeks.

Client will obtain an average of 7 hours of sleep per night within 4 weeks.

Implementation

Steps

1. Have Mr. Murphy moved to a room at the end of the hall. Match with roommate who is also alert and oriented.
2. Arrange for client to have a CD player with earphones, to play music of his choice when first going to sleep.
3. Discourage frequent daytime napping; instead replace it with regular exercise (e.g., have Mr. Murphy propel down hallways in wheelchair [5 minutes, 4 times each day]).
4. Have an egg crate mattress placed over bed mattress. Have staff position client with extra pillows before bedtime.

Rationale

Matching roommates with similar nighttime behaviors and daytime routines can reduce sleep disruption (Ancoli-Israel, 1997).

Soothing music blocks out sounds from care-giving environment and reduces anxiety, promoting relaxation (Pope, 1995).

Increases likelihood of client feeling fatigued and ready for sleep at bedtime.

Increases comfort of sleeping position, enhancing relaxation, which can promote a sleep state.

Evaluation

Ask Mr. Murphy to use a visual analog scale to rate the quality of his sleep at the end of each week.

Ask Mrs. Murphy to evaluate her preceptions of Mr. Murphy's level of fatigue.

Have Mr. Murphy report on the time he estimates falling asleep and the number of awakenings at night.

Ask Mr. Murphy at the end of 4 weeks to keep a record for a week of the length of time he estimates sleeping.

Defining characteristics are shown in bold type.

It is important for the plan of care to include strategies that fit the client's living environment and lifestyle. An effective plan includes outcomes established over a realistic time frame that focus on the goal of improving the quality of sleep. This type of plan may require many weeks to accomplish.

In a health care setting, the nurse plans treatments or routines to give the client more time to rest. For example, the nurse might turn and reposition a client at the same time a treatment like suctioning is to be performed, to limit the number of nurse-client contacts. In a nursing home the nurse may plan rest periods around the activities of other residents. All staff caring for the client should know the plan so that they can cluster activities at times to reduce awakenings.

The nature of a sleep disturbance determines whether referrals to additional health care providers are necessary. For example, if a sleep problem is related to a situational crisis or emotional problem, the nurse may refer the client to a psychiatric clinical nurse specialist, pastoral care professional, or clinical psychologist for counseling. When chronic insomnia is the problem, a medical referral or referral to a sleep center can be beneficial.

▉ Implementation

Nursing interventions for improving the quality of a person's sleep are largely focused on health promotion. When a client becomes hospitalized, the differences in nursing care in an acute care setting focus on managing the environment and trying to support the client's normal sleep habits. When clients enter long-term care or nursing home environments, special considerations are needed to promote adequate sleep and rest.

Health promotion.
Clients need adequate sleep and rest to maintain active and productive lifestyles. The nurse performs specific interventions to promote a person's normal sleep and rest pattern.

Environmental controls. All clients require a sleeping environment with a comfortable room temperature and proper ventilation, minimal noise, a comfortable bed, and proper lighting. Infants sleep best when the room temperature is 18° to 21° C (65° to 69.8° F) at night. Cribs should be positioned away from open windows or drafts. The infant is covered with a light, warm blanket. Healthy infants should be placed on their side or back when being put to sleep (American Academy of Pediatrics, 1992). This position has been shown to reduce the incidence of SIDS. There seems to be a greater incidence of SIDS in infants who are positioned prone, on their stomachs. Children and adults vary more in regard to comfortable room temperature but usually sleep best in cooler environments. Some prefer to sleep without covers. Older adults may require extra blankets or covers. Many older clients sleep wearing socks (Box 32-5).

BOX 32-5
Gerontological Nursing Practice

Sleep-wake pattern
- Maintain a regular rising time.
- Eliminate naps unless they are a routine part of the schedule.
- If naps are used, limit to 20 minutes or less twice a day.
- Avoid extremes of sleep, that is, becoming excessively sleepy on the weekends.
- Go to bed when sleepy.
- Use relaxation techniques to promote sleep.
- If unable to sleep in 15 to 30 minutes, get out of bed.

Environment
- Sleep where you sleep best.
- Keep noise to minimum; use soft music to mask noise if necessary.
- Use night-light, and keep path to bathroom free of obstacles.
- Set room temperature to preference; use blankets and socks to promote warmth.

Medications
- Use sedatives and hypnotics as last resort and then only short-term if absolutely necessary.
- Adjust medications being taken for other conditions and look for drug interactions that may cause insomnia or EDS.

Physiological/illness factors
- Elevate head of bed and provide extra pillows as preferred.
- Use analgesics 30 minutes before bed to ease aches and pains.
- Use therapeutics to control symptoms of chronic conditions as prescribed.

Distracting noise needs to be eliminated or reduced so that the bedroom is as quiet as possible. This is not always easy when a family consists of several members. In the home the TV or the ringing of the telephone may disrupt a client's sleep. The family becomes important participants in care when each has different schedules for going to sleep. It may require the cooperation of several people living with the client to reduce noise. Some clients sleep better with familiar inside noises, such as the hum of a ceiling fan.

The bed and mattress should provide support and comfortable firmness. A bed board can be placed under the mattress to add support. Sometimes extra pillows help a person to position more comfortably in bed. The position of the bed in the room may also make a difference for some clients.

For any client prone to confusion or falls, safety is critical. In the home a small night-light might assist the client in orienting to the room environment before arising to go to the bathroom. Beds set lower to the floor may reduce the risk of falls when a person stands. Clutter should be removed from the path a client uses to walk from the bed to the bathroom. If a client needs help in ambulating from the bed to the bathroom, a small bell at the bedside can be used to call family members.

Clients vary in regard to the amount of light that they prefer at night. Infants and older adults sleep best in softly lit rooms. Light should not shine directly on their eyes. Small table lamps or night-lights prevent total darkness. For older adults, this reduces the chance of confusion when arising from bed. If streetlights shine through windows or when clients nap during the day, heavy shades, drapes, or slatted blinds are helpful.

Promoting bedtime routines. Bedtime routines relax clients in preparation for sleep. It is important for persons to go to sleep when they feel fatigued or sleepy. Going to bed while fully awake and thinking about concerns can cause insomnia and interfere with the bed as a stimulus for sleep. To develop good sleep habits at home, clients and their bed partners should learn techniques that promote sleep and conditions that interfere with sleep (Box 32-6).

Newborns and infants benefit from quiet activities such as holding them snugly in blankets, talking or singing softly, and gently rocking. A bedtime routine (e.g., same hour for bedtime or quiet activity) used consistently helps young children avoid delaying sleep. Toddlers and preschoolers may be too excited and full of energy to go to bed. Patterns of preparing for bedtime need to be reinforced. Reading stories, allowing children to sit in a parent's lap while listening to music or prayer, and coloring are routines that can be associated with preparing for bed.

Adults need to avoid excessive mental stimulation just before bedtime. Reading a light novel, watching a relaxing television program, or listening to music helps a person relax. Relaxation exercises can induce calm (see Chapter 33). Guided imagery and praying may also induce sleep.

Promoting comfort. People fall asleep only after feeling comfortable and relaxed. The nurse can recommend and use several measures to promote comfort (Box 32-7). Minor irritants can keep persons awake. Diapers should be changed before placing infants in bed. Soft cotton nightclothes keep infants or small children warm and comfortable. An extra blanket can prevent chilling when one tries to fall asleep.

Clients who suffer painful illnesses can try a variety of measures at home to promote comfort. Application of dry or moist heat, use of supportive dressings or splints (see Chapter 38), and proper positioning with the use of extra pillows for support can be very helpful. For clients with temporary acute pain (e.g., following surgery), it may be advantageous to the client and bed partner to let the client sleep alone until the pain subsides.

For clients with physical illness, the nurse can help them learn ways to control symptoms that disrupt sleep. For example, a client with respiratory abnormalities should sleep with two pillows or in a semisitting position to ease the effort to breathe. The client may benefit from taking prescribed bronchodilators before sleep to prevent airway obstruction.

Promoting activity. In the home it may help to encourage clients to stay physically active during the day so that they are more likely to sleep at night. Increasing daytime activity lessens problems with falling asleep. Rigorous exercise should always be planned at least several hours before bedtime.

Exercise is believed to be beneficial to older adults by improving nighttime sleep. However, individuals with chronic diseases that influence their functional abilities are likely to have limited activity (Lueckenotte, 1996). The nurse must recommend activities that are safe for older clients to perform. Walking, swimming, and cycling on a stationary bike are excellent for those clients with limited physical impairment. Repetitions of sit-to-stand or transferring and up to 5 minutes of walking or wheelchair propulsion are excellent for those with physical limitations (Alessi and others, 1995). Weight lifting

---

BOX 32-6

Client Teaching for Sleep Hygiene Habits

- Caution client against sleeping long hours during weekends or holidays to prevent disturbance of normal sleep-wake cycle.
- Explain that if possible, the bedroom should not be used for intensive studying, snacking, TV watching, or other nonsleep activity, besides sex.
- Explain that client should try to avoid worrisome thinking when going to bed and should use relaxation exercises.
- If client has trouble falling asleep, advise to get out of bed and do some quiet activity until feeling sleepy enough to go back to bed.
- Instruct client to avoid heavy meals for 3 hours before bedtime; a light snack may help.

Box 32-7

Comfort Measures for Promoting Sleep

Encourage client to wear loose-fitting nightwear.

Instruct family on ways to position client and support dependent body parts to protect pressure points and aid muscle relaxation.

Have client void before going to bed.

Instruct family on technique for giving client a back massage.

If client is excessively diaphoretic or becomes incontinent, change the bed linens.

using light weights (e.g., 2 to 5 lb) is also excellent to build upper body strength and endurance.

Stress reduction. When clients feel emotionally upset, they should be urged to try not to force sleep. Otherwise, insomnia often develops, and soon bedtime is associated with the inability to relax. A client who has difficulty falling asleep can be helped by getting up and pursuing a relaxing activity rather than staying in bed and thinking about sleep. When the emotional problem is ongoing and the client finds little relief, the nurse should encourage referral to an appropriate counselor.

Children often have problems going to bed and falling asleep. Toddlers often become fearful as a result of separation from parents. Preschoolers commonly have trouble falling asleep because of excess activity and stimulation (Wong, 1995). Preschoolers also have bedtime fears (fear of the dark or strange noises), awaken during the night, or have nightmares. After nightmares, parents should enter children's rooms immediately and talk to them briefly about their fears to provide a cooling-down period. Comforting children while they lie in their own bed can be reassuring. Keeping a light on in the room may also help. Usually experts do not recommend that a child be allowed to sleep with parents; however, cultural traditions may cause families to approach sleep practices differently. For example, Hispanic and Asian families often practice co-sleeping, in which children are allowed to sleep with parents or siblings to lessen the child's anxiety and promote a sense of security.

Bedtime snacks. Some persons enjoy bedtime snacks, whereas others cannot sleep after eating. A dairy product snack such as warm milk or cocoa that contains L-tryptophan may help to promote sleep. A full meal before bedtime can often cause gastrointestinal upset and interfere with the ability to fall asleep.

Clients should avoid drinking excess fluids or ingesting caffeine before bedtime. Coffee, tea, cola, and chocolate will cause a person to stay awake or awaken throughout the night. Alcohol can interrupt sleep cycles and reduce the amount of deep sleep. Coffee, tea, colas, and alcohol act as diuretics, causing **nocturia.**

Infants require special measures to minimize nighttime awakenings for feedings. Wong (1995) recommends offering the last feeding as late as possible. A gradual reduction in the amount of formula or duration of breast feeding can also help. Infants should not be given bottles in bed because of the risk of choking and aspiration.

Pharmacological approaches to promoting sleep. Many of the drugs clients take to manage symptoms are associated with causing insomnia. CNS stimulants such as amphetamines, nicotine, terbutaline, theophylline, and pemoline (Cylert) should be used sparingly and under medical management (McKenry and Salerno, 1995). Withdrawal from CNS depressants such as alcohol, barbiturates, and tricyclic antidepressants (amitriptyline, imipramine, doxepin, and triazolam [Halcion]) can also cause insomnia and must be managed carefully.

Sleep medications can help a client if used correctly. However, long-term use of antianxiety, sedative, or hypnotic agents can disrupt sleep and lead to more serious problems. One group of drugs considered to be relatively safe are the benzodiazepines (Table 32-2). These medications do not cause general CNS depression like **sedatives** or **hypnotics** do. Appropriate administration is acute and short-term use (no longer than 2 to 3 weeks) (Ancoli-Israel, 1997).

The use of benzodiazepines in the older adult population is potentially dangerous because of the drug's tendency to remain active in the body for a longer time. This means the drugs can potentially interact with other agents (Lueckenotte, 1996). Short-acting benzodiazepines (oxazepam, lorazepam, temazepam) at the lowest possible dose are recommended. Initial doses should be small, and increments are added gradually, based on client response, for a limited time.

Melatonin is a hormone produced in the brain that helps control circadian rhythms (Ancoli-Israel, 1997). It is a popular nutritional supplement in the United States used to aid sleep. Research regarding the long-term effects of melatonin is inconclusive. Melatonin is usually sold in 3-mg tablets, but the body produces less than 0.5 mg. The nurse should caution clients about the timing of ingestion and the dose taken.

The use of nonprescription sleeping medications is not advisable. Over the long term, these drugs can lead to further sleep disruption even when they initially seem effective. The nurse can help clients use behavioral and proper sleep hygiene measures to establish sleep patterns that do not require the use of drugs.

Regular use of any sleep medication can lead to tolerance, and withdrawal can then cause rebound insomnia. All clients should understand the possible side effects of sleep medications. Routine monitoring of client response to sleeping medications is important.

Managing specific sleep disturbances. Clients who suffer specific sleep disturbances will likely benefit from the health promotion strategies discussed so far. However, there are also therapies unique to the specific type of sleep disturbance.

Weight loss can be effective for the client with obstructive sleep apnea. It is important for the client to follow an appropriate weight reduction plan (see Chapter 34) and to keep the weight off. In milder cases of obstructive sleep apnea, body position during sleep can be effective. Ancoli-Israel (1997) recommends a simple measure of having clients keep off their backs during sleep by sewing a pocket into the back of their nightshirt and inserting a tennis ball into the pocket.

Acute care. The nursing interventions described for health promotion are applicable to a client requiring

TABLE 32-2
Pharmacology of Antiinsomnia Agents

Generic Name	Trade Name	Onset of Action (min)	Oral Dosage* (mg)	Indications
Alprazolam	Xanax	15-60	0.25-0.5 (3 times daily)	Anxiety
Diazepam	Valium	15-45	5-10 at bedtime	Sleep disorder
Flurazepam	Dalmane Apo-Flurazepam	15-45	15-30 at bedtime	Sleep disorder
Lorazepam	Ativan Apo-Lorazepam	15-60	1-4 at bedtime	Anxiety, sleep disorder
Oxazepam	Serax Zapex	45-90	10-30 (3-4 times daily)	Anxiety
Temazepam	Restoril	25-27	15-30 at bedtime	Sleep disorder
Triazolam	Halcion	15-30	0.125-0.25 at bedtime	Sleep disorder
Zolpidem	Ambien	15-45	10-20 at bedtime	Sleep disorder

*Smaller dosages may be prescribed for older adult clients.

acute care. The nature of the acute care setting requires the nurse to be creative in finding ways to maintain the client's normal sleep pattern.

Managing environmental stimuli. The ability to control noise in the hospital environment can be very challenging. Since many clients spend only a short time in hospitals, staff often forget the importance of establishing good sleep conditions. Box 32-8 outlines options for the nurse to use in reducing room noise.

In the hospital setting, the nurse should plan care to avoid awakening clients. The nurse can help by scheduling assessments, treatments, procedures, and routines

---

Box 32-8
Control of Noise in the Hospital

Close doors to the client's room when possible.
Keep doors to work areas on unit closed when in use.
Reduce volume of nearby telephone and paging equipment.
Wear rubber-soled shoes. Avoid clogs.
Turn off bedside oxygen and other equipment that is not in use.
Turn down alarms and beeps on bedside monitoring equipment.
Turn off room TV and radio unless client prefers soft music.
Avoid abrupt loud noise such as flushing a toilet or moving a bed.
Keep necessary conversations at low levels, particularly at night.
Conduct conversations and reports in a private area away from client rooms.

---

for times when clients are awake. For example, a client who has had surgery should have the surgical dressing changed, be repositioned, receive a pain medication, and have a set of vital signs completed before retiring for the night. Medications should be given and blood drawn during waking hours when possible. The nurse should plan with the radiology department and other services to schedule therapies at intervals that give clients time to rest. Whenever it becomes necessary to awaken a client, it should be done as soon as possible so that the client can fall back to sleep quickly.

Safety. Safety precautions are important for clients who awaken during the night to use the bathroom and for those with excessive daytime sleepiness. Beds should be set lower to the floor to lessen the chance of the client's falling when first standing. Clutter should be removed and equipment moved from the path a client uses to walk from the bed to the bathroom. If a client needs assistance in ambulating from the bed to the bathroom, the call light should always be within the client's reach. The nurse should be sure the client knows how to turn the light on correctly.

Clients who experience daytime sleepiness can fall asleep while sitting up in a chair or wheelchair. The nurse should position clients so that they will not fall out of the chair when sleeping. Elevating the client's feet on a small bench or an overturned wastebasket will prevent the client from tipping over. A pillow placed in the client's lap might offer some support. If a client enjoys leaning over an overbed table while sitting in a chair, be sure the table is locked and secure. Use of safety belts is considered to be a restraint and should be avoided (see Chapter 28).

Comfort measures. One way the nurse can make the client more comfortable in an acute setting is by providing personal hygiene before bedtime. A warm bath or shower can be very relaxing. Clients restricted to bed should be offered the opportunity to wash their face and hands. Toothbrushing and care of dentures also help to prepare the client for sleep. Clients should void before retiring so they are not kept awake by a full bladder. While a client prepares for bed, the nurse can help to position the client off any potential pressure sites.

Compared with beds at home, hospital beds are harder and of a different height, length, and width. Keeping beds clean and dry and in a comfortable position may help clients relax. Many hospitals offer egg crate mattresses for client comfort (see Chapter 38). These support surfaces offer little in the way of pressure sore prevention but do provide an extra layer of comfortable support.

Removal of irritating stimuli is another way the nurse can improve the client's comfort for a restful sleep. Changing or removal of moist dressings, repositioning drainage tubings, reapplying wrinkled thromboembolic hose, and changing tape on nasogastric tubes eliminate constant irritants to the client's skin. When an IV site becomes irritated and painful, reinsertion of the IV is usually recommended (see Chapter 31). Clients who are incontinent should have the perineal or anal area cleaned thoroughly. Diaphoretic clients will benefit from a cool sponging.

Restorative care. The quality of sleep in a long-term care or nursing home environment is often fragmented. Residents of a nursing home often suffer chronic disease, incontinence, and dementia and take multiple medications, all of which can disrupt sleep. Psychotropic medications are commonly used in nursing homes, with some evidence of a change in normal diurnal variation in sleep (Alessi and others, 1995). Schnelle and others (1993) found noise, light, and repositioning of nursing home residents during linen changes as factors that caused clients to awaken, often for periods of 4 minutes or longer. Besides care activities, nursing home residents themselves can be very disruptive by crying out loudly to roommates or nursing staff.

In the long-term care environment, many clients are requiring rehabilitation or ongoing supportive care. The nature of their illnesses and treatment requirements can pose problems for attaining restful sleep. For example, clients who are ventilator dependent will likely get brief periods of sleep throughout the day rather than prolonged sleep because of disruptions from ventilator alarm sounds, sounds of air movement through airway tubing, and the need for occasional suctioning.

Maintaining activity. General recommendations to improve sleep in older adults have often suggested increasing daytime activity or exercise (National Institutes of Health Consensus Development Conference, 1991). Stevenson and Topp (1990) studied the effects of long-term exercise in older adults residing in the community and found improved self-reported sleep. However, in a study of extremely frail older adults residing within a nursing home, Alessi and others (1995) did not find an improvement in sleep as a result of physical activity. Alessi and others (1995) acknowledged that the clients in their study suffered from complex problems, all of which could have negated the benefits of exercise. The general benefits of activity and exercise—improved activity endurance, improved mobility, and improved sense of well-being—may prove to be beneficial to those older adults who are not institutionalized and thus not exposed to repetitive environmental distractions.

In the restorative care setting, the nurse should try to limit the time clients spend in bed. In the nursing home meals should be served in the resident dining area. Otherwise clients should be up in a chair for meals as well as for personal hygiene activities. It is also important to keep the residents involved in social activities planned at the nursing home (e.g., card playing, arts and crafts, sing-alongs). Regular exercise (e.g., walking or wheelchair propulsion down a hallway) keeps the clients active and stimulated. It is also ideal to limit naps to once a day for 30 minutes or less (Ancoli-Israel, 1997).

Clients with dementia often have disrupted sleep-wake cycles. They often become easily fatigued and experience periods of insomnia (Lueckenotte, 1996). In this situation activities and visits may need to be shortened to allow the client to maintain an adequate energy level. If the client awakens during the night, keeping the lights at a low level and using soothing techniques such as quiet music or a back rub can promote sleep.

Reducing sleep disruption. Knowing the many factors that can disrupt sleep in clients who reside in restorative care settings, the nurse must find ways to make the environment more conducive to sleep. As in the case of the acute care setting, noise control is critical. Often staff within a nursing home naturally speak louder because of residents' difficulties with hearing. Walking up close to a client and talking in a normal but clear voice will likely improve the client's hearing and reduce the chance of awakening a nearby roommate. Training nurse's aides to be more sensitive to the sources of noise that disrupt clients' sleep can be very useful.

Evaluation

Client care. Evaluation of therapies designed to promote sleep and rest must be individualized. Clients in relatively good health may not need as much sleep as clients whose physical conditions are poor.

If the nurse has established realistic goals of care, the expected outcomes become guidelines for evaluating the client's progress and response to interventions. Evaluative measures may be used shortly after a therapy has been tried (e.g., observing if a client falls asleep after reducing room noise and light). Other evaluative measures may be used after a client awakens from sleep (e.g., asking a client to describe the number of awakenings during the night). Together the client and bed partner can usually provide accurate information. If the client lives or sleeps alone, reliability of evaluation can be questioned.

When expected outcomes are not met, the nurse revises nursing measures based on the client's needs or preferences. Finding an effective therapy depends on the client's sleep disturbance, age, and normal sleep pattern. The nurse documents the client's response to sleep therapies so that a continuum of care can be maintained.

Client expectations.

The nurse will review the progress in the plan of care with the client and determine if the client's expectations were met. Does the client believe the nurse's interventions were helpful and useful? Did the nurse incorporate the client's typical sleep routine into the plan of care? For the hospitalized client, did the staff avoid unnecessary interruptions and give the client a chance to rest? The client's perceptions are valuable sources of information regarding the overall success in improving the quality of the client's sleep.

Key Terms

advanced sleep phase syndrome	narcolepsy
biological clocks	nocturia
bruxism	NREM sleep
bulbar synchronizing region (BSR)	REM sleep
cataplexy	reticular activating system (RAS)
circadian rhythm	sedatives
hypnotics	sleep
insomnia	sleep apnea
	sleep deprivation

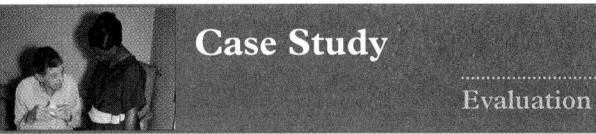

Case Study

Evaluation

After 4 weeks at the nursing home, Anna has successfully been able to have Mr. Murphy transferred to a new room and has been monitoring his progress. He has been in the new room for 2 weeks. Anna asks Mr. Murphy, "Tell me how our plan to improve your sleep has been working. Have the music and headphones been helpful?" Mr. Murphy replies, "Well, it has helped to be down here at the end of the hall. It still is a bit noisy, especially if the nurses are working with people across the way. I have used the headphones the last 2 weeks, and they have helped me relax and fall asleep in about 20 or 30 minutes." Anna questions Mr. Murphy further and learns that he is awakening 2 or 3 times during the night. However, during the last week he estimated getting about 6 hours of sleep, an improvement from a month ago. Mr. Murphy also reports that the staff have usually been good about reminding him to do his daily exercises with the wheelchair. He dislikes staying in his room and has tried to exercise as much as possible.

Anna decides to revise the care plan, adding an intervention for placing a sign on the client's door at night asking staff to keep the door closed. Mr. Murphy's sleep is improving, and Anna selects an additional measure aimed at reducing awakenings.

Anna wants to know Mr. Murphy's level of satisfaction with her care. She asks, "Have I met your expectations so far? If not, tell me how I can better help you." Mr. Murphy replies, "You've been great. I know you can't make this place like home. There is so much to think about when you are here. I think about my wife a lot." Anna responds, "Tell me more. What do you mean there is so much to think about?" Anna recognizes that sleep can be altered by psychological and physical stressors. She decides to reassess Mr. Murphy to determine if additional nursing interventions might be appropriate.

Documentation Note

Client reports some improvement in overall sleep quality. Able to fall asleep within 20 to 30 minutes using headphones with music. Reports sleeping approximately 6 hours per night. Continues to experience reawakenings, resulting from noise in outside hallway. Recommend closing room door at night to reduce noise further. Client has begun to admit thinking about his wife and possibly other concerns. Will explore further with him.

■ Key Concepts

Sleep is believed to provide physiological and psychological restoration.

The 24-hour sleep-wake cycle is a circadian rhythm that influences physiological function and behavior.

The control and regulation of sleep depends on a balance between CNS regulators.

During a typical night's sleep a person passes through four to six complete sleep cycles. Each sleep cycle contains three NREM stages of sleep and a period of REM sleep.

The number of hours of sleep needed by each person to feel rested is variable.

Long-term use of sleeping pills may lead to difficulty in initiating and maintaining sleep.

The hectic pace of a person's lifestyle, emotional and psychological stress, and alcohol ingestion disrupt the sleep pattern.

An environment with a darkened room, reduced noise, comfortable bed, and good ventilation promotes sleep.

The most common type of sleep disorder is insomnia, which is characterized by the inability to fall asleep, to remain asleep during the night, or to go back to sleep after awakening earlier than is desired.

Only a client can report whether sleep is restful.

When using environmental controls to promote sleep, the nurse should consider the usual characteristics of the client's home environment and normal lifestyle.

Noise can disrupt sleep and enhance pain perception.

A bedtime routine of relaxing activities prepares a person physically and mentally for sleep.

Pain or other symptom control is essential to promote the ability to sleep.

One of the most important nursing interventions for promoting sleep is establishing periods for uninterrupted sleep and rest.

■ Critical Thinking Activities

1. Mrs. Riley is a 66-year-old woman who comes to the community health clinic every 6 months for management of her hypertension. During this visit she reports the following to the nurse: "I am having more difficulty falling asleep. During the last month I bet I got up at least twice every night. My husband is convinced something is wrong. I still go to bed about the same time, around 10 PM, and I awaken around 6 AM." What would your analysis be of this client's assessment? How might you proceed further?

2. Edward Pena is a 34-year-old businessman who comes to the physician's office complaining of being very sleepy during the day. He has noticed the problem for about 3 months. He states, "If I'm lucky, I get about 4 or 5 hours of sleep each night." He spends most of the workweek flying to various cities across the country. His day begins at 5 AM and often does not end until 7 PM or later. He admits that his eating habits are erratic; sometimes he does not have a meal until 8 or 9 at night. He drinks coffee during the day to keep him going. Mr. Pena likes to play golf on weekends but exercises little during the week. Last month his boss had a long talk with Mr. Pena after hearing that he had fallen asleep during a business meeting. This was the second time it had occurred. Mr. Pena is asking if he might be able to try a sleeping pill to help him sleep. What might be Mr. Pena's problem? What recommendations might you make to help him sleep?

3. Explain the value of having a client complete a visual analog scale that rates quality of sleep.

References

Alessi CA and others: Does physical activity improve sleep in impaired nursing home residents? *J Am Geriatr Soc* 43:1098, 1995.

American Academy of Pediatrics: Positioning and SIDS: AAP Task Force on Infant Positioning and SIDS, *Pediatrics* 79:1122, 1992.

American Sleep Disorders Association: *The international classification of sleep disorders: diagnostic and coding manual,* Rochester, NY, 1990, Allen Press.

Anch AM and others: *Sleep: a scientific perspective,* Englewood Cliffs, NJ, 1988, Prentice-Hall.

Ancoli-Israel, S: Sleep problems in older adults: putting myths to bed, *Geriatrics* 52(1):20, 1997.

Berman TM and others: Sleep disorders: take them seriously, *Patient Care* 24:85, © 1990, Medical Economics.

Born J and others: The significance of sleep onset and slow wave sleep for nocturnal release of growth hormone (GH) and cortisol, *Psychoneuroendocrinology* 13:233, 1988.

Campbell SS, Dawson D: Aging young sleep: a test of the phase advance hypothesis of sleep disturbances in the elderly, *J Sleep Res* 1:205, 1992.

Carskadon MA: Patrons of sleep and sleepiness in adolescents, *Pediatrician* 17:5, 1990a.

Carskadon MA: Sleep disturbances. In Friedman SB and others, editors: *Comprehensive adolescent health care,* St. Louis, 1990b, Mosby.

Close SJ: Assessment of sleep in hospital patients: a review of methods, *J Adv Nurs* 13:501, 1988.

Close SJ: Post-operative patients' views of sleep, pain, and recovery, *J Clin Nurs* 1(2):83, 1992.

Douglas AB and others: Historical data base questionnaires, sleep and life cycle diaries. In Laughton EM, Broughton RJ, editors: *Medical monitoring in the home and work environment,* New York, 1990, Raven Press.

Gillis AM, Flemmons WN: Cardiac arrhythmias during sleep. In Kryzer MH and others, editors: *Principles and practices of sleep medicine,* ed 2, Philadelphia, 1994, WB Saunders.

Griffin JP: The impact of noise on critically ill people, *Holistic Nurs Pract* 6(4):53, 1992.

Hauri P, Linde S: *No more sleepless nights,* New York, 1990, Wiley.

Karni A et al: Dependence on REM sleep of overnight improvement of a perceptual skill, *Science* 265:679, 1994.

Landis CA: Arrhythmias and sleep pattern disturbances in cardiac patients, *Prog Cardiovasc Nurse* 3:73, 1988.

Leger D: The cost of sleep-related accidents: a report for the National Commission on Sleep Disorders Research, *Sleep* 17(1):84, 1994.

Lueckenotte A: *Gerontologic nursing,* St. Louis, 1996, Mosby.

McKenry LM, Salerno E: *Mosby's pharmacology in nursing,* ed 19, St. Louis, 1995, Mosby.

Mendleson WB: Neuroendocrinology and sleep. In *Human sleep: research and clinical care,* New York, 1987, Plenum.

National Commission on Sleep Disorders Research: *Wake up America: a national sleep alert,* vol 3, 1993.

National Institutes of Health Consensus Development Conference: The treatment of sleep disorders of older people, *Sleep* 14:169, 1991.

Naylor MW, Aldrich MS: Approach to the patient with disordered sleep. In Kryger MH and others, editors: *Principles and practice of sleep medicine,* ed 2, Philadelphia, 1994, WB Saunders.

Parkinson D: Strategies for helping parents: overcoming sleep problems in babies and toddlers, *Professional Care Mother Child* 4:215, 1994.

Pope DS: Music, noise, and the human voice in the nurse-patient environment, *Image J Nurs Sch* 27(4):291, 1995.

Robinson CR: Impaired sleep. In *Pathophysiological phenomena in nursing: human responses to illness,* ed 2, Philadelphia, 1993, WB Saunders.

Schnelle JF and others: The nighttime environment, incontinence care, and sleep disruption in nursing homes, *J Am Geriatr Soc* 41:910, 1993.

Sleep Research Society: *Brain mechanisms of sleep and wakefulness: basics of sleep behavior,* Rochester, Minn, 1993, UCLA & Sleep Research Society.

Stevenson JS, Topp R: Effects of moderate and low intensity long-term exercise by older adults, *J Res Nurs Health* 13:209, 1990.

Webb WB: Technical comments: the cost of sleep-related accidents: a reanalysis, *Sleep* 18(4):276, 1995.

Webster RA, Thompson DR: Sleep in hospital, *J Adv Nurs* 11:447, 1986.

Wong DL: *Whaley and Wong's nursing care of infants and children,* ed 5, St. Louis, 1995, Mosby.

Wood AM: A review of literature relating to sleep in hospital with emphasis on the sleep of the ICU patient, *Intensive Crit Care Nurs* 9:129, 1992.

Zorick F: Insomnia. In Kryger MH and others, editors: *Principles and practice of sleep medicine,* ed 2, Philadelphia, 1994, WB Saunders.

33

Comfort

OBJECTIVES

Mastery of content in this chapter will enable the student to:

- Define the key terms listed.
- Discuss common misconceptions about pain.
- Describe the physiology of pain.
- Identify components of the pain experience.
- Discuss the three phases of behavioral responses to pain.
- Explain how the gate control theory relates to selecting nursing therapies for pain relief.
- Assess a client experiencing pain.
- Develop appropriate nursing diagnoses for a client in pain.
- Describe guidelines for selecting and individualizing pain therapies.
- Describe applications for use of nonpharmacological pain therapies.
- Discuss nursing implications for administering analgesics.
- Describe interventions for the relief of acute pain following operative or medical procedures.
- Describe the sequence of activities related to pain management in cancer clients.
- Successfully evaluate a client's response to pain therapies.

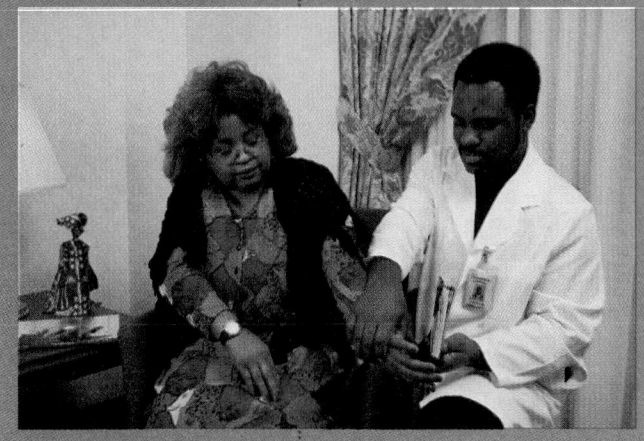

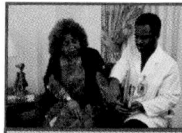

Case Study

....
Mrs. Ellis

Mrs. Ellis is a 70-year-old black female with hypertension, diabetes, and rheumatoid arthritis. She has been receiving home visits following a recent hospitalization for the control of her diabetes. Her current health priority is the discomfort and disability associated with her rheumatoid arthritis. Her hands and feet are severely deformed by the arthritis. The pain in her feet has become so severe that Mrs. Ellis can often only walk short distances. The pain interferes with sleep and reduces her energy both physically and emotionally; therefore she remains at home. She has lived alone since her husband's death 6 years ago.

Jim is a 26-year-old sophomore nursing student assigned to do home visits with the community health nurse. Jim has had the opportunity to conduct assessments, perform procedures, and teach health promotion with a variety of clients with various illnesses over the past 6 weeks. This is Jim's first experience with a client with severe chronic pain.

SCIENTIFIC KNOWLEDGE BASE

Comfort

Comfort is a concept central to the art of nursing. Each individual brings physiological, social, spiritual, psychological, and environmental characteristics that influence how comfort is interpreted and experienced.

Comfort is experienced in the following four contexts:

Physical—Pertaining to bodily sensations
Social—Pertaining to interpersonal, family, and societal relationships
Psychospiritual—Pertaining to internal awareness of self and meaning in life
Environmental—Pertaining to the external background of human experience (e.g., light, noise, temperature)

An understanding of comfort gives the nurse a larger range of choices when selecting pain therapies. Pain management is more than administering analgesics. The nurse must first understand how the pain experience affects a client's comfort level and then use therapies that meet the unique needs of clients (Jurf and Nirschl, 1993).

Nature of Pain

Pain is more than a single sensation caused by a specific stimulus. It is subjective and highly individualized.

The person experiencing pain is the only authority on it. According to McCaffery and Beebe (1989), "Pain is whatever the experiencing person says it is, existing whenever he says it does."

Pain is a protective physiological mechanism, resulting from a harmful stimulus. A client with a sprained ankle avoids bearing full weight on the foot to prevent further injury. Pain can also be a warning of tissue damage, which should be the nurse's first consideration when assessing pain (Jurf and Nirschl, 1993). Clients unable to feel sensations, such as after spinal cord injury, are unaware of pain-inducing injuries.

Health care personnel often hold prejudices against clients in pain. Unless clients have objective signs of pain, a nurse may not believe they are uncomfortable. The extent to which nurses make assumptions about clients in pain influences their nursing assessment and can seriously limit their ability to offer pain relief (Walker, 1994). Too often, nurses allow misconceptions about pain (Box 33-1) to affect their willingness to intervene (McCaffery and Ferrell, 1996). Many nurses even avoid acknowledging a client's pain because of their own fear of the outcome of their interventions and denial that the client is having pain.

Physiology of Pain

Pain is a complex mixture of physical, emotional, and behavioral reactions. An understanding of the three components of pain, **reception, perception, and reaction,** helps the nurse recognize factors that cause pain, symptoms that accompany pain, and the rationale and actions of therapies.

Reception. Any cellular damage caused by thermal, mechanical, chemical, or electrical stimuli (Table 33-1) results in the release of pain-producing substances. Exposure to painful stimuli releases substances

---

Box 33-1
Common Biases and Misconceptions About Pain

Drug abusers and alcoholics overreact to discomforts.
Clients with minor illnesses have less pain than those with severe physical alterations.
Administering analgesics regularly leads to clients' tolerance and drug dependence.
The amount of tissue damage in an injury accurately indicates pain intensity.
Health care personnel are the best authorities on the nature of pain.
Psychogenic pain is not real.
Illness and its associated suffering are an inevitable part of aging.
Severe pain can be controlled only by narcotics.

TABLE 33-1
Examples of Physical Sources of Pain

Type of Stimulus	Source	Pathophysiological Process
Mechanical	Alteration in body fluids	Edema distending body tissues
	Duct distention	Overstretching of duct's narrow lumen (e.g., passage of kidney stone through ureter)
	Space-occupying lesion (tumor)	Irritation of peripheral nerves by growth of lesion within confined space
Chemical	Perforated visceral organ	Chemical irritation by secretions on sensitive nerve endings (e.g., ruptured appendix, duodenal ulcer)
Thermal	Burn (heat or extreme cold)	Inflammation or loss of superficial layers of epidermis, causing increased sensitivity of nerve endings
Electrical	Burn	Skin layers burned with muscle and subcutaneous tissue injury, causing injury to nerve endings

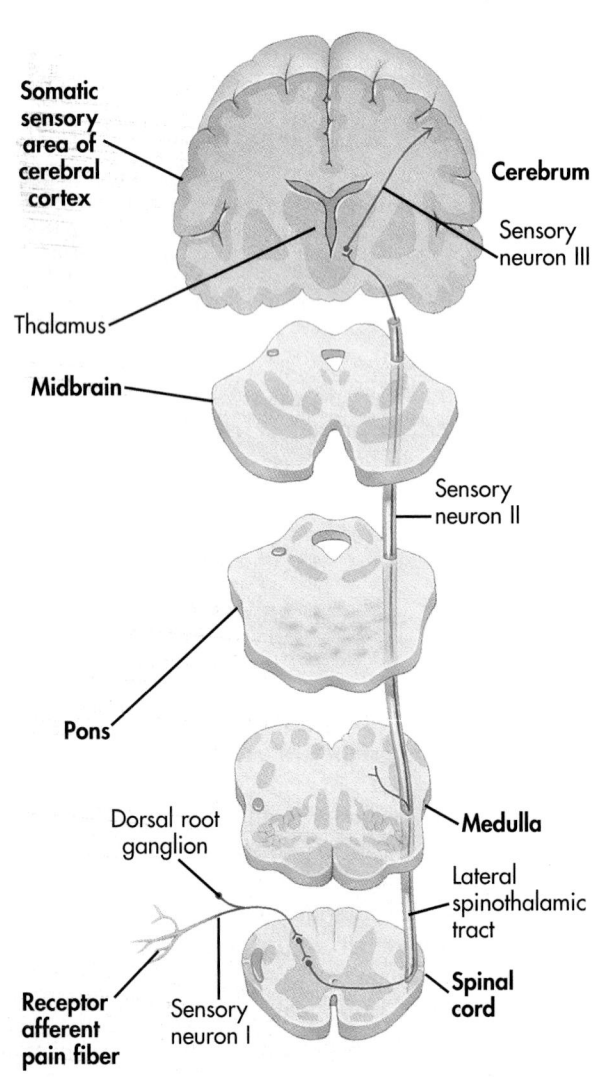

Figure 33-1. Spinothalamic pathway that conducts pain stimuli.

such as histamine, bradykinin, and potassium, which combine with receptor sites on **nociceptors** (receptors that respond to harmful stimuli) to initiate the neural transmission associated with pain (Bonica, 1990; Jurf and Nirschl, 1993).

Nerve impulses resulting from the painful stimulus travel along afferent peripheral nerve fibers. Two types of peripheral nerve fibers conduct painful stimuli: the fast, myelinated A-delta fibers and the small, slow unmyelinated C fibers. The A fibers send sharp, localized, and distinct sensations. The small C fibers relay impulses that are poorly localized, visceral, and persistent (Puntillo, 1988; Willens, 1996). For example, after stepping on a nail, a person initially feels a sharp localized pain, which is the result of A-fiber transmission. Within a few seconds the pain becomes more diffuse and widespread until the whole foot aches because of C fiber innervation.

A-delta and C fibers transmit impulses from the periphery to the dorsal horn of the spinal cord where an excitatory neurotransmitter, substance P, is released. This causes a synaptic transmission from the afferent (sensory) peripheral nerve to spinothalamic tract nerves. Pain stimuli travel through nerve fibers in the spinothalamic tracts, cross to the opposite side of the spinal cord, and then travel up the spinal cord. Figure 33-1 shows the normal pain reception pathway. After the pain impulse ascends the spinal cord, information is sent quickly to higher centers in the brain.

A protective reflex response also occurs with pain reception (Figure 33-2). A fibers send sensory impulses to the spinal cord, where they synapse with spinal motor neurons. The motor impulses travel via a reflex arc along efferent nerve fibers back to a peripheral muscle near the stimulation site. Muscle contraction leads to a protective withdrawal from the source of pain. When superficial fibers in the skin are stimulated, a person moves away from the pain source. If internal tissue such as muscle becomes stimulated, tightening and guarding of muscles occur.

Pain reception requires an intact peripheral nervous system and spinal cord. Common factors that disrupt pain reception include trauma, drugs, tumor growth, and metabolic disorders.

Neuroregulators. Neuroregulators are substances that affect the sending of nerve stimuli (Box 33-2). **Neurotransmitters** such as substance P send electrical impulses across the synaptic cleft between two nerve fibers. They either excite or inhibit nerve transmission. **Neuromodulators** such as **endorphins** modify neuron activity without directly transferring a nerve signal through a **synapse**. They are believed to act indirectly by increasing and decreasing the effects of neurotransmitters. Pain perception is influenced by the balance of neurotransmitters and the descending pain-control fibers originating from the cerebral cortex.

Gate control theory of pain. Researchers know there is no specific pain center in the nervous system. The gate control theory gives the nurse a conceptual basis for pain-relief measures. The gate control theory of Melzack and Wall (1965) suggests that pain impulses can be regulated or even blocked by gating mechanisms along the central nervous system. The gating mechanism occurs within the spinal cord and sites within the thalamus, reticular formation, and limbic system (Melzack and Wall, 1988; Raj, 1994). The theory suggests that pain impulses pass through when the gate is

---

Box 33-2
Neurophysiology of Pain: Neuroregulators

Neurotransmitters
Substance P
Found in the pain neurons of the dorsal horn (excitatory peptide)
Needed to transmit pain impulses from the periphery to higher brain centers
Causes vasodilation and edema

Serotonin
Released from the brainstem and dorsal horn to inhibit pain transmission

Prostaglandins
Increase sensitivity to pain

Neuromodulators
Endorphins and Dynorphins
Are the body's natural supply of morphine-like substances
Activated by stress and pain
Located within the brain, spinal cord, and gastrointestinal tract
Cause analgesia when they attach to opiate receptors in the brain

Bradykinin
Released from plasma that leaks from surrounding blood vessels at the site of tissue injury
Binds to receptors on peripheral nerves, increasing pain stimuli

---

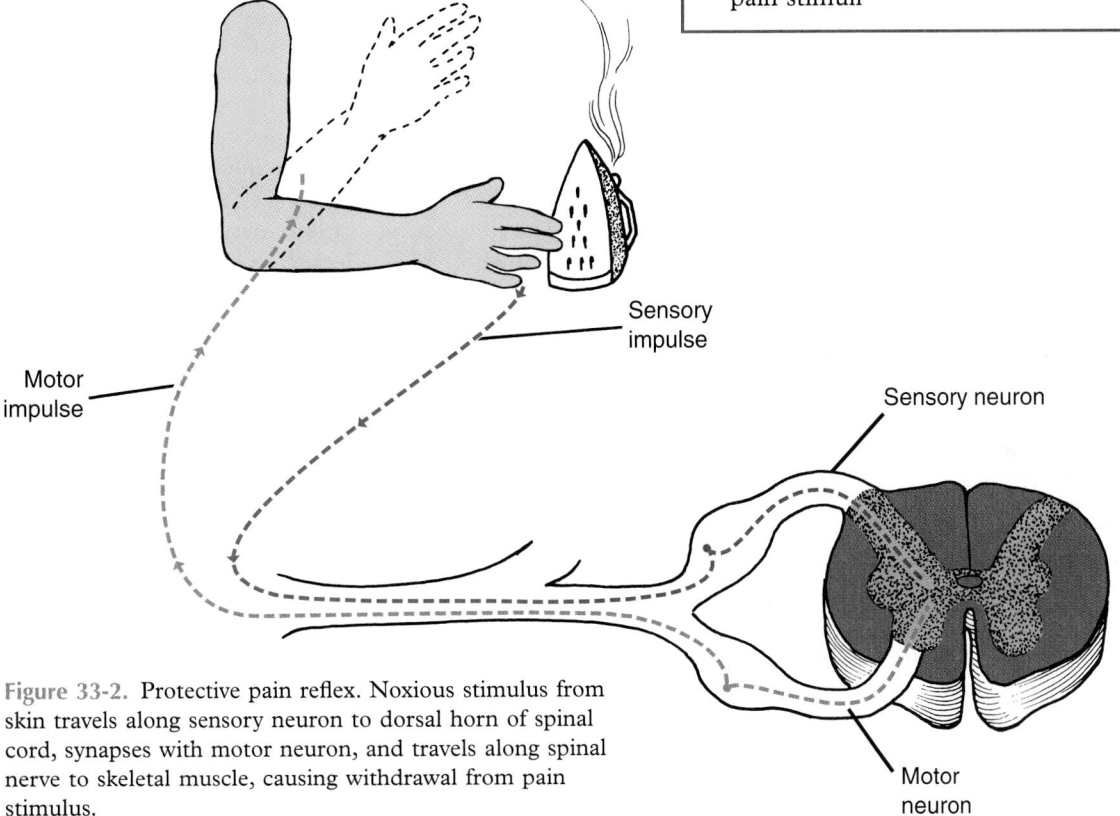

Figure 33-2. Protective pain reflex. Noxious stimulus from skin travels along sensory neuron to dorsal horn of spinal cord, synapses with motor neuron, and travels along spinal nerve to skeletal muscle, causing withdrawal from pain stimulus.

open and not while it is closed. Closing of the gate is the basis for pain-relief therapies. For example, distraction, counseling, and placebo techniques are ways to release endorphins.

Perception.   Perception is the point at which a person is aware of pain. Meinhart and McCaffery (1983) describe three interactional systems of pain perception as sensory-discriminative, motivational-affective, and cognitive-evaluative (Box 33-3). A client's neurological function can easily influence the pain experience. Any factor that interrupts or influences normal pain reception or perception affects the client's awareness and response to pain. Some therapies also influence pain perception and response. For example, analgesics, sedatives, and anesthetics depress the central nervous system. The nurse should assess the neurological status of a client at risk for being insensitive to pain to provide preventive care.

Reaction.   The reaction to pain is the physiological and behavioral responses that occur after pain is perceived (e.g., crying, moving away from the painful stimulus).

Box 33-3
Interactional Systems of Pain Perception

Sensory-Discriminative

Nerve transmission occurs between the thalamus and sensory cortex.

A person perceives the location, severity, and character of pain.

Factors that lower consciousness decrease pain perception.

Factors that increase the awareness of stimuli (e.g., anxiety, sleep deprivation) increase pain perception.

Motivational-Affective

Interaction between the reticular formation and limbic system results in pain perception.

The reticular formation creates a defensive response, causing a person to interrupt or avoid pain stimuli.

The limbic system controls emotional response and coping with pain.

Cognitive-Evaluative

Higher cortical centers in the brain influence perception.

Culture, experience with pain, and emotions influence a person's evaluation of the pain experience.

Helps a person to interpret the intensity and quality of pain so that action can be taken.

Physiological responses.   As pain impulses travel up the spinal cord toward the brainstem and thalamus, the autonomic nervous system is stimulated as part of the stress response. Pain of low to moderate intensity and superficial pain cause the flight-or-fight reaction of the general adaptation syndrome (see Chapter 22). Stimulation of the sympathetic branch of the autonomic nervous system results in the physiological responses summarized in Table 33-2. If pain is unrelenting, severe, or deep, typically involving visceral organs, the parasympathetic nervous system goes into action. Sustained physiological responses to pain could cause serious harm. Except in cases of severe traumatic pain, which may place a client into shock, most clients adapt, with physical signs returning to normal. Thus a client in pain will not always have physical signs (McCaffery and Ferrell, 1996).

Behavioral responses.   The phases of a pain experience are anticipation, sensation, and aftermath (Meinhart and McCaffery, 1983). Anticipation occurs before pain is perceived. A person knows pain will occur. Therefore anticipation allows a person to learn about pain and its relief through instruction and support. Nurses are important in helping clients during the anticipatory phase. An example involves the nurse explaining the stinging sensation of a needle-stick. Proper explanation helps clients control their anxiety. In cases in which clients are too fearful, anticipation of pain can heighten pain perception.

Sensation of pain occurs when pain is felt. People react to pain in different ways. A person's tolerance to pain is the point at which there is an unwillingness to accept pain of greater severity or duration. Tolerance depends on attitudes, motivation, and values. The client with high pain tolerance is able to endure severe pain without assistance. Often a nurse must encourage such a client to accept pain-relieving measures. In contrast, a client with low tolerance may seek relief before pain occurs. The nurse is often more than willing to attend to the client whose pain tolerance is high. Yet it is unfair to ignore the needs of a client unable to tolerate even minor pain.

Typical body movements and facial expressions that indicate acute pain include clenching the teeth, holding the painful part, and bent posture. The nurse soon learns to recognize patterns of behavior that reflect pain. However, lack of pain expression does not mean the client is not having pain. Unless a client openly reacts to pain, it is difficult to assess the nature and extent of the discomfort. The nurse helps the client communicate the pain response more effectively.

The aftermath phase occurs when pain is reduced or stopped. Even though the source of pain is controlled, a client may still require the nurse's attention. During the aftermath, clients may have physical symptoms such as chills, nausea, vomiting, anger, or depression. If a

TABLE 33-2
Physiological Reactions to Pain

Response	Cause or Effect
Sympathetic Stimulation*	
Dilation of bronchial tubes and increased respiratory rate	Provides increased oxygen intake
Increased heart rate	Provides increased oxygen transport
Peripheral vasoconstriction (pallor, elevation in blood pressure)	Elevates blood pressure with shift of blood supply from periphery and viscera to skeletal muscles and brain
Increased blood glucose level	Provides additional energy
Diaphoresis	Controls body temperature during stress
Increased muscle tension	Prepares muscles for action
Dilation of pupils	Affords better vision
Decreased gastrointestinal motility	Frees energy for more immediate activity
Parasympathetic Stimulation†	
Pallor	Causes blood supply to shift away from periphery
Muscle tension	Results from fatigue
Decreased heart rate and blood pressure	Results from vagal stimulation
Rapid, irregular breathing	Causes body defenses to fail under prolonged stress of pain
Nausea and vomiting	Causes return of gastrointestinal function
Weakness or exhaustion	Results from expenditure of physical energy

*Pain of low to moderate intensity and superficial pain.
†Severe or deep pain.

client has pain again and again, aftermath responses can become serious health problems.

•••••••••NURSING KNOWLEDGE BASE....

Acute and Chronic Pain

Minor discomforts such as the ache of overexercised muscles or the burning discomfort of eye strain rarely cause a person to seek health care. The pain nurses most often observe in clients includes acute, chronic malignant, and chronic nonmalignant pain (National Institutes of Health, 1986). Acute pain follows acute injury, disease, or types of surgery and has a rapid onset, varies in intensity (mild to severe), and lasts briefly. Acute pain warns people of impending injury or disease. It eventually resolves with or without treatment after a damaged area heals.

Clients in acute pain are frightened, anxious, and expect relief quickly. The time sequence of acute pain usually results in a willingness by health team members to treat acute pain aggressively. However, conflict between nurse and client may arise if the nurse does not provide quick relief. Acute pain is self-limiting, and the client therefore knows an end is in sight.

Acute pain seriously threatens a client's recovery by hampering the client's ability to become active and involved in self-care. It may cause complications such as physical and emotional exhaustion, immobility, sleep deprivation, and pulmonary complications (Lazzara, 1993). Client education and rehabilitation may be delayed and hospitalization prolonged if acute pain is not controlled. After acute pain is relieved, the client can direct full attention toward recovery.

Chronic pain is prolonged, varies in intensity, and usually lasts more than 6 months (McCaffery, 1986; Fulton, 1996). Chronic pain caused by uncontrolled cancer or its treatment or other progressive disorders is called **intractable pain** (malignant pain). It can last until death.

Chronic nonmalignant pain such as low back pain results from nonprogressive or healed tissue injury. However, the pain is ongoing and often does not respond to treatment. Frequently the cause is unknown. In chronic pain, endorphins often cease to function.

Health care workers are usually less willing to treat chronic pain as aggressively as acute pain. However, the AHCPR reports that up to 90% of the 8 million Americans who have cancer can have their pain managed with relatively simple means (Jacox and others, 1994). Too often these clients are undertreated.

Clients with chronic pain often have periods of **remissions** (partial or complete disappearance of symptoms) and **exacerbations** (increases in severity). This unpredictability frustrates the client, often leading to depression. Chronic pain is a major cause of psychological and physical disability, leading to problems such as job loss, inability to perform simple daily activities, sexual dysfunction, and social isolation.

The client with chronic pain often does not show overt symptoms and does not adapt to the pain but seems to suffer more with time because of physical and mental exhaustion. Symptoms of chronic pain include fatigue, insomnia, anorexia, weight loss, withdrawal, depression, hopelessness, and anger.

Caring for the client with chronic pain is an unusual challenge. The nurse should not become frustrated or offer any false hope for a cure. The nurse must minimize or reduce the client's perception of pain.

Factors Influencing Pain

The nurse considers all factors affecting the client in pain to accurately assess the client's pain and to select appropriate pain therapies.

Age. Developmental differences influence how children and older adults react to pain. Young children have trouble understanding pain and the procedures that nurses administer that may cause pain. Young children without full vocabularies also have difficulty verbally describing and expressing pain to parents or care givers. Children's temperaments affect how they cope with pain. Children often describe procedures as the most distressing aspect of disease or hospitalization.

Children are grossly undermedicated for pain. When comparing children with adults having the same medical diagnoses, children received fewer medication doses. In addition, analgesic doses are often too small or given too infrequently to be effective (Ochsenreither and Cubina, 1996). The nurse must understand a child's response to pain. For example, the nurse observes children who cannot yet speak for behavioral changes such as irritability, loss of appetite, unusual quietness, disturbed sleep patterns, restlessness, and rigid posturing (Jacox and others, 1994). If a behavior such as crying changes after a child receives an analgesic, it was probably caused by pain.

Pain is not a natural part of aging. However, older adults often suffer acute and chronic painful disease, which is frequently taken for granted or underestimated. Older adults can suffer serious loss of functional status as a result of pain. Mobility, self-care activities, socialization, and activity tolerance can all be reduced (Walker, 1994). A client with cognitive impairment may have trouble recalling pain experiences and providing detailed explanations (Eiman and others, 1996).

The ability of older adults to interpret pain can be complicated by multiple diseases and vague symptoms affecting similar parts of the body. When older clients have more than one source of pain, a nurse must gather detailed assessments. Different diseases can cause similar symptoms.

Gender. Generally, men and women do not differ significantly in pain responses. However, cultural influences on gender may produce different expressions of pain (e.g., making it acceptable for a little boy to be brave and not cry, whereas a little girl in the same situation may cry). In a review of pain literature, Vallerand (1995) reported that men had a higher pain **threshold** and pain **tolerance** than women. Women reported more arthritis, facial pain, and migraine headache pain, whereas men experienced more cluster headache, backache, and cardiac pain.

Culture. Culture influences how people perceive the causes of and learn to react to and express pain. Italian, Jewish, black, and Spanish-speaking persons smile readily and use facial expressions and gestures to communicate pain or displeasure (Giger and Davidhizar, 1995). In contrast, Irish, English, and Northern European persons tend to have less facial expression and are less responsive, especially to strangers such as professional care givers. Understanding cultural background, socioeconomic status, and personal characteristics helps the nurse more accurately assess pain and its meaning for clients (Jurf and Nirschl, 1993; Bozeman, 1996).

Meaning of pain. The meaning a client associates with pain affects the pain experience. Clients perceive pain differently if it suggests a threat, loss, punishment, or challenge. The degree and quality of pain perceived by a client are related to the meaning of pain (Bozeman, 1996).

Attention. The degree to which a client focuses on pain influences pain perception. Increased attention has been associated with increased pain, whereas distraction has been associated with decreased pain. Nurses apply this concept in pain-relief therapies such as listening to music and rhythmical breathing (Jurf and Nirschl, 1993). By focusing a client's attention and concentration on other stimuli, the nurse places pain on the periphery of awareness. Usually, increased tolerance for pain lasts only during the time of distraction (McCaffery and Beebe, 1989).

Anxiety. Elevated anxiety levels cause an increase in pain perception. In addition, pain may also cause anxiety. Autonomic arousal patterns are similar in pain and anxiety (Good, 1995). Emotionally healthy persons are usually able to tolerate moderate or even severe pain better than those less stable emotionally.

Fatigue. Fatigue heightens pain perception. This intensifies pain and decreases coping abilities (Jurf and

Nirschl, 1993). Pain is often experienced less after restful sleep than at the end of a tiring day.

Previous experience.

Previous pain experience does not necessarily mean a client will accept pain more easily in the future. Frequent episodes of pain without relief or bouts of severe pain may produce anxiety or fear. In contrast, experiences with the same type of pain that has successfully been relieved makes it easier for the client to interpret the pain sensation. As a result, the client is better prepared to take steps to relieve the pain.

A client who has had no experience with pain may have an impaired ability to cope with it. The nurse should prepare such a client with a clear explanation of the type of pain that will be experienced and methods to reduce it (Ferrell and Rhiner, 1994).

Coping style.

The experience of pain can be lonely. Frequently clients feel a loss of control over their environments or the outcome of events. Coping style thus influences the ability to deal with pain. Clients with internal loci of control perceive themselves as having personal control over their environments and the outcome of events. They ask questions, desire information, and like choices of treatment. In contrast, clients with external loci of control perceive other factors in their environments, such as nurses, as being responsible for the outcome of events. These clients tend to be less demanding, follow directions, and take a passive stance in managing their pain. They want specific instructions but may become anxious if too much information is given or they are expected to assume responsibility for their care (Courts, 1996). Those with internal loci of control report less severe pain than those with external loci. This concept is applied in the use of **patient-controlled analgesia (PCA).**

Family and social support.

A client often depends on the support and assistance of spouse, family, or friends when coping with pain. Although pain still exists, the presence of a loved one can minimize loneliness and fear. Clients of different sociocultural groups have different expectations of people to whom they complain about pain. Absent family or friends can often make the pain experience more stressful. The presence of parents is especially important for children in pain.

CRITICAL THINKING IN CLIENT CARE

Synthesis

Because the experience of pain is both unique and dynamic, critical thinking requires synthesis of knowledge about the client's pain and experience from the client's perspective. In addition, the nurse brings previous experience, intellectual attitudes, and professional standards when partnering with the client in an attempt to ease the client's suffering.

Knowledge.

It is important for the nurse to apply knowledge regarding the physiology of pain, along with the physiology of any underlying disease processes, to understand the client's pain response and the types of interventions best suited for pain management. Knowledge and application of communication skills will enhance the thoroughness of a pain assessment. Once the nurse has a clear picture of the physiological nature of a client's condition, synthesis of knowledge regarding the client's psychological and sociocultural perspective becomes critical for an individualized approach to care. In addition, an understanding of pharmacology will equip the nurse to collaborate with the physician in selecting certain pain therapies.

Experience.

Caring for clients who have pain is an important part of a nurse's clinical experience. Because pain is so common, the nurse soon learns that clients vary widely in their expressions of pain, the degree pain affects their behaviors, and the actions they take to find relief. Such experience should sensitize the nurse to the personal nature of pain. Furthermore, the nurse's own experience with pain emphasizes the importance of having someone who is supportive and understanding. Reflecting on the experiences of caring for those in pain helps the nurse to search for better approaches for each new client encountered.

Attitudes.

Critical thinking attitudes ensure that the nurse makes decisions that are fair and responsible. When a client is in pain, perseverance is often needed to find an approach that will offer the client some degree of relief. Quick solutions often can simply aggravate a client's discomfort. The nurse must learn as much as possible about the client's pain, try various interventions, and continue different approaches until an effective one is discovered. The nurse's integrity ensures an openness to new information and approaches that other members of the team might be able to offer.

Standards.

The application of intellectual standards is particularly important when attempting to acquire an accurate pain assessment. A clear, precise, and accurate description of the client's pain is essential. The nurse makes sure that information related to factors influencing the client's pain is relevant and complete. The nurse must also be fair and listen to all sources, including client, family, and friends, who have been affected by the client's experience to gain a clear picture of what pain means for the client.

Professional standards, such as those developed by the Agency for Health Care Policy and Research

(AHCPR) and the World Health Organization (WHO), all of which are discussed more thoroughly later in the chapter, provide valuable guidelines for pain management. The nurse applies these standards when making decisions about pain therapies. The standards are established by nursing and other health care experts to improve the quality of care to those in pain.

NURSING PROCESS

▪ Assessment

Accurate and factual pain assessment is necessary for judging clients' progress and response, arriving at proper nursing diagnoses, and selecting appropriate therapies. Pain assessment is one of the most common and one of the most difficult activities a nurse performs. The nurse assesses the pain experience from the client's perspective. It is important to carefully interpret pain cues and remember that psychological and physical components of pain influence the reaction to it.

The AHCPR has established specific guidelines for assessing clients who are to have surgery or other procedures. The focus is planning successful pain-management therapies before pain is experienced. Because it involves a collaborative approach, the AHCPR pain treatment flow chart (Figure 33-3) provides a useful conceptual approach to acute pain control in general. Clients must understand that informed reporting of pain is valuable and necessary if the health care team is to manage pain in an individualized and effective way.

Nurses must be sensitive to a client's level of discomfort. If pain is acutely severe, it is unlikely the client can provide a detailed description. During an episode of acute pain, the nurse primarily assesses how the client feels, determining physiological responses to pain and the location, severity, and quality of pain. A more thorough pain assessment takes time and should be done when the client becomes more alert and attentive. Physical reassurance may have analgesic qualities.

For clients with chronic pain, assessment may best be focused on the emotional impact and the meaning of the pain experience, as well as on its history and context (NIH, 1986). For clients with chronic nonmalignant pain, assessment should include level of function, because it may be impossible to achieve complete pain relief. The AHCPR recommends that families of cancer clients learn how to assess pain so as to promote continuity of effective pain management (Jacox and others, 1994). In the home setting, family members' involvement in pain assessment offers the client and family control over the pain experience (Box 33-4). The nurse should be aware of possible errors in pain assessment. Bias (overestimating or underestimating level of pain), vague or unclear assessment questions, and use of unreliable or invalid pain-assessment tools will not provide

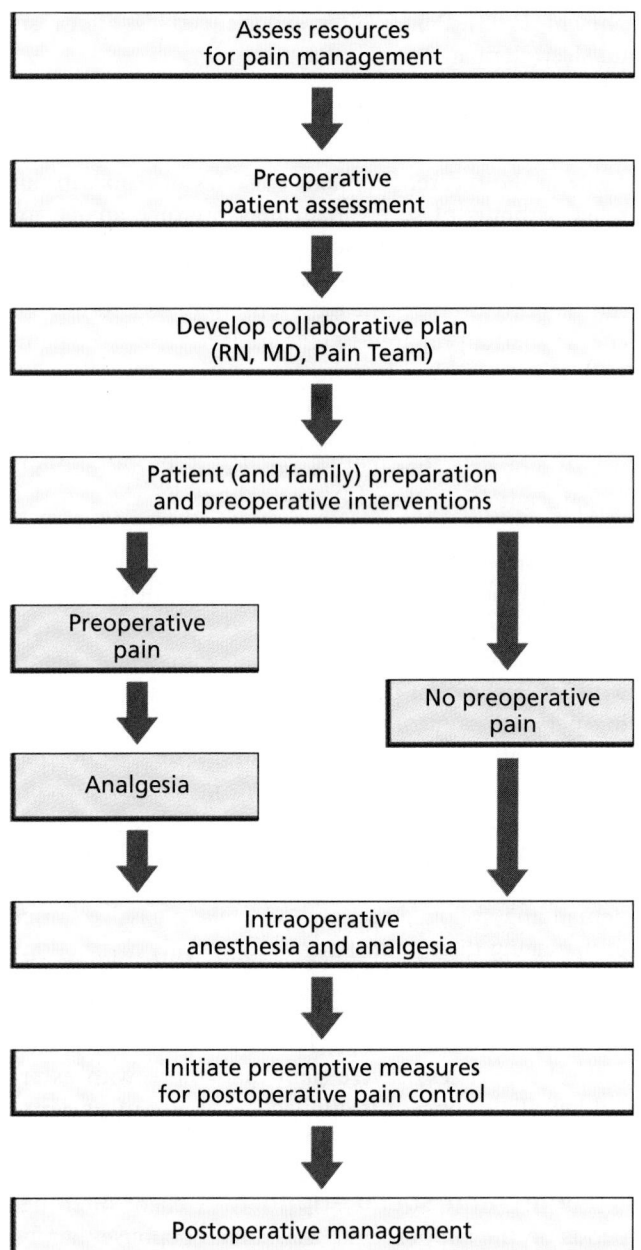

Figure 33-3. Pain treatment flow chart: preoperative and intraoperative phases. (From AHCPR: Acute pain management guideline panel: *Acute pain management in infants, children and adolescents: operative or medical procedures and trauma,* Clinical practice guideline, AHCPR Pub. No. 92-0032, Rockville, Md, February 1992, AHCPR, PHS, USDHHS.)

accurate data (McCaffery and Ferrell, 1996; Willens, 1996). The nurse should recognize clients who do not provide complete, pertinent, or accurate pain information.

Client's expression of pain. Clients often fail to report or discuss pain (McCaffery and Ferrell, 1996). To complicate assessment, nurses frequently believe that clients will report pain if they have it. A nurse

Box 33-4
Routine Clinical Approach to Pain Assessment and Management "ABCDE"

A   *A*sk about pain regularly.
    *A*ssess pain systematically.
B   *B*elieve the client and family in their report of pain and what relieves it.
C   *C*hoose pain control options appropriate for the client, family, and setting.
D   *D*eliver interventions in a timely, logical, and co-ordinated fashion.
E   *E*mpower clients and their families.
    *E*nable them to control their course to the greatest extent possible.

From Jacox A and others: *Management of cancer pain*, Clinical practice guideline No. 9, AHCPR Pub. No. 94-0592, Rockville, Md, March 1994, AHCPR, USDHHS, PHS.

TABLE 33-3
Implications of Pain Assessment for Nursing Interventions

Assessment Criteria	Nursing Interventions
Onset and duration	Administer analgesics so that peak action occurs when pain is most acute (e.g., during dressing change or exercise therapy).
Location	Position client off affected area. Apply local treatments (e.g., elastic bandage and splinting) directly over painful site.
Severity	Change or revise interventions, depending on success of one intervention.
Precipitating or aggravating factors	Avoid activities that cause or aggravate pain. Teach client or family to avoid same activities.
Relief measures	Use measures that client uses to relieve pain, as long as they are safe and appropriate.

should ask about pain regularly. A client must trust a nurse and perceive the nurse's willingness to help before discussing pain openly. The nurse should learn verbal or nonverbal ways that the client communicates discomfort.

Clients unable to communicate effectively often require special attention during assessment. Children, developmentally delayed persons, psychotic clients, clients with dementia, and non–English-speaking clients all require different approaches. Cognitively impaired clients require simple assessment approaches involving close observation of behavior. If a client speaks a different language, a family member or interpreter may be needed. Clients in pain often confide in only one person (Willens, 1996).

Classification of the pain experience.
It helps to know the phase of pain clients are undergoing, because it influences not only clients' symptoms but also the types of therapies most likely to relieve pain. Clients in the anticipatory phase such as those scheduled for diagnostic procedures or surgery may appear anxious or fearful, or they may ask questions about upcoming pain. Studies have shown that providing clients with physiological coping (positioning, deep breathing), sensory information (description of discomforts to be expected), and procedural information leads to clients with fewer complications, reporting less pain, and using less analgesia (AHCPR, 1992).

Clients who are sensing pain, especially severe pain, want fast relief. These clients may demonstrate more intense responses to the pain, such as crying or guarding the painful area, or they may have increases in their vital signs. After the pain has been relieved, the nurse

must assess carefully for physical and psychological effects.

The nurse assesses if the client's pain is acute or chronic. If the pain is acute in nature, a detailed assessment of pain characteristics is needed. With chronic pain the nurse determines if it is intermittent, persistent, or limited.

Characteristics of pain.
Characteristics of pain can be detailed only by the client. Client self-report to assess pain characteristics is the single most reliable indicator of the existence and intensity of pain and any related discomfort (NIH, 1986).

Onset and duration. The nurse asks questions to determine the onset, duration, and time sequence of pain. When did the pain begin? How long has it lasted? Does it occur at the same time each day? How often does it recur?

It may be easier to diagnose the nature of pain by identifying time factors. The onset of sudden and severe pain is easier to assess than gradual, mild discomfort. Knowing the time cycle of a client's pain helps the nurse to intervene before the pain occurs or worsens (Table 33-3).

Location. To assess pain location, the nurse asks the client to point to all areas of discomfort. To localize the pain more specifically, the client traces the area from the most severe point outward. This is difficult to do if pain is diffuse, involves several sites, or involves large parts of the body. A drawing showing the location of pain can be used as a baseline if the pain changes. The nurse uses anatomical landmarks and descriptive terminology to record pain location (e.g., "Pain is in the right upper abdominal quadrant"). Pain classified by location may be superficial or cutaneous, deep or visceral, localized or diffuse, or referred or radiating (Table 33-4).

Severity. The most subjective characteristic of pain may be its severity or intensity. Clients are often asked to describe pain as mild, moderate, or severe. However, the meaning of these terms differs for the nurse and client.

Descriptive scales measure pain severity objectively (Figure 33-4). A verbal descriptor scale (VDS) consists of a line with three- to five-word descriptors equally spaced along the line. The nurse shows the client the scale and asks the client to determine the current intensity of pain. In addition, the nurse asks how much the pain hurts at its worst and how much it hurts at its best. A numerical rating scale (NRS) requires clients to rate pain on a scale of 0 to 10. The scales work best when assessing an individual client's pain intensity before and after therapeutic interventions. When scales

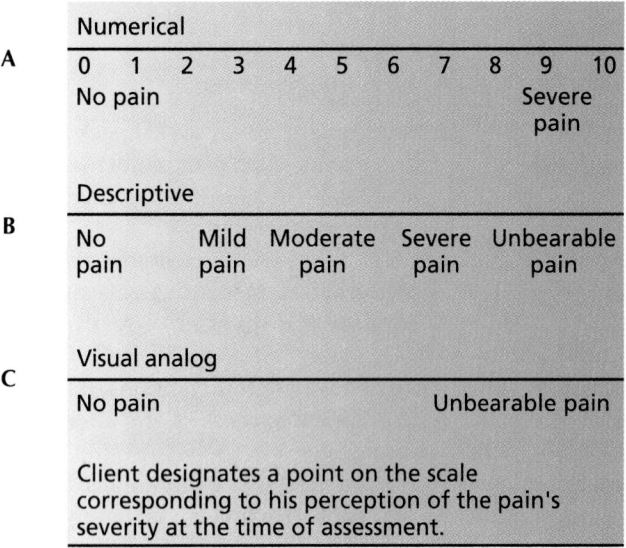

Figure 33-4. Sample pain scales. **A,** Numerical; **B,** descriptive; **C,** visual analog.

TABLE 33-4
Classification of Pain by Location

Location	Characteristics	Examples of Causes
Superficial or Cutaneous Pain resulting from stimulation of skin	Pain is of short duration and is localized. It usually is sharp sensation.	Needle-stick; small cut or laceration
Deep Visceral Pain resulting from stimulation of internal organs	Pain is diffuse and may radiate in several directions. Duration varies, but it usually lasts longer than superficial pain. Pain may be sharp, dull, or unique to organ involved.	Crushing sensation (e.g., angina pectoris); burning sensation (e.g., gastric ulcer)
Referred Common in visceral pain because many organs themselves have no pain receptors; entrance of sensory neurons from affected organ into same spinal cord segment as neurons from areas where pain is felt	Pain is felt in part of body separate from source of pain and may assume any characteristic.	Myocardial infarction, which may cause referred pain to jaw, left arm, and left shoulder; kidney stones, which may refer pain to groin
Radiating Sensation of pain extending from initial site of injury to another body part	Pain feels as though it travels down or along body part. It may be intermittent or constant.	Low back pain from ruptured intravertebral disk; pain radiates down leg from sciatic nerve irritation

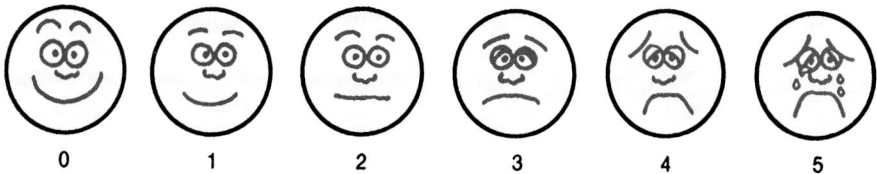

Figure 33-5. Faces Scale. (From Wong DL, Baker CM: Pain in children: comparison of assessment scales, *Oklahoma Nurs* 33[1]:8, 1988a.)

are used to rate pain, a 10-cm (4-inch) baseline is recommended (AHCPR, 1992; Willens, 1996).

A visual analog scale (VAS) consists of a straight line without labeled subdivisions. The straight line shows a continuum of intensity and has labeled endpoints. A client indicates pain by marking the appropriate point on the VAS. This scale gives the client total freedom to identify pain severity. The VAS may be a more sensitive measure of pain severity, because clients mark at any point on the continuum rather than having to choose one word or number (Mottola, 1993).

Several pain scales have been developed to assess pain in children. Wong and Baker (1988b) developed a Faces Scale to assess pain in children (Figure 33-5). The scale consists of six cartoon faces ranging from a very happy, smiling face for "no pain" to increasingly less happy faces to a final sad, tearful face for "worst pain." Children as young as 3 years of age can use the scale. Researchers are beginning to test the Faces Scale with older adults. The advantage is that clients do not have to interpret the meaning of numbers or adjectives. The faces more clearly and quickly depict the concept of pain or discomfort (Willens, 1996).

A unique tool designed to measure pain intensity in children is the Oucher pain scale developed by Beyer and others (1992). The "Oucher" consists of two separate scales: a 0 to 100 scale on the left for older children (Figure 33-6) and a six-picture photographic scale on the right for younger children. Photographs of the face of a child (in increasing levels of discomfort) are designed to cue children into understanding what pain is and its severity. A child merely points to the selection, thus simplifying the task of describing the pain.

A pain scale should be designed so it is easy to use and not time consuming for clients. If a client can easily read and understand a scale, the description of pain should be more accurate. Descriptive scales are useful not only in assessing the severity of pain but also in evaluating changes in a client's condition. The nurse does not use pain scales to compare one client with another.

Quality. Another subjective characteristic of pain is quality. When assessing the quality of pain, the nurse should not provide descriptive words for the client. Assessment is more accurate if a client can describe the sensation in his or her own words after open-ended questions. For example, the nurse might say, "Tell me

what your pain feels like." The only time the nurse offers to list descriptive terms is when the client cannot describe pain. The qualities of pricking, burning, and aching are useful to describe pain initially (McCaffery and Beebe, 1989). Later the client may choose more descriptive terms.

There is some consistency in the way clients describe certain types of pain. The pain of a myocardial infarction is often described as crushing or viselike, whereas the pain of a surgical incision is often described as sharp

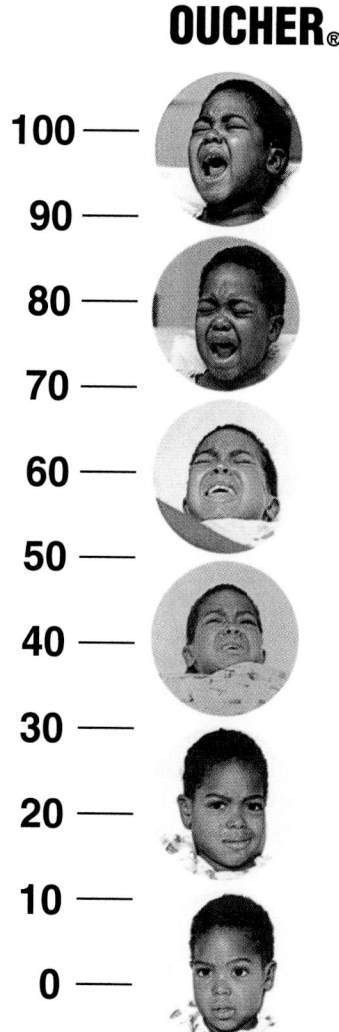

Figure 33-6. Oucher pain scale. (© Beyer, Denyes 1990. Used with permission.)

and stabbing. When the descriptions fit the pattern forming in the nurse's assessment, a clearer analysis can be made of the nature and type of pain.

Pain pattern. Many factors affect the character of pain. It helps to assess specific events or conditions that precipitate or aggravate pain. The nurse asks the client to describe activities that cause pain, such as physical activity, coffee or alcohol ingestion, urination, swallowing, or emotional stress. The nurse may ask the client to demonstrate actions that cause painful responses such as coughing or turning in a certain manner. After identifying specific factors, it is easier to plan interventions to avoid worsening the pain (Willens, 1996).

Relief measures. The nurse should know if a client has an effective way for relieving pain such as changing position, using ritualistic behavior (pacing, rocking, rubbing), eating, or applying heat or cold to the painful site. In the home, the nurse must be sure relief measures are used safely. Assessment of relieving factors should also include identifying practitioners (e.g., internist, chiropractor, faith healer) whose services the client has sought. Clients with chronic pain are more likely to try alternative health care methods (Courts, 1996).

Concomitant symptoms. Concomitant symptoms are those that often occur with pain, including nausea, headache, dizziness, urge to urinate, constipation, and restlessness. Certain types of pain have predictable symptoms. For example, severe rectal pain often causes constipation. These symptoms can be as much a problem to a client as the pain itself.

Physical signs and symptoms. When a client has pain, the nurse should assess vital signs, conduct a focused physical examination, and observe for autonomic nervous system involvement (see Table 33-2). In the case of cancer clients, a neurological examination (see Chapter 24) is especially important (Jacox and others, 1994). Physiological signs can reveal pain in a client who tries not to complain or admit pain. There is no predictable level or extent of change in a client's condition that indicates pain.

At the onset of acute pain, the heart and respiratory rates and blood pressure increase. The nurse compares vital sign values with baseline measurements recorded before onset. A change in vital signs is significant, but the nurse should take into account all signs and symptoms before determining that pain is the cause. The nurse should not confuse signs and symptoms of pain with other pathological changes. The nurse performs an assessment based on the client's pain history. The painful area should be examined to see if palpation or manipulation of the site increases pain (Jacox and others, 1994). During a general overview, the nurse observes for cues indicating pain (e.g., posturing, restricting limb movement, guiding a painful area).

If pain is unrelieved, the nurse looks for signs of physical exhaustion. Decreasing vital sign values indicate parasympathetic nerve response. The client be-

comes less responsive to stimuli within the environment. The nurse should measure vital signs more often if the client's condition deteriorates.

Behavioral effects. When clients have pain, the nurse assesses their verbalization, vocal response, facial and body movements, and social interaction (Box 33-5). A verbal report of pain is a vital part of assessment. The nurse must be willing to listen and understand. Many clients cannot verbalize discomfort because of an inability to communicate. In these cases the nurse must be alert for behaviors that indicate pain. Nurses must watch for subtle indicators of pain in nonalert older adults such as withdrawal or restlessness. Subtle facial expressions or body movements often reveal more about the character of pain than vocalizations. In addition, some nonverbal expressions characterize sources of pain. For example, chest pain causes a client to grab or hold the chest.

Influence on activities of daily living. Pain is a stressful event that can alter lifestyle and psychological well-being. By recognizing the effects of pain on a client, the nurse can identify more clearly the nature and implications of the pain. Clients who live with daily pain are less able to participate in routine activities. Assessment reveals the extent of the disability and the adjustments that will be necessary for participation in self-care (Box 33-6).

Client expectations. Clients rely on their care givers to recognize and alleviate their physical discomfort (Gerteis and others, 1993). This may involve using a skilled and caring approach, trying a variety of comfort measures, and serving as an advocate for the client. Research by Gerteis and others (1993) has shown that from the point of view of clients and families, what matters most is when care givers go out of their way for them. A caring nurse is one perceived to tailor care to the individual's needs. The nurse should always ask

---

Box 33-5
Behavioral Indicators of the Effects of Pain

Vocalizations
Moaning, crying, screaming, and gasping

Facial Expressions
Grimace, clenched teeth, wrinkled forehead, tightly closed or opened eyes or mouth, and lip biting

Body Movement
Restlessness, immobilization, muscle tension, increased hand and finger movements, pacing activities, and rhythmic or rubbing motions

Social Interaction
Avoidance of conversation or social contacts, focus only on activities for pain relief, reduced attention span

Box 33-6
Assessing the Influence of Pain on Activities of Daily Living

Sleep
Does the client have difficulty in falling asleep?
Does pain awaken the client at night?
Are sleeping pills or other aids needed?

Hygiene
Does pain hinder the client's ability to use eating utensils or bathe, dress, or perform other hygiene measures independently?
Are family members or friends available or needed to assist?

Sexual Function
Do physical conditions such as arthritis or back pain prevent the client from assuming usual positions during intercourse?
Does pain or fatigue reduce the client's desire for sex?
Are clients fearful that pain will increase as a result of intercourse?

Home Management and Work Activities
Is the client able to perform usual housework chores?
Is physical activity required in the job, and is activity now limited by pain?
If pain is related to emotional stress, does the job involve tension-filled decision making?
Must the client stop activities momentarily to relieve pain?

Social Activities
Does the client regularly socialize?
To what extent has pain disrupted activities?

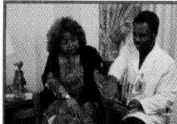

Case Study
Synthesis in Practice

Jim prepares for tomorrow's home health visit with Mrs. Ellis. He reviews what he has learned about the gate control theory, the physiology of chronic pain, and the pathophysiology of rheumatoid arthritis. This allows him to anticipate the need to carefully assess to what extent pain limits Mrs. Ellis' ability to walk and use her upper extremities. Jim plans to assess the location, duration, and aggravating and relieving factors influencing Mrs. Ellis' pain, as well as any behavioral symptoms he might observe. He also wants to use a VAS to establish a baseline for the severity of the pain, as well as any behavioral systems he observes. Because Mrs. Ellis is 70, Jim reviews gerontological principles and knows he must take time to establish a trusting relationship with the client so as to encourage a complete description of the pain experience. Jim recalls pain descriptions and symptoms communicated to him by previous clients and the various interventions they used to relieve their pain. He also remembers his own experiences with pain after suffering a broken arm during a soccer game. This experience will sensitize him to the personal and dynamic nature of each individual's pain experience.

Jim considers the AHCPR guidelines for the management of chronic pain. He wants to be careful in clarifying with Mrs. Ellis the extent to which the chronic arthritic pain and the acute exacerbations have impacted her life. If Jim is to help her with pain relief and health promotion activities, he must learn as much as he can about Mrs. Ellis' lifestyle and the support systems that are available for her. If she is reportedly living alone, Jim wants to assess if family or friends who can offer assistance live nearby.

---

clients what they expect regarding their comfort needs. This might include asking clients not only what interventions they might prefer but also how they should be administered. It is also important to understand if clients expect full pain relief or if they simply hope to have their discomfort reduced. When clients ask the nurse for assistance because of pain, they typically expect nurses to respond promptly.

Successful critical thinking requires a synthesis of knowledge, experience, information gathered from clients, and critical thinking attitudes and standards. Clinical judgments require the nurse to anticipate what information is needed, analyze the data, and make decisions regarding client care. The client expects competent and informed care. Jim incorporates previous knowledge and experience in providing care for Mrs. Ellis.

■ Nursing Diagnosis

Accurate nursing diagnoses for clients in pain result from thorough data collection and analysis (see nursing diagnoses box). An accurate diagnosis is made after reviewing clusters of defining characteristics. In the example of the diagnosis of *pain,* the nurse may assess the client's withdrawal from communication, rigid posturing, moaning, and verbalization of discomfort. In contrast, the diagnosis of *anxiety* may be made by observing a client's facial tension and appearance, poor eye contact, restlessness, and verbalization of feeling scared. The two diagnoses have similar defining characteristics, but the nurse sorts out patterns to reveal *pain* versus *anxiety.*

The related factor for the diagnostic statement focuses on the specific nature of the client's problem. *Pain related to physical trauma* and *pain related to natural child-birth processes* require very different nursing interventions. Successful identification of related factors ensures that nursing therapies will be directed toward relieving the client's discomfort.

NURSING DIAGNOSES FOR CLIENTS WITH PAIN

Anxiety
Coping, ineffective individual
Hopelessness
Injury, risk for
Mobility, impaired physical
Pain
Pain, chronic
Self-care deficit; bathing/hygiene, dressing/
    grooming, feeding
Sexual dysfunction
Sleep pattern disturbance

Planning

The nurse develops an individualized plan of care for each nursing diagnosis identified (see care plan). The nurse and client set realistic expectations for pain relief and the degree of pain relief to expect. The client should understand that complete pain relief cannot be guaranteed, but it will be attempted. Goals are to be individualized and realistic with measurable outcomes. For example, if a client's baseline assessment reveals a pain severity consistently between 7 and 8 on a VAS, a realistic goal is for the client to achieve improved comfort with the outcome of reaching a reduction in pain severity to a 4 or 5 on the scale.

In the home, the nurse will plan to use some of the client's remedies, as long as they are safe. This might require the nurse to assess the home environment carefully to be sure there are no obvious risks to the client. For example, a client might wish to use a heating pad, but the nurse discovers on examination that the electrical cord is frayed and damaged.

It is always important to remember that a successful plan of care requires development of a therapeutic relationship with the client and a focus on education re-

---

CASE STUDY NURSING CARE PLAN

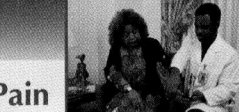

Chronic Pain

Assessment

When Jim enters Mrs. Ellis' four-room apartment, he finds the home to be in some disarray. Mrs. Ellis is sitting in a recliner in her living room, with clothing on the floor and soiled dishes on a nearby table. Mrs. Ellis reports that the **pain** she has been experiencing has **made it** very **difficult to walk between rooms.** She is able to get to the bathroom, but it does cause her to become fatigued. Her **pain is constant and localized in the joints of her hands, knees, and feet.** When Jim shows her a VAS, Mrs. Ellis **rates the pain at the level of 5 on a scale of 0-10.** Jim asks how she would rate the **pain when** it is **most severe,** and Mrs. Ellis **rates the pain at 9.** She currently takes aspirin for the pain. The pain continues to **prevent her from being able to fall asleep,** and when she does fall asleep, she **often reawakens at night.** She has begun to have some "burning in the stomach" when she takes the aspirin. Jim asks her to stand and walk with him to the kitchen. She is **able to stand with much difficulty** and has an **unsteady gait.** Jim asks if Mrs. Ellis has friends or neighbors available who can assist her, and Mrs. Ellis responds, "I hate to be a bother, although my next door neighbor has offered to help in the past."

Nursing Diagnosis

Chronic pain related to rheumatoid arthritis.

Planning

Goals

Client will achieve a sense of pain relief within
    1 week.
Client will ambulate with less discomfort on self-
    report within 14 days.

Expected Outcomes

Client will report pain at 3 on a scale of 0 to 10 fol-
    lowing relaxation therapy and heat application.
Client will demonstrate ability to rise to standing po-
    sition without assistance within 1 week.
Client will demonstrate ability to walk from room to
    room with steady gait in 2 weeks.

CASE STUDY NURSING CARE PLAN—cont'd

Implementation

Steps	Rationale
1. Confer with client's physician regarding possibility of nonsteroidal antiinflammatory drugs (NSAIDs) for pain relief.	Aspirin can cause irritation of gastric mucosa with bleeding or ulceration. Replacement with NSAID provides better analgesic and antiinflammatory properties with fewer gastrointestinal disturbances. Caution is necessary with older adults (McKenry and Salerno, 1995).
2. Have client take analgesics approximately 30 minutes before client begins ambulation, self-care activities, or goes to sleep. Instruct client to take medication with a light snack or meal and a full glass of water. During instruction, tell client the drug will relieve pain.	Medication will exert peak effect when client begins activities. Administration with meals and water reduces chance of gastrointestinal upset. An added placebo effect is brought into play when client's attention is focused on action and purpose of analgesic. Then medication is taken with assurance that it will work (McCaffery, 1996; Salerno, 1996).
3. Have client place a sturdy stool in shower stall and run warm water continuously over joints of hands and feet.	Heat reduces pain by improving blood flow and reducing stiffness of inflamed tissues.
4. Have client apply moist, warm compresses to joints of hands three times a day.	Cutaneous stimulation may activate mechanoreceptor A-beta fibers, thus inhibiting transmission of pain by releasing inhibitory neurotransmitters.
5. Refer client to physical therapist to determine possible use of a walker or other assistive devices.	

Evaluation

Observe client's ability to stand and walk from living room to kitchen.

Ask if client experiences discomfort during dressing and bathing activities.

Observe client perform dressing and/or bathing as appropriate, noting range of motion.

Ask client to rate pain on a scale of 0 to 10 and compare with baseline assessment. Use after nursing therapies are administered.

Defining characteristics are shown in bold type.

garding pain. The nurse can best help by seeing the client as a total person, listening carefully to concerns, attending promptly to his or her needs, and respecting any response to pain. In a successful nurse-client relationship, the nurse recognizes that the client knows more about his or her own pain and its relief.

The client who understands pain will be better prepared to cope with discomfort. A client can better prepare for an impending painful experience, such as postoperative pain or a diagnostic test, after being properly informed. However, for some clients, early warning can be a problem. Highly anxious or fearful clients often become irrational and are unable to learn. If clients seem unlikely to benefit from advanced preparation, it is best to explain invasive procedures a short time before they occur.

When developing the care plan, the nurse selects priorities based on the client's level of pain and its effect on the client's condition. For acute severe pain, it is important to provide quick relief. Analgesics can be very effective. After a client gains some relief from pain, the nurse plans other therapies such as relaxation or the application of heat to enhance the effect of analgesics.

A comprehensive plan includes a variety of resources for pain control, such as family and friends. The family may need to administer care in the home and thus be prepared to assess the client's pain and administer therapies safely. In an acute care setting the family must understand the nature and extent of the client's pain and the choice of therapies. Family members or friends who show a disinterest or prejudice toward pain can impede the client's recovery. Additional resources available include nurse specialists, physical therapists, and occupational therapists. An oncology nurse specialist knows therapies for chronic, malignant pain. Physical therapists can plan exercises that strengthen muscle groups and lessen pain. Occupational therapists may devise splints to support painful body parts.

■ Implementation

The nature of pain and the extent to which it affects an individual's physical and psychosocial well-being determine the choice of pain-relief therapies. Nurses administer and monitor therapies ordered by physicians for pain relief and independently use pain-relief measures that complement those prescribed by a physician. Client remedies are often most successful, especially when the client has already had experience with pain. Generally, the least invasive or safest therapy should be tried first. If there is doubt about a nursing therapy, the nurse should consult a physician.

Regardless of the type of therapies used, the nurse's ability to show caring toward a client can maximize pain control. Pain can be minimized through caring behaviors such as gentle handling and touch. Burnside (1988) suggests that two types of touching, task-oriented and affective, can be effective with clients. Task-oriented touching occurs when a nurse takes a client's blood pressure or helps the client walk. Affective is less routine and is intended to show concern, such as giving a client a hug. Often one can combine task-oriented and affective touching (e.g., placing a hand on the client's shoulder while administering a tablet). Simply sitting and holding a client's hand, allowing a client to move at his or her own speed, speaking in a soft tone of voice, and staying with a client for a time after a procedure are all caring behaviors. The nurse's use of nonverbal expressions to reinforce words of encouragement and support also convey caring. When a nurse can successfully convey compassion, maintain the client's dignity, and consistently strive to minimize discomfort or suffering, pain-relieving measures will be more successful.

Health promotion.

Because pain is such a common health problem, the nurse will find many opportunities to assist clients with pain-relief therapies. When providing pain-relief measures, the nurse chooses therapies suited to the client's unique pain experience. McCaffery (1979) suggests guidelines for individualizing pain therapy (Box 33-7).

Maintaining wellness. Measures that promote a sense of well-being to minimize or avoid discomfort include warm baths, thorough personal hygiene measures, and a schedule of adequate rest. Chapter 32 discusses the effect pain can have on a client's sleep pattern and ways to promote better sleep habits. The nurse should also help the client find ways to plan rest periods before participating in exhaustive activities. Clients with chronic pain should rest before any social activities in the home.

Pain can disable and immobilize a person enough to impair the ability to perform self-care activities. As a result the client might also experience social isolation, depression, and changes in self-concept. Change in function can mean a significant loss to a client. The nurse helps clients and families learn to discuss their feelings about the loss so as to find ways to cope with pain and the lifestyle it imposes (see Chapter 21).

Box 33-7
Guidelines for Individualized Pain Therapy

Use different types of pain-relief measures. This produces an additive effect in reducing pain and allows for changes in the character of pain.

Provide pain-relief measures before pain becomes severe. It is easier to prevent severe pain than to relieve it after it occurs.

Use measures the client believes are effective. The client's beliefs may make pain therapy successful, so include those remedies unless they are harmful.

A client may have ideas about measures to use and times to use them. Consider the client's ability or willingness to participate in pain-relief measures.

Suggest measures that require little physical effort for clients unable to actively assist with pain therapy because of fatigue or altered levels of consciousness. Do not force participation.

Choose pain-relief measures on the basis of client behavior that reflects the severity of pain. Never administer a potent analgesic for mild pain. Only the client can determine the potency of an effective therapy.

If a therapy is ineffective at first, encourage the client to try it again before abandoning it. Client anxiety or doubt may prevent therapy from relieving pain, or the measure may require adjustment or practice to become effective.

Keep an open mind about ways to relieve pain. Rejecting nonconventional therapy leads to mistrust. Be sure all therapies are safe.

Keep trying. When efforts at pain relief fail, do not abandon the client but reassess the situation and consider alternative therapies.

Protect the client. Pain therapy should not cause more distress than the pain itself; the nurse wants to relieve pain without disabling the client mentally, emotionally, or physically.

Educate the client about pain. The nurse should explain the cause of pain, times when analgesics can be given, and alternative therapies.

Pain from an injury or disabling illness may limit a client's mobility. In this case health promotion is aimed at retaining function. The nurse instructs clients and families on the proper use of elastic bandages, braces, and splints that protect body parts. If crutches or other assistive devices are needed, the nurse ensures that they are used safely and properly (see Chapter 37). When a client has chronic, disabling pain it can be helpful for the nurse to instruct family on proper positioning techniques and ways to assist the client with ambulation.

The nurse may refer clients who have difficulty eating, bathing, grooming, and dressing to an occupational therapist. Some agencies may require a physician's order to ultimately initiate occupational therapy. Devices designed to maintain function, even when finger movement or grasp is impaired, can help. The therapist can attach eating utensils, a comb, or a toothbrush to extension devices that have enlarged handles or splints for easy use. Clothing fasteners made of Velcro tape allow clients to remove or apply clothing by themselves.

A client with pain may avoid sexual activity. The need for sexual warmth is not negated by pain. Clients can learn to express themselves sexually by assuming alternative positions during intercourse and learning more about ways to make their partner feel sexually stimulated. Nurses should caution clients that some pain medications can decrease libido and potency.

Nonpharmacological pain-relief measures. One of the most basic nursing responsibilities is protecting the client from harm. A number of nonpharmacological therapies that lessen the reception and perception of pain can be used in any health care setting. Similarly, these therapies can be used in combination with pharmacological measures. The AHCPR guidelines for acute pain management (1992) cite nonpharmacological interventions to be appropriate for clients who:

Find such interventions appealing

Express anxiety or fear

May benefit from avoiding or reducing drug therapy

Are likely to experience and need to cope with a prolonged interval of postoperative pain

Have incomplete pain relief after use of pharmacological therapies

In the case of cancer clients, the nurse evaluates the effects of nonpharmacological measures to ensure pain relief occurs so that clients are not excluded from use of pharmacological therapies as needed.

Reducing pain reception and perception. One simple way to promote comfort is by removing or preventing painful stimuli (Box 33-8). Many of these measures are easy for family members to learn. Removing stimuli is especially important for clients who are immobilized or unable to sense discomfort. Pain can also be prevented by anticipating painful activities (e.g., ambulation, turning). Before performing a procedure the nurse considers the client's condition, aspects of the procedure that are painful, and ways to avoid causing pain. It takes only simple consideration of the client's comfort and a little extra time to avoid pain-producing situations.

Cutaneous stimulation. Cutaneous stimulation is the stimulation of the skin to relieve pain. A massage (Box 33-9), warm bath, ice bag, and **transcutaneous electrical nerve stimulation (TENS)** are simple ways to reduce pain perception. The specific way in which cutaneous stimulation works is unclear. One suggestion is

---

> ### Box 33-8
> ### Controlling Painful Stimuli in the Client's Environment
>
> Tighten and smooth wrinkled bed linen.
> Position client off tubing or other equipment.
> Loosen constricting bandages (unless applied as pressure dressing).
> Change wet dressings or bed linen.
> Position client correctly.
> Check temperature of hot or cold applications, including bath water.
> Lift client up in bed; do not pull.
> Position client correctly on bed pan.
> Avoid exposing skin or mucous membranes to irritants (e.g., diarrheal stool, wound drainage).
> Prevent urinary retention by keeping Foley catheters patent and free flowing.
> Prevent constipation with fluids, diet, and exercise.

---

that it releases endorphins. The gate control theory suggests that cutaneous stimulation activates larger, faster A-beta sensory nerve fibers. This decreases pain transmission through small-diameter A-delta and C fibers. Synaptic gates close to the transmission of pain impulses.

An advantage to cutaneous stimulation is that the measures can be used in the home, giving clients and families some control over pain symptoms and treatment. The proper use of cutaneous stimulation can reduce pain perception and help to reduce muscle tension that might otherwise increase pain. When using cutaneous stimulation methods, the nurse eliminates sources of environmental noise, helps the client to assume a comfortable position, and explains the purpose of the therapy. Cutaneous stimulation should not be used directly on sensitive skin areas (e.g., burns, bruises, skin rashes, inflammation, underlying bone fractures) (Meintz, 1995).

Cold and heat applications (see Chapter 38) relieve pain and promote healing. When using any form of heat or cold application, the nurse instructs the client to avoid injury to the skin. Especially at risk are clients with spinal cord or other neurological injury, older adults, and confused clients.

Another form of cutaneous stimulation sometimes called *counterstimulation* is TENS, involving stimulation of the skin with a mild electrical current passed through external electrodes. It requires a physician's order. The TENS unit (Figure 33-7) consists of a battery-powered transmitter, lead wires, and electrodes. The electrodes are placed directly over or near the site of pain. Hair or skin preparations should be removed before attaching the electrodes. When a client feels pain, the transmitter is turned on and a buzzing or tingling sensation is created. The tingling sensation can be applied until pain relief is achieved. TENS is useful in managing postoperative pain and in reducing pain caused by postoperative procedures (e.g., removing drains) (Stanik-Hutt, 1993; Courts, 1996). It is easy to use and is contraindicated for only a few clients.

Distraction. With meaningful sensory stimuli, a client can ignore or become unaware of pain. Pleasurable stimuli cause the release of endorphins. Distraction directs a client's attention to something else and thus can reduce the awareness of pain and even increase tolerance. Distraction may work best for short, intense pain lasting a few minutes such as during an invasive proce-

---

Box 33-9

Procedural Guidelines for Techniques for Massage and Backrub

1. Based on client assessment, decide on performing massage on one or more body parts.
2. Help client to assume comfortable lying or sitting position.
3. Dim room lights and/or turn on soft music.
4. Massage each body part at least 10 minutes.
   Hands: Make contact with the client's skin, first with one hand and then the other. Using both hands, slowly open the client's palm, gliding your fingers over the palmar surface. While supporting the hand, use both thumbs to apply friction to the palm and use them in a circular motion to stretch the palm outward. Massage each finger outward and then separately, using a corkscrewlike motion from base of finger to the tip. With thumb and finger, knead each small muscle in the client's fingers. Glide hands smoothly from fingertips to wrists. Repeat for other hand.
   Arms: Use a gliding stroke to massage from the client's wrist to forearm. With thumb and forefinger of both hands, knead muscles from forearm to shoulder. Continue kneading biceps, deltoid, and triceps muscles. Finish with gliding strokes from the wrist to the shoulder.
   Neck: Support the neck at the hairline with one hand and massage up it with a gliding stroke. Knead muscles on one side. Switch hands to support neck and knead other side. Stretch the neck slightly, with one hand at the top and the other at the bottom.
   Back: Begin at sacral area and massage in circular motion (Figure 33-8) while moving upward from buttocks to shoulders. Use a firm, smooth stroke over the scapula. Continue in one smooth stroke to upper arms and laterally along sides of back down to iliac crests. Use long, gliding strokes along muscles of spine. Knead any muscles that feel tense or tight.
5. At end of massage have client relax, taking slow, deep breaths.

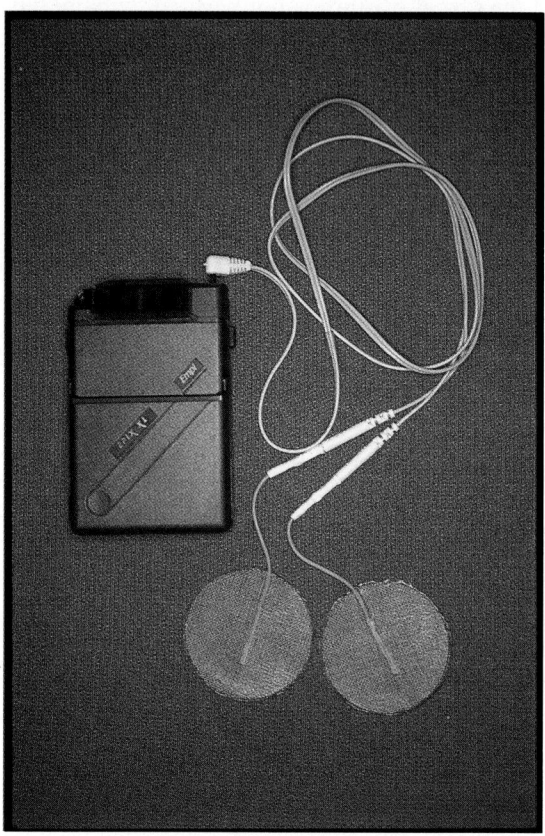

Figure 33-7. TENS unit.

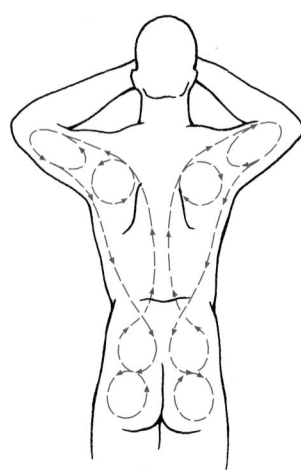

Figure 33-8. Back massage pattern.

dure or while waiting for an analgesic to work. Useful forms of distraction include singing, praying, listening to music, describing photos out loud, telling jokes, and playing games.

Relaxation. The ability to relax physically promotes mental relaxation. **Relaxation** techniques provide clients with self-control when pain occurs, reversing the physical and emotional stress of pain. Clients who use relaxation techniques successfully go through physiological and behavioral changes (e.g., decreased pulse and blood pressure and decreased muscle tension). Relaxation strategies include simple relaxation, imagery, and music-assisted relaxation. Relaxation and imagery techniques can be simple and have been successful in reducing self-reported pain and analgesic use (McCaffery and Beebe, 1989; Stanik-Hutt, 1993). The techniques require periodic reinforcement through encouragement and coaching (AHCPR, 1992).

For effective relaxation the client needs to participate and cooperate. Relaxation techniques are taught only when the client is not in acute discomfort and thus is able to concentrate. The nurse explains the technique in detail and notes that it may take several training sessions before clients can effectively minimize pain. Relaxation training can be practiced indefinitely and usually has no side effects. The nurse describes common sensations that the client may experience (e.g., a decrease in temperature, a feeling of heaviness, numbness of a body part). The client uses these sensations as feedback. Acting as a coach, the nurse guides the client slowly through the steps of the exercise. The environment should be free of noises or other irritating stimuli. The client should sit in a comfortable chair in good alignment or lie in bed. A light sheet or blanket keeps the client warm and comfortable. Relaxation may be done alone or with guided imagery.

In **guided imagery,** the client creates an image in the mind, concentrates on that image, and gradually becomes less aware of pain. Initially the nurse asks the client to think of a pleasant scene or experience that promotes using all senses. The client describes the image, and the nurse records it so that it can be used later. The nurse uses only specific information given by the client and makes no changes in the image. The following is an example of a portion of a guided imagery exercise:

Imagine yourself lying on a cool bed of grass with the sounds of rushing water from a nearby stream. It's a warm, balmy day. You turn to see a patch of blue wildflowers in bloom and can smell their fragrance.

The nurse sits close enough to the client to be heard but is not intrusive. A calm, soft voice helps the client to focus more completely on the suggested image. While relaxing, the client focuses on the image, and it becomes unnecessary for the nurse to speak continuously. If the client shows signs of agitation, restlessness, or discomfort, the nurse should stop the exercise and begin later when the client is more at ease.

Progressive relaxation exercises involve a combination of controlled breathing exercises and a series of contractions and relaxations of muscle groups. The client begins by breathing slowly and diaphragmatically, allowing the abdomen to rise slowly and the chest to expand fully. Often a client closes the eyes to focus on the exercise. When the client establishes a regular breathing pattern, the nurse coaches the client to locate any area of muscular tension, think about how it feels, tense the muscles fully, and then completely relax them. This creates the sensation of removing all discomfort and stress. Gradually the client can relax the muscles without first tensing them. After the client achieves full relaxation, pain perception is lowered, and anxiety toward the pain experience becomes minimal.

If the client becomes agitated or uncomfortable, the nurse stops the exercise. If the client reports having difficulty relaxing only part of the body, the nurse slows the progression of the exercise and concentrates on the tensed body part. The client may stop the exercise at any time. With practice, the client can learn to perform relaxation exercises independently. Relaxation techniques are particularly effective for chronic pain, labor pains, and relief of procedure-related pain. The techniques are less effective for episodes of acute or severe pain.

Anticipatory guidance. Modifying anxiety directly associated with pain relieves pain and adds to the effects of other pain-relief measures. Moderate anxiety can help when a client anticipates pain. Clients can learn what is to be expected during a painful event. The AHCPR (1992) reports that giving clients detailed descriptions of all medical procedures, expected postoperative discomfort, and instruction aimed at decreasing treatment- and mobility-related pain can decrease self-reported pain, analgesic use, and postoperative length of stay. Clients should receive sufficient procedural and sensory information (e.g., prick of a needle during blood draw, burning during urinary catheter insertion) to satisfy their interest and enable them to assess, evaluate, and communicate pain (Jurf and Nirschl, 1993; Woodin, 1993).

Acute care.
In the acute care setting nurses will care for clients with acute pain and chronic pain. The additional effects of other symptoms and multiple treatments can make pain management complex. The nurse's ability to make appropriate decisions depends on a critical thinking approach.

Pharmacological pain therapy. Several pharmacological agents provide pain management. All require a physician's order. The nurse's judgment in the use of medications with or without other pain therapies ensures the best pain relief possible. A systematic approach ensures quick response on the part of care givers to client discomfort.

Analgesics. **Analgesics** are the most common method of pain relief. Although analgesics can effectively relieve pain, nurses and physicians tend to undertreat clients because of incorrect drug information, concerns about addiction, anxiety over errors in judgment while using narcotic analgesics, and administration of less medication than was ordered. Nurses must understand the drugs available for pain relief and their pharmacological effects (Hekmat and others, 1994; McCaffery and Ferrell, 1996). Clients need to be reassured that fears of addiction are unfounded.

The three types of analgesics are nonnarcotic and nonsteroidal antiinflammatory drugs (NSAIDs), **narcotic** analgesics or opioids, and adjuvants or coanalgesics (Table 33-5). NSAIDs are effective in treating mild to moderate pain. One exception is ketorolac

(Toradol), which is an injectable analgesic NSAID that is comparable to morphine in efficacy (McKenry and Salerno, 1995). NSAIDs act by inhibiting the synthesis of **prostaglandins** and by inhibiting the cellular responses during inflammation. Most NSAIDs act on peripheral nerve receptors to diminish transmission and reception of pain stimuli. One exception, acetaminophen, acts on central nervous system prostaglandins. Opioid or narcotic analgesics are generally used for severe pain. They act on the central nervous system to produce a combination of depressing and stimulating effects. Adjuvants such as sedatives, antianxiety agents, and muscle relaxants enhance pain control or relieve other symptoms associated with pain, such as depression and nausea. They may be given alone or with analgesics.

Narcotic analgesics such as morphine act on higher centers of the brain and spinal cord by binding with opiate receptors to modify perception of and reaction to pain. Morphine is a derivative of opium. It raises the pain threshold (reducing pain perception), reduces anxiety and fear (components of the reaction to pain), and induces sleep. Morphine and other narcotic analgesics can depress vital nervous system functions such as respirations. Clients may also have side effects such as nausea, vomiting, constipation, and altered mental processes. Characteristics of an ideal analgesic include the following:

1. Rapid onset
2. Prolonged effectiveness
3. Effectiveness in all age-groups
4. Oral and parenteral use
5. Lack of severe side effects
6. Nonaddicting nature
7. Inexpensive

The proper use of analgesics requires careful assessment, application of pharmacological principles (see Chapter 26), and common sense (Box 33-10). Responses to analgesics are highly individualized. An NSAID may be as effective as a potent narcotic for some clients, or an orally administered analgesic may bring the same relief as an injectable form. Nurses must remain familiar with comparative doses of different analgesics. In addition, nurses on succeeding shifts must know the route of administration most effective for a client so that controlled, sustained pain relief is achieved.

Children require careful calculation of drug doses. Equianalgesic charts that convert recommended adult doses to children's doses are available. These charts consider age and body size. Older adults also require special considerations (Box 33-11).

Patient-controlled analgesia. Clients benefit from having control over pain therapy. When clients depend on nurses for analgesia, an erratic cycle of alternating

TABLE 33-5
Analgesics and Indications for Therapy

Drug Category	Indications
Nonnarcotic Analgesics	
Acetaminophen (Tylenol, Datril)	Mild postoperative pain; fever, rheumatic and nonrheumatic inflammation
Acetylsalicylic acid (aspirin)	
Choline magnesium trisalicylate (Trilisate)	
NSAIDs	
Ibuprofen (Motrin, Nuprin)	Dysmenorrhea, muscle aches, vascular headaches, rheumatoid arthritis, soft tissue injury, gout
Naproxen (Naprosyn)	
Indomethacin (Indocin)	
Tolmetin (Tolectin)	
Piroxicam (Feldene)	
Ketorolac (Toradol)	Postoperative and traumatic pain
Narcotic Analgesics, Opioids	
Meperidine (Demerol)	Postoperative pain, severe traumatic pain, cancer pain (EXCEPTION: Demerol not given for cancer pain), myocardial infarction
Methylmorphine (codeine)	
Morphine sulfate (Morphine)	
Fentanyl (Sublimaze)	
Butorphanol (Stadol)	
Hydromorphone HCl (Dilaudid)	
Adjuvants	
Amitriptyline (Elavil)	Anxiety, depression, nausea, vomiting
Hydroxyzine (Vistaril)	
Chlorpromazine (Thorazine)	
Diazepam (Valium)	

Box 33-10
Nursing Principles for Administering Analgesics

Know the Client's Previous Response to Analgesics

Determine whether relief was obtained.

Ask whether a nonnarcotic was as effective as a narcotic.

Identify previous doses and routes of administration to avoid undertreatment.

Determine whether the client has allergies.

Select Proper Medications When More Than One Is Ordered

Use NSAIDs or milder narcotics for mild to moderate pain.

The concurrent use of opioids and NSAIDs often provides for more effective analgesics than either drug class alone.

Use of NSAIDs can help reduce opioid side effects.

In older adults, avoid combinations of narcotics.

Remember that morphine and hydromorphone are the narcotics of choice for long-term management of severe pain.

Know that injectable medications act quicker and can relieve severe, acute pain within 1 hour and that oral medication may take as long as 2 hours to relieve pain.

For chronic pain, give an oral drug for longer, more sustained relief.

Know the Accurate Dosage

Remember that doses at the upper end of normal are generally needed for severe pain.

Adjust doses, as appropriate, for children and older clients.

Dosage typically requires adjustment over time.

Know the comparative potencies of analgesics (refer to drug manual or pharmacy) in oral and injectable form.

Assess the Right Time and Interval for Administration

Administer analgesics as soon as pain occurs and before it increases in severity.

Do not give analgesics only on "as needed" schedules. An around-the-clock administration schedule is best.

Give analgesics before pain-producing procedures or activities.

Know the average duration of action for a drug and the time of administration so that the peak effect occurs when pain is most intense.

Choose the Right Route

Intravenous and oral routes are preferred.

Intramuscular administration should be avoided, because this route can be painful and absorption is not reliable.

---

pain and analgesia often occurs (Lazzara, 1993). The client feels pain and asks for a drug, but the nurse may be unable to give it promptly. Within 1 hour analgesia finally occurs, but pain relief may last only ½ hour and the client may be sedated as long as 1 hour. Then the client feels pain again, and the cycle starts over.

PCA is a safe method for postoperative, traumatic, labor and delivery, sickle cell crisis, and cancer pain management that most clients prefer to intermittent injections (Timmons and Bower, 1993). It is a drug-delivery system that allows clients to administer pain medications when they want them. It has been an effective form of pain management with the elderly and with children as young as 10 years of age (Egbert and others, 1993; Lazzara, 1993). Systemic PCA usually involves intravenous drug administration, but it can also be given subcutaneously. PCA uses portable infusion pumps containing a chamber for a syringe (Figure 33-9, A) or specifically designed devices like the wristwatch (Figure 33-9, B) that deliver a small preset dose of medication (usually morphine). To receive a dose, the client pushes a button attached to the PCA

device. The system is designed to deliver no more than a specified number of doses either every hour or every 4 hours (depending on pump) to avoid overdoses. A typical PCA prescription relies on a series of "loading" doses (e.g., 3 to 5 mg of morphine, repeated every 5 minutes until initial postoperative pain diminishes). A low-dose basal infusion (0.5 to 1 mg/hr) at night allows uninterrupted sleep. On-demand doses typically add 1 mg of morphine every 6 minutes, with a total hourly limit of 10 mg (AHCPR, 1992). Most pumps have locked safety systems to prevent tampering. Even though a dose can be released only over a select number of minutes, a small bell alarms each time the client pushes the button. The bell acts as a placebo (Timmons and Bowers, 1993). The client believes a dose is delivered with each ring.

Benefits of PCA include clients having control over pain, pain relief not depending on nurse availability, clients tending to take less medication, and small doses of narcotics delivered at short intervals stabilizing serum drug concentrations for sustained pain relief (Lazzara, 1993). Client preparation and teaching are

> ### Box 33-11
> ### Gerontological Nursing Practice
>
> In older adults there is fear that pain will result in crippling and forced dependency.
>
> Older adults are at high risk for pain-inducing situations.
>
> Several pain-producing conditions may coexist.
>
> The potential for lowered pain tolerance exists with diminished adaptive capacity.
>
> Changes in peripheral vascular function, skin, and transmission of pain impulses place the older adult at risk for being unable to sense pain (Ebersole and Hess, 1994).
>
> When administering analgesics, nurses should confer with physicians regarding proper dosing. Clients may be susceptible to side effects of narcotics because of changes in serum proteins, liver and renal function, and a reduction in cardiac output.
>
> The risk for gastric and renal toxicity from NSAIDs is increased among older adults.
>
> Older adults are more sensitive to the analgesic effects of opioid drugs as they experience a higher peak and longer duration of pain relief.
>
> Pain is *not* normal with aging. Presence of pain requires aggressive assessment and management.

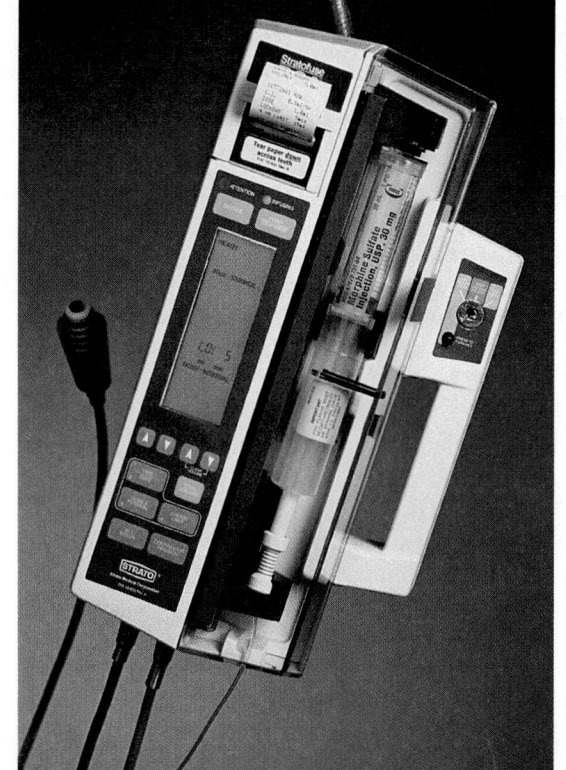

A

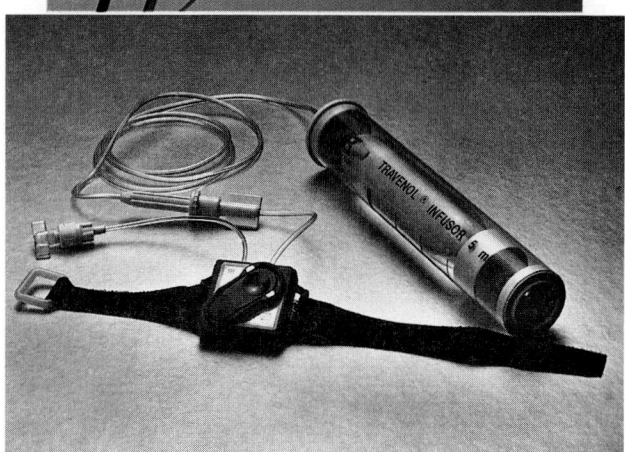

B

Figure 33-9. PCA devices. **A,** Computerized pump; **B,** wristwatch device. (Courtesy Baxter Healthcare Corp, Irvine, Calif.)

critical to the safe and effective use of PCA (Box 33-12) (Timmons and Bower, 1993). Clients must be able to understand the use of the equipment and be physically able to locate and press the button to deliver the dose (Lazzara, 1993).

Nurses must check the intravenous line and PCA device regularly to ensure proper functioning. Certain pumps keep track of accumulative dosage and print out the information on demand. Drug doses must be carefully documented, and any narcotics that are wasted or unused must be recorded (see Chapter 26). Successful implementation of PCA into nursing practice requires that nurses accept pain as a subjective and personal experience (Lazzara, 1993; Fulton, 1996). Use of PCA in practice can give the nurse and client more flexibility in pain management.

Placebos. A **placebo** is a dose form that contains no pharmacologically active ingredient but may relieve pain. Commonly used placebos are normal saline, sterile water, and sugar. The pharmacy prepares placebos in forms (e.g., tablets) that make them look like medications. A doctor's order is required. When the placebo is administered correctly, the client is convinced that it will provide pain relief. A nurse can also use a "placebo effect" when administering analgesics by telling clients that the drug will act to reduce pain. Belief that a medication will work and trust in the nurse increases the likelihood of pain relief. The nurse administers the placebo as though it were an actual pain medication, assesses the pain carefully, and evaluates the placebo's effects.

Local anesthetics. **Local anesthesia** is the loss of sensation to a localized body part. Physicians use local anesthesia while suturing a wound, moving a painful body part, delivering an infant, and performing some surgery. The nurse is responsible for protecting the client from injury or other adverse effects. Local anesthetics have fewer risks than general anesthetics, which cause loss of consciousness and depress vital functions.

Client Teaching for Preparation for Patient-Controlled Analgesia

- Teach the use of PCA before surgery so that the client can understand how to use it after awakening from anesthesia. (Confused and unresponsive clients; clients with a history of narcotic abuse, neurological disease, or impaired renal or pulmonary function; and those unable to press the delivery button are not candidates for PCA).
- Instruct clients on the purpose of PCA, operating instructions, expected pain relief, precautions, and potential side effects (IVNS, 1990), emphasizing that the client controls medication therapy.
- Explain that the pump prevents risks of overdose.
- Tell family members or friends that they should not operate the PCA device for the client.
- Have the client demonstrate use of the PCA delivery button.

The drugs produce temporary loss of sensation by inhibiting nerve conduction; they also block motor and autonomic functions when administered as nerve blocks. Typically a client loses sensation in small sensory nerves before losing motor function; conversely, motor activity returns before sensation.

Local anesthetics can cause side effects, depending on their absorption. Itching, burning of the skin, and a localized rash are common with topical application. Application to vascular mucous membranes may cause systemic effects such as a change in heart rate. Injection increases the risk of systemic effects.

The nurse provides emotional support to clients receiving local anesthesia by explaining insertion sites and warning clients that they will temporarily lose sensory function. Autonomic function (bowel and bladder control) may also be temporarily lost. To reassure the client, the nurse explains application of the anesthetic and the sensations experienced. Injection can be painful unless the physician first numbs the injection site. The nurse prepares clients for such discomfort. Before a client receives an anesthetic, the nurse checks for allergies. To monitor systemic effects, the nurse assesses blood pressure and pulse. Spinal anesthesia may also cause respiratory changes.

After administration of a local anesthetic the nurse protects the client from injury until full sensory and motor function return. Pain is a protective mechanism. Until a local anesthetic is absorbed and metabolized, the client must be careful in using an anesthetized body part. Clients can easily injure themselves without knowing it.

Epidural analgesia. Epidural analgesia is a form of local anesthesia and an effective therapy for the treatment of postoperative, trauma, chronic, and cancer pain (Naber and others, 1994). It permits control or reduction of severe pain without the sedative effects of narcotics. Epidural analgesia can be short or long term, depending on the client's condition and life expectancy. Short-term therapy is used for pain after intrathoracic, abdominal, and orthopedic surgery. Long-term therapy is used for intractable pain in the lower part of the body. Naber and others (1994) describe the following advantages of epidural analgesia:

Production of excellent analgesia
Occurrence of minimal sedation
Longer-lasting pain relief with fewer narcotic doses
Facilitation of early ambulation
Avoidance of repeated injections
No significant effect on sensation
Little effect on blood pressure or heart rate
Fewer pulmonary complications, or improved pulmonary function

Epidural analgesia is administered into the spinal epidural space usually while the client is in the operating room or in a postanesthesia care unit (Woodin, 1993). A physician inserts the catheter into the level of the vertebral interspace nearest to the area requiring analgesia or at the L4 to L5 space depending on physician preference. Once the catheter is advanced into the epidural space (Figure 33-10) and the needle is removed, the remainder of the catheter is secured with an occlusive dressing and taped up the back of the client (Naber and others, 1994). If the catheter is only temporary, it is connected to tubing positioned along the spine and over the client's shoulder. The end of the catheter can then be placed on the client's chest for the nurse's access. Permanent catheters may be tunneled through the skin and exit at the client's side (Figure 33-11).

The catheter is connected to a continuous **epidural infusion** pump or a port or reservoir, or it is capped off for bolus injections. To reduce the risk of accidental epidural injection of drugs intended for intravenous use, it helps to place a brightly colored intermittent injection cap on the catheter tubing. Labeling the catheter "epidural catheter" also helps. Continuous infusions must be administered through electronic infusion devices for proper control (Woodin, 1993). Because of the catheter location, strict surgical aseptic technique is needed to prevent a serious and potentially fatal infection. Physicians are notified immediately of any signs or symptoms of infection or pain at the insertion site (Naber and others, 1994).

Narcotics used commonly for epidural analgesia include preservative-free morphine sulfate, fentanyl, methadone, and meperidine. Morphine has a long-lasting effect but also causes more side effects. The medications block transmission of pain stimuli in the spinal cord (Naber and others, 1994).

Nursing implications for managing epidural analge-

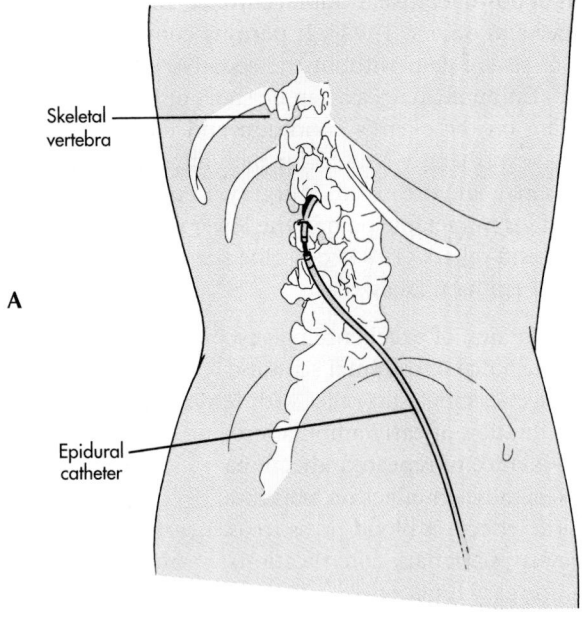

A

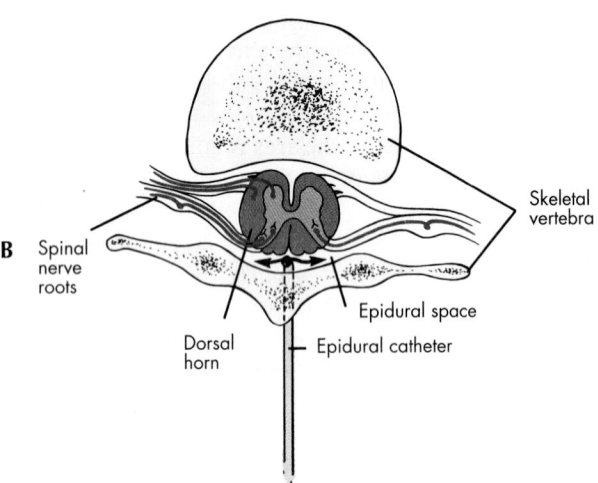

B

Figure 33-10. **A,** Epidural catheter insertion. **B,** Anatomical drawing of epidural space.

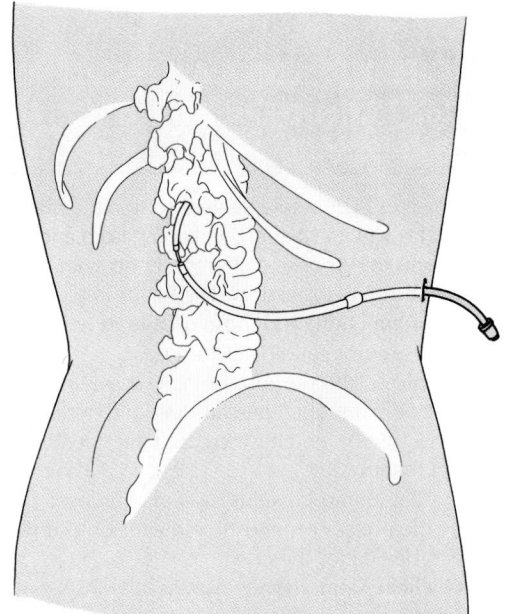

Figure 33-11. Tunneled epidural catheter.

sia are numerous (Table 33-6). Monitoring for drug effects differs, depending on if infusions are intermittent or continuous. Complications of epidural narcotic use include respiratory depression (rare), nausea and vomiting, urinary retention, constipation, and pruritis. When clients are started on epidural analgesia, monitoring occurs as often as every 15 minutes, including assessment of respiratory rate, respiratory effort, and skin color. Pulse oximetry may be used. If a client remains stable, monitoring can move to every hour. Clients should be informed about the potential for respiratory depression and instructed to notify a nurse if breathing difficulty develops. If respiratory depression develops, the infusion is turned off immediately.

Clients with intractable pain. Intractable pain cannot be permanently relieved. It can become so debilitating that clients will try anything to gain relief. The AHCPR released clinical practice guidelines for the

management of cancer pain (Jacox and others, 1994). The guidelines are designed to treat cancer pain in a more comprehensive and aggressive manner. Similiarly, they provide clients and families more options for pain relief. Figure 33-12 is a flow chart depicting cancer pain management from assessment to various treatment measures. The best choice of treatment often changes as the client's condition and the characteristics of pain change. Both nonpharmacological and pharmacological therapies can be beneficial (Ferrell and Rhiner, 1994).

Administering analgesics to treat cancer-related pain requires applying principles different from those used to treat acute pain. The WHO (1990) recommends a three-step approach to managing cancer pain (Figure 33-13). Therapy begins with NSAIDs and/or adjuvants and then progresses to strong opioids if pain persists. When a client with cancer first has pain, it is best to begin with a higher dosage than will be needed for relief. The physician can slowly decrease the dosage to the amount needed, thus giving the client immediate relief. Side effects of analgesia are aggressively treated so analgesia can be continued. Terminally ill clients with prolonged pain develop a tolerance to analgesics. They thus require higher dosages to attain pain relief. Higher dosages are not lethal, because clients also develop tolerance to life-threatening side effects (Ferrell and Rhiner, 1994). Tolerance does not prevent the side effect of constipation.

For clients with cancer, the aim of drug therapy is to anticipate and minimize pain rather than cure it. It is therefore necessary to give required dosages regularly. Prescribing analgesics on an as-needed basis for cancer

TABLE 33-6

Nursing Care of Clients With Epidural Infusions

Goal	Actions
Prevent catheter displacement	Secure catheter (if not connected to implanted reservoir) carefully to outside skin
Maintain catheter function	Check external dressing around catheter site for dampness or discharge (Leak of cerebrospinal fluid may develop)
	Use transparent, adhesive dressing to aid inspection
	Inspect catheter for breaks
Prevent infection	Use strict aseptic technique when caring for catheter
	Do not routinely change dressing over site
	Change tubing every 24 hours
Monitor for respiratory depression	Monitor vital signs, especially respirations, per policy
	Pulse oximetry and apnea monitoring may be used
Prevent undesirable complications	Assess for pruritis (itching) and nausea and vomiting
	Administer antiemetics as ordered
Maintain urinary and bowel function	Monitor intake and output
	Assess for bladder and bowel distention
	Assess for discomfort, frequency, and urgency

clients is ineffective and causes more suffering. Analgesics are needed even when pain, nausea, and other symptoms subside. Regular administration maintains blood levels for ongoing pain control.

Transdermal drug systems administer drugs such as fentanyl over predetermined rates up to 24 hours. This is useful when clients are unable to take drugs orally. Self-adhesive patches release the drug slowly over time, achieving effective analgesia. Caution is needed in administering transdermal patches to clients who are hyperthermic. Hyperthermia causes more rapid drug absorption.

Analgesics in the form of suppositories may be given rectally when clients have nausea and vomiting or are fasting before or after surgery (Jacox and others, 1994). The route is contraindicated if clients have diarrhea or if cancerous lesions involve the anus or rectum.

Another measure to treat severe intractable cancer pain is morphine given by continuous intravenous drip or intermittently by a PCA pump. Continuous infusions provide improved, uniform pain control because lower dosages are used (Lazzara, 1993). Thus there are fewer side effects. The total daily dosage may be less than with regular intramuscular injections.

Continuous-drip morphine is given in acute care settings and the home. Morphine mixed in intravenous solution is delivered by an infusion control pump to ensure safe and accurate administration. Each agency has guidelines for morphine dose and infusion rates. The drug can cause numerous side effects that require the nurse's ongoing assessment. Adjuvant drugs such as antiemetics, corticosteroids, anticonvulsants, neuroleptics, biphosphonates, and calcitonin (bone pain) or an-

tidepressants may be needed to enhance pain control and prevent side effects (Jacox and others, 1994).

When a client is first placed on continuous-drip morphine, it is essential that an intravenous access is patent and the intravenous site is without complications (see Chapter 31). To prevent overdose and central nervous system depression, the nurse records baseline blood pressure and respiratory rates before the infusion begins. After the infusion starts, the nurse monitors vital signs as often as every 15 to 30 minutes for the first few hours until the client gains relief at a constant dosage. If blood pressure or respirations decrease, the infusion rate is reduced according to the physician's order or agency policy. If the client shows signs of severe respiratory depression, the physician will order the infusion discontinued. The narcotic antagonist naloxone (Narcan) should be available to reverse respiratory depression (Lazzara, 1993; Salerno, 1996).

Restorative care. Clients in need of restorative care for pain usually are suffering chronic or intractable pain that is unrelenting. The nurse continues to use nonpharmacological measures that are effective for individual clients. However, additional pharmacological measures are designed to give a client better long-term pain control. The focus in restorative care is to use a comprehensive approach in supporting the client and family.

Morphine infusions. In the home or extended care settings, clients may use ambulatory infusion pumps for narcotic infusions. The pumps are lightweight, compact (about the size of a transistor radio), and allow free movement. The pump is battery powered

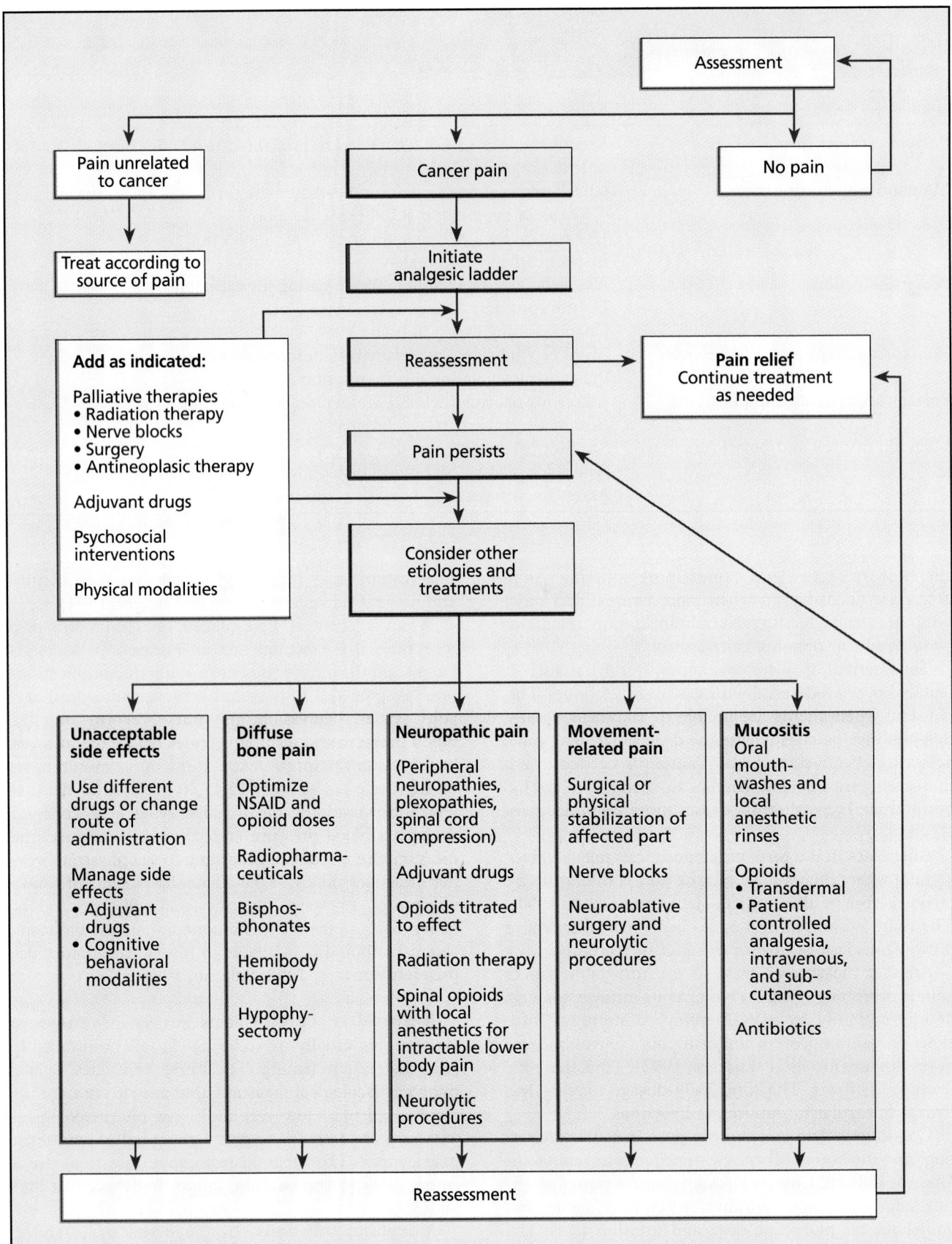

Figure 33-12. Flowchart: continuing pain management in patients with cancer. (From Jacox A and others: *Management of cancer pain,* Clinical practice guideline No. 9, AHCPR Pub. No. 94-0592, Rockville, Md., March 1994, AHCPR, USDHHS, PHS.)

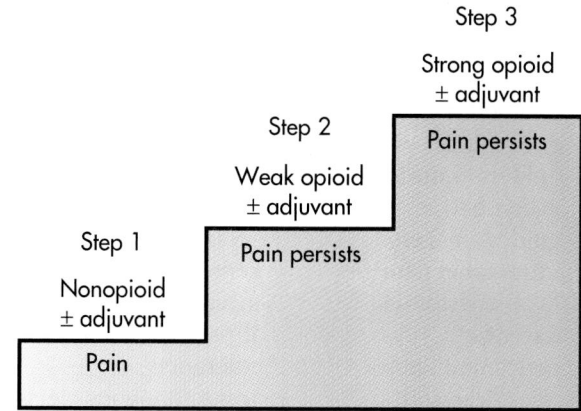

Step 3
Strong opioid
± adjuvant

Step 2
Weak opioid
± adjuvant

Pain persists

Step 1
Nonopioid
± adjuvant

Pain persists

Pain

Figure 33-13. WHO analgesic ladder is a three-step approach to using drugs in cancer pain management. ± *adjuvant,* with or without adjuvant medications. (From World Health Organization: *Cancer pain relief and palliative care,* Report of a WHO expert committee, WHO Technical Report Series No. 804, Geneva, Switzerland, 1990, WHO.)

and worn in a pouch attached to a belt or harness. The bag of medication and intravenous fluid fits inside the pump. A dose of morphine, delivered continuously over 24 hours, is usually slowly infused into a central venous catheter either by way of a peripherally inserted central catheter (PICC) or a more traditional subclavian placed catheter. Both catheters can be left in place for an extended period of time. The pumps differ from PCA devices, which deliver only small, preset doses of medication. The client and family learn to manage the pump, observe for drug side effects, and maintain function of the central venous catheter (Box 33-13). Because the client is initially managed on morphine in the hospital before going home, the risk of side effects is not as great unless the client or family member increases dosages. A home health nurse makes routine visits to be sure the client manages the pump correctly.

Hospice. Hospices are programs to care for the terminally ill (see Chapter 21). *Hospice* in Latin means *a place to rest.* Hospices are often affiliated with hospitals. The programs help terminally ill clients continue to live at home in comfort and privacy with the help of a health care team. Pain control is a priority. Clients receive the proper dosage and forms of analgesics to provide pain relief. Families learn to monitor the client's symptoms and become primary care givers.

Pain clinics. Pain clinics have evolved to provide pain management for a variety of clients. A comprehensive pain center can treat clients in the hospital or in outpatient clinics. Nurses, physicians, physical therapists, and dietitians collaborate to find the most effective pain-relief therapies. Diverse therapies, as well as research into new treatments, are among the center's services (Miller and others, 1996).

Client Teaching for Ambulatory Infusion Pumps

- Tell client and family to observe for the following side effects: dizziness or fainting, nausea, vomiting, slow and shallow respirations, constipation, mood changes, euphoria, inability to empty bladder fully, dry mouth, weakness, agitation, tremors, strange dreams.
- Instruct family on how to administer naloxone (Narcan) intramuscularly to reverse respiratory depression.
- Teach client and family how to keep central venous catheter patent, maintain pump flow rate, and irrigate the catheter routinely with heparin flush.
- Tell client how to prevent air from entering central venous catheter and to clamp catheter when infusion has stopped.
- Explain how to prevent infection at catheter site and to keep site clean with soap and water.
- Have client follow a preventive bowel routine using stool softeners, laxatives, dietary fiber, hydration, and routine exercise.
- Warn client against wearing pump in shower or submerging in bathtub. Device can be temporarily disconnected during shower or placed in a plastic bag hung outside shower or tub.
- During sleep, keep the pump on the bed or adjacent nightstand. During lovemaking, the pump can be set to the side so it does not interfere with closeness and intimacy.
- Instruct the client and family on the purpose of the pump alarms and how to respond when they go off.
- Keep a 24-hour emergency telephone number nearby.

▪ Evaluation

Client care. With regard to pain management, the client is the source for evaluating outcomes. The client is the only one who will know if the severity of pain has lessened and which therapies are most successful in bringing relief. To evaluate the effectiveness of nursing interventions, comparisons are made with baseline pain assessments to evaluate if the severity and other characteristics of pain have changed (Woodin, 1993). For example, the nurse will readminister a VAS after a therapy to see if pain severity decreases. Similarly, the nurse evaluates whether the client's response to pain (e.g., positioning and body movements, ability to socialize or perform self-care) has changed. Outcomes are compared with expected outcomes to determine the client's health status. Continuous evaluation allows the nurse to determine whether new or revised therapies are required and if new nursing diagnoses have developed.

Client expectations. If a nurse has successfully developed a good relationship with a client, subtle behaviors often indicate the level of a client's satisfaction. When the nurse has successfully made a client feel more comfortable, often a gentle smile, a sigh of relief, or reaching out for the nurse's hand can convey the client's gratitude. However, it is important for the nurse to *ask* the client if his or her expectations of care have been met. For example, asking the client, "Can you tell me if you feel we have done all we can to make you feel comfortable?" or "Are you happy with the way we are trying to relieve your pain?" goes a long way toward showing the client a commitment to his or her needs. If a client's expectations have not been met, then the nurse needs to spend more time understanding the client's desires. Working closely with the client will enable the nurse to redefine those expectations that can be realistically met within the limits of the client's condition and treatment.

Key Terms

analgesics	perception
cutaneous stimulation	placebo
endorphins	prostaglandins
epidural infusion	reaction
exacerbations	reception
guided imagery	relaxation
intractable pain	remissions
local anesthesia	synapse
narcotic	threshold
neuromodulator	tolerance
neurotransmitters	transcutaneous electrical nerve stimulation (TENS)
nociceptors	
pain	
patient-controlled analgesia (PCA)	

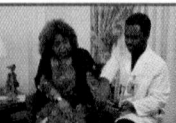

Case Study

Evaluation

After 2 weeks, Jim returns to evaluate Mrs. Ellis' progress. Mrs. Ellis reports that she has seen her physician and has been referred to physical therapy for heat therapy and fitting for supportive splints. In addition, the physician has prescribed NSAIDs for her acute exacerbations and to reduce her gastrointestional irritation. She reports that she is falling asleep more easily if she takes the medicine 30 minutes before going to bed. When Jim asks her to rate her current level of pain, she rates it a 3 on a scale of 0 to 10. Mrs. Ellis also notes that during the last week, the pain never felt worse than a rating of about 5. During the visit she gets up to walk to the kitchen. Jim notes that although it takes her time to stand, she walks with a steadier stride. She is trying ambulating with a walker that the physical therapist recommended. Jim asks if Mrs. Ellis has thought of anyone whom she could call when she needs assistance. Mrs. Ellis mentions that she has confided in a neighbor, who has offered to take her shopping and to church as needed. Mrs. Ellis is also pleased to report that her Bible study group is going to have a covered dish dinner and meet at her house so she will not have to be on her feet so much.

Documentation Note

Client reports reduction in severity of pain and improvement in ability to fall asleep with use of NSAIDs. Appears less fatigued and is ambulating with a steadier gait, using walker. Initiated social contacts and identified neighbor as support system. Will evaluate effectiveness of heat therapy and supportive devices at next visit.

■ Key Concepts

Pain, a protective mechanism that warns a person of tissue injury, is completely subjective. Misconceptions about pain can lead to undertreatment.

Knowledge of the three components of the pain experience—reception, perception, and reaction—provides the nurse with guidelines for determining relief measures.

The pain experience is influenced by a client's age, sex, anxiety, culture, experience, and the meaning of pain.

A client's pain tolerance influences the nurse's perceptions of the seriousness of the discomfort.

The difference between acute and chronic pain involves the duration of discomfort, physical signs and symptoms, and the client's perceptions regarding relief.

Pain scales are used to objectively evaluate the severity of pain and the effectiveness of pain therapies.

The client's family and friends can be a key resource in pain assessment.

The nurse individualizes pain therapy by collaborating closely with the client, using assessment findings, trying a variety of therapies, and maintaining the client's well-being.

Eliminating sources of painful stimuli is a basic nursing measure for promoting comfort.

Nonpharmacological cutaneous therapies are effective in altering client perception of pain, promoting muscle relaxation, and giving the client control over pain experienced.

Using a regular schedule for analgesic administration is more effective than an as-needed schedule.

A PCA device gives clients pain control with a low risk of overdose.

The nurse's primary role in caring for a client who receives local anesthesia is protecting the client from injury.

The aim of therapy for cancer clients is to anticipate and prevent pain rather than treat it.

The most serious side effect of morphine infusions is respiratory depression, which can be reversed with intravenous Narcan.

Evaluation of pain therapy requires consideration of the changing character of pain, response to therapy, and the client's perceptions of a therapy's effectiveness.

■ Critical Thinking Activities

1. Mrs. Wiegand is a 76-year-old married woman who comes to the outpatient clinic with complaints, in her words, of severe burning pain in her hands and wrists. She has been diagnosed with arthritis for more than 1 year. What type of questions might you ask of Mrs. Wiegand to assess how this pain has affected her lifestyle?

2. Mr. Jasper and Mr. Stern are clients experiencing back pain. Mr. Jasper's pain resulted from a fall from a ladder 48 hours ago. Mr. Stern's pain has been bothering him for more than 8 months with no known cause. As the nurse caring for both clients, how might you anticipate differences in assessment and treatment?

3. Consider the previous example of Mr. Stern. What might influence your approach to assessment if Mr. Stern were 39 versus 80 years of age?

4. Ms. Rogers is receiving morphine by way of a PCA device following abdominal surgery for a hysterectomy. During your assessment, you note Ms. Rogers to be more drowsy and her respirations have decreased from 16 a minute to 10. What actions should you take?

5. Mr. Lake is a 45-year-old man who experienced a traumatic injury to his left arm following an industrial accident 24 hours ago. His arm is in a very bulky dressing, and pain is aggravated when he lies on his left side. He has an intravenous line with a continuous infusion of intravenous fluids in his right arm. What nonpharmacological pain-relief measures might be helpful for Mr. Lake?

References

AHCPR: Acute pain management guideline panel: *Acute pain management in infants, children and adolescents: operative or medical procedures and trauma,* Clinical practice guideline, AHCPR Pub. No. 92-0032, Rockville, Md, February 1992, AHCRP, PHS, USDHHS.

Beyer JE and others: The creation, validation, and continuing development of the Oucher: a measure of pain intensity in children, *J Pediatr Nurs* 7(5):335, 1992.

Bonica J: *The management of pain,* ed 2, Philadelphia, 1990, Lea & Febiger.

Bozeman M: Cultural aspects of pain management. In Salerno E, Williams J, editors: *Pain management handbook: an interdisciplinary approach,* St. Louis, 1996, Mosby.

Burnside I: *Nursing and the aged,* ed 3, St. Louis, 1988, Mosby.

Courts N: Nonpharmacologic approaches to pain. In Salerno E, Williams J, editors: *Pain management handbook: an interdisciplinary approach,* St. Louis, 1996, Mosby.

Ebersole P, Hess P: *Toward healthy aging,* ed 3, St. Louis, 1994, Mosby.

Egbert A and others: Effects of patient-controlled analgesia on postoperative anxiety in elderly men, *Am J Crit Care* 2(2):118, 1993.

Eiman M and others, Geriatric pain management. In Salerno E, Williams J, editors: *Pain management handbook: an interdisciplinary approach,* St. Louis, 1996, Mosby.

Ferrell B, Rhiner M: Managing cancer pain: a three-step approach, *Nurse 94* 24:57, 1994.

Fulton T: Nurses' adoption of a patient-controlled analgesia approach, *West J Nurs* Res 18(4):383, 1996.

Gerteis M and others: *Through the patient's eyes,* San Francisco, 1993, Jossey-Bass.

Giger JN, Davidhizar RE: *Transcultrual nursing: assessment and intervention,* ed 2, St. Louis, 1995, Mosby.

Good M: Relaxation techniques for surgical patients, *Am J Nurs* 95(5):38, 1995.

Hekmat N and others: Preventive pain management in the postoperative hand surgery patient, *Orthop Nurs,* 13(3):37, 1994.

Intravenous Nurses Society: Intravenous nusing standards of practice, *J Intravenous Nurs* 5:70, 1990.

Jacox A and others: *Management of cancer pain,* Clinical practice guideline No. 9, AHCPR Pub. No. 94-0592, Rockville, Md, March 1994, AHCPR, USDHHS, PHS.

Jurf J, Nirschl A: Acute postoperative pain management: a comprehensive review and update, *Crit Care Nurs Q* 16(1): 8, 1993.

Lazzara D: Patient-controlled analgesia in the intensive care unit, *Crit Care Nurs Q* 16(1):26, 1993.

McCaffery M: *Nursing management of the patient with pain,* ed 2, Philadelphia, 1979, Lippincott.

McCaffery M: *Pain: assessment and intervention in nursing practice,* course syllabus, St. Louis, 1986, Barnes Hospital.

McCaffery M, Beebe A: *Pain: clinical manual for nursing practice,* St. Louis, 1989, Mosby.

McCaffery M, Ferrell B: Correcting misconceptions about assessment and use of opioid analgesics: educational strategies aimed at public concerns, *Nurs Outlook* 44(4):184, 1996.

McKenry LM, Salerno E: *Mosby's pharmacology in nursing,* ed 19, St. Louis, 1995, Mosby.

Meinhart N, McCaffery M: *Pain: a nursing approach to assessment and analysis,* Norwalk, Conn, 1983, Appleton-Century-Crofts.

Meintz S: Whatever became of the back rub? *RN* 58(4):49, 1995.

Melzack R, Wall P: Pain mechanisms: a new theory, *Science* 150:971, 1965.

Melzack R, Wall P: *The challenge of pain,* Harmondsworth, 1988, Penguin.

Miller B and others: Team approach to pain management. In Salerno E, Williams J, editors: *Pain management handbook: an interdisciplinary approach,* St. Louis, 1996, Mosby.

Mottola C: Measurement strategies: the visual analogue scale, *Decubitus* 6(5):56, 1993.

Naber L and others: Epideral analgesia for efficient pain control, *Crit Care Nurs,* 14(5):69, 1994.

National Institutes of Health Consensus Development Panel: New gains against pain, *Emerg Med,* November 1986.

Ochsenreither J Cubina M: Pediatric pain management. In Salerno E, Williams J, editors: *Pain management handbook: an interdisciplinary approach,* St. Louis, 1996, Mosby.

Puntillo K: The phenomenon of pain and critical care nursing, *Heart Lung* 17:262, 1988.

Raj P: *Practical management of pain,* ed 2, St. Louis, 1994, Mosby.

Salerno E: Pharmacologic approaches. In Salerno E, Williams J, editors: *Pain management handbook: an interdisciplinary approach,* St. Louis, 1996, Mosby.

Stanik-Hutt J: Strategies for pain management in traumatic thoracic injuries, *Crit Care Nurs Clin North Am* 5(4):713, 1993.

Timmons M, Bower F: The effect of structured preoperative teaching on patients' use of patient-controlled analgesia (PCA) and their management of pain, *Orthop Nurs* 12(1): 23, 1993.

Vallerand A: Gender differences in pain, *Image J Nurs Sch* 27(3):235, 1995.

Walker J: Caring for elderly people with persistent pain in the community: a qualitative perspective on the attitudes of patients and nurses, *Health Soc Care* 2(4):221, 1994.

Willens J: Introduction to pain management. In Salerno E, Williams J, editors: *Pain management handbook: an interdisciplinary approach,* St. Louis, 1996, Mosby.

Wong DL, Baker CM: Pain in children: comparison of assessment scales, *Oklahoma Nurs* 33(1):8, 1988a.

Wong DL, Baker CM: Pain in children: comparison of assessment scales, *Pediatr Nurs* 14(1):9, 1988b.

Woodin L: Cutting postop pain, *RN* 56(8):26, 1993.

World Health Organization: *Cancer pain relief and palliative care,* Report of a WHO expert committee, WHO Technical Report Series No. 804, Geneva, Switzerland, 1990, WHO.

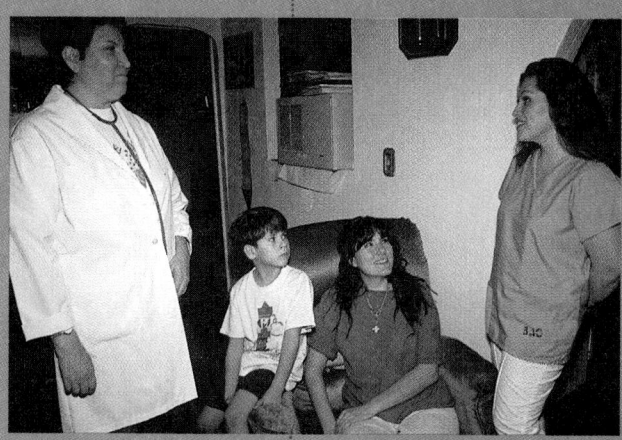

CHAPTER

34

Nutrition

OBJECTIVES

Mastery of content in this chapter will enable the student to:

- Define the key terms important in basic nutrition.
- List the six categories of nutrients and explain why each is necessary for nutrition.
- Explain the importance of a balance between energy intake and output.
- List the end products of carbohydrate, protein, and lipid metabolism.
- Explain the significance of saturated, unsaturated, and polyunsaturated lipids in nutrition.
- Describe the basic food groups (using the food guide pyramid) and their value in planning meals for good nutrition.
- Explain recommended daily allowances (RDAs).
- Discuss the major areas of nutritional assessment.
- Identify nutritional problems and describe a client at risk for these problems.
- State the goals of enteral nutrition.
- Describe the procedure for initiating and maintaining tube feedings.
- State the goals of total parenteral nutrition.
- Describe the procedure for initiating and maintaining total parenteral nutrition.

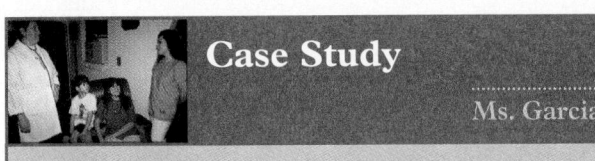

Case Study

Ms. Garcia

Ms. Garcia is a 24-year-old Hispanic single mother who is being seen at home by the nurse. She has inflammatory bowel disease (IBD) and has recently had an operation to remove a segment of her small intestine. Ms. Garcia has had IBD for 10 years, but this is her first surgical procedure. She lives with a roommate and her 5-year-old son in a second-story apartment. Ms. Garcia's roommate works part-time and helps with child care for Ms. Garcia in exchange for buying their groceries and preparing meals. Ms. Garcia's parents live in another state, and her father has had a stroke. Although Ms. Garcia's mother came to visit during her hospitalization for the surgery, she had to return home to care for Ms. Garcia's father. Ms. Garcia works at a fast-food restaurant, from which she has taken several weeks off for her surgery. Ms. Garcia's physician has ordered home nursing visits to assess the status of her abdominal wound and to determine how well she is eating. Ms. Garcia's weight had dropped by 15 lb before the operation, and she is currently about 10% below her ideal weight.

Shawneen Bott is a senior nursing student who is in her home health nursing rotation. Shawneen is single and 22 years of age. She has seen other home care patients with her preceptor, but Ms. Garcia is the closest to her own age. Shawneen is a little nervous about this visit because she will be performing her first independent assessment and treatment with observation by her nursing preceptor, Robyn Sandstrom.

Nutrition is a basic component of health. Nutrition is essential for normal growth and development, tissue maintenance and repair, cellular metabolism, and organ function. An adequate supply of nutrients is needed for essential functions of cells.

Scientific principles regarding nutrition and the role of various nutrients in metabolism and health form a basis for the nutritional plan of care that nurses develop with their clients. Disease processes, age, gender, and activity can affect utilization of nutrients and nutritional requirements. Pharmaceutical agents prescribed to treat disease can also interact with nutrients and foods.

SCIENTIFIC KNOWLEDGE BASE

Principles of Nutrition

The body requires food to provide energy for all functions including movement, maintenance of body temperature, growth and development, cellular metabolism, synthesis and repair of tissues, and organ function. Metabolism refers to all of the biochemical and physiological processes by which the body maintains itself.

The gastrointestinal system comprises a number of organs and structures that enable the body to nourish itself through the ingestion of food. Each organ or structure in the gastrointestinal tract has a specific function aimed toward preparing food for the digestion and absorption of its nutrients. Only through breaking food substances down during the digestive process can nutrients be successfully absorbed. The nutrients are then transported through the blood to organs for metabolic processes to occur.

Digestion. The process of **digestion** begins in the mouth, where mastication, or chewing, breaks down food into smaller particles, and amylase in saliva begins to break down starches. Mucus lubricates food particles for their passage through the esophagus into the stomach. Churning movements of the stomach mix food particles with hydrochloric acid. The most significant absorption of nutrients occurs in the small intestine. Digestive proteins in the gastrointestinal system act on food particles to break them into a simpler form. Most nutrients are digested and absorbed in the small intestine; the large intestine absorbs electrolytes and water, thus helping to maintain the body's electrolyte balance (see Chapter 36).

Absorption. The small intestine is the primary site of **absorption** of simple nutrients. It is lined with villi, which project into the lumen and greatly increase the surface area available for absorption. Cholesterol, vitamins E and K, folic acid, riboflavin, and thiamin are absorbed in the upper duodenum; glucose, amino acids, and fats are absorbed in the lower duodenum and upper jejunum, and sucrose, lactose, and maltose are absorbed in the lower jejunum and ileum.

Intestinal contents move by peristaltic action into the large intestine. Water is the only nutrient absorbed from the large intestine. Other nutrients remaining in the intestinal contents when they reach the large intestine are excreted as waste products. When intestinal motility is increased, such as in diarrhea, the body loses nutrients that move through the small intestine too quickly for complete absorption.

Metabolism. Nutrients are transported through the circulatory system to body tissues. Through **metabolism,** nutrients are converted into necessary substances for cell function. Carbohydrates, protein, and fat produce chemical energy and maintain a dynamic balance of tissue buildup and breakdown. The chemical energy produced by metabolism is converted to other types of energy by different tissues. Muscle contraction involves mechanical energy, the nervous system involves electrical energy, and the mechanisms of heat production involve thermal energy. These forms of energy all originate in metabolism.

Absorbed nutrients are carried to the liver, where major metabolic processes occur. The liver also regulates energy through its control of glucose metabolism. **Glucose** is the primary fuel for the body. The liver and muscles store glucose in the form of **glycogen** via a process called **glycogenesis. Lipogenesis** stores excess glucose as fat. Insulin and glucagon act as regulatory hormones to promote glucose storage or use. Insulin promotes glucose utilization, and glucagon promotes glucose storage. During states where energy needs exceed glycogen storage, the body breaks down fat and amino acids for conversion to glucose via a process called **gluconeogenesis.**

The basal metabolic rate (BMR) represents the energy needs of a person at rest after awakening. Energy balance occurs when energy requirements equal energy intake. In general, when a person's energy needs are exceeded or are insufficient, the person gains weight or loses weight, respectively.

The two basic types of metabolism are anabolism and catabolism. **Anabolism** is the production of more-complex chemical substances by synthesis of nutrients. **Catabolism** is the breakdown of body tissues into simpler substances. Although catabolism produces some energy, both processes require energy, which must be provided from food or stored sources.

Storage. The body's major form of stored energy is fat in the adipose tissue. Glycogen is stored in small reserves in liver and muscle tissue, and protein is stored in muscle mass. When the body's energy requirements exceed the energy supplied, stored energy is used; unused energy is stored, principally in fat.

Fat-soluble vitamins are also stored in limited reserves (6 to 8 months) and are released to meet the body's needs when not provided sufficiently by dietary intake. A high intake of fat-soluble vitamins can result in vitamin toxicity. Water-soluble vitamins are minimally stored (3 to 5 days) and therefore must be provided by daily intake.

Elimination. The intestinal contents move through the large intestine by peristalsis (see Chapter 36). As the material moves toward the rectum, water is absorbed into the mucosa. The end products of digestion include cellulose and similar fibrous substances the body is unable to digest. Sloughed cells from the intestinal walls, mucus, digestive secretions, water, and microorganisms are also eliminated.

Nutrients. Found in foods, **nutrients** provide the substances necessary for body function. Energy needs are met by the metabolism of carbohydrates, lipids, and, if necessary, protein. Vitamins and minerals do not provide energy, but they are necessary in the chemical reactions that produce energy. Water is essential to life. It acts as a chemical fluid to transport substances, it provides a fullness to tissues, and it helps to maintain body temperature.

Carbohydrates. Carbohydrates are composed of carbon, hydrogen, and oxygen. They are starches and sugars obtained mainly from plant foods; the only important source of animal carbohydrate is the lactose in milk (milk sugar). Carbohydrates may contribute as much as 90% of the total caloric intake in parts of the world where grains are a major ingredient of every meal.

Proteins. Proteins are made of hydrogen, oxygen, carbon, and nitrogen, and their most basic forms are amino acids. **Amino acids** are the most important components of proteins in the human body. They are essential for synthesis of body tissue in growth, maintenance, and repair. Some amino acids cannot be synthesized by the body and can only be obtained in food; these are the essential amino acids. Protein can be used as a source of energy, providing 4 kcal/g.

Protein foods tend to be expensive, and their contribution to total caloric intake is usually higher in affluent families and developed countries. Protein intake is of particular importance during periods of rapid growth and after disease and injury.

The required daily allowance of protein ranges from 2.2 g/kg body weight for infants under 6 months to 56 g for males over 15 years. Most healthy people require only about 0.8 g/kg body weight. In disease, protein requirements can double or triple, such as for major burns. Pregnant women require an additional 30 g and lactating women an additional 20 g above the usual daily need.

Nutrition experts believe that the intake of protein in America is generally greater than required. Protein foods are expensive to buy and produce, and meats, whole milk, cheese, and eggs contain significant amounts of saturated fatty acids and cholesterol. Nutritional guidelines recommend reducing saturated fats and cholesterol in the diet along with increasing complex carbohydrates from fruits, vegetables, and whole grains (USDA, 1990, 1995).

Lipids. Lipid is a comprehensive term applied to compounds that are insoluble in water but soluble in organic solvents such as ethanol and acetone. Lipids include fats that are solid at room temperature and oils that are liquid at room temperature. Lipids are composed of carbon, hydrogen, and oxygen.

Approximately 98% of the lipids in foods and 90% of the lipids in the human body are in the form of triglycerides. High blood levels of certain lipoproteins have been linked to cardiovascular diseases.

A **saturated fatty acid** contains as much hydrogen as it can hold. An **unsaturated fatty acid** can take up another hydrogen atom, and a **polyunsaturated fatty**

acid can take up many more hydrogen atoms and become hydrogenated fat. Ingestion of saturated fatty acids appears to increase blood cholesterol levels. Ingestion of unsaturated fatty acids has a minimal effect on blood cholesterol. Polyunsaturated fatty acids appear to lower blood cholesterol levels. Fatty acids are usually not purely saturated, unsaturated, or polyunsaturated. Most animal fats have high proportions of saturated fatty acids; most vegetable fats have higher amounts of unsaturated and polyunsaturated fatty acids (e.g., safflower oil is about 75% polyunsaturated, olive oil about 25%).

Fat is the body's form of stored energy. The metabolism of 1 g of lipid yields 9 kcal (38 J), more than twice the energy provided by carbohydrates or proteins. Lipids account for 35% to 45% of the American diet. Nutritional guidelines recommend a reduction of lipid intake to about 30% (10% saturated lipids and 20% polyunsaturated lipids) of the total caloric intake (American Heart Association, 1996a, b).

Vitamins. Vitamins are organic substances present in small amounts in foods and are essential for normal metabolism because they serve as coenzymes in cellular enzyme reactions. The body is unable to synthesize vitamins in the required amounts and depends on dietary intake. The National Research Council reviews new research and periodically revises the recommended allowances for vitamins and other nutrients. Although contained in many foods, vitamins are affected by processing, storage, and preparation. Vitamin content is usually highest in foods that are fresh and used quickly after minimal exposure to heat, air, or water. Vitamins are classified as water soluble and fat soluble (Table 34-1).

Water-soluble vitamins cannot be stored in the body and must be taken in daily. It was once assumed that because water-soluble vitamins are not stored in the body, toxicity was not a problem with these vitamins. However, studies of people who took megadoses of vitamin C and vitamin B_6 indicate that toxicity can occur. Vitamins are used as catalysts in biochemical reactions. When there is enough of a vitamin to meet the catalyst demands, the rest of the vitamin supply acts as a free chemical and may be toxic to the body.

Fat-soluble vitamins can be stored in the body, and therefore daily intake is not needed. However, with the exception of vitamin D, these vitamins should be provided by dietary intake. Toxicity to some fat-soluble vitamins, usually the result of megadoses of synthetic vitamins, has been recognized.

Controversy exists over the safety and need for vitamin supplementation. In general, vitamin needs appear to be modestly increased in the following conditions: pregnancy and lactation (A, C, D, B complex including folate), oral contraceptive use (B complex, C), aging (C, thiamine, riboflavin, pyridoxine), weight reduction diets less than 1200 kcal, strenuous exercise (riboflavin),

smoking (vitamin C), alcohol consumption (B complex, C), and caffeine consumption (B complex, C). Disease can pro-duce increased needs or the inability to store or excrete certain vitamins.

Minerals. Minerals are inorganic elements that act as catalysts in biochemical reactions. Minerals are classified as macrominerals when the daily requirement is 100 mg or more and microminerals when less than 100 mg is needed daily. Because the required amount of microminerals is usually very small or a trace, they are also called trace elements (see Table 34-1). In addition to the microminerals in Table 34-2, arsenic, nickel, silicon, tin, vanadium, boron, aluminum, and cadmium play unidentified roles in nutrition (see also Chapter 31).

Water. Water is an important nutrient because the function of cells depends on a fluid environment. A lean person's body contains a higher percentage of water than an obese person's body. Infants have the greatest percentage of total body weight as water; older adults have the least. Infants and older adults are most vulnerable to water deprivation or water loss. Body water is stored in two compartments: the extracellular fluid (e.g., plasma, tissue fluid, secretory fluid) and the intracellular fluid (e.g., all water inside cells).

Fluid needs are met by the ingestion of liquids and solid foods such as fresh fruits and vegetables and by water produced when food is oxidized during digestion. In a healthy individual, the fluid intake from all sources equals the fluid output through elimination, respiration, and sweating. An ill person can have an increased need for fluids, as is the case with an increased body temperature or hypermetabolic state. In addition, an ill person can have a decreased ability to manage body fluids, as is the case in a client with cardiopulmonary or renal disease.

Thirst is a protective mechanism that alerts the oriented person to the need for fluids. Thirst is a less reliable guide for infants and confused clients. These clients are usually unable to communicate that they are thirsty.

Foundations of Nutrition

A number of agencies and organizations in the United States regularly publish and update dietary guidelines. The guidelines change as nutritional research discovers new knowledge. Some guidelines are intended to provide information and education for the general public about a healthful diet. Organizations whose missions are the reeducation in incidence or management of specific diseases publish nutritional guidelines specific to those diseases.

Food guide pyramid. The pyramid was designed as a basic guide for buying food and meal preparation (Figure 34-1). This basic plan provides for diets ranging from 1600 to 2800 kcal/day (USDA, 1992). The pyramid suggests that an individual select most of

TABLE 34-1
Characteristics of Nutrients

Nutrient	Functions	Results of Deficiency	Results of Excess	Sources
Water-Soluble Vitamins				
C (ascorbic acid)	Production of collagen, integrity of capillary walls, formation of red blood cells, metabolism of amino acids, reduction of iron salts, protection of other vitamins from oxidation	Scurvy, poor wound healing, bleeding gums, loose teeth, bruising	Kidney stones, scurvy on withdrawal, urinary tract infection	Citrus fruits, potatoes, cabbage, tomatoes, broccoli, strawberries, cantaloupe, green peppers
Vitamin B complex B_1 (thiamine)	Component of enzymes, carbohydrate oxidation	Beriberi (rare), polyneuritis, mental confusion, muscular weakness, ataxia, tachycardia, cardiac enlargement	Rapid pulse, headaches, weakness, irritability, insomnia	Pork, fish, eggs, poultry, dried beans, whole grains, wheat germ, oatmeal, bread, pasta
B_2 (riboflavin)	Metabolism of nutrients, essential for growth, oxidation and reduction of fat, carbohydrates, and proteins	Ariboflavinosis: cracks at mouth corners, scaly desquamation of skin around mouth, eye irritation, glossitis, photophobia	Ulcer, elevated blood glucose level, increased uric acid levels in blood	Milk, whole grains, green vegetables, liver
Niacin	Essential for protein use, glycolysis, fat synthesis, tissue repair	Pellagra: weakness, anorexia, lassitude, indigestion; severe pellagra: dermatitis, diarrhea, dementia	Ulcer, liver dysfunction, elevated blood glucose level, increased blood uric acid levels, diarrhea, nausea, flushing	Meats, dairy products, whole grains, cereals, tuna
B_6	Metabolism of nutrients, synthesis of nonessential amino acids, conversion of tryptophan to niacin, proper function of blood and cells of central nervous system	Gastrointestinal upsets, irritability, weakness, nervousness, convulsions, anemia, skin lesions	Reverses antiparkinsonian effects of levodopa; megadoses: peripheral nerve damage, loss of sensation, numbness, awkward gait, depression	Whole grains, liver, fish, poultry, green beans, nuts, meats, potatoes
Folacin, folic acid	Metabolism of some amino acids, maturation of red blood cells	Macrocytic anemia	Diarrhea, insomnia, irritability; potentially harmful because body is able to store folacin	Liver, green leafy vegetables, meat, fish, poultry, whole grains
B_{12} (cobalamin)	Manufacture of enzymes essential to metabolism of nutrients, nucleic acid, and folic acid; proper function of cells of bone marrow, gastrointestinal tract, and nervous system	Absence of intrinsic factor in gastric juice preventing absorption of vitamin B_{12} and resulting in pernicious anemia, neurological disorders	None known	Milk, eggs, cheese, meat, fish, poultry, foods of animal origin (plant foods contain no vitamin B_{12})

Data from Grant JA, Kennedy-Caldwell C: *Nutritional support in nursing*, New York, 1988, Grune & Stratton; Whitney EN and others: *Understanding normal and clinical nutrition*. St. Paul, 1991, West; and Committee on Dietary Allowances, Food and Nutrition Board, National Academy of Sciences, National Research Council: *Estimated safe and adequate daily dietary intakes*, Washington, DC, 1989.

Continued

TABLE 34-1

Characteristics of Nutrients—cont'd

Nutrient	Functions	Results of Deficiency	Results of Excess	Sources
Pantothenic acid	Metabolism of nutrients, synthesis of cholesterol and steroid hormones, activity of adrenal cortex	None known	Increased need for thiamine, occasional diarrhea, water retention	Meats, whole grain cereals, legumes
Biotin	Synthesis of fatty acids, use of glucose, metabolism of protein, use of vitamin B_{12} and folic acid	Produced by ingestion of large amounts of raw egg whites that contain protein substance avidin, which binds biotin to itself	None known	Liver, kidneys, dark green vegetables, egg yolk, green beans
Fat-Soluble Vitamins				
A (retinol, retinal, and retinoic acid)	Growth and maintenance of epithelial tissue, maintenance of visual acuity in dim light	Night blindness, rough scaly skin, dry mucous membranes, decreased resistance to infection, faulty tooth and bone development	Nausea, vomiting, abdominal pain, and growth failure in children; weight loss in adults; megadoses: hair loss, bone swelling and tenderness, joint pain, hepatomegaly, splenomegaly, headache	Whole milk, whole milk products, eggs, green leafy vegetables, yellow fruits and vegetables
D (cholecalciferol, engosterol)	Absorption and use of calcium in bone and tooth development	Rickets and delayed dentition in children, osteomalacia in adults	Megadoses: loss of appetite, vomiting, diarrhea, fatigue, growth failure, drowsiness, kidney stones	Sunlight, fortified milk, fortified margarines, fish liver oils
E (tocopherol)	Protection of vitamins A and C and polyunsaturated fatty acids from oxidation, synthesis of heme	Increased hemolysis of red blood cells and macrocytic anemia in premature infants	Interference with the use of vitamins A and K, prolonged prothrombin time, intestinal irritability, fatigue, dizziness	Vegetable oils, green leafy vegetables, milk, eggs, meats, cereals
K	Essential to prothrombin formation and blood clotting	Hemorrhagic disease of the newborn, prolonged clotting time in adults	Hyperbilirubinemia in infants, vomiting in adults	Green leafy vegetables, synthesis in gastrointestinal tract

Mineral	Functions	Deficiency Symptoms	Toxicity Symptoms	Food Sources
Macrominerals				
Calcium	Formation of teeth and bones, contraction of muscle fibers, transmission of nerve impulses, activation of enzymes, permeability of cell membranes, coagulation of blood, cardiac function	Tingling of fingers and around the mouth, muscle cramps, carpopedal spasm, tetany, convulsions, stunted growth, bone loss in adults, pathological fractures	Relaxed skeletal muscles, deep bone pain, kidney stones, cardiac irregularities	Milk, milk products, leafy green vegetables, fish
Magnesium	Supports function of B vitamins; use of calcium, potassium, and protein; maintenance of electrical activity in nerves and muscles	Neuromuscular irritability, disorientation, confusion, leg cramps, hallucinations, tachycardia, convulsions, hypertension	Lethargy, respiratory dysfunction, coma, death	Whole grains, fish, nuts, legumes, green vegetables
Phosphorus	Formation of bone and teeth, activation of B vitamins, transfer of energy within cells, promotion of normal muscle and nerve activity, metabolism of carbohydrates, regulation of acid-base balance, transmission of hereditary traits	Hemolytic anemia, defective white blood cell function, delayed clotting, bone pain, pathological fractures	Erosion of jaw, calcium loss	Pork, beef, dried peas and beans, dairy products
Microminerals				
Copper	Essential to hemoglobin formation, cofactor in synthesis of phospholipids, formation and activity of some enzymes, synthesis of prostaglandin	Abnormal blood cell development in infants, bone demineralization	Headache, dizziness, heartburn, weakness, nausea, vomiting, diarrhea, Wilson's disease	Liver, kidney, shellfish, nuts, raisins
Fluoride	Formation of teeth, prevention of dental caries	Poor dental health	Mottling, pitting, and discoloration of tooth enamel	Fluoridated water, seafood, toothpaste, mouthwash gels
Iodine	Basic component of thyroid hormones	Cretinism in infants, simple goiter in children and adults, depressed thyroid function	Toxic goiter	Iodized salt, seafood, food additives, dough oxidizers, dairy disinfectants, coloring agents
Iron	Essential to the formation of hemoglobin, synthesis of vitamins, purines, and antibodies	Anemia, fatigue, weakness, lethargy, lowered immunity	Hemosiderosis, acute iron poisoning from accidental ingestion in infants and children: cramps, abdominal pain, nausea, vomiting, black stools, cirrhosis	Liver, lean meats, whole grains, enriched breads and cereals, green vegetables
Zinc	Connective tissue integrity, involvement in immune response, formation of enzymes	Impaired wound healing, decreased sensations of taste and smell, delayed growth	Anemia, fever, nausea, vomiting, muscle pain, weakness, decreases calcium absorption	Oysters, liver, meats, poultry, legumes, nuts

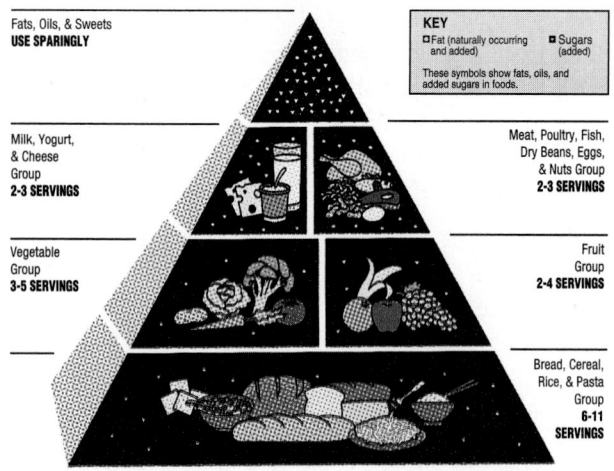

Figure 34-1. Food guide pyramid. (From U.S. Department of Agriculture: *USDA's food guide pyramid,* USDA Human Nutrition Information Pub No. 249, Washington, DC, 1992, U.S. Government Printing Office.)

Box 34-1
Dietary Guidelines for Americans

Eat a variety of foods.
Balance the food you eat with physical activity.
Maintain or improve your weight.
Choose a diet with plenty of grain products, vegetables, and fruits.
Choose a diet low in fat, saturated fat, and cholesterol.
Choose a diet moderate in sugars.
Choose a diet moderate in salt and sodium.
If you drink alcoholic beverages, do so in moderation.

Data from USDA and USDHHS: *Nutrition and your health: dietary guidelines for Americans,* USDA/DHHS Home and Garden Bull No. 232, Washington, DC, 1990, U.S. Government Printing Office; U.S. Department of Agriculture, Agricultural Research Service, Dietary Guidelines Committee, 1995: *Report of the dietary guidelines advisory committee on the dietary guidelines for Americans,* Springfield, Va, 1995, National Technical Information Service.

the day's selections from the grain group (6 to 11 servings), the vegetable group (3 to 5 servings), and the fruit group (2 to 4 servings). Selections should include 2 to 3 servings per day from the milk group and from the meat group (which includes dry beans and nuts). The fats, oils, and sweets group is to be used sparingly.

Recommended daily allowances. The Committee on Dietary Allowances of the Food and Nutrition Board of the National Academy of Sciences has published a list of **recommended daily allowances (RDAs)** since 1943. The RDAs are the level of intake of essential nutrients considered, in the judgment of the committee and on the basis of scientific knowledge, to be adequate to meet the nutritional needs of healthy people.

Other dietary guidelines. In 1990 the U.S. Department of Health and Human Services (USDHHS) and the Public Health Service (PHS), after a 4-year consensus process, published *Healthy People 2000: National Health Promotion and Disease Prevention Objectives.* The report defines national goals or objectives to be met in this decade to increase the proportion of Americans who live long, healthy lives. Nutrition-related goals for the year 2000 include increasing intake of fruits, vegetables, and grain products and reducing sodium consumption. In 1995 a special focus was placed on consistency with the food guide pyramid and the nutrition facts label (USDA, 1995) (Box 34-1).

NURSING KNOWLEDGE BASE

Nutrition themes are present in most of our society. We celebrate holidays and events with food, bring food to those who are grieving, use food for medicinal purposes,

recognize cultural food differences, incorporate food into family traditions and rituals, associate appearance with eating behaviors, abstain from or recognize foods in religious beliefs and practices, and associate certain foods and dining practices with socioeconomic status.

For most people, food has sociological and psychological significance. The significance varies with each individual. In attempting to impact eating patterns, the nurse must understand how the client's values, beliefs, and attitudes about food affect food purchase, preparation, and intake. Nurses must also be cognizant of their own values, beliefs, and attitudes about food.

Nutritional requirements vary according to client's developmental needs. Individuals differ in caloric and nutrient requirements by stage of development, activity levels, conditions such as pregnancy and lactation, and the presence of disease. A summary of factors that influence dietary patterns and needs is presented in Box 34-2.

Alternative Food Patterns

Many people follow special patterns of food intake based on religion, cultural background, ethics, health beliefs, personal preference, or concern for the efficient use of land to produce food. Such special diets are not necessarily more or less nutritional than diets based on the food guide pyramid or other nutritional guidelines because good nutrition depends on a balanced intake of all required nutrients. A common dietary pattern is the vegetarian diet, which is the consumption of a diet consisting predominantly of plant foods. Vegetarians may be ovolactovegetarians, who avoid meat, fish, and poultry but eat eggs and milk, or lactovegetarians, who drink milk but avoid eggs. Vegans eat only foods of plant origin and should supplement their diets with vitamin B_{12} and carefully choose foods to ensure that their diets are adequate in Vitamin D and calcium and varied enough to ensure ingestion of essential amino acids.

Developmental Needs

Nutrient and kilocalorie needs are unique to the individual's developmental stage. Maturation of the gas-trointestinal system, periods of rapid growth and development, alterations in digestion and absorption, activity level, and pregnancy affect nutrient and energy needs.

⋯CRITICAL THINKING IN CLIENT CARE

Synthesis

Critical thinking enables the nurse to synthesize information gathered from knowledge, experience, attitudes, and standards. The end result of critical thinking will be the nurse's judgments and subsequent interventions. Examples of how the nurse might use critical thinking to develop the nutritional plan of care are presented in each section.

Knowledge. Application of knowledge from nutritional principles and the basic and social sciences forms the nurse's knowledge base related to nutritional care. The interplay of information derived from interviewing and observing the client and the responses obtained during nursing interventions will guide the nurse toward application of knowledge. For example, the client may report a dietary pattern of avoiding a food such as cabbage. This pattern could arise from physiological discomfort (gas-forming food), psychological issues (forced to eat cabbage as a child), sociological reasons (associated with lower socioeconomic class), ethnicity (not readily available in the country of origin), teaching- or learning-related reasons (never taught how to prepare cabbage), or mythology (a food that contains harmful chemicals). The nurse will need to explore the client's dietary patterns with acceptance and open-mindedness to discover the unique reasons for the client's eating behaviors.

Experience. People's dietary patterns are based on multiple factors. Just as the nurse's clients are influenced by multiple factors to develop dietary practices, so too has the nurse been influenced. Individuals who have nutritional or health problems often need to change their long-standing dietary practices to enhance health. In assisting a client to change dietary patterns, nurses may draw on examples from their own experience. Perhaps the nurse has attempted to change a dietary practice or has a family member who requires a special diet. Previous experiences with therapeutic diets or behavioral changes may assist the nurse to identify nursing interventions that will be successful for the client.

Attitudes. Open-mindedness is a critical thinking skill that is beneficial during nutritional assessment and counseling. Nurses encounter clients whose dietary practices are dramatically different from their own yet provide a nutritionally balanced diet. In addition, nurses encounter clients whose dietary patterns are not healthful but whose beliefs and values about food are dramatically different from those of the nurse. To develop effective interventions for these clients, the nurse may recommend practices that would be personally difficult but may be quite effective for the client. Open-mindedness requires nurses to step out of their own realm of experience to attempt to understand the collective experience of the client.

Standards. When assisting clients to adjust to changes in nutritional patterns, the nurse incorporates standards from the recommended daily allowances (RDAs), American Heart Association, or other professional organizations. Because food holds strong symbolic values and is closely associated with nurturing, ethical issues in health care have arisen around the withdrawal or withholding of specialized feeding (Burck, 1996). As part of an advanced directive, clients are asked if they wish to have nutrition or hydration as a means of life support. Advanced directives make the client's wishes known and have become a standard area of assessment for clients in the hospital and in the home care setting.

NURSING PROCESS AND NUTRITION

▪ Assessment

Nutritional screening is part of the nurse's initial assessment of the client. If the client is found to be at risk for nutritional problems (Box 34-3), the nurse may conduct a more in-depth nutritional assessment with the assistance of a nutritionist. The intent of the nutritional assessment, as outlined by the American Society

for Parenteral and Enteral Nutrition (ASPEN, 1995), is as follows:

1. Establish baseline subjective and objective nutrition parameters.
2. Identify specific nutritional deficits.
3. Determine nutritional risk factors.
4. Establish nutritional needs.
5. Identify medical and psychosocial factors that may influence the prescription and administration of nutritional support.

The nutritional assessment consists of nursing health assessment and physical examination, observation, medical record review (if available), and laboratory data.

In addition to the general nursing health assessment and physical examination (Chapter 24), the nurse can obtain a more specific diet history (Box 34-4) to assess the client's actual or potential nutritional needs. The diet history focuses on habitual intake of food and liquids and information about preferences, allergies, and digestive problems. When interviewing the client about dietary practices, the nurse should ask open-ended questions that encourage the client to elaborate. For example, the nurse may ask a client who reports that she avoids dairy products, "What caused you to avoid dairy products?" The client's answer to this question may lead to physiological, psychological, sociological, religious,

---

Box 34-3

Nutritionally-at-Risk Adult Clients

Involuntary loss or gain of ≥10% of usual body
  weight within 6 months
                    or
≥5% of usual body weight in 1 month
20% over or under ideal body weight
Presence of chronic disease or increased metabolic
  requirements
Altered diets or diet schedules
Inadequate nutrient intake for >7 days

Data from ASPEN Board of Directors: Standards for nutrition support: hospitalized patients, *NCP* 10:208, 1995.

Box 34-4

Information in a Diet History

Name
Age
Present weight
Usual weight
Recent weight changes
Height
Number of meals and snacks a day
Person who prepares meals
Food preferences, allergies, and aversions
Foods that cause indigestion, diarrhea, or gas
Chewing or swallowing difficulties
Use of dentures
Usual bowel movements
Dietary problems
Use of medications
  Prescribed
  Over-the-counter
  Recreational
History of diseases, surgeries, or weight problems
Level of physical activity
Appetite changes
Type, time, and size of usual meals
Personal crises

cultural, or food preference factors that can be further explored.

Clients at risk for nutritional problems.

A client with a condition that interferes with the ability to ingest, digest, or absorb adequate nutrients should be considered at risk. Congenital anomalies and surgical revisions of the gastrointestinal tract interfere with normal function. Clients fed only by intravenous infusion of 5% to 10% dextrose are at risk for nutritional deficiencies. Older adults, infants, or the malnourished are at greatest risk. Common conditions and pathophysiology that place clients at nutritional risk are summarized in Box 34-3.

Client expectations.

Clients who require assistance with nutritional problems can have a variety of expectations. Clients with impairments in upper arm mobility may expect assistance with a range of activities, such as preparing the meal, setting up the meal tray or plate, or being fed. Another client may expect information on the availability and use of assistive devices, used to increase a client's independence with meals. Clients who have impaired vision need to be taught how to feed themselves. It is also important for the nurse to learn what the client expects in terms of resuming a normal diet or learning to adjust to a therapeutic diet.

Identifying the client's expectations for nutritional management is just as important as assessing for nutritional alterations. The client and family need to be able to continue nutritional interventions in the home or community-based environment.

Diet history.

A detailed record can be kept of food intake over 3 days that represents the client's typical pattern, including a weekend day. This record allows the nurse to calculate the client's nutritional intake and to compare it with the RDAs. The nurse should carefully instruct the client in how to record the specific type of food and the amount ingested. If a scale is not available for determining the weight of solid foods, the nurse should assist the client to accurately estimate portion size. The nurse also gathers information about the client's activity level to determine energy need. The energy need is compared to actual caloric intake. The nurse attempts to elicit clients' expectations about their nutritional health and encourages clients to participate in developing the nutritional plan of care.

Examination.

The nurse examines the client for signs of actual or potential nutritional alterations (Table 34-2). The skin and hair are primary areas that reflect nutrient deficiencies. The nurse should be alert for rashes, dry scaly skin, poor skin turgor, skin lesions, hair loss, easily pluckable hair, hair without luster, and an unhealthy scalp.

Anthropometry.

Anthropometry is a system of measurement of the size and makeup of the body at specific body sites. Anthropometric measurements that aid in identifying nutritional problems may include measurement of wrist circumference, mid–upper-arm circumference, and triceps skinfold.

Unless contraindicated, height and weight measurements should be obtained during admission to the hospital or on entry into an outpatient care setting. If possible, the client should be weighed at about the same time each day, on the same scale, and with the same amount of clothing. Height and weight can be compared with the usual measurements and with standards for normal height-weight relationships.

Laboratory values.

Laboratory values useful in nutritional assessment include complete blood count, albumin, transferrin, prealbumin, electrolytes, blood urea nitrogen, creatinine, glucose, and triglycerides. A low red blood cell count and depressed hemoglobin value may indicate anemia. The hemoglobin, hematocrit, and blood urea nitrogen values also help to reflect the state of hydration. Decreased serum levels of albumin and transferrin identify protein-calorie malnutrition. Reduced levels of albumin and transferrin in adults can indicate a visceral protein deficit.

Urinary nitrogen excretion is obtained by collecting a 24-hour urine sample for nitrogen. Nitrogen excretion measured in the urine plus a factor added for nitrogen losses from the gastrointestinal and pulmonary systems can be used to estimate the amount of protein needed to achieve a positive **nitrogen balance.**

• •

Successful critical thinking requires a synthesis of knowledge, experience, information gathered from clients, and critical thinking attitudes and standards. Clinical judgments require the nurse to anticipate what information is needed, analyze the data, and then make decisions regarding client care. The client expects competent and informed care. Shawneen incorporates previous knowledge and experience in providing care for Ms. Garcia.

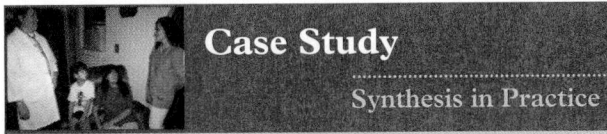

Case Study
Synthesis in Practice

As Shawneen prepares to assess Ms. Garcia, she recalls information about nutrition and its affect on wound healing. She will focus assessment on Ms. Garcia's weight, recent weight loss, elimination patterns, and discomfort. Shawneen knows that it is important to assess for fluid balance as well.

Shawneen knows that consulting with a dietitian to further assess Ms. Garcia's nutritional status and

Continued

TABLE 34-2
Clinical Signs of Nutritional Status

Body Area	Signs of Good Nutrition	Signs of Poor Nutrition
General appearance	Alert, responsive	Listless, apathetic, cachectic
Weight	Normal for height, age, body build	Overweight or underweight (special concern for underweight)
Posture	Erect, arms and legs straight	Sagging shoulders, sunken chest, humped back
Muscles	Well-developed, firm, good tone, some fat under skin	Flaccid, poor tone, undeveloped, tender, "wasted" appearance, cannot walk properly
Nervous control	Good attention span, not irritable or restless, normal reflexes, psychologic stability	Inattentive, irritable, confused, burning and tingling of hands and feet (paresthesia), loss of position and vibratory sense, weakness and tenderness of muscles (may result in inability to walk), decrease or loss of ankle and knee reflexes
Gastrointestinal function	Good appetite and digestion, normal regular elimination, no palpable (perceptible to touch) organs or masses	Anorexia, indigestion, constipation or diarrhea, liver or spleen enlargement
Cardiovascular function	Normal heart rate and rhythm, no murmurs, normal blood pressure for age	Rapid heart rate (above 100 beats/minute, tachycardia), enlarged heart, abnormal rhythm, elevated blood pressure
General vitality	Endurance, energetic, sleeps well, vigorous	Easily fatigued, no energy, falls asleep easily, looks tired, apathetic
Hair	Shiny, lustrous, firm, not easily plucked, healthy scalp	Stringy, dull, brittle, dry, thin and sparse, depigmented, can be easily plucked
Skin (general)	Smooth, slightly moist, good color	Rough, dry, scaly, pale, pigmented, irritated, bruises, petechiae
Face and neck	Skin color uniform, smooth, healthy appearance, not swollen	Greasy, discolored, scaly, swollen, skin dark over cheeks and under eyes, lumpiness or flakiness of skin around nose and mouth
Lips	Smooth, good color, moist, not chapped or swollen	Dry, scaly, swollen, redness and swelling (cheilosis), or angular lesions at corners of the mouth or fissures or scars (stomatitis)
Mouth, oral membranes	Reddish pink mucous membranes in oral cavity	Swollen, boggy oral mucous membranes
Gums	Good pink color, healthy, red, no swelling or bleeding	Spongy, bleed easily, marginal redness, inflamed, gums receding
Tongue	Good pink color or deep reddish in appearance, not swollen or smooth, surface papillae present, no lesions	Swelling, scarlet and raw, magenta color, beefy (glossitis), hyperemic and hypertrophic papillae, atrophic papillae
Teeth	No cavities, no pain, bright, straight, no crowding, well-shaped jaw, clean, no discoloration	Unfilled caries, absent teeth, worn surfaces mottled (fluorosis), malpositioned
Eyes	Bright, clear, shiny, no sores at corner of eyelids, membranes moist and healthy pink color, no prominent blood vessels or mound of tissue or sclera, no fatigue circles beneath	Eye membranes pale (pale conjunctivae), redness of membrane (conjunctival injection), dryness of infection, Bitot's spots, redness and fissuring of eyelid corners (angular palpebritis), dryness of eye membrane (conjunctival xerosis), dull appearance of cornea (corneal xerosis), soft cornea (keratomalacia)
Neck (glands)	No enlargement	Thyroid enlarged
Nails	Firm, pink	Spoon-shaped (koilonychia), brittle, ridged
Legs and feet	No tenderness, weakness, or swelling; good color	Edema, tender calf, tingling, weakness
Skeleton	No malformations	Bowlegs, knock-knees, chest deformity at diaphragm, beaded ribs, prominent scapulas

Data from Williams SR: Nutritional guidance in prenatal care. In Worthington-Roberts BS and others: *Nutrition in pregnancy and lactation*, St. Louis, 1985, Mosby.

Continued from p. 953

assist with nutritional interventions will be beneficial. The dietitian will use data from Shawneen's initial nursing assessment and assist Shawneen to collect further nutritional-related information.

Experience has taught Shawneen that economic and cultural preferences will also affect how food is chosen, purchased, and prepared. She will need to be creative in teaching Ms. Garcia to adjust to a new diet.

Nursing Diagnosis

Following assessment, the nurse clusters relevant defining characteristics to determine whether actual or potential nutritional problems exist (see nursing diagnoses box). An alteration can occur when a nutrient is not ingested in sufficient quantity, is poorly digested, or is incompletely absorbed or when total daily caloric needs are deficient or excessive.

Nurses should be cautious in their diagnosis of nutritional excess. The obese client can actually have nutrient deficiencies and may require supplements or specialized nutritional support during episodes of acute illness. The assessment should elicit dietary patterns that have contributed to the obesity and will require careful scrutiny for adequacy of all food groups. Patterns such as inadequate fruit and vegetable intake can be present. The nursing diagnosis should be as precise as possible. Related factors must be accurate so that the nurse can select appropriate interventions. For example, a diagnosis of *fluid volume deficit related to vomiting* will require different interventions from *fluid volume deficit related to anorexia*.

NURSING DIAGNOSES FOR CLIENTS WITH NUTRITIONAL ALTERATIONS

Aspiration, risk for
Body image disturbance
Diarrhea
Fatigue
Fluid volume deficit
Nutrition, altered: less than body requirements
Nutrition, altered: more than body requirements
Nutrition, altered: risk for more than body requirements
Self-care deficit, feeding
Tissue perfusion, altered: gastrointestinal

Planning

The identification of clients at risk for nutritional problems should result in a care plan that will prevent or minimize nutritional problems. The client and family need to collaborate in the care plan. Since food purchase and preparation may involve family members, the nutritional plan of care might not succeed without their involvement and understanding of nutritional goals (Box 34-5). Other professionals who may assist the nurse to develop the nutritional plan of care include the nutritionist, nutritional support clinical nurse specialist, pharmacists, and physicians.

A list of diets commonly used for hospitalized clients is provided in Table 34-3. In the hospital or home care setting, some clients with physiological conditions that cause more severe cases of malnutrition may require enteral tube feeding or parenteral nutrition to meet fluid, electrolyte, and nutritional needs.

Enteral tube feeding can be administered into the stomach or intestines via a tube inserted through the nose (nasogastric or nasointestinal), an endoscopically placed tube (PEG), a surgically inserted tube (gastrostomy or jejunostomy), or a tube inserted using radiography (RAG).

In **parenteral nutrition (PN),** a solution consisting of glucose, amino acids, lipids, minerals, electrolytes, trace elements, and vitamins is given through an indwelling peripheral or central venous catheter.

A general goal for nutritional alterations is to improve the client's nutritional status. If the nutritional diagnosis is *altered nutrition, less than body requirements,* the outcome will be for the client to gain weight or to ingest

BOX 34-5
Client Teaching For Altered Nutrition

- Instruct client about how to accurately record a 3-day diet record: explain the importance of recording all foods, brands of specific processed foods, time of day that foods were ingested, food preparation method (e.g., fried, boiled), and the amount of food ingested. Assist client to accurately estimate portion sizes.
- Review finds of 3-day diet record with client to identify patterns and areas for enhancing nutritional intake.
- Involve client in planning alternative dietary patterns and food choices.
- Help client to assess and incorporate meal preferences and budgetary limitations into diet.
- Teach client how to incorporate menu planning in weekly shopping lists. Involve family members if client does not do the shopping.
- Teach creativity within the guidelines of prescribed diets (using seasonings, different preparation techniques, incorporating ethnic foods as able).

TABLE 34-3
Hospital Therapeutic Diets

Diet	Description
Regular	Is ordered for patients requiring no specific modifications. Generally, allows patients to select their food choices based on normal nutritional requirements for patient's age, sex, and activity level.
Clear-liquid	Allows clear, bland liquids, such as chicken broth, gelatin, and apple juice, that leave little residue and are easily absorbed. Is commonly ordered for short-term use (24 to 48 hours) after episodes of vomiting, diarrhea, or surgery.
Full-liquid	Consists of foods that liquefy at room or body temperature and are easily digested and absorbed. Includes foods allowed on clear-liquid diet plus milk and some milk-containing foods, such as creamed, strained soups. Is commonly ordered before or after surgery for patients who are acutely ill from infection or for patients who cannot chew or tolerate solid foods.
Pureed	Includes easily swallowed foods that do not require chewing. May be ordered for patients with head and neck abnormalities or who have had surgery.
Mechanical or dental-soft	Consists of foods that do not need chewing, such as chopped or ground foods. Avoids tough meats, nuts, bacon, and fruits with tough skins or membranes. May be ordered for patients who have chewing problems caused by lack of teeth or sore gums.
Soft	Includes foods that are low in fiber, easily digested, easy to chew, and simply cooked. Does not permit fatty, rich, and fried foods. Is sometimes referred to as *low-fiber diet.*
High-fiber	Includes sufficient amounts of indigestible carbohydrate to relieve constipation, increase gastrointestinal motility, and increase stool weight. May be ordered for patients with diverticulosis or irritable bowel syndrome.
Sodium-restricted	Allows low levels of sodium and may include a 4-g (no added salt), 2-g (moderate), 1-g (strict), or 500-mg (very strict) diet. May be ordered for patients with congestive heart failure, renal failure, cirrhosis, or hypertension.
Prudent (low-cholesterol)	Is ordered to reduce high serum lipid levels. Reduces cholesterol intake to 300 mg daily and fat intake to 30% to 35% by eliminating or reducing fatty foods.
Diabetic	Is ordered as essential treatment for patients with diabetes mellitus. Provides patients with exchange list of foods recommended by American Diabetes Association, which allows patient to select set amount of food from basic food groups.

From Cole G: *Foundations of nursing,* ed 2, St. Louis, 1995, Mosby.

adequate nutrients in a certain category. The nutritional goal for **obesity** will involve interventions to assist the client to safely achieve weight reduction. Specific, individualized goals will be determined by assessing the behaviors that have led to the nutritional alteration and teaching new behaviors that will enable the client to achieve an adequate nutritional status.

Weight gain or loss of $\frac{1}{2}$ to 1 lb/wk is a realistic level for clients who are underweight or overweight. Clients often have unrealistic expectations about nutritional repletion or dieting in reference to weight gain or loss. The nurse assists clients to understand this concept by asking them to reflect on their rate of weight gain or loss. Changes in weight usually have occurred over months or years unless an acute illness has occurred. When clients do not see rapid achievement of weight goals, they may become discouraged. The nurse assists clients to view nutritional repletion or weight loss as a long-term rather than a short-term goal. Short-term goals may involve achieving calorie or nutrient targets on a daily or weekly basis.

▪ Implementation

Health promotion. Nurses can play a major role in promoting healthy dietary practices. Using tools such as the food guide pyramid, the nurse can assist clients with food choices, menu planning, and dietary patterns. The nurse can also educate clients about food labels and their meaning. An area of particular importance is education about product claims that can be misleading; "reduced fat" foods may still have significant amounts

CASE STUDY NURSING CARE PLAN

Nutrition

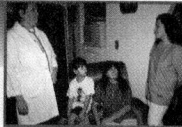

Assessment

Ms. Garcia's diet history reveals that she is **below her estimated caloric requirement by 800 kcal/day** and **protein intake is 10 g below her required need.** She tries to eat three meals a day but cannot because of **the feeling of fullness. Milk and milk products cause abdominal cramping.** Ms. Garcia enjoys foods from her **Hispanic heritage, such as beans, corn, tortillas, tomatoes, soups, yellow vegetables, and rice.** On physical examination Ms. Garcia does exhibit some signs of nutritional deficiency. Her **albumin, transferrin, and prealbumin levels are slightly below normal, she is 20% below ideal body weight, and she complains of feeling weak.** She would like to gain weight and has requested assistance in identifying appropriate foods.

Nursing Diagnosis

Altered nutrition: less than body requirements related to inadequate intake of calories and proteins.

Planning

Goal

Client will achieve ideal body weight (8-12 weeks).

Expected Outcomes

Client will gain $\frac{1}{2}$ to 1 lb/wk.

Client will not report cramping or diarrhea.

Client's albumin, transferrin, and prealbumin will begin to return to normal.

Implementation

Steps

1. Use lactose-free oral supplements, $1\frac{1}{2}$ kcal/ml, between or with meals. Choose flavors that appeal. Take three cans per day.

2. Ms. Garcia will provide her roommate with a list of "favorite foods" so that these can be included in the food purchases.

3. Ms. Garcia will eat six small meals instead of trying to eat three large ones.

4. Ms. Garcia will weigh herself 3 times per week. She will notify Shawneen if her weight does not increase after two weight recordings or if she loses weight.

Rationale

The formula is lactose free and is available in multiple flavors. The oral supplement will also provide supplemental protein and vitamins. Three cans per day will provide 750 to 1125 extra calories.

Appealing foods are more likely to be ingested.

Spreading intake out over the day may assist client to ingest more.

Periodic weight recordings will assist client to see progress and will alert family if the interventions are not working.

Evaluation

Weigh Ms. Garcia on a weekly basis.

Review Ms. Garcia's use of the oral supplements and frequent meals.

Measure laboratory values at 6-week intervals.

Defining characteristics are shown in bold type.

of fat, "lite" foods may still contain considerable calories, and "low cholesterol" may not mean low fat.

An increasing percentage of Americans are overweight, and many people who attempt to lose weight are unsuccessful or gain weight again after completing a diet. Fad diets abound, and bookstores are filled with best-selling diet books. Some weight reduction methods lack scientific validity, and some are dangerous. The nurse has an opportunity to educate the client about lifelong eating habits.

Acute care. Ill or debilitated clients usually have poor appetites. The nurse is involved in the daily care of the client and monitors the client's nutritional status. Nurses can help by displaying interest in the client's intake, by understanding the influences that reduce appetite, and by planning interventions to increase intake.

One of the most disruptive influences on intake in acute care is diagnostic testing. Some blood and radiographic studies require the client to fast. Therefore the client's food is usually withheld until the client returns from the test or the testing is completed. Mealtimes are disrupted, and sometimes clients are too fatigued to eat or experience discomfort related to the test. Stress also influences intake. Clients who are worried about their families, finances, employment, or illness may not be able to eat or eat enough to compensate for the effect of stress on metabolism.

Medications also affect intake and in some cases the utilization of nutrients. Medications can affect the sensations of taste or smell, and as a result food is not appetizing. Medications can also cause nausea or vomiting; the client is anorexic as a result of the nausea, or the nutrients are lost. In addition, medications such as insulin and thyroid hormones can affect metabolism. Nurses keep these factors in mind when designing measures to promote nutrition.

Food presentation is a factor in appetite. Hot foods that are cold or cold foods that are warm are not appetizing. Overcooked or undercooked foods are unappealing. A meal tray precariously balanced on a crowded, soiled overbed table does not enhance the meal. Clients who are bothered by food odors may need the nurse to remove the cover from hot food before the tray is brought into the room. Attention to details in food presentation, meal scheduling, and the client's difficulties with food may enhance a client's intake. A nurse can help to stimulate a client's appetite through environmental adaptations, consultation with a diet therapist, special diets and food preferences, and client and family counseling.

Providing a comfortable environment. Nurses should provide an environment conducive to eating. The client's room should be free of reminders of treatments and odors. Mouth care should be provided when necessary to remove unpleasant tastes. The client should be positioned comfortably so that the meal can be more enjoyable. If a client refuses a portion of the meal, every effort should be made to replace it with a suitable alternative.

Assisting clients with feeding. Nurses can improve client feeding by carefully protecting clients' dignity and actively involving them. Any material used to protect clothing should be referred to as a napkin, not a bib. The nurse should allow the client time to empty the mouth after every spoonful, attempting to match the speed of feeding to the client's readiness and asking frequently about the rate. The nurse should also allow clients to direct the order in which they wish to eat food items. Mealtime is a good time for nurses to instruct clients about the selection of appropriate foods and the importance of a balanced diet.

Disabled clients. Clients with disabilities that interfere with independent food intake should be allowed to do as much as possible for themselves. When necessary, the nurse should prepare the tray, cutting food into bite-sized pieces, buttering bread, and pouring liquids. Special eating utensils should be used. Some disabled clients may become tired from their efforts to feed themselves. The nurse should determine whether this client is still hungry and needs assistance. The results of self-feeding should be evaluated on the basis of food intake. Success should be recognized and commended. The nurse who finds a way to aid the disabled client to eat more independently should share this information by incorporating it into the care plan.

Providing enteral tube feedings. Enteral nutrition (EN) refers to nutrients given via the intestinal tract. This includes blended foods, modular formulas, and chemically defined formulas. Oral diets provide a safe and economical method of meeting nutritional needs and are the preferred method if the client's gastrointestinal tract is functional. For clients with eating difficulties, EN may be indicated.

Studies have demonstrated a beneficial effect of enteral feedings over parenteral routes. Postoperative feeding by the enteral route can help reduce sepsis and enhance the immune response, and EN is also preferable to total parenteral nutrition (TPN) in protecting intestinal mucosal cells (Kudsk and others, 1992).

Tube feedings. When the client cannot ingest, chew, or swallow food but can digest and absorb nutrients, a feeding tube is placed nasally into the stomach or small intestine or surgically into the stomach or jejunum (Skills 34-1 and 34-2). Intestinal tubes may reduce the risk of aspiration of formula into the lungs during enteral feeding and may be necessary when gastric emptying is delayed.

Traditional bedside methods of testing placement of small-bore feeding tubes, such as injection of air, are ineffective. The most reliable method is the radiographic verification, but it is costly. Therefore other methods to test placement such as pH testing are used.

Text continued on p. 962

Inserting a Small-Bore Nasoenteric Tube for Enteral Feedings

Delegation Considerations

This skill requires problem solving and knowledge application unique to a professional nuse. For this reason, delegation of this skill to unlicensed assistive personnel is inappropriate.

Equipment

- Nasogastric or nasointestinal tube (8 to 12 Fr) with guidewire or stylet
- 60-ml or larger Luer-Lok or catheter-tip syringe
- Hypoallergenic tape and tincture of benzoin
- pH indicator strip
- Glass of water and straw
- Emesis basin
- Safety pin
- Rubber band
- Towel
- Facial tissues
- Clean gloves
- Suction equipment in case of aspiration
- Penlight to check placement in nasopharynx
- Tongue blade

STEPS	RATIONALE
1. Assess client for the need for enteral tube feeding: NPO or insufficient intake for more than 5 days, functional gastrointestinal (GI) tract, unable to ingest sufficient nutrients.	Identifying clients who need tube feedings before they become nutritionally depleted may help to prevent complications related to malnutrition.
2. Assess client for appropriate route of administration:	Evaluates nares for patency.
a. Close each nostril alternately, and ask client to breathe.	Nares may be obstructed. Assessment determines which naris to use.
b. Assess for gag reflex.	Identifies ability to swallow and risk of aspiration.
c. Inspect nares for any irritation or obstruction.	
d. Review client's medical history for nasal problems and risk of aspiration.	Nurse may seek physician's order to change route of nutritional support or to place tube past the stomach into the intestine with increased risk of aspiration.
3. Review physician's order for type of tube and enteral feeding schedule.	Procedure and tube feedings require a physician's order.
4. Wash hands.	Reduces transfer of microorganisms.
5. Explain procedure to client.	Reduces anxiety and helps client to assist in insertion.
6. Stand on same side of bed as naris for insertion, and assist client to high Fowler's position unless contraindicated. Place pillow behind head and shoulders.	Allows easier manipulation of tube. Fowler's position reduces risk of aspiration and promotes effective swallowing.
7. Place bath towel over chest. Keep facial tissues within reach.	Prevents soiling of gown. Insertion of tube may produce tearing.
8. Determine length of tube to be inserted and mark with tape:	Length approximates distance from nose to stomach in 98% of clients. For duodenal or jejunal placement, an additional 20 to 30 cm is required.
a. Traditional method: measure distance from tip of nose to earlobe to xiphoid process of sternum (see illustration, p. 960).	
9. Prepare nasogastric or nasointestinal tube for intubation:	
a. Plastic tubes should not be iced.	Tubes will become stiff and inflexible, causing trauma to mucous membranes.
b. Inject 10 ml of water from 30-ml or larger Luer-Lok or catheter-tip syringe into the tube.	Aids in guidewire or stylet insertion.
c. Make certain that guidewire is securely positioned against weighted tip and that both Luer-Lok connections are snugly fitted together.	Promotes smooth passage of tube into GI tract. Improperly positioned stylet can induce serious trauma.

Continued

········ **Skill 34-1—cont'd**
Inserting a Small-Bore Nasoenteric
Tube for Enteral Feedings

STEPS	RATIONALE
10. Cut tape 10 cm (4 inches) long.	
11. Put on clean gloves.	Reduces transmission of microorganisms.
12. Dip tube with surface lubricant into glass of water.	Activates lubricant to facilitate passage of tube into naris to GI tract.
13. Insert tube through nostril to back of throat (posterior nasopharynx). Aim back and down toward ear.	Natural contours facilitate passage of tube into GI tract and reduces gagging by client.
14. Flex client's head toward chest after tube has passed through nasopharynx.	Closes off glottis and reduces risk of tube entering trachea.

CRITICAL DECISION POINT

Encourage client to swallow by giving small sips of water or ice chips when possible. Advance tube as client swallows. Rotate tube 180 degrees while inserting.

15. Emphasize need to mouth breathe and swallow during the procedure.	Helps facilitate passage of tube and alleviates client's fears during the procedure.
16. Advance tube each time client swallows until desired length has been passed. Do not force tube. If resistance is met or client starts to cough, choke, or become cyanotic, stop advancing the tube and pull tube back.	Reduces discomfort and trauma to client.
17. Check for position of tube in back of throat with penlight and tongue blade.	Tube may be coiled, kinked, or entering trachea.
18. Perform measures to verify placement of tube:	
a. Inject 30 ml of air into the tube, and aspirate GI contents with a syringe.	Obtain GI contents to determine proper placement (Metheny and others, 1993).
b. Measure pH of aspirated GI contents (see illustration) (Metheny and others, 1993) (see box).	Gastric sites usually have a pH range of 1 to 4. Intestinal sites have a pH of greater than 6.

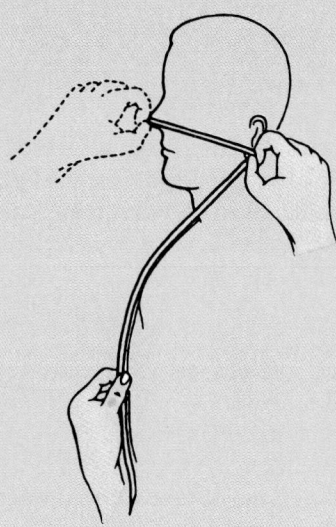

Step 8a

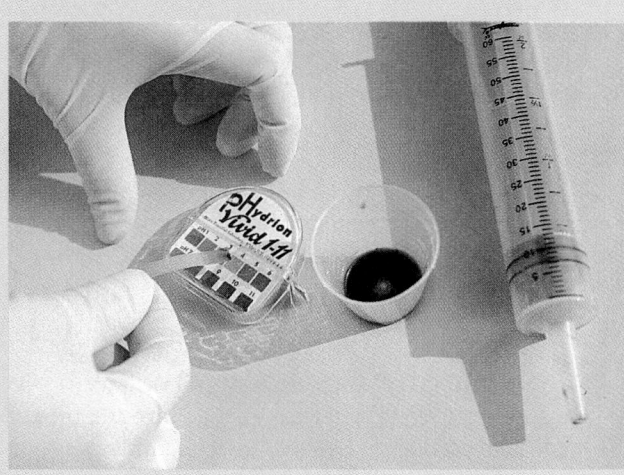

Step 18b

STEPS   **RATIONALE**

Obtaining GI Fluid for pH Measurement, Large- and Small-Bore Feeding Tubes: Bolus and Continuous Feeding

- Flush tube with 30 ml of warm water after medications or completed feedings.
- Wait 1 hour after feeding or medications.
- Plan pH testing at times when continuous feedings may be withheld, such as for chest physical therapy or avoidance of medication interaction.

- Flush tube with 30 ml of air.
- Aspirate GI contents.
- If unable to aspirate GI contents, reposition client to allow tip of tube to rest in GI fluid. Flush tube with 30 ml of air, and attempt to aspirate.

Modified from Metheny N and others: Effectiveness of pH measurements in predicting feeding tube placement, *Nurs Res* 38(5):285, 1989.

CRITICAL DECISION POINT

Auscultation is no longer considered a reliable method for verification of tube placement because a tube inadvertently placed in the lungs, pharynx, or esophagus can transmit a sound similar to that of air entering the stomach (Metheny and others, 1990a; Chang and others, 1982).

19. Apply tincture of benzoin or other skin adhesive on tip of client's nose and tube. Allow to dry.

20. Remove gloves, and secure tube with tape, avoiding pressure on naris.
    a. Split one end of tape lengthwise 5 cm (2 inches). Place the intact end of tape over bridge of client's nose. Wrap each of the 5-cm strips around tube as it exits nose (see illustrations).

Helps tape adhere better. Protects skin.

A properly secured tube allows the client more mobility and prevents trauma to nasal mucosa.
Securing tape to nares prevents tissue necrosis.

Continued

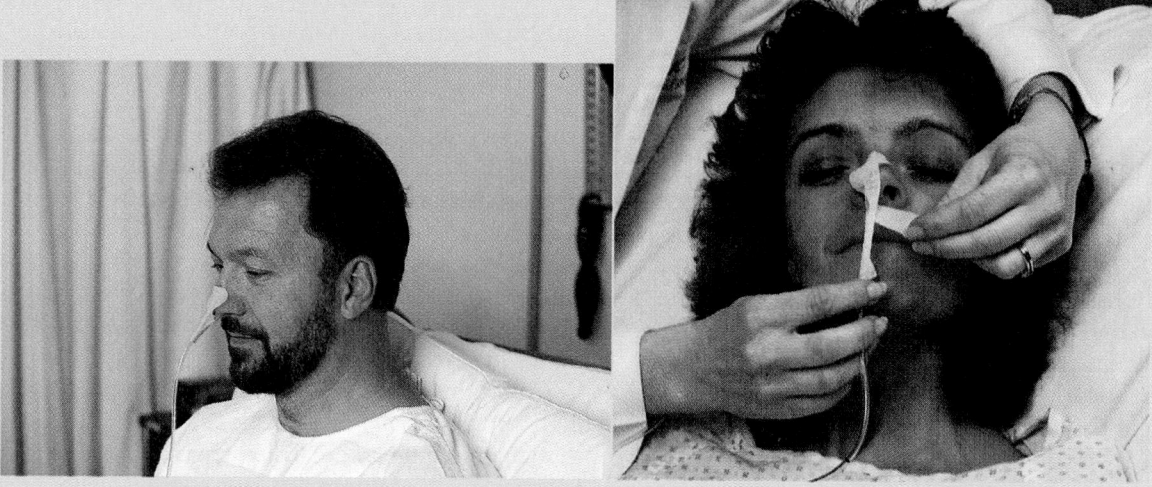

Step 20a

Skill 34-1—cont'd
Inserting a Small-Bore Nasoenteric Tube for Enteral Feedings

STEPS	RATIONALE
b. Fasten end of nasogastric tube to client's gown by looping rubber band around tube in slip knot. Pin rubber band to gown.	Reduces traction on the naris if tube moves.
21. For intestinal placement, position client on right side when possible until radiological confirmation of correct placement has been verified. Otherwise, assist client to a comfortable position.	Promotes passage of the tube into the small intestine (duodenum or jejunum).

CRITICAL DECISION POINT
Leave guidewire or stylet in place until correct position is ensured by x-ray film. Never attempt to reinsert partially or fully removed guidewire or stylet while feeding tube is in place.

22. Obtain x-ray film of abdomen.	Placement of tube is verified by x-ray examination (Metheny, 1988).
23. Apply gloves, and administer oral hygiene (see Chapter 29). Cleanse tubing at nostril.	Promotes client comfort and integrity of oral mucous membranes.
24. Remove gloves, dispose of equipment, and wash hands.	Reduces transmission of microorganisms.
25. Inspect naris and oropharynx for any irritation after insertion.	If insertion was difficult, irritation of naris or oropharynx may have occurred.
26. Ask if client feels comfortable.	Evaluates client's level of comfort.
27. Observe client for any difficulty breathing or gagging.	Malposition of the tube may cause these symptoms.

Recording and Reporting
- Record and report type and size of tube placed, location of distal tip of tube, client's tolerance of procedure, pH value, and confirmation of tube position by x-ray.

Home Care Considerations
- Placement may be verified on the basis of pH recordings. A small amount of water may be instilled via the feeding tube while the client is carefully observed for coughing or gagging.
- The client and care provider should be instructed to report pH values that fall outside of an established range and to report any difficulties that occur during the feeding.

Some clients will have a more permanent device, such as a gastrostomy tube or a jejunostomy tube, placed for EN (Skill 34-3). A **gastrostomy feeding tube** is a long, hollow, flexible tube inserted into the stomach during surgery or by endoscopic placement (Figure 34-2, p. 968). A **jejunostomy tube** is a large-bore tube surgically inserted into the jejunum.

The formula used for tube feedings must be nutritionally adequate, tolerated by the client, and delivered at a rate and volume that is appropriate for the area of the gastrointestinal tract where the feeding occurs. A wide variety of commercial products are available for tube feedings. Most are ready to use and provide standard nutritional content in approximately 1500 ml. The formulas differ in osmolarity, digestibility, caloric density, viscosity, nutrient content, and electrolyte content. Generally physicians choose EN formulas on the basis of the type and amount of protein, the caloric density, and the presence of any disease state that requires a specific formula (e.g., hepatic or renal disease, diabetes, critically ill or burned clients).

Clients may be maintained indefinitely on tube feedings, which can provide all the essential nutrients. Although cramping and diarrhea are associated with tube feedings, these symptoms usually subside when the flow rate of the solution is reduced or a formula containing

Text continued on p. 968

Administering Enteral Feedings
via Nasoenteric Tubes

Delegation Considerations

Administration of enteral tube feeding via nasogastric tube is a procedure that can be delegated to unlicensed assistive personnel.

- The professional nurse should verify tube placement before the feeding and establish patency of the tube by flushing it with water.
- The nurse should also ensure that the client is sitting upright in a chair or in bed and instruct the assistive personnel to infuse the feeding slowly.
- Unlicensed personnel should be instructed to report any difficulty infusing the feeding or any discomfort voiced by the client.

Equipment

- Disposable feeding bag and tubing or ready-to-hang system
- 30-ml or larger Luer-Lok or catheter-tip syringe
- Stethoscope
- pH indicator strip
- Infusion pump (required for intestinal feedings): use pump designed for tube feedings
- Prescribed enteral feedings
- Gloves
- Equipment to obtain blood glucose by fingerstick

STEPS	RATIONALE
1. Assess client's need for enteral tube feedings: impaired swallowing, decreased level of consciousness, head or neck surgery, facial trauma, surgeries of upper alimentary canal.	Identify clients who need tube feedings before they become nutritionally depleted.
2. Auscultate for bowel sounds before feeding.	Absent bowel sounds may indicate decreased ability of GI tract to digest or absorb nutrients.
3. Obtain baseline weight and laboratory values. Assess client for fluid volume excess or deficit, electrolyte abnormalities, and metabolic abnormalities such as hyperglycemia.	Enteral feedings are to restore or maintain a client's nutritional status. Provides objective data to measure effectiveness of feedings.
4. Verify physician's order for formula, rate, route, and frequency. Laboratory data and bedside assessments, such as finger-stick blood glucose measurement, are also ordered by the physician.	Tube feedings, laboratory tests, and bedside tests must be ordered by physician.
5. Explain procedure to client.	Well-informed client is more cooperative and at ease.
6. Wash hands.	Reduces transmission of microorganisms.
7. Prepare feeding container to administer formula:	
a. Have tube feeding at room temperature.	Cold formula may cause gastric cramping and discomfort because the liquid is not warmed by mouth and esophagus.
b. Connect tubing to container as needed or prepare ready-to-hang container.	Tubing must be free of contamination to prevent bacterial growth.
c. Shake formula container well, and fill container and tubing with formula (see illustration, p. 964).	Filling the tubing with formula prevents excess air from entering GI tract.
8. Place client in high Fowler's position, or elevate head of bed 30 degrees.	Elevated head helps prevent aspiration.
9. Determine tube placement:	
a. Aspirate gastric contents to check for gastric residual (see illustration, p. 964). Return aspirated contents to stomach unless the volume exceeds 150 ml.	Presence of gastric secretions indicates that the distal end of the tube is in the stomach. Residual volume indicates if gastric emptying is delayed. Delayed gastric emptying may be reflected by 150 ml or more remaining in the client's stomach.
b. Measure pH of aspirated GI contents.	Gastric contents usually have a pH range of 1 to 4. Intestinal sites have a pH of greater than 6 (Metheny and others, 1993).

Continued

Administering Enteral Feedings via Nasoenteric Tubes

STEPS	RATIONALE

CRITICAL DECISION POINT

Auscultation is no longer considered a reliable method for verification of placement of tube because air in tube inadvertently placed in lungs, pharynx, or esophagus can transmit sound similar to that of air entering stomach (Metheny and others, 1990a, 1990b; Chang and others, 1982).

10. Initiate feeding:
    a. Bolus or intermittent feeding:
       (1) Pinch proximal end of the feeding tube.   Prevents air from entering client's stomach.
       (2) Remove plunger from syringe and attach barrel of syringe to end of tube.
       (3) Fill syringe with measured amount of formula. Release tube and hold syringe high enough to allow it to empty gradually by gravity, refill; repeat until prescribed amount has been delivered to the client.
       (4) If feeding bag is used, hang feeding bag on an IV pole. Fill bag with prescribed amount of formula, and allow bag to empty gradually over at least 30 minutes.   Gradual emptying of tube feeding by gravity from syringe or feeding bag reduces risk of abdominal discomfort, vomiting, or diarrhea induced by bolus or too-rapid infusion of tube feedings.
    b. Continuous-drip method (see illustration):
       (1) Hang feeding bag and tubing on IV pole.   Continuous feeding method is designed to deliver prescribed hourly rate of feeding. This method reduces risk of abdominal discomfort. Clients who receive continuous drip feedings should have residuals checked every 4 hours and tube placement verified.

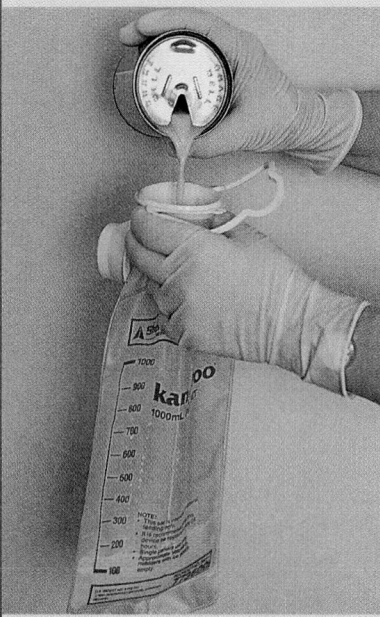

Step 7c

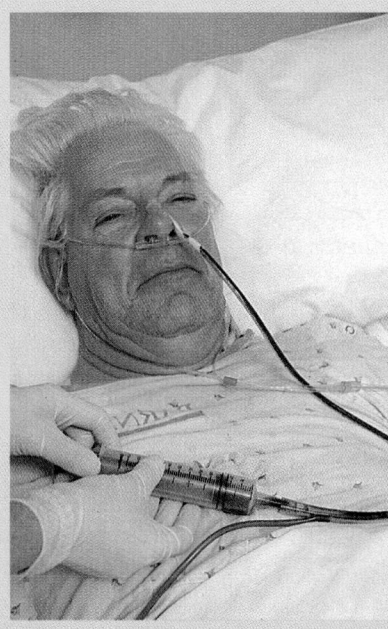

Step 9a

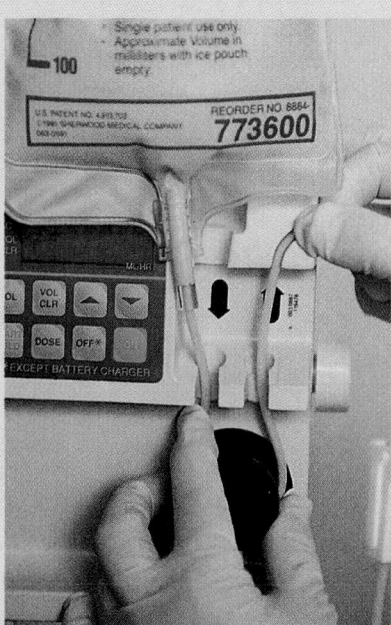

Step 10b

STEPS	RATIONALE
(2) Connect distal end of tubing to the proximal end of the feeding tube.	
(3) Connect tubing through infusion pump and set rate.	
11. Advance tube feeding gradually (see box).	Tube feedings should be advanced gradually to prevent diarrhea and gastric intolerance to formula.

Advancing the Rate of Tube Feeding

Intermittent

1. Start formula at full strength for isotonic formulas (300 to 400 mOsm) or diluted to isotonicity.
2. Infuse formula over at least 20 to 30 minutes via syringe or feeding container.
3. Begin feedings with no more than 150 to 250 ml at one time. Increase by 50 ml per feeding per day to achieve needed volume and calories in six to eight feedings.

Continuous

1. Start formula at full strength for isotonic formulas (300 to 400 mOsm) or diluted to isotonicity.
2. Begin infusion rate at 30 to 50 ml/hr.
3. Advance rate by 10 to 20 ml/hr per day to target rate if tolerated.

STEPS	RATIONALE
12. When tubing feedings are not being administered, cap or clamp the proximal end of the feeding tube.	Prevents air from entering stomach between feedings.
13. Administer water via feeding tube as ordered with diluted formula.	Provides client with source of water to help maintain fluid and electrolyte balance.
14. Rinse bag and tubing with warm water whenever feedings are interrupted.	Rinsing bag and tubing with warm water clears old tube feedings and reduces bacterial growth.
15. Measure amount of aspirate (residual) every 4 hours.	Evaluates tolerance of tube feeding.
16. Monitor finger-stick blood glucose every 6 hours until maximum administration rate is reached and maintained for 24 hours.	Alerts nurse to client's tolerance of glucose.
17. Monitor intake and output every 24 hours.	Intake and output are indications of fluid balance or fluid volume excess or deficit.
18. Weigh client daily until maximum administration rate is reached and maintained for 24 hours; then weigh client 3 times per week.	Weight gain is indicator of improved nutritional status; however, sudden gain of more than 2 lb in 24 hours usually indicates fluid retention.
19. Observe return of normal laboratory values.	Improving laboratory values (i.e., albumin, transferrin, and prealbumin) indicate an improved nutritional status.

Recording and Reporting

- Record amount and type of feeding, client's response to tube feeding, patency of tube, and any side effects. Report client's tolerance and adverse effects.

Home Care Considerations

- Ask client or care provider about any symptoms or discomfort during enteral feedings. Reinforce instruction to contact nurse if symptoms or discomfort occurs.

Delegation Considerations

Administration of enteral tube feeding via a gastrostomy or jejunostomy tube or a jejunal tube is a procedure that can be delegated to unlicensed assistive personnel.

- The professional nurse should verify tube placement before the feeding and establish patency of the tube by flushing it with water.
- The nurse should also ensure that the client is sitting upright in a chair or in bed and instruct the assistive personnel to infuse the feeding slowly.
- Unlicensed personnel should be instructed to report any difficulty infusing the feeding or any discomfort voiced by the client.

Equipment

- Disposable feeding container or ready-to-hang bag
- 30-ml or larger Luer-Lok or catheter-tip syringe
- Formula
- Infusion pump: use pump designed for tube feedings
- pH indicator strips
- Stethoscope
- Gloves
- Equipment to obtain blood glucose by fingerstick

STEPS	RATIONALE
1. Assess client's need for enteral tube feedings (see Skill 34-2): impaired swallowing, decreased level of consciousness, surgeries of upper alimentary tract, need for long-term enteral nutrition.	Identifies clients who need tube feedings before they become nutritionally depleted. Enteral feeding preserves the function and mass of the gut, promotes wound healing, diminishes hypermetabolism in burn injuries, and may decrease infection in critically ill clients (Zaloga, 1994).
2. Auscultate for bowel sounds before feeding. Consult physician if bowel sounds are absent.	Absence of bowel sounds may indicate decreased or absent peristalsis and increased risk of aspiration or abdominal distention.
3. Obtain baseline weight and laboratory values.	Enteral feedings are to restore or maintain nutritional status. Provides objective data to measure effectiveness of feedings.
4. Verify physician's order for formula, rate, route, and frequency.	Tube feedings must be ordered by physician.
5. Explain procedure to client.	Well-informed client is more cooperative and feels more at ease.
6. Prepare feeding container to administer formula: a. Have tube feeding at room temperature.	Cold formula may cause gastric cramping and discomfort because the liquid is not warmed by mouth and esophagus.
b. Connect tubing to container as needed, or prepare ready-to-hang bag.	Tubing must be free of contamination to prevent bacterial growth.
c. Fill container and tubing with formula.	Placement of formula through tubing prevents excess air from entering gastrointestinal tract.
7. Elevate head of bed 30 to 45 degrees.	Elevating client's head helps prevent chance of aspiration.
8. Verify tube placement: **A. Gastrostomy tube:** (1) Aspirate gastric secretions, and check pH. Return aspirated contents unless the volume exceeds 150 ml. (2) Measure gastric residual.	Gastric pH should range from 1 to 4.
B. Jejunostomy tube: (1) Aspirate gastric secretions, and check pH.	Presence of intestinal fluid indicates that end of tube is in small intestine (i.e., duodenum or jejunum). Generally the intestinal residual is very small (30 ml or less). If fluid tests acidic on pH test or volume of residual is large (more than 30 ml), displacement of the tube into the stomach may have occurred.

STEPS	RATIONALE
9. Flush with 30 ml of water.	
10. Initiate feedings:	Usually gastrostomy and jejunostomy feedings are given continuously to ensure proper absorption.
A. Syringe feedings:	However, initial feedings may be given by bolus to
(1) Pinch proximal end of gastrostomy tube.	assess client's tolerance to formula. See Skill 34-2
(2) Remove plunger and attach barrel of syringe to end of tube, then fill syringe with formula.	for guidelines to advance enteral feedings.
(3) Allow syringe to empty gradually. Refill until prescribed amount has been delivered to client.	
B. Continuous drip method:	
(1) Fill feeding container with enough formula for 4 hours of feeding.	
(2) Hang container on IV pole, and clear tubing of air.	
(3) Thread tubing on pump according to manufacturer's directions.	
(4) Connect tubing to end of feeding tube.	
(5) Begin infusion at prescribed rate.	
11. Assess skin around tube exit site. The skin around the tube should be cleansed daily with warm water and mild soap. Dressings around the exit site are not recommended.	Report any drainage, redness, swelling, or displacement of the tube to the physician.
12. Dispose of supplies, and wash hands.	Prevents transmission of microorganisms.
13. Measure the amount of aspirate (residual) every 4 hours.	Evaluates tolerance of tube feeding.
14. Monitor finger-stick blood glucose every 6 hours until maximum administration rate is reached and maintained for 24 hours.	Alerts nurse to client's tolerance of glucose.
15. Monitor intake and output every 24 hours.	Intake and output are indications of fluid balance or fluid volume excess.
16. Weigh client daily until maximum administration rate is reached and maintained for 24 hours; then weigh client 3 times per week.	Weight gain is indicator of improved nutritional status; however, a sudden gain of more than 2 lb in 24 hours usually indicates fluid retention.
17. Observe return of normal laboratory values.	Improving laboratory values (albumin, transferrin, prealbumin) indicate an improved nutritional status.
18. Inspect site for signs of pressure.	Enteral tubes can cause uncomfortable pressure areas on client's nares.

Recording and Reporting

- Record amount and type of feeding and client's response to tube feeding, patency of tube, and any side effects.
- Report to oncoming nursing staff: type of feeding, status of feeding tube, client's tolerance, adverse effects.

Home Care Considerations

- Ask client or care provider about any symptoms or discomfort during enteral feeding. Reinforce instruction to contact nurse if symptoms or discomfort occur.
- Instruct client or care provider in how to care for gastrostomy or jejunostomy tube site and symptoms to report.

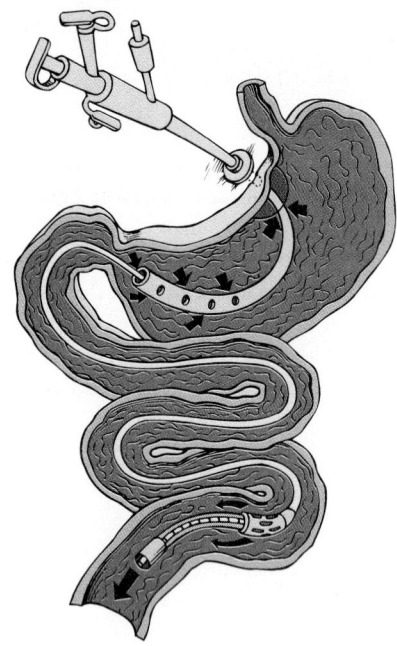

Figure 34-2. Endoscopic insertion of jejunostomy tube.

fiber is used. Stools will be softer when the client receives a liquid formula; however, more than three liquid stools per day or large watery stools would constitute diarrhea while on tube feeding.

Providing PN. PN is a complex form of therapy that provides daily nutritional requirements by the intravenous route. PN is chosen when the gastrointestinal system cannot be used or when the gastrointestinal tract cannot tolerate EN in an amount to provide adequate nutrients and calories. The complications of PN can be reduced by meticulous care of the venous access device, a gradual increase in the administration rate of PN over several hours or days, careful assessment of laboratory parameters for metabolic or electrolyte abnormalities, and assessment of fluid balance.

PN solutions that contain 10% dextrose or greater are hyperosmolar (i.e., highly concentrated) and as a result are infused through central venous lines. The solution itself is tailored to the client's specific nutritional needs but typically contains all major nutrients.

Lipid emulsions are often added to the dextrose and amino acid mixture to form what is called a total nutrient admixture. Some clients, however, may receive lipid emulsions separate from the other solution. Lipid emulsions provide fat as a nutrient to prevent essential fatty acid deficiencies and supplemental calories.

Some clients cannot receive lipids at all during an acute illness or can only receive a limited amount because they have elevated triglyceride levels. The lipids can be administered via a peripheral line or through the central line. Because lipid emulsions provide a more conducive environment for bacterial and fungal growth, the container should not be administered beyond

12 hours from the time it was started (Crocker and others, 1984). The lipid emulsion or total nutrient admixture should not be used if it appears to have an oil or cream layer or if it has separated.

The recommended initial infusion rate for a fat emulsion infused separately from PN is 1 ml/min. Reactions to this emulsion can include dyspnea, cyanosis, allergy, nausea, vomiting, headache, chest pain, back pain, pressure over the eyes, or dizziness. If symptoms appear, the nurse should stop the infusion and notify the physician. If the client tolerates the fat emulsion, the rate can gradually be increased as ordered by the physician.

Initiating PN. PN with concentrated dextrose requires an intravascular catheter threaded into a central vein such as the jugular or subclavian. Nurses assist in the procedure for inserting a central venous catheter, and specially trained nurses insert peripherally inserted central catheters. A chest x-ray film is used to confirm the location of the central venous catheter. Clients may have a long-term central venous access device, such as a tunneled catheter or an implanted port.

Before beginning an infusion, the nurse verifies the solution prepared by the pharmacy with the physician's order. An infusion pump is used to administer PN. The solution is typically started at a low rate, such as 40 to 60 ml/hr, and gradually advanced over several hours or a day to the goal rate. Most hospitalized clients receive the PN over 24 hours. When clients receive PN at home, they usually give the solution over 12 to 16 hours.

Caring for the client receiving PN. Nursing care for the client receiving PN is based on four major nursing goals: (1) preventing infection; (2) maintaining the PN system; (3) preventing metabolic, electrolyte, or fluid balance complications; and (4) assessing the client's readiness for EN or discharge planning for home PN.

Primary methods to prevent infection include asepsis during central venous catheter insertion, meticulous care of the central venous catheter, use of an in-line filter on the IV tubing, and care to avoid contaminating tubing connections. If possible, the PN line should be reserved for PN only because multiple uses can increase the risk of bacterial contamination. No other solutions, except lipid emulsions, should be infused through the PN line.

Clients receiving PN have laboratory measurements monitored regularly. Capillary blood glucose testing or urine glucose testing occurs during the initiation of PN to assess for metabolic tolerance (Table 34-4). The nurse should be alert for changes in vital signs or fluid balance, **hyperglycemia** or glucosuria, or any unusual symptoms and report them to the physician. An increased temperature may be an early sign of infection and should be reported to the physician.

Restorative care

Diet therapy in disease management. Dietary intake patterns that result in good nutrition must often

TABLE 34-4

Interventions for Preventing Metabolic Complications of TPN

Intervention	Rationale
Weigh client daily.	Documents that the client is maintaining or gaining weight and has a proper fluid balance.
Record intake and output.	Provides database for ongoing fluid balance assessment.
If client is allowed oral intake, maintain calorie count of foods eaten.	Provides data needed to calculate TPN caloric requirement.
Test urine or blood every 4 to 6 hours to measure glucose.	Determines whether client is excreting glucose in the urine and an insulin supplement may be needed.
Obtain blood samples for measurement of iron, transferrin, and white blood cells.	Evaluates cellular nutritional status.
Continually assess fluid and electrolyte status.	Provides for early detection of circulatory overload or dehydration.
Maintain infusion rate as ordered. Do not speed or slow infusion unless instructed by the physician or a severe complication occurs.	Prevents hyperglycemia, osmotic diuresis, hypoglycemia, and fluid overload.

be modified for clients with specific diseases. Diet modifications are necessary to correspond with the body's ability to metabolize certain nutrients, to correct nutritional deficiencies, and to eliminate harmful foods from the diet. In all cases, the nurse works with the physician and diet therapist when planning and implementing modified diets.

Home care. Specialized nutrition therapies, such as EN and PN, may need to be continued beyond the hospital setting to the home care setting. In home care, nurses are often the only care provider who sees the client on a regular basis. Home care nurses teach clients or care givers how to administer PN or EN, assess the client for tolerance of the nutrition prescription, and evaluate the client's progress toward nutritional goals.

📭 Evaluation

Client care. The value of the nurse's activities in meeting the client's nutritional needs is measured by an ongoing evaluation. Adequate time should be allowed to test a nursing approach to a problem.

Evaluation of clinical progress can include objective data, such as weight gain or improved laboratory parameters, or subjective data, such as the client's reporting improvement in food choices or in self-reporting improved intake. When clinical progress does not occur, the nurse determines whether the interventions were not effective, were not done or accepted by the client, were not realistic or appropriate, or were affected by unanticipated or unidentified factors.

If outcomes are not met, the nurse reassesses the client to determine if important data were missed. Clients may need reeducation if essential skills or knowledge has been forgotten or misunderstood. The

nurse should also attempt to validate that the client is in agreement with the goals and is willing and able to follow the nutritional plan of care.

Client expectations. Clients do not always enter the health care system as willing participants. Often, entry into the health care system is associated with some type of loss. Clients may agree to interventions because they feel powerless. Because nutritional interventions so often depend on the client's willingness and ability to change behavior patterns and learn new patterns, the interventions may not be successful if the client is not fully committed to the new behaviors. The client may also find it difficult to change behavior and may be less motivated with the passage of time.

Most clients respond well to the opportunity to make informed choices. The nurse should explain the health reasons for the behavioral change and give the client options for how the change may be achieved. Education may need to be provided in several brief sessions to maximize retention of information (see Box 34-5).

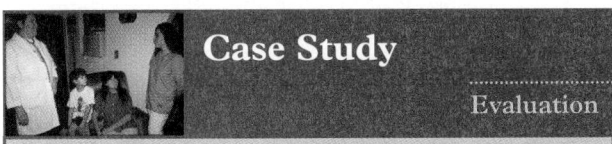

Case Study
Evaluation

Shawneen sees Ms. Garcia on a home visit 3 weeks after her teaching session. She contacted Ms. Garcia and asked her to keep a 3-day food intake record before the visit. During the home visit, Shawneen notes that Ms. Garcia has gained 4 lb. Her 3-day food intake indicates use of the nutritional supplement and improved protein intake. Ms. Garcia tells

Continued

Shawneen that her appetite has improved and that she is usually able to finish a small meal. She still is bothered by milk products if she has more than 8 oz at a time.

Shawneen advises Ms. Garcia to continue the current plan of care and emphasizes that her slow, consistent weight gain is appropriate. She consults with Ms. Garcia about a visit in another 3 weeks and asks Ms. Garcia to call her if Ms. Garcia's symptoms return or her weight gain stops.

Documentation Note
Ms. Garcia visited in her home. Weight gain of 4 lb in 3 weeks. Counseled to continue with new eating habits and to continue to avoid more than 8 oz of milk products. Rescheduled visit in 3 weeks.

Key Terms

absorption
amino acids
anabolism
anthropometry
carbohydrates
catabolism
digestion
enteral nutrition (EN)
gastrostomy feeding
  tube
gluconeogenesis
glucose
glycogen
glycogenesis
glycogenolysis
hyperglycemia
jejunostomy tube

lipid
lipogenesis
metabolism
minerals
nitrogen balance
nutrients
obesity
parenteral nutrition
  (PN)
polyunsaturated fatty
  acid
proteins
recommended daily
  allowances (RDAs)
saturated fatty acid
unsaturated fatty acid
vitamins

■ Key Concepts

Nutrients needed by the body to carry out vital functions are water, carbohydrates, proteins, lipids, vitamins, and minerals.

Body weight is maintained when food intake equals energy requirements.

Proteins are essential for growth, maintenance, and repair.

Essential amino acids and the essential fatty acids must be supplied by dietary intake because the body is unable to synthesize them from other ingested substances.

Digestion is the mechanical and chemical process by which food is broken down into its simplest form for absorption. Digestion and absorption occur mainly in the small intestine.

Recommended daily allowances, another basis for diet selection, were formulated for population groups, not individuals.

Guidelines for dietary change advocate reduced intake of fat, saturated fat, salt, refined sugar, and cholesterol and increased intake of complex carbohydrates and fiber.

Age affects the requirements for essential nutrients. Periods of rapid growth increase the need for protein, vitamins, and minerals.

Because improper nutrition can affect all body systems, nutritional assessment includes a review of the total physical assessment.

Proper feeding techniques can protect the dependent client from loss of dignity and self-esteem.

Special hospital diets alter the composition, texture, digestibility, and residue of foods to suit the client's particular needs.

Tube feedings can be used for clients who are unable to ingest food but are able to digest and absorb foods.

Enteral nutrition may protect intestinal structure and function and enhance immunity.

Total parenteral nutrition supplies essential nutrients in appropriate amounts to support life through the introduction of a concentrated nutrient solution into a large central vein or the right atrium of the heart.

Evaluation of the outcomes of nursing intervention in the area of nutritional support is essential to revise, update, or continue nursing activities.

Critical Thinking Activities

1. You are completing a nursing history for a 24-year-old client who has diabetes. The client is slightly underweight and tells you that he is vegetarian and eats no animal products including fish, eggs, and milk. What information about his diet would you need to determine whether it is adequate in calories and protein? What laboratory tests would reflect protein status? What physical assessment findings might suggest inadequate protein intake?

2. Mrs. Evans is 75 years of age and lives alone. She receives a social security check, which pays for her rent and utilities with about $100 a month left over. She has arthritis and has difficulty ambulating more than about 50 feet at a time. How might Mrs. Evans' situation affect her nutritional status?

3. While giving Mr. Orzo a bath, you notice that his PN solution looks odd. There is a small yellow layer at the top of the bag. Mr. Orzo is receiving lipids, amino acids, and dextrose in a single solution. What could this layer indicate, and what should you do first?

References

ASPEN Board of Directors: Standards for nutrition support: hospitalized patients, *NCP* 10:208, 1995.

American Heart Association Science Advisory and Coordinating Committee: Dietary guidelines for Americans. *Circulation* 94:1795, 1996a.

American Heart Association Science Advisory and Coordination Committee: Fish consumption, fish oil, lipids, and coronary heart disease, *Circulation* 94:2347, 1996b.

Burck R: Feeding, withdrawing, and withholding: ethical perspectives, *NCP* 11:243, 1996.

Chang J and others: Inadvertent endobronchial intubation with nasogastric tube, *Arch Otolaryngol* 108:528, 1982.

Cole G: Foundation of nursing, ed 2, St. Louis, 1996, Mosby.

Committee on Dietary Allowances, Food and Nutrition Board, National Academy of Sciences, National Research Council: *Estimated safe and adequate daily dietary intakes,* Washington, DC, 1989.

Crocker K and others: Microbial growth comparisons of five commercial parenteral lipid emulsions, *JPEN J Parenter Enteral Nutr* 8:391, 1984.

Grant JA, Kennedy-Caldwell C: *Nutritional support in nursing,* New York, 1988, Grune & Stratton.

Kudsk KA and others: Enteral vs parenteral feeding: effects on septic morbidity following blunt and penetrating abdominal trauma, *Ann Surg* 215:503, 1992.

Metheny N: Measures to test placement of nasogastric and enteral feeding tubes: a review, *Nurs Res* 37(6):323, 1988.

Metheny N and others: Effectiveness of pH measurements in predicting feeding tube placement, *Nurs Res* 38(5):285, 1989.

Metheny N and others: Detection of inadvertent respiratory placement of small-bore feeding tubes: a report of 10 cases, *Heart Lung* 19(6):631, 1990a.

Metheny N and others: Effectiveness of the auscultatory method in predicting feeding tube location, *Nurs Res* 39(5):262, 1990b.

Metheny N and others: Effectiveness of pH measurements in predicting feeding tube placement: an update, *Nurs Res* 42:324, 1993.

U.S. Department of Agriculture: *USDA's food guide pyramid,* USDA Human Nutrition Information Service Pub No. 249, Washington, DC, 1992, U.S. Government Printing Office.

U.S. Department of Agriculture: *Report of the dietary guidelines advisory committee on the dietary guidelines for Americans,* Springfield, Va, 1995, National Technical Information Service.

U.S. Department of Agriculture and U.S. Department of Health and Human Services: *Nutrition and your health: dietary guidelines for Americans,* USDA/USHHS Home and Garden Bull No. 232, Washington, DC, 1990, U.S. Government Printing Office.

Whitney EN and others: *Understanding normal and clinical nutrition.* St. Paul, 1991, West.

Williams SR: Nutritional guidance in prenatal care. In Worthington-Roberts BS and others: *Nutrition in pregnancy and lactation,* St. Louis, 1985, Mosby.

Zaloga G: Timing and route of nutritional support. In Zaloga G, editor: *Nutrition and critical care,* St. Louis, 1994, Mosby.

35

Urinary Elimination

OBJECTIVES

Mastery of content in this chapter will enable the student to:

- Define the key terms listed.
- Explain the function of each organ in the urinary system.
- Describe the process of urination.
- Identify factors that commonly influence urination.
- Compare and contrast common alterations in urination.
- Obtain a nursing history from a client with an alteration in urination.
- Describe physical assessment techniques used to assess urinary elimination.
- Describe characteristics of normal and abnormal urine.
- Describe nursing implications of common diagnostic tests of the urinary system.
- Identify nursing diagnoses relevant to the urinary system.
- Discuss nursing measures to assist the client with urinary elimination.
- Describe nursing measures to control incontinence.
- Discuss nursing measures to reduce urinary tract infections.
- Apply or insert an external or indwelling catheter.

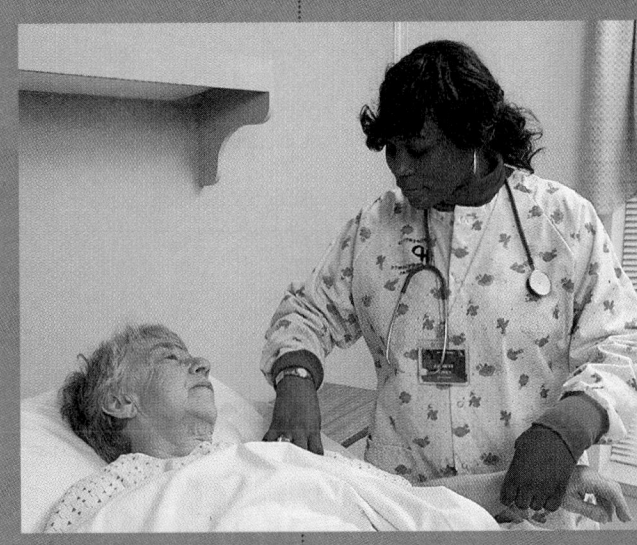

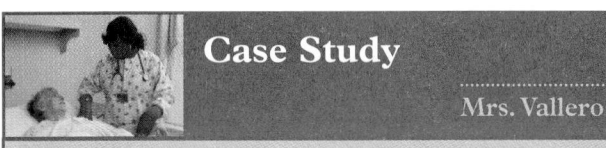

Case Study

....
Mrs. Vallero

Mrs. Vallero is an 85-year-old woman who is lying in her hospital bed. It is 9:30 AM. She has been in the hospital for 2 days for acute pneumonia. At the 7 AM report you learned her catheter and IV were removed yesterday at 4 PM after she was taking fluids without nausea and her output totaled 2000 ml. Her total input yesterday was 3400 ml: 2000 ml IV and 1400 ml oral. At 12 AM Mrs. Vallero was found to be incontinent of a small amount of urine and was complaining of lower abdominal pain. She was catheterized at 1 AM for 1100 ml of pale, clear yellow urine after the physician was called. The physician ordered "single catheterization now and times one." Today at 8 AM, she ate one slice of toast, half of her scrambled eggs, and 400 ml of fluids. She says she has not gone to the bathroom this morning but has "dribbled some."

Mrs. Stone is a 43-year-old divorced mother of two daughters. Mrs. Stone is a sophomore nursing student in her sixth week of clinical rotation at a community hospital. She was in the hospital as a client at the birth of her daughters. At the birth of her second child a year ago she had a cesarean section and had a urinary catheter in for 2 days.

Normal elimination of urinary wastes is a function most people take for granted. When the urinary system fails to function properly, virtually all body systems can be affected. Clients with alterations in urinary elimination may also be affected by resulting body image problems. The nurse provides understanding and sensitivity to the client's needs. With any client who has urinary elimination problems, the nurse must identify problems and acceptable solutions.

SCIENTIFIC KNOWLEDGE BASE

Knowledge from the biological and social sciences helps the nurse to identify actual and potential urinary tract problems that the client might encounter. A thorough understanding of related information helps the nurse to provide complete and competent care to the client with altered elimination.

Urinary Elimination

Urinary elimination depends on the function of the kidneys, ureters, bladder, and urethra. The kidneys remove wastes from the blood and urine. The ureters transport urine from the kidneys to the bladder. The bladder holds urine until the urge to urinate develops. The urine leaves the body through the urethra. All these organs must be intact and functional for the successful removal of urinary wastes.

Kidneys. The kidneys are reddish-brown, bean-shaped organs that lie on either side of the vertebral column behind the abdominal peritoneum and against the deep muscles of the back. The kidneys are level with the twelfth thoracic and third lumbar vertebrae. Normally the left kidney is 1.5 to 2 cm ($^6/_{10}$ to $^8/_{10}$ inch) higher than the right because of the anatomical position of the liver.

The functional units called **nephrons** remove waste products from the blood and regulate water and electrolyte concentrations in body fluids. The kidneys can efficiently filter the blood of waste products in part because of their high blood flow, which represents approximately 25% of the cardiac output. Blood reaches nephrons through the renal artery, which branches into smaller arteries, eventually becoming the afferent arterioles that directly supply the nephrons. A cluster of capillaries forms the **glomerulus,** which is the initial site of urine formation.

The glomerular capillaries filter water and glucose, amino acids, urea, uric acid, creatine, and major electrolytes. Normally, 180 L of blood filters through the nephrons each day. Protein does not normally filter through the glomerulus. Therefore, protein in the urine, **proteinuria,** is a sign of glomerular injury.

However, not all glomerular filtrate is excreted as urine. Approximately 99% is reabsorbed into the plasma. When the filtrate leaves the glomerulus, it passes through a system of tubules in which water and glucose, amino acids, uric acid, sodium, potassium, and bicarbonate ions are selectively reabsorbed into plasma. Hydrogen and potassium ions and ammonia are secreted into the tubules and become a part of the urine.

The normal range of urine production is 1 to 2 L/day (McCance and Huether, 1994). Fluid intake and body temperature may affect urine production. Urine is usually 95% water and 5% solutes. These solutes include electrolytes and organic solutes like urea, uric acid, creatinine, and ammonia.

Ureters. Urine leaves the tubules and enters collecting ducts that transport it to the renal pelvis. A ureter is attached to each kidney pelvis and carries urinary wastes into the bladder. Ureters are long, tubular structures, 25 to 30 cm (10 to 12 inches) long and 1.25 cm ($^1/_2$ inch) in diameter in the adult. They extend behind the peritoneum to join at the floor of the bladder in the pelvic cavity. Urine draining from the ureters to the bladder is sterile.

Three layers of tissue form the wall of the ureter. The inner layer is a mucous membrane that lines the renal tubules and urinary bladder. The mucous lining is an excellent medium for the growth and spread of microorganisms. The middle layer consists of smooth muscle fibers; it helps to transport urine through the ureters by peristaltic waves. An outer layer of fibrous connective tissue supports the ureters.

Peristaltic waves cause the urine to enter the bladder in spurts rather than steadily. To prevent urine from returning to the ureters, a small flaplike fold of mucous membrane acts as a valve and covers the juncture of the ureters and bladder. An obstruction within the ureters, such as a kidney stone (renal calculus), results in strong peristaltic waves that attempt to move the obstruction into the bladder. At the same time a reflex response causes the renal arterioles to constrict to reduce urine production in the kidney on the affected side.

Bladder. The urinary bladder is a hollow, distensible, muscular organ that is a reservoir for urine. When empty, the bladder lies in the pelvic cavity behind the symphysis pubis. In the male the bladder rests against the rectum posteriorly, and in the female it rests against the anterior wall of the uterus and vagina.

The bladder's shape changes as it fills with urine. Normally it holds approximately 600 ml of urine. When the bladder is full, its superior surface expands up into a dome and pushes above the symphysis pubis. A greatly distended bladder, one with 1000 ml or more, may reach the umbilicus. In a pregnant woman the fetus pushes against the bladder, causing a feeling of fullness and reducing its capacity.

Urethra. Urine travels from the bladder through the urethra and passes to the outside of the body through the urethral meatus. Mucous membrane lines the urethra, and urethral glands secrete mucus into the urethral canal. Thick layers of smooth muscle surround the urethra. In women the urethra is approximately 4 to 6.5 cm ($1\frac{1}{2}$ to $2\frac{1}{2}$ inches) long. The external urethral sphincter, located about halfway down the urethra, permits voluntary flow of urine. This short length in women and girls provides an easy access for microorganisms. In men the urethra, which is also a passageway for cells and secretions from reproductive organs, is 20 cm (8 inches) long. It has three sections: the prostatic urethra, the membranous urethra, and the penile urethra.

Act of Urination

Urination, **micturition,** and **voiding** are all terms for the process by which urine is expelled from the urinary bladder. The desire to urinate can be sensed when the bladder contains only a small amount of urine (150 to 200 ml in an adult and 50 to 100 ml in a child). As the volume of urine increases, the bladder wall stretches, sending sensory impulses for the sacral reflex (S2 to S4). The detrusor muscle contracts and the internal

urethral sphincter relaxes so that urine may enter the urethra, although voiding does not yet occur. As the bladder contracts, nerve impulses travel to the midbrain and cerebral cortex. A person is thus conscious of the need to urinate. If the person chooses not to void, the external urinary sphincter remains contracted, and the micturition reflex is inhibited. However, when a person is ready to void, the external sphincter relaxes, the micturition reflex stimulates the detrusor muscle to contract, and urination occurs.

Factors influencing urination. Normal urinary elimination can be affected by physiologic factors, psychosocial conditions, and diagnostic or treatment-induced factors (Box 35-1). Knowledge of these factors enables the nurse to anticipate possible elimination problems.

Common urinary elimination problems. The most common urinary problems involve disturbances in micturition. These disturbances result from impaired bladder function, obstruction to urine outflow, or an inability to voluntarily control micturition. Some clients may have permanent or temporary changes in the normal pathway of urination. For example, the client with a **urinary diversion** may have special problems because urine drains through an artificial opening (stoma) on the abdominal wall.

Urinary retention. **Urinary retention** is an accumulation of urine in the bladder because the bladder is unable to partially or completely empty. The client who retains 25% of total bladder capacity is experiencing urinary retention. Total bladder capacity is calculated by adding the amount voided to the residual volume (the amount left in the bladder after urination) (Gray, 1992). Urine collects in the bladder, stretching its walls and causing feelings of pressure, discomfort, tenderness over the symphysis pubis, restlessness, and diaphoresis. Key assessments include an absence of urinary output over several hours and a distended bladder. The client under the influence of anesthesia or analgesia may perceive only pressure, but the alert client has worsening discomfort resulting in severe pain as the bladder distends beyond its normal capacity. In urinary retention, the bladder may hold more than 1000 ml of urine.

Eventually, retention with outflow may develop. Pressure in the bladder builds so that the external urethral sphincter is unable to hold back urine. The sphincter opens to allow a small volume of urine (25 to 60 ml) to escape, after which the bladder pressure falls enough to allow the sphincter to close. The client may void or be incontinent of small amounts of urine 2 or 3 times an hour with no relief of distention or discomfort. Retention with incontinence is sometimes referred to as overflow incontinence (Gray, 1992). Bladder spasms may occur with voiding and lead to acute discomfort.

Slow urine production can cause retention by filling

Box 35-1
Factors Influencing Urinary Elimination

Growth and Development

Infants and young children cannot concentrate urine and reabsorb water effectively.

Children cannot control urination voluntarily until 18 to 24 months.

A child must be able to recognize the feeling of bladder fullness, to hold urine for 1 to 2 hours, and to communicate the sense of urgency to a parent.

With age, the ability to concentrate urine declines and the frequency of urination increases.

The process of aging may impair micturition.

Problems of mobility sometimes make it difficult for older adults to reach the toilet or bedside commode in time.

Chronic diseases, such as multiple sclerosis or stroke, alter urinary patterns.

Sociocultural Factors

Cultural and gender norms vary on the privacy or publicness of urination. North Americans expect toilet facilities to be private, whereas some European cultures accept communal toilet facilities.

Social expectations (e.g., school recesses) influence the time of urination.

Psychological Factors

Anxiety and stress do not affect the characteristics of urine but may affect a sense of urgency and increase the frequency of urination.

Anxiety may prevent complete urination because tension makes it difficult to relax abdominal muscles.

Personal Habits

Privacy and adequate time to urinate are usually important to most people. Some people need distractions to relax.

Muscle Tone

Weak abdominal and pelvic floor muscles impair bladder contraction and control of the external sphincter.

Decreased muscle tone may be caused by immobility, childbirth, or trauma.

Muscle tone may also be lost with continuous drainage of urine through an indwelling catheter.

Fluid Intake

If fluids, electrolytes, and solutes are balanced, increased fluid intake increases urine production.

Alcohol stops the release of antidiuretic hormones, thus promoting urine production.

Fluids containing caffeine increase urinary output frequency.

Foods with high fluid content, such as fruits and vegetables, may increase urine production.

Pathological Conditions

Diabetes mellitus and multiple sclerosis cause neuropathies that alter bladder function.

Rheumatoid arthritis, degenerative joint disease, and parkinsonism slow or hinder physical activity and interfere with urination.

Acute renal disease reduces urine volume; chronic renal disease initially increases volume of poorly concentrated urine.

Febrile conditions reduce the amount of urine but increase its concentration.

Spinal cord injuries interrupt voluntary bladder emptying.

Surgical Procedures

The stress response to surgery reduces the amount of urinary output to increase circulatory fluid volume.

Anesthetics and pain-killing drugs slow the filtration rate and reduce urinary output.

Local trauma during lower abdominal and pelvic surgery may obstruct urine flow, so indwelling catheters may be needed.

Medications

Diuretics prevent reabsorption of water and certain electrolytes, and urinary output increases.

Some drugs also change the color of urine (e.g., amitriptyline turns it blue-green, and methyldopa turns it red; warfarin sodium turns it orange, and indomethacin turns it green).

Medications may affect the ability to relax and empty the bladder.

Diagnostic Examinations

Following intravenous pyelograms, monitor client for complications such as hypersensitivity reactions and acute renal failure.

Cystoscopy may cause localized edema of the urethral passageway and bladder sphincter spasm, resulting in urinary retention and the passing of red or pink urine.

the bladder gradually, thus preventing activation of the stretch receptors. After distending beyond a certain point, the bladder cannot contract. Retention can occur because of many other factors (Table 35-1).

Lower urinary tract infections. Urinary tract infections account for 40% of hospital-acquired (**nosocomial**) infections in the United States (Palmer and others, 1996). Most of these infections are directly due to catheterization. **Bacteriuria** (bacteria in the urine) is often inevitable once a retention catheter is inserted (Warren, 1994). The catheter is a source of injury to the mucosa, thus allowing bacterial invasion. It is important to keep catheterization at a minimum because bacteriuria may lead to the spread of organisms into the bloodstream (**urosepsis**) and kidneys, especially in the severely compromised client.

Microorganisms can enter the urinary tract through the urethral meatus or the bloodstream. However, the ascending route through the urethra is more common. Bacteria inhabit the vagina in women and the distal urethra and external genitalia in men and women. Organisms enter the urethral meatus easily and travel up the inner mucosal lining to the bladder. Women are more susceptible to urinary tract infection because of the proximity of the anus to the urethral meatus and be-

cause of a short urethra. In the male the length of the urethra and the antibacterial substance in prostatic secretions reduce the risk of urinary tract infection.

In a healthy person with good bladder function, organisms are flushed out during voiding. However, bladder distention reduces blood flow to the mucosal and submucosal layer, and tissues become more susceptible to bacteria. **Residual urine,** urine that remains in the bladder after urination, is an ideal site for microorganism growth. Table 35-1 summarizes the predisposing causes of lower urinary tract infection.

Clients with urinary tract infections often have pain or burning during urination (**dysuria**) and urgency. An irritated bladder causes a frequent and urgent sensation of the need to void. Fever, chills, nausea and vomiting, and malaise may develop. Irritation to bladder and urethral mucosa may result in blood-tinged urine (hematuria). The urine appears concentrated and cloudy because of bacteria. The older adult with urinary tract infection may exhibit an alteration in mental status such as acute confusion (Foreman and Zane, 1996). If infection spreads to the kidneys (pyelonephritis), fever, flank pain, tenderness, and chills are common symptoms.

Urinary incontinence. Urinary incontinence is the loss of control over micturition. It may be tempo-

TABLE 35-1
Causes of Urinary Elimination Disorders

Disorder	Causes
Urinary Retention	
Urine flow is obstructed; urine accumulates in bladder. Low fluid intake can lead to retention.	Prostate gland enlargement, fecal impaction, pregnancy in third trimester, urethral stricture or edema after childbirth, and urethral edema after surgery or diagnostic examination may obstruct urine flow.
	Spinal cord and peripheral nerve trauma and degeneration of peripheral nerves (e.g., diabetic neuropathy) alter sensory and motor innervation.
	Emotional anxiety and muscle tension may alter ability to relax sphincters.
	Medications (anesthetics and narcotics).
Lower Urinary Tract Infection	
Microorganisms may be introduced resulting in bacterial spread, causing inflammation of bladder muscle.	Kinked or blocked urethral catheter and urinary retention can cause obstruction of urine flow.
	Poor perineal hygiene, frequent sexual intercourse, ingredients in bubble baths, improperly handled diagnostic instruments, improperly sterilized instruments, and contaminated urine receptacles can cause spread of bacteria.
Urinary Incontinence	
Incontinence involves incompetent or weakened sphincter and loss of control of voiding.	Multiple childbirths, pelvic organ surgery, and removal of prostate gland can weaken sphincter.
	Mental confusion, sedatives or analgesics, spinal cord injury, bladder spasm, and bladder atrophy can cause loss of voiding control.

rary or permanent. The client cannot control the external urethral sphincter. Leakage may be continuous or intermittent. Nurses may be the professional to whom clients will reveal their incontinence. Therefore the nurse must be sensitive to this problem, which is thought to occur in some settings like nursing homes in 50% of the population (Colling, 1994). There are five types of incontinence (Table 35-2). The causes of incontinence vary by type.

Incontinence is a common problem that can develop in people of every age (*Consumer Version: Clinical Practice Guidelines,* 1996). It is a myth that incontinence is caused by aging. However, Webb (1994) notes that urinary incontinence, particularly stress and urge incontinence, is not uncommon in younger women and often goes undiagnosed. The annual cost of incontinence for clients in the community and in nursing homes is over $10 million annually (Urinary Incontinence Guideline Panel, 1992). Urinary incontinence has an impact on body image and social interaction. Clothing becomes wet with urine, and the accompanying odor adds to embarrassment. Clients with this problem often avoid physical and social activities.

Older adults are more susceptible to incontinence

TABLE 35-2
Types of Urinary Incontinence

Description	Causes	Symptoms
Total		
Total uncontrollable and continuous loss of urine	Neuropathy of sensory nerves Trauma or disease of spinal nerves or urethral sphincter Fistula between bladder and vagina	Constant flow of urine at unpredictable times Nocturia Lack of awareness of bladder filling or incontinence
Functional		
Involuntary unpredictable passage of urine in client with intact urinary and nervous systems	Change in environment Sensory, cognitive, or mobility deficits	Strong urge to void with loss of urine before reaching appropriate receptacle
Stress		
Increased intraabdominal pressure causing leakage of small amount of urine	Coughing, laughing, vomiting, or lifting with full bladder Obesity Full uterus pressing against bladder during third trimester of pregnancy Incompetent bladder outlet Weak pelvic musculature	Dribbling of urine with increased intraabdominal pressure Urinary urgency Frequency
Urge		
Involuntary passage of urine after strong sense of urgency to void	Decreased bladder capacity Irritation of bladder stretch receptors Alcohol or caffeine ingestion Increased fluid intake	Urinary urgency Abnormal frequency (more often than every 2 hours) Bladder contracture or spasm Nocturia Voiding in small (less than 100 ml) or in large (more than 550 ml) amounts
Reflex		
Involuntary loss of urine occurring at somewhat predictable intervals when specific bladder volume is reached	Upper spinal cord injury or disease involving area above reflex arc, blocking cerebral awareness Lower spinal cord injury blocking impulses to reflex arc	Lack of awareness of bladder filling No urge to void Uninhibited bladder contraction or spasm at regular intervals

because of functional limitations and the environment in which they live. An older person with restricted mobility has a greater chance of being incontinent because of the inability to reach toilet facilities in time. Low-set chairs and beds raised well above the floor may be obstacles for the older adult who must get up to reach a toilet. An older adult who has difficulty undoing buttons or manipulating zippers faces another obstacle. The older adult with chronic health problems may lack the energy to walk very far at one time, and if there is only one toilet in the home, the distance may be too far for the client with urge incontinence. Continued episodes of incontinence can create skin breakdown. Acidic urine is irritating to the skin. The client who has frequent incontinence is especially at risk for pressure ulcers (see Chapter 38).

Urinary Diversions

With surgery it is possible to divert the drainage of urine from a diseased or dysfunctional bladder. There are two classifications for urinary diversions: continent and incontinent. A **ureterostomy** (an incontinent diversion) is any surgical procedure that creates stomas on the outer abdominal wall for urine drainage. Typically the client with a ureterostomy has had the bladder removed surgically because of a malignant growth, birth defects, or a spinal cord injury. A ureterostomy may be the preferred treatment for chronic incontinence.

Figure 35-1 illustrates several types of ureterostomies. The ileal loop or conduit, which has been commonly used for the last 40 years, involves separating a loop of intestinal ileum with its blood supply intact. The surgeon implants the ureters into the ileum, which becomes an outlet for urine drainage. The ileum is not a reservoir. The remaining ileum is reconnected to the rest of the digestive tract.

A ureterostomy involves bringing the end of one or both ureters to the abdominal surface. To avoid the need for two collecting devices, a transureterostomy connects the ureters and brings one out through the abdominal wall.

The client with a ureterostomy must wear a stomal pouch continuously because there is no sphincter control for regulation of urine flow. Because of continuous urinary drainage, the client must maintain skin integrity. Any obstruction within a ureterostomy may lead to serious fluid and electrolyte alterations.

In the last 10 years continent urinary reservoirs (CUR) have become a viable option for some clients requiring a urinary diversion. This procedure done surgically results in a **continent pouch** or reservoir formed from a bowel segment. Clients self-catheterize the pouch to achieve continence. Kock, Indiana, Mainz, and Miami pouches are common types of these diversions (Razor, 1993).

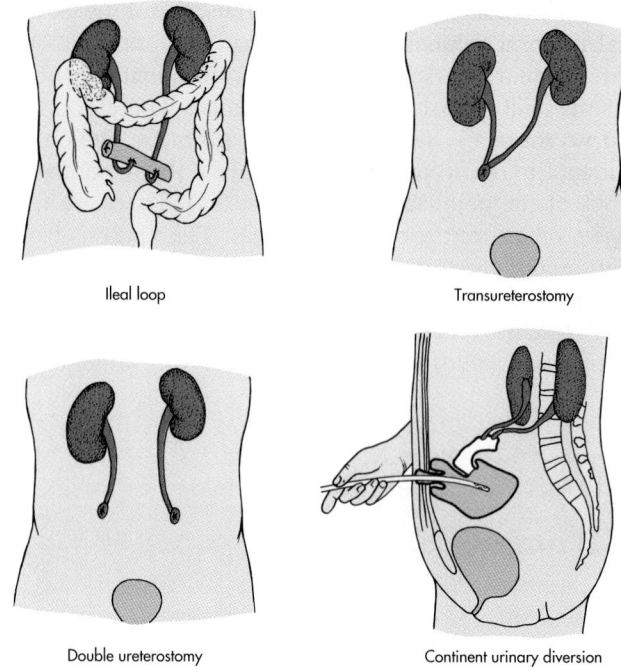

Ileal loop

Transureterostomy

Double ureterostomy

Continent urinary diversion

Figure 35-1. Types of urinary diversions.

A urinary diversion poses threats to body image. The client may wear an artificial device to collect urine and must learn to manage it. The client with a continent device must learn to self-catheterize the internal pouch that holds urine. The client with a urinary diversion can wear normal clothing, engage in any physical activity, travel, and have sexual relations.

⋯NURSING KNOWLEDGE BASE

Urinary elimination is a natural and often private process that may require physiological and psychological assistance from the nurse. Therefore, providing nursing care for a client with potential or actual urinary problems requires that the nurse have an understanding beyond anatomy and physiology. The nurse must be knowledgeable about concepts such as infection control, hygiene measures, growth, and development and also be sensitive to the client's psychosocial needs when a urinary problem develops.

Infection Control and Hygiene

The urinary tract is a common site for infection, and therefore the nurse uses principles of infection control to prevent the onset and spread of urinary tract infections and to promote the treatment of infections that do occur (see Chapter 25). Urinary tract infections are often caused by *Escherichia coli,* and the infections can occur anywhere along the urinary tract from the urethra to the kidneys. Urinary tract infections that occur after admission to a health care facility are called nosocomial infections. The reason for most nosocomial infections is lack of hand washing.

Principles of medical and surgical asepsis must be meticulously followed when carrying out procedures involving the urinary tract or external genitalia. Any instrumentation on the urinary tract such as catheterization requires the use of sterile technique. Procedures that involve manipulation of the perineum such as perineal care or examination of the genitalia requires the use of medical asepsis.

Developmental Considerations

The neonate should void within 24 hours after birth. In the neonate and infant, urination is a voiding response and is produced when the bladder fills. As the child reaches the age of 2 or 3, the neuromuscular and cognitive functions develop to the point where the child can facilitate and inhibit control of the bladder, and toilet training is usually begun. Many children attain bladder control by age 3, but daytime accidents and nocturnal enuresis may continue until the age of 5 (see Chapter 20).

As we age, changes occur in both the male and female that may contribute to the development of voiding problems. In the male, prostate enlargement may start after age 40 and continue until the 80s, thus producing problems with frequency. In the female, childbearing and hormonal levels may influence urination. Changes associated with pregnancy often produce urinary frequency and urgency. With repeated deliveries or hormone changes after menopause, temporary or permanent changes can occur that result in decreased perineal muscle tone. These changes may lead to urgency and stress incontinence (see Chapter 20). Hormonal changes may also contribute to an increased susceptibility to infection. Decreased levels of estrogen tend to cause the urethral mucosa to become thinner and more fragile and consequently more easily traumatized and infected (Penn and others, 1994).

Psychosocial Implications

Self-concept, culture, and sexuality are all closely related concepts that may be affected. Self-concept changes as we develop over our life span and includes one's body image, self-esteem, roles, and identity (see Chapter 16). Little children may not want to urinate on the toilet because they don't want to flush part of themselves away. Gender influences the position we use to urinate. Males tend to stand to urinate, and females assume a sitting position. Culture may influence how urination is talked about and how much privacy is needed. It may be considered improper in some cultures for a male to ask a female client about private matters such as urination (see Chapter 18).

CRITICAL THINKING IN CLIENT CARE

Synthesis

In caring for clients with altered patterns of elimination, the nurse synthesizes knowledge, draws from experience, applies critical thinking attitudes, and is knowledgeable about the standards of practice. Practical experience and knowledge from scientific and nursing domains assist in providing individualized nursing care for these clients.

Knowledge. The nurse must incorporate knowledge from a number of sources. It is important that the nurse understand normal urinary elimination changes caused by pathological conditions and changes associated with age, gender, and improper hygiene practices. A comprehensive view of a client's situation allows the nurse to make the most accurate decisions in client care. Information regarding a client's fluid balance and knowledge of medication will further complement the nurse's knowledge base.

When clients have changes in their fluid balance, this also impacts elimination patterns. In addition, these changes can increase the clients' risks for impairments in urination related to infection, incontinence, or retention.

Experience. Previous and personal experience provides the nurse with a basis for determining elimination needs. Perhaps the nurse has cared for a previous client who was incontinent. The nurse may have had personal experience of a Foley catheter insertion when a child was delivered by cesarean section. Perhaps the nurse or a close personal friend experienced a urinary tract infection and the burning, urgency, and hesitancy associated with it. Last, when caring for previous clients, experience has taught the nurse that voiding patterns are individual and that to find out about voiding patterns the nurse must ask clients about their usual patterns of elimination.

Attitude. Elimination needs of clients are individual and very personal. Flexibility and creativity are needed to establish elimination schedules and interventions. The nurse must consider the client's preferences first in setting elimination practices and priorities. Perseverance and client advocacy enables the nurse to respond promptly to the client's need to adapt to altered urinary elimination.

Standards. Because urination is often a private matter, the nurse must be concerned about protecting the client's privacy. In addition, it is important that the nurse adhere to the standards of medical and surgical asepsis. Interventions to restore urinary elimination may be invasive. Adherence to standards of asepsis reduces risk of infection.

NURSING PROCESS AND ALTERATIONS IN URINARY ELIMINATION

▪ Assessment

To identify a urinary elimination problem and gather data for a care plan, the nurse obtains a nursing history, performs a physical assessment, assesses the client's urine, and reviews information from diagnostic tests and examinations.

Nursing history. The nurse synthesizes information from the scientific and the nursing knowledge base to gather a history. The nursing history includes a review of the client's elimination patterns and symptoms of urinary alterations, as well as the following assessment of factors that may be affecting the ability to urinate normally.

Pattern of urination. Ask the client about daily voiding patterns, including frequency and times of day, normal volume at each voiding, and history of recent changes. Frequency varies among individuals. Most people void an average of 5 or more times a day. The client who voids frequently during the night may have renal or cardiovascular disease. Information about the pattern of urination is necessary to establish a baseline of comparison.

Symptoms of urinary alterations. Certain symptoms of alterations may occur in more than one type of urinary disorder. During assessment, the nurse asks the client about the symptoms listed in Table 35-3. The nurse also assesses whether the client is aware of conditions or factors that precipitate or aggravate symptoms.

Factors affecting urination. The nurse summarizes factors in the client's history that normally affect urination. These factors include the following:

1. Medications, including over-the-counter drugs, may affect fluid and electrolyte balance. Diuretics are successfully used to regulate fluid balance; however, side effects can further potentiate fluid and electrolyte imbalances. Narcotic analgesics may cause urinary retention. Anesthetics can temporarily depress renal function.
2. Consider the client's mobility status as it influences access to toileting facilities. Assessments that should be made include use of walking aids, distance to the toilet, ability to remove clothing or to get in and out of the bathroom, and lighting.
3. Environmental barriers in the home or health care setting may prevent the client from accessing the toilet. The client may need an elevated toilet seat, grab bars, or a portable commode (Smith, 1994).
4. Sensory restrictions (e.g., clients with visual problems who may have trouble reaching toilet facilities) may hamper self-toileting. If the client has difficulty with hand coordination, the nurse assesses the type of clothing and the client's ease in using clothing fasteners.
5. Past illness such as urinary tract infection or surgery increases the risk for recurrent problems. Chronic diseases (e.g., multiple sclerosis) that impair bladder function require the nurse to consider preventive care measures. Clients returning from surgery often have difficulty voiding the first few hours until the effects of anesthesia diminish.
6. The presence of urinary diversion will directly affect urinary elimination. If the client has a urinary diversion, the nurse assesses its type, location, and function. The condition of surrounding skin and usual methods for management (presence of appliance or pouch, type of skin care products and application) should also be assessed. If the client has an incontinent diversion, the methods and frequency of appliance changes and the type of nighttime drainage system are assessed. Additionally, in the client with a CUR the frequency and type of catheters used must be determined.
7. Personal habits may inhibit urination or put the client at risk for infection. If a client is hospitalized, the nurse assesses the extent to which personal habits are altered. Privacy is often difficult to accomplish in a health care setting, particularly if a client must use a bedpan (see Chapter 36) or a urinal. The nurse assesses the client's knowledge and practices of perineal hygiene (see Chapter 29).
8. Clients recovering from major surgery and suffering critical illness or disability often have an indwelling catheter to aid urinary drainage and provide a measurement of urinary output. A catheter places a client at risk for infection.
9. Fluid intake is directly related to urinary output. A client's physical condition affects the frequency with which the nurse monitors fluid intake (see Chapter 31). Regular intake and output (I&O) measurements help to assess a client's overall fluid balance. Clients who have urinary tract infections and are experiencing urgency, burning, and frequency may mistakenly decrease their fluid intake to try to fix the symptoms.
10. Consider the client's age when assessing micturition habits. Toilet training and enuresis are concerns that arise in the toddler and preschooler. In the adult, increasing age may bring disease and physiological changes that predispose to incontinence.

TABLE 35-3
Common Symptoms of Urinary Alterations

Description	Causes or Associated Factors
Urgency Feeling of the need to void immediately	Full bladder Inflammation or irritation to bladder mucosa from infection Incompetent urethral sphincter Psychological stress
Dysuria Painful or difficult urination	Bladder inflammation Trauma or inflammation of urethra
Frequency Voiding at frequent intervals	Increased fluid intake Bladder inflammation Increased pressure on bladder (e.g., pregnancy or psychological stress)
Hesitancy Difficulty in initiating urination	Prostate enlargement Anxiety Urethral edema
Polyuria Voiding large amount of urine	Excess fluid intake Diabetes mellitus or insipidus Use of diuretics
Oliguria Diminished urinary output in relation to fluid intake	Dehydration Renal failure Urinary tract obstruction Increased secretion of antidiuretic hormone (ADH)
Nocturia Urination, particularly excessive, at night	Excess intake of fluids (especially coffee or alcohol before bedtime) Renal disease Cardiovascular disease
Dribbling Leakage of urine despite voluntary control of micturition	Urine retention from incomplete bladder emptying Stress incontinence
Hematuria Presence of blood in urine	Neoplasms of kidney, certain glomerular diseases, infections of kidneys or bladder, traumatic injury to urinary structure, calculi, blood dyscrasia
Retention Accumulation of urine in bladder, with inability of bladder to empty	Urethral obstruction, bladder inflammation, decreases in sensory activity, neurogenic bladder, prostate enlargement after anesthesia, side effects of certain medications (e.g., anticholinergics, antispasmodics, antidepressants)
Residual Urine Volume of urine remaining in bladder after voiding (volumes of 100 ml or more)	Inflammation or irritation of bladder mucosa from infection, neurogenic bladder, prostatic enlargement, trauma or inflammation of urethra

Client expectations. Note the client's responses to questions about urination. Does the client seem hesitant or embarrassed? Psychosocial factors such as culture or sexuality may be influencing the client's response. In addition, ask the client what he or she expects from care. Does the client expect the infection to be resolved? Does the woman who has stress incontinence expect this condition to be relieved?

Does the client have expectations about urination or catheterization? Since urination is often considered a private matter, clients may find it difficult to be asked about their voiding habits. The postoperative client or client taking medications that affect urination may become concerned that something is wrong when asked every couple of hours if they have voided. Clients receiving intravenous fluids may not realize that they may have an increased need for urination. Urinary catheters may indicate to some that the client is very ill and not recognize that urinary catheters are used for diagnosis and monitoring for a variety of clients.

Physical assessment

Skin and mucosa. The nurse assesses the skin's hydration status by noting texture and turgor. The nurse also assesses the skin around periurethral tissues and stomas for excoriation, drainage, and tenderness. Urinary incontinence, fluid imbalance, and electrolyte disturbances increase the risk for skin breakdown. Assessment of the oral mucosa also reveals whether hydration is adequate. To assess urinary function, the nurse examines the kidneys, bladder, and urethral meatus (see Chapter 24).

Kidneys. If the kidneys become infected or inflamed, flank pain typically develops. The nurse can assess for tenderness early in the disease by percussing the costovertebral angle (the angle formed by the spine and twelfth rib). Inflammation of the kidney results in pain on percussion.

Bladder. Normally the bladder rests below the symphysis pubis and cannot be examined by the nurse. When distended, the bladder rises above the symphysis pubis at the midline of the abdomen and just below the umbilicus. When the nurse applies light pressure to the bladder, the client may feel tenderness or even pain. Palpation may also cause the urge to urinate.

Urethral meatus. The female client assumes a dorsal recumbent position to provide full exposure of the genitalia. The nurse uses the gloved nondominant hand to retract the labial folds to see the urethral meatus. There is normally no discharge from the meatus. Drainage may indicate infection. The nurse notes the color and consistency of drainage. A clear, watery drainage is probably urine.

The male's urethral meatus is normally a small opening at the tip of the penis. A hypospadias is a congenitally formed opening of the urethra on the undersurface of the penis. The nurse inspects the meatus for discharge and inflammation. It may be necessary to retract the foreskin in uncircumcised males to see the meatus.

Assessment of urine. The assessment of urine involves measuring the client's fluid intake and urinary output and observing the characteristics of the urine.

Intake and Output. When clients have altered or impaired urinary elimination, their I&O are measured to help monitor fluid and electrolyte balance. Although often written as part of a physician's order, placing a client on I&O may be a nurse's or physician's judgment (see Chapter 31). Placing a client on I&O measurements requires cooperation and assistance from the client and family. Intake measurements must include all oral liquids and semiliquids, all enteral feedings through nasogastric, gastrostomy, or jejunostomy tubes, and all parenteral fluids like intravenous solutions, blood components, and parenteral nutrition (see Chapter 31).

The nurse is responsible for accurate recording. Measurements are kept throughout the day and totaled every 8 hours, but the nurse may determine that more frequent measurements are required. Marking the I&O when the client has voided or eaten is often a task that is delegated. Before delegating this task, the nurse should inform the care provider what the metric conversions are for common liquid, holding containers such as coffee cups and milk cartons and ensure that the care provider knows aseptic principles relating to body fluids. The nurse should caution the care provider to be sensitive to the privacy needs of the clients and clarify what should be reported to the nurse about I&O, such as changes in color, amount, or odor of urine or presence and frequency of incontinence and inform the care provider about the amount of assistance the client requires to use the urinal and if standing is permitted.

Urinary output is a key indicator of kidney function. A change in urine volume is a significant indicator of fluid imbalance or kidney disease. For example, in a catheterized postoperative client, hourly urinary output provides an indirect measure of circulating volume. If the urinary output falls below 30 ml/hr, the nurse must notify the physician and assess for other signs of shock.

The nurse assesses urine volume by measuring with a **graduated measuring container** (receptacle for volume measurement) the client's output that has been collected in a bedpan, urinal, **urine hat** (a receptacle that fits inside the commode), or catheter bag. It is critical that each client have an individual measuring container with name and room number marked on it and that only one graduate be used for each client. Transmission of microorganisms occurs when equipment is used for other clients.

Special urometers attach to catheter drainage tubing and are a convenient means of measuring urine volume on a regular basis. A urometer holds 100 to 200 ml of urine. After measuring urine from a urometer, the nurse can drain the cylinder into the urinary drainage bag or into a receptacle for disposal. If a precise measurement of fluid intake is needed from the client who is at home, the nurse may ask the client to show a commonly used glass or cup on which the intake estimate is based.

Characteristics. The nurse inspects the client's urine for color, clarity, and odor. How frequently the nurse monitors urinary output is based on the client's condition. Minor changes are monitored and documented. In a client with a known urinary tract infection who has had a slight sediment in the urine, this information would be monitored for improvement and recorded. Unexpected changes such as the appearance of blood in the urine **(hematuria)** should alert the nurse to assess for associated signs and symptoms and report the information to the physician.

Color. Normal urine ranges in color from a pale straw color to amber, depending on its concentration. Urine is usually more concentrated in the morning. As the person drinks more fluids, it becomes less concentrated.

Bleeding from the kidneys or ureters usually causes urine to become dark red; bleeding from the bladder or urethra usually causes a bright red urine. Drugs can also change the urine's color. Beets, rhubarb, and blackberries may cause red urine. Special dyes used in intravenous diagnostic studies are eventually excreted by the kidneys and discolor the urine. Dark amber urine may be the result of high concentrations of bilirubin (urobilinogen) in clients with liver disease. The nurse reports unexpected color changes to the physician.

Clarity. Normal urine appears transparent at the time of voiding. Urine that stands several minutes in a container becomes cloudy. Freshly voided urine in clients with renal disease may appear cloudy because of protein concentration. Urine also appears thick and cloudy as a result of bacteria.

Odor. Urine has a characteristic ammonia odor. The more concentrated the urine, the stronger the odor. As urine remains standing (e.g., in a collection device), more ammonia breakdown occurs, and the odor becomes stronger.

Testing. The nurse is frequently responsible for collecting urine specimens for laboratory testing. The type of test determines the method of collection. All specimens are labeled with the client's name, date, and time of collection. Table 35-4 lists routine urinary analysis and specific nursing interpretations for each.

Specimen collection. The nurse collects several types of urine specimens for testing.

Urinalysis sample. A simple urinalysis does not require a sterile urine specimen. The client may void into a clean urine cup, a urinal, or a bedpan. The client must void before defecating so that feces do not contaminate it. If a woman is menstruating, the nurse

---

TABLE 35-4
Routine Urinalysis Values

Measurement (Normal Value)	Interpretation
pH (4.6 to 8.0)	pH level helps to indicate acid-base balance. Urine that stands for several hours becomes alkaline from bacterial invasion. If pH is alkaline, selected antibiotics (e.g., neomycin and streptomycin) are more effective against urinary tract infections.
Protein (up to 8 mg/100 ml)	Protein is normally not present in urine. It is seen in renal disease because damage to glomerular membrane allows protein to enter urine. However, temporary presence of protein can occur after strenuous exercise, exposure to cold, or psychological stress.
Glucose (not normally present)	Diabetic clients have glucose in urine because of inability of tubules to reabsorb high serum glucose concentrations (over 180 mg/100 ml). Ingestion of high concentrations of glucose may cause some to appear in urine of healthy persons.
Ketones (not normally present)	With poor control of diabetes, clients experience breakdown of fatty acids. End product of fatty acid metabolism is ketones. Clients with dehydration, starvation, or excessive aspirin ingestion also have ketonuria.
Blood (up to two red blood cells)	Damage to glomerulus or tubules may cause blood cells to enter urine. Trauma or disease of lower urinary tract also causes hematuria.
Specific gravity (1.01 to 1.03)	Specific gravity tests measure concentration of particles in urine. High specific gravity reflects concentrated urine, and low specific gravity reflects diluted urine. Dehydration, reduced renal blood flow, and increase in ADH secretion elevate specific gravity. Overhydration and inadequate ADH secretion reduce it.

makes note of this on the specimen requisition in case red blood cells appear. The nurse transfers the urine to the proper container and sends it to the laboratory.

Clean-voided or midstream specimen. To obtain a specimen relatively free of the microorganisms growing in the lower urethra, the nurse instructs the client on the method for obtaining a clean-voided specimen. Female and male clients are given a sterile urine cup, sterile disinfectant wipes, and clean gloves. The cup and disinfectant wipes are often prepackaged together. The package usually contains instructions, but the client should be instructed on how to wash and how to collect the specimen. Anxiety, difficulty or inability to read, or language barriers may prohibit the client from fully comprehending the instructions independently.

The woman should wipe from the meatus toward the rectum. The man cleans the meatus in a circular motion moving from the meatus up the glans penis. The nurse cautions the client against wiping repeatedly with the contaminated cloth. The client receives a sterile urine cup. The nurse instructs the client to allow the first part of the urine stream to be discarded. The initial stream cleans or flushes the urethral orifice and meatus of resident bacteria. During the midstream or middle portion of voiding, the nurse or client collects the specimen. Immediately after obtaining the specimen the nurse places a sterile top securely over the container and sends it to the laboratory for testing. Urine specimens must reach the laboratory within 1 hour of collection or be refrigerated. Urine that stands in a container at room temperature can grow bacteria.

Sterile specimen. Another method for collecting a sterile urine specimen for culture is by catheterizing a client or by obtaining the specimen from an indwelling catheter. Urine specimens should not be collected for culture from urine drainage bags unless it is the first urine drained into a new sterile bag. Bacteria grow rapidly in drainage bags and would give a false measurement of bacteria.

During catheterization the nurse collects the specimen as soon as urine flows from the catheter's end. After filling the sample container, the nurse withdraws the catheter or connects the newly inserted indwelling catheter to a drainage tube (Skill 35-1).

If a client already has an indwelling catheter, the nurse uses a sterile syringe to withdraw urine. Most urine drainage tubes have special ports referred to as sampling ports to withdraw specimens. If there is no sampling port, it is safe to insert a needle directly into the end of a self-sealing rubber catheter. However, Silastic, plastic, or silicone catheters are not self-sealing. A 3- to 5-ml syringe with a 1-inch needle (21 to 25 gauge) is best to prevent creation of a hole in the catheter port. Some companies have mass produced catheters with a sampling port that accepts most plastic or blunt cannulas (needleless) to reduce the risk of needle-stick. Read the manufacturer's instructions to determine if the catheter tubing in use accepts blunt cannulas.

First the nurse clamps the tubing about 3 inches below the sampling port, allowing fresh sterile urine to collect in the tube. The nurse then wipes the port with a disinfectant swab. Insertion of the needle at a 30-degree angle ensures entrance into the catheter lumen. The nurse withdraws 3 ml for a culture (Figure 35-2). While aspirating urine, the nurse must be careful not to raise the tubing, which would cause urine to return to the bladder.

After obtaining the specimen, the nurse transfers the urine into a sterile container using sterile aseptic technique and places it in a plastic pouch or bag per agency policy for transportation to the laboratory. The laboratory requisition should indicate the way the specimen was collected. The site from which the specimen was obtained should be inspected periodically to check that the catheter is not leaking.

Twenty-four-hour urine specimen. Some tests of renal function and urine composition require a 24-hour collection of urine. The nurse indicates the starting time on the gallon container and on the laboratory requisition and discards the first sample. The 24-hour collection period begins after the first specimen is discarded. The client then collects all urine voided in 24 hours. Any missed specimens make the results inaccurate, and the test must be restarted. The nurse should remind the client to void before defecating so that urine is not contaminated by feces. The laboratory should be consulted for instructions. The client should void the last specimen as close as possible to the end of the 24-hour period.

Urine collection in children. Specimen collection from infants and children is often difficult. Preschool children and toddlers have difficulty voiding on request. Offering a young child fluids 30 minutes before requesting a specimen may help. The nurse must use terms for urination that the child can understand. A young child may be reluctant to void in unfamiliar receptacles. A potty chair is usually more effective. The

Text continued on p. 992

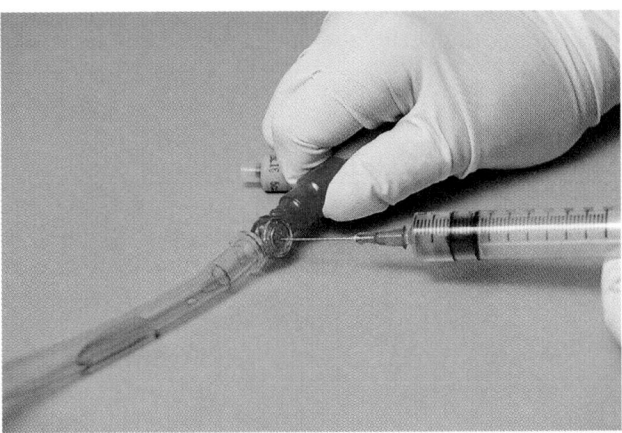

Figure 35-2. Urine specimen collection; aspiration from a collection port in drainage tubing of an indwelling catheter.

Inserting a Straight or Indwelling Catheter

Delegation Considerations
Catheterization is not typically delegated to unlicensed assistive personnel. It may be delegated in some settings.

The skill of catheterization requires problem solving and knowledge application unique to a professional nurse. Unlicensed assistive personnel may measure drainage from the catheter and provide perineal care. Unlicensed assistive personnel must be told to report specific abnormal findings to the nurse.

Equipment
- Catheterization kit containing the following sterile items:
  Gloves (extra pair optional)
  Drapes, one fenestrated
  Lubricant
  Antiseptic cleansing solution
  Cotton balls
  Forceps
  Prefilled syringe with sterile water to inflate balloon of indwelling catheter
  Catheter of correct size and type for procedure (i.e., intermittent or indwelling)
  Sterile drainage tubing with collection bag and multipurpose tube holder or tape, safety pin, and elastic band for securing tubing to bed if client is bed-bound (for indwelling catheter)
  Receptacle or basin (usually bottom of catheterization tray)
  Specimen container
- Blanket

STEPS	RATIONALE
1. Assess status of client:	
a. Time of last urination by asking client, checking I&O flow sheet, or palpating the bladder.	Bladder fullness may be detected with deep palpation above the symphysis pubis.
b. Level of awareness or developmental stage.	Reveals client's ability to cooperate and level of explanation needed.
c. Mobility and physical limitations of client.	Affect way that nurse positions client.
d. Client's gender and age.	Determines catheter size: 8 to 10 Fr is generally used for children, 14 to 16 Fr is indicated for women, 12 Fr may be considered for young girls, and 16 to 18 Fr is used for male clients unless larger size is ordered by physician.
e. Distended bladder.	Causes pain. Can indicate need to insert catheter if client is unable to void independently.
f. Assess perineum for erythema, drainage, and odor.	Determines condition of perineum.
g. Any pathological condition that may impair passage of catheter (i.e., enlarged prostate gland in men).	Obstruction prevents passage of catheter through urethra into bladder.
h. Allergies.	Determines allergy to antiseptic, tape, latex, and lubricant. Betadine allergies are common; if the client is unaware of allergy, ask if allergic to shellfish.
2. Review client's medical record, including physician's order and nurses' notes.	Determines purpose of inserting catheter: preparation for surgery, urinary irrigations, collection of sterile urine specimen, or measurement of residual urine. Assess for previous catheterization, including catheter size, response of client, and time of last catheterization.
3. Assess client's knowledge of the purpose for catheterization.	Reveals need for client instruction.
4. Explain procedure to client.	Promotes cooperation.
5. Arrange for extra nursing personnel to assist as necessary.	Client may be unable to assume positioning for procedure.

Continued

.... *Skill 35-1—cont'd*
Inserting a Straight or Indwelling Catheter

STEPS	RATIONALE
6. Begin monitoring I&O.	Catheterized clients are at risk for urinary complications.
7. Wash hands.	Reduces transmission of microorganisms.
8. Close curtain or door.	Offers privacy, reduces embarrassment, and aids in relaxation during procedure.
9. Raise bed to appropriate working height.	Promotes use of proper body mechanics.
10. Facing client, stand on left side of bed if right-handed (on right side if left-handed). Clear bedside table and arrange equipment.	Successful catheter insertion requires nurse to assume comfortable position with all equipment easily accessible.
11. Raise side rail on opposite side of bed, and put side rail down on working side.	Promotes client safety.
12. Place waterproof pad under client.	Prevents soiling of bed linen.
13. Position client:	Provides good visualization of perineal structures.
A. Female client:	
(1) Assist to dorsal recumbent position (supine with knees flexed). Ask client to relax thighs so the hip joints can be externally rotated.	Legs may be supported with pillows to reduce muscle tension and promote comfort.
(2) Position female client in side-lying (Sims') position with upper leg flexed at knee and hip if unable to be supine. If this position is used, nurse must take extra precautions to cover rectal area with drape during procedure to reduce chance of cross-contamination.	This alternate position is used if client cannot abduct leg at hip joint (e.g., if client has arthritic joints). Also, this position may be more comfortable for client. Support client with pillows if necessary to maintain position.
B. Male client:	
(1) Assist to supine position with thighs slightly abducted.	Comfortable position for client that aids in visualization.
14. Drape client:	
A. Female client:	
(1) Drape with bath blanket. Place blanket diamond fashion over client, with one corner at client's neck, side corners over each arm and side, and last corner over perineum.	
B. Male client:	
(1) Drape upper trunk with bath blanket, and cover lower extremities with bed sheets, exposing only genitalia.	Avoids unnecessary exposure of body parts and maintains client's comfort.
15. Wearing disposable gloves, wash perineal area with soap and water as needed; dry.	Reduces microorganisms near urethral meatus and allows further opportunity to visualize perineum and landmarks.
16. Remove and discard gloves; wash hands.	
17. Position lamp to illuminate perineal area. (When using flashlight, have assistant hold it.)	Permits accurate identification and good visualization of urethral meatus.
18. Open package containing drainage system; place drainage bag over edge of bottom of bed frame, and bring drainage tube up between side rail and mattress (indwelling catheter only).	Permits accurate identification and good visualization of urethral meatus.

STEPS	RATIONALE
19. Open catheterization kit according to directions, keeping bottom of container sterile.	Prevents transmission of microorganisms from table or work area to sterile supplies. The materials in the kit are ordered in sequence of use.
20. Apply sterile gloves (see Chapter 25).	Allows nurse to handle sterile supplies without contamination.
21. Organize supplies on sterile field. Open inner sterile package containing catheter. Pour sterile antiseptic solution into correct compartment containing sterile cotton balls. Open packet containing lubricant. Remove specimen container (lid should be loosely placed on top) and prefilled syringe from collection compartment of tray, and set them aside on sterile field.	Maintains principles of surgical asepsis and organizes work area.
22. Before inserting indwelling catheter, test balloon by injecting fluid from prefilled syringe into balloon port (see illustrations).	Checks integrity of balloon. Do not use the catheter if the balloon does not inflate or leaks.
23. Lubricate 2.5 to 5 cm (1 to 2 inches) of catheter for women and 12.5 to 17.5 cm (5 to 7 inches) for men.	
24. Apply sterile drape:	
A. Female client:	
(1) Allow top edge of drape to form cuff over both hands. Place drape down on bed between client's thighs. Slip cuffed edge just under buttocks, taking care not to touch contaminated surface with gloves.	Outer surface of drape covering hands remains sterile. Sterile drape against sterile gloves is sterile.
(2) Pick up fenestrated sterile drape, and allow it to unfold without touching an unsterile object. Apply drape over perineum, exposing labia and being sure not to touch contaminated surface.	Maintains sterility of work surface.

Continued

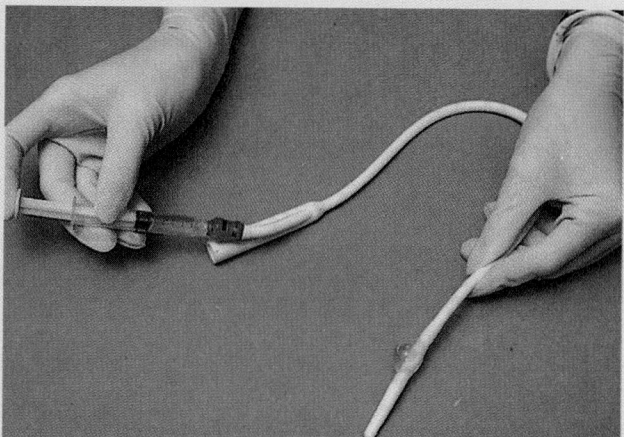

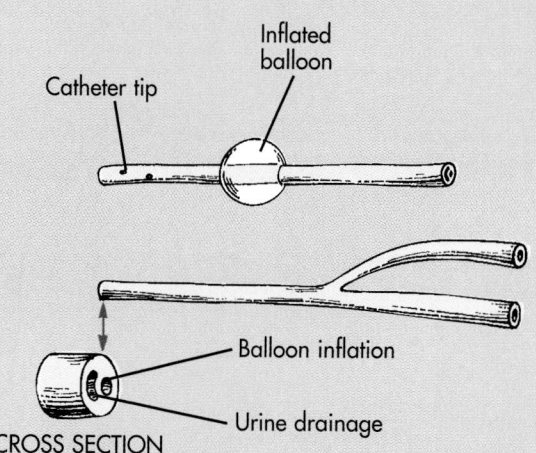

Inflated balloon

Catheter tip

Balloon inflation

Urine drainage

CROSS SECTION

Step 22

Skill 35-1—cont'd
Inserting a Straight or Indwelling Catheter

STEPS	RATIONALE
B. Male client:	
(1) Two methods are used for draping depending on preference. *First method:* apply drape over thighs and under penis without completely opening fenestrated drape. *Second method:* Apply drape over thighs just below penis. Pick up fenestrated sterile drape, allow it to unfold, and drape it over penis with fenestrated slit resting over penis.	Maintains sterility of work surface.
25. Place sterile tray and contents on sterile drape between thighs. Open specimen container.	Provides easy access to supplies during catheter insertion. Maintains aseptic technique during procedure.
26. Cleanse urethral meatus:	
A. Female client:	
(1) With nondominant hand, carefully retract labia to fully expose urethral meatus. Maintain position of nondominant hand throughout procedure.	Full visualization of urethral meatus is provided. Full retraction prevents contamination of urethral meatus during cleansing.
(2) Using forceps in sterile dominant hand, pick up cotton ball saturated with antiseptic solution and clean perineal area, wiping front to back from clitoris toward anus. Using a new cotton ball for each area, wipe along the far labial fold, near labial fold, and directly over center of urethral meatus.	Cleansing reduces number of microorganisms at urethral meatus. Use of single cotton ball for each wipe prevents transfer of microorganisms. Preparation moves from area of least contamination to that of most contamination. Dominant hand remains sterile.
B. Male client:	
(1) If client is not circumcised, retract foreskin with nondominant hand. Grasp penis at shaft just below glans. Retract urethral meatus between thumb and forefinger. Maintain nondominant hand in this position throughout procedure.	Accidental release of foreskin or dropping of penis during cleansing requires process to be repeated because area has become contaminated.

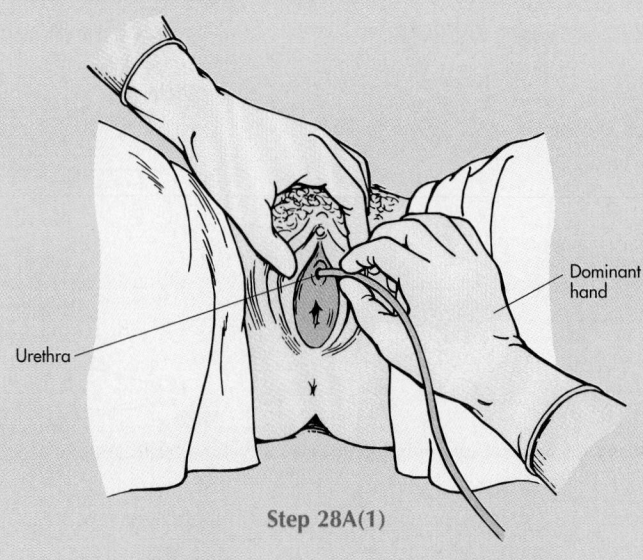

Urethra

Dominant hand

Step 28A(1)

STEPS	RATIONALE
(2) With dominant hand, pick up cotton ball with forceps and clean penis. Move it in circular motion from urethral meatus down to base of glans. Repeat cleansing three more times, using clean cotton ball each time.	Reduces number of microorganisms at urethral meatus and moves from areas of least to most contamination. Dominant hand remains sterile.
27. Pick up catheter with gloved dominant hand 7.5 to 10 cm (3 to 4 inches) from catheter tip. Hold end of catheter loosely coiled in palm of dominant hand (optional: may grasp catheter with forceps).	
28. Insert catheter:	
A. Female client:	
(1) Ask client to bear down gently as if to void, and slowly insert catheter through urethral meatus (see illustration).	Relaxation of external sphincter aids in insertion of catheter.
(2) Advance catheter a total of 5 to 7.5 cm (2 to 3 inches) in adult or until urine flows out catheter's end. When urine appears, advance catheter another 2.5 to 5 cm (1 to 2 inches). Do not force against resistance.	Female urethra is short. Appearance of urine indicates that catheter tip is in bladder or lower urethra. Advancement of catheter ensures bladder placement.

CRITICAL DECISION POINT

If no urine appears, check if catheter is in vagina. If misplaced, leave catheter in vagina as landmark indicating where not to insert, and insert another.

(3) Release labia and hold catheter securely with nondominant hand. Inflate balloon if retention catheter is used (see box).	Bladder or sphincter contraction may cause accidental expulsion of catheter.

Continued

Inflation of Balloon for Indwelling Catheter

Inflate balloon of indwelling catheter with amount of fluid recommended by the manufacturer.

a. While holding catheter with nondominant hand at urethral meatus, take end of catheter and place it between first two free fingers of nondominant hand.

b. With free dominant hand, attach syringe to injection port at end of catheter.

c. Slowly inject total amount of solution. If client complains of sudden pain, aspirate solution and advance catheter farther.

d. After inflating balloon, release catheter and pull gently to feel resistance. Then move catheter slightly back into bladder. Inflation of balloon anchors catheter tip in place above bladder outlet to prevent removal of catheter (see illustrations).

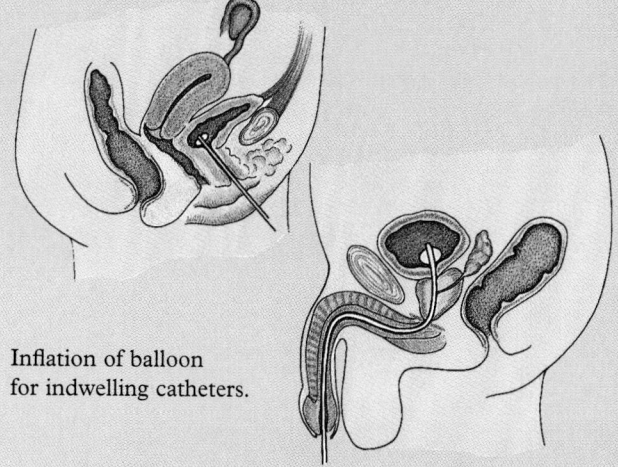

Inflation of balloon for indwelling catheters.

Skill 35-1—cont'd
Inserting a Straight or Indwelling Catheter

STEPS	RATIONALE
B. Male client:	
(1) Lift penis to position perpendicular to client's body and apply light traction (see illustration).	Straightens urethral canal to ease catheter insertion.
(2) Ask client to bear down as if to void, and slowly insert catheter through urethral meatus.	Relaxation of external sphincter aids in insertion of catheter.
(3) Advance catheter 17 to 22.5 cm (7 to 9 inches) in adult or until urine flows out catheter's end. If resistance is felt, withdraw catheter; do not force it through urethra. When urine appears, advance catheter another 2.5 to 5 cm (1 to 2 inches).	The adult male urethra is long. It is normal to meet resistance at the prostatic sphincter. When resistance is met, nurse should hold catheter firmly against sphincter without forcing catheter. After a few seconds, the sphincter relaxes and the catheter is advanced. Appearance of urine indicates catheter tip is in bladder or urethra. Further advancement of catheter ensures proper placement.
(4) Lower penis and hold catheter securely in nondominant hand. Place end of catheter in urine tray receptacle. Inflate balloon if retention catheter is used (see box on p. 989).	Catheter may be accidentally expelled by bladder or urethral contraction. Collection of urine prevents soiling and provides output measurement.
(5) Reduce (or reposition) the foreskin.	Paraphimosis (retraction and constriction of the foreskin behind the glans penis) secondary to catheterization may occur if foreskin is not reduced.
29. Collect urine specimen as needed. Fill specimen cup or jar to desired level (20 to 30 ml) by holding end of catheter in dominant hand over cup.	Allows sterile specimen to be obtained for culture analysis.

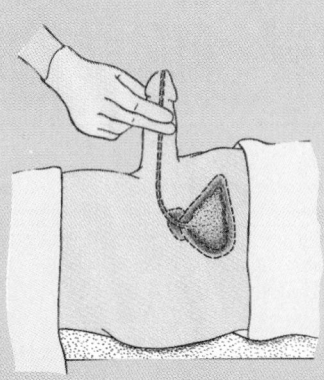

Step 28B(1)

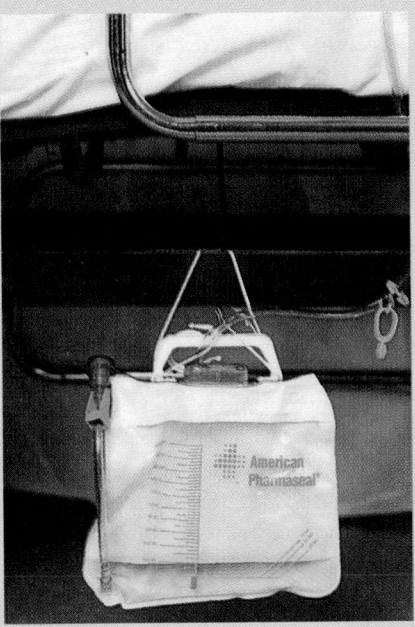

Step 32

STEPS	RATIONALE
30. Allow bladder to empty fully (about 800 to 1000 ml) unless institution policy restricts maximal volume of urine to drain with each catheterization. Check institution policy before beginning catheterization; some agencies restrict maximal amount of urine that can be drained off at one time. This amount may vary from 800 to 1000 ml.	There is no limit to the amount of urine that can be drained. (Williams and others, 1993; Sueppel, 1995). As always the nurse should monitor the client's condition, and if vital signs change or if pain or bleeding occurs, temporarily stop the flow of urine and continue when the client's condition warrants. Retained urine may serve as a reservoir for growth of microorganisms.
31. Remove straight, single-use catheter:	
a. Withdraw catheter slowly but smoothly until removed.	Minimizes discomfort to client.
32. Attach end of retention catheter to collecting tube of drainage system (see illustration). Drainage bag must be below level of bladder; do not place bag on side rails of bed.	Establishes closed system for urine drainage.
33. Anchor catheter:	
A. Female client:	
(1) Secure catheter tubing to inner thigh with strip of nonallergenic tape (commercial multipurpose tube holders with a Velcro strap are available). Allow for slack so movement of thigh does not create tension on catheter (see illustration).	Anchoring catheter to inner thigh reduces pressure on urethra, thus reducing possibility of tissue injury in this area.
B. Male client:	
(1) Secure catheter tubing to top of thigh or lower abdomen (with penis directed toward chest). Allow slack in catheter so movement does not create tension on catheter (see illustration).	Anchoring catheter to lower abdomen reduces pressure on urethra at junction of penis and scrotum, thus reducing possibility of tissue injury in this area.

Continued

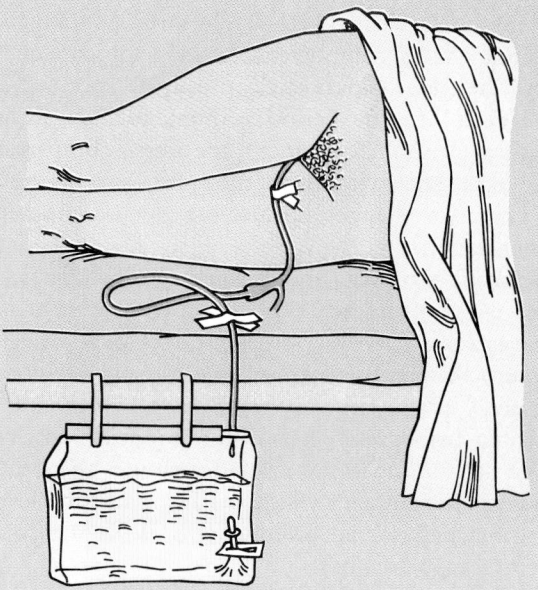

Step 33A(1)

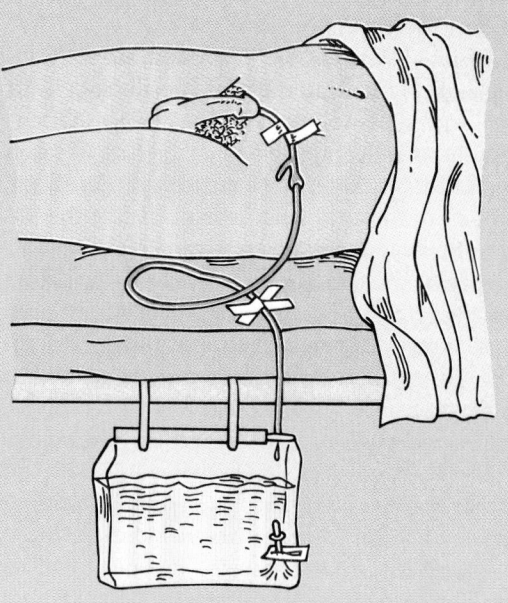

Step 33B(1)

Inserting a Straight or Indwelling Catheter

STEPS	RATIONALE
34. Assist client to comfortable position. Wash and dry perineal area as needed.	Maintains comfort and security.
35. Remove gloves, and dispose of equipment, drapes, and urine in proper receptacles.	Reduces transmission of microorganisms.
36. Wash hands.	Reduces spread of microorganisms.
37. Palpate bladder.	Determines if distention is relieved.
38. Ask about client's comfort.	Determine if client's sensation of discomfort or fullness has been relieved.
39. Observe character and amount of urine in drainage system.	Determines if urine is flowing adequately.
40. Determine that there is no urine leaking from catheter or tubing connections.	Prevents injury to client's skin.

Recording and Reporting

- Report and record type and size of catheter inserted, amount of fluid used to inflate balloon, characteristics of urine, amount of urine, reasons for catheterization, specimen collection if appropriate, and client's response to procedure and teaching concepts.
- Initiate I&O records.
- If catheter is definitely in bladder and no urine is produced within an hour, absence of urine should immediately be reported to physician.

Home Care Considerations

- Clients who are at home may use a leg bag during the day and switch to a large-volume bag at night so that sleep can remain uninterrupted.
- Clients may catheterize themselves at home on an intermittent basis using clean technique.

---

nurse must use special collection devices for infants or toddlers who are not toilet trained. Clear, plastic, single-use bags with self-adhering material can be attached over the child's urethral meatus.

Common urine tests. Common urine tests include urinalysis, measurement of specific gravity, urine culture, and glucose and ketone levels. Often the nurse's role in collecting specimens is that of teaching. The nurse should identify what preparation (if any) is needed before the test, what is expected of the patient during the test, and any posttest care.

Urinalysis. The laboratory performs urinalysis on a routine or clean-voided specimen or on a specimen obtained from a catheter. Table 35-4 lists normal values. The urinalysis is a screening test for renal disease, metabolic disorders, lower urinary tract alterations, and fluid imbalances. For a quick screening, the nurse can perform certain portions of the urinalysis with special reagent strips. The nurse dips the strips into urine and watches for a color change, which indicates the presence of protein, blood, sugar, ketones, and other solutes. The nurse can also perform a specific gravity test in the clinic or hospital unit.

Glucose and ketones. An accurate measurement of glucose and ketones always requires a double-voided specimen. A Keto-Diastix or Multistix reagent strip easily detects glucose and ketone. The strips contain chemicals that change color when exposed to glucose and ketone. The nurse dips a stick in a urine specimen and pulls it out. After the period recommended by the manufacturer (10 to 15 seconds), the nurse compares the color of the stick with that of the color chart on the bottle. The color change indicates the glucose and ketone concentration.

Specific gravity. To measure specific gravity, the nurse uses a urinometer and cylinder. The urinometer has a specific gravity scale at the top and a weighted mercury bulb at the bottom. The nurse pours a urine specimen into a clean dry cylinder and suspends the weighted urinometer in it. The concentration of dissolved substances in the urine determines the depth at which the urinometer will float. The point the level of urine reaches on the urinometer scale is the specific gravity measurement.

Urine culture. A urine culture simply requires a sterile sample of urine. It takes approximately 72 hours before the laboratory can report significant findings of bacterial growth. If bacteria are present, an additional test for sensitivity determines the antibiotics that will be effective or ineffective.

Diagnostic examinations.

The urinary system is one of the few organ systems amenable to accurate diagnostic study by radiographic techniques. The two approaches for visualizing urinary structures, namely direct and indirect techniques, can be quite simplistic or very complex, requiring extensive nursing interventions. These procedures are further subdivided into invasive and noninvasive categories.

Noninvasive procedures

Abdominal roentgenogram. Abdominal roentgenogram, also referred to as plain film, KUB, or flat plate of the abdomen, is commonly used to assess the gross structures of the urinary tract for abnormalities. It can be used to determine size, parity, shape, and location of the kidneys, ureters, and bladder structures. It is also useful in visualizing calculi or tumors in these organs. In addition, the ribs or other surrounding support structures can be assessed for fractures or abnormalities. The lack of positive findings on the roentgenogram does not rule out the possibility of abnormalities in the urinary tract. The nursing implications for clients undergoing this procedure include explanation of the procedure and alleviation of client anxiety. No special bowel preparation is usually indicated.

Intravenous pyelogram. To view the entire urinary system and to assess some renal function excretory urogram or intravenous pyelogram (IVP) is done. Although these procedures are noninvasive, the IVP does require that the client receive an intravenous injection of a radiopaque dye. Because the kidneys and ureters lie behind the intestines, it is necessary that the client receive a bowel preparation before the procedure.

Nursing implications before the test include recognizing clients at risk for alterations in renal function as a result of the intravenous injection of the contrast material. Any client with preexisting renal insufficiency is at risk. Older adults in particular are prone to the nephrotoxic effects of these substances because of their propensity for volume depletion during bowel preparation. Appropriate nursing assessment of volume status before this procedure is of utmost importance (see Chapter 31).

Additional nursing implications before the test are as follows:

1. Assess the client for allergy: intravenous contrast materials; shellfish or iodine allergy, which may predict allergies to the IVP dye.
2. Have the client take a cathartic on the evening before the test.
3. Explain that the client is usually NPO after midnight.
4. Explain that facial flushing is normal during dye injection and that the client may feel dizzy, warm, or nauseous.
5. Explain that an intravenous infusion for dye injection is started before the test.
6. Explain that the test involves x-ray studies taken at several intervals and that the client will void near the end of the test.

Nursing implications after the test are as follows:

1. Ensure that the client resumes a normal diet.
2. Encourage fluid intake to minimize dehydration caused by fasting and to avoid the potential nephrotoxic effects of the contrast material.
3. Explain to the client to watch for itching, rash, or hives, which indicate delayed hypersensitivity to IVP dye.
4. Monitor I&O, or explain to the client to report decreased or absent urination.

Renal scan. Renal scans allow indirect visualization of urinary tract structures after an intravenous injection of radioactive isotopes. The isotope can be detected without the need of bowel preparation. A very low dosage of radioisotope is used, and its half-life is short. Therefore no precautions against radioactive exposure are needed.

Except for the venipuncture, the procedure is painless. The scanning procedure is completed in approximately 1 hour. Information pertaining to renal blood flow, anatomical structures, and their excretory function can be obtained from this procedure. This procedure is indicated for clients unable to receive IVP dyes.

Nursing implications before the test include the following:

1. Explain that the radioisotope is injected intravenously through an existing IV line or needle.
2. Explain that the client will feel no discomfort but must lie still.
3. Explain that there is no risk of radioactive exposure.

Computerized axial tomography. Computerized axial tomography is a computerized x-ray procedure that is used to obtain detailed images of structures within a selected plane of the body. With this procedure, it is possible to visualize abnormal pathology such as tumors, obstructions, retroperitoneal masses, and lymph node enlargement. Although this procedure is noninvasive, in some examinations oral and/or intravenous contrast material is used to enhance the areas under study.

Renal ultrasound. Ultrasonography is a painless noninvasive diagnostic tool in the assessment of urinary disorders. It makes use of high-frequency, inaudible sound waves that reflect off tissue. The ultrasound is used to identify gross renal anatomy and structural abnormalities of the kidneys or lower urinary tract. Such abnormalities as tumors or cysts in the kidney are easily identified with this procedure.

Invasive procedures

Endoscopy. Endoscopy is the visualization of organs with the aid of a telescope or fiber-optic imaging. To view the interior of the bladder and urethra, the physician performs a cystoscopy. This is the most common of the three procedures. The cystoscope looks like a urinary catheter, although it is not as flexible. It is inserted through the urethra. The procedure is painful during instrument insertion. Unless the client lies still, the bladder may be perforated. Local, spinal, or general anesthesia may be administered. Because the test requires insertion of a foreign object into a sterile cavity, the client receives large amounts of fluids (intravenously or orally) before and during the procedure to maintain a continuous urine flow and to flush out bacteria. Antibiotics may also be administered intravenously. During the test, urine and tissue specimens may be collected.

Nursing implications before the test include the following:

1. Observe the client signing an informed consent form.
2. Perform a bowel preparation or enema, or administer a cathartic on the evening before the test.
3. If local anesthetic will be used, encourage intake of oral fluids.
4. If general anesthetic is to be used, ensure that the client is NPO after midnight.
5. Since this procedure is considered a minor surgical procedure, a preoperative checklist may need to be completed (see Chapter 40).
6. Explain that insertion of the cystoscope is similar to insertion of a urethral catheter.
7. Explain the importance of lying still during the test.
8. Explain that an intravenous line will be started to give fluids during the test.
9. Administer a sedative or analgesic per the physician's orders.

Nursing implications after the test include the following:

1. Instruct the client to remain in bed as ordered.
2. Assess for signs of urinary retention and first voiding.
3. Observe characteristics of urine, noting bloody or cloudy urine.
4. Encourage increased fluid intake, and monitor I&O.
5. Observe for fever, dysuria, or a drop in blood pressure.
6. Administer medications to alleviate bladder spasms and/or lower back pain.

In addition to complete visual inspection of the bladder and urethra through the cystoscope, retrograde pyelography may also be performed. During this procedure the physician passes a small catheter through the cystoscope into the bladder that allows catheterizing of the ureters and renal pelvis. Urine specimens are then collected separately from each ureter. Radiopaque dye can be instilled into the renal pelvis while serial x-ray films are taken to examine the filling of the renal collecting system. Invasive examinations to visualize the bladder and urethra include retrograde cystograms, voiding cystourethrogram, and cystourethrogram. All of these studies involve the instillation of a radiopaque fluid into the bladder via a catheter (urethral or suprapubic). Serial x-ray films taken during these procedures will provide information regarding abnormalities in bladder mucosa, demonstrate vesicoureteral reflux, provide information regarding bladder function, and provide an assessment of the size and shape of the ureters. Nursing implications for this procedure are the same as those for the cystoscopy procedure.

Arteriogram (angiogram). The renal angiogram is an invasive radiographic procedure with radiopaque contrast material that outlines the vascular supply to the kidneys. Most frequently this procedure evaluates the arterial system; however, techniques to investigate the venous system (venogram) are available. Pretest nursing implications are similar to those for the IVP. Clients may be given a narcotic or antianxiety agent for relaxation before the examination.

Nursing implications after the angiogram include the following:

1. Monitor the client's vital signs hourly until stability is verified, and then advance the intervals to every 2 hours, then every 4 hours.
2. Ensure that the client maintains bed rest for 4 to 8 hours.
3. Check pulses and assess the circulation in the cannulated extremity.
4. Observe for bleeding, increased tenderness, or hematoma formation at the catheter insertion site for 24 hours.
5. Maintain a pressure dressing over the site for 24 hours.
6. Observe the client for possible delayed reactions to the contrast material.
7. Monitor the client's I&O, and report abnormalities in urine volume to the physician.

Urodynamic testing. Urodynamic testing is a group of tests that measure transport, elimination, and storage of urine in the lower urinary tract. The tests do not cause much pain, but they do require catheterization. A contraindication to testing is a urinary tract infection. Care after the procedures includes teaching the client the signs and symptoms of infection and to report to the physician if any of those signs and symptoms appear.

....

Successful critical thinking requires a synthesis of knowledge, experience, information gathered from clients, and critical thinking attitudes and standards. Clinical judgments require the nurse to anticipate what information is needed, to analyze the data, and then to make decisions regarding client care. The client expects competent and informed care. Mrs. Stone incorporates previous knowledge and experience in providing care for Mrs. Vallero.

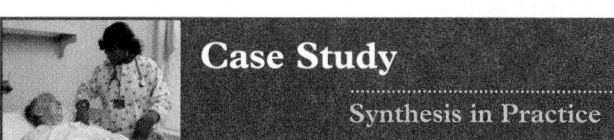

Case Study

Synthesis in Practice

As Mrs. Stone prepares to assess the client, she remembers that urinary problems are common in the elderly but that age alone does not cause incontinence. She recalls that clients with urinary retention may leak urine and therefore be misdiagnosed as incontinent. She knows clients generally should void at least every 6 to 8 hours and that Mrs. Vallero's problems last night with urination, her recent catheterization, and her decreased mobility since hospitalization could predispose her to retention or incontinence. In addition, she knows she will need to assess if Mrs. Vallero feels the urge to urinate, if she has gone to the bathroom to try to urinate, and to find out more about her normal urination patterns at home.

Previous clinical experience has taught Mrs. Stone that palpation of the abdomen can cause some discomfort. Mrs. Vallero grimaces slightly when her abdomen is palpated and says she's only got a little "dolor."

Because pneumonia and bed rest have left Mrs. Vallero in a weakened state, Mrs. Stone must be flexible and creative in designing a plan of care to meet the client's elimination needs. This plan needs to incorporate scheduled voiding, oral fluids, and increased physical activity.

▪ Nursing Diagnosis

The nurse's thorough assessment of the client's urinary function may identify defining characteristics that support actual or risk for elimination problems. Identification of the defining characteristics leads the nurse to select an appropriate diagnostic label. When the nurse is first using nursing diagnosis or is not sure what diagnoses to select, it is very helpful to read the definition of the diagnosis and to examine whether there is a match between the data collected and the defining character-

▪ NURSING DIAGNOSES FOR CLIENTS WITH INCONTINENCE

Body image disturbance
Incontinence, functional
Incontinence, reflex
Incontinence, stress
Incontinence, total
Incontinence, urge
Infection, risk for
Knowledge deficit
Pain
Self-care deficit, toileting
Skin integrity, impaired, risk for
Urinary elimination, altered
Urinary retention

istics. This step is also very helpful when the nursing diagnosis is based on incontinence.

There are five recognized diagnoses for incontinence (see nursing diagnoses box), and it is not easy for the beginning student to make a decision without looking for a match between data and defining characteristics. The differentiation between stress and urge incontinence is a common problem. In both, the client has an involuntary loss of urine, but the accuracy of data collection helps to identify the correct diagnosis. If the client loses urine after sneezing or coughing, then the diagnosis is stress incontinence. If the client reports that there was a strong urge to urinate just before the incontinence occurred, then the diagnosis is urge incontinence.

Associated problems require interventions that often have no direct effect on urinary elimination. For example, when the client has a *toileting self-care deficit related to limited lower extremity mobility,* appropriate nursing interventions provide the client a means of easy access to toileting facilities. However, if the nurse identifies the related factors in the aforementioned example to be loss of voluntary control of micturition, interventions would be selected to prevent incontinence. It is important to identify the correct related factors for a given nursing diagnosis because this will affect the selection of the appropriate nursing interventions.

▪ Planning

The nurse and client work together to establish ways of maintaining client involvement in nursing care and to maintain normal elimination patterns when possible (see care plan on p. 996). Reinforcement of good health habits that are already followed improves the likelihood for compliance with the plan of care. The nurse determines any assistive devices that will be required and the client's educational needs. Return demonstrations of psychomotor and self-care skills are performed by the

CASE STUDY NURSING CARE PLAN

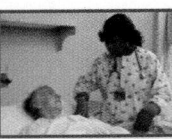

Urinary Retention

Assessment

Mrs. Vallero is **unable to void after catheter removal.** She has been catheterized once and 1100 ml of urine obtained. She complains of **dribbling** and being unable to urinate. She was **incontinent** on the last shift of a **small amount of urine.** The nursing assessment reveals a **distended bladder.**

Nursing Diagnosis

Urinary retention related to detrusor inadequacy secondary to catheterization.

Planning

Goal

Client will have normal micturition with complete bladder emptying by 2/28.

Expected Outcomes

Client will void within 8 hours.
Client will void 300 ml or more with each voiding.
Client's urine remains clear yellow.
Client is free of discomfort during voiding.
Client's bladder remains nondistended.

Implementation

Steps

1. Have client attempt voiding at regularly scheduled times.
2. Have client use bladder compression (Credé's method) during voiding.
3. Allow client to sit on toilet for 15 minutes to encourage second voiding.

4. Encourage fluids of 2000 ml/day.

Rationale

Training bladder can help reduce dribbling (Ebersole and Hess, 1994).
Credé's method helps to stimulate micturition and promotes bladder emptying.
Sitting on the toilet facilitates the use of the abdominal muscles and gravity to promote voiding.
Adequate fluids are necessary to ensure perfusion of the kidneys.

Evaluation

Measure and observe color of each voided specimen.
Palpate client's bladder every 4 hours and after each voiding.
Ask client about sensation to void, bladder fullness, and discomfort when voiding.

---

client to ensure adherence to procedures and accuracy in their performance.

Significant others are also included in planning and in teaching sessions. The nurse must identify who will be involved with the care of the client at home. The nurse's active and thoughtful role in planning these interventions will result in the client's progress toward improved urinary elimination.

In the hospital, planning care also includes preparations for discharge. The need for home health services should be explored and appropriate referrals made. Planning should include consideration of the client's home environment and normal elimination routines. The nurse should enlist the assistance of other disciplines in this planning process (e.g., social services) to explore family financial resources or other influences that may affect the discharge process. Community re-

sources like ostomy support groups for clients with incontinent diversions may be used.

Client-centered goals and outcomes should be established in collaboration with the client. A realistic client goal may be that the client has normal micturition with complete bladder emptying within 1 month. To achieve this goal, a number of outcomes may be identified; for example, the client will ingest at least 2000 ml of fluids per day, empty the bladder within 1 hour of drinking, and have less than 50 ml of residual urine within 1 month. Problems develop when the goal and outcomes are established without adequate assessment and collaboration with the client. The nurse may have assumed that the client can swallow and that the client understands why complete bladder emptying is desirable.

Box 35-2
Urinary Elimination Health Promotion/Restoration Activities

Adequate Hydration

A client with normal renal function who does not have heart disease or alterations requiring fluid restriction should drink 2000 to 2500 ml of fluid daily.

Micturition Habits

Ensure client comfort and privacy.
Allow sufficient time to void (at least 30 minutes).
Integrating the client's habits into the care plan fosters a more normal voiding pattern.
Offer the client use of toilet facilities if possible, avoiding bedpans.
Ensure access to toilet facilities.
Assist the client in the appropriate position for voiding (i.e, females—sitting, males—standing).

Personal Hygiene

Instruct female clients to cleanse the perineum and urethra from front to back after each voiding and bowel movement.
Clients prone to urinary tract infections should be encouraged to shower instead of bathe.

Complete Bladder Emptying

Clients who have difficulty starting or stopping the urine stream may benefit from exercises to strengthen pelvic muscles.

Credé's method of manual bladder compression helps to stimulate urination and manually expels urine when bladder tone is reduced.
Drug therapy alone or in conjunction with other therapies can be useful for treating problems of incontinence and retention.

Infection Prevention

Ensure adequate fluid intake.
Encourage good hand washing.
Prevent breaks in closed catheter drainage systems.
Follow tips for preventing infection in catheterized clients.
Teach client how to keep urine acidic. Acid urine tends to inhibit growth of microorganisms. Meats, eggs, whole-grain breads, cranberries, and prunes increase urine acidity.

Skin Integrity

The skin is the first barrier of defense.
The normal acidity of urine is irritating to the skin.
Washing with mild soap and warm water is the best way to remove urine from the skin.
After performing hygiene, dry clothing should be applied immediately on incontinent client.
Clients with external urinary devices should receive assistance in selecting appliances that fit appropriately. They should also be taught preventive skin care measures.

Implementation

Clients should know basic mechanisms for urine production and voiding. The nurse focuses on client education, normal micturition, complete bladder emptying, prevention of infection, skin integrity, and comfort.

Health promotion. Success of therapies aimed at optimizing normal urinary elimination depends in part on successful client education (Box 35-2). The nurse instructs clients about their specific elimination problems. For example, a client who practices poor hygiene will benefit from learning about normal sterility of the urinary tract and ways to prevent bacterial invasion of the urinary tract. It may also be useful to discuss the basic mechanism for urine production and voiding for clients with elimination alterations. Knowledge of factors that promote normal urine production and voiding can also help. Health promotion skills should always be the initial focal point of teaching (Box 35-3).

The nurse can easily incorporate teaching during delivery of care. For example, if the nurse is attempting to

---

BOX 35-3
Client Teaching for Urinary Elimination Problems

- Instruct client or care giver about observations to make regarding urinary output.
- Provide clients with pertinent signs and symptoms of infections.
- Frequently remind ambulatory clients about intake and output measurements.
- Reinforce correct perineal hygiene measures to reduce the risk of urinary tract infection.
- Determine client's knowledge of medications and provide instruction on medications that affect urination, color of urine, and urine volume.
- Instruct client and care giver regarding health promotion measures to prevent infection.

increase the client's fluid intake, a good time to discuss benefits is while giving fluids with medications or meals. The nurse may be more successful in teaching about perineal hygiene during a bath or while giving catheter care. The nurse can easily include family members in informal discussions.

Normal micturition

Stimulating the micturition reflex. The client's ability to void depends on feeling the urge to urinate, on being able to control the urethral sphincter, and on being able to relax. The nurse can foster relaxation and stimulate the reflex to void by helping clients to assume the normal position for voiding.

Females are better able to void in a squatting position. This position promotes contraction of the pelvic and intraabdominal muscles that assist in sphincter control and bladder contraction. If the client cannot use a toilet, the nurse positions her on a bedpan or bedside commode.

The male client voids more easily in the standing position. At times it may be necessary for one or more nurses to assist the male client to stand. If the client cannot reach a toilet, he may stand at the bedside and void into a **urinal** (a plastic or metal receptacle for urine) (Figure 35-3). Always determine mobility status before standing a client to void.

If the client is unable to stand at the bedside, the nurse may need to assist him to use the urinal in bed. When possible, the client should hold the urinal and position the penis in the urinal. If the client needs assistance, the nurse should position the penis completely within the urinal and hold the urinal in place or assist the client to hold the urinal. Make sure the penis is placed completely within the urinal to avoid urine spills.

Once the client has finished voiding, the nurse should remove the urinal and wash and dry the penis to prevent growth of microorganisms and to aid in preventing skin breakdown.

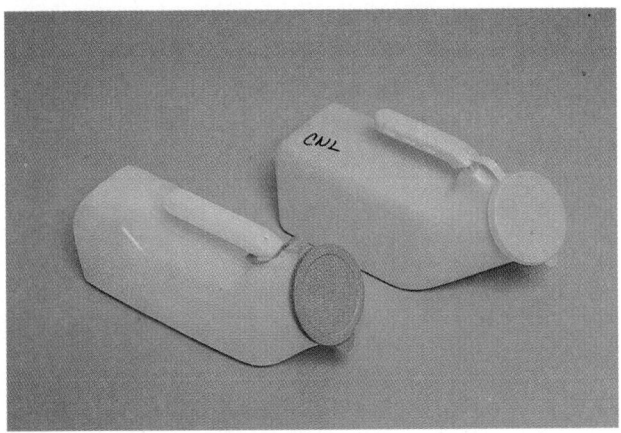

Figure 35-3. Types of male urinals.

Other measures to promote normal micturition include the use of sensory stimuli (e.g., turning running water on, putting a client's hand in a pan of warm water, or stroking the female client's inner thigh). Each tends to promote relaxation and the reflex to void.

Maintaining elimination habits. Many clients follow set routines of normal voiding. In a hospital or long-term care facility, the nurse's routines may conflict with those of the client. Integrating the client's habits into the care plan fosters a more normal voiding pattern.

The client should be given privacy and not be rushed. The nurse must assess the times when a client normally voids and offer the opportunity to use a toilet at those times. The nurse must also respond in a timely manner to the client's urge to urinate. Delay in assisting the client to the bathroom may interfere with normal micturition. Research has shown that promptly assisting clients to toileting facilities reduces incontinence when the clients were able to perceive the urge to void (Penn and others, 1994). Older adults may also require other special interventions owing to the aging process (Box 35-4).

Privacy is essential for normal voiding. If the client cannot reach the bathroom, the nurse makes sure the bedside area is private. In the home, the debilitated client may prefer using a bedside commode enclosed behind a partition or room divider. Some clients are embarrassed by the sound of voiding. Running water or flushing the toilet masks the sound effectively. Young children are often unable to void in the presence of persons other than parents.

Comfort is an important factor in facilitating voiding. Therefore activities that increase client comfort may aid urination. If the client typically uses special measures to void (e.g., reading or listening to music), the nurse should encourage their continued use at home and, when possible, in the health care setting. There are a number of commodes on the market that have arms or adjustable heights that make access not only easier but possible in some cases (Smith, 1994). Toilet seat extenders are used for clients with arthritis or after a total hip replacement to aid the client in sitting and in rising off the toilet.

The nurse should encourage appropriate personal hygiene including hand washing and perineal care (see Chapters 25 and 29). Genitourinary infections are second only to respiratory infections. Bacteria are the most common cause of these infections, and *E. coli* invasion through the urethra is the most frequent organism and route (Gray, 1992).

Maintaining adequate fluid intake. A simple method of promoting normal micturition is maintenance of a good fluid intake. A client with normal renal function who does not have heart disease or alterations requiring fluid restriction should drink 2000 to 2500 ml of fluid daily. When fluid intake is increased, excreted

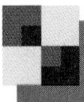

- The older client may experience urinary incontinence problems as a result of mobility problems or neurological impairments. The nurse should be aware of these problems and arrange scheduled toileting and promote access to toileting facilities.
- Older clients may be prone to physiological urinary retention as a result of diminished bladder muscle tone, capacity, and contractility (Penn and others, 1994). This may increase their risk toward large postvoid residuals with a concomitant risk of frequent infections. Teaching sessions should include techniques to stimulate the voiding reflex, as well as provide for complete bladder emptying and prevention from infections.
- Older clients may also experience delayed sensations to void, resulting in urgency. The nurse educates the client regarding any factor that interferes with the client's perceptions to void (e.g., medications, emotional disturbances, or decreased fluid intake).
- Older adults experience the following physiological changes that make them more prone to incontinence. During teaching sessions, the nurse considers these normal physiological changes to plan appropriate interventions:

    Decreased renal blood flow secondary to decreased cardiac output.

    Decreased ability to concentrate urine secondary to decrease in nephron mass.

    Decreased tone of the pelvic floor muscles.
- Older adults in institutionalized settings (e.g., hospitals, nursing homes) are at the greatest risk for experiencing incontinence problems.
- Older adults may also experience sensory alterations such as diminished vision, which may delay attempts to locate toilet facilities (Ebersole and Hess, 1994). During teaching sessions, the nurse orients clients to their environment with special emphasis on the location of toileting facilities, bedpans or urinals, and assistive devices (e.g., walkers, call light).

TABLE 35-5
Treatment Options for Incontinence

Type	Treatments
Total	Protective undergarments
	External or internal catheters
	Artificial sphincter
Functional	Bladder training
	Protective undergarments
	Environmental alterations
	Indwelling and external catheters
	Skin care
Stress	Conditioning (Kegel) exercises
	Estrogen replacement
	Alpha-adrenergic agonists
	Surgery
	Intravaginal electrical stimulation
	Bladder neck suspension surgery
	Artificial sphincter
	Penile clamp
Urge	Anticholinergic drug therapy
	Biofeedback
	Treatment of associated urinary tract infection
	Treatment of associated vaginitis
	Incontinence garments
Reflex (upper moto-neuron lesion)	Intermittent self-catheterization
	Bladder training
	Electrical stimulation

urine flushes out solutes or particles that may collect in the urinary system. Because a client probably is not accustomed to drinking 2500 ml of water daily, the nurse should offer fluids the client prefers. At home it may help to set a schedule for drinking fluids (e.g., with meals or medications). A simple trick is to encourage the client to drink a cup of water after voiding. Voiding becomes a natural cue to drinking fluids. A rigid schedule is not needed. To prevent nocturia, fluids should be avoided 2 hours before bedtime.

Promotion of bladder emptying. Clients with urinary retention and incontinence are frequently unable to empty the bladder. Incontinence is a major nursing challenge. Choosing from a variety of treatment options, the client and nurse work together to design interventions that promote continence or control wetness (Table 35-5).

Strengthening pelvic floor muscles. Clients who have difficulty starting and stopping the urine stream may benefit from exercises to strengthen pelvic muscles. The client may practice Kegel exercises anytime and anywhere. The client first learns to feel the pelvic muscles. The client does this with each voiding.

Then while sitting or standing, the client tries to tighten the muscles around the anus without tensing leg, buttock, or abdominal muscles. This maneuver allows the client to identify the posterior muscles of the pelvic floor.

Modified sit-ups may also aid bladder control by strengthening the abdominal muscles. Starting with a few at a time and gradually increasing the number of repetitions will improve pelvic muscle strength.

Manual bladder compression. By manually compressing the walls of the bladder, a person can improve bladder emptying. Credé's method helps to stimulate micturition and manually expels urine when bladder tone is reduced. The client places both hands flat on the abdomen below the umbilicus and above the symphysis pubis with the fingers pointed down toward the bladder's dome. The client compresses the hands downward against the bladder's walls while tightening the perineum, contracting the abdominal wall, and holding the breath. When urine is in the bladder, Credé's compression causes the sensation of bladder fullness. The maneuver also promotes bladder emptying by relaxing the urethral sphincter.

Drug therapy. Drug therapy alone or in conjunction with other therapies can be useful for treating problems of incontinence and retention. Drugs are used to increase bladder emptying (e.g., retention), bladder capacity (e.g., urge incontinence), and sphincter tone (e.g., stress incontinence).

When the bladder empties, the detrusor muscle contracts in response to stimulation. Incomplete bladder emptying results from impaired innervation or weakness of the detrusor muscle. As a result, the client experiences retention and overflow incontinence. Therapy with cholinergic drugs is aimed at increasing bladder contraction and improving emptying. Bethanechol (Urecholine) stimulates nerves to increase bladder wall contraction and relax the sphincter. It can be given subcutaneously or orally. Alpha-adrenergic agents such as phenoxybenzamine can also be used to improve bladder emptying. The effect of the drug can be augmented by using Credé's method or other measures for stimulating micturition.

If urine is in the bladder, **urge incontinence** may occur as a result of hyperactivity of the bladder muscle that suddenly increases pressure. Uncontrolled bladder contractions may be caused by local irritants such as stones or infection. Anticholinergic drugs (e.g., propantheline) reduce incontinence by blocking contractility of the bladder. These drugs should be used with caution in clients with heart disease, glaucoma, high blood pressure, kidney and liver disease, and urinary retention. Direct smooth-muscle relaxants may also be used. These drugs work by decreasing the contractility of the bladder. Oxybutynin is a commonly used drug in this category. Client instructions are similar to those for propantheline (Urinary Incontinence Guideline Panel, 1992).

To treat stress incontinence, alpha-adrenergic drugs may be used. Phenylpropanolamine is the drug commonly used. This medication along with pelvic strengthening exercises has been found to work in some women. Estrogen therapy has also been used to decrease stress incontinence (Urinary Incontinence Guideline Panel, 1992).

Acute care.
Often clients need care in hospitals, clinics, or their homes for urinary conditions of sudden onset. One of the most frequent treatments is urinary catheterization.

Catheterization. **Catheterization** of the bladder involves introducing a rubber or plastic tube through the urethra and into the bladder. The catheter provides a continuous flow of urine in clients unable to control micturition or in clients with obstructions. Because bladder catheterization carries a high risk of urinary tract infection, the nurse first relies on other interventions to empty the bladder.

Types of catheterization. Intermittent catheterizations and indwelling catheterization are the two forms of catheter insertion. With the intermittent technique, a single-use straight catheter is introduced for a short period to drain the bladder (5 to 10 minutes). When the bladder is empty, the nurse removes the catheter. Intermittent catheterization can be repeated as necessary. An indwelling or Foley catheter remains in place until a client is able to void completely and voluntarily. It may be necessary to change indwelling catheters periodically.

The single-use straight catheter has a single lumen with a small opening approximately 1.3 cm ($\frac{1}{2}$ inch) from the tip. Urine drains from the tip, through the lumen, and to a receptacle. An indwelling Foley catheter has a small inflatable balloon that encircles the catheter just below the tip. When inflated, the balloon rests against the bladder outlet to anchor the catheter in place. The indwelling catheter also has as many as two or three separate lumens within the body of the catheter. One lumen drains urine through the catheter to a collecting tube. A second lumen carries sterile water to and from the balloon when it is inflated or deflated. A third (optional) lumen may be used to instill fluids or drugs into the bladder. A three-lumen catheter is most often inserted when irrigations of the catheter are anticipated. These three-way catheters are often used with male clients who have had a transurethral resection of the prostate.

Indications for use. When the need for catheterization is short term or to minimize infection in clients chronically unable to void, the intermittent method is best. Intermittent catheterization is indicated in the following situations:

1. For immediate relief of acute bladder distention
2. For long-term management of clients with incompetent bladders
3. To obtain a sterile urine specimen
4. To assess for residual urine after voiding
5. To instill a medication

Done correctly, intermittent catheterization has a lower risk of infection than indwelling catheterization. However, if a client requires frequent intermittent catheterization, an indwelling catheter may be preferable. Indwelling catheterization is indicated in the following situations:

1. Obstruction to urine outflow

2. Clients undergoing surgical procedures involving the urinary tract or surrounding structures
3. To prevent urethral obstruction from blood clots
4. To accurately record output in critically ill or comatose clients
5. To prevent skin breakdown in incontinent comatose clients
6. To provide continuous or intermittent bladder irrigations

Catheter insertion. Urethral catheterization requires a physician's order. The nurse must use strict sterile technique (see Chapter 25). The steps for inserting an indwelling and a single-use straight catheter are the same. The difference lies in the procedure taken to inflate the indwelling catheter balloon and secure the catheter. The nurse can collect needed specimens while inserting an indwelling catheter. Skill 35-1 lists steps for performing female and male urethral catheterization.

Closed drainage systems. After an indwelling catheter is inserted, it is necessary to maintain a closed urinary drainage system to minimize the risk of infection. Urinary drainage bags are plastic and can hold approximately 2000 ml of urine. The bag should hang on the bed frame without touching the floor. When the client ambulates, the nurse or client carries the bag below the level of the client's bladder. The nurse should never raise a drainage bag and tubing above the level of the client's bladder. Urine in the bag and tubing is a medium for bacteria, and infection can develop if urine is allowed to reflux (return to the bladder).

Most drainage bags contain an antireflux valve to prevent urine from reentering the drainage tubing and contaminating the bladder. A spigot at the base of the bag provides a means for the nurse to empty the bag. The spigot should always be clamped, except during emptying, and tucked into the protective pouch at the bag's side.

Some urinary drainage bags have special urometers between the collection tubing and bag. The **urometer** is a clear graduated cylinder that measures small volumes (100 to 200 ml) of urine. The urometer is useful for clients requiring frequent urinary output measurements. The nurse simply notes the volume of urine in the urometer and opens the valve that allows urine from the urometer to enter the drainage bag. When urine from the drainage bag is measured, it is best to use a separate graduated receptacle for accuracy.

To keep the drainage system patent the nurse checks for kinks or bends in the tubing, avoids positioning the client on drainage tubing, prevents tubing from becoming dependent, and observes for clots or sediment that may occlude the tubing.

Routine catheter care. Clients with indwelling catheters require specific perineal hygiene care to reduce the risk of urinary tract infection. Any secretions or encrustation at the catheter insertion site must be completely removed. Perineal care and the cleansing of the first 2 inches of the catheter every 8 hours are minimally expected. These measures are often referred to as catheter care. The use of powders or lotions on the perineum is contraindicated because of the risk of growth of microorganisms, which may ascend the urinary tract. Clients who are catheterized and who are incontinent of stool will need cleaning after bowel movements.

Provide perineal care (see Skill 29-2), and assess the urethral meatus and surrounding tissues for inflammation, swelling, and discharge. Note the amount, color, odor, and consistency of discharge to determine local infection and status of hygiene.

Replace, as necessary, the adhesive tape or multipurpose tube holder that anchors the catheter to the client's leg or abdomen, and remove adhesive residue from the skin. Secure the catheter, thus reducing the risk of the catheter's being pulled on and exposing the portion that was in the urethra. This also prevents drag on the catheter and avoids pressure from the balloon on the bladder floor. Replace the urinary tubing and collection bag if necessary, adhering to principles of surgical asepsis. The urinary tubing and collection bag should be changed if there are signs of leakage, odor, or sediment buildup. Check the drainage tubing and bag to ensure that no tubing loops hang below the level of the bladder, the tube is coiled and secured onto the bed linen, the tube is not kinked or clamped, and the drainage bag is positioned on the bed frame.

Removal of indwelling catheter. Removal of a retention catheter is a skill requiring clean technique. If the retention catheter balloon is not fully deflated, its removal can result in trauma and subsequent swelling of the urethral meatus, and urinary retention can occur. If the catheter was in place for more than several days, the client may experience dysuria resulting from inflammation of the urethral canal. Because of decreased bladder muscle tone, the client may urinate frequently or experience urinary retention.

Before removing a catheter, the nurse checks agency policy or the physician's orders to determine if a sterile specimen is required. To remove a catheter, the nurse requires a clean disposable towel, clean gloves, and a sterile syringe the same size as the volume of solution within the catheter's inflated balloon. The end of each catheter contains a label that denotes the volume of solution (5 to 30 ml) within a balloon. The nurse positions the client in the same position as during catheterization.

Remove the adhesive tape or Velcro tube anchoring the catheter. Cleanse any residue from the skin, and insert the hub of the syringe into the inflation valve (balloon port). Aspirate the entire amount of fluid used to inflate the balloon, and then pull the catheter out smoothly and slowly to prevent trauma to urethral mucosa. If resistance is met as the catheter is pulled, stop because the balloon is probably still inflated. Wrap the contaminated catheter in a waterproof pad, and unhook the collection bag and drainage tubing from the bed. Provide perineal care following removal, and document the removal.

The catheter causes inflammation of the urethral canal. The nurse notes the time and amount of the client's first void. Often the client's I&O are monitored until voiding is established. If more than 8 hours elapse before the client voids, it may be necessary to catheterize the client again to determine if there is a blockage, retention, or suppression of urine. If the volume of urine voided is small, residual urine may be in the bladder.

Alternatives to catheterization. To avoid the risks associated with catheters inserted through the urethra, alternatives for urinary drainage exist. **Suprapubic catheters** are inserted surgically into the bladder through the lower abdomen above the symphysis pubis (Figure 35-4). While most successfully used for short time periods with clients who have had gynecological and bladder surgery, the suprapubic catheter may be used in elderly males who require a long-term alternative to urinary catheterization. As with indwelling urinary catheters, the suprapubic catheter predisposes the client to urinary tract infections, but the incidence may be lower. Spread of infection to the kidneys may require removing the catheter. The advantages of a suprapubic catheter for clients are that they may void naturally when the catheter is clamped and it is more comfortable (Warren, 1994). Daily care will depend on policy, but the cleaning and dressing of the site are similar to care of any surgical drain (see Chapter 40).

The condom catheter is suitable for incontinent or comatose male clients who still have complete and spontaneous bladder emptying (Skill 35-2).

The condom catheter poses little risk of infection. Infections, however, can result from buildup of secretions around the urethra, trauma to the urethral meatus, or buildup of pressure in the outflow tubing.

The nurse should change a condom catheter daily to check for skin irritation. The nurse cleans the urethral meatus and penis thoroughly with each catheter change. Twisting of the condom at the drainage tube attachment irritates the skin and obstructs urine outflow. The drainage tubing must be checked frequently for patency. For a man with a retracted foreskin, maintaining the intactness of a conventional condom catheter may prove difficult. Special devices are available to help alleviate this problem (Figure 35-5). Manufacturers' guidelines for product application should be consulted.

External incontinence devices for women are more difficult to design and fit (Smith, 1994). Women may wear the newer absorbent pads and adult disposable undergarments. However, wearers of these disposable undergarments report skin irritation, odor, and increased infection rate. For the active incontinent woman, these devices are options that can promote more independence.

Restorative care. Returning to normal micturition often means preventing complications from treatment. Many restorative functions are related to preventing infection after catheterization, promoting comfort, and preventing skin breakdown if the client is incontinent.

Preventing infection. Maintaining a closed urinary drainage system is important in infection control. A break in the system can lead to introduction of microorganisms. Sites at risk are at the place of catheter insertion, drainage bag, spigot, tube junction, and junction of tube and bag (Figure 35-6). In addition, the nurse monitors the patency of the system to prevent pooling of urine. Urine in the drainage bag is an excellent medium

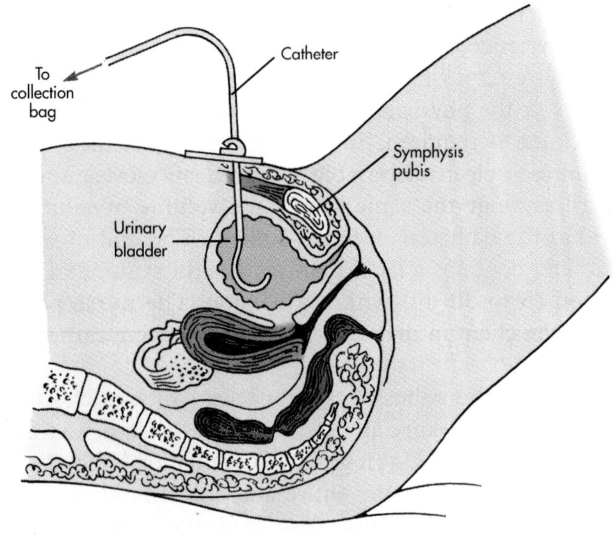

Figure 35-4. Placement of suprapubic catheter above the symphysis pubis. (From Elkin M and others: *Nursing interventions and clinical skills*, St. Louis, 1996, Mosby.)

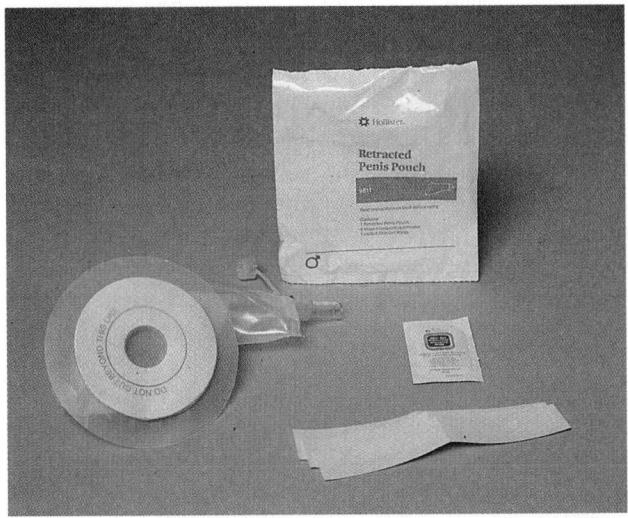

Figure 35-5. Retracted penis-pouch external urinary device.

Applying a Condom Catheter

Delegation Considerations

The skill of applying a condom catheter can be delegated to unlicensed assistive personnel.

- Ensure that care provider knows Standard Precaution guidelines relating to body fluids.
- Caution care provider to be sensitive to the privacy needs of the client.
- Clarify that skin of penile shaft is intact and free from swelling, redness, or open lesions before condom catheter is applied.
- Clarify the care provider's understanding of how to apply the adhesive strip that secures the condom catheter.

Equipment

- Condom catheter kit
    Rubber condom sheath (appropriate size)
    Strip of elastic adhesive
    Skin preparation
- Urinary collection bag with drainage tubing or leg bag and straps
- Basin with warm water and soap
- Towels and washcloths
- Bath blanket
- Nonsterile disposable gloves
- Scissors and/or safety razor

STEPS	RATIONALE
1. Assess urinary elimination patterns, client's ability to voluntarily urinate, and continence.	Clients who are incontinent are at risk for skin breakdown.
2. Assess mental status of client so appropriate teaching related to condom catheter can be implemented.	Some male clients may be incontinent only at night. Teaching can be implemented to instruct client on self-application.
3. Assess condition of penis.	Provides baseline to compare changes in condition of skin after condom catheter application.
4. Assess client's knowledge of the purpose of a condom catheter.	Reveals need for client instruction.
5. Explain procedure to client.	Reduces anxiety and promotes cooperation.
6. Arrange for extra nursing personnel to assist with moving dependent client.	Promotes client safety and proper use of body mechanics by nurse.
7. Wash hands.	Reduces transmission of microorganisms.
8. Provide privacy by closing room door or bedside curtain.	Maintains client's self-esteem.
9. Raise bed to appropriate working height. Raise side rail on opposite side of bed, and lower side rail on working side.	Promotes use of good body mechanics and client safety.
10. Assist client into supine position. Place bath blanket over upper torso. Fold sheets so lower extremities are covered; only genitalia should be exposed.	Promotes comfort; draping prevents unnecessary exposure of body parts.
11. Prepare urinary drainage collection bag and tubing (see illustration). Clamp off drainage bag port. Secure collection bag to bed frame; bring drainage tubing up through side rails onto bed. Prepare leg bag for connection to condom if necessary.	Provides easy access to drainage equipment after condom catheter is in place.

Continued

Step 11

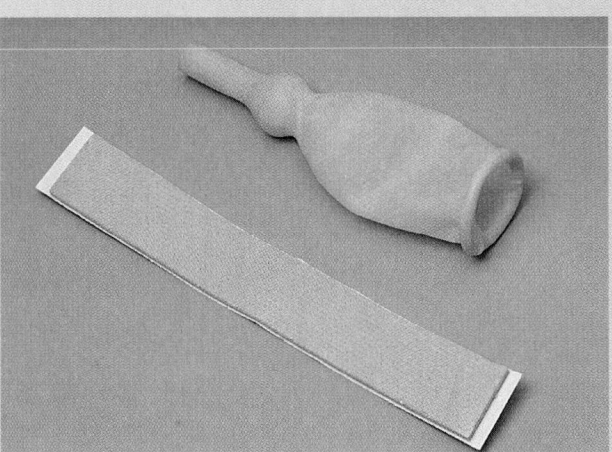

⋯⋯⋯ Skill 35-2—cont'd
Applying a Condom Catheter

STEPS	RATIONALE
12. Apply disposable gloves. Provide perineal care (see Skill 29-2), and dry thoroughly.	Removes irritating secretions. Rubber sheath of condom rolls onto dry skin more easily.
13. Clip hair at base of penis. In some cases shaving the hair at the base of the penis may be necessary.	Hair adheres to condom and is pulled during condom removal or may get caught in rubber as condom catheter is applied.
14. Apply skin preparation to penis, and allow to dry. If client is uncircumcised, return foreskin to normal position.	Skin preparation has an alcohol base. Evaporation is necessary to prevent irritation.
15. With nondominant hand, grasp penis along shaft. With dominant hand, hold condom sheath at tip of penis and smoothly roll sheath onto penis.	Prepares penis for easy condom placement.

CRITICAL DECISION POINT

Allow 2.5 to 5 cm (1 to 2 inches) of space between tip of glans penis and end of condom catheter (see illustration).

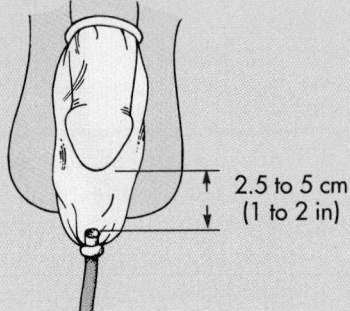

2.5 to 5 cm (1 to 2 in)

16. Spiral wrap penile shaft with strip of elastic adhesive. With some brands of catheters the adhesive strip is applied before the condom is applied. Do not use any tape because it may impede circulation.	Condom must be secured firmly so it is snug and stays on but not tight enough to cause constriction of blood flow. Strip should be spiral wrapped and not overlap itself. Tapes other than that provided by manufacturer will not provide the flexibility needed for spiral wrap and may impair circulation to the penis.
17. Connect drainage tubing to end of condom catheter. Be sure condom is not twisted. Catheter can be connected to large-volume bag or leg bag (see illustration).	Allows urine to be collected and measured. Keeps client dry. Twisted condom obstructs urine flow.
18. Place excess coiling of tubing on bed, and secure to bottom sheet.	Promotes free drainage of urine.
19. Place client in safe, comfortable position. Lower bed, and place side rails accordingly.	Promotes safety and comfort.

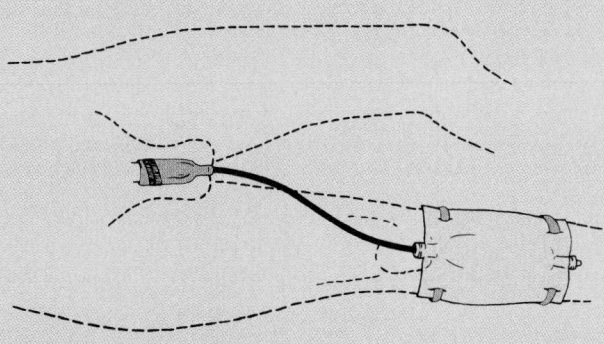

Step 17

STEPS	RATIONALE
20. Dispose of contaminated supplies, and wash hands.	Reduces spread of microorganisms.
21. Observe urinary drainage.	Determines if normal voiding is occurring.
22. Inspect penis with condom catheter in place within 30 minutes after application. Look for swelling and discoloration, and ask client if there is any discomfort.	Determines if catheter has been applied incorrectly.
23. Remove and change condom and inspect skin on penile shaft for signs of breakdown or irritation at least daily when hygiene is performed and when condom is reapplied.	Indicates if condom or urine is causing irritation or if adhesive is too restrictive. Frequent assessment of circulation of glans penis is important to determine if condom has been applied too tightly.

Recording and Reporting

- Report and record pertinent information: condom application, condition of skin, voiding pattern.
- Monitor I&O as indicated.

Home Care Considerations

- If leg bag is used, assess leg every 8 hours for circulatory impairment. Switch to a drainage bag at night.
- Teach client that a collection bag that fills completely may put unnecessary tension on the catheter and contribute to problems keeping the catheter intact (Smith, 1994).

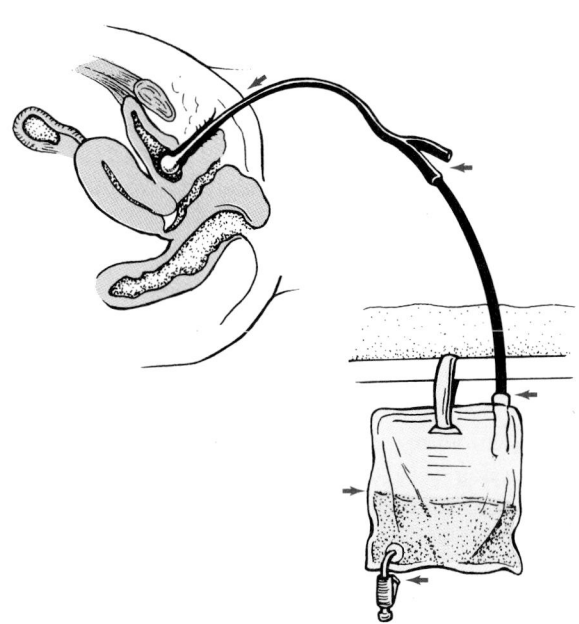

Figure 35-6. Potential sites for introduction of infection.

for microorganism growth. Bacteria can travel up drainage tubing to grow in pools of urine. Therefore it is important to prevent the abnormal backward flow of urine **(urinary reflux).** If this urine flows back into the bladder, an infection will probably develop. Box 35-5 gives suggestions for ways to prevent infections in catheterized clients.

Promotion of comfort. Clients with urinary alterations can be uncomfortable as a result of the symptoms of urinary problems. Frequent or unpredictable voiding, dysuria, and painful distention are sources of discomfort.

The incontinent client gains comfort from having clean, dry clothing. When stress incontinence is the problem, a protective pad or sanitary belt offers protection against soiling. Wet clothing adheres to the skin and can cause rubbing and irritation.

Dysuria may be relieved by giving urinary analgesics that act on the urethral and bladder mucosa. Phenazopyridine helps to relieve dysuria, burning, and itching. It comes combined with sulfonamide antibiotics in preparations such as Azo Gantanol and Azo Gantrisin. The sulfonamide provides additional antibacterial action. Clients taking drugs with phenazopyridine should be aware that their urine may appear orange and their clothing may be stained. They must drink large amounts of fluids to prevent toxicity from the sulfonamides and to maintain optimal flow through the urinary system.

Box 35-5
Tips for Preventing Infection in Catheterized Clients

Follow good hand-washing techniques.

Do not allow the spigot on the drainage bag to touch a contaminated surface.

Do not open the drainage system at connection points to obtain specimens or measure urine.

If the drainage tubing becomes disconnected, do not touch the ends of the catheter or tubing. Wipe the ends of the tube with antiseptic solution before reconnecting.

Each client should have a separate receptacle for measuring urine to prevent cross-contamination.

Prevent pooling of urine and reflux of urine into the bladder. Avoid raising the drainage bag above the level of the bladder.

Avoid allowing any dependent loops of tubing.

If it is necessary to raise the bag during transfer of the client to a bed or stretcher, clamp the tubing.

Before client exercises or ambulates, drain all urine from tubing into bag.

Avoid prolonged clamping or kinking of the tubing (except during bladder conditioning).

Empty the drainage bag at least every 8 hours.

Remove the catheter as soon as possible after conferring with physician.

Tape the catheter to secure it in place, noting specific guidelines regarding the male client's taping procedure.

Perform routine perineal hygiene every shift and after defecation.

Always ask clients about allergies to sulfa before giving these drugs.

If the client has local discomfort from an inflamed urethra, a warm sitz bath may provide pain relief. The warm water soothes inflamed tissues near the urethral meatus by improving blood supply. The client is often relaxed after a sitz bath, so voiding occurs easily. The client should be encouraged to void in the sitz bath if the urge occurs (see Chapter 29).

The pain of distention cannot be relieved unless the client is able to empty the bladder. Methods for stimulating micturition may be the only sources of pain relief.

Maintenance of skin integrity. The normal acidity of urine is irritating to the skin. When urine becomes alkaline, encrustation or precipitate collects on the skin, fostering breakdown. Continuous exposure of the skin to urine leads to gradual maceration and excoriation. Washing with mild soap and warm water is the best way to remove urine from the skin. Body lotion keeps the skin moisturized and provides a barrier to the urine.

Clients who wet their clothing should receive a clean set of clothes after each voiding.

When the skin becomes irritated or inflamed, the physician may prescribe a cream or spray containing steroids to reduce inflammation (e.g., triamcinolone [Kenalog]). If fungal growth develops, the antifungal drug nystatin (Mycostatin), available in cream or powder form, is effective.

The client with a ureterostomy has a special hygiene problem because urine drains from the ostomy site continuously. The drainage pouch or appliance frequently becomes moist and slips from the skin. Continual oozing of urine around the stoma causes skin breakdown. Skin barriers provide a layer of protection between the skin and ostomy pouch. When urine leaks, it frequently covers the outer skin barrier. An enterostomal therapist can help the client select an ostomy appliance that fits snugly against the skin's surface around the stoma (see Chapter 36).

◼ Evaluation

Client care. To evaluate the care plan the nurse uses the expected outcomes developed during planning to determine whether interventions were effective. This evaluation process is a dynamic one. The nurse uses this information to monitor the client's progress and direct future interventions. The optimal goal is the client's ability to urinate voluntarily without dysuria, urgency, or frequency. The client's urine should be an amber color, clear, without abnormal constituents, and within the normal range of pH and specific gravity.

The nurse can also evaluate specific outcomes designed to demonstrate normal urinary function and prevent complications of urinary alterations. Has the client's intake been at least 2000 ml? Is the bladder distended? Is there less than 50 ml of residual urine on the second voiding? Does urinary output equal fluid intake? Are there a reduced number of incontinent episodes? Is the urine culture showing negative bacterial growth? Does the client use correct hand-washing techniques? Are there any areas of skin breakdown around the perineum, stoma, or condom?

As nurses become more comfortable with the roles of client advocate and primary nurse, the delivery of quality care becomes a paramount goal. To this end, nurses are actively involved in developing methods to systematically evaluate the nursing process. Nursing research is being conducted to validate nursing interventions. Quality improvement is evolving as a tool to evaluate nursing care delivery. Its goal is to ensure the delivery of competent, state-of-the-art nursing care with positive outcomes for each client.

Client expectations. Control over urination is taken for granted until it is lost. Clients report that it is degrading and they feel like a baby when they lose control over voiding. To that end, evaluation of care from the incontinent client's standpoint centers around maintaining a level of dryness that is personally satisfactory. Clients want to have control, and to that outcome they should be able to express confidence in utilizing triggering mechanisms to initiate voiding.

In clients who have a urinary tract infection, pain, urgency, and frequency rule their life. Clients who have an infection will be satisfied with their care if they can report an absence or decrease in their symptoms. Can the client void without dysuria? Can the client sleep and carry out activities of daily living with lessened or no discomfort?

For all clients with urinary problems, lack of privacy is a potential issue. Did they feel that staff were considerate, and did the staff protect their privacy? Clients will also evaluate whether they were included in the planning of their care. Were they able to tell you the important information about their habits? Did you consider that information when you suggested a plan of care or implemented an intervention?

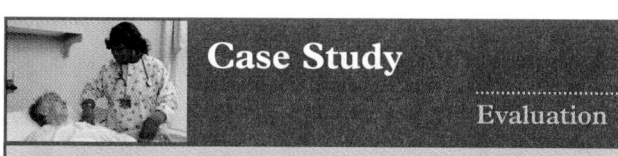

Case Study

Evaluation

Mrs. Stone and her instructor talk with Mrs. Vallero and explain that she probably needs to be catheterized again. She asks to try to "go" and nods to the bathroom. Mrs. Stone suggests that she sit for at least 15 minutes and leave the water running in the sink. The nurse also shows Mrs. Vallero how to push on her abdomen after she is sitting in the bathroom. Mrs. Vallero was able to void after 5 minutes.

Documentation Note
Client moved slowly to the bathroom. Her gait was steady, slow, and slightly stooped. Breathing was even and non-labored, and as she sat on the toilet, she said, "I'm ready." Mrs. Vallero used manual bladder compression and turned the water on in the sink. She voided 1300 ml of clear, pale yellow urine. Stated that she felt her bladder was empty. Client returned to bed. No bladder distention to palpation.

Key Terms

bacteriuria	stress incontinence
catheterization	suprapubic catheter
continent pouch	total incontinence
dysuria	urge incontinence
functional incontinence	ureterostomy
glomerulus	urinal
graduated measuring	urinary diversion
container	urinary incontinence
hematuria	urinary reflux
micturition	urinary retention
nephrons	urine hat
nosocomial	urometer
proteinuria	urosepsis
reflex incontinence	voiding
residual urine	

■ Key Concepts ■

Micturition or voiding is influenced by voluntary control from higher brain centers and involuntary control from the spinal cord.

Symptoms common to urinary disturbances include urgency, dysuria, polyuria, oliguria, and difficulty in starting the urinary stream.

When collected properly, a clean-voided urine specimen does not contain bacteria picked up from the urethral meatus.

A client can better understand the importance of perineal hygiene by knowing that the urinary tract is normally sterile.

Methods of promoting the micturition reflex assist clients in sensing the urge to urinate and controlling urethral sphincter relaxation.

An increased fluid intake results in urine formation that flushes particles and solutes from the urinary system.

Incontinence is classified as acute, urge, stress, overflow, or functional. Each type of incontinence has specific nursing interventions.

An indwelling urinary catheter remains in the bladder for an extended period, making the risk of infection greater than with intermittent catheterization.

Closed drainage systems deliver sterile solutions and medication to the bladder. Strict asepsis is necessary when caring for a client with a closed bladder drainage system.

Because urine drains almost continuously from a ureterostomy, there is risk of skin breakdown around a stoma site.

A primary function of the elimination process is fluid balance.

Critical Thinking Activities

1. Six hours after removal of an indwelling catheter you are checking on your client and she states her bladder feels full. She says she has only minimal incisional discomfort (1 on pain scale of 1 to 5) and demands client-controlled analgesia of morphine. The patient is 1 day post total abdominal hysterectomy and bilateral salpingo-oophorectomy. This is the second postoperative day. Her I&O balanced in the first 24 hours. She has no intravenous fluids and has had 1000 ml of oral intake this day. At 11 AM when her Foley catheter was removed, there was 700 ml in the bag. She has a midline dressing on her lower abdomen and no drainage tubes. What assessments would you make to determine bladder status? What interventions would you implement to enhance urination?

2. You are on a home visit to a client who is using a condom catheter. His wife, who is the care giver, tells you the "darn thing never stays on." What problems might cause the condom not to stay on? What assessments of the client do you need to make to determine the cause? If the catheter was applied incorrectly by the wife, what steps can be taken to ensure she understands how to do the procedure?

References

Colling J: An update on the AHCPR guideline implementation, *Nurse Pract Forum* 5(3):134, 1994.

Consumer version: clinical practice guidelines, AHCPR Publication No. 92-0038, Rockville, Md, 1996, Agency for Health Care Policy and Research, Public Health Services, U.S. Department of Health and Human Services.

Ebersole P, Hess P: *Toward health aging,* ed 4, St. Louis, 1994, Mosby.

Elkin M and others: *Nursing interventions and clinical skills,* St. Louis, 1996, Mosby.

Foreman M, Zane D: Nursing strategies for acute confusion in elders, *Am J Nurs* 96(4):44, 1996.

Gray M: *Genitourinary disorders,* St. Louis, 1992, Mosby.

McCance KL, Huether SE: *Pathophysiology: the biologic basis for disease in adults and children,* ed 2, St. Louis, 1994, Mosby.

Palmer S and others: *Infection control,* El Paso, Tex, 1996, Skidmore-Roth.

Penn C and others: Assessment of urinary incontinence, *J Gerontol Nurs* 22(1):8, 1994.

Razor B: Continent urinary reservoirs, *Semin Oncol Nurs* 9(4):272, 1993.

Smith D: Devices for continence, *Nurse Pract Forum* 5(3):186, 1994.

Sueppel C: Rapid or slow decompression, *Urol Nurs* 15(2):64, 1995.

Urinary Incontinence Guideline Panel: *Urinary incontinence in adults: clinical practice guidelines,* AHCPR Publication No. 92-0038, Rockville, Md, March 1992, Agency for Health Care Policy and Research, Public Health Services, U.S. Department of Health and Human Services.

Warren J: Catheter-associated bacteriuria in long term care facilities, *Infection Control Hosp Epidemiol* 15(8):557, 1994.

Webb ML: Urinary incontinence in younger women, *Nurse Pract Forum* 5(3):164, 1994.

Williams M and others: Urinary retention in hospitalized women, *J Gerontol Nurs* 19(2):7, 1993.

36

Bowel Elimination

OBJECTIVES

Mastery of content in this chapter will enable the student to:

- Define the key terms listed.
- Discuss the role of gastrointestinal organs in digestion and elimination.
- Explain the physiology of normal defecation.
- List and discuss psychological and physiological factors that influence the elimination process.
- Describe common physiological alterations in elimination.
- Assess a client's elimination pattern.
- Perform a guaiac test for occult blood.
- List nursing diagnoses related to alterations in elimination.
- Describe nursing implications for common diagnostic examinations of the gastrointestinal tract.
- Administer an enema.
- List nursing measures aimed at promoting normal elimination and defecation.
- Discuss the relationship between the structure and function of a bowel diversion and nursing care required.

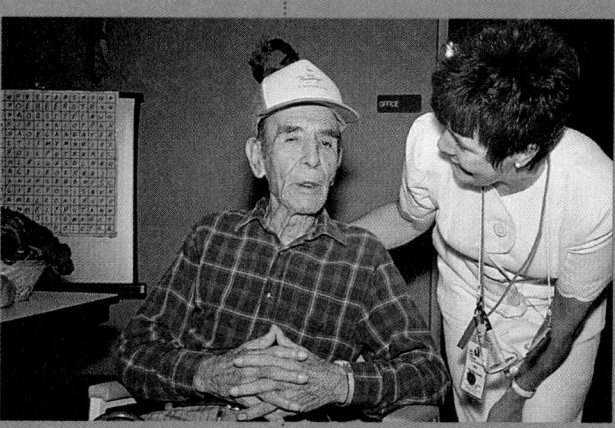

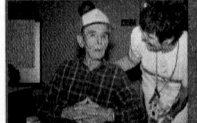

Case Study

Residing in the assisted living wing of one of the four local long-term care centers, Mario Gutierrez busies himself in his small garden plot. He is 82 years old, widowed, and has lived in this particular area of the care center for over 3 years. His family, with whom he is quite close, is scattered across the country. One niece lives in the same town. Mr. Gutierrez feels he is in good health. He believes that as long as he eats green chili peppers every day, he will remain healthy. His diet also consists of flour and corn tortillas, beans, and rice. He likes most meats, but he prefers chicken and asado (pork). For breakfast he usually has huevos rancheros. He has been hospitalized only twice, once for the flu and once for placement of a pacemaker. He presently takes only three medications: digoxin, Zestril, and Metamucil.

This afternoon, Mr. Gutierrez has telephoned his niece for the fourth time. The complaint is always the same: Mr. Gutierrez's bowels are "locked up and haven't moved in the last 2 days." He had eaten a big meal last night and was now "all bloated." His niece tried to explain about eating, bowel habits, and methods of facilitating bowel movements, but in exasperation reminded Mr. Gutierrez that the nursing student was coming later this afternoon and he could talk to the student about his problem.

Vickie, a 45-year-old married mother of two sons, is Mr. Gutierrez's nursing student. Vickie's oldest son is a freshman at the same community college she is attending; the other is a sophomore in high school. Her husband, Roger, is very supportive of her being in school. Vickie has been seeing Mr. Gutierrez once a week for 5 weeks as a portion of a home health clinical experience. They have developed a good rapport. Mr. Gutierrez's self-identified problems with his bowels is a frequent topic of conversation.

Regular bowel elimination is essential for the maintenance of a healthy body state. Although often considered a common and expected occurrence in the older adult, individuals of any age can experience changes in intestinal elimination. These changes may be the result of illness, diagnostic testing, or surgical intervention. Alterations in intestinal elimination can be responsive to both preventive and supportive nursing care.

SCIENTIFIC KNOWLEDGE BASE

Anatomy and Physiology of the Gastrointestinal Tract

The gastrointestinal (GI) tract is a series of hollow mucous membrane–lined muscular organs that begin at the mouth and end at the anal orifice. The functions of the GI tract are to prepare food products for use by the body's cells and to promote the absorption of fluid and nutrients. The GI tract is a complex system, and changes in any one area can alter total body functioning.

Mouth. The mouth mechanically and chemically breaks down nutrients into usable size and form. The teeth **masticate** food, breaking it down into a size suitable for swallowing. Saliva, produced by the salivary glands in the mouth, dilutes and softens the **bolus** of food in the mouth for easier swallowing. Digestion begins in the mouth and ends in the small intestine.

Esophagus. As food enters the upper esophagus, it passes through the upper esophageal sphincter, a circular muscle that prevents air from entering the esophagus and food from refluxing into the throat. The bolus of food travels down the esophagus and is pushed along by slow peristaltic waves. **Peristalsis** propels food through the length of the GI tract.

The bolus of food moves down the esophagus and reaches the cardiac sphincter, which lies between the esophagus and the upper end of the stomach. The sphincter prevents reflux of stomach contents back into the esophagus.

Stomach. The stomach performs three tasks, including the storage of the swallowed food and liquid; the mixing of food, liquid, and digestive juices; and the emptying of its contents into the small intestine. The stomach produces and secretes hydrochloric acid (HCl), mucus, the enzyme pepsin, and intrinsic factor. Pepsin and HCl facilitate the digestion of protein. Mucus protects the stomach mucosa from acidity and enzyme activity. The intrinsic factor is essential in the absorption of vitamin B_{12}.

Small intestine. Movement within the small intestine, occurring by both **segmentation** and peristalsis (Figure 36-1), facilitates both digestion and absorption. Approximately 7 to 10 L of liquid **chyme** moves through on an average day. Reabsorption in the small intestine is so efficient that by the time the chyme reaches the end of the small intestine, it is more paste-like in consistency, with a volume of 600 to 800 ml (Phipps and others, 1995). The small intestine is divided into three sections: the duodenum, the jejunum, and the ileum.

Segmentation

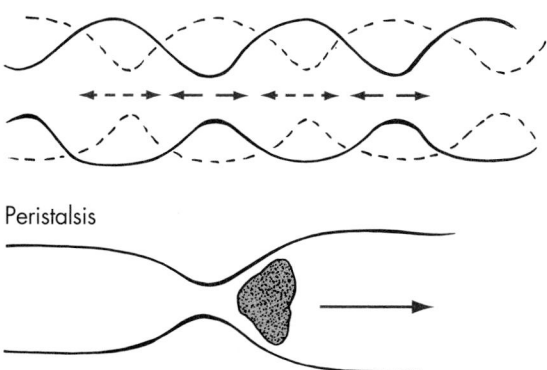

Peristalsis

Figure 36-1. Segmented and peristaltic waves.

The duodenum, which is approximately 2 feet long, continues to process the chyme from the stomach. The second section, the jejunum, is approximately 5 feet long and has the primary function of absorption of carbohydrates and proteins. The ileum, which is approximately 12 feet long, specializes in the absorption of water, fats, and bile salts. Most nutrients and electrolytes are absorbed in the small intestine. Nutrients are almost entirely absorbed by the duodenum and jejunum. The ileum absorbs certain vitamins, iron, and bile salts.

If small intestine function is impaired, the digestive process is greatly altered. Conditions such as inflammation, surgical resection, or obstruction can disrupt peristalsis, reduce the area of absorption, or block the passage of chyme. Electrolyte and nutrient deficiencies then develop.

Large intestine. The lower GI tract is called the *large intestine* (**colon**) because it is larger in diameter than the small intestine. However, its length (1.5 to 1.8 m [5 to 6 feet]) is much shorter. The larger intestine is divided into the cecum, colon, and rectum. The large intestine is the primary organ of bowel elimination.

Chyme enters the large intestine by waves of peristalsis through the ileocecal valve, a circular muscle layer that prevents regurgitation. The colon is divided into the ascending, transverse, descending, and sigmoid colons. The colon's muscular tissue allows it to accommodate and eliminate large quantities of waste and gas (**flatus**). There are four functions of the colon: absorption, protection, secretion, and elimination. A large volume of water (up to 2.5 L) and significant amounts of sodium and chloride are absorbed by the colon daily. The amount of water absorbed from chyme depends on the speed at which colonic contents move. Chyme is normally a soft, formed mass. If peristalsis is abnormally fast, there is less time for water to be absorbed and the stool will be watery. If peristaltic contractions

slow down, water continues to be absorbed and a hard mass of stool forms, resulting in constipation.

The secretory function of the colon aids in electrolyte balance. Bicarbonate is secreted in exchange for chloride. About 4 to 9 mEq of potassium is also released daily. Serious alterations in colon function (e.g., diarrhea) can cause electrolyte disturbances.

Slow peristalic contractions move contents through the colon. Intestinal content is the main stimulus for contraction. Mass peristalsis pushes undigested food toward the rectum. These mass movements occur only three or four times daily, with the strongest during the hour after mealtime.

The rectum is the final portion of the large intestine. Normally the rectum is empty of waste products (**feces**) until just before defecation. The rectum contains vertical and transverse folds of tissue that may help to temporarily hold fecal contents during **defecation.** Each fold contains an artery and veins that can become distended from pressure during straining. This distention can result in hemorrhoid formation.

Anus. Feces and flatus are expelled from the rectum through the anal canal and anus. Contraction and relaxation of the internal and external sphincters, innervated by sympathetic and parasympathetic stimuli, aid in the control of defecation. The anal canal is richly supplied with sensory nerves that help to control continence.

Defecation. The physiological factors critical to bowel function and defecation include normal GI tract function, sensory awareness of rectal distention and rectal contents, voluntary sphincter control, and adequate rectal capacity and compliance (Doughty, 1996). Normal defecation begins with movement in the left colon moving stool toward the anus. When stool reaches the rectum the distention causes relaxation of the internal sphincter, and an awareness of the need to defecate is created. If the individual determines the time for defecation is not right, the external sphincter is voluntarily contracted, closing the anus, and defecation is delayed. At the time of defecation, the external sphincter relaxes and abdominal muscles contract, increasing intrarectal pressure and forcing the stool out (Doughty, 1996). Pressure can be exerted to expel feces through a voluntary contraction of the abdominal muscles while maintaining forced expiration. This is termed **Valsalva maneuver.** This will assist in stool passage. Clients with cardiovascular disease, glaucoma, increased intracranial pressure, or a new surgical wound can be placed at further risk with this maneuver and should be cautioned to avoid straining to pass the stool. Normal defecation is painless, resulting in passage of soft, formed stool. See Box 36-1 for other factors influencing elimination and defecation.

Box 36-1
Factors Influencing Bowel Elimination

Age

Infants have a smaller stomach capacity, less secretion of digestive enzymes, and more rapid intestinal peristalsis. The ability to control defecation does not occur until 2 to 3 years of age.

Adolescents experience rapid growth of the large intestine and increased secretion of HCl.

Older adults have decreased chewing ability. Partially chewed food is not digested as easily. Peristalsis declines, and esophageal emptying slows. Absorption by the intestinal mucosa is impaired. Muscle tone in the perineal floor and anal sphincter weakens, causing difficulty in controlling defecation (Box 36-2).

Diet

Regular daily food intake promotes peristalsis.

High-fiber foods, raw fruits, cooked fruits, greens (cabbage and spinach), raw vegetables, and whole grains (cereals and breads) promote peristalsis and defecation by creating bulk (Yen, 1995).

Low-fiber foods (pasta, lean meats, and milk) slow peristalsis.

Gas-producing foods (broccoli, cauliflower, onions, and dried beans) can stimulate peristalsis.

Persons with lactose intolerance lack the enzyme lactose, which is needed to digest the simple sugars in milk. Such intolerance can lead to diarrhea and cramping.

Position During Defecation

Squatting allows a person to lean forward, exert intraabdominal pressure, and contract thigh muscles to normally defecate.

Older adults or those with arthritis may be unable to rise from a toilet seat.

Immobilized clients, required to use a bedpan while lying, cannot contract muscles to defecate.

Pregnancy

As pregnancy advances and the fetus enlarges, pressure is exerted on the rectum. Constipation commonly occurs.

Diagnostic Tests

Certain examinations involving visualization of GI structures require the emptying of bowel contents. NPO status, bowel evacuants, and enema administration to cleanse the bowel before a test are factors that interfere with normal elimination.

Barium examinations require ingestion of barium, a mixture that can harden and cause serious constipation unless eliminated soon after a test.

Fluid Intake

Fluid liquefies intestinal contents for easier passage.

Hot beverages and fruit juices soften stool and increase peristalsis.

Large quantities of milk may slow peristalsis and cause constipation.

Activity

Immobilization depresses colon motility, and regular physical exercise promotes peristalsis.

Psychological Factors

Stress, anxiety, or fear can initiate parasympathetic impulses, causing acceleration of digestion and peristalsis. Diarrhea and gaseous distention may result.

Emotional depression can decrease peristalsis and lead to constipation.

Personal Habits

Personal habits such as failing to respond to the need to defecate and lack of privacy interfere with normal elimination patterns and can lead to constipation.

Hospitalized clients often share toilet facilities or use bedpans or bedside commodes. The resulting embarrassment causes them to ignore the urge to defecate.

Pain

Hemorrhoids, rectal surgery, and abdominal surgery may cause a client to suppress defecation because of pain; constipation develops.

Medications

Laxatives and cathartics soften stool and promote peristalsis.

Antidiarrheal agents inhibit peristalsis.

Narcotic analgesics, opiates, and anticholinergic drugs depress peristalsis and can cause constipation.

Antibiotics alter normal bowel flora and can produce diarrhea.

Drugs that contain iron may turn the stool black. Antacids may cause a white discoloration. Anticoagulants may result in frank or occult blood in the stool.

Surgery and Anesthesia

General anesthetics temporarily halt peristalsis.

Surgery involving bowel manipulation temporarily stops peristalsis (paralytic ileus) for 24 to 48 hours.

Common Bowel Elimination Problems

Alteration in bowel elimination can result from a variety of factors. Some of the more common alterations are discussed in the paragraphs that follow.

Constipation. **Constipation** is defined as having fewer bowel movements than normal with the difficult passage of hard, dry feces (Lueckenotte, 1996). Common causes of constipation include changes in diet, medications, inflammation, environmental factors (unavailability of toilet facilities, lack of privacy), and lack of knowledge about regular bowel habits. In the older adult, it is usually diet related, most commonly a lack of fiber (Gibson and others, 1995). Regardless of etiology, intestinal motility slows, causing prolonged exposure of the fecal mass to the intestinal walls. Fecal water continues to be absorbed, leaving little to soften and lubricate the stool (Lueckenotte, 1996).

Constipation can be a significant threat to well-being. Straining during defecation is contraindicated for clients with cardiovascular problems or for those who have had recent abdominal or rectal surgery. Clients who exert effort to pass a stool experience Valsalva maneuver, a forced expiratory effort against a closed airway. The action traps the blood in the chest; upon relaxing, blood rushes to the heart, overloading the heart. This can result in cardiac dysrhythmias or angina. It also increases intraabdominal pressure, leading to stress on suture lines.

Impaction. **Fecal impaction** results from unrelieved constipation. It is a collection of hardened feces, wedged in the rectum, that cannot be expelled. Clients at greatest risk for impaction include those who are confused or unconscious, badly constipated, or those who have experienced an interruption in nerve supply to the bowel. An obvious sign of impaction is the inability to pass a stool for several days, despite a repeated urge to defecate. When a continuous oozing of diarrheal stool develops in such a client, impaction should be suspected. **Anorexia,** abdominal distention and cramping, and rectal pain may occur.

Diarrhea. **Diarrhea** is an increased frequency in the passage of loose stools. A variety of conditions cause diarrhea (Table 36-1).

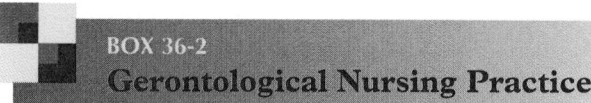

TABLE 36-1
Conditions That Cause Diarrhea

Condition	Physiological Effects
Emotional stress (anxiety)	Increased intestinal motility
Intestinal infection (streptococcal or staphylococcal enteritis)	Inflammation of intestinal mucosa, increased mucus secretion in colon
Food allergies	Reduced digestion of food elements
Food intolerance (greasy foods, coffee, alcohol, spicy foods)	Increased intestinal motility, increased mucus secretion in colon
Tube feedings	Hyperosmolarity of some enteral solutions results in diarrhea, because hyperosmolar fluids draw fluids into the gastrointestinal tract
Medications	
Iron	Irritation of intestinal mucosa
Antibiotics	Suprainfection allowing overgrowth of normal flora, inflammation and irritation of mucosa
Laxatives (short term)	Increased intestinal motility
Colon disease (colitis, Crohn's disease)	Inflammation and ulceration of intestinal walls, reduced absorption of fluids, increased intestinal motility
Surgical alterations	
Gastrectomy	Loss of reservoir function of stomach, improper absorption because food is moved into duodenum too quickly
Colon resection	Reduced size of colon, reduced amount of absorptive surface

---

BOX 36-2
Gerontological Nursing Practice

- Maintenance of a proper diet, including the appropriate intake of fluid and bulk. Fiber (4 to 6 g, which is equal to 3 to 4 tablespoons of bran per day) is recommended to reduce the risk of constipation (Gibson and others, 1995).
- Proper body position to facilitate bowel evacuation.
- Education concerning the dangers of excessive laxative/cathartic use for bowel elimination. Excessive use of these medications may cause an atony of the colon, further contributing to chronic constipation (Lueckenotte, 1994). Instruct clients that if their stool is soft and passes easily, it is not necessary to have a bowel movement daily. If clients should miss a daily movement, it does not mean that they are constipated and require a laxative.
- Instruct clients that changes in dietary intake can cause transient changes in bowel elimination patterns. Also, changes in RDA include a decrease in calories because of a decrease in metabolic rate and an increase in calcium. Clients should also avoid tobacco products and large amounts of alcohol (Lueckenotte, 1996).

Fluid and electrolyte imbalances can result from diarrhea. Older adults and the very young are at the greatest risk. Because of the irritating effects of the intestinal contents, persistent diarrhea readily leads to skin breakdown in the buttocks and perianal region.

The aim of treatment is first to maintain adequate hydration (Lueckenotte, 1996). Parenteral replacement of fluids may be necessary if the client is at risk for fluid and electrolyte imbalance. Intervention is then aimed toward identifying and correcting causative factors. Depending on the cause, antispasmodic or antidiarrheal medications may be used to slow peristalsis.

Incontinence. **Fecal incontinence** is the involuntary passage of stool. Any condition that impairs function or control of the anal sphincter may cause fecal incontinence. Conditions creating frequent, loose, large-volume, watery stools also predispose to incontinence.

In many situations, the client is mentally alert but physically unable to avoid defecation. Loss of control over intestinal elimination may be associated with feelings of inadequacy or guilt. Like diarrhea, incontinence predisposes the client to skin breakdown.

Flatulence. Flatulence is one of the most common GI disorders. It refers to a sensation of bloating and abdominal distention that is accompanied by excess gas. The accumulation of gas forces the diaphragm up and reduces lung expansion (Phipps and others, 1995).

Hemorrhoids. **Hemorrhoids** are masses of dilated blood vessels that lie beneath the lining of the skin in the anal mucosa. Increased venous pressure resulting from straining at defecation, pregnancy, congestive heart failure, and chronic liver disease can lead to the development of hemorrhoids. Passage of hard stool can cause hemorrhoidal tissue to stretch and bleed. Hemorrhoidal tissue can become inflamed and tender, and clients may complain of itching and burning. Because pain worsens during defecation, the client may ignore the urge to defecate, resulting in constipation.

Bowel diversions. Certain diseases prevent the normal passage of intestinal contents throughout the small and large bowel. The treatment for these disorders may result in the need for a temporary or permanent artificial opening (**stoma**) in the abdominal wall. Surgical openings may be created in the ileum (ileostomy) or colon (colostomy) with the end of the intestine brought through the abdominal wall to create the stoma.

Depending on the type of surgical procedure done, the client will either have no control over when fecal material exits the stoma (incontinent ostomy) or will have control (continent ostomy).

Incontinent ostomies. The location of the ostomy determines stool consistency. For example, an ileos-

tomy bypasses the entire large intestine, creating frequent, liquid stools. The sigmoid colostomy emits near-normal stool. The location of an ostomy depends on the client's medical problem and general condition.

Loop colostomies are usually temporary large stomas constructed in the transverse colon (Figure 36-2). The surgeon pulls a loop of bowel onto the abdomen. A plastic rod, bridge, or rubber catheter is temporarily placed under the bowel loop to keep it from slipping back. The surgeon then opens the bowel and sutures it to the skin of the abdomen. The loop ostomy has two openings through the stoma. The proximal end drains stool while the distal portion drains mucus.

The end colostomy consists of one stoma formed from the proximal end of the bowel with the distal portion of the GI tract either removed or sewn closed

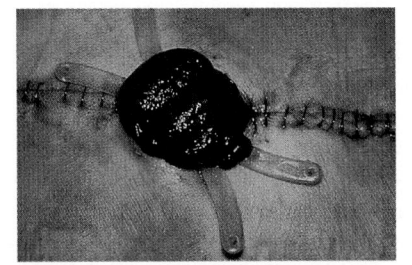

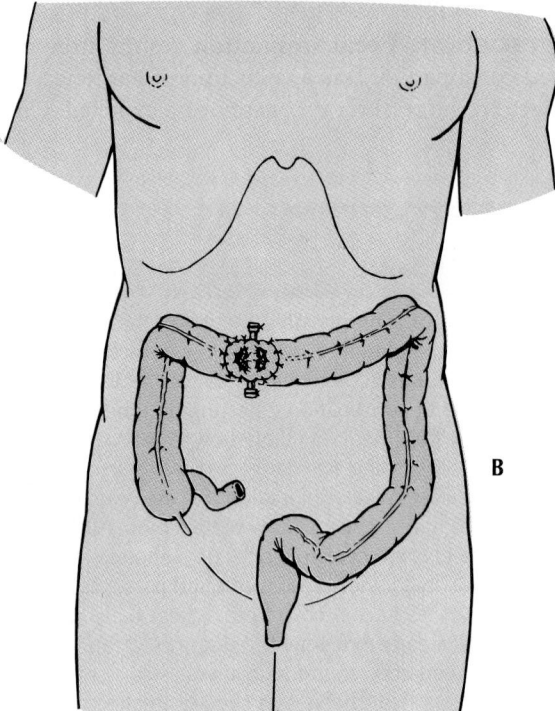

Figure 36-2. A, A transverse loop colostomy supported with a flexible red rubber catheter. (Courtesy Hollister, Inc., Libertyville, Ill.) **B,** Abdominal view of loop colostomy in transverse colon. (From Hampton BG, Bryant RA: *Ostomies and continent diversions: nursing management,* St. Louis, 1992, Mosby.)

(called *Hartmann's pouch*) and left in the abdominal cavity. End colostomies are a surgical treatment for colorectal cancer. In such cases the rectum also might be removed. Client's with diverticulitis often have a temporary end colostomy constructed with a Hartmann's pouch (Figure 36-3).

Unlike the loop colostomy, the bowel is surgically severed in a double-barrel colostomy (Figure 36-4) and the two ends are brought out onto the abdomen. The double-barrel colostomy consists of two distinct stomas: the proximal functioning stoma and the distal nonfunctioning stoma.

Ostomies that emit frequent semisolid or liquid stools (e.g., ileostomy) create a management challenge. A pouch must always be worn because of the continuous oozing of liquid stool. The pouch must be emptied, washed, and, if a two-piece ostomy system is being used, even replaced throughout the day. Skin care is vital to prevent exposure to fecal irritants.

A colostomy in the transverse or sigmoid colon needs less frequent emptying of the pouch. Although some clients might choose to not always wear a pouch, most with sigmoid colostomies do, even though bowel movements may occur only once or twice daily.

Continent ostomies. Certain types of surgery may provide continence for select colectomy clients. These continent ostomies are also called *continent diversions* or *continent reservoirs*. In an ileoanal pull-through, the colon is removed and the ileum is anastomosed or connected to an intact anal sphincter (Dalton-Loehner and Connor, 1989).

A newer surgical procedure based on the ileoanal pull-through is the ileoanal reservoir (IAR), also called a *restorative proctocolectomy* (Beitz, 1994). In this proce-

dure the client has no permanent external stoma and therefore does not need to wear an ostomy pouch. Clients have an internal pouch created from their ileum. These ileum pouches can be constructed in various configurations. The end of the pouch is sewn or anastomosed to the anus (Figure 36-5). The client may have a temporary ostomy until the surgically created pouch has healed. When healing has occurred and the client has successfully learned Kegel exercises to strengthen the pelvic floor, the temporary ostomy is removed. The client then has bowel movements from only the anal area.

The Kock continent ileostomy is another new type of continent ostomy (Rolstad and Hoyman, 1992). An internal reservoir or pouch is created from a piece of the client's small intestine. Part of the pouch is brought out onto the client's abdomen as an enteral stoma. At the end of the internal part of the pouch is a one-way nipple valve, which is how continence is accomplished. This valve only allows fecal contents to drain from the pouch when an external catheter is intermittently placed into the stoma.

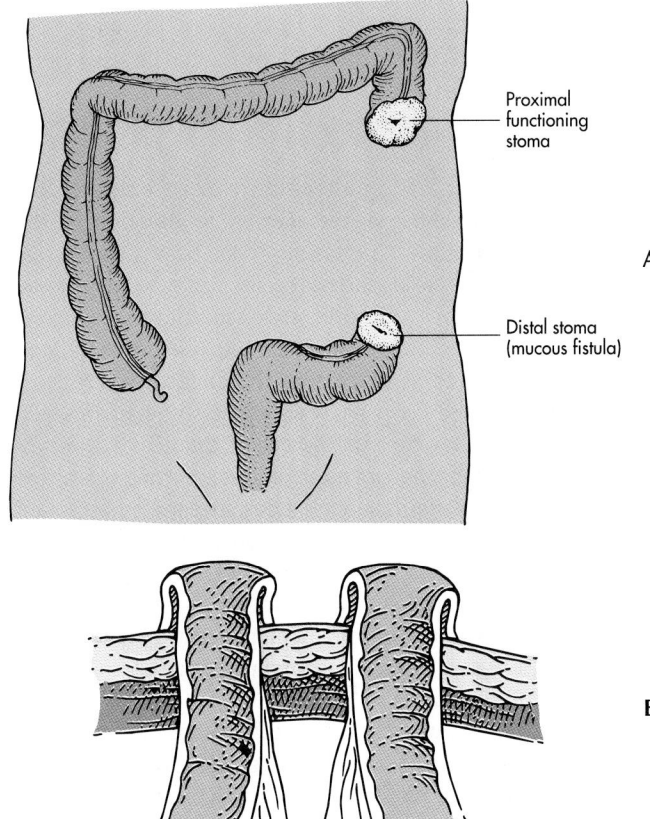

A

B

Figure 36-4. Double-barrel colostomy. **A,** Double-barrel colostomy in the descending colon. **B,** Cross sectional view of double-barrel stoma. (From Hampton BG, Bryant RA: *Ostomies and continent diversions: nursing management,* St. Louis, 1992, Mosby.)

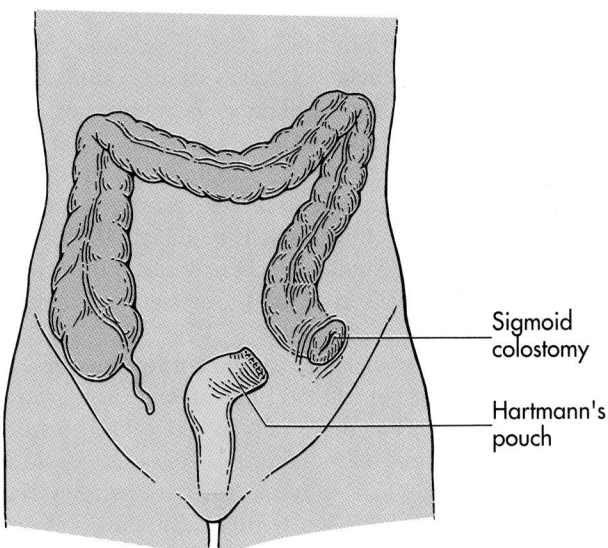

Sigmoid colostomy

Hartmann's pouch

Figure 36-3. Sigmoid colostomy. Distal bowel is oversewn and left in place to create Hartmann's pouch. (From Hampton BG, Bryant RA: *Ostomies and continent diversions: nursing management,* St. Louis, 1992, Mosby.)

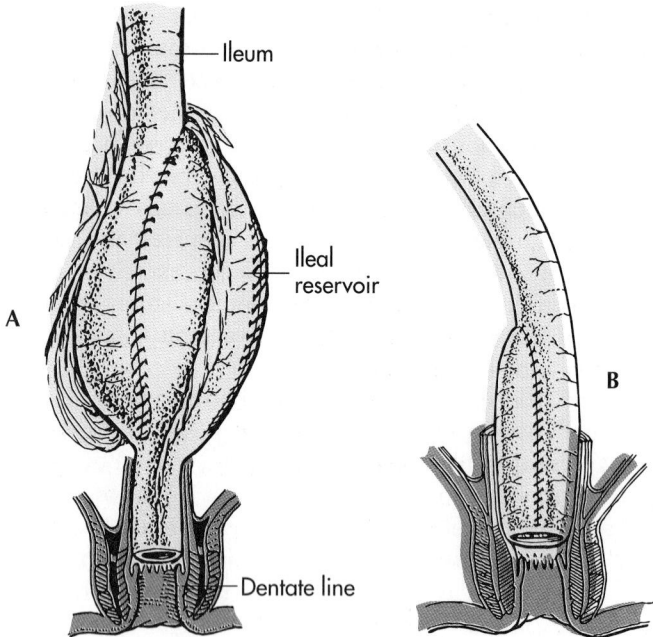

Figure 36-5. Ileoanal reservoirs (IAR). **A,** S-shaped configuration. **B,** J-shaped configuration. (From Hampton BG, Bryant RA: *Ostomies and continent diversions: nursing management,* St. Louis, 1992, Mosby.)

NURSING KNOWLEDGE BASE

Any bowel elimination alteration can be embarrassing for a client. Because of the sensitivity many clients experience regarding elimination of the bowel with its associated sounds and odors, nurses must be very sensitive to their own communication techniques, especially the nonverbal. Changes in facial expression or gagging can be perceived as disgust by the client. Awareness of the client's need for privacy should also be addressed.

Clients with a chronic disease of the GI system have endured numerous hospitalizations, perhaps multiple surgeries, and significant changes in eating habits and lifestyles. They are often on complicated medication regimens that are also taxing both physically and financially. Their desire for wellness may lead them to consider alternative forms of medical treatment. It is important for the nurse to remain accepting of clients' health care choices.

An ostomy causes serious body image changes, with clients perceiving a stoma as a form of mutilation. Even though clothing conceals the ostomy, the client feels different. The idea of being different or not a whole person can affect the client's social interaction with others, resulting in isolation. Some clients experience difficulty in maintaining or initiating normal sexual relations. One important factor in the client's acceptance of this change in body functioning is the ability to control fe-

cal secretions. Foul odors, spillage, leakage of liquid stools, and the inability to regulate bowel movements further place the client at risk for loss of self-esteem.

CRITICAL THINKING IN CLIENT CARE

Synthesis

As the nurse begins the problem-solving process of caring for a client experiencing elimination problems, it becomes important to reflect on the knowledge, experience, and standards of care that will improve client outcomes. Assuming the proper attitudes of critical thinking will also ensure a well-designed, individualized approach to care.

Knowledge. The nurse reflects on knowledge regarding normal anatomy and physiology of the GI tract, as well as knowledge regarding specific GI alterations. This information will help the nurse more accurately focus the nursing assessment and identify alterations when they exist. Even insignificant alterations in bowel elimination can produce significant health problems for the client. For example, diarrhea can lead to electrolyte imbalances, dehydration, and rectal soreness.

Abdominal pain is one of the most common complaints of clients who seek health care. The nurse must apply knowledge of the nature of pain (see Chapter 33) and pain assessment to accurately analyze elimination problems.

Functional bowel disorders make up the most frequently reported GI complaints. Nurses should understand and consider the psychological aspects associated with these diseases to provide appropriate care (Caudell, 1994).

The intake of certain foods is often reflective of the client's culture or beliefs. Foods in various cultures have different status relating to religion, availability, cost, and tradition. For example, among Hispanic Americans certain hot foods are utilized for conditions producing fever, and cold foods are used for disorders such as cancer or headache (Giger and Davidhizar, 1995). The nurse should understand the client's cultural heritage and the role diet plays in health promotion and maintenance.

A final area of knowledge, important for the nurse to synthesize during clinical decision making, is gerontological principles. Far too often, an older adult's problems with intestinal elimination are discounted as an everyday complaint. The nurse must remember that what might appear at the outset to be quite insignificant can be a major problem to the client physically and psychologically.

Experience. Elimination alterations are common for many clients who seek health care. In the acute care environment numerous variables, including diet changes, medications, fluid restrictions, and diagnostic tests, can cause major alterations to bowel function. The nurse can provide better care to clients by reflecting on those experiences involving clients with similar alterations and similar lifestyle habits affecting elimination.

Attitudes. A nurse will apply all of the attitudes of critical thinking when caring for a client with elimination problems. Creativity comes into play, especially when adjustments are needed in the client's diet and exercise planning. Similarly, perseverance is important in selecting effective diet therapies and in finding the best appliances for ostomy clients. Confidence is an important factor in providing care to clients with bowel diversions or resections. Often these clients are very sick and in much pain. The nurse's confidence with moving and positioning the client, handling stomal supplies, and managing pain will place the client at ease and facilitate the recovery process.

Standards. To establish regular bowel habits, clients require consistency in bowel care and training. It is possible to establish regular bowel habits by setting standards for appropriate nutritional and elimination support. Regardless of age or disease state, maintenance of bowel functioning and integrity is essential to well-being.

When assessing a client's abdominal pain, findings should be specific, clear, precise, and accurate. Although the intellectual standards for critical thinking apply to all symptoms, thorough pain assessment is critical. A multitude of problems can be detected on the basis of the nature of abdominal pain. Physicians will collaborate with the nurse on the basis of his or her assessment to identify the appropriate medical diagnosis.

Clients with alterations in bowel elimination, especially incontinence, can be at risk for ridicule and shame on the part of some health care providers. This may be especially true for providers with limited educational experience, to whom the task of client hygiene is often delegated. It is the responsibility of the nurse to make certain such individuals understand the needs of these clients and attend to their needs in a respectful way.

NURSING PROCESS AND ALTERATIONS IN BOWEL ELIMINATION

The needs and problems of clients experiencing alterations in bowel elimination are distinct and numerous. The nurse must incorporate several assessment skills and utilize appropriate communication techniques throughout the entire care planning process.

▪ Assessment

Assessment of bowel elimination requires the nurse to review any complaints the client may have affecting the GI system. Because the client's chewing ability, recent intake of both solids and liquids, personal eating habits, and level of stress all influence bowel functioning, this information should be included in the review (Barkauskas and others, 1994).

Health history. In determining the client's bowel habits, the nurse will remember "normal" is unique to each individual. The nurse applies this knowledge in preparing questions for the client interview to determine the presence and extent of GI alterations. Family members can help if the client is unable to provide necessary information.

Areas typically assessed in the history include the following (Barkauskas and others, 1994):

1. Determine the time of the last bowel movement and if any changes in elimination patterns have occurred. Ask client to make suggestions as to the basis for any change.
2. Client's description of usual characteristics of stool. The nurse determines whether the stool is normally watery or formed, soft or hard, and the typical color. The client also describes a normal stool's shape.
3. Appetite, recent change in eating patterns, and change in weight (amount of loss or gain).
4. Identification of routines followed to promote normal elimination. Examples are drinking hot liquids, using a laxative, eating specific foods, or taking time to defecate during a certain part of the day.
5. Assessment of the use of artificial aids at home, for example, the use of enemas, laxatives, or special foods before having a bowel movement. The nurse asks how often the client uses them.
6. Presence and status of artificial orifices. If the client has an ostomy, the nurse assesses the frequency of fecal drainage, character of feces, type of appliance used, and methods used to maintain the ostomy's function.
7. Daily diet history, including the client's dietary preferences. Is mealtime regular or irregular, and are certain foods eaten infrequently?
8. Description of daily fluid intake. This includes the type and amount of fluid. The client may have to estimate the amount using common household measurements.
9. History of surgery or illnesses affecting the GI tract. This information can often help to explain symptoms, the potential for maintaining or restoring a normal elimination pattern, and whether there is a family history of cancer involving the GI tract.

10. Medication history. Determine whether the client takes medications that might alter defecation or fecal characteristics.
11. Emotional state. Observation of emotions, tone of voice, and mannerisms can reveal significant behaviors indicating stress.
12. History of exercise. Obtain a description of the type and amount of daily exercise.
13. History of pain or discomfort. Ask the client whether there is a history of abdominal or anal pain. The location and nature of pain can help to locate the source of a problem (see Chapter 33).
14. Social history. If the client is not independent in bowel management, determine methods and degree of assistance required.

Physical assessment.   The nurse assesses the status of GI function to detect factors that may affect elimination and to gather data regarding the client's elimination problems. Table 36-2 summarizes some of the assessments to include in the examination of bowel function (Doughty, 1992). The nurse will conduct an examination of the oral cavity, abdomen, and anus and rectal canal (see Chapter 24).

After completion of the anal assessment, the nurse directly inspects feces on the glove for several characteristics (Table 36-3). If there are no feces on the glove, the nurse asks the client to describe a typical stool, noting recent changes. The client or primary care giver is the most knowledgeable about changes. The nurse should also determine whether the client passes an unusual amount of or little flatus.

Laboratory and diagnostic examinations

Laboratory tests.   Several laboratory tests are available to assist in diagnosing problems within the GI system, including the following blood tests:

Total bilirubin—a degraded product of hemoglobin is excreted in the bile. Obstruction in the biliary tract contributes primarily to a rise in direct values.

Alkaline phosphatase—an enzyme found in many tissues. Obstructive biliary tract disease may cause significant elevation.

Amylase—an enzyme secreted by the pancreas. Damage to these cells causes the enzymes to be absorbed into the blood.

Protein—a measure of nutrition. Malnourished clients have greatly deceased levels of blood protein.

Carcinoembryonic antigen (CEA)—a protein. It is typically elevated in persons with colorectal tumors.

Analysis of fecal contents can also detect alterations in GI functioning. Bacteria can easily be acquired by a person who handles a specimen improperly. Standard precautions must be followed for anyone coming in contact with the specimen (see Chapter 25). The client is often capable of obtaining the specimen without assistance if properly instructed. The client must understand that feces cannot be mixed with urine or water. The client defecates into a clean, dry bedpan or special container that is placed under the toilet seat.

Laboratory tests for blood in the stool and stool cul-

TABLE 36-2
Focused Physical Examination for Bowel Function Evaluation

Parameter	Assessment Strategy
Chewing	Inspect condition of teeth and gums. Poor dentition or poorly fitting dentures influence the ability to chew.
Mobility	*In ambulatory clients*—Observe gait; determine need for assistive devices or personnel. *In wheelchair-bound clients*—Note degree of needed assistance to transfer from chair to commode or toilet.
Dexterity	Ask client to demonstrate hand motions that would be required to insert suppository or perform digital stimulation (e.g., grasping a pencil, rotation of forefinger).
Anal sphincter function	Inspect anus at rest. Then perform digital examination while asking client to contract and relax sphincter followed by Valsalva maneuver. The inability to sense rectal distention, to voluntarily contract anus, or to "bear down" is indicative of impaired function.
Abdominal muscle contractility	Instruct client to "bear down" (or to push against the examiner's hand) while lightly palpating the abdominal wall. Check for presence, volume, and consistency of stool in rectum. The presence of large amounts of stool is indicative of decreased sensation and/or impaired emptying.

Data from Doughty D: A step-by-step approach to bowel training, *Progressions* 4(2):18, 1992.

TABLE 36-3
Fecal Characteristics

Characteristic	Normal	Abnormal	Abnormal Cause
Color	Infant: yellow; adult: brown	White or clay	Absence of bile
		Black or tarry (melena)	Iron ingestion or upper GI bleeding
		Red	Lower GI bleeding, hemorrhoids, ingestion of beets
		Pale with fat	Malabsorption of fat
		Translucent mucus	Spastic constipation, colitis, excess straining
		Bloody mucus	Neoplasm or inflammation
Odor	Pungent; affected by food type	Noxious change	Blood in feces or infection
Consistency	Soft, formed	Liquid	Diarrhea, reduced absorption
		Hard	Constipation
Frequency	Varies: infant 5 to 8 times daily (breastfed) or 1 to 3 times daily (bottle fed); adult daily or 2 to 3 times a week	Infant more than 6 times daily or less than once every 1 to 2 days; adult more than 3 times a day or less than once a week	Hypomotility or hypermotility
Amount	150 g per day (adult)		
Shape	Resembles diameter of rectum	Narrow, pencil shaped	Obstruction, rapid peristalsis
Constituents	Undigested food, dead bacteria, fat, bile pigment, cells lining intestinal mucosa, water	Blood, pus, foreign bodies, mucus, worms	Internal bleeding, infection, swallowed objects, irritation, inflammation
		Excess fat	Malabsorption syndrome, enteritis, pancreatic disease, surgical resection of intestine

tures require only a small sample. Minimum abrasions of the intestinal mucosa are thought to cause blood loss of 1 to 3 ml daily in feces (Barkauskas and others, 1994). Blood loss of over 50 ml appears as **melena.** To detect quantities less than 50 ml, laboratory analysis is needed. The nurse collects approximately an inch of formed stool or 15 to 30 ml of liquid diarrheal stool. Tests for measuring the output of fecal fat require the client to collect stools for 3 to 5 days. All fecal material must be saved throughout the test period. Some tests require a chemical preservative.

After obtaining a specimen, the nurse tightly seals the container, completes laboratory requisition forms, and records all specimen collections in the client's medical record. The nurse avoids delays in sending specimens to the laboratory. Some tests require the stool to be warm. When stool specimens are allowed to stand at room temperature, bacteriological changes that alter test results can occur.

A common fecal test is the **guaiac test,** which measures microscopic amounts of blood in the feces (Box 36-3). It is a useful diagnostic screening test for colon cancer (Box 36-4). One positive result does not confirm GI bleeding. The test should be repeated at least three times while the client refrains from eating meat, poultry, fish, turnips, and horseradish and using certain drugs such as steroids, iron, and salicylate. Agencies differ on the performance of this test. The JCAHO requires nurses to be tested for competency in performing guaiac tests.

Diagnostic examinations. A variety of radiological and diagnostic tests are utilized with the client experiencing alterations in the GI system. The preparation and the test itself are often quite unpleasant for the client. See Box 36-5 for an explanation of these tests.

Client expectations.
When the nurse assesses the client's expectations of care it may be helpful to anticipate the client's need for privacy and respect. Bowel elimination problems can be embarrassing. The nurse should be able to ask the client what is important to ensure that care is given in a personal and professional way.

Because there is a direct link between nutrition and bowel elimination, the nurse must consider the client's cultural choices of dietary components. Concessions may need to be made on certain food selections. Methods of preparation may also be a concern, especially if tradition and cost are deciding factors.

Box 36-3

Procedural Guidelines for Measuring Occult Blood in the Stool

1. Explain purpose of test and ways client can assist. Client can collect own specimen if possible.
2. Wash hands.
3. Apply clean, disposable gloves.
4. Use tip of wooden applicator (see illustration) to obtain a small portion of uncontaminated stool specimen.

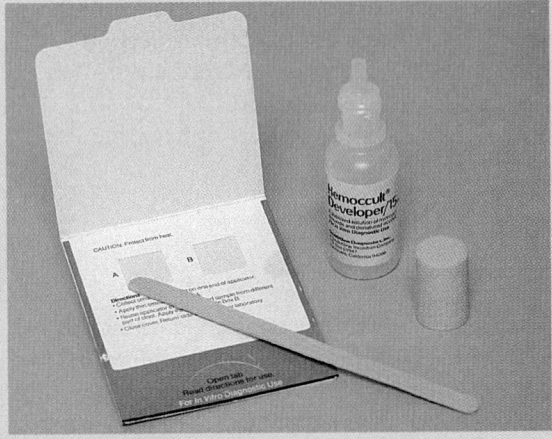

Step 4

5. Perform hemoccult slide test:
   a. Open flap of slide and, using a wooden applicator, thinly smear stool in first box of the guaiac paper. Apply a second fecal specimen from a different portion of the stool to slide's second box (see illustration).

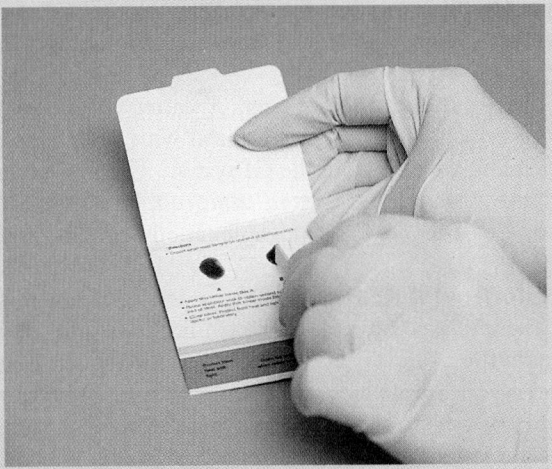

Step 5a

   b. Close slide cover and turn the packet over to reverse side (see illustration). Open cardboard flap and apply two drops of developing solution on each box of guaiac paper.

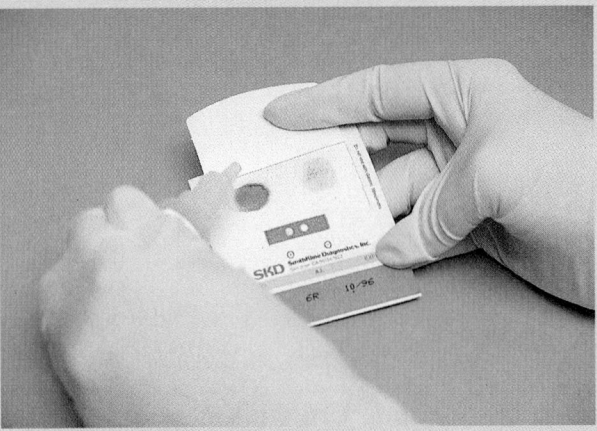

Step 5b

   c. Assess the color of the guaiac paper after 30 to 60 seconds.
   d. Dispose of test slide in proper receptacle.
6. Wrap wooden applicator in paper towel, remove gloves, and dispose in proper receptacle.
7. Wash hands.
8. Record results of test; note any unusual fecal characteristics.

Box 36-4
Screening for Colon Cancer

Risk Factors
Age: over 50
Family history: colorectal cancer or polyps
Cultural: colorectal cancer is one of the most frequently occurring cancers among elderly blacks
History of inflammatory bowel disease (colitis or Crohn's disease)
Living in urban area
Diet: high intake of fats and low fiber intake

Warning Signs
Change in bowel habits
Rectal bleeding

Screening Tests
Digital rectal examination every year after age 40
Guaiac test for occult blood every year after age 50
Endoscopy every 3 to 5 years after age 50, after two annual negative examinations

From American Cancer Society: *Colon and rectal cancer—1996*, Atlanta, 1996, The Society.

When determining the client's expectations, be sure to consider his or her normal bowel pattern. The client may wish to have activities planned so that normal routines can be maintained. If what is "normal" to the client is unhealthy or could promote negative health practices, the nurse must first meet the client's educational needs.

Box 36-5
Radiographic and Diagnostic Tests

Plain Film of Abdomen/Kidneys, Ureter, Bladder

A simple x-ray film of the abdomen requiring no preparation.

Upper GI/Barium Swallow

An x-ray examination using an opaque contrast medium (barium) to examine the structure and motility of the upper GI tract, including pharynx, esophagus, and stomach. May be extended as a "small bowel follow through" to examine the duodenum and small bowel.

Client must be NPO at midnight the night before the examination.

Client must remove all jewelry or other metallic objects.

After the test, client must increase fluids to facilitate passage of barium.

Upper Endoscopy

An endoscopic examination of the upper GI tract allowing more direct visualization through a lighted fiber-optic tube that contains a lens, forceps, and brushes for biopsy.

Preparation is similar to that of the upper GI.

Light sedation is required.

Barium Enema

An x-ray examination using an opaque contrast medium to examine the lower GI tract.

Preparation includes NPO at midnight, a bowel prep such as magnesium citrate, and in some instances enemas to empty out any remaining stool particles.

Ultrasound

A technique that uses high-frequency sound waves to echo off body organs, creating a picture.

Preparation depends on the organ to be visualized and may include NPO or no prep.

Colonoscopy

An endoscopic examination of the colon with the use of colonoscope inserted into the rectum.

Preparation is similar to that of a barium enema: clear liquids the day before and then some form of bowel cleanser, such as GoLytely. Enemas until clear may also be ordered. Light sedation is required.

Flexible Sigmoidoscopy

An examination of the interior of the sigmoid colon through the use of a flexible or rigid lighted tube.

Preparation is similar to that of a barium enema or colonoscopy. Light sedation is required.

Computerized Tomography Scan

An x-ray examination of the body from many angles utilizing a scanner analyzed by a computer.

Preparation may be NPO, or nothing may be required.

The client must be informed of the need to lie very still. If claustrophobia is a problem, light sedation may be utilized.

Magnetic Resonance Imaging

A noninvasive examination that uses magnet and radio waves to produce a picture of the inside of the body.

Preparation is NPO 4 to 6 hours before examination.

No metallic objects are allowed in the room, including metal objects on clothes.

....

Successful critical thinking requires a synthesis of knowledge, experience, information gathered from clients, and critical thinking attitudes and standards. Clinical judgments require the nurse to anticipate what information is needed, to analyze the data, and then make decisions regarding client care. The client expects competent and informed care. Vickie incorporates previous knowledge and experience in providing care for Mr. Gutierrez.

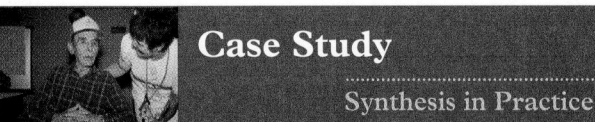

Case Study

Synthesis in Practice

When Vickie prepared to conduct an assessment of Mr. Gutierrez, she reflected back on experiences with other clients in the home setting. She recalled one client in particular who had elimination problems resulting from a diet consisting mainly of high-fat and high-carbohydrate foods. She thought that her involvement with that client would likely help in the care of Mr. Gutierrez.

Vickie also reviewed her class notes on the anatomy and physiology of the GI system. Given Mr. Gutierrez's age, Vickie focused on reviewing the physiological changes that aging produces within the GI system. These changes include loss of teeth, taste bud atrophy, decreased secretion of gastric acid, and a slight decrease in small intestine motility (Lueckenotte, 1996).

Vickie will need to do a thorough assessment of Mr. Gutierrez's dietary intake over the last few days. Being familiar with Mr. Gutierrez's Hispanic heritage, Vickie anticipates certain food preferences and will need to assess these. Vickie knows Mr. Gutierrez does not like the food served at the long-term care center and frequently requests "home cooked" tortillas and green chili peppers from his niece.

The symptoms Mr. Gutierrez exhibits, no bowel movement in 2 days and a feeling of bloating, can be associated with several different problems. Vickie plans the assessment to be thorough and precise, being sure to rule out any abdominal discomfort or other symptoms that can be expected from elimination problems. Because problems with bowel elimination have been an ongoing concern for Mr. Gutierrez, Vickie will need perseverance as she begins to identify nursing diagnoses and outline goals of care. Vickie will need to avoid preconceived ideas regarding constipation in older adults. She must remain open to all the possibilities concerning changes in GI functioning.

Nursing Diagnosis

The nurse gathers data from the nursing assessment and analyzes clusters of defining characteristics to identify relevant nursing diagnoses (see nursing diagnoses box). Reflecting on each of the data sources is necessary in determining the correct diagnosis. Selected defining characteristics can apply to more than one diagnosis, so the nurse must be clinically skillful in seeing the patterns that reveal the diagnosis that best fits the client's situation. For example, a client may report not having a bowel movement for several days. This defining characteristic may apply to the diagnosis of *constipation*, as well as *perceived constipation*. The difference is that on examination the client with *constipation* has a dry, hard stool with abdominal or rectal fullness. In contrast, the client with *perceived constipation* has expectation of having a stool daily, and in fact the stools can be quite normal.

It is important to establish the correct *"related to"* factor for a diagnosis. For example, for the diagnosis of *constipation* the nurse must distinguish between nutritional imbalance, exercise, medications, and emotional problems as causative factors. Selection of the correct etiology for the diagnosis ensures the appropriate nursing interventions will be implemented.

Planning

After nursing diagnoses are identified, the nurse and client set goals and expected outcomes to direct interventions. The care plan should incorporate the client's elimination routines or habits as much as possible and reinforce those which promote health. The plan must also take into consideration preexisting health concerns. For example, if the client is at risk for the development of congestive heart failure, increasing fluid intake must be tailored to the client's ability to safely handle the volume of fluid.

Defecation patterns vary among individuals. For this reason, the nurse and client work together to plan effective interventions (see care plan). What may be a re-

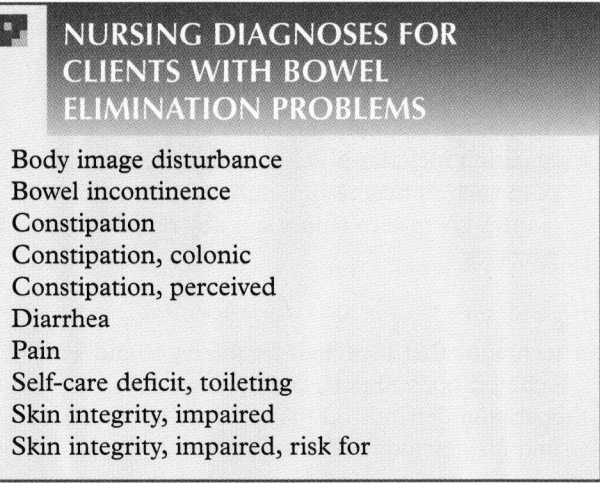

NURSING DIAGNOSES FOR CLIENTS WITH BOWEL ELIMINATION PROBLEMS

Body image disturbance
Bowel incontinence
Constipation
Constipation, colonic
Constipation, perceived
Diarrhea
Pain
Self-care deficit, toileting
Skin integrity, impaired
Skin integrity, impaired, risk for

CASE STUDY NURSING CARE PLAN

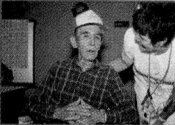

Bowel Elimination

Assessment

From their first visit, Vickie and Mr. Gutierrez have been able to communicate without difficulty. Mr. Gutierrez complains of feeling **"full of gas"** but hasn't "passed any wind," perhaps in the last 2 days. Because of the feeling of fullness Mr. Gutierrez also states, "I really **haven't felt like eating today** and I need to move my bowels. I took a laxative last night, and I think I need an enema." Vickie confirms that Mr. Gutierrez had his **last bowel movement 3 days ago.** The **stool was brown in color and hard-formed.** On examination of the abdomen Vicki finds **hypoactive bowel sounds** in all four quadrants. A medication history shows that Mr. Gutierrez frequently resorts to taking laxatives. An assessment of Mr. Gutierrez's diet reveals a high intake of corn tortillas and cheese and a low intake of fruits. His stove has not been working well, and he has been unable to prepare rice and beans, which he enjoys. On the basis of the nursing history, Vickie estimates Mr. Gutierrez normally drinks about 1200 ml of fluid daily.

Nursing Diagnosis

Constipation related to less than adequate fluid and dietary intake and chronic laxative use.

Planning

Goal

Client will establish and maintain a normal defecation pattern within 1 month.

Expected Outcomes

Client will have a bowel movement within 48 hours.

Client's abdomen will be soft, nondistended, and nontender within 24 hours.

Client will pass soft, formed stools at least every 3 days.

Implementation

Steps

1. Instruct client on a weekly menu plan, including foods high in fiber: posole, beans and rice, tomatoes, and wheat tortillas.

2. Consult with client's niece and long-term care center to have client's stove repaired.

3. Educate client about use of liquids to promote softening of stool and defecation; have client drink fluids of choice (1 glass every 2 hours during the day).

4. Have client take time to defecate 1 hour after breakfast or other meal, until a regular time becomes established.

Rationale

High-fiber foods increase peristalsis, improving movement of intestinal contents through the GI tract. The need for laxatives is also reduced (Gibson and others, 1995).

Cooking facilities are necessary for preparation of selected food preferences.

Fluids keep fecal mass soft and increase stool bulk, causing increase in colon peristalsis (Phipps and others, 1996).

Gastrocolic reflex normally occurs approximately 1 hour after breakfast, resulting in mass movement of colon contents (Lueckenotte, 1996).

Evaluation

Ask client to keep a diary of foods and fluids ingested for 1 week and review.

Ask client to describe the effect fluids and high-fiber foods have on elimination.

Ask client to describe frequency and character of stool.

Palpate abdomen for distention and tenderness.

Defining characteristics are shown in bold type.

alistic time frame to establish a normal defecation pattern for one client might be very different for another. Involvement of the family in the plan of care is also important. When clients are disabled or debilitated, family often become the primary care givers. Client and family education is important to promote understanding of ways to establish normal bowel function.

Other health team members can be important resources for the client. The nurse often refers the client to a dietitian to plan a nutritionally balanced diet that incorporates the client's food preferences and lifestyle. A clinical nurse specialist or enterostomal therapist can provide guidance in the care and management of ostomy sites and problems involving incontinence or skin breakdown. If access to proper nutrition is a concern, community organizations that deliver meals to the home or that provide transportation for clients can be beneficial. In many institutions, members of the health care team collaborate in developing a critical pathway for client care. A pathway offers recommended clinical interventions throughout the course of a client's treatment (Figure 36-6).

The nurse will establish realistic goals and outcomes for the client's care. The outcomes provide measurable behaviors or physiological responses that indicate progress toward the goal of a normal elimination pattern. Nursing interventions are designed to achieve the outcomes of care.

▪ Implementation

Health promotion activities. The factors that normally promote bowel elimination become the nurse's interventions for helping clients to develop normal bowel habits.

Diet. Depending on the client's elimination problem, specific foods are recommended to ensure proper nutrient intake and normal defecation (Box 36-6). There is increasing evidence indicating that low fat intake and increases in dietary fiber and bulk-forming foods reduce the client's risks of colorectal cancers, digestive diseases, and other cancers. Assisting clients and their families in different food preparation practices, new menus, and healthy snacking can help to reduce the risks of GI disease. Consideration must be given to whether a client can afford the foods recommended. In addition to solid foods, the nurse encourages the client to drink 2000 to 3000 ml of fluids daily, if not contraindicated by other medical conditions.

Exercise. An age-related exercise program also assists clients in maintaining healthy bowel patterns. Regular exercise, three to five times a week, promotes normal GI motility. Examples of exercise include walking, cycling, or swimming. A client experiencing a period of immobilization from illness should ambulate as soon as possible. Clients restricted to bed may benefit from active range-of-motion exercises.

Box 36-6
Dietary Recommendations for Elimination Problems

Constipation

Increase intake of high-fiber foods. Added fluids should accompany increase in fiber intake.
  Vegetables (dried beans, brussels sprouts, corn, peas, and potatoes)
  Fruits (apples with peels, raisins, and prunes)
  Cereals (bran and whole wheat) and whole grain breads
For the older adult with poor dentition, offer chopped, not pureed, foods. Add extra chopped vegetables to soups.
Persons with difficulties in swallowing need mashed, not pureed, foods. Liquids such as fruit juices and hot tea are beneficial.

Diarrhea

Avoid spicy or high-fiber foods.
If client is lactose intolerant, avoid the use of milk and milk products.
Increase intake of low-fiber foods: chicken, fish, lean beef, pasta, and milk products.
If diarrhea causes serious fluid loss, replace with water, weak tea, gelatin, plain soda, and bouillon.

Flatulence

Avoid gas-producing foods: cauliflower, broccoli, brussels sprouts, onions, dried beans and lentils, and beer.

Ostomies

Remember that the location of an ostomy determines the type of diet needed for regular evacuation. Initially place clients on low-fiber diets to avoid irritation to mucosa and stomal obstruction. Add high-fiber foods one at a time over a period of several weeks. Maintain a high fluid intake. Remind ostomy clients to eat slowly and chew food well when on low-fiber diets.
Avoid foods that may cause blockage: blackberries and raspberries, oranges, red apples with tough skins, bing cherries, large quantities of corn, Chinese bean sprouts in large amounts, stringy beef, popcorn, and hot dogs with heavy skins.

BARNES	**CARE PATH® 550** **MAJOR SMALL & LARGE** **BOWEL PROCEDURE**				1

SERVICE	PHYSICIAN		
PRIMARY NURSE	PRIMARY NURSE		
DC DATE	ADM DATE	DATE OF SURGERY **A-8**	

Problem Number	PATIENT PROBLEMS / NURSING DIAGNOSES
#1	ALTERATION IN COMFORT RELATED TO ABDOMINAL SURGERY
#2	ALTERATION IN BOWEL ELIMINATION RELATED TO ABDOMINAL SURGERY
#3	ALTERATION IN SKIN INTEGRITY RELATED TO ABDOMINAL INCISION AND RECOVERY FROM SURGERY
#4	LACK OF KNOWLEDGE RELATED TO HOSPITALIZATION AND SURGICAL PROCEDURE
#5	ALTERATION IN BODY IMAGE RELATED TO ABDOMINAL SURGERY AND OSTOMY

* IF APPROPRIATE

#	1, 2, 3	3, 4, 5	4	4	1, 4
	ASSESSMENT / MONITORING	**CONSULTS**	**PROCEDURES / TEST**	**TREATMENT**	**ACTIVITY**
DAY 1 PRE OP	Assessment: Nursing Admission lab results Monitoring: VS routine O₂ saturation x1 I & O	Nurse specialist (if ostomy is a consideration).	CBC, 6, 12, PT, PTT T & C x2 units (admission labs) EKG ≥ 40 years old CXR ≥ 50 years old UA with micro *Mark ostomy site	Antithrombolytic stockings Mechanical bowel preparation	UAL
DAY 2 DOS	Assessment: Wound/dressing q 4 hrs. Bowel function q 4 hrs. Stoma appearance q 4 hrs. Pulmonary status q 2 hrs. Comfort level q 2 hrs. Braden score x1 Patency of tubes and characteristics of drainage q 8 hrs. IV patency & site appearance q 8 hrs. Fall risk factors Monitoring: VS q 1 hr. x 2 q 2 hrs. x2 then q 4 hrs. I & O q 4 hrs. O₂ saturation x1 x2	Respiratory Therapy for O₂		Antithrombolytic stockings O₂ to maintain O₂ saturation ≥ 92% Oral care q 4 hrs. Assist with Incentive Spirometer and TCDB q 2 hrs. Gastric decompression and tube irrigation	Bedrest
DAY 3 POD 1	Assessment: Wound/dressing q 4 hrs. Bowel function q 4 hrs. Stoma appearance q 4 hrs. Pulmonary status q 2 hrs. Comfort level q 2 hrs. Braden score x1 Patency of tubes and characteristics of drainage q 8 hrs. IV patency & site appearance q 8 hrs. Fall risk factors Lab results **O₂ saturation ≥ 92%** Monitoring: VS q 4 hrs. I & O q 8 hrs. Room air O₂ saturation x1 x2	Social Work Respiratory (if O₂ or tx needed) Nurse specialist (if ostomy placed).	CBC, 6	Antithrombolytic stockings Oral care q 4 hrs. Assist with Incentive Spirometer q 2 hrs. Gastric decompression and tube irrigation d/c foley d/c O₂	Up in chair with assist x1 x2 x3 Ambulate in room with assist x1 x2 Bed bath
DAY 4 POD 2	Assessment: Wound/dressing q 4 hrs. Bowel function q 4 hrs. Stoma appearance q 4 hrs. Pulmonary status q 2 hrs. Comfort level q 2 hrs. Braden score x1 Patency of tubes and characteristics of drainage q 8 hrs. IV patency & site appearance q 8 hrs. Fall risk factors Lab results **Voiding without difficulty (UO ≥ 240 cc q 8 hrs.)** Monitoring: VS q 4 hrs. I & O q 8 hrs.	Dietary screening		Antithrombolytic stockings Oral care q 4 hrs. Assist with Incentive Spirometer q 2 hrs. Gastric decompression and tube irrigation *Abdominal wound wet to dry dressing Change TID	Up in chair with assist x1 x2 x3 Ambulate in room with assist x1 x2 Bed bath

SIGNATURE	INIT.	SIGNATURE	INIT.	SIGNATURE	INIT.

Figure 36-6. Example of a portion of a care path for major small and large bowel procedure. (Courtesy Barnes-Jewish Hospital, St. Louis.)

Timing and privacy. One of the most important habits a nurse can teach a client regarding bowel habits is to take time for defecation. Ignoring the urge to defecate and not taking time to defecate completely are common causes of constipation. To establish regular bowel habits, a client must know when the urge to defecate normally occurs.

Defecation is most likely to occur an hour after meals. If attempts are made to defecate during the time when mass colonic peristalsis occurs, the chances of success are great. If a client is restricted to bed or requires assistance in ambulating, the nurse should recommend use of a bedside commode or a bedpan or have a care giver help the client to reach the bathroom. Prompt assistance is needed before the urge disappears.

Clients may have previously established routines to assist them with defecation. When clients become hospitalized, health promotion habits can become disrupted. The nurse should encourage clients to maintain as many of these regular practices as they are able. Privacy is often a concern for all clients. Health care providers often walk in and out of rooms without knocking, and many clients may reside in semiprivate rooms or living areas. The nurse must remain acutely aware of the client's need for modesty and privacy.

Promotion of normal defecation. To help clients evacuate contents normally and without discomfort the nurse recommends interventions that stimulate the defecation reflex or increase peristalsis. One way to promote defecation is by having the client assume a squatting position during defecation. Squatting increases pressure on the rectum and facilitates use of intraabdominal muscles. Clients who have difficulty in squatting because of muscular weakness or mobility limitations benefit from the use of elevated toilet seats. Regular toilets are too low for clients unable to lower themselves to a squatting position because of joint or muscle-wasting diseases or those who have had abdominal surgery. With an elevated seat, less effort is needed to sit or stand.

Acute care. When clients become acutely ill, the GI system is often one of the first systems to be affected. Simple changes in activity levels, sleeping patterns, diet, and medications directly impact regular bowel habits. Surgical intervention can create additional elimination problems for the acute care client. Sensitivity to the client's need for the provision of as much self-care as possible will assist the client in coping with the changes.

Medications. Medications can initiate and facilitate stool passage. **Cathartics** and **laxatives** have the short-term action of emptying the bowel. These agents are also used in bowel evacuation for clients undergoing GI tests and abdominal surgery. Although the terms *cathartic* and *laxative* are often used interchangeably, cathartics have a stronger effect on the intestines.

Although the oral route is more commonly used, cathartics prepared as suppositories are more effective because of their stimulant effect on the rectal mucosa. Cathartic suppositories such as bisacodyl (Dulcolax) may act within 30 minutes. The nurse should give the suppository shortly before the client's usual time to defecate or immediately after a meal.

The nurse teaches clients about the potential harmful effects of repeated use of laxatives. The client should understand that laxatives and cathartics are not meant for long-term maintenance of bowel function.

Cathartics are classified by the method by which the agent promotes defecation. Stimulant cathartics cause local irritation to the intestinal mucosa and inhibit reabsorption of water in the large intestine. Intestinal irritation increases intestinal motility. The rapid movement of feces causes retention of water in the stool. The drugs can cause formation of a soft to fluid stool in 6 to 8 hours. Clients tend to abuse stimulants more than other cathartics. Overuse leads to loss of intestinal tone.

Saline or osmotic agents contain a salt preparation not absorbed by the intestines. The cathartic draws water into the fecal mass. This osmotic action increases the bulk of the intestinal contents and enhances lubrication. Rapid bowel evacuation may occur in 1 to 3 hours. Magnesium hydroxide (Milk of Magnesia) and sodium phosphate (Phospho-Soda) are saline cathartics. Clients with impaired kidney function should avoid using these drugs because of the toxic buildup of magnesium.

Wetting agents or stool softeners are detergents that lower the surface tension of feces, allowing penetration by water and fat. These drugs also inhibit absorption of water by the intestines. The fecal mass becomes large and soft, preventing the client from straining during defecation. Commonly used wetting agents are dioctyl sodium sulfosuccinate (Colace) and dioctyl calcium sulfosuccinate (Surfak).

Bulk-forming cathartics consist of cellulose and polysaccharides that absorb water and increase solid intestinal bulk. The fecal bulk stretches the intestinal walls, stimulating peristalsis. Passage of stool will occur in 12 to 24 hours. Bulk laxatives are the least irritating and safest of all cathartics. Clients should be encouraged to take bulk cathartics with plenty of liquids.

Lubricants soften the fecal mass, thus easing the strain of defecation. Clients with painful hemorrhoids particularly benefit from a lubricant. The only lubricant laxative available is mineral oil. Regular use of mineral oil interferes with absorption of the fat-soluble vitamins A, D, E, and K. The drug can also cause a dangerous form of pneumonia if aspirated.

For clients with diarrhea, the most effective antidiarrheal agents are opiates. Antidiarrheal agents decrease intestinal muscle tone to slow the passage of feces. As a result, more water is absorbed by intestinal walls. Antidiarrheal agents should be used with caution, because opiates are habit forming.

Enemas. An **enema** is instillation of a preparation into the rectum and sigmoid colon. An enema is given primarily to promote defecation by stimulating peristalsis. The volume of fluid instilled breaks up the fecal mass, stretches the rectal wall, and initiates the defecation reflex. Enemas are also given as a vehicle for drugs that exert a local effect on rectal mucosa.

The most common use for an enema is temporary relief of constipation. Other indications include removing impacted feces; emptying the bowel before diagnostic tests, surgery, or childbirth; and beginning a program of bowel training. Clients should be discouraged from relying on enemas to maintain bowel regularity. Enemas do not treat the cause of constipation. As with laxative abuse, frequent use destroys normal defecation reflexes.

Cleansing enemas promote complete evacuation of feces from the colon. They act by stimulating peristalsis through the infusion of a large volume of solution or through local irritation of the colon's mucosa. Cleansing enemas include tap water, normal saline, low-volume hypertonic saline, and soapsuds solution. Each solution exerts a different osmotic effect, causing the movement of fluids between the colon and interstitial spaces beyond the intestinal wall. Infants and children can tolerate only normal saline, because they are at risk for fluid imbalance.

Tap water is hypotonic and exerts a lower osmotic pressure than fluid in interstitial spaces. After infusion into the colon, tap water escapes from the bowel lumen into interstitial spaces. The net movement of water is low; the infused volume stimulates defecation before large amounts of water leave the bowel. Tap water enemas should not be repeated, because water toxicity or circulatory overload can develop if large amounts of water are absorbed.

Physiologically, normal saline is the safest solution to use because it exerts the same osmotic pressure as fluids in interstitial spaces around the bowel. The volume of infused saline stimulates peristalsis. Giving saline enemas does not create the danger of excess fluid absorption. If prepared saline is not available at home, 500 ml (1 pint) of tap water mixed with 1 teaspoon of table salt can be substituted.

Hypertonic solutions infused into the bowel exert osmotic pressure that pulls fluids out of interstitial spaces. The colon fills with fluid, and the resultant distention promotes defecation. Clients unable to tolerate large volumes of fluid benefit most from this type of enema. A hypertonic solution of 120 to 180 ml (4 to 6 ounces) is usually effective. The Fleet's enema is most commonly used.

Soap solution may be added to tap water or saline to create the additional effect of intestinal irritation. Only pure castile soap is safe. Harsh soaps or detergents can cause serious bowel inflammation. The recommended ratio of soap to solution is 5 ml (1 teaspoon) of castile soap to 1000 ml of warm water or saline.

A physician may order a high or low cleansing enema. The terms *high* and *low* refer to the height from which and hence the pressure with which the fluid is delivered. High enemas are given to cleanse the entire colon. A low enema cleans only the rectum and sigmoid colon. After the enema is infused, the client is asked to turn from the left lateral to the dorsal recumbent, then over to the right lateral position. The position change ensures fluid reaches the large intestine.

Oil-retention enemas lubricate the rectum and colon. The feces absorb the oil and become softer and easier to pass. To enhance action of the oil, the client retains the enema for several hours if possible.

Carminative enemas provide relief from gaseous distention. They improve the ability to pass flatus. An example of a carminative enema is MGW solution, which contains 30 ml of magnesium, 60 ml of glycerin, and 90 ml of water.

A return-flow enema, or **Harris flush,** is a mild colonic irrigation that helps to expel flatus. The nurse first administers a small amount (100 to 200 ml) of mild enema solution into the rectum and colon. Then the nurse lowers the enema container to allow the solution to flow back through the rectal tube and into the container. Repeating this process several times aids in reducing flatus and promoting peristalsis.

Certain enemas or enema administrations contain drugs. An example is polystyrene sodium sulfonate (Kayexalate), used to treat clients with dangerously high serum potassium levels. Skill 36-2 on p. 1036 outlines the steps for enema administration.

The physician often orders "enemas till clear," which means that the enema is repeated until the client passes fluid that is clear and contains no fecal material. It may be necessary to give as many as three enemas, but the nurse should caution the client against using more than three. Excess enema use seriously depletes fluids and electrolytes. If the enema fails to return a clear solution after three times, the physician should be notified. When an enema is given to a child, it helps to have a parent assist. The child should be able to see the equipment for the procedure.

Giving an enema to a client who is unable to contract the external sphincter can cause difficulties. The nurse gives the enema with the client positioned on the bedpan. Giving the enema with the client sitting on the toilet is unsafe, because the curved rectal tubing can abrade the rectal wall.

Impaction removal. For clients with an impaction, the fecal mass may be too large to be passed voluntarily. If enemas fail, the nurse must break up the fecal mass with the fingers and remove it in sections. The procedure can be very uncomfortable for the client. Excess rectal manipulation may cause irritation to the mucosa, bleeding, and stimulation of the vagus nerve, which can result in a reflex slowing of the heart rate. Because of the procedure's potential complications, in many institutions only physicians are allowed to remove impactions digitally. If the nurse performs the procedure, a physician's order is necessary (Box 36-7).

Positioning on bedpan.

A client restricted to use of a bedpan for defecation will usually need assistance. Sitting on a bedpan can be uncomfortable and awkward. The nurse should help to position the client comfortably. Two types of bedpans are available. The regular bedpan, made of metal or hard plastic, has a curved smooth upper end and a sharp-edged lower end and is about 5 cm (2 inches) deep. A fracture pan, designed for clients with body or leg casts or for whom the semi-Fowler's position is contraindicated, has a shallow upper end about 1.3 cm (½ inch) deep (Figure 36-7).

The upper end of either pan fits under the buttocks toward the sacrum, with the lower end just under the upper thighs. The pan should be high enough so that feces enter it. The most important element for the nurse to consider in positioning the client is preventing muscle strain and discomfort. A client should never be placed on a bedpan and then left with the bed flat unless activity restrictions demand it. This forces the client to hyperextend the back to lift the hips onto the pan (Figure 36-8, *top*). It may be necessary to have the bed flat when placing the client on a bedpan. Then the nurse should raise the head of the bed 30 to 45 degrees (Figure 36-8, *bottom*). Clients who have overhead trapeze frames can easily lift themselves by grasping the trapeze bar. Box 36-8 describes steps in assisting a client with a bedpan.

For the more mobile client, a bedside commode can

Box 36-7

Procedural Guidelines for Digital Removal of Stool

1. Explain the procedure and help the client to lie on the left side with knees flexed and back toward the nurse.
2. Drape the trunk and lower extremities with a bath blanket and place a waterproof pad under the buttocks. Keep a bedpan next to the client.
3. Apply disposable gloves and lubricate the index finger of dominant hand with lubricating jelly.
4. Gently insert the index finger into the rectum and advance the finger slowly along the rectal wall toward the umbilicus.
5. Gently loosen the fecal mass by massaging around it. Work the finger into the hardened mass.
6. Work the feces downward toward the end of the rectum. Remove small pieces at a time and discard into bedpan.
7. Reassess the client's heart rate and look for signs of fatigue. Stop the procedure if the heart rate drops significantly or the rhythm changes.
8. Continue to remove feces, and allow the client to rest at intervals.
9. After completion, offer a washcloth and towel to wash and dry the buttocks and anal area. Assist as needed.
10. Remove bedpan and dispose of feces. Remove gloves by turning them inside out, then discard.
11. Assist client to toilet or clean bedpan if urge to defecate develops.
12. Wash hands. Record results of disimpaction by describing fecal characteristics.
13. Follow procedure with enemas or cathartics as ordered by physician.

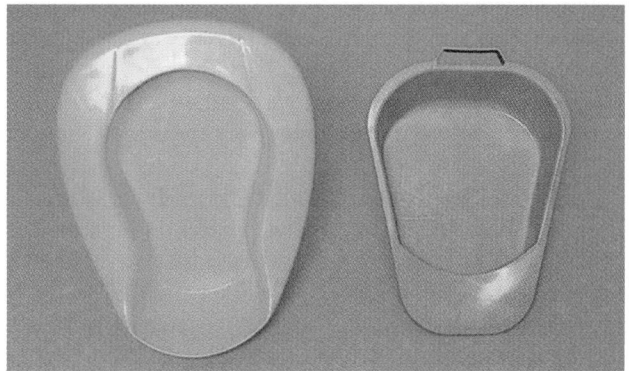

Figure 36-7. Types of bedpans. *From left,* regular bedpan and fracture bedpan.

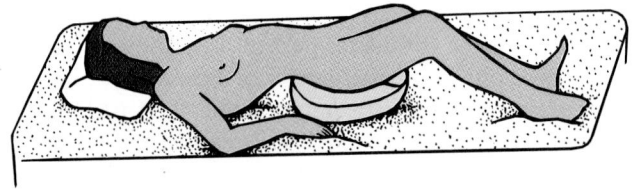

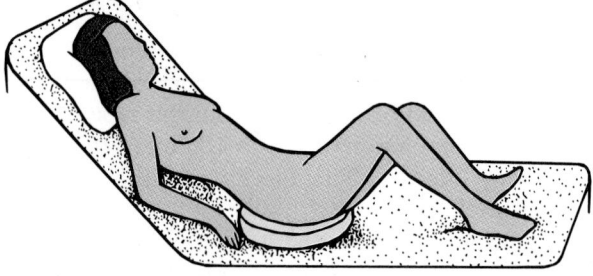

Figure 36-8. Positions on a bedpan. *Top,* Improper positioning of client. *Bottom,* Proper position reduces client's back strain.

Box 36-8

Procedural Guidelines for Assisting Client On and Off a Bedpan

1. Assess the client's level of mobility, strength, ability to help, and presence of any condition (e.g., orthopedic) that may interfere with use of a bedpan.
2. Explain the technique you will use in turning and positioning to the client.
3. Offer the bedpan at a time that coincides with the duodenocolic or mass peristaltic reflex.
4. Wash and dry hands and apply disposable gloves.
5. Close the room curtain for privacy.
6. If metal bedpan is used, hold it under warm running water for a couple of minutes, then dry.
7. Raise the bed to a comfortable working height and be sure client is positioned high in bed with head elevated 30 degrees (unless contraindicated). Raise the side rail opposite the side where the nurse is standing.
8. Fold back top linen to client's knees.
9. Assist with positioning: Instruct client to bend knees and place weight on heels. Place your hand, palm up, under client's sacrum, resting elbow on mattress. Then have client lift hips while you slip bedpan into place with other hand.
10. Dependent client: Lower head of bed flat and have client roll onto side opposite nurse. Apply powder lightly to lower back and buttocks. Place bedpan firmly against buttocks and push down into mattress with open rim toward client's feet. Keeping one hand against bedpan, place other hand around client's fore-

hip (see illustration). Ask client to roll onto pan, flat on bed. With client positioned comfortably, raise head of bed 30 degrees.

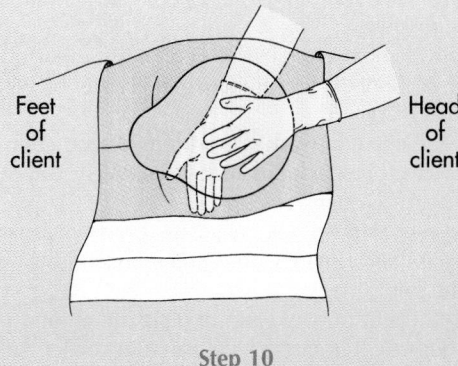

Feet of client

Head of client

Step 10

11. Place rolled towel under lumbar curve of client's back.
12. Place call light and toilet tissue within client's reach, and keep side rails up as needed.
13. Remove bedpan as client lifts hips up or as client carefully rolls off pan and to side. Hold pan firmly as client moves.
14. Assist in cleansing anal area. Wipe from pubic area toward anus. Replace top covers.
15. If a specimen or intake and output are collected, do not dispose of tissue in bedpan.
16. Have client wash and dry hands.
17. Empty pan's contents, dispose of gloves, and wash hands.
18. Inspect stool for color, amount, consistency, odor, or presence of abnormal substances.

be a safe, effective alternative to a bedpan. Its use is less exhausting and allows the client to assume a more "normal" or "familiar" position for defecation.

Restorative care. As the client recovers and is able to return home or to an extended care facility, establishment of regular elimination patterns must begin again. Bowel retraining is one essential step in regaining independence.

Bowel training. The client with incontinence is unable to maintain bowel control. A bowel training program can help some clients, especially those who still have some neuromuscular control, to achieve normal defecation. The training program involves setting up a daily routine. By attempting to defecate at the same time each day and using measures that promote defeca-

tion, the client gains control of bowel reflexes. The program requires time, patience, and consistency. The physician determines the client's physical readiness and ability to benefit from bowel training.

Ostomy care. A client with a temporary or permanent bowel diversion has unique elimination needs. The client with an incontinent **ostomy** wears a pouch or appliance to collect stool emitted from the stoma. Meticulous skin care is needed to prevent liquid stool from irritating skin around a stoma (Box 36-9).

Some clients irrigate their ostomies to establish regular bowel elimination. The muscular quality of the colon allows it to be safely irrigated with a relatively large volume of water or saline. The irrigation acts like an enema, distending the bowel and stimulating peristalsis. Only specific equipment for irrigating an ostomy

Client Teaching for Stoma Care (Conventional Incontinent Ileostomy)

- Teach the client that the drainage from the stoma site is very irritating to skin tissues and that contact should be avoided if at all possible. If contact occurs, thorough cleansing with soap and water should be performed as soon as possible.
- Teach the client to avoid use of alcohol to cleanse around a stoma. Alcohol dilates capillaries and causes bleeding of the stomal margin.
- Instruct the client to wash skin with mild soap and water or commercial preparations such as PeriWash. Pat or blot dry the skin thoroughly.
- Tell the client not to use creams or ointments on peristomal skin, because they prevent the pouch from adhering to the skin.
- Teach the client to avoid use of peroxide around or on stoma, because it irritates tissue (Paulford-Lecher, 1995).
- If yeast infections develop, instruct the client to wash thoroughly but gently, pat dry, and apply medically prescribed Kenalog spray and Mycostatin topical powder to irritated skin.
- Teach the client to routinely inspect the appearance of the stoma and surrounding skin. (The stoma should be moist, shiny, and dark pink to red.) Bleeding around the stoma should be minimal. Tell the client to report excess bleeding, abnormal color, or edema to the nurse or physician.
- Teach the client how to select and apply a skin barrier and pouch. Include length of wear.
- Teach the client how to empty and change the pouch. It should be emptied when one-third to one-half full.
- Teach the client methods of reducing odor.
- Tell the client to carry ostomy supplies at all times.

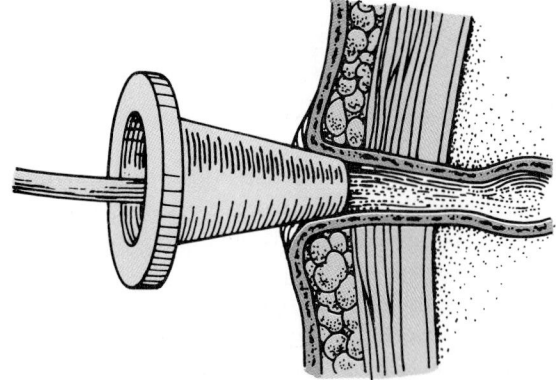

Figure 36-9. Ostomy irrigation cone inserted into stoma.

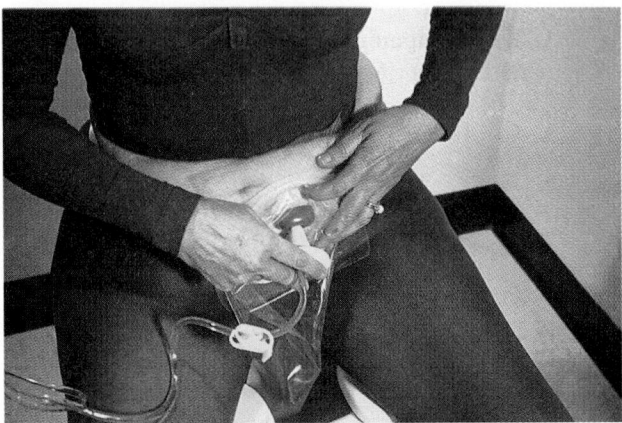

Figure 36-10. Client irrigating ostomy using irrigation sleeve.

should be used. *Never* use an enema set to irrigate an ostomy. The shape of the stoma requires the use of a special cone-tipped irrigating tube (Figure 36-9). Care must be taken to avoid trauma to the stoma or bowel. Clients typically use warm tap water to cleanse the bowel. The physician recommends when to begin irrigations and their frequency. Eventually clients develop their own schedules. With irrigation some clients gain greater freedom without the need to wear a stomal pouch continuously.

Most clients prefer sitting on the toilet during irrigation. Because the stoma has no sphincter, the irrigation solution begins to drain when the cone is removed. The client wears a long plastic irrigating sheath (Figure 36-10) or bag that extends from the stoma down into the toilet. The irrigating solution (500 to 1000 ml tepid saline or water) is instilled over 15 minutes and then allowed to drain from the stoma into the toilet without soiling the skin. It may take up to an hour for feces and solution to be totally expelled. After the

greatest portion has passed, the client may choose to close the bottom of the sheath and wear it as a bag until drainage stops.

A client with an ostomy can suffer a change in body image. The appearance of the stoma and accompanying body odors can cause psychological stress. For the client with a new ostomy, it is important for the nurse to promote independence and acceptance of the ostomy. Early involvement in self-care promotes the client's independence. Even simple tasks such as holding pieces of equipment during stomal pouching can help the client begin to adjust to bodily changes. Many clients benefit from the information and encouragement from ostomy support groups.

Incontinent ostomies require a pouch to collect feces. An effective pouching system protects the skin, contains feces, and is comfortable and inconspicuous. A person wearing a pouch should feel secure to participate in any activity. Many pouching systems are available.

A pouching system consists of a pouch and skin barrier. Pouches come in disposable or reusable one- and two-piece systems. Skin barriers include wafers, pastes, powders, and a liquid film that is applied to the skin around the stoma. A good skin barrier protects the skin

Text continued on p. 1035

Pouching an Ostomy

Delegation Considerations

The skill of pouching an ostomy, especially a newly established ostomy, requires problem solving and knowledge application unique to a professional nurse. Delegation is inappropriate. Pouching of an established ostomy can be delegated to assistive personnel.

- Assist care provider in selecting appropriate pouch and skin barrier.
- Inform care provider of the signs of stomal and peristomal skin changes that should be reported to an RN.
- Have care provider monitor and report characteristics and volume of ostomy output.

Equipment

- Pouch, clear drainable colostomy/ileostomy in correct size for two-piece system or custom cut-to-fit one-piece type with attached skin barrier
- Pouch closure device, such as clamp
- Adhesive remover (optional)
- Clean disposable gloves
- Deodorant
- Gauze pads or washcloth
- Towel or disposable waterproof barrier
- Basin with warm tap water
- Scissors
- Skin barrier such as sealant wipes or wafer
- Tape or ostomy belt

STEPS	RATIONALE
1. Auscultate for bowel sounds.	Documents presence of peristalsis.
2. Observe skin barrier and pouch for leakage and length of time in place. Depending on type of pouching system used (such as with an opaque pouch), the nurse may have to remove the pouch to fully observe the stoma. Clear pouches permit the viewing of the stoma without their removal.	May indicate need for different type of pouch or sealant.
3. Observe stoma for color, swelling, trauma, and healing; stoma should be moist and reddish-pink. Assess type of stoma. Stomas can be flush with the skin or be a budlike protrusion on the abdomen (see illustration for a normal bud stoma).	Stoma characteristics should be one of the factors to consider when selecting an appropriate pouching system.
4. Measure the stoma with each pouching change. Follow pouch manufacturer's directions and measuring guide as to which pouch to use based on client's stoma size.	Determines correct size equipment, preventing trauma to stoma.
5. Observe abdominal incision (if present).	Relationship to stoma determines proper placement of pouch.

Continued

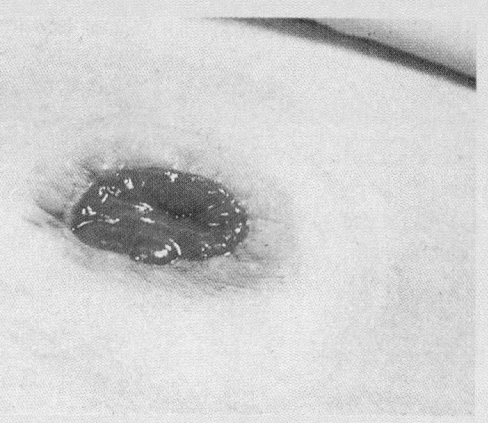

Step 3 (Courtesy Hollister, Inc., Libertyville, Ill.)

Pouching an Ostomy

STEPS	RATIONALE
6. Observe effluent from stoma and keep a record of intake and output. Ask client about skin tenderness.	
7. Avoid unnecessary changing of the entire pouching system. A one-piece pouch with attached skin barriers or the skin barrier of a two-piece pouching system should be changed every 3 to 7 days, *not* daily.	Pouches should be emptied when one-third to one-half full, because the weight of contents may dislodge the skin seal, and ostomy drainage is irritating to the skin. Also, pouches collect flatus (gas), which needs to be expelled because it can disrupt the skin seal.

CRITICAL DECISION POINT

Do not put holes in pouch for flatus to escape.

STEPS	RATIONALE

8. Assess abdomen for best type of pouching system to use. Consider:
  a. Contour and peristomal plane
  b. Presence of scars, incisions
  c. Location and type of stoma
	Determines pouching system selection and need for other equipment.

9. Assess the client's self-care ability to determine the best type of pouching system to use.	Clients who have difficulty using their hands or who have limited vision may find a one-piece system or a precut pouch and skin barrier more desirable to use; others prefer being able to keep the skin barrier in place for several days, changing just the pouch, and therefore prefer the two-piece system.
10. After skin barrier and pouch removal, assess skin around stoma, noting scars, folds, skin breakdown, and peristomal suture line if present.	Determines need for barrier paste to increase adherence of pouch to skin or to fill in irregularities.
11. Determine client's emotional response and knowledge and understanding of an ostomy and its care.	Assists in determining extent to which client is able to participate in care and need for teaching and information clarification.
12. Explain procedure to client; encourage client's interaction and questions.	Lessens anxiety and promotes client's participation.
13. Assemble equipment and close room curtains or door.	Optimizes use of time; conserves client's and nurse's energy. Provides privacy.
14. Position client either standing or supine and drape. If seated, position either on or in front of the toilet.	When client is supine, fewer wrinkles allow for ease of application of pouching system; maintains client's dignity.
15. Wash hands and put on disposable gloves.	Reduces transmission of microorganisms.
16. Place towel or disposable waterproof barrier under the client.	Protects bed linen.
17. Remove used pouch and skin barrier gently by pushing the skin away from the barrier. An adhesive remover may be used to facilitate removal of the skin barrier.	Reduces trauma; jerking irritates the skin and can cause tears.
18. Cleanse peristomal skin gently with warm tap water using gauze pads or clean washcloth; do not scrub the skin; dry completely by patting the skin with gauze or towel.	Avoid use of soap, because it leaves a residue on the skin that interferes with pouch adhesion to the skin. Skin must be as dry as skin barrier; pouch does not adhere to wet skin. If blood appears on the gauze pad, do not be alarmed; the stoma, if rubbed, may ooze some blood from the cleaning process. Bleeding into the pouch is abnormal. The stoma's surface is a highly vascular mucous membrane.

STEPS	RATIONALE
19. Measure the stoma for correct size of pouching system needed using the manufacturer's measuring guide (see illustration).	Ensures accuracy in determining correct pouch size needed. Stoma shrinks and does not reach usual size for 6 to 8 weeks.
20. Select appropriate pouch for client based on client assessment. With a custom cut-to-fit pouch, use an ostomy guide to cut opening on the pouch ¹⁄₁₆ to ⅛ inch larger than stoma before removing backing. Prepare pouch by removing backing from barrier and adhesive (see illustration). With ileostomy, apply thin circle of barrier paste around opening in pouch; allow to dry.	The paste facilitates seal and protects skin. Size of pouch opening keeps drainage off skin and lessens risk of damage to stoma during peristalsis or activity. Pouch and skin barrier are changed whenever leaking. Can also be changed before or after tub bath or shower. Stool is alkaline and this irritates the skin; fecal bacteria can colonize on the skin and increase risk of infection. Change when client is comfortable; before a meal is better, because this avoids increased peristalsis and chance of evacuation during the pouch change.
21. Apply the skin barrier and pouch. If creases next to stoma occur, use barrier paste to fill in; let dry 1 to 2 minutes.	

CRITICAL DECISION POINT

If client has surgical incision near stoma, the skin barrier may have to be trimmed for fit.

    A. For one-piece pouching system:
      (1) Use skin sealant wipes on skin directly under adhesive skin barrier or pouch; allow to dry. Press the adhesive backing of the pouch and/or skin barrier smoothly against the skin, starting from the bottom and working up and around the sides.

Continued

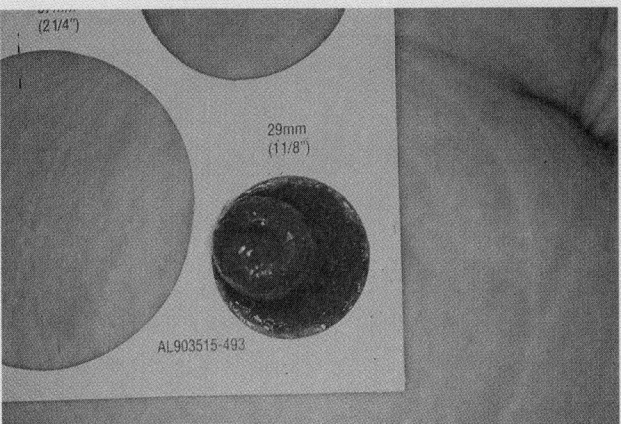

Step 19

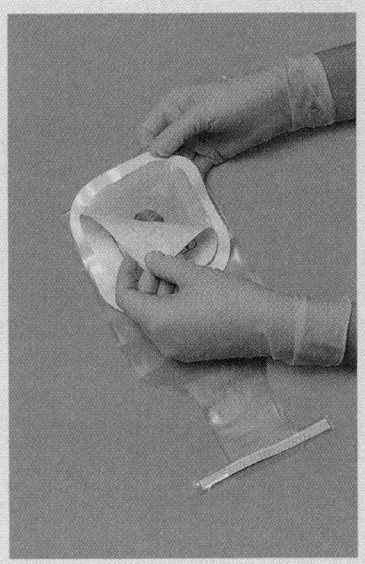

Step 20

STEPS	RATIONALE
(2) Hold pouch by barrier, center over stoma, and press down gently on barrier; bottom of pouch should point toward client's knees.	
(3) Maintain gentle finger pressure around the barrier for 1 to 2 minutes.	
B. For two-piece pouching system:	
(1) Apply flange (barrier with adhesive) as in steps above for one-piece system. Then snap on pouch and maintain finger pressure.	Creates wrinkle-free, secure seal; decreases irritation from the adhesive on skin.
22. Apply nonallergic paper tape around the pectin skin barrier in a "picture frame" method. Half of the tape should be on the skin barrier and half on the client's skin. Some clients may prefer a belt attached to the pouch for extra security rather than tape.	"Picture framing" the pectin skin barrier adds to the security of keeping the pouch system attached securely.

CRITICAL DECISION POINT

Be sure belt is not too tight by placing two fingers between belt and skin.

23. Although many ostomy pouches are odor-proof, some nurses and clients like to put a small amount of ostomy deodorant into the pouch. Do not use "home remedies," such as aspirin, to control ostomy odor.	Aspirin or other substances can harm the stoma.
24. Fold bottom of drainable open-ended pouches up once and close using a closure device such as a clamp (or follow manufacturer's instructions for closure).	Maintains secure seal to prevent leaking.
25. Properly dispose of old pouch and soiled equipment. Consider spraying deodorant in room if needed.	Lessens odors in room.
26. Remove gloves and wash hands.	Reduces transmission of microorganisms.
27. Change pouch every 3 to 7 days unless leaking; pouch can remain in place for tub bath or shower; after bath, pat adhesive dry.	Avoids unnecessary trauma to skin from too frequent changes. Drying ensures adhesion of pouch.
28. Ask if client feels discomfort around stoma.	Determines presence of skin irritation.
29. Note appearance of stoma around skin and existing incision (if present) while pouch is removed and skin is cleansed. Reinspect condition of skin barrier and adhesive.	Determines condition of tissues and progress of healing. Determines presence of leaks.
30. Auscultate bowel sounds and observe characteristics of stool.	Determines return of peristalsis and bowel elimination.
31. Observe client's nonverbal behaviors as pouch is applied. Ask if client has any questions about pouching.	May indicate emotional response to stoma and readiness for teaching. Determines level of understanding of procedure.

Recording and Reporting

- Chart type of pouch and skin barrier applied.
- Record amount and appearance of stool, texture, condition of peristomal skin, and sutures.
- Report any of the following to the charge nurse and/or physician:

   Abnormal appearance of stoma, suture line, peristomal skin, character of output, absence of bowel sounds.

   No flatus in 24 to 36 hours and no stool by third day.

- Document abdominal distention and excessive tenderness, nature of bowel sounds.
- Record client's level of participation and need for teaching.

Home Care Considerations

- Evaluate the client's home toileting facilities. This includes presence of adequate toileting facilities, flushable toilet, and number and location of toilets.
- Caution the client that most ostomy pouches and barriers cannot be flushed down the toilet; they clog the system. Dispose of used ostomy pouch according to local sanitation regulations.
- Instruct client to use a washcloth or any soft material to cleanse around stoma.

and prevents irritation from repeated pouch removal.

The pouch is changed when there is little drainage from the ostomy (e.g., before meals or at bedtime). The client should participate in the procedure as much as possible. The client must learn to recognize the normal appearance of a stoma. Skill 36-1 describes the steps for pouching an ostomy.

Care of hemorrhoids. Many clients experience discomfort as a result of alterations in elimination. The client with hemorrhoids has pain when hemorrhoidal tissues are directly irritated from passage of hard stool. The primary goal for the client with hemorrhoids is soft-formed stools. Proper diet, fluids, and regular exercise improve the likelihood of soft stools. Local heat provides temporary relief to swollen hemorrhoids. A sitz bath is the most effective means of heat application. To prevent trauma to tissues, the nurse must use caution when inserting rectal thermometers, suppositories, or rectal tubes. A generous amount of lubricating jelly reduces friction. Often the client is better able to insert an object safely into the rectum. The nurse should never attempt to force an object into the rectum without full view of the anus.

Flatulence. Flatulence can also cause discomfort. Air swallowing increases flatus. The client can reduce the amount of air swallowed by not drinking carbonated beverages, not using straws for drinking, and not chewing gum or hard candies.

When flatulence results in abdominal cramping, ambulation promotes the passage of flatus. Having the client walk down the hall may be enough to stimulate peristalsis and relieve gas. When conservative measures fail, flatulence can be relieved by insertion of a rectal tube. The client assumes a side-lying position while the nurse inserts the tube in the same manner as for an enema (Skill 36-2). Because fluid is not instilled into the bowel, the nurse can advance the tube to reach areas where flatus has accumulated (15 cm or 6 inches in an adult and 5 to 10 cm or 2 to 4 inches in a child). If the client complains of pain with tube placement or resistance is met, the nurse should discontinue the procedure and notify the client's physician.

After inserting the tube, the nurse instructs the client to lie quietly in bed. To prevent the tube from being dislodged, the nurse tapes it to a buttock. A gauze dressing or waterproof pad placed around the open end of the rectal tube catches any liquid fecal material. Continual use of rectal tubes can cause irritation and eventual excoriation of the anus and rectal mucosa. A rectal tube should not remain in place longer than 30 minutes. The physician will determine the frequency with which the tube can be inserted. If flatulence persists, the nurse notifies the physician.

Maintenance of skin integrity. The client with diarrhea or fecal incontinence is at risk for skin breakdown when fecal contents remain on the skin. The same problem exists for the client with a colostomy that drains liquid stool. Liquid stool is usually acidic and contains digestive enzymes. Irritation from repeated wiping with toilet tissue aggravates skin breakdown. Cleansing the skin after soiling helps but may result in more breakdown unless the skin is thoroughly dried.

The nurse should instruct the client about cleansing the anal area with mild soap and water after each passage of stool. When caring for a debilitated, incontinent client who is unable to ask for assistance, the nurse should check frequently for defecation. The anal areas can be protected with petrolatum jelly, zinc oxide, or

Administering a Cleansing Enema

Delegation Considerations

The skill of administering an enema can be delegated to unlicensed assistive personnel.

- Inform and assist care provider in proper way to position clients who have mobility restrictions.
- Caution care provider about transmission of pathogens.
- Inform care provider about how to position clients who also have therapeutic equipment present, such as drains, intravenous catheters, or traction.
- Inform care provider regarding signs and symptoms of client not tolerating the procedure, and when it must be stopped.

Equipment

- Disposable gloves
- Water-soluble lubricant
- Waterproof, absorbent pads
- Bath blanket
- Toilet tissue
- Bedpan, bedside commode, or access to toilet
- Wash basin, washcloths, towel, and soap
- IV pole

Enema bag administration

- Enema container
- Tubing and clamp (if not already attached to container)
- Appropriate size rectal tube:
  - Adult: 22 to 30 Fr
  - Child: 12 to 18 Fr
- Correct volume of warmed solution:
  - Adult: 750 to 1000 ml
  - Child:
    - 150 to 250 ml, infant
    - 250 to 350 ml, toddler
    - 300 to 500 ml, school-age child
    - 500 to 700 ml, adolescent

Prepackaged enema

- Prepackaged enema container with rectal tip

STEPS	RATIONALE
1. Assess status of client: last bowel movement, normal bowel patterns, hemorrhoids, mobility, external sphincter control, abdominal pain.	Determines factors indicating need for enema and influencing the type of enema used.
2. Assess for presence of increased intracranial pressure, glaucoma, or recent rectal or prostate surgery.	Conditions contraindicate use of enemas.
3. Determine client's level of understanding of purpose of enema.	Allows nurse to plan for appropriate teaching measures.
4. Check client's medical record to clarify the rationale for the enema.	Determines purpose of enema administration: preparation for special procedure or relief of constipation.
5. Review physician's order for enema.	Order by physician is required. Determines number and type of enema to be given.
6. Collect appropriate equipment.	
7. Correctly identify client and explain procedure.	Information promotes client cooperation and reduces anxiety.
8. Assemble enema bag with appropriate solution and rectal tube.	
9. Wash hands and apply gloves.	Reduces transmission of microorganisms.
10. Provide privacy by closing curtains around bed or closing door.	Reduces embarrassment for client.
11. Raise bed to appropriate working height for nurse: raise side rail on opposite side.	Promotes good body mechanics and client safety.
12. Assist client into left side-lying (Sims') position with right knee flexed. Children may also be placed in dorsal recumbent position.	Allows enema solution to flow downward by gravity along natural curve of sigmoid colon and rectum, thus improving retention of solution.

CRITICAL DECISION POINT

If client is suspected of having poor sphincter control, position on bedpan.
Client will have difficulty retaining enema solution.

STEPS	RATIONALE
13. Place waterproof pad under hips and buttocks.	Prevents soiling of linen.
14. Cover client with bath blanket, exposing only rectal area, clearly visualizing anus.	Provides warmth, reduces exposure of body parts, and allows client to feel more relaxed and comfortable.
15. Place bedpan or commode in easily accessible position. If client will be expelling contents in toilet, ensure that toilet is free. (If client will be getting up to bathroom to expel enema, place client's slippers and bathrobe in easily accessible position.)	Used in case client is unable to retain enema solution.
16. Administer enema:	
A. Prepackaged disposable container:	
(1) Remove plastic cap from rectal tip. Tip is already lubricated, but more jelly can be applied as needed.	Lubrication provides for smooth insertion of rectal tube without causing rectal irritation or trauma.
(2) Gently separate buttocks and locate rectum. Instruct client to relax by breathing out slowly through mouth.	Breathing out promotes relaxation of external rectal sphincter.
(3) Insert tip of bottle gently into rectum. Adult: 7.5 to 10 cm (3 to 4 inches) Child: 5 to 7.5 cm (2 to 3 inches) Infant: 2.5 to 3.75 cm (1 to 1½ inches)	Gentle insertion prevents trauma to rectal mucosa.
(4) Squeeze bottle until all of solution has entered rectum and colon. Instruct client to retain solution until the urge to defecate occurs, usually 2 to 5 minutes.	Hypertonic solutions require only small volumes to stimulate defecation.
B. Enema bag:	
(1) Add warmed solution to enema bag: warm tap water as it flows from faucet, place saline container in basin of hot water before adding saline to enema bag, check temperature of solution with bath thermometer or by pouring small amount of solution over inner wrist.	Hot water can burn intestinal mucosa. Cold water can cause abdominal cramping and is difficult to retain.
(2) Raise container, release clamp, and allow solution to flow long enough to fill tubing.	Removes air from tubing.
(3) Reclamp tubing.	Prevents further loss of solution.
(4) Lubricate 6 to 8 cm (3 to 4 inches) of tip of rectal tube with lubricating jelly.	Allows smooth insertion of rectal tube without risk of irritation or trauma to mucosa.
(5) Gently separate buttocks and locate anus. Instruct client to relax by breathing out slowly through mouth.	Breathing out promotes relaxation of external anal sphincter.
(6) Insert tip of rectal tube slowly by pointing tip in direction of client's umbilicus (see illustration on p. 1038). Length of insertion varies: Adult: 7.5 to 10 cm (3 to 4 inches) Child: 5 to 7.5 cm (2 to 3 inches) Infant: 2.5 to 3.75 cm (1 to 1½ inches)	Careful insertion prevents trauma to rectal mucosa from accidental lodging of tube against rectal wall. Insertion beyond proper limit can cause bowel perforation.

Continued

Skill 36-2—cont'd
Administering a Cleansing Enema

STEPS	RATIONALE
(7) Hold tubing in rectum constantly until end of fluid instillation.	Bowel contraction can cause expulsion of rectal tube.
(8) Open regulating clamp and allow solution to enter slowly with container at client's hip level.	Rapid instillation can stimulate evacuation of rectal tube.
(9) Raise height of enema container slowly to appropriate level above anus: 30 to 45 cm (12 to 18 inches) for high enema, 30 cm (12 inches) for regular enema, 7.5 cm (3 inches) for low enema.	Allows for continuous, slow instillation of solution. Raising container too high causes rapid instillation and possible painful distention of colon. High pressure can cause rupture of bowel in infant.
(10) Lower container or clamp tubing if client complains of cramping or if fluid escapes around rectal tube.	Temporary cessation of instillation prevents cramping, which may prevent client from retaining all fluid, altering effectiveness of enema.
(11) Clamp tubing after all solution is instilled.	Prevents entrance of air into rectum.
17. Place layers of toilet tissue around tube at anus and gently withdraw rectal tube.	Provides client's comfort and cleanliness.
18. Explain to client that feeling of distention is normal. Ask client to retain solution as long as possible while lying quietly in bed. (For infant or young child, gently hold buttocks together for a few minutes.)	Solution distends bowel. Length of retention varies with type of enema and client's ability to contract rectal sphincter. Longer retention promotes more effective stimulation of peristalsis and defecation.
19. Discard enema container and tubing in proper receptacle or rinse out thoroughly with warm soap and water if container is to be reused.	Reduces transmission and growth of microorganisms.
20. Assist client to bathroom or help to position client on bedpan.	Normal squatting position promotes defecation.
21. Observe character of feces and solution (caution client against flushing toilet before inspection).	

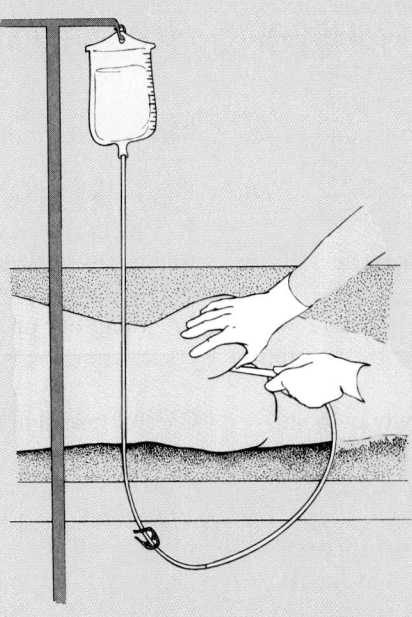

Step 16B(6)

STEPS	RATIONALE

CRITICAL DECISION POINT

When enemas are ordered "until clear," observe contents of solution passed. Return is "clear" when no solid fecal material exists, but solution may be colored.

STEPS	RATIONALE
22. Assist client as needed to wash anal area with warm soap and water (if nurse administers perineal care, use gloves).	Fecal contents can irritate skin. Hygiene promotes client's comfort.
23. Remove and discard gloves and wash hands.	Reduces transmission of microorganisms.
24. Inspect color, consistency, amount of stool, and fluid passed.	Determines if stool is evacuated or fluid is retained. Note abnormalities such as presence of blood or mucus.
25. Assess condition of abdomen; cramping, rigidity, or distention can indicate a serious problem.	Determines if distention is relieved. Excess volume can distend or perforate the bowel.

Recording and Reporting

▪ Record type and volume of enema given and characteristics of results.
▪ Report failure of client to defecate to physician.

Home Care Considerations

▪ For clients who require enemas for bowel preparation at home, instruct family not to exceed recommended fluid volume levels or number of enemas. Encourage family about the need for slow administration of warmed fluid.
▪ Instruct family about the negative side effects of tap water enemas.

other barrier ointments that hold moisture in the skin, preventing drying and cracking. Yeast infections of the skin can develop easily. Baby powder or cornstarch should not be used, because they have no medicinal properties and they frequently cake on the skin and become difficult to remove.

Evaluation

Client care. For the client with alterations in bowel elimination, the effectiveness of nursing interventions is measured by the success of meeting the client's expected outcomes and goals of care. Optimally, the client will be able to eliminate soft-formed stools regularly. In addition, the client will gain the information necessary to establish a normal elimination pattern.

The nurse evaluates success of the plan by having the client describe his or her elimination pattern following therapy. The nurse will focus on evaluating the character of the client's stool. A return to a more normal, regular elimination pattern can take time. The nurse will also reexamine the client periodically. A soft, nondistended abdomen is a desirable finding.

For the client with an ostomy, success at self-care and the ability to care for the ostomy appliances will be evaluated. The nurse must inspect skin integrity around the stoma site, looking for a reduction in inflammation around the stoma. The evaluation might also include observing the client change an ostomy pouch or perform an irrigation. The nurse will evaluate the output or functioning of the ostomy or reservoir as well. In addition, the client's self-esteem must be considered and can be evaluated by the client's response to and willingness to care for the ostomy.

Client expectations. Using client expectations identified previously, the nurse will determine the client's level of satisfaction with nursing care. Does the client feel that the nurse provided care respectfully, offering privacy and support when necessary? Is the client satisfied with the elimination pattern established? Are stools easier to manage? What worked, and what did not?

The nurse's goal for the ostomy client is to achieve a realistic level of self-care and to maintain or reinforce a healthy body image. When discussing these issues with the client, the nurse should determine if his or her nursing care helped the client accept the ostomy. Were expectations of the client unrealistic? Did the client feel like a partner in care? Learning about the client's level of satisfaction with care can go a long way toward helping future clients.

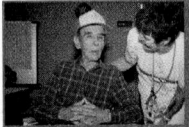

Case Study

Evaluation

Vickie returns to see Mr. Gutierrez 2 weeks later. Vickie is eager to determine if Mr. Gutierrez has made any changes in his diet and how his problems with bowel elimination have been progressing. Vickie is also anxious to learn if the niece has assisted in having Mr. Gutierrez's stove repaired.

Mr. Gutierrez tells Vickie that he has been eating bran cereal in the morning, has been eating rice and/or beans for dinner, and has added one fruit each day to his diet. He has been walking twice a day through the long-term care center. Although he doesn't have a bowel movement each day, his stools are much softer and easier to pass and he says he is less concerned. He has not taken a laxative for a stool since last talking with Vickie.

Documentation Note

Client's problem with bowel elimination is improving. The client's abdomen is soft and nondistended; bowel sounds normal and audible in all quadrants. Per teaching plan, client has altered eating habits to include more fiber, fruit, and fluids. Niece assisted in having stove repaired. Although client's concern over bowel habits has not ceased, the client does state he feels "in better control" and has decreased laxative use.

Key Terms

anorexia	flatus
bolus	guaiac test
cathartics	Harris flush
chyme	hemorrhoids
colon	laxatives
constipation	masticate
defecation	melena
diarrhea	ostomy
enema	peristalsis
fecal impaction	segmentation
fecal incontinence	stoma
feces	Valsalva maneuver

■ Key Concepts

A primary function of the elimination process is fluid balance.

Mechanical breakdown of food elements, GI motility, and selective absorption and secretion of substances by the large intestine influence the character of feces.

Food high in fiber content and an increased fluid intake keep feces soft.

Regular use of laxatives can lead to constipation.

The greatest danger from diarrhea is fluid and electrolyte imbalance.

The location of an ostomy influences the consistency of stool.

Assessment of an elimination pattern should focus on bowel habits, an analysis of factors that normally influence defecation, a review of recent changes in elimination, and a physical examination.

A guaiac test is recommended for clients who take anticoagulants, who have a bleeding disorder or GI disorder causing bleeding, or who are at risk for colon cancer.

Indirect and direct visualization of the lower GI tract requires cleansing of the bowel before the procedure.

The nurse should consider frequency of defecation, fecal characteristics, and effect of foods on GI function when selecting a diet promoting normal elimination.

Proper positioning on a bedpan allows the client to assume a position similar to squatting without experiencing muscle strain.

Cathartics or laxatives should be administered shortly before the usual time of defecation.

Proper administration of an enema is the slow instillation of the proper volume of a warm solution.

Proper selection and use of ostomy pouch systems protects peristomal skin.

A continent ostomy provides control over when fecal material exits.

Irrigation of an ostomy follows the same principles as an enema administration, except that a special irrigating tube is needed and the client cannot control passage of feces.

Dangers during digital removal of stool include traumatizing the rectal mucosa and promoting vagal stimulation.

Skin breakdown can occur after repeated exposure to liquid stool. This is especially true in clients with a stoma.

Critical Thinking Activities

1. While fulfilling your community service responsibility of taking blood pressures at the senior citizens' center, one of the clients tells you that this morning after he had a bowel movement, he noticed bright red blood on the toilet tissue. What further data would you need to gather?

2. An elderly woman with complaints of constipation tells you high-fiber foods are just too expensive. What would you advise?

3. This is your first day of caring for a bedridden, comatose, 87-year-old man. In reviewing his chart, you can find no entry of a bowel movement for the past 10 days. How would you proceed with your bowel assessment?

References

American Cancer Society: *Colon and rectal cancer—1996,* Atlanta, 1996, The Society.

Barkauskas VH and others: *Health and physical assessment,* St. Louis, 1994, Mosby

Beitz JM: The ileoanal reservoir: an alternative ileostomy, *J Wound Ostomy Continence Nurs* 21(3):120, 1994.

Caudell KA: Psychophysiological factors associated with irritable bowel syndrome, *Gastroenterol Nurs,* 17(2):61, 1994.

Dalton-Loehner D, Connor P: Beyond ileostomy: surgery for a normal life, *RN* 52:29, 1989.

Doughty D: A physiologic approach to bowel training, *J Wound Ostomy Continence Nurs,* 23(1):46, 1996.

Doughty D: A step-by-step approach to bowel training, *Progressions* 4(2):18, 1992.

Gibson CJ and others: Effectiveness of bran supplement on the bowel management of elderly rehabilitation clients, *J Gerontol Nurs* (10):21, 1995.

Giger JN, Davidhizar RE: *Transcultural nursing: assessment and intervention,* ed 2, St. Louis, 1995, Mosby.

Hampton BG, Bryant RA: *Ostomies and continent diversions: nursing management,* St. Louis, 1992, Mosby.

Lueckenotte AG: *Gerontologic nursing,* St. Louis, 1996, Mosby.

Lueckenotte AG: *Pocket guide to gerontologic assessment,* ed 2, St. Louis, 1994, Mosby.

Paulford-Lecher N: Getting your client started with an ostomy pouch, *Nurs 95* 25(4):32L, 1995.

Phipps WJ and others: *Medical-surgical nursing,* ed 5, St. Louis, 1995, Mosby.

Rolstad BS, Hoyman K: Continent diversion and reservoirs: In Hampton BG, Bryant RA: *Ostomies and continent diversions: nursing management,* St. Louis, 1992, Mosby.

Yen PK: Digestive dilemmas, *Geriatric Nurs* 16(3):141, 1995.

Clients With Special Needs

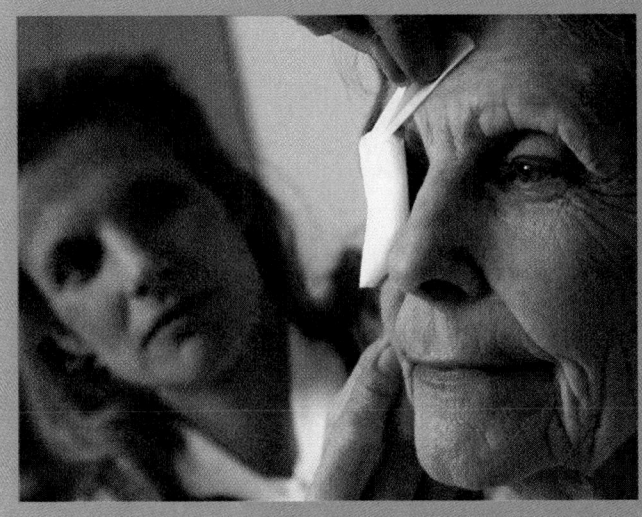

UNIT

7

Immobility

OBJECTIVES

Mastery of content in this chapter will enable the student to:

- Define the key terms listed.
- Describe mobility and immobility.
- Discuss the benefits and hazards of bed rest.
- Identify changes in metabolic rate associated with immobility.
- Describe physical changes associated with immobility.
- Describe musculoskeletal changes associated with immobility.
- Discuss factors that contribute to pressure ulcer formation.
- Describe psychosocial and developmental effects of immobilization.
- Complete a nursing assessment of an immobilized client.
- Develop a nursing care plan for an immobilized client.
- List appropriate nursing interventions for an immobilized client.
- State evaluation criteria for the immobilized client.

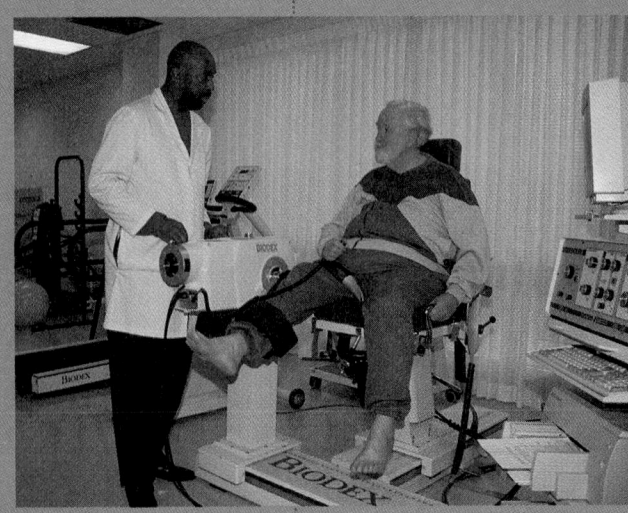

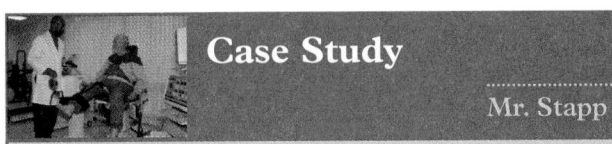

Case Study
Mr. Stapp

Bob Stapp is a 54-year-old man who is being admitted to the rehabilitation center after a bilateral total knee replacement 3 days ago. Mr. Stapp is expecting to be at the center about 10 days, when he will go home and continue therapy on an outpatient basis. He says his health is good, except he has a "bit of sugar" and "can't seem to lose that 50 pounds the doc wants me to." He plans to return to work in the steel mill, where he has worked for 28 years, as soon as he gets the doctor's okay. His postoperative course has been as expected.

Mark Weber is a 52-year-old nursing student who is completing the second half of his first clinical experience in nursing. He is a retired fireman, divorced, and has a son who is also in nursing school at a nearby college. It is his first day at the center; he spent the first half of his clinical experience on an orthopedic unit in a community hospital. Mark has never taken care of someone who is his same age.

SCIENTIFIC KNOWLEDGE BASE

Mobility

Mobility is a person's ability to move around freely in his or her environment. It serves many purposes, including expressing emotion, self-defense, attaining basic needs, performing recreational activities, and completing **activities of daily living (ADLs),** those activities of physical self-care such as bathing, dressing, and eating. In addition, mobility assists in maintaining the body's normal physiological activities. To maintain normal physical mobility, the nervous, muscular, and skeletal systems of the body must be intact, functioning, and used regularly. Although we all welcome a rare day to lie in bed and rest, the person who is immobile is predisposed to developing a wide variety of complications. Factors that contribute to the amount of disability include the degree of **immobility** (inability to move around freely), length of immobilization, severity of the illness, emotional state of the client, and the client's premorbid physical condition.

A decline in the client's mobility status may result from many types of health problems. Clients with certain illnesses, injuries, or surgeries may experience a period of immobilization as a result of changes in medical and physical status. Immobilization can also be used therapeutically to limit the movement of the whole body or a body part, and clients may have ambulation restrictions.

Mobility is often essential to the client's perception of health. Mobility is not simply the ability to move but is a complex interaction among the physical and psychosocial resources of the client and the resources in the environment. The aspects of the individual include motor skills, biological and psychological health, and sensory-perceptual capacity. Complete, unrestricted mobility requires voluntary motor and complete sensory control of all body regions. It also requires an environment that enables movement. Nurses may see clients at any point on the mobility-immobility continuum.

Mobility may be taken for granted until it is lost. Many of our bodily functions rely on mobility for optimum functioning. The benefits of mobility are often not appreciated until immobility is imposed or until functioning is decreased because mobility has declined.

Bed Rest

Bed rest is an intervention in which the client is restricted to bed for therapeutic reasons. Bed rest has different meanings among nurses, physicians, and other health care professionals. When bed rest is prescribed, the limitations on mobility should be explicit. Most often clarification of bathroom privileges is needed. The general objectives of bed rest include the following:

1. Reducing physical activity and the oxygen needs of the body
2. Allowing ill or debilitated clients to rest and regain strength
3. Preventing further injury to traumatized structures (e.g., spinal and vertebral injury)

Bed rest has physiological and psychological benefits only if the client finds it restful and if the client can freely move and change positions. Clients resistant to bed rest may actually expend more energy in fighting it than they would if allowed to move from bed to chair.

Clients with a wide variety of conditions are placed on bed rest. The duration of bed rest depends on the type and nature of the illness or injury and the client's prior state of health. The risks and benefits of bed rest must be weighed for each client.

Immobility

Immobility occurs when a client is unable to independently move or change positions or movement is restricted for medical reasons. The effects of immobility are systemic and functional. No body system is immune to the effects of immobility. In a classic study, Deitrick and others (1948) found that even young healthy men put on bed rest had physiological problems. Periods of immobility or prolonged bed rest can cause major physiological and psychological effects, which can be gradual or immediate and can vary from client to client. The greater the extent and the longer the duration of immobility, the more pronounced the consequences. The client with complete mobility restrictions is continually at risk for the hazards of immobilization (Box 37-1). Nursing care and education are directed toward minimizing these hazards because it is generally easier to prevent the complications than to treat or cure them.

Immobility may be the result of either physical inactivity or physical restriction of movement. Physical inactivity may occur as a response to severe pain or as a result of sensory changes reducing the physical stimulus to move. Immobility may also be a result of cognitive-emotional changes, such as depression, or a result of a treatment, such as prescribed bed rest. Physical restriction or limitation of movement, such as by cast, traction, or restraints, results in an imposed reduction of movement. Both inactivity and restricted movement may cause changes in body position and posture that result in a loss of the body's ability to adapt to such changes. The degree of the client's immobility depends on the interaction of the conditions present.

Clients who are partially mobile usually have a motor or sensory impairment in a region of the body or a therapeutic restriction (e.g., a casted extremity). A partial loss of mobility may be temporary (e.g., the result of a fracture) or permanent (e.g., the result of paralysis). In some cases the restriction of mobility benefits the client's recovery, such as with a casted extremity. The hazards associated with partial mobility depend on the degree and duration of immobilization and the client's previous condition. The resulting hazards are usually temporary and resolve shortly after complete mobility is restored. Generally clients who are relatively healthy before immobilization are more likely to have complete mobility restored.

Physiological effects. Each body system is at risk for impairments resulting from immobility. The severity of the impairment depends on the client's age, overall mental and physical health, and the degree of immobility. Frail older adult clients with chronic illnesses develop pronounced effects of immobility more quickly than do younger clients. For a frail older adult client who has a stroke and is immobile, the impairments developing from the immobility can occur within a few days. Often it is complications that occur secondary to immobility such as sepsis and pneumonia that explain most deaths during the second and third week following a stroke (Moore, 1994).

Immobility disrupts normal metabolic functioning, including the metabolic rate and the metabolism of car-

---

Box 37-1
Hazards of Immobility

Physiological Effects
Metabolic System

Decreased basal metabolic rate (BMR)
Altered carbohydrate, fat, and protein metabolism
Fluid and electrolyte imbalances
Increased bone resorption
Gastrointestinal disturbances

Respiratory System

Decreased hemoglobin levels
Reduced lung expansion
Respiratory muscle weakness
Stasis of secretions

Cardiovascular System

Orthostatic hypotension
Increased cardiac workload
Thrombus formation

Musculoskeletal System

Loss of endurance
Decreased muscle mass
Atrophy
Decreased stability
Joint contractures
Disuse osteoporosis

Integumentary System

Pressure ulcer formation

Urinary System

Renal calculi
Decreased urinary output
Urinary stasis
Urinary tract infection

Psychosocial Effects

Depression
Behavioral changes
Altered sleep-wake cycles
Decreased coping abilities
Increased isolation
Sensory deprivation

Developmental Effects

Decreased progression through developmental tasks
Increased dependence

bohydrates, fats, and proteins. It can also cause fluid and electrolyte imbalances, problems with bone metabolism, and gastrointestinal disturbances.

Changes in metabolic rate. Decreased mobility results in a decrease in the basal metabolic rate (BMR). The client's BMR falls in response to the decreased energy requirement of body cells, which is directly related to cellular oxygen demands. However, fever or wound healing may increase the BMR because these conditions increase cellular oxygen requirements (McCance and Huether, 1994).

Changes in metabolism of carbohydrates, fats, and proteins. As bed rest continues, pancreatic activity decreases, as does the body's ability to tolerate glucose. Insulin production is not enough to lower serum glucose levels. As proteins are metabolized, nitrogen is produced as an end product. Nitrogen balance provides a reliable indicator of protein use by the body. A **negative nitrogen balance** exists when the excretion of nitrogen from the breakdown of protein exceeds intake. A negative nitrogen balance predisposes the client to problems with wound healing and normal tissue growth. Decreased mobility results in increased percentage of body fat and the loss of lean body mass.

Fluid and electrolyte imbalances. Because the client is in a recumbent position, major shifts in blood volume occur. During bed rest the client may initially lose an additional average of 600 ml/day (Rubin, 1988). This **diuresis** (increased urine excretion) occurs as a result of the changes of increased blood flow to the kidneys and the expanded circulating blood volume. Excretion of electrolytes through the skin and urinary system is also a potential risk.

Bone metabolism. There is an increased excretion of calcium in the urine during bed rest (Deitrick and others, 1948). The probable source of this calcium is **bone resorption** (bone loss). Normally the kidneys are able to excrete excess calcium. However, if the kidneys are unable to respond appropriately, **hypercalcemia** (excessive calcium in the blood) results. Hypercalcemia may further lead to the formation of kidney stones.

Gastrointestinal changes. Although impairments in gastrointestinal functioning vary in clients, the symptoms are related to decreased motility. Activity stimulates peristalsis. The immobile client is at risk for constipation from lack of activity and from hypercalcemia, which depresses peristalsis. Constipation may be so severe that fecal impaction may occur (Figure 37-1). The client who is impacted may have no bowel movements or may have liquid stool that passes around the area of impaction (see Chapter 36).

Respiratory changes. When a client assumes a recumbent position, the lungs shift position a full 90 degrees. This shift in lung position and body fluids, along with the pressure of the abdominal contents pushing against the diaphragm, causes a change in lung volume (Rubin, 1988). Respiratory problems occurring with

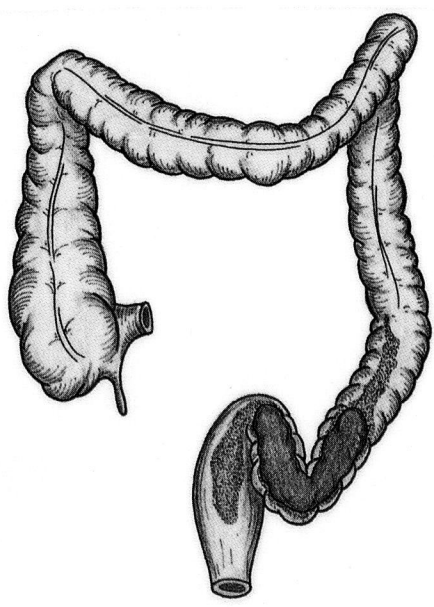

Figure 37-1. Fecal impaction with liquid stool passing around impaction.

immobility are caused by decreased hemoglobin, decreased lung expansion, generalized respiratory muscle weakness, and stasis of secretions.

Because of the diuretic response to bed rest, hypovolemia may result, causing transient elevations in hematocrit values on or about the eight day of immobilization. Red blood cell mass and hemoglobin levels decline (Rubin, 1988).

Immobilization decreases lung expansion. Changes in the client's position alter ventilation and the distribution and blood flow through the lung. In the sidelying position, for example, the dependent lung is less effectively oxygenated. Thus turning and positioning are critical.

Limited physical activity and metabolic changes result in weakened respiratory muscles. Thus the work of breathing increases, causing a proportional decline in the client's ability to cough productively. Ultimately the distribution of mucus in the bronchi increases, particularly when the client is in the supine, prone, or lateral position (Figure 37-2). Mucus accumulates in the dependent regions of the bronchial tube, and because mucus is an excellent medium for bacterial growth, hypostatic bronchopneumonia may result. Pneumonia that results from fluid accumulation as a result of inactivity is called **hypostatic pneumonia.**

With decreased lung expansion and weakened respiratory muscles, secretions stagnate or pool in the dependent lung regions (Figure 37-3). In addition, cilia become unable to move the secretions from the respiratory tract. Thus the potential increases for pneumonia and atelectasis. **Atelectasis** is a collapse of the alveoli that prevents the normal exchange of oxygen and carbon dioxide.

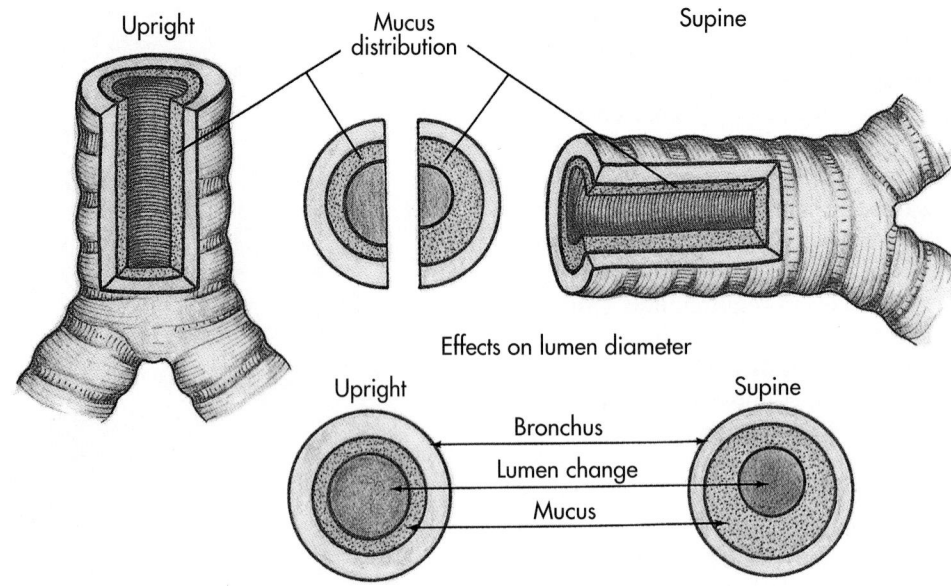

Upright   Mucus distribution   Supine

Effects on lumen diameter

Upright   Supine

Bronchus

Lumen change

Mucus

Figure 37-2.   Effect of recumbency and gravity on distribution of respiratory tract mucus of bronchiolar lumen.

Cardiovascular changes. The cardiovascular system is also affected by immobilization. Orthostatic hypotension occurs in the client on bed rest, but it may also occur in clients with prolonged sitting. **Orthostatic hypotension** is a drop of 15 mm Hg or more in systolic blood pressure when the client rises from a lying or sitting position to a standing position. In the immobilized client, there is decreased circulating fluid volume, pooling of blood in the lower extremities, and decreased autonomic response. These result in decreased venous return, central venous pressure, and stroke volume and a drop in systolic blood pressure when the client stands (McCance and Huether, 1994).

Increased cardiac workload is demonstrated by rate changes. Prolonged bed rest increases the resting heart rate 4 to 15 beats/min. When the immobilized client is asked to do physical activity such as with range-of-motion (ROM) exercises or ADLs, this increased rate is more pronounced. As the workload of the heart increases, so does its oxygen consumption. The heart therefore works harder and less efficiently during prolonged rest.

Immobile clients are at risk for deep venous thrombosis (DVT). A **thrombus** is an accumulation of platelets, fibrin, clotting factors, and cellular elements of the blood attached to the interior wall of a vein or artery, sometimes occluding the lumen of the vessel (Figure 37-4). A number of factors predispose to venous thrombi: hypovolemia, tissue injury, surgery, and clotting abnormalities. In addition, the weight of the legs on the bed compresses the blood vessels of the calves, causing stasis and injury to vessel linings. Another problem in the venous system is the loss of the pumping action of the skeletal muscles. Normally calf

muscles aid venous return by pumping blood through the legs back to the heart. However, this mechanism is reduced when the client is on bed rest or has a cast on a leg. Clients with large abdomens such as women who are pregnant or obese clients are at greater risk for DVT because of compression of the veins in the groin (Nunnelee, 1995).

Venous thrombi put the client at risk for pulmonary emboli, a life-threatening complication. Pulmonary emboli are clots that have moved in the venous system, blocking a portion of the pulmonary artery system and thus disrupting blood flow to the lungs. Immobilized surgical and older adult clients are at high risk for developing pulmonary emboli.

Musculoskeletal changes. Restricted mobility leads to loss of strength and endurance, decreased muscle mass, and decreased stability or balance. A decline in skeletal muscle strength can ultimately reduce the debilitated client's return to the premorbid functioning (Kasper and others, 1993).

Muscle strength is lost when muscles are inactive. The rate of decline will vary with the degree of immobility but may be rapid as mobility and weight bearing are restricted (Kasper and others, 1996). These effects can be devastating to clients who are marginally functioning at their ADLs.

Reduced endurance results when clients are immobile from changes in muscle strength and altered cardiovascular functioning. Because of the increased cardiac workload, muscle endurance is decreased as a result of the decreased ability of the cardiopulmonary system to meet the oxygen needs of the tissue. In addition, because of the metabolic changes, the client loses lean body mass, which is composed partially of muscle.

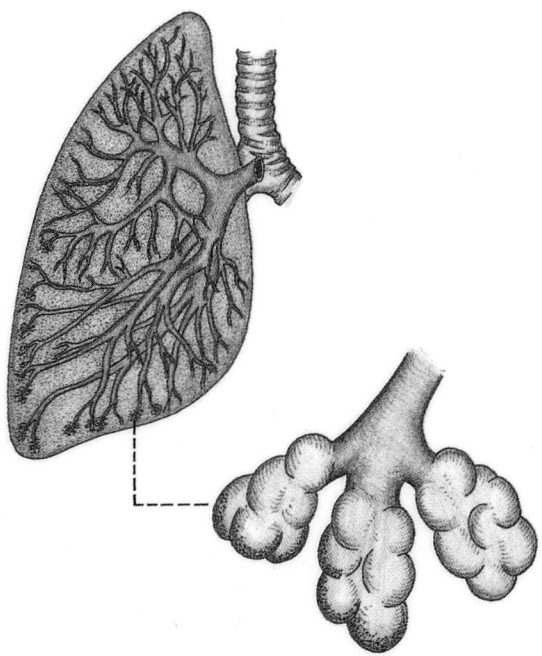

Figure 37-3. Pooling of secretions in dependent regions of lungs in supine position.

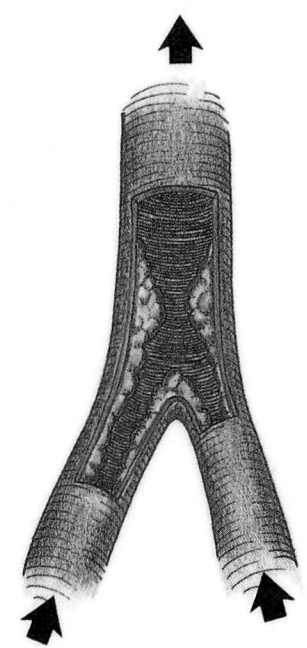

Figure 37-4. Thrombus formation in vessel.

Therefore the reduced muscle mass is unable to sustain prolonged activity without fatigue.

Muscle mass decreases from metabolic causes and disuse. As immobility continues and the muscles are not exercised, muscle mass continues to decrease. The muscle atrophies, and the size of the muscle decreases. The leg muscles appear to be the most affected by immobility, which accounts in part for the difficulty the older client may have in getting up out of a chair after periods of bed rest.

Decreased stability is the result of loss of endurance, decreased muscle mass, and joint abnormalities. Therefore clients are unable to move steadily, and their risk for falling increases.

Immobilization causes two skeletal changes. A **joint contracture** is abnormal and may result in permanent contraction of a joint characterized by flexion and fixation. It is caused by disuse, atrophy, and shortening of muscle fibers and surrounding joint tissues. When a contracture occurs, the joint cannot maintain its full range of joint motion, leaving it in a nonfunctional position (Figure 37-5). Foot-drop contracture (Figure 37-6) results in the foot being permanently fixed in plantar flexion. Ambulation is difficult with the foot in this position.

The second skeletal change is **disuse osteoporosis,** a disorder characterized by bone resorption secondary to immobility. Osteoporosis is the result of impaired calcium metabolism. Because immobilization results in bone resorption, bone tissue is less dense, and osteoporosis results. The client is at risk for **pathological fractures,** a type of fracture that occurs as a result of bone weakness.

Integument changes. The direct effect of pressure on the skin by immobility is compounded by the changes in metabolism that accompany immobility. Older adult clients and clients with paralysis have a greater risk for developing pressure ulcers. Pressure affects cellular metabolism by decreasing or obliterating tissue circulation. When a client lies in bed or sits in a chair, the weight of the body is on bony prominences. The longer the pressure is applied, the longer the period of **ischemia** and therefore the greater the risk of skin breakdown (Figure 37-7) (see Chapter 38). Any break in the skin's integrity is difficult to heal in the immobilized client. Preventing a pressure ulcer is much less expensive than treating one (Helme, 1994).

Tissue metabolism depends on the body's receipt of oxygen and nutrients from the blood supply and the elimination of metabolic wastes. Any factor that interferes with this process affects cellular metabolism and, as a result, the function or life of the cell.

Urinary elimination changes. Urine flows out of the renal pelvis and into the ureter and bladder because of gravitational forces when the client is upright. When the client is recumbent, the kidneys and ureters move toward a more level plane, and urine formed by the kidney must enter the bladder against gravity. Because the peristaltic contractions of the ureters are insufficient to overcome gravity, the renal pelvis may fill before urine enters the ureters (Figure 37-8). This condition, called urinary stasis, increases the client's risk of urinary tract infection and renal calculi. **Renal calculi** are calcium stones that lodge in the renal pelvis and pass through the ureters (Figure 37-9).

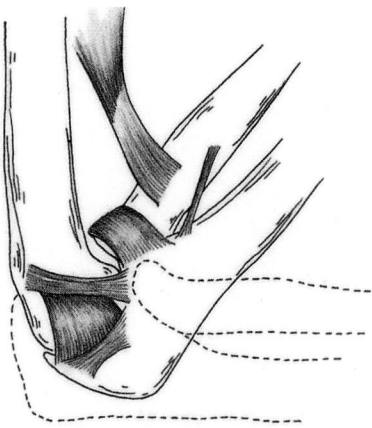

Figure 37-5. Flexion contracture of elbow resulting in permanent flexion of joint. Normally the elbow is able to extend to a 90-degree angle *(dotted line)* and to a 180-degree angle *(not shown)*.

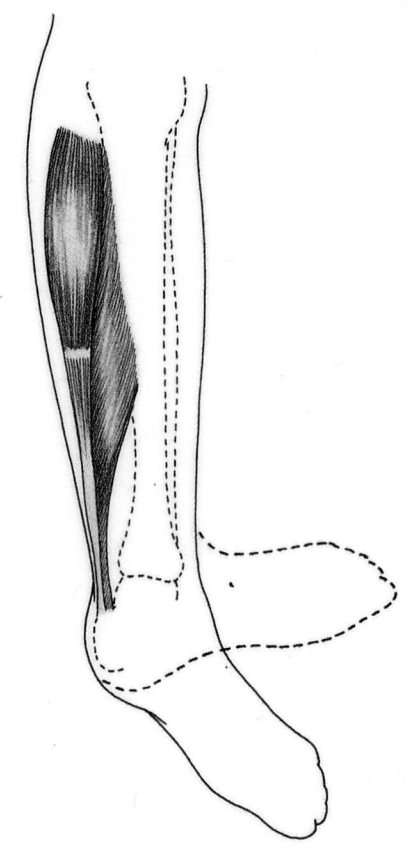

Figure 37-6. Foot-drop. Ankle is fixed in plantar flexion.

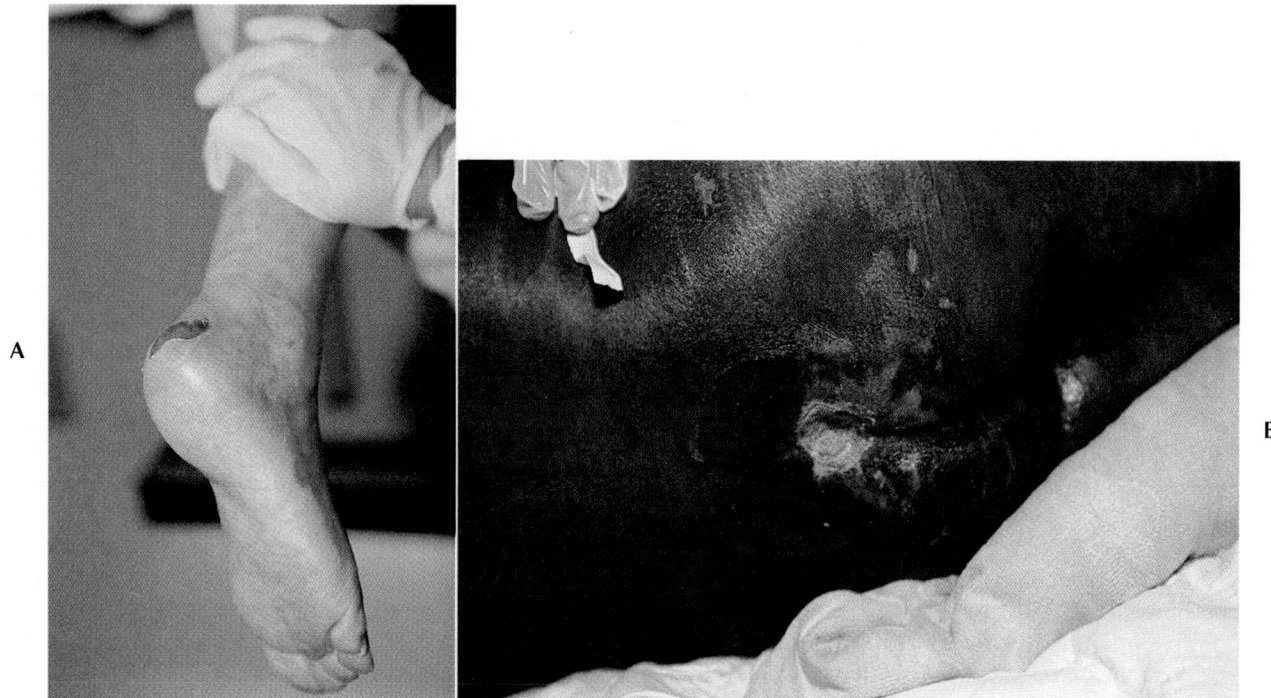

Figure 37-7. **A,** Formation of pressure sore on heel. **B,** Pressure ulcer with tissue necrosis on coccyx.

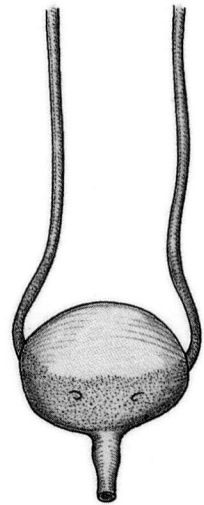

Figure 37-8.   Stasis of urine.

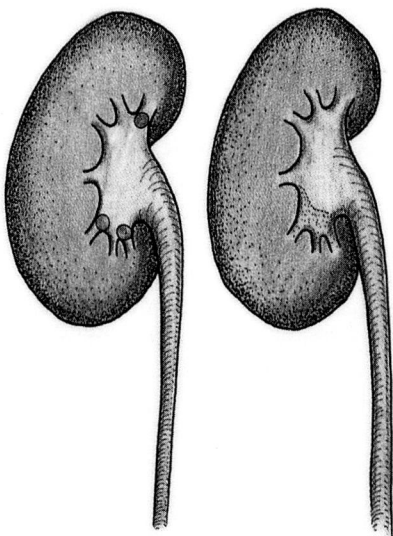

Figure 37-9.   Renal calculi in renal pelvis.

During the initial period of immobility, urine volume is increased secondary to fluid shifts and a natural diuresis (Deitrick and others, 1948). As immobility continues, fluid intake diminishes, and other causes such as fever increase the risk of dehydration. Because of these factors, urinary output declines on or about day 5 or 6. The urine then produced is usually highly concentrated. This concentrated urine increases the risk for calculi formation and infection.

Immobility also increases the risk of incontinence. Barriers such as side rails, distant bathrooms, and lack of staff to help with toileting make incontinence a problem particularly for the older adult client (see Chapter 35).

⋯⋯⋯⋯NURSING KNOWLEDGE BASE⋯

Monitoring or assisting clients with mobility is basic to nursing. Concepts that relate to mobility such as movement, exercise and rest, and posture are soundly grounded in many nursing theories. The nurse caring for the client who is immobile needs to recognize that immobilization may lead to a variety of psychosocial responses and influence the development of the client. In addition, the nurse caring for the client who is immobile needs good assessment skills. Since mobility is a function of intact neurological and musculoskeletal systems, the nurse must draw on assessments to fully understand the client's initial condition as well as to monitor and evaluate care (see Chapter 24).

Psychosocial Effects

Immobilization may lead to emotional, intellectual, sensory, and sociocultural responses. The most common emotional changes are depression, behavioral changes, sleep-wake disturbances, and impaired coping.

The immobilized client can become depressed be-

cause of changes in role, self-concept, independence, and other factors. Depression is an affective disorder characterized by exaggerated feelings of sadness, melancholy, dejection, worthlessness, emptiness, and hopelessness out of proportion to reality.

The immobilized client requires constant nursing care. Because of physiological hazards, the client cannot be allowed to sleep for 8 hours without a change of position or other nursing care. Disruption of normal sleeping patterns can further cause behavioral changes. Nursing interventions should be used to ensure the client receives sufficient sleep (see Chapter 32). The client who is on bed rest and is able to change position during sleep does not require continuous physical nursing care directed at reducing the hazards of immobility. Unless other treatment activities are required during the night, the care plan for the physiologically stable client on bed rest can provide for uninterrupted sleep.

Long-term immobility or bed rest can affect usual coping patterns. Such a client may withdraw and become passive. The passive client allows nurses to provide care but is not interested in increasing independence or involvement in care. Early in the care of an immobilized client the nurse should assess the client's normal coping mechanisms. The nurse then designs a nursing care plan that will allow the client to continue to use these coping abilities or will help the client develop new ones.

Developmental Effects

More developmental changes tend to be associated with immobility in the very young and in the older adult. The immobilized young or middle-age adult may experience few, if any, developmental changes. However, there are exceptions, such as a mother who has complications at childbirth and as a result cannot interact with the newborn as expected.

When the infant, toddler, or preschooler is immobilized, it is usually because of trauma or the need to correct a congenital skeletal abnormality. Prolonged immobilization can delay the child's motor skill and intellectual development. Nurses caring for immobilized children should plan activities that provide physical and psychosocial stimuli. Other activities focus on the specific effects of immobilization.

Immobilization of older adult clients increases their physical dependence on others and accelerates functional losses in physiological systems. Immobilization of an older adult client usually results from a degenerative disease, neurological trauma, or a chronic illness. For some clients, immobilization occurs gradually and progressively, whereas for others—especially those who have had a stroke—immobilization is sudden. When providing nursing care for an older adult client, the nurse should develop a care plan that encourages the client to perform as many self-care activities as possible, thereby maintaining the highest level of functional mobility. Blair (1995) points out that nurses may inadvertently contribute to a client's loss of mobility by providing unnecessary help with ADLs.

CRITICAL THINKING IN CLIENT CARE

Synthesis

The nurse draws information from a variety of sources when determining care with a client. The nurse must understand what sources are being used in order to validate and prioritize nursing care for the immobilized client. The client's needs are multiple, and by integrating knowledge and experience the nurse is able to determine the needs as well as focus on the nonphysiological areas that impact on the client and family.

Knowledge. Drawing on previous information from pathophysiology, the nurse is able to anticipate the types of limitations in mobility clients may have. These limitations may be the direct results of musculoskeletal alteration or may be the results of deconditioning resulting from a chronic health problem. Knowledge of physical assessment techniques enable the nurse to determine the exact extent of any limitations. To fully anticipate the functional needs of the client with impaired mobility, the nurse must assess the client's developmental stage to determine current functional and mobility status, as well as to determine the health care needs of the client.

The use of proper body mechanics is important for the nurse and client alike to assist the client to turn, position, and transfer safely. Knowledge from physiology enables the nurse to observe for complications of immobility and intervene appropriately. Further, teaching is an important role in the rehabilitation process because the client's rehabilitation work needs to be vigorously maintained when returning home.

Experience. The nurse may have taken care of other clients who have had mobility restrictions. These experiences help the nurse to anticipate client needs such as pain control, positioning, and support of activities of daily living. Visits to a physical therapy unit in the hospital or in a community setting can increase a nurse's experiential base. In addition, the nurse can use experience from a personal exercise plan to help the client improve mobility status during health promotion activities, acute care, or rehabilitation.

Attitude. The nurse must be creative in designing solutions to improve the client's mobility status. The nurse may confer with other health care providers to determine the setting in which the care is best provided. Collaboration and creativity establish an individualized rehabilitation program. The nurse must reflect on the nurse's own perceptions of the client's mobility status. Self-reflection enables the nurse to act as a client advocate to encourage the client's motivation to improve mobility status, as well as identifying ways in which the family can also participate.

Standards. The nurse promotes client independence while adhering to the prescribed rehabilitation plan and maintaining client safety. The nurse recognizes the client's physical limitations and the emotional stress associated with impaired mobility. Concern and compassion for the client help to establish and maintain the client's self-confidence, independence, and self-respect.

The nurse knows that the synthesis of knowledge, experience, attitudes, and standards into the plan of care for a client with impaired mobility is important in developing an individualized care plan for the client. Such a plan of care will help to prevent complications, promote rehabilitation, and promote a timely return of clients to their home.

NURSING PROCESS AND IMMOBILITY

▪ Assessment

The assessment includes the client's present mobility, information about pre-illness functioning, and the potential effects of immobility.

Mobility. Assessment of the client's mobility focuses on range of joint motion, muscle strength, activity tolerance, gait, and posture. Chapter 27 describes the normal ROM for all joints in the body. Observation during ADLs enables the nurse to estimate the client's fatigability, muscle strength, and ROM.

Finally, observing the client's posture while sitting

and standing and assessing gait help the nurse to determine the type of assistance the client may require to change positions or transfer from bed to chair. This information helps the nurse to assess the client's overall level of mobility and coordination.

Risks and indicators of immobility.

The nurse assesses immobilized clients for physiological changes resulting from immobility. A head-to-toe physical assessment (see Chapter 24) allows the nurse to assess the physical function. It also includes a review of psychosocial and developmental dimensions.

Physiological condition.

The nurse assesses those body systems most likely to be affected by immobility. During this assessment the nurse is mindful of normal functioning as well as expected changes attributable to the client's developmental stage.

Metabolic system. When assessing the client's metabolic functioning, the nurse uses **anthropometric measurements** (body measures of height, weight, and skinfolds) to evaluate muscle atrophy. Intake and output records and laboratory data assist in evaluating fluid and electrolyte status. A client's nutritional status is assessed to determine risk for nitrogen imbalance. A client whose mobility is restricted may have a reduced appetite, altered gastrointestinal function, and a reduced capacity to self-feed.

Anorexia occurs commonly in immobilized clients. The nurse should assess food intake and the environment for unpleasant odors or noises that may interfere with appetite. Nutritional imbalances can be avoided if the nurse learns the client's previous dietary patterns and food preferences early in the immobilization (see Chapter 34).

Anthropometric measurements include height, weight, mid–upper-arm circumference, and triceps skinfold measurements. Ideally this assessment should be done early in the period of immobilization and should be repeated at regular intervals. Assessment of height and weight is discussed in Chapter 24. A decrease in mid–upper-arm circumference, measured in centimeters, or triceps skinfolds, measured in millimeters, indicates a decline in muscle mass. After the initial assessment this measurement may be done every 2 to 4 weeks depending on the client's age, premorbid condition, and the amount of immobility.

If an immobilized client has a wound, the speed of healing indicates how well nutrients are delivered to the tissues for use (see Chapter 38). The normal progression of wound healing indicates that the metabolic needs of the injured tissues are being met.

Respiratory system. A respiratory assessment should be performed every 2 hours for acutely ill clients with restricted activity. The nurse should inspect chest wall movements and auscultate the entire lung region to identify regions of diminished breath sounds. Ausculta-

tion for adventitious lung sounds should focus on the dependent lung field because pulmonary secretions tend to move to these lower regions. If a client has an atelectatic area, breath sounds may be asymmetrical. A complete respiratory assessment identifies the presence of secretions and can be used to determine nursing interventions necessary to maintain optimal respiratory function.

Cardiovascular system. The cardiovascular assessment of the immobilized client includes monitoring blood pressure, apical and peripheral pulses, and observing the venous system. Because of the risk for orthostatic hypotension, blood pressure should be measured, particularly when the client switches from lying to a sitting or standing position. In this way the client's ability to tolerate postural changes can be assessed.

Recumbency increases the cardiac workload and results in an increased pulse rate. In some clients, particularly the older adult, the heart may not be able to tolerate the increased workload, and a form of cardiac failure may develop. Monitoring the client's peripheral pulses allows the nurse to evaluate the heart's ability to pump the blood throughout the body. The absence of a peripheral pulse, particularly one that was previously present, should be documented and reported after a complete circulatory assessment is made (see Chapter 24).

Edema may indicate the heart's inability to handle the increased workload. Because fluid moves to dependent body regions, assessment of the immobilized client should include the sacrum, legs, feet, and hips. If the heart is unable to tolerate the increased cardiac workload, the peripheral body regions such as the hands, feet, nose, and earlobes will be colder than the central body regions.

Finally the nurse assesses the venous system for DVT. To assess for DVT, the nurse should remove the client's elastic stockings once every 8 hours and observe the calves for redness, warmth, and tenderness. The nurse should ask the client about calf pain. The nurse may also ask the client to dorsiflex the foot and assess for the presence of calf pain. Calf pain on dorsiflexion (positive Homans' sign) may indicate DVT. Homans' sign is not reliable, however, and as many as half of all clients with DVT will have a negative Homans' sign (Nunnelee, 1995).

In addition, calf and thigh circumferences should be measured daily in clients at high risk for developing thrombi. DVT can also occur in the thigh. To measure circumferences, the nurse marks a point on each of the client's calves and thighs 10 cm from the midpatella. The circumferences are measured each day using the marks as a reference point for placing the tape measure. One-sided edema can be an early as well as the only clue to DVT (Nunnelee, 1995).

Musculoskeletal system. The major musculoskeletal abnormalities identified during assessment include decreased muscle strength, loss of muscle tone and mass, and contractures. Clients with musculoskeletal injuries or chronic conditions require careful palpation of joints and extremities to reduce discomfort. Because immobilized clients are weakened, the nurse must determine if difficulty in moving joints is the result of fatigue or decreased range of joint motion.

Skin integrity. The nurse must continually assess the skin for signs of pressure ulcer formation. The client with sensorimotor impairments, the chronically ill client in long-term care, the client with diminished mental status, the incontinent client in any setting, the orthopedic client, and the multiple-trauma client are at high risk for developing pressure ulcers.

The nurse should look for specific factors such as sensory loss and anemia (see Chapter 24) when assessing clients at risk for pressure ulcer formation. When assessing the client's skin, the nurse should view all pressure points to determine whether they are adequately protected and the skin is not exposed to body fluids. Last, the nurse assesses the client's nutritional status and observes for signs of infection that increase the risk for pressure ulcers (see Chapter 38).

Elimination system. The client's elimination status should be evaluated on each shift, and the total intake and output should be evaluated every 24 hours (see Chapter 31). The nurse should determine that the client is receiving the correct amount and type of fluids orally or parenterally.

Assessment of elimination should also include auscultation for bowel sounds, the frequency and consistency of bowel movements, and the client's usual urine and bowel elimination patterns. Accurate assessment and documentation enable the nurse to intervene before fecal impaction occurs and may also prevent urine incontinence. Elimination assessment should be done minimally at the beginning and end of each shift.

Psychosocial condition. Changes in psychosocial status usually occur slowly and are often overlooked by health care personnel. The nurse should observe for changes in emotional status (e.g., depression). The nurse also observes for behavioral changes (e.g., cooperative clients who become argumentative or modest clients who begin to expose themselves repeatedly). The nurse should try to determine the reasons for such behavioral alterations to identify specific nursing therapies. Continual communication with the family is vital because they may identify and report changes in personality that staff may not recognize.

Changes in the client's sleep-wake cycle such as difficulty falling asleep or frequent awakenings must be identified and corrected (see Chapter 32). Many sleep disruptions can be prevented or minimized with an assessment of prior sleep habits and early intervention when problems are suspected. Finally, the nurse should observe for changes in the use of normal coping mechanisms to adapt to immobilization. Decreasing coping ability may cause the client to become disoriented, confused, or depressed or to experience other behavioral changes.

Development. Assessment of the immobilized client should include developmental considerations to ensure that all needs are identified. With a young child the nurse determines where the child was developmentally prior to immobilization and whether the child is able to meet developmental tasks and is progressing normally. Development may regress or be slowed because of immobilization. By identifying a child's overall developmental needs, the nurse can design nursing therapies to maintain normal development. When developmental delays are temporary, the nurse may also need to assure the parents.

Developmental assessment is as important with the older adult client as with the young child. The nursing assessment enables the nurse to determine the older adult client's ability to meet needs independently. A decline in developmental functioning prompts investigation to determine the reasons the change occurred and the interventions necessary to restore the client to an optimal level of function (see Chapter 20).

Client expectations. Clients with impaired mobility may have certain expectations of the care provider. For example, some clients may expect to be challenged to improve their level of independence. This is particularly true of clients in the rehabilitative phase of their illness or injury. On the other hand, a client's physiological condition may contraindicate such independence in function. Clients may agree or disagree with their physical limitations and expect their care givers to do the same. In knowing the client's expectations, the nurse is able to identify when care may be modified to meet these expectations, know when teaching is needed to explain why care cannot be modified, or be a compassionate listener to clients who cannot be as mobile as they wish.

....

Successful critical thinking requires a synthesis of knowledge, experience, information gathered from clients, and critical thinking attitudes and standards. Clinical judgments require the nurse to anticipate what information is needed, to analyze the data, and then to make decisions regarding client care. The client expects competent and informed care. Mark Weber incorporates previous knowledge and experience in providing care for Mr. Stapp.

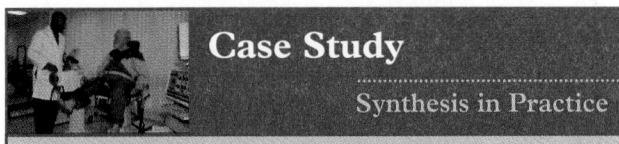

Case Study

Synthesis in Practice

As Mark prepares for an assessment on Mr. Stapp, he reviews the pathophysiology regarding the hazards of immobility. He gathers knowledge about knee replacement surgery and the expected postoperative physical therapy and rehabilitative measures. During a previous clinical experience, Mark cared for a client who was recently diagnosed with diabetes mellitus. He knows that the presence of diabetes mellitus can affect Mr. Stapp's postoperative status in several ways. Wound healing is slower in clients with diabetes. In addition, because Mr. Stapp will be participating in a physical exercise program to increase knee mobility, his caloric requirements may need to change and his blood sugar levels need to be monitored.

Mark knows that he needs to respect Mr. Stapp's need to be independent and desire to participate in rehabilitation. Although Mark and his client are close in age, he knows that Mr. Stapp has his own life goals. He approaches this clinical experience with energy and creativity; he plans to implement individualized care to increase Mr. Stapp's mobility status and progression through rehabilitation.

 NURSING DIAGNOSES FOR CLIENTS WITH IMMOBILITY

Activity intolerance
Airway clearance, ineffective
Breathing pattern, ineffective
Constipation, colonic
Coping, ineffective individual
Disuse syndrome, risk for
Fluid volume deficit, risk for
Gas exchange, impaired
Infection, risk for
Mobility, impaired physical
Skin integrity, impaired, risk for
Sleep pattern disturbance
Social isolation
Tissue perfusion, altered: peripheral, risk for
Urinary elimination, altered

Nursing Diagnosis

An immobilized or partially immobilized client may have one or more nursing diagnoses (see nursing diagnoses box). The two diagnoses most directly related to mobility problems are *impaired physical mobility* and *risk for disuse syndrome*. *Impaired physical mobility* is used for the client who demonstrates functional limitations but is not completely immobile. On the other hand, the client who is immobile and is at risk for multisystem pathophysiology because of the unavoidable inactivity should be considered at *risk for disuse syndrome*. Beyond these diagnoses the list of potential diagnoses is extensive because immobility affects multiple body systems. Many alterations in physiological, sociocultural, and developmental functioning are related to immobility. Often these problems are interrelated, and it is imperative that nursing care focus on all dimensions.

Assessment reveals clusters of data that indicate whether a client is at risk or if a problem exists. Assessment also identifies pertinent defining characteristics that support the diagnostic label and probable cause of the diagnosis. Locating the probable cause of the diagnosis, based on assessment data, is important to planning client-centered goals and subsequent nursing interventions that will best help the client.

Impaired physical mobility related to bed rest would require slightly different interventions than *impaired physical mobility related to pain in the left shoulder*. The first diagnosis would require interventions aimed at keeping the client as mobile as possible and encouraging the client to do self-care and ROM in bed. The second diagnosis would require the nurse to assist the client with comfort measures so the client would then be willing and more able to move. In both situations the nurse

would explain the importance of activity to healthy body functioning.

Immobility may lead to complications like pulmonary emboli or pneumonia. If these conditions develop, the nurse will collaborate with the physician or nurse practitioner for prescribed therapy to intervene. The nurse is alert for these potential complications and works to prevent them.

Planning

Clients at risk for hazards of immobility require nursing care plans directed at meeting their actual and potential needs (see care plan on p. 1056). In addition, the nurse must develop client-centered goals aimed at preventing or reducing the hazards of immobility. Care planning is individualized to the client, taking into consideration the client's most immediate needs. The immediacy of any problem is determined by the effect the problem has on the client's mental and physical health.

The nurse may need the help of another health team member such as a physical or occupational therapist when considering mobility needs. These factors are important for clients in institutional and home settings. Discharge planning is begun when a client enters the health care system. Anticipating the client's discharge from an institution, a referral may be necessary to help the client remain mobile or regain mobility at home.

Because many of the skills associated with care of the immobile are delegated, such as turning and applying elastic stockings, it may be easy for the nurse to overlook the potential complications of immobility until they occur. Therefore the nurse must be vigilant in monitoring the client, reinforcing prevention techniques, and supervising UAP in carrying out activities aimed at preventing immobility complications.

The care plan is developed with the client and

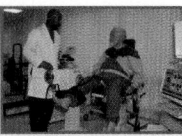

CASE STUDY NURSING CARE PLAN

Skin Care

Assessment

Mr. Bob Stapp, a 54-year-old client, is admitted to the rehab hospital after bilateral **total knee replacements (TKR).** He has a history of smoking. He is **50 lb overweight.** He does not use his incentive spirometer. He is to **start physical therapy this afternoon.** He is able to **transfer himself with help to a chair from the bed and can stand on his own with the aid of a walker.** He has **50-degree flexion of his knee.**

Nursing Diagnosis

Impaired immobility related to mobility restrictions secondary to bilateral TKR.

Planning

Goal

Client will remain free of complications of immobility.

Expected Outcomes

Client's calf diameters will remain within 1 cm of baseline by 3/12.

Client's lung fields will remain clear.

Client's skin will remain dry and intact.

Implementation

Steps	Rationale
1. Administer low-dose heparin as ordered.	Administration of low-dose heparin has shown reductions in risk of vein thrombosis (Nunnelee, 1995).
2. Apply intermittent compression stockings, and remove them each shift for hygiene.	Application increases venous tone, improving venous return, and reduces venous stasis (Nunnelee, 1995).
3. Reinforce antiembolic exercises hourly while awake.	
4. Reinforce use of incentive spirometer every 2 hours while awake.	
5. Instruct client to shift position every ½ hour while awake.	
6. Ask client to report any numbness or burning over pressure areas such as the heels of the feet.	
7. Keep heels off the bed by placing a pad under the lower legs.	Using a thin pad under the lower legs raises the heel just enough so that a paper can slide between the heels and the bed, reducing the pressure on the heels, so that blood flow is optimized (AHCPR, 1994).

Evaluation

Measure calves daily; report any increases in dimensions.
Perform circulatory assessment to extremities every shift.
Auscultate lung fields every shift.
Observe skin condition daily.

Defining characteristics are shown in bold type.

significant others based on one or more client-centered goals. Goals, like diagnoses, must be prioritized and are mutually set with the client and family. Rehabilitation is most effective when clients are active in their own care. A family who does too much or too little in an attempt to help the client may seriously impede the progress of the client. Watching a family member walk slowly and using effort may seem cruel, so the family may excessively perform tasks that clients need to learn how to do for themselves.

Implementation

Nursing interventions for the completely or partially immobilized client focus on health promotion and prevention of the hazards of immobility. In the acute care setting, specific interventions are designed to reduce the impact of immobility on the client, and thus reduce complications of immobility to the body systems.

Health promotion. Structured exercise programs for immobile clients can enhance their feelings of well-being as well as their endurance, strength, and health. The advantages of exercise can be seen with coronary clients, who are traditionally bed-bound when first admitted to the hospital. Exercise is recommended preoperatively for clients expected to have mobility restrictions after surgery. Special care units for older adult clients have been developed in some acute care hospitals that focus on mobility and exercise from the moment the client is admitted to the unit.

Disuse and disease may account for much of the functional decline in the older adult population. Therefore the older adult client need not accept muscle deterioration as inevitable, and the nurse must be alert to preventing further disuse while the client is ill.

Nurses can contribute to promoting health for many types of clients by encouraging or starting managed exercise programs (Box 37-2). Even hospitalized clients can be encouraged to do stretching, ROM, and light walking within the limits of their condition. Postopera-

---

Box 37-2

Procedural Guidelines for Assisting Clients to Exercise

1. Teach clients breathing skills to help reduce anxiety and to fully oxygenate tissues and expand lungs.
2. Always know client's limitations.
3. Do not force a muscle or a joint during exercise.
4. Let each client move at own pace.
5. Keep a record of the client's progress, and provide feedback as client exercises.
6. Posture, body alignment, and good body mechanics should be maintained during exercise.
7. Monitor vital signs before, during, and after exercise.
8. Stop exercising if client has pain, shortness of breath, or a change in vital signs.
9. Clients should wear shoes and comfortable clothing.
10. Know what the client's mobility skills were prior to hospitalization.
11. Be aware of any medical limitations (e.g., weight-bearing status, untreated fracture, cardiovascular disease).

---

tive ambulation might be more enticing if others also participate. A lounge area can be used for ROM exercises where music and company may make the task more interesting to both client and nurse. Distances walked should be measured in feet and yards instead of "walked to the nurses' station and back to room."

Metabolic system. A dietary plan of carbohydrates, proteins, and fats is designed to meet the client's needs. Carbohydrates are needed to meet energy requirements. Proteins are necessary for tissue repair. Fats prevent further breakdown of nutritional stores. The specific caloric and diet prescription is determined from the nutritional assessment in collaboration with a registered dietitian (see Chapter 34).

Respiratory system. Nursing interventions for the respiratory system are aimed at promoting expansion of the chest and lungs, preventing stasis of pulmonary secretions, and maintaining a patent airway.

Promoting expansion of the chest and lungs. The nurse can counteract reduced chest expansion with several interventions. A healthy adult resting in bed will change position once every 11 to 12 minutes. Changing the client's position allows the dependent lung to expand. This maintains the elastic recoil property of the lungs and clears the dependent lung of pulmonary secretions. The minimum suggested timing for turning is every 2 hours, but that may not be enough. The nurse must judge the client's particular situation to determine the frequency of position changes. The most effective position in bed for lung expansion is high Fowler's, but in this position the client may still be susceptible to hazards. The client in this position tends to slide down in bed, which increases risk for skin breakdown due to shearing force. The tendency to slide may also decrease lung expansion, and this, with pooling of secretions in the bases, may lead to pneumonia.

Preventing stasis of pulmonary secretions. Stagnant secretions accumulating in the bronchi and lungs of the immobilized or bed-bound client may lead to the growth of bacteria and the subsequent development of pneumonia. The stagnation of secretions can be reduced by changing the client's position at least every 2 hours. This change rotates the dependent lung, mobilizing the secretions.

The immobile client should take in a minimum of 2000 ml/day, if not contraindicated, to help keep mucociliary clearance normal. In clients free from infection and with adequate hydration, pulmonary secretions will appear thin, watery, and clear. The client can easily remove the secretions with coughing. Without adequate hydration the secretions are thick and tenacious and difficult to remove. Encouraging fluids also benefits in helping with bowel and urine elimination and aids in maintaining circulation and skin integrity. Older adults with restricted mobility have specific hydration needs and require assistance in meeting those needs (Box 37-3).

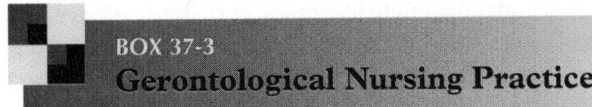

Perhaps the best method for preventing pulmonary secretions is **chest physiotherapy.** The use of positioning techniques drains secretions from specific segments of the bronchi and lungs into the trachea and helps the client expel the secretions by coughing. Chest physiotherapy is a precise procedure requiring specific nursing skills (see Chapter 30). This therapy may also be carried out by respiratory or physical therapists.

Cardiovascular system. Nursing therapies are designed to minimize or prevent orthostatic hypotension, increased cardiac workload, and thrombus formation.

Reducing orthostatic hypotension. After bed rest, clients usually have an increased pulse rate, a decrease in pulse pressure, and an increase in fainting in response to a tilting or an erect posture (Roper, 1996). The nurse attempts to get the client out of bed as soon as the physical condition allows it, even if the move is only to a chair. This activity maintains muscle tone and increases venous return. **Isometric exercises,** those activities that involve muscle tension without muscle shortening, do not have any beneficial effect on preventing orthostatic hypotension but may improve activity tolerance.

When getting the client from a supine position into a chair, the nurse moves the client gradually. The nurse first obtains baseline blood pressure and pulse with the client in the supine position (Roper, 1996). The nurse then raises the client to a high Fowler's position and measures blood pressure and pulse again to detect decreases in blood pressure or elevations in pulse. The nurse remains with the client in the high Fowler's position for a few moments to allow the body to adapt. The nurse continually monitors the client for dizziness or light-headedness and whether spots are seen. Then the nurse has the client sit at the side of the bed with the feet on the floor. If there is no dizziness, the nurse as-

sists the client to a chair. When getting an immobile client up for the first time, the nurse should get the assistance of at least one other person. This is a precautionary step. The client would still be expected to do as much of the transfer as the condition allows.

Preventing thrombus formation. Positioning techniques help reduce pressure to the skin. Proper positioning used with other therapies (e.g, heparin and elastic stockings) helps reduce thrombus formation. When positioning clients, the nurse uses caution to prevent pressure on the posterior knee and deep veins in the lower extremities. Client teaching should include avoiding crossing the legs, not sitting for prolonged periods of time, not wearing tight clothing that constricts the legs or waist, not putting pillows under the knees, and avoiding massaging the legs.

Range-of-joint-motion exercises reduce the risk of contractures but may also aid in preventing thrombi (see Chapter 27). Activity causes contraction of the skeletal muscles, which in turn exerts pressure on the veins to promote venous return, thereby reducing venous stasis. Specific exercises that help prevent thrombophelebitis are ankle pumps, foot circles, hip rotation, and knee flexion. Ankle pumps, sometimes called calf pumps, include alternating plantar flexion and dorsiflexion. Foot circles require the client to rotate the ankle. This can be done by instructing the client to make the letters of the alphabet with the feet. Inward and outward rotation of the hip can be done while the client is supine (lying on back) or sitting. Knee flexion involves alternately extending and flexing the knee. These exercises that are aimed at preventing thrombus are sometimes referred to as antiembolic exercises and should be done hourly while awake.

Musculoskeletal system. The immobilized client must exercise to prevent excessive muscle atrophy, decreased endurance, and joint contractures. The amount of activity required to prevent physical disuse syndromes is only about 2 hours in a 24-hour period, but it should be scheduled regularly throughout the day. The best method to prevent complications from impaired mobility is to encourage ambulation.

If the client is unable to move any part or all of the body, the nurse must perform passive range-of-joint-motion exercises for all immobilized joints at least 3 or 4 times a day unless contraindicated medically. If one extremity is paralyzed, the client can be taught to perform self-ROM.

Clients on bed rest should have active range-of-joint-motion exercises incorporated into the daily schedule (see Chapter 27). These exercises can be incorporated into ADLs (Box 37-4).

The best nursing intervention is establishing an individualized progressive exercise program. A progressive exercise program gradually increases the client's physical activity to reverse the deconditioning associated with immobility. Progressive exercise programs are used

Box 37-4

Box 37-4
Incorporating Active Range-of-Joint-Motion Exercises Into Activities of Daily Living

Nodding head "yes" exercises *neck* (flexion).

Shaking head "no" exercises *neck* (rotation).

Moving right ear to right shoulder exercises *neck* (lateral flexion).

Moving left ear to left shoulder exercises *neck* (lateral flexion).

Reaching to turn on overhead light exercises *shoulder* (extension).

Reaching to bedside stand for book exercises *shoulder* (extension).

Scratching back exercises *shoulder* (hyperextension).

Rotating shoulders toward chest exercises *shoulder* (abduction).

Rotating shoulders toward back exercises *shoulder* (adduction).

Eating, bathing, shaving, and grooming exercise *elbow* (flexion and extension).

All activities requiring fine motor coordination, such as writing and eating, exercise *fingers* and *thumb* (flexion, extension, abduction, adduction, and opposition).

Walking exercises *hip* (flexion, extension, and hyperextension).

Moving to side-lying position exercises *hip* (flexion, extension, and abduction).

Moving from side-lying position exercises *hip* (extension and adduction).

Rolling feet inward exercises *hip* (internal rotation).

Rolling feet outward exercises *hip* (external rotation).

Walking exercises *knee* (flexion and extension).

Moving to and from a side-lying position exercises *knee* (flexion and extension).

Walking exercises *ankle* (dorsiflexion and plantar flexion).

Moving toe toward head of bed exercises *ankle* (dosiflexion).

Moving toe toward foot of bed exercises *ankle* (plantar flexion).

Walking exercises *toes* (extension and hyperextension).

Wiggling toes exercises *toes* (abduction and adduction).

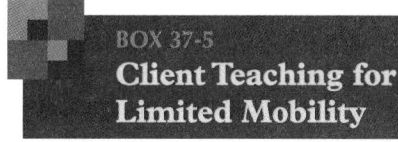

BOX 37-5
Client Teaching for Limited Mobility

- Explain the need for position changes at regular intervals based on client needs.
- Demonstrate passive and active range-of-joint-motion exercises.
- Describe the risk factors for pressure sores.
- Describe early warning signs of immobility (e.g., continued erythema over a bony prominence) so interventions can be developed to prevent worsening of the condition.
- Discuss activities to reduce the psychosocial problems of immobilization.
- Encourage the client's participation in care and decision making.
- Explain the need to maintain fluid and nutrition intake.
- Explain the need for isometric and isotonic exercises while on bed rest.

program, and the nurse would reinforce the specific exercise program.

Skin integrity. Early identification of high-risk clients aids the nurse in preventing pressure ulcers. Interventions aimed at prevention are positioning, skin care, and the use of pressure relief devices. The immobilized client's position should be changed according to the client's activity level, perceptual ability, and daily routines (see Chapter 38). The time a client sits uninterrupted in a chair should be limited to 1 hour or less, but this time interval is individualized. The client should be repositioned frequently because uninterrupted pressure will cause skin breakdown. The nurse should teach clients who are able to shift their weight every 15 minutes. Chair-bound clients should have a pressure-reducing device for the chair (AHCPR, 1994).

Elimination system. Nursing interventions for maintaining optimal urinary functioning are directed toward keeping the client well hydrated without causing bladder distention and the reflux of urine into the ureters and, in some instances, the renal pelvis. Adequate hydration helps to prevent renal calculi and urinary tract infections. The client should void dilute urine that is comparable to the amount of intake. If the client is also incontinent, the nurse modifies the care plan so the increased urinary output does not cause skin breakdown.

To prevent bladder distention, the nurse assesses the frequency and amount of urinary output. A client who continually dribbles urine and whose bladder is distended has reflex incontinence. If the immobilized client does not have voluntary control of bladder elimination, bladder retraining may be necessary. If the client experiences bladder distention, the nurse may be

for clients with musculoskeletal, neurological, cardiopulmonary, renal, and other chronic diseases. Teaching is an important aspect for clients with limited mobility (Box 37-5). Depending on the setting and resources available, the nurse may want to refer the client for physical therapy. The therapist may set up the exercise

required to insert a straight catheter or an indwelling Foley catheter (see Chapter 35).

The nurse must also record the frequency and consistency of bowel movements. A diet rich in fruits and vegetables can help to facilitate normal peristalsis. If a client is unable to maintain normal bowel patterns, the nurse may initiate a bowel training program and the physician may order stool softeners, cathartics, or enemas (see Chapter 36).

Psychosocial problems. The nurse should anticipate changes in psychosocial status to intervene with preventive measures. The nurse can provide routine and informal socialization for the client. Nursing activities are planned to give the client opportunities to interact with the staff. If possible, the client should be placed in a room with other mobile clients. If the client must remain in a private room, staff members are asked to visit with the client periodically throughout the client's waking hours.

The nurse also provides stimuli to maintain the client's orientation and to entertain the client. Bedside chats at appropriate moments orient the client to the schedule of nursing activities, meals, and visiting hours. Books from the hospital library help to occupy the client. If the client's condition permits it, the client can participate in craft activities.

Clients should be encouraged to wear their glasses or artificial teeth and to shave or apply makeup. These are normal activities through which people maintain body image. In addition, the client should be encouraged to perform as much self-care as possible. Hygiene and grooming articles should be kept within easy reach so the client can attend to personal needs.

Nursing care between 10 PM and 7 AM should be scheduled to minimize sleep interruptions. The balance between rest and the physiological effects of bed rest must be weighed. Assessments may be kept to a minimum in a stable client who is able to turn in bed unassisted. More seriously ill clients may need medications, assessments, and skin care during the night. Nursing care should be coordinated to prevent as many interruptions as possible.

Finally, the nurse should observe the client for failure to cope with restricted mobility. If the nursing care plan is not improving the client's coping patterns, outside assistance may be required. Recommendations of consultants should be incorporated into the care plan.

Developmental changes. Nursing care should stimulate the client mentally as well as physically, particularly with a young child. Play activities can be incorporated into the nursing care plan. Puzzles, for example, can help to develop fine motor skills. An immobilized child should be placed in a room with children of the same age who are not immobilized, unless a contagious disease is present.

Immobilization or restricted mobility of an older adult may require complex care and innovative approaches from the nurse. It is not uncommon for older adult clients to have one or more chronic illnesses. Because of deconditioning associated with age and chronic illness, older adults are at high risk for the hazards of immobility.

Inactive older adults are at risk for cognitive changes and depression as a result of immobilization, chronic illnesses, and medications. Therefore the nurse should focus on activities to promote cognitive awareness of the client's surroundings (see Chapter 39). If the client has pictures and cards in the room, the nurse should inquire about them. Families can be asked about factual information relating to these items so that the staff can reinforce information with clients as needed. Explanations should be given before starting care and the client encouraged to make decisions about care.

Nursing care should be planned to allow the older adult client to perform as many ADLs as possible. Frail older adult clients may need their position changed every hour instead of every 2 hours and may need more frequent range-of-joint-motion exercises. Not only are older adults more susceptible to the hazards of immobility, but the consequences of immobility appear more quickly and become severe more rapidly.

Acute care. Clients in acute care settings may demonstrate some problems associated with prolonged immobility, such as impaired respiratory status, orthostatic hypotension, and impaired skin integrity. In these clients nursing interventions are designed to reduce the impact of immobility on body systems and prepare the client for the restorative phase of care. These interventions are used in combination with those outlined in the health promotion section to return the client to an optimal level of function.

Respiratory system. The nurse should encourage the client to deep breathe and cough every 1 to 2 hours while awake. Alert clients can be taught to deep breathe or yawn every hour. This action expands all lobes of the lungs and prevents atelectasis. Coughing reduces the stasis of pulmonary secretions. Some immobile clients, particularly after surgery, should use an incentive spirometer to aid in deep breathing (see Chapter 30).

Postoperative pain medications can depress the respiratory center so the rate of respiration or expansion of the lungs is decreased. The client may be drowsy as a result of the medication. Therefore the nurse should actively reinforce coughing and deep breathing exercises and encourage early ambulation.

If abdominal binders or rib supports are required, they should be removed every 2 hours to allow the client to breathe deeply. Binders must be assessed for correct positioning and adjusted as necessary to prevent interference with respirations. Often clients will wear the binder only when ambulating. Specific physician instructions for the use of binders will vary.

Maintaining a patent airway. Immobilized clients and those on bed rest are generally weakened. If the weakness progresses, the cough reflex gradually becomes inefficient. If the client is too weak or unable to cough up secretions, the nurse must maintain a patent airway by using suctioning techniques (see Chapter 30). This may involve oral or nasotracheal suctioning, as well as suctioning of artificial airways. The stasis of secretions in the lungs may be life-threatening for an immobilized client because hypostatic bronchopneumonia can easily develop. Dislodging and mobilizing stagnant secretions reduce the risk of pneumonia. Assessment findings indicating this condition include productive cough with greenish-yellow sputum, fever, and pain on breathing.

Cardiovascular system. The nurse uses interventions to reduce cardiac workload, which is increased by immobility. When a client moves up in bed or strains on defecation, a Valsalva maneuver occurs. When using this maneuver, the client holds the breath and strains, increasing intrathoracic pressure, which decreases venous return and cardiac output. When the strain is released, venous return and cardiac output immediately increase, and systolic blood pressure and pulse pressure rise. These pressure changes produce a reflex bradycardia that may be associated with sudden cardiac death in clients with heart disease. The nurse teaches the client to breathe out while moving or being lifted up in bed to avoid straining.

Interventions that reduce the risk of thrombus formation in the immobilized client include leg exercises, encouraging fluids, and position changes. Preoperative clients are instructed on exercise before surgery (see Chapter 40). Other interventions such as intermittent pneumatic compression devices require a physician's order.

When DVT is suspected, it should be reported immediately. The leg should be elevated, with no pressure on the area of the leg with the suspected thrombus. The family, client, and all health care personnel should be instructed not to massage the area because the thrombus may be dislodged.

Elastic stockings aid in maintaining pressure on the muscles of the lower extremities and are believed to promote venous return. The stockings must be applied properly (Skill 37-1) and removed and reapplied at least once a shift. In addition, the stockings should always be clean and dry, and it may be necessary for the client to have two pairs. Clients often come to the hospital with stockings they have worn for years. These must be assessed to see if the client is wearing them correctly and if they fit properly. Properly applied stockings are snug and smooth. Clients may roll these stockings at the knee because of poor fit and thus constrict venous return. An important teaching point is that clients should be told not to roll stockings.

Intermittent pneumatic compression (IPC) provides rhythmic, external extremity compression through inflatable "stockings" or "boots." These devices, sometimes referred to as pulsating antiembolic stockings (PAS), are effective in reducing DVT in general surgical high-risk clients with malignant disease and clients with orthopedic or neurological conditions (Roper, 1996). In postoperative clients these compression stockings are kept on until the client is ambulatory.

Immobilized clients are frequently placed on low-dose heparin therapy to minimize the risk of venous thromboembolism. Heparin is an anticoagulant and thus suppresses clot formation. This therapy requires a physician's order. The medication is usually administered every 8 to 12 hours. The usual route of administration is subcutaneous injection. Because of the action of this medication, the nurse must continually assess the client for signs of bleeding (e.g., increased bruising, guaiac-positive stools, and bleeding gums). These risks exist, although most clients do not experience side effects.

Musculoskeletal system. Some orthopedic and neurological conditions require more frequent passive ROM exercises to restore the injured joint or extremity to maximal function. Clients with such conditions may use automatic equipment for passive range-of-joint-motion exercises. The machine referred to as CPM, or continuous passive motion, moves the extremity within a prescribed range for a specific period. This method is beneficial when the client must gradually increase ROM of a particular joint.

Restorative care. The goal of restorative care for the client who is immobile is to maximize functional mobility and independence and reduce residual functional deficits such as impaired gait and decreased endurance. The focus in restorative care is not only on ADLs that relate to physical self-care but also on **instrumental activities of daily living (IADLs).** IADLs are activities that are necessary to be independent in society beyond eating, grooming, transferring, and toileting and include such skills as shopping, preparing meals, banking, and taking medications.

The nurse uses many of the same interventions as described in the health promotion and acute care sections, but the emphasis is on working collaboratively with clients and their significant others and with other health care professionals. The emphasis is on facilitating the client's return to maximal functional ability in both ADLs and IADLs so that quality of life is enhanced. Intensive specialized therapy such as occupational or physical therapy is common. The client in an institution will likely go to the therapy department 2 to 3 times a day. The nurse's role is to work collaboratively with these professionals and reinforce exercises and teaching done. Common items used to help adapt to mobility limitations include walkers, canes, wheelchairs, and assistive devices such as toilet seat extenders, reaching sticks, special silverware, and clothing with Velcro closures.

.... Skill 37-1
Applying Elastic Stockings

Delegation Considerations

The skill of applying elastic stockings can be delegated to unlicensed assistive personnel. The following information is needed when delegating this skill:

- Avoid activities that promote venous stasis (e.g., crossing legs, wearing garters, or elevating legs on pillows).
- When possible, elevate legs to improve venous return.
- Do not massage legs.

- Elevate legs before applying stockings.
- Avoid wrinkles in the stockings.
- Observe for allergic reactions, skin irritation, and thrombophlebitis.

Equipment
- Tape measure
- Talcum powder
- Elastic support stockings

STEPS	RATIONALE

1. Assess client for risk factors in Virchow's triad to determine need for elastic stockings:
  a. *Hypercoagulability:* all clients with clotting disorders, fever, dehydration, pregnancy and first 6 weeks postpartum if the woman was confined to bed, and oral contraceptive use (especially if client smokes)
  b. *Venous wall abnormalities:* local trauma, orthopedic surgeries, major abdominal surgery, varicose veins, atherosclerosis
  c. *Blood stasis:* immobility, obesity, pregnancy
	Potential candidates for elastic stockings are clients who have an alteration in one of the elements of Virchow's triad (Bright and Georgi, 1992; von Rueden and Harris, 1995).

2. Observe for signs, symptoms, and conditions that might contraindicate use of elastic stockings: a. Dermatitis or open skin lesion.	Elastic stockings may aggravate skin condition or cause it to spread. Also, physician may want medication and dressing applied to lesion.
b. Recent skin graft.	Continuous pressure is necessary to keep graft adherent to recipient bed, but pressure should not be so firm as to cause death of graft.
c. Disproportionately large thighs.	Elastic stockings may not fit correctly, causing excessive pressure and constriction around thighs, thereby reducing venous return (Phipps, 1995).
d. Decreased circulation in lower extremities as evidenced by cyanotic, cool extremities.	Elastic stockings may further impede circulation.
3. Obtain physician's order.	May be needed for legal or reimbursement reasons.
4. Assess client's or care giver's understanding of application of elastic stockings.	Identifies potential educational needs of client or care giver.
5. Assess and document the condition of client's skin and circulation to the legs (i.e., presence of pedal pulses, edema, discoloration of the skin, temperature, lesions, or cuts).	Identifies a baseline for skin integrity and quality of peripheral pulses in lower extremities.
6. Explain procedure and reasons for applying stockings.	Reduces anxiety and encourages client cooperation.
7. Use tape measure to measure client's legs to determine proper stocking size.	Stockings must be measured according to manufacturer's directions. Elastic stockings come in two lengths: knee length and thigh length. The choice of length depends on physician's order.

STEPS	RATIONALE

CRITICAL DECISION POINT

Compare client's measurements with the manufacturer's sizing chart. If too large, stockings will not adequately support extremities. If too small, stockings may impede circulation. The optimum stocking pressure is 20 to 30 mm Hg at the ankle, decreasing to 8 mm Hg at the middle to upper thigh. This change in pressure produces the greatest increase in venous flow velocity that is both safe and practical (Bright and Georgi, 1992).

STEPS	RATIONALE
8. Wash hands.	Reduces transmission of microorganisms.
9. Position client in supine position. Elevate head of bed to comfortable level.	Promotes good body mechanics for nurse. Client position eases application. Also, the stockings should be applied before standing to prevent stagnation of blood in lower extremities. If client has been standing, client should sit in chair or lie in bed for 15 minutes with legs elevated before applying elastic stockings (Bright and Georgi, 1992).
10. After legs are cleansed, apply small amount of talcum powder to legs and feet, provided client does not have sensitivity to talcum powder.	Talcum powder reduces friction and allows for easier application of stockings.
11. Apply stockings:	
a. Turn elastic stocking inside out by placing one hand into sock, holding toe of sock with other hand, and pulling (see illustration).	Allows easier application of stocking.
b. Place client's toes into foot of elastic stocking, making sure that sock is smooth (see illustration).	Wrinkles in sock can impede circulation to lower region of extremity (Bright and Georgi, 1992).
c. Slide remaining portion of sock over client's foot, being sure that the toes are covered. Make sure the foot fits into the toe and heel position of the sock. Sock will now be right side out (see illustration, p. 1064).	If toes remain uncovered, they will become constricted by elastic and their circulation can be reduced.

Continued

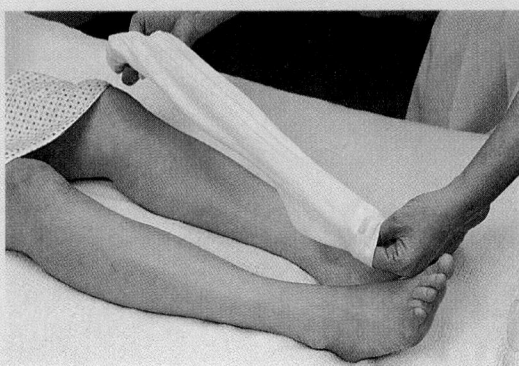

Step 11a

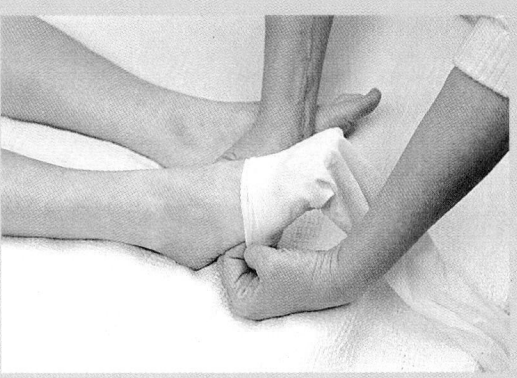

Step 11b

Skill 37-1—cont'd
Applying Elastic Stockings

STEPS	RATIONALE
d. Slide sock up over client's calf until sock is completely extended. Be sure sock is smooth and no ridges are present (see illustration).	Ridges impede venous return and can counteract overall purpose of elastic stocking (Bright and Georgi, 1992).
e. Instruct client not to roll socks partially down.	Rolling sock partially down has a constricting effect and can impede venous return.
12. Reposition client to position of comfort, and wash hands.	Maintains proper body alignment and promotes comfort. Reduces transmission of microorganisms.
13. Inspect stocking to make sure there are no wrinkles or binding at top of stocking.	Wrinkles lead to increased pressure and alter circulation.
14. Observe client's reaction to stockings.	Ensures client is adapting to stockings and is not experiencing any discomfort from stockings.
15. Observe client or care giver apply stockings.	Determines ability to perform skill accurately.
16. Remove stockings at least once a shift, and assess skin and circulatory status.	Stockings may shift or be too tight, and this step ensures skin and circulation are intact.

Recording and Reporting
- Record date and time of stocking application and stocking length and size in nurses' notes (flow sheet may be used).
- Record condition of skin and circulatory assessment including pulses, temperature, sensation, movement, capillary refill, and calf circumference at application and each shift.
- Report changes indicating a decline in circulation.

Home Care Considerations
- Instruct clients to have two pairs of stockings—one pair to wear, the other to wash.
- Instruct clients that if there are weight changes greater than 10 lb, stockings should be remeasured.
- Remind clients to put on stockings prior to getting up for the morning or sitting for prolonged periods. As the day progresses, leg swelling may increase and may make stocking application difficult. (It may be helpful to remind clients that they may have noticed this swelling when wearing shoes.)

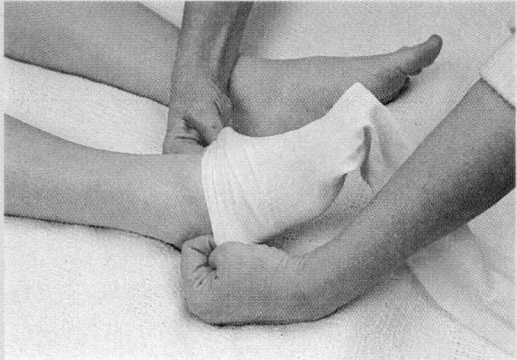

Step 11c

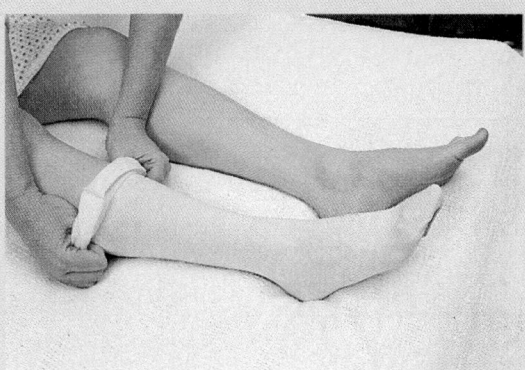

Step 11d

Restorative care is carried out in a variety of settings for the client who has mobility limitations. The site of care depends on the level of care needed, the amount and frequency of care required, and the types of care that are available in a geographical area. Long-term care refers to a variety of supportive care services that are provided clients who have lost the ability for some aspect of self-care. The term *long-term care* is somewhat misnamed, however, since the restorative care services that a client requires may be from several weeks to years. After a total knee replacement it is not unusual for a client to move from the acute care setting to a restorative care setting such as a nursing home or a rehabilitation hospital or to a rehabilitative unit at the same hospital where acute care was provided. Restorative care may also take place at home. The client may go from a hospital to a nursing home to home or go directly home from a hospital. The client may receive care in the home by a professional or make outpatient visits to the therapists' offices.

Evaluation

Client care. All nursing interventions for reducing the risks of immobility are evaluated by comparing the client's actual response to the expected outcomes for each goal. If expected outcomes are not achieved, the nurse will need to revise the care plan. The success in meeting each outcome is based on the use of evaluative measures such as ROM status, exercise tolerance, and fluid intake.

The nurse can also evaluate specific outcomes designed to demonstrate normal function of specific subsystems and to prevent complications in those systems. Are the lungs clear? Is the client performing leg exercises regularly? Are bowel sounds present? Are bowels remaining soft, formed, and regular? Are there any areas of skin breakdown around pressure points? Does the client remain injury free?

Client expectations. Movement is often taken for granted until it is lost. Clients who are immobile and dependent on others for some or all of their needs can become overly dependent or try to do too much themselves too early. It is a difficult task finding the interdependent balance between independence and dependence. Clients will want control over their mobility that is personally satisfactory. For clients who are completely dependent on others for care, control over how and when things are done may be very important. Do they feel they are treated with dignity? Do care givers treat them as adults? Clients who are dependent on others for care may see their demands as the only control they have over their life.

For most clients with mobility problems, lack of control is often a major issue. Do they feel staff were considerate, and did staff protect their privacy? Were their preferences taken into consideration when planning care? Did care givers talk to them or ignore them? It is helpful to remember that lack of movement is often associated with punishment in our society. Children are given "time-outs," teens are "grounded," and criminals are jailed. It is therefore important to recognize that immobility may lead to fear, anger, grief, withdrawal, or hostility. Whether the nurse is sensitive to these reactions and helps the client work through them or responds negatively to the client can make a big difference in the client's outcome.

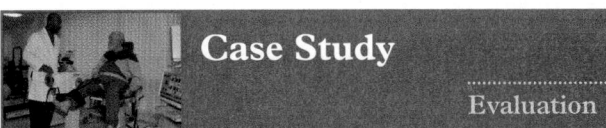

Case Study
Evaluation

It has been 2 weeks since Mark Weber began to care for Mr. Stapp. Mr. Stapp's independence has increased greatly. He now has 110 degrees of flexion and 100 degrees of extension in his knees, and he is able to transfer independently and do his ROM exercises. He is planning to go home over the weekend. He is scheduled to return to his surgeon's office in 1 week.

During rehabilitation, Mr. Stapp concentrated on increasing his exercise while monitoring his caloric intake. During the acute and restorative care he lost a total of 15 lb. He has worked out a diet with the dietitian at the center and will show this to his private medical physician, whom he is scheduled to visit in 1 month. Mr. Stapp has set a 30-lb goal for weight loss.

Documentation Note
Mr. Stapp discharged today. He received his prescriptions and follow-up appointments with his orthopedic surgeon and private medical physician. He received instruction on specific exercises to increase his knee mobility. He was met by his son and escorted by wheelchair to his son's car.

Key Terms

activities of daily living (ADLs)	**instrumental activities of daily living (IADLs)**
anthropometric measurements	**ischemia**
atelectasis	**isometric exercises**
bed rest	**joint contracture**
bone resorption	**mobility**
chest physiotherapy	**negative nitrogen balance**
disuse osteoporosis	**orthostatic hypotension**
diuresis	**pathological fracture**
hypercalcemia	**renal calculi**
hypostatic pneumonia	**thrombus**
immobility	

▪ Key Concepts

Normal physical mobility depends on intact and functioning nervous and musculoskeletal systems.

The risk of disabilities related to immobilization depends on the extent and duration of the immobilization.

Immobility may result from illness or trauma or may be prescribed for therapeutic reasons; in any case it presents hazards in the physiological, psychological, and developmental dimensions.

Pressure ulcers are one of the most common physiological hazards of immobility, but the nurse can take actions to prevent or treat them.

Effects of immobility include depression, behavioral changes, changes in the sleep-wake cycle, decreased coping abilities, and developmental effects.

Assessment focuses on range of joint motion, musculoskeletal status, and complete physical examination for potential adverse effects in all body systems, as well as psychosocial and developmental effects.

After identifying nursing diagnoses, the nurse plans and implements interventions to prevent or minimize the hazards and complications of immobilization.

Adequate hydration measures can reduce immobility-related complications in the respiratory and elimination systems.

Proper positioning techniques reduce the risk of contractures.

The primary evaluation criterion for nursing care in the developmental dimension for immobilized clients is the prevention of any measurable decline in functioning or delay in development.

Early mobilization helps to decrease the effects of bed rest.

▪ Critical Thinking Activities

1. You are caring for an 80-year-old female client who is admitted to a nursing home for rehabilitation after a fractured hip. She was in good health and independent until she fell. What evaluative measures should you make to ensure that she is getting proper lung expansion while she is in the nursing home undergoing rehabilitation?

2. The client you are caring for is on complete bed rest and has a history of thrombophlebitis. You ask the client during your assessment if she is doing her leg exercises. She replies, "No, I don't need to. I have these fancy stockings." She raises her legs and shows you intermittent compression stockings. What do you reply?

3. Mrs. Williams is a client you are seeing in her home after her laparoscopic-assisted vaginal hysterectomy. She has been home for 2 hours since she was released from the surgery center. What assessments must you make on this initial visit?

References

Agency for Health Care Policy and Research (AHCPR): *Treating pressure sores: consumer guide,* Clinical Practice Guidelines, No. 15, Rockville, Md, 1994, U.S. Department of Health and Human Services.

Blair C: Combining behavior management and mutual goal setting to reduce physical dependency in nursing home residents, *Nurs Res* 44(3):160, 1995.

Bright LD, Georgi S: Peripheral vascular disease: is it arterial or venous, *Am J Nurs* 92(9):34, 1992.

Deitrick JE and others: Effects of immobilization upon various metabolic and physiologic functions of normal men, *Am J Med* 4:3, 1948.

Helme T: Position changes for residents in long-term care, *Adv Wound Care* 7(5):57, 1994.

Kasper C and others: Alterations in skeletal muscle related to impaired physical mobility: an empirical model, *Res Nurs Health* 16:265, 1993.

Kasper C and others: Alterations in skeletal muscle related to short-term impaired physical mobility, *Res Nurs Health* 19:133, 1996.

McCance KL, Huether SE: *Pathophysiology: the biologic basis for disease in adults and children,* ed 2, St. Louis, 1994, Mosby.

Moore K: Stroke: the long road back, *RN* 57(3):50, 1994.

Phipps WJ and others: *Medical-surgical nursing,* ed 5, St. Louis, 1995, Mosby.

Nunnelee J: Minimize the risk of DVT, *RN* 58(12):28, 1995.

Roper M: Back to basics: assessing orthostatic vital signs, *Am J Nurs* 96(8):43, 1996.

Rubin M: The physiology of bedrest, *Am J Nurs* 88:50, 1988.

von Rueden KT, Harris JR: Pulmonary dysfunction related to immobility in the trauma patient, *AACN Clin Issues* 6(2): 212, 1995.

Skin Integrity and Wound Care

OBJECTIVES

Mastery of content in this chapter will enable the student to:

- Define the key terms listed.
- Describe risks and contributing factors for pressure ulcer development.
- List the four stages of pressure ulcers.
- Discuss the body's response during each phase of the wound healing process.
- Classify a wound according to the state of skin integrity, severity, cleanliness, and descriptive qualities.
- Differentiate healing by primary and secondary intention.
- Discuss common complications of wound healing.
- Explain factors that impair or promote normal wound healing.
- Describe the purposes of and precautions taken with applying bandages and binders.
- Describe the purposes and precautions when applying topical solutions to wounds.
- Describe the differences in therapeutic effects of heat and cold.
- Complete an assessment for a client with impaired skin integrity.
- List nursing diagnoses associated with impaired skin integrity.
- Develop a nursing care plan for a client with impaired skin integrity.
- State evaluation criteria for a client with impaired skin integrity.

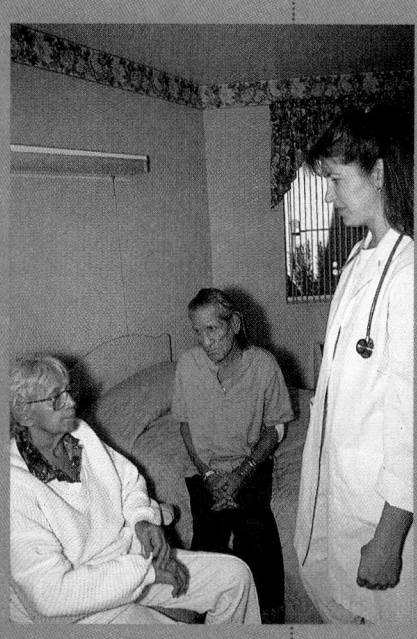

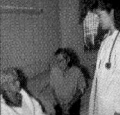

Case Study

....
Mr. Ahmed

Mr. Omar Ahmed, a 76-year-old accountant, has once again been admitted to the hospital, this time for treatment of his pneumonia. Before his admission he had been unable to eat and had lost more than 20 lbs over the last 2 months. Three years ago he had coronary artery bypass surgery. As a precaution, he has been put on telemetry monitoring. He also has hypertension and non–insulin-dependent diabetes mellitus (NIDDM). His mobility is limited because of his weakness, difficulty breathing, and acutely ill state. Mr. Ahmed is retired. He lives in a one-family home with his wife, Natalie. Their children and grandchildren live nearby and visit often. On admission his skin is intact. He complains that his "bottom hurts" from lying in bed. He has a temperature of 101° F, and he is diaphoretic.

Lynda Abraham is a junior nursing student who is doing 2 days a week of her clinical experience for her medical-surgical nursing course on Mr. Ahmed's medical nursing unit. This is her first hospital-based clinical practice.

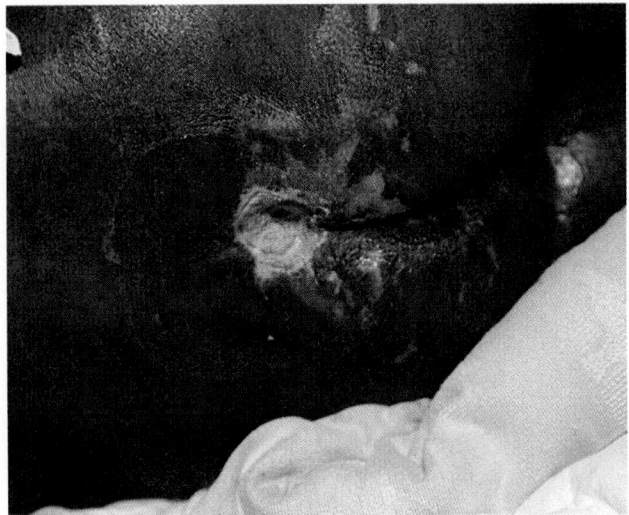

Figure 38-1.   Pressure ulcer with tissue necrosis.

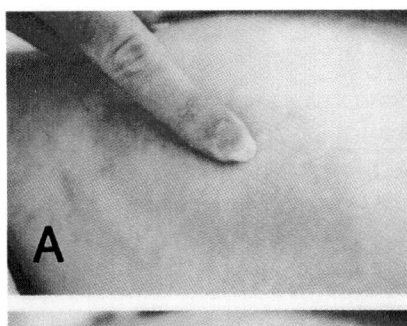

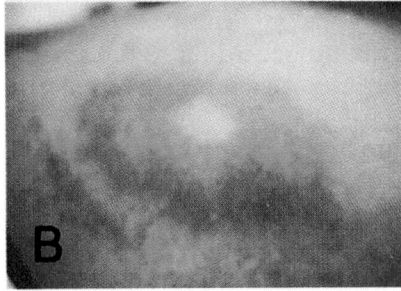

Figure 38-2.   **A,** Reactive hyperemia. **B,** Blanches with fingertip pressure.

············ SCIENTIFIC
KNOWLEDGE BASE

Pressure Ulcers

Pressure ulcer (formerly called *pressure sore, decubitus ulcer,* or *bedsore*) is the preferred term used to describe impaired skin integrity (Figure 38-1) from pressure (AHCPR, 1992, 1994; Maklebust and Sieggreen, 1996). An ill client experiencing decreased mobility, impaired neurological functioning, decreased sensory perception, or decreased circulation is at risk for pressure ulcer development.

Tissue ischemia is the localized absence of blood or a major reduction of blood flow resulting from mechanical obstruction (Pires and Muller, 1991). The reduction in blood flow causes blanching. **Blanching** is seen when the normal red tones of the lightly pigmented skin are absent. Tissue damage occurs when the capillary closing pressure exceeds the normal range of 16 to 32 mm Hg (Kosiak, 1959; Maklebust and Sieggreen, 1996).

After a period of ischemia the skin can undergo one of two hyperemic changes. In lightly pigmented clients, **normal reactive hyperemia** (redness) is the visible effect of localized vasodilation, the body's normal response to lack of blood flow to the underlying tissue (Figure 38-2, *A*). The area blanches with fingertip pres-

sure (Figure 38-2, *B*). When a client is lying or sitting, the weight of the body is placed on bony prominences. When the pressure is removed, there is a period of reactive hyperemia, or a sudden increase in blood flow to the region. Reactive hyperemia, which lasts less than 1 hour, is a compensatory response; it is effective only if the pressure on the skin is removed before tissue necrosis or damage occurs. **Abnormal reactive hyperemia** is an excessive vasodilation and **induration** in response to pressure. The skin appears bright pink to red. The induration is an area of localized edema under the skin. Abnormal reactive hyperemia (Figure 38-3)

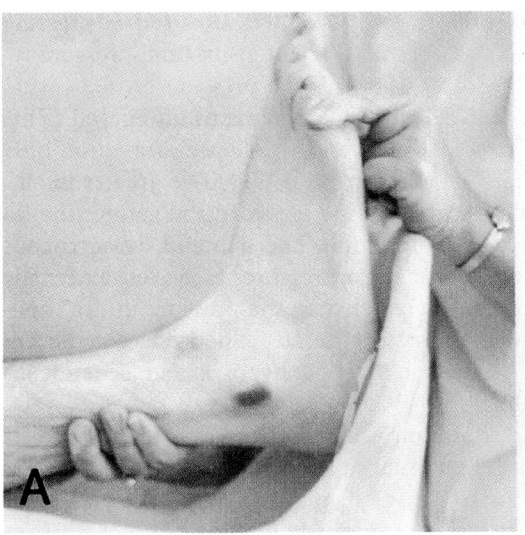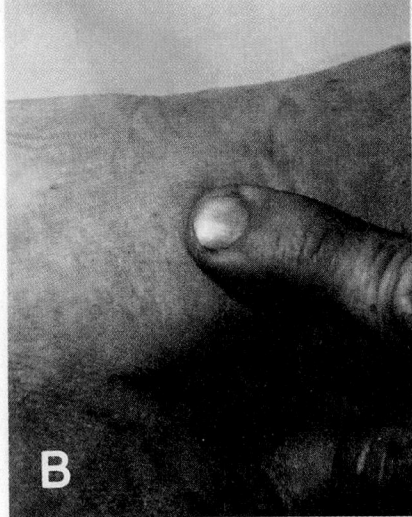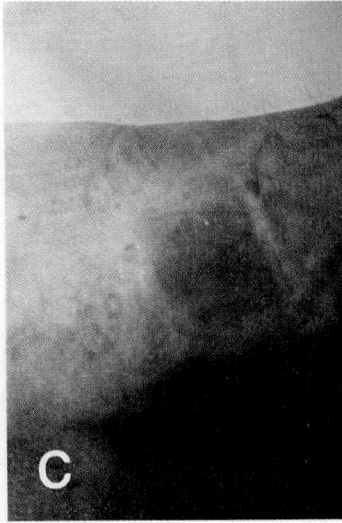

Figure 38-3. **A,** Abnormal reactive hyperemia. **B** and **C,** In abnormal reactive hyperemia the area is much darker than the surrounding skin and does not blanch with fingertip pressure.

can last more than 1 hour, up to 2 weeks after the removal of pressure (Pires and Muller, 1991).

There are structural differences in black skin, such as decreased elastin and increased and dilated superficial blood vessels (Montagna and others, 1993). Clients with darkly pigmented skin have no change in skin color of their intact skin. Therefore in clients with dark skin there is no blanching of their skin when pressure occurs over a bony prominence (Bennett, 1995).

Contributing factors to pressure ulcer formation.

In addition to prolonged pressure, additional factors can further increase the client's risk for pressure ulcer development. These include shearing force, friction, moisture, nutrition, infection, impaired peripheral circulation, obesity, and age.

Shearing force. **Shearing force** is the pressure exerted against the skin when a client is moved or repositioned in bed by being pulled or being allowed to slide down in bed (Figure 38-4). When a shearing force is present, the skin and subcutaneous layers adhere to the surface of the bed, and the layers of muscle and even the bones slide in the direction of body movement. The underlying tissue capillaries are compressed and severed by the pressure. As a result, minute layers of bleeding and necrosis occur deep within the tissues. Subcutaneous fat is more vulnerable to the effects of shearing and the resultant pressure from the underlying bony structure. Eventually a tract opens to the skin to allow drainage from the necrotic area.

Friction. **Friction** is an injury to the skin that has the appearance of an abrasion. Friction results from two surfaces rubbing against one another. The body surfaces most at risk to friction are the elbows and heels,

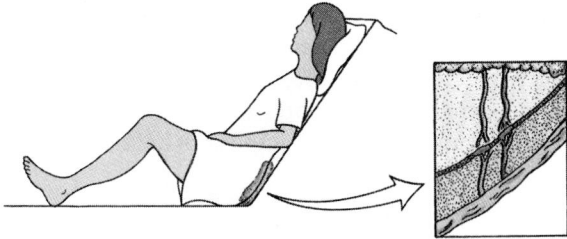

Figure 38-4.   Shearing force exerted against sacral area.

because abrasion of these surfaces occurs when they are rubbed against the sheets during repositioning. Injury from friction is shallow without necrosis and is limited to the epidermis (Bryant and others, 1992).

Moisture. Moisture on the skin increases the risk of ulcer formation. Moisture reduces the skin's resistance to other physical factors such as pressure or shearing force. Moisture can originate from wound drainage, perspiration, incontinence, vomitus, and condensation from humidified oxygen-delivery systems. The susceptibility to pressure ulcer formation increases with the duration of the exposure to moisture (Jeter and Lutz, 1996).

Nutrition. Poor nutrition increases the risk of pressure ulcer formation by causing atrophy and a decrease in subcutaneous tissue (Strauss and Margolis, 1996). Because of these changes, less tissue is present to serve as padding between the skin and underlying bone (Breslow and others, 1993). Therefore the effects of pressure are increased on remaining tissue. The client can have protein deficiency and negative nitrogen balance and have an inadequate intake of vitamin C

(Himes, 1997). Poor nutritional status may be overlooked if the client has a weight equal to or above the ideal body weight (IBW).

Poor nutrition alters fluid and electrolyte balance. In clients with severe protein loss, hypoalbuminemia (serum albumin below 3 g/100 ml) leads to a shift of fluid from the extracellular fluid volume to the tissues, resulting in edema (Breslow and others, 1993). **Edema** increases the affected tissue's risk for pressure ulcers. The blood supply to the edematous tissue is decreased, and waste products remain because of the changing pressures in the capillary circulation and capillary bed. **Anemia** increases risk for pressure ulcer formation, because the decreased levels of hemoglobin reduce the oxygen-carrying capacity of the blood and the amount of oxygen available to tissues.

A healthy adult client requires 0.8 g of protein per kilogram every 24 hours; however, in the presence of a wound this requirement must increase (Bryant and others, 1992). Continuous assessment of physical and laboratory data can alert the nurse to changes in nutritional status.

Cachexia is generalized ill health and malnutrition, marked by weakness and emaciation. It is usually associated with severe diseases such as cancer and end-stage cardiopulmonary or renal diseases. This condition increases the client's risk for pressure ulcers. Basically the cachectic client has lost the adipose tissue necessary to protect bony prominences from pressure.

Infection. Infection results from the presence of pathogens in the body. A client with an infection usually has a fever. Infection and fever increase the metabolic needs of the body, making an already hypoxic tissue more susceptible to ischemic injury. In addition, fever results in diaphoresis and increased skin moisture, which further predispose the client to skin breakdown.

Impaired peripheral circulation. Impaired peripheral circulation is related to pressure ulcer development. With decreased circulation the tissue becomes hypoxic and more susceptible to ischemic damage. Impaired circulation occurs in clients who have peripheral vascular diseases, are in shock, spend prolonged periods of time on hard operating room tables, or are receiving vasopressor-type medications.

Obesity. Obesity can speed pressure ulcer development. Adipose tissue in small quantities protects the skin by cushioning bony prominences against pressure. However, adipose tissue is poorly vascularized, and the adipose and underlying tissues are more susceptible to ischemic damage. When excessive adipose is present, the client is more susceptible to pressure ulcers.

Age. Pressure ulcer development occurs more frequently in clients over 65 years of age. There is a greater incidence of pressure ulcer development in this population (Kane and others, 1994).

Pathogenesis of pressure ulcers. A pressure ulcer occurs as a result of an intensity-time-pressure relationship (Stotts, 1988). If the pressure on the tissues is greater than 32 mm Hg and remains unrelieved to the point of hypoxia, the vessels collapse and thrombose (develop a clot) (Bergstrom, 1992). The greater the intensity and duration of the pressure, the greater the incidence of ulcer formation. The skin and subcutaneous tissue can tolerate some pressure. However, externally applied pressure greater than the pressure in the capillary bed decreases or obliterates blood flow to adjacent tissues. These tissues become hypoxic, and ischemic injury results.

Second, duration influences the detrimental effects of pressure. Low-intensity pressures over a long period of time can be just as damaging to the tissue as high-intensity pressure over short periods of time (Bryant and others, 1992). If the pressure is relieved before the critical point, circulation to the affected tissues is restored through reactive hyperemia. The coccyx-sacral areas, heels, and elbows are the most susceptible (Maklebust and Sieggreen, 1996).

Last, tissue tolerance to pressure determines ulcer development. Tissue tolerance is influenced by the ability of the skin and underlying structures to work together to offset the load (pressure) from the surface of the tissues to the underlying skeleton (Bryant and others, 1992). The effect of pressure can be increased by unequal distribution of body weight.

Stages of pressure ulcers. Pressure ulcers may occur initially in the superficial layers of the skin. In 1992 the AHCPR's Pressure Ulcer Guideline Panel revised the classification of pressure ulcers (AHCPR, 1992). These staging definitions were developed to classify a pressure ulcer based on the depth of tissue destroyed.

I. Nonblanchable erythema of the intact skin, the heralding lesion of skin ulceration, occurs (Figure 38-5, *A*).

II. Partial-thickness skin loss involves epidermis and/or dermis. Ulcer is superficial and presents clinically as an abrasion, blister, or shallow crater (Figure 38-5, *B*).

III. Full-thickness skin loss involves damage or necrosis of subcutaneous tissue that may extend down to but not through the underlying fascia. Ulcer presents clinically as a deep crater with or without undermining of adjacent tissue (Figure 38-5, *C*).

IV. Full-thickness skin loss occurs with extensive destruction, tissue necrosis, or damage to muscle, bone, or supporting structures (Figure 38-5, *D*).

A necrotic pressure ulcer cannot be staged until it is debrided, because the depth of the wound bed and tissue type cannot be visualized initially (AHCPR, 1994).

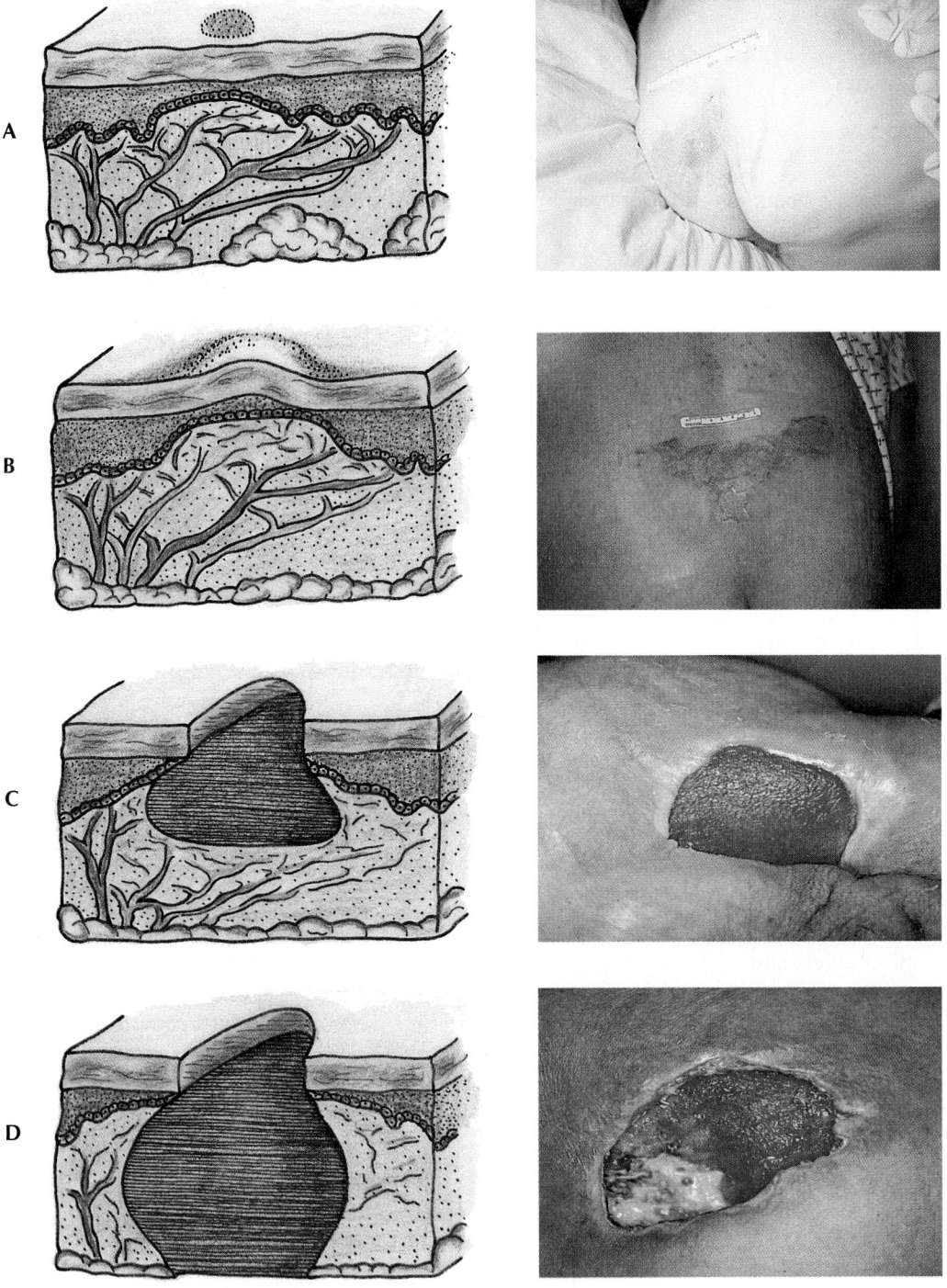

Figure 38-5.   **A,** Stage I pressure ulcer. **B,** Stage II pressure ulcer. **C,** Stage III pressure ulcer. **D,** Stage IV pressure ulcer. (Courtesy Laurel Wiersema-Bryant, RN, MSN, Clinical Nurse Specialist, Barnes Hospital, St. Louis, Mo.)

TABLE 38-1
Wound Classifications

Type and Description	Causes	Implications for Healing
Status of Skin Integrity		
Open wound involving break in skin or mucous membranes	Trauma by sharp object (e.g., surgical incision, venipuncture, gunshot wound)	Exposes body to invasion by microorganisms Loss of blood and body fluids through wound Reduces function of body part
Closed wound involving no break in skin integrity	Part of body being struck by blunt object Twisting, straining, or deceleration force against body (e.g., bone fracture or tear of visceral organ)	May predispose person to internal hemorrhage Reduces function of affected body part
Cause		
Intentional wound resulting from therapy	Surgical incision Introduction of needle into body part	Usually performed under aseptic technique, which minimizes chances of infection Wound edges usually smooth and clean
Unintentional wound occurring unexpectedly	Traumatic injury (e.g., knife wound, burn, pressure ulcer)	Occurs under unsterile conditions Wound edges often jagged
Severity of Injury		
Superficial wound involving only epidermal layer of skin	Result of friction applied to skin surface (e.g., abrasion, first-degree burn)	Creates risk of infection Does not involve underlying injury to tissues or organs Blood supply to area intact
Penetrating wound involving break in epidermal skin layer and dermis and deeper tissues or organs	Foreign object or instrument entering deep into body tissues, usually unintentional (e.g., gunshot wound, stab wound)	High risk of infection because foreign object is contaminated May cause internal and external hemorrhage Damage to organs causes temporary or permanent loss of function
Perforating penetrating wound in which foreign object enters and exits internal organ	Same as penetrating wound	High risk of infection Nature of injury depends on organ perforated: Lung—compromised oxygenation Major vessel—serious hemorrhage Intestine—contamination of abdominal cavity by feces
Cleanliness		
Clean wound containing no pathogenic organisms	Surgical wound that does not enter the gastrointestinal tract, respiratory tract, or oropharyngeal cavity	Low risk of infection
Clean-contaminated wound made under aseptic conditions but involving entrance into body cavity that normally harbors microorganisms	Surgical wound entering gastrointestinal or respiratory tract or oropharyngeal cavity	Greater risk of infection than with clean wound
Contaminated wound existing under conditions in which presence of micororganisms is likely	Open, traumatic wounds Surgical wound in which break in asepsis occurred	Tissues often not healthy and show inflammation High risk of infection

TABLE 38-1
Wound Classifications—cont'd

Type and Description	Causes	Implications for Healing
Infected wound involving bacterial organisms in wound site	Any wound that does not properly heal and grows organisms Old traumatic wound Surgical incision into area infected (e.g., ruptured bowel)	Wound presents signs of infection (e.g., inflammation, purulent drainage, skin separation)
Colonized wound containing micro-organisms (usually multiple)	Chronic wound (e.g., vascular wound or stasis or pressure ulcer)	Wound healing slow High risk of infection
Descriptive Qualities		
Laceration: tearing of tissues with irregular wound edges	Severe traumatic injury (e.g., knife wound, industrial accident involving machinery, tissues cut by broken glass)	Wound usually created by contaminated object Depth determines other complications
Abrasion: superficial wound involving scraping or rubbing of skin's surface by friction	Fall (e.g., skinned knee or elbow) Dermatological procedure for removing scar tissue	Painful from exposure of superficial nerves Deeper tissues uninvolved Risk of infection from exposure to contaminated surface
Contusion: closed wound caused by blow by blunt object; contusion by bruise characterized by swelling, discoloration, and pain	Bleeding in underlying tissues caused by blunt force against body part	More severe if internal organ contused May cause temporary loss of function of body part Localized bleeding into tissues may form hematoma, or collection of blood

Do not use the staging system to measure pressure ulcer healing (NPUAP, 1995).

Wounds and Wound Classifications

The integument or skin is the body's protective barrier against injury and disease-causing organisms and is a sensory organ for pain, temperature, and touch. Injury to the skin causes risks to safety and initiates a complex healing response.

Wound classifications help to define the risks and care implications associated with particular types of wounds (Table 38-1). It is important to know the etiology of the wound, which will determine the type of treatment and risks.

Wound Healing Process

The process of wound healing involves an orderly series of integrated physiological responses. The process is basically the same for all acute wounds but is affected by multiple factors (Box 38-1). A wound with little or no tissue loss, such as a clean surgical incision, heals by **primary intention.** The skin edges **approximate,** or close together, and the risk of infection developing is slight. In contrast, a wound involving loss of tissue such as a severe laceration or a chronic wound such as a pressure ulcer heals by **secondary intention.** The edges do not close, increasing the risk for infection and loss of tissue function. There are also instances in which a surgical wound is initially closed in the deep tissue layers; however, the subcutaneous fat and skin layers are left open. This method of wound closure is called *delayed primary intention.* The wound heals with a layer of granulation tissue at the edges and base, and several days after the initial wounding the wound edges are brought together with sutures or adhesive closures and the wound goes on to heal by primary intention.

Healing by primary intention. The healing process occurs in three stages.

Inflammatory phase. The inflammatory phase begins immediately after the injury; lasts about 4 days; and includes hemostasis, inflammation, and epithelial cell migration. During hemostasis (termination of bleeding), injured blood vessels constrict. Fibronectin, a glycoprotein found in acute wounds, binds to platelets and **fibrin** to form the initial clot that fills in the tissue defect

Box 38-1
Factors Influencing Wound Healing

Age

Blood circulation and oxygen delivery to the wound, clotting, inflammatory response, and phagocytosis may be impaired in the very young and the elderly. Risk of infection is greater.

Cell growth and differentiation in reconstruction are slower with advancing age.

Scar tissue is more taut and less pliable, increasing the risk of altered body part function in older adults.

Nutrition

Tissue repair and infection resistance depend on balanced diet. Surgery, severe wounds, serious infections, and preoperative nutritional deficits increase nutritional requirements.

Obesity

The less abundant supply of blood vessels in fatty tissue impairs delivery of nutrients and cellular elements needed for healing.

Suturing of adipose tissue is more difficult. If the wound heals by secondary intention, dehiscence or evisceration and subsequent infection are greater.

Extent of Wound

Deeper wounds with more tissue loss heal more slowly and by secondary intention and thus are more vulnerable to complications.

Oxygenation

Reduced oxygen delivery to the wound inhibits repair.

Low arterial oxygen tension alters the synthesis of collagen and the formation of epithelial cells.

A wound heals more slowly when local blood flow is reduced and the wound is not exposed to oxygen.

The low hemoglobin levels exhibited in severe anemia reduce oxygenation and impede tissue repair.

Smoking

Functional hemoglobin levels decrease; oxygen release in the tissues is impaired.

Immunosuppression

Reduced immune response contributes to poor healing.

Cortisone depresses fibroblast activity and capillary growth and thereby impairs wound closure.

Because steroids mask an inflammatory response, the nurse may not be able to detect early signs of inflammation or infection.

Chemotherapeutic drugs and certain cancerous diseases interfere with leukocyte production and the immune response.

Diabetes Mellitus

The diabetic client has small vessel disease that impairs tissue perfusion; thus oxygen delivery may be poor.

An elevated blood glucose level impairs macrophage function.

Risk of infection is increased because of poor wound healing.

Radiation

Radiotherapy, which eventually results in fibrosis and vascular scarring, interferes with postoperative wound healing when surgery is delayed more than 4 to 6 weeks and irradiated tissues have become fragile and poorly perfused.

Wound Stress

Sustained stress (e.g., vomiting, abdominal distention, coughing) disrupts wound layers and tissue repair.

(Wysocki, 1992). During the inflammatory phase, complex chemical reactions result in white blood cells that enter the wound and begin wound cleansing. These phagocytic cells remove cellular debris and protect the wound from bacterial invasion. Then epithelial cells migrate from the wound margins toward the base of the clot or scab until, after about 48 hours, a thin layer of epithelial tissue forms over the wound to exclude infectious organisms and toxic materials.

Proliferative reconstruction phase. Reconstruction begins on the third or fourth day after injury and lasts from 2 to 3 weeks. Monocytes that have become

macrophages continue to clear the wound of unwanted debris (destructive process), and fibronectin promotes fibroblast migration and cells that synthesize collagen (Wysocki, 1992). **Collagen** can be found as early as the second day and is the main component of scar tissue. As reconstruction progresses, new capillary networks form to provide oxygen and nutrients for the continued synthesis and support of collagen. As collagen fibers and capillary networks continue to synthesize and increase in size (proliferate), the wound begins to close with new tissue. The amount of scar tissue formed is influenced by the degree of stress on the wound. As the tensile strength of the wound increases, the risk of wound separation or rupture is less likely. After 15 to 20 days the wound can resist normal stress such as tension or twisting. Impairment of healing during this stage usually results from factors such as age, anemia, hypoproteinemia, and zinc deficiency.

Maturation phase. Maturation, the final stage of healing, may take more than a year, depending on the depth and extent of the wound. The collagen scar continues to gain strength for several months but will remain weaker and lighter in color than the tissue it replaces.

An important concept in wound healing is that the stages of wound healing, although progressive, do not occur in a linear fashion. A normally healing wound could simultaneously be in all three stages of wound healing. The stages described previously provide a model for acute wound healing.

Healing by secondary intention.

When tissue loss in a wound is extensive, healing takes longer. Inflammation is often chronic, and tissue defects become filled with fragile granulation tissue rather than collagen. **Granulation tissue** is a form of connective tissue (scar) that has a more abundant blood supply than collagen. Because the wound is larger, it takes much longer to fill and the amount of connective tissue scarring is larger. Formulation of granulation tissue occurs at the same time as wound contraction. The tissue and skin surrounding the defect are mobilized and pulled together, thus reducing the size of the defect (Bryant and others, 1992). Contraction speeds healing because it reduces the amount of scar tissue required for repair. The degree of contraction is limited by the mobility of surrounding tissue (Bryant and others, 1992). In some areas of the body, such as wounds on the face, sternum, and anterior lower leg, contraction gives poor cosmetic results. Wound contraction is not the same as a contracture or deformity resulting from muscle shortening and joint fixation. Special attention should be paid to maintaining joint mobility when a wound has occurred within a joint to prevent or minimize cosmetic deformities or flexion contractures.

Complications of Wound Healing

Wound healing is not without complications. When caring for clients with wounds, the nurse must observe the healing process while observing for complications.

Hemorrhage. Bleeding from an acute wound is normal during and immediately after initial trauma, but **hemostasis** usually occurs within several minutes. Hemorrhage occurring later indicates a slipped surgical suture, a dislodged clot, infection, or the erosion of a blood vessel by a foreign object (e.g., a drain). Hemorrhage may be external or internal. Symptoms of internal bleeding are hypovolemic shock and swelling of the affected body part. A **hematoma** is a localized collection of blood underneath tissues, often appearing as a bluish swelling or mass. External hemorrhaging may be more obvious, because dressings covering the wound soon become saturated with blood. Surgical drains also drain blood.

Infection. Bacterial wound infection inhibits healing by increasing tissue damage and altering the healing process. The chances of wound infection are greater when the wound contains dead or necrotic tissue, when foreign bodies are in or near the wound, and when the blood supply and local tissue defenses are reduced.

A contaminated or traumatic wound infection may develop within 2 to 3 days; a surgical wound infection may develop within 4 to 5 days. Locally, drainage may be yellow, green, or brown and may be odorous, depending on the causative organism. The wound edges may appear tense, swollen, painful, and with redness extending beyond the immediate wound edge. Systemic signs include fever, general malaise, and an elevated white blood cell count.

Dehiscence. When an acute wound fails to heal properly, the layers of skin and tissue may separate. This most commonly occurs before collagen formation (3 to 11 days after injury). **Dehiscence** is the partial or total separation of layers of skin and tissue above the fascia in a wound that is not healing properly. Obese clients have a high risk for dehiscence because of constant strain on their wounds and the poor vascularity of fatty tissue. Dehiscence occurs most often in abdominal surgical wounds after a sudden strain such as coughing, vomiting, or sitting up in bed. Clients often report feeling as though something has given way. When serosanguineous drainage increases from a wound, the nurse should be alert for dehiscence.

Evisceration. Evisceration occurs when wound layers separate, and visceral organs may protrude through the wound opening. It is a medical emergency requiring placement of sterile towels soaked in sterile saline over the extruding tissues to reduce chances of bacterial invasion and drying before surgical repair occurs.

Fistulas. A **fistula** is an abnormal passage between two organs or between an organ and the outside of the body. A surgeon may create a fistula for therapeutic purposes (e.g., making an opening between the stomach and the outer abdominal wall to insert a gastrostomy tube for feeding). Most fistulas result from poor wound healing caused by trauma, infection, radiation exposure, or disease such as cancer. Fistulas increase the risks of infection, fluid and electrolyte imbalances, and skin breakdown from chronic drainage.

NURSING KNOWLEDGE BASE

A major aspect of nursing care is the maintenance of skin integrity and wound care. Impaired skin integrity can occur from prolonged pressure, irritation of the skin, or immobility, leading to the development of pressure ulcers.

Prediction and prevention.
Prevention and treatment of pressure ulcers are major nursing priorities. In 1992 AHCPR developed guidelines for care of adult clients at risk for pressure ulcers. Predictive instruments for pressure ulcer development can identify those clients at highest risk for pressure ulcers. Clients with little risk for pressure ulcer development are spared the unnecessary expense of preventive treatments and the risk of complications.

One reliable tool is the Braden Scale. The Braden Scale is composed of six subscales: sensory perception, moisture, activity, mobility, nutrition, and friction and shear (Table 38-2). A hospitalized adult with a score of 16 or below is considered at risk. In older clients, a score of 17 or 18 may be a more efficient prediction of risk (Braden and Bergstrom, 1992). This instrument is highly reliable in the identification of clients at greatest risk for pressure ulcers (Bergstrom and others, 1987a, 1987b; Capobianco and McDonald, 1996).

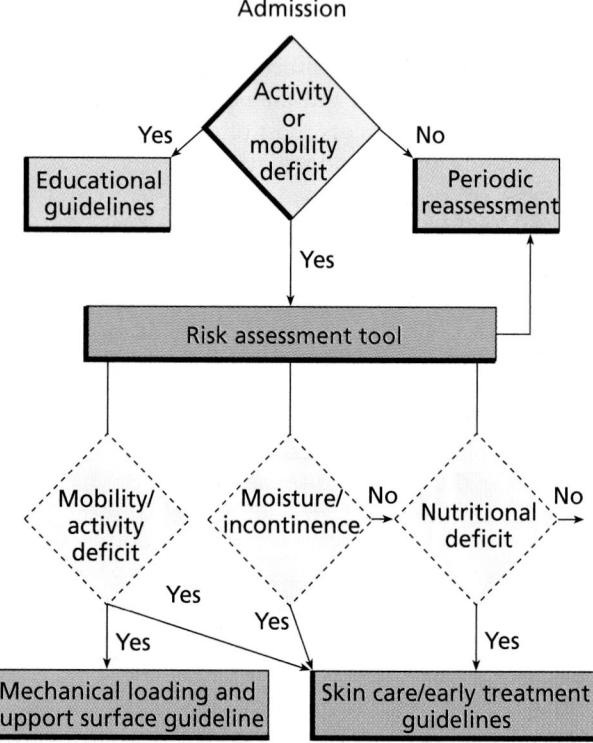

Figure 38-6. Pressure ulcer prediction and prevention algorithm. (From Agency for Health Care Policy and Research: *Pressure ulcers in adults: prediction and prevention,* Pub. No. 92-0047, Rockville, Md, 1992, U.S. Department of Health and Human Services, Public Health Service.)

Additional instruments, such as the Gosnell, Knoll, and Norton Scale are also effective in pressure ulcer prediction. The overall objective of predictive instruments is to effectively and efficiently identify those clients with the greatest risk for pressure ulcer development. From this and using the AHCPR algorithm (Figure 38-6), risk identification and plan of care is devised. Lyder (1996) has raised the issue of the limitations of these pressure ulcer risk assessment scales in minority clients, since the tools were not developed involving clients with darkly pigmented skin.

Prevention.
Prevention of pressure ulcers is a priority in caring for clients and is not limited to clients with restrictions in mobility. Impaired skin integrity is not a problem in healthy, immobilized individuals but is a serious and potentially devastating problem in the ill or debilitated client (AHCPR, 1992). Using the AHCPR (1992) algorithm (see Figure 38-6) can be useful in caring for clients at risk for pressure ulcers.

CRITICAL THINKING IN CLIENT CARE

Synthesis

Clients who have pressure ulcers or chronic wounds require competent nursing care that integrates information from all health-related sciences. Nurses are able to draw from knowledge and experience to incorporate appropriate standards of practice into the management of the client's wound.

Knowledge.
Performing a pressure ulcer risk assessment requires the nurse to use one of the validated risk assessment tools. Knowing normal physiology and the impact of pressure on the skin enables the nurse to practice preventive nursing measures. In addition, knowledge of the normal healing pattern helps the nurse to recognize alterations requiring intervention. In choosing interventions, the nurse must consider the type of wound, the pain associated with it, conditions that affect healing, and the client's psychological well-being.

Experience.
By observing the normal characteristics of a healing wound, the nurse can assess how the client's wound is healing. This is especially important when the client has some factors that may impede wound healing, such as peripheral vascular disease, poor nutrition, or reduced mobility.

The nurse is better able to assess a client's wound by being able to draw from experience and recognize normal characteristics of wound healing. When caring for a client who develops problems with wound healing, the nurse learns the clinical signs of complications. This is especially important when caring for a client with

TABLE 38-2
Braden Scale for Predicting Pressure Sore Risk

	1 Point	2 Points	3 Points	4 Points
Sensory Perception Ability to respond meaningfully to pressure-related discomfort	**Completely limited:** Unresponsive (does not moan, flinch, or grasp) to painful stimuli because of diminished level of consciousness or sedation. **or** Limited ability to feel pain over most of body surface.	**Very limited:** Responds only to painful stimuli. Cannot communicate discomfort except by moaning or restlessness. **or** Has a sensory impairment that limits the ability to feel pain or discomfort over half of body.	**Slightly limited:** Responds to verbal commands but cannot always communicate discomfort or need to be turned. **or** Has some sensory impairment, which limits ability to feel pain or discomfort in 1 or 2 extremities.	**No impairment:** Responds to verbal commands. Has no sensory deficit that would limit ability to feel or voice pain or discomfort.
Moisture Degree to which skin is exposed to moisture	**Constantly moist:** Skin is kept moist almost constantly by perspiration, urine, etc. Dampness is detected every time patient is moved or turned.	**Very moist:** Skin is often, but not always, moist. Linen must be changed at least once a shift.	**Occasionally moist:** Skin is occasionally moist, requiring an extra linen change approximately once a day.	**Rarely moist:** Skin is usually dry; linen requires changing only at routine intervals.
Activity Degree of physical activity	**Bedfast:** Confined to bed.	**Chairfast:** Ability to walk severely limited or nonexistent. Cannot bear own weight and/or must be assisted into chair or wheelchair.	**Walks occasionally:** Walks occasionally during day, but for very short distances, with or without assistance. Spends majority of each shift in bed or chair.	**Walks frequently:** Walks outside the room at least twice a day and inside room at least once every 2 hours during waking hours.
Mobility Ability to change and control body position	**Completely immobile:** Does not make even slight changes in body or extremity position without assistance.	**Very limited:** Makes occasional slight changes in body or extremity position but unable to make frequent or significant changes independently.	**Slightly limited:** Makes frequent though slight changes in body or extremity position independently.	**No limitations:** Makes major and frequent changes in position without assistance.

Instructions: Score client in each of the six subscales. Maximum score is 23, indicating little or no risk. A score of ≤16 indicates "at risk"; ≤9 indicates high risk.

Continued

TABLE 38-2
Braden Scale for Predicting Pressure Sore Risk—cont'd

	1 Point	2 Points	3 Points	4 Points
Nutrition Usual food intake pattern	**Very poor:** Never eats a complete meal. Rarely eats more than one third of any food offered. Eats 2 servings or less of protein (meat or dairy products) per day. Takes fluids poorly. Does not take a liquid dietary supplement. **or** Is NPO and/or maintained on clear liquids or IVs for more than 5 days.	**Probably inadequate:** Rarely eats a complete meal and generally eats only about half of any food offered. Protein intake includes only 3 servings of meat or dairy products per day. Occasionally will take a dietary supplement. **or** Receives less than optimal amount of liquid diet or tube feeding.	**Adequate:** Eats over half of most meals. Eats a total of 4 servings of protein (meat, dairy products) each day. Occasionally will refuse a meal, but will usually take a supplement if offered. **or** Is on a tube-feeding or TPN regimen that probably meets most of nutritional needs.	**Excellent:** Eats most of every meal. Never refuses a meal. Usually eats a total of 4 or more servings of meat and dairy products. Occasionally eats between meals. Does not require supplements.
Friction and Shear	**Problem:** Requires moderate to maximal assistance in moving. Complete lifting without sliding against sheets is impossible. Frequently slides down in bed or chair, requiring frequent repositioning with maximal assistance. Spasticity, contractions, or agitation leads to almost constant friction.	**Potential problem:** Moves feebly or requires minimal assistance. During a move skin probably slides to some extent against sheets, chair, restraints, or other devices. Maintains relatively good position in chair or bed most of the time but occasionally slides down.	**No apparent problem:** Moves in bed and in chair independently and has sufficient muscle strength to sit up completely during move. Maintains good position in bed or chair at all times.	

darkly pigmented skin (Box 38-2). Reflecting on such experience prepares the nurse to assess wounds more accurately.

Attitudes. The nurse must be observant when caring for an acutely ill client; at times assessment for skin breakdown may be overlooked because of other perceived priorities by the nurse, such as respiratory or cardiac status. The nurse is the client advocate and ensures that meticulous skin assessment and pressure ulcer prevention measures are incorporated into the plan of care. Skin assessment is important whenever a client's health status changes (AHCPR, 1992, 1994).

In the immediate postoperative period, clients may require well-thought-out modifications of dressing care techniques. The dressing may not be changed, but the nurse is responsible for ensuring that the dressing remains dry and intact. With knowledge about pressure

Box 38-2
Box 38-2
Assessment Tips for Examining Intact Dark Skin

Assess Skin Color

Appears darker than surrounding skin (purplish/blue hue)

May have a purplish/bluish hue

Importance of Lighting Source

Use natural or halogen light

Avoid fluorescent lamps

Assess Skin Temperature

When first touched, skin will feel warm compared to surrounding area

Later this will be replaced by an area of coolness, which is a sign of tissue devitalization

Assess for Edema/Fluid

May be taut, shiny, or indurated; edema may occur with induration of more than 15 mm in diameter

---

ulcers, wounds, and normal wound healing, the nurse can find creative measures to reduce the risks of impaired skin integrity and promote wound healing.

Standards. The 1992 and 1994 clinical guidelines written by the AHCPR are the standards of care for clients with pressure ulcers (Murphy, 1996). A summary of the AHCPR prevention points compiled by NPUAP can be found in Box 38-3.

Standard protocols for surgical wounds include cleaning primary intention wounds with a skin cleaner and covering the wound with a dressing. The skin cleaners, dressing material used, and frequency of dressing change vary by agency policy.

NURSING PROCESS

Assessment

Baseline and continual assessment data provide critical information about the client's skin integrity and the increased risk for pressure ulcer development or impaired wound healing.

Pressure ulcers. Assessment for pressure ulcers (Skill 38-1) is not limited to the skin but must also include the underlying tissue and muscle. Pressure ulcers have multiple etiological factors. Baseline and continual assessment data can provide critical information about the client's skin integrity and increased risk for pressure ulcer development.

Predictive measures. The predictive instruments increase the nurse's early detection of clients at greatest

risk for ulcer development. It is best to use predictive instruments to assess risks for impaired skin integrity in those clients who are immobilized, malnourished, incontinent, or paralyzed. Prompt identification of such clients enables nurses to individualize costly resources to appropriate clients and reduce their risk.

Skin. Assessment for tissue pressure indicators includes visual and tactile inspection of the skin (Pires and Muller, 1991). Baseline assessment determines the client's normal skin characteristics and any actual or potential areas of breakdown. This is especially important with high risk clients. The skin of an older adult client is more fragile and has an increased risk for skin breakdown (Box 38-4). The nurse pays particular attention to areas exposed to casts, traction, or splints. The frequency of systematic pressure assessment should occur at least once a day on those clients at greater risk for pressure ulcer development (AHCPR, 1992). Assessment also depends on the schedule of appliance application and the skin's response to the external pressure (Figures 38-7 and 38-8).

When hyperemia is noted, the nurse documents its location, size, and color and reassesses the area after 1 hour. If the nurse suspects abnormal reactive hyperemia, outlining the affected area with a marker makes reassessment easier. Another early warning sign of pressure damage is a blister or pimple over the weight-bearing area with possible hyperemia. Pires and Muller (1991) report that a frequently overlooked sign of early pressure is a scabbing over of the weight-bearing areas in the absence of trauma (Figure 38-9). All of these signs are very early indicators of impaired skin integrity, but damage to the underlying tissue may be more progressive. The nurse palpates the tissues adjacent to the observed area to acquire further data about induration and the damage to the skin and underlying tissues.

The nurse assesses clients with lightly pigmented skin for blanching with return to normal skin tones. The nurse also notes changes in color, temperature, and hardness of the surrounding skin and tissues (Pires and Muller, 1991).

The nurse includes visual and tactile inspection over the body areas most frequently at risk for pressure ulcer development (Figure 38-10). When a client lies in bed or sits in a chair, body weight is heavily placed on certain bony prominences. Body surfaces subjected to the greatest weight or pressure are at greatest risk for decubitus ulcer formation.

Mobility. Assessment includes documenting level of mobility, the potential effects of impaired mobility on skin integrity, and data regarding the quality of muscle tone and strength. For example, the nurse determines whether the client can lift the weight off the ischial tuberosities and can roll the body to a side-lying position. The client may have adequate range of motion (ROM) to independently move into a more protective

Text continued on p. 1084

> ### Box 38-3
> ## Pressure Ulcer Prevention Points
>
> ### Risk Assessment
>
> 1. Consider all bed- or chair-bound persons, or those whose ability to reposition is impaired, to be at risk for pressure ulcers.
> 2. Select and use a method of risk assessment, such as the Norton scale or the Braden Scale, that ensures systematic evaluation of individual risk factors.
> 3. Assess all at-risk clients at the time of admission to health care facilities and at regular intervals thereafter.
> 4. Identify all individual risk factors (decreased mental status, moisture, incontinence, nutritional deficits) to direct specific preventive treatments. Modify care according to the individual factors.
>
> ### Skin Care and Early Treatment
>
> 1. Inspect the skin at least daily, and document assessment results.
> 2. Individualize bathing frequency. Use a mild cleansing agent. Avoid hot water and excessive friction.
> 3. Assess and treat incontinence. When incontinence cannot be controlled, cleanse skin at time of soiling, use a topical moisture barrier, and select underpads or briefs that are absorbent and provide a quick drying surface to the skin.
> 4. Use moisturizers for dry skin. Minimize environmental factors leading to dry skin, such as low humidity and cold air.
> 5. Avoid massage over bony prominences.
> 6. Use proper positioning, transferring, and turning techniques to minimize skin injury due to friction and shear forces.
> 7. Use dry lubricants (cornstarch) or protective coverings to reduce friction injury.
> 8. Identify and correct factors compromising protein/calorie intake and consider nutritional supplementation/support for nutritionally compromised persons.
> 9. Institute a rehabilitation program to maintain or improve mobility/activity status.
> 10. Monitor and document interventions and outcomes.
>
> ### Mechanical Loading and Support Surfaces
>
> 1. Reposition bed-bound persons according to appropriate turning schedule (see Skill 38-1, Step 9b).
> 2. Use a written repositioning schedule.
> 3. Place at-risk persons on a pressure-reducing mattress/chair cushion. Do not use donut-type devices.
> 4. Consider postural alignment, distribution of weight, balance and stability, and pressure relief when positioning persons in chairs or wheelchairs.
> 5. Teach chair-bound persons, who are able, to shift weight every 15 minutes.
> 6. Use lifting devices (e.g., trapeze or bed linen) to move rather than drag persons during transfer and position changes.
> 7. Use pillows or foam wedges to keep bony prominences such as knees and ankles from direct contact with each other.
> 8. Use devices that totally relieve pressure on the heels (e.g., place pillows under the calf to raise the heels off the bed).
> 9. Avoid positioning directly on the trochanter when using the side-lying position (use the 30° lateral inclined position).
> 10. Elevate the head of the bed as little (maximum 30° angle) and for as short a time as possible.
>
> ### Education
>
> 1. Implement educational programs for the prevention of pressure ulcers for all levels of health care providers, clients, family, and caregivers.
> 2. Include information on:
>   a. Etiology of and risk factors for pressure ulcers
>   b. Risk assessment tools and their application
>   c. Skin assessment
>   d. Selection/use of support surfaces
>   e. Individualized programs of skin care
>   f. Positioning to decrease risk of tissue breakdown
>   g. Accurate documentation of pertinent data
>
> Data from National Pressure Ulcer Advisory Panel: Pressure ulcers incidence, economics, risk assessment, Consensus Development Conference Statement, *Decubitus* 2(2):24, 1989.

Assessment for Risk of Pressure Ulcer Development

Delegation Considerations

Assessment of adults for risk of pressure ulcers requires problem solving and knowledge application unique to professional nursing. For this procedure delegation is not appropriate. Instruct unlicensed personnel to report any changes in skin integrity to nurse immediately.

Equipment
- Risk assessment tool
- Documentation record
- Body chart or tracing film and/or camera

STEPS	RATIONALE
1. Identify client's risk for pressure ulcer formation:	Determines need to administer preventive care and use topical agents for existing ulcers.
a. Paralysis or immobilization caused by restrictive devices	Client is unable to turn or reposition independently.
b. Sensory loss	Client feels no discomfort from pressure.
c. Circulatory disorders	Reduce perfusion of skin's tissue layers.
d. Decreased level of consciousness, sedation, or anesthesia	Client is unable to perceive pressure to turn or reposition independently.
e. Shearing force	Causes skin and underlying subcutaneous layers to adhere to surface of bed. Trauma occurs to underlying tissues.
f. Moisture: incontinence, perspiration, wound drainage, or vomitus	Reduces skin's resistance to pressure from shearing force.
g. Malnutrition	Can lead to weight loss, muscle atrophy, and reduced tissue mass. Less tissue is available to pad between skin and underlying bone. Poor protein, vitamin, and caloric intake limit wound-healing capabilities.
h. Anemia	Decreased hemoglobin level reduces oxygen-carrying capacity of blood and amount of oxygen available to tissues.
i. Infection	Causes increase in metabolic demands of tissues. Accompanying diaphoresis leaves skin moist.
j. Obesity	Poorly vascularized excess adipose tissue is more susceptible to pressure. Body weight against bony prominences places underlying skin at risk for breakdown.
k. Cachexia	Causes loss of adipose tissue that protects bony prominences from pressure.
l. Hydration: edema or dehydration	Edematous tissue has decreased blood supply and thereby is less tolerant of pressure, friction, and shearing force. Dehydrated skin is less elastic, and skin turgor is poor.
m. Older adulthood	Skin is less elastic and drier; tissue mass is reduced.
n. Existing pressure ulcers	Limits surfaces available for position changes, placing available tissues at increased risk.

Continued

Assessment for Risk of Pressure Ulcer Development

STEPS	RATIONALE
2. Assess condition of skin over regions of pressure. Look for the following characteristics:	
a. Normal or abnormal reactive hyperemia lasting less than 1 hour	May indicate that tissue was under pressure. Normal reactive hyperemia is normal physiological response to hypoxemia. In dark-skinned persons, skin that was under pressure will appear darker than surrounding skin and may even take on purplish hue (Pires and Muller, 1991; Bennett, 1995).
	Affected area blanches at fingertip pressure (Pires and Muller, 1991).
	Abnormal reactive hyperemia lasts longer than 1 hour. Surrounding tissue does not blanch (Pires and Muller, 1991).
b. Blanching	Blanching is a normal, expected response.
c. Induration	Localized edema beneath the skin surface; induration commonly occurs with abnormal reactive hyperemia (Pires and Muller, 1991).
d. Pallor and mottling	Persistent hypoxia in tissues that were under pressure is an abnormal physiological response.
e. Absence of superficial skin layers	Represents early pressure ulcer formation.
f. Scabs, blisters, or pimples	Early signs of skin damage, but damage to underlying tissue may be more progressive (Pires and Muller, 1991).
3. Assess client for areas of potential pressure:	Clients at high risk have multiple sites of pressure necrosis.
a. Nares	Pressure can occur from nasogastric tube or nasal O_2 cannula.
b. Tongue, lips	Oral airway and endotracheal tube are high-risk locations.
c. Intravenous sites (especially long-term access sites)	Stress occurs at catheter exit sites.
d. Drainage tubes	There is stress against tissue at exit site.
e. Foley catheter	There is pressure against labia, especially with edema.
4. Observe client for preferred positions when in bed or chair.	Weight of body will be placed on bony prominences. Contractures (flexion and fixation of joint) may result in pressure exerted in unexpected places. Phenomenon is best assessed through observation.
5. Observe client's mobility and ability to initiate and assist with position changes.	Potential for friction and shear increases when client is completely dependent for position changes.
6. Obtain risk score:	Risk score depends on instrument used and predicts client's need for preventive care (AHCPR, 1992).
a. Braden Scale (see Table 38-3)	

STEPS	RATIONALE
7. Assist client to change position.	Avoid positions that place the client directly on an area of existing ulceration. It may be helpful to use a schedule for position changes.
Use the following positions: a. Supine b. Prone c. 30-degree lateral (see Figure 38-13)	Achieved with one pillow under shoulder and one pillow under leg on the same side. Protects sacrum and trochanters.
8. Palpate any area of discoloration or mottling. Skin temperature changes may be an important early indicator of a stage I (see Figure 38-5) pressure ulcer in clients with darkly pigmented skin (Bennett, 1995).	Early detection of pressure indicates need for more frequent position changes.
9. Monitor length of time any area of discoloration persists:	In lightly pigmented clients, redness usually persists for half of time hypoxia occurred. For example, redness lasts 15 min, so hypoxia lasted approximately 30 min.
a. Determine appropriate turning interval, which should be (turning interval − hypoxia time = suggested interval)	For example, turning interval is 2 hours, hypoxia time is 30 min (2 hr − 30 min = 1½ hr suggested turning interval).
b. Use pressure-relief device, if indicated	Short turning intervals (e.g., 1 to 2 hours) may not be realistic. Therefore use of device is recommended.
10. Obtain nutritional assessment data, including serum albumin level, total protein level, hemoglobin level, and IBW percentage.	Poor nutritional status decreases skin's and underlying tissue's tolerance to pressure, friction, and shearing force (AHCPR, 1994).
11. Assess client's and family's understanding of risks for pressure ulcers.	Provides opportunity to begin prevention education (Ayello, 1993, 1995).
12. Observe client's skin for areas at risk for change in color or texture.	Enables the nurse to evaluate success of prevention techniques.
13. Observe tolerance of client for position change.	Position changes may interfere with client's sleep and rest pattern.
14. Compare subsequent risk assessment scores.	Provides ongoing comparison of client's risk level to facilitate appropriateness of care plan.

Recording and Reporting
- Record client's risk score.
- Record appearance of skin under pressure.
- Describe positions, turning intervals, pressure-relieving support devices, and other prevention measures.
- Report any need for additional consultations for the high-risk client.

Home Care Considerations
- The 30-degree lateral and prone positions may be useful at night to prolong the time between position changes, resulting in less sleep disruption for the client and care giver.
- Pressure-relief maneuvers must be customized for the independent client. The individual may find a watch with a timer, even or odd hours, and television commercials helpful in remembering to complete pressure-relief techniques.

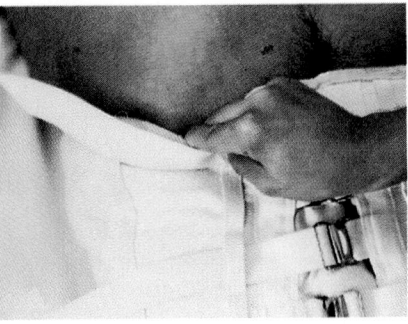

Figure 38-7.   Benign devices such as this corset may result in scabbing or blistering, resulting from external pressure.

position. Finally, the nurse notes the client's activity tolerance (see Chapter 37).

Nutritional status. An assessment of the client's nutritional status should be done at least every 3 months as an integral part of the initial assessment data for clients at risk for impaired skin integrity (AHCPR, 1994) (Box 38-5; see Chapter 34). Total protein levels are also correlated with pressure ulcer development. Total protein levels below 5.4 g/100 ml decrease colloid osmotic pressure, which leads to interstitial edema and decreased oxygen to the tissues. Edema decreases the skin and underlying tissue's tolerance to pressure, friction, and shearing force.

The nurse assesses wounds at the time of injury; before the initiation of treatment; and after therapy, when the wound is relatively stable. Each condition requires different observations and actions.

Wounds. The assessment of a client's wound varies from one health care setting to another. It is important that the nurse be thorough in this assessment and accurately collect pertinent data. The nurse assesses wounds at the time of injury, before initiation of treatment, and after therapy. Each condition requires different observations and actions.

Emergency setting. In an emergency the type of wound determines the criteria for inspection. After a client's cardiopulmonary status is stabilized (see Chapter 30), the nurse inspects the wound for bleeding. An **abrasion** is usually superficial with little bleeding but some weeping (plasma leakage from damaged capillar-

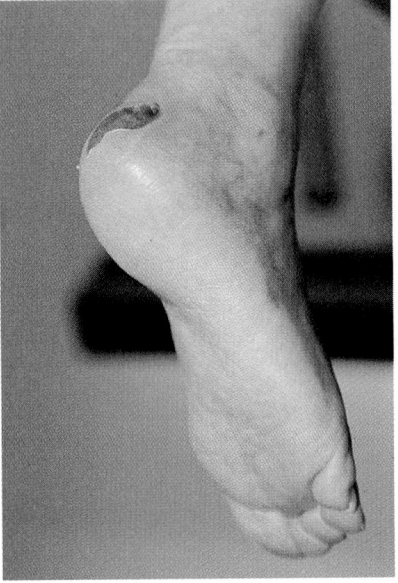

Figure 38-8.   Formation of pressure ulcer on heel resulting from external pressure from mattress of bed.

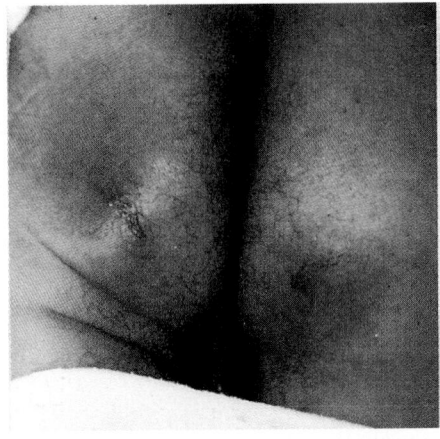

Figure 38-9.   Scabbing over bony prominences is a sign of excessive pressure.

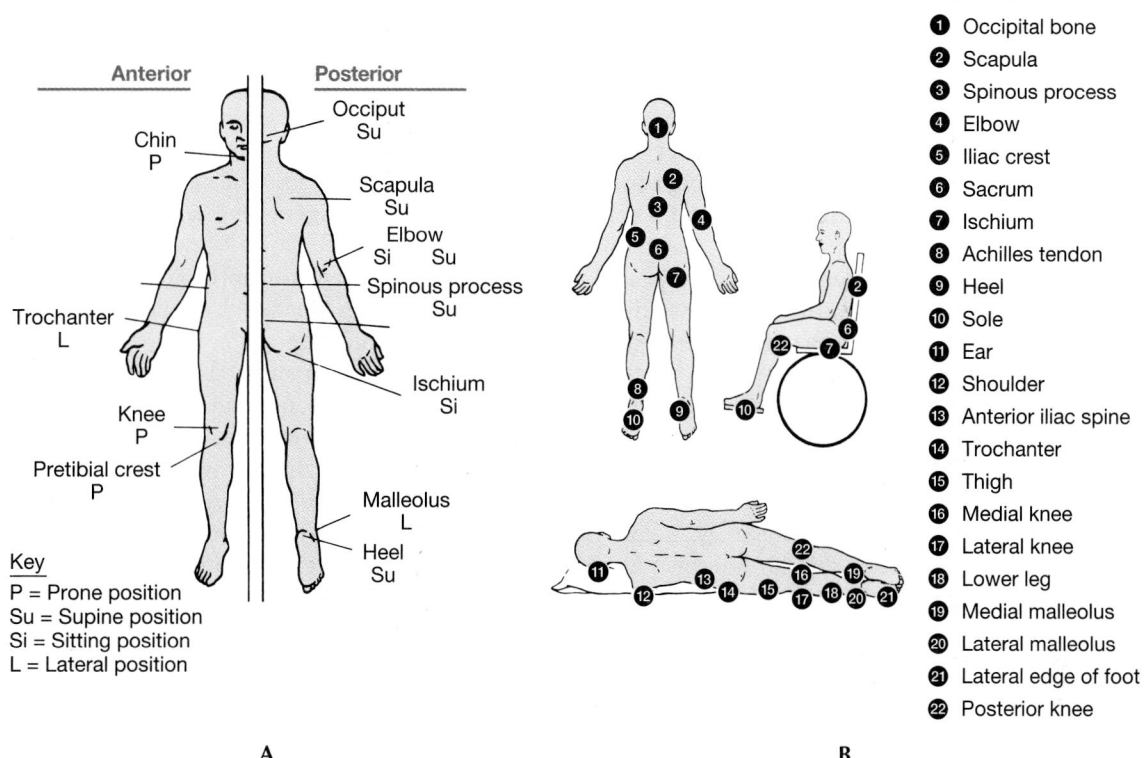

Figure 38-10.   **A,** Bony prominences most frequently underlying pressure ulcers. **B,** Pressure ulcer sites. (From Trelease CC: *Ostomy/Wound Manage* 20:46, 1988.)

ies). The depth and location of a **laceration,** a torn, jagged wound, affect the extent of bleeding, with serious bleeding possible in lacerations greater than 5 cm (2 inches) long or 2.5 cm (1 inch) deep.

Puncture wounds bleed in relation to the depth and size of the wound; internal bleeding and infection are the primary dangers. The nurse next inspects the wound for contaminant material such as soil, broken glass, shreds of cloth, and foreign substances clinging to penetrating objects. The nurse then assesses the size of the wound and the need for suturing or surface protection. When the injury is the result of trauma from a dirty penetrating object, the nurse asks if the client has received a tetanus toxoid injection within the last year.

Stable setting. Once an acute wound is stable after surgery or treatment, the nurse assesses its progress toward healing. If the wound is covered by a dressing that the physician has written orders not to change, the nurse inspects only the dressing and any external drains. Should a dressing appear saturated with drainage, the nurse may reinforce the secondary dressing pending a definitive response and orders from the physician. Saturated dressings provide an excellent environment for bacterial growth, and the physician will need to be informed of the color, odor, and estimate of drainage amount.

When a dressing change is planned, it may help to administer an analgesic at least 30 minutes before

---

Box 38-5

Nutritional Assessment and Management of Pressure Ulcers: AHCPR 1994 Treatment Guideline Recommendations

Ensure adequate dietary intake to prevent malnutrition to the extent that this is compatible with the individual's wishes.

Perform an abbreviated nutritional assessment, as defined by the Nutrition Screening Initiative, at least every 3 months for individuals who are unable to take food by mouth or who experience an involuntary change in weight.

Encourage dietary intake or supplementation if an individual with a pressure ulcer is malnourished. If dietary intake continues to be inadequate, impractical, or impossible, nutritional support (usually tube feeding) should be used to place the client into positive nitrogen balance (approximately 30 to 35 calories/kg/day and 1.25 to 1.50 g of protein/kg/day) according to goals of care.

Give vitamin and mineral supplements if deficiencies are confirmed or suspected.

exposing a wound. The nurse must avoid accidentally removing or displacing underlying drains.

The nurse first inspects the appearance of the wound, noting the approximation of wound edges, the presence of exudate, the condition of underlying tissue in an open wound, and signs of dehiscence, evisceration, or infection. The nurse also notes **ecchymosis,** skin discoloration or bruising caused by blood leakage into subcutaneous tissues after trauma to underlying vessels. The outer edges of a wound normally appear inflamed for the first 2 to 3 days, but this slowly disappears. If infection develops, the wound edges usually become brightly inflamed, warm, tender, and swollen.

The nurse next assesses the character of wound drainage by noting the amount, color, odor, and consistency. The amount of drainage depends on the location and extent of the wound and can be measured by comparing the weights of wet and dry dressings. A rule of thumb is 1 g of drainage equals 1 ml. Another simple method for estimating the volume of wound drainage is to report the number and type of dressings used and saturated over what interval of time. The color and consistency of drainage vary, depending on its components. Types of drainage include the following:

1. Serous: clear, watery plasma
2. Sanguineous: fresh bleeding
3. Serosanguineous: pale, more watery, a combination of plasma and red cells, may be blood-streaked
4. Purulent: thick, yellow, green, or brown, indicating the presence of dead or living organisms and white blood cells

If the drainage has a pungent or strong odor, an infection is likely. The nurse objectively documents the integrity of the wound and the character of drainage, describing the appearance by observable characteristics.

The presence of drains is another important assessment criterion. A drain is used in a surgical wound if a large amount of drainage is expected and if keeping wound layers closed is especially important, because accumulated fluid under the tissues prevents closure. A drain may lie under a dressing, extend through a dressing, or be connected to a drainage bag or suction apparatus. A pin or clip through a Penrose drain prevents it

from slipping farther into a wound (Figure 38-11). As wound drainage decreases, the physician slowly withdraws the drain or leaves orders for the nurse to withdraw the drain a specified length over several days. The nurse first observes the security of the drain and its location with respect to the wound. Next the nurse notes the character and amount of drainage if there is a collecting device (Figure 38-12). The nurse pays particular attention to the flow of drainage through the tubing and notifies the physician of any sudden decrease that might indicate a blocked drain or an increase indicating bleeding or infection.

In the case of a surgical wound, the nurse inspects the staples, sutures, or wound closures for irritation and notes whether the closures are intact. The nurse may choose to count sutures when the physician has removed a portion of them. After the first few days when normal swelling around closures usually has subsided, continued swelling may indicate overly tight closures, which can cause wound separation or dehiscence. Early suture removal reduces formation of defects along the suture line and minimizes chances of unattractive scar formation.

When a wound exhibits swelling or separation of its

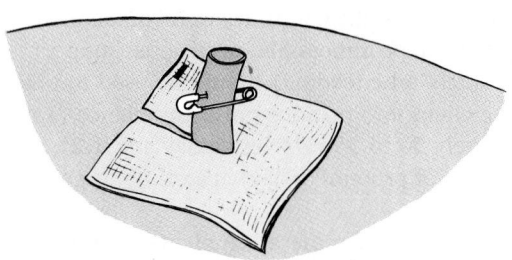

Figure 38-11. Penrose drain.

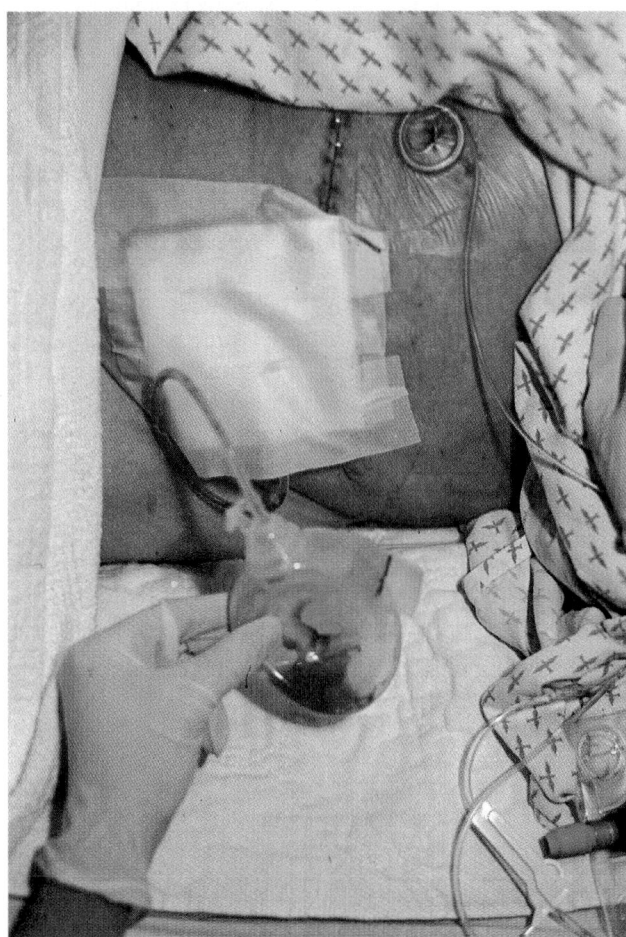

Figure 38-12. Jackson-Pratt drainage tubes and reservoir.

edges, the nurse can use light palpation to detect localized areas of tenderness or collection of drainage. Wearing sterile gloves, the nurse gently applies the fingertips along the wound edges. If pressure causes fluid to be expressed from the wound, the nurse notes the character of the drainage and collects it for culturing if necessary. Sensitivity to such palpation is normal, but extreme tenderness may indicate infection.

Pain assessment is an important component of wound assessment for detecting complications and planning future wound care (Rook, 1996). Serious discomfort during inspection or palpation of the wound suggests underlying problems, whereas discomfort related to dressing removal or application calls for administration of analgesics before future dressing changes.

Wound cultures. If the nurse detects purulent or suspicious-looking drainage, a **wound culture** may be ordered by the physician. The nurse should never collect a wound culture sample from old drainage, because resident colonies of bacteria grow in exudate. The nurse first cleans the wound to remove skin flora. Aerobic organisms grow in superficial wounds exposed to the air, and anaerobic organisms tend to grow within body cavities. To collect an aerobic specimen the nurse inserts a sterile swab from a culturette tube into wound secretions, returns the swab to the culturette tube, caps the tube, and crushes the inner ampule so that the medium for organism growth coats the swab tip. The nurse then sends the labeled specimen to the laboratory immediately. To collect an anaerobic specimen deep in a body cavity, the nurse uses a sterile syringe tip to aspirate visible drainage from the inner wound, expels any air from the syringe, and injects contents into a special vacuum container with culture medium. In some institutions, the nurse may place a cork over the needle to prevent entrance of air and sends the syringe to the lab. The AHCPR (1994) guidelines recommend using the needle aspiration technique rather than the quantitative swab technique (Box 38-6).

Client expectations. When clients have a pressure ulcer or a chronic wound, their course of treatment is usually costly and lengthy. Because the client must be involved with the wound care management, it is important to know the client's expectations. A client who unrealistically expects rapid wound healing may be easily discouraged and not adhere to the treatment regimen. Likewise, a client who knows that the process is lengthy may unrealistically expect the area to heal without scarring. Knowing these expectations assists the nurse in providing individualized care and helping the client modify expectations when needed.

••••••••••••••••••••••••••

Successful critical thinking requires a synthesis of knowledge, experience, information gathered from clients, and critical thinking attitudes and standards. Clinical judgments require the nurse to anticipate what information is needed, to analyze the data, and to then make decisions regarding client care. The client expects competent and informed care. Lynda Abraham incorporates previous knowledge and experience in providing care for Mr. Ahmed.

Box 38-6

Recommendations for Standardized Techniques for Wound Cultures

Needle Aspiration Procedure

Clean intact skin with an antimicrobial solution. Allow it to dry.

Insert the needle through the client's skin while maintaining adequate *negative* pressure in the syringe.

When doing the aspiration culture technique, it is essential to probe two to four areas when obtaining the culture.

Quantitative Swab Procedures

Clean the wound surface with a nonantimicrobial. Allow to dry.

Swabbing of the wound should be to a 1 × 2 cm area. Enough pressure needs to be used so that fluid is expressed from the wound tissue.

Data from Stotts NA: Determination of bacterial burden in wounds, NPUAP Proceedings 1995, *Adv Wound Care* 8(4):28, 1995.

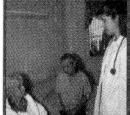

Case Study

Synthesis in Practice

When Ms. Abraham returns the next day, she finds that Mr. Ahmed has a small 1 × 2 inch (2.5 × 5 cm) × ⅛ inch deep shallow wound on his sacrum. There is no necrotic tissue, and the wound bed has beefy red tissue. When Ms. Abraham prepares to conduct a skin assessment on Mr. Ahmed, she recalls information about the pathogenesis of pressure ulcers and guidelines for skin assessment for clients with darkly pigmented skin. She will focus on determining changes in Mr. Ahmed's skin integrity.

Ms. Abraham observed care of a stage IV pressure ulcer during an experience in an extended care facility. From that experience she increased her knowledge about the debilitating effects of pressure ulcers. In addition, she was able to practice skin assessment techniques during her clinical experience in the extended care facility.

◪ Nursing Diagnosis

A client with actual or high risk for *impaired skin integrity* may also have one or more nursing diagnoses related to the condition. Assessment reveals clusters of data that indicate whether an actual or a risk for *impaired skin integrity* exists. After gathering appropriate assessment data, the nurse clusters defining characteristics to establish nursing diagnoses. For example, the destruction of the skin's surface clearly allows the nurse to diagnose *impaired skin integrity*. The identification of nursing diagnoses related to wound healing helps the nurse to anticipate the need for supportive or preventive care (see nursing diagnoses box).

The nurse assesses related factors contributing to each diagnostic statement. These related factors become the focus of the nurse's interventions. For example, the client with *impaired skin integrity related to a surgical incision* requires a different set of interventions than the client with *impaired skin integrity related to pressure and nutritional deficiency*. The client whose surgical incision causes drainage will require different and perhaps more frequent skin cleansing and dressings chosen to contain more drainage.

◪ Planning

The nurse plans therapeutic interventions for clients with actual or potential risks to skin integrity (see care plan). These therapies are designed according to severity of risks to the client, and the plan is individualized according to developmental stage and level of health. In addition, the nurse must develop client-centered goals aimed at preventing or reducing impaired skin integrity. Care planning is individualized to the client, taking into consideration the client's most immediate needs.

Other client factors to be considered when setting priorities include everyday activities and family factors. The nurse may need the help of another health team member, such as a physical or occupational therapist, when considering mobility needs. These factors are important for clients in institutional and home settings. Discharge planning is begun when a client enters the health care system. Anticipating the client's discharge from an institution, a referral to a skilled nursing care facility or home health agency may be necessary to help the client remain or regain mobility at home.

With the trend toward earlier discharge from health care settings, it is important to consider the client's plan for discharge. Clients and their families may need to continue the objectives of wound management after discharge. Thus they may need to discuss the likelihood of the client returning home, returning home with the assistance of home nursing, or transferring to a skilled nursing facility for more care and observation.

◪ Implementation

Health promotion and prevention of pressure ulcers. Once risk factors are identified, the nurse then reduces environmental factors that accelerate pressure ulcer formation, such as high room temperature (causing diaphoresis), moisture, or wrinkled bed linen.

Early identification of high-risk clients and their risk factors aids the nurse in preventing pressure ulcers.

TABLE 38-3
A Quick Guide to Prevention

Risk Factor	Nursing Interventions
Immobility	Establish individualized turning schedule.
	Reduce shear and friction.
	Provide pressure-relief surface.
Inactivity	Provide assistive devices to increase activity.
Incontinence	Assess need for incontinence management.
	Clean and dry skin after soiling.
Malnutrition	Provide adequate nutritional and fluid intake.
	Consult dietitian for nutritional evaluation.
Diminished sensation, decreased mental status	Assess client's and family's ability to provide care.
	Educate care giver regarding pressure ulcer prevention.
Impaired skin integrity	Avoid pressure.
	Do not use donut-shaped cushions.
	Lubricate skin.
	Do not massage red areas.
	Do not use heat lamps.

Data from Maklebust J, Sieggreen M: *Pressure ulcers: guidelines for prevention and nursing management,* West Dundee, Ill, 1991, S-N Publications.

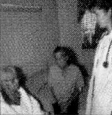

CASE STUDY NURSING CARE PLAN

Skin Integrity and Wound Care

Assessment

Mr. Ahmed is **febrile and has limited activity tolerance.** He **does not tolerate position changes or sitting out of bed; he wants to stay in a semi-Fowler's position at all times.** He complains of **a painful, burning sensation in his sacral region.** On inspection, **reactive hyperemia remains for a period of greater than 1 hour. His hypoxia time is 30 minutes. A 1 × 2 inch open area is present; serous drainage is noted.** On palpation, **underlying skin is soft and indurated.**

Nursing Diagnosis

Impaired skin integrity related to pressure on bony prominence in sacral region.

Planning

Goal

Injury to skin and underlying tissue resulting from pressure on bony prominence will be reduced within 2 to 4 weeks.

Expected Outcomes

Wound will decrease in size by 2/21.

Wound drainage will be reduced by 2/19.

Reactive hyperemia to surrounding tissue will remain within normal limits.

Implementation

Steps

1. Reposition client every 90 min. Turning interval: 120 min − 30 min hypoxia time = 90 min.

2. Apply dressing to wound.

3. Place client on an egg crate mattress.

Rationale

Repositioning removes pressure and allows normal hyperemic response. Frequency of turning is based on initial assessment (Maklebust, 1991).

Dressings protect underlying skin and remove drainage from surface of wound (Maklebust, 1991).

Clients with pressure ulcer development are at greater risk for new ulcers and need preventive measures to prevent ulcer progression (NPUAP, 1989).

Evaluation

Measure wound size daily.

Observe the color and amount of drainage with each dressing change.

Observe and time the duration of reactive hyperemia after each position change.

Palpate underlying and adjacent tissues after each position change.

Defining characteristics are shown in bold type.

Prevention minimizes the impact that risk factors or contributing factors may have on pressure ulcer development. Table 38-3 outlines some nursing interventions for the prevention of pressure ulcers. Three major areas of nursing interventions for prevention of pressure ulcers are hygiene and topical skin care, use of the 30-degree lateral position, and the use of therapeutic beds and mattresses.

Hygiene and topical skin care. The nurse must keep the client's skin clean and dry. In this initial line of defense for preventing skin breakdown, the client's skin must be continually assessed by nurses. In addition, the types of products available for skin care are numerous, and their uses need to be matched to the specific needs of the client (Maklebust and Sieggreen, 1996).

When the skin is cleaned, soaps are avoided. Soaps and alcohol-based lotions cause drying and leave an alkaline residue. The alkaline residue discourages the growth of normal skin bacteria, thus promoting an overgrowth of opportunistic bacteria, which can then enter an open wound.

After the skin is cleansed and completely dried, protective moisturizer should be applied to keep the epidermis well lubricated but not oversaturated. Cornstarch is a dry lubricant and helps to reduce friction. A & D, Unicare, and Pericare are bland, water-repellent ointments that protect the skin from moisture (AHCPR, 1992). In addition, these ointments are easily cleansed from the skin. When using any water-repellent ointment, the nurse must completely clean the area on a routine basis. Ointment, when left in place too long, can be a medium for bacteria and can cause further skin problems such as **maceration** and infection.

When the client's skin is exposed to body fluids such as urine, bowel, or wound drainage, the area should be cleansed, and a skin barrier containing petrolatum (e.g., Vaseline) or zinc oxide is applied. These barriers protect the skin from excessive moisture and toxins from urine or stool.

When clients are incontinent, absorptive underpads such as adult diapers or incontinence briefs can be used. Those products drain moisture away from the client's skin. The proper absorptive garments have a quilted lining and contain a polymer filling. The newer products also lubricate the skin, as well as protect from moisture. These absorptive underpads (Senecare and Silopad [Silipos Silicone Technology, NY]) are placed in direct contact with the skin. As the client moves, the skin is lubricated, friction is reduced, and excess moisture is absorbed into the pad (Marchand and Lidowski, 1993). When providing skin care to the incontinent client, the health care team must also assess and treat the causes of incontinence (see Chapter 35).

Positioning. Positioning interventions are designed to reduce pressure and shearing force to the skin. The immobilized client's position should be changed according to activity level, perceptual ability, and daily routines (Bergstrom and others, 1987a, 1987b). Therefore a standard turning interval of 1½ to 2 hours may

not prevent pressure sore development in some clients. The Wound Ostomy Continence Nurses (WOCN) Association and AHCPR recommend reducing shear by keeping the client's head of bed below the 30-degree angle, using assistive devices when turning or transferring clients, using the bed gatch or footboard, and using the 30-degree lateral position (Figure 38-13) (Bryant and others, 1992; Marchand and Lidowski, 1993).

When the client can sit in a chair, the time should be limited to 2 hours or less. Again, the exact time interval is individualized (see Skill 38-1). However, the nurse should not allow the client to sit for a period longer than the recommended time interval that was calculated during assessment. Thus if the timing interval is every 1½ hours, the client should remain in a sitting position less than every 1½ hours. In the sitting position, the pressure on the ischial tuberosities is greater than when in the supine position. In addition, a high-risk client sitting in a chair should be taught or assisted to shift weight every 15 minutes. Shifting weight provides short-term relief to the ischial tuberosities. A client should also sit on gel or an air cushion to redistribute weight so that it is not all on the ischium. Rigid and donut-shaped cushions are contraindicated because they reduce blood supply to the area, resulting in wider areas of ischemia (AHCPR, 1992).

After the client is repositioned, the nurse reassesses the skin and observes for normal reactive hyperemia and blanching. *The reddened areas should never be massaged.* This change in practice is a result of nursing research (AHCPR, 1992). Massaging the reddened areas increases breaks in the capillaries in the underly-

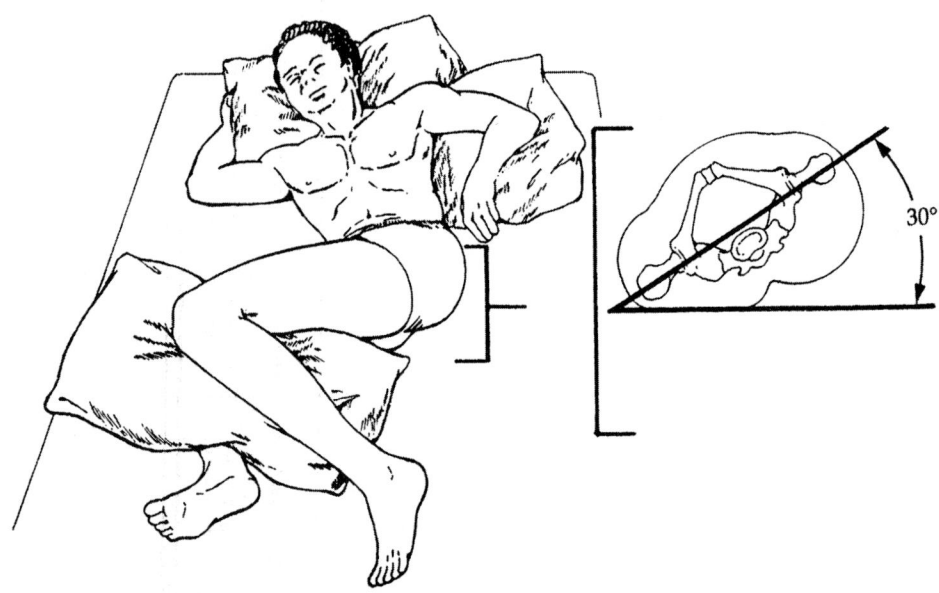

Figure 38-13. Thirty-degree lateral position to avoid pressure points. (From Bryant RA, and others: Pressure ulcer. In Bryant RA, editor: *Acute and chronic wounds: nursing management*, St. Louis, 1992, Mosby.)

ing tissues and increases the risk of pressure ulcer formation.

Therapeutic beds and mattresses. A variety of special beds and mattresses have been designed to reduce the hazards of immobility to the skin and musculoskeletal system. However, none eliminates the need for meticulous nursing care. No single device eliminates the effects of pressure on the skin.

When selecting specialty beds, the nurse must thoroughly assess clients' needs (Box 38-7). A flow diagram (Figure 38-14) assists the nurse in clinical decision making. In addition, Table 38-4 lists the specific device and pertinent nurse alerts for using the equipment safely. Clients and families need to be taught the reason for and proper use of the beds or mattresses (Box 38-8). When used correctly, these mattresses and specialty beds assist in reducing pressure ulcers in high-risk clients.

Acute care

Pressure ulcers. In addition to removing all pressure from the affected area and keeping pressure from the area, cleanliness of the ulcer area and all skin surfaces is essential (Skill 38-2). Maintaining cleanliness may be extremely difficult with incontinent, feverish, or confused clients.

Moisture in and around an area of skin breakdown can cause further ulceration and infection. Many products are available for the care of pressure ulcers (Table 38-5). Before instituting treatment measures, the nurse must thoroughly assess the client's pressure ulcer and determine the correct dressing based on the stage of ulcer development.

The nurse cleans the affected area to (1) remove bacterial and surface contaminants and (2) protect the healing area. All pressure ulcers are considered contaminated or colonized wounds (AHCPR, 1994). Therefore the nurse must select appropriate solutions. Caution is needed, because antiseptics can damage tissues unprotected by the dermis and may inactivate some drugs. The ulcer should be cleansed with normal saline rather than cytotoxic skin cleaning solutions that kill the fibroblasts needed to heal the pressure ulcer (AHCPR, 1994).

An ulcer that has necrotic tissue or eschar or shows signs of sloughing must be debrided by a physician. **Eschar** is a thick, leathery devitalized necrotic tissue. **Sloughing** is the shedding of loose, stringy necrotic tissue as the result of skin ulceration. **Debridement** is the removal of devitalized tissue so that healthy tissue can regenerate.

For reddened areas or areas of broken skin integrity, skin care products that lubricate and protect, stimulate circulation, and promote wound healing are recommended. When the ulcer is pink with granulation tissue throughout, a dressing is indicated to promote healing. A clean, moist environment promotes migration of epithelial cells across the ulcer surface.

Nutritional status. Maintaining adequate protein intake, serum albumin, and hemoglobin levels is important in treatment of pressure ulcers (see Chapter 34).

Increased protein intake, two to four times above the daily recommended requirement, helps rebuild epidermal tissue. Increased caloric and protein intakes help promote healing of pressure ulcers (Breslow and others, 1993). Increased intake of vitamin C promotes protein synthesis and tissue repair (AHCPR, 1994).

A low hemoglobin level decreases delivery of oxygen to the tissues and leads to further ischemia.

Box 38-7
AHCPR 1994 Support Surface Recommendations

Assess all clients with existing pressure ulcers to determine their risk for developing additional pressure ulcers. If the client remains at risk, use a pressure-reducing surface.

Use a static support surface if a client can assume a variety of positions without bearing weight on a pressure ulcer and without "bottoming out."

Use a dynamic support surface if the client cannot assume a variety of positions without bearing weight on a pressure ulcer, if the client fully compresses the static support surface, or if the pressure ulcer does not show evidence of healing.

If a client has large stage III or stage IV pressure ulcers on multiple turning surfaces, a low–air-loss bed or an air-fluidized bed may be indicated.

When excess moisture on intact skin is a potential source of maceration and skin breakdown, a support surface that provides air flow can be important in drying skin and preventing additional pressure ulcers.

BOX 38-8
Client Teaching for Therapeutic Beds and Mattresses

- Explain the reasons for the client's reduced mobility.
- Teach basic preventive care measures to reduce the hazards to the client's skin.
- Demonstrate how to optimize the client's safety by reducing risk of falls, using proper body mechanics, and using the equipment correctly.
- Teach client how to maintain optimal independence and mobility.
- Teach client that fluid intake must increase, and determine which type and amount of fluids are appropriate.

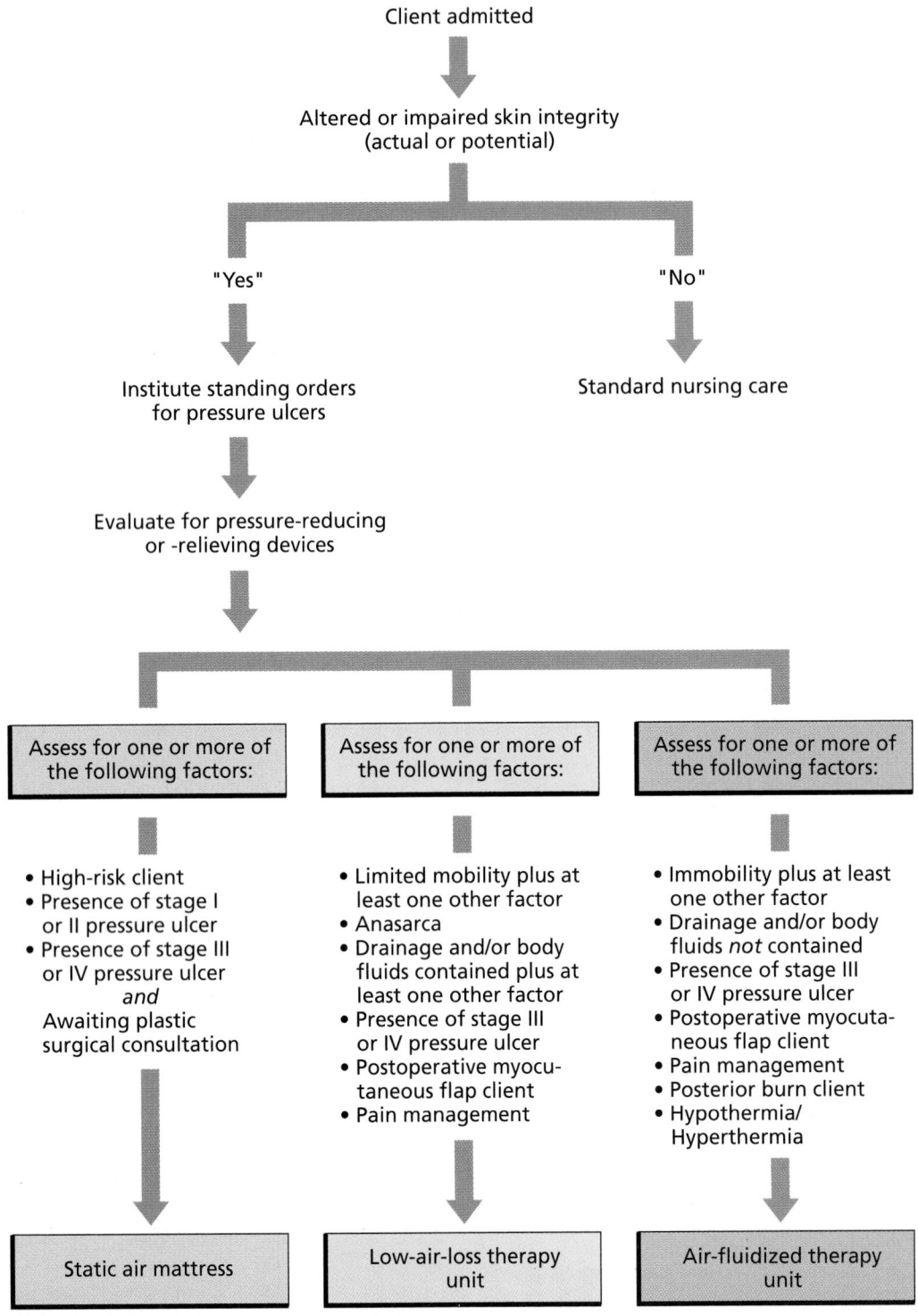

Figure 38-14. Flow diagram for ordering specialty beds. (From Thomas C: *Ostomy/Wound Manage* 23:51, 1989.)

Wounds

First aid for wounds. In an emergency setting the nurse uses first aid measures for wound care. Under more stable conditions the nurse is able to use a variety of interventions for wound healing. When a client suffers a traumatic wound, first aid interventions include promoting hemostasis, cleansing the wound, and protecting the wound from further injury.

Hemostasis. After assessing the type and extent of the wound, the nurse controls bleeding of a laceration by applying direct pressure on the wound with a sterile or clean dressing, such as a washcloth. After bleeding subsides, an adhesive bandage strip or gauze dressing taped over the laceration allows skin edges to close and a blood clot to form. If a dressing becomes saturated with blood, the nurse adds another layer of dressing,

TABLE 38-4

Surface Types by Purpose and Advantages

Type	Examples	Purpose	Advantages	Disadvantages	Notes
Foam overlay	Geomatt Biogard	Pressure reduction, comfort	Low cost, ease of use, many sizes	Hot, traps moisture, life is limited, loses pressure reduction with use	Usually one-client use; washing removes flame-retardant chemicals; ease of use at home
Foam replacement	MaxiFloat DeCube Comfortex	Pressure reduction, comfort	Reduced bed height, reduces nursing time, multiple client use	High initial cost, difficult to evaluate when effectiveness is lost	Some have removable sections (cubes); may be rented or purchased
Fluid overlay	Lotus	Pressure reduction, comfort	Easily cleaned, multiple client use, readily available	Heavy, leaks with puncture, cannot raise head of bed	May be rented or purchased; baffled systems control motion
Air overlay	Sofcare Roho KoalaKare	Pressure relief	Ease of setup, single- or multiple-use products available	Lack of comfort, damaged by sharp objects, requires monitoring for inflation	May be rented or purchased; adapts to multiple settings
Low air loss	KinAir Flexicair Mediscus	Pressure relief	Ease of use, seat deflates for transfer, company offers support staff	Portable blowers are noisy, surface may be slippery, noisy	Generally rented; home unit is available
Air fluidized	Clinitron Fluidair Skytron	Pressure relief	Reduced friction and shear, facilitates control of high drainage, company offers support staff	Coughing may be less effective, heavy, circulating air may dehydrate, transfers are difficult	Available for home, but may be too heavy
Kinetic	Rotokinetic treatment table	Movement, skeletal stability	Mobilize secretions, skeletal stability, supports traction, company offers support staff	Must be kept in rotation or no pressure reduction, shearing if client position is not correct	Must be in rotation 21 hours/day, now available as low-air-loss version
Bariatric	Burke	Management of morbidly obese, staff safety	Facilitates client independence, converts to a chair	Width is standard so surface may not accommodate turning	Requires addition of special mattress and overlay for pressure relief

continues to apply pressure, and elevates the affected part. Serious lacerations should be sutured by a physician in an emergency clinic or hospital.

A puncture wound is allowed to bleed to remove dirt and other contaminants. If a penetrating object such as a knife blade is in a client's body, removal could cause massive, uncontrolled bleeding. The nurse may apply pressure around the object but not on it or on adjacent tissues.

Cleansing. Gentle cleansing of a wound removes contaminants that serve as sources of infection. However, vigorous cleaning can cause bleeding or further injury. For abrasions, minor lacerations, and small puncture wounds the nurse first rinses the wound in running

Treating Pressure Ulcers

Delegation Considerations

Treatment of pressure ulcers requires problem solving and knowledge application unique to professional nursing. For this procedure delegation is not appropriate. Instruct unlicensed personnel to report changes in skin integrity to the nurse immediately. In some states and practice settings, *nonsterile* dressing application may be delegated to others for chronic, established wounds where the protocol has been evaluated and designated by a professional nurse.

Equipment
- Disposable gloves (clean)
- Goggles and cover gown
- Plastic bag for dressing disposal
- Measuring device (tape measure)
- Cotton-tipped applicators
- Camera and tracing film (optional)
- Topical cleansing agent (see Table 38-6)
- Sterile solution container
- Washbasin, washcloths, towels
- Dressing of choice (see Table 38-5)
- Skin protectant
- Hypoallergenic tape (if needed)
- 35-ml syringe with 19-gauge needle
- Documentation records (e.g., graph paper)

STEPS	RATIONALE
1. Assess the client's level of comfort and need for pain medication.	Dressing change procedure is better tolerated if pain is controlled.
2. Determine if client has allergies to topical agents.	Topical agents may cause localized skin reactions.
3. Review physician's order for topical agent or dressing (in many cases physician follows nurse's recommendation for pressure ulcer care).	Ensures that proper medication and treatment are administered.
4. Wash hands and apply clean gloves. Close room door or bedside curtains.	Reduces transmission of microorganisms and prevents accidental exposure to body fluids.
5. Position client to allow dressing removal.	Area should be accessible for dressing change.
6. Assess pressure ulcer and surrounding skin to determine ulcer stage (see Figure 38-5).	Assessment of a pressure ulcer should be comprehensive (Ayello, 1996).
a. Note color, moisture, and appearance of skin around ulcer and of ulcer itself.	
b. Measure two maximum perpendicular diameters.	Skin condition may indicate progressive tissue damage. Provides an objective measure of wound size. May influence size and type of dressing selected. Surface area = length × width
c. Measure depth of pressure ulcer using sterile cotton-tipped applicator or other device that will allow measurement of wound depth.	Depth measure is important for determining wound volume. While surface area adequately represents tissue loss in stage I and II ulcers, volume more adequately represents tissue loss in deeper stage III and IV wounds. Volume = 2(L × D) + 2(W × D) + (L + D)
d. Measure depth (D) of undermining skin by lateral tissue necrosis. Use a cotton-tipped applicator and gently probe under skin edges.	Undermining represents the loss of the underlying tissue (subcutaneous and muscle) to a greater extent than the skin (see illustration). Undermining may indicate progressive tissue necrosis.
7. Wash skin around ulcer gently with warm water and rinse area thoroughly with water.	Reduces number of resident bacteria. Soap can be irritating to skin.
8. Gently dry skin thoroughly by patting lightly with towel.	Retained moisture causes maceration of skin layers.
9. Change to sterile gloves (check agency policy).	Aseptic technique must be maintained during cleansing, measuring, and application of dressings. Refer to institutional policy regarding use of clean or sterile gloves.

STEPS	RATIONALE
10. Cleanse ulcer thoroughly with normal saline or cleansing agent: a. Use irrigating syringe for deep ulcers. b. Cleansing in the shower may be done with a hand-held shower head.	Removes wound debris. Previously applied enzymes may require soaking for removal.
11. Apply topical agents, as prescribed: a. Enzymes: (1) Apply thin, even layer of ointment over necrotic areas of ulcer only. Do not apply enzyme to surrounding skin. (2) Apply gauze dressing directly over ulcer. (3) Tape securely in place. b. Hydrocolloid beads or paste: (1) Fill ulcer defect to approximately half of the total depth with hydrocolloid beads or paste. (2) Cover with hydrocolloid dressing; extend dressing 1 to 1½ inches beyond edges of wound. c. Hydrogel agents: (1) Cover surface of ulcer with Hydrogel using applicator or gloved hand.	Topical agents should be changed as wound heals or worsens. Thick layer of ointment is not necessary. Thin layer absorbs and acts more effectively. Excess medication can irritate surrounding skin. Enzyme can cause burning, paresthesia, and dermatitis to surrounding skin. Protects wound. Prevents bacteria from entering wound. Hydrocolloid beads or paste assists in absorbing wound drainage. Highly draining wounds are best treated with hydrocolloid beads or granules. Maintains wound humidity. May be left in place 7 days. Not effective on dry eschar (Bryant and others, 1992). Provides maintenance of wound humidity while absorbing excess drainage. May be used as carrier for topical agents.

Continued

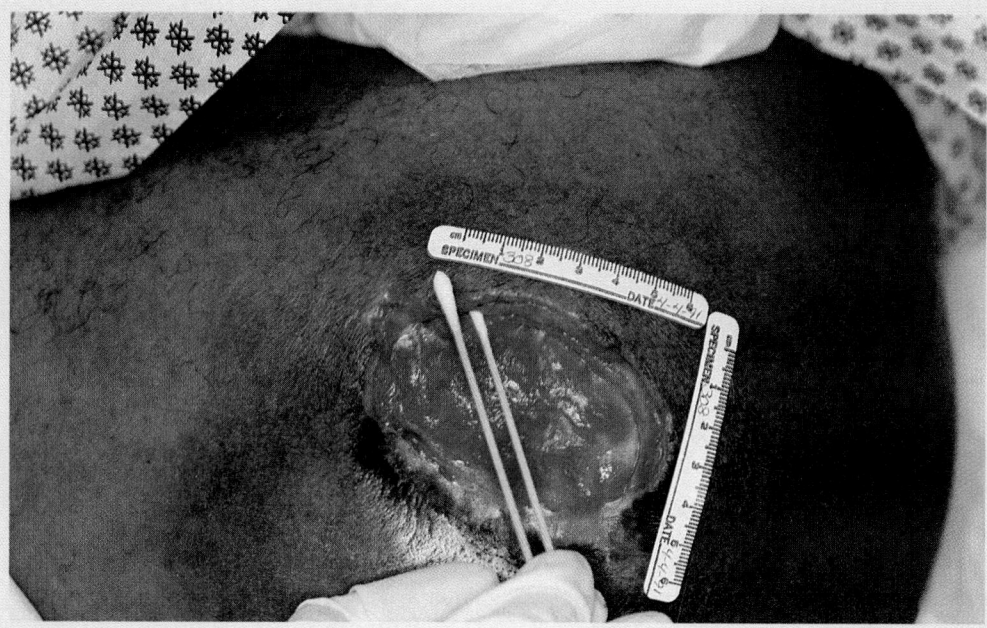

Step 6d

STEPS	RATIONALE
(2) Apply dry fluffy gauze or hydrocolloid or transparent dressing over gel to completely cover ulcer.	Holds Hydrogel against wound surface; is absorbent.
d. Calcium alginates:	
(1) Pack wound with alginate using applicator or gloved hand.	Provides maintenance of wound humidity while absorbing excess drainage.
(2) Apply dry gauze, foam, or hydrocolloid over alginate.	Holds alginate against wound surface.
12. Reposition client comfortably off pressure ulcer.	Avoids accidental removal of dressings.
13. Remove gloves and dispose of soiled supplies. Wash hands.	Reduces transmission of microorganisms.

CRITICAL DECISION POINT

A clean pressure ulcer should show evidence of some healing within 2 to 4 weeks.

14. Observe skin surrounding ulcer for inflammation, edema, and tenderness.	Contact dermatitis may result from exposure to certain topical agents. Without proper preventive care, ulcer can spread to involve neighboring tissue.
15. Inspect dressings and exposed ulcer, observing for drainage, foul odor, and tissue necrosis. Monitor client for signs and symptoms of infection, including fever and elevated white blood cell count.	Ulcers can become infected.
16. Compare subsequent ulcer measurements.	Allows comparison of serial measurements to assess wound healing. It is helpful to plot surface area and volume measurements on graph paper.
17. Do *not* use the pressure ulcer staging system to measure pressure ulcer healing (NPUAP, 1995).	

Recording and Reporting

- Record appearance of ulcer in client's record.
- Describe type of topical agent used, dressing applied, and client's response.
- Report any deterioration in ulcer appearance to nurse in charge or physician.

Home Care Considerations

- Cost can be a factor. Some clients have more time than financial resources. They may choose a less expensive treatment option such as dressing material, especially if there is no third-party reimbursement.
- "Disposal of contaminated dressings in the home should be done in a manner consistent with local regulations."
- Discuss need for home pressure-relief surface or bed.

water, cleans it with mild soap and water, and may apply an over-the-counter antiseptic. When a laceration is bleeding profusely, the nurse should only brush away surface contaminants and concentrate on hemostasis until the client can be cared for in a clinic or hospital.

Protection. Regardless of whether bleeding has stopped, the nurse protects the wound by applying sterile or clean dressings and immobilizing the body part. A light dressing applied over minor wounds prevents entrance of microorganisms. In the case of small abrasions, it is acceptable to leave the wound open to air so that a scab can form.

The more extensive the wound, the larger the bandage required. In the home a clean towel or diaper may be the best dressing. A bulky dressing applied with pressure minimizes movement of underlying tissues and

TABLE 38-5

Treatment Options by Ulcer Stage

Ulcer Stage	Ulcer Status	Dressing*	Comments	Expected Change	Adjuvant
I	Intact	None Film, adherent Hydrocolloid	Allows visual assessment. Protects from shear. May not allow visual assessment.	Resolves slowly without epidermal loss over 7 to 14 days.	Turning schedule. Support hydration. Nutritional support. Silicone-based lotion to decrease shear. Pressure-relief mattress or chair cushion.
II	Clean	Composite Hydrocolloid Hydrogel sheet	Viasorb, film plus Telfa. Exudry. Limits shear. Change every 7 days if occlusive seal. Absorbent, requires secondary dressing of gauze or adherent film.	Heals through re-epithelialization and epithelial budding.	See previous stage. Manage incontinence.

III	Clean	Hydrocolloid
		Hydrogel
		
		Exudate absorbers
		  Calcium alginate
		  Wound pastes
		
		Gauze, fluffy
		Growth factors
		Adherent film
			See stage II.
			Apply ¼-inch thick, cover with gauze or hydrocolloid.
			Change when strike through is noted on secondary dressing. Cover with gauze or hydrocolloid.
			Use with normal saline.
			Use with gauze.
			Will facilitate softening of eschar.
				Heals through granulation and reepithelialization. (NOTE: Does not become a stage II ulcer as it heals.)	See previous stages.
					Electrical stimulation.
					Evaluate pressure-relief needs.
					
					See previous stages.
					Surgical consult for debridement.

	Eschar	Hydrocolloid Gauze plus ordered solution None	Will facilitate softening of eschar. Absorb drainage. Rarely, if eschar is dry and intact, no dressing is used, allowing eschar to act as physiological cover.	Eschar will lift at the edges as healing progresses. Cross-hatching central area of eschar with a small blade will facilitate release from center.	Surgical consult for closure.
IV	Clean	Hydrogel Hydrocolloid plus hydrocolloid paste/beads Calcium alginate Gauze Growth factors	See stage III Clean. See stage III Clean; critical to treat areas of undermining.	Heals through granulation and re-epithelialization. Because of contraction, surface may close more rapidly than base, leaving wound cavity.	See stages I, II, and III Clean.
	Eschar	See stage III Eschar	See stage III Clean. Pack deeply undermined ulcers. Use with gauze.	See stage III Eschar.	See stage III Eschar.

NOTE: As with *all* occlusive dressings, wound should *not* be clinically infected.

helps to immobilize the entire body part. A bandage or cloth wrapped around a penetrating object should immobilize it adequately.

Dressings. The use of dressings requires an understanding of wound healing, as well as factors influencing healing. A variety of dressing materials are commercially available. Unless a dressing is suited to the characteristics of a wound, the dressing can hinder wound repair.

The choice of dressings and the method of dressing a wound influence healing. The proper dressing should not allow a draining wound to become overly dry with extensive scab formation. When this occurs, the dermis dehydrates and crusts. As a result, a barrier forms against normal epidermal cell growth, leaving a depression or defect in the new epidermal surface. Furthermore, dryness may increase discomfort. Ideally a dressing leaves a wound slightly moist to promote normal epidermal cell migration. The dressing should also absorb drainage to prevent pooling of exudate that may promote bacterial growth and to prevent wound drainage from coming into contact with intact skin.

For surgical wounds that heal by primary intention, dressings are commonly removed as soon as drainage stops. The primary dressing placed in the operating room is frequently removed by the physician 2 to 3 days postoperatively. This coincides with initial epithelialization, so when the primary dressing is removed the risk of infection is less. In contrast, when the nurse dresses an open wound healing by secondary intention, the dressing material becomes a means for mechanically removing exudate and debriding necrotic tissue.

Purposes. A dressing may serve several purposes. It discourages exposure to microorganisms. However, if a wound has minimal drainage, the natural formation of a fibrin seal eliminates the need for a dressing. A pressure dressing promotes hemostasis by exerting localized, downward pressure over an actual or potential bleeding site and fosters normal healing by eliminating dead space in underlying tissues. The nurse must assess skin color, pulses in distal extremities, client comfort, and any changes in sensation to ensure that pressure dressings do not interfere with circulation.

A dressing also promotes healing by absorbing drainage, preventing drying of the wound surface, and debriding the wound. Contact dressings may stick to underlying tissue; removal of such dressings disturbs healing surfaces but also cleans debris, exudate, and necrotic tissue from wounds that require debridement.

A firmly taped or wrapped dressing supports or immobilizes a body part, minimizing movement of the underlying incision and traumatized tissues. A dressing also serves to protect the client from seeing the wound, which may be unpleasant and cause anxiety. Finally, a dressing promotes thermal insulation to the wound surface and protects it from the dehydrating effects of air.

Types. Dressings vary by type of material and mode of application (dry, wet to dry, and moist). They should be easy to apply, comfortable, and made of materials that promote wound healing.

Gauze dressings are the most common type. They do not interact with wound tissues and thus cause little wound irritation. Gauze is available in different textures and in squares, rectangles, and rolls of various lengths and widths. Gauze dressings are best used for exudative wounds, wounds with dead space or sinus tracts, and wounds with a combination of exudate and necrotic tissue (Bryant and others, 1992). The nurse applies dry gauze such as a 4×4 pad or Telfa to wounds with moderate drainage.

For wounds requiring debridement, a wet-to-dry dressing may be effective. The nurse moistens the contact dressing and applies it as a single layer against the wound surface. Moistening the contact layer increases the ability of the gauze to collect exudate and wound debris. Another dry layer of a fluffy, absorbent gauze is then applied. This type of dressing should be removed abruptly from the wound surface during the dressing change procedure and may be quite painful. Increasing awareness and acceptance of moist wound healing encourages the use of a moist dressing that must remain damp along the wound surface. It is critical that the first layer remain damp, because wounds heal more quickly and autolytic debridement is enhanced in a moist environment. Autolysis involves the breakdown of necrotic tissue provided by the body's own white blood cells. If a moist dressing begins to dry, it must be changed.

Another type of dressing is a self-adhesive, transparent film, a synthetic permeable membrane that acts as a temporary second skin. It has several advantages. It adheres to undamaged skin to contain exudate and minimize wound contamination. It also serves as a barrier to external fluids and bacteria yet still allows the wound to breathe. It promotes a moist environment that speeds epithelial cell growth. It also permits visualization of the wound.

Hydrocolloid and hydrogel dressings are occlusive (hydrocolloid) and semiocclusive (hydrogel) dressings that contain hydroactive particles. Both are moldable, easy to apply, and may increase comfort (Regan, 1992). Hydrocolloid and hydrogel dressings are autolytic because they maintain wound humidity, slowly liquefy necrotic debris, and provide protective cushioning. The occlusive hydrocolloid dressings are not recommended for infected wounds, but they may protect clean wounds from secondary infection (Bryant and others, 1992). This type of dressing is most useful on shallow to moderately deep dermal ulcers. An advantage of many of the specialty dressings is that they need to be changed less frequently than traditional gauze dressings, often as infrequently as once or twice weekly. This minimizes disruption of the healing wound tissues, maintains a moist wound healing environment, and allows valuable nursing time to be spent on other care issues.

Changing dressings. To prepare for changing a dressing, the nurse must know the type of dressing, any underlying drains or tubing used, and the type of supplies needed for wound care. The nurse can adjust the type and amount of dressings if the character or amount of drainage changes or if a wound becomes deeper. Notifying the physician of any change is essential.

The physician's order for changing a dressing should indicate the dressing type, frequency of changing, and solutions or ointments to be applied. An order to "reinforce dressing p.r.n." (add dressings without removing existing ones) is common immediately after surgery, when the physician does not want accidental disruption of the suture line or loss of hemostasis. A client's medical or operating room record usually reveals whether drains are present. After the initial dressing change, the nurse communicates on the care plan the type of dressing materials and solutions to use, as well as the type and location of drains.

The nurse uses aseptic technique during dressing change procedures (see Chapter 25). Also essential is ensuring that the client understands the steps of the procedure beforehand so less anxiety is experienced, describing normal signs of the healing process, and offering to answer questions about the procedure or wound.

If wound care is needed in the home, the nurse must demonstrate dressing changes to the client and family and then provide an opportunity for practice. In the home, wound healing stabilizes so that sterile technique is usually unnecessary. However, clients must learn clean technique. The client should be able to change a dressing independently or with assistance from a family member before discharge unless home health care is to be provided. Skill 38-3 outlines the steps for changing dry and wet-to-dry dressings.

Securing dressings. The nurse uses tape, ties, or bandages and cloth binders to secure a dressing over a wound site. The choice of anchoring depends on the wound size, location, drainage, frequency of dressing changes, and the client's level of activity. The nurse most often uses strips of tape to secure dressings if the client is not allergic to them. Nonallergenic paper, plastic, and woven fabric tapes minimize skin reactions. More skin tears occur with silk tape as compared to soft cloth tape. Adhesive tape, the most likely anchor to cause skin irritation, adheres well to the skin's surface, whereas elastic adhesive tape compresses closely around pressure bandages and permits more movement of a body part (O'Brien and Reilly, 1995).

Tape is available in various widths; the nurse chooses a size that sufficiently secures the dressing. The tape should cross the dressing and adhere to several inches of skin on each side. When securing the dressing, the nurse presses the tape gently, exerting pressure away from the wound. Tape is never applied over irritated skin. An adhesive skin barrier wafer such as a hydrocol-loid dressing may be applied to the skin around the wound so that the tape is secured to the skin barrier wafer rather than to sensitive skin. To remove tape safely, the nurse loosens the tape ends and gently pulls the outer end toward the wound, parallel to the skin, applying light traction to the skin away from the wound.

To avoid repeated removal of tape from sensitive skin, the nurse can secure dressings with reusable Montgomery ties (Figure 38-15). Each tie consists of a long strip; half contains an adhesive backing to apply to the skin, and the other half folds back and contains a cloth tie to be tied across a dressing and untied at dressing changes. A large, bulky dressing may require two or more sets of Montgomery ties. To provide even support to a wound and immobilize a body part, the nurse may apply elastic gauze or cloth bandages and binders over a dressing.

Comfort measures. Any wound can be painful, depending on the extent of tissue injury. The nurse uses several techniques to minimize discomfort. Careful removal of tape, gentle cleansing of wound edges, and careful manipulation of dressings and drains minimize stress on sensitive tissues. Turning and positioning also reduce strain. Administration of analgesic medications

Text continued on p. 1104

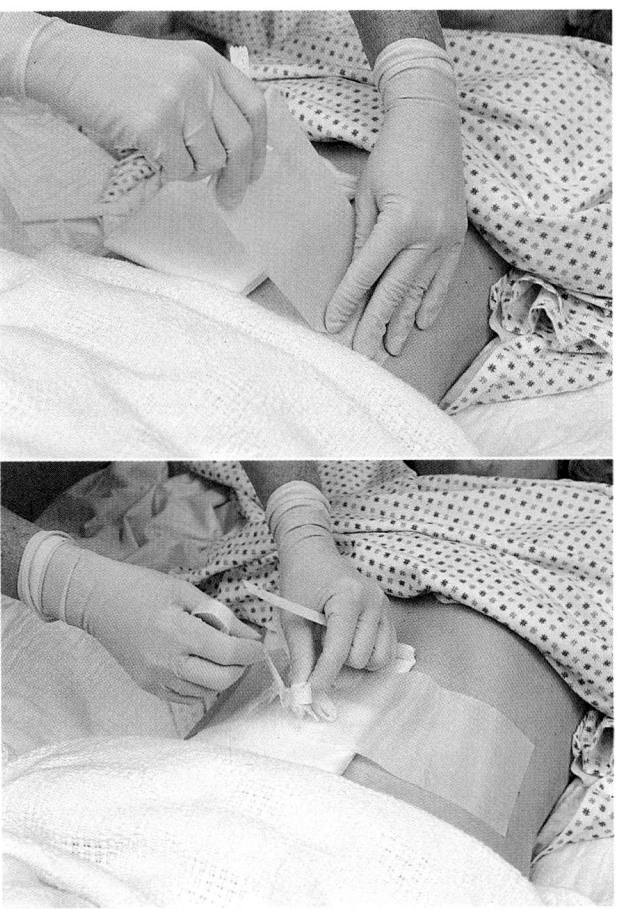

Figure 38-15. Montgomery ties.

········ **Skill 38-3**

Applying Dry and Wet-to-Dry Moist Dressings

Delegation Considerations

Controversy about delegating wound care to other personnel exists. All nurses should check their specific state practice act as to what interventions are considered within the scope of nursing practice and which can be delegated to others, including unlicensed assistive personnel. In some states, aspects of wound care such as dressing change can be delegated. This may include the changing of dressings using *clean* technique for chronic wounds. The care of acute new wounds and those that require sterile technique for dressing change generally remain within the domain of professional nursing practice. The *assessment* of the wound remains within the scope of the professional nurse even if the dressing change is delegated to others.

Equipment

- Sterile gloves
- Dressing set (sterile), scissors, forceps
- Sterile drape (optional)
- Variety of gauze dressings and pads
- Fine mesh gauze (wet-to-dry only)
- Sterile basin
- Antiseptic ointment (optional)
- Cleansing solution
- Sterile solution (wet-to-dry only)
- Clean, disposable gloves
- Tape, ties, or bandage as needed
- Waterproof bag
- Extra gauze dressings, Surgipads, or ABD pads
- Bath blanket
- Adhesive remover (optional)
- Disposable mask (optional)
- Moisture-proof gown (optional)
- Goggles (optional)

STEPS	RATIONALE
1. Assess size and location of wound to be dressed.	Assists nurse to plan for proper type and amount of supplies needed. Alerts nurse when assistance is needed to hold dressings in place.
2. Assess client's level of comfort.	Removal of dry dressing can be painful; client may require pain medication (Rook, 1996).
3. Review medical orders for dressing change procedure.	Indicates type of dressing or applications to use.
4. Explain procedure to client and instruct client not to touch wound area or sterile supplies.	Decreases anxiety. Sudden, unexpected movement on client's part could result in contamination of wound and supplies.
5. Close room or cubicle curtains and windows.	Provides privacy and reduces airborne microorganisms.
6. Position client comfortably and drape with bath blanket to expose only wound site.	Provides access to the wound, yet minimizes unnecessary exposure.
7. Place disposable bag within reach of work area. Fold top of bag to make cuff.	Ensures easy disposal of soiled dressings. Prevents soiling of bag's outer surface.
8. Apply face mask and protective eyewear, if required, and wash hands thoroughly.	Reduces transmission of pathogens to exposed tissues. Protects nurse from splashes.
9. Put on clean, disposable gloves and remove tape, bandage, or ties.	Prevents transmission of infectious organisms from soiled dressings to nurse's hands.
10. Remove tape: pull parallel to skin; pull toward dressing; remove remaining adhesive from skin.	Pulling tape toward dressing reduces stress on suture line or wound edges.
11. With gloved hand carefully remove gauze dressings one layer at a time, taking care not to dislodge drains or tubes. Keep soiled undersurface away from client's sight.	Appearance of drainage may be upsetting to client. Removal of one layer at a time reduces the chance of accidental removal of underlying drains.
a. If dressing sticks on a wet-to-dry dressing, do not moisten it; instead gently free dressing and alert client of potential discomfort.	Wet-to-dry dressing should debride wound.

STEPS	RATIONALE
12. Observe character and amount of drainage on dressing and appearance of wound.	Provides estimate of drainage amount and assessment of wound's condition.
13. Dispose of soiled dressings in disposable bag.	Reduces transmission of microorganisms.
14. Remove gloves by pulling them inside out. Dispose in bag.	Prevents contact of nurse's hands with material on gloves.
15. Open sterile dressing tray or individually wrapped sterile supplies. Place on bedside table (see illustration).	Sterile dressings remain sterile while on or within sterile surface. Preparation of supplies prevents break in technique during dressing change.
16. Apply dressing:	
A. Dry dressing:	
(1) Open bottle of solution (if ordered) and pour into sterile basin.	Keeps supplies sterile.
(2) Apply sterile gloves.	Allows handling of sterile supplies without contamination.
(3) Inspect wound for appearance, drains, drainage, and integrity. Avoid contact with contaminated material.	Indicates status of wound healing.
(4) Cleanse wound with solution:	
(a) Use separate swab for each cleansing stroke.	Prevents contamination of previously cleaned area.
(b) Clean from least contaminated area to most contaminated.	Prevents introduction of organisms into wound.
(5) Use dry gauze to swab in same manner as Step 16A(4) to dry wound.	Reduces excess moisture, which could eventually harbor microorganisms.
(6) Apply antiseptic ointment if ordered, using same technique as for cleansing.	Helps to reduce growth of microorganisms. Ointment may be applied to dressing if direct application causes discomfort.
(7) Apply dry sterile dressings to incision or wound:	
(a) Apply loose, woven gauze as contact layer.	Promotes proper absorption of drainage.

Continued

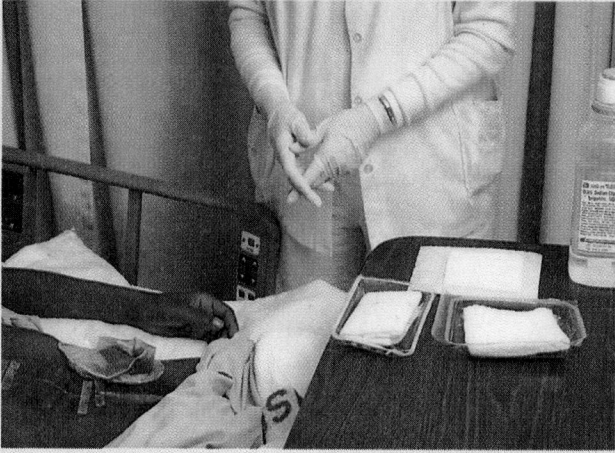

Step 15

Applying Dry and Wet-to-Dry Moist Dressings

STEPS	RATIONALE
(b) Cut 4 × 4 gauze flat to fit around drain, if present. Precut gauze is also available.	Secures drain and promotes drainage absorption at site.
(c) Apply second layer of gauze.	Protects wound from microorganisms.
(d) Apply thicker woven pad.	Protects wound from external environment.
B. Wet-to-dry dressing:	
(1) Pour prescribed solution into sterile basin and add fine-mesh gauze.	Contact layer must be totally moistened to increase dressing's absorptive abilities.
(2) Apply sterile gloves.	Allows handling of sterile supplies without contamination.
(3) Inspect wound for color, character of drainage, type of sutures, and drains (see illustration).	Provides assessment of wound healing.
(4) Cleanse wound with prescribed antiseptic solution or normal saline. Clean from least to most contaminated area.	Assists in debridement and cleanses wound of debris.
(5) Apply moist fine-mesh gauze as a single layer directly onto wound surface. If wound is deep, gently pack gauze into wound with forceps until all wound surfaces are in contact with moist gauze (see illustrations).	Absorbs drainage and adheres to debris. Wound should be loosely packed to facilitate wicking of drainage into absorbent outer layer of dressing.
(6) Apply dry, sterile 4 × 4 gauze over wet gauze.	Pulls moisture from wound.
(7) Cover with ABD pad, Surgipad, or gauze.	Protects wound from the entrance of microorganisms.
17. Apply tape over dressing, Kling roll (for circumferential dressings), or Montgomery ties. For application of Montgomery ties (see Figure 38-15):	Secures dressing in place.
a. Expose adhesive surface of tape on end of each tie.	Montgomery tie allows for frequent dressing changes without removal of adhesive tape.

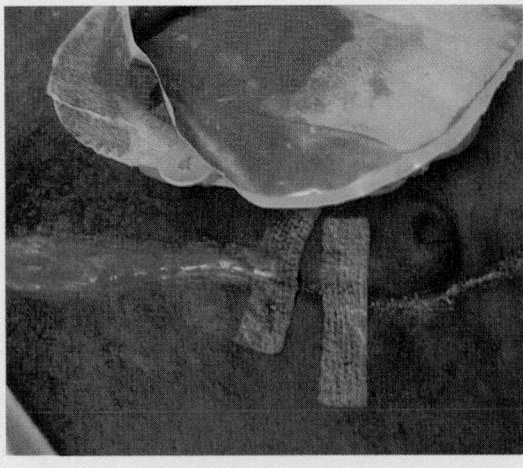

Step 16B (3)

STEPS	RATIONALE
b. Place ties on opposite sides of dressing.	
c. Place adhesive directly on skin or use skin barrier.	
d. Secure dressing by lacing ties across it.	Ensures dressing remains intact and covers wound.
18. Remove gloves and dispose in bag. Remove mask and eyewear.	Reduces transmission of infection.
19. Assist client to comfortable position.	Promotes client's sense of well-being. Enhances comfort.
20. Dispose of supplies and wash hands.	Reduces transmission of infection.

Recording and Reporting

- Report brisk, bright red bleeding or evidence of wound dehiscence or evisceration to physician immediately.
- Report wound appearance and characteristics of drainage at shift change.
- Record wound appearance, color, presence and characteristics of exudate, type and amount of dressings used, and tolerance of client to procedure.
- Write date and time dressing applied on tape in ink (not marker).

Home Care Considerations

- More expensive specialty dressings may be used, because they decrease the frequency of dressing changes.
- Clean dressings may also be used in the home setting.
- Disposal of contaminated dressings in the home should be done in a manner consistent with local regulations.

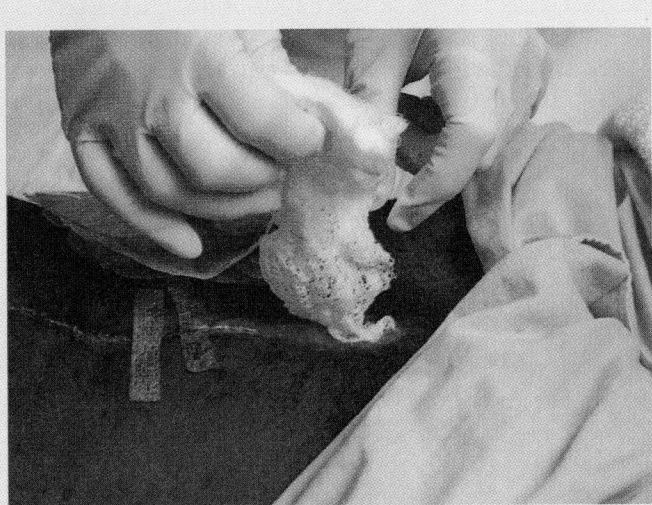

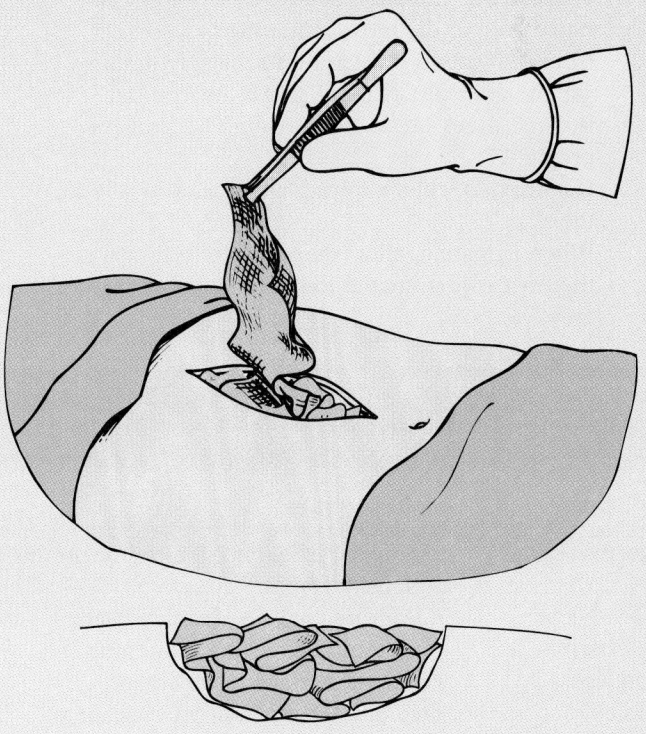

Step 16B (5)

30 to 60 minutes before dressing changes (depending on a drug's time of peak action) also reduces discomfort (Rook, 1996) (see Chapter 33).

Cleansing wounds and drain sites. Although a moderate amount of wound exudate promotes epithelial cell growth, the physician may order cleansing of a wound or drain site if a dressing does not properly absorb drainage or if an open drain deposits drainage onto the skin. Wound cleansing requires good hand washing and aseptic techniques (see Chapter 25). The nurse may apply antiseptics locally to intact skin to remove pathogens or use irrigation to remove debris. The most effective antiseptic solutions for skin cleansing are tincture of chlorhexidine (Hibiclens) and the iodophors such as Betadine, which act against bacteria as they remain on the skin.

Hydrogen peroxide should not be used in the presence of granulation tissue or as an irrigating solution for deep wounds. The use of hydrogen peroxide in deep wounds or blind cavities may result in air embolus (Lineaweaver and others, 1985). Normal saline is not irritating to wounded tissues and is one of the best solutions to use for wound cleansing and irrigation (Table 38-6).

The basic principles of wound cleaning are to remove bacteria and surface contaminants and to protect the healing wound (Bryant and others, 1992). When cleansing surgical or traumatic wounds, the nurse applies antiseptic solutions with sterile gauze or by irrigation. The following principles are important when cleaning an incision or the area around a drain:

1. Cleanse in a direction from the least contaminated area to the most contaminated, such as from the wound or incision to the surrounding skin or drain site (Figure 38-16) or from an isolated drain site to the surrounding skin (Figure 38-17).
2. Use friction when applying antiseptics locally to the skin.
3. When irrigating, allow the solution to flow from the least contaminated to the most contaminated area.

Wound irrigations. Irrigations are a special means of cleansing wounds of exudate and debris. The nurse uses an irrigating syringe to flush the area with a constant flow of solution. Irrigations are useful for cleaning open deep wounds or sensitive or inaccessible body parts. Through irrigations, cleansing or locally acting medications can be applied to an affected area. The nurse administers the prescribed solution (usually normal saline) at body temperature to enhance comfort and provide local cleansing application.

When irrigating clean proliferative wounds, the nurse uses sterile technique and an irrigation system with a safe pressure (4 to 15 psi) to prevent trauma to the newly formed granulation tissue (AHCPR, 1994). An example of a safe wound cleansing and irrigation system is a 35-ml syringe and a 19-gauge needle, which has a psi of 8. This method provides an ideal solution pressure for cleansing wounds while minimizing tissue trauma (Figure 38-18). The syringe tip should be over but not sticking into the wound, and fluid should not flow over a contaminated area before entering the wound (Figure 38-19). Skill 38-4 lists steps for wound irrigation.

Suture care. A surgeon closes a wound by bringing the edges as close together as possible to reduce the formation of scar tissue while minimizing trauma and tension and controlling bleeding. Sutures are threads or wires made of silk, steel, cotton, nylon, and polyester (Dacron) and are used to sew body tissues together. Dacron sutures minimize scar formation. Steel staples, a type of outer skin closure, are frequently used because they result in less trauma to tissues while providing extra strength (Figure 38-20). It is also common to see wounds closed with Steri-strips, a sterile butterfly tape applied along both sides of a wound to keep the edges closed (Figure 38-21).

Sutures are placed within tissue layers in deep wounds and superficially to complete wound closure. Deeper sutures are usually made of an absorbable material that disappears in several days. Sutures are foreign bodies and thus capable of causing local inflammation.

Policies vary at institutions as to who may remove sutures. If the nurse removes sutures, a physician's order

TABLE 38-6
Cleansing Agents

Solution	Indications	Implications
Normal saline	Useful for irrigation of clean or noninfected wound.	May be used under gentle pressure (35-ml syringe with 19-gauge needle) to assist in wound debridment.
Cara-Klenz PharmaClens	Cleansers used for cleaning dead, necrotic tissue and secretions.	Assists in removal of necrotic tissue and does not delay wound healing.
Safclens	Nonionic surfactant detergent.	Topical agent useful for cleansing wounds.
Biolex	Detergent, surfactant for cleansing wounds.	Topical agent for cleansing wounds.

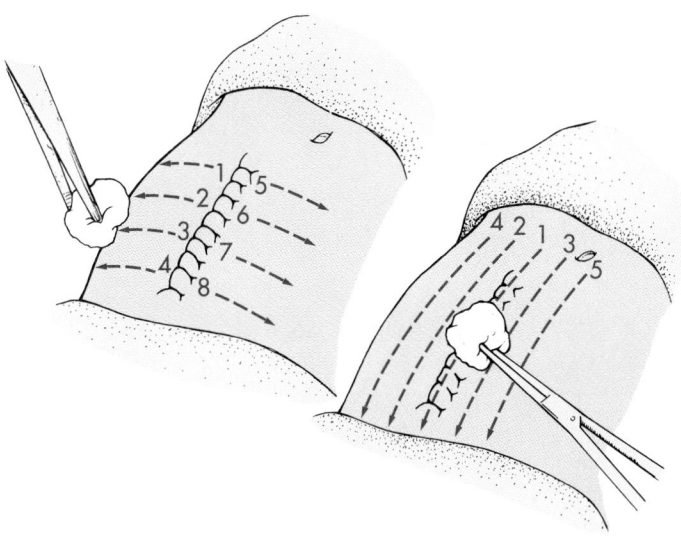

Figure 38-16. Methods for cleansing wound site.

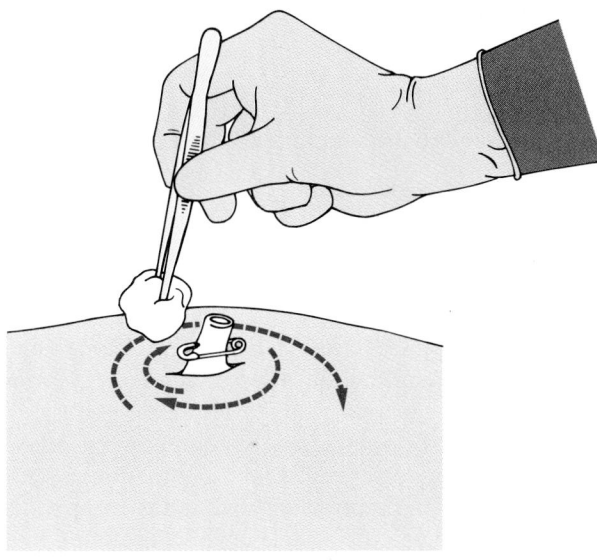

Figure 38-17. Cleansing of drain site.

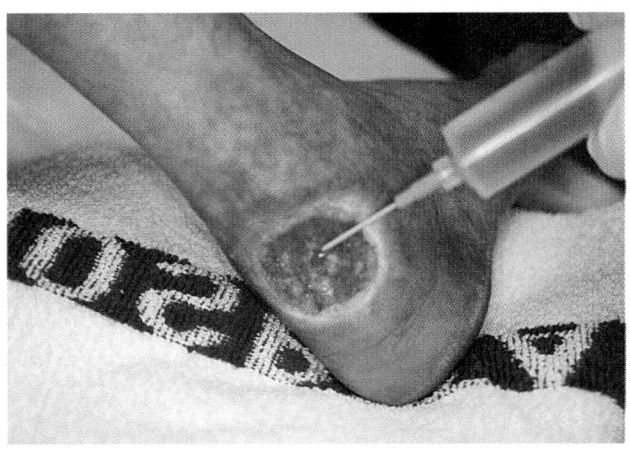

Figure 38-18. Wound irrigation by 35-ml syringe and 19-gauge catheter to facilitate removal of necrotic slough.

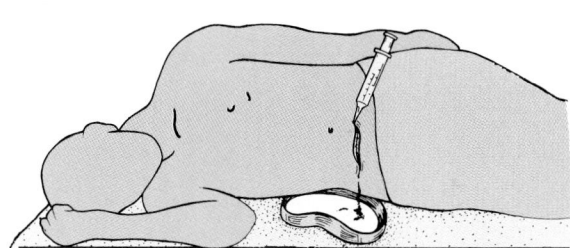

Figure 38-19. Position of client for abnormal wound irrigation.

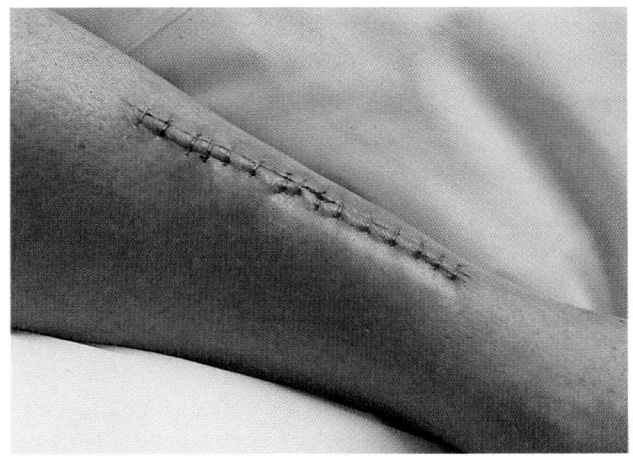

Figure 38-20. Wound sutured with staples.

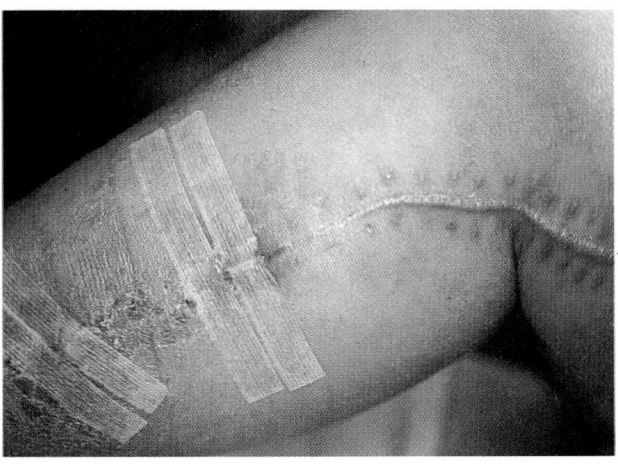

Figure 38-21. Steri-strips placed over incision for closure.

Skill 38-4
Performing Wound Irrigations

Delegation Considerations

Check institutional policy and the state's nurse practice act regarding which wound care interventions can be delegated to unlicensed assistive personnel. The skill of wound irrigation requires problem solving and knowledge application unique to a professional nurse, particularly regarding the assessment of any wounds and care of acute new wounds. However, cleansing of chronic wounds using *clean* technique can be delegated to assistive personnel. In this situation, instruct staff on what to report when a wound is cleansed. Assistive personnel must also know how to use clean technique to avoid cross-contamination from irrigation syringes and equipment.

Equipment

- Irrigant/cleansing solution (volume 1.2 to 2 times the estimated wound volume)
- Irrigation delivery system depending on amount of pressure desired:
  Sterile irrigation 35-ml syringe with sterile soft angiocath or 19-gauge needle (AHCPR, 1994) *or* Hand-held shower or whirlpool
- Clean gloves
- Sterile gloves
- Waterproof underpad, if needed
- Dressing supplies
- Disposable waterproof bag
- Gown, if risk of spray
- Goggles, if risk of spray

STEPS	RATIONALE
1. Assess client's level of pain. Administer prescribed analgesic 30 to 45 minutes before starting wound irrigation procedure.	Discomfort may be related directly to wound or indirectly to muscle tension or immobility. Increased comfort level permits client to move more easily and be positioned to facilitate wound irrigation.
2. Review medical record for physician's prescription for irrigation of open wound and type of solution to be used.	Open wound irrigation requires medical order including type of solutions to use.
3. Assess recent recording of signs and symptoms related to client's open wound: a. Condition of skin and wound b. Elevation of body temperature c. Drainage from wound (amount, color) d. Odor e. Consistency of drainage f. Size of wounds, including depth, length, and width	Data are used as baseline to indicate change in condition of wound. May indicate response to infection. Amount will decrease as healing takes place. Strong odor indicates infectious process. Leukocytes produce thick drainage. Determines stage of healing.
4. Explain procedure of wound irrigation and cleansing.	Information will reduce client's anxiety.
5. Position client comfortably to permit gravitational flow of irrigating solution through wound and into collection receptacle (see Figure 38-19). Position client so that wound is vertical to collection basin.	Directing solution from top to bottom of wound and from clean to contaminated area prevents further infection. Positioning client during planning stage provides bed surfaces for later preparation of equipment.
6. Warm irrigation solution to approximate body temperature.	Warmed solution increases comfort and reduces vascular constriction response in tissues.
7. Wash hands.	Reduces transmission of microorganisms.
8. Form cuff on waterproof bag and place it near bed.	Cuffing helps to maintain large opening, thereby permitting placement of contaminated dressing without touching refuse bag itself.
9. Close room door or bed curtains.	Maintains privacy.
10. Apply gown and goggles if needed.	Protects nurse from splashes or sprays of blood and body fluids.

STEPS	RATIONALE
11. Put on clean gloves and remove soiled dressing and discard in waterproof bag. Discard gloves.	Reduces transmission of microorganisms.
12. Prepare equipment; open sterile supplies.	
13. Put on sterile gloves.	
14. To irrigate wound with wide opening:	
a. Fill 35-ml syringe with irrigation solution.	Flushing wound helps remove debris and facilitates healing by secondary intention.
b. Attach 19-gauge needle or angiocath (see Figure 38-19).	Provides ideal pressure for cleansing and removal of debris.
c. Hold syringe tip 2.5 cm (1 inch) above upper end of wound and over area being cleansed.	Prevents syringe contamination. Careful placement of the syringe prevents unsafe pressure of the flowing solution.
d. Using continuous pressure, flush wound; repeat Steps 15a, b, and c until solution draining into basin is clear.	Clear solution indicates all debris has been removed.
15. To irrigate deep wound with very small opening:	
a. Attach soft angiocatheter to filled irrigating syringe.	Catheter permits direct flow of irrigant into wound. Expect wound to take longer to empty when opening is small.
b. Lubricate tip of catheter with irrigating solution; then gently insert tip of catheter and pull out about 1 cm (½ inch).	Removes tip from fragile inner wall of wound.
c. Using slow, continuous pressure, flush wound.	

CRITICAL DECISION POINT

CAUTION: **Splashing may occur during this step.**

d. Pinch off catheter just below syringe while keeping catheter in place.	Avoids contamination of sterile solution.
e. Remove and refill syringe. Reconnect to catheter and repeat until solution draining into basin is clear.	
16. To cleanse wound with hand-held shower:	Useful for clients able to shower with assistance or independently. May be accomplished at home. A shower table is helpful for bed-bound or acutely ill clients.
a. With client seated comfortably in shower chair, adjust spray to gentle flow; water temperature should be warm.	
b. Cover shower head with clean washcloth if needed.	
c. Shower for 5 to 10 minutes with shower head 12 inches (30 cm) from wound.	

CRITICAL DECISION POINT

Consider culturing a wound if it has a foul, purulent odor; inflammation surrounds the wound; a nondraining wound begins to drain; or client is febrile.

Continued

········ Skill 38-4—cont'd
Performing Wound Irrigations

STEPS	RATIONALE
17. Obtain cultures, if needed, after cleansing with nonbacteriostatic saline.	Routine culturing of open wounds is not recommended by AHCPR (1994). They recommend using quantitative bacterial cultures (tissue biopsy or wound fluid by needle aspiration) rather than swab cultures, which often detect only surface bacterial contaminants.
18. Dry wound edges with gauze; dry client if shower or whirlpool is used.	Prevents maceration of surrounding tissue from excess moisture.
19. Apply appropriate dressing (see Skill 38-2).	Maintains protective barrier and healing environment for wound.
20. Remove gloves, and if worn, mask, goggles, and gown.	Prevents transfer of microorganisms.
21. Assist client to comfortable position.	
22. Dispose of equipment and soiled supplies. Wash hands.	Reduces transmission of microorganisms.
23. Assess type of tissue in the wound bed.	Identifies wound healing progress and determines type of wound cleansing needed.
24. Inspect dressing periodically.	Determines client's response to wound irrigation and need to modify plan of care.
25. Evaluate skin integrity.	Determines if extension of wound has occurred.
26. Observe client for signs of discomfort.	Client's pain should not increase as a result of wound irrigation.
27. Observe for presence of retained irrigant.	Retained irrigant is a medium for bacterial growth and subsequent infection.

Recording and Reporting
- Record wound irrigation and client response on progress notes.
- Immediately report any evidence of fresh bleeding, sharp increase in pain, retention of irrigant, or signs of shock to attending physician.
- At change of shift, report expected and unexpected outcomes that have actually occurred.

Home Care Considerations
- Teach client and care giver how to make normal saline, especially if cost is an issue. Normal saline can be made by using 2 teaspoons of salt in 1 liter (1 quart) of boiling water (Barr, 1995).
- Tell client and care giver that because normal saline has no preservatives, it should be thrown out 24 to 48 hours after it is first opened or made (Barr, 1995).

is required. The nurse must be familiar with the types of suture methods (Figure 38-22). The nurse should never pull the visible contaminated portion of the suture through underlying tissue because infection could result.

Drainage evacuation. When drainage interferes with healing, drainage evacuation can be achieved by using a drain or a drainage tube with continuous suction. **Drainage evacuators** are convenient, portable units that connect to tubular drains within a wound bed and exert a safe, constant, low-pressure vacuum to remove and collect drainage (see Figure 38-12). The nurse ensures that suction is exerted and that all con-

nection points between the evacuator and tubing are intact. The evacuator collects drainage that the nurse assesses for volume and character. When the evacuator fills, the nurse measures output by emptying the contents into a graduated cylinder and immediately resets the evacuator to apply suction. Special skin barriers, similar to those used with ostomies (see Chapters 33 and 34), may be applied around drain sites. The soft, waferlike, plastic barriers are applied to the skin with adhesive. If drain sites are leaking, drainage then flows on the barrier but not directly onto the skin.

Bandages and binders. A simple gauze dressing is often not enough to immobilize or provide support to a

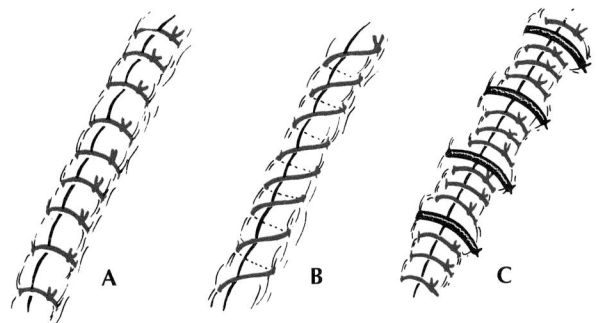

Figure 38-22. Examples of suturing methods. **A,** Intermittent. **B,** Continuous. **C,** Retention.

wound. **Bandages** and **binders** applied over or around dressings can provide extra protection and therapeutic benefits by creating pressure over a body part, immobilizing a body part, supporting a wound, reducing or preventing edema, securing a splint, or securing dressings.

Bandages are available in rolls of various widths and materials including gauze, elasticized knit, elastic webbing, flannel, and muslin. Gauze bandages are lightweight and inexpensive, mold easily around contours of the body, and permit air circulation to underlying skin to prevent maceration. Elastic bandages conform well to body parts but can also be used to exert pressure over a body part.

Binders are bandages made of large pieces of material to fit a specific body part. An arm sling and a breast binder are two examples of binders.

Principles for applying bandages and binders.
Correctly applied bandages and binders do not cause injury to underlying or nearby body parts or create discomfort for the client. Before applying a bandage or binder, the nurse should perform the following steps:

1. Inspect the skin for abrasions, edema, discoloration, or exposed wound edges
2. Cover exposed wounds or open abrasions with a sterile dressing
3. Assess the condition of underlying dressings and change them if they are soiled
4. Assess the skin of underlying body parts and parts that will be distal to the bandage for signs of circulatory impairment (coolness, pallor or cyanosis, diminished or absent pulses, swelling, numbness, and tingling) to provide a means for comparing changes in circulation after bandage application

Table 38-7 outlines the principles of bandage and binder application. After a bandage is applied, the nurse assesses, documents, and immediately reports any changes in circulation, comfort level, body function such as ventilation, and skin integrity. The nurse who applies a bandage can loosen or readjust it as necessary, but the nurse should seek an order before loosening or removing a bandage applied by the physician. The nurse explains to the client that any bandage or binder will feel relatively firm or tight, assesses the bandage carefully to be sure it is applied properly and is provid-

TABLE 38-7

Principles for Bandage and Binder Application

Principle	Rationale
Position body part to be bandaged in comfortable position of normal anatomical alignment.	Bandages cause restriction in movement. Immobilization in normal functioning position reduces risks of deformity or injury.
Prevent friction between and against skin surfaces by applying gauze or cotton padding.	Skin surfaces in contact with each other (e.g., between toes or under breasts) can rub against each other to cause abrasion or chafing. Bandages over bony prominences may rub against skin to cause breakdown.
Apply bandages securely to prevent slippage during movement.	Friction between bandage and skin can cause skin breakdown.
When bandaging extremities, apply bandage first at distal end and progress toward trunk.	Gradual application of pressure from distal toward proximal portion of extremity promotes venous return and minimizes risk of edema or circulatory impairment.
Apply bandages firmly, with equal tension exerted over each turn or layer. Avoid excess overlapping of bandage layers.	Equal tension prevents unequal pressure distribution over bandaged body part. Localized pressure causes circulatory impairment.
Position pins, knots, or ties away from wound or sensitive skin areas.	Pins and ties used to secure bandages and binders can exert localized pressure and irritation.

ing therapeutic benefit, and replaces bandages as they become soiled.

Binder application. Binders are especially designed for the body part to be supported. The most common types of binders are the breast binder, abdominal binder, T binder, and sling (Skill 38-5).

Breast binder. A breast binder looks like a tight-fitting sleeveless vest. It conforms to the shape of the chest wall and is available in different sizes. Breast binders can provide support after breast surgery or exert pressure to reduce lactation after childbirth. Chest expansion should be unimpaired, but if pulmonary secretions increase, the nurse must encourage active pulmonary hygiene exercises.

Abdominal binder. An abdominal binder supports large incisions that are vulnerable to stress when the client moves or coughs. It is a rectangular piece of cotton or elasticized material with many tails attached to the two longer sides or long extensions on each side to surround the abdomen (Figure 38-23). Skill 38-5 describes steps for an abdominal binder application.

T binders. A T binder looks like the letter T (Figure 38-24) with either a single or double tail. T binders secure rectal or perineal dressings. The belt of the binder fits securely around the waist, with the tail passing between the legs from back to front. T binders are easily soiled and require frequent changing. Irritation to the urethra or scrotum must be avoided.

Slings. Slings support arms with muscular sprains or fractures. A commercially made sling consists of a long sleeve that extends to the elbow and a strap that fits around the neck. In the home a large triangular piece of cloth can be used as a sling. The client may sit or lie supine for a sling application (Figure 38-25). The nurse instructs the client to bend the affected arm, bringing the forearm straight across the chest. The open sling fits under the client's arm and over the chest, with the base of the triangle under the wrist and the triangle's point at the elbow. One end of the sling fits around the back of the neck. The nurse brings the other end up over the affected arm while supporting the extremity. The nurse ties the two ends at the side of the neck so that the knot does not press against the cervical spine. The loose fold at the elbow can be folded evenly around the elbow and pinned. The lower arm should always be supported at a level above the elbow to prevent the formation of dependent edema.

Bandage application. Rolls of bandage can secure or support dressings over irregularly shaped body parts. Each roll has a free outer end and a terminal end at the center. The rolled portion of the bandage is its body, and its outer surface is placed against the client's skin or dressing. Skill 38-6 describes the steps for applying an elastic bandage. The nurse may use a variety of bandage turns depending on the body part to be bandaged (Table 38-8).

Heat and cold therapy. The local application of heat and cold to an injured body part provides

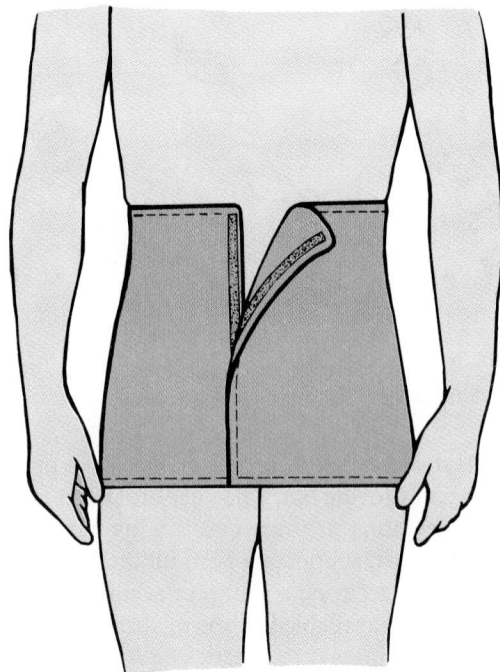

Figure 38-23.   Abdominal binder secured with Velcro.

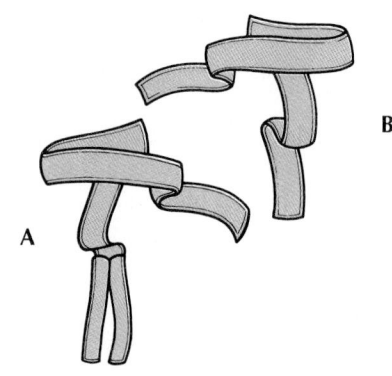

Figure 38-24.   T binders. **A,** Double T (male). **B,** Single T (female).

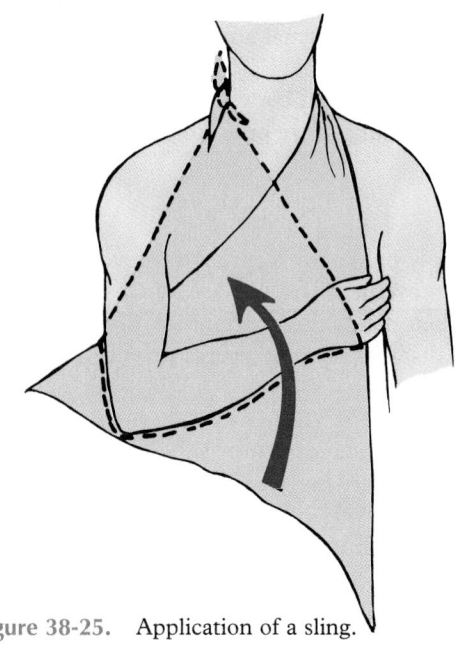

Figure 38-25.   Application of a sling.

Applying an Abdominal, T, or Breast Binder

Delegation Considerations

The skills of applying a binder (abdominal, T, or breast) can be delegated to unlicensed assistive personnel.

- Be sure personnel are competent to perform procedures.
- The nurse should complete an assessment of the client's ability to breathe deeply, cough effectively, and move independently; of skin for irritation/abrasion; of incision/wound and dressing; and of comfort level before a binder or sling is applied for the first time.
- The nurse should evaluate the client's response to binder application.

Equipment

- Gloves, if wound drainage is present.
- Abdominal binder:
    Correct size cloth/elastic straight binder
    Safety pins (unless Velcro closure or metal fasteners are attached): six to eight safety pins are usually adequate for abdominal binders
- T and double-T binders:
    Correct size binder
    Safety pins: two pins for T binder; three pins for double-T binder
- Breast binder:
    Correct size binder
    Safety pins (approximately 12) unless Velcro closure is attached

STEPS	RATIONALE
1. Observe client with need for support of thorax or abdomen. Observe ability to breathe deeply and cough effectively.	Baseline assessment determines client's ability to breathe and cough. Impaired ventilation of lung can lead to alveolar atelectasis and inadequate arterial oxygenation.
2. Review medical record if medical prescription for particular binder is required and reasons for application.	Application of supportive binders may be used on nursing judgment. In some situations, physician input is required.
3. Inspect skin for actual or potential alterations in integrity. Observe for irritation, abrasion, skin surfaces that rub against each other, or allergic response to adhesive tape used to secure dressing.	Actual impairments in skin integrity can be worsened with application of a binder. Binder can cause pressure and excoriation.
4. Inspect any surgical dressing.	Dressing replacement or reinforcement precedes application of any binder.

CRITICAL DECISION POINT

Dressing should be clean and dry, and incision/wound should be entirely covered by dressing.

5. Assess client's comfort level, using analog scale of 0 to 10 (see Chapter 33) and noting any objective signs and symptoms.	Data will determine effectiveness of binder placement.

CRITICAL DECISION POINT

Expect client in moderate-to-severe pain to have diaphoresis, tachycardia, and elevated blood pressure.

6. Gather necessary data regarding size of client and appropriate binder.	Ensures proper fit of binder.
7. Explain procedure to client.	Promotes client's understanding and cooperation.
8. Teach skill to client or significant other.	Reduces anxiety and ensures continuity of care after discharge.

Continued

Applying an Abdominal, ⊤, or Breast Binder

STEPS	RATIONALE
9. Wash hands and apply gloves (if likely to contact wound drainage).	Reduces transmission of microorganisms.
10. Close curtains or room door.	Maintains client's comfort and dignity.
11. Apply binder.	
A. Abdominial binder:	
(1) Position client in supine position with head slightly elevated and knees slightly flexed.	Minimizes muscular tension on abdominal organs.
(2) Fanfold far side of binder toward midline of binder.	Reduces time client remains in uncomfortable position.
(3) Instruct and assist client to roll away from nurse toward raised side rail while firmly supporting abdominal incision and dressing with hands.	Reduces pain and discomfort.
(4) Place fanfolded ends of binder under client.	Permits placement and centering of binder with minimal discomfort.
(5) Instruct or assist client to roll over folded ends.	
(6) Unfold and stretch ends out smoothly on far side of bed.	Maintains skin integrity and comfort.
(7) Instruct client to roll back into supine position.	Facilitates chest expansion and adequate wound support when the binder is closed.
(8) Adjust binder so that supine client is centered over binder using symphysis pubis and costal margins as lower and upper landmarks.	Centers support from binder over abdominal structures, which reduces incidence of decreased lung expansion.

CRITICAL DECISION POINT

Cover any exposed areas of an incision or wound with sterile dressing.

(9) Close binder. Pull one end of binder over center of client's abdomen. While maintaining tension on that end of binder, pull opposite end of binder over center and secure with Velcro closure tabs, metal fasteners, or horizontally placed safety pins (see Figure 38-23).	Provides continuous wound support and comfort.
(10) Assess client's comfort level.	Helps determine effectiveness of binder placement.
(11) Adjust binder as necessary.	Promotes comfort and chest expansion.
B. Single-⊤ and double-⊤ binders (see Figure 38-24):	
(1) Assist client to dorsal recumbent position, with lower extremities slightly flexed and hips rotated slightly outward.	Minimizes muscular tension on perineal organs.
(2) Have client raise hips and place horizontal band around client's waist (or above iliac crests) with vertical tails extending past buttocks. Overlap waistband in front and secure with safety pins.	Permits placement of binder. Secures binder around client.

STEPS	RATIONALE
(3) Complete binder application:	
(a) T binder: Bring remaining vertical strip over perineal dressing and continue up and under center front of horizontal band. Bring ends over waistband and secure all thicknesses with safety pin.	Single-T and double-T binders provide support to perineal muscles and organs and help maintain placement of perineal or suprapubic dressing.
(b) Double-T binder: Bring remaining vertical strips over perineal or suprapubic dressing with each tail supporting one side of scrotum and proceeding upward on either side of penis. Continue drawing ends behind and then downward in front of horizontal band. Secure all thicknesses with one horizontally placed safety pin.	
(4) Assess client's comfort level with client in lying, sitting, and standing positions. Readjust front pins and tails as necessary, ensuring that tails are not too tight. Increase padding if any area rubs against surrounding tissues.	Determines efficacy of binder to maintain dressings and support perineal structures.

CRITICAL DECISION POINT

Binder should hold perineal or suprapubic dressing in place as the client ambulates without applying pressure to urethra or scrotum.

STEPS	RATIONALE
(5) Instruct client regarding removal of binder before defecating or urinating and need to replace binder after performing these bodily functions.	Cleanliness of binder reduces infection risk.
C. Breast binder:	
(1) Assist client in placing arms through binder's armholes.	Eases binder placement process.
(2) Assist client to supine position in bed.	Supine positioning facilitates normal anatomical position of breasts; facilitates healing and comfort.
(3) Pad area under breasts if necessary.	Prevents skin contact with undersurface.
(4) Using Velcro closure tabs or horizontally placed safety pins, secure binder at nipple level first. Continue closure process above and then below nipple line until entire binder is closed.	Horizontal placement of pins may reduce risk of uneven pressure or localized irritation.
(5) Make appropriate adjustments, including individualizing fit of shoulder straps and pinning waistline darts to reduce binder size.	Maintains support to client's breasts.
(6) Instruct and observe skill development in self-care related to reapplying breast binder.	Self-care is integral aspect of discharge planning. Skin integrity and comfort level goals are ensured.

Continued

. . . . Skill 38-5—cont'd
Applying an Abdominal, T, or Breast Binder

STEPS	RATIONALE
12. Remove gloves and wash hands.	Prevents cross-infections.
13. Observe site for skin integrity, circulation, and characteristics of the wound. (Periodically remove binder and surgical dressing to assess wound characteristics.)	Determines that binder has not resulted in complication to skin, wound, or underlying organs.
14. Assess comfort level of client, using analog scale of 0 to 10 and noting any objective signs and symptoms.	Binders should not increase discomfort.
15. Assess client's ability to ventilate properly, including deep breathing and coughing.	Identifies any impaired ventilation and potential pulmonary complications.
16. Identify client's need for assistance with activities such as hair combing, dressing, and ambulating.	Mobility of upper extremities may be limited depending on severity and location of incision.

Recording and Reporting
- Report any skin irritation to nurse at between-shift report.
- Record application of binder, condition of skin, circulation, integrity of dressing, and client's comfort level.
- Report ineffective lung expansion to physician immediately.

Home Care Considerations
- Abdominal, T, and breast binders are washable and are placed over a line to dry.
- Instruct care giver to avoid excessive pressure with binder application.

---

therapeutic benefits. Before using these therapies, however, the nurse must understand normal body responses to local temperature variations, assess the integrity of the body part, determine the client's ability to sense temperature variations, and ensure proper operation of equipment. The nurse is legally responsible for the safe administration of all heat and cold applications.

Body responses to heat and cold. Exposure to heat and cold can cause systemic and local responses. Systemic responses occur through heat loss mechanisms (sweating or vasodilation) or mechanisms promoting heat conservation (vasoconstriction or piloerection) and heat production (shivering) (see Chapter 23). Local responses to heat and cold occur through stimulation of temperature-sensitive nerve endings within the skin.

The body's adaptive ability creates the major problem in protecting clients from injury resulting from temperature extremes. A person initially feels an extreme change in temperature but within a short time hardly notices the temperature variation. This phenomenon can be dangerous, because a person insensitive to heat and cold extremes can suffer serious tissue injury. The nurse must recognize clients most at risk for injuries from heat and cold applications (Table 38-9).

Local effects of heat and cold. Heat and cold stimuli create different physiological responses. The choice of heat or cold therapy depends on the local responses desired for wound healing (Table 38-10).

Heat generally is therapeutic. If heat is applied for 1 hour or more, however, blood flow is reduced by a reflex vasoconstriction as the body attempts to control heat loss from the area. The periodic removal and reapplication of local heat will restore vasodilation. Continuous exposure to heat damages epithelial cells, causing redness, localized tenderness, and even blistering of the skin.

Prolonged exposure of the skin to cold results in a reflex vasodilation. The cell's inability to receive adequate blood flow and nutrients results in tissue ischemia. The skin initially takes on a reddened appearance, followed by a bluish-purple mottling with numbness and a burning type of pain. Tissues can actually freeze from exposure to extreme cold.

Factors influencing heat and cold tolerance. The body's response to heat and cold therapies depends on the following factors:

1. *Duration of application.* A person is better able to tolerate short exposures to any temperature extremes.

TABLE 38-8
Types of Bandage Turns

Type	Description	Purpose or Use
Circular	Bandage turn overlapping previous turn completely	Anchors bandage at the first and final turn; covers small part (finger, toe)
Spiral	Bandage ascending body part with each turn overlapping previous one by one-half or two-thirds width of bandage	Covers cylindrical body parts such as wrist or upper arm
Spiral—reverse	Turn requiring twist (reversal) of bandage halfway through each turn	Covers cone-shaped body parts such as the forearm, thigh, or calf; useful with nonstretching bandages such as gauze or flannel
Figure eight	Oblique overlapping turns alternately ascending and descending over bandaged part; each turn crossing previous one to form figure eight	Covers joints; snug fit provides excellent immobilization
Recurrent	Bandage first secured with two circular turns around proximal end of body part; half turn made perpendicular up from bandage edge; body of bandage brought over distal end of body part to be covered with each turn folded back over on itself	Covers uneven body parts such as head or stump

········ Skill 38-6
Applying an Elastic Bandage

Delegation Considerations

The application of an elastic bandage can be delegated to unlicensed assistive personnel.
- Be sure personnel are trained on application of elastic bandages.
- The nurse should completely assess the client's wound and distal extremity circulation before and after bandage application.

Equipment
- Correct width and number of bandages
- Safety pins, clips, or adhesive tape
- Disposable gloves, if wound drainage is present

STEPS	RATIONALE
1. Inspect skin for alterations in integrity as indicated by abrasions, discoloration, chafing, or edema. (Look carefully at bony prominences.)	Altered skin integrity contraindicates the use of elastic bandages.
2. Inspect surgical dressing.	Surgical dressing replacement or reinforcement precedes application of any bandage.
3. Observe adequacy of circulation (distal to bandage) by noting surface temperature, skin color, and sensation of body parts to be wrapped.	Comparison of area before and after application of bandage is necessary to ensure continued adequate circulation. Impairment of circulation may result in coolness to touch when compared with opposite side of body, cyanosis or pallor of skin, diminished or absent pulses, edema or localized pooling, and numbness or tingling of part.
4. Review medical record for specific orders related to application of elastic bandage. Note area to be covered, type of bandage required, frequency of change, and previous response to treatment.	Specific prescription may direct procedure, including factors such as extent of application (e.g., toe to knee, toe to groin) and duration of treatment.
5. Identify client's and primary care giver's present knowledge level of skill if bandaging will be continued at home.	Ensures that planning and teaching are individualized.
6. Explain procedure to client.	Increased knowledge promotes cooperation and reduces anxiety.
7. Teach skill to client or significant other.	Reduces anxiety and ensures continuity of care after discharge.
8. Wash hands and apply gloves if drainage is present.	Reduces transmission of microorganisms.
9. Close room door or curtains.	Maintains client's comfort and dignity.
10. Assist client to assume comfortable, anatomically correct position.	Maintains alignment. Prevents musculoskeletal deformity.

CRITICAL DECISION POINT

Bandages applied to lower extremities are applied before client sits or stands. Elevation of dependent extremities for 20 minutes before bandage application will enhance venous return.

STEPS	RATIONALE
11. Hold roll of elastic bandage in dominant hand and use other hand to lightly hold beginning of bandage at distal body part. Continue transferring roll to dominant hand as bandage is wrapped.	Maintains appropriate and consistent bandage tension.

CRITICAL DECISION POINT

Toes or finger tips should be visible for follow-up circulatory assessment.

STEPS	RATIONALE
12. Apply bandage from distal point toward proximal boundary using variety of turns to cover various shapes of body parts (see Table 38-8).	Bandage is applied in manner that conforms evenly to body part and promotes venous return.
13. Unroll and very slightly stretch bandage.	Maintains uniform bandage tension.
14. Overlap turns by one-half to two-thirds width of bandage roll.	Prevents uneven bandage tension and circulatory impairment.
15. Secure first bandage with clip or tape before applying additional rolls.	
a. Apply additional rolls without leaving any uncovered skin surface. Secure last bandage applied.	Prevents wrinkling or loose ends.
16. Remove gloves if worn and wash hands.	Reduces transmission of microorganisms.
17. Assess distal circulation when bandage application is complete and at least twice during 8-hour period.	Early detection and management of circulatory impairment ensures healthy neurovascular status.
a. Observe skin color for pallor or cyanosis.	
b. Palpate skin for warmth.	
c. Palpate pulses and compare bilaterally.	
d. Ask if client is aware of pain, numbness, tingling, or other discomfort.	Neurovascular changes indicate impaired venous return.
e. Observe mobility of extremity.	Determines if bandage is too tight, which restricts movement, or determines if joint immobility is attained.
18. Have client demonstrate bandage application.	Return demonstration documents learning.

Recording and Reporting
- Document condition of wound, integrity of dressing, application of bandage, circulation, and client's comfort level.
- Report any changes in neurological or circulatory status to nurse in charge or physician.

Home Care Considerations
- Instruct client or care giver not to make bandages too tight, which interferes with circulation.
- Elastic bandages that are used to reduce swelling are best applied to the feet in the morning, before getting out of bed.
- Always remove an elastic bandage daily and inspect skin beneath it.

TABLE 38-9

Conditions That Increase Risk of Injury From Heat and Cold Application

Condition	Risk Factors
Very young; older adults	Thinner skin layers in children and older adults increase risk of burns; older adults have reduced sensitivity to pain.
Open wounds, broken skin, stomas	Subcutaneous and visceral tissues are more sensitive to temperature variations; they also contain no temperature and fewer pain receptors.
Areas of edema or scar formation	There is reduced sensation to temperature stimuli because of thickening of skin layers from fluid buildup or scar formation.
Peripheral vascular disease (e.g., diabetes, arteriosclerosis)	Body's extremities are less sensitive to temperature and pain stimuli because of circulatory impairment and local tissue injury; cold application would further compromise blood flow.
Confusion or unconsciousness	There is reduced perception of sensory or painful stimuli.
Spinal cord injury	Alterations in nerve pathways prevent reception of sensory or painful stimuli.
Abscessed tooth or appendix	Infection is highly localized; application of heat may cause rupture with spread of microorganisms systemically.

TABLE 38-10

Therapeutic Effects of Heat and Cold Applications

Physiological Response	Therapeutic Benefit	Examples of Conditions Treated
Heat Therapy		
Vasodilation	Improves blood flow to injured body part	Inflamed or edematous body part
Reduced blood viscosity	Promotes delivery of nutrients and removal of wastes	New surgical wound
		Infected wound
Reduced muscle tension	Lessens venous congestion in injured tissues	Arthritis or degenerative joint disease
Increased tissue metabolism		Localized joint pain or muscle strains
	Improves delivery of leukocytes and antibiotics to wound site	Low back pain
Increased capillary permeability		Menstrual cramping
	Promotes muscle relaxation	Hemorrhoidal, perianal, and vaginal inflammation
	Reduces pain from spasm or stiffness	Local abscesses
	Increases blood flow	
	Provides local warmth	
	Promotes movement of waste products and nutrients	
Cold Therapy		
Vasoconstriction	Reduces blood flow to injured site, preventing edema formation	Immediately after direct trauma (e.g., sprains, strains, fractures, and muscle spasms)
Local anesthesia		
Reduced cell metabolism	Reduces inflammation	
	Reduces localized pain	Superficial laceration or puncture wound
Increased blood viscosity	Reduces oxygen needs of tissues	Minor burn
	Promotes blood coagulation at injury site	Suspected malignancy in area of injury or pain
Decreased muscle tension	Relieves pain	After injections
		Arthritis or joint trauma

2. *Body part.* The neck, inner aspect of the wrist and forearm, and perineal regions are more sensitive to temperature variations. The foot and the palm of the hand are less sensitive.
3. *Damage to body surface.* Exposed skin layers are more sensitive to temperature variations.
4. *Prior skin temperature.* The body responds best to minor temperature adjustments.
5. *Body surface area.* A person is less tolerant of temperature changes over a large area of the body.
6. *Age and physical condition.* The very young and old are most sensitive to heat and cold. If a client's physical condition reduces the reception or perception of sensory stimuli, the tolerance to temperature extremes is high, but the risk of injury is also high.

Assessment for temperature tolerance. Before applying heat or cold therapies, the nurse first observes the area to be treated so that therapy-related skin changes can later be evaluated. Alterations in skin integrity, such as abrasions, open wounds, edema, bruising, bleeding, or localized areas of inflammation, increase the risk of thermal injury. The nurse identifies conditions that contraindicate heat or cold therapy. Heat should not be applied over an active area of bleeding (risk of continued bleeding) or an acute localized inflammation such as appendicitis (risk of rupture). If the client has cardiovascular problems, it is unwise to apply heat to large portions of the body, because massive vasodilation may disrupt blood supply to vital organs. Cold is contraindicated if the site of injury is edematous or the client has impaired circulation or is shivering (may intensify shivering and reduce blood flow).

The nurse also assesses the client's sensory function and ability to recognize when heat or cold becomes excessive. If a client has peripheral vascular disease, the nurse particularly observes circulation to the extremities. If a client is confused or unresponsive, the nurse checks skin integrity frequently after therapy begins.

Finally, the nurse assesses the condition of all equipment used, checking for cracked cords, frayed wires, damaged insulation, exposed heating components, leaks, and evenness of temperature distribution.

Client education and safety. Before application of heat or cold therapy, the client should understand its purpose, the symptoms of temperature exposure, and the precautions taken to prevent injury. Box 38-9 provides hints for safely applying heat and cold therapy.

Applying heat and cold. A prerequisite to using heat or cold application is a physician's order, which should include the body site to be treated and the type, frequency, and duration of application. The correct temperature to use for heat and cold applications varies according to agency policy.

Box 38-9
Safety Suggestions for Applying Heat or Cold Therapy

Explain to the client the sensations to be felt during the procedure.
Instruct the client to report changes in sensation or discomfort immediately.
Provide a timer, clock, or watch so that the client can help the nurse to time the application.
Keep the call light within the client's reach.
Refer to the institution's policy and procedure manual for safe temperatures.
Do not allow the client to adjust temperature settings.
Do not allow the client to move an application or place his or her hands on the wound site.
Do not place the client in a position that prevents movement away from the temperature source.
Do not leave unattended a client who is unable to sense temperature changes or move from the temperature source.

Choice of moist or dry. Heat and cold applications can be administered in dry or moist forms. The type of wound or injury, location of the body part, and presence of drainage or inflammation are considered when selecting dry or moist applications. Table 38-11 summarizes advantages and disadvantages of both.

Warm moist compresses. For open wounds, sterile, warm, moist compresses improve circulation, relieve edema, and promote concentration of pus and drainage. A **compress** is a piece of gauze dressing moistened in a prescribed warmed solution. A pack is a larger cloth or dressing applied to a larger body area.

Heat from warm compresses evaporates quickly. To maintain a constant temperature, the nurse must change the compress frequently or apply a warm aquathermic pad or waterproof heating pad over the compress. Because moisture conducts heat, any device's temperature setting should be lower for a moist compress than for a dry application. A layer of plastic wrap or a dry towel can also be used to insulate the compress and retain heat. Moist heat promotes vasodilation and evaporation of heat from the skin's surface. For this reason a client may feel chilly. The nurse controls drafts and keeps the client covered with a blanket or robe. Skill 38-7 describes the steps for applying a warm compress.

Warm soaks. Immersion of a body part in a warmed solution promotes circulation, lessens edema, increases muscle relaxation, and can provide a means to debride wounds and apply medicated solution. A soak can also be accomplished by wrapping the body part in dressings and saturating them with the warmed solution.

TABLE 38-11
Choice of Dry or Moist Applications

Advantages	Disadvantages
Moist Applications	
Moist application reduces drying of skin, softens wound exudate, and comforms well to body area being treated.	Prolonged exposure can cause maceration of skin. Moist heat will cool rapidly because of moisture evaporation.
Moist heat penetrates deeply into tissue layers.	Moist heat creates greater risk for burns to skin, because moisture conducts heat.
Warm, moist heat does not promote sweating and insensible fluid loss.	
Dry Applications	
Dry heat has less risk of burns to skin than moist applications.	Dry heat increases body fluid loss through sweating.
Dry application does not cause skin maceration.	Dry applications do not penetrate deep into tissues.
Dry heat retains temperature longer, because it is not influenced by evaporation.	Dry heat causes increased drying of skin.

The nurse positions the client comfortably, places waterproof pads under the area to be treated, and heats the solution to the client's tolerance. The nurse checks the temperature by placing a small amount of solution on the forearm. After immersing the body part, the nurse covers the container and extremity with a towel to reduce heat loss. It is usually necessary to remove the cooled solution and the body part and add heated solution after about 10 minutes. The problem is to keep the solution at a constant temperature. Never add a hotter solution while the body part remains immersed. After any soak, the nurse dries the body part thoroughly to prevent maceration.

Sitz bath. The client who has had rectal surgery or an episiotomy during childbirth or who has painful hemorrhoids or vaginal inflammation may benefit from a **sitz bath,** a bath in which only the pelvic area is immersed in warm fluid. The client sits in a special tub or chair or in a basin that fits on the toilet seat so that the legs and feet remain out of the water. Immersing the entire body causes widespread vasodilation and negates the effect of local heat to the pelvic area.

The desired temperature for a sitz bath depends on whether the purpose is to promote relaxation or to clean a wound. It may be necessary to carefully add hot water during the procedure, which usually lasts 20 minutes. A disposable basin contains an attachment that resembles an enema bag and allows the gradual introduction of warmer water.

The nurse should prevent overexposure by draping bath blankets around the client's shoulders and thighs and controlling drafts. The client should be able to sit in the basin or tub with feet flat on the floor and without pressure on the sacrum or thighs. Because exposure of a large portion of the body to heat causes extensive va-

sodilation, the nurse should assess the client's pulse and facial color and ask whether the client feels light-headed or nauseated.

Aquathermia (water-flow) pads. The aquathermia (water-flow) pad (Figure 38-26) is useful for treating muscle sprains and areas of mild inflammation or edema. The unit consists of a waterproof plastic or rubber pad connected by two hoses to an electrical control unit that has a heating element and motor. Distilled water circulates through hollowed channels within the pad to the control unit where water is heated or cooled (depending on temperature setting). Although the units are safer than the conventional heating pad, the nurse should still check for equipment malfunctions. The temperature setting is fixed by inserting a plastic key into the temperature regulator. If the water in the unit runs low, the nurse simply adds distilled water to the reservoir at the top of the control unit.

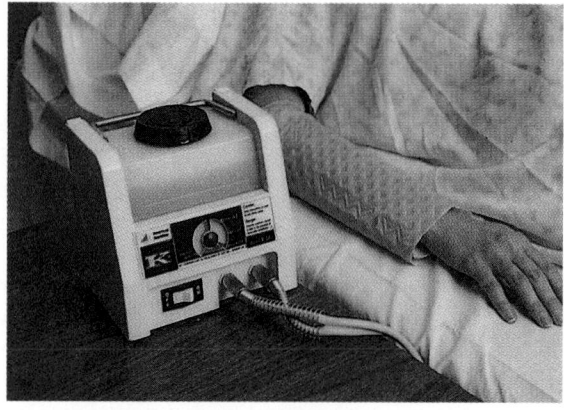

Figure 38-26.   Aquathermia pad.

Applying a Moist Hot Compress to an Open Wound

Delegation Considerations

This skill can be delegated to unlicensed assistive personnel.

- Ensure care giver can perform skill competently.
- Caution care giver to maintain proper temperature of application during the duration of treatment.
- Caution care giver to keep application in place for only the length of time specified in the physician's orders.
- Have care giver notify the nurse when treatment is complete so that an evaluation of client's response can be made.

Equipment

- Prescribed solution warmed to appropriate temperature
- Sterile gauze dressings or commercially prepared compresses
- Sterile container for solution
- Dry bath towel
- Disposable gloves
- Sterile gloves
- Waterproof pad
- Ties or tape
- Aquathermia or heating pad (optional)
- Bath blanket

STEPS	RATIONALE
1. Refer to physician's order for type of compress, location and duration of application, desired temperature, and institutional policies regarding temperature of compress.	Ensures safe and correct application.
2. Inspect condition of exposed skin and wound on which compress is to be applied.	Provides baseline to determine changes in skin during heat application.

CRITICAL DECISION POINT

Very thin or damaged skin is more susceptible to injury from heat. Nonintact skin and drainage from wounds are indications to wear gloves.

3. Assess client's extremities for sensitivity to temperature and pain by measuring light touch, pinprick, and temperature sensation.	Clients insensitive to heat or cold sensations must be monitored closely during treatment.

CRITICAL DECISION POINT

Diabetic clients, victims of stroke, and clients with peripheral neuropathy are particularly at risk for thermal injury.

4. Refer to medical record to identify any systemic contraindications to heat application.	Heat causes vasodilation, which aggravates active bleeding. Heat applied to localized area of acute inflammation or tumor may cause rupture or activate cell growth.
5. Assemble equipment and supplies.	Organization of supplies prevents unnecessary delays in the procedure.
6. Explain steps of procedure and purpose to client. Describe sensations to be felt, such as decreasing warmth and wetness. Explain precautions to prevent burning.	Minimizes client's anxiety and promotes cooperation during the procedure.
7. Close door and bedside curtains.	Decreases drafts, thus decreasing the transmission of microorganisms. Provides for client privacy.

Continued

.... Skill 38-7—cont'd
Applying a Moist Hot Compress to an Open Wound

STEPS	RATIONALE
8. Assist client in assuming comfortable position in proper body alignment, and place waterproof pad under area to be treated.	Compress remains in place for several minutes. Limited mobility in uncomfortable position causes muscular stress. Pad prevents soiling of bed linen.
9. Expose body part to be covered with compress and drape client with bath blanket.	Prevents unnecessary cooling and exposure of body part.
10. Wash hands.	Reduces transmission of microorganisms.
11. Prepare compress:	Ensures orderly procedure.
a. Pour solution into sterile container.	
b. If using portable heating source, warm solution. Commercially prepared compresses may remain under infrared lamp until just before use. Open sterile packages and drop gauze into container to become immersed in solution.	Compresses must retain warmth for therapeutic benefit.

CRITICAL DECISION POINT

Temperature must be tested by applying sterile solution to nurse's forearm (without contaminating solution).

c. Adjust temperature of aquathermia pad (if needed).	
12. Apply disposable gloves. Remove any existing dressing covering wound. Dispose of gloves and dressings in proper receptacle.	Reduces transmission of microorganisms.
13. Assess condition of wound and surrounding skin. Inflamed wound appears reddened, but surrounding skin is less red in color.	Provides baseline to determine skin changes following compress application.

CRITICAL DECISION POINT

If skin surrounding wound is reddened, application may be contraindicated.

14. Apply sterile gloves.	Allows nurse to manipulate sterile dressing and touch open wound.
15. Pick up one layer of immersed gauze, wring out any excess solution, and apply it lightly to open wound.	Excess moisture macerates skin and increases risks of burns and infection. Skin is sensitive to sudden change in temperature.
16. In a few seconds, lift edge of gauze to assess for redness.	Increased redness indicates burn.
17. If client tolerates compress, pack gauze snugly against the wound. Be sure all wound surfaces are covered by hot compress.	Packing of compress prevents rapid cooling from underlying air currents.
18. Cover moist compress with dry sterile dressing and bath towel. If necessary, pin or tie in place. Remove sterile gloves.	Dry sterile dressing will prevent transfer of microorganisms to wound via capillary action caused by moist compress. Towel insulates compress to prevent heat loss.

STEPS	RATIONALE
19. Apply aquathermic or waterproof heating pad over towel (optional). Keep it in place for desired duration of application.	Provides constant temperature to compress.
20. If an aquathermia pad is *not* used to maintain temperature of application, change hot compress using sterile technique every 5 minutes or as ordered during duration of therapy.	Prevents cooling and maintains therapeutic benefit of compress.
21. After prescribed time, apply disposable gloves and remove pad, towel, and compress. Reassess wound and condition of skin, and replace dry sterile dressing as ordered.	Continued exposure to moisture will macerate skin. Prevents entrance of microorganisms into wound site.
22. Assist client to preferred comfortable position.	Maintains client's comfort.
23. Dispose of equipment and soiled compress. Wash hands.	Reduces transmission of microorganisms.
24. Inspect affected area covered by compress and heating pad every 5 to 10 minutes.	Assists in determining effects of application.
25. Ask every 5 to 10 minutes if client notices any unusual burning sensation not felt before application.	It may be difficult to assess burn merely by color changes if wound is inflamed or drainage is present.
26. Have client explain and demonstrate application.	Evaluates client's understanding of and ability to perform procedure.

Recording and Reporting

- Record type, location, and duration of application. Note solution and temperature.
- Describe condition of wound and skin before and after treatment, as well as client's response to therapy.
- Describe any instructions given and client's ability to explain and perform procedure.
- Report unusual findings to nurse in charge or physician.

Home Care Considerations

- When necessary, assess availability of primary care givers to assist clients in application of compress, their understanding of purpose of procedure, and their willingness to comply with procedure and not leave client with compress in place beyond prescribed time limit.
- Assess physical environment to determine existence of adequate facilities to prepare hot compress and provide for sterile technique.

To avoid burning the client's skin, the nurse folds a thin cloth or pillowcase over the heating pad; tape, ties, or a gauze roll holds the pad in place. Pins are never used. The nurse checks the skin frequently for signs of burning. An application should last only 20 to 30 minutes, and the client must not lie on the pad.

Commercial hot packs. Commercially prepared, disposable hot packs apply warm, dry heat to an injured area. Striking, kneading, or squeezing the pack mixes chemicals that release heat. Package directions recommend the time for heat application.

Hot water bottles. The hot water bottle is an economical means of applying heat to an injured body part. Many clients use them in the home. Nurses must give clients and family members the following instructions about the safe use of water bottles:

1. Ensure no leaks. Fill the bottle with tap water, secure the cap, and turn the bottle upside down.
2. Use warm tap water.
3. Fill the bag only two-thirds full, expel air at the top, and secure the cap. The bag is then easier to mold over a body part.
4. Wipe off moisture on the outside of the bag.
5. Never apply a water bottle directly to the skin surface. Cover it with a towel or pillowcase.
6. Keep the bottle in place for 20 to 30 minutes.

Electric heating pads. Another conventional form of heat therapy is the heating pad, an electric coil enclosed within a waterproof pad covered with cotton or flannel cloth. The pad is connected to an electric cord that has a temperature-regulating unit for a high, medium, or low setting. Nurses should advise clients to avoid using the high setting and to never lie on the pad. Another precaution to note is that a safety pin inserted through a pad can result in an electrical shock.

Cold moist compresses. The procedure for applying cold moist compresses is the same as that for warm compresses. Cold compresses should be applied for 20 minutes at a temperature of 15° C (59° F) to relieve inflammation and swelling. They may be clean or sterile. The nurse observes for adverse reactions such as burning or numbness, mottling of the skin, redness, extreme paleness, or a bluish skin discoloration.

Cold soaks. The procedure for preparing cold soaks and immersing a body part is the same as for warm soaks. The desired temperature for a 20-minute soak is 15° C (59° F). The nurse takes precautions to protect the client from chilling.

Ice bag or collar. For a client who has a muscle sprain, localized hemorrhage, or hematoma or has undergone dental surgery, an ice bag is ideal to prevent edema formation, control bleeding, and anesthetize the body part. Proper use of the bag requires the following:

1. Fill the bag with water, secure the cap, invert to check for leaks, and pour out the water.

2. Fill the bag two-thirds full with crushed ice so that the bag can mold easily over a body part.
3. Release air from the bag by squeezing its sides before securing the cap (because excess air interferes with conduction of cold).
4. Wipe off excess moisture.
5. Cover the bag with a flannel cover, towel, or pillowcase.
6. Apply the bag to the injury site for 30 minutes; the bag can be reapplied in an hour.

Commercial cold packs. Commercially prepared single-use ice packs come in various sizes and shapes. When the pack is squeezed or kneaded, an alcohol-based solution is released inside to create the cold temperature. The soft outer coverings can usually be safely applied directly to the skin surface.

Restorative care. Healing for a pressure ulcer or a chronic wound care is lengthy and requires continuity of care from the acute care setting to the restorative care setting. In this setting many of the principles and interventions detailed in the acute care section are used. The nurse needs to continue diligent assessment to identify those clients at risk for impaired skin integrity and institute preventive measures as needed.

Despite the nurse's efforts with wound care, wound healing will not occur if the client is malnourished. Tissue repair requires more protein, carbohydrates, fats, vitamins, minerals, water, and oxygen than normal tissue metabolism (see Chapter 34). In addition, the delivery of nutritional substances to tissues depends on a healthy circulatory system. Malnutrition causes an insufficient supply of the necessary nutritional elements and alterations in blood vessel integrity. The nurse therefore works closely with dietitians to provide a well-balanced diet and educates the client about the importance of good dietary habits (see Chapter 34). For clients weakened or debilitated by illness, supportive nutritional therapies may become necessary. The surgical client who is well nourished and has no complications requires at least 0.8 g of protein per kilogram daily for nutritional maintenance (Konstantinides, 1992). Supplemental tube feedings (enteral feedings) introduce nutrients directly into the gastrointestinal tract. If a client is unable to tolerate enteral feedings, the physician may order parenteral (intravenously administered) nutrition.

The client with a wound that restricts mobility or has the potential to compromise the function of a joint may require additional physical and/or occupational therapy. The nurse works closely with the physical therapist in monitoring the client's activity and tolerance for exercise. It is important to optimize activity within the client's physical limitations and return function as rapidly as possible.

Some chronic wounds are the result of underlying

pathology that may continue long after wound healing occurs.

▪ Evaluation

Client care. Nursing interventions for reducing and treating pressure ulcers are evaluated by determining the client's response to nursing therapies and by determining whether each goal was achieved. The optimal goals are to prevent injury to the skin and tissues, reduce injury to the skin and underlying tissues, and restore skin integrity. The nurse also evaluates specific interventions designed to promote skin integrity and to teach the client and family to reduce future threats to skin integrity (Box 38-10). The nurse also evaluates the client's and family's need for additional support services and initiates the referral process. Specific recommendations for clients with pressure ulcers in the home setting are summarized in Box 38-10.

Client expectations. The client and care giver understand how to prevent or treat pressure ulcers. Helping them understand the content in the AHCPR consumer version of the prevention and treatment guidelines is helpful. Clients may enter into the wound healing phase with unrealistic expectations regarding duration of care. The nurse needs to collect evaluation data about the client's perception of wound care management. Clients with chronic wounds are often cared for in their home settings and have certain expectations about their level of comfort, lifestyle, independence, and privacy. Therefore, the nurse must determine from the client whether his or her expectations were respected and met.

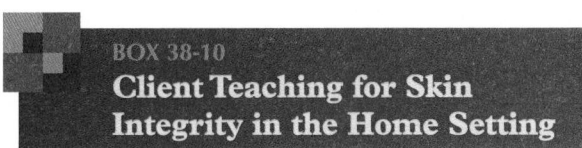

BOX 38-10
Client Teaching for Skin Integrity in the Home Setting

Assessment

▪ Assessment and documentation [of the pressure ulcer] should be carried out at least weekly, unless there is evidence of deterioration, in which case both the pressure ulcer and the client's overall management must be reassessed immediately. In the home setting, this may require the assistance of the client and family because weekly assessment by health care providers is not always feasible.

Ulcer Care—Dressings

▪ Consider care giver time when selecting a dressing.

  In the home setting, care givers may choose more expensive dressing materials to reduce the frequency of dressing changes.

Infection Control

▪ Clean dressing may also be used in the home setting. Disposal of contaminated dressings in the home should be done in a manner consistent with local regulations.

  Clean dressings, as opposed to sterile ones, are recommended for home use. The "no-touch" technique can be used for dressing changes. This technique is a method of changing surface dressings without touching the wound or the surface of any dressing that might be in contact with the wound. Adherent dressings should be grasped by the corner and removed slowly, whereas gauze dressings can be pinched in the center and lifted off.

  The Environmental Protection Agency recommends that soiled dressings be placed in securely fastened plastic bags before being added to other household trash. Have client check local regulations.

Modified from Agency for Health Care Policy and Research Panel for the Treatment of Pressure Ulcers in Adults: *Treatment of pressure ulcers: clinical practice guidelines,* No. 15, Pub. No. 95-0653, Rockville, Md, 1994, U.S. Department of Health and Human Services, Public Health Service.

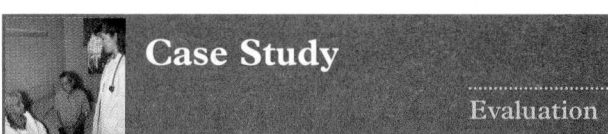

Case Study
Evaluation

Lynda Abraham has completed her clinical experience with Mr. Ahmed. His pressure ulcer is still present, but it is reduced in size and is healing. No other sites of abnormal reactive hyperemia were assessed, and the rest of his skin remains intact. He is going to be discharged to his home in 2 days. Lynda has taught Mr. Ahmed's wife how to do the dressing changes, as well as how to assess her husband's skin for signs of increased risk for or actual further skin breakdown. On her last day of this clinical experience, Lynda has prepared to refer her client to a home care agency. Lynda, with the help of her instructor, has devised a plan of care for the home; Lynda and her instructor are meeting with the home health nurse today when she visits Mr. and Mrs. Ahmed in the hospital.

Documentation Note

Small amount of serous drainage from stage II pressure ulcer on his sacrum. Wound is 1 × 1 inch (2.5 × 2.5 cm) × 1/8 inch deep, with beefy red tissue. Mrs. Ahmed cleansed the wound with normal saline and applied a hydrocolloid dressing. She maintained aseptic technique. During the dressing change she correctly assessed her husband's skin. She reminds her husband to change his position every 1 1/2 to 2 hours. Awaiting visit from home care nurse.

Key Terms

abnormal reactive
  hyperemia
abrasion
anemia
approximate
bandages
binders
blanching
cachexia
collagen
compress
debridement
dehiscence
drainage evacuators
ecchymosis
edema
eschar
evisceration
fibrin

fistula
friction
granulation tissue
hematoma
hemostasis
induration
laceration
maceration
normal reactive hyper-
  emia
pressure ulcer
primary intention
secondary intention
shearing force
sitz bath
sloughing
tissue ischemia
wound culture

References

Agency for Health Care Policy and Research: *Pressure ulcers in adults: prediction and prevention,* Pub. Nos. 92-0047, 92-0050, Rockville, Md, 1992, U.S. Department of Health and Human Services, Public Health Service.

Agency for Health Care Policy and Research Panel for the Treatment of Pressure Ulcers in Adults. *Treatment of pressure ulcers: clinical practice guidelines,* No. 15, Pub. No. 95-0653, Rockville, Md, 1994, U.S. Department of Health and Human Services, Public Health Service.

Ayello EA: A critique of AHCPR's "Preventing pressure ulcers—a patient's guide" as a written instruction tool, *Decubitus* 6:44, 1993.

Ayello EA: Critique of AHCPR's consumer guide "treating pressure sores," *Adv Wound Care* 8(5):18, 1995.

Barr JE: Principles of wound cleansing, *Ostomy/Wound Manage* 41(17A suppl):465, 1995.

Bennett MA: Report of the Task Force on the implications for darkly pigmented intact skin in the prediction and prevention of pressure ulcers, *Adv Wound Care* 8(6):34, 1995.

Bergstrom N: A research agenda for pressure ulcer prevention, *Decubitus* 5(5):22, 1992.

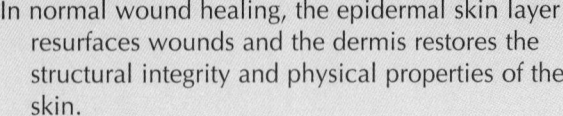

■ Key Concepts

In normal wound healing, the epidermal skin layer resurfaces wounds and the dermis restores the structural integrity and physical properties of the skin.

A clean surgical incision with little tissue loss heals by primary intention.

Healing by primary intention proceeds through three stages: inflammation, proliferation, and maturation.

When there is extensive tissue loss, a wound heals by secondary intention.

The chances of wound infection are greater when the wound contains dead or necrotic tissue, when foreign bodies lie on or near the wound, and when blood supply and tissue defenses are reduced.

Physical stress from vomiting, coughing, or sudden muscular contraction can cause separation of wound edges.

Wound assessment requires a description of the appearance of the wound, palpation of the area, and information regarding character of drainage, drains and wound closures, and pain.

Wound drains remove secretions within tissue layers to promote wound closure.

The nurse never collects a wound culture from old drainage.

Principles of wound first aid include control of bleeding, cleansing, and protection.

The layers of a dry dressing protect the wound edges, absorb drainage, and prevent entrance of bacteria.

The wet-to-dry dressing mechanically removes dead tissue and wound exudate to debride the wound.

When cleaning wounds or drain sites, the nurse cleans from the least to most contaminated area, away from wound edges.

A bandage or binder should be applied in a manner that does not impair circulation or irritate the skin.

The safe use of heat or cold therapy requires an assessment of the client's sensory function, identification of risk factors, and understanding of the physiological effects of heat and cold.

An acute sprain, fracture, or bruise responds best to cold applications.

Warm applications are effective for improving circulation to wound sites and promoting muscle relaxation.

The choice of moist or dry applications depends on the type of wound, location of body part, and presence of drainage or inflammation.

Critical Thinking Activities

1. You are teaching a client's family how to irrigate the midabdominal wound that is healing by secondary intention. The spouse states, "I always thought it was best to paint the wound with povidone-iodine to prevent infection." How should you respond to the spouse? What is the rationale behind your response? What does the spouse need to know about irrigating the wound?

2. A client has two Jackson-Pratt drainage collectors on the right side of the abdomen. What nursing assessments should be made to ensure proper functioning of this system? Can any aspects of care for this type of drain collector be delegated? Explain the rationale for your answer.

3. Your 85-year-old black male client is admitted to the hospital with a diagnosis of left cerebral vascular accident. He has right-sided weakness, and he cannot turn or walk without using his walker and another person's assistance. He also has difficulty swallowing, and he is incontinent of urine.
   a. What risk factors, if any, for pressure ulcers does this client have?
   b. What characteristics should the nurse assess to monitor for a stage I pressure ulcer?
   c. How should this be accomplished?

Bergstrom N and others: A clinical trial of the Braden Scale for predicting pressure sore risk, *Nurs Clin North Am* 22(2):417, 1987a.

Bergstrom N and others: The Braden Scale for predicting pressure sore risk, *Nur Res* 36:205, 1987b.

Braden B, Bergstrom N. In Bryant RA, editor: *Acute and chronic wounds: nursing management,* St. Louis, 1992, Mosby.

Breslow RA and others: The importance of dietary protein in healing pressure ulcers, *J Am Geriatr Soc* 41:357, 1993.

Bryant RA and others: Pressure ulcer. In Bryant RA, editor: *Acute and chronic wounds: nursing management,* St. Louis, 1992, Mosby.

Capobianco ML, McDonald DD: Factors affecting the predictive validity of the Braden Scale, *Adv Wound Care* 9(6):32, 1996.

Ebersole P, Hess P: *Toward healthy aging: human needs and nursing response,* ed 4, St. Louis, 1994, Mosby.

Goodridge DM: Pressure ulcer risk assessment tools: what's new for gerontological nurses, *J Gerontol Nurs* 19(1):23, 1993.

Himes D: Nutritional supplements in the treatment of pressure ulcers: practical perspectives, *Adv Wound Care* 10(1):30, 1997.

Jeter KF, Lutz JB: Skin care in the frail, elderly, dependent, incontinent patient, *Adv Wound Care,* 9(1):29, 1996.

Kane RL and others: *Essentials of clinical geriatrics,* ed 3, New York, 1994, McGraw-Hill.

Konstantinides NN: Principles of nutritional support. In Bryant RA, editor: *Acute and chronic wounds: nursing management,* St. Louis, 1992, Mosby.

Kosiak M: Etiology and pathology of ischemic ulcers, *Arch Phys Med Rehabil* 40:62, 1959.

Lineaweaver W and others: Topical antimicrobial toxicity, *Arch Surg* 120:267, 1985.

Lyder CH: Examining the inclusion of ethnic minorities in pressure ulcer prediction studies, *J WOCN* 23:257, 1996.

Maklebust J, Sieggreen M: *Pressure ulcers: guidelines for prevention and nursing management,* West Dundee, Ill, 1991, S-N Publications.

Maklebust J, Sieggreen M: *Pressure ulcers: guidelines for prevention and nursing management,* ed 2, Springhouse, Pa, 1996, Springhouse.

Marchand AC, Lidowski H: Reassessment of the use of genuine sheepskin for pressure ulcer prevention and treatment, *Decubitus* 6(1):44, 1993.

Montagna W and others: Black skin—structure and function, San Diego, 1993, Academic Press.

Murphy RN: Legal and practical impact of clinical practice guidelines on nursing and medical practice, *Adv Wound Care* 9(5):31, 1996.

National Pressure Ulcer Advisory Panel: Pressure ulcers incidence, economics, risk assessment, Consensus Development Conference Statement, *Decubitus* 2(2):24, 1989.

National Pressure Ulcer Advisory Panel: Position on reverse staging of pressure ulcers, *Adv Wound Care* 8(6):32, 1995.

O'Brien JM, Reilly NJ: Comparison of tape products on skin integrity, *Adv Wound Care* 8(6):26, 1995.

Pires M, Muller A: Detection and management of early tissue pressure indicators: a pictorial essay, *Progressions* 3(3):3, 1991.

Regan MB: The use of intrasite gel in healing open sternal wounds, *Ostomy/Wound Manage* 38(3):15, 1992.

Rook JL: Wound care pain management, *Adv Wound Care* 9(6):24 1996.

Stotts NA: Predicting pressure ulcer development in surgical patients, *Heart Lung* 17(6):641, 1988.

Stotts NA: Determination of bacterial burden in wounds, NPUAP Proceedings 1995, *Adv Wound Care* 8(4):28, 1995.

Strauss EA, Margolis DJ: Malnutrition in patients with pressure ulcer: morbidity, mortality, and clinically practical assessments, *Adv Wound Care* 9(5):37, 1996.

Thomas C: Specialty beds: decision-making made easy, *Ostomy/Wound Manage* 23:51, 1989.

Trelease CC: Developing standards for wound care, *Ostomy/Wound Manage* 20:46, 1988.

Wysocki AB: Fibronectin in acute and chronic wounds, *J ET Nurs* 19:166, 1992.

Sensory Alterations

OBJECTIVES

Mastery of content in this chapter will enable the student to:

- Define the key terms listed.
- Differentiate among the processes of reception, perception, and reaction to sensory stimuli.
- Discuss common causes and effects of sensory alterations.
- Discuss common sensory changes that occur with aging.
- Identify factors to assess in determining sensory status.
- Describe behaviors indicating sensory alterations.
- Develop a care plan for clients with visual, auditory, tactile, speech, gustatory, and olfactory alterations.
- Describe nursing interventions that promote effective communication with clients who have sensory alterations.
- Describe conditions in the health care agency or client's home that can be adjusted to promote meaningful sensory stimulation.
- Discuss ways to maintain a safe environment for clients with sensory alterations.

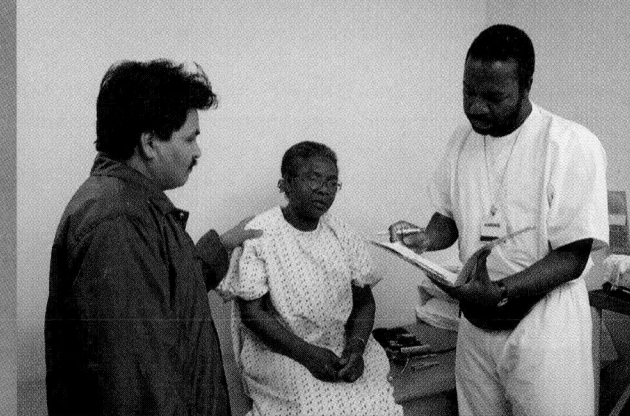

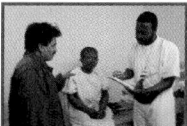
Case Study
Mrs. Alicea

Mrs. Alicea is a 73-year-old woman who is visiting the senior health center for her routine 6-month checkup. She has been visiting the senior center on a regular basis for the past 8 years. Mrs. Alicea has lived alone since her husband died 1 year ago. She lives in a small, single-story, four-room home a few miles away from the health center. Her son, Rico, lives 5 minutes away. Rico drives Mrs. Alicea to her health care visits. Six months ago, Mrs. Alicea reported a progressive hearing loss. Today, as she enters the clinic she reports, "Having trouble seeing."

Peter Morris is a 33-year-old junior nursing student assigned to the senior health center. He is learning to conduct assessments and to develop health promotion plans for visiting clients. Peter is married and has two children. For the past month, Peter has been working at the center and participating in teaching health promotion activities. He is enjoying this rotation as he is learning more about geriatric clients and recognizing that they are very independent and capable of productive lifestyles.

Part of the uniqueness of human beings is the ability to sense various stimuli caused by changes in their internal and external environment, perceive and organize those stimuli, and respond appropriately. The sense organs of sight (**visual**), hearing (**auditory**), touch (**tactile**), smell (**olfactory**), taste (**gustatory**), and balance function to produce the special senses and to initiate reflexes important for homeostasis. The body also has a **proprioceptive** sense of its position and movement in space. Meaningful stimuli from sensory organs allow a person to learn about the environment and are necessary for healthy functioning and normal development of the sensory organs. When sensory function is altered, the client's ability to relate to and function within the environment changes drastically. The nurse must understand and help to meet the needs of clients with sensory alterations, as well as recognize clients most at risk for developing sensory problems. The nurse helps clients with sensory alterations learn to react safely and effectively in their environment.

SCIENTIFIC KNOWLEDGE BASE

Normal Sensation
Normally, the nervous system continually receives thousands of bits of information from sensory nerve organs, relays the information through appropriate channels, and integrates the information into a meaningful response. The nervous system must be intact for sensory stimuli to reach appropriate brain centers and for the individual to perceive the sensation. After interpreting the significance of a sensation, the person can react to the stimulus.

Reception, perception, and reaction comprise any sensory experience (see Chapter 33). Reception begins with stimulation of a nerve cell called a *receptor,* which is usually specifically designed for only one type of stimulus. Once a nerve impulse is created, it travels along pathways to the spinal cord or directly to the brain. Sensory nerve pathways usually cross over to send stimuli to opposite sides of the brain.

The actual perception or awareness of unique sensations depends on the receiving region of the cerebral cortex, where specialized brain cells interpret the quality and nature of the sensory stimuli. When the person becomes conscious of the stimuli and receives the information, perception takes place. Perception includes an integration and interpretation of the stimuli based on the person's experiences.

A person usually reacts to stimuli that are most meaningful or significant at the time. It is impossible to react to each of the multiple stimuli entering the nervous system. The brain is normally capable of discarding or storing sensory information to prevent sensory bombardment. After continued reception of the same stimulus, however, a person stops responding, and the sensory experience goes unnoticed. This adaptability phenomenon occurs with most sensory stimuli.

The balance between sensory stimuli entering the brain and those that actually reach conscious awareness maintains a person's well-being. If an individual attempts to react to every stimulus within the environment or if the variety and quality of stimuli are lacking, sensory alterations occur.

Types of Sensory Alterations
Many factors influence the capacity to receive or perceive sensations (Box 39-1). The types of sensory alterations commonly seen by the nurse are **sensory deficits, sensory deprivation,** and **sensory overload.** When a client suffers from more than one sensory alteration, the ability to function and relate effectively within the environment is seriously impaired.

Sensory deficits. A defect in the normal function of sensory reception and perception is a sensory deficit (Box 39-2). As a result a client may not be able to receive certain stimuli (e.g., blindness, deafness) or the stimuli are distorted (e.g., blurred vision from cataracts, abnormal taste sensation from xerostomia). A sudden sensory loss such as that caused by injury or as a side effect to medications (Box 39-3) can cause fear, anger, and feelings of helplessness. The client may withdraw socially to cope with the sensory loss. The client's safety

Box 39-1
Factors That Influence Sensory Function

Age
Infants

Binocular vision begins at 6 weeks of age and is well established by 4 months. During the second year of life, the infant can discriminate shapes, objects, and colors. A neonate will initially respond generally to loud noises. Within a year the infant can locate sounds. Hearing loss in infants can occur from a variety of prenatal and postnatal conditions.

Children

Refractive errors are the most common types of visual disorders in children and can be treated with corrective lenses. More serious visual impairment affects a child's ability to play and socialize. A blind child cannot imitate others.

Adults

Visual changes during adulthood include presbyopia (inability to focus on near objects) and the need for glasses for reading (ages 40 to 50).

Older Adults

Hearing changes include decreased hearing acuity, speech intelligibility, and pitch discrimination, which is referred to as *presbycusis*.

Low-pitched sounds are heard the best, but it is difficult to hear conversation over background noise.

It is also difficult to discriminate the consonants (*f, z, s, th, ch, p, k, t,* and *g*). Vowels that have a low pitch are easier to hear. Speech sounds are garbled, and there is a delayed reception and reaction to speech.

A decrease in active sebaceous glands causes the cerumen to become dry and completely obstruct the external auditory canal (Thompson and Wilson, 1996).

Reduced visual fields, increased glare sensitivity, impaired night vision, reduced accommodation, reduced depth perception, and reduced color discrimination are also experienced by older adults. They require three times as much light to see objects as they did when they were in their twenties (Ebersole and Hess, 1994).

Older adults experience olfactory changes, including a loss of cells in the olfactory bulb of the brain and a decrease in the number of sensory cells in the nasal lining (Ebersole and Hess, 1994). This change begins around age 50. Reduced sensitivity to odors is common.

Aging causes taste buds to atrophy, to lose efficiency in relaying flavor, and to reduce in number (Ebersole and Hess, 1994). Reduced taste discrimination is common.

Proprioceptive changes include an increased difficulty with balance, spatial orientation, and coordination (age 60). Older adults cannot avoid obstacles as quickly, nor are they able to prevent an accident from happening to themselves when fast action is needed. The automatic response to protect and brace oneself when falling is slower (Ebersole and Hess, 1994).

Older adults experience tactile changes, including declining sensitivity to pain, pressure, and temperature.

Medications

Many medications cause **ototoxicity,** which may affect hearing, balance, or both. The most common symptom reported is **tinnitus.** Ototoxicity causes a progressive or continuing hearing loss. Most clients are not aware it is occurring (McKenry and Salerno, 1995).

Environment

Excessive environmental stimuli (e.g., noise from hospital equipment, staff conversation) can result in sensory overload, marked by confusion, disorientation, and inability to make decisions. Restricted environmental stimulation (e.g., bed rest and isolation) can lead to sensory deprivation. Poor quality of environment (e.g., reduced lighting, narrow walkways, background noise) can worsen sensory impairment.

Preexisting Illnesses

Peripheral vascular disease can cause reduced sensation in the extremities and impaired cognition. Chronic diabetes can cause reduced vision or blindness or peripheral neuropathy. Some neurological disorders such as stroke impair sensory reception.

Smoking

Chronic tobacco use can atrophy the taste buds and affect olfactory function.

Noise Levels

Constant exposure to high noise levels can cause hearing loss.

Box 39-2
Common Sensory Deficits

Visual

Presbyopia—A gradual decline in the ability of the lens to accommodate or to focus on close objects. Individual is unable to see near objects clearly.

Cataract—Cloudy or opaque areas in part or all of the lens that interfere with passage of light through the lens. Cataracts usually develop gradually, without pain, redness, or tearing in the eye.

Dry eyes—Result when tear glands produce too few tears. Common in older adults and resulting in itching, burning, or even reduced vision.

Open-angle glaucoma—An increase in intraocular pressure caused by an obstruction to the normal flow of aqueous humor through Schlemm's canal. Causes progressive pressure against the optic nerve, resulting in visual field loss, decreased visual acuity, and a halo effect around the eyes, if untreated.

Diabetic retinopathy—Pathological changes occur in the blood vessels of the retina resulting in decreased vision or vision loss.

Senile macular degeneration—Condition in which the macula (specialized portion of the retina responsible for central vision) loses its ability to function efficiently. First signs may include blurring of reading matter, distortion or loss of central vision, and distortion of vertical lines.

Hearing

Presbycusis—A common progressive hearing disorder in older adults.

Cerumen accumulation—Buildup of ear wax in the external auditory canal. Cerumen, which is normally absorbed in a younger person's ear, becomes hard and collects in the canal and causes a conduction deafness.

Balance

Dizziness and disequilibrium—Common condition in older adulthood, usually resulting from vestibular dysfunction. Frequently an episode of vertigo or disequilibrium is precipitated by change in position of the head to the rest of the body.

Taste

Xerostomia—Decrease in salivary production that leads to thicker mucus and a dry mouth. Can interfere with the ability to eat and leads to appetite and nutritional problems.

Neurological

Peripheral neuropathy—Disorder of the peripheral nervous system. Commonly caused in older adults by diabetes, Guillain-Barré syndrome, and neoplasms (Ebersole and Hess, 1994). Symptoms include numbness and tingling of the affected area and stumbling gait.

Stroke—Cerebrovascular accident caused by clot, hemorrhage, or emboli affecting blood vessel leading to or within the brain. Creates altered proprioception with marked incoordination and imbalance. Loss of sensation and motor function in extremities controlled by the affected area of the brain also occurs.

---

is threatened because of an inability to respond normally to stimuli in the environment. When a deficit develops gradually or when considerable time has passed since the onset of an acute sensory loss, the client learns to rely on unaffected senses. Some senses may even become more acute to compensate for an alteration. For example, a blind client often develops an acute sense of hearing. Clients with sensory deficits may change their behaviors in adaptive or maladaptive ways.

Sensory deprivation. When an inadequate quality or quantity of stimulation impairs perception, sensory deprivation occurs. A person suffers from inadequate cerebral cortical arousal. Three types of sensory deprivation (Ebersole and Hess, 1994) are reduced sensory input such as hearing loss, elimination of order or meaning from input such as that which occurs from

confusion, and restriction of the environment such as bed rest that produces monotony and boredom.

The effects of sensory deprivation can be far reaching (Box 39-4). Behaviors in children are often demonstrated by a higher-than-normal level of anxiety that leads to restlessness, difficulty with problem solving, and depression (Wong, 1995). In adults the symptoms of sensory deprivation can easily cause nurses or physicians to believe that a client is psychologically ill, confused, suffering from severe electrolyte imbalance, or under the influence of psychotropic drugs.

Sensory overload. When a person receives multiple sensory stimuli and the brain cannot perceptually disregard or selectively ignore some stimuli, sensory overload occurs. Because of the multitude of stimuli leading to overload, the person no longer perceives the

Box 39-3
Medications Reported to Cause Ototoxicity

Antibiotics
Aminoglycosides
Minocycline
Vancomycin

Diuretics
Ethacrynic acid
Furosemide
Bumetanide
Torsemide

Cardiac Drugs
Class Ia antidysrhythmics
Quinidine
Procainamide
Disopyramide

Analgesics
NSAIDs
Aspirin
Ibuprofen
Naproxen

Antineoplastic Agents
Bleomycin
Cisplatin
Dactinomycin
Mechlorethamine

From: Lilley LL, Auker R: *Pharmacology and the nursing process*, St. Louis, 1996, Mosby.

Box 39-4
Effects of Sensory Deprivation

Cognitive
Reduced capacity to learn, inability to solve problems, poor task performance, disorientation, bizarre thinking, regression

Affective
Boredom, restlessness, increased anxiety, emotional lability, increased need for physical stimulation and socialization

Perceptual
Reduced attention span, disorganized visual and motor coordination, temporary loss of color perception, disorientation, confusion of sleeping and waking states

···NURSING KNOWLEDGE BASE

A better understanding of the effects sensory changes have on individuals and the types of interventions that can minimize alterations improves the level of care clients receive. The U.S. Bureau of the Census (1990) has projected that by the year 2000, the number of persons 85 and older is expected to be 34.8 million. Because the older adult population experiences a diversity of sensory alterations, it is important for nurses to remain informed of new nursing knowledge about this population.

Chen (1994) studied the relationship of hearing loss, loneliness, and self-esteem. A significant positive relationship was found between the hearing impaired and loneliness and between hearing impairment and self-esteem. The more severe a hearing impairment, the more likely it was that an individual suffered loneliness and reduced self-esteem. Findings from this study reveal the importance for nurses to assess how a sensory deficit such as hearing loss influences the client's self-esteem and social relationships.

Blake (1993) notes that older adults, who are more functionally impaired, are at a higher risk for depressive symptoms and disorders. Visual, hearing, and tactile deficits often lead to withdrawal from social activities, which in turn can contribute to depression. The risk of depression, social isolation, and low self-esteem increases when a functional impairment interferes with the person's ability to participate in enjoyable and meaningful activities (Miller, 1994).

Nursing is concerned with not only managing the problems of clients with sensory alterations but also preventing sensory alterations. Excessive noise is a common cause of sensory overload. Heitz and others (1992)

environment in a way that makes sense. Overload prevents meaningful response by the brain, thoughts race, attention moves in many directions, and restlessness occurs. As a result, the client can demonstrate panic, confusion, aggressiveness, and combativeness. Sleep loss is common. Overload thus causes a state similar to that associated with sensory deprivation.

The acutely ill client may easily develop sensory overload. One common causative factor is noise. Add to the effects of noise the constant monitoring of clients and the nursing activities of turning, repositioning, and administering treatments; it becomes clear that critically ill clients are literally bombarded with stimuli. Some clients are more sensitive to sensory overload than others. Behavioral changes associated with sensory overload can easily be confused with mood swings or simple disorientation. The point at which stimuli become enough to tax a client's endurance changes according to level of fatigue, attitude, and physical well-being.

found that human voices were often mentioned as disturbing noises by hospitalized clients. The voices of nurses in the hallways and at the nurses' station were particularly irritating when clients wished to sleep. Clients who listened to music through earphones had less sensory stimulation and thus required less pain medication than those who did not listen to music (Heitz and others, 1992).

CRITICAL THINKING IN CLIENT CARE

Synthesis

As a nurse applies the nursing process for clients with sensory alterations, information from a variety of sources must be analyzed and integrated. The nurse learns to anticipate the kind of information needed so that good clinical judgments can be made. A combination of past client care experiences and the application of scientific and nursing knowledge assist the nurse in selecting an individualized plan of care for the client.

Knowledge. A variety of factors contribute to sensory alterations. Knowledge of those factors, the normal components of a sensory experience, and anatomy and physiology help the nurse to understand how a particular alteration affects a client's function. When nurses are able to identify the characteristics demonstrated by clients with sensory alterations and the interventions that are best suited to minimize those alterations, a comprehensive plan of care can be implemented.

Depending on the nature of the client's problem, the nurse relies on knowledge of communication principles (see Chapter 13) to select the best method to communicate and interact with clients. Clients with hearing impairment, for example, require different communication approaches to ensure a complete and accurate nursing assessment is obtained. Emotional support may be needed when caring for clients with sensory alterations.

Because a variety of medications can affect sensory function, it is also important for the nurse to have a good knowledge of pharmacology. Being able to anticipate the side effects of medications can allow the nurse to prepare clients for possible sensory changes.

Experience. Most of us have experienced some degree of alteration in sensory function either personally or in interacting with family and friends. Previous personal and clinical experiences with individuals who have had sensory alterations enable the nurse to better anticipate the type of care measures a client will require. How do individuals adapt to hearing aids and glasses? What adjustments do they make to function safely in their homes? Are different communication techniques necessary when speaking with individuals with hearing impairment? Such experiences will help the nurse incorporate successful nursing interventions when caring for clients with sensory alterations.

Attitudes. Creativity may be necessary to generate solutions to problems created by a client who experiences an alteration in sensation. A client living in a nonstimulating home environment may experience sensory deprivation. The nurse must consider different environmental changes to introduce meaningful stimuli that can induce a more normal sensory experience. Similarly, clients with sensory deficits need to make adjustments within their home environments to reduce the risk of injury. With the knowledge gained regarding how sensory alterations change sensory perception, the nurse can find creative ways to help clients make changes for a safer home setting.

Standards. Learning to adjust to sensory impairment is possible. An important ethical standard to follow when assisting clients with sensory alterations is preservation of autonomy. Autonomy means the person is reasonably independent and self-governing in decision making (see Chapter 11). For the client to regain independence, the nurse must not override autonomy with the principle of beneficence (the duty to do good for someone). Nurses need to remember that although professionals believe they know what is best the client has to live with the sensory alteration and adapt to the consequences of his or her own choices.

NURSING PROCESS

Assessment

When assessing clients with or at risk for sensory alterations, the nurse considers all factors that influence sensory function, particularly age. The nurses collects a complete history that assesses the client's current sensory status, the degree to which a sensory deficit affects the client's lifestyle, self-care ability, psychosocial adjustment, health promotion habits, and safety. The assessment must also focus on the quality and quantity of environmental stimuli.

Clients at risk. A nurse learns to include sensory assessment as a priority for clients at risk for sensory alterations. The older adult is obviously in a high-risk group because of normal physiological changes associated with aging. Older clients often underreport certain sensory changes, assuming that they are a part of aging (Ebersole and Hess, 1994).

Clients who are immobilized by bed rest, physical encumbrances (e.g., casts, traction), or chronic disability are unable to experience all the normal sensations of free movement. Such a condition can lead to sensory deprivation. The nurse remains alert for any behavioral changes common to deprivation. Another group at risk includes clients isolated in a health care setting or at home. For example, the client in isolation as a result of active tuberculosis is often restricted to a private hospital room and is unable to enjoy normal interactions with visitors.

A hospital environment is full of sensory stimuli. A healthy person can change an environment or seek a different one. As a result of illness or hospitalization, a client is often confined to an unfamiliar and unresponsive environment. This does not mean that all hospitalized clients experience sensory overload. However, the nurse must assess more carefully those clients subjected to high stress levels (e.g., ICU environment, long-term hospitalization, multiple therapies).

Sensory status.
The nursing history allows for assessment of the nature and characteristics of any sensory alteration. This includes the type and extent of sensory impairment, the onset and duration of symptoms, and whether there are factors that aggravate or relieve symptoms. Often the nurse can observe such characteristics by watching the client perform routine activities of daily living in the home or health care setting. For example, observing the client eating may reveal problems with vision. The nurse asks the client to describe the sensory deficit. For example:

Are you currently having any difficulty seeing, hearing, sensing touch, or maintaining balance?
Describe your visual/hearing loss for me.
Explain how your ability to feel things has changed.
How long have you been experiencing a visual problem?
When did you begin to feel numbness in your legs?
What factors allow you to hear conversations more easily?

Assessment of the client's self-rating for sensory deficit is also useful. Janken and Cullinan (1990) found that a client's self-rating for hearing was one of the most important defining characteristics for accurately diagnosing auditory sensory perceptual alteration. The nurse can simply ask the client, "Rate your hearing as excellent, good, fair, poor, or bad."

Client's lifestyle.
Based on a client's self-rating, the nurse may explore more fully the client's perception of a sensory loss. This provides a more in-depth look at how the client's quality of life has been influenced. The nurse can ask the client to describe any problems resulting from a sensory loss.

It is important to consider how a given sensory alteration affects the client's ability to retain social relationships, continue performing at work or school, and function within the home setting.

Socialization.
The amount and quality of contact with supportive family members or significant others determine whether a client with sensory alterations becomes isolated. The nurse assesses if a client lives alone and whether family, friends, or neighbors frequently visit. The absence of visitors to the hospital or long-term care facility creates a sense of monotony that contributes to social isolation.

The nurse needs to assess the client's social skills and level of satisfaction in the support given by family and friends. Is the client satisfied with the support made available by friends? Does the family offer support when the client requires assistance as a result of sensory loss? The long-term effects of sensory alterations can significantly influence family dynamics and a client's willingness to remain active in society.

Self-care management.
A client's functional abilities can be separated into two categories: activities of daily living (ADLs) and instrumental activities of daily living (IADLs). If a sensory alteration impairs a client's functional abilities, there are implications for planning discharge from a health care setting and in providing resources within the home. The nurse can assess self-care and functional status by gathering the following information:

Can the client with altered vision prepare a meal, bathe safely using hot water, or write a check?
Does a client's loss of balance prevent rising from a toilet seat safely or descending a row of stairs?
Can the client with diminished tactile perception button a shirt or dress?
If a client with a sensory alteration withdraws and avoids social contact, does the client retain interest in self-grooming?

The nurse considers the activities the client normally engages in for self-care and then determines to what extent the sensory alteration impairs function.

Psychosocial adjustment.
Nursing history can also reveal any recent changes in a client's behavior. Frequently family and friends are the best resources for this information. The client may be unaware of or unwilling to discuss such changes. The nurse determines if the client has displayed any recent mood swings (e.g., outbursts of anger, depression, fear, irritability). Sensory alterations may also cause changes in the client's orientation and ability to concentrate. Difficulty in communicating or avoidance of conversation can develop when clients have hearing deficits.

Health promotion practices.
It is important for the nurse to assess the daily routines clients follow in maintaining sensory function. The information learned will help determine the client's need for education or

referral to appropriate resources. The nurse asks the following questions:

What type of ear and eye care is incorporated into daily hygiene practices?

Are safety glasses or shields used for those individuals who participate in sports, recreational activities, or those who work in settings where eye injury is a possibility?

Does the client know how to properly care for eyeglasses, contact lenses, or hearing aids (see Chapter 29)?

Are the devices in proper working order?

When was the last time the client had an eye examination or hearing screening?

Environment. The client's environment can either minimize or heighten sensory alterations. In some cases the environment is the cause of the problem. The nurse assesses the quality and quantity of stimuli within the health care setting and home environment, looking for factors that pose risks or that require adjustment to ensure the client's safety.

Hazards. The home environment should be a place that is healthy, comfortable, and safe. When a client has a sensory alteration, it may become necessary to make changes in a person's home environment. The nurse must first assess the home setting for the presence of any hazards that increase the risk for injury. A home safety checklist is usually available in most home health agencies for the nurse to complete. The nature of a client's sensory alteration makes certain features of the home more hazardous than others. For example, clients with visual problems will require more changes in lighting than perhaps those with a hearing deficit. Clients with hearing deficits may require safety alarms with visual signals.

In a health care setting, the nurse should assess for any factors that create dangers to the client. For example, a client's room in the hospital should be assessed for clutter, unnecessary equipment, and obstacles in the path leading to the client's bathroom. The nurse should be sure to ask the client about any barriers or obstacles the client perceives as potentially dangerous.

Meaningful stimuli. Meaningful stimuli reduce the incidence of sensory deprivation. In the home care setting the nurse checks for bright colors, comfortable furnishings, adequate lighting, good ventilation, and clean surroundings. The nurse also observes the home environment for presence of stimuli, such as pets, family pictures, television, and a clock or calendar. In a health care setting, the nurse notes if clients have roommates or visitors. A client can also become disoriented in a barren environment that gives few signals for normal sensory perception. The presence or absence of meaningful stimuli influences alertness and the ability to participate in self-care.

Amount of stimuli. Excessive environmental stimuli can cause sensory overload. In an acute care setting, the nurse assesses the level of care required. The frequency of observations, tests, and procedures may be stressful to the client. The location of a client's room may be near repetitive or loud noises (e.g., nurses' station or supply room). There may be an abundance of equipment that creates noise in the client's room. Moreover, a roommate who persistently talks or continuously keeps lights or a television on can contribute to sensory overload. Clients in pain, traction, or restricted by a cast may also be at risk for excessive stimulation.

Communication methods. Clients with existing sensory deficits often develop alternative ways of communicating. The nurse must understand the client's method of communication to interact effectively with the client. A deaf or hearing-impaired client may read lips, use sign language, use a hearing aid, or read and write notes. The visually impaired client learns to detect voice tones and inflections to acquire the emotional tone of a conversation.

Physical examination. Clients with known or suspected sensory deficits resulting from visual and hearing losses, spinal cord injury, or peripheral neuropathies will require complete and detailed sensory examinations. Chapter 24 explains the examination approaches and techniques to use. Table 39-1 summarizes client behaviors reflecting sensory deficits.

An assessment of mental status is valuable if the nurse suspects sensory deprivation. Observation of the client during history taking, physical examination, or care can provide data that reveal key client behaviors. The nurse will observe the client's physical appearance and behavior, measure cognitive ability, and assess the client's emotional stability. The nurse should remember that factors other than sensory deprivation or overload may cause impaired perception (e.g., medications, pain, electrolyte imbalances).

Client expectations. Whenever the nurse conducts an assessment for a client's plan of care, it is necessary to also review the client's expectations. It is always important to remember that some clients enter the health care system willingly, whereas others experience confusion or unfamiliarity with health care agencies. Many clients may have a definite plan as to how they want their care delivered. In relation to clients with sensory alterations, maintaining a regimen for the care of assistive devices (e.g., glasses, hearing aids) can be important. The client may expect the nurse to either perform care or provide equipment for the client so that devices can be properly cared for regularly. Asking the client what he or she expects helps the nurse to know if special communication approaches are necessary or if the client simply wants to be treated with respect. Frequently clients may request family members or friends

TABLE 39-1
Behaviors Indicating Sensory Deficits

Behavior Indicating Deficit (Children)	Behavior Indicating Deficit (Adults)
Vision	
Self-stimulation, including eye rubbing, body rocking, sniffing or smelling, arm twirling; hitching (using legs to propel while in sitting position) instead of crawling	Poor coordination, squinting, underreaching or over-reaching for objects, persistent repositioning of objects, impaired night vision, accidental falls
Hearing	
Frightened when unfamiliar people approach, no reflex or purposeful response to sounds, failure to be awakened by loud noise, slow or absent development of speech, greater response to movement than to sound, avoidance of social interaction with other children	Blank looks, decreased attention span, lack of reaction to loud noises, increased volume of speech, positioning of head toward sound, smiling and nodding of head in approval when someone speaks, use of other means of communication such as lip reading or writing, complaints of ringing in ears
Touch	
Inability to perform developmental tasks related to grasping objects or drawing, repeated injury from handling of harmful objects (e.g., hot stove, sharp knife)	Clumsiness, overreaction or underreaction to painful stimulus, failure to respond when touched, avoidance of touch, sensation of pins and needles, numbness
Smell	
Difficult to assess until child is 6 or 7 years old, difficulty discriminating noxious odors	Failure to react to noxious or strong odor, increased body odor, increased sensitivity to odors
Taste	
Inability to tell whether food is salty or sweet, possible ingestion of strange-tasting things	Change in appetite, excessive use of seasoning and sugar, complaints about taste of food, weight change
Position Sense	
Clumsiness, extraneous movement, excessive arm swinging in those with hyperactivity or learning difficulty	Poor balance and spatial orientation, shuffling gait, reduced response to brace self when falling, more precise and deliberate movements

to be involved in their care. The nurse can begin this assessment by simply asking, "For you to feel like you are receiving the best care, what do you expect from me and the other nurses?" or "Now that I better understand what affects your ability to see/hear, what do you expect in the care we will be providing you?"

....

Successful critical thinking requires a synthesis of knowledge, experience, information gathered from clients, and critical thinking attitudes and standards. Clinical judgments require the nurse to anticipate what information is needed, to analyze the data, and to then make decisions regarding client care. The client expects competent and informed care. Peter incorporates previous knowledge and experience in providing care for Mrs. Alicea.

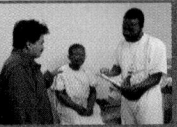

Case Study
....
Synthesis in Practice

As Peter prepares to conduct an assessment of Mrs. Alicea, he recalls what he has learned about the pathophysiology of eye disorders. The "warning signs" of eye problems is the area Peter will focus on, determining which if any of the signs Mrs. Alicea has experienced. Because Mrs. Alicea reportedly has a hearing and visual loss, Peter will consider the communication approaches best suited for conducting a successful assessment. It will be helpful for Peter to position himself so that Mrs. Alicea can see his face clearly. Peter must also speak slowly and enunciate words clearly, giving time for Mrs. Alicea to respond to questions. Avoidance of questions answered by "yes" or "no" will require Mrs. Alicea to provide more detailed answers, ensuring the questions are heard correctly.

Peter also recognizes the need to respect Mrs. Alicea's cultural background and to explore the role Rico plays in supporting his mother. Is Rico the primary individual who offers assistance with IADLs or other activities? Geissler's (1994) research of the Hispanic culture finds that the traditional clients of all socioeconomic and educational levels use biomedical and folk health systems. Family interdependence takes precedence over independence. Thus Rico may play a key role in Mrs. Alicea's ability to maintain self-care. Hispanic clients value health practitioners who are informal and friendly and who include family members in the interactions. Taking time to listen is also important. Giger and Davidhizar (1994) note that when being interviewed, Mexican Americans may engage in "small talk" before discussing the serious aspect of the interview. Providing time for small talk will often facilitate accomplishing the nurse's goal of gathering a complete assessment. Finally, Mexican Americans tend to use diplomacy and tactfulness when communicating with others. Self-disclosure is reserved for those whom the individual knows well. It will thus be important for Peter to spend time in conveying a sense of caring and respect for Mrs. Alicea to be successful with the assessment.

Peter's own grandmother has bilateral cataracts. Peter has witnessed how his grandmother has made adaptations around her home to continue activities she enjoys. Similarly, Peter has learned in class that a variety of adaptations can be made to maximize the sensory functions a client still has. Peter will plan to discover if Mrs. Alicea has made any adaptations in her home environment. Creativity will be an important attitude to exercise.

Nursing Diagnosis

After assessment, the nurse reviews all available data and looks for patterns of defining characteristics suggestive of a health problem relating to sensory alterations (see nursing diagnoses box). For example, the advanced age of a client, apathy, the client's inattentiveness during conversations, and the client's self-rating of hearing as "poor" are all defining characteristics for the nursing diagnosis *sensory/perceptual alteration, auditory* (Janken and Cullinan, 1990). The nurse validates findings to ensure accuracy of the diagnosis. For example, a colleague may be asked to examine the auditory canal or the nurse may discuss further with the client the self-rating for hearing to confirm the nursing diagnosis.

 NURSING DIAGNOSES FOR CLIENTS WITH SENSORY ALTERATIONS

Hopelessness
Injury, risk for
Self-care deficit, bathing/hygiene
Self-care deficit, dressing/grooming
Sensory/perceptual alterations, auditory, tactile, gustatory, olfactory
Social interaction, impaired
Social isolation
Thought processes, altered

The nurse determines the factor that likely causes the client's health problem. In the previous example, impacted cerumen is the etiology for the client's hearing alteration. For a client with impacted cerumen, regular irrigations of the ear canal have the potential for improving auditory perception (Thompson and Wilson, 1996). In contrast, if the client's auditory alteration was related to hearing loss from nerve deafness, nursing interventions of alternative communication methods would be more successful in minimizing the hearing impairment.

Planning

The plan of care (see care plan) depends on the nurse's assessment of the client's perception and acceptance of the sensory alteration, as well as the extent to which the client has adjusted to the sensory loss. The nurse tries to provide care that will enable the client to adapt to the health care setting and to the home. The client must actively participate in choosing therapies for the plan of care. Family members are also encouraged to assist. Clients who have sensory alterations at the time of entering a health care setting are usually most informed about how to adapt interventions to their lifestyles. The visually impaired in particular need to control whatever part of their care they can.

Priorities of care must be set with regard to the extent a sensory alteration affects a client. Safety is a top priority. The client can assist in prioritizing by choosing aspects of care that are most important. For example, the client may prefer to learn more about ways to communicate more effectively or about adaptive methods that will enable participation in a favorite hobby.

Some sensory alterations are short term. Appropriate interventions are thus likely to be only temporary. Sensory alterations such as permanent visual loss require long-term goals. Sometimes it becomes necessary for the client to make major changes in the way self-care activities, communication, and socialization are performed.

When developing a care plan, the nurse reviews all

CASE STUDY NURSING CARE PLAN

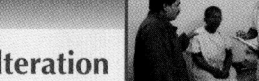

Sensory Alteration

Assessment

Mrs. Alicea comes to the clinic reporting **"having trouble seeing,"** especially with **"having a hard time judging distances between objects, which seems worse at night."** Peter spends 20 minutes speaking with Mrs. Alicea and finds the client needs to have questions repeated several times. Mrs. Alicea **cannot judge steps clearly** and has also noticed **a sensitivity to glare.** In addition, when the client tries to read or sew, her **vision is blurred even with glasses.** On physical examination, Mrs. Alicea's corneas appear opaque and there is a **reduction in accommodation.** Her external auditory canals are free from cerumen. Motor function and peripheral sensation appear intact. Mrs. Alicea reports that it has been about 2 years since she has been to an eye doctor. Peter also speaks with Rico, Mrs. Alicea's son. Peter recalls the importance of inspecting the home of a client with a sensory alteration for safety hazards. Rico has made a safety environmental check but asks Peter for any tips he has considering Mrs. Alicea's condition.

Nursing Diagnosis

Risk for injury related to visual alterations.

Planning

Goal

Client's home environment is safe and free of hazards within 4 weeks.

Expected Outcomes

Client will report a decreased difficulty with depth perception with 4 weeks.

Client and son will make recommended changes to home environment within 4 weeks.

Implementation

Steps

1. Recommend son install a nonglare work surface in the kitchen area.
2. Explain use of a pocket magnifier and offer list of locations where one can be purchased.
3. Have client make appointment with ophthalmologist within next month.

4. Teach son methods to improve environmental safety such as installation of handrails along stairs, secure carpeting, removal of throw rugs, and painting edge of stairs.
5. Recommend son install incandescent lights in the home.

Rationale

Magnifier can enlarge visual images when reading or doing close work.

Older adults should have routine eye examinations at least annually. Client is presenting symptoms of cataracts.

A decrease in visual acuity and depth perception can place the client at risk for falls in the presence of environmental hazards (Miller, 1994).

Proper illumination will improve the client's visual acuity.

Evaluation

Ask client and son to discuss changes made in the home to reduce environmental hazards.

Have client describe perception of risk for accidents in the home.

Defining characteristics are shown in bold type.

resources available to clients. The family can play a key role in providing meaningful stimulation and learning ways to help a client adjust to any limitations. Referral to resources such as occupational therapists, social service, and speech therapists ensures a multidisciplinary approach. There are also numerous community-based resources and organizations whose volunteers assist deaf, blind, and sensorially impaired clients and their families.

Implementation

Nursing interventions involve the client and family so that a safe, pleasant, and stimulating sensory environment can be maintained. Effective interventions help the client with sensory alterations to function safely with existing deficits and to continue a normal lifestyle.

Health promotion. Good sensory function begins with prevention. When clients enter primary care settings, the nurse reviews common-sense approaches for reducing risk of sensory loss.

Screening and prevention. The prevention of visual impairment in children requires appropriate screening (Wong, 1995). Three recommended interventions include screening for rubella and syphilis in women who are considering pregnancy, adequate prenatal care to prevent premature birth with the danger of exposure of the infant to excessive oxygen, and periodic screening of all children for congenital blindness and visual impairment caused by **refractive errors** and strabismus. Children should receive immunizations early for rubella (see Chapter 25).

The most common visual problem in childhood is nearsightedness. The nurse's role is one of detection and referral. Parents must know signs suggesting visual impairment (e.g., failure to react to light, reduced eye contact from the infant). Any signs should be reported to a physician immediately. School nurses usually conduct routine vision testing of school-age and adolescent children.

Trauma is a common cause of blindness in children. Penetrating injury from propulsive objects or penetrating wounds are just some examples. Parents and children require counseling on ways to avoid eye trauma. Safety equipment can be found in most sports shops and department stores.

For adults, routine screening of visual function is necessary to detect problems early. This is especially true of glaucoma, which can lead to permanent visual loss if left undetected. The American Academy of Ophthalmology (1993) recommends regular medical eye examinations every 3 to 5 years if a client is age 39 and over. Examinations should occur every 1 to 2 years if there is a family history of glaucoma, if the client is of African descent, if the client has had a serious eye injury, or if the client is taking steroid medications.

Adults are at risk for eye injury when playing sports and working in jobs involving exposure to chemicals or flying objects. The Occupational Safety and Health Administration has guidelines for safety in the workplace. Employers must have employees wear eye goggles and/ or use equipment that reduces risk of injury. Nurses play a role in reinforcing eye safety.

Hearing impairment is one of the most common disabilities in the United States. Children at risk include those with a family history of childhood hearing impairment, perinatal infection (rubella, herpes, cytomegalovirus), low birth weight, chronic ear infection, and Down syndrome. Nurses should advise pregnant women to seek early prenatal care, avoid ototoxic drugs, and seek testing for syphilis and rubella.

Children with chronic middle ear infections, a common cause of impaired hearing, should receive periodic auditory testing. Exposure to loud noise is also a risk factor for hearing loss. The nurse advises both children and parents to take precautions when involved in activities associated with high-intensity noise. Earplugs and earphones can block high-decibel sounds.

Guidelines for hearing screening for adults are variable. If a client works or lives in an environment where there is a high noise level, annual screening is recommended. The most important thing for adults to understand is to not accept hearing loss as a natural part of aging. Once a client reports a hearing loss, it is important to have regular testing.

Use of assistive aids. Health maintenance for clients with sensory deficits requires appropriate use of assistive aids and good, routine hygiene. A client who wears corrective lenses, eyeglasses, or hearing aids should make sure they are kept clean, accessible, and functional (see Chapter 29). A family member or friend should also know how to clean an assistive aid.

The greatest risk from contact lens wear is serious eye infection. Infrequent lens disinfection, contamination of lens storage cases and contact lens solutions, and use of homemade saline increases a client's risk. The nurse must reinforce proper lens care in any health maintenance discussion.

There are now a wide variety of hearing aids that enhance a person's hearing ability and can be cosmetically acceptable. Chapter 29 summarizes the care of hearing aids. A person is a candidate for a hearing aid depending on the perception of the need for hearing help, the attitude toward the hearing problem, and motivation to seek solutions (Cunningham and Ganzel, 1991). The nurse can give clients useful information on the benefits of wearing a hearing aid. Having a family member or friend support the use of the aid can improve adherence. Thompson and Wilson (1996) warn that older adults fitted with hearing aids often avoid their use in social situations because of the extraneous noise they cause or because batteries can become nonfunctional.

Promoting meaningful stimulation. The nurse can help clients make adjustments so that their

BOX 39-5
Client Teaching for Promoting Sensory Stimulation

- The effect of glare can be reduced by eliminating waxed floors and shiny surfaces exposed to bright sunlight, installing tinted glass or sheer curtains over large windows, and using soft and diffused lighting.
- Teach client to use assistive devices to improve visual acuity (e.g., pocket magnifiers, telescopic lens eyeglasses, large-print books).
- Recommend introducing brighter colors (e.g., red, orange, yellow) into the home environment so that differentiations can be made in surfaces and room objects.
- Explain that clients can maximize hearing function or minimize hearing loss through use of amplification on TVs or radios, alarm clocks that activate a flashing light, and use of recorded music in low-frequency sound.
- Instruct clients on ways to promote sense of taste through good oral hygiene, serving well-seasoned and differently textured foods, avoiding blending or mixing foods, and chewing food thoroughly.
- Recommend ways to enhance the sense of smell: sniffing food before eating, removing unpleasant odors from the environment, and introducing pleasant smells as mild room deodorizers or fragrant flowers.

environment becomes more stimulating (Box 39-5). This is best done when the nurse considers the normal physiological changes that accompany sensory deficits. For example, with aging the pupil loses the ability to adjust to light. The resultant increased sensitivity to glare can be reduced by techniques that reduce entrance of bright light into the person's living environment. Older adults often experience hearing loss from the formation of impacted cerumen, which thickens and builds up in the ear canal. Use of ear drops or local irrigation can remove hardened cerumen and improve the client's hearing. Irrigation of the canal with tepid water in a 60-ml syringe will remove cerumen. Lewis-Cullinan and Janken (1990), in a study involving 226 clients, found improvement in the hearing test scores in 75% of the ears irrigated.

Clients with reduced tactile sensation usually have the impairment over a limited portion of their bodies. The nurse can stimulate existing function by providing touch therapy. If the client is willing to be touched, hair brushing and combing, a backrub, and touching of the arms or shoulders increase tactile contact. Turning and positioning can also improve the quality of tactile sensation.

Creating a safe environment. When sensory function becomes impaired, individuals become less secure within their home and working environments. Security is necessary for a sense of independence. The nurse makes recommendations for improving safety within a client's living environment without restricting the client's independence. The nature of an actual or potential sensory loss determines the safety precautions taken.

Visual adaptations. Safety is a factor if a client has a reduction in any of the following: visual acuity, peripheral vision, adaptation to the dark, and depth perception. With reduced peripheral vision a client cannot see panoramically. Older adults with reduced adaptation to the dark require three times as much light to see objects as they did as young adults. With reduced depth perception, a person cannot see how far away objects are located.

The home safety assessment helps the nurse identify hazards within the client's living environment. Clutter such as footstools or electrical cords should be removed. Furniture should be arranged so that a client can move about easily without fear of tripping or running into objects. All flooring should be kept in good repair, and throw rugs should be removed. Stairwells should have securely fastened banisters or handrails extending the full length of the stairs.

Front and back entrances to the home and work areas must be properly lighted. Families should be encouraged to have lights with higher wattage and wider illumination installed. Fluorescent lighting should be avoided. A light switch should be located at the top and bottom of stairwells.

Driving can be a safety hazard for older adults. A sensitivity to glare can be a special problem during night driving. Reduced peripheral vision may prevent a driver from seeing a car in an adjacent lane. Reduced vision, complicated by a decrease in reaction time, reduced hearing, and decreased strength in the legs and arms, can seriously limit an older adult's driving skills. Box 39-6 summarizes driving tips for clients with visual limitations.

The inability to see visual contrast can be a problem in being able to see dials or controls on electrical appliances and equipment. Color contrasts (e.g., tape, paint, nail enamel) can be used to highlight dials. The nurse should tour the client's home to find opportunities for color coding.

Hearing adaptations. It is important for an individual to hear environmental sounds such as an alarm clock or doorbell. Such alarms can be amplified or changed to a more low-pitched, buzzerlike sound. There are also sound lamps that respond with light to the sounds of babies crying, smoke detectors, and burglar alarms. Signaling devices allow a deaf person greater independence. Family and friends who call the client regularly should learn to let the phone ring for a longer period.

Smell and tactile adaptations. A reduced sensitivity to odors means the client may be unable to smell leaking gas, a smoldering cigarette, fire, or tainted food. The client should use smoke detectors and take precautions such as checking ashtrays or placing cigarette

Box 39-6
Driving Tips for Older Adults

Drive in familiar areas
Do not drive during rush hour
Drive defensively
Avoid driving at dusk or night
Go slow, but not too slow
Keep the car in good working condition

Box 39-7
Communication Methods for the Hearing Impaired

Get the client's attention. Do not startle the client when entering the room. Do not approach a client from behind. Be sure the client knows you wish to speak.

Face the client and stand or sit on the same level. Be sure your face and lips are illuminated to promote lip reading. Do not speak with something in your mouth. Keep your hands away from your mouth.

If the client wears glasses, be sure they are clean so that your gestures and face can be seen. If the client wears a hearing aid, make sure it is in place and working.

Speak slowly and articulate clearly. Older adults may take longer to process verbal messages. Use a normal tone of voice and inflections of speech. Refrain from speaking with something in your mouth.

When you are not understood, rephrase rather than repeat the conversation.

Use visible expressions. Speak with your hands, your face, and your eyes.

Do not shout. Loud sounds are usually higher pitched and may impede hearing by accentuating vowel sounds and concealing consonants. If speaking loudly is necessary, speak in lower tones.

Talk toward the client's best or normal ear.

Use written information to enhance the spoken word.

Do not restrict a deaf client's hands. Never have intravenous lines in both of the client's hands if the preferred method of communication is sign language.

Avoid eating, chewing, or smoking while speaking.

Avoid speaking from another room or while walking away.

butts in water. The client should also learn to check dates on food packages and inspect the appearance of food.

When clients have reduced tactile sensation, caution is necessary in the use of water bottles or heating pads (see Chapter 38). The temperature on the home water heater should be no higher than 120° F.

Communication. It is important for individuals to be able to interact with people around them. Sensory deficits can create a sense of isolation. The nature of a sensory loss influences the methods and styles of communication the nurse uses.

The client with a hearing impairment can speak normally but needs family and friends to use special approaches to hear what they communicate more clearly. A deaf client can have serious speech alterations. Clients may use sign language, use lip reading, write with pad and pencil, or learn to use a computer for communication (Box 39-7).

Client instruction is an important aspect of communication. There are teaching booklets available in large print for clients with visual loss. The client who is blind may require more frequent and detailed verbal explanations. The visually impaired can also learn by listening to audiotapes or by reading booklets printed in braille. Clients with hearing impairment may benefit from written instructional materials and visual teaching aids (e.g., posters, graphs). Demonstrations by the nurse can also be helpful.

Acute care. Some clients enter acute care settings for the therapeutic management of sensory deficits (e.g., acute eye infection), and some clients in acute care settings have preexisting sensory problems. Safety is an obvious priority. It also becomes important to know the extent of any sensory impairment before the acute episode of illness so that the nurse can appropriately support self-care activities for the client.

Orientation to the environment. Clients with sensory impairments require a complete orientation to their care setting. Reorientation to the environment includes ensuring name tags on uniforms are visible, addressing the client by name, explaining the client's location (especially if clients have been transported for tests), and frequently including time and date in conversations. Short and simple repeated explanations help to reduce confusion. The nurse can encourage family and friends not to argue with or contradict a confused client but to explain calmly their location, identity, and time of day.

Clients with serious visual impairments must feel comfortable in knowing the boundaries of their environment. Normally we see physical boundaries within a room. The visually impaired touch the boundaries to make them real (Norris, 1989). The client needs to walk through a room and feel the walls to establish a sense of direction. The nurse explains objects within the room, such as chairs or equipment. The client may need to re-orient frequently with the nurse describing the location of key items (e.g., call light). It is helpful when approaching a blind client to do so from the front.

It is important to keep all objects in the same position and place. After moving an object even a short distance, it no longer exists for a blind person. Simply moving a chair can create a safety hazard. The nurse asks the client where to arrange objects so that ambulating can be easier. Traffic patterns such as to the bathroom should be kept clear.

Safety measures. The client with recent visual impairment often requires help with walking. The nurse should stand at the client's nondominant side approximately one step in front (Figure 39-1). The client uses the nondominant hand to grasp the nurse's elbow or upper arm. The nurse walks one half step ahead and slightly to the client's side. The client's shoulder should be directly behind the nurse's shoulder. The nurse describes the course of movement and ensures that obstacles have been removed. It is important to relax and walk at a comfortable pace. The nurse warns the client when approaching doorways or narrow spaces. A client with visual impairment should not be left alone in an unfamiliar area.

A visually impaired client who spends time in bed should have a call light nearby. Necessary objects such as water and facial tissue should be placed in front of the client to prevent falls caused by reaching over side rails. The nurse ensures the client's glasses are clean and easy to reach. A night-light in the room or bathroom can help reduce falls. The light reduces the time required for the eyes to adapt to the dark.

A client with a hearing impairment may have difficulty hearing the sounds that occur in a typical care setting such as an intravenous pump alarm, malfunctioning suction machine, or instructions from a visiting x-ray technician. The nurse should make more frequent visits to the bedside. Never restrict both arms of deaf or hearing-impaired clients with intravenous lines or restraints. It is wise to place notes on the intercom at the nurses' station, on the client's chart, and at the bedside if the client is hard of hearing or blind.

Controlling sensory stimuli. The nurse can reduce sensory overload by organizing the client's care plan to control excessive stimuli. Combining activities such as dressing changes, bathing, and vital sign assessment in one visit prevents the client from becoming overly fatigued. The client also needs scheduled time for rest and quiet. Coordination with laboratory and radiology departments can reduce the time needed for tests and examinations. The nurse may encourage a family member to sit quietly with a client or involve the client in an undemanding repetitive activity such as combing hair.

The nurse tries to control extraneous noise in and around a client's room, such as television volume and visitors. Routine nursing procedures should be performed as quietly as possible. Bedside equipment not in use, such as suction and oxygen equipment, should be turned off. Nursing staff should also try to control laughter or conversation at the nurses' station. Nurses should allow clients to close room doors.

In addition to controlling excess stimuli, the nurse tries to introduce meaningful stimulation. Making the environment pleasing and comfortable can go a long way in preventing or minimizing sensory alterations. Box 39-8 summarizes tips for introducing stimuli into a care environment.

Restorative care. After a client has experienced a sensory loss, it becomes important to understand the implications of the loss and to make adjustments needed to continue a normal lifestyle. Many of the interventions previously discussed under health promotion, such as adapting the environment, can be used after a client leaves an acute care setting.

Promoting self-care. A client who has undergone surgery for a sensory deficit needs specific instructions and support to return to the home environment. Most clients undergo same-day surgical procedures (see Chapter 40). Family members or friends should understand the way the client's sensory impairment will affect normal ADLs. The client's family can be more supportive when they understand sensory deficits and

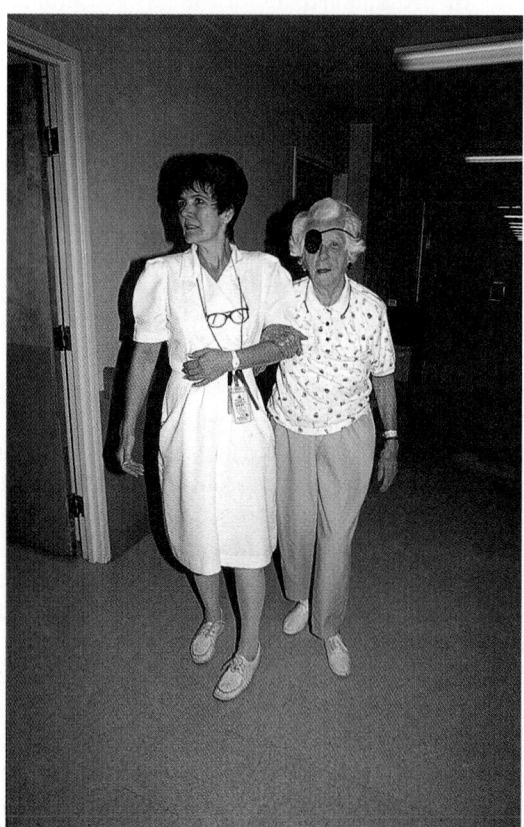

Figure 39-1. Nurse assists visually impaired client with ambulation.

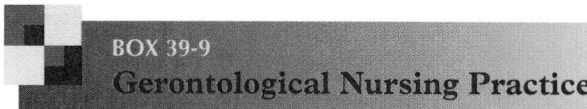

Box 39-8
Introducing Stimuli Into the Care Setting

Visual

Open the drapes to the client's room.

Raise the head of the bed and draw back dividing curtains or partitions.

Provide attractive decorations on tables or cabinets, such as fresh flowers, plants, a picture, or greeting cards.

Provide talking books and large-print reading material.

Auditory

Sit down and speak with the client. Make the conversation meaningful.

Turn on a radio with the type of music the client enjoys.

A favorite radio or television program can be stimulating.

Taste and Smell

Provide attractive, taste-appealing meals. Be sure tableware and glasses are clean. Foods meant to be served warm should be warm, and cold foods should be cold.

Provide a variety of textures, aromas, and flavors to enhance the client's appetite.

BOX 39-9
Gerontological Nursing Practice

- Assist in recommending alterations in living arrangements if physical isolation is a factor.
- Give older adults extra time to communicate.
- Assist clients in keeping contact with people important to them.
- Encourage and facilitate some socialization (Cookfair, 1996).
- Help clients acquire information about mutual help groups.
- Arrange for security escort services as needed.
- Link clients with religious organizations attuned to the social needs of older adults.
- Bring a pet into the home.

the types of factors that worsen or lessen sensory problems. There are resources within a community that provide information to assist clients with personal care needs. The American Foundation for the Blind, American National Red Cross, and National Association for Speech and Hearing are some examples.

There are a number of simple ways to help sensorially impaired clients continue independent self-care activity. A visually impaired client's meals can be set up as though food on the plate and condiments, salad, or drinks around the plate are numbers on the face of a clock. The client can become oriented to the items after the family member explains each item's location. Similarly, the client with a recent visual impairment may need assistance in arranging self-care items such as clothing, hygiene and food supplies, and utensils to continue managing daily care activities.

The client with a visual impairment needs assistance in reaching toilet facilities safely. Safety bars should be installed near the toilet. A bar that is a different color from the wall is easier to see. Towels should never be placed on safety bars to interfere with a person's grasp.

If tactile sense is decreased, the client can dress more easily with zippers or Velcro strips, pullover sweaters or blouses, and elasticized waists. If the client has a partial paralysis and reduced sensation, the affected side should be dressed first. A client may also need assistance with basic grooming such as brushing, combing, and shampooing hair.

Socialization. Interacting with others can become a burden for many clients. Asking people to continuously repeat what they say is both embarrassing and exhausting for a client with a hearing loss. Clients often lose the motivation to engage in social activities. As a person withdraws from interaction, a sense of loneliness can develop. The nurse can introduce therapies to reduce loneliness, particularly for older adult clients (Box 39-9). Family members must learn to focus on a person's ability to interact rather than the person's disability. It should not be assumed, for example, that a person who has difficulty hearing does not wish to speak.

▪ Evaluation

Client care. When caring for the client with a sensory alteration, the nurse evaluates whether care measures improve or at least maintain a client's ability to interact and function within the environment. The nurse adapts evaluation measures to the client's sensory deficit to determine whether actual outcomes are the same as expected outcomes. For example, the nurse will be sure a client with a hearing deficit can hear the nurse's queries about responses to treatment. When expected outcomes have not been achieved, there may be a need to change interventions or add new ones, such as altering the client's environment.

If nursing care has been directed at improving or maintaining sensory acuity, the nurse evaluates the integrity of the sensory organs and the client's ability to perceive stimuli. This may involve a simple vision or hearing assessment, for example, or asking the client to perform a self-care skill. When client teaching is designed to improve a client's sensory function, it is important to determine whether the client is following recommended therapies. Asking the client to explain or demonstrate a newly learned self-care skill is an effective evaluative measure.

Client expectations. It is important for the nurse to learn if the client perceives his or her care to have been satisfactorily provided. Any type of sensory deficit can be embarrassing and a threat to a person's self-image. Does the client feel comfortable in relating to the nurse, given the presence of a sensory deficit? Was the client able to maintain a regimen for care of assistive devices? Did the client perceive the nurse as exhibiting a caring, professional approach? Asking the client if nursing care successfully met his or her expectations will be valuable knowledge when the nurse cares for other clients with similar sensory problems.

sual acuity and sensitivity to glare. Son has been very supportive in making necessary home environment changes and plans to make additional ones. Client has set an appointment with ophthalmologist within next 2 weeks.

Key Terms

gustatory	**sensory deprivation**
olfactory	**sensory overload**
ototoxicity	**tactile**
proprioceptive	**tinnitus**
refractive errors	**visual**
sensory deficits	

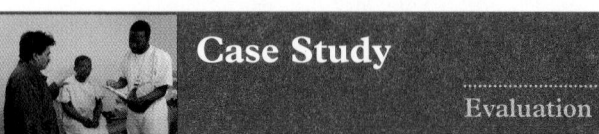

Case Study

Evaluation

One month has passed since Mrs. Alicea's last visit to the senior health care center. With Mrs. Alicea's arrival to the clinic, Peter sits down and talks with both the client and her son Rico. He learns that Mrs. Alicea is no longer having difficulty with glare, because Rico changed the lights in the house to incandescent bulbs. Rico also reports that he plans to install some sheer curtains Mrs. Alicea chose last week, to hang over the large window in the living room. Mrs. Alicea also tells Peter that Rico has made a "few changes around the house," including rearranging furniture, securing the rugs, installing a handrail to the basement, and removing extension cords. After purchasing a magnifier at a local drug store, Mrs. Alicea is able to read the newspaper more easily.

On examination, Mrs. Alicea's visual acuity continues to reveal blurring when she tried to read an informational pamphlet. Her pupils continue to respond slowly to accommodation. Peter inquires as to whether Mrs. Alicea has made an appointment with her ophthalmologist. She confirms that the appointment is scheduled within the next 2 weeks.

Overall, Mrs. Alicea confides, "I think I have been helped with the ideas we talked about last time. I feel a little better about getting around the house and doing the things I like to do." When asked if he has noticed any changes in his mother's actions, Rico states, "She seems less fearful of possibly falling."

Documentation Note
Client visited clinic this morning as scheduled. Has implemented measures at home to improve her vi-

References

American Academy of Ophthalmology: *Cataract,* San Francisco, 1993, American Academy of Ophthalmology.

Blake DG: *Depression in late life,* ed 2, St. Louis, 1993, Mosby.

Chen HL: Hearing in the elderly: relation of hearing loss, loneliness, and self-esteem, *J Gerontol Nurs* 20(6):22, 1994.

Cookfair JM: *Nursing care in the community,* ed 2, St. Louis, 1996, Mosby.

Cunningham DR, Ganzel TM: Hearing aids: how they work and whom they help, *Hosp Med* 41:71, 1991.

Ebersole P, Hess P: *Toward healthy aging,* ed 4, St. Louis, 1994, Mosby.

Geissler E: *Pocket guide to cultural assessment,* St. Louis, 1994, Mosby.

Giger JN, Davidhizar RE: *Transcultural nursing: assessment and intervention,* ed 2, St. Louis, 1995, Mosby.

Heitz L and others: Effect of music therapy in the postanesthesia care unit: a nursing intervention, *J Post Anesth Nurs* 7:22, 1992.

Janken JK, Cullinan CL: Auditory sensory/perceptual alteration: suggested revision of defining characteristics, *Nurs Diagn* 1(4):147, 1990.

Lewis-Cullinan C, Janken JK: Effect of cerumen removal on the hearing ability of geriatric patients, *J Adv Nurs* 15:594, 1990.

Lilley LL, Auker R: *Pharmacology and the nursing process,* St. Louis, 1996, Mosby.

McKenry LM, Salerno E: *Mosby's pharmacology in nursing,* ed 19, St. Louis, 1995, Mosby.

Miller CA: *Nursing care of older adults: theory and practice,* ed 2, Philadelphia, 1994, Lippincott.

Norris RM: Common sense tips for working with blind patients, *Am J Nurs* 89:360, 1989.

Thompson JM, Wilson SF: *Health assessment for nursing practice,* St. Louis, 1996, Mosby.

U.S. Bureau of the Census: *Statistical abstract of the United States,* Washington, DC, 1990, The Bureau.

Wong DL: *Whaley and Wong's nursing care of infants and children,* ed 5, St. Louis, 1995, Mosby.

▪ Key Concepts ▪▪

Sensory reception involves the stimulation of sensory nerve fibers and the transmission of impulses to higher centers within the brain.

Because a client learns to rely on unaffected senses after a sensory loss, the nurse designs interventions to preserve function of these senses.

Sensory deprivation results from an inadequate quality or quantity of sensory stimuli.

Aging results in a gradual decline of acuity in all senses.

Environmental stimuli in a hospital, such as an intensive care unit, place a client at risk for sensory overload.

The extent of support from family members and significant others can influence the quality of sensory experiences.

Assessment of sensory function includes a physical examination and measurement of functional abilities.

The presence of cerumen in the external auditory canal is a common cause of hearing loss in older adults.

A client's self-rating of hearing is an important defining characteristic for auditory sensory perceptual alteration.

Sensory losses can create loneliness and impair the ability to socialize.

An assessment of environment includes identifying hazards, sources of meaningful stimulation, and the amount of stimuli.

Prenatal screening and childhood immunization are critical in preventing sensory alterations in the newborn and child.

The care plan for clients with sensory alterations should include participation by family members.

A blind client must learn boundaries within the environment to ambulate safely.

Clients with existing sensory deficits can learn alternative ways to communicate.

Nursing care for clients with sensory alterations includes using stronger sensory stimuli, compensating with other senses, and modifying the environment to maximize remaining sensory function.

To prevent sensory overload the nurse controls stimuli, orients the client to the environment, and promotes rest by minimizing interruptions.

▪ Critical Thinking Activities ▪▪

1. Mrs. Wilson, 72 years of age, attends the clinic for regular checkups every 6 months. During a routine conversation, she states, "I am not seeing as well these days." Discuss three symptoms clients experience with aging. What strategies can you use to assist Mrs. Wilson to see better?

2. Mr. Thomas is a 72-year-old client who exhibits a blank, dull affect; a hesitancy to communicate; and a tendency to speak loudly when spoken to. Physical examination should be focused on what potential problem area for this client?

3. Mrs. Tillis lives in a two-room apartment on the second floor. During your home visit you notice there is a single light over the stairwell. The client's apartment is painted in a dull gray, with throw rugs throughout. Mrs. Tillis is 80 years of age and lives alone. What recommendations might you make to improve the safety of Mrs. Tillis' environment?

40

Surgical Client

OBJECTIVES

Mastery of content in this chapter will enable the student to:

- Define the key terms listed.
- Explain the concept of perioperative nursing care.
- Differentiate between classifications of surgery and types of anesthesia.
- List factors to include in the preoperative assessment of a surgical client.
- Design a preoperative teaching plan.
- Prepare a client for surgery.
- Explain the differences in caring for the client undergoing outpatient surgery versus the client undergoing inpatient surgery.
- Describe intraoperative factors that can affect a client's postoperative course.
- Identify factors to include in the assessment of a client in postoperative recovery.
- Describe the rationale for nursing interventions designed to prevent postoperative complications.

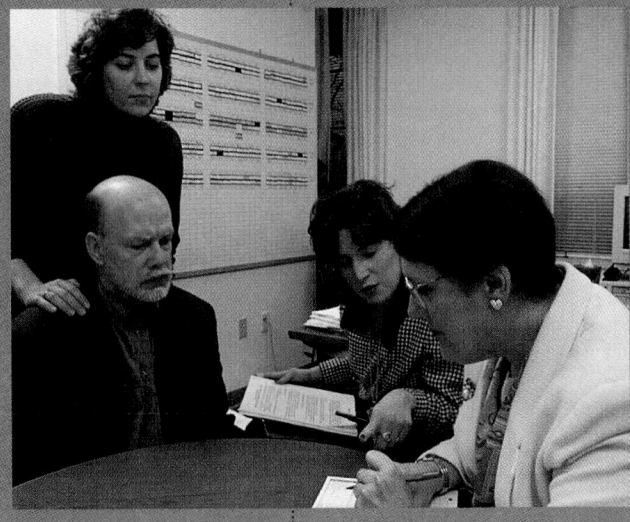

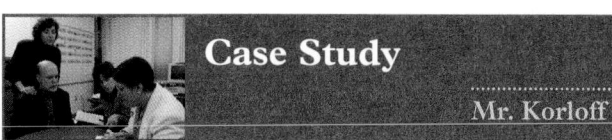

Case Study

Mr. Korloff

Mr. Korloff is a 53-year-old man who has been experiencing abdominal pain for 2 months. Following a series of diagnostic tests, he is now scheduled for an elective laparoscopic cholecystectomy. Mr. Korloff is originally from Russia and has lived in the United States for 20 years. He speaks English quite well but still has a Russian accent. He is a vice president for an international business firm. He is widowed and has two adult daughters, both of whom were born in Russia before coming to the United States. The daughters are married and live in the same neighborhood as Mr. Korloff.

Sue Collins is a nursing student assigned to the preadmission center at the local hospital where she has been working for 2 weeks. She is completing her last clinical rotation and will be graduating in 1 month. Sue is 30 years old, married, and with no children. She plans to seek employment in a hospital on a general surgery floor after graduation. Sue's father recently had surgery for prostate cancer.

Surgery is performed in a variety of settings, including hospitals, ambulatory surgery centers, clinics, physicians' offices, and even mobile units. Minor surgeries are performed on an **outpatient** basis, with the client entering the setting, undergoing surgery, and being discharged the same day. Most clients undergoing major surgery enter the setting as outpatients for preoperative screening and testing and are admitted to the hospital after surgery. Only clients requiring extensive preoperative care are admitted to the hospital before surgery. Regardless of the setting in which they work, nurses must understand the principles of caring for perioperative clients.

SCIENTIFIC KNOWLEDGE BASE

Classification of Surgery

Surgical procedures are classified according to the client's admission status, urgency, and purpose of surgery (Table 40-1). For example, a breast biopsy, done for diagnostic purposes, would be classified as urgent and done on an outpatient basis. The classification indicates to the nurse the type of preparation and care a client might require.

Surgical Risk Factors

Knowledge regarding the physiology of stress (see Chapter 21) and risk factors that may affect how a client

responds to the stress of surgery is necessary to anticipate client needs for preoperative preparation and teaching and postoperative care. A study by Brooks-Brunn (1997) identified six risk factors that have a significant association with postoperative pulmonary complications, specifically pneumonia and atelectasis. These factors include the following: age 60 or greater, impaired preoperative cognitive function, smoking history within the past 8 weeks, body mass index of 27 or greater, history of cancer, and an incision site that was either above the umbilicus or both above and below the umbilicus.

Age. Very young and older clients are at greater surgical risk as a result of an immature or a declining physiological status. Maintaining the client's normal body temperature is a concern during surgery. When compared with an adult, an infant has proportionately greater surface area and less subcutaneous fat, placing these clients at risk for wide temperature variations. In addition, general anesthetics can inhibit shivering, a protective reflex to maintain body temperature, and can cause vasodilation, which results in heat loss. During surgery, an infant also has difficulty in maintaining a normal circulatory blood volume. The total blood volume of infants is considerably less than that of older children and adults, creating a risk for both dehydration and overhydration.

With advancing age a client's physical capacity to adapt to the stress of surgery is hampered because of deterioration of certain body functions. Table 40-2 summarizes physiological factors that place older adult clients at risk for surgery.

Nutrition. Normal tissue repair and resistance to infection depend on adequate nutrition. Surgery intensifies the need for nutrients. Postoperatively, a client requires adequate calories to ensure a positive nitrogen balance (see Chapter 34). A malnourished client is prone to improper wound healing, reduced energy stores, and infection after surgery.

Obesity. An obese client usually has reduced ventilatory and cardiac function and has difficulty in resuming normal physical activity. The position required on the operating table for surgery may further limit the obese client's ventilation. A body mass index of 27 or greater significantly increases the incidence of postoperative pulmonary complications (Brooks-Brunn, 1997). To calculate the index, divide the client's weight in kilograms by the height in meters squared.

Excess weight placed on skin over bony prominences may restrict blood flow and result in skin impairment. The obese client is susceptible to poor wound healing and wound infection because of the structure of fatty tissue, which contains a poor blood supply. The fatty tissue structure slows the delivery of essential nutrients, antibodies, and enzymes needed for healing. It is also

TABLE 40-1
Examples of Classifications for Surgical Procedures

Type	Description	Example
Seriousness		
Major	Involves extensive reconstruction or alteration in body parts; poses great risks to well-being	Coronary artery bypass, colon resection, removal of larynx, resection of lung lobe
Minor	Involves minimal alteration in body parts; often designed to correct deformities	Cataract extraction, facial plastic surgery, skin graft, tooth extraction
Urgency		
Elective	Is performed on basis of client's choice; is not essential and may not be necessary for health	Bunionectomy, facial plastic surgery, hernia repair, breast reconstruction
Urgent	Is necessary for client's health, may prevent additional problems from developing	Excision of cancerous tumor, removal of gallbladder for stones, vascular repairs
Emergency	Must be done immediately to save life or preserve function of body part	Repair of perforated appendix, control of internal hemorrhaging
Purpose		
Diagnostic	Is surgical exploration that allows physician to confirm diagnosis; may involve removal of tissue for further diagnostic testing	Exploratory laparotomy (incision into peritoneal cavity to inspect abdominal organs), breast mass biopsy
Palliative	Relieves or reduces intensity of disease symptoms; will not produce cure	Colostomy, debridement of necrotic tissue, resection of nerve roots
Reconstructive	Restores function or appearance to traumatized or malfunctioning tissues	Internal fixation of fractures, scar revision
Transplant	Is performed to replace malfunctioning organs or structures	Kidney, cornea, or liver transplant; total hip replacement

often difficult to close the surgical wound of an obese client because of the thick adipose layer. The risk for dehiscence is increased because of these factors (see Chapter 38).

Radiotherapy. The client with cancer will often undergo radiotherapy before surgery to reduce the size of the cancerous tumor so it can be removed surgically. Radiation causes fibrosis and vascular scarring in the radiated area. This causes tissues to become fragile and poorly oxygenated. Ideally, the surgeon waits to perform surgery 4 to 6 weeks after the completion of radiation treatments.

Fluid and electrolyte balance. The body responds to surgery as a form of trauma. As a result of the adrenocortical stress response, hormonal reactions cause sodium and water retention and potassium loss within the first 2 to 5 days after surgery. Protein breakdown creates a negative nitrogen balance. The severity of the stress response influences the degree of fluid and electrolyte imbalance. The more extensive the surgery, the more severe the stress. Clients with preexisting renal, gastrointestinal, or cardiovascular problems are at greater risk.

Preexisting medical conditions. Previous illnesses can influence the client's ability to tolerate anesthesia and surgery and to reach full recovery (Table 40-3). Many conditions affect normal healing processes.

Allergies. Allergies to medications, topical agents used to prepare the skin for surgery, and latex can create significant risks for the surgical client. An allergic response to any agent can be potentially fatal, depending on the severity of the response. Latex allergies are on the rise. Latex is used to make a variety of medical products, including gloves. A latex allergy may be manifested as contact dermatitis with redness, inflammation, and blisters; as contact urticaria with pruritus, redness, and swelling; or as anaphylaxis (Redmond, 1996).

Medications. Prescription or over-the-counter medications may have adverse effects on the client undergoing surgery. Medications may affect cardiac and circulatory function, pulmonary function, healing and metabolic processes, and the client's ability to respond to stress (Table 40-4).

TABLE 40-2
Physiological Factors That Place Older Adult Clients at Risk for Surgery

Alterations	Risks	Nursing Implications
Cardiovascular		
Degenerative change in myocardium and valves	Reduces cardiac reserve	Assess baseline vital signs.
Rigidity of arterial walls and reduction in sympathetic and parasympathetic innervation to heart	Predisposes client to postoperative hemorrhage and rise in systolic and diastolic blood pressure	Instruct client on techniques for performing leg exercises and proper turning.
Increase in calcium and cholesterol deposits within small arteries; arterial walls thickened	Predisposes client to clot formation in lower extremities	
Pulmonary		
Rib cage stiffens and enlarges	Reduces vital capacity	Instruct client on proper technique for coughing and deep-breathing exercises.
Reduced diaphragm excursion	Greater residual capacity or volume of air left in lung after normal breath increases, reducing amount of new air brought into lungs with each inspiration	
Lung tissue less distensible; alveoli enlarged	Reduces blood oxygenation	
Renal		
Reduced blood flow to kidneys	Increases danger of shock when blood loss occurs	Determine baseline urinary output for 24 hours.
Reduced glomerular filtration rate and excretory times	Limits ability to remove drugs or toxic substances	
Reduced bladder capacity	Voiding frequency increases, and larger amount of urine stays in the bladder after voiding	Instruct client to notify nurse immediately when sensation of bladder fullness develops.
	Sensation of need to void may not occur until bladder is filled	Keep call light or bedpan within easy reach.
Neurological		
Sensory losses, including reduced tactile sense, increased pain tolerance	Client less able to respond to early warning signs of surgical complications	Orient client to surrounding environment. Observe for nonverbal signs of pain.
Decreased reaction time	Client becomes confused easily after anesthesia	
Metabolic		
Lower basal metabolic rate	Reduces total oxygen consumption	
Reduced number of red blood cells and hemoglobin levels	Reduces ability to carry adequate oxygen to tissues	Administer necessary blood products.
Change in total amounts of body potassium and water volume	Greater risk for fluid or electrolyte imbalance	Monitor electrolyte levels.

Smoking habits. The client who smokes is at a greater risk for postoperative pulmonary complications than a nonsmoker. The chronic smoker has an increased amount of thickened mucous secretions in the lungs. General anesthetics further stimulate these pulmonary secretions. The smoker has difficulty expectorating the secretions because of decreased ciliary action.

Smoke also causes local irritation to the tracheobronchial mucosa.

Alcohol and controlled substance use. Habitual use of alcohol and controlled substances predisposes the client to adverse reactions to anesthetic agents. The client also experiences a cross-tolerance

TABLE 40-3

Medical Conditions That Increase the Risks of Surgery

Type of Condition	Reason for Risk
Bleeding disorders (thrombocytopenia, hemophilia)	Disorders increase risk of hemorrhaging during and after surgery.
Diabetes mellitus	Diabetes increases susceptibility to infection, impaired wound healing, and decreased glucose tolerance. Fluctuating blood levels may cause central nervous system (CNS) malfunction during anesthesia.
Heart disease (recent myocardial infarction, dysrhythmias, congestive heart failure)	Stress of surgery causes increased demands on myocardium to maintain cardiac output. General anesthetic agents depress cardiac function.
Upper respiratory infection	Infection increases risk of respiratory complications during anesthesia (e.g., pneumonia and spasm of laryngeal muscles).
Cancer	Alters immune response and energy reserves.
Liver disease	Liver disease alters metabolism and elimination of drugs administered during surgery and impairs wound healing and clotting time because of alterations in protein metabolism.
Fever	Fever predisposes client to fluid and electrolyte imbalances and may indicate underlying infection.
Chronic respiratory disease (emphysema, bronchitis, asthma)	Respiratory disease reduces client's means to compensate for acid-base alterations. Anesthetic agents reduce respiratory function, increasing risk for severe hypoventilation.
Immunological disorders	Immunological disorders increase risk of infection and delay wound healing after surgery.
Abuse of street drugs	Persons abusing drugs may have underlying disease (human immunodeficiency virus [HIV]/hepatitis) and altered wellness, which affect healing.

TABLE 40-4

Drugs With Special Implications for the Surgical Client

Drug Class	Effects During Surgery
Antibiotics	Potentiate action of anesthetic agents
Antidysrhythmics	Can reduce cardiac contractility and impair conduction during anesthesia
Anticoagulants	Alter normal clotting factors and thus increase risk of hemorrhaging
	Should be discontinued at least 48 hours preoperatively
	Can further alter clotting mechanisms if commonly used medications (e.g., aspirin and ibuprofen) are used
Anticonvulsants	Can alter metabolism of anesthetic agents after long-term use of certain anticonvulsants (e.g., phenytoin [Dilantin] and phenobarbital)
Antihypertensives	Interact with anesthetic agents to cause bradycardia, hypotension, and impaired circulation
	Inhibit synthesis and storage of norepinephrine in sympathetic nerve endings
Corticosteroids	With prolonged use, cause adrenal atrophy, which reduces body's ability to withstand stress
	Can temporarily increase doses before and during surgery
Insulin	Diabetic client's need for insulin preoperatively is reduced because client fasts
	Can increase dose requirements postoperatively because of stress response and intravenous administration of glucose solutions
Diuretics	Potentiate electrolyte imbalances (particularly potassium) after surgery

to anesthetic drugs, necessitating higher-than-normal doses.

Cognitive function. A client with impaired cognitive function may be unable to follow instructions and participate in either preoperative teaching or postoperative care activities. A client's recovery is facilitated when the client is able to actively participate in postoperative care.

Incision Site

The pain of an abdominal incision decreases the ability of the client to maintain full lung expansion and resume activity. Pain causes the client to splint respirations and to thus breathe less deeply. Pain also limits the degree to which the client is willing to cough, which is so important in keeping the airways clear. If the abdominal incision is extensive, the client's ability to turn, position, and transfer from bedside to chair can also be slowed or limited.

NURSING KNOWLEDGE BASE

Perioperative nursing refers to the role of the nurse caring for clients during the preoperative, intraoperative, and postoperative phases of a client's surgical experience. The concept of perioperative nursing stresses the importance of providing continuity of care for the surgical client using the nursing process. In some hospitals, perioperative nurses assess a client's health status preoperatively, identify specific client needs, teach and counsel, attend to the client's needs in the operating room, and then follow the client's recovery. However, in other institutions, different nurses care for the surgical client during each phase of the surgical experience. Involving a perioperative nurse in all phases of the surgical experience ensures continuity of care for the client. The nurse's major responsibility is safe, consistent, and effective nursing care during each phase of surgery.

CRITICAL THINKING IN CLIENT CARE

Synthesis

Clients react to surgery in different ways. The perioperative nurse must be able to use critical thinking based on knowledge, previous experience, and client assessment to anticipate problems preoperatively and be prepared to aggressively intervene during surgery and postoperatively.

Knowledge. It is essential for the perioperative nurse to have a strong knowledge base in anatomy and physiology, principles of aseptic technique (see Chapter 25), pharmacology, and teaching-learning principles (see Chapter 15). Anticipation of potential complica-

tions during the perioperative experience requires the nurse to understand the effect on body systems that the procedure and drugs will have, in addition to the normal stress response. The role of the perioperative nurse in infection control is based in microbiology and knowledge of the immune system and aseptic technique. Effective **preoperative teaching** is accomplished when the nurse assesses the client's and family's readiness and ability to learn and is knowledgeable about the surgical procedure and body's responses to the stressors of surgery.

Experience. Personal experience with surgery helps the nurse to understand the anxiety of the client and family, as well as to explain some of the physical sensations that the client may experience. Previous experiences with surgical clients enable the nurse to anticipate questions that may be asked by the client and family and to help focus preoperative teaching. In addition, past experiences will help the nurse to recognize physiological changes in clients more quickly so that preventive measures can be initiated early.

Attitudes. One of the principal roles of the perioperative nurse is that of client advocate. When a client consents to surgery and receives an anesthetic agent that alters the level of consciousness, the responsibility for protection of the client is given to health care providers. The perioperative nurse is accountable to the client for maintaining the rights of the client when the client cannot speak on his or her own behalf.

Perioperative nurses must also be creative in developing plans of care that incorporate clients' individual differences. For example, positioning a client on the operating table who is obese requires an understanding of correct anatomical position and the physiology of pressure ulcer development. The perioperative nurse must assess the client and use the most appropriate padding and positioning techniques to prevent injury.

Discipline is also an important attitude when caring for surgical clients. The surgical client will experience numerous routines necessary both for preparation for surgery and for an efficient and optimal recovery. The nurse must systematically adhere to the standards of care that are established in ensuring high-quality care for the client.

Standards. The application of critical thinking intellectual standards is important for the surgical client, particularly if the client has preexisting physical or psychological factors that might influence the outcomes of surgery. The nurse must be very precise, accurate, and complete in gathering assessment data and use a logical, relevant, and deeply thought-out approach in making clinical decisions. The client's condition can change quickly, requiring the nurse to look for significant change and to respond appropriately as needed.

The Association of Operating Room Nurses (AORN) has established standards of practice for nurses practicing in the operating room. The standards cover practices that ensure safety of the client, appropriate monitoring and evaluation, infection-control practices, and timely and effective nursing interventions. The perioperative nurse is responsible for maintaining these standards (AORN, 1996).

PREOPERATIVE SURGICAL PHASE

Surgical clients enter the health care setting in different stages of health. A client may enter the facility feeling relatively healthy while awaiting elective surgery or may be in much distress when facing emergency surgery. Many tests and procedures may be needed to ensure that surgery is indicated and that the client is in optimum condition for surgery. During these tests and procedures the client meets many health care personnel, all of whom play a role in care and recovery. Family members or friends also play an important role by providing support through their presence, but they also face many of the same stressors as the client.

Clients may undergo preoperative preparation several days before the day of surgery. Preadmission testing may be done in the hospital, physician's office, or outpatient laboratory. With this testing completed, the client usually enters the hospital the day surgery is performed. Many hospitals have special outpatient or "ambulatory" surgery units, where clients come to the hospital, undergo surgery, and return home on the same day. Outpatient surgery is also performed in freestanding clinics and ambulatory surgery centers. The more traditional preoperative routine involves the client entering the hospital the day before surgery. Regardless of the method of entry into the health care setting, the nurse must be able to properly prepare the client for surgery.

The nurse's role in the preoperative surgical phase is to assess the client's physical and emotional well-being, recognize the degree of surgical risk, coordinate diagnostic tests, and identify nursing diagnoses reflecting client and family needs. This information is then used to develop and implement a plan of care to prepare the client physically, mentally, and spiritually for surgery and to communicate pertinent information to surgical team members.

NURSING PROCESS

▪ Assessment

The nurse's assessment of the surgical client establishes a normal baseline for the client and alerts the nurse to special needs and potential intraoperative and post-operative complications (e.g., infection, impaired skin integrity).

Nursing history. The nurse obtains a history with key elements that pertain to the surgical client's risks and needs. In the ambulatory surgical setting, the history may be less involved than that collected when the client is hospitalized the evening before surgery. If a client is unable to relate all the necessary information, the nurse interviews family members or significant others.

Medical history. A review of the client's medical history should include past illnesses and the primary reason for seeking medical care. Candidates for ambulatory surgery should also be screened for major medical conditions that may increase the risk for complications. If a client is at increased risk, surgery as an outpatient may not be advisable.

Previous surgeries. Past experience with surgery can reveal potential physical and psychological responses to a procedure and alert the nurse to special needs and risk factors. Complications such as anaphylaxis or **malignant hyperthermia** (see Chapter 22) during previous surgery alert the nurse to the need for preventive measures and availability of emergency equipment. A history of postoperative complications such as persistent vomiting or excessive pain alerts the nurse to the possible need for different medications. Reports of severe anxiety before a previous surgery may identify the need for additional emotional support and preoperative teaching.

Medication history. The nurse will review whether the client is taking any medications that might predispose him or her to surgical complications. If a client regularly uses prescription or over-the-counter medications, the physician may decide to temporarily discontinue the drugs before surgery or adjust the dosages. Clients should be instructed to ask the physician if they should take their usual medications the morning of surgery. If the client is undergoing inpatient surgery, all prescription drugs taken before surgery are automatically discontinued after surgery unless reordered.

Allergies. If one or more allergies exist, the client receives an allergy identification band to be worn during the surgery and until the client is discharged. The nurse also makes sure that the front of the client's chart has an allergy alert label listing all allergies. A client must be carefully screened for a previous latex allergy.

Smoking habits. The client who smokes is at a greater risk for postoperative pulmonary complications than a nonsmoker. After surgery, the client will have greater difficulty clearing the airways of mucous secretions and is at increased risk for **laryngospasm.** The nurse will use this information to plan aggressive postoperative pulmonary hygiene.

Alcohol and controlled substance use. The surgical team must be aware of the use of alcohol and controlled substances by clients to be prepared for adverse reactions, such as withdrawal, that may occur during surgery. The physician and nurse must also be alert for an increased need for postoperative analgesics.

Client expectations. It is important to identify the client's and family's perceptions and expectations regarding surgery, recovery, and the nursing and medical staff. This information provides the nurse with information to plan interventions for teaching and emotional preparation, as well as provides the basis for evaluation of care. For example, clients may have expectations regarding pain control and the use of pain medications. Clients prepared to experience pain and taught the proper use of pain-relief measures require less medication (Meeker, 1994).

Clients and family members may often have misconceptions about surgery. It is important to discuss with them their understanding of the purpose of the tests, the possible outcomes, and the persons responsible for informing them of results and providing follow-up care.

The nurse faces an ethical dilemma when a client is unaware of the real reason for surgery. The nurse should confer with the physician before revealing specific information related to the medical diagnosis to prevent confusion and to alert the physician that clarification may be needed. When a client is well prepared and knows what to expect, the nurse reinforces the client's knowledge.

Family support. The nurse determines the extent of the client's support from family members or friends. Surgery often results in temporary disability that often requires direct care and assistance from significant others during recovery. The client cannot always immediately assume the same level of physical activity and often returns home with dressings to change or exercises to perform. The nurse needs to determine the client's home environment and factors that may interfere with postoperative restrictions or care activities.

Occupation. Surgery may result in physical alterations that hinder or prevent a person from returning to work. The nurse assesses the client's occupational history to anticipate the effects surgery might have on convalescence and eventual work performance. This prepares the nurse to explain any restrictions the client may have when returning to work. When a client is unable to return to a previous line of work, the nurse may refer the client to a social worker to obtain knowledge of job-training programs or help in seeking economic assistance.

Feelings. Surgery causes anxiety for most clients. They often feel that they have little control over the situation. The family may be concerned about the ability of the client to return to a productive life and the impact recovery will have on the family.

The nurse may be able to detect the client's feelings about having surgery from both verbal and nonverbal cues. A client who is fearful may ask many questions or be very quiet, may seem uneasy when strangers enter the room, or may actively seek the company of friends and relatives.

It is often difficult to assess feelings thoroughly when ambulatory surgery is scheduled. The nurse usually has limited time for establishing a relationship with the client. In most outpatient surgical programs, the nurse telephones the client at home before surgery or interviews the client during a preadmission testing visit. For hospital inpatients, the nurse should choose a time for discussion after preliminary admitting or diagnostic tests have been completed. The nurse explains it is normal to have fears and concerns. The client's ability to share these feelings depends in part on the nurse's willingness to ask questions, listen, be supportive, and clarify misconceptions.

Cultural factors. Cultural differences in the use of both verbal and nonverbal communication require the nurse to validate interpretation of cues with the client and family. This is especially important after the nurse conducts the initial preoperative assessment and then looks for changes in the client's status after surgery. For example, clients from Asian cultures may remain silent out of respect, not fear, and individuals from Central and South America are used to having many family members and friends surrounding them and helping to express their needs.

Response to the stress of surgery may differ among cultures, particularly depending on their locus of control. Individuals who believe a relationship exists between actions and outcomes have an internal locus of control and thus act to influence future behaviors and situations (Giger and Davidhizar, 1995). Such individuals will be more likely to respond to preoperative instruction and take steps to be active in the recovery process. Individuals who believe efforts and outcomes are unrelated have an external locus of control and view the future as the result of chance or fate. Such individuals might have little motivation to participate in postoperative recovery activities. Those cultures that subscribe to an external locus of control tend to be fatalistic and may include Mexican Americans, Appalachians, and Puerto Ricans (Giger and Davidhizar, 1995). Whites and blacks are believed to fall within both the internal and external locus-of-control orientations. Some American Indians, Chinese Americans, and Japanese Americans are more or less in harmony with nature and have beliefs that fall outside the locus-of-control concept.

Coping resources. Assessment of feelings and self-concept helps to reveal whether the client has the ability to cope with the stress of surgery. It is also valuable to ask the client about stress management. If the client has had previous surgery, the nurse determines the behaviors that helped to resolve past tension or nervousness, including reliance on support from family. The nurse may instruct the client on relaxation exercises (see Chapter 33), which can help to control anxiety.

Body image. Surgical removal of a diseased tissue often leaves permanent disfigurement or alteration in body function. Concern over mutilation, change in sexuality, or loss of a body part compounds a client's fears. Individuals react differently, depending on age, culture, occupation, self-image, and degree of self-esteem.

The nurse should encourage clients to express concerns. The client facing even temporary disability or sexual dysfunction requires understanding and support. Discussions about sexuality, for example, should be held with the client's sexual partner so he or she can gain a shared understanding of how to cope with limitations in sexual function.

Physical examination.

The nurse conducts a partial or complete physical examination (see Chapter 24), depending on the setting and nature of the surgery. The assessment focuses on findings related to the client's medical history and on body systems that will be affected by anesthesia and surgery.

General survey. Gestures and body movements may reflect energy or weakness caused by illness. Height and body weight are important indicators of nutritional status and are used to calculate medication dosages. Preoperative assessment of vital signs provides a baseline with which to compare alterations that occur during and after surgery. Anesthetic agents typically depress all vital functions; however, adverse drug reactions may include elevations in heart rate and blood pressure. Preoperative assessment of vital signs is also important in ruling out fluid and electrolyte abnormalities (see Chapter 31).

An elevated temperature is cause for concern. If the client has an underlying infection, surgery may be postponed until the infection has been treated. An elevated body temperature also alters drug metabolism and increases the risk of fluid and electrolyte imbalance.

Head and neck. The condition of oral mucous membranes reveals the level of hydration. Dehydration increases the risk for the development of serious fluid and electrolye imbalances during surgery. During the oral examination, loose or capped teeth must be identified because they can become dislodged during endotracheal intubation. Dentures must be noted so that they can be protected from loss or damage.

Inspection of the soft palate and nasal sinuses can reveal sinus drainage indicative of respiratory or sinus infection. To rule out the possibility of local or systemic infection, the nurse palpates for cervical lymph node enlargement. The nurse also inspects the jugular veins for distention. Excess fluid within the circulatory system or failure of the heart to contract efficiently may lead to jugular vein distention. A client with heart disease is at risk for cardiovascular complications during surgery.

Integument. The nurse carefully inspects the client's skin overlying all body parts, especially bony prominences. During surgery a client must lie in a fixed position, often for several hours. If the client's skin shows signs of pressure over bony prominences, the nurse must be sure he or she is not positioned over that area. A client is suceptible to skin breakdown if the skin is thin, dry, or has poor turgor (see Chapter 38).

Thorax and lungs. A decline in ventilatory function, assessed through breathing pattern and chest excursion, may place the client at risk for respiratory complications. Serious pulmonary congestion may cause postponement of surgery. Narrowing of the airways, as occurs with chronic obstructive pulmonary disease and identified by the presence of wheezing on auscultation of the lungs, would increase the risk of airway obstruction because of bronchospasm related to endotracheal intubation and anesthesia (Brooks-Brunn, 1995).

Heart and vascular system. If the client has heart disease, assessment of the apical pulse is important. After surgery the nurse will compare the rate and rhythm of the pulse with preoperative baselines.

Assessment of peripheral pulses and the color and temperature of extremities is particularly important for the client undergoing vascular surgery, surgery on an extremity using a tourniquet, or when constricting bandages or casts will be applied to an extremity after surgery. Postoperative color changes, change in sensation, or development of a weak or absent pulse in a client who had adequate circulation before surgery indicates impaired circulation. Prior vascular surgery with implanted grafts, such as arteriovenous shunts for hemodialysis, should be noted to plan for modified surgical positioning.

Abdomen. Alteration in gastrointestinal function after surgery may result in decreased or absent bowel sounds and distention. The nurse should know whether the client is simply obese or the abdomen has become distended. Assessment of preoperative bowel sounds and normal elimination pattern is useful as a baseline. If surgery requires manipulation of portions of the gastrointestinal tract or if a general anesthetic is used, normal peristalsis may not return and bowel sounds will be absent or diminished for several days.

Neurological status. A client's level of consciousness will change as a result of general anesthesia. However, after the effects of anesthesia disappear, the client should return to the preoperative level of responsiveness.

Spinal or epidural anesthesia causes temporary paralysis of the lower extremities. The nurse should be aware of preexisting weakness or impaired mobility of the lower extremities to avoid becoming alarmed when full motor function does not return immediately after the procedure.

Risk factors.

Various conditions and factors increase the risk for physical problems during surgery. Knowledge of risk factors (see p. 1147) will enable the nurse to take necessary precautions in planning care.

Diagnostic screening. Before a client has surgery, diagnostic tests are ordered to screen for preexisting abnormalities. Clients scheduled for elective surgery undergo these tests as an outpatient on or before the morning of surgery. If tests reveal severe problems, the surgeon or anesthesiologist may cancel surgery until the condition is stabilized.

The nurse is responsible for coordinating the completion of tests and for verifying that the client is prepared properly. The nurse also reviews diagnostic results as they become available, alerting physicians to findings and planning appropriate therapy.

Screening tests depend on the condition of the client and the nature of the surgery. However, routine screening tests may include a complete blood count (CBC), serum electrolyte analysis, coagulation studies, serum creatinine test, blood type and cross-match, urinalysis, a 12-lead electrocardiogram, and a chest x-ray study (Table 40-5).

Complete blood count. A CBC is an analysis of a peripheral venous blood specimen that measures red blood cell count, white blood cell count, platelet count, hemoglobin concentration, and hematocrit. An abnormal CBC may indicate many alterations (e.g., anemia, blood coagulation alterations) that place the client at risk for cardiovascular and pulmonary complications or infection. The etiology of the abnormality must be identified and may require treatment before surgery.

Serum electrolyte analysis. Analysis of serum electrolyte levels (see Chapter 31) also requires the collection of a peripheral venous blood sample. Because of the potential for fluid and electrolyte imbalances during and after surgery, the surgeon screens preoperative electrolyte levels to determine whether electrolyte replacement is necessary preoperatively.

Coagulation study. The ability of blood to clot or coagulate is essential to minimize the risk of hemorrhaging. Prothrombin time (PT), partial thromboplastin time (PTT), and platelet counts are routine tests for clotting ability. Coagulation studies allow the nurse and physician to identify clients at risk for bleeding tendencies and thrombus formation.

Serum creatinine test. A serum creatinine test assesses renal function. Creatinine is the by-product of muscle metabolism. The body excretes a constant amount of creatinine through the kidneys, which is an excellent measure of the glomerular filtration rate. A rise in creatinine level can be a sensitive indicator of renal failure.

Urinalysis. Analysis of a urine specimen consists of screening for urinary tract infection, renal disease, and diabetes mellitus. The nurse assists the client in collecting a clean voided specimen (see Chapter 35). The urinalysis measures urine color, pH, and specific gravity. It also determines the presence of protein, glucose, ketones, and blood.

Chest x-ray study. A chest x-ray examination allows the physician to examine the condition of the heart and lungs before surgery. The x-ray reveals the overall size and shape of the heart, presence of lung lesions and chest wall abnormalities, and position of the diaphragm and aorta. If abnormalities are detected, surgery may be postponed until the condition is stabilized or different types and dosages of anesthetic agents may be used.

Type and cross-match. If the client is at risk for intraoperative blood loss, the physician orders a blood specimen for type and cross-matching. This test enables the laboratory to determine blood type and prepare blood products to match the client's blood. The surgeon orders the number and form of blood units to have available during surgery. An option frequently used for elective surgery is for the client to donate blood in advance of surgery. The client can then receive his or her own autologous blood, if replacement is necessary (see Chapter 31).

Additional screening tests. If a client is over age 40 or has heart disease, an electrocardiogram (ECG) is ordered. It involves the painless application of electrodes to the chest and extremities. An ECG measures the heart's electrical activity to determine whether heart rate and rhythm and other factors are normal. Depending on the type of surgery, a variety of additional diagnostic tests for specific anatomical structures and physiological functions may be ordered.

TABLE 40-5
Common Laboratory Test Values

Test	Normal Values*
Sodium (Na)	136-145 mEq/L
Potassium (K)	3.5-5.0 mEq/L
Chloride (Cl)	90-110 mEq/L
Bicarbonate (CO)	22-26 mEq/L
Creatinine	0.7-1.5 mg/dl
Hemoglobin (Hgb)	12-18 g/dl
Hematocrit (Hct)	37%-52%
Prothrombin time (PT)	11.0-12.5 seconds
Partial thromboplastin time (PTT)	30-40 seconds
Platelet count	150,000-400,000/mm

From Pagana KD, Pagana TJ: *Diagnostic testing and nursing implications: a case study approach*, ed 4, St. Louis, 1994, Mosby.
*Normal ranges vary slightly among laboratories.

Successful critical thinking requires a synthesis of knowledge, experience, information gathered from clients, and critical thinking attitudes and standards. Clinical judgments require the nurse to anticipate what information is needed, to analyze the data, and to then make decisions regarding client care. The client expects competent and informed care. Sue incorporates previous knowledge and experience in providing care for Mr. Korloff.

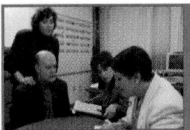

Case Study

Synthesis in Practice

As Sue prepares to conduct the preadmission assessment of Mr. Korloff, she will recall what she has learned regarding risk factors for clients undergoing surgery. Mr. Korloff has had a history of heart disease in the past, according to the referral note. Five years ago he was treated for a cardiac dysrhythmia but has had no further problems. Sue will plan to question Mr. Korloff thoroughly about any potential cardiac symptoms.

Sue's knowledge of laparoscopic surgery will help her anticipate the types of postoperative problems Mr. Korloff is likely to develop, such as food intolerance and abdominal or referred pain from the carbon dioxide gas used during laparoscopy. Sue's knowledge regarding family dynamics, particularly within the Russian culture, will assist her in assessing the level of involvement of Mr. Korloff's daughters in his preparation and care. Russian Americans typically have strong family ties and values. The father usually plays a primary role in the function of the family. It will be important to assess Mr. Korloff's opinions about surgery first and then work to include the family.

Sue's experience with her own father after surgery will help her to explain some of the sensations that Mr. Korloff can expect, such as a sore throat from the endotracheal tube used for administering anesthesia. She will also need to draw on her experiences with clients she cared for after laparoscopic cholecystectomies during her previous rotation on a general surgery floor. She will be able to inform Mr. Korloff and his daughters that he will have intravenous fluids infusing until he is able to tolerate oral fluids and that he will likely experience only mild discomfort. Mr. Korloff will be able to get out of bed the evening of surgery, and if all goes well he will likely be discharged the next day.

▪ Nursing Diagnosis

The nurse clusters defining characteristics gathered during assessment to identify nursing diagnoses and related factors for the client and family (see nursing diagnosis box). The diagnoses establish direction for care that will be provided during one or all surgical phases. For example, a client's restlessness, poor eye contact, and expressed concern about the results of surgery in-

■ NURSING DIAGNOSES FOR THE PREOPERATIVE CLIENT

Airway clearance, ineffective
Anxiety
Coping, ineffective family: compromised
Coping, ineffective individual
Decisional conflict
Fear
Fluid volume deficit
Hopelessness
Knowledge deficit
Nutrition, altered: less than body requirements
Nutrition, altered: more than body requirements
Powerlessness
Role performance, altered
Skin integrity, impaired, risk for
Sleep pattern disturbance

dicate the diagnosis of *anxiety*. However, the assessment must be validated to avoid misdiagnosis. In the assessment above, restlessness may also indicate pain.

A diagnosis and its related factors provide the nurse with direction toward specific interventions likely to be effective. The related factors must be accurate to avoid inappropriate interventions. For example, *anxiety related to knowledge deficit of perioperative routines* will require the nurse to offer thorough instruction preoperatively and immediately postoperatively. However, *anxiety related to threat of altered role performance* will require counseling and coaching during postoperative recovery. If the threat is real, a social worker may be necessary.

Preoperatively, nursing diagnoses may focus on the intraoperative and postoperative risks a client may face. Preventive care is essential to manage the surgical client effectively. The nature and type of surgery, as well as the client's health status, suggest defining characteristics for many nursing diagnoses.

▪ Planning

It is essential to include the client, family, and primary care giver before surgery. Involving the client early minimizes surgical risks and postoperative complications. Structured preoperative teaching reduces the amount of anesthesia and postoperative pain medication needed, decreases the occurrence of postoperative urinary retention, promotes an earlier return to normal oral intake, and decreases length of hospital stay (Meeker, 1994). Clients informed about the surgical experience are less likely to be fearful and are able to prepare for expected outcomes.

For the ambulatory surgical client, the preoperative planning phase usually occurs in the outpatient surgery setting before or on the morning of surgery. Ideally, it begins in the home. This gives the client time to think about the surgical experience, make necessary physical preparations (e.g., altering diet or discontinuing medication use), and ask questions about postoperative procedures. Well-planned, preoperative care ensures the client is well informed and able to actively participate during recovery. The family or significant others may also play an active supportive role for the client.

Planning may also require referral to other members of the health care team. Clients who will require aggressive pulmonary rehabilitation, such as those undergoing thoracic surgery, may be referred to a respiratory therapist. Many clients and their families benefit from referral to a chaplain, particularly when a child is undergoing surgery or the procedure is an emergency or is life threatening.

The plan of care begins in the preoperative phase and is modified during the intraoperative and postoperative phases (see care plan on p. 1158). The goals of preoperative care include understanding the physiological and psychological responses to surgery, understanding intraoperative and postoperative events, and remaining free of surgical wound infection. Outcomes established for each goal of care provide behavioral targets to gauge the client's progress.

▪ Implementation

Preoperative nursing interventions provide the client with an understanding of surgery and prepare the client physically and psychologically for the surgical intervention.

Informed consent. A surgeon cannot legally perform surgery or an anesthesiologist cannot administer an anesthetic until a client understands the need for the procedure and the steps involved, risks, expected results, and alternative treatments. Chapter 12 summarizes issues and guidelines for informed consent. All consent forms must be signed before the nurse administers preoperative medications. Ideally, a surgeon obtains consent before a client is admitted to the hospital or ambulatory surgery center.

Health promotion. Health promotion activities during the preoperative phase focus on prevention of complications, health maintenance, and rehabilitation.

Preoperative teaching. Structured preoperative teaching has proven benefits (Lindeman and VanAernam, 1971; Oetker-Black, 1993; Roach and others, 1995). Preoperative teaching provided in a structured format using teaching and learning principles has a positive influence on clients' recovery. Structured teaching can influence postoperative factors such as the following:

1. *Ventilatory function.* Teaching improves the ability to cough and deep breathe effectively.
2. *Physical functional capacity.* Teaching improves the ability to ambulate and resume activities of daily living.

3. *Sense of well-being.* Clients who are prepared for surgery experience less anxiety and report a greater sense of psychological well-being.
4. *Length of hospital stay.* Structured preoperative teaching can reduce the client's length of hospital stay.
5. *Anxiety about pain and amount of pain medication needed for comfort.* Clients who learn about pain and ways to relieve it are less anxious about the pain, ask for what they need, and actually require less pain medication.

The most effective type of teaching program for surgical clients is planned, so all clients receive the same information (Lindeman and VanAernam, 1971). This is made easier by a flow sheet that outlines the standards for preoperative preparation. Today, because many clients are not admitted to the hospital before surgery, preoperative teaching may occur in the home, physician's office, or preadmission unit (Graham and others, 1996). Printed literature and videotapes are made available to clients. Preoperatively, nurses may call clients the evening before surgery to clarify questions.

Including family members and significant others in preoperative preparation is valuable. They are frequently the coaches for postoperative exercises when the client returns from surgery. If family members and significant others do not understand routine postoperative events, their anxiety can increase and heighten the client's fears or concerns. Their misunderstanding and anxiety can be reduced with thoughtful preparation. However, if the client does not wish them to be included, the request for privacy should be respected.

Timing. Preoperative teaching is best when initiated the week before admission and reinforced immediately before surgery. Teaching performed when the client is less anxious will result in more effective learning. Anxiety and fear are barriers to learning. The nurse assesses the surgical client's readiness and ability to learn (see Chapter 15). If the client is capable and receptive to learning, the nurse presents information in a logical sequence beginning with preoperative events and advancing to intraoperative and postoperative routines. Preoperative teaching checklists give nurses useful guidelines for presenting clients with comprehensive instructions.

Content. Preoperative teaching should include information to assist the client, family, and significant others to prepare for the surgical experience and participate in the plan of care. The nurse should first assess their level of understanding about the surgery, perioperative routines, and expectations and then provide the information discussed in the following sections:

Surgical procedure. After the surgeon has explained the basic purpose of the surgical procedure and its steps, the client may ask the nurse additional questions. The nurse is careful to avoid saying anything that

CASE STUDY NURSING CARE PLAN

Surgery

Assessment

As Mr. Korloff enters the preadmission center for his testing, Sue greets him and his daughters. She explains the need to gather a history and asks Mr. Korloff if he wishes to have his daughters join him. He smiles and says, "Yes, my daughters will be my nurses for a few days." Sue asks Mr. Korloff what he has been told regarding the preoperative procedures and postoperative recovery. Mr. Korloff **states that he knows very little about the surgery.** His doctor explained that the procedure is safe, but he knows few specifics. He **asks if he will have an intravenous line, where his daughters can wait, and if he will be awake during the surgery.** The nursing staff report that **Mr. Korloff's daughters have been calling on the phone and asking many questions about intraoperative and postoperative events.**

Nursing Diagnosis

Knowledge deficit regarding implications of surgery (cholecystectomy) related to first surgical experience and inadequate preparation.

Planning

Goal

Client will understand intraoperative and postoperative events before the day of surgery.

Expected Outcomes

Client and his daughters will describe events that commonly occur in the holding area and operating room on the day before surgery.

Client and his daughters will describe routine postoperative nursing procedures on the day of admission.

Client and his daughters will describe ways to participate in postoperative care on the day of admission.

Implementation

Steps

1. Send Mr. Korloff a copy of the teaching booklet *Your Surgical Experience.* Arrange time to call at home and answer any questions on booklet's content.

2. Provide planned teaching session for Mr. Korloff and his daughters after preadmission testing. Explain events that will occur in holding area (e.g., insertion of intravenous line and vital sign check) and in operating room (e.g., positioning and anesthesia). Use visual aids to assist Mr. Korloff's understanding of the laparoscopic procedure.

3. Provide planned teaching session on day of admission with Mr. Korloff and his daughters to explain common events that occur after surgery and demonstrate postoperative exercises included in the teaching booklet.

Rationale

Clients who are prepared for surgery experience less anxiety and report a greater sense of psychological well-being (Meeker, 1994).

Teaching focused on information client will need to know on morning of admission will decrease anxiety and allow client and family to better participate in care (Meeker, 1994).

Preoperative teaching improves client's ability to ambulate, participate in care activities, and resume activities of daily living after surgery. Demonstration is an effective method in teaching psychomotor skills (Meeker, 1994).

Evaluation

Ask Mr. Korloff and his daughters to identify the basic purpose of the surgery and changes to expect afterward.

Ask Mr. Korloff and his daughters to identify routine types of postoperative monitoring and treatment.

Ask Mr. Korloff to state the most frightening aspect of surgery for him.

Have Mr. Korloff perform postoperative exercises.

Defining characteristics are shown in bold type.

contradicts the surgeon's explanation. One way to avoid contradictions is to first ask what the client has been told. If the client has little or no understanding about the surgery, the nurse refers the client back to the surgeon for additional information.

Preoperative routines. Certain preoperative routines are expected and should be explained to the client and family. Any diagnostic tests that remain to be done should be completed. For example, the client may need to have a chest x-ray. Knowing what tests are planned will increase the client's sense of control.

The anesthesiologist will visit with the client to complete a preanesthesia assessment. The client and family need to know about this visit, so that the family can plan to be present if they have questions or are needed to provide additional information.

The client and family must understand that the client can have no oral intake (either food or liquids) for approximately 4 to 8 hours before surgery, unless explicitly specified by the anesthesiologist or surgeon. During the use of general anesthesia, the muscles relax and gastric contents can reflux into the esophagus. The anesthetic eliminates the client's ability to gag. Therefore the client is at risk for aspiration of food or fluids from the stomach into the lungs. The physician's orders will provide further guidance for routines to be explained to the client (e.g., intravenous therapy, preoperative medications, insertion of a urinary catheter).

Intraoperative routines. The scheduled operative time is only an anticipated time, because other surgeries may be scheduled first. Unanticipated delays may occur for many unharmful reasons. It must be emphasized that this time is a rough estimate, and the actual time could be much longer. Family members should be told where to wait and be informed that the surgeon will speak to them when the surgery has been completed. Excessive delays are communicated to the family.

Postoperative routines. The client and family want to know about postoperative events. If they understand routine postoperative vital sign monitoring, they are less likely to worry when nurses perform these assessments. The nurse can also explain if the client is to have intravenous lines, dressings, or drainage tubes. It is important to neither overprepare nor underprepare the client and family. The nurse cannot predict all of the client's requirements, and a client may be misinformed about a therapy that may not be initiated. Contradictions between the nurse's explanations and reality can cause anxiety.

Some hospitals use CareMaps or critical paths (Figure 40-1) as a plan for the anticipated sequence of postoperative events. These maps are helpful teaching aids, because they indicate the expected postoperative course following a specific surgery.

Sensory preparation. The nurse should provide the client with information about sensations typically experienced before, during, and after surgery. Prepara-tory information helps clients anticipate the steps of a procedure and form a realistic image of the surgical experience. When events occur as predicted, the client is better able to cope and attend to the experiences. For example, the operating room is very bright. A cuff for a noninvasive blood pressure monitor will be applied to the client's arm. This monitor may make a hum and a beep, and the cuff tightens around the client's arm. Informing the client about these and other sensations in the operating room will reduce anxiety before the client is anesthetized, which will help to decrease the amount of anesthetic needed for induction. Other postoperative sensations the nurse describes include blurred vision from ophthalmic ointment, dryness of the mouth or the sensation of a sore throat resulting from an endotracheal tube, pain at the incision site, tightness of the dressings, and feeling cold.

Pain relief. One of the surgical client's greatest fears is pain. The family is also concerned for the client's comfort. Preoperative preparation regarding pain and pain control can help the client to cope with the pain. Patient-controlled analgesia (PCA) is commonly used and provides the client with control over pain. The client needs to know how to operate the pump and the importance of administering medication as soon as pain becomes persistent (see Chapter 33). Analgesics will not provide adequate pain relief if the client waits until the pain becomes excruciating before using or requesting an analgesic. The nurse should encourage the client to use analgesics as needed and not be fearful of any dependence.

If epidural, intramuscular, or oral analgesics will be used, the client needs to know the schedule for these drugs. The client should be encouraged to inform nurses as soon as pain becomes a persistent discomfort. The client should also know it takes time for a drug to act and that all the discomfort will rarely be eliminated. The nurse also informs the client and family of other therapies available for pain relief.

Postoperative exercises.

Every preoperative teaching program includes explanation and demonstration of the five postoperative exercises: diaphragmatic breathing, incentive spirometry, controlled coughing, turning, and leg exercises (Skill 40-1).

Diaphragmatic breathing improves lung expansion and oxygen delivery without using excess energy. The client learns to use the diaphragm during deep breathing to take slow, deep, and relaxed breaths. Eventually the client's lung volume improves. Deep breathing also helps to clear any anesthetic gases from the airways.

To facilitate deep breathing the physician often orders an incentive spirometer for the client (see Chapter 30). Incentive spirometry encourages forced inspiration. The therapy is effective in preventing atelectasis postoperatively. Incentive spirometry helps to reinflate collapsed alveoli and remove secretions.

BARNES	**CARE PATH® 540** **TOTAL MASTECTOMY WITH** **MALIGNANCY WITHOUT CC**

SERVICE		PHYSICIAN	
PRIMARY NURSE		PRIMARY NURSE	
DC DATE	ADM DATE	DATE OF SURGERY	**A-8**

Problem Number	PATIENT PROBLEMS / NURSING DIAGNOSES
#1	ALTERATION IN COMFORT
#2	ALTERATION IN COPING
#3	ALTERATION IN SELF-CONCEPT
#4	LACK OF KNOWLEDGE

#	1, 2	2, 3	1	1, 3	1
	ASSESSMENT / MONITORING	CONSULTS	PROCEDURES / TEST	TREATMENT	ACTIVITY
DAY 1 DOS	VS q 4 hrs x1 x2 x3 x4 x5 x6 I & O Pain Control Dressing / JP patency and drainage Ability to void Circulation Emotional response / family coping	Social Work		JP to bulb suction Incentive Spirometer / TCDB Avoid trauma to extremity	Up with assist to bathroom in PM
DAY 2 POD 1	VS q 8 hrs. if stable x1 x2 x3 I & O Pain Control Dressing / JP patency and drainage **Voiding without difficulty** Circulation Emotional response / family coping	Social Work visit Reach to Recovery		JP to bulb suction **Uses Incentive Spirometer** **independently** Avoid trauma to extremity	Up as tolerated with assist if needed

SIGNATURE	INIT.	SIGNATURE	INIT.	SIGNATURE	INIT.

540

1

Figure 40-1. Portion of care path for total mastectomy with malignancy. (Courtesy Barnes-Jewish Hospital, St. Louis, Mo.)

	1	3, 4	2, 3, 4	2, 3	
MEDS / IVS	NUTRITION	PATIENT / FAMILY EDUCATION	DISCHARGE PLANNING	PSYCHOSOCIAL/ EMOTIONAL/ SPIRITUAL NEEDS	INITIALS (SEE KEY AT BOTTOM)
IVF IM Analgesics Antibiotic if ordered	Clear liquid. Advance as tolerated to diet as prior to admission	Nursing: Pain control Positioning / mobility TCDB Incentive Spirometer Diet IV JP Primary Nursing	**Pt./family verbalizes understanding of Care Path.** **Plan of care has been mutually set with pt./family.**		
DC IVF when tolerating PO well DC IM analgesics Start oral analgesics **Pain controlled with oral analgesics**	**Tolerating diet as prior to admission**	Social Work: Assess resource needs Initiate education re: dx, prosthesis, support groups Nursing: Arm protection S/S infection BSE	Social Work: Complete high risk screening	Social Work: Assess counseling needs Initiate support Nursing: Therapeutic emotional care	

BARNES CARE PATH® 540 TOTAL MASTECTOMY WITH MALIGNANCY WITHOUT CC — 2 — A-8

PATIENT PROBLEMS / NURSING DIAGNOSES

Figure 40-1, cont'd   Portion of care path for total mastectomy with malignancy.

Teaching Postoperative Exercises

Delegation Considerations
The skill of teaching postoperative exercises requires problem solving and knowledge application unique to a professional nurse. Unlicensed assistive personnel can reinforce and assist clients to perform postoperative exercises.

Equipment
- Pillow (optional; used to splint surgical incision when coughing)
- Incentive spirometer
- Elastic stocking or sequential compression stockings

STEPS	RATIONALE
1. Assess client's risk for postoperative respiratory complications: identify presence of chronic pulmonary condition (e.g., emphysema or asthma); any condition that affects chest wall movement, such as obesity or abdominal or thoracic surgery; history of smoking; and presence of reduced hemoglobin.	With general anesthesia lungs are not fully inflated during surgery; cough reflex is suppressed, and mucus collects within airway passages. Postoperatively, inadequate lung expansion can increase risk for atelectasis and pneumonia if chronic lung conditions are present. Smoking damages ciliary clearance and increases mucus secretion. A reduced hemoglobin level can lead to reduced oxygen delivery.

CRITICAL DECISION POINT
Observe and report to physician if client has had a cold or upper respiratory infection within past week.

2. Assess client's ability to cough and deep breathe by placing hand on client's abdomen, having client take a deep breath, and observing movement of shoulders, chest wall, and abdomen. Measure chest excursion during a deep breath. Ask client to cough after taking a deep breath.	Reveals maximum potential for chest expansion and ability to cough forcefully; serves as baseline to measure client's ability to perform exercises postoperatively. Diaphragmatic breathing allows for lung expansion and improved ventilation and increases blood oxygenation. Coughing loosens secretions and removes the secretions from the pulmonary alveoli.
3. Assess client's risk for postoperative thrombus formation (elderly, immobilized clients are most at risk). Observe for a positive Homans' sign (which may or may not be present) by monitoring calf pain when dorsiflexing the client's foot with the knee flexed. Observed for calf pain, redness, swelling, or vein distention.	Following general anesthesia, circulation is slowed, and when rate of blood flow is slowed, there is a greater tendency for clot formation. Immobilization results in decreased muscular contraction in lower extremities, which promotes venous stasis.

CRITICAL DECISION POINT
If calf tenderness is present, notify the physician and do not manipulate the extremity any further. Antiembolism stockings or pneumatic compression cuffs may be ordered.

4. Assess client's ability to move independently while in bed.	Clients confined to bed rest, even for limited periods, will need to turn regularly. Determines existence of any mobility restrictions.
5. Assess client's willingness and capability to learn exercises; note factors such as attention span, anxiety, level of consciousness, and language level.	Ability to learn depends on readiness, ability, and learning environment.

STEPS	RATIONALE

6. Assess family members' or significant other's willingness to learn and to support client postoperatively.

Family member or significant other can coach clients on exercise performance.

7. Assess client's medical orders preoperatively and postoperatively.

May require adaptations in way exercises are performed.

8. Teach diaphragmatic breathing:

  a. If possible, assist client to a comfortable semi-Fowler's or high Fowler's position with knees flexed. If client chooses to sit, assist to side of bed or to upright position in chair.

Upright position facilitates diaphragmatic excursion.

  b. Stand or sit facing client.

Client will be able to observe breathing exercises performed by nurse.

  c. Instruct client to place palms of hands across from each other, down, and along lower borders of anterior rib cage; place tips of third fingers lightly together (see illustration). Demonstrate for client.

Position of hands allows client to feel movement of chest and abdomen as diaphragm descends and lungs inside chest wall expand.

  d. Have client take slow, deep breaths, inhaling through nose, and pushing abdomen against hands. Tell client to feel middle fingers separate as client inhales. Explain that client will feel normal downward movement of diaphragm during inspiration. Explain that abdominal organs descend and chest wall expands. Demonstrate for client.

Slow, deep breaths prevent panting or hyperventilation. Inhaling through nose warms, humidifies, and filters air. Explanation and demonstration focus on normal ventilatory movement of chest wall. Client learns to understand how diaphragmatic breathing feels.

  e. Avoid using chest and shoulders while inhaling, and instruct client in same manner.

Using auxiliary chest and shoulder muscles during breathing increases useless energy expenditures and does not promote full lung expansion.

  f. Take a slow, deep breath and hold for count of 3, and then slowly exhale through mouth as if blowing out a candle (pursed lips). Explain that client will feel middle fingertips touch as chest wall contracts.

Allows for gradual expulsion of air.

Continued

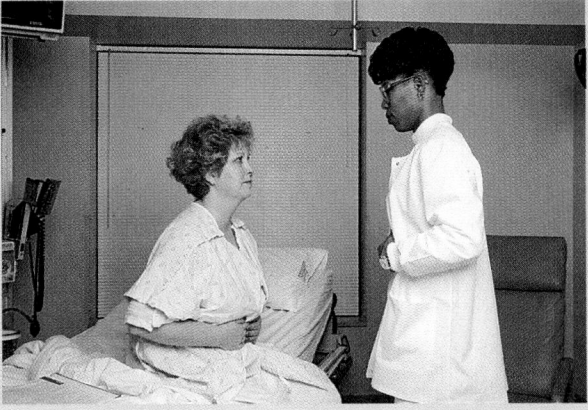

Step 8c

.... **Skill 40-1—cont'd**
Teaching Postoperative Exercises

STEPS	RATIONALE
g. Repeat breathing exercise three to five times.	Allows client to observe slow, rhythmical breathing pattern.
h. Have client practice exercise. Client is instructed to take 10 slow, deep breaths every 2 hours while awake during postoperative period until mobile.	Repetition of exercise reinforces learning. Regular deep breathing will prevent postoperative complications.
9. Teach incentive spirometry:	
a. Wash hands.	Reduces transmission of microorganisms.
b. Instruct client to assume semi-Fowler's or high Fowler's position.	Promotes optimal lung expansion during respiratory maneuver.

CRITICAL DECISION POINT

Client can usually be positioned upright with head of bed elevated postoperatively. If client must remain flat in bed, stress that exercises can still be performed.

c. Demonstrate to client how to place mouthpiece so that lips completely cover mouthpiece (see illustration).	Demonstration is reliable technique for teaching psychomotor skill and enables client to ask questions.
d. Instruct client to inhale slowly and maintain constant flow through unit. When maximal inspiration is reached, client should hold breath for 2 to 3 seconds and then exhale slowly. Number of breaths should not exceed 10 to 12 per minute (Dettenmeier, 1992).	Maintains maximal inspiration and reduces risk of progressive collapse of individual alveoli. Slow breathing prevents or minimizes pain from sudden pressure changes in chest (Dettenmeier, 1992).
e. Instruct client to breathe normally for short period.	Prevents hyperventilation and fatigue.
f. Have client repeat maneuver until goals are achieved.	Ensures correct use of spirometer.
g. Wash hands.	Reduces transmission of microorganisms.

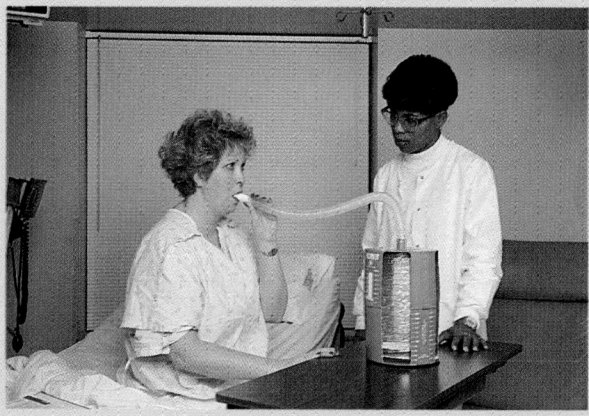

Step 9c

STEPS	RATIONALE
10. Teach controlled coughing:	
a. Explain importance of maintaining an upright position.	Position facilitates diaphragm excursion and enhances thorax expansion.
b. Demonstrate coughing. Take two slow, deep breaths, inhaling through nose and exhaling through mouth.	Deep breaths expand lungs fully so that air moves behind mucus and facilitates effects of coughing.
c. Inhale deeply a third time and hold breath to count of 3. Cough fully for two to three consecutive coughs without inhaling between coughs. (Tell client to push all air out of lungs.)	Consecutive coughs help remove mucus more effectively and completely than one forceful cough.

CRITICAL DECISION POINT

Coughing may be contraindicated after brain, spinal, or eye surgery.

d. Caution client against just clearing throat instead of coughing. Explain that coughing will not cause injury to incision.	Clearing throat does not remove mucus from deeper airways. Postoperative incisional pain makes it harder to cough effectively.
e. If surgical incision is to be either abdominal or thoracic, teach client to place pillow over incisional area and place hands over pillow to splint incision. During breathing and coughing exercises, press gently against incisional area for splinting or support.	Surgical incision cuts through muscles, tissues, and nerve endings. Deep breathing and coughing exercises place additional stress on suture line and cause discomfort. Splinting incision with hands or pillow provides firm support and reduces incisional pulling.
f. Client continues to practice coughing exercises, splinting imaginary incision. The client is instructed to cough two to three times every 2 hours while awake.	Value of deep coughing with splinting is stressed to effectively expectorate mucus with minimal discomfort.
g. Instruct client to examine sputum for consistency, odor, amount, and color changes.	Sputum consistency, odor, amount, and color changes may indicate the presence of a pulmonary complication such as pneumonia.

CRITICAL DECISION POINT

For clients with preexisting pulmonary disease, know the character of sputum.

11. Teach turning:	
a. Instruct client to assume supine position toward right side of bed.	Positioning begins on right side of bed so that turning to left side will not cause client to roll toward bed's edge.
b. Have client place the left hand over incisional area to splint it.	Splinting incision supports and minimizes pulling on suture line during turning.
c. Instruct client to keep left leg straight and flex right knee up and over left leg.	Straight leg stabilizes the client's position. Flexed right leg shifts weight for easier turning.

CRITICAL DECISION POINT

Clients who have had back surgery or vascular repair may be restricted from flexing their legs or turning or may need assistance for positioning.

Continued

Teaching Postoperative Exercises

STEPS	RATIONALE
d. Have client grab left side rail with right hand, pull toward left, and roll onto left side.	Pulling toward side rail reduces effort needed for turning.
e. Instruct client to turn every 2 hours while awake.	Reduces risk of vascular and pulmonary complications.
12. Teach leg exercises:	
a. Have client assume supine position in bed. Demonstrate leg exercises by performing passive range-of-motion exercises and simultaneously explaining exercise.	Provides normal anatomical position of lower extremities.

CRITICAL DECISION POINT

If client's surgery involves one or both extremities or if vascular alteration is present, surgeon must order leg exercises in postoperative period.

b. Rotate each ankle in complete circle. Instruct client to draw imaginary circles with big toe. Repeat five times.	Leg exercises maintain joint mobility and promote venous return.
c. Alternate dorsiflexion and plantar flexion by moving both feet up and down. Direct client to feel calf muscles contract and relax alternately (see illustration).	Stretches and contracts gastrocnemius muscles.
d. Client continues leg exercises by alternately flexing and extending knees. Repeat five times (see illustration).	Contracts muscles of upper legs and maintains knee mobility.
e. Client alternately raises each leg straight up from bed surface, keeping legs straight. Repeat five times.	Promotes contraction and relaxation of quadriceps muscles.
f. Have client continue to practice exercises at least every 2 hours while awake. Client is instructed to coordinate turning and leg exercises with diaphragmatic breathing, incentive spirometry, and coughing exercises.	Repetition of exercise sequence reinforces learning. Establishes routine for exercises that develops habit for performance. Sequence of exercises should be leg exercises, turning, breathing, and coughing.

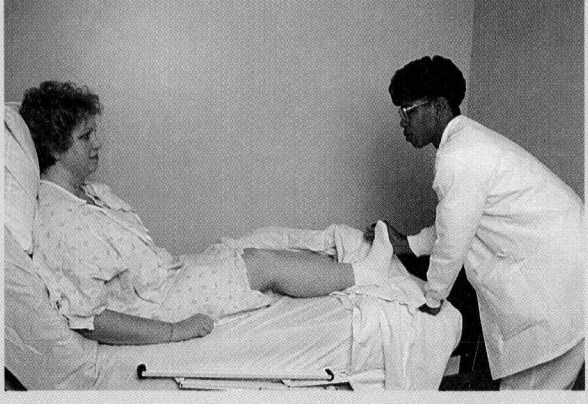

Step 12c

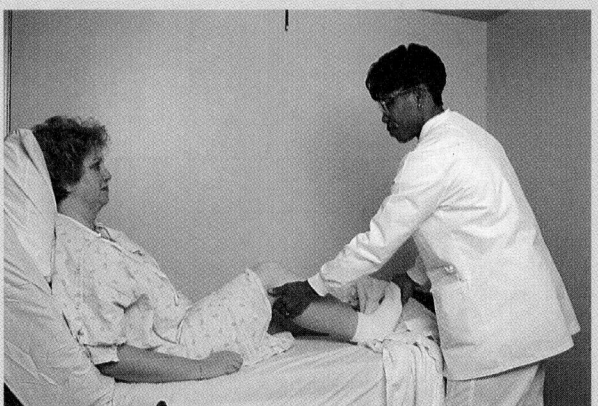

Step 12d

STEPS	RATIONALE
13. Observe client performing all four exercises independently.	Provides opportunity for practice and return demonstration of exercises. Ensures client has learned correct technique.
14. Observe family members' or significant other's ability to coach client.	Family member or significant other can assist positively or interfere with correct technique.
15. Evaluate client's chest excursion.	Determines degree of lung expansion.
16. Auscultate client's lungs.	Breath sounds reveal if airways are clear.
17. Assess for Homans' sign.	Negative sign indicates no venous thrombosis.

Recording and Reporting

- Record which exercises have been demonstrated to client and whether client can perform exercises independently or not.
- Record physical assessment findings in nurse's notes or flow sheet.
- Report any problems client has in practicing exercises to nurse assigned to client on next shift.

Home Care Considerations

- Client who practice exercises in the home will not have an incentive spirometer available. Focus on this portion of instruction once the client enters the surgical waiting area, before any analgesia or preanesthetic is given.

Coughing assists in removing retained mucus in the airways. A deep, productive cough is more beneficial than merely clearing the throat. The client must anticipate postoperative discomfort and understand the importance of coughing, even when it is difficult. The nurse also teaches the client to splint an abdominal incision to minimize pain during coughing. Nurses direct clients to cough and deep breathe at least every hour while awake until ambulating frequently (Brooks-Brunn, 1995).

Leg exercises and turning improve blood flow to the extremities and thus reduce stasis and the potential for clot formation and subsequent pulmonary emboli. Contraction of lower leg muscles promotes venous return, making it difficult for clots to form. Turning also helps to mobilize pulmonary secretions and increases ventilation and perfusion to the lungs (Brooks-Brunn, 1995). The nurse encourages the client to perform leg exercises and turn at least every 2 hours while awake.

After explaining each exercise, the nurse demonstrates it. The nurse then acts as a coach, guiding the client through each exercise.

Activity resumption. The type of surgery a client undergoes affects the speed with which normal physical activity and regular eating habits can be resumed. The nurse explains that it is normal for the client to progress gradually in activity and eating. If the client tolerates activity and diet well, activity levels will progress more quickly.

Promotion of nutrition. The surgical client is vulnerable to fluid and electrolyte imbalances as a result of inadequate preoperative intake, excessive fluid losses during surgery, and the stress response. A client usually takes nothing by mouth after midnight before the morning of surgery to reduce risks of vomiting and aspirating emesis during surgery. The nurse should instruct the client to eat and drink sufficient amounts before fasting to ensure adequate fluid and nutrition intake. The client's diet should include foods high in protein, with sufficient amounts of carbohydrates, fat, and vitamins. The nurse instructs the client and family members regarding preoperative fasting requirements and oral medication use. The nurse notifies the surgeon and anesthesiologist as soon as possible if the client eats or drinks during the fasting period.

For hospitalized clients, all fluids and solid foods are removed from the client's bedside and a sign is posted over the bed to alert hospital personnel and family members about fasting restrictions. The nurse instructs the client to rinse the mouth with water or mouthwash and brush the teeth as long as no water is swallowed. Oral medications may be taken with sips of water if ordered by the physician. The dietary department should be notified to cancel meals.

A client who is at home the evening before surgery must understand the importance of not taking food or fluids and be willing to follow restrictions.

Promotion of rest. Rest is essential for normal healing. Anxiety about surgery can easily interfere with the ability to relax or sleep. The underlying condition necessitating surgery may be painful, further impairing rest.

The client may feel like part of an assembly line during the preoperative surgical phase. Frequent visits by staff members, diagnostic testing, and physical preparation for surgery consume a large amount of time, and the client has few opportunities to reflect on events. The nurse makes sure that the client feels like an individual. The client and family need time to express feelings about surgery either together or separately. The client's level of anxiety influences the frequency of discussions, and the nurse encourages expression of these concerns.

The nurse should attempt to make the client's environment quiet and comfortable. Frequently, the physician orders a sedative-hypnotic or antianxiety agent for the night before surgery. Sedative-hypnotics (e.g., flurazepam [Dalmane]) affect and promote sleep. Antianxiety agents (e.g., alprazolam [Xanax] and diazepam [Valium]) act on the cerebral cortex and limbic system to relieve anxiety.

An advantage to ambulatory surgery or same-day surgical admissions is that the client is able to sleep at home the night before surgery. The client will probably get more rest in a familiar environment.

Acute care.

The degree of preoperative physical preparation depends on the client's health status, the surgery to be performed, and the surgeon's preferences. A seriously ill client will receive more supportive care than the client facing a less serious elective procedure.

Minimize risk of surgical wound infection. The risk of developing a surgical wound infection is determined by the amount and type of microorganisms contaminating a wound, susceptibility of the host, and condition of the wound at the end of the operation. All three factors interact, determining the risk for infection.

The skin is a favorite site for microorganisms to grow and multiply. Without proper skin preparation, the risk of postoperative wound infection is high. Bathing with an antimicrobial soap (e.g., chlorhexidine) the evening before surgery is believed to effectively reduce the incidence of postoperative wound infections (Larsen, 1993). Some physicians may order clients to bathe or shower more than once, whereas others may have clients give special attention to cleansing the proposed operative site. If the surgical procedure involves the head, neck, or upper chest area, the client may also be required to shampoo the hair. Frequently, skin preparation includes hair removal from the surgical site. This is done as close to the time of surgery as possible (AORN, 1996).

Prevention of bowel incontinence and contamination. The client may receive a bowel preparation if surgery involves the lower gastrointestinal system. Ma-

nipulation of portions of the gastrointestinal tract during surgery results in absence of peristalsis for 24 hours and sometimes longer. Enemas and cathartics cleanse the gastrointestinal tract to prevent postoperative constipation or incontinence during surgery. An empty bowel reduces risk of injury to the intestines and minimizes contamination of the operative wound in case a portion of the bowel is incised or opened. Chapter 36 summarizes enema administration.

Interventions on day of surgery. On the morning of surgery the nurse completes the routine procedures discussed in the following sections before releasing the client for surgery.

Documentation. Before the client goes to the operating room, the nurse checks the medical record to be sure all pertinent laboratory and test results are present. The nurse checks all consent forms for completeness and accuracy of information. A preoperative checklist (Figure 40-2) provides guidelines for ensuring completion of all nursing interventions. The nurse also checks the nurse's notes to be sure documentation is current. This is especially important if the client experienced unpredicted problems the night before surgery.

Assessment of vital signs. The nurse makes a final assessment of vital signs. If the preoperative vital signs are abnormal, surgery may need to be postponed. Therefore the nurse notifies the physician of abnormalities before sending the client to surgery.

Hygiene. Basic hygiene measures remove skin contamination and increase the client's comfort. If the client is unwilling to take a complete bath, a partial bath is refreshing and removes irritating secretions or drainage from the skin. Because the client cannot wear personal nightwear to the operating room, the nurse provides a clean hospital gown and instructs the client to remove all other articles of clothing, including undergarments. After having nothing by mouth throughout the night, the client usually has a very dry mouth. The nurse may offer mouthwash and toothpaste, again cautioning the client not to swallow water.

Preparation of hair and removal of cosmetics. During surgery the anesthesiologist positions the client's head to put an endotracheal tube into the airway (see Chapter 30). This may involve manipulation of the hair and scalp. To avoid injury, the nurse asks the client to remove hairpins or clips. Clients should also remove hairpieces or wigs. Long hair can be braided. The client will be asked to wear a disposable hat to contain hair before entering the operating room.

During and after surgery the anesthesiologist and nurses assess skin and mucous membranes to determine the client's level of oxygenation and circulation. A pulse oximeter is usually applied to a finger to monitor oxygen saturation of the blood. For these reasons, all makeup (lipstick, powder, blush, and nail polish) and artificial fingernails should be removed to expose normal skin and nail coloring. Anything in or around the

A-1c PREOPERATIVE/PREPROCEDURAL CHECKLIST

● File with other A-1c's of same date. ●

PROCEDURE: _____

DATE OF PROCEDURE: _____

1. Place initials in appropriate box: YES, NO, N/A (not applicable, or was not ordered). Each item must have an entry.
2. Explain any "No." This can be done in the space after the item or in the "Comments" section. Use back of form, if needed.
3. To give more information on any item, use the space after the item. If more space needed, use the "Comments" section or back of form.

DATE

HOSP. NO.

NAME

BIRTHDATE

ADDRESS

IF NOT IMPRINTED, PLEASE PRINT DATE, HOSP. NO., NAME AND LOCATION

YES	NO	N/A	
			Special Information (e.g., blind, O₂, combative)
			Preoperative orders written.
			(If "NO", Dr. _____ notified at _____ date/time.)
			Consent complete and in medical record.
			Allergies (or NKA) labelled on cover of medical record.
			Specify Allergies:
			Isolation label on cover of medical record. Specify type:
			Ordered lab results in medical record.
			Urinalysis results in medical record.
			Chest x-ray completed. (Report in medical record: Yes ___ No ___)
			EKG in medical record.
			Type and cross/screen (circle) done. Date drawn:
			History and physical in medical record.
			Forms complete and in medical record:
			1. Nursing documentation with assessment, VS, and wt./ht.
			2. IV Solution Administration Cardex.
			3. Medication Administration Cardex.
			Addressograph plate on cover of medical record. All volumes to procedure, if required.

COMMENTS:

			Blood band on patient and legible. Specify location ___ and blood band # ___
			Identification band on patient and legible. Specify location:
			Bathed and in proper attire.
			Nail polish, makeup, and hairpins removed.
			Jewelry removed. Specify item(s) removed and disposition:
			Prosthesis removed: hearing aid, dentures, eye glasses, contact lenses (circle).
			Other: Disposition:
			Anti-embolism stockings on.
			Sequential compression device sleeves on and controller to OR.
			NPO since:
			Teaching completed and documented.
			Preps/tests completed as ordered. Specify:
			Voided/catheterized (circle). Time:
			Medication(s) given.
			Medication(s)/article(s) sent with patient. Specify:

COMMENTS:

Date	Initials	Signature and Title of Individuals Filling Out Form
Date	Initials	Signature of RN Sending Patient to Procedure

41006/4-93/H7528   **THE UNIVERSITY OF IOWA HOSPITALS AND CLINICS**

Side tabs: A 1c / B CLIN. NOTES / C LABORATORY / D X-RAY EXAM / E CONSULTATION / F SPEC. EXAM / G THERAPY / H PATHOLOGY / I DIAGNOSIS

Figure 40-2. Preoperative/preprocedural checklist. (Courtesy University of Iowa Hospitals and Clinics, Iowa City, Iowa.)

eye may irritate or injure the eye during surgery. Therefore contact lenses, false eyelashes, and eye makeup must also be removed. Glasses usually remain in the room or are given to the family immediately before the client enters the operating room.

Removal of prostheses. It is easy for any type of prosthetic device to become lost or damaged during surgery. The client must remove for safekeeping all removable prosthetics. If the client has a brace or splint, the nurse checks with the physician to determine whether it should remain with the client, to be reapplied after surgery.

Although hearing aids, dentures, and eyeglasses must be removed, this should not be done until immediately before the client is taken to surgery. Allowing the client to wear these aids facilitates communication and increases the client's sense of control. The nurse should refer to the institution's policies for clarification.

Having dentures in place provides a better seal for ventilation during intubation in the operating room. Therefore in some settings, dentures are left in place until after the first stages of anesthesia. For many clients, removing dentures is embarrassing. Therefore if the dentures are to be removed before surgery, privacy should be offered. Dentures, placed in special containers, are labeled with the client's name for safekeeping to prevent breakage. The client is assessed for loose teeth. A broken tooth can become dislodged during insertion of an endotracheal tube and obstruct the airway.

In some agencies nurses inventory and secure all prosthetic devices. It is also common for nurses to give prosthetics to family members or significant others or to keep the devices at the client's bedside.

Preparation of bowel and bladder. The client may require an enema or cathartic the morning of surgery. If so, it should be given at least 1 hour before the client is scheduled to leave, allowing time for the client to defecate without rushing.

The bladder is not prepared until the morning of surgery. The nurse instructs the client to void just before entering the operating room. If the client is unable to void, a notation should be entered on the preoperative checklist. An empty bladder minimizes incontinence and injury to the bladder during surgery. An empty bladder also makes abdominal organs more accessible during surgery.

Application of antiembolism stockings. Many physicians order **antiembolism stockings** for wear during surgery. Designed to support the lower extremities, they maintain compression of small veins and capillaries. The constant compression forces blood into larger vessels, thus promoting venous return and preventing venous stasis. When correctly sized and properly applied, antiembolism stockings can reduce the risk of thrombi (see Chapter 37). Pneumatic antiembolism stockings are also used for promoting venous return. These stockings are attached to an air pump that inflates and deflates the stockings, applying intermittent pressure sequentially from the ankle up the leg (Box 40-1).

Promotion of client's dignity. During preoperative preparations, care can become depersonalized unless the nurse maintains the client's privacy and reduces sources of anxiety. Ambulatory and same-day surgical admission clients often must sit in a waiting room before surgery. To protect clients' modesty, the nurse allows clients to wear underclothes when possible and provides cover robes. Hospitalized clients should be ensured privacy by closing room curtains or doors during preoperative preparation. Family may be allowed to stay until the client is transported to the operating room.

Performing special procedures. A client's condition may warrant special interventions before surgery. The surgeon's orders inform nurses of the need to start intravenous infusions, insert a Foley catheter or **nasogastric** (NG) **tubes** (Skill 40-2), or administer medications.

Safeguarding valuables. If a client has valuables, the nurse turns them over to family members or secures

---

Box 40-1

Procedural Guidelines for Application of Antiembolism Stockings and Sequential Compression Stockings

Antiembolism Stockings

1. Measure client for the proper size stocking (see product directions). With client standing, measure from gluteal fold to the floor and measure circumference of largest part of calf.
2. With client lying down, invert the stocking out over the foot (Figure 40-3, *A*). Hold the section of the heel and toe and slip the stocking over the client's foot (Figure 40-3, *B* and *C*).
3. With the foot smoothly applied, ask the client to raise the foot and ease the stocking snugly up over the leg (Figure 40-3, *D*). Be sure it is applied smoothly without wrinkles.

Sequential Compression Stockings

1. Measure client for proper size stocking by measuring around the largest part of the client's thigh.
2. Place a protective stockinette over the client's leg.
3. Wrap the stocking around the leg, starting at the ankle, with the opening over the patella (Figure 40-4).
4. Attach the stockings to the insufflator, and verify that the intermittent pressure is between 35 and 45 mm Hg.

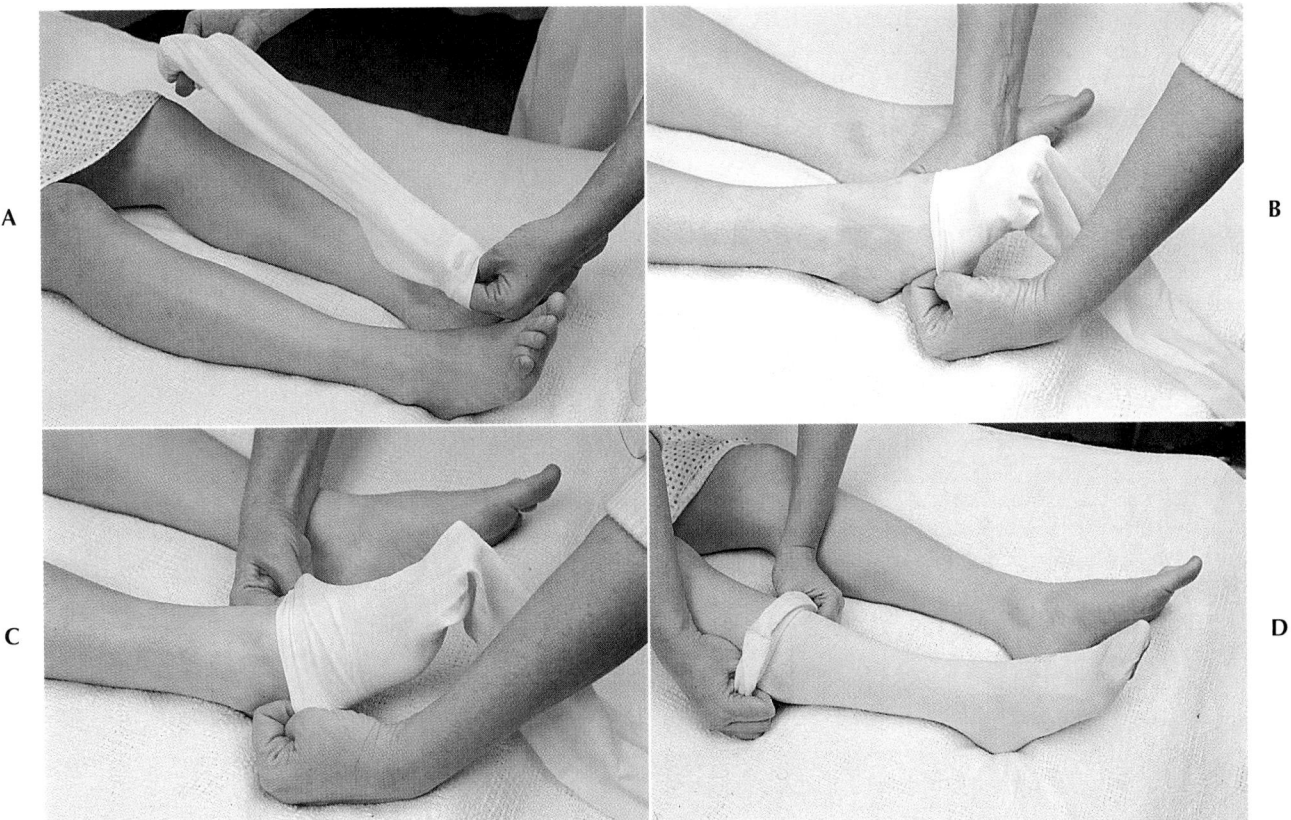

Figure 40-3. **A,** Nurse turns stocking inside out, over foot of stocking. **B,** Nurse applies stocking over foot up to heel. **C,** Stocking is applied smoothly over heel. **D,** Stocking is pulled up evenly over leg.

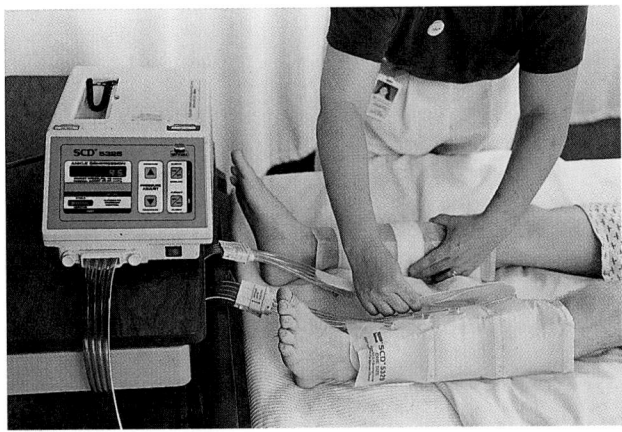

Figure 40-4. Application of sequential compression stockings.

them for safekeeping. Many facilities require clients to sign a release to free the institution of responsibility for lost valuables. Valuables can usually be stored and locked in a designated location. Clients are often reluctant to remove wedding rings or religious medals. A wedding band can be taped in place; however, care should be taken not to create a tourniquet with the tape. If there is a risk that the client will experience swelling of the hand or fingers, the band should be removed. Many hospitals allow clients to pin religious medals to their gowns or tuck them into the cap covering their hair, although the risk of loss increases.

Administering preoperative medications. Typically, the physician orders preoperative drugs to be given before the client leaves for the operating room. The nurse provides all nursing care measures before giving the drugs. Because the drugs cause sedation, the side rails should be in the up position, the bed in the low position, and the call bell within easy reach for the client. The client should be instructed to remain in bed until the surgical nursing assistant or transporter arrives to take the client to the operating room and to call for assistance if there is a need to get out of bed. The client should be warned to anticipate drowsiness and dry mouth, although the drugs usually do not induce sleep.

▪ Evaluation

Evaluation of the preoperative goals and outcomes of the plan of care begins before surgery and extends into the postoperative period, providing direction for future

Inserting and Maintaining a Nasogastric Tube

Delegation Considerations

The skill of inserting and maintaining the NG tube requires problem solving and knowledge application unique to a professional nurse. Unlicensed assistive personnel may measure and record the drainage from the NG tube and provide oral and nasal hygiene and comfort measures.

Equipment

- No. 14 or no. 16 Fr NG tube (smaller-lumen catheters are not used for decompression in adults because they must be able to remove thick secretions)
- Water-soluble lubricating jelly
- pH test strips (measure gastric aspirate acidity)
- Tongue blade
- Flashlight
- Asepto bulb or catheter-tipped syringe
- 1-inch (2.5-cm) wide hypoallergenic tape
- Safety pin and rubber band
- Clamp, drainage bag, or suction machine or pressure gauge if wall suction is to be used
- Bath towel
- Glass of water with straw
- Facial tissues
- Normal saline
- Tincture of benzoin (optional)
- Disposable gloves

STEPS	RATIONALE
1. Inspect condition of client's nasal and oral cavity.	Baseline condition of nasal and oral cavity determines need for special nursing measures for oral hygiene after tube placement.
2. Ask if client has had history of nasal surgery and note if deviated nasal septum is present.	Nurse should insert tube into uninvolved nasal passage. Procedure may be contraindicated if surgery is recent.
3. Palpate client's abdomen for distention, pain, and rigidity. Auscultate for bowel sounds.	Baseline determination of level of abdominal distention later serves as comparison once tube is inserted.
4. Assess client's level of consciousness and ability to follow instructions.	Determines client's ability to assist in procedure.

CRITICAL DECISION POINT

If client is confused, disoriented, or unable to follow commands, obtain assistance from another staff member to insert the tube.

5. Check medical record for surgeon's order, type of NG tube to be placed, and whether tube is to be attached to suction or drainage bag.	Procedure requires physician's order. Adequate decompression depends on NG suction.
6. Prepare equipment at the bedside. Have a 2- to 3-inch piece of tape ready with one end split in half.	
7. Identify client and explain procedure.	Identification prevents error of placing tube in wrong client. Explanation gains client's cooperation and lessens possibility that client will remove tube.
8. Wash hands and put on disposable gloves.	Reduces transmission of microorganisms.
9. Position client in high Fowler's position with pillows behind head and shoulders. Raise bed to a horizontal level comfortable for the nurse.	Promotes client's ability to swallow during procedure. Good body mechanics prevent injury to nurse or client.
10. Pull curtain around the bed or close room door.	Provides privacy.

STEPS	RATIONALE
11. Stand on client's right side if right-handed, left side if left-handed.	Allows easiest manipulation of tubing.
12. Place bath towel over client's chest; give facial tissues to client.	Prevents soiling of client's gown. Tube insertion through nasal passages may cause tearing and coughing with increased salivation.
13. Instruct client to relax and breathe normally while occluding one naris. Then repeat this action for other naris. Select nostril with greater air flow.	Tube passes more easily through naris that is more patent.

14. Measure distance to insert tube:
  a. Traditional method: measure distance from tip of nose to earlobe to xiphoid process (see illustration).
  b. Hanson method: first mark 50-cm point on tube, then do traditional measurement. Tube insertion should be to midway point between 50 cm (20 inches) and traditional mark.
	Tube should extend from nares to stomach; distance varies with each client.

15. Mark length of tube to be inserted with small piece of tape placed so it can easily be removed.	Marks amount of tube to be inserted from nares to stomach.
16. Cut a 10-cm (4-inch) piece of tape. Split one end down the middle lengthwise 5 cm (2 inches). Place on bed rail or bedside table.	Tape will be used after tube insertion to anchor the tube securely.
17. Curve 10 to 15 cm (4 to 6 inches) of end of tube tightly around index finger, then release.	Curving tube tip aids insertion and decreases stiffness of tube.
18. Lubricate 7.5 to 10 cm (3 to 4 inches) of end of tube with water-soluble lubricating jelly.	Minimizes friction against nasal mucosa and aids insertion of tube.
19. Alert client that procedure is to begin.	Decreases client anxiety and increases client cooperation.

Continued

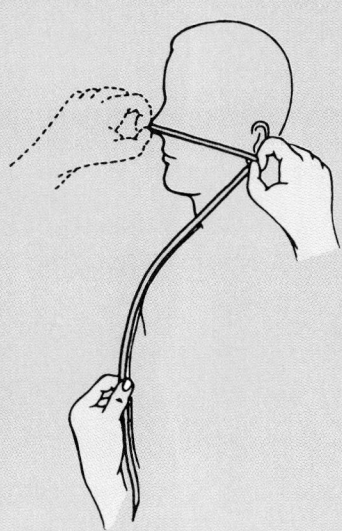

Step 14a

Skill 40-2—cont'd
Inserting and Maintaining a Nasogastric Tube

STEPS	RATIONALE
20. Initially instruct client to extend neck back against pillow; insert tube slowly through naris with curved end pointing downward (see illustration).	Facilitates initial passage of tube through naris and maintains clear airway for open naris.
21. Continue to pass tube along floor of nasal passage, aiming down toward ear. When resistance is felt, apply gentle downward pressure to advance tube (do not force past resistance).	Minimizes discomfort of tube rubbing against upper nasal turbinates. Resistance is caused by posterior nasopharynx. Downward pressure helps tube curl around corner of nasopharynx.
22. If resistance is met, try to rotate the tube and see if it advances. If still resistant, withdraw tube, allow client to rest, relubricate tube, and insert into other naris.	Forcing against resistance can cause trauma to mucosa. Helps relieve client's anxiety.

CRITICAL DECISION POINT

If unable to insert tube in either naris, stop procedure and notify physician.

23. Continue insertion of tube until just past nasopharynx by gently rotating tube toward opposite naris.	
a. Stop tube advancement, allow client to relax, and provide tissues.	Relieves client's anxiety; tearing is natural response to mucosal irritation, and excessive salivation may occur because of oral stimulation.
b. Explain to client that next step requires that client swallow. Give client glass of water unless contraindicated.	Sipping of water aids passage of NG tube into esophagus.
24. With tube just above oropharynx, instruct client to flex head forward, take a small sip of water, and swallow. Advance tube 2.5 to 5 cm (1 to 2 inches) with each swallow of water. If client is not allowed fluids, instruct to dry swallow or suck air through straw. Advance tube with each swallow.	Flexed position closes off upper airway to trachea and opens esophagus. Swallowing closes epiglottis over trachea and helps move the tube into the esophagus. Swallowing water reduces gagging or choking. Water can be removed later from stomach by suction.

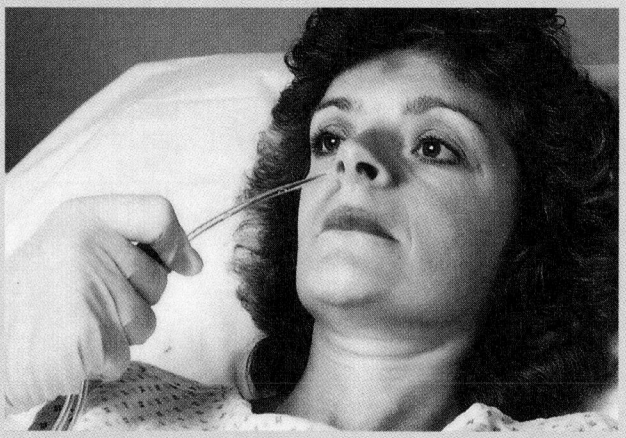

Step 20

STEPS	RATIONALE
25. If client begins to cough, gag, or choke, withdraw slightly and stop tube advancement. Instruct client to breathe easily and take sips of water.	Tubing may accidentally enter larynx and initiate cough reflex. Gaging is eased by swallowing water. Risk for aspiration increases if vomiting occurs.

CRITICAL DECISION POINT

If vomiting occurs, assist client in clearing airway; oral suctioning may be needed. Do not proceed until airway is cleared.

26. If client continues to cough during insertion, pull tube back slightly.	Tube may enter larynx and obstruct airway.
27. If client continues to gag, check back of pharynx using flashlight and tongue blade.	Tube may coil around itself in back of throat and stimulate gag reflex.
28. After client relaxes, continue to advance tube desired distance.	Tip of tube should be within stomach to decompress properly.
29. Once tube is correctly advanced, remove tape used to mark length of tube and place the prepared split tape with nonsplit side on nose. Anchor with one of split ends while checking tube placement.	Tube should be partially anchored before placement is checked.
30. Checking tube placement:	
a. Ask client to talk.	Client is unable to talk if NG tube has passed through vocal cords.
b. Inspect posterior pharynx for presence of coiled tube.	Tube is pliable and can coil up in back of pharynx instead of advancing into esophagus.
c. Draw up 10 to 20 ml of air into catheter-tipped syringe and attach to end of tube. Auscultate over left upper quadrant of abdomen while quickly injecting air into tube.	A whooshing or gurgling sound may indicate tube is correctly placed in stomach; however, sounds transmitted by insufflation of air may also be transmitted from pleural space to upper abdomen, giving false impression of placement (Metheny, 1988; Metheny and others, 1990).

CRITICAL DECISION POINT

This method used alone is not considered the most effective in determining placement of tube in stomach and should be used with other methods to accurately assess tube placement, such as x-ray examination. Check institutional policy for preferred methods for checking tube placement.

d. Aspirate gently back on syringe to obtain gastric contents, observing color (see illustration, p. 1176).	Gastric contents are usually cloudy and green, but may be off-white, tan, bloody, or brown in color. Aspiration of contents provides means to measure fluid pH and thus determine tube tip placement in gastrointestinal tract.
e. Measure pH of aspirate with color-coded pH paper with range of whole numbers 1 to 11 (see illustration, p. 1176).	Gastric aspirates have decidedly acidic pH values, preferably 4 or less, compared with intestinal aspirates, which are usually greater than 4, or respiratory secretions, which are usually greater than 5.5 (Metheny and others, 1993; Metheny and others, 1994).

.... Skill 40-2—cont'd
Inserting and Maintaining
a Nasogastric Tube

STEPS	RATIONALE

CRITICAL DECISION POINT

Be sure to use gastric (Gastrocult) pH test and not Hemoccult test.

f. If tube is not in stomach, advance another 2.5 to 5 cm (1 to 2 inches) and repeat steps, 30c, d, and e to check tube position.	Tube must be in stomach to provide decompression.
31. Anchoring tube:	
a. After tube is properly inserted and positioned, either clamp end or connect it to drainage bag or suction machine.	Drainage bag is used for gravity drainage. Intermittent suction is most effective for decompression. Client going to the operating room often has tube clamped.
b. Tape tube to nose; avoid putting pressure on nares.	Prevents tissue necrosis. Tape anchors tube securely.
(1) Before taping tube to nose, apply small amount of tincture of benzoin to lower end of nose and allow to dry (optional). Be sure top end of tape over nose is secure.	Benzoin prevents loosening of tape if client perspires.

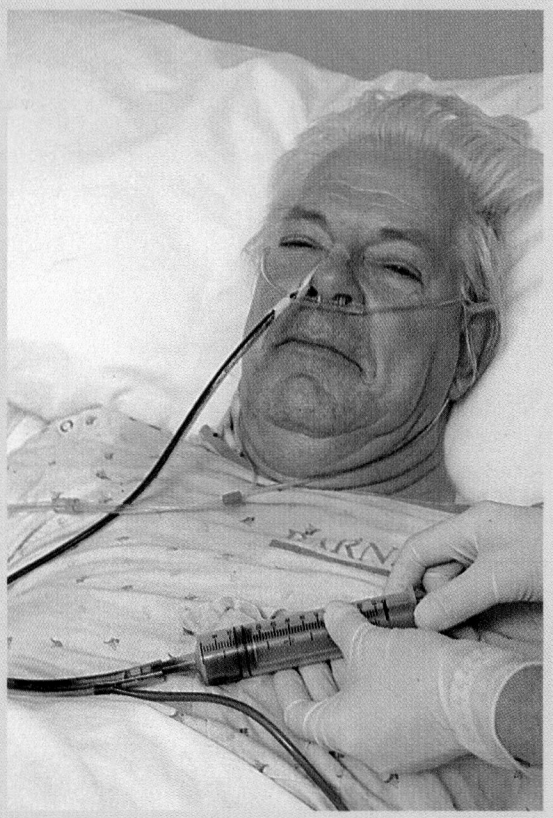

Step 30d

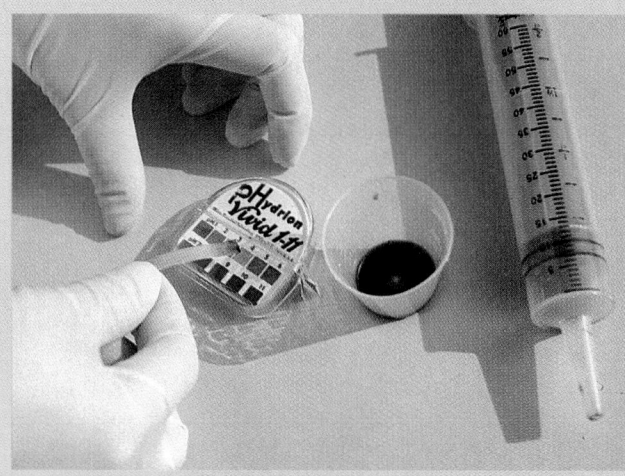

Step 30e

STEPS	RATIONALE
(2) Carefully wrap two split ends of tape around tube (see illustration).	
(3) Alternative: Apply tube fixation device using shaped adhesive patch (see illustration).	
c. Fasten end of NG tube to client's gown by looping rubber band around tube in slip knot. Pin rubber band to gown (provides slack for movement).	Reduces pressure on the nares if tube moves.
d. Unless physician orders otherwise, head of bed should be elevated 30 degrees.	Helps prevent esophageal reflux and minimizes irritation of tube against posterior pharynx.
e. Explain to client that sensation of tube should decrease somewhat with time.	Adaptation to continued sensory stimulus.
f. Remove gloves and wash hands.	Reduces transmission of microorganisms.
32. Tube irrigation:	
a. Wash hands and put on gloves.	Reduces transmission of microorganisms.
b. Check for tube placement in stomach (see Step 30). Reconnect NG tube to connecting tube.	Prevents accidental entrance of irrigating solution into lungs.
c. Draw up 30 ml of normal saline into Asepto or catheter-tipped syringe.	Use of saline minimizes loss of electrolytes from stomach fluids.
d. Clamp NG tube. Disconnect from connection tubing and lay end of connection tubing on towel.	Reduces soiling of client's gown and bed linen.
e. Insert tip of irrigating syringe into end of NG tube. Remove clamp. Hold syringe with tip pointed at floor and inject saline slowly and evenly. Do not force solution.	Position of syringe prevents introduction of air into vent tubing, which could cause gastric distention. Solution introduced under pressure can cause gastric trauma.

Continued

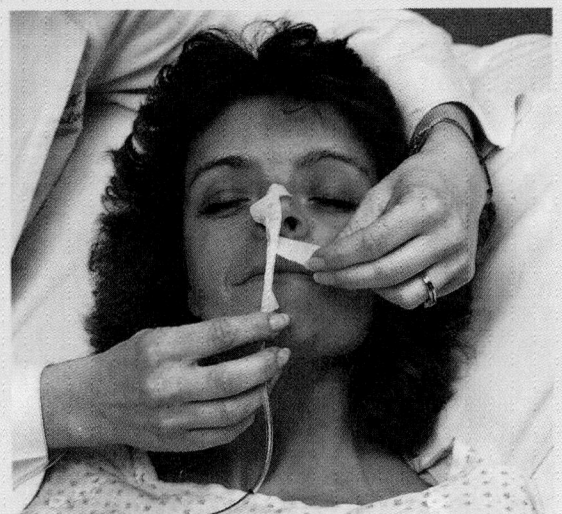

Step 31b(2)

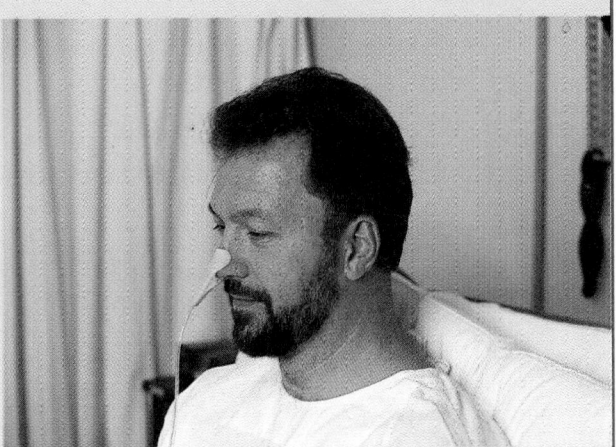

Step 31b(3)

.... Skill 40-2—cont'd
Inserting and Maintaining a Nasogastric Tube

STEPS	RATIONALE

CRITICAL DECISION POINT

Do not introduce saline through blue colored "pigtail" air vent of Salem sump tube.

f. If resistance occurs, check for kinks in tubing. Turn client onto left side. Repeated resistance should be reported to surgeon.	Tip of tube may lie against stomach lining. Repositioning on left side may dislodge tube away from the stomach lining. Buildup of secretions will cause distention.
g. After instilling saline, immediately aspirate or pull back slowly on syringe to withdraw fluid. If amount aspirated is greater than amount instilled, record the difference as output. If amount aspirated is less than amount instilled, record the difference as intake.	Irrigation clears tubing, so stomach should remain empty. Fluid remaining in stomach is measured as intake.
h. Reconnect NG tube to drainage or suction. (If solution does not return, repeat irrigation.)	Reestablishes drainage collection; may repeat irrigation or repositioning of tube until NG tube drains properly.
i. Remove gloves and wash hands.	Reduces transmission of microorganisms.

33. Discontinuation of NG tube:

a. Verify order to discontinue NG tube.	Physician's order required for procedure.
b. Explain procedure to client and reassure that removal is less distressing than insertion.	Minimizes anxiety and increases cooperation. Tube passes out smoothly.
c. Wash hands and apply disposable gloves.	Reduces transmission of microorganisms.
d. Turn off suction and disconnect NG tube from drainage bag or suction. Remove tape from bridge of nose and unpin tube from gown.	Have tube free of connections before removal.
e. Stand on client's right side if right-handed, left side if left-handed.	Allows easiest manipulation of tube.
f. Hand the client facial tissue; place clean towel across chest. Instruct client to take and hold a deep breath.	Client may wish to blow nose after tube is removed. Towel may keep gown from getting soiled. Airway will be temporarily obstructed during tube removal.
g. Clamp or kink tubing securely and then pull tube out steadily and smoothly into towel held in other hand while client holds breath.	Clamping prevents tube contents from draining into oropharynx. Reduces trauma to mucosa and minimizes client's discomfort. Towel covers tube, which can be an unpleasant sight. Holding breath helps to prevent aspiration.
h. Measure amount of drainage and note character of content. Dispose of tube and drainage equipment.	Provides accurate measure of fluid output. Reduces transfer of microorganisms.
i. Clean nares and provide mouth care.	Promotes comfort.
j. Position client comfortably and explain procedure for drinking fluids, if not contraindicated.	Depends on physician's order. Sometimes clients are NPO for up to 24 hours. When fluids are allowed, the order usually begins with a small amount of ice chips each hour and increases as client is able to tolerate more.

STEPS	RATIONALE
34. Clean equipment and return to proper place. Place soiled linen in utility room or proper receptacle.	Proper disposal of equipment prevents spread of microorganisms and ensures proper exchange procedures.
35. Remove gloves and wash hands.	Reduces transmission of microorganisms.
36. Observe amount and character of contents draining from NG tube. Ask if client feels nauseated.	Determines if tube is decompressing stomach of contents.
37. Palpate client's abdomen periodically, noting any distention, pain, and rigidity and auscultate for the presence of bowel sounds. Turn off suction while auscultating.	Determines success of abdominal decompression and the return of peristalsis. The sound of the suction apparatus may be transmitted to abdomen and be misinterpreted as bowel sounds.
38. Inspect condition of nares and nose.	Evaluates onset of skin and tissue irritation.
39. Observe position of tubing.	Determines if tension is being applied to nasal structures.
40. Ask if client feels sore throat or irritation in pharynx.	Evaluates level of client's discomfort.

Recording and Reporting

- Record in nurse's notes time and type of NG tube inserted, client's tolerance of procedure, confirmation of placement, character of gastric contents, pH value, and whether tube is clamped or connected to drainage device.

- Record in nurse's notes and/or flow sheet amount and character of contents draining from NG tube every shift, unless ordered more frequently by physician.

interventions. The client's surgery may be an emergency, or procedures may be required up until the time the client is taken to surgery. This leaves little time for evaluation. For some measures, such as those to prevent infection, evaluation is done postoperatively when the outcome can be determined.

Client care. The nurse determines if the client and family have adequate preoperative preparation by asking the client to describe the surgical procedure, its purpose, and the postoperative care that will be performed. The client's understanding of the physiological and psychological responses to surgery are evaluated by having the client and family describe the reasons for postoperative exercises and spirometry. Adequacy of preoperative teaching is evaluated by having the client demonstrate exercises. Anxiety is evaluated by monitoring pulse and blood pressure, facial expressions, and verbal interactions. In addition, the nurse can ask the client if he or she remains anxious or fearful of any aspect of the surgery.

Client expectations. The nurse determines if the client's and family's expectations have been met up to this point. This involves spending time talking with the client and family to learn if they are satisfied with their preparation and the approach used by the nursing staff. For example, a client might expect that his or her spouse will be involved in all preoperative preparations or that a physician will speak with him or her personally. Knowing this information assists the nurse in improving the client's satisfaction with care. In emergent situations, this may become more difficult to evaluate. The family may become the focus of the evaluation if the client is unable to respond or is in a condition that prevents a meaningful discussion.

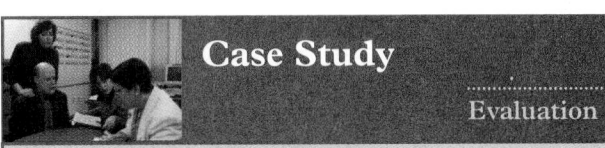

Case Study

Evaluation

It is the morning of Mr. Korloff's surgery, and Sue is admitting him to the hospital with the assistance of one of his daughters. She checks that the informed consent has been signed and witnessed and completes his physical assessment, which focuses on

Continued

Continued from p. 1179

assessing breath sounds, condition of his skin, and vital signs. Sue also completes the preoperative checklist. She asks Mr. Korloff if he has any questions about the nature or purpose of the surgery. Sue also reviews with Mr. Korloff and his daughter the events that will occur in the holding area and the **postanesthesia care unit** (PACU). She asks if they are frightened or anxious about any aspect of the procedure or routine, and she addresses their concerns. Sue then reviews with Mr. Korloff the exercises that were in the booklet he received in the mail. Sue has Mr. Korloff demonstrate coughing and deep breathing, while reinforcing its importance once surgery is over. Mr. Korloff is then provided with a hospital gown and cover-up and shown to the changing area. After he has removed his clothes and put on the hospital gown, Mr. Korloff and his daughter are accompanied to the holding area.

Documentation Note

Client admitted for scheduled laparoscopic cholecystectomy. BP 142/84, P 88, R 18, T 98.9° F. Lungs are clear to auscultation bilaterally with normal excursion. Skin warm and dry; no evidence of lesions. Client remained NPO during the night. Reviewed instructions on postoperative exercises, and client is able to demonstrate coughing and deep breathing. Daughters will be in waiting area during procedure.

Transport to the Operating Room

Personnel in the **operating room** notify the nursing unit when it is time for surgery. In many hospitals a nursing assistant or transporter brings a stretcher for transporting the client. The transporter checks the client's identification bracelet against the client's medical record to be sure the correct person is going to surgery. When a client is to be transported by a stretcher, the nurses and transporter assist the client to safely transfer from bed to stretcher. If able, the ambulatory surgery client may walk to the operating room, providing more control over the event.

The family is provided an opportunity to visit before the client is transported to the operating room. The nurse then directs the family to the appropriate waiting area. If the client has been hospitalized before surgery and will be returning to the same nursing unit, the nurse prepares the bed and room for the client's return. The nurse will be better prepared for postoperative care if the room is readied before the client's return.

A postoperative bedside unit should include the following:

1. Sphygmomanometer, stethoscope, and thermometer
2. Emesis basin
3. Clean gown
4. Washcloth, towel, and facial tissues
5. Intravenous pole
6. Suction equipment
7. Oxygen equipment
8. Extra pillows for positioning
9. Bed pads to protect bed linen from drainage
10. Intravenous pump
11. PCA pump

Holding area. In many hospitals the client enters a preanesthesia care unit (PSCU) (sometimes called a holding area) outside the operating room, where the nurse completes the preoperative preparations. Nurses in the PSCU are usually part of the operating room staff and wear surgical scrub suits.

The nurse, nurse anesthetist, or anesthesiologist will insert an intravenous catheter into the client's vein to establish a route for fluid replacement and intravenous drugs. A large-bore intravenous catheter is used for optimal infusion of all fluids, including blood and blood products. Preoperative medications are administered.

If hair around the surgical site needs to be removed, this is done in a private area near the operating room immediately before surgery. AORN-recommended practices include the use of clippers for preoperative hair removal. Clippers minimize the risk of irritation and small cuts, which predispose the client to infection (AORN, 1996). The nurse should consult the physician's order sheet and the institution's policy and procedure manual.

⋯INTRAOPERATIVE SURGICAL PHASE

Care of the client during surgery requires careful preparation and knowledge of the events that will occur during the surgical procedure.

Nurse's Role During Surgery

The nurse usually assumes one of two roles in the operating room: **circulating nurse** or **scrub nurse.** The circulating nurse cares for the client while in the operating room by completing another preoperative assessment, establishing and implementing the intraoperative plan of care, evaluating the care, and providing for the continuity of care postoperatively. The circulating nurse assists the anesthesiologist or nurse anesthetist with endotracheal intubation, calculating blood loss and urinary output, and administering blood. This nurse monitors sterile technique and a safe operating room environment, assists the surgeon and scrub nurse by operating nonsterile equipment and providing additional instruments and supplies, and maintains accurate and complete written records.

The scrub nurse is responsible for maintaining a sterile field during the surgical procedure and adhering to strict surgical asepsis (see Chapter 25). This nurse assists with applying surgical drapes and provides the surgeon with instruments, sponges, sutures, and other supplies.

Admission to the Operating Room

The circulating nurse transfers the client to the operating room. The client is usually still awake and will notice nurses and physicians wearing complete surgical masks, protective eyewear, and gowns. The staff members carefully transfer the client to the operating table, being sure the stretcher and table are locked in place. After the client is on the table, the nurse fastens a safety strap around the client's legs.

NURSING PROCESS

▣ Assessment

The circulating nurse or nurse in the PSCU conducts a special preoperative assessment to verify the client is ready for surgery and to use as a basis for planning intraoperative care. The client is asked his or her name, and this is compared with the identification band and chart. The nurse reviews consent forms, allergies, medical history, physical assessment findings, and test results. The nurse verifies with the client what surgery is to be performed and the surgical site. A brief assessment of key body systems is performed. Special attention is also paid to the psychological comfort of the client.

▣ Nursing Diagnosis

Preoperative nursing diagnoses are reviewed and, based on this assessment, modified to individualize the care plan for the client in the operating room. Additional diagnoses and related factors are added based on the client's condition, specific surgical intervention, and method and type of anesthesia used (see nursing diagnosis box). These diagnoses provide direction for both intraoperative and postoperative care of the client.

▣ Planning

Some goals of preoperative care extend into the intraoperative phase. These include remaining free of infection and achieving psychological and physical comfort. Additional goals include maintaining skin integrity, therapeutic body temperature, and fluid and electrolyte balance. Achievement of the goals will be measured through outcomes, such as the presence of intact skin, without redness or irritation; body temperature within the client's normal range; stable vital signs; adequate

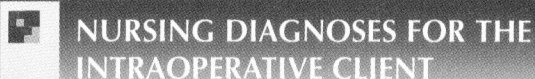

NURSING DIAGNOSES FOR THE INTRAOPERATIVE CLIENT
Aspiration, risk for
Fluid volume deficit
Gas exchange, impaired
Infection, risk for
Injury, risk for
Skin integrity, impaired, risk for
Thermoregulation, ineffective
Tissue perfusion, altered
Urinary elimination, altered

urinary output; and electrolyte values within the normal range.

▣ Implementation

A major focus of intraoperative care is to prevent injury and complications related to anesthesia, surgery, positioning, and equipment used. The nurse acts as an advocate for the client during surgery. The client's dignity and rights are protected at all times.

Acute care

Physical preparation. After securing the client's safety, the circulating nurse completes the physical preparation. The nurse applies small, plastic electrodes on the chest and extremities for continuous electrocardiographic monitoring during surgery. A monitor displays the heart's electrical activity. Next, the nurse applies a blood pressure cuff around the client's arm to allow the anesthesiologist to measure the blood pressure while using both hands to ventilate the client. A pulse oximeter probe is attached to the client's finger or earlobe, allowing measurement of the oxygen saturation in the blood and an evaluation of ventilation.

Psychological support. Entering the operating room is stressful for most clients. The nurse reassures the client and should remain at the client's side until after anesthesia is induced. Offering a hand to hold is often helpful. If the client is awake during surgery, this support is given throughout the surgical procedure.

Introduction of anesthesia. The nature and extent of a client's surgery and the client's current physical status influences the type of anesthesia administered in surgery. It is most important for the nurse to know the complications to watch for after anesthesia has been administered to a client.

General anesthesia. Under **general anesthesia** all sensation and consciousness is lost, muscles relax, and amnesia is experienced. General anesthesia is used for major procedures requiring extensive tissue manipulation.

The greatest risks from general anesthesia are the side effects, including cardiovascular depression or irritability, respiratory depression, and liver and kidney damage.

Regional anesthesia. **Regional anesthesia** results in loss of sensation in an area of the body by anesthetizing sensory pathways. This type of anesthesia is given by infiltration and local application (see Chapter 33). Administration techniques include peripheral nerve blocks and spinal, epidural, and caudal blocks.

There are risks involved with infiltrative anesthetics, particularly in the case of spinal anesthesia. The client may experience a sudden fall in blood pressure, and respiratory paralysis may develop. The client requires careful monitoring during and immediately after regional anesthesia.

Local anesthesia. Local anesthesia involves loss of sensation at the desired site by inhibiting peripheral nerve conduction. Local anesthesia is commonly used for minor procedures performed in ambulatory surgery. Local anesthetics are also administered to clients receiving general anesthesia. Long-acting local anesthetics are sometimes injected into the incision at the end of the client's surgery for postoperative pain relief.

The nurse supports the client by explaining procedures, encouraging questions, and warning the client when unpleasant sensations will be experienced. In some settings, music is provided to mask unpleasant sounds and to promote relaxation.

Positioning. Ideally the client's position during surgery provides good access to and exposure of the operative site and sustains adequate circulatory and respiratory function. It should not impair neuromuscular structures or skin integrity. The client's comfort and safety must be considered. When general anesthesia is used, the nursing personnel and surgeon usually do not position the client until the stage of complete relaxation.

It is sometimes difficult to understand why clients may feel discomfort after surgery. Normal range of motion is maintained by the alert person by pain and pressure receptors. If a joint is extended too far, pain stimuli warn that muscle and joint strain are too great. In a client who is anesthetized, normal defense mechanisms cannot guard against joint damage, muscle stretch, and strain. The client's muscles are so relaxed that it is relatively easy to place the client in a position he or she normally could not assume while awake. The client often remains in a given position for several hours. Once the client awakens, musculoskeletal pain can be significant.

Prevention of infection. Prevention of infection is a primary responsibility of perioperative nurses. Both the circulating and scrub nurse closely monitor surgical asepsis (see Chapter 25) and correct any breaks in sterile technique. Standard precautions are also followed to protect clients and staff members from possible infections.

Once the client is positioned, the circulating nurse prepares the skin for the surgical incision. An antimicrobial solution is applied to the skin (e.g., chlorhexidine or povidone-iodine) to reduce the microorganisms normally located on the skin and to minimize their entry into the surgical wound (Larson, 1993). The scrub nurse and the surgeon apply sterile surgical drapes to create a sterile field for the surgical procedure.

Prevention of injury. Prevention of injury to the client is an extremely important part of the nurse's role. The scrub and circulating nurses, together, count all of the sponges, needles, and instruments brought to the sterile field. This is done before the first incision is made and at the completion of the procedure. During the procedure, a close count of these items is maintained by the perioperative nurses to prevent accidental loss of any item inside the surgical wound. The nurse who fails to accurately count items can be held legally accountable and found negligent if a client is injured by a misplaced item (see Chapter 12). The perioperative nurse must also be aware of the risks to the client when using special equipment (e.g., electrosurgical cautery and lasers) and implement additional interventions to protect the client. If electrosurgical cautery is used, the nurse applies a grounding pad to the client to protect against burns. Lasers pose an increased risk of fire and client injury. The laser beam generates intense heat and can be reflected. Of particular concern is the oxygen-rich environment of the airway. Specific protective measures are taken to protect the client and operating room staff during laser surgery (e.g., using water-soaked drapes and sponges, nonreflective instruments, and eye protection). If laser surgery is near the airway, a special endotracheal tube is used.

Maintenance of fluid and electrolyte balance. Maintenance of fluid and electrolyte balance is the responsibility of the nurse and the anesthesiologist or nurse anesthetist. Blood loss and urinary and NG drainage are monitored during surgery; intravenous solutions are administered to replace lost fluids and may be supplemented by blood products if necessary.

Temperature control. The client's temperature is continuously monitored throughout surgery. The perioperative nurse may give special attention to the older adult to prevent heat loss. The room should be kept warm (18° to 21° C, or 65° to 70° F) until the surgical drapes are in place. A warming blanket may be placed under the client. A reflective hat or blanket may be used to prevent heat loss. Some hospitals use a warm air blanket under the surgical drapes. Irrigating solutions and blood are warmed before administration.

Documentation of intraoperative care. During the intraoperative phase, the nursing staff continue the established plan of care and modify it as needed. Throughout the surgical procedure, the circulating nurse keeps an accurate record of client care activities and procedures performed by operating room personnel; this record provides useful data for the nurse who cares for the client postoperatively.

Evaluation

Many interventions implemented during the intraoperative phase are evaluated postoperatively, because complications (e.g., infection) can arise days after surgery.

Client care. At the end of the surgical procedure, the nurse performs a postoperative evaluation of the client. The nurse inspects the skin under the grounding pad and areas of the skin where pressure may have been exerted by equipment or because of positioning. Thermoregulation is monitored by measurement of body temperature during the procedure and immediately postoperatively. Vital signs are obtained and lung sounds are auscultated to assess pulmonary and fluid and electrolyte status.

Client expectations. A client not receiving general anesthesia should be questioned frequently during the procedure regarding pain, numbness, and perceived temperature. This will help to determine if adequate analgesia is being maintained and if the client is comfortable in regard to position and temperature.

When the client is undergoing major surgery, it can be very important to keep the family informed. Typically, family members want to know if surgery is progressing without problems. Many hospitals provide phones within waiting areas that allow nursing staff to reach families and to explain the progress of the surgery. Nursing staff on the surgical nursing division can also stop by the waiting area to make sure that families are not in need of additional information or support.

POSTOPERATIVE SURGICAL PHASE

Postoperative care of the client is challenging because of complex physiological changes. To assess the client's postoperative condition the nurse relies on information from the preoperative nursing assessment and on information regarding the surgical procedure and events occurring during surgery. Good clinical decision making requires the nurse to be skilled at noticing change. A variation from the norm may indicate the onset of complications.

The postoperative course involves two phases: the immediate **recovery** period and **convalescence.** For an ambulatory surgical client the immediate recovery period normally lasts only 1 to 2 hours, and convalescence will occur at home. For a hospitalized client the immediate postoperative period may last a few hours, with convalescence taking 1 or more days depending on the extent of surgery and the client's response.

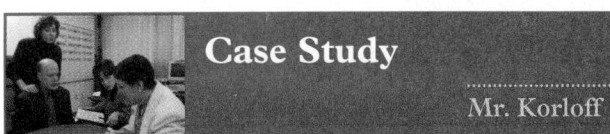

Case Study

Mr. Korloff

Mr. Korloff's surgery is completed, and he is being transferred to the PACU. Sue has requested that she accompany Mr. Korloff into the PACU. He received general anesthesia, and the procedure was uneventful. Mr. Korloff did not receive any blood or blood products. He did receive Ringer's lactate solution intravenously via a catheter in the left lower forearm. Small gauze dressings were applied to the four small abdominal puncture wounds. At this time, the priorities are to maintain Mr. Korloff's vital signs and airway, which is established with an oral airway, and to protect him from injury during transport to the PACU.

NURSING PROCESS

Assessment

Immediately after surgery, the client is transferred to the PACU, formerly called the recovery room, for close monitoring (Figure 40-5). Before the arrival of the client, the PACU nurse receives a report from the surgical team in the operating room to determine the client's general status and the need for special equipment and nursing care.

When the client enters the PACU, the nurse performs a rapid assessment of the respiratory and circulatory status of the client and attaches electronic monitors. Then the nurse and members of the surgical team confer about the client's status. During this report, the client is continuously monitored. The report includes a review of anesthetic agents given so the PACU nurse can anticipate the course of recovery. A report on intravenous fluids and blood products given during surgery alerts the nurse to the fluid and electrolyte balance. The perioperative nurse reports any allergies or drainage devices and whether the client had any surgical complications, such as excessive blood loss. The surgeon often reports any special concerns (e.g., whether the client is at risk for hemorrhage or infection). After reviewing events occurring in the operating room, the PACU nurse then conducts a focused assessment of the client's status. After this initial assessment, the nurse evaluates blood pressure and other key observations every 15 minutes or more frequently if indicated. Based on these assessments the plan of care is modified to meet the immediate needs of the client.

Respiration. The nurse assesses the quality of the client's respirations and the patency of the airway. A

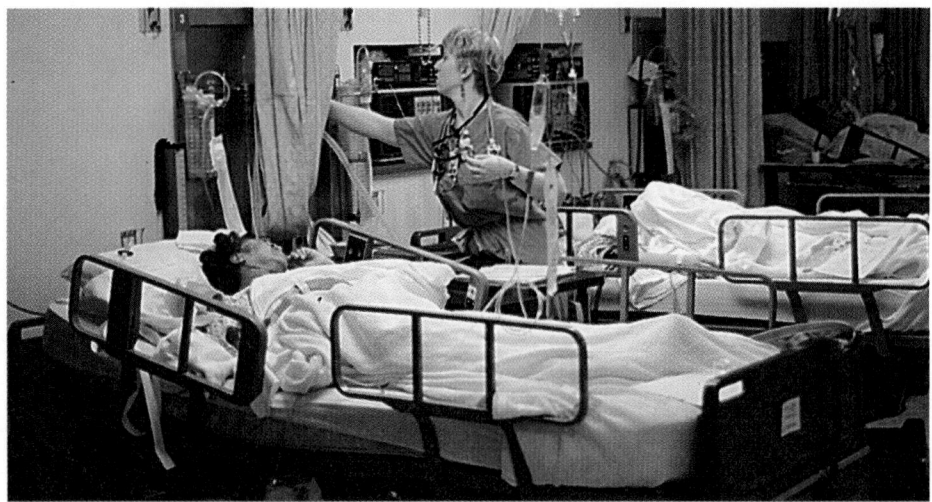

Figure 40-5. Nurse in PACU.

client receiving a general anesthetic often has an artificial airway in place when arriving in the PACU. Certain anesthetic agents may continue to cause respiratory depression. Thus the nurse is especially alert for slow, shallow breathing. The nurse assesses respiratory rate, rhythm, depth of ventilation, symmetry of chest wall movement, breath sounds, and color of mucous membranes. Lung sounds are auscultated to identify any abnormalities such as rales, wheezing, or decreased breath sounds. If breathing is unusually shallow, placement of the nurse's hand over the client's face or mouth allows the nurse to feel exhaled air. Pulse oximetry is used to continuously monitor the oxygen saturation of the blood (see Chapter 23).

Circulation. The client is at risk for cardiovascular complications from blood loss at the surgical site, side effects of anesthesia, electrolyte imbalances, and depression of normal circulatory regulating mechanisms. Continuous electrocardiographic monitoring can detect rhythm and rate disturbances. Careful assessment of heart rate and rhythm and blood pressure reveals the client's cardiovascular status. The nurse compares preoperative vital signs with postoperative values to determine the client's status.

The nurse assesses circulatory perfusion by noting the color of nail beds and skin. Procedures that impair circulation, such as vascular surgery, use of a tourniquet, or application of casts or tight dressings, require the nurse to assess peripheral pulses distal to the site of surgery, tourniquet, or cast.

The PACU nurse must always be alert to the amount of bleeding that occurs after surgery and the possibility of hemorrhage. Blood loss may occur externally through a drain or incision or internally within the surgical wound. Either type of hemorrhage may manifest itself first by restlessness and then by a fall in blood pressure; elevated heart and respiratory rate; thready pulse; and cool, clammy, pale skin.

Temperature control. The operating room environment is cool, and the client's depressed level of body function results in a lowering of metabolism and fall in body temperature. When clients begin to awaken, they may complain of feeling cold and uncomfortable. Shivering may not be a sign of hypothermia but rather a side effect of certain anesthetic agents. The nurse measures body temperature to provide direction for interventions.

Neurological function. On arrival in the PACU the client is usually drowsy and reacting to verbal commands. However, drugs, electrolyte and metabolic changes, pain, and emotional factors influence level of consciousness. Normally as anesthetic agents are metabolized, the client's reflexes return, muscle strength is regained, and a normal level of orientation returns. The nurse can easily check for pupillary and gag reflexes (see Chapter 24). If a client has had surgery involving a portion of the neurological system, the nurse will conduct a more thorough neurological assessment.

Skin integrity and condition of the wound. The PACU nurse assesses the condition of the client's skin. A rash may indicate a drug sensitivity or allergy. Abrasions or petechiae may result from inadequate padding during positioning or restraining that injured skin layers. Burns or serious injury to the skin should be communicated by an incident report. Most surgical wounds are covered with a dressing that protects the wound site and collects drainage. The nurse observes the amount, color, odor, and consistency of drainage on dressings and estimates the amount of drainage by noting the number of saturated gauze sponges.

Genitourinary function. A spinal anesthetic may prevent the client from feeling bladder fullness or distention and cause urinary retention for up to 6 to 8 hours. The nurse palpates the lower abdomen just above the symphysis pubis for bladder distention. A full bladder can be painful and is often the cause of a client's restlessness, agitation, or high blood pressure in the PACU. If the client has a Foley catheter (see Chapter 35), there should be a continuous flow of urine of at least 30 ml/hr in adults. The nurse observes the color and odor of urine. Surgery involving portions of the urinary tract normally causes bloody urine for at least 12 to 24 hours.

Gastrointestinal function. Anesthetic agents slow gastrointestinal motility and may cause nausea. In addition, manipulation of the intestines during abdominal surgery further impairs peristalsis. A nurse will normally hear faint or absent bowel sounds in all four quadrants during the immediate recovery phase. Inspection of the abdomen rules out distention that may be caused by the accumulation of gas. Distention may develop if internal bleeding occurs in a client who has had abdominal surgery. If an NG tube is in place, the nurse assesses the patency of the tube and the color and amount of any drainage.

Fluid and electrolyte balance. Because of the surgical client's risk for fluid and electrolyte abnormalities, the nurse assesses the hydration status and monitors cardiac and neurological function for signs of electrolyte alterations (see Chapter 31). The nurse inspects the intravenous catheter insertion site to be sure it is patent and no signs of infiltration are present. It is important that a good venous access is available in case the client requires fluid replacement. The physician orders a prescribed solution and rate for each intravenous infusion.

Monitoring and accurate recording of intake and output helps to assess the fluid and electrolyte balance, as well as renal and cardiac function. The nurse measures all sources of output, including urine, gastric drainage, and wound drainage, and consults with the physician if appropriate.

Comfort. As a client awakens from general anesthesia, the sensation of discomfort can become prominent. Pain can be perceived before full consciousness is regained. Acute incisional pain causes the client to become restless and may cause changes in vital signs. It is difficult for clients to begin coughing and deep-breathing exercises when they have pain, particularly if there is an abdominal or chest incision. The client who had regional or local anesthesia usually does not experience pain initially, because the incisional area is still anesthetized. The PACU nurse must be skilled at assessing levels of pain (see Chapter 33) and be alert to the client's need for pain medication.

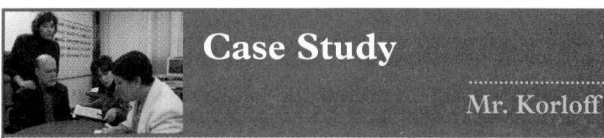

Case Study
Mr. Korloff

Sue begins an assessment of Mr. Korloff as soon as he enters the PACU. She inspects the intravenous site and finds it without inflammation or tenderness. Ringer's lactate continues to run at 100 ml/hr. Sue's assessment continues as follows: temperature 98.6° F; apical pulse 82, strong and regular; respirations 22 with some labored breathing; blood pressure 122/70; O_2 saturation 90% by pulse oximeter; lungs clear on auscultation with oxygen running at 2 L by nasal cannula; skin pale without bruises or burns; abdominal dressings dry and intact; oral airway in place. Sue asks Mr. Korloff to spit out the airway, which he does without difficulty. Mr. Korloff grimaces while Sue helps him to turn, and she asks if he is in pain. He responds that he has some discomfort in his right shoulder and feels as though it is hard to get his breath. Sue knows from her preparation that laparoscopic surgery requires insufflation of the gas CO_2 into the abdominal cavity. The gas can cause referred pain, and it can irritate the phrenic nerve and cause some difficulty breathing. Sue assists Mr. Korloff to Sims' position (left side with right knee flexed) to help move the gas pocket away from the diaphragm. Five minutes later he reports breathing with less effort and denies discomfort. Sue continues to monitor vital signs every 5 minutes until respirations stabilize and then every 15 minutes until Mr. Korloff is released from the PACU.

Documentation Note

Sue documents her assessment findings, interventions, and Mr. Korloff's response to these interventions. She uses a graph to plot vital signs. Using the graph allows Sue to easily identify a trend in Mr. Korloff's status.

▪ Nursing Diagnosis

Based on the postanesthesia assessment and reports given by the operating room nurse, surgeon, and anesthesiologist, postoperative nursing diagnoses are identified for the client. These diagnoses give direction to the continuing care of the client in the PACU (see nursing diagnosis box).

It is important to analyze and validate data and cluster findings to identify correct nursing diagnoses. For example, a finding of restlessness could be related to *pain, urinary retention, altered tissue perfusion,* or *anxiety.*

NURSING DIAGNOSES FOR THE POSTOPERATIVE CLIENT

Activity intolerance
Airway clearance, ineffective
Body image disturbance
Breathing pattern, ineffective
Communication, impaired verbal
Fluid volume deficit, risk for
Infection, risk for
Mobility, impaired physical
Pain
Role performance, altered
Urinary elimination, altered

Further assessment and clustering of findings would lead to the correct diagnosis.

Planning

Because of the critical nature of the immediate postoperative period, the plan of care always involves close monitoring of the client and frequent assessments. Goals of care for the client during this period include returning the client to normal physiological functioning without complications and maintaining physical and psychological comfort. Outcomes include stable vital signs within the client's normal range, patent airway, palpable peripheral pulses, oxygen saturation over 95%, an intact incision with minimal wound drainage, and balanced intake and output. The client should also be awake and oriented to the PACU environment with the ability to move all extremities and verbalize pain relief and decreased anxiety.

Implementation

Respiration. Following general anesthesia, the client often has an oral or nasal airway inserted to maintain a patent airway until regular breathing at a normal rate resumes. This airway is not taped in place. As respiratory function returns, the nurse will ask the client to expel the airway. The client's ability to do so signifies a return of a normal gag reflex.

One of the nurse's greatest concerns is airway obstruction resulting from aspiration of emesis, accumulation of mucous secretions in the pharynx, or swelling or spasm of the larynx. The following measures maintain airway patency:

1. Position the client on one side with the face down and the neck slightly extended. A small, folded towel supports the head. Neck extension prevents occlusion of the airway at the pharynx. When the face is kept turned downward, the tongue moves forward and mucous secretions flow out of the mouth instead of accumulating in the pharynx. If the nature of the surgery prevents turning the client on one side, the head of the bed is slightly elevated and the client's neck slightly extended, with the head turned to the side. Never position the client with arms over or across the chest, because this reduces maximum chest expansion.

2. Suction the artificial airway and oral cavity for mucous secretions as necessary. Care must be taken to avoid continually eliciting the gag reflex, which might cause vomiting. Before removing an airway, the back of the airway should be suctioned so that mucous plugs and secretions are not retained.

3. Begin any coughing and deep-breathing exercises as soon as the client can respond to instructions.

4. Administer oxygen as ordered, by mask or nasal prongs. In many PACU settings, oxygen is routinely administered.

Circulation. The nurse must be aware of changes in blood pressure or heart rate. The physician may have written an order indicating which changes are to be reported. However, the nurse must use judgment and notify the physician when there is a significant change or a continuous trend in vital signs. If hemorrhage is external, the nurse should observe for increased bloody drainage on dressings or through drains. If a dressing becomes saturated, the blood will ooze down the client's sides and collect in a pool under bedclothes. When hemorrhage is internal, the operative site becomes swollen and tight, and a hematoma may develop. The first signs of suspected hemorrhaging should be reported to the physician immediately. The nurse closely monitors vital signs until the client's condition stabilizes.

Temperature control. The client is usually cool when arriving in the PACU. Therefore the nurse provides specially warmed blankets or other warming devices (e.g., a hot air blanket). Increasing body warmth causes the client's metabolism to rise and circulatory and respiratory functions to improve.

Neurological functioning. Deep breathing and coughing will help to expel retained anesthetic gases and promote return of the client's level of consciousness. The nurse arouses the client by calling his or her name in a moderate tone of voice, noting whether the client responds appropriately. If the client remains asleep or unresponsive, the nurse attempts arousal through touch or by gently moving a body part. If a painful stimulus is needed to arouse the client, the nurse should notify the anesthesiologist. Orientation to the PACU environment is important in maintaining alertness. The nurse explains that surgery is completed and describes all procedures and nursing measures performed.

Wound and dressing care.
Dressings should be left in place to reduce the risk of infection. The PACU nurse may simply add an extra layer of gauze on top of the original dressing if drainage develops. Notify the physician if bleeding is excessive. In certain types of surgery, the physician may choose to use no dressing at all.

Gastrointestinal function.
To minimize nausea the nurse avoids sudden movement of the client. If the client has an NG tube, the nurse maintains the tube patency. Occlusion of an NG tube causes the accumulation of gastric contents in the stomach. Because stomach emptying slows under anesthesia, the accumulated contents cannot escape, and nausea and vomiting develop. Normally a client does not receive fluids to drink in the PACU because of the risk of vomiting. A moist cloth or swab is sometimes used to relieve dryness of the client's lips and mouth.

Genitourinary function.
A full bladder is painful and can cause the client to be restless or agitated. If the bladder becomes distended, the nurse will probably need to obtain a physician's order to insert a catheter. If a catheter is already in place and urinary output is less than 30 ml/hr in an adult client, the nurse notifies the surgeon.

Fluid and electrolyte balance.
The client's only source of fluid intake immediately after surgery is intravenously; therefore it is important to maintain patency of the infusion (see Chapter 31). The client may also receive blood products, depending on the amount of blood lost during surgery.

Comfort.
The anesthesiologist or nurse anesthetist orders medications for pain management in the PACU. Intravenous opioid analgesics, such as morphine sulfate, are the drugs of choice for the immediate postoperative period (AHCPR, 1992). The nurse administers morphine intravenously, titrating it until pain relief is achieved. Morphine may depress vital signs and level of consciousness. However, a low blood pressure may be caused by acute pain. In such a situation an analgesic may improve vital sign values. The PACU nurse is skilled at determining the proper dose of an analgesic.

Postanesthesia care in ambulatory surgery.
The postanesthesia care of ambulatory surgery clients occurs in two phases, in two separate areas of the surgical unit. Phase I is essentially the same as described for hospitalized clients. Phase II, however, prepares the client for discharge and self-care. The client receiving only local anesthesia may be admitted directly to the Phase II area. In Phase II, clients are encouraged to gradually sit up on the stretcher or recliner and begin to take ice chips or sips of water after regaining full alertness.

Phase II postanesthesia care occurs in a room equipped with medical recliner chairs, side tables, and footrests. Kitchen facilities for preparing light snacks and beverages are located in the area, along with bathrooms. The Phase II environment promotes the client's and family's comfort and well-being until discharge. The nurse monitors clients but not at the same intensity as in Phase I. In Phase II the nurse initiates postoperative teaching with clients and family members (Box 40-2). After the client's condition becomes stable, he or she is discharged.

▪ Evaluation

The PACU nurse continuously evaluates the effectiveness of interventions. The client's condition can change quickly. The nurse may need to increase frequency of select interventions or choose totally new interventions. If evaluation reveals the client is recovering from anesthesia, the physician will discharge the client from the PACU.

Client care.
Evaluation of the client's return to normal physiological functioning is determined by the nurse's frequent assessment of vital signs, pulse oximetry readings, peripheral pulses, wound drainage, and intake and output. The nurse uses the Glasgow Coma Scale (see Chapter 24) to evaluate level of consciousness and asks the client to move all extremities. Significant changes in any findings are reported to the surgeon.

Client expectations.
Pain is subjective and therefore must be validated with the client. The nurse asks the client to rate pain relief on a pain scale and further validates this with assessment of vital signs, facial expressions, and positioning posture. If pain relief is not

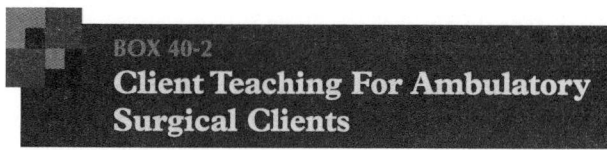

BOX 40-2
Client Teaching For Ambulatory Surgical Clients

- Physician's office telephone number (24-hour answer)
- Surgery center's telephone number
- Follow-up appointment, date, time
- Review of prescribed medications
- Guidelines related to specific surgery
    Dressing and wound care
    Activity restrictions
- Guidelines related to anesthesia
    Dietary
    Activity restrictions
- Warning signs of complications

adequate the nurse should ask the anesthesiologist or nurse anesthetist to change the dosage or type of medication ordered. Evaluation of the client's level of anxiety must also be validated. Nonverbal behavior, blood pressure, and heart rate may indicate the presence or absence of anxiety. The nurse should validate this by asking about the client's feelings and concerns. Further explanations may be required to decrease anxiety.

Discharge From the PACU

The nurse evaluates a client's readiness for discharge from the PACU on the basis of achieved outcomes. If the client's condition is still unstable after 2 to 3 hours, the anesthesia provider may transfer the client to an intensive care unit (ICU). When a hospitalized client's condition stabilizes, it is time for transfer from the PACU to the postoperative nursing unit. Nursing care focuses on returning the client to a functional level of wellness as soon as possible.

The client discharged from the PACU is transported to the postoperative unit on a stretcher. Staff members assist in safely transferring the client to a bed. The PACU nurse reviews the client's course and the PACU record with the nurse caring for the client postoperatively. This report includes a review of physician orders requiring attention. Before the PACU nurse leaves, the unit nurse takes a complete set of vital signs to compare with postanesthesia findings. Minor vital sign variations normally occur after transporting the client. In some settings, when the client is stable, a transporter may take the client to the postoperative unit. In this situation the PACU nurse telephones a report to the nurse on the postoperative unit.

The preoperative nurse usually advises the family to remain in the waiting room while the client is in the operating room and the PACU, so the surgeon can report to them at the end of the surgery. Under special circumstances a family member may visit the client in the PACU. In some facilities a parent may remain with a pediatric client in the PACU to provide emotional support. If the client's stay in the PACU is extended, the nurse can explain that the client is being held longer for observation.

Communication with the family while the client is in the operating room and PACU is very important. Progress reports reduce the anxiety of family members (Leske, 1993). However, while the client is in surgery the nurse should confer with the surgeon before giving progress reports to the family. When the surgery is complete, the surgeon reports to the family the client's status, the results of surgery, and the occurrence of any complications. The nurse should listen to the family's concerns and feelings and assess the ability of the family to cope with this information.

···NURSING PROCESS

▪ Assessment

Once the client arrives at the postoperative unit and the first set of vital signs has been measured, the nurse's assessment includes an initial check of the client's general condition, level of consciousness, condition of dressings and drains, intravenous fluid status, comfort level, and skin integrity. The physical measurements and observations that were performed in the PACU are continued on the postoperative unit. Vital sign routines vary among agencies but may involve assessing the client at least every 15 minutes the first hour, every 30 minutes for 1 to 2 hours, every hour for 4 hours, and then every 4 hours. Assessments may be more frequent, depending on the client's condition. If the client appears normal during the initial assessment, the nurse should not assume that further monitoring is unnecessary. A client's condition can change rapidly. A nurse is guilty of neglect when failing to follow the assessment schedule. The nurse documents the initial assessment and makes entries in the nurse's notes. Vital signs, intravenous fluid intake, and urinary output are entered on flow sheets. The initial findings are a baseline for identifying any postoperative changes.

After the nurse completes the first assessment of the client and has attended to the immediate needs, the family is allowed to visit. The nurse should explain the purpose of postoperative procedures. The family will want to know how the client is doing. The nurse tells them when vital signs are stable and the client seems to be awakening without difficulty. The family should know that the client will fall in and out of sleep for most of the day. The nurse should also remind the family that frequent assessments of the client's condition are to be expected, and if the client had spinal anesthesia, loss of sensation and movement in the extremities can remain for several hours.

▪ Nursing Diagnosis

The nurse determines the status of previous problems identified and clusters new relevant data to identify additional postoperative diagnoses (see nursing diagnosis box on p. 1186). Previously defined diagnoses such as *risk for impaired skin integrity* may continue as a postoperative problem. For example, an older adult client who has had lengthy abdominal surgery and who has a preexisting problem of dehydration and malnutrition is *at risk for impaired skin integrity*. However, client problems can also change. *Risk for impaired skin integrity* can change to *impaired skin integrity* if a skin tear develops.

▪ Planning

During the convalescent phase, the nurse has much information to use for planning the client's care. Postoperative physical assessment data compared with data from the preoperative nursing history allow the nurse to plan specific nursing interventions. The surgeon's postoperative orders also provide guidelines. Typical postoperative orders include the following:

1. Frequency of special assessments
2. Types of intravenous fluids and rate of infusion
3. Postoperative drugs
4. Oxygen therapy or incentive spirometry
5. Dietary restrictions
6. Level of activity the client is allowed to resume
7. Positioning in bed
8. Intake and output
9. Laboratory tests and x-ray studies
10. Special directions

The nurse considers effects of the stress of surgery and limitations imposed when establishing goals of care for the client. Likewise, the nurse considers goals of care established during the preoperative and intraoperative phases, such as achieving physical and psychological comfort and return of normal physiological function. Additional goals include adequate wound healing without the presence of infection and the client's return to a functional state of health and maintenance of self-concept.

Case Study

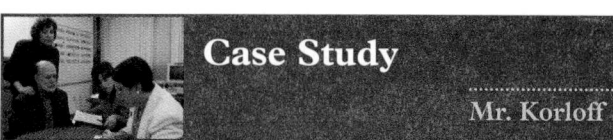

Mr. Korloff

It is the evening of the day of Mr. Korloff's surgery. Mr. Korloff has been transferred to the nursing division for an overnight stay because of his previous cardiac history. He performs deep-breathing and coughing exercises and uses the incentive spirometer as ordered. Because he is ambulating frequently in the hall, with the assistance of his daughters, he is not performing postoperative leg exercises. The intravenous fluids were discontinued just before he left the PACU. Mr. Korloff was able to tolerate a clear liquid diet and had adequate bowel sounds. He rates his pain as 5 on a 10-point scale, continuing to note some discomfort in the shoulder area. His pain has been controlled with an oral pain medication, acetaminophen, which he receives every 3 to 4 hours. His vital signs are within normal limits compared to preoperative values, and his lungs are clear on auscultation. The four small abdominal puncture wounds are without drainage or redness.

▪ Implementation

Acute care. Nursing interventions are directed at preventing complications so that the client returns to the highest level of functioning possible. Failure of the client to become actively involved in recovery adds to the risk of complications developing (Table 40-6). Critical thinking again is important, because the nurse must consider the interrelationship of all body systems and the effect of therapies that are provided.

Maintaining respiratory function. To prevent respiratory complications the nurse begins aggressive pulmonary hygiene measures immediately. The following measures promote expansion of the lung:

1. Encourage diaphragmatic breathing exercises at least every hour while the client is awake. Maximal inspirations lasting 3 to 5 seconds open alveoli.
2. Instruct the client to use an incentive spirometer for maximum inspiration (see Chapter 30).
3. Encourage early ambulation. Walking causes the client to assume a position that does not restrict chest wall expansion and stimulates an increased respiratory rate and circulation.
4. Assist clients who are restricted to bed to turn side-to-side every 1 to 2 hours while awake and to sit when possible. Turning permits expansion of the lungs, mobilizes secretions, and improves circulation. Sitting causes lowering of abdominal organs, thus facilitating diaphragmatic movement and lung expansion.

The following measures promote the removal of pulmonary secretions:

1. Encourage coughing exercises at least every 2 hours while the client is awake, and maintain pain control to promote a full productive cough.
2. Provide oral hygiene to expectorate mucus. Oral mucosa becomes dry when the client is allowed nothing by mouth or placed on limited fluid intake.
3. Initiate postural drainage, percussion, and orotracheal or nasotracheal suction for clients too weak or unable to cough (Brooks-Brunn, 1995) (see Chapter 30).

Preventing circulatory stasis. Early measures directed at preventing circulatory complications prevent venous stasis. The following measures promote normal venous return and peripheral blood flow:

1. *Encourage clients to perform leg exercises at least every hour while awake unless contraindicated by surgery.*
2. *Apply elastic antiembolism stockings as ordered by the physician.* The stockings should be removed every 8 hours and left off for 1 hour.
3. *Apply pneumatic sequential compression stockings.*

TABLE 40-6
Postoperative Complications

Complication	Cause
Respiratory System	
Atelectasis is collapse of alveoli with retained mucous secretions.	Inadequate lung expansion Anesthesia, analgesics, and immobilized position preventing full lung expansion Greater risk in clients with upper abdominal surgery who have pain during inspiration and repress deep breathing
Pneumonia is inflammation of alveoli caused by infectious process; it may involve one or several lobes of lung, and development in lower dependent lobes of lung is common in immobilized surgical client.	Poor lung expansion with retained secretions Common resident bacteria in respiratory tract, *Diplococcus pneumoniae,* which causes most cases of pneumonia
Hypoxia is inadequate concentration of oxygen in arterial blood. Signs and symptoms include restlessness, dyspnea, high blood pressure, tachycardia, diaphoresis, and cyanosis.	Respirations depressed by anesthetics or analgesics Increased retention of mucus with impaired ventilation because of pain or poor positioning
Pulmonary embolism is embolus blocking pulmonary artery and disrupting blood flow to one or more lobes of lung.	Same factors that lead to formation of thrombus or embolus High risk to immobilized surgical client with preexisting circulatory or coagulation disorders
Circulatory System	
Hemorrhage is loss of large amount of blood externally or internally in short period of time.	Slipping of suture or dislodged clot at incisional site Clients with coagulation disorders are at greater risk
Hypovolemic shock is inadequate perfusion of tissues and cells from loss of circulatory fluid volume.	In surgical client, usually caused by hemorrhage
Thrombophlebitis is inflammation of vein often accompanied by clot formation; leg veins are most commonly affected.	Venous stasis aggravated by prolonged sitting or immobilization Trauma to vessel wall and hypercoagulability of blood increasing risk of vessel inflammation
Thrombus is formation of clot attached to interior wall of a vein or artery, which can occlude vessel lumen.	Venous stasis (see *thrombophlebitis*) and vessel trauma
Embolus is piece of thrombus that has dislodged and circulates in bloodstream until it lodges in another vessel, commonly lungs, heart, or brain.	Venous injury common after surgery of legs, abdomen, pelvis, and major vessels Thrombi also forming from increased coagulability of blood
Gastrointestinal System	
Abdominal distention is retention of air within intestines.	Slowed peristalsis from anesthesia, bowel manipulation, or immobilization
Constipation is infrequent passage of stools; it is not a concern immediately after surgery, especially if client has preoperative bowel preparation. After client resumes solid diet, failure to pass stool within 48 hours is a problem.	Slowed peristalsis (see *distention*) and delay in resuming normal diet
Nausea and vomiting are symptoms of improper gastric emptying or chemical stimulation of vomiting center.	Severe pain, abdominal distention, fear, medications, eating or drinking before peristalsis returns, initiating gag reflex
Genitourinary System	
Urinary retention is involuntary accumulation of urine in bladder as result of loss of muscle tone.	Effects of anesthesia and narcotic analgesics Local manipulation of tissues around bladder and edema interfering with bladder tone

TABLE 40-6
Postoperative Complications—cont'd

Complication	Cause
Integumentary System	
Wound infection is invasion of deep or superficial wound tissues by pathogenic microorganisms.	Contamination of wound after surgery Contaminated wound before surgical exploration
Wound dehiscence is separation of wound edges at suture line.	Malnutrition, obesity, preoperative radiation to surgical site, old age, poor circulation to tissues Unusual strain on suture line from coughing
Wound evisceration is protrusion of internal organs and tissues through incision. It usually occurs 6 to 8 days after surgery.	See *dehiscence* Client with dehiscence at risk for developing evisceration
Skin breakdown.	Prolonged immobilization and pressure

Compressed air inflates the padded plastic stocking systematically from ankle to calf to thigh and then deflates, promoting venous return and reducing venous stasis.

4. *Encourage early ambulation.* Most clients are ordered to ambulate the evening of surgery, depending on the severity of surgery and the client's condition. The degree of activity allowed progresses as the client's condition improves. Before ambulation, the nurse assesses vital signs. Abnormalities may contraindicate ambulation. If vital signs are normal, the nurse first assists the client to sit on the side of the bed. Dizziness is a sign of postural hypotension (see Chapter 23). A recheck of blood pressure determines whether ambulation is safe. The nurse assists with ambulation by standing at the client's side and assisting with equipment. During the first few times out of bed, the client may be able to walk only a few feet. Tolerance should improve each time. The nurse evaluates the client's tolerance to activity, periodically assessing pulse rate.

5. *Avoid positioning the client in a manner that interrupts blood flow to the extremities.* While in bed, the client should not have pillows or rolled blankets placed under the knees. Compression of the popliteal vessels can cause a thrombus to form. When sitting in a chair, the client should elevate the legs on a footstool, avoiding hyperextension of the knee. The client should never be allowed to sit with one leg crossed over the other.

6. *Give anticoagulant drugs as ordered.* Physicians often order small doses of anticoagulants, such as heparin, for clients at greatest risk for thrombus formation. Orthopedic clients often receive low doses of aspirin for anticoagulation.

7. *Promote adequate fluid intake orally or intravenously.* Adequate hydration prevents the concentration of platelets and red blood cells. When the plasma volume is low, these cells may form small clots within blood vessels. Adequate hydration also promotes tissue healing.

Promoting normal elimination and adequate nutrition. Interventions for preventing gastrointestinal complications promote the return of normal elimination and faster resumption of normal nutritional intake. It takes several days for a client who has had surgery on gastrointestinal structures to resume a normal dietary intake. Normal peristalsis may not return for 2 to 3 days. In contrast, the client whose gastrointestinal tract is unaffected directly by surgery must simply endure the effects of anesthesia before resuming dietary intake. The following measures promote return of normal elimination:

1. *Assess for return of peristalsis.* The nurse routinely auscultates the abdomen to detect the return of normal bowel sounds (see Chapter 24). The nurse asks whether the client is passing flatus, an important sign indicating normal bowel function.

2. *Maintain a gradual progression in dietary intake.* Immediately after surgery, a client receives only intravenous fluids. Once the physician orders a normal diet, the nurse first provides clear liquids such as water, apple juice, or tea after nausea subsides. Overloading with large amounts of fluids may lead to distention and vomiting. If the client tolerates liquids without nausea, the diet is advanced to full liquids, followed by a light diet of solid foods, and finally a regular diet, stressing the importance of foods that are high in protein and vitamin C. Clients who have had abdominal surgery are usually not allowed anything by mouth (NPO) the first 24 to 48 hours.

3. *Promote ambulation and exercise.* Physical activity stimulates a return of peristalsis. The client who suffers abdominal distention and "gas pain" will often obtain relief while walking.

4. *Maintain an adequate fluid intake.* Fluids keep fecal material soft for easy passage.
5. *Administer fiber supplements, stool softeners, enemas, rectal suppositories, and rectal tubes as ordered.* Constipation or distention can develop postoperatively.

The following measures assist the client to maintain an adequate dietary intake:

1. Remove sources of noxious odors.
2. Assist the client to sit (if possible) during mealtime to minimize pressure on the abdomen.
3. Provide small servings of nonspicy food.
4. Provide frequent oral hygiene to eliminate dryness and bad tastes in the mouth.
5. Provide meals when the client is rested and free from pain. A client will often lose interest in eating if mealtime has been preceded by exhausting activities such as ambulation or postoperative exercises. When a client has pain, the associated nausea causes a loss of appetite.

Promoting urinary elimination. The depressant effects of anesthesia and analgesics impair the sensation of bladder fullness. If bladder tone is reduced, the client has difficulty initiating urination. Clients who undergo surgery of the urinary system frequently have Foley catheters inserted until voluntary control of urination returns. The following measures promote normal urinary elimination (see Chapter 35):

1. *Assist the client to assume normal positions for voiding.*
2. *Check the client frequently for the need to void.* The feeling of bladder fullness and urgency to void is often sudden, and the nurse must respond promptly when the client calls for assistance.
3. *Assess for bladder distention.* If a client does not void within 8 hours of surgery, it may be necessary to insert a straight urinary catheter. Continued difficulty may require a Foley catheter, although the risk for urinary tract infection increases.
4. *Monitor intake and output.* If the client's urine is dark, concentrated, and less than 30 ml/hr, a physician should be notified. A client can easily become dehydrated as a result of fluid loss from the surgical wound, decreased intake, and increased fluid requirements.

Promoting wound healing. A surgical wound undergoes considerable stress during convalescence. Inadequate nutrition, impaired circulation, and metabolic alterations increase the risk for delayed healing. A wound may also undergo considerable physical stress (e.g., strain on sutures from coughing, vomiting, distention, and movement of body parts). A critical time for wound healing is 24 to 72 hours after surgery (see Chapter 38). If a wound becomes infected, it usually occurs 3 to 6 days after surgery. The nurse uses aseptic technique during dressing changes and wound care. Surgical drains must remain patent so that accumulated secretions are removed from the incision site. Ongoing observation of the wound identifies early signs and symptoms of infection.

Promoting rest and comfort. A surgical client's pain increases as the effects of anesthesia wear off. The client becomes more aware of surroundings and more perceptive of discomfort. The incisional area may be only one source of pain. Irritation from drainage tubes, tight dressings, or casts and the muscular strains caused from positioning on the operating room table can cause discomfort.

Pain can significantly slow recovery. The client becomes reluctant to perform necessary postoperative exercises. The nurse should assess pain thoroughly. It should not be assumed that the pain is incisional in origin. When the client requests pain medication, the nature and character of the pain should be determined. Clients have the most surgical pain during the first 24 to 48 hours after surgery. The nurse should provide analgesics as often as allowed during this time. Chapter 33 reviews treatment options for acute surgical pain.

Maintaining self-concept. The appearance of wounds, bulky dressings, and extruding drains and tubes threatens a client's self-concept. The nature of the surgery may also create a permanent change in body image. If surgery leads to impairment in body function, the client's role within the family can change significantly. The nurse should observe the client for alterations in self-concept. Clients may show a revulsion toward their appearance by refusing to look at an incision or carefully covering dressings with bedclothes. The fear of not being able to return to a functional role in the family may even cause the client to avoid participating in the care plan.

The family can play an important role in efforts to improve the client's self-concept. The family should be accepting of the client's needs and still encourage independence. The following measures maintain the client's self-concept:

1. *Provide privacy* during dressing changes or wound inspection by closing room curtains and draping client so that only the dressing and incisional area are exposed.
2. *Maintain the client's hygiene.* A complete bath the first day after surgery can make the client feel renewed. The nurse offers a clean gown and washcloth when the gown becomes soiled. The nurse keeps the client's hair neatly combed and offers frequent oral hygiene, especially for the client who is allowed nothing by mouth.
3. *Prevent drainage sets from overflowing.* Typically the drainage sets are measured every 8 hours for output recording.

4. *Maintain a pleasant environment.* The nurse should store or remove all unused supplies and keep the bedside orderly and clean.

5. *Offer opportunities for the client to discuss feelings about appearance.* Clients worry about permanent scarring. A client is more apt to look at an incision several days after surgery when healing is occurring and the client begins to gain energy and a feeling of well-being. When the client chooses to look at an incision for the first time, the area should be clean. Eventually the client should be able to care for the incision site by applying simple dressings or bathing.

6. *Give the family opportunities to discuss ways to promote the client's self-concept.* Encouraging independence can be difficult for a family member who has a strong desire to assist the client in any way. By knowing about the appearance of a wound or incision, family members can be supportive during dressing changes. The topic or tone of a conversation can also help family members to distract a client from dwelling on fears and concerns.

Restorative care. Other activities that are involved in postoperative care are to promote return to a functional state of health. Throughout the postoperative convalescent period the nurse promotes the client's independence and active participation in care. When a client is in pain or suffers from postoperative complications, there is little motive for self-care. The goals a nurse sets for a client's involvement must be realistic. It is unrealistic for the nurse to involve the client if movement is highly restricted or if participation increases the discomfort.

The nurse should keep the client and family informed of progress made toward recovery. Many clients become depressed if they think recovery is slow. The nurse explains the length of time expected to reach a level of maximal recovery. When using a CareMap, the nurse may show the client's progress compared with the CareMap and explain any alterations. Surgery may also cause permanent physical limitations that will require time for the client to accept.

The nurse plans care daily, keeping in mind the ultimate goals for recovery. From the moment the client enters the hospital, the nurse anticipates and plans for the client's return home.

Involvement of family members in the care plan can facilitate early discharge and adequate care at home. The nurse instructs family members about care activities. If family members are unable to assist the client, the nurse works with the physician, social worker, or discharge planner to make plans for home care.

Evaluation

The nurse evaluates effectiveness of care on the basis of expected outcomes resulting from nursing interven-

tions. The nurse can evaluate the ambulatory surgical client's outcomes by making a postoperative telephone call to the client's home. The call, usually placed 24 hours after surgery, reassures the client that the nurse is concerned and allows the nurse to evaluate the progress of recovery. In the inpatient setting the nurse monitors the client's progress over several days. The use of evaluative measures determines whether outcomes are achieved.

Client care. The nurse evaluates the client's clinical progress by observing the client's participation in postoperative exercises, self-care activities, and ambulation. Physiological functioning is evaluated through the continuous assessment of vital signs, breath sounds, peripheral pulses, bowel sounds, and urinary output. Wound healing is evaluated by assessing for redness and drainage from the incision.

Client expectations. Adequate preoperative preparation and teaching not only affect the speed of recovery but also help the client and family to set realistic expectations regarding the outcomes of surgery and postoperative care. Physical and psychological comfort are typical expectations of clients and families. Achievement of this goal is determined by having the client use a pain scale to evaluate pain relief, observing the client's participation in care, discussing the client's expectations regarding recovery, and observing nonverbal signs that may indicate anxiety. Client self-concept can be evaluated by observing the client's willingness to assume increasing responsibility for self-care, wanting to inspect the incision, and asking for and repeating discharge instructions. Information regarding home care options should be made available to clients and families.

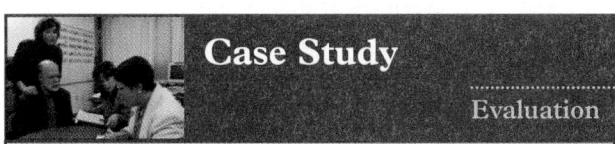

Case Study

Evaluation

Mr. Korloff progressed well and is ready for discharge the day after surgery. He expresses relief that everything went well so that he will be able to return to work, hopefully by next week. Sue has been able to follow the client and continue to care for him on the surgical division. Sue explains how to remove the gauze on the puncture sites and to bathe and shower tomorrow. Symptoms the client and family should be observant for are redness, swelling, bile-colored drainage or pus from the abdominal wounds, severe abdominal pain, nausea, vomiting, and fever or chills. Any of these symptoms should be reported to Mr. Korloff's physician immediately. His daughters observed the puncture sites and are able to identify symptoms of complications. Mr. Korloff is ready for discharge and plans to stay with one of his daughters over the weekend. Sue has coordinated through the physician's office a time for Mr. Korloff's follow-up appointment.

Documentation Note
Sue documents Mr. Korloff's readiness for discharge as follows: Abdominal puncture sites dry and intact, without redness. Discharge teaching provided to client and daughters. Repeated signs and symptoms of complications; wound care instructions; activity restrictions; and follow-up appointment time, date, and place.

Key Terms

antiembolism stockings	outpatient
circulating nurse	perioperative nursing
convalescence	postanesthesia care
general anesthesia	unit
laryngospasm	preoperative teaching
malignant hyper-	recovery
thermia	regional anesthesia
nasogastric tube	scrub nurse
operating room	

▪ Key Concepts

Perioperative nursing is professional nursing care afforded the surgical client before, during, and after surgery.

In addition to the nature of nursing care provided, previous illnesses and past surgeries influence the ability to tolerate surgery.

Older adult clients are at surgical risk from their declining physiological status.

All medications taken before surgery are automatically discontinued after surgery unless a physician reorders the drugs.

Family members are important in assisting clients with physical limitations and in providing emotional support during the postoperative recovery.

Preoperative assessment of vital signs and physical findings provides an important baseline with which to compare postoperative assessment data.

A client's feelings about surgery can have a significant impact on relationships with nursing staff and the client's ability to participate in care.

Surgical removal of a body part may permanently alter body image and sexuality.

Nursing diagnoses of the surgical client may pose implications for nursing care during one or all phases of surgery.

Primary responsibility for informed consent rests with the surgeon.

Structured preoperative teaching positively influences postoperative recovery.

If hair around the incision must be removed, it should be clipped as close as possible to the time of surgery to minimize infection.

In ambulatory surgery, nurses must use the limited time available to educate clients, assess their health status, and prepare them for surgery.

The responsibility of nurses within the operating room focuses on protecting the client from potential harm.

Assessment of the postoperative client centers on the body systems most likely to be affected.

Because a surgical client's condition may change rapidly during recovery, the nurse monitors the client's status at least every 15 minutes.

The PACU nurse reports to the nurse on the postoperative unit information pertaining to the client's current physical status and risk for postoperative complications.

From the time of admission, the nurse plans for the surgical client's discharge.

Critical Thinking Activities

1. Mr. Wilson is a 76-year-old client admitted for a fractured hip. He has a history of emphysema. What risk does Mr. Wilson face as a result of surgery, and why?
2. Mary is the nurse working in the preadmission center for surgical services. She is interviewing Mrs. Rice, who states that she has been taking one baby aspirin every day to help with her circulation. Why is this important for Mary to document?
3. Angie is a nursing student assigned to Mrs. Lyons, a 45-year-old woman who is recovering from surgery for a colon resection. It is the third day af-ter surgery, and Mrs. Lyons' NG tube was removed yesterday afternoon. During her morning rounds, Angie is assessing Mrs. Lyons and finds that her abdomen is distended. What might this indicate?
4. Mr. Pulley had a colon resection yesterday and has a midline incision that extends from the xiphoid process to the symphysis pubis. Carmen has been assigned as his nurse and assesses rales when auscultating his lungs. What information regarding Mr. Pulley's incision must Carmen consider in planning interventions to address the nursing diagnosis of *ineffective airway clearance?*

References

AHCPR, Acute Pain Management Guideline Panel: *Acute pain management in infants, children, and adolescents: operative or medical procedures and trauma,* Clinical practice guideline, AHCPR Pub. No. 92-0032, Rockville, Md, 1992, Agency for Health Care Policy and Research, PHS, USDHHS.

Association of Operating Room Nurses: *Standards and recommended practices,* Denver, 1996, AORN.

Brooks-Brunn JA: Postoperative atelectasis and pneumonia, *Heart Lung* 24(2):94, 1995.

Brooks-Brunn JA: Surgery—protecting the lungs, *Reflections* 23(1):16, 1997.

Dettenmeier PA: *Pulmonary nursing care,* St. Louis, 1992, Mosby.

Giger JN, Davidhizar RE: *Transcultural nursing: assessment and intervention,* St. Louis, 1995, Mosby.

Graham K and others: Preadmission strategies: reducing the length of preoperative stay, *Leadership* Jan/Feb:7, 1996.

Larson E and others: Effects of a protective foam on scrubbing and gloving, *Am J Infect Control* 21(6)297, 1993.

Leske JS: *Effects of "progress reports" on anxiety levels of elective surgical patients' family members.* Paper presented at Midwest Nursing Research Society: Nursing Research and its Multidisciplinary Dimensions, March 27-30, 1993.

Lindeman C, VanAernam B: Nursing intervention with the presurgical patient: the effects of structured and unstructured preoperative teaching, *Nurs Res* 20:319, 1971.

Meeker B: Preoperative patient education: evaluating postoperative patient outcomes, *Patient Ed Couns* 23:41, 1994.

Metheny N: Measures to test placement of nasogastric and nasointestinal feeding tubes: a review, *Nurs Res* 37:324, 1988.

Metheny N and others: Effectiveness of the auscultatory method in predicting feeding tube location, *Nurs Res* 39:262, 1990.

Metheny N and others: Effectiveness of pH measurements in predicting feeding tube placement: an update, *Nurs Res* 42(6):324, 1993.

Metheny N and others: Visual characteristics of aspirates from feeding tubes as a method for predicting tube location, *Nurs Res* 43(5):282, 1994.

Oetker-Black S: Preoperative preparation, *AORN J* 57(4): 1402, 1993.

Pagana KD, Pagana TJ: *Diagnostic testing and nursing implications: a case study approach,* ed 4, St. Louis, 1994, Mosby.

Redmond MC: Latex allergy: recognition and perioperative management, *J Post Anesth Nurs* 11(1):6, 1996.

Roach J and others: A preoperative assessment and education program: implementation and outcomes, *Patient Ed Couns* 25:83, 1995.

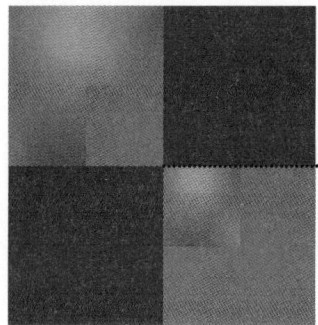

Common Abbreviations

NOTE: Abbreviations in common use can vary widely from place to place. Each institution's list of acceptable abbreviations is the best authority for its records.

°C	degrees centigrade
°F	degrees Fahrenheit
μg	microgram
μm	micrometer
ℨ	dram
@	at

A

aa	of each
ABG	arterial blood gas
ac	before meals
ad lib	freely as desired
ADL	activities of daily living
Ag	silver, antigen
AIDS	acquired immunodeficiency syndrome
ALS	amyotrophic lateral sclerosis
AM	morning
ama	against medical advice
AMI	acute myocardial infarction
amp	ampule
ARC	AIDS-related complex
ARDS	adult respiratory distress syndrome
AS	aortic stenosis
ASD	atrial septal defect

B

Ba	barium
BE	barium enema
bid	two times a day
BM, bm	bowel movement
BMR	basal metabolic rate
BP	blood pressure
BPH	benign prostatic hypertrophy
BRP	bathroom privileges
BSA	body surface area
BUN	blood urea nitrogen

C

c̃	with
c/o	complains of
Ca	calcium, cancer, carcinoma
CAD	coronary artery disease
cap	capsule
CAT	computed axial tomography
cath	catheter, catheterize
CBC	complete blood count
CBR	complete bed rest
CC	chief complaint
cc	cubic centimeter
CCU	coronary care unit, critical care unit
CDC	Centers for Disease Control and Prevention
CEA	carcinoembryonic antigen
CFT	complement-fixation test
cg	centigram
CHF	congestive heart failure
CHO	carbohydrate
Cl	chlorine
cm	centimeter
cm³	cubic centimeter
CNS	central nervous system
CO	carbon monoxide
CO₂	carbon dioxide
COPD	chronic obstructive pulmonary disease
CPK	creatine phosphokinase
CPR	cardiopulmonary resuscitation
CSF	cerebrospinal fluid
CT	computed tomography
CVA	cerebrovascular accident, costovertebral angle
CVP	central venous pressure

D

D&C	dilation and curettage
D5W	5% dextrose in water
db, dB	decibels
dc	discontinue
DIC	disseminated intravascular coagulation
diff	differential blood count
dil	dilute
DJD	degenerative joint disease
dl	deciliter
DM	diastolic murmur
DNR	do not resuscitate
DOE	dyspnea on exertion
dx, Dx	diagnosis

E

EBV	Epstein-Barr virus
ECF	extracellular fluid
ECG	electrocardiogram
ECHO	echocardiography
ECT	electroconvulsive therapy
EDC	estimated date of confinement
EDD	estimated date of delivery
EEG	electroencephalogram
EKG	electrocardiogram
elix	elixer
EMG	electromyogram
ENG	electronystagmography
ER	emergency room
ERG	electroretinogram
ESRD	end-stage renal disease
EST	electroshock therapy

F

℥	fluid ounce
FANA	fluorescent antinuclear antibody test
FBS	fasting blood sugar
Fe	iron
FEV	forced expiratory volume
FHR	fetal heart rate
FRC	functional residual capacity
FSH	follicle-stimulating hormone
FUO	fever of unknown origin
Fx, fx	fracture, fractional urine test

G

g, gm, Gm	gram
Gc, GC	gonococcus
GI	gastrointestinal
gr	grain
grav I, II, III, etc.	pregnancy one, two, three, etc.
gt, gtt	drop, drops
GTT	glucose tolerance test
GU	genitourinary
GYN, Gyn	gynecological

H

H_2O	water
h	hour
H^+	hydrogen ion
h/o	history of
H&P	history and physical examination
HAV	hepatitis A virus
Hb	hemoglobin
HBAg	hepatitis B antigen
HBV	hepatitis B virus
Hct, HCT	hematocrit
HDL	high-density lipoprotein
Hg	mercury
Hgb	hemoglobin
HIV	human immunodeficiency (AIDS) virus
HLA	human lymphocyte antigen
HSV2	herpes simplex virus, type 2

I

I&O	intake and output
IC	inspiratory capacity
ICP	intracranial pressure
ICU	intensive care unit
IDDM	insulin-dependent diabetes mellitus
IE	immunoelectrophoresis
Ig	immunoglobulin
IgA, etc.	immunoglobulin A, etc.
IM	intramuscular
IOP	intraocular pressure
IPPB	intermittent positive pressure breathing
IV	intravenous
IVP	intravenous push; intravenous pyelogram
IVU	intravenous urogram

J

JRA	juvenile rheumatoid arthritis

K

K	potassium
kg	kilogram
KUB	kidney, ureters, and bladder (radiograph)
KVO	keep vein open

L

L	liter
L&A	light and accommodation
LBBB	left bundle branch block
LE	lupus erythematosus
LGV	lymphogranuloma venereum
LLL	left lower lobe
LLQ	left lower quadrant
LMP	last menstrual period
LNMP	last normal menstrual period

LP	lumbar puncture	para I, II, etc.	unipara, bipara, etc.
LUL	left upper lobe	PAT	paroxysmal atrial tachycardia
LUQ	left upper quadrant	pc	after meals
LVH	left ventricular hypertrophy	PCG	phonocardiogram
		P_{CO_2}	partial pressure of carbon dioxide
M		PCP	pulmonary capillary pressure, phencyclidine
m	meter	PCV	packed cell volume
m, min, ♍	minum	PCWP	pulmonary capillary wedge pressure
MAP	mean arterial pressure		
mcg	microgram	PD	interpupillary distance; postural drainage
MCH	mean corpuscular hemoglobin		
MCHC	mean corpuscular hemoglobin concentration	PE	pulmonary embolism, physical examination
MCV	mean cell volume, mean corpuscular volume	PEEP	positive end expiratory pressure
		PEG	pneumoencephalography
mg	milligram	per	through, by way of
Mg	magnesium	PERRLA	pupils equal, round, and reactive to light and accommodation
MG	myasthenia gravis		
MI	myocardial infarction	PET	positron emission tomography
MICU	medical intensive care unit	PG	prostaglandin
ml	milliliter	pH	hydrogen ion concentration (acidity and alkalinity)
mm	millimeter		
mm³	cubic millimeter	PID	pelvic inflammatory disease
mm Hg	millimeters of mercury	PKU	phenylketonuria
MRI	magnetic resonance imaging	PM	postmortem
MS	multiple sclerosis	PM	evening
MW	molecular weight	PMS	premenstrual syndrome
		PND	paroxysmal nocturnal dyspnea, postnasal drip
N			
N	nitrogen	P_{O_2}	partial pressure of oxygen
Na	sodium	PO, po	orally
NICU	neonatal intensive care unit	PPD	purified protein derivative
NIH	National Institutes of Health	ppm	parts per million
nm	nanometer	prn	when required, as often as necessary
NMR	nuclear magnetic resonance		
NPO	nothing by mouth	PT	physical therapy; prothrombin time
NS	normal saline	PTT	partial thromboplastin time
		PUO	pyrexia of unknown origin
O		PVC	premature ventricular contraction
O_2	oxygen		
OD	right eye; optical density; overdose	**Q**	
OL	left eye	q	every
OOB	out of bed	q2h	every 2 hours
ORIF	open reduction and internal fixation	q3h	every 3 hours
		q4h	every 4 hours
OS	left eye	qd	every day
OT	occupational therapy	qh	every hour
OTC	over-the-counter	qid	four times a day
ou	both eyes	qn	every night
oz, ℥	ounce	qod	every other day
		qns	quantity not sufficient
P			
P&A	percussion and auscultation	**R**	
Pa_{CO_2}	partial pressure of carbon dioxide (arterial blood)	R/O	rule out
		RBBB	right bundle branch block
Pa_{O_2}	partial pressure of oxygen (arterial blood)	RBC	red blood cell

RDS	respiratory distress syndrome
Rh+	positive Rh factor
Rh−	negative Rh factor
RHD	rheumatic heart disease
RLL	right lower lobe
RLQ	right lower quadrant
RML	right middle lobe
ROM	range of motion
ROS	review of systems
RS	Reiter's syndrome
RSV	Rous sarcoma virus
RUL	right upper lobe
RUQ	right upper quadrant
Rx	take; treatment

S

$\bar{s}$	without
SB	sternal border
SC	subcutaneous
sib	sibling
SICU	surgical intensive care unit
SIDS	sudden infant death syndrome
Sig	write on label
SLE	systemic lupus erythematosus
sol	solution, dissolved
sos	if necessary
sp gr, SG, sg	specific gravity
SQ, subq	subcutaneous
SR	sedimentation rate
ss	half
SSS	sick sinus syndrome, specific soluble substance, short-stay surgery
stat	immediately
STD	sexually transmitted disease
STS	serologic test for syphilis
susp	suspension
SV	stroke volume

T

T_3	triiodothyronine
T_4	tetraiodothyronine
T&A	tonsillectomy and adenoidectomy
TAB	typhoid and paratyphoid A and B
TAH	total abdominal hysterectomy

TAT	tetanus antitoxin; thematic apperception test
TB, TBC	tuberculosis
TBG	thyroxin-binding globulin
TG	triglyceride
TIA	transient ischemic attack
TIBC	total iron-binding capacity
tid	three times a day
TKO	to keep open
TLC	total lung capacity; thin layer chromatography
TPN	total parenteral nutrition
TPR	temperature, pulse, and respirations
tr, tinct	tincture
TST	triple sugar iron test
TSH	thyroid-stimulating hormone

U

UA	urinalysis
UGI series	upper gastrointestinal series
UIBC	unsaturated iron-binding capacity
URI	upper respiratory infection
US	ultrasound
UTI	urinary tract infection

V

V&T	volume and tension
VC	vital capacity
VD	venereal disease
VDA	visual discriminatory acuity
VDH	valvular disease of the heart
VDRL	Venereal Disease Research Laboratory
VLDL	very low-density lipoprotein
VS	vital signs
VSD	ventricular septal defect
V_T	tidal volume

W

W/V	weight/volume
WBC	white blood cell, white blood count
WNL	within normal limits
WR	Wassermann reaction

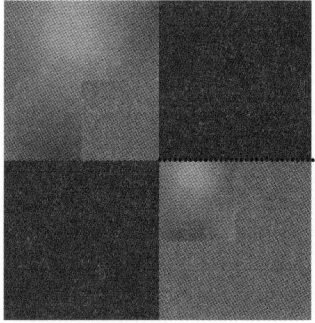

Glossary

abduction Movement of a limb away from the body.

abnormal reactive hyperemia Hyperemia over a pressure site lasting longer than 1 hour following removal of pressure; surrounding skin does not blanch.

abrasion Scraping or rubbing away of epidermis; may result in localized bleeding and later weeping of serous fluid.

absorption Passage of drug molecules into the blood. Factors influencing drug absorption include route of administration, ability of the drug to dissolve, and conditions at the site of absorption.

accessory muscles Muscles in the thoracic cage that assist with respiration.

accommodation The process of responding to the environment through new activity and thinking and changing the existing schema or developing a new schema to deal with the new information. A toddler whose parent consistently corrected him when he called a horse a "doggie" accommodates and forms a new schema for horses.

accountability State of being answerable for one's actions—the professional nurse answers to herself, the client, the profession, the employing institution, and society for the effectiveness of nursing care performed.

acculturation Process of intercultural borrowing between diverse peoples, resulting in new and blended patterns.

acne Inflammatory, papulopustular skin eruption, usually occurring on the face, neck, shoulders, and upper back.

acromegaly Chronic metabolic condition caused by overproduction of growth hormone and characterized by gradual, marked enlargement and elongation of bones of the face, jaw, and extremities.

active listening Listening attentively with the whole person—mind, body, and spirit. It includes listening for main and supportive ideas, acknowledging and responding, giving appropriate feedback, and paying attention to the other person's total communication, including the content, the intent, and the feelings expressed.

active range of motion (ROM) The range of movement through which a joint can be moved without assistance.

active strategies of health promotion Activities that depend on the client being motivated to adopt a specific health program.

active transport Movement of materials across the cell membrane by means of chemical activity that allows the cell to admit larger molecules than would otherwise be possible.

activities of daily living (ADLs) Activities usually performed in the course of a normal day in the client's life, such as eating, dressing, bathing, brushing the teeth, or grooming.

activity tolerance Kind and amount of exercise or work that a person is able to perform.

actual loss A loss of an object, person, body part or function, or emotion that is overt and easily identifiable.

actual nursing diagnosis A judgment that is clinically validated by the presence of major defining characteristics.

acuity charting Mechanism by which entries describing client care activities are made over a 24-hour period. The activities are then translated into a rating score or acuity score that allows for a comparison of clients who vary by severity of illness.

acute care Pattern of health care in which a client is treated for an acute episode of illness, for the sequelae of an accident or other trauma, or during recovery from surgery.

acute illness Illness characterized by symptoms that are of relatively short duration, are usually severe, and affect the functioning of the client in all dimensions.

adaptation Process by which changes occur in any of a person's dimensions in response to stress.

adduction Movement of a limb toward the body.

adolescence The period in development between the onset of puberty and adulthood. It usually begins between 11 and 13 years of age.

adult day care centers A facility for the supervised care of older adults, providing such activities as meals and socialization during specified day hours.

advanced practice nurse A registered professional nurse who has been educated at the master's level, has completed advanced physical assessment and pharmacology, and is certified in an area of expertise. Includes clinical nurse specialists, nurse practitioners, nurse midwives, and certified registered nurse anesthetists.

advanced sleep phase syndrome Common in older adults, a disturbance in sleep manifested as early waking in the morning with an inability to get back to sleep. It is believed that this syndrome is caused by advancing of the body's circadian rhythm.

adventitious sounds Abnormal lung sounds heard with auscultation.

adverse effect Harmful or unintended effect of a medication, diagnostic test, or therapeutic intervention.

advocacy Process whereby a nurse objectively provides clients with the information they need to make decisions and supports the clients in whatever decisions they make.

afebrile Without fever.

affective learning Acquisition of behaviors involved in expressing feelings in attitudes, appreciations, and values.

afterload The resistance to left ventricular ejection; the work the heart must overcome to fully eject blood from the left ventricle.

AHCPR Agency for Health Care Policy and Research, which synthesizes research and develops standards of practice.

air pollution Contamination of the environmental atmosphere with substances known as pollutants that are not normally found in the air.

airway resistance The pressure difference between the mouth, nose, or other airway opening and the alveoli.

alarm reaction The mobilization of the defense mechanisms of the body and mind to cope with a stressor. The initial stage of the general adaptation syndrome.

aldosterone A mineralocorticoid steroid hormone produced by the adrenal cortex with action in the renal tubule to regulate sodium and potassium balance in the blood.

Allen's test A test that assesses the patency of the radial artery. It is performed routinely prior to sampling for an arterial blood gas. The client's hand is formed into a fist while the nurse compresses the ulnar artery. Compression of the ulnar artery is continued while the fist is opened. If blood perfusion through the radial artery is adequate, the hand should flush and resume normal pinkish coloration.

alopecia Partial or complete loss of hair; baldness.

Alzheimer's disease Disease of the brain parenchyma that causes a gradual and progressive decline in cognitive functioning.

AMBULARM A device used for the client who climbs out of bed unassisted and is in danger of falling. This device is worn on the leg and signals when the leg is in a dependent position such as over the side rail or on the floor.

ambulatory health services Health services provided on an outpatient basis to those who visit a hospital or other health care facility.

amino acid An organic compound of one or more basic groups and one or more carboxyl groups. Amino acids are the building blocks that construct proteins and the end products of protein digestion.

anabolism Constructive metabolism characterized by conversion of simple substances into more complex compounds of living matter.

analgesic Relieving pain; drug that relieves pain.

analogies Resemblances made between things otherwise unlike.

anaphylactic reaction A hypersensitive condition induced by contact with certain antigens.

anemia Disorder characterized by a decrease in hemoglobin of the blood.

aneurysms Localized dilations of the wall of a blood vessel, usually caused by atherosclerosis, hypertension, or a congenital weakness in a vessel wall.

angina pectoris Episodic chest pain caused most often by myocardial anoxia, resulting from atherosclerosis of the coronary arteries. Pain radiates down the inner aspect of the left arm and is often accompanied by feeling of suffocation and impending death.

angiography A radiographic visualization of the internal anatomy of the heart and blood vessels after the introduction of a radiopaque contrast medium.

angiotensin A polypeptide occurring in the blood causing vasoconstriction, increased blood pressure, and the release of aldosterone from the adrenal cortex.

anion gap The difference between the concentrations of serum cations and anions, determined by measuring the concentrations of sodium cations and chloride and bicarbonate anions.

anions Negatively charged electrolytes.

anorexia Lack or loss of appetite resulting in the inability to eat.

anthropometric measurements Body measures of height, weight, and skinfolds to evaluate muscle atrophy.

anthropometry Measurement of various body parts to determine nutritional and caloric status, muscular development, brain growth, and other parameters.

antibodies Immunoglobulins, essential to the immune system, that are produced by lymphoid tissue in response to bacteria, viruses, or other antigens.

anticipatory grief Grief response in which the person begins the grieving process before an actual loss.

anticipatory guidance The psychological preparation of a person to help relieve fear and anxiety of an event expected to be stressful, such as the preparation of a child for surgery.

antidiuretic hormone (ADH) A hormone that decreases the production of urine by increasing the reabsorption of water by the renal tubules. ADH is secreted by cells of the hypothalamus and stored in the posterior lobe of the pituitary gland.

antiembolic stockings Elasticized stockings that prevent formation of emboli and thrombi, especially after surgery or during bed rest.

antigen Substance, usually a protein, that causes the formation of an antibody and reacts specifically with that antibody.

antipyretic Substance or procedure that reduces fever.

Apgar score The evaluation of an infant's physical condition, usually performed 1 minute and again 5 minutes after birth, based on a rating of five factors that reflect the infant's ability to adjust to extrauterine life.

aphasia Abnormal neurological condition in which language function is defective or absent; related to injury to speech center in cerebral cortex, causing receptive or expressive aphasia.

apical pulse The heartbeat taken with the bell or diaphragm of a stethoscope placed on the apex of the heart.

apnea Cessation of airflow through the nose and mouth.

apocrine gland Large, deep exocrine glands located in the axillary, anal, genital, and mammary areas of the body; secrete sweat having a strong odor.

apothecary system System of measurement; basic unit of weight is a grain. Weights derived from the grain are the gram, ounce, and pound. The basic measure for fluid is the minim. The fluidram, fluid ounce, pint, quart, and gallon are measures derived from the minim.

approximate To come close together, as in the edges of a wound.

arcus senilis An opaque ring, gray to white in color, that surrounds the periphery of the cornea. The condition is caused by deposits of fat granules in the cornea. Occurs primarily in older adults.

asepsis Absence of germs or microorganisms.

assault Unlawful threatening or inflicting of harm on another.

assertive communication A type of communication based on a philosophy of protecting individual rights and responsibilities. It includes the ability to be self-directive in acting to accomplish goals and advocate for others.

assessment First step of the nursing process; activities required in the first step are data collection, data validation, data sorting, and data documentation. The purpose is to gather information for health problem identification.

assimilation To become absorbed into another culture and to adopt its characteristics.

associative play A form of play in which a group of children participate in similar or identical activities without formal organization, direction, interaction, or goals.

atelectasis Collapse of alveoli, preventing the normal respiratory exchange of oxygen and carbon dioxide.

atherosclerosis Common arterial disorder characterized by yellowish plaques of cholesterol, lipids, and cellular debris in the inner layers of the walls of the large- and medium-sized arteries.

atrioventricular (AV) node A portion of the cardiac conduction system located on the floor of the right atrium; it receives electrical impulses from the atrium and transmits them to the bundle of His.

atrophied Wasted or reduced size or physiological activity of a part of the body caused by disease or other influences.

attachment Initial psychosocial relationship that develops between parents and the neonate.

attentional set Internal state of the learner that allows focusing and comprehension.

auditory Related to, or experienced through, hearing.

auscultation Method of physical examination; listening to the sounds produced by the body, usually with a stethoscope.

auscultatory gap Disappearance of sound when obtaining a blood pressure; typically occurs between the first and second Korotkoff's sounds.

authority The right to act in areas where an individual has been given and accepts responsibility.

autologous transfusion A procedure in which blood is removed from a donor and stored for a variable period before it is returned to the donor's own circulation.

automated speech recognition Voice-recognition computer technology that allows an individual to speak and enter data into a computer through voice tones.

autonomy Ability or tendency to function independently.

autopsy Postmortem examination performed to confirm or determine the cause of death.

bacteriuria Presence of bacteria in the urine.

balance Position when the person's center of gravity is correctly positioned so that falling does not occur.

bandages Available in rolls of various widths and materials including gauze, elasticized knit, elastic webbing, flannel, and muslin. Gauze bandages are lightweight and inexpensive, mold easily around contours of the body, and permit air circulation to underlying skin to prevent maceration. Elastic bandages conform well to body parts but can also be used to exert pressure over a body part.

basal cell carcinoma A malignant, epithelial cell tumor that begins as a papule and enlarges peripherally, developing a central crater that erodes, crusts, and bleeds. Metastasis is rare.

basal metabolic rate (BMR) Amount of energy used in a unit of time by a fasting, resting subject to maintain vital functions.

basic human needs Needs for things, such as food, water, safety, and love, that people require to maintain vital functions.

battery Legal term for touching of another's body without consent.

bed boards Boards placed under the mattress of a bed that provide extra support to the mattress surface.

bed rest Placement of the client in bed for therapeutic reasons for a prescribed period.

beneficence The doing or active promotion of doing good. One of the four principles of the ethical theory of deontology.

bereavement Response to loss through death; a subjective experience that a person suffers after losing a person with whom there has been a significant relationship.

binder Bandages made of large pieces of material to fit specific body parts.

bioethics A branch of ethics within the field of health care.

biological clock Cyclical nature of body functions; functions controlled from within the body are synchronized with environmental factors; same meaning as biorhythm.

biotransformation The chemical changes that a substance undergoes in the body, such as by the action of enzymes.

blanching Whitening of the skin from pressure, vasoconstriction, or hypotension.

body image Persons' subjective concept of their physical appearance.

body mechanics Coordinated efforts of the musculoskeletal and nervous systems to maintain proper balance, posture, and body alignment.

bolus Round mass of chewed food ready to be swallowed.

bonding The parents' emotional tie to their child that usually develops soon after birth as a result of their interaction.

bone resorption Destruction of bone cells and release of calcium into the blood.

borborygmi Audible abdominal sounds produced by hyperactive intestinal peristalsis.

brachial pulse Rhythmic beating palpated over the brachial artery.

bradycardia Slower than normal heart rate; heart contracts fewer than 60 times per minute.

bradypnea An abnormally slow rate of breathing.

bronchoscopy Visual examination of the tracheal and bronchial tree using a flexible fiberoptic bronchoscope.

bruit Abnormal sound or murmur heard while auscultating an organ, gland, or artery.

bruxism Grinding of teeth during sleep.

buccal Of or pertaining to the inside of the cheek or the gum next to the cheek.

buccal cavity Consists of the lips surrounding the opening of the mouth, the cheeks running along the side walls of the cavity, the tongue and its muscles, and the hard and soft palate.

buffer Substance or group of substances that can absorb or release hydrogen ions to correct an acid-base imbalance.

bulbar synchronizing region (BSR) Area in the pons and medial forebrain region releasing serotonin from specialized cells believed to aid in sleep.

bundle of His A portion of the cardiac conduction system that arises from the distal portion of the atrioventricular (AV) node and extends across the AV groove to the top of the intraventricular septum, where it divides into right and left bundle branches.

cachexia Malnutrition marked by weakness and emaciation, usually associated with severe illness.

capitation A payment mechanism in which a provider (e.g., health care network) receives a fixed amount of payment per enrollee.

carbohydrates Dietary classification of foods comprising sugars, starches, cellulose, and gum.

carbon monoxide Colorless, odorless, poisonous gas produced by the combustion of carbon or organic fuels.

cardiac catheterization A diagnostic procedure in which a catheter is introduced into a large vein, usually of an arm or leg, and threaded through the circulatory system to the heart.

cardiac index (CI) The adequacy of the cardiac output for an individual. It takes into account the body surface area (BSA) of the client.

cardiac output Volume of blood expelled by the ventricles of the heart, equal to the amount of blood ejected at each beat, multiplied by the number of beats in the period of time used for computation (usually 1 minute).

cardiopulmonary rehabilitation Actively assisting the client to achieve and maintain an optimal level of health through controlled physical exercise, nutrition counseling, relaxation and stress management techniques, prescribed medications and oxygen, and compliance.

cardiopulmonary resuscitation (CPR) Basic emergency procedures for life support consisting of artificial respiration and manual external cardiac massage.

care To feel concern or interest in one who has sorrow or difficulties.

care management A care delivery model that structures accountability for client outcomes within a unit or area of care. Typically one care giver coordinates care from admission through discharge within an acute care setting.

CareMap A multidisciplinary collaborative treatment plan that details the series of interventions and anticipated outcomes for specific clients of a selected case type across a course of treatment or hospital stay. A trademark and concept of The Center for Case Management, South Natick, Massachusetts.

case management Organized system for delivering health care to an individual client or group of clients across an episode of illness and/or a continuum of care; includes assessment and development of a plan of care, coordination of all services, referral, and follow-up; usually assigned to one professional.

case management plan A one- to two-page multidisciplinary integrated care plan for the problems, key interventions, and expected outcomes of the client with a specific disease or condition.

cataplexy Condition characterized by sudden muscular weakness and loss of muscle tone.

cathartics Drugs that act to promote bowel evacuation.

catheterization Introduction of a catheter into a body cavity or organ to inject or remove fluid.

cations Positively charged electrolytes.

center of gravity Midpoint or center of the weight of a body or object.

centigrade Denotes temperature scale in which 0 degrees is the freezing point of water and 100 degrees is the boiling point of water at sea level; also called Celsius.

centralized management An organizational management structure that has a single administrator leading an organization, with subordinate administrators overseeing responsibilities for each department.

certification A process in which an individual, an institution, or an educational program is evaluated and recognized as meeting certain predetermined standards.

certified nurse-midwives (CNM) Nurse who is educated in midwifery and possesses certification in accordance with criteria of the American College of Midwives.

certified registered nurse anesthetist (CRNA) A nurse who has received advanced training in an accredited program in anesthesiology. They provide surgical anesthesia under the guidance and supervision of an anesthesiologist.

cerumen Yellowish or brownish waxy secretion produced by sweat glands in the external ear.

change-of-shift reports Reports that occur between two scheduled nursing work shifts. Nurses communicate information about their assigned clients to nurses working on the next shift of duty.

chancre A skin lesion or venereal sore (usually primary syphilis) that begins at the site of infection as a papule and develops into a red, bloodless, painless ulcer with a scooped-out appearance.

channels Method used in the teaching-learning process to present content: visual, auditory, taste, smell. In the communication process, a method used to transmit a message: visual, auditory, touch.

charting by exception (CBE) A charting methodology in which data are entered only when there is an exception from what is normal or expected. Reduces time spent documenting in charting. It is a shorthand method for documenting normal findings and routine care.

chest percussion Striking of the chest wall with a cupped hand to promote mobilization and drainage of pulmonary secretions.

chest physiotherapy (CPT) Group of therapies used to mobilize pulmonary secretions for expectoration.

chest tube A catheter inserted through the thorax into the chest cavity for removing air or fluid, used following chest or heart surgery or pneumothorax.

chronic illness Illness that persists over a long period of time and affects physical, emotional, intellectual, social, and spiritual functioning.

chyme Viscous, semifluid contents of the stomach present during digestion of a meal, which eventually pass into the intestines.

circadian rhythm Repetition of certain physiological phenomena within a 24-hour cycle.

circulating nurse Assistant to the scrub nurse and surgeon whose role is to provide necessary supplies, dispose of soiled instruments and supplies, and keep an accurate count of instruments, needles, and sponges used.

circumduction Movement of the arm in full circle; includes all movements of the shoulder ball-and-socket joint.

civil law Statutes concerned with protecting a person's rights.

client adherence Clients and families must invest time in carrying out the required home treatments.

client advocate Role of the nurse to protect the client's human and legal rights and provide assistance in asserting those rights if the need arises.

client-centered goal Specific measurable objective designed to reflect the client's highest level of wellness and independence in function.

climacteric Physiological, developmental change that occurs in the

male reproductive system between the ages of 45 to 60.

clinical criteria Objective or subjective signs and symptoms, clusters of signs and symptoms, or risk factors.

clinical nurse specialists (CNSs) Nurses prepared at the graduate level and who practice in a specialty area of nursing.

clubbing A bulging of the tissues at the nail base that is due to insufficient oxygenation at the periphery resulting from conditions such as chronic emphysema and congenital heart disease.

code of ethics Formal statement that delineates a profession's guidelines for ethical behavior; a code of ethics sets standards or expectations for the professional to achieve.

cognitive appraisal The extent to which individuals perceive a stressful situation as a challenge or an obstacle that exceeds their capacity to cope.

cognitive learning Acquisition of intellectual skills that encompass behaviors such as thinking, understanding, and evaluating.

collaboration Process in which a nurse works with other health care providers and the client to develop a plan of care to address the client-identified care needs, as well as those identified by the professional team.

collaborative interventions Therapies that require the knowledge, skill, and expertise of multiple health care professionals.

collagen Substance that combines to form the white, glistening, inelastic fibers of tendons, ligaments, and fasciae.

colloid osmotic pressure An abnormal condition of the kidney caused by the pressure of concentrations of large particles, such as protein molecules, that will pass through a membrane.

colon Portion of the large intestine from the cecum to the rectum.

common law One source for law that is created by judicial decisions as opposed to those created by legislative bodies (statutory law).

communicable disease Any disease that can be transmitted from one person or animal to another by direct or indirect contact, or by vectors.

communication Ongoing, dynamic series of events that involves the transmission of meaning from sender to receiver.

competence A specific range of skills necessary to perform a task.

complete bed bath Bath in which the entire body of a client is washed in bed.

compliance Person's fulfillment of the prescribed course of treatment.

complicated bereavement A prolongation or abnormal expression of bereavement.

compress Soft pad of gauze or cloth used to apply heat, cold, or medications to the surface of a body part.

computer-based client records (CBCR) A comprehensive computerized system utilized by all health care practitioners to permanently store information pertaining to a client's health status, clinical problems, and functional abilities.

concentration Relative content of a component within a substance or solution.

concentration gradient A gradient that exists across a membrane separating a high concentration of a particular ion from a low concentration of the same ion.

conceptual model A set of global or general ideas about the individuals, groups, populations, situations, or events of interest to a discipline.

concrete operation A thought process based on concrete rather than abstract points of reference.

conjunctivitis A highly contagious eye infection. The crusty drainage that collects on eyelid margins can easily spread from one eye to the other.

connotative meaning The shade or interpretation of a word's meaning influenced by the thoughts, feelings, or ideas people have about the word.

consensus decision making A group process involving all participants, with the outcome being a decision that all members can agree with and support.

conservation The ability to recognize that the amount or quantity of a substance remains the same even when its shape or appearance changes.

constipation Condition characterized by difficulty in passing stool or an infrequent passage of hard stool.

consultation Process in which the help of a specialist is sought to identify ways to handle problems in client management or in the planning and implementing of programs.

contaminated Process by which an object becomes unclean or unsterile.

continent pouch Urine reservoir formed from a bowel segment.

continuing education Formal educational programs designed to further the knowledge, skills, and professional attitudes of practicing nurses.

convalescence Period of recovery after an illness, injury, or surgery.

coordination A process that a nurse uses to ensure that the client's plan of care is carried out in an organized manner with appropriate use of resources.

coping mechanisms Psychological adaptive behaviors learned through experience and used to manage stress.

cough A sudden, audible expulsion of air from the lungs. The person breathes in, the glottis is partially closed, and the accessory muscles of expiration contract to expel the air forcibly.

counseling Implementation method that helps the client recognize and manage stress and that facilitates interpersonal relationships between the client and the family, significant others, or the health care team.

crackles Fine bubbling sounds heard on auscultation of the lung; produced by air entering distal airways and alveoli, which contain serous secretions.

crime Act that violates a law and that may include criminal intent.

criminal law Concerned with acts that threaten society but may involve only an individual.

crisis intervention Use of therapeutic techniques directed toward helping a client resolve a particular and immediate problem.

critical pathways Tools used in managed care that incorporate the treatment interventions of care givers from all disciplines who nor-

mally care for a client. Designed for a specific care type, a pathway is used to manage the care of a client throughout a projected length of stay.

critical period of development A specific time period when the environment has its greatest effect on a specific aspect of an individual's development

critical thinking The active, purposeful, organized, cognitive process used to carefully examine one's thinking and the thinking of other individuals.

cultural phenomena Cultural variables that have the ability to impact the health of clients.

cultural values Values adopted as a result of the social setting in which a person lives.

culture Nonphysical traits, such as values, beliefs, attitudes, and customs, that are shared by a group of people and passed from one generation to the next.

cutaneous stimulation Stimulation of a person's skin to prevent or reduce pain perception. A massage, warm bath, hot and cold therapies, and transcutaneous electric nerve stimulation are some ways to reduce pain perception.

cyanosis Bluish discoloration of the skin and mucous membranes caused by an excess of deoxygenated hemoglobin in the blood or a structural defect in the hemoglobin molecule.

data, actions, client response (DAR) The format used in focus charting for recording client information.

data analysis Logical examination of and professional judgment about client assessment data; used in the diagnostic process to derive a nursing diagnosis.

data clustering Categorizing of related data into groups.

data collection Part of the assessment step of the nursing process when all pertinent subjective and objective information about the client is gathered. Data collection includes the nursing history, physical examination, laboratory data and diagnostic tests, and information from health team members and the client's family and significant others.

data documentation A thorough and accurate documentation of facts is necessary when recording client data. If an item is not recorded, it is lost and unavailable to anyone researching the client's medical record. If specific information is not given, the reader is left with only general impressions.

death Cessation of life as indicated by the absence of heartbeat or respiration. Legally, death is total absence of activity in the brain and central nervous, cardiovascular, and respiratory systems.

debridement Removal of dead tissue from a wound.

decentralized management An organizational philosophy that brings decisions down to the level of the staff. Individuals best informed about a problem or issue participate in the decision-making process.

decision making A process involving critical appraisal of information that results from recognition of a problem and ends with the generation, testing, and evaluation of a conclusion. Comes at the end of critical thinking.

defamation of character Communication disseminated about a person that injures that persons's reputation.

defecation Passage of feces from the digestive tract through the rectum.

defendant Individual or organization against whom legal charges are brought forth in a court of law.

defense mechanisms Coping mechanisms that regulate emotional distress and thus protect a person from anxiety and stress.

defining characteristics Related signs and symptoms or clusters of data that support the nursing diagnosis.

dehiscence Separation of a wound's edges, revealing underlying tissues.

dehydration or fluid volume deficit Excessive loss of water from the body tissues, accompanied by a disturbance of body electrolytes.

delegation The process of assigning another member of the health care team to be responsible for aspects of client care; for example, assigning nurse assistants to bathe a client.

dementia   Irreversible mental state characterized by decreased intellectual function, changes in personality, impaired judgment, and often changes in affect as a result of permanently altered cerebral metabolism.

denial   An unconscious refusal to admit an unacceptable idea.

denotative meaning   Is shared by individuals who use a common language. The word "baseball" has the same meaning for all individuals who speak English, but the word "code" denotes cardiac arrest primarily to health-care providers.

dental caries   Abnormal destructive condition in a tooth caused by a complex interaction of food, especially starches and sugars, with bacteria that form dental plaque.

dentin   An ivory substance harder than bone. Dentin surrounds a tooth's pulp cavity. A layer of enamel covers the upper portion of each tooth at the crown.

deontology   A traditional theory of ethics that proposes to define actions as right or wrong based on the characteristics of fidelity to promises, truthfulness, and justice. The conventional use of ethical terms such as justice, autonomy, beneficence, and nonmaleficence constitutes the practice of deontology.

dermis   Sensitive vascular layer of the skin directly below the epidermis composed of collagenous and elastic fibrous connective tissues that give the dermis strength and elasticity.

detoxify   To remove the toxic quality of a substance; the liver acts to detoxify chemicals in drug compounds.

development   Qualitative or observable aspects of the progressive changes one makes in adapting to the environment.

developmental crises   Crises associated with normal and expected phases of growth and development, e.g., the response to menopause. Same as maturational crises.

diagnostic process   Mental steps (data clustering and analysis, problem identification) that follow assessment and lead directly to the formulation of a diagnosis.

diagnostic reasoning   A process that enables an observer to assign meaning and to classify phenom-ena in clinical situations by integrating obervations and critical thinking.

diagnosis-related groups   Group of clients classified to establish a mechanism for health care reimbursement based on length of stay; classification is based on the following variables: primary and secondary diagnosis, comorbidities, primary and secondary procedures, and age.

diaphoresis   Secretion of sweat, especially profuse secretion associated with an elevated body temperature, physical exertion, or emotional stress.

diaphragmatic breathing   Respiration in which the abdomen moves out while the diaphragm descends on inspiration.

diarrhea   Increase in the number of stools and the passage of liquid, unformed feces.

diastole   Period of time between contractions of the atria or the ventricles during which blood enters the relaxed chambers.

diastolic pressure   The minimum level of blood pressure measured between contractions of the heart.

diffusion   Movement of molecules from an area of high concentration to an area of lower concentration.

digestion   Breakdown of nutrients by chewing, churning, mixing with fluid, and chemical reactions.

dignity   The person's ability to maintain a self-concept as a person of value.

direct care provider   Role of the nurse to assist the client to regain health through the healing process. The nurse provides a holistic approach to care, including treatments and skills, the impact of illness on the client/family, and spiritual and social well-being.

discharge planning   Activities directed toward identifying future proposed therapy and the need for additional resources before and after returning home.

disinfection   Process of destroying all pathogenic organisms, except spores.

disuse osteoporosis   Reductions in skeletal mass routinely accompanying immobility or paralysis.

diuresis   Increased rate of formation and excretion of urine.

documentation   Written entry into the client's medical record of all pertinent information about the client. These entries validate the client's problems and care and exist as a legal record.

dorsalis pedis pulse   Rhythmic beating palpated over the dorsalis pedis artery.

dorsiflexion   Flexion toward the back.

drainage evacuators   Convenient portable units that connect to tubular drains lying within a wound bed and exert a safe, constant, low-pressure vacuum to remove and collect drainage.

drug rehabilitation centers   An agency that provides long-term care for a gradual return to the community of a person with a chemical or drug dependency.

dysmenorrhea   Painful menstruation.

dyspnea   Sensation of shortness of breath.

dysrhythmia   Deviation from the normal pattern of the heartbeat.

dysuria   Painful urination resulting from bacterial infection of the bladder and obstructive conditions of the urethra.

ecchymosis   Discoloration of the skin or bruise caused by leakage of blood into subcutaneous tissues as a result of trauma to underlying tissues.

eccrine glands   Two types of sweat glands; eccrine glands are present throughout the body and promote cooling by evaporation of their secretions.

echocardiography   Diagnostic procedure that uses ultrasonic waves for studying the structure and motion of the heart.

ectropion   Eversion of the eyelid, exposing the conjunctival membrane and part of the eyeball.

eczema   Superficial dermatitis of unknown cause.

edema   Abnormal accumulation of fluid in interstitial spaces of tissues.

egocentric   A developmental characteristic wherein a toddler is only able to assume the view of his or her own activities and needs.

electrocardiogram   A graphic record of the electrical activity of the myocardium.

electrolyte   Element or compound that, when melted or dissolved in water or other solvent, dissociates into ions and can carry an electrical current.

emerging majority Aging and the low birth rate in the European majority and youth combined with the high reproductive rate among Asians, African Americans, Hispanics, and Native Americans are shifting the population and people of color.

empathy Understanding and acceptance of a person's feelings and the ability to sense the person's private world.

empowerment A management technique that fosters the growth and development of individual staff members so that they become less and less dependent on their work leader. Empowerment helps staff to make decisions confidently on their own.

endogenous infections Infections produced within a cell or organism.

endorphins Naturally occurring neuropeptides composed of amino acids and secreted within the central nervous system to reduce pain.

endoscope Instrument used to visualize the interior of body organs and cavities with an endoscope.

enema Procedure involving introduction of a solution into the rectum for cleansing or therapeutic purposes.

enteral nutrition (EN) Provision of nutrients through the gastrointestinal tract when the client cannot ingest, chew, or swallow food but can digest and absorb nutrients.

entropion A condition in which the eyelid turns inward toward the eye.

epidermis Outer layer of the skin that has several thin layers of skin in different stages of maturation; shields and protects the underlying tissues from water loss, mechanical or chemical injury, and penetration by disease-causing microorganisms.

epidural infusion A type of nerve block anesthesia in which an anesthetic is intermittently or continuously injected into the lumbosacral region of the spinal cord.

erythema Redness or inflammation of the skin or mucous membranes that is a result of dilation and congestion of superficial capillaries; sunburn is an example.

eschar Scab or dry crust that results from excoriation of the skin.

ethic of care The delivery of health care based on ethical principles and standards of care.

ethical dilemma A dilemma existing when the right thing to do is not clear. Resolution requires the negotiation of differing values among those involved in the dilemma.

ethical principles A set of guidelines for a profession's expectations and standards of behavior for its members.

ethics Principles or standards that govern proper conduct.

ethnicity Cultural group's sense of identification associated with the group's common social and cultural heritage.

ethnocentrism Tendency of members of one cultural group to view the members of other cultural groups in terms of the standards of behavior, attitudes, and values of their own group.

eupnea Normal respirations that are quiet, effortless, and rhythmical.

euthanasia Deliberately bringing about the death of a person who has an incurable disease or condition, either actively, by administering a lethal drug, or passively, by withholding treatment and allowing the person to die.

evaluation Determination of the extent to which established client goals have been achieved.

evisceration Protrusion of visceral organs through a surgical wound.

exacerbations Increases in the seriousness of a disease or disorder as marked by greater intensity in signs or symptoms.

excoriation Injury to the skin's surface caused by abrasion.

exercise stress test An evaluation of the client's cardiopulmonary endurance during physical activity. An electrocardiogram and analysis of respiratory function is usually performed during the test.

exhaustion stage Phase that occurs when the body can no longer resist the stress; when the energy necessary to maintain adaptation is depleted.

exogenous infection Infection originating outside an organ or part.

exostosis An abnormal benign growth on the surface of a bone.

expected outcomes Expected conditions of a client at the end of therapy or of a disease process, including the degree of wellness and the need for continuing care, medications, support, counseling, or education.

expressive aphasia Inability to name common objects or to express simple ideas in words or writing.

extended care facility An institution devoted to providing medical, nursing, or custodial care for an individual over a prolonged period of time, such as during the course of a chronic disease or during the rehabilitation phase after an acute illness.

extension Movement by certain joints that increases the angle between two adjoining bones.

extracellular fluids Portion of body fluids composed of the interstitial fluid and blood plasma.

exudate Fluid, cells, or other substances that have been slowly discharged from cells or blood vessels through small pores or breaks in cell membranes.

Fahrenheit Denotes temperature scale in which 32 degrees is the freezing point of water and 212 degrees is the boiling point of water at sea level.

faith More than a set of beliefs but a way of relating to self, others, and a Supreme Being.

family Group of interacting individuals composing a basic unit of society.

family as client Nursing perspective in which the family is viewed as a unit of interacting members having attributes, functions, and goals separate from those of the individual family members.

family as context Nursing perspective in which the primary focus of care is on an individual within a family.

family as system Based on a systems theory framework whereby the family is viewed as an open system with boundaries, self-regulating mechanisms, subsystems, and suprasystems all affecting the family unit.

family forms Patterns of people considered by family members to be included in the family.

family functioning Processes families use to achieve their goals.

family hardiness   The internal strengths and durability of the family unit; characterized by a sense of control over the outcome of life events and hardships, a view of change as beneficial and growth-producing, and an active rather than passive orientation in responding to stressful life events.

family health   Determined by the effectiveness of the family's structure, the processes that the family uses to meet its goals, and internal and external resources.

febrile   Pertaining to or characterized by an elevated body temperature.

fecal impaction   Accumulation of hardened fecal material in the rectum or sigmoid colon.

fecal incontinence   Inability to control passage of feces and gas from the anus.

feces   Waste or excrement from the gastrointestinal tract.

feedback   Process in which the output of a given system is returned to the system.

felony   Crime of a serious nature that carries a penalty of imprisonment or death.

feminist ethic   An ethical approach that focuses on relationships of those involved in an ethical dilemma rather than traditional abstract principles of deontology.

femoral pulse   Rhythmic beating palpated over the femoral artery.

fertilization   The union of the male and female gametes to form a zygote from which an embryo develops.

fever   Elevation in the hypothalamic set-point, so that body temperature is regulated at a higher level.

fibrin   Protein product formed from the action of thrombin on fibrinogen in the clotting process.

fibrocystic breast disease   A benign condition characterized by lumpy painful breasts and sometimes nipple discharge. Symptoms are more apparent before the menstrual period. Known to be a risk factor for breast cancer.

fidelity   The agreement to keep a promise.

fight-or-flight response   The total physiologic response to stress that occurs during the alarm reaction stage of the general adaptation syndrome. Massive changes in all body systems prepare a human being to choose to flee or to remain and fight the stressor.

filtration   The straining of fluid through a membrane.

fistula   Abnormal passage from an internal organ to the body surface or between two internal organs.

flatus   Intestinal gas.

flow sheet   Document on which frequent observations or specific measurements are recorded.

fluid overload   Excess extracellular fluid volume.

fluid volume deficit (FVD)   A fluid and electrolyte disorder caused by failure of the body's homeostatic mechanisms to regulate the retention and excretion of body fluids. The condition is characterized by decreased output of urine, high specific gravity of urine, output of urine that is greater than the intake of fluid in the body, hemoconcentration, and increased serum levels of sodium.

fluid volume excess   A fluid and electrolyte disorder characterized by an increase in fluid retention and edema, resulting from failure of the body's homeostatic mechanisms to regulate the retention and excretion of body fluids.

focus charting   A charting methodology for structuring progress notes according to the focus of the note, for example, symptoms and nursing diagnosis. Each note includes data, actions, and client response.

FOCUS-PDCA   Acronym for a process improvement model that includes nine steps: find a process to improve, organize a team, clarify knowledge of the process, understand sources of process variation, select the process improvement, and then plan, do, check, and act on the improvement. A multidisciplinary team familiar with a process of care participates in the FOCUS-PDCA activity.

food poisoning   Toxic processes resulting from the ingestion of a food contaminated by toxic substances or by bacteria-containing toxins.

foot boots   Soft, foot-shaped devices designed to reduce the risk of footdrop, by maintaining the foot in dorsiflexion.

footdrop   An abnormal neuromuscular condition of the lower leg and foot, characterized by an inability to dorsiflex, or evert, the foot.

friction   Effects of rubbing or the resistance that a moving body meets from the surface on which it moves; a force that occurs in a direction to oppose movement.

functional health patterns   A method for organizing assessment data based on the level of client function in specific areas, for example, mobility.

functional illiteracy   An inability to read or comprehend above a fifth-grade level.

functional incontinence   Involuntary, unpredictable loss of urine.

functional nursing system   Method of client care delivery in which each staff member is assigned a task that is completed for all clients on the unit.

gait   Manner or style of walking, including rhythm, cadence, and speed.

gastrostomy feeding tube   The insertion of a feeding tube, through a stoma, into the stomach for the purpose of providing enteral nutrition.

gender identity   Individual's sense of being feminine or masculine that develops from infancy.

general adaptation syndrome (GAS)   Generalized defense response of the body to stress, consisting of three stages: alarm, resistance, and exhaustion.

general anesthesia   Intravenous or inhaled medications that cause the client to lose all sensation and consciousness.

geriatrics   Branch of health care dealing with the physiology and psychology of aging and with the diagnosis and treatment of diseases affecting older adults.

gerontology   The study of all aspects of the aging process and its consequences.

gingiva   Gum of the mouth; a mucous membrane with supporting fibrous tissue that overlies the crowns of unerupted teeth and encircles the necks of those teeth that have erupted.

global aphasia   Abnormal neurological condition in which language function is defective or absent, affecting the client's ability to understand and to speak.

glomerulus   Cluster or collection of capillary vessels within the kidney involved in the initial formation of urine.

gluconeogenesis Formation of glucose or glycogen from substances that are not carbohydrates, such as protein or lipid.

glycogen Polysaccharide that is the major carbohydrate stored in animal cells.

glycogenolysis Catabolism of glycogen into glucose, carbon dioxide, and water.

goals Desired results of nursing actions, set realistically by the nurse and client as part of the planning stage of the nursing process.

Good Samaritan Laws Legislation enacted in some states to protect health care professionals from liability in rendering emergency aid, unless there is proven willful wrong or gross negligence.

graduated measuring container Receptacle for volume measurement.

granulation tissue Soft, pink, fleshy projections of tissue that form during the healing process in a wound not healing by primary intention.

graphic user interface Mechanism whereby user accesses computer functions through trackball, touch pads, mouse, and icons.

grief Form of sorrow involving the person's thoughts, feelings, and behaviors, occurring as a response to an actual or perceived loss.

grieving process Sequence of affective, cognitive, and physiological states through which the person responds to and finally accepts an irretrievable loss.

growth The measurable or quantitative aspect of an individual's increase in physical dimensions as a result of an increase in cell number. Indicators of growth include changes in height, weight, and sexual characteristics.

guaiac test Test of feces for the presence of occult (hidden) blood.

guided imagery Method of pain control in which the client creates a mental image, concentrates on that image, and gradually becomes less aware of pain.

gustatory Pertaining to the sense of taste.

hand rolls A roll of cloth that keeps the thumb slightly adducted and in opposition to the fingers.

hand-wrist splints Splints individually molded for the client to maintain proper alignment of the thumb, slight adduction of the wrist, and slight dorsiflexion.

Harris flush A return flow enema that helps to expel flatus.

healing Holistic or three-dimensional phenomenon that results in the restoration of balance or harmony to the body, mind, and spirit.

health Dynamic state in which individuals adapt to their internal and external environments so that there is a state of physical, emotional, intellectual, social, and spiritual well-being.

health belief Client's personal beliefs about levels of wellness, which can motivate or impede participation in changing risk factors, participating in care, and selecting care options.

health belief model Conceptual framework that describes a person's health behavior as an expression of the person's health beliefs.

health care problems Any conditions or dysfunctions that the client experiences as a result of illness or treatment of an illness.

health care team All those people, departments, and ancillary services that collectively render care and services to the client.

health maintenance Beliefs and practices include such phenomena as daily health-related activities, diet, exercise, rest, and clothing.

health maintenance organization (HMO) A type of group health care practice that provides basic and supplemental health maintenance and treatment services to voluntary enrollees who prepay a fixed periodic fee that is set without regard to the amount or kind of services received.

health promotion model Defines health as a positive, dynamic state, not merely the absence of disease. The health promotion model emphasizes well-being, personal fulfillment, and self-actualization rather than reacting to the threat of illness.

health protection Beliefs and practices include the use of special health-related activities, such as food taboos; exercise—special, seasonal activities; clothing—protective items worn daily, etc.

health restoration Activities include necessary diet changes, rest, special clothing, etc. The health maintenance, protection, and restoration beliefs and practices that may be found among people from different ethnocultural backgrounds is infinite.

health traditions Data include health and healing beliefs and practices, nutritional variables, and food practices.

health-healing/disordering model A conceptual map that denotes the concept of health, which incorporates both healing and disordering processes as aspects of health.

health-illness continuum Scale by means of which a person's level of health can be described, ranging from high-level wellness to severe illness. The scale takes into account the presence of risk factors.

heat exhaustion An abnormal condition caused by depletion of body fluid and electrolytes resulting from exposure to intense heat or the inability to acclimatize to heat.

heat stroke Continued exposure to extreme heat raising the core body temperature to 47° C (105° F) or higher.

hematemesis Vomiting of blood indicating upper gastrointestinal bleeding.

hematoma Collection of blood trapped in the tissues of the skin or an organ.

hematuria Abnormal presence of blood in the urine.

hemolysis Breakdown of red blood cells and release of hemoglobin that may occur following administration of hypotonic intravenous solutions, causing swelling and rupture of erythrocytes.

hemoptysis Coughing up blood from the respiratory tract.

hemorrhoids Permanent dilation and engorgement of veins within the lining of the rectum.

hemostasis Termination of bleeding by mechanical or chemical means or by the coagulation process of the body.

hemothorax Accumulation of blood and fluid in the pleural cavity between the parietal and visceral pleurae.

heritage assessment Data include client's age, ethnic origin, race, place of birth, religion, and identification with a given heritage.

heritage consistency Theoretical model that assesses a client's acculturation to a new culture on a continuum.

hernia Protrusion of an organ through an abnormal opening in the muscle wall of the cavity that surrounds it.

holistic Of or pertaining to the whole, considering all factors.

Holter monitor A device for making prolonged electrocardiograph recordings on a portable recorder while the client continues normal daily activities.

home IV therapies The delivery of intravenous (IV) therapy to the client in the home, usually provided by professional nurses through home care agencies.

homeostasis State of relative constance in the internal environment of the body, maintained naturally by physiological adaptive mechanisms.

homophobia The fear of or prejudice against homosexuals.

hope Confident, yet uncertain, expectation of achieving a future goal.

hospice System of family-centered care designed to help terminally ill persons be comfortable and maintain a satisfactory lifestyle throughout the terminal phase of their illness.

humidification The process of adding water to gas.

humor A coping strategy based on an individual's cognitive appraisal of a stimulus that results in behavior such as smiling, laughing, or feelings of amusement that lessen emotional distress.

hydrocephalus An abnormal accumulation of cerebrospinal fluid in the ventricles of the brain.

hydrostatic pressure A pressure caused by a liquid.

hypercapnia Greater than normal amounts of carbon dioxide in the blood; also called hypercarbia.

hypercarbia Greater than normal amounts of carbon dioxide in the blood; also called hypercapnia.

hyperextension A position of maximal extension of a joint.

hyperglycemia Elevated serum glucose levels.

hypertension Disorder characterized by an elevated blood pressure persistently exceeding 150/90 mm Hg.

hyperthermia Situation in which body temperature exceeds the set-point.

hypertonic The situation in which one solution has a greater concentration of solute than another solution; therefore the first solution exerts greater osmotic pressure.

hypertonicity Excessive tension of the arterial walls or muscles.

hyperventilation Respiratory rate in excess of that required to maintain normal carbon dioxide levels in the body tissues.

hypervolemia Increase in the amount of fluid in the circulating blood volume.

hypnotics Class of drug that causes insensibility to pain and induces sleep.

hypoglycemia Reduced serum glucose levels.

hypostatic pneumonia Pneumonia that results from fluid accumulation as a result of inactivity.

hypotension Abnormal lowering of blood pressure that is inadequate for normal perfusion and oxygenation of tissues.

hypothermia Abnormal lowering of body temperature below 93° F or 35° C, usually caused by prolonged exposure to cold.

hypotonic A situation in which one solution has a smaller concentration of solute than another solution; therefore the first solution exerts less osmotic pressure.

hypotonicity Reduced tension of the arterial walls or muscles.

hypoventilation Respiratory rate insufficient to prevent carbon dioxide retention.

hypovolemia An abnormally low circulating blood volume.

hypoxia Inadequate cellular oxygenation that may result from a deficiency in the delivery or use of oxygen at the cellular level.

iatrogenic infection Infection caused by a treatment or diagnostic procedure.

identity A component of self-concept characterized by one's persisting consciousness of being oneself, separate and distinct from others.

idiosyncratic reactions An individual sensitivity to effects of a drug caused by inherited or other bodily constitution factors.

illness Abnormal process in which any aspect of a person's functioning is diminished or impaired as compared with that person's previous condition.

illness behavior Ways in which people monitor their bodies, define and interpret their symptoms, take remedial actions, and use the health care system.

illness prevention Health education programs or activities directed toward protecting clients from threats or potential threats to health and toward minimizing risk factors.

immobility Inability to move about freely, caused by any condition in which movement is impaired or therapeutically restricted.

immunity The quality of being insusceptible to or unaffected by a particular disease or condition.

implementation Initiation and completion of the nursing actions necessary to help the client achieve health care goals.

incentive spirometer resistive breathing device (ISRBD) One method for respiratory muscle training, resistive breathing is achieved by placing a restrictive breathing device into a volume-dependent incentive spirometer.

incentive spirometry Method of encouraging voluntary deep breathing by providing visual feedback to clients of the inspiratory volume they have achieved.

incident report Confidential document that describes any client accident while the person is on the premises of a health care agency.

Independent Practice Association (IPA) A prepaid health service system in which office-based physicians contract for the care of clients on a prenegotiated fee-for-service basis.

induration Hardening of a tissue, particularly the skin, because of edema or inflammation.

inference Taking one proposition as a given and guessing that another proposition follows.

infiltration Dislodging an intravenous catheter or needle from a vein into the subcutaneous space.

inflammation Protective response of body tissues to irritation or injury.

inflammatory response Localized response to trauma to prevent the spread of infection and to promote wound healing.

informed consent Process of obtaining permission from a client to perform a specific test or procedure, after describing all risks, side effects, and benefits.

infusion   Introduction of fluid into the vein, giving intravenous fluid over time.

infusion pump   Device that delivers a measured amount of fluid over a period of time.

inhalation   Method of medication delivery through the client's respiratory tract. The respiratory tract provides a large surface area for drug absorption. Inhalation can be through the nasal or oral route.

inhalers   Aerosol sprays, mists, or powders that penetrate lung airways, which the client inhales through the mouth.

injection   Parenteral administration of medication; four major sites of injection: subcutaneous, intramuscular, intravenous, and intradermal.

insomnia   Condition characterized by chronic inability to sleep or remain asleep through the night.

inspection   Method of physical examination by which the client is visually systematically examined for appearance, structure, function, and behavior.

instillation   To cause to enter drop by drop, or very slowly.

instrumental activities of daily living (IADLs)   Activities that are necessary to be independent in society beyond eating, grooming, transferring, and toileting and include such skills as shopping, preparing meals, banking, and taking medications.

integument   Skin and its appendages: hair, nails, and sweat and sebaceous glands.

interdependent interventions   Actions carried out by the nurse in collaboration with another health care professional.

interdisciplinary   Representation of the various professional disciplines that are involved in a particular work issue or clinical practice problem.

Internet   An electronic superhighway, which is a vast network over telephone and cable lines.

interpersonal communication   Exchange of information between two persons or among persons in a small group.

interstitial fluid   Fluid that fills the spaces between most of the cells of the body and provides a substantial portion of the liquid environment of the body.

interview   Organized, systematic conversation with the client designed to obtain pertinent health-related subjective information.

intracellular fluid   Liquid within the cell membrane.

intractable pain   Pain not easily relieved, such as that occurring with some types of cancer.

intradermal   Injection given between layers of the skin, into the dermis. Injections are given at a 5- to 15-degree angle.

intramuscular (IM)   Injections given into muscle tissue. The intramuscular route provides a fast rate of absorption that is related to the muscle's greater vascularity. Injections are given at a 90-degree angle.

intraocular   Method of medication delivery that involves inserting a medication disk, similar to a contact lens, into the client's eye.

intrapersonal communication   Communication that occurs within an individual; for example, persons "talk with themselves" silently or form an idea in their own mind.

intravascular   Fluid contained within the vessels of the circulatory system.

intravascular fluid   Pertaining to fluids circulating within blood vessels of the body.

intravenous   Injection directly into the bloodstream. Action of the drug begins immediately when given intravenously.

invasion of privacy   Release of personal information (e.g., health records, financial statements, or employment history) without the person's permission.

ions   Electrically charged particles including anions and cations.

irrigation   Process of washing out a body cavity or wounded area with a stream of fluid.

ischemia   Decreased blood supply to a body part, such as skin tissue, or to an organ, such as the heart.

isometric exercises   Activities that involve muscle tension without muscle shortening, do not have any beneficial effect on preventing orthostatic hypotension, but may improve activity tolerance.

isotonic   The situation in which two solutions have the same concentration of solute; therefore both solutions exert the same osmotic pressure.

jaundice   Yellow discoloration of the skin, mucous membranes, and sclera, caused by greater than normal amounts of bilirubin in the blood.

jejunal feeding tube   The insertion of a feeding tube, usually by the nasal route, and allowing the tube to pass into the client's jejunum for the purpose of providing enteral nutrition.

joint contracture   An abnormality that may result in permanent condition of a joint, is characterized by flexion and fixation, and is caused by disuse, atrophy, and shortening of muscle fibers and surrounding joint tissues.

joints   Connections between bones; classified according to structure and degree of mobility.

judgment   The ability to form an opinion or draw sound conclusions.

justice   The ethical standard of fairness.

Kardex   Trade name for card-filing system that allows quick reference to the particular need of the client for certain aspects of nursing care.

Korotkoff sounds   Sounds heard during the taking of blood pressure using a sphygmomanometer and stethoscope.

kyphosis   An exaggeration of the posterior curvature of the thoracic spine.

laceration   Torn, jagged wound.

land pollution   The depositing of trash and other hazardous wastes on and in the soil that cause contamination of the soil and ground water.

language   A code that conveys specific meaning as words are combined.

laryngospasm   A sudden uncontrolled contraction of the laryngeal muscles, which in turn decreases airway size.

laxative   Drug that acts to promote bowel evacuation.

leadership   To influence the behavior of others toward the accomplishment of common goals.

leadership styles   Clusters of behaviors that characterize the manner in which a manager uses interpersonal behaviors to influence accomplishment of a work unit's goals. Examples include directing, coaching, supporting, and delegating.

learning Acquisition of new knowledge and skills as a result of reinforcement, practice, and experience.

learning objective Written statement that describes the behavior a teacher expects from an individual following a learning activity.

left-sided heart failure An abnormal condition characterized by impaired functioning of the left ventricle due to elevated pressures and pulmonary congestion

leukoplakia Thick, white patches observed on oral mucous membranes.

libel Written false statement about persons that may injure their reputation.

licensed practical nurse (LPN) Also known as the licensed vocational nurse (LVN), or in Canada, registered nurse's assistant (RNA); trained in basic nursing skills and the provision of direct patient care.

life-saving measure Independent, dependent, or interdependent nursing intervention that is implemented when a client's physiological or psychological status is threatened.

lipids Compounds that are insoluble in water but soluble in organic solvents.

lipogenesis The process during which fatty acids are synthesized.

living wills Instruments by which a dying person makes wishes known.

local adaptation syndrome (LAS) Localized response of tissue, an organ, or a system that occurs as a direct reaction to stress.

local anesthesia Loss of sensation at the desired site of action.

lordosis An increased lumbar curvature.

loss Absence of a significant other, object, or state of health to which the person must adapt through the grieving process.

lymphocyte One type of leukocyte developing in the bone marrow; responsible for synthesizing antibodies and T cells that attack antigens.

maceration Softening and breaking down of skin from prolonged exposure to moisture.

malignant hyperthermia An autosomal dominant trait characterized by often fatal hyperthermia in affected people exposed to certain anesthetic agents.

malnutrition Any nutritional disorder such as unbalanced, insufficient, or excessive diet or impaired absorption, assimilation, or utilization of food.

malpractice Injurious or unprofessional actions that harm another.

malpractice insurance A type of insurance to protect the health care professional. In case of a malpractice claim, the insurance pays the award to the plaintiff.

managed care A health care system in which there is administrative control over primary health care services. Redundant facilities and services are eliminated, and costs are reduced. Preventive care and health education are emphasized.

management The process that involves planning, organizing, directing, and controlling of work activities to achieve a functional and productive work group.

masticate To chew or tear food with the teeth while it becomes mixed with saliva.

maturation The genetically determined biological plan for growth and development. Physical growth and motor development are a function of maturation.

maturational crises Same as developmental crises. Those crises associated with normal and expected phases of growth and development, e.g., the response to menopause.

maturational loss Loss, usually of an aspect of self, resulting from the normal changes of growth and development.

Medicaid State medical assistance to people with low incomes, based on Title XIX of the Social Security Act. States receive matching federal funds to provide medical care and services to people meeting categorical and income requirements.

medical asepsis Procedures used to reduce the number of microorganisms and prevent their spread.

medical diagnosis Formal statement of the disease entity or illness made by the physician.

medical record Client's chart; a legal document.

Medicare A federally funded national health insurance program in the United States for people over 65 years of age. The program is administered in two parts. Part A provides basic protection against costs of medical, surgical, and psychiatric hospital care. Part B is a
vouintary medical insurance program financed in part from federal funds and in part from premiums contributed by people enrolled in the program.

medication abuse A maladaptive pattern of recurrent medication use.

medication allergy An adverse reaction to a medication such as rash, chills, or gastrointestinal disturbances. Once a drug allergy occurs, the client can no longer receive that particular medication.

medication dependence A maladaptive pattern of medication use in the following patterns: using excessive amounts of the medication, increased activities directed toward obtaining the medication, withdrawal from professional or recreational activities, etc.

medication error Any event that could cause or lead to a client's receiving inappropriate drug therapy or failing to receive appropriate drug therapy.

medication interaction The response when one drug modifies the action of another drug. The interaction can potentiate or diminish the actions of another drug, or it may alter the way a drug is metabolized, absorbed, or excreted.

melanoma A group of malignant neoplasms, primarily of the skin, that are composed of melanocytes. Common in fair-skinned people having light-colored eyes and in persons who have had a sunburn.

melena Abnormal black, sticky stool containing digested blood; indicative of gastrointestinal bleeding.

menarche Onset of a girl's first menstruation.

menopause The physiologic cessation of ovulation and menstruation that typically occurs during middle adulthood in women.

menstrual cycle Recurring cycle of changes in the ovaries and hormone levels involving the development of an egg, ovulation, and implantation of the egg or sloughing of the corpus luteum and lining. The cycle can be divided into proliferative and secretory phases by uterine changes or follicular, ovulation, and luteal phases based on ovarian activity.

message Information sent or expressed by sender in the communication process.

metabolic acidosis Abnormal condition of high hydrogen ion concentration in the extracellular fluid caused by either a primary increase in hydrogen ions or a decrease in bicarbonate.

metabolic alkalosis Abnormal condition characterized by the significant loss of acid from the body or by increased levels of bicarbonate.

metabolism Aggregate of all chemical processes that take place in living organisms, resulting in growth, generation of energy, elimination of wastes, and other functions concerned with the distribution of nutrients in the blood after digestion.

metacommunication system Dependent not only on what is said but also on the relationship to the other person involved in the interaction. It is a message that conveys the sender's attitude toward the self and the message and the attitudes, feelings, and intentions toward the listener.

metastasize The spread of tumor cells to distant parts of the body from a primary site, e.g., lung, breast, or bowel.

metered dose inhaler A device designed to deliver a measured dose of an inhalation drug.

metric system Logically organized decimal system of measurement; metric units can easily be converted and computed through simple multiplication and division. Each basic unit of measurement is organized into units of 10.

microorganisms Microscopic entities capable of carrying on living processes, such as bacteria, viruses, and fungi.

micturition Urination; act of passing or expelling urine voluntarily through the urethra.

milliequivalent per liter (mEq/L) Number of grams of a specific electrolyte dissolved in 1 liter of plasma.

mind-body interaction Belief that a person's state of mind can have a negative or beneficial effect on level of health.

minerals Inorganic elements essential to the body because of their role as catalysts in biochemical reactions.

misdemeanor Lesser crime than a felony; the penalty is usually a fine or imprisonment for less than 1 year.

mobility Person's ability to move about freely.

morals Personal conviction that something is absolutely right or wrong in all situations.

motivation Internal impulse that causes a person to take action.

mourning A psychological process of reaction activated by an individual to assist in overcoming a great personal loss.

murmurs Blowing or whooshing sounds created by changes in blood flow through the heart or by abnormalities in valve closure.

muscle tone Normal state of balanced muscle tension.

myocardial contractility The measure of stretch of the cardiac muscle fiber. It can also affect stroke volume and cardiac output. Poor contraction decreases the amount of blood ejected by the ventricles during each contraction.

myocardial infarction Necrosis of a portion of cardiac muscle caused by obstruction in a coronary artery.

myocardial ischemia A condition that results when the supply of blood to the myocardium from the coronary arteries is insufficient to meet the oxygen demands of the organ.

myotonia Any condition in which a muscle or a group of muscles does not readily relax after contracting.

NANDA North American Nursing Diagnosis Association, organized in 1973, which formally identifies, develops, and classifies nursing diagnoses.

narcolepsy Syndrome involving sudden sleep attacks that a person cannot inhibit; uncontrollable desire to sleep may occur several times during a day.

narcotic Drug substance, derived from opium or produced synthetically, that alters perception of pain and that with repeated use may result in physical and psychological dependence.

nasogastric tube Tube passed into the stomach through the nose for the purpose of emptying the stomach of its contents or for delivering medication and/or nourishment.

nebulization Process of adding moisture to inspired air by the addition of water droplets.

necrotic Of or pertaining to the death of tissue in response to disease or injury.

negative health behaviors Practices actually or potentially harmful to health, such as smoking, drug or alcohol abuse, poor diet, and refusal to take necessary medications.

negative nitrogen balance Condition occurring when the body excretes more nitrogen than it takes in.

negligence Careless act of omission or commission that results in injury to another.

neonate Stage of life from birth to 1 month of age.

nephrons Structural and functional units of the kidney containing renal glomeruli and tubules.

neuromodulator A substance that alters transmission of nerve impulses.

neurotransmitter Chemical that transfers the electrical impulse from the nerve fiber to the muscle fiber.

nitrogen balance Relationship between the nitrogen taken into the body, usually as food, and the nitrogen excreted from the body in urine and feces. Most of the body's nitrogen is incorporated into protein.

nociceptors Somatic and visceral free nerve endings of thinly myelinated and unmyelinated fibers. They usually react to tissue injury but may also be excited by endogenous chemical substances.

nocturia Urination at night; can be a symptom of renal disease or may occur in persons who drink excessive amounts of fluids before bedtime.

nocturnal enuresis Incontinence of urine during the night.

noise pollution Noise level in an environment when it becomes uncomfortable to its inhabitants.

nonmaleficence The fundamental ethical agreement to do no harm. Closely related to the ethical standard of beneficence.

nonshivering thermogenesis Occurs primarily in neonates. Because neonates cannot shiver, a limited amount of vascular brown adipose tissue present at birth can be metabolized for heat production.

nonverbal communication Communication using expressions, gestures, body posture, and positioning rather than words.

normal reactive hyperemia   Hyperemia over a pressure site lasting 1 hour or less following removal of pressure; surrounding skin does blanch.

normal sinus rhythm (NSR)   The wave pattern on an electrocardiogram that indicates normal conduction of an electrical impulse through the myocardium.

nosocomial infections   Infections acquired during hospitalization or stay in a health care facility.

NPUAP   National pressure ulcer advisory panel.

NREM sleep   Abbreviation for non–rapid eye movement sleep, which occurs during the first four stages of normal sleep.

nurse administrator   A nurse who manages client care and specific nursing services within a health care agency. Positions range from middle management, such as the nurse manager or supervisor, to upper management, such as associate director, director, or vice president.

nurse educator   A nurse who primarily practices in schools of nursing and staff development departments of health care institutions.

nurse practice acts   Statutes enacted by the legislature of any of the states or by the appropriate officers of the districts or possessions that describe and define the scope of nursing practice.

nurse practitioners (NPs)   Nurses with advanced education who focus their practice in primary care settings, such as ambulatory care, private practice, or community-based settings. A significant percentage of primary care encounters extend beyond the boundaries of medicine and demand the expertise of the nurse. The nurse practitioner is able to establish a collaborative provider-client relationship.

nurse researcher   Usually a doctorally prepared nurse who investigates problems to improve nursing care, further define and expand the scope of nursing, or validate nursing care practices.

nurse-initiated interventions   The response of the nurse to the client's health care needs and nursing diagnoses. This type of intervention is "an autonomous action based on scientific rationale that is executed to benefit the client in a predicted way related to the nursing diagnosis and client-centered goals.

nursing care plan   Written outline, or schema, that includes identification of the client's expected outcomes for problem resolution and specific interventions and nursing orders. The care plan, a legal document that is part of the client's chart, documents and ensures use of the nursing process.

nursing diagnosis   Formal statement of an actual or potential health problem that nurses can legally and independently treat. The second step of the nursing process, during which the client's actual and potential unhealthy responses to an illness or condition are identified.

nursing health history   Data collected about a client's present level of wellness, changes in life patterns, sociocultural role, and mental and emotional reactions to illness.

nursing interface   A mechanism for nurses to access information on computerized systems.

nursing intervention   Nursing action performed to prevent harm from occurring to a client or to improve the mental, emotional, physical, or social function of a client.

nursing process   Systematic problem-solving method by which nurses individualize care for each client. The five steps of the nursing process are assessment, diagnosis, planning, implementation, and evaluation.

nutrients   Foods that contain elements necessary for body function, including water, carbohydrates, proteins, fats, vitamins, and minerals.

nystagmus   Involuntary, rhythmic movements of the eyes; the oscillations may be horizontal, vertical, rotatory, or mixed. May be indicative of vestibular, neurological, or vascular disease.

obesity   Abnormal increase in the proportion of fat cells, mainly in the viscera and subcutaneous tissues of the body.

object permanence   A developmental task involving recognition that an object or person out of sight still exists.

objective data   Information that can be observed by others; free of feelings, perceptions, prejudices.

olfactory   Pertaining to the sense of smell.

oncotic pressure   The total influence of the protein on the osmotic activity of plasma fluid.

operating room   (1) A room in a health care facility in which surgical procedures requiring anesthesia are performed. (2) Informal: a suite of rooms or an area in a health care facility in which patients are prepared for surgery, undergo surgical procedures, and recover from the anesthetic procedures required for the surgery.

ophthalmic   Drugs given into the eye, in the form of either eye drops or ointments.

opthalmoscope   An instrument used to illuminate the structures of the eye in order to examine the fundus, which includes the retina, choroid, optic nerve disk, macula, fovea centralis, and retinal vessels.

oral hygiene   Condition or practice of maintaining the tissues and structures of the mouth.

orthopnea   Abnormal condition in which a person must sit or stand up to breathe comfortably.

orthostatic hypotension   Abnormally low blood pressure occurring when a person stands up.

osmolality   The concentration or osmotic pressure of a solution expressed in osmoles or milliosmoles per kilogram of water.

osmolarity   The osmotic pressure of a solution expressed in osmoles or milliosmoles per kilogram of the solution.

osmole   The quantity of a substance in solution in the form of molecules, ions, or both (usually expressed in grams) that has the same osmotic pressure as one mole of an ideal nonelectrolyte.

osmoreceptors   A neuron in the hypothalamus that is sensitive to the fluid concentration in the blood plasma and regulates the secretion of antidiuretic hormone.

osmosis   Movement of a pure solvent through a semipermeable membrane from a solution with a lower solute concentration to one with a higher solute concentration.

osmotic pressure   Drawing power for water, which depends on the number of molecules in the solution.

osteoporosis   A disorder characterized by abnormal rarefaction of bone, occurring most frequently in postmenopausal women, in sedentary or immobilized individuals, and in clients on long-term steroid therapy.

ostomy Surgical procedure in which an opening is made into the abdominal wall to allow the passage of intestinal contents from the bowel (colostomy) or urine from the bladder (urostomy).

otoscope An instrument, with a special ear speculum, used to examine the deeper structures of the external and middle ear.

ototoxicity Having a harmful effect on the eighth cranial (auditory) nerve or the organs of hearing and balance.

outcome/outcome indicators Condition of a client at the end of treatment, including the degree of wellness and the need for continuing care, medication, support, counseling, or education.

outliers Clients with extended lengths of stay beyond allowable inpatient days or costs.

outpatient Client who has not been admitted to a hospital but receives treatments in a clinic or facility associated with the hospital.

oximeter, oximetry A device used to measure oxyhemoglobin in the blood.

oxygen saturation The amount of hemoglobin fully saturated with hemoglobin, given as a percent value.

pain Subjective, unpleasant sensation caused by noxious stimulation of sensory nerve endings.

palliative Relating to treatment designed to relieve or reduce intensity of uncomfortable symptoms but not to produce a cure.

pallor Unnatural paleness or absence of color in the skin.

palpation Method of physical examination whereby the fingers or hands of the examiner are applied to the client's body for the purpose of feeling body parts underlying the skin.

palpitations Bounding or racing of the heart associated with normal emotions or a heart disorder.

Papanicolaou (Pap) smear A painless screening test for cervical cancer. Specimens are taken of squamous and columnar cells of the cervix.

parallel play A form of play among a group of children, primarily toddlers, in which each one engages in an independent activity that is similar but not influenced by or shared with the others.

paralytic ileus Usually temporary paralysis of intestinal wall that may occur after abdominal surgery or peritoneal injury and that causes cessation of peristalsis. Leads to abdominal distention and symptoms of obstruction.

parenteral administration Giving medication by a route other than the gastrointestinal tract.

parenteral nutrition (PN) The administration of a nutritional solution into the vascular system.

partial bed bath Bath in which body parts that might cause the client discomfort if left unbathed (that is, face, hands, axillary areas, back, and perineum) are washed in bed.

parturition The process of giving birth.

passive range of motion (ROM) The range of movement through which a joint is moved with assistance.

passive strategies of health promotion Activities that involve the client as the recipient of actions by health care professionals.

pathogens Microorganisms capable of producing disease.

pathological fractures Fractures resulting from weakened bone tissue; frequently caused by osteoporosis or neoplasms.

patient-controlled analgesia (PCA) Drug delivery system that allows clients to self-administer analgesic medications when they want.

patient-focused care A care delivery model with a multidisciplinary focus. Cross-trained care givers form self-governed teams to assume responsibility for the work process that delivers care to clients. A typical patient-focused care unit has its own admitting, pharmacy, laboratory, and radiology areas.

peak expiratory flow rate (PEFR) The maximal flow rate, measured in liters, that can be generated during a forced expiratory maneuver.

perceived loss A loss that is less obvious to the individual experiencing it. Although easily overlooked or misunderstood, a perceived loss results in the same grief process as an actual loss.

perception Persons' mental image or concept of elements in their environment, including information gained through the senses.

perceptual biases Human tendencies that interfere with accurately perceiving and interpreting messages from others.

perceptual bound thinking Cognitive stage of development for preschoolers, characterized by the child's tendency to judge persons, objects, and events by their outward appearance or what seems to be. For example, two nickels are perceived to be more than a dime.

percussion Method of physical examination whereby the location, size, and density of a body part is determined by the tone obtained from the striking of short, sharp taps of the fingers.

perfusion (1) Passage of a fluid through a specific organ or an area of the body. (2) Therapeutic measure whereby a drug intended for an isolated part of the body is introduced via the bloodstream.

perineal care Procedure prescribed for cleaning the genital and anal areas as part of the daily bath or after various obstetrical and gynecological procedures.

perioperative nursing Refers to the role of the operating room nurse during the preoperative, intraoperative, and postoperative phases of surgery.

peristalsis Rhythmic contractions of the intestine that propel gastric contents through the length of the gastrointestinal tract.

peritonitis Inflammation of the peritoneum produced by bacteria or irritating substances introduced into the abdominal cavity by a penetrating wound or perforation of an organ in the gastrointestinal tract or the reproductive tract.

PERRLA Acronym for "pupils equal, round, reactive to light, accommodative"; the acronym is recorded in the physicial examination if eye and pupil assessments are normal.

petechiae Tiny purple or red spots that appear on skin as minute hemorrhages within dermal layers.

pharmacokinetics Study of how drugs enter the body, reach their site of action, are metabolized, and exit from the body.

phlebitis Inflammation of a vein.

physical examination   Assessment of the client's body using the techniques of inspection, auscultation, palpation, and percussion for the purpose of determining physical abnormalities.

physician-initiated interventions   Based on the physician's response to a medical diagnosis, the nurse responds to the physician's written orders.

PIE note   Problem-oriented medical record; the four interdisciplinary sections are the data base, problem list, care plan, and progress notes.

placebo   Dosage form that contains no pharmacologically active ingredients but may relieve pain through psychological effects.

plaintiff   Individual who files formal charges against an individual or organization for a legal offense.

planning   The process of designing interventions to achieve the goals and outcomes of health care delivery.

plantar flexion   A toe-down motion of the foot at the ankle.

pleural friction rub   Adventitious lung sound caused by inflamed parietal and visceral pleura rubbing together on inspiration.

pneumothorax   Collection of air or gas in the pleural space.

point of maximal impulse (PMI)   Point where the heartbeat can most easily be palpated through the chest wall.

poison   Any substance that impairs health or destroys life when ingested, inhaled, or absorbed by the body in relatively small amounts.

poison control center   One of a network of facilities that provides information regarding all aspects of poisoning or intoxication, maintains records of their occurrence, and refers clients to treatment centers.

pollutant   A harmful chemical or waste material discharged into the water or atmosphere.

polypharmacy   The use of a number of different drugs by a client who may have one or several health problems.

polysomnogram   Monitoring device that involves placement of electrodes on the scalp, face, chin, and legs to measure brain waves, eye movements, and muscle activity; used to diagnose sleep disorders.

polyunsaturated fatty acid   Fatty acid that has two or more carbon double bonds.

positive health behaviors   Activities related to maintaining, attaining, or regaining good health and preventing illness. Common positive health behaviors include immunizations, proper sleep patterns, adequate exercise, and nutrition.

possible nursing diagnosis   A judgment that describes a suspected problem for which there are insufficient data currently available.

postanesthesia care unit   An area adjoining the operating room to which surgical clients are taken while still under anesthesia.

postural drainage   Use of positioning along with percussion and vibration to drain secretions from specific segments of the lungs and bronchi into the trachea.

postural hypotension   Abnormally low blood pressure occurring when an individual assumes the standing posture; also called orthostatic hypotension.

posture   Position of the body in relation to the surrounding space.

preadolescence   The transitional developmental stage that occurs between childhood and adolescence.

precertification   Preliminary screening process used by third-party payers to approve use of health care services by enrollees of a health plan.

preferred provider organization (PPO)   Group of physicians or a hospital that provides company employees and their dependents with comprehensive health services at a discount.

preload   The volume of blood in the ventricles at the end of diastole, immediately before ventricular contraction.

prenatal care   The health care provided the mother and fetus before childbirth.

preoperational thought   Children can think about things not physically present by using mental representations but are limited by their inability to use logic.

preoperative teaching   Instruction regarding a client's anticipated surgery and recovery given before surgery. Instruction includes, but is not limited to, dietary and activity restrictions, anticipated assessment activities, postoperative procedures, and pain relief measures.

prescriptions   Written directions for a therapeutic agent (e.g., medication, drugs).

pressure ulcer   Inflammation, sore, or ulcer in the skin over a bony prominence.

preventive nursing actions   Nursing actions directed toward preventing illness and promoting health to avoid the need for primary, secondary, or tertiary health care.

primary intention   Primary union of the edges of a wound, progressing to complete scar formation without granulation.

primary nursing system   A method of nursing practice in which the client's care is managed, for the duration, by one nurse, who directs and coordinates other nurses and health care personnel. When on duty, the primary nurse cares for the client directly.

primary prevention   First contact in a given episode of illness that leads to a decision regarding a course of action to prevent worsening of the health problem.

prioritization   Act of listing nursing diagnoses in their order of importance of client health and well-being.

proactivity   Characteristic of one who always takes action, seeks opportunity, and asserts oneself.

problem identification   One of the steps of the diagnostic process in which the client's health care problem is recognized as a result of data analysis based on professional knowledge and experience.

problem solving   A methodical, systematic approach to explore conditions and develop solutions, including analysis of data, determination of causative factors, and selection of appropriate actions to reverse or eliminate the problem.

problem-oriented medical record (POR or POMR)   Method of recording data about the health status of a client that fosters a collaborative problem-solving approach by all members of the health care team.

process indicators   Specific measures that evaluate the manner in which care is delivered (e.g. correct procedure for dressing changes).

productive cough A sudden expulsion of air from the lungs that effectively removes sputum from the respiratory tract and helps clear the airways.

professionalism Conduct or qualities that characterize or mark a professional person.

professional standards review organizations (PSROs) Focuses on evaluation of nursing care provided in a health care setting. The quality, effectiveness, and appropriateness of nursing care for the client is the focus of evaluation.

prone Position of the client lying facedown.

prospective payment Procedure by which the federal government sets rates for hospitals in advance for treatment of specific illnesses.

prostaglandins Potent hormone-like substances that act in exceedingly low doses on target organs. They can be used to treat asthma and gastric hyperacidity.

protector Role of the nurse to help maintain a safe environment for the client and take steps to prevent injury and protect the client from possible adverse effects of diagnostic or treatment measures.

protein Any of a large group of naturally occurring, complex, organic nitrogenous compounds. Each is composed of large combinations of amino acids containing the elements carbon, hydrogen, nitrogen, oxygen, usually sulfur, and occasionally phosphorus, iron, iodine, or other essential constituents of living cells. Protein is the major source of building material for muscles, blood, skin, hair, nails, and the internal organs.

proteinuria Presence in the urine of abnormally large quantities of protein, usually albumin. Persistent proteinuria is usually a sign of renal disease or renal complications of another disease, or hypertension or heart failure.

protocol Written and approved plan specifying the procedures to be followed during an assessment or in providing treatment.

provider The individual or agency that provides health care services to clients.

psychomotor learning Acquisition of ability to perform motor skills.

ptosis Abnormal condition of one or both upper eyelids in which the eyelid droops, caused by weakness of the levator muscle or paralysis of the third cranial nerve.

puberty Developmental period of emotional and physical changes, including the development of secondary sex characteristics and the onset of menstruation and ejaculation.

public communication The interaction of one individual with large groups of people.

pulmonary function test A procedure for determining the capacity of the lungs to exchange oxygen and carbon dioxide efficiently.

pulse deficit Condition that exists when the radial pulse is less than the ventricular rate as auscultated at the apex or seen on an electrocardiogram. The condition indicates a lack of peripheral perfusion for some of the heart contractions.

pulse pressure The difference between the systolic and diastolic pressures, normally 30 to 40 mm Hg.

Purkinje network A complex network of muscle fibers that spread through the right and left ventricles of the heart and carry the impulses that contract those chambers almost simultaneously.

pursed-lip breathing Deep inspiration followed by prolonged expiration through pursed lips.

pyrexia Abnormal elevation of the temperature of the body above 37° C (98.6° F) because of disease. Same as fever.

pyrogens Substances that cause a rise in body temperature, as in the case of bacterial toxins.

quality improvement The monitoring and evaluation of processes and outcomes in health care or any other business to identify opportunities for improvement.

quality indicator A quantitative measure of an important aspect of care that determines whether quality of service conforms to requirements or standards of care.

range of motion The range of movement of a joint, from maximum extension to maximum flexion, as measured in degrees of a circle.

rapid eye movement (REM) sleep Stage of sleep in which dreaming and rapid eye movements are prominent; important for mental restoration.

Raza-Latina A popular term used as a reference group name for people of Latin-American descent.

reaction Component of the pain experience that may include both physiological responses such as in the general adaptation syndrome and behavioral responses.

reactive hyperemia Condition characterized by an increased blood flow to part of the body, as in the inflammatory response, local relaxation of arterioles, or obstruction of the outflow of blood from an area.

reality orientation Therapeutic modality for restoring an individual's sense of the present.

receiver Person to whom message is sent during the communication process.

reception Neurophysiological components of the pain experience, in which nervous system receptors receive painful stimuli and transmit them through peripheral nerves to the spinal cord and brain.

receptive aphasia Abnormal neurological condition in which language function is defective because of an injury to certain areas of the cerebral cortex; specifically, language is not understood.

recommended daily allowances (RDAs) Suggested or recommended amounts of various nutrients used in planning diets.

record Written form of communication that permanently documents information relevant to health care management.

rectocele A bulging of the posterior vaginal wall, caused by prolapse of the rectum.

referent Factor that motivates a person to communicate with another individual.

reflection A process of thinking back or recalling an event to discover the meaning and purpose of that event. Useful in critical thinking.

reflex incontinence Involuntary loss of urine occurs with some predictability.

reflex pain response Reflected, involuntary withdrawal of a body part away from a noxious or painful stimulus.

refractive error Defect in the ability of the lens of the eye to focus light, such as occurs in nearsightedness and farsightedness.

regional anesthesia   Loss of sensation in an area of the body supplied by sensory nerve pathways.

registered professional nurse   Health care professional who has completed a course of study at an accredited school of nursing and has passed a licensure examination administered by NCLEX or the Canadian Nurses' Association Testing Service.

regression   A return to an earlier developmental stage or behavior.

regressive behavior   A defense mechanism whereby an individual resorts to a more primitive or earlier way of doing things. For example, instead of dealing with a stressful situation, a person chooses to stay in bed.

regulatory agencies   Local, state, province, or national agencies that inspect and certify health care agencies as meeting specified standards. These agencies can also determine the amount of reimbursement for health care delivered.

rehabilitation   Restoration of an individual to normal or near-normal function following a physical or mental illness, injury, or chemical addiction.

reinforcement   Provision of a contingent response to a learner's behavior that increases the probability of the behavior's recurring.

related factor   Any condition or event that accompanies or is linked with the client's health care problem.

relative humidity   Amount of moisture in the air as compared with the maximum amount that the air could contain at the same temperature.

relaxation   Act of being relaxed or less tense.

religion   The belief in a divine or superhuman power or powers to be obeyed and worshiped as the creator and ruler of the universe.

reminiscence   Recalling the past for the purpose of assigning new meaning to past experiences.

remissions   Partial or complete disappearances of the clinical and subjective characteristics of chronic or malignant disease; remission may be spontaneous or the result of therapy.

renal calculi   Calcium stones in the renal pelvis.

renin   A proteolytic enzyme, produced by and stored in the juxtaglomerular apparatus that surrounds each arteriole as it enters a glomerulus. The enzyme affects the blood pressure by catalyzing the change of angiotensinogen to angiotensin, a strong repressor.

report   Transfer of information from the nurses on one shift to the nurses on the following shift. Report may also be given by one of the members of the nursing team to another health care provider, for example, physician or therapist.

residual urine   Volume of urine remaining in the bladder after a normal voiding; the bladder normally is almost completely empty after micturition.

resistance stage   Third stage of the stress response, when the person attempts to adapt to the stressor. The body stabilizes, hormone levels stabilize, and heart rate, blood pressure, and cardiac output return to normal.

respiratory acidosis   Abnormal condition characterized by increased arterial carbon dioxide concentration, excess carbonic acid, and increased hydrogen ion concentration.

respiratory alkalosis   Abnormal condition characterized by decreased arterial carbon dioxide concentration and decreased hydrogen ion concentration.

respite care   Short-term health services to dependent older adults either in their home or in an institutional setting.

responsibility   Carrying out duties associated with a particular role.

restorative care   Health care settings and services where clients who are recovering from illness or disability receive rehabilitation and supportive care.

restraints   Devices to aid in the immobilization of a client or client's extremity.

reticular activating system (RAS)   Group of specialized nerve cells located in the brainstem, upper spinal cord, and cerebral cortex.

return demonstration   Demonstration after the client has first observed the teacher and then practiced the skill in mock or real situations.

rhonchi   Abnormal lung sound auscultated when the client's airways are obstructed with thick secretions.

right-sided heart failure   An abnormal condition that results from impaired functioning of the right ventricle characterized by venous congestion in the systemic circulation.

risk factor   Any internal or external variable that makes a person or group more vulnerable to illness or an unhealthy event.

risk nursing diagnosis   Describes human responses to health conditions/life processes that may develop in a vulnerable, individual, family, or community.

role   Set of behaviors by means of which a person participates in a social group.

sandbags   Sand-filled plastic tubes that can be shaped to body contours. They can mobilize an extremity or maintain body alignment.

saturated fatty acid   Fatty acid in which each carbon in the chain has an attached hydrogen atom.

scientific method   A codified sequence of steps used in the formulation, testing, evaluation, and reporting of scientific ideas.

scientific rationale   Reason, based on supporting literature, why a specific nursing action was chosen.

scintigraphy   A diagnostic technique that produces a photographic recording that shows the distribution and intensity of radioactivity in various tissues and organs after the administration of a radiopharmaceutical.

scoliosis   A lateral spinal curvature.

scrub nurse   Registered nurse or operating room technician who assists surgeons during operations.

seamless care delivery   A delivery of health care model that eliminates fragmentation of health care services. Clients are able to enter a system and receive a continuum of services when they need it, with minimal inconvenience and with a limited number of health professionals involved.

sebum   Normal secretion of the sebaceous glands of the skin; when combined with sweat, forms a moist, oily, acidic film that protects the skin from drying.

secondary intention   Wound closure in which the edges are separated, granulation tissue develops to fill the gap, and finally, epithelium grows in over the granulation, producing a larger scar than results with primary intention.

secondary prevention Level of preventive medicine that focuses on early diagnosis, use of referral services, and rapid initiation of treatment to stop the progress of disease processes.

sedatives Medications that produce a calming effect by decreasing functional activity, diminishing irritability, and allaying excitement.

segmentation Alternating contraction and relaxation of gastrointestinal mucosa.

self-concept Complex, dynamic integration of conscious and unconscious feelings, attitudes, and perceptions about one's identity, physical being, worth, and roles; how a person perceives and defines self.

self-directed work team A work team whereby the members establish goals, implement an action plan, and take accountability for outcomes or results.

self-esteem Feeling of self-worth characterized by feelings of achievement, adequacy, self-confidence, and usefulness.

sender Person who initiates interpersonal communication by conveying a message.

sensible water loss Loss of fluid from the body through the secretory activity of the sweat glands and the exhalation of humidified air from the lungs.

sensorimotor period The development phase of childhood encompassing the period from birth to 2 years of age.

sensory deficit Defect in the function of one or more of the senses, resulting in visual, auditory, or olfactory impairments.

sensory deprivation State in which stimulation to one or more of the senses is lacking, resulting in impaired sensory perception.

sensory overload State in which stimulation to one or more of the senses is so excessive that the brain disregards or does not meaningfully respond to stimuli.

seriation The cognitive skill of being able to arrange a series of objects in succession by size.

serum half-life Time needed for excretion processes to lower the serum drug concentration by half.

sexual dysfunction Inability or difficulty in sexual functioning caused by physiological or psychological factors or both.

sexual orientation Clear, persistent erotic preference for a person of one sex or the other.

sexual response cycle Phases of biological sexual response: excitement, plateau, orgasm, and resolution, as defined by Masters and Johnson.

sexuality "A function of the total personality . . . concerned with the biological, psychological, sociological, spiritual and culture variables of life . . ." (Sex Information and Education Council of the United States, 1980).

shared governance An organized, systematic approach to decision making that enables all levels of nurses to participate in the resolution of clinical, professional, and administrative practice issues.

shearing force Friction exerted when a person is moved or repositioned in bed by being pulled or allowed to slide down in bed.

side effects Any reaction or consequence that results from medication or therapy.

side rails Bars positioned along the sides of the length of the bed or stretcher to reduce the client's risk of falling.

sinoatrial (SA) node Called the "pacemaker of the heart" because the origin of the normal heartbeat begins at the SA node. The SA node is in the right atrium next to the entrance of the superior vena cava.

situational leadership A comprehensive management approach that takes into account the style of the leader, maturity of the work group, and the situation needing management.

situational loss Loss of a person, thing, or quality resulting from a change in a life situation, including changes related to illness, body image, environment, and death.

sitz bath Bath in which only the hips or buttocks are immersed in fluid.

skilled nursing facility An institution or part of an institution that meets criteria for accreditation established by the sections of the Social Security Act that determine the basis for Medicaid and Medicare reimbursement for skilled nursing care, including rehabilitation and various medical and nursing procedures.

slander Utterance of a false statement about another that harms that person's reputation.

sleep State marked by reduced consciousness, diminished activity of the skeletal muscles, and depressed metabolism.

sleep apnea The cessation of breathing for a time during sleep.

sleep deprivation Condition resulting from a decrease in the amount, quality, and consistency of sleep.

sloughing Shedding of dead tissue cells.

SOAP note Progress notes that focus on a single client problem and include subjective and objective data, analysis, and planning; most often used in the POMR.

socialization Process of being raised within a culture and acquiring the characteristics of the given group.

solute A substance dissolved in a solution.

solution Mixture of one or more substances dissolved in another substance. The molecules of each of the substances disperse homogeneously and do not change chemically. A solution may be a liquid, gas, or a solid.

solvent Any liquid in which another substance can be dissolved.

source record Organization of a client's chart so that each discipline (e.g., nursing, medicine, social work, or respiratory therapy) has a separate section in which to record data. Unlike POMR, the information is not organized by client problems. The advantage of a source record is that care givers can easily locate the proper section of the record in which to make entries.

sphygmomanometer Device for measuring the arterial blood pressure that consists of an arm or leg cuff with an air bladder connected to a tube and a bulb for pumping air into the bladder and a gauge for indicating the amount of air pressure being exerted against the artery.

spiritual distress State of being out of harmony with a system of beliefs, a Supreme Being, or God.

spiritual well-being An individual's spirituality that enables a person to love, have faith and hope, seek meaning in life, and nurture relationships with others.

spirituality Spiritual dimension of a person, including the relationship with humanity, nature, and a Supreme Being.

standardized care plans Written care plans used for groups of clients that have similar health care problems.

standards of care The minimum level of care accepted to ensure high quality of care to clients. Standards of care define the types of therapies typically administered to clients with defined problems or needs.

standards of practice Provide the client with assurance that they are receiving high-quality nursing care, the nurses know how to provide the care, and there are measures to determine if the care meets the established standards and expected outcomes.

standing order Written and approved documents containing rules, policies, procedures, regulations, and orders for the conduct of client care in various stipulated clinical settings.

statutory law Of or related to laws enacted by a legislative branch of the government.

stenosis An abnormal condition characterized by the constriction or narrowing of an opening or passageway in a body structure.

sterilization (1) Rendering a person unable to produce children; accomplished by surgical, chemical, or other means. (2) A technique for destroying microorganisms using heat, water, chemicals, or gases.

stoma Artificially created opening between a body cavity and the body's surface; for example, a colostomy, formed from a portion of the colon pulled through the abdominal wall.

stratum corneum Horny outermost layer of skin, composed of dead cells converted to keratin, which continually flakes away.

stress Physiological or psychological tension that threatens homeostasis or a person's psychological equilibrium.

stress incontinence Involuntary loss of urine due to increase abdominal pressure, e.g., sneezing, coughing.

stressor Any event, situation, or other stimulus encountered in a person's external or internal environment that necessitates change or adaptation by the person.

striae Streaks or linear scars that result from rapid development of tension in the skin.

stroke volume The amount of blood ejected by the ventricles with each contraction. It can be affected by the amount of blood in the left ventricle at the end of diastole (preload), the resistance to left ventricular ejection (afterload), and myocardial contractility.

structure indicators Evaluate the structure or systems for delivering care, e.g., percentage of staff on nights, compliance in checking emergency cart contents, and nurses' attendance at required courses.

subacute care Level of medical specialty care provided to clients who need a greater intensity of care than that provided in a skilled nursing facility but who do not require acute care.

subcutaneous Injection given into the connective tissue, under the dermis. The subcutaneous tissue absorbs drugs more slowly than those injected into muscle. Injections are usually given at an angle of 45 degrees.

subcutaneous layer Continuous layer of connective tissue over the entire body between the skin and the deep fascia.

subjective data Information gathered from client statements; the client's feelings and perceptions. Not verifiable by another except by inference.

sublingual A route of medication administration in which the medication is placed underneath the client's tongue.

supine Position of the client in which the client is resting on the back.

suppression A psychological defense mechanism that defers the full expression of emotion through the performance of activities. It allows a person to function under stress until the presence of supportive persons makes the expression of emotions safe.

suprapubic catheter Catheter surgically inserted through abdomen into bladder.

surfactant The chemical produced in the lung by alveolar type 2 cells that maintains the surface tension of the alveoli and keeps them from collapsing.

surgical asepsis Procedures used to eliminate any microorganisms from an area. Also called sterile technique.

symbolic communication The use of an image, object, or action to represent something else and to help convey meaning, which is established by the symbol's association, resemblance, or conventional or personal use.

sympathy Concern, sorrow, or pity felt by the nurse for the client in which the nurse personally identifies with the client's needs. Sympathy is a subjective look at another person's world that prevents a clear perspective of all sides of the issues confronting that person.

synapse Region surrounding the point of contact between two neurons or between a neuron and an effector organ.

syncope A brief lapse in consciousness caused by transient cerebral hypoxia.

syndrome diagnosis A diagnostic label given to a distinct cluster of nursing diagnoses that frequently go together and present a clinical picture.

synergistic effect When two drugs act synergistically, the effect of the two drugs combined is greater than the effect that would be expected if the individual effects of the two drugs acting alone were added together.

systolic pressure The pressure exerted in the aorta and large arteries during systolic contraction of the left ventricle. Indicated during blood pressure measurement at the point when sound can first be heard during deflation of the blood pressure cuff.

tachycardia Rapid regular heart rate ranging between 100 and 150 beats per minute.

tachypnea An abnormally rapid rate of breathing.

tactile   Relating to the sense of touch.

tactile fremitus   A tremulous vibration of the chest wall during breathing that is palpable on physical examination.

task-oriented behavior   Actions involving a person's cognitive abilities in an attempt to solve problems, resolve conflicts, and gratify the person's needs in order to reduce or avoid stress.

teaching   Implementation method used to present correct principles, procedures, and techniques of health care; to inform clients about their health status; and to refer clients and family to appropriate health or social resources in the community.

teaching-learning process   An interaction between the teacher and learner in which specific learning objectives are presented; provides the organizational structure and framework for client education.

team building   Development of a group of multidisciplinary health care professionals who work together to solve a health-related problem, e.g., critical pathways, quality indicators.

team nursing   A decentralized system in which the care of a client is distributed among the members of a team. The charge nurse delegates authority to a team leader, who must be a professional nurse.

team nursing system   Method of client care delivery in which a small group of staff together provide client care to an assigned number of clients.

teratogens   Chemical or physiological agents that may produce adverse effects in the embryo or fetus.

territoriality   Persistent attachment of a person to a specific area or space.

tertiary prevention   Activities directed toward rehabilitation rather than diagnosis and treatment.

therapeutic communication   Process in which the nurse consciously influences a client or helps the client to a better understanding through verbal and/or nonverbal communication.

therapeutic effect   The desired benefit of a medication, treatment, or procedure.

thermoregulation   Internal control of body temperature.

third-party payers   Health insurance plans that reimburse for health care services rendered to clients.

thoracentesis   Surgical perforation of the chest wall and pleural space with a needle for the aspiration of fluid or to obtain a specimen for diagnostic or therapeutic purposes.

threshold   Point at which a person first perceives a painful stimulus as being painful.

thrill   A continuous palpable sensation like the purring of a cat.

thrombus   Accumulation of platelets, fibrin, clotting factors, and the cellular elements of the blood attached to the interior wall of a vein or artery, sometimes occluding the lumen of the vessel.

time orientation   Value that a client places on promptness, future planning, and keeping appointments, which are important in the planning of long-term care and self-care discharge therapies.

tinnitus   Ringing heard in one or both ears.

tissue ischemia   The point at which tissues receive insufficient oxygen and perfusion.

tolerance   Point at which a person is not willing to accept pain of greater severity or duration.

tort   Act that causes injury for which the injured party can bring civil action.

total incontinence   Total uncontrollable continuous loss of urine.

toxic effect   An effect of a medication that results in an adverse response.

traditional approach   Ancient ethnocultural and religious beliefs and practices that have been handed down through the generations.

transcutaneous electrical nerve stimulation (TENS)   Technique in which a battery-powered device blocks pain impulses from reaching the spinal cord by delivering weak electrical impulses directly to the skin's surface.

transdermal disk   Medication delivery device in which the medication is saturated on a waferlike disk, which is affixed to the client's skin. This method ensures that the client receives a continuous level of medication.

transfer report   Verbal exchange of information between care givers when a client is moved from one nursing unit or health care setting to another. The report includes information necessary to maintain a consistent level of care from one setting to another.

transfusion reaction   A systemic response by the body to the administration of blood incompatible with that of the recipient.

trapeze bar   Metal triangular-shaped bar that can be suspended over a client's bed from an overhanging frame; permits clients to move up and down in bed while in traction or some other encumbrance.

triangulation   Complaining to a third party rather than confronting the problem or expressing concerns directly to the source. It lowers team morale and is often contagious.

trimester   Referring to one of the three phases of pregnancy.

trochanter roll   Rolled towel support placed against the hips and upper leg to prevent external rotation of the legs.

turgor   Normal resiliency of the skin caused by the outward pressure of the cells and interstitial fluid.

unlicensed assistive personnel   Category of health care providers such as nurse assistants or technicians who are unlicensed and who have limited formal education. This individual is trained in basic client care and assists the registered nurse with client care. This may include activities of daily living, vital signs, assistance with meals, simple wound care, assisting with ambulation, discontinuing intravenous peripheral lines, and insertion and care of indwelling or intermittent Foley catheters.

unsaturated fatty acid   Fatty acid in which an unequal number of hydrogen atoms are attached and the carbon atoms attach to each other with a double bond.

ureterostomy   Diversion of urine away from a diseased or defective bladder through an artificial opening in the skin.

urge incontinence   Involuntary loss of urine after a strong urgency to void.

urinal   Receptacle for collecting urine.

urinary incontinence Inability to control urination.

urinary reflux Abnormal, backward flow of urine.

urinary retention Retention of urine in the bladder; condition frequently caused by a temporary loss of muscle function.

urine hat Receptacle for collecting urine that fits toilet.

urometer A device for measuring frequent and small amounts of urine from an indwelling urinary catheter system.

urticaria An itchy skin eruption characterized by transient wheals of varying shapes and sizes with well-defined erythematous margins and pale centers.

user interface Traditional mechanism whereby a user of a computer accesses functions and information via a keyboard and monitor.

utilitarianism An ethic that proposes that the value of something is determined by its usefulness. The greatest good for the greatest number of people constitutes the guiding principle for action in a utilitarian model of ethics.

validation Act of confirming, verifying, or corroborating the accuracy of assessment data or the appropriateness of the care plan.

Valsalva maneuver Any forced expiratory effort against a closed airway, such as when an individual holds the breath and tightens the muscles in a concerted, strenuous effort to move a heavy object or to change positions in bed.

value Personal belief about the worth of a given idea or behavior.

values clarification Technique for clarifying values, developed by Louis Raths; process designed to give an individual the opportunity to find meaning and significance in personal values.

valvular heart disease An acquired or congenital disorder of a cardiac valve characterized by stenosis and obstructed blood flow or valvular degeneration and regurgitation of blood.

variance The unexpected event that occurs during client care and that is different from what is predicted on a CareMap. Variance or exceptions are interventions or outcomes that are not achieved as anticipated. Variance may be positive or negative.

vascular access device Catheters, cannulas, or infusion ports designed for long-term, repeated access to the vascular system.

vasoconstriction Narrowing of the lumen of any blood vessel, especially the arterioles and the veins in the blood reservoirs of the skin and abdominal viscera.

vasoconstrictor Nerves or stimulation of dilator nerves.

vasodilation An increase in the diameter of a blood vessel caused by inhibition of its vasoconstrictor nerves or stimulation of dilator nerves.

venipuncture Technique in which a vein is punctured transcutaneously by a sharp rigid stylet (such as a butterfly needle), a cannula (such as an angiocatheter that contains a flexible plastic catheter), or a needle attached to a syringe.

ventilation Respiratory process by which gases are moved into and out of the lungs.

ventricular gallop An abnormal low-pitched extra heart sound (S_4) heard in early diastole.

verbal communication The sending of messages from one individual to another or to a group of individuals through the spoken word.

vertigo A sensation of dizziness or spinning.

vibration Fine, shaking pressure applied by hands to the chest wall only during exhalation.

virtual reality A virtual environment that is a computer-simulated world that changes in response to a person's actions.

virulence A very pathogenic or rapidly progressive condition.

visual Related to, or experienced through, vision.

vital signs Temperature, pulse, respirations, and blood pressure.

vitamins Organic compound essential in small quantities for normal physiological and metabolic functioning of the body. With few exceptions, vitamins cannot be synthesized by the body and must be obtained from the diet or dietary supplements.

vocal fremitus Vibration of the chest wall as the person speaks or sings that allows the person's voice to be heard by the examiner during auscultation of the chest with a stethoscope.

voiding The process of urinating.

volunteer agencies Not-for-profit health care agencies established within a community to meet specific needs.

water pollution Contamination of lakes, rivers, and streams by industrial pollutants.

wellness Dynamic state of health in which an individual progresses toward a higher level of functioning, achieving an optimum balance between internal and external environments.

wellness nursing diagnosis A clinical judgment about an individual, group, or community in transition from a specific level of wellness to a higher level of wellness.

wellness-illness model Describes the relationship between health, disease, wellness, and illness as distinct parts of a process involving the changing person in the changing world. In this model, health is viewed as an objective process characterized by stability, balance, and integrity of functioning.

wheezes Adventitious lung sound caused by a severely narrowed bronchus.

work redesign Formal process used to analyze the work of a certain work group and to change the actual structure of the jobs performed.

wound culture Specimen collected from a wound to determine the specific organism that is causing an infectious process.

Z-track injection A technique for injecting irritating preparations into muscle without tracking residual medication through sensitive tissues.

zygote Fertilized ovum created by joining of the ovum and sperm.

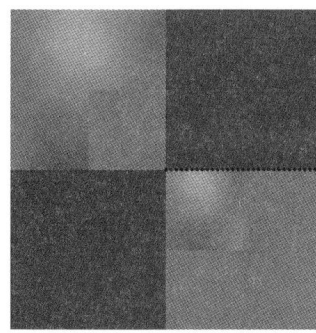

Index